D1251094

# Hypertension

A Companion to Brenner and Rector's
*The Kidney*

DREXEL UNIVERSITY
HEALTH SCIENCES LIBRARIES
HAHNEMANN LIBRARY

# Hypertension

A Companion to Brenner and Rector's
*The Kidney*

Second Edition

## SUZANNE OPARIL, M.D.

Director, Vascular Biology and Hypertension Program
Division of Cardiovascular Diseases

Professor of Medicine, Physiology, and Biophysics
University of Alabama at Birmingham
Birmingham, Alabama

## MICHAEL A. WEBER, M.D.

Associate Dean for Clinical Research and Professor of Medicine
State University of New York Health Science Center at Brooklyn
Brooklyn, New York

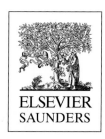

ELSEVIER
SAUNDERS

**ELSEVIER**
**SAUNDERS**

The Curtis Center
170 S Independence Mall W 300E
Philadelphia, Pennsylvania 19106

WJ
300
K44
2004
Comp.OW

**HYPERTENSION: A COMPANION TO BRENNER AND RECTOR'S
THE KIDNEY**

0-7216-0258-4

Copyright © 2005, Elsevier Inc. All rights reserved.

No part of this publication may be reproduced or transmitted in any form or by any means, electronic or mechanical, including photocopying, recording, or any information storage and retrieval system, without permission in writing from the publisher. Permissions may be sought directly from Elsevier's Health Sciences Rights Department in Philadelphia, PA, USA: phone: (+1) 215 238 7869, fax: (+1) 215 238 2239, e-mail: health-permissions@elsevier.com. You may also complete your request on-line via the Elsevier homepage (http://www.elsevier.com), by selecting 'Customer Support' and then 'Obtaining Permissions'.

---

**NOTICE**

Medicine is an ever-changing field. Standard safety precautions must be followed, but as new research and clinical experience broaden our knowledge, changes in treatment and drug therapy may become necessary or appropriate. Readers are advised to check the most current product information provided by the manufacturer of each drug to be administered to verify the recommended dose, the method and duration of administration, and contraindications. It is the responsibility of the treating physician, relying on experience and knowledge of the patient, to determine dosages and the best treatment for each individual patient. Neither the publisher nor the editor assumes any liability for any injury and/or damage to persons or property arising from this publication.

---

Previous edition copyrighted 2000

**Library of Congress Cataloguing-in-Publication Data**
Hypertension : a companion to Brenner and Rector's the kidney / [edited by] Suzanne Oparil, Michael A.
   Weber.—2nd ed.
     p. ; cm.
   Companion v. Brenner and Rector's the kidney / edited by Barry M. Brenner. 7th ed. c2004.
   Includes bibliographical references and index.
   ISBN 0-7216-0258-4
     1. Hypertension. I. Oparil, Suzanne. II. Weber, Michael A. III. Brenner & Rector's the kidney.
   [DNLM: 1. Hypertension—therapy. 2. Antihypertensive Agents—therapeutic use.
   3. Hypertension—complications. 4. Hypertension—physiopathology. 5. Life Style. WG 340
   H99426 2005]
   RC685.H8H76783 2005
   616.1'32—dc22

2004051303

*Acquisitions Editor: Susan F. Pioli*
*Developmental Editor: Kim J. Davis*
*Publishing Services Manager: Joan Sinclair*

**Working together to grow
libraries in developing countries**

www.elsevier.com | www.bookaid.org | www.sabre.org

**ELSEVIER**    BOOK AID International    Sabre Foundation

Printed in China.

Last digit is the print number: 9 8 7 6 5 4 3 2 1

# Contributors

Roland Asmar, M.D.
Medical Director
Department of Cardiology
The Cardiovascular Institute
Paris, France
*Clinical Applications of Arterial Stiffness in Hypertension*

Jan N. Basile, M.D.
Professor of Medicine
Division of General Internal Medicine/Geriatrics
Medical University of South Carolina
Lead Physician-Primary Care
Ralph H. Johnson VA Medical Center
Charleston, South Carolina
*Hypertension in the Elderly*

D.G. Beevers
Professor
Department of Medicine
University of Birmingham
City Hospital
Birmingham, England
*The LIFE Study*

Lawrence J. Beilin, M.D. (Lond), M.B.B.S., F.R.C.P., F.R.A.C.P.
Professor of Medicine
School of Medicine and Pharmacology
University of Western Australia
West Australian Institute for Medical Research
Perth, Western Australia
*Alcohol and Hypertension*

Grzegorz Bilo, M.D.
Department of Clinical Medicine, Prevention and Applied Biotechnology
University of Milano-Bicocca
Second Cardiology Unit
S. Luca Hospital, IRCCS Instituto Auxologico Italiano
Milan, Italy
*Prognostic and Diagnostic Value of Ambulatory Blood Pressure Monitoring*

Henry R. Black, M.D.
Associate Vice President for Research
Chairman, Department of Preventive Medicine
Rush University Medical Center
Attending Physician
Rush University Medical Center
Chicago, Illinois
*The Concept of Total Risk*

Guido Boerrigter, M.D.
Instructor of Medicine
Mayo Clinic College of Medicine
Cardiology Fellow
Division of Cardiovascular Diseases
Department of Internal Medicine
Mayo Clinic
Rochester, Minnesota
*Endothelin in Hypertension*

Lee R. Bone, R.N., M.P.H.
Associate Professor
Department of Health Policy and Management
The Johns Hopkins University Bloomberg School of Public Health
Baltimore, Maryland
*Community Outreach*

Hans Brunner
University of Lausanne
Lausanne, Switzerland
*The VALUE Trial*

John C. Burnett, Jr., M.D.
Professor of Medicine and Physiology
Mayo Clinic College of Medicine
Director for Research
Director, Cardiorenal Research Laboratory
Division of Cardiovascular Diseases
Department of Internal Medicine
Mayo Clinic and Foundation
Rochester, Minnesota
*Endothelin in Hypertension*

David A. Calhoun, M.D.
Associate Professor of Medicine
Vascular Biology and Hypertension Program
University of Alabama at Birmingham
Birmingham, Alabama
*Resistant Hypertension*

Vito M. Campese, M.D.
Professor of Medicine, Physiology and Biophysics
Chief, Division of Nephrology and Hypertension
Keck School of Medicine
University of Southern California
Los Angeles, California
*Natriuretic Peptides*

**Robert M. Carey, M.D., M.A.C.P.**
Harrison Distinguished Professor of Medicine
Department of Medicine
University of Virginia Health System
Charlottesville, Virginia
*The Angiotensin Receptors: AT₁ and AT₂*

**J. Jaime Caro, M.D.C.M., F.R.C.P.C., F.A.C.P.**
Adjunct Professor
Department of Medicine
McGill University
Montreal, Quebec, Canada
Scientific Director
Caro Research Institute
Concord, Massachusetts
*Current Prescribing Practices*

**Oscar A. Carretero, M.D.**
Professor of Medicine
Henry Ford Health Sciences Center
Detroit, Michigan
Case Western Reserve University
Cleveland, Ohio
Division Head
Department of Hypertension and Vascular Research
Henry Ford Hospital
Detroit, Michigan
*The Kallikrein-Kinin System as a Regulator of Cardiovascular and Renal Function*

**Mark C. Chappell, Ph.D.**
Associate Professor
Hypertension and Vascular Disease Center
Wake Forest University School of Medicine
Winston-Salem, North Carolina
*Angiotensin-(1-7)*

**George S. Chrysant, M.D.**
Interventional Cardiologist
Integris Baptist Medical Center
Associate Director
Oklahoma Cardiovascular and Hypertension Center
Oklahoma City, Oklahoma
*Ischemic Heart Disease in Hypertension*

**Jeffrey A. Cutler, M.D., M.P.H.**
Senior Scientific Advisor
Division of Epidemiology and Clinical Applications
National Heart, Lung, and Blood Institute
Bethesda, Maryland
*The Blood Pressure Lowering Treatment Trialists' Collaboration (BPLTTC)*

**Björn Dahlöf, M.D., Ph.D., F.A.C.C.**
Associate Professor
Department of Medicine
Göteborg University
Sahlgrenska University Hospital/östra
Medical Advisor
Scandinavian CRI
Göteborg, Sweden
**The LIFE Study**

**Alexandre A. da Silva, Ph.D.**
Instructor
Department of Physiology and Biophysics
University of Mississippi Medical Center
Jackson, Mississippi
*Obesity and Hypertension: Impact on the Cardiovascular and Renal Systems*

**Ulf de Faire, M.D., Ph.D.**
Professor
Division of Epidemiology, IMM
Karolinska Institute
Professor
Department of Cardiology
Karolinska University Hospital
Stockholm, Sweden
*The LIFE Study*

**Maria Carolina Delgado, M.D.**
Research Investigator
Department of Internal Medicine
Division of Cardiovascular Medicine
University of Michigan Medical Center
Ann Arbor, Michigan
*Pathophysiology of Hypertension*

**Richard B. Devereux, M.D.**
Professor
Department of Medicine
Weill Medical College of Cornell University
Attending Physician
Department of Medicine
New York Presbyterian Hospital
New York, New York
*The LIFE Study*

**Joseph A. Diamond, M.D., F.A.C.C.**
Associate Professor
Department of Medicine
Albert Einstein College of Medicine
Bronx, New York
Director of Nuclear Cardiology
Department of Cardiology
Long Island Jewish Medical Center
New Hyde Park, New York
*Left Ventricular Hypertrophy, Congestive Heart Failure, and Coronary Flow Reserve Abnormalities in Hypertension*

**Donald J. DiPette, M.D.**
Chair, Department of Medicine
Texas A&M University College of Medicine and
Scott & White Hospital
Temple, Texas
*Vasodilator Peptides: CGRP, Substance P, and Adrenomedullin*

**Debra I. Diz, Ph.D.**
Professor
Hypertension and Vascular Disease Center
Wake Forest University School of Medicine
Winston-Salem, North Carolina
*Angiotensin-(1-7)*

Jonathan M. Edelman, M.D.
Executive Director
Department of Clinical Development
Merck and Company, Inc.
West Point, Pennsylvania
*The LIFE Study*

William J. Elliott, M.D., Ph.D.
Professor of Preventive Medicine, Internal Medicine, and
Pharmacology
Department of Preventive Medicine
Rush Medical College
Attending Physician
Rush University Medical Center
Chicago, Illinois
*The Concept of Total Risk*

Steffan Enkman, M.Sc.Pharm.
Novartis Pharma
Basel, Switzerland
*The VALUE Trial*

Bonita Falkner, M.D.
Professor of Medicine and Pediatrics
Thomas Jefferson University
Philadelphia, Pennsylvania
*Hypertension in Children*

William L. Fan, M.D.
Fellow
Division of Nephrology
Department of Medicine
Duke University Medical Center
Durham, North Carolina
*Dietary Approaches to Hypertension Management: The DASH
Studies*

Robert R. Fenichel, M.D., Ph.D.
Lecturer
Department of Medicine
Georgetown University Medical School
Washington, DC
*How Antihypertensive Drugs Get Approved in the United States*

Carlos M. Ferrario, M.D., F.A.C.C., F.A.C.A.
Professor and Director
Hypertension and Vascular Disease Center
Wake Forest University School of Medicine
Winston-Salem, North Carolina
*Angiotensin-(1-7)*

Stanley S. Franklin, M.D.
Clinical Professor of Medicine
Associate Medical Director
UCI Heart Disease Prevention Program
Department of Medicine
University of California, Irvine College of Medicine
Irvine, California
*Epidemiology of Hypertension*
*New Interpretations of Blood Pressure: The Importance of Pulse
Pressure*

Edward D. Freis, M.D.
Professor Emeritus
Department of Medicine
Georgetown University School of Medicine
Senior Medical Investigator
Department of Medicine
Veterans Administration Hospital
Washington, DC
*A History of Hypertension Treatment*

William H. Frishman, M.D., M.A.C.P.
Barbara and William Rosenthal Professor and Chair
Department of Medicine
New York Medical College
Director of Medicine
Westchester Medical Center
Valhalla, New York
*β-Adrenergic Blockers*

Edward D. Frohlich, M.D.
Alton Ochsner Distinguished Scientist
Ochsner Clinic Foundation
Professor, Department of Medicine and Physiology
Louisiana State University School of Medicine
Clinical Professor of Medicine and Adjunct Professor
Department of Pharmacology
Tulane University School of Medicine
New Orleans, Louisiana
*Direct-Acting Smooth Muscle Vasodilators and Adrenergic
Inhibitors*

John W. Funder, M.D., Ph.D.
Professor
Department of Medicine
Monash University
Senior Fellow
Prince Henry's Institute of Medical Research
Clayton, Victoria, Australia
Professorial Fellow
Department of Neuroscience
University of Melbourne
Parkville, Victoria, Australia
*Aldosterone and Mineralocorticoids*

Frej Fyhrquist
Professor of Medicine
Minerva Institute for Medical Research
Biomedicum Helsinki
Helsinki, Finland
*The LIFE Study*

Gerardo Gamba, M.D., Ph.D.
Molecular Physiology Unit
Department of Nephrology and Mineral Metabolism
Instituto Nacional de Ciencias Médicas y Nutrición Salvador
Zubirán
Department of Genomic Medicine and Environmental
Toxicology
Instituto de Investigaciones Biomédicas
Universidad Nacional Autónoma de México
Tlalpan, Mexico City, Mexico
*Diuretics: Mechanisms of Action*

Apoor S. Gami, M.D.
**Assistant Professor of Medicine**
**Division of Cardiovascular Diseases**
**Mayo Clinic College of Medicine**
**Rochester, Minnesota**
*Obstructive Sleep Apnea and Hypertension*

Haralambos Gavras, M.D., F.R.C.P.
**Professor**
**Department of Medicine**
**Boston University School of Medicine**
**Chief**
**Hypertension and Atherosclerosis Section**
**Boston Medical Center**
**Boston, Massachusetts**
*ACE Inhibitor Trials: Effects in Hypertension*

Irene Gavras, M.D.
**Professor**
**Department of Medicine**
**Boston University School of Medicine**
**Attending Physician**
**Hypertension and Atherosclerosis Section**
**Boston Medical Center**
**Boston, Massachusetts**
*ACE Inhibitor Trials: Effects in Hypertension*

Todd W. B. Gehr, M.D.
**Chairman of Nephrology**
**Professor of Medicine**
**Virginia Commonwealth University**
**Medical College of Virginia Hospitals**
**Richmond, Virginia**
*Hypertension in Patients on Renal Replacement Therapy*
*Angiotensin-Converting Enzyme Inhibitors*

Gilbert W. Gleim, Ph.D.
**Associate Director**
**Department of Medical Communications**
**Merck Research Laboratories**
**West Point, Pennsylvania**
*The LIFE Study*

John E. Hall, Ph.D.
**Guyton Professor and Chairman**
**Department of Physiology and Biophysics**
**University of Mississippi Medical Center**
**Jackson, Mississippi**
*Obesity and Hypertension: Impact on the Cardiovascular and
Renal Systems*

Donna S. Hanes, M.D.
**Assistant Professor and Director of Clinical Education**
**Department of Medicine, Division of Nephrology**
**University of Maryland Hospital**
**Baltimore, Maryland**
*Renal Protection in Chronic Kidney Disease*

Stephen B. Harrap, M.B.B.S., Ph.D., F.R.A.C.P.
**Professor and Head**
**Department of Physiology**
**University of Melbourne**
**Victoria, Australia**
*Blood Pressure Genetics*

Katherine E. Harris, Dr.PH
**Director**
**Department of Clinical Biostatistics**
**Merck and Company, Inc.**
**West Point, Pennsylvania**
*The LIFE Study*

Erhard Haus, M.D., Ph.D.
**Professor**
**Department of Anatomic and Clinical Pathology**
**University of Minnesota**
**Minneapolis, Minnesota**
**Pathologist**
**Department of Anatomic and Clinical Pathology**
**Regions Hospital**
**HealthPartners Medical Group**
**St. Paul, Minnesota**
*Chronotherapeutics in the Treatment of Hypertension*

Ramon C. Hermida, Ph.D.
**Professor, Bioengineering and Chronobiology**
**Laboratories**
**University of Vigo**
**Vigo, Spain**
*Chronotherapeutics in the Treatment of Hypertension*

Martha N. Hill, Ph.D., R.N., F.A.A.N
**Dean and Professor**
**The Johns Hopkins University**
**School of Nursing**
**Baltimore, Maryland**
*Nursing Clinics in the Management of Hypertension
Community Outreach*

Hans Ibsen, M.D., D.M.Sci.
**University of Copenhagen**
**Department of Medicine**
**Glostrup University Hospital**
**Glostrup, Denmark**
*The LIFE Study*

Hope Intengan, Ph.D.
**Metabolic Research Unit/Diabetes Center**
**University of California at San Francisco**
**San Francisco, California**
*Remodeling of Resistance Arteries in Hypertension*

Joseph L. Izzo, Jr., M.D.
**Professor**
**Departments of Medicine and Pharmacology**
**Head, Clinical Pharmacology Division**
**Vice Chair, Department of Medicine**
**State University of New York at Buffalo**
**Buffalo, New York**
*The Sympathetic Nervous System in Acute and Chronic Blood
Pressure Elevation*

Garry L. R. Jennings, M.D., F.R.C.P., F.R.A.C.P.
**Professor and Director**
**Baker Heart Research Institute**
**Melbourne, Australia**
*Exercise and Hypertension*

Ernest F. Johnson III, M.D.
Fellow
Division of Nephrology
Case Western Reserve University
Cleveland, Ohio
*Management of Hypertension in Black Populations*


Colin I. Johnston, M.D., M.B.B.S., F.R.A.C.P., F.A.H.A.
Professor
Department of Medicine
Monash University
Senior Principal Research Fellow
Baker Heart Research Institute
Melbourne, Australia
*Angiotensin Converting Enzymes: Properties and Function*


Daniel W. Jones, M.D.
Vice Chancellor for Health Affairs and Dean
School of Medicine
University of Mississippi Medical Center
Jackson, Mississippi
*Obesity and Hypertension: Impact on the Cardiovascular and
Renal Systems*
*Pheochromocytoma: Detection and Management*


Stevo Julius, M.D., M.D. (Hon), Sc.D.
Professor of Medicine and Physiology
Frederick G.L. Huetwell Professor of Hypertension
Department of Internal Medicine
Division of Hypertension
The University of Michigan Health System
Ann Arbor, Michigan
*The LIFE Study*
*The VALUE Trial*
*Main Results from VALUE*
*Clinical Outcome Trials of Hypertension with Angiotensin
Receptor Blockers*


William B. Kannel, M.D., M.P.H.
Professor of Medicine and Public Health
Department of Preventive Medicine
Boston University School of Medicine
Boston, Massachusetts
Framingham Study
NHLBI/Boston University
Framingham, Massachusetts
*Coronary Atherosclerotic Sequelae of Hypertension*


Khurshed A. Katki, Ph.D.
Instructor
Department of Medicine
Texas A&M University
Research Scientist
Scott & White Memorial Hospital
Temple, Texas
*Vasodilator Peptides: CGRP, Substance P, and
Adrenomedullin*


Sverre E. Kjeldsen, M.D., Ph.D., F.A.H.A.
Adjunct Professor
Department of Internal Medicine
University of Michigan
Ann Arbor, Michigan
Chief Physician
Department of Cardiology
Ullevaal University Hospital
Oslo, Norway
*The LIFE Study*
*The VALUE Trial*
*Main Results from VALUE*


Thomas R. Kleyman, M.D.
Professor of Medicine
Chief, Renal-Electrolyte Division
Department of Medicine
University of Pittsburgh
Pittsburgh, Pennsylvania
*Diuretics: Mechanisms of Action*


Mark A. Knepper, M.D., Ph.D.
Laboratory of Kidney and Electrolyte Metabolism
National Heart, Lung and Blood Institute
National Institutes of Health
Bethesda, Maryland
*Diuretics: Mechanisms of Action*


Panagiotis Kokkoris, M.D.
Endocrinologist
Department of Endocrinology, Diabetes and
Metabolism
Hellenic Air Force General Hospital
Athens, Greece
*Obesity in Hypertension: The Role of Diet and Drugs*


John B. Kostis, M.D.
John G. Detwiler Professor of Cardiology
Professor of Medicine and Pharmacology
Chairman, Department of Medicine
UMDNJ-Robert Wood Johnson Medical School
Chief of Medical Service
Department of Medicine
Robert Wood Johnson University Hospital
New Brunswick, New Jersey
*Angiotensin II Receptor Antagonists*


Lawrence R. Krakoff, M.D.
Professor
Department of Medicine
Mount Sinai School of Medicine
New York, New York
Chief
Department of Medicine
Englewood Hospital and Medical Center
Englewood, New Jersey
*Initial Evaluation and Follow-Up Assessment*

Krister J. Kristianson, Ph.D.
**Director for Clinical Research**
**Merck Research Laboratories**
**Scandinavian Operations**
**Sollentuna, Sweden**
*The LIFE Study*

Jay J. Kuo, Ph.D.
**Instructor**
**Department of Physiology and Biophysics**
**University of Mississippi Medical Center**
**Jackson, Mississippi**
*Obesity and Hypertension: Impact on the Cardiovascular and Renal Systems*

Jay Lakkis, M.D.
**Fellow in Nephrology**
**Department of Medicine**
**University of Maryland School of Medicine**
**Baltimore, Maryland**
*Diabetes Mellitus and the Cardiovascular Metabolic Syndrome: Reducing Cardiovascular and Renal Events*

John H. Laragh, M.D.
**Director of the Cardiovascular Center**
**New York Hospital**
**Cornell University Medical Center**
**New York, New York**
*The VALUE Trial*

David M. Levine, M.D., Sc.D, M.P.H.
**Samsung Professor of Medicine, Public Health and Nursing**
**Department of Medicine**
**Johns Hopkins University**
**Johns Hopkins Hospital**
**Baltimore, Maryland**
*Community Outreach*

Kathleen C. Light, Ph.D.
**Professor**
**Department of Psychiatry**
**University of North Carolina School of Medicine**
**Chapel Hill, North Carolina**
*Environmental and Psychosocial Stress in Hypertension Onset and Progression*

Lars H. Lindholm, M.D., Ph.D.
**Professor and Chair**
**Department of Public Health and Clinical Medicine**
**Umea University Hospital**
**Umea, Sweden**
*The LIFE Study*

Jiankang Liu, M.D., Ph.D.
**Postdoctoral Fellow**
**Department of Physiology and Biophysics**
**University of Mississippi Medical Center**
**Jackson, Mississippi**
*Obesity and Hypertension: Impact on the Cardiovascular and Renal Systems*

Thomas F. Lüscher, M.D.
**Professor and Head of Cardiology**
**University Hospital**
**Zurich, Switzerland**
*Endothelium in Hypertension: Nitric Oxide*

Giuseppe Mancia, M.D.
**Head, Department of Clinical Medicine, Prevention and Applied Biotechnologies**
**University of Milano-Bicocca**
**Head, Unit of Clinica Medica**
**St. Gerardo Hospital**
**Chairman, Centro Intrauniversitario Fisiologia Clinica e Ipertensione**
**Milan, Italy**
*Prognostic and Diagnostic Value of Ambulatory Blood Pressure Monitoring*

George A. Mansoor, M.D., F.R.C.P.
**Associate Professor**
**Center for Cardiology and Cardiovascular Biology**
**University of Connecticut Health Center**
**Attending Physician**
**John Dempsey Hospital**
**Farmington, Connecticut**
*White-Coat Hypertension*

David A. McCarron, M.D.
**Visiting Professor**
**Department of Nutrition**
**University of California, Davis**
**Davis, California**
**President**
**Academic Network, LLC**
**Portland, Oregon**
*Diet: Micronutrients*

Heather L. McGuire, M.D.
**Fellow**
**Division of Nephrology**
**Department of Medicine**
**Duke University Medical Center**
**Durham, North Carolina**
*Dietary Approaches to Hypertension Management: The DASH Studies*

Gordon T. McInnes, M.D., B.Sc.
**Professor of Clinical Pharmacology**
**Division of Cardiovascular and Medical Sciences**
**University of Glasgow**
**Consultant Physician**
**Department of Acute Medicine**
**Western Infirmary**
**Glasgow, United Kingdom**
*The VALUE Trial*
*Critical Assessment of Hypertension Guidelines*

Ellen G. McMahon, Ph.D.
**Regional Medical and Research Specialist**
**Pfizer, Inc.**
**New York, New York**
*Mineralocorticoid Receptor Antagonists*

Renee P. Meyer, M.D.
Assistant Professor of Medicine
Department of Internal Medicine/Geriatrics
Medical University of South Carolina
Geriatrics and Extended Care
Ralph H. Johnson VA Medical Center
Charleston, South Carolina
*Hypertension in the Elderly*

Nancy Houston Miller, B.S.N.
Associate Director
Stanford Cardiac Rehabilitation Program
Stanford University School of Medicine
Palo Alto, California
*Nursing Clinics in the Management of Hypertension*

Mitra K. Nadim, M.D.
Assistant Professor of Clinical Medicine
Associate Director, Hypertension Center
Division of Nephrology
University of Southern California
Los Angeles, California
*Natriuretic Peptides*

Shawna D. Nesbitt, M.D., M.S.
Assistant Professor
Medical Director, Parkland Hospital Hypertension Clinic
Department of Internal Medicine
University of Texas Southwestern Medical Center
Dallas, Texas
*Clinical Outcome Trials of Hypertension with Angiotensin Receptor Blockers*

Joel M. Neutel, M.D.
Associate Professor of Medicine
University of California, Irvine
Irvine, California
Director of Research
Orange County Research Center
Tustin, California
*Fixed Combination Antihypertensive Therapy*

Markku S. Nieminen, M.D., Ph.D., F.A.C.C., F.E.S.C.
Professor and Chief
Division of Cardiology
University Central Hospital
Helsinki, Finland
*The LIFE Study*

Jürg Nussberger, M.D.
Professor of Medicine
Faculté de Biologie et de Médecine
Hospices Cantonaux
Professor of Medicine
Division of Hypertension and Vascular Medicine
Centre Hospitalier Universitaire Vaudois
Lausanne, Vaud, Switzerland
*Renin Inhibitors*

Per Omvik, M.D., Ph.D.
Vice Dean and Professor
Department of Internal Medicine
University of Bergen
Professor
Department of Cardiology
Haukeland University Hospital
Bergen, Norway
*The LIFE Study*

Suzanne Oparil, M.D., F.A.C.C.
Director
Vascular Biology and Hypertension Program
Division of Cardiovascular Diseases
Professor of Medicine, Physiology, and Biophysics
University of Alabama at Birmingham
Birmingham, Alabama
*The Antihypertensive and Lipid-Lowering to Prevent Heart Attack Trial (ALLHAT)*
*The LIFE Study*
*Ischemic Heart Disease in Hypertension*

Lionel H. Opie, M.D., D.Phil., D.Sc.
Director, Hatter Institute
Faculty of Health Sciences
University of Cape Town
Senior Physician, Hypertension Clinic
Department of Medicine
Groote Schuur Hospital
Cape Town, South Africa
*Calcium Channel Blockers: Controversies, Lessons, and Outcomes*

Lars Osterberg, M.D.
Clinical Assistant Professor of Medicine
Stanford University School of Medicine
Stanford, California
Chief of General Internal Medicine
VA Palo Alto Health Care System
Palo Alto, California
*Medication Adherence for Antihypertensive Therapy*

Gianfranco Parati, M.D., F.A.H.A., F.E.S.C.
Professor
Department of Clinical Medicine, Prevention and Applied Biotechnology
University of Milano-Bicocca
Head, Second Cardiology Unit
S. Luca Hospital, IRCCS Istituto Auxologico Italiano
Milan, Italy
*Prognostic and Diagnostic Value of Ambulatory Blood Pressure Monitoring*

Krista A. Payne, M.Ed., B.A. (Hons)
Senior Researcher
Caro Research
Montreal, Quebec, Canada
*Current Prescribing Practices*

Ole Lederballe Pedersen, M.D., D.M.Sci.
**Associate Professor**
**Department of Clinical Pharmacology**
**University of Aarhus**
**Aarhus, Denmark**
**Consultant**
**Department of Medicine**
**Sygehus Viborg**
**Viborg, Denmark**
*The LIFE Study*

Robert A. Phillips, M.D., Ph.D., F.A.C.C., F.A.H.A.
**Professor**
**Department of Medicine**
**New York University School of Medicine**
**Chairman**
**Department of Medicine**
**Lenox Hill Hospital**
**New York, New York**
*Left Ventricular Hypertrophy, Congestive Heart Failure and*
*Coronary Flow Reserve Abnormalities in Hypertension*

Xavier Pi-Sunyer, M.D., M.P.H.
**Professor of Medicine**
**Columbia University College of Physicians and Surgeons**
**Chief**
**Division of Endocrinology, Diabetes and Nutrition**
**St. Luke's-Roosevelt Hospital Center**
**New York, New York**
*Obesity in Hypertension: The Role of Diet and Drugs*

Francis Plat, M.D.
**Vice President**
**Cardiovascular Research and Development**
**Novartis Pharmaceuticals Corporation**
**Basel, Switzerland**
*The VALUE Trial*

James L. Pool, M.D.
**Professor**
**Departments of Medicine and Pharmacology**
**Baylor College of Medicine**
**Houston, Texas**
*α-Adrenoceptor Blockers*

Francesco Portaluppi, M.D.
**Associate Professor of Internal Medicine**
**Department of Clinical and Experimental Medicine**
**University of Ferrara**
**Director, Hypertension Center**
**St. Anna Hospital**
**Ferrara, Italy**
*Chronotherapeutics in the Treatment of Hypertension*

L. Michael Prisant, M.D., F.A.C.C., F.A.H.A.
**Professor of Medicine**
**Director of Hypertension and Clinical Pharmacology**
**Department of Medicine**
**Medical College of Georgia**
**Augusta, Georgia**
*Calcium Antagonists*

Ian B. Puddey, M.D., M.B.B.S., F.R.A.C.P.
**Professor**
**School of Medicine and Pharmacology**
**University of Western Australia**
**Nedlands, Western Australia**
*Alcohol and Hypertension*

Satish R. Raj, M.D.
**Instructor**
**Departments of Medicine and Pharmacology**
**Vanderbilt University**
**Attending Physician**
**Autonomic Dysfunction Center**
**Vanderbilt University Medical Center**
**Nashville, Tennessee**
*Orthostatic Hypotension and Autonomic Dysfunction*
*Syndromes*

Gerald M. Reaven, M.D.
**Professor of Medicine**
**Division of Cardiovascular Medicine**
**Stanford University School of Medicine**
**Stanford, California**
*The Role of Insulin Resistance and Compensatory*
*Hyperinsulinemia in Patients with Essential*
*Hypertension*

Scott T. Reeves, M.D., M.B.A., F.A.C.C., F.A.S.E.
**Professor**
**Department of Anesthesia and Perioperative Medicine**
**Medical University of South Carolina**
**Charleston, South Carolina**
*Anesthesia and Hypertension*

Alain Reinberg, M.D., Ph.D.
**Directeur de Recherches**
**National Center for Scientific Research**
**Unité de Chronobiologie**
**Foundation A. de Rothschild**
**Paris, France**
*Chronotherapeutics in the Treatment of Hypertension*

Ira W. Reiser, M.D.
**Clinical Associate Professor of Medicine**
**Department of Medicine**
**State University of New York Health Science Center at**
**Brooklyn**
**Attending Physician**
**Division of Nephrology and Hypertension**
**Department of Medicine**
**The Brookdale University Hospital and Medical Center**
**Brooklyn, New York**
*Renovascular Hypertension: Diagnosis and Treatment*

Timothy L. Reudelhuber, Ph.D.
**Director**
**Laboratory of Molecular Biochemistry of**
**Hypertension**
**Clinical Research Institute of Montreal (ICRM)**
**Montreal, Quebec, Canada**
*Renin*

Molly E. Reusser, M.A.
**Technical Writer**
**Academic Network**
**Portland, Oregon**
*Diet: Micronutrients*

J.G. Reves, M.D.
**Vice President for Medical Affairs**
**Dean, College of Medicine**
**Medical University of South Carolina**
**Charleston, South Carolina**
*Anesthesia and Hypertension*

Nour-Eddine Rhaleb, Ph.D., F.A.H.A.
**Associate Professor of Medicine**
**Department of Physiology**
**Wayne State University**
**Senior Scientist**
**Departments of Internal Medicine, Hypertension, and**
**Vascular Research**
**Henry Ford Hospital**
**Detroit, Michigan**
*The Kallikrein-Kinin System as a Regulator of Cardiovascular*
*and Renal Function*

David Robertson, M.D.
**Elton Yates Professor of Medicine, Pharmacology, and**
**Neurology**
**Vanderbilt University**
**Nashville, Tennessee**
*Orthostatic Hypotension and Autonomic Dysfunction*
*Syndromes*

Edward J. Roccella, Ph.D., M.P.H.
**Coordinator, Office of Prevention, Education and Control**
**National Heart, Lung and Blood Institute**
**Bethesda, Maryland**
*The National High Blood Pressure Education Program*

Peter Rudd, M.D.
**Professor**
**Department of Medicine**
**Stanford University**
**Stanford, California**
*Medication Adherence for Antihypertensive Therapy*

Michael C. Ruddy, M.D.
**Clinical Associate Professor**
**Department of Medicine**
**UMDNJ-Robert Wood Johnson Medical School**
**New Brunswick, New Jersey**
**Chief, Section of Nephrology**
**Department of Medicine**
**University Medical Center at Princeton**
**Princeton, New Jersey**
*Angiotensin II Receptor Antagonists*

Luis Miguel Ruilope, M.D.
**Chief, Hypertension Unit**
**12 de Octubre Hospital**
**Carretera de Andalucia**
**Madrid, Spain**
*Vasopeptidase Inhibitors*

Ernesto L. Schiffrin, M.D., Ph.D., F.R.C.P.C., F.A.C.P.
**Professor of Medicine**
**University of Montreal**
**Director, CIHR Multidisciplinary Research Group on**
**Hypertension and Hypertension Clinic**
**Clinical Research Institute of Montreal**
**Staff, Division of Internal Medicine**
**Hôtel-Dieu Hospital of the University of Montreal Hospital**
**Centre (CHUM)**
**Montreal, Quebec, Canada**
*Remodeling of Resistance Arteries in Hypertension*
*Endothelin Antagonists*

John A. Schirger, M.D.
**Instructor of Medicine**
**Mayo Clinic College of Medicine**
**NIH Cardiology Fellow**
**Division of Cardiovascular Disease**
**Mayo Clinic**
**Rochester, Minnesota**
*Endothelin in Hypertension*

M. Anthony Schork, Ph.D.
**Emeritus Professor**
**Department of Biostatistics**
**University of Michigan**
**Ann Arbor, Michigan**
*The VALUE Trial*

Alexander M. M. Shepherd, M.D., Ph.D., F.A.H.A.
**Professor and Chief**
**Division of Clinical Pharmacology**
**Departments of Medicine and Pharmacology**
**University of Texas Health Science Center at San Antonio**
**San Antonio, Texas**
*Pharmacokinetics of Antihypertensive Drugs*

Domenic A. Sica, M.D., F.A.C.P.
**Professor of Medicine and Pharmacology**
**Department of Medicine**
**Virginia Commonwealth University**
**Chairman, Section of Clinical Pharmacology and Hypertension**
**Division of Nephrology**
**Virginia Commonwealth University**
**Richmond, Virginia**
*Hypertension in Patients on Renal Replacement Therapy*
*Angiotensin-Converting Enzyme Inhibitors*

Helmy M. Siragy, M.D., F.A.C.P., F.A.H.A.
**Professor of Medicine and Endocrinology**
**Director of the Hypertension Center**
**University of Virginia**
**Charlottesville, Virginia**
*The Angiotensin Receptors: $AT_1$ and $AT_2$*

Beverly A. Smith, B.S.N.
**Associate Director**
**Global Cardiovascular Clinical Development**
**Novartis Pharmaceuticals Corporation**
**East Hanover, New Jersey**
*The VALUE Trial*

Michael H. Smolensky, Ph.D.
Professor
Department of Environmental and Occupational Medicine
School of Public Health
University of Texas-Houston Health Science Center
Houston, Texas
*Chronotherapeutics in the Treatment of Hypertension*

Steven Snapinn, Ph.D.
Senior Director
Department of Biostatistics
Amgen, Incorporated
Thousand Oaks, California
*The LIFE Study*

Virend K. Somers, M.D., D.Phil.
Professor of Medicine
Divisions of Cardiovascular Diseases and Hypertension
Mayo Clinic College of Medicine
Rochester, Minnesota
*Obstructive Sleep Apnea and Hypertension*

Lukas E. Spieker, M.D.
Department of Cardiology
University Hospital
Zurich, Switzerland
*Endothelium in Hypertension: Nitric Oxide*

Samuel Spitalewitz, M.D.
Associate Professor of Clinical Medicine
Department of Medicine
State University of New York Health Science Center at Brooklyn
Attending Physician and Physician-in-Charge of the Renal and Hypertension Clinics
The Brookdale University Hospital and Medical Center
Brooklyn, New York
*Renovascular Hypertension: Diagnosis and Treatment*

Pelle Stolt, Ph.D.
Novartis AG
Basel, Switzerland
*The VALUE Trial*
*Main Results from VALUE*

Scott C. Supowit, Ph.D.
Associate Professor
Department of Medicine
Texas A&M University System Health Science Center School of Medicine
Temple, Texas
*Vasodilator Peptides: CGRP, Substance P, and Adrenomedullin*

Laura P. Svetkey, M.D., M.H.S.
Professor
Department of Medicine
Director, Duke Hypertension Center
Director of Clinical Studies
Sarah W. Stedman Nutrition and Metabolism Center
Duke University Medical Center
Durham, North Carolina
*Dietary Approaches to Hypertension Management: The DASH Studies*

Sandra J. Taler, M.D.
Associate Professor of Medicine
Mayo Clinic College of Medicine
Department of Internal Medicine
Division of Nephrology and Hypertension
Mayo Clinic
Rochester, Minnesota
*Hypertension in Pregnancy*

Lakshmi S. Tallam, Ph.D.
Instructor
Department of Physiology
University of Mississippi Medical Center
Jackson, Mississippi
*Obesity and Hypertension: Impact on the Cardiovascular and Renal Systems*

E. Ann Tallant, Ph.D.
Associate Professor
Hypertension and Vascular Disease Center
Wake Forest University School of Medicine
Winston-Salem, North Carolina
*Angiotensin-(1-7)*

Chris Tikellis, Ph.D., B.Sc. (Hons)
Department of Diabetic Complications
Baker Heart Research Institute
Melbourne, Australia
*Angiotensin-Converting Enzymes: Properties and Function*

Fiona Turnbull, M.B.Ch.B., F.A.F.P.H.M.
Senior Research Fellow
Heart and Vascular Division
The George Institute for International Health
University of Sydney
Sydney, Australia
*The Blood Pressure Lowering Treatment Trialists' Collaboration (BPLTTC)*

Donald G. Vidt, M.D.
Consultant
Department of Nephrology and Hypertension
Cleveland Clinic Foundation
Cleveland, Ohio
Professor of Medicine
College of Medicine and Public Health
Ohio State University
Columbus, Ohio
*Management of Hypertensive Emergencies and Urgencies*

Ralph E. Watson, M.D., F.A.C.P.
Associate Professor of Medicine
Director, Hypertension Clinic
College of Human Medicine
Michigan State University
East Lansing, Michigan
*Vasodilator Peptides: CGRP, Substance P, and Adrenomedullin*

Michael A. Weber, M.D.
Associate Dean for Clinical Research and Professor of Medicine
State University of New York Health Science Center at Brooklyn
Brooklyn, New York
*The VALUE Trial*
*Main Results from VALUE*

Hans Wedel
Professor
Department of Biostatistics and Epidemiology
Nordic School of Public Health
Gothenburg, Sweden
*The LIFE Study*

Alan B. Weder, M.D.
Professor
Department of Internal Medicine
Division of Cardiovascular Medicine
University of Michigan Medical Center
Ann Arbor, Michigan
*Pathophysiology of Hypertension*

Myron H. Weinberger, M.D.
Professor of Medicine
Hypertension Research Center
Indiana University School of Medicine
Indianapolis, Indiana
*Initial Choices in the Treatment of Hypertension*
*Aggressive Blood Pressure Targets: Developing Effective Algorithms*

Matthew R. Weir, M.D.
Professor of Medicine
Director
Division of Nephrology
University of Maryland School of Medicine
Baltimore, Maryland
*Renal Protection in Chronic Kidney Disease*
*Diabetes Mellitus and the Cardiovascular Metabolic Syndrome: Reducing Cardiovascular and Renal Events*

William B. White, M.D.
Professor of Medicine and Chief
Division of Hypertension and Clinical Pharmacology
University of Connecticut School of Medicine
Medical Director, Clinical Trials Unit
University of Connecticut Health Center
Farmington, Connecticut
*White-Coat Hypertension*

Marion R. Wofford, M.D., M.P.H.
Associate Professor
Department of Medicine
University of Mississippi Medical Center
Jackson, Mississippi
*Pheochromocytoma: Detection and Management*

Nathan D. Wong, Ph.D., F.A.C.C.
Professor and Director
Heart Disease Prevention Program
Division of Cardiology
Department of Medicine
University of California, Irvine
Irvine, California
*Epidemiology of Hypertension*

Jackson T. Wright, Jr., M.D., Ph.D.
Professor
Department of Medicine
Case Western Reserve University
Program Director, General Clinical Research Center
Director, Clinical Hypertension Program
University Hospitals of Cleveland
Cleveland, Ohio
*The Antihypertensive and Lipid-Lowering Treatment to Prevent Heart Attack Trial (ALLHAT)*
*Management of Hypertension in Black Populations*

Xiao-Ping Yang, M.D.
Senior Staff Scientist
Hypertension Research Division
Department of Internal Medicine
Henry Ford Hospital
Detroit, Michigan
*The Kallikrein-Kinin System as a Regulator of Cardiovascular and Renal Function*

William F. Young, Jr., M.D.
Professor of Medicine
Mayo Clinic College of Medicine
Division of Endocrinology and Metabolism
Mayo Clinic
Rochester, Minnesota
*Adrenal Cortex Hypertension*

Alberto Zanchetti
Professor of Medicine
Centro di Fisiologia Clinica e Hypertension
University of Milan
Scientific Director
Instituto Auxologico Italiano
Milan, Italy
*The VALUE Trial*

Huawei Zhao, M.D.
Research Associate
Department of Pharmacology and Toxicology
Michigan State University
East Lansing, Michigan
*Vasodilator Peptides: CGRP, Substance P, and Adrenomedullin*

# Preface

Creating a comprehensive book on hypertension is a demanding task, particularly for the numerous contributors who provide chapters giving detailed descriptions of the most current information in their fields. For this reason, we were both highly gratified by the enthusiastic acceptance and wide distribution of the first edition of this book.

Now, 4 years later, the dedication and generosity of our professional colleagues have allowed us to produce this second edition. In some ways, it might have been tempting simply to add some updates to the original volume; after all, many of the chapters from the earlier edition remain highly relevant and contemporary. But, despite our earlier success, we have decided to entirely re-cast this publication. The last few years have seen not only the completion of a number of important and high-impact clinical trials in hypertension but also the emergence of new attitudes toward the scientific infrastructure and the clinical priorities of hypertension. We believe that the effort involved in creating this new book has been fully worthwhile.

Major trials that have been recently completed have been allocated chapters in this volume. These include two studies done in high-risk hypertensive patients, both comparing the relatively new angiotensin receptor blockers against older, more established drug classes. The Losartan Intervention For Endpoint Reduction (LIFE) trial compared the angiotensin receptor blocker, losartan, with the β-blocker, atenolol, and concluded that the angiotensin receptor blocker was significantly more efficacious in preventing strokes in hypertensive patients who are at high risk due to the presence of electrocardiographic evidence of left ventricular hypertrophy. The Valsartan Antihypertensive Long-term Use Evaluation (VALUE) trial compared the angiotensin receptor blocker, valsartan, with the calcium channel blocker, amlodipine. This study was confounded because the protocol resulted in achievement of somewhat unequal blood pressures in the two treatment groups. Importantly, VALUE emphasized that blood pressure control, perhaps more than any other factor, is the key to preventing major events and mortality in hypertension. Both the LIFE and VALUE trials also provided evidence that the angiotensin receptor blockers may have the added benefit of preventing or at least delaying the appearance of new-onset diabetes, an important attribute considering the worldwide epidemic of the triad of obesity, insulin resistance, and the cardio-metabolic syndrome.

Two trials, the Irbesartan Diabetic Nephropathy Trial (IDNT) and Reduction of Endpoints in Non-Insulin Dependent Diabetes Mellitus with the Angiotensin II Antagonist Losartan (RENAAL), were performed in patients with diabetic nephropathy and demonstrated that—for the same effects on blood pressure—angiotensin receptor blockers were more efficacious than other drug classes in preventing further deterioration of renal function and progression to end-stage renal disease. Apart from the importance of these results, and their implications for therapy, the studies have had the additional effect of focusing attention on the interaction of hypertension and diabetes.

One of the most noted events since the first edition was the publication of the Antihypertensive and Lipid-Lowering treatment to prevent Heart Attack Trial (ALLHAT). This large-scale trial, conducted primarily in the United States across a diverse population of high-risk hypertensive patients, compared the effects on fatal and nonfatal coronary events (as well as other relevant secondary endpoints) of treatments based on a thiazide-like diuretic, a dihydropyridine calcium channel blocker, and an angiotensin-converting enzyme (ACE) inhibitor. The three treatments had virtually identical effects on the primary coronary outcomes, but the diuretic had advantages with respect to some of the secondary endpoints, at least in some high-risk subgroups of patients.

The study was greeted with criticism from an array of experts who argued that its conclusions were influenced by artifacts of the study design that favored the diuretic, particularly in terms of achieving blood pressure control, and that there was no creditable basis for claiming superiority—or, for that matter, even economic advantage—for the thiazide when the full cost of therapy beyond drug acquisition was taken into account. This broad-based skepticism regarding the interpretation of ALLHAT has diluted its impact on hypertension practice, although it still remains a subject of much discussion and debate. A particularly interesting finding of ALLHAT was that the incidence of new-onset diabetes during the trial was significantly higher with the diuretic than with the other drugs, although during the relatively short-term follow-up of these patients there was no indication that having diabetes increased their risk of cardiovascular events. In this edition of our book, the authors of ALLHAT present their results as a chapter and provide an interesting discussion.

More than ever, hypertension is characterized by a wide array of issues at the molecular, physiologic, clinical, and population levels. A review of our contents will indicate that we have left very few stones unturned in our quest to provide a broad and contemporary view of hypertension. Right now, in the clinical arena, there is a particularly strong focus on the importance of blood pressure control. Although this goes back to the very origins of our understanding of hypertension as a clinical condition, compelling new data have made us more aware than ever that achieving aggressive target blood pressure levels during treatment may represent the single most important benefit that we can provide our patients. Throughout this book the message of blood pressure control across hypertension in its many clinical manifestations is addressed consistently by the authors.

Another contemporary issue in hypertension is the dramatically growing prevalence of the metabolic syndrome and its frequent outcome, type 2 diabetes mellitus. Even the lay public is now aware that there is a worldwide problem of obesity, perhaps exaggerated by the more physically passive and sedentary lifestyles that so many people have adopted. Most worrying, children even more than adults appear to have fallen victim to the dual problems of increased calories and decreased activity. A consequence of this is that not only is the prevalence of hypertension increased, but also it is likely to be associated with concomitant problems of obesity, lipid disorders, and glucose intolerance. Our readers will find these issues addressed in several places throughout this book. We are working hard to understand the pathophysiology, clinical characteristics, and optimal management for this important and highly prevalent syndrome.

Diabetes mellitus, particularly type 2, is increasing dramatically in incidence and is frequently part of the hypertension story. It would be easy to blame this on the aging of our populations in North America and Western Europe, but the unfortunate fact is that children and young adults are also now prone to this disorder. Currently, we equate diabetes with the presence of cardiovascular disease; in fact, most of our colleagues in endocrinology simply regard type 2 diabetes as being equivalent to coronary disease in creating cardiovascular risk. A small consolation is that we are getting a better idea of how differing therapies and approaches to management might provide some measure of protection for our patients who have diabetes and certainly for those who have this condition in association with hypertension and renal involvement. Once more, several chapters in this edition will provide insights and recommendations for understanding and managing this all-too-common problem.

The sophisticated readers of a book of this type are already aware that creating guidelines for the management of hypertension or other medical conditions can be as much a political as a scientific process. Ultimately, their recommendations to some extent represent the compromises of a group of experts, with disparate interpretations of scientific, clinical, and practical issues, attempting to achieve a consensus. Despite the differences among the specific recommendations produced by organizations or agencies around the world, they all recognize that control of blood pressure in all countries is far from optimal and that aggressive reduction of blood pressure remains the primary objective of treatment. There is also a growing agreement among the guidelines that starting therapy with combination drug treatment—which previously had been regarded as an imprecise or even shot-gun approach to hypertension—may in fact be desirable as a means to more effectively and rapidly achieve blood pressure control in patients whose pretreatment blood pressures are excessively elevated.

A quick review of the chapters in this book will reveal the various categories or sections into which we have placed them. Section 1 provides interesting background information on hypertension: its history, chiefly from a clinical perspective, and the role of an official organization—the National High Blood Pressure Education Program—in disseminating information to the American public about the importance of diagnosing and treating hypertension; and, of course, there is a chapter on the epidemiology of this very common condition.

Given the wide variety of regulatory systems and structural factors that influence blood pressure, Section 2 describes pathophysiology and is relatively large and comprehensive. A number of chapters deal with the renin-angiotensin-aldosterone system, including renin itself, the various forms of angiotensin, angiotensin-converting enzyme, angiotensin receptors, aldosterone, and selective mineralocorticoid receptors. There is strong evidence that this system not only plays a major role in blood pressure control, but also contributes to several mechanisms that

appear to accelerate atherosclerosis and other forms of hypertension and related target organ damage. This information lays the ground work for later chapters that describe the growing role of drugs that interrupt the renin-angiotensin-aldosterone system in managing hypertension as well as other cardiovascular and renal diseases.

Complementary to the renin axis is the sympathetic nervous system, which clearly is also pivotal in governing blood pressure. Increased sympathetic activity appears to be a major mediator of the blood pressure effects of obesity and other metabolic disorders that predispose to the development of hypertension. Other important vasoactive mediators, including the natriuretic peptides, the vasodilator peptides and the kallikrein-kinin system are also discussed in detail. Our section on pathophysiology emphasizes the endothelium, and looks at the importance of early structural changes in the microcirculation, as well as the stiffness of larger arteries. A chapter on the metabolic syndrome lays the foundation for important clinical issues discussed elsewhere in the book.

The transition to these more clinical issues requires, first of all, an understanding of the concept of total risk, particularly as hypertension is just one of the contributors to cardiovascular events and mortality. There is little doubt, however, that hypertension is a major antecedent to coronary events and to heart failure. These relationships are discussed in Section 3, which deals with target organ damage and cardiovascular events. The connection between blood pressure and the kidney is particularly strong, and this Section contains an important chapter that delineates how preventing the progression of renal disease depends highly on blood pressure control as well as other strategies. It is fascinating how, even at this relatively advanced stage of our understanding of hypertension, we are still seeking better ways of interpreting the blood pressure itself: which component or derivative of the blood pressure is the most important prognostically, and which should be the primary target of treatment?

After Section 4 explores blood pressure both from a diagnostic and mechanistic point of view, Section 5 goes on to describe the general principles of treating hypertension. The early chapters in this Section report the findings of major clinical trials in hypertension and related areas, including those that were discussed above, and review major meta-analyses looking at the comparative effects of antihypertensive drugs on major cardiovascular outcomes. Commentaries on current prescribing practices in hypertension and some of the highlights and controversies arising from published hypertension guidelines are included, as well as discussion of some innovative approaches to managing hypertension, including nursing clinics and community outreach programs. Getting patients to take their medications, one of the hardest tasks in hypertension, is also dealt with here.

We have taken a broader view of hypertension treatment than consideration of drug therapy alone, and Section 6 contains detailed chapters on lifestyle modifications. These include discussions of micronutrients, special diets involving adjustments in macro- and micronutrients that appear to affect blood pressure, and thoughtful reviews of the mechanisms as well as the challenges of management of obesity in hypertension. Further chapters deal with the relationship between alcohol and hypertension, the role of physical activity in prevention and treatment, and a careful look at the common concomitant diagnosis of diabetes.

Section 7 considers some contemporary issues in the use of antihypertensive agents: how best to choose the initial drug for treating hypertension, the pharmacokinetics of the major antihypertensive drugs, the growing role of fixed combination antihypertensive agents, and the concept of chronotherapeutics in which drugs are designed to exert maximal effects during the early morning hours when patients may be at greatest risk of cardiovascular events.

Circumstances that can affect the selection of antihypertensive drugs, including the presence of concomitant conditions and the special needs of different populations, are discussed in Section 8. Particular focus is directed toward the special needs of patients with such conditions as diabetes or the metabolic syndrome, chronic kidney disease, and coronary heart disease. Optimal strategies for treating African American patients, the elderly and children, as well as the special requirements of treating hypertension in pregnancy are considered in depth. The challenges associated with treatment-resistant hypertension and orthostatic hypotension are also dealt with here.

There is always strong interest in the properties of individual drugs, and Section 9 gives detailed information regarding all the currently used antihypertensive drug classes. Potential new classes are also considered, including endothelin antagonists, vasopeptidase inhibitors and renin inhibitors. We have also included a chapter describing the process by which the United States Food and Drug Administration approves new antihypertensive agents.

The final part of the book, Section 10, deals with secondary hypertension and special circumstances that can affect the management of hypertension. Beyond the most important secondary forms of hypertension, including aldosterone excess, renovascular disease and pheochromocytoma, we have included chapters on obstructive sleep apnea and the special requirements of general anesthesia in hypertensive patients, as well as management of patients with hypertensive emergencies. In view of the ever more aggressive blood pressure targets recommended by contemporary guidelines, our final chapter offers strategies and treatment algorithms for achieving this ambitious goal.

Our most important task is to thank our many colleagues who labored so hard to write contemporary and incisive chapters for this book. Thanks to their efforts, readers will now have access to a comprehensive and detailed review of hypertension as we understand it today. We would also like to thank Susan Pioli and Kim Davis at our publisher, Elsevier, who have worked so closely with us in dealing with the time-consuming and complicated issues of producing a work of this magnitude. Finally, we are delighted to acknowledge Lorraine Wilson at the Downstate College of Medicine in Brooklyn, NY, and Carla Segars at the University of Alabama, Birmingham, for their outstanding administrative support and commitment in completing this task.

**Suzanne Oparil, M.D.**
**Michael A. Weber, M.D.**

# Preface to the First Edition

Results of recent population surveys have underscored the enormity of the health problem posed by elevated blood pressure. With a prevalence of 20% of the adult population worldwide, high blood pressure increases the cardiovascular risk of billions of people. Careful analyses of cohort data have shown that this increased risk pertains not only to persons with frank hypertension by traditional definitions but also to those with blood pressures at the higher end of the "normal" range. The risk of cardiovascular disease is directly and linearly related to both systolic and diastolic blood pressure, although the slope of this relationship is steeper for systolic than for diastolic pressure. Recent analyses have shown that elevated pulse pressure may carry the worst prognosis of all, particularly among the elderly.

The risk of elevated blood pressure is clearly modifiable with appropriate and aggressive antihypertensive treatment. Results of recent randomized clinical trials have reinforced the concept that lowering blood pressure can prevent morbidity and mortality due to cardiovascular diseases, including stroke, congestive heart failure, myocardial infarction, and end-stage renal disease. Further, these studies have shown that lowering blood pressure to more aggressive target levels confers relatively greater benefit in those persons at highest risk, including diabetics and persons with renal insufficiency accompanied by proteinuria.

Despite the impressive successes of controlled clinical trials in preventing hypertension-related cardiovascular events, the incidence of heart failure and end-stage renal disease has increased dramatically since the early 1980s. A major contributor to this trend is inadequate control of blood pressure in the population. Hypertension control rates are disappointing (only 27% in the United States and much lower in other industrialized countries, for example, 6% in the United Kingdom) and have declined in recent years.

The challenge to the practicing physician, then, is to translate the promising results of clinical trials into everyday practice. Impediments to this effort include nonadherence to prescribed medical regimens by patients, failure to communicate the need for treatment by providers, the cost of care, failure to prescribe medications in adequate doses, and the requirement for multidrug regimens to achieve adequate control in most patients. Hope for the future lies in innovative health care delivery systems that utilize nurses, pharmacists, and other nonphysician providers, increased emphasis on adherence-enhancing measures, and reliance on referral to hypertension specialists for the care of complex and resistant patients. The team approach to care of hypertensive patients also facilitates implementation of lifestyle modification measures, including novel dietary programs, that can reduce blood pressure.

Broader recognition by health care providers of the need to treat to lower goal blood pressures and by the health care delivery system of the importance of successful antihypertensive treatment should yield immediate benefit. Results of randomized controlled trials currently in progress will yield insights into whether specific antihypertensive drugs are more—or less—effective than others in preventing morbid and mortal cardiovascular events. These studies should provide definitive answers to the question of whether blood pressure reduction per se fully accounts for the benefits of antihypertensive treatment or whether the mechanism of action of antihypertensive drugs also has a bearing on outcomes.

Interesting questions and controversies remain. High blood pressure rarely exists as a solitary abnormality. Metabolic changes such as lipid disorders and insulin resistance, often associated with obesity, are common in hypertensive patients. In addition, cardiovascular findings, including changes in the structure and function of the left ventricle or stiffening of the arteries, as well as evidence for renal hyperfiltration, are also part of this syndrome. Since these findings can be detected in the apparently normotensive offspring of patients with hypertension, the issue of how and when to best evaluate those at risk of hypertension and its consequences becomes important. Another ongoing question: Although randomized clinical trials with hard endpoints are critical to hypertension guideline writers and policy makers, how can practicing physicians best judge the true effectiveness of treatment in their own individual patients? Can surrogate endpoints like regression of left ventricular hypertrophy, improvement in arterial compliance, or reduction in proteinuria be regarded as legitimate guideposts in patient management?

The science of vascular biology has become a critical part of hypertension. Changes in the endothelium and in the structure and function of the arterial wall are critical in determining the cardiovascular prognosis of patients with this condition. The renin-angiotensin-aldosterone system, together with the many other vasoactive peptides and substances with which it interacts, has become an important therapeutic target as well as a subject of basic scientific interest. There is now an active ongoing search for links between these vascular and clinical findings and the underlying genetic variations and abnormalities that are responsible for them.

It could be anticipated that application of knowledge gained from the human genome project and other studies of the inheritance of high blood pressure and related comorbid conditions will lead to better understanding of the pathophysiology of essential hypertension and to the selection of more effective, targeted antihypertensive therapy based on the genotype of the patient.

This entirely new book is intended to be a useful reference for clinicians who provide care for hypertensive patients, for scientists who are studying the pathobiology of blood pressure control and hypertension-related target organ disease, and for health care planners from academia, industry, and government. The volume begins with a brief history of clinical hypertension and an overview of the epidemiology of hypertension worldwide. Sections 2 and 3 emphasize contemporary issues in the pathophysiology of blood pressure elevation and its cardiovascular complications and target organ damage, as well as common comorbid conditions, such as obesity and insulin resistance. A particularly novel aspect of these sections is the discussion of primary arterial pathology and arterial stiffness in the pathogenesis of hypertension, providing a mechanistic basis for the recent emphasis on pulse pressure as a predictor of cardiovascular morbidity and mortality in hypertensive subjects. Consideration of target organ damage and cardiovascular complications, as well as blood pressure level per se, as components of total cardiovascular risk is presented as a critical factor in deciding when and how aggressively to treat the patient with elevated blood pressure.

Section 4 on diagnosis emphasizes the importance of accurate blood pressure measurement, including the role of ambulatory and self-measurement of blood pressure in guiding antihypertensive therapy, as well as the complex issue of white-coat hypertension. Section 5 on general considerations in antihypertensive treatment focuses on a number of contemporary issues, including use of outcome data from recent clinical trials in making therapeutic decisions. A critical assessment of hypertension treatment guidelines and their impact on office practice is presented. Current prescribing practices, as well as the cost-effectiveness of antihypertensive therapy in a managed care setting, are discussed. Novel systems for delivering antihypertensive therapy, including nursing clinics and community outreach programs, and for optimizing compliance with antihypertensive medication occupy prominent positions in this section.

Section 6 deals with lifestyle modification in the prevention and treatment of hypertension. It discusses the value of a balanced diet rich in fruits, vegetables, and low-fat dairy products, for example, the Dietary Approaches to Stop Hypertension (DASH) diet, as well as weight reduction, increased physical activity, and moderation of alcohol consumption as primary or adjunctive therapy in hypertensive patients.

Section 7 outlines general considerations for the initial choice of antihypertensive drug treatment, including low-dose fixed-combination therapy, and the role of chronotherapeutics in treatment decisions. Special considerations in the treatment of hypertensive patients with comorbid conditions, particularly insulin resistance, diabetes, ischemic heart disease, and renal disease, as well as in special patient groups, including women, the elderly, and Blacks, are discussed in Section 8. Chapters on resistant hypertension and orthostatic hypotension round out this section.

The process of antihypertensive drug registration in the United States is described in Section 9, which also includes detailed consideration of antihypertensive drug actions by class. New antihypertensive drug classes, including endothelin antagonists, renin inhibitors, and the vasopeptidases, which combine neutral endopeptidase and angiotensin-converting enzyme–inhibiting properties, as well as the established classes, are discussed here.

Section 10 emphasizes recent advances in the diagnosis and treatment of secondary hypertension. Obstructive sleep apnea, a recently recognized and important cause of hypertension, is highlighted. Anesthesia in the hypertensive patient and the treatment of hypertensive emergencies, specialized areas that often baffle clinicians, are discussed in this section. The volume ends with a set of tables listing the antihypertensive drugs currently available in the United States.

We thank the contributing authors for their scholarly and extremely contemporary treatment of important topics in hypertension pathophysiology, diagnosis, and therapy. We also express our appreciation to Richard Zorab, Jennifer Shreiner, and the production staff at W.B. Saunders Company for their expertise and diligent attention to detail in the preparation of this text.

**Suzanne Oparil, M.D.**
**Michael A. Weber, M.D.**

# Contents

# SECTION 1

# Background and History

## Chapter 1

# A History of Hypertension Treatment

**Edward D. Freis**

Much of the early history of hypertension was collected by Ruskin and presented in his book entitled *Classics in Arterial Hypertension*.[1] This book is the primary source of my review of the opinions of the ancient physicians. Prior to the twentieth century there were no clinical instruments for measuring blood pressure noninvasively. However, the presence of a high blood pressure had long been recognized by the degree of "hardness" of the pulses (difficulty in obliterating the pulse by manually compressing the radial artery).

The first known reference to increased tension within the arterial system was made in a Chinese book written about 2600 B.C. entitled *The Yellow Emperor's Classic of Internal Medicine*.[2] The author stated "Nothing surpasses the examination of the pulse, for with it errors cannot be committed. In order to examine whether Yin or Yang predominates one must distinguish a gentle pulse and one of low tension from a hard and pounding pulse." He further stated that "The heart influences the force which fills the pulse with blood. If too much salt is eaten in food, the pulse hardens." He also described a syndrome closely resembling hypertensive cardiac failure, stating that "when the pulse is abundant but tense and hard like a cord there are dropsical swellings."

A medical textbook from the Ashurbanipal Library at Nineveh (669-626 B.C.) advised that apoplexy be treated with venesection and cupping, which reduces blood pressure. The *Pulse Classic of Wang* (280 A.D.) stated that in apoplexy the pulse should be superficial and slow. If it is firm rapid and large there is danger." Leeches were a popular treatment for apoplexy in ancient times. Some of the ancient Chinese texts recommend acupuncture or venesection for hardening of the pulse.[1]

In Roman medicine, Cornelius Celsus[3] wrote that increased rate and tension of the pulse occurs with exercise, passion, and even the doctor's arrival (the Roman version of the "White Coat" phenomenon).

The Chinese and Arabic cultures considered that overeating and overexcitability were harmful. The Arabian textbook called *The Therapy* warned: "Nothing is more harmful to an aged person than to have a clever cook and a beautiful concubine." Obesity was considered to be dangerous by Hippocrates, who stated it was associated with sudden death[4] (metabolic syndrome). Hippocrates correctly believed that apoplexy caused paralysis and both resulted from plethora of the brain. He also was the first to find that head wounds of the brain caused paralysis on the opposite side of the body. He recommended

bleeding in patients with stroke, a treatment used until the eighteenth century.

Galen (131-201 A.D.) was the great medical authority until the eighteenth century. But he was often wrong. For example, he denied that stroke was associated with a hard pulse, that is, hypertension.[5] He also failed to believe that blood circulates from arteries to veins. Autopsies were forbidden until the seventeenth century.[6] This held back the growth of medical knowledge for hundreds of years.

## MEDICAL ADVANCES DURING AND AFTER THE RENAISSANCE

Thomas Young, who lived in the early eighteenth century, was a scientific phenomenon, making important discoveries in diverse fields of science, including theories of light and visual accommodation, color vision, a partial translation of the Rosetta stone, and also became fluent in seven different languages.

Young's studies on the arterial system were remarkable. In 1808, in his Croonian Lecture,[7] he stated, "that pressure of the blood at the beginning of the great trunk of the aorta is kept up without noticeable loss down to the branches of the lower order". In studies in dogs he discovered that the fall in systolic blood pressure from the aorta to arteries as small as 200 μm in diameter was approximately 16 mm Hg. Sugiura and Freis measured the systolic pressure drop in dogs using modern equipment.[8] We found it to average 17 mm Hg, confirming Young's finding of 1808.

Richard Bright in 1836 was the first to describe Bright's disease, an inflammatory disease of the kidneys now known as acute glomerular nephritis, which he described as including inflammation and hardening of the kidneys, fullness and hardness of the pulse (hypertension), and albuminuria.[9] Bright benefited from the contributions of previous investigators. Aetios in the sixth century A.D. described a sclerosis of the kidneys associated with oliguria, hematuria, and edema. Cotugo first described albuminuria in 1770.[1] Cardiac hypertrophy with widespread sclerosis of the arteries was described by Morgagni at autopsy.[1]

Bright brought these and his own observations together and illustrated them with anecdotal case presentations. He later expanded these observations to include reduced specific gravity of the urine with increased urea, as well as apoplexy, serositis, hypertrophy of the left ventricle, and stroke. Most importantly, he listed scarlatina as a possible cause of acute glomerulonephritis. He also noted thickening of the walls of small arteries in the kidneys and throughout the body in chronic glomerulonephritis.

In 1872 Gull and Sutton[10] observed that chronic Bright's disease was due to a primary, generalized deposition of hyaline fibrosis of the arterioles and capillaries. These changes resulted in hypertrophy of the left ventricle and contracted kidneys. In 1874 Mahomed, also in England, was the first to indicate that generalized arteriolar disease frequently occurred without preceding renal disease.[11] In 1876 Gowers[12] described the constricted arterioles in the optic fundi of patients with generalized arteriolar disease using an ophthalmoscope invented by Helmholtz 25 years earlier.

Sir Clifford Allbutt popularized the concept of hypertensive disease. In 1895 he presented his views on "senile plethora and hyperpiesia" as a generalized disease of the small arteries, which was separate from glomerulonephritis.[13] In addition, he separated hypertensive arteriolar disease from atherosclerosis of the large arteries. These could occur together or separately. In Germany, the generalized arteriolar disease was called *hypertenonie essential* meaning *primary hypertension*.[14] However, in English speaking countries it was translated to mean *essential hypertension*.[15] The latter suggested that the term *essential* indicated that the elevation of blood pressure was a compensatory reaction of the cardiovascular system to overcome ischemia of the tissue caused by constricted arterioles. Misinterpretation helped to discourage any attempts to lower the blood pressure by developing antihypertensive drugs.

## QUANTITATING BLOOD PRESSURE

Stephen Hales, an eighteenth century parson, is credited for being the first person to measure blood pressure in a living animal. To do so he tied a horse to a fallen-down wooden gate. He then inserted a sharpened brass tube into a carotid artery. Using the windpipe of a goose, he connected the brass tube to a vertical glass tube held aloft by an assistant.[16] The pulsating column of blood rose to a height of 8 feet, 8 inches initially and then gradually declined to two feet, at which point the animal died.

Fifty years later Poiseuille[17] introduced the mercury hydrometer, which greatly reduced the height of the column needed for measuring the blood pressure. Carl Ludwig[18] in 1864 added a float to the top of the mercury column in Poiseuille's hydrometer, with a horizontal arm lightly touching a smoked drum. The pressure wave of the arterial pulse was then recorded on a slowly revolving smoked drum.

For clinical purposes, however, a simple noninvasive method for measuring blood pressure that could be used on humans was needed. Because hypertension usually has no symptoms, the only way to detect the disease and measure its severity is to use some kind of indirect method.

The early attempts were not very accurate and estimated the systolic blood pressure only. Von Basch[19] used the mercury manometer attached to a rubber bulb placed on the radial artery. He then compressed the artery slowly with the bulb until the pulse was obliterated. Only the systolic pressure could be measured by this method (read off the mercury manometer). In 1889 Von Hemlhotz made some improvement on the Von Bosch instrument, which he used to first diagnose coarctation of the aorta by measuring the systolic blood pressure in the radial and temporal arteries compared with that in the dorsalis pedis artery.

An important advance was made by Riva-Rocci, who invented the inflatable rubber cuff to occlude the brachial artery in the upper arm.[20] He could only measure the systolic blood pressure, which he did by inflating and then slowly deflated the cuff until he could feel the first pulse detected at the radial artery. To obtain better accuracy, Von Recklinghausen increased the width of the cuff from 5 to 14 cm.[21]

The greatest advance was made by a Russian Army officer, Nikolai Sergeyevich Korotkov[22] in 1905. Using the inflatable rubber cuff, he listened with a stethoscope over the brachial artery. After he inflated the cuff to obliterate the pulse, he slowly deflated it while listening with the stethoscope over the brachial artery just below the cuff. He proved that the first sound heard was at the systolic blood pressure and the point where the sounds disappeared represented the diastolic blood pressure. It was not long before every doctor's office contained a blood pressure manometer.

## THE TREATMENT OF HYPERTENSION— EARLY ATTEMPTS

In 1897 Tigerstedt and Bergman in Sweden discovered a pressor protein in the kidney, which they called renin.[23] This led in 1934 to another important discovery by Goldblatt[24]: Constriction of a renal artery caused an increased secretion of renin, which resulted in hypertension. Six years later Page and Helmer[25] and Braun-Menendez[26] simultaneously discovered angiotensin, a polypeptide formed by the action of circulating renin. The active form of angiotensin is a powerful pressor substance. These fundamental discoveries had important clinical consequences, including the diagnosis and surgical treatment of renovascular hypertension and the development of angiotensin-converting enzyme (ACE) inhibitors and angiotensin receptor blockers (ARBs), pharmacologic agents of great importance in the treatment of cardiovascular diseases, including hypertension.

## LOW-SODIUM DIETS

In 1905 two French medical students, Ambard and Beaujard[27] were the first to promote the concept that the cause of hypertension was salt in the diet. They thought the culprit was chloride rather than sodium. They claimed some success in reducing blood pressure by restricting salt.

In the 1940s Kempner demonstrated that a diet of plain rice, fruit and vitamin tablets was effective in reducing blood pressure in patients with severe or even malignant hypertension. All other foods, including salt, were forbidden. Kempner maintained 100% compliance by forcing the patients to live for 100 days confined to special dormitories. Kempner thought that the success of his diet was due to the lack of protein, but two other investigators, Watkin et al.[28] and Murphy,[29] both found that the effectiveness of Kempner's diet was due to its extremely low sodium content of only 20 to 30 mEq/day,[30] much lower than the moderate restriction that is used today to approximately 80 mEq/day. The antihypertensive effectiveness of the lesser degree of sodium restriction is controversial.[31-36] The much greater sodium restriction in the Kempner diet reduced plasma and extracellular fluid volume by an amount similar to that produced by thiazide diuretics.[37,38] This suggests that the antihypertensive effects of both the Kempner rice diet and thiazide diuretics are volume dependent. These observations also suggest that sodium restriction may not be very effective unless it is reduced to the point of lowering plasma and extracellular volume.[28,29,38,39]

## SURGICAL SYMPATHECTOMY

At the turn of the century it was already known that the excitation of the sympathetic nervous system caused a rise in blood pressure and, therefore, it was thought that removal of the sympathetic ganglia might control hypertension. The first operation to remove part of the sympathetic ganglia in order to treat hypertension was carried out in Germany by Bruening[40] in 1923. Sympathectomy was later carried out by American surgeons, especially Peet[41] and Smithwick[42] in the 1940s, but it was a major debilitating, painful operation only justified in severe hypertension. However, the operation stimulated the development of drugs that inhibited the sympathetic nervous system by blocking transmission of sympathetic nerve activity through the autonomic ganglia. These ganglion blocking agents, such as tetraethylammonium,[43] hexamethonium,[44] pentaquine,[45] and bretylium,[46] did reduce blood pressure and reversed signs and symptoms of malignant hypertension, but the side effects of autonomic blockade were too great to justify use of these drugs except in patients with severe hypertension. Nevertheless, these early studies demonstrated that antihypertensive drugs were beneficial and stimulated the search for agents that had fewer side effects.

## EARLY ANTIHYPERTENSIVE DRUG TREATMENT

Sodium thiocyanate was introduced as a drug treatment for hypertension by Treupel and Edinger[47] in 1900 and later by Hines in 1946.[48] It was not very effective in reducing blood pressure and was potentially toxic.

The prevailing opinion of physicians during the period between 1920 and 1970 was that hypertension was a disease of the small arteries and the arterioles, resulting in restricted blood flow. They believed that in order to maintain a normal blood supply to the tissues, compensatory adjustments had to be made by the body to raise the blood pressure in order to restore normal blood flow through the narrowed channels.

P.D. White, perhaps the premier cardiologist of his day, wrote in 1931: "Hypertension may be an important compensatory mechanism which should not be tampered with even were it certain that we could control it." This opinion persisted[49] in leading medical centers until the early 1970s except for patients with malignant hypertension. The first effective drug treatment of patients with severe, including malignant, hypertension was suggested to me by James Shannon, then with Squibb Company Research in 1946. I gave the antimalarial drug pentaquine to 17 patients with severe hypertension, 3 of them in the malignant phase of the disease.[45] Because of dis-

turbing side effects, the drug was not acceptable for clinical use. However, it lowered blood pressure and reduced several of its complications, including neuroretinitis, congestive heart failure, and headache in the patients with malignant hypertension. There was no improvement in renal failure. Nevertheless, this study demonstrated that reduction of blood pressure with a drug could reduce organ damage. Therefore, it was a stimulus for developing antihypertensive drugs with fewer side effects. Page and Taylor[50] reported in 1949 that pyrogen treatment reduced blood pressure and improved signs and symptoms in malignant hypertension, but it had too many side effects for regular clinical use.

The ganglion blocking drugs were introduced by Acheson and Moe,[51] who found that tetraethylammonium blocked autonomic nerve transmission in animals. In 1947 Lyons[43] used the drug in patients. While the drug reduced blood pressure, the effect was too short to be used in treatment, and intravenous administration was required. Hoobler[52] found that tetraethylammonium abolished the skin temperature gradient from the foot to the umbilicus, as occurs in a sympathectomized extremity, thereby proving that the blood pressure effect was likely due to sympathetic nerve blockade.

Longer-acting ganglion blockers soon appeared, the prime example being hexamethonium.[53] In 1950 Restall and Smirk[54] published on the treatment of severe hypertension with two or three subcutaneous injections per day of hexamethonium. Despite orthostatic hypotension and a great number of other side effects, they reported regression of neuroretinitis, reduction of heart size, and clearing of the signs of heart failure.

## RESERPINE, HYDRALAZINE, AND THIAZIDE DIURETICS

Reserpine is still a useful antihypertensive drug. Several Veterans Administration Cooperative studies[55,56] demonstrated that the customary dose of 0.25 mg could be reduced to 0.1 mg per day without losing much if any antihypertensive effectiveness but with great reduction in side effects. Addition of a thiazide diuretic to reserpine in a 0.1 mg dose provided excellent blood pressure control with very few side effects. Because both drugs are inexpensive, they could be made available in third world countries as 1 tablet daily of either reserpine or a diuretic alone or in a fixed-dose combination tablet of reserpine with a thiazide diuretic. A fixed-dose combination of reserpine, hydralazine, and chlorothiazide with the brand name of "Ser-Ap-Es" was the most widely used treatment for hypertension in the 1960s to 1980 until other newer brand name drugs appeared.

Around 1980, a steady bombardment of U.S. physicians with questionable data about the toxicity of thiazide diuretics, especially deadly cardiac arrhythmias due to drug-induced hypokalemia, new onset diabetes, and increased serum cholesterol, convinced many physicians that thiazides are dangerous drugs. Sales of diuretics plummeted while sales of the new more expensive classes of drugs took over. Several physicians, including myself, wrote articles defending the diuretics, but to no avail until the early 1990s, when controlled clinical outcome trials in elderly patients demonstrated that diuretics are not toxic. Importantly, the ALLHAT study,[57] carried out in more than 42,000 older patients with hypertension plus at least one other cardiovascular risk factor, demonstrated that thiazides are more effective than ACE inhibitors or calcium channel blockers in controlling blood pressure and reducing many of the cardiovascular complications of hypertension.

Chlorothiazide, the first thiazide diuretic, was discovered by Beyer and Sprague. It reduced extracellular volume to the same degrees as a strict low-salt diet, similar to a strict rice diet.[38] Thiazide diuretics were effective in controlling blood pressure in approximately 50% of patients, and also enhanced the antihypertensive effects of other drugs. This unique action has made possible the success of small-dose fixed dose combination drugs, one of the constituents being a diuretic.[58]

When first administered, the thiazides reduce blood pressure by lowering cardiac output, but after several weeks of continued treatment, cardiac output returns to pretreatment levels and total peripheral resistance falls to maintain the reduction in blood pressure.[59] It is interesting that Ledingham,[60] Borst,[61] and Guyton[62] all observed the opposite effect during salt-loading hypertension. The early elevation of blood pressure with salt loading was due to an increased cardiac output, which after a month or more converted to a normal cardiac output, the hypertension being maintained by an increased total peripheral resistance. This has been called "delayed autoregulation" for the salt-loading hypertension[62] and "reverse autoregulation"[63] in the response to the diuretics. The mechanism is unknown.

## β-ADRENERGIC BLOCKING DRUGS

Prichard and Gilliam[63] were the first to demonstrate the effectiveness of β-blockers in reducing blood pressure and preventing its complications, as demonstrated in several controlled trials. β-Blockers were especially effective when combined with a diuretic. The various types of β-blockers are discussed in other chapters.

## ACE INHIBITORS, ANGIOTENSIN RECEPTOR BLOCKERS, AND THE CALCIUM CHANNEL BLOCKERS

ACE inhibitors were developed in the late 1970s[64] and their close cousins, the angiotensin receptor blockers (ARBs), were developed about a decade later. They are major drug classes that block the actions of the renin-angiotensin system. These drugs and the calcium channel blockers are relatively recent important additions to the armamentarium of antihypertensive drugs and will be discussed in greater detail in other chapters.

## CONTROLLED CLINICAL TRIALS

A most important advance with regard to prevention of cardiovascular complications in patients with hypertension was made possible by the new availability of methods for the prospective, unbiased evaluation of the efficacy and safety of antihypertensive drug treatment in preventing cardiovascular complications in patients with essential hypertension.

Until 1970 there were two schools of thought regarding antihypertensive treatment in patients with systolic/diastolic essential hypertension. The opinion of most, in part based on autopsy evidence, was that hypertension was an adaptive response to provide adequate blood flow through the narrowed arteriolar channels in hypertension. Therefore, reducing the blood pressure would only make matters worse.[49] The opposing school, which was much smaller in numbers, believed that the constriction of the arterioles was due to unknown causes. It was further believed that it was the elevated blood pressure that caused the hyaline sclerosis of the arteriolar walls. This hypothesis further proposed that the complications of hypertension, such as accelerated atherosclerosis, were due to the elevated blood pressure. In fact, all of these complications such as myocardial infarction, heart failure, stroke, and renal damage, were consequences of the stresses induced by the hypertension. Isolated systolic hypertension was rightly considered to be caused by loss of distensibility of the elastic proximal aorta due to aging, but was not considered to be a subject of interest for antihypertensive drug treatment until some years later.

The first multiclinic prospective controlled double blind trial designed to determine unequivocally whether drug treatment was safe and effective was carried out by the Veterans Administration Cooperative Study Group. The results were reported in 1967 for the subgroup with severe hypertension (baseline diastolic blood pressures of 115 to 129 mm Hg)[65] and in 1970 for the patients with mostly moderate hypertension.[66] The prevention of morbidity and mortality was so great in the treated patients with severe hypertension compared with the placebo group that the study was discontinued in those severely hypertensive patients after approximately 1 year. The results for the patients with moderate (and a few with mild) hypertension, including those with pretreatment diastolic blood pressure between 90 and 114 mm Hg, were reported in 1970. The risk of developing a major cardiovascular complication over a 5-year period was significantly reduced with active treatment (combination of chlorothiazide, reserpine, and hydralazine) compared with placebo. The greatest reductions in the treated patients were in the incidence of stroke and heart failure. While the trend was favorable in the subgroup with mild hypertension, the sample size of the mild group (baseline diastolic blood pressure of 90/109 mm Hg) was too small to be statistically significant.

The Medical Research Council (MRC) trial[67] in 1985 and other trials[68,69] were large enough and well enough controlled to determine that drug treatment is also effective in preventing complications in patients with mild hypertension. Subsequent trials have found that the further the blood pressure is reduced (to <140/90 mm Hg), the greater is the prevention of complications[70,71] down to <130/80 mm Hg in patients with diabetes and chronic renal disease.

Other clinical trials, including the Systolic Hypertension in the Elderly Program (SHEP),[72] demonstrated that antihypertensive treatment was equally or even more effective in preventing cardiovascular complications in elderly patients with isolated systolic hypertension as in middle-aged patients with both systolic and diastolic hypertension.

## SUMMARY

It has been approximately 80 years since the Actuarial Society of America published their breakthrough book *Blood Pressure Study of 1925* that described the high mortality in mild and moderate hypertension due to cardiovascular complications.[73]

In 1905 Korotkov provided an instrument for making the measurement of blood pressure clinically possible. Hypertensive hormones and neurotransmitters such as renin, angiotensin, norepinephrine, epinephrine, and aldosterone, were discovered by 1950. Yet only a small fraction of patients had hypertension due to abnormalities in any of these mediators. Hypertension of unknown cause, so-called essential hypertension, is by far the most common form of hypertension occurring in humans.

Because autopsy studies showed that essential hypertension is associated with sclerotic thickening of the arteriolar walls, producing narrowed channels of the arterioles, it was formerly believed that elevated blood pressure was a compensatory reaction to provide normal blood flow through the narrowed arterial channels. Therefore, no attempts to reduce blood pressure were undertaken. However, controlled clinical trials beginning around 1970 proved that reduction of blood pressure with antihypertensive drugs significantly reduced cardiovascular complications.

In recent years it has been shown that the lower the blood pressure, the better, down to an optimal level of 120/80 mm Hg. The only way to accomplish this is to use combinations of antihypertensive drugs in adequate dosage. Currently doctors are being advised to be more aggressive even with those who have only mild hypertension and to use diet, exercise, and drugs such as statins to reduce the associated atherosclerosis.

We have come a long way during the past 100 years. We have learned to measure blood pressure, and recognize the risks for complications of hypertension and reduce them with antihypertensive drugs and other treatment.

## References

1. Ruskin A. Classics in Arterial Hypertension. Springfield, IL, Charles C Thomas, 1956.
2. Nei Ching. Yellow Emperor's Classic of Internal Medicine, Books 2-9. Published between 2698 and 2598 B.C.
3. Celsus AAC De Re Medicina, 3 vols. Translated by W Spencer. London, Heinemann, 1935-1938.
4. Hippocrates. Genuine Works of Hippocrates, 2 vols. Translated by F Adams. London, Sydenham Society, 1849.
5. Galen C. Introduction in Pulsus and Teuthram. Interpreted by M Gregory. London, Guliel Rovillius, 1959.
6. Wepfer JJ. Observations Anatomicae ex Cadaveribus eorum quos sustilit Apoplexia. Cum Exercitatione de ejus Loco Affecto. Shaffhausen. Johann Casper Suterus, 1658.
7. Young TJ. The Croonian Lecture: On the functions of the heart and arteries. Philos Trans R Soc Lond 1:1-31 1809.
8. Sugiura T, Freis ED. Pulse pressure in small arteries. Circ Res 11:838-842, 1962
9. Bright R. Cases and observations, illustrative of renal disease accompanied with the secretion of albuminous urine. Guy's Hosp Rep 1:338-379, 1836.
10. Gull WW, Sutton HG. On the pathology of the morbid state commonly called chronic Bright's disease with contracted kidney ("arteriocapillary fibrosis"). Med Chir Trans Lond 65: 273-326, 1872.
11. Mahomed FA. Chronic Bright's disease without albuminuria. Guy's Hosp Rep 25:295-416, 1881.
12. Gowers W. The state of the arteries in Bright's disease. Br Med J 2:743-745, 1876.
13. Allbutt TC. Senile plethora or high arterial pressure in elderly persons. Transaction of the Hunter Society 1895-1896, 77th session, 1896; pp 38-57.
14. Frank O. Ein neues optisches fermanometer. Z Biol 82:49-57, 1925.
15. Janeway TC. Guide to the Use of Sphygmomanometer. New York, D Appleton, 1904.
16. Hales S. Statistical Essays: Containing Hemostatics; or an Account of Some Hydraulick and Hydrostatistical Experiments Made on the Blood and Blood-vessels of Animals. London, Innys and Manby, 1933.
17. Poiseuille JLM. Recherches expérimental sur le movement des liquides dans les tubes de tres petites diametres. Arch Gen Med 550-554, 1828.
18. Ludwig C. Beitraege zur Kenntniss des einflusses der respirations-bewegungeb aug den Blutlauf im Aortensysteme. Arch Anat Physiol Wissen Med (Muller's Arch) 242-302, 1847.
19. von Basch S. Ueber die Messung des Blutdrucks beim Menschen. Z Klin Med 2:79-96, 1880.
20. Riva-Rocci S. Un nuovo sfigmomanometro. Gaza Med Torino 47:981-1001, 1896.
21. von Recklinghausen H. Uber blutdruckmessung beim menschen. Arch Exp Pathol Pharmak 46:78, 1901.
22. Korotkov NS. K voprosu metodakh uzsledovaniya krovyanovo davleniya. [A contribution to the problem of methods for the determination of blood pressure]. Izvestiya Imperatorskoi Voenno-Meditsinskoy Akademii (Rep ImperMil-Med Acca St Petersburg). 11:365-367, 1905.
23. Tigerstedt R. Bergman PG. Niere und kreislauf. Scand Arch Physiol 7-8:223-271, 1897-1898.
24. Goldblatt H. Lynch T, Hanzal RF, et al. Studies on experimental hypertension. I. The production of persistent elevation of systolic blood pressure by means of renal ischemia. J Exp Med 59:347-379, 1934.
25. Page IH, Helmer OM. A crystalline pressor substance (angiotonin) resulting from the reaction between renin and renin-activator. J Exp Med 71:495-520, 1940.
26. Braun-Menendez EJ, Fasciolo C, Le Loir F, et al. The substance causing renal hypertension. J Physiol (Lond) 98:283-298, 1940.
27. Ambard L, Beaujard E. Causes de l'hypertension artérielle. Arch Gen Med 1:520-533, 1904.
28. Watkin DM, Fraeb HF, Hatch FT, et al. Effects of diet in essential hypertension. II. Results with unmodified Kempner rice diet in 50 hospitalized patients. Am J Med 9:441-448, 1950.
29. Murphy RJF. The effect of "Rice Diet" on plasma volume and extracellular fluid space in hypentensive subjects. J Clin Invest 29:912-920, 1950.
30. Kempner W. Treatment of kidney disease and hypentensive vascular disease with Rice Diet. II. N Carolina Med J 5:273-274, 1944.
31. MacGregor GA, Markandu ND, Best FE, et al. Double-blind randomised crossover trial of moderate sodium restriction in essential hypertension. Lancet 1:351-355, 1982.
32. Parijis J, Joosens JV, Van der Linden L, Vestrecken G, et al. Moderate sodium restriction and diuretics in the treatment of hypertension. Am Heart J 85:22-34, 1973.
33. Morgan T, Adam W, Gillies A, et al. Hypertension treated by salt restriction. Lancet 1:227-230, 1978.
34. Richards AM, Nicholls MG, Espiner EA, et al. Blood-pressure response to moderate sodium restriction and to potassium supplementation in mild essential hypertension. Lancet 1: 757-761, 1984.
35. Watt GC, Edwards C, Hart JT, et al. Dietary sodium restriction for mild hypertension in general practice. Br Med J 286:432-435, 1983.
36. Silman AJ, Mitchell P, Locke C, et al. Evaluation of the effectiveness of a low sodium diet in the treatment of mild to moderate hypertension. Lancet 1:1179-1182, 1983.
37. Dustan HP, Cumming GR, Corcoran AC, et al. A mechanism of chlorothiazide-enhanced effectiveness of antihypertensive ganglioplegic drugs. Circulation 19:360-365, 1959.
38. Wilson IM, Freis ED. Relationship between plasma and extracellular fluid volume depletion and the antihypertensive effect of chlorothiazide. Circulation 20:1028-1036, 1959.

39. Beard T, Cooke HM, Gray WR, et al. Randomised controlled trial of a no-added-sodium diet for mild hypertension. Lancet 2:455-458, 1982.

40. Bruening F. Die operative behandlung der angina pectoris durch exstirpation des halsbrutstsympathicus und bemerkungen ueber die operative behandlung der abnormen blutdrucksgerung. Klin Wochenschr 236:270-276, 1947.

41. Peet MM. Results of bilateral supradiaphragmatic splanchnicectomy for arterial hypentension. N Engl J Med 236:270-276, 1947.

42. Smithwick RH, Thompson JE. Splanchnicectomy for essential hypertension; results in 1,266 cases. JAMA 152:1501-1504, 1953.

43. Lyons RH, Moe GK, Neligh RM, et al. The effects of blockade of the autonomic ganglia in man with tetraethylammonium. Am J Med Sci 123:315-323, 1947.

44. Smirk FH. Practical details of the methonium treatment of high blood pressure. NZ Med J 49:637-643, 1950.

45. Freis ED, Wilkins RW. Effects of pentaquine in patients with hypertension. Proc Soc Exp Biol Med 64:731-736, 1947.

46. Freis ED. Bretylium and guanethidine: Two new drugs producing specific blockade of the sympathetic nervous system. Heart Bull 9:88-89, 1960.

47. Truepel G, Edinger A. Utersuchungen uber rhodan-verbindungen. Munchen Med Wchnschr 16:717-767, 1900.

48. Hines EA. The thiocyanates in the treatment of hypertensive disease. Med Clin North Am 30:869-877, 1946.

49. Goldring W, Chasis H. Antihypertensive drug therapy: An appraisal. *In* Ingelfinger FJ, Relamn AS, Finland M (eds). Controversies in Internal Medicine. Philadelphia, WB Saunders, 1966; pp 83-91.

50. Page IH, Taylor RD. Pyogens in the treatment of malignant hypertension. Mod Concepts Cardiovasc Dis 18:51-52, 1949.

51. Acheson GH, Moe GK. The action of tetraethylammonium ion on the mammalian circulation. J Pharmacol Exp Ther 87:220-226, 1946.

52. Hoobler SW, Malton SD, Ballatine TH Jr, et al. Studies on vasomotor tone. I. Effect of the tetraethylammonium ion on the peripheral blood flow of normal subjects. J Clin Invest 28:638-647, 1949.

53. Schnaper HW, Johnson RL, Tuohy ED, et al. The effect of hexamethonium as compared to procaine or metycaine lumbar block on the blood flow to the foot of normal subjects. J Clin Invest 30:786-791, 1951.

54. Restall PA, Smirk FH. Treatment of high blood pressure with hexamethonium iodide. NZ Med J 49:206-209, 1950.

55. Veterans Administration Cooperative Study Group on Antihypertensive Agents. Comparsion of propranolol and hydrochlorothiazide for the initial treatment of hypertension. II. Results of long-term therapy. JAMA 248:2471-2477, 1982.

56. Veterans Administration Cooperative Study on Antihypertensive Agents. A double-blind control study of antihypertensive agents: I. Comparative effectiveness of reserpine, reserpine and hydralazine, and three ganglionic blocking agents, chlorisondamine, mecamyamine, and pentolinium tartrate. Arch Intern Med 106:81-96, 1960.

57. The ALLHAT Collaborative Research Group. Major outcomes in high-risk hypertensive patients randomized to angiotensin-converting enzyme inhibitor or calcium channel blocker vs. diuretic. The Antihypertensive and Lipid-Lowering Treatment to Prevent Heart Attack trial (ALLHAT). JAMA 288:2981-2997, 2002.

58. Freis ED. Improving treatment effectiveness. Arch Int Med 159:2317-2326, 1979.

59. Shah S, Khatri I, Freis ED. Mechanism of antihypertensive effect of thiazide diuretics. Am Heart J 95:611-618, 1978.

60. Ledingham JM, Cohen RD. The role of the heart in the pathogenesis of renal hypertension. Lancet 186:979-981, 1963.

61. Borst JGG, Borst-De Geus A. Hypertension explained by Starling's theory of circulatory homoeostasis. Lancet 1:677-682, 1963.

62. Guyton AC, Coleman TG, Cowley AW, et al. A systems analysis approach to understanding long-range anterial blood pressure control and hypertension. Circ Res 35:139, 1974.

63. Prichard BNC, Gillam PMS. Use of propranolol (Inderal) in treatment of hypertension. Br Med J 5411:725-727, 1964.

64. Ondetti MA, Rubin B, Cushman DW. Design of specific inhibitors of angiotensin-converting enzyme: New class of orally active antihypertensive agents. Science 196:441-447, 1977.

65. Veterans Administration Cooperative Study Group on Antihypertensive Agents. Effects of treatment on morbidity in hypertension: Results in patients with diastolic blood pressure averaging 115 through 129 mmHg. JAMA 202:1028-1034, 1967.

66. Veterans Administration Cooperative Study Group on Antihypertensive Agents. Effects of treatment on morbidity in hypertension: Results in patients with diastolic blood pressure averaging 90 through 114 mmHg. JAMA 213:143-152, 1970.

67. MRC trial of treatment of mild hypertension: principal results. Medical Research Council Working Party. Br Med J 291:97-104, 1985.

68. The Australian therapeutic trial in mild hypertension. Report by the Management Committee. Lancet 1:1261-1267, 1980.

69. Five-year findings of the hypertension detection and follow-up program. I. Reduction in mortality of persons with high blood pressure, including mild hypertension. Hypertension Detection and Follow-up Program Cooperative Group. JAMA 242:2562-2571, 1979.

70. Chobanian AV, Bakris G, Black HR, et al. and the National Blood Pressure Education Program Coordinating Committee. The Seventh Report of the Joint National Committee on Prevention, Detection, Evaluation, and Treatment of High Blood Pressure. JAMA 289:2560-2571, 2003.

71. Hansson L, Zanchetti A, Carruthers SG, et al. Effects of intensive blood-pressure lowering and low-dose aspirin in patients with hypertension: Principal results of the Hypertension Optimal Treatment (HOT) randomized trial. Lancet 351:1755-1762, 1998.

72. Prevention of stroke by antihypertensive drug treatment in older persons with isolated systolic hypertension. Final results of the Systolic Hypertension in the Elderly Program (SHEP). SHEP Cooperative Research Group. JAMA 265:3255-3262, 1991.

73. Actuarial Society of America. Blood Pressure Study of 1925. New York, Actuarial Society of America and Association of Life Insurance Medical Directors, 1925.

# The National High Blood Pressure Education Program

## Edward J. Roccella

## PROGRAM ORIGIN

Published in 1965, the Report of the Commission on Heart Disease, Cancer, and Stroke contains the recommendations of the subcommittee on hypertension. It calls for a nationwide increase in screening and treatment of high blood pressure.[1] Unfortunately, after publication of the report, no initiative was launched to address the problem, even though actuarial studies showed a clear relationship between rising blood pressure and increased chance of death, and several epidemiologic studies had reported a relatively high prevalence of hypertension in the U.S. population, with only a small percentage receiving adequate treatment.[2,3] Although the report appeared to be ahead of its time, what was lacking was clear evidence regarding the benefits of lowering raised arterial pressure. That evidence soon came in a dramatic fashion with the 1967, 1970, and 1972 publications of the Veterans Administration Cooperative Study on the Treatment of Hypertension.[4-6]

## LANDMARK MEETING

In April 1972, Elliott L. Richardson, then Secretary of the Department of Health, Education, and Welfare, met with Mrs. Mary Lasker, a longtime supporter of biomedical research and lobbyist for improving the nation's health; Mr. Michael Gorman, of the National Committee Against Mental Illness; Ms. Deeda Blair, a philanthropist associate of Mrs. Lasker; and Dr. Michael DeBakey, a noted cardiovascular surgeon. The purpose of their meeting was to convince Secretary Richardson that the moment had arrived for the federal government to take the initiative and begin a nationwide effort to reduce high blood pressure. During the meeting with the Secretary, Mrs. Lasker outlined the extraordinary findings of the soon-to-be-landmark Veterans Administration Cooperative Study on the Treatment of Hypertension, which was supported in part by the Lasker Foundation and conducted by Dr. Edward Freis. She emphasized that this science was not being applied in clinical practice and the nation was experiencing unprecedented rates of heart attack and stroke. Secretary Richardson was especially responsive to the suggestion to launch a national campaign to detect and treat hypertension. His father, a distinguished surgeon in Boston at the Massachusetts General Hospital, had suffered a career-ending stroke that was attributed to uncontrolled high blood pressure and had spent the remaining 15 years of his life in a wheelchair. Secretary Richardson directed Dr. Theodore Cooper, Director of the then National Heart and Lung Institute (NHLI) to develop a national plan of action.

The fortunate temporal coincidence of a proven medical intervention, the active interest of major philanthropists and a noted cardiovascular surgeon, a favorable public policy position, and a personal interest of the key policymaker led to a rapid decision—the establishment of the National High Blood Pressure Education Program (NHBPEP), which was launched officially in July 1972. This education program was designed and implemented by the then NHLI staff to raise public awareness and stimulate blood pressure screening and treatment throughout the nation. Adding to the support for the NHBPEP was the enactment by Congress, on September 19, 1972, of the National Heart, Blood Vessel, Lung and Blood Act of 1972 (Public Law 92-423). This Act became the legislative basis for the NHBPEP by calling for expanded efforts in the areas of information dissemination and public and professional education, with special emphasis on certain areas, including hypertension.

Concurrently, Mrs. Lasker, Dr. DeBakey, and Dr. Malcolm Todd from the American Medical Association developed articles of incorporation to form Citizens for the Treatment of High Blood Pressure, a private-sector group that would work in tandem with the NHLI effort. Citizens would use its private-sector platform and join with the NHLI to focus its efforts on creating a national consciousness regarding high blood pressure as a medical problem. Early in 1973, Citizens encouraged Congress to enact legislation creating hypertension project grants for state health departments. Eventually passed in 1975, this legislation provided $120 million to the states for hypertension screening and control over a period of a decade. Congress later gave large demonstration grants to seven states to test the research hypothesis that maximal screening and detection would reduce the prevalence of high blood pressure. Another important function of Citizens was to stimulate private-sector resources to address this large public health problem. The NHLI and other federal agencies could not provide all the funding needed to implement these initiatives. Armed with solid data regarding the significance of hypertension, Citizens and NHLI staff worked to push innovative programs, such as financial support from the life insurance industry for health education programs for high blood pressure detection and control. Demonstration programs on the cost-effectiveness of hypertension screening and control were conducted at worksites.[7,8] The spirited collaboration of the people involved launched and then vitalized the NHBPEP program over the years, contributing immensely to advancement of the health of the American people.

The National High Blood Pressure Education Program by Edward J. Roccella, Ph.D., is in the Public Domain.

## PROGRAM TENETS

### Strong Science Base

From the inception of the NHBPEP, the program planners recognized the need to ground the program activities to a strong science base. The congressional act that established the program mandated the need to translate health information into positive action because research results were not being used to improve the public's health. Large-scale community-based education programs and messages would not go forward unless there was a scientific rationale and data to support them.

### Achieving Consensus

It is reasonable to expect that different people might have different points of view regarding the interpretation of data generated in research studies. From the beginning, the opinions of professional and voluntary societies—such as the American College of Cardiology, the American Heart Association, the American Hospital Association, the American Medical Association, the American Osteopathic Association, the National Medical Association, and the National Kidney Foundation—were actively sought. All points of view would be heard. It became clear that differences of opinion needed to be resolved so that the health and medical professions could provide clear and consistent messages to the public, patients, and practicing physicians. To avoid confusion, the program needed to speak with one voice. For example, at the time, hypertension was defined in various ways. Some suggested that hypertension was defined as systolic blood pressure (SBP) of 100 mm Hg plus one's age, whereas others defined it as diastolic blood pressure (DBP) greater than 105 mm Hg. Thus, consensus became another critical program tenet.

To achieve consensus among the major scientific, professional, voluntary societies and federal agencies, the NHBPEP Coordinating Committee was formed to serve as a policymaking body.[9] This committee has now grown to represent 39 professional and voluntary societies and 7 federal agencies. Its purpose is to review the scientific evidence, develop clear messages, agree on national priorities, and then develop and implement program activities. Each of the member organizations brings a different perspective to the hypertension arena. Some organizations have a clinical perspective; others have strong interests in subsets of the population, such as minorities, who experience an unusually high burden of the consequences of hypertension; and yet others have a population-wide or public health interest. The representatives participating in the Coordinating Committee are selected by their parent organizations, not by the NHBPEP. The intent of this approach is to increase the probability that consensus, once adopted, will have credibility and be widely implemented by the Coordinating Committee member organizations.

### Evaluation

A third program tenet has been evaluation of activities. The approach of the NHBPEP always has been geared toward evaluation as an early step prior to implementation. Defining a problem before implementation—using outcome data to the extent that resources, opportunity, and the state-of-the-art permit—is a core planning tenet for the program. Evaluation data include national baseline surveys of the public's knowledge, attitudes, and reported behavior; surveys of physicians' response to hypertension therapy selection and management; and data on prescribing patterns and patient visits. Other efforts include gathering and analyzing data on hypertension prevalence and control rates as well as trends in morbidity and mortality rates for stroke, coronary heart disease (CHD), heart failure, and end-stage renal disease (ESRD). This information helps track program progress and is useful in identifying program deficits and planning future direction and activities.

## MASS MEDIA EFFORTS

To reach the many different people in the United States with high blood pressure, education messages require that the target audience be partitioned in various ways. The audience to be reached is divided into those who are unaware of their condition; those who are aware but are doing little, if anything, to control their blood pressure; those who are aware, treated, and controlled but who need reinforcement to stay on therapy; and those who are aware, were treated, but dropped out of care and require advice and motivation to reenter treatment. Those without hypertension are candidates for primary prevention messages, or they may reinforce needed action by friends or relatives who do have elevated blood pressure. The target audiences can be further segmented by sex, race, age, ethnicity, and other factors. For all these different groups, high blood pressure may have different meanings. Accordingly, the messages and skills required, as well as the channels of communication and even the language spoken, may be different. Figures 2–1 and 2–2 are examples of messages designed to reach different audiences.

### Leveraging Program Resources

A multitude of communication channels and activities must be used to reach the many target populations with the NHBPEP's science- and consensus-based messages. Program partners are called upon to adapt existing materials and distribute them to their constituents. The American Medical Association, the American Heart Association, the National Kidney Foundation, the International Society of Hypertension in Blacks, and city, county, and state health departments have developed their own print, radio, and television high blood pressure education materials aimed at various target audiences. The National Heart, Lung, and Blood Institute (NHLBI) program staff developed a unique semi-preproduced television program on hypertension, called "Silent Killer," and successfully marketed it to a number of television and radio talk shows. The product was packaged as a kit and contained film clips and a script that could be used verbatim or as a guide for the local television host with questions and answers allowing dialog among the host and guests—usually local physicians and nurses. More than 5000 kits were distributed throughout the nation. In collaboration with Safeway grocery stores, a high blood pressure message was printed on grocery bags. More than 1 million shopping bags were distributed with messages encouraging Americans to control their hypertension.

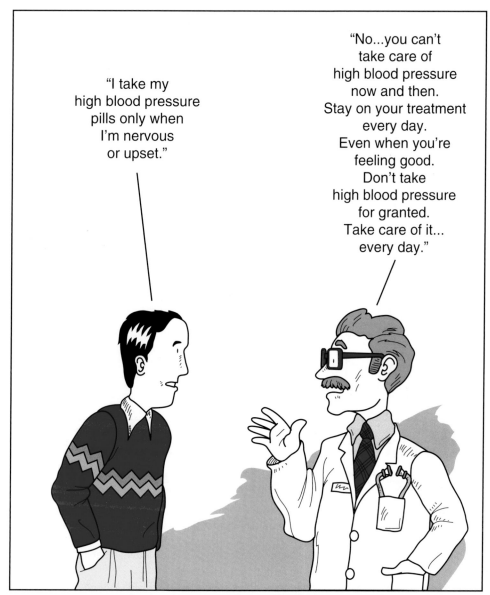

**Figure 2-1** A public service message on high blood pressure education and prevention targeting individuals with hypertension.

## HIGH BLOOD PRESSURE EDUCATION MONTH

Another highly visible program strategy designed to stimulate community-based action and sustain interest in hypertension is High Blood Pressure Education Month, which is May of each year. Each year, a kit of program-planning materials is designed, produced, and distributed to state and local health departments, community hospitals, voluntary health organizations, and civic groups. The kit contains suggested print ads, camera-ready artwork, suggested newspaper articles, community activity ideas, and heart-healthy recipes. It also features proclamations to be signed by governors, mayors, or local dignitaries declaring May as National High Blood Pressure Education Month and recommending that citizens get their blood pressure measured and, if needed, treated and controlled. Participating organizations are encouraged to put their names on the materials to increase their own visibility and to work harder to disseminate the message.

High Blood Pressure Education Month also encourages communities to conduct education and screening programs at churches.[10] This forum became a successful way to reach African Americans, who have a high prevalence of hypertension and risk of cardiovascular disease. A program-planning guide was developed to provide direction for health

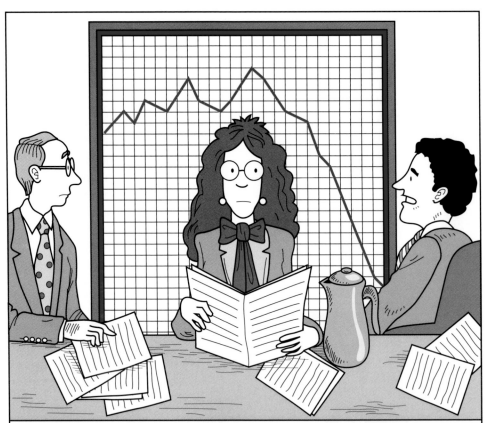

**Figure 2–2** A message on high blood pressure education and prevention targeting businesses and their employees.

professionals to reach out to religious congregations to implement programs to reduce the risk of cardiovascular disease.[11] In an effort to reach men, a planning guide was created to develop high blood pressure education and screening programs at sporting events.[12] Hypertension screening and education programs were conducted at professional baseball and hockey games, at high school football games, golf tournaments, and basketball games.

## THE JOINT NATIONAL COMMITTEE REPORTS

When the U.S. Congress passed a law creating the NHLI (now the National Heart, Lung, and Blood Institute [NHLBI]) and directing its function—to improve the health of the people of the United States through the conduct of research, investigations, experiments, and demonstrations relating to the cause, prevention, and methods of diagnosis and treatment of diseases of the heart and circulation—it also indicated that the obligation to the public would not be fulfilled even if and when every research project was completely successful. The Institute was directed to develop and implement methods of public and professional education in disease prevention and control. This directive is completely compatible with the responsibility of the NHBPEP. The translation of research results into practice is a natural complement to the research program, and the NHBPEP facilitates this process.

One important tool that the NHBPEP has fostered is the development of clinical guidelines and working group reports.[13-35] These guidelines are developed in partnership with the Coordinating Committee member organizations. The first clinical guideline was titled the Joint National Committee (JNC) on the Detection, Evaluation, and Treatment of High Blood Pressure, which published its report in 1977.[29] The JNC report was designed to bring order to a then-chaotic situation regarding hypertension management. At that time many clinicians were of the opinion that elevated blood pressure was needed to perfuse the organs of the body and there was little reason to lower blood pressure. Thus, the important findings of Freis and colleagues were not being applied to practice. In addition, there was confusion regarding whether to use the fourth or fifth Korotkoff sound to measure DBP and regarding which drug to use as the initial therapy for treating hypertension. The first JNC document provided consensus regarding key hypertension detection and control issues, with clinical recommendations based on the available scientific evidence. In making their recommendations, the JNC reports have evolved to address difficult questions, such as the cutpoints to be used to define hypertension, which antihypertensive drugs should be used first and why, and careful assessment of absolute versus relative risk of cardiovascular disease and what this means to the responsible physician. Through the years, the program produced seven JNC reports at approximately 4- to 5-year intervals, each report building on the evidence and making recommendations to the practicing community.[29-35] The JNC reports have been a critical component of the NHBPEP. The intent has always been to synthesize the available scientific evidence and then to unify the positions of member organizations and send one clear message. One challenge has been to achieve consensus among the many organizations on the Coordinating Committee. Having the many organizations on the Coordinating Committee agree on strategies to prevent and manage hypertension and to speak with one voice helps to bring clear messages and guidance to the health professionals. The JNC documents demonstrate that different disciplines can agree when the focus is on the common good.

## RESULTS OF THE NATIONAL HIGH BLOOD PRESSURE EDUCATION PROGRAM

A variety of methods have been used to measure program impact. Process measures employed included the number of health education activities, materials produced and distributed, news articles written, people having their blood pressure measured, antihypertensive drug sales, and reported changes in behavior. In the early days of the NHBPEP, the evaluation process was rudimentary at best. With insight and gradual maturing overtime, it became clear that what really mattered were changes leading to improvement in health status and outcome.

Table 2–1 shows the changes in hypertension prevalence during the last 40 years. In the first three-point estimates, the age-adjusted hypertension prevalence remained fairly stable, with approximately 40% of the population reporting blood pressures >140/90 mm Hg or taking antihypertensive medication. Then, during the 1980s, the prevalence of hypertension declined. While the reason for this reduction is subject to discussion, some of this decline is associated with activities that encouraged the American public to take action, such as increasing fruit and vegetable consumption and decreasing sodium intake. The increase in the prevalence of hypertension from 1999 to 2000 may be attributed in part to the national obesity epidemic.[36] Figure 2–3 describes changes in mean arterial blood pressure associated with NHBPEP activities. It is clear that the average blood pressure for the nation has declined. This decline is associated with a reduction in mortality. Table 2–2 describes trends in the public's awareness of hypertension as reported in the National Health and Nutrition Examination Survey for adults ages 18 to 74. Awareness rates have substantially improved from half to nearly three fourths of the hypertensive population.

In addition to increasing the public's awareness about hypertension, the NHBPEP also appears to have interested scientists and clinical investigators to seek more information about the condition and has stimulated interest in hypertension research. Figure 2–4 shows the number of reported citations from the National Library of Medicine's PubMed database accessed by using the search terms *hypertension* and *clinical trials*, indicating that high blood pressure research and subsequent publications have grown steadily.

Table 2–2 shows that high blood pressure treatment and control rates have improved rather remarkably in the years since creation of the NHBPEP. Blood pressure was controlled

**Table 2-1** Hypertension among Persons 20 to 74 Years of Age, Both Genders, and All Races: United States, 1960-1962, 1971-1974, 1976-1980, 1988-1994, and 1999-2000*

| | Percent of Population (Standard Error) | | | | |
| --- | --- | --- | --- | --- | --- |
| | 1960-62 | 1971-74 | 1976-80 | 1988-94 | 1999-2000 |
| Both Sexes | 38.1 | 39.8 | 40.4 | 23.9 (0.6) | 28.7 (1.6) |
| Male | 41.3 | 43.9 | 45.2 | 26.4 (0.9) | 29.8 (1.9) |
| Female | 35.0 | 35.8 | 35.8 | 21.4 (0.7) | 27.5 (1.7) |

From US Department of Health and Human Services, National Center for Health Statistics. A chartbook of trends in the health of Americans, 2002.
*Age adjusted to the 2000 standard population. Excludes pregnant women.

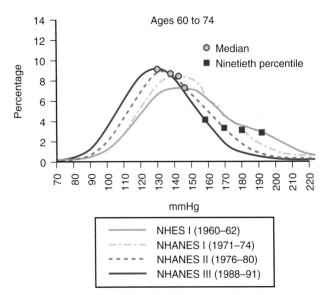

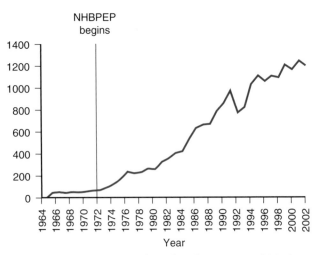

**Figure 2–4** Hypertension clinical trial citations–PubMed Search.

**Figure 2–3** Smoothed weighted frequency distribution, median, and 90th percentile of SBP for ages 60 to 74 years, United States, 1960 to 1991. (From Burt VL, Cutler JA, Higgins M, et al. Trends in the prevalence, awareness, treatment, and control of hypertension in the adult US population. Data from the health examination surveys, 1960 to 1991. Hypertension 26(1):60-69, 1995.)

in more than 34% of the hypertensive population in 1999 to 2000. Because hypertension is the primary antecedent of congestive heart failure, the decrease in prevalence, reduction in mean arterial pressures, and improvement of hypertension control rates suggest that the prevalence of heart failure should also decrease. Figure 2–5 shows the age-adjusted prevalence of heart failure by race and sex for persons ages 25 to 74 over the years since the NHBPEP began. The prevalence of heart failure in this population has declined in both races and in both sexes. Because hypertension is also associated with ESRD, the decline in average blood pressure and improvement in the hypertension control rate should also decrease the incidence of ESRD. While ESRD has been increasing, Figure 2–6, which shows the incidence rates by primary diagnosis, indi-

cates that hypertension is no longer as great a contributor to this condition as diabetes.

Large-scale clinical trials have shown that controlling hypertension will reduce CHD and stroke regardless of race or gender. Figures 2–7 and 2–8 show 60% and 50% declines in age-adjusted mortality for stroke and CHD, respectively, during the last 30 years. These declines are seen in both genders and races. It should be noted that the decline in CHD and stroke preceded the advent of the NHBPEP. Figure 2–9 shows age-adjusted stroke mortality rates beginning with 1960. If a regression line is plotted for the years 1960 to 1971 and then cast forward, the expected rates of stroke mortality can be plotted. However, beginning at the point of NHBPEP inception, the observed rates were much lower than expected and many more people who were projected to die of stroke were alive. The precise contribution of the NHBPEP to improving this disease outcome will never be known, but it is hoped the steady decline in deaths from stroke and CHD will continue in synchrony with the efforts of the NHBPEP. The NHBPEP is clearly the dividend of a very worthwhile investment promulgated by Mrs. Lasker and colleagues. The nation owes its gratitude to these

**Table 2–2** Trends in Awareness, Treatment, and Control of High Blood Pressure, 1976-2000

| | National Health and Nutrition Examination Survey (Percent*) | | | |
|---|---|---|---|---|
| | **1976-80**[1] | **1988-91**[1] | **1991-94**[2] | **1999-2000**[3] |
| Awareness | 51 | 73 | 68 | 70 |
| Treatment | 31 | 55 | 54 | 59 |
| Control[†] | 10 | 29 | 27 | 34 |

[1]Data from Burt VL, Cutler JA, Higgins M, et al. Trends in the prevalence, awareness, treatment, and control of hypertension in the adult US population. Data from the health examination surveys, 1960 to 1991. Hypertension 26:60-69, 1995.
[2]Data from the sixth report of the Joint National Committee on Prevention, Detection, Evaluation, and Treatment of High Blood Pressure. Arch Intern Med 157:2413-2446, 1997.
[3]Unpublished data computed by M. Wolz, National Heart, Lung, and Blood Institute.
*Percent of adults age 18 to 74 years with systolic blood pressure (SBP) of 140 mm Hg or greater, diastolic blood pressure (DBP) of 90 mm Hg or greater, or taking antihypertensive medication.
[†]SBP below 140 mm Hg and DBP below 90 mm Hg and taking antihypertensive medication.

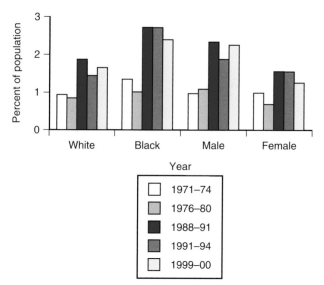

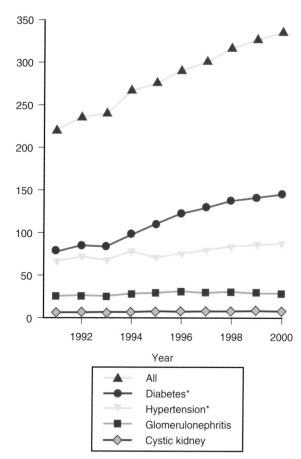

**Figure 2-5** Prevalence of CHF by race and gender, ages 25 to 74, United States, 1971-1974 to 1999-2000. Age adjusted to 2000 U.S. census population. Note: White and Black in 1999-2000 excludes Hispanics. (From National Heart, Lung, and Blood Institute. Morbidity and Mortality: 2002 Chart Book on Cardiovascular, Lung, and Blood Disease. Accessed September 2003, http://www.nhlbi.nih.gov/resources/docs/cht-book.htm and 1999-2000 unpublished data computed by M. Wolz and T. Thom, National Heart, Lung, and Blood Institute. June 2003.)

*These disease categories were treated as being mutually exclusive.

**Figure 2-6** Trends in incident rates of end-stage renal disease (ESRD) by primary diagnosis adjusted for age, gender, and race. (From United States Renal Data System. 2002. Figure 1.14. Accessed September 2003 http://www.usrds.org/slides.htm.)

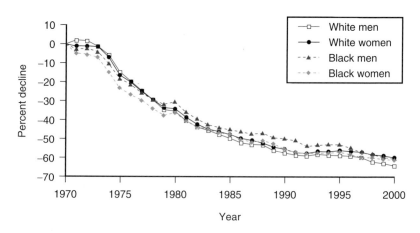

**Figure 2-7** Percent decline in age-adjusted mortality rates for stroke by gender and race: United States, 1970 to 2000. (Prepared by T. Thom, National Heart, Lung, and Blood Institute from Vital Statistics of the United States National Center for Health Statistics. Death rates are age adjusted to the 2000 U.S. census population.)

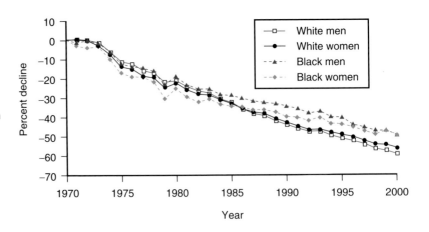

**Figure 2–8** Percent decline in age-adjusted mortality rates for coronary heart disease (CHD) by gender and race: United States, 1970 to 2000. (Prepared by T. Thom, National Heart, Lung, and Blood Institute from Vital Statistics of the United States, National Center for Health Statistics. Death rates are age adjusted to the 2000 U.S. census population.)

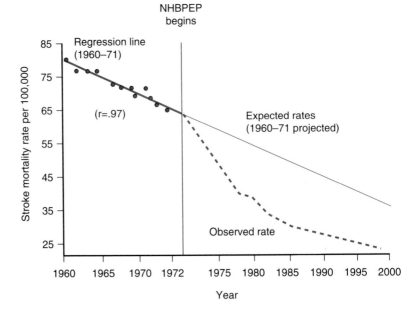

**Figure 2–9** Age-adjusted stroke mortality rates. Expected rates from a regression line of best fit to observed rates 1960 to 1971 are projected to 2000 and compared with observed rates 1972 to 1998. (From National Center for Health Statistics.)

distinguished individuals who translated their vision into action. One can only wonder what would have been without their initiative.

## References

1. United States President's Commission on Heart Disease, Cancer and Stroke: Report to the President: A national program to conquer heart disease, cancer and stroke. Washington, DC, U.S. Government Printing Office, 1965.
2. Society of Actuaries. Build and Blood Pressure Study 1959. Volumes I and II. Chicago, IL, Society of Actuaries, 1960.
3. Thompson KJ: Some observations on the development and course of hypertensive vascular disease. Proceedings of the 38th Annual Meeting, Medical Section, American Life Convention, June 15-17. 1950; pp. 85-112.
4. Effects of Treatment on Morbidity in Hypertension. Results in patients with diastolic blood pressures averaging 115 through 129 mm Hg. JAMA 202(11):1028-1034, 1967.
5. Effects of treatment on morbidity in hypertension. II. Results in patients with diastolic blood pressure averaging 90 through 114 mm Hg. JAMA 213(7):1143-1152, 1970.
6. Effects of treatment on morbidity in hypertension. 3. Influence of age, diastolic pressure, and prior cardiovascular disease; further analysis of side effects. Circulation. 45(5):991-1004, 1972.
7. Foote A, Erfurt JC. Controlling hypertension: A cost-effective model. Prev Med 6(2):319-343, 1977.
8. Foote A, Erfurt, JC. Hypertension control at the work site: Comparison of screening and referral alone, referral and follow-up, and on-site treatment. N Engl J Med 308(14):809-813, 1983.
9. National Heart, Lung, and Blood Institute and National High Blood Pressure Education Program. National High Blood Pressure Education Program, Coordinating Committee. Accessed August 19, 2003. Available from http://www.nhlbi.nih.gov/about/nhbpep/index.htm
10. National Heart, Lung, and Blood Institute, National High Blood Pressure Education Program. National High Blood Pressure Education Month. Accessed August 19, 2003. Available from http://hin.nhlbi.nih.gov/nhbpep_kit/
11. National Heart, Lung, and Blood Institute and Office of Prevention, Education and Control. Working with religious congregations: A guide for health professionals. NIH Pub. No. 97-4058. Bethesda, MD, National Institutes of Health, National Heart, Lung, and Blood Institute, Office of Prevention, Education, and Control, 1997; pp. 1-44.

12. National Heart, Lung, and Blood Institute and Office of Prevention, Education and Control. The Sports Guide: NHLBI Planning Guide for Cardiovascular Disease Risk Reduction Projects at Sporting Events. NIH Pub No. 96-3802. Bethesda, MD, National Institutes of Health, National Heart, Lung, and Blood Institute, Office of Prevention, Education, and Control, 1996.

13. Phillips SJ, Whisnant JP. Hypertension and the brain. The National High Blood Pressure Education Program. Arch Intern Med 152(5):938-945, 1992.

13. National High Blood Pressure Education Program Working Group on Hypertension Control in Children and Adolescents. Update on the 1987 task force report on high blood pressure in children and adolescents: A working group report from the National High Blood Pressure Education Program. Pediatrics 98(4):649-658, 1996.

14. Task Force on Blood Pressure Control in Children. National Heart, Lung, and Blood Institute, Bethesda, MD. Report of the Second Task Force on Blood Pressure Control in Children—1987. Pediatrics79(1):1-25, 1987.

15. Report of the Task Force on Blood Pressure Control in Children. Pediatrics 59(5):I-II, 797-820, 1977.

16. Sowers JR, Reed J. 1999 Clinical advisory treatment of hypertension and diabetes. J Clin Hypertens (Greenwich) 2(2): 132-133, 2000.

17. National High Blood Pressure Education Program Working Group. Report on hypertension in diabetes. Hypertension 23(2):145-158; discussion 159-160, 1994.

18. National High Blood Pressure Education Program Working Group. Report on hypertension in the elderly. Hypertension 23(3):275-285, 1994.

19. Smith LH, Drach G, Hall P, et al. National High Blood Pressure Education Program (NHBPEP) review paper on complications of shock wave lithotripsy for urinary calculi. Am J Med 91(6):635-641, 1991.

20. National High Blood Pressure Education Program Working Group. Report on high blood pressure in pregnancy. Am J Obstet Gynecol 183(1):S1-S22, 2000.

21. National High Blood Pressure Education Program Working Group. Report on high blood pressure in pregnancy. Am J Obstet Gynecol 163(5):1691-1712, 1990.

22. Whelton PK, He J, Appel LJ, et al. National High Blood Pressure Education Program Coordinating Committee. Primary prevention of hypertension: Clinical and public health advisory from the National High Blood Pressure Education Program. JAMA 288(15):1882-1888, 2002.

23. National High Blood Pressure Education Program Working Group. Report on primary prevention of hypertension. Arch Intern Med 153(2):186-208, 1993.

24. National High Blood Pressure Education Program Working Group. 1995 update of the working group reports on chronic renal failure and renovascular hypertension. Arch Intern Med 156(17):1938-1947, 1996.

25. National High Blood Pressure Education Program Working Group. Report on hypertension and chronic renal failure. Arch Intern Med 151(7):1280-1287, 1991.

27. National High Blood Pressure Education Program Working Group. Report on ambulatory blood pressure monitoring. Arch Intern Med 150(11):2270-2280, 1990.

28. Chobanian AV, Hill, M. National Heart, Lung, and Blood Institute workshop on sodium and blood pressure: A critical review of current scientific evidence. Hypertension 35(4): 858-863, 2000.

29. Report of the Joint National Committee on Detection, Evaluation, and Treatment of High Blood Pressure. A cooperative study. JAMA 237(3):255-261, 1977.

30. The 1980 report of the Joint National Committee on Detection, Evaluation, and Treatment of High Blood Pressure. Arch Intern Med 140(10):1280-1285, 1980.

31. The 1984 report of the Joint National Committee on Detection, Evaluation, and Treatment of High Blood Pressure. Arch Intern Med 144(5):1045-1057, 1984.

32. The 1988 report of the Joint National Committee on Detection, Evaluation, and Treatment of High Blood Pressure. Arch Intern Med 148(5):1023-1038, 1988.

33. The fifth report of the Joint National Committee on Detection, Evaluation, and Treatment of High Blood Pressure (JNC V) Arch Intern Med 153(2):154-183, 1993.

34. The sixth report of the Joint National Committee on Prevention, Detection, Evaluation, and Treatment of high blood pressure. Arch Intern Med 157(21):2413-2446, 1997.

35. Chobanian AV, Bakris GL, Black HR, et al. National Heart, Lung, and Blood Institute Joint National Committee on Prevention, Detection, Evaluation, and Treatment of High Blood Pressure. The seventh report of the Joint National Committee Prevention, Detection, Evaluation and Treatment of High Blood Pressure: The JNC 7 Report. JAMA 289(19):2560-2572, 2003. [Epub 2003 May 14]

36. Flegal, KM, Carroll MD, Ogden CL, Johnson CL. Prevalence and Trends in Obesity Among US Adults, 1999-2000. JAMA 288(14):1723-1727, 2002.

# Epidemiology of Hypertension
## Nathan D. Wong, Stanley S. Franklin

Approximately 50 million individuals in the United States and 1 billion worldwide are affected by hypertension.[1] There are, however, important differences in prevalence between populations and ethnic groups.[2-4] Although there is a dramatic age-related increase in the prevalence of hypertension, several important cardiovascular risk factors, particularly obesity, nutrient intake, physical activity, and diabetes also relate to the likelihood of hypertension. The Framingham Heart Study has estimated that individuals normotensive at age 55 years have a 90% lifetime risk of developing hypertension.[5] Hypertension represents a potent risk factor for cardiovascular, peripheral vascular, and renal disease[6-10] (Figure 3–1). The higher the blood pressure, the greater is the likelihood of myocardial infarction, heart failure, stroke, and kidney disease. This chapter reviews the prevalence and natural history of hypertension, the risk factors associated with the development of hypertension, the cardiovascular risks associated with hypertension, and the extent of treatment and control of hypertension.

## CLASSIFICATION OF HYPERTENSION

Blood pressure (BP) is continuously distributed with a skewed normal distribution and without distinct separation between normotensive and hypertensive values. It has been suggested that the cutpoint for hypertension is best defined as the level of arterial BP at which the benefits of intervention exceed those of inaction. Over the decades the classification of hypertension has changed as a result of (1) the decrease in severity of hypertension over the past half century, (2) the improvement in the efficacy and side effect profile of antihypertensive medications, and (3) the recognition of the continuum of cardiovascular risk across all levels of BP. This has resulted in a gradual reduction in the lower limits of target BP for therapeutic intervention.

The most recent definition of hypertension as released by the Seventh Report of the Joint National Committee on Prevention, Detection, Evaluation, and Treatment of High Blood Pressure (JNC 7)[1] is a systolic blood pressure (SBP) ≥140 mm Hg or diastolic blood pressure (DBP) ≥90 mm Hg, which simplifies hypertension classification by including only stage 1 (SBP 140-159 mm Hg or DBP 90-99 mm Hg) or stage 2 (SBP 160 mm Hg or higher or DBP 100 mm Hg or higher) (Table 3–1). Perhaps the most important change is the new classification of "prehypertension" (SBP 120-139 mm Hg or DBP 80-89 mm Hg), which combines the normal and high-normal categories of the previous JNC VI report, in recognition of the fact that even these levels of BP confer an increased risk of the development of hypertension[11] and future cardiovascular events.[12] Individuals with prehypertension may require health-promoting lifestyle modification to prevent the development of future hypertension and cardiovascular disease.

## PREVALENCE OF HYPERTENSION

The Fourth National Health and Nutrition Examination Survey[4] (NHANES IV) showed an overall prevalence of hypertension (140 mm Hg SBP or greater or 90 mm Hg DBP or greater, or on antihypertensive medication) of 28.7% in 1999-2000, which varied from 7.2% in those aged 18 to 39 years to 65.4% in those aged 60 years and older, and which was greater in women (30.1%) than in men (27.1%). Noteworthy is the fact that since 1988-1991 the prevalence of hypertension has increased significantly in women and in all age groups, although most dramatically in those aged 60 and older, who experienced an increase in prevalence from 57.9% in 1988-1991 to 65.4% in 1999-2000 (Figure 3–2). Moreover, in the United States, prevalence of hypertension is greatest among non-Hispanic Blacks and least among Mexican Americans[4] (Figure 3–3).

Compared with the United States, data primarily from the past decade have shown that the prevalence of hypertension is similar in Canada, but is markedly higher in European countries (44% overall, 55% in Germany)[3] (Figure 3–4). The specific reasons for such substantial geographic variation in hypertension prevalence are not entirely clear, but differences in nutrient intake, obesity, physical activity, alcohol intake, environmental toxins, psychosocial stressors, and genetic susceptibility have been suggested.[13]

## CHARACTERISTICS OF HYPERTENSION AS A RISK FACTOR

Numerous epidemiologic studies have consistently shown a relation of increased BP to risk of cardiovascular disease. The relationship is *strong, continuous, and graded* without any distinct threshold level; it is present both in men and in women, in younger and older adults, and in those with and without known coronary heart disease (CHD); it is present in different countries and in different ethnic and racial groups. As with other risk factors, there is evidence of *tracking of BP*, which refers to the stability of BP over time in an individual in relation to his or her peers. Of note, however, there is evidence of *disparate rather than parallel tracking of BP*, whereby an individual in the upper quintile or decile of BP will have a much steeper age-BP relationship than one in the lower quintile or decile of BP. Although the lability of BP is directly related to age and severity of hypertension, suggesting that it may also relate to cardiovascular risk, when other risk factors are accounted for by multivariate analysis, risk is largely unaffected by lability of BP. It is the average BP over the day and night cycle, not lability, that determines cardiovascular risk.

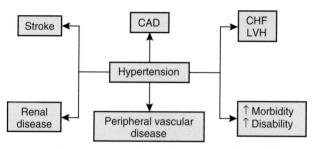

**Figure 3–1** Hypertension: A significant CV and renal disease risk factor. Adapted from the National High Blood Pressure Education Program Working Group. Arch Intern Med 153: 186-208, 1993.

**Table 3–1** Blood Pressure Classification According to JNC 7

| BP Classification | SBP mm Hg | DBP mm Hg |
|---|---|---|
| Normal | <120 and | <80 |
| Prehypertension | 120–139 or | 80–89 |
| Stage 1 Hypertension | 140–159 or | 90–99 |
| Stage 2 Hypertension | ≥160 or | ≥100 |

Data from Chobanian AV, Bakris GL, Black HR, et al. The Seventh Report of the Joint National Committee on Prevention, Detection, Evaluation, and Treatment of High Blood Pressure. The JNC 7 Report. JAMA 289:2560-2572, 2003.

## CARDIOVASCULAR COMPLICATIONS OF HYPERTENSION

Early reports by the Framingham Heart Study demonstrated that hypertension, SBP, and DBP are risk factors for CHD,[9, 10] helping dispel a longstanding belief that the common variety of hypertension was a benign condition essential for ade-quate perfusion of peripheral tissues. A 36-year follow-up from the Framingham Heart Study showed that hypertension is associated with twofold to fourfold increases in risk for the development of CHD, stroke, peripheral artery disease, cardiac failure, and overall cardiovascular events in both men and women.[14] The Seven Countries Study provided strong ecologic study evidence demonstrating a direct relation of SBP and DBP within 16 communities to CHD death rates, showing a doubling in risk for every increment of 10 mm Hg in the population's median SBP.[6] Among middle-aged men screened in the Multiple Risk Factor Intervention Trial (MRFIT), a direct relation of increasing SBP and DBP with CHD mortality over 11.6 years was shown.[7] Moreover, a pooling of results from 418,343 persons initially free of CHD showed CHD mortality to begin increasing at levels of DBP above 73 mm Hg and to increase more than fivefold between levels of 73 and 105 mm Hg.[15] A meta-analysis has further emphasized the importance of increasing risk above nor-motensive levels, showing that starting at an SBP/DBP of 115/75 mm Hg, cardiovascular mortality doubles with each increment of 20/10 mm Hg throughout the BP range.[16] In the Framingham Heart Study, more than a third of those with high-normal BP (130-139 mm Hg SBP or 85-89 mm Hg DBP) developed hypertension in the next 4 years (Figure 3–5).[11] Compared with those with "optimal" BP of <120 mm Hg SBP and <80 mm Hg DBP, those with high-normal BP also had nearly a threefold greater incidence of developing major cardiovascular events in the next 12 years (Figure 3–6).[12]

Left ventricular hypertrophy (LVH) is a particularly important independent risk factor for cardiovascular disease, and is the response of the heart to chronic pressure and/or volume overload. Hypertension often precedes the development of LVH. The Framingham Heart Study has demonstrated the highest (versus lowest) quartile of left ventricular mass to be associated with a fourfold increased risk of cardiovascular events in women and a threefold increased risk of events in

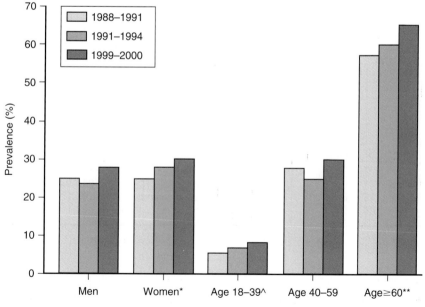

**Figure 3–2** Trends in prevalence of hypertension in the U.S. population, by sex and age group, 1988-2000. Data from Hajjar I, Kotchen TA. Trends in prevalence, awareness, treatment, and control of hypertension in the United States, 1988-2000. JAMA 290:199-206, 2003.

^ *p* = .05, * *p* = .03, ** *p* = .002 for change from 1988 to 2000; analyses by gender are age-adjusted to 2000 U.S. population.

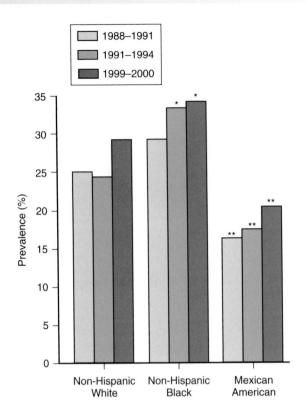

**Figure 3-3** Trends in prevalence of hypertension in the U.S. population, by race/ethnicity, 1988-2000. Data from Hajjar I, Kotchen TA. Trends in prevalence, awareness, treatment, and control of hypertension in the United States, 1988-2000. JAMA 290:199-206, 2003.

* *p* <.01, ** *p* <.001, compared with non-Hispanic Whites within given time period; no significant trends across time periods within gender; analyses are age-adjusted to 2000 U.S. population.

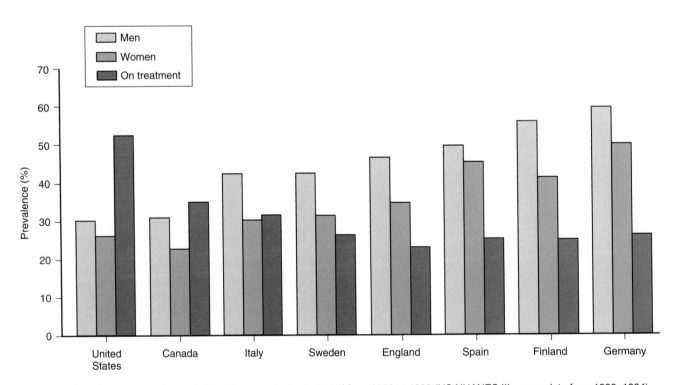

Based on surveys of 1823 to 23,129 respondents conducted from 1986 to 1999 (US NHANES III survey data from 1988–1994).

**Figure 3-4** Hypertension prevalence and treatment among persons 35-64 years old in 6 European countries, Canada, and the United States. Adapted from Wolf-Maier K et al. Hypertension prevalence and blood pressure levels in 6 European countries, Canada, and the United States. JAMA 289:2363-2369, 2003.

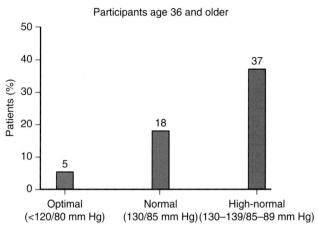

**Figure 3–5** Year progression to hypertension: The Framingham Heart Study. Data from Vasan RS, Larson MG, Leip EP, et al. Assessment of frequency of progression to hypertension in non-hypertensive participants in the Framingham Heart Study. Lancet 358:1682-1686, 2001.

men.[17,18] It has been well demonstrated that aggressive control of hypertension can prevent the development or induce regression of LVH.[19]

The incidence of stroke and peripheral arterial disease also increases dramatically with increasing BP, particularly SBP. Stroke incidence is approximately three times greater in persons with stage 2 systolic hypertension (160 mm Hg or greater) and 50% higher in those with stage 1 systolic hypertension (140-159 mm Hg) compared with those with BP below these levels. From a 50-year follow-up of the Framingham Heart Study, elevated midlife BP during the prior 10 years is associated with a significant 1.7-fold increase in the risk of stroke per standard deviation increment in women and a 1.9-fold increase in risk per standard deviation increment in men at age 60.[20] Of those experiencing stroke, 30% have stage 1 hypertension and 40% stage 2 hypertension (with half of this latter group having SBP of 180 mm Hg or

greater). Framingham has also shown peripheral arterial disease (intermittent claudication) risk to increase dramatically by approximately threefold in men and more than fourfold in women from the first through fifth quintiles of SBP, and approximately twofold across quintiles of DBP.[21]

Finally, the relation of increasing BP levels to incidence of end-stage renal disease (ESRD) is well documented. MRFIT showed the multivariate-adjusted relative risk of ESRD to be 1.7 in men for every 16 mm Hg increment in SBP. Baseline SBPs of >140 mm Hg were associated with a fivefold to sixfold greater risk for the development of ESRD compared with SBPs below 117 mm Hg.[22] Risk of developing ESRD is graded and continuous throughout the entire distribution of BP above optimal. Even persons with high-normal BP have approximately a twofold greater risk of developing ESRD and those with stage 2 hypertension have a sixfold or greater risk of developing ESRD compared with those with optimal BP.[22]

## AGE-RELATED INFLUENCES ON BLOOD PRESSURE AND RELATION TO CORONARY HEART DISEASE RISK

Approximately 25% of persons with hypertension are younger than 50 years old, with the remaining 75% 50 years old or older; 45% of all persons with hypertension are 50 to 69 years of age.[23] Application of JNC 7 BP categories to recently released 1999-2000 data from NHANES IV shows that among adults younger than the age of 50, nearly 30% are prehypertensive. Prevalence of hypertension (SBP ≥140 mm Hg or DBP ≥90 mm Hg or reporting hypertension medication use) increases dramatically by age, accounting for 7% of subjects aged 18 to 29, 16.6% of those aged 30 to 39, 33% of those aged 40 to 49, and 54% of those aged 50 to 59 years. By the seventh decade of life, approximately 70% are hypertensive, increasing to more than 80% in those aged 80 and older. After age 60, less than 20% of persons have BP in the normal range (<120 mm Hg SBP and >80 mm Hg DBP) (Figure 3–7).

Of particular interest is the transition of hypertension subtype with increasing age among those untreated for hypertension. From NHANES 1999-2000 data, the predominant

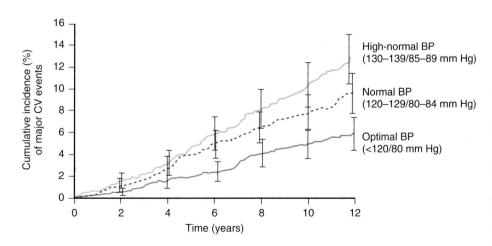

**Figure 3–6** Impact of high-normal BP on risk of major cardiovascular events in men. These events are defined as death resulting from cardiovascular disease: recognized myocardial infarction (MI), stroke, or congestive heart failure. Adapted from Vasan RS, Larson MG, Leip EP, et al. Impact of high-normal blood pressure on the risk of cardiovascular disease. N Engl J Med 345:1291-1297, 2001.

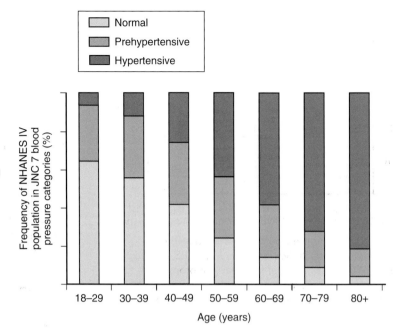

**Figure 3-7** Distribution of blood pressure categories in the JNC 7 guidelines among population in NHANES 1999-2000 by age.

*p* <.0001 comparing distribution of blood pressure categories across age groups

form of hypertension among those younger than 40 years old is isolated diastolic hypertension (IDH) (SBP <140 mm Hg and DBP ≥90 mm Hg), which accounts for 60% of those with hypertension in this age group (Figure 3–8). During ages 40 to 49 there are roughly equal proportions of IDH (SBP <140 mm Hg and DBP ≥90 mm Hg) and systolic-diastolic hypertension (SDH) (SBP ≥140 mm Hg and DBP ≥90 mm Hg), which together account for three fourths of persons with hypertension. Beginning at age 50, the most predominant form of hypertension is isolated systolic hypertension (ISH), accounting for more than 75% of those with hypertension aged 50 to 59, approximately 80% of hypertension in those aged 60 to 69,

and approximately 90% of those with hypertension aged 70 years or older (see Figure 3–8). Thus, ISH is the most common subtype of hypertension and SBP is less likely to be under control than DBP.[24] Because guidelines classify hypertension on the basis of which component (SBP or DBP) is in the higher category, the majority of persons with hypertension can be defined based on (or "upstaged" by) SBP, leading to a 94% accurate classification of BP by assessment of SBP alone. In contrast, among those aged 18 to 49 years, 65% of individuals with untreated hypertension in the NHANES III population were upstaged by DBP alone.[24] This indicates SBP is the more important overall determinant of upstaging of untreated

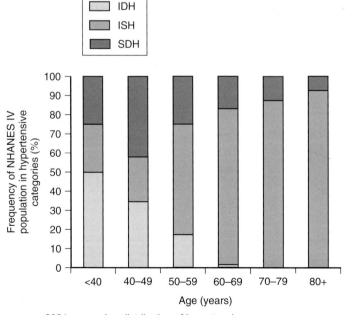

**Figure 3-8** Distribution of hypertension subtype in the untreated hypertensive population in NHANES 1999-2000 by age.

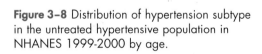

*p* <.0001 comparing distribution of hypertension groups across age categories

hypertension and hence eligibility for therapy in the population, because the great majority of individuals with untreated or inadequately treated hypertension are 50 years of age or older, with an 80% prevalence of ISH.[24]

Both cross-sectional[25] and longitudinal population studies[26] demonstrate that SBP rises from adolescence through most of adulthood, whereas DBP initially increases with age, but levels off at ages 50 to 55 and decreases after ages 60 to 65. Thus pulse pressure (PP), defined by the difference between peak SBP and end-diastolic BP, increases after ages 50 to 55, a change that is accelerated from the ages of 60 to 65 and older. The rise in SBP and DBP up to ages 50 to 55 can best be explained by the dominance of peripheral vascular resistance. In contrast, after the sixth decade of life (1) increasing PP and decreasing DBP are surrogate measurements for central elastic artery stiffness; (2) central arterial stiffness overrides increased systemic vascular resistance and becomes the dominant hemodynamic factor in both normotensive and hypertensive individuals, as manifested by an increase in SBP, a decrease in DBP, and hence, a rise in PP; and (3) hypertension, left untreated, may accelerate stiffening of elastic arteries, which, in turn, may set up a vicious cycle of worsening hypertension and further increases in elastic artery stiffness.[26]

## BLOOD PRESSURE COMPONENTS AS PREDICTORS OF RISK

An increased SBP alone has been well documented to be associated with increased risks of CHD, myocardial infarction, kidney failure, stroke, heart failure, and peripheral vascular disease (Table 3–2).[22,27-30] In the MRFIT study, whereas those with the highest SBP had the highest risk of CHD mortality, a particularly increased risk was observed for those with the highest SBP (>160 mm Hg) in conjunction with the lowest diastolic BP (<70 mm Hg) and, therefore, the highest PP (Figure 3–9).[27]

Moreover, in the Framingham cohort, future CHD risk in those ages 50 and older and free of clinical cardiovascular disease was inversely correlated with DBP at any level of SBP ≥120 mm Hg, suggesting that PP was an important component of risk.[31] This suggests that PP may be useful as an adjunct to SBP in predicting risk. A strong independent association of higher levels of SBP and lower levels of DBP with thoracic aortic calcium, an indicator of atherosclerosis, is evidence of the significance of increased PP in the etiology of arterial stiffness and atherosclerosis.[32] Numerous other reports have also shown that at a given level of SBP, there is an inverse relation of CHD risk with DBP, indicating PP as superior to the reference SBP in predicting total and cardiovascular mortality and CHD risk.[33-37]

Additional information relating BP indices to CHD risk emerged from the Framingham Heart Study when individuals younger than 50 years of age were examined.[38] In this younger group, DBP was a more powerful predictor of CHD risk than SBP; PP was not predictive. With increasing age there was a continuous, graded shift from DBP to SBP and eventually to PP as predictors of CHD risk. From age 60 and older, when considered with SBP,[38] DBP was negatively related to CHD risk, so PP emerged as the best predictor. The bias in favoring DBP over SBP as a risk factor by earlier generations of physicians may, in part, be due to the emphasis on hypertension as a young person's condition. However, with the aging of the population over the past half-century, hypertension has become largely a condition affecting older persons with ISH.

**Table 3–2** Relative Risks of Cardiovascular and Renal Diseases Associated with Elevated Systolic Blood Pressure

| Disease | Relative Risk |
|---------|---------------|
| Kidney failure (ESRD) | ≥2.8 |
| Stroke | ≥2.7 |
| Heart failure | ≥1.5 |
| Peripheral vascular disease | ≥1.8 |
| Myocardial infarction* | =1.6 |
| Coronary artery disease | ≥1.5 |

Adapted from Kannel WB. Risk stratification in hypertension: New insights from the Framingham Study. Am J Hypertens 13:3S-10S, 2000; Perry HM Jr et al. Early predictors of 15-year end-stage renal disease in hypertensive patients. Hypertens 25(part 1):587-594, 1995; Klag MJ et al. Blood pressure and end-stage renal disease in men. N Engl J Med 334:13-18, 1996; Nielsen WB et al. A significant risk factor of cerebral apoplexy and acute myocardial infarction. A prospective population based study. Ugeskr Laeger158:3779-3783, 1996; Neaton JD et al. Serum cholesterol, blood pressure, cigarette smoking, and death from coronary heart disease: Overall findings and differences by age for 316,099 white men. Arch Intern Med 152:56-64, 1992.
ESRD, end-stage renal disease; SBP ≥165 mm Hg.
*Men only.

SBP VERSUS DBP IN RISK OF CHD MORTALITY

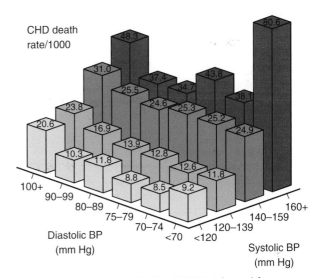

**Figure 3–9** SBP-associated risks: MRFIT. Adapted from Neaton JD, Wentworth D. Serum cholesterol, blood pressure, cigarette smoking, and death from coronary heat disease: Overall findings and differences by age for 316,099 white men. Arch Intern Med 152:56-64, 1992.

## IMPACT OF OTHER CARDIOVASCULAR RISK FACTORS AND TARGET ORGAN DAMAGE

Hypertension is usually accompanied by other cardiovascular risk factors and is metabolically linked to dyslipidemia, glucose intolerance, abdominal obesity, and hyperinsulinemia. Only about 20% of the time does hypertension occur in isolation. About half of the persons with hypertension have two or more other accompanying risk factors. The clustering of other CHD risk factors adds to the importance of hypertension as a risk factor. For example, in a hypothetical 55-year-old adult with hypertension, the estimated 10-year risk of CHD is expected to increase fourfold to fivefold from the additional impact of several other CHD risk factors.[14] Both traditional and new cardiovascular risk factors from JNC 7, as well as examples of target organ damage, are listed in Box 3–1.[1] The following have been added to the traditional risk factors of age, family history of hypertension, cigarette smoking, diabetes mellitus, and dyslipidemia: (1) obesity (body mass index $\geq 30$ kg/m$^2$), (2) physical inactivity, and (3) microalbuminuria (50-300 mg of urinary albumin/24 hours). The European Society of Hypertension[39] has added elevated high-sensitivity C-reactive protein (>3 mg/L) as a risk factor. The presence of one or more of these risk factors greatly increases the rationale for more intensive treatment to BP goal levels, as well as consideration of therapy at lower cutpoints. This is demonstrated well by data from the Multiple Risk Factor Intervention trial, showing a substantial additive impact of type 2 diabetes on the risk of CHD conferred by increasing SBP levels (Figure 3–10).[40]

**Box 3–1** Cardiovascular Risk Factors and Target Organ Damage

**Major Risk Factors**
- Hypertension*
- Cigarette smoking
- Obesity (BMI $\geq 30$ kg/m$^2$)*
- Physical inactivity
- Dyslipidemia*
- Diabetes mellitus*
- Microalbuminuria or estimated GFR <60 ml/min
- Age (>55 years for men, >65 years for women)
- Family history of premature cardiovascular disease (men <55 years or women <65 years)

**Target Organ Damage**
- Heart (left ventricular hypertrophy, angina or prior myocardial infarction, prior coronary revascularization, or heart failure)
- Brain (stroke or transient ischemic attack)
- Chronic kidney disease
- Peripheral arterial disease
- Retinopathy

Adapted from Chobanian AV, Bakris GL, Black HR, et al. The Seventh Report of the Joint National Committee on Prevention, Detection, Evaluation, and Treatment of High Blood Pressure. The JNC 7 Report. JAMA 289:2560-2572, 2003.
*Components of the metabolic syndrome.
BMI, body mass index; GFR, glomerular filtration rate.

## SIGNIFICANCE OF HYPERTENSION IN THE METABOLIC SYNDROME

There is general agreement that people with the metabolic syndrome are at increased risk of developing cardiovascular disease and diabetes (see Chapter 13).[41] Indeed, the cluster of abnormalities associated with the metabolic syndrome are probably more important than any single risk factor in predisposing to CHD. According to the Third Report of the National Cholesterol Education Program Expert Panel on Detection, Evaluation, and Treatment of High Blood Cholesterol in Adults (ATP III),[41] the metabolic syndrome is defined as consisting of three or more of the following abnormalities: waist circumference >102 cm in men and >88 cm in women (abdominal obesity); serum triglycerides level $\geq 150$ mg/dl (1.69 mmol/L); high-density lipoprotein (HDL) cholesterol level <40 mg/dl (1.04 mmol/L) in men and <50 mg/dl (1.29 mmol/L) in women; BP $\geq 130/85$ mm Hg or being treated for hypertension; and a fasting serum glucose level of 110 mg/dl (6.1 mmol/L) or higher. (Some experts recommend separating diabetes from this definition, because specific treatment goals for BP and hypercholesterolemia exist for diabetics who should be treated as having a CHD risk equivalent.) (See Table 3–3.)

One study of U.S. adults with the metabolic syndrome reported that more than 80% of those satisfying these criteria (excluding those with diabetes who are universally considered high risk, warranting aggressive clinical management) had elevated triglycerides, low HDL cholesterol, and elevated BP. In this sample, 83% of men and 87% of women with the metabolic syndrome had elevated BP (SBP/DBP of 130/85 mm Hg or higher, or on treatment) consistent with the ATP III criteria (Figure 3–11).[42] Approximately one fourth of U.S. adults have the metabolic syndrome (including those with diabetes), although this varies dramatically with age, with prevalence increasing to near 40% in older age groups.[43] There is also great variation in risk among those with the metabolic syndrome; most women are at low or intermediate risk, whereas most men are at intermediate or high global risk (>20% calculated risk of CHD in the next 10 years), the latter of which would constitute a CHD risk-equivalent by ATP III standards.[42] Moreover, projections have estimated that BP control, ideally to optimal levels, and preferably combined (lipid and BP) risk factor management, can prevent the vast majority of CHD events.[42]

## RELATIVE VERSUS ABSOLUTE RISK ASSESSMENT AND PROJECTION OF TREATMENT BENEFIT

Over the past several decades, there has been a gradual evolution from the use of *relative risk* to *absolute risk* as the basis of deciding whom and when to treat. Relative risk quantifies the likelihood of future cardiovascular events in a "hypertensive" population in comparison with a "normotensive" reference population, with impact most frequently expressed as a risk ratio (RR). In contrast, absolute risk imparts information as to the expected absolute incidence of cardiovascular deaths or morbid events. In calculating absolute risk, one must not only include hypertension as a risk factor, but also age, gender, and all other major cardiovascular risk factors that commonly cluster with hypertension[1,43] (see Chapter

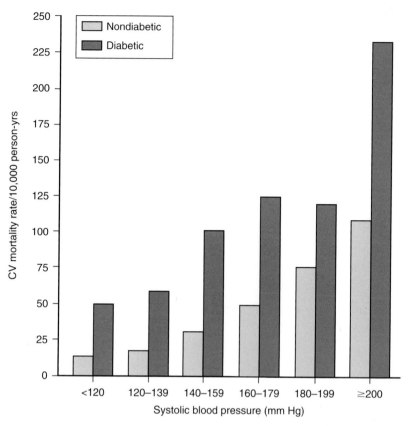

**Figure 3–10** MRFIT: Association between systolic blood pressure and cardiovascular (CV) death in type 2 diabetes. Adapted from Stamler J et al. Diabetes, other risk factors, and 12-yr cardiovascular mortality for men screened in the Multiple Risk Factor Intervention Trial. Diabetes Care 16:434-444, 1993.

21). Over the past decade there have been many national and international guidelines for antihypertensive therapy that have used absolute risk in varying degrees to assist physicians in decision making.

**Table 3–3** Criteria for the Metabolic Syndrome (without diabetes)*

| Risk Factor | Defining Level |
|---|---|
| Abdominal obesity† | |
| Waist circumference‡ | |
|    Men | >102 cm (>40 in) |
|    Women | >88 cm (>35 in) |
| Triglyceride | ≥150 mg/dl |
| High-density lipoprotein cholesterol | |
|    Men | <40 mg/dl |
|    Women | <50 mg/dl |
| Blood pressure | ≥130/≥85 mm Hg or treated |
| Fasting glucose§ | ≥110 mg/dl |

Modified from the executive summary of the third Report of the National Cholesterol Education Program (NCEP) Expert Panel on Detection, Evaluation, and Treatment of High Blood Cholesterol in Adults (Adult Treatment Panel III). JAMA 285:2486-2497, 2001.
*Diagnosis is established when three or more of these risk factors are present.
†Abdominal obesity is more highly correlated with metabolic risk factors than is ↑ body mass index.
‡Some men develop metabolic risk factors when circumference is only marginally increased.
§Some experts recommend separating out those with diabetes, those with a fasting glucose of 126 mg/dl, because clear guidelines for these persons exist.

In trying to estimate absolute benefit in terms of preventable CHD events from control of hypertension, one can apply absolute risk estimates obtained from Framingham algorithms to the general U.S. population of adults with hypertension.[44] This calculation suggests that treatment of the U.S. population with hypertension (30-74 years of age) to a nominal goal of <140 mm Hg SBP and <90 mm Hg DBP could prevent approximately 19% of CHD events in men and 31% of CHD events in women in the next 10 years. Treatment to an idealized goal of <120 mm Hg SBP and <80 mm Hg DBP could prevent 37% and 56% of CHD events, respectively.[44] The long-term value of sustained antihypertensive treatment has also been estimated from a secular trend study from Framingham involving three successive cohorts between the ages of 50 and 59 years in 1950, 1960, and 1970.[45] After adjusting for risk factors, there was as much as a 60% reduction in cardiovascular mortality in those receiving antihypertensive therapy for 20 years compared with their untreated counterparts.

## GLOBAL RISK STRATIFICATION

Based on the results of considerable outcome data, there is consensus that antihypertensive medications should be used as part of therapy in all high-risk patients.[1,39] These would include individuals with persistent stage 2 hypertension BP (≥160/100 mm Hg) and those with stage 1 hypertension BP (≥140-159/90-99 mm Hg) or prehypertension BP (≥120-139/80-89 mm Hg) with associated risk factors or cardiovascular disease. The latter two BP categories encompass those individuals with (1) hypertensive target organ involvement (LVH, microalbuminuria [50-300 mg albuminuria/24 hours], mild increase in serum creatinine [1.3-1.5 mg/dl in men and

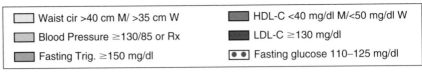

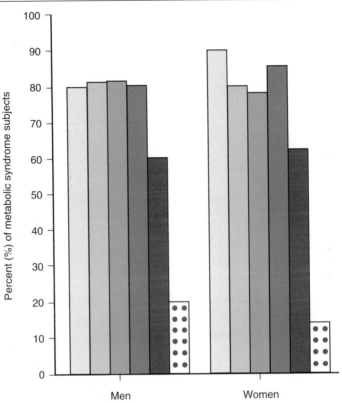

**Figure 3–11** Prevalence of selected risk factors in U.S. adults with the metabolic syndrome (without diabetes). Adapted from Wong ND, Pio J, Franklin SS, L'Italien GJ, Kamath T, Williams R. Preventing heart disease by nominal and optimal control of blood pressure and lipids in persons with the metabolic syndrome. Am J Cardiol 91:1421-1426, 2003.

1.2-1.4 mg/dl in women], and grade 3 or 4 retinopathy [retinal hemorrhages/exudates and papilledema, respectively]); (2) associated clinical conditions (CHD, heart failure, stroke, renal impairment [serum creatinine of >1.5 mg/dl in men and >1.4 mg/dl in women], peripheral vascular disease); or (3) diabetes with or without vascular complications.

On the other hand, there is considerable disagreement about when to supplement lifestyle treatment measures with antihypertensive therapy in individuals with stage 1 hypertension (140-159/90-99 mm Hg) without associated risk factors or cardiovascular disease. To date, there have been no definitive trials to assess the benefit of treatment in this group, which represents the largest single category within the hypertensive population: Ogden et al.[46] found that in the NHANES III adult hypertensive population, 20.7% had complicated hypertension, 31.3% had uncomplicated but stage 2 hypertension, 5% had stage 1 hypertension without additional risk factors, and 43% had uncomplicated stage 1 hypertension with at least one or more additional risk factors.

## ACCURACY OF CURRENT RISK ASSESSMENT FOR UNCOMPLICATED MILD HYPERTENSION

JNC 7 guidelines[1] suggest that every individual with uncomplicated stage 1 hypertension who does not respond to lifestyle modification promptly be started on antihypertensive therapy.

In contrast, the European Society of Hypertension guidelines[39] stress the importance of assessing global risk and then complementing lifestyle modification with drug therapy in the presence of moderate to high risk. This type of assessment requires that the number and severity of risk factors in an individual be used to calculate the likelihood of future CHD events by multivariate assessment, similar to that based on the Framingham risk equations. According to these criteria, in the presence of a 10-year risk of hard CHD events of >20%, based on Framingham risk equations and designated a CHD risk equivalent by the Third Adult Treatment Panel of the National Cholesterol Education Program,[41] therapeutic intervention should be considered for those with SBP of 130 to 159 mm Hg and DBP of 80 to 89 mm Hg as it is for others in this range with diabetes or target organ damage. In the presence of an intermediate risk (e.g., 10-year 6%-20% risk), consideration can be given for using noninvasive screening tests for the detection of subclinical cardiovascular disease to further stratify risk.[47]

Data from NHANES adults surveyed in 1999-2000 show that a substantial proportion of persons with hypertension is at intermediate risk (6%-20% estimated 10-year risk of CHD). By the sixth decade of life, more than 40% are at high risk (>20% 10-year risk of CHD, including those with known CHD, stroke, or peripheral vascular disease); by the eighth decade of life this rises to more than 60% of persons with hypertension (Figure 3–12). Approximately 60% of males and 40% of females with hypertension are at high risk of CHD based on these estimates.

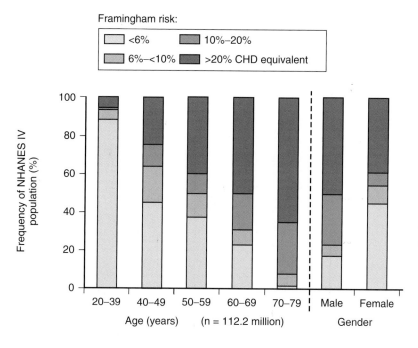

Framingham risk:

- □ <6%
- ▤ 6%–<10%
- ▨ 10%–20%
- ▩ >20% CHD equivalent

Frequency of NHANES IV population (%)

Age (years)  (n = 112.2 million)  Gender

**Figure 3–12** Distribution of Framingham Risk in the NHANES 1999-2000 Hypertensive Population by Age and Gender. People with diabetes, prior cardiovascular disease (CHD, MI, stroke, CHF), or peripheral vascular disease (PVD) were treated as CHD equivalents.

Noninvasive subclinical disease measures, including carotid artery intimal medial thickness (IMT) measured by ultrasound, ankle brachial index, coronary artery calcium, echocardiographic left ventricular mass, and left ventricular global systolic function (ejection fraction), have been shown to have reasonable sensitivity and reproducibility in detecting subclinical atherosclerotic disease and also show predictive value over and above standard assessment of risk factors. If evidence of significant subclinical disease is revealed (e.g., coronary calcium score >400, ankle brachial index <0.90, or carotid artery IMT ≥1 mm), one can make the case for stratification of treatment to the next highest level (e.g., as a CHD risk equivalent), warranting lower cutpoints for treatment initiation or BP goal.[47] For example, the Assessment of Prognostic Risk Observational Survey (APROS) study[48] found that 53% of patients previously classified as mild or medium risk by the World Health Organization/ International Society of Hypertension were reclassified as high risk (10-year risk ≥20%) after LVH was found on echocardiography and/or significant increased diffuse or focal carotid artery IMT was found by ultrasound examination.

However, the prognostic utility and cost-benefit considerations of using noninvasive screening tests in selected intermediate-risk population groups have yet to be determined, and no consensus regarding such screening currently exists for the general population of hypertensives. Therefore, clinical judgment based on a thorough office-based examination and global risk assessment remains the primary basis on which to decide when antihypertensive therapy should be added to lifestyle measures in uncomplicated prehypertension and stage 1 hypertension.

## HYPERTENSION AWARENESS, TREATMENT, AND CONTROL RATES

Since 1988-1991, there have been no significant improvements in awareness of hypertension in men (from 63% in 1988-1991 to 66% in 1999-2000) and actually a trend toward lesser awareness in women (from 75% in 1998-1991 to 71% in 1999-2000).[4] Although a trend toward improvements in awareness among Mexican Americans has been noted, no significant improvements were seen in any other ethnic group.

Treatment rates, however, have improved from 52.4% to 58.4% (p = .007) overall due to improvements in treatment rates in men (44.5%-54.3%, p <.001) but not in women (60.1%-62.0%, p = .24) (Figures 3–13 and 3–14).[4] Rates of treatment have improved significantly in non-Hispanic whites and non-Hispanic Blacks, but only marginally in Mexican Americans, during this time period.

Significant improvement in control of hypertension, both among those treated and among all with hypertension, have also been seen in men, but not in women during this time period. In 1999-2000, approximately 60% of men being treated had their hypertension controlled to <140/90 mm Hg compared with less than 50% of women (see Figures 3–13 and 3–14). Women, older persons, and Mexican Americans tended to have the lowest rates of hypertension control. The improvement in control rates for men exclusively resulted from substantial improvements in control in non-Hispanic white men (from 20.7% in 1988-1991 to 36.5% in 1999-2000), without any significant change in men of other race/ethnic groups.[4] The reasons for the poorer treatment and control rates in women are not well understood. The poorer control

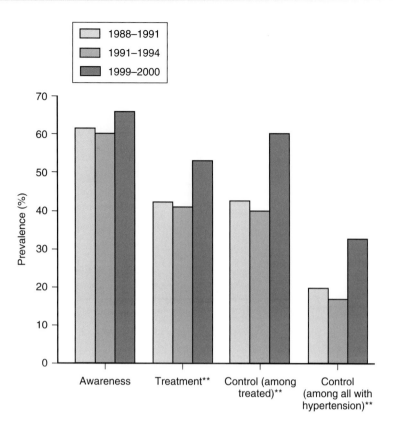

**Figure 3-13** Trends in awareness, treatment, and control among men with hypertension, U.S. population, 1988-2000. Adapted from Hajjar I, Kotchen TA. Trends in prevalence, awareness, treatment, and control of hypertension in the United States, 1988-2000. JAMA 290:199-206, 2003.

** *p* <.001 for change from 1988 to 2000

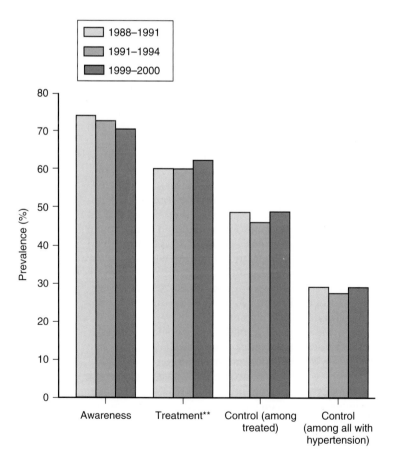

**Figure 3-14** Trends in awareness, treatment, and control among women with hypertension, U.S. population, 1988-2000. Adapted from Hajjar I, Kotchen TA. Trends in prevalence, awareness, treatment, and control of hypertension in the United States, 1988-2000. JAMA 290:199-206, 2003.

**No significant changes in awareness, treatment, or control from 1988 to 2000

rates in older persons, despite universal health insurance (Medicare) for those aged 65 and older, may in part be a reflection of greater severity of their hypertension, particularly ISH. It has been noted that improving hypertension treatment and control in women, the elderly, Mexican Americans, and persons with diabetes will have a significant impact on overall control rates, and unless hypertension control rates improve, the 50% target for hypertension control by 2010 will not be met.[4]

Although hypertension treatment rates are far from optimal in the United States (52.5%), they are substantially higher than in European countries (26.8%) (see Figure 3–4). This has been attributed to lower thresholds for treatment in the United States, increasing the numbers of treated cases, and lowering the mean BP in the population.[3]

## POPULATION VERSUS HIGH-RISK APPROACHES FOR PREVENTION

Prevention of complications of hypertension requires concerted efforts of both population and high-risk approaches.[49] The former involves efforts of public health education, the media, communitywide alliances, and legislation promoting healthful policies, in an effort to gradually reduce morbidity and mortality in the population from shifting the population distribution of BPs downward (or prevent their upward trends). The latter requires intensive one-on-one clinical management of patients with preexisting hypertension to reduce individual risks of cardiovascular, renal, and other complications. Efforts of governmental, community, and healthcare providers cooperating together are vital to successfully prevent and manage hypertension and its consequences.

## SUMMARY

Hypertension is associated with a twofold to fourfold increased risk of CHD, stroke, peripheral vascular disease, and renal disease. Increased SBP is strongly associated with increases in risk, even when diastolic pressure is normal; a high PP further increases risk. An increase in risk of developing of hypertension and cardiovascular events begins among persons in the prehypertension range of BP. Three out of four persons with hypertension are age 50 or older, and by the age of 80, more than 65% of the population will have hypertension, as currently defined. Over the past 15 years, prevalence has increased among women and older persons, but treatment and control have improved only among men. ISH is the predominant form of hypertension after the sixth decade of life, whereas diastolic hypertension is the most common form before the age of 50. Hypertension is seldom a lone cardiovascular risk factor; it tends to cluster with additional risk factors as part of the metabolic syndrome. Appropriate risk stratification of persons with hypertension involves a combined approach of an office-based examination and global risk assessment. In intermediate-risk persons with hypertension, subclinical disease screening may be useful to identify candidates for more intensive treatment. For both primary and secondary prevention, treatment of all significant risk factors, as opposed to treating only hypertension, will result in the largest reduction in cardiovascular risk.

## References

1. Chobanian AV, Bakris GL, Black HR, et al. The Seventh Report of the Joint National Committee on Prevention, Detection, Evaluation, and Treatment of High Blood Pressure. The JNC 7 Report. JAMA 289:2560-2572, 2003.
2. The WHO Monica Project: Risk factors. Int J Epidemiol 18:S46-S55, 1989.
3. Wolf-Maier K, Cooper RS, Banegas JR, et al. Hypertension prevalence and blood pressure levels in 6 European countries, Canada, and the United States. JAMA 289:2363-2369, 2003.
4. Hajjar I, Kotchen TA. Trends in prevalence, awareness, treatment, and control of hypertension in the United States, 1988-2000. JAMA 290:199-206, 2003.
5. Vasan RS, Beiser A, Seshadri S, et al. Residual lifetime risk for developing hypertension in middle-aged women and women: The Framingham Heart Study. JAMA 287:1003-1010, 2002.
6. Keys A. Seven Countries: A Multivariate Analysis of Death and Coronary Heart Disease. Cambridge, MA, Harvard University Press, 1980.
7. Stamler J, Stamler R, Neaton JD. Blood pressure, systolic and diastolic, and cardiovascular risks: US population data. Arch Intern Med 153:598-615, 1993.
8. McMahon S, Peto R, Cutler J, et al. Blood pressure, stroke, and coronary heart disease: Part 1. Prolonged differences in blood pressure: Prospective observational studies corrected for the regression dilution bias. Lancet 335:765-774, 1990.
9. Kannel WB, Dawber TR, Kahan A, et al. Factors of risk in development of coronary heart disease: Six year follow-up experience—The Framingham Study. Ann Intern Med 55:33-50, 1961.
10. Kannel WB, Gordon T, Schwartz MR. Systolic versus diastolic blood pressure and risk of coronary heart disease: The Framingham Study. Am J Cardiol 27:335-345, 1971.
11. Vasan RS, Larson MG, Leip EP, et al. Assessment of frequency of progression to hypertension in non-hypertensive participants in the Framingham Heart Study. Lancet 358:1682-1686, 2001.
12. Vasan RS, Larson MG, Leip EP, et al. Impact of high-normal blood pressure on the risk of cardiovascular disease. N Engl J Med 345:1291-1297, 2001.
13. Kotchen TA, Kotchen JM. Regional variation in blood pressure: Environment or genes? Circulation 96:1071-1073, 1997.
14. Kannel WB, Wilson PWF. Cardiovascular risk factors and hypertension. *In* Izzo JL, Black HR (eds): Hypertension Primer, 3rd ed. Dallas, TX, American Heart Association, 2003.
15. McMahon S, Peto R, Cutler J, et al. Blood pressure, stroke, and coronary heart disease: Part 1. Prolonged differences in blood pressure: Prospective observational studies corrected for the regression dilution bias. Lancet 335:765-774, 1990.
16. Lewington S, Clarke R, Qizilbash N, et al. Age-specific relevance of usual blood pressure to vascular mortality. Lancet 287:1003-1010, 2002.
17. Levy D. Left ventricular hypertrophy risk. *In* Izzo JL, Black HR (eds). Hypertension Primer, 3rd ed. Dallas, TX, American Heart Association, 2003.
18. Levy D, Garrison RJ, Savage DD, et al. Prognostic implications of echocardiographically determined left ventricular mass in the Framingham Heart Study. N Engl J Med 322:1561-1566, 1990.
19. Matthew J, Sleight P, Lonn E, et al. for the Heart Outcomes Prevention Evaluation (HOPE) Investigators. Reduction of cardiovascular risk by regression of electrocardiographic markers of left ventricular hypotrophy by the angiotensin-converting enzyme inhibitor ramipril. Circulation 102:1615-1621, 2001.
20. Wolf PA. Cerebrovascular risk. *In* Izzo JL, Black HR (eds). Hypertension Primer, 3rd ed. Dallas, TX, American Heart Association, 2003.
21. Kannel WB, McGree DL. Update on some epidemiologic features of intermittent claudication: The Framingham Study. J Am Geriatr Soc 33:13-18, 1985.

22. Klag MJ, Whelton PK, Randall BL, et al. Blood pressure and end-stage renal disease in men. N Engl J Med 334:13-18, 1996.

23. Franklin SS. Aging and hypertension: The assessment of blood pressure indices in predicting coronary heart disease. J Hypertension 17(Suppl 5):S29-S36, 1999.

24. Franklin SS, Jacobs MJ, Wong ND, et al. Predominance of isolated systolic hypertension among middle-aged and elderly US hypertensives—Analysis based on NHANES III. Hypertension 37:869-874, 2001.

25. Burt VL, Whelton P, Roccella EJ, et al. Prevalence of hypertension in the US adult population: Results from the Third National Health and Nutrition Examination Survey, 1988-1991. Hypertension 25:305-313, 1995.

26. Franklin SS, Gustin W, Wong ND, et al. Hemodynamic patterns of age-related changes in blood pressure: The Framingham Heart Study. Circulation 96:308-315, 1997.

27. Neaton JD Wentworth D. Serum cholesterol, blood pressure, cigarette smoking, and death from coronary heart disease. Overall findings and differences by age for 316,099 white men. Arch Intern Med 152:56-64, 1992.

28. Perry HM Jr, Miller JP, Fornoff JR, et al. Early predictors of 15-year end-stage renal disease in hypertensive patients. Hypertension 25(4 Pt 1):587-594, 1995.

29. Nielsen WB, Vestbo J, Jensen GR. Isolated systolic hypertension: A significant risk factor of cerebral apoplexy and acute myocardial infarction. A prospective population based study. Ugeskr Laeger 158:3779-3783, 1996.

30. Kannel WB. Risk stratification in hypertension: New insights from the Framingham Study. Am J Hypertens 13(1 Pt 2):3S-10S, 2000.

31. Franklin SS, Khan SA, Wong ND, et al. Is pulse pressure useful in predicting risk for coronary heart disease? The Framingham Heart Study. Circulation 100:354-360, 1999.

32. Wong ND, Sciammarella M, Arad Y, et al. Relation of thoracic aortic and aortic valve calcium to coronary artery calcium and risk assessment. Am J Cardiol 92:951-955, 2003.

33. Benetos A, Safar M, Rudnichi A, et al. Pulse pressure: A predictor of long-term cardiovascular mortality in a French male population. Hypertension 30:1410-1415, 1997.

34. Verdecchia P, Schillaci G, Borgione C, et al. Ambulatory pulse pressure: A potent predictor of total cardiovascular risk in hypertension. Hypertension 32:983-988, 1998.

35. Staessen JA, Gasowski, Wang JG, et al. Risks of untreated and treated isolated systolic hypertension in the elderly meta-analysis of outcome trials. Lancet 104:865-872, 2000.

36. Dart AM, Kingwell BA. Pulse pressure—A review of mechanisms and clinical relevance. J Am Coll Cardiol 37:975-984, 2001.

37. Van Bortel LMAB, Struijker-Boudier HAJ, Safar ME. Pulse pressure, arterial stiffness, and drug treatment of hypertension. Hypertension 38:914-921, 2001.

38. Franklin SS, Larson MG, Khan SA, et al. Does the relation of blood pressure to coronary heart disease risk change with aging? The Framingham Heart Study. Circulation 103:1245-1249, 2001.

39. Guidelines Committee. 2003 European Society of Hypertension-European Society of Cardiology guidelines for the management of arterial hypertension. J Hypertens 21:1011-1053, 2003.

40. Stamler J, Vaccaro O, Neaton JD, et al. Diabetes, other risk factors, and 12-yr cardiovascular mortality for men screened in the Multiple Risk Factor Intervention Trial. Diabetes Care 16:434-444, 1993.

41. Executive Summary of the Third Report of the National Cholesterol Education Program (NCEP) Expert Panel on Detection, Evaluation, and Treatment of High Blood Cholesterol in adults (Adult Treatment Panel III). JAMA 285:2486-2497, 2001.

42. Wong ND, Pio J, Franklin SS, et al. Preventing heart disease by nominal and optimal control of blood pressure and lipids in persons with the metabolic syndrome. Am J Cardiol 91:1421-1426, 2003.

43. Ford ES, Giles WH, Dietz WH. Prevalence of the metabolic syndrome among US adults: Findings from the Third National Health and Nutrition Examination Survey. JAMA 287:356-359, 2002.

44. Wong ND, Thakral G, Franklin SS, et al. Preventing heart disease by controlling hypertension: Impact of hypertensive subtype, stage, age, and gender. Am Heart J 145(5):888-895, 2003.

45. Sytkowski PA, D'Agostino RB, Belanger AJ, et al. Secular trends in long-term sustained hypertension, long-term treatment, and cardiovascular mortality. Circulation 93:697-703, 1996.

46. Ogden LG, He J, Lydick E, et al. Long-term absolute benefit of lowering blood pressure in hypertensive patients according to the JNC VI risk stratification. Hypertension 35:539-543, 2000.

47. Wilson PWF, Smith SC, Blumenthal RS, et al. 34th Bethesda Conference: Task force #4—How do we select patients for atherosclerosis imaging? J Am Coll Cardiol 41:1898-1906, 2003.

48. Cuspidi C, Ambrosioni E, Mancia G, et al. Role of echocardiography and carotid ultrasonography in stratifying risk in patients with essential hypertension: The assessment of prognostic risk observational survey. J Hypertens 20:1307-1314, 2002.

49. Pearson TA. Primary prevention. *In* Wong ND, Black HR, Gardin JM (eds). Preventive Cardiology. New York, Mc-Graw Hill, 2000.

# Pathophysiology

## Chapter 4

# Pathophysiology of Hypertension
## Maria Carolina Delgado, Alan B. Weder

Regulation of blood pressure is one of the most complex of physiologic functions, dependent on the integrated actions of cardiovascular, renal, neural, and endocrine systems. Hypertension is a disorder of the average level about which blood pressure is regulated, and although it is of clinical importance because chronically elevated blood pressure damages the heart, blood vessels, and kidneys, at least in its early stages hypertension does not cause obvious disturbances of cardiovascular function. Most of the functional cardiovascular derangements of hypertension arise from the compensatory mechanisms elevated blood pressure provokes (e.g., vascular and ventricular hypertrophy) or from its contribution to vascular damage (e.g., atherosclerosis and nephrosclerosis). Investigating the pathophysiology of hypertension therefore means understanding the mechanisms of normal blood pressure control and seeking evidence of subtle abnormalities that precede (or at least coincide with) the rise of blood pressure to hypertensive levels.

Because hypertension represents a quantitative dysfunction of the highly interactive elements of the cardiovascular system, traditional reductionist research modes are unlikely to yield more than fragments of the answer to the question of what causes hypertension.[1-3] Pathophysiologic thinking is one such reductionist approach. Essentially mechanistic and concerned largely with the immediate or proximate causes of disease, such research seeks to identify the structures and functions that result in elevated blood pressure. Pathophysiologic studies have been of great value in describing the underlying causes of differences between hypertensives and normotensives but less successful in identifying root causes of hypertension. To address causality, findings gathered in the physiologic investigation of cardiovascular control systems will need to be integrated into broader frameworks: The value of evolutionary research for organizing the findings derived from pathophysiologic research has been pointed out before.[4] The goal of evolutionary thinking is to understand how heritable traits affect reproductive success, and ultimately to describe not only the fundamental genetic complement underpinning hypertension but also the environmental factors necessary for expression of the phenotype and the physiologic processes mediating the interaction of genes and environment. Each such complement of genes, each set of environmental exposures, and each history of their interaction will be unique, so that a truly comprehensive description of the pathophysiology of hypertension will probably never be possible. But by integrating broad frames such as evolution into our

pathophysiologic thinking, we are likely to get a better understanding of ultimate causation.

This introduction attempts to lay out some of the broad principles of cardiovascular regulation that are relevant to a consideration of the pathophysiology of essential hypertension. We do not aim to summarize the mechanisms to be explored in detail by experts in the succeeding chapters of this volume but rather to demonstrate how complex the task of formulating an integrated pathophysiologic picture of hypertension is likely to be. We begin by emphasizing three fundamental features of blood pressure control:

1. Blood pressure regulation is flexible and responsive to local organ perfusion requirements.
2. Blood pressure regulation is integrated into overall cardiovascular-renal function to serve total-body homeostasis.
3. The level at which blood pressure is regulated changes throughout a patient's life history.

## BLOOD PRESSURE CONTROL AND LOCAL NEEDS

At its most basic level, blood pressure provides the driving force that moves blood through the vascular system. Because maintenance of this function is absolutely critical to life, it is not surprising that natural selection has favored organisms that have evolved mechanisms that contribute to blood pressure stability. Nor is it unexpected that such mechanisms are powerful and highly redundant, providing ample "backup" to cope with changes in environmental factors, including electrolyte intake, physical activity, threats, and trauma. Indeed, it would be remarkable if the situation were otherwise.

All mammals have fundamentally the same circulatory system, so blood pressure control systems are likely to be highly evolutionarily conserved across species, and it may therefore not seem surprising that mean arterial blood pressure in the aortic root is essentially constant in mammals, about 100 mm Hg.[5] This constancy is in contrast to many anatomic features (e.g., heart weight) and physiologic functions (e.g., heart rate) that are scaled to average body mass across a wide range of species sizes.[6] In many cases, unscaled variables (i.e., those not related to body size) are con strained by fundamental and invariant physical or chemical features important to life, such as diffusion distances. Because several other critical aspects of circulatory function are similarly unscaled, notably capillary and red blood cell diameters, it seems plausible to assume that blood pressure is part of a system finely adapted in many ways to ensure optimal delivery of metabolic substrates at the tissue level. The level of blood pressure characteristic of mammals as an adaptation of their particular body plan is evidenced by the differing average blood pressure levels found in other animals. Birds, for example, operate at a higher average blood pressure level than do mammals, and the reasons for the difference are not clear.[6]

Whereas the constancy of blood pressure in mammals might seem to imply rigidity of function, nothing could be further from the truth. An example of naturally elevated blood pressure in a nonhuman mammalian species is instructive in demonstrating how flexible blood pressure regulation can be. Giraffes have evolved to occupy an ecologic niche of arboreal feeding by means of selection for an extreme elongation of the neck (selection pressure may have been multifunctional [e.g., male-male competition]). Although closely related to the other ruminants, where blood pressure averages the expected value of about 100 mm Hg mean, giraffes demonstrate extraordinarily high blood pressures at the level of the heart, with estimates of resting blood pressure of 180 mm Hg[7] to greater than 300 mm Hg.[8]

Elevated blood pressure in these animals serves to maintain blood flow to the brain, so that blood pressure level at the base of the skull is about 100 mm Hg. The cardiovascular system has accommodated the particular structural adaptations of giraffe anatomy by altering force generation at the left ventricle and thus aortic root pressure to provide precisely the energy necessary to drive blood to the brain. It is theoretically possible for natural selection to have altered the structural plan of the giraffe body to one in which the brain migrated to a more central body location and therefore could operate at a "normal" systemic blood pressure. However, such an adaptation would involve wrenching changes in the established body plan and ontologic course of vertebrate development that would undoubtedly be difficult to fashion. Nature usually shapes its adaptations conservatively. The giraffe's neck, for instance, although markedly different in appearance from that of the taxonomically related cow, nonetheless contains the same seven cervical vertebrae. In meeting the cardiovascular demand imposed by its anatomic adaptation, rather than redesigning the system, it is more efficient to draw on built-in features of the cardiovascular repertoire—notably the ability to regulate average blood pressure level—and to use those features to match the specific circulatory demands imposed by neck elongation. Thus although generally fixed within a narrow range in mammals, when necessary, blood pressure can be maintained indefinitely at a markedly increased level when critical local needs require it.

The giraffe illustrates an important principle of blood pressure control: Blood pressure level is flexible and responsive to important physiologic needs (e.g., brain perfusion). From the viewpoint of the fitness of the organism in terms of natural selection, this functional trade-off of high blood pressure for optimal brain perfusion is perfectly reasonable, even if some adverse consequences flow from the compromise. The adaptationist paradigm holds that, in general, natural selection favors any individual or suite of novel features (in the case of

the giraffe, a long neck and the attendant elevated pressure) when the net impact of such changes is favorable in terms of reproductive success of the affected individual's genes. Importantly, not every preserved element need be in itself adaptive. Thus, whereas employing high blood pressure as a way of matching circulatory function to an unusual anatomic situation is an elegant solution to an adaptive challenge, it does not imply that giraffes do not pay a price for maintaining high aortic root pressures. They evidence a large number of pathologic effects of high blood pressure, including massive left ventricular hypertrophy (LVH) and extraordinary arterial vascular smooth muscle hypertrophy in the limbs.[9,10] It seems likely that such cardiovascular adaptations are potentially deleterious, but any such adverse consequences are more than balanced by the advantages of a long neck on overall fitness.

## BLOOD PRESSURE CONTROL AND INTEGRATED CARDIOVASCULAR-RENAL FUNCTION

In addition to providing perfusion to the brain, blood pressure plays a key role in the optimization of other organ and whole-body functions. Starling recognized as long ago as 1909 that total-body sodium and water balance is regulated in part by renal arterial perfusion pressure.[11] This concept was further characterized by subsequent investigators, most notably by Guyton et al., who proposed that blood pressure and sodium homeostasis are related through the mechanism of pressure natriuresis: When perfusion pressure increases, renal sodium output increases and extracellular fluid and blood volumes contract by an amount sufficient to return arterial blood pressure to its baseline.[12,13] Guyton characterized the relationship between natriuresis and mean arterial blood pressure by a pressure-natriuresis curve characteristic of each individual, which is shifted to a higher value on the pressure axis when hypertension is chronically sustained.[13]

In most normotensives, that curve is very steep, because blood pressure differs very little at extremes of sodium intake. In some normotensives and in a greater proportion of hypertensives, the slope of the curve is diminished, meaning that blood pressure varies continuously with differences in salt intake. Such individuals are said to be "salt-sensitive."[14]

Although the phenomenon of salt-sensitivity is often characterized as a primary isolated defect in pressure-natriuresis and while that deficiency surely underlies the volume responsiveness of blood pressure in patients with advanced renal insufficiency, more subtle renal dysfunctions also may be important.[15] One such physiologic mechanism recently proposed as contributing to renal physiologic and structural changes causing salt-sensitivity is a resetting of the set-point of tubuloglomerular feedback.[16]

Mammalian kidneys accurately match glomerular filtration to tubular sodium excretion by regulating afferent and efferent glomerular arteriolar resistance in response to distal tubular chloride load (Figure 4–1). Responses of glomerular filtration rate over a wide range of distal tubular load are described by a nonlinear function referred to as the tubuloglomerular function (TGF) curve.[17] TGF is a classic negative feedback loop, serving to control whole-body homeostasis. Thus, when the macula densa senses a decrease in sodium (NaCl) delivery to

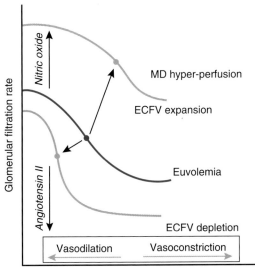

**Figure 4–1** The relation between the GFR and the distal sodium (NaCl) delivery, as expressed in tubular glomerular feedback (TGF). A resetting of the operating point downward and to the left occurs in depletion of the extracellular fluid volume (ECFV) (i.e., dehydration). A resetting of the operating point upward and to the right occurs in expansion of the ECFV or in a sustained increase in the delivery of NaCl to the distal tubules (i.e., tubular hyperperfusion of the macula densa [MD]), under euvolemic condition. The vascular tone (vasodilation or vasoconstriction) of the afferent arterioles is the main mechanism of the change in the GFR. Resetting of the TGF operating point is largely dependent on the balance between the levels of angiotensin II, extracellular adenosine, and nitric oxide in the vicinity of the glomerular arterioles. Resetting of the set-point has been proposed to result in chronically elevated glomerular filtration and promote renal damage. (From Aviv A, Hollenberg NK, Weder A. Sodium glomerulopathy: Tubuloglomerular feedback and renal injury in African Americans. Kidney Int 65(2): 361-368, 2004.)

the distal tubule, a signal is relayed to the afferent arteriole to dilate, resulting in increased glomerular capillary hydrostatic pressure and increased glomerular filtration rate. If as hypothesized, the TGF curve is displaced such that at a given distal tubular load a higher glomerular filtration rate is required to maintain normal whole-body sodium homeostasis, the chronic increase in glomerular capillary pressure could result in renal damage, which could in turn further depress pressure natriuresis and lead to a cycle of increasing salt-sensitivity of blood pressure and progressive renal injury. Such a sequence is consistent with the results of the African American Study of Kidney Disease and Hypertension, in which angiotensin-converting enzyme inhibitors and β-blockers, drugs that affect renin-dependent mechanisms, presumably including afferent arteriolar resistance and thus glomerular capillary pressure, slowed the progression of renal disease more effectively than a calcium channel blocker.[18] Interestingly, more aggressive control of systemic hypertension did not significantly affect the progression of renal damage and TGF, suggesting that local intrarenal hemodynamic factors are more important than systemic blood pressure as a cause of renal damage in this population. TGF

resetting, by triggering a pathophysiologic cascade compromising whole-body sodium metabolism, may necessitate increased reliance on a flexible compensatory system, blood pressure, resulting in a salt-sensitive pressure–natriuresis curve. Salt-sensitivity of blood pressure thus serves a critical biologic need, the maintenance of sodium balance in the face of a disorder of another important physiologic regulator of sodium balance, TGF. The point to be remembered is that cardiovascular-renal homeostatic mechanisms are highly integrated and redundant.

## CHANGING THE SET-POINT: GROWTH, DEVELOPMENT, AND HYPERTENSION

As pointed out in 1978 by Sir George Pickering, *hypertension* is defined by an arbitrary division in the continuous blood pressure distribution.[19] Two sets of definitions are commonly used, one for adults and one for children and adolescents. Adult levels exceeding a threshold of usually 140 mm Hg systolic or 90 mm Hg diastolic in the United States are defined as being *hypertensive*. Such cut-points are based largely on tradition rather than on any biologic significance of the values. In childhood, hypertension is defined as a blood pressure exceeding the 95th percentile for age,[20] another arbitrary division that results in a constantly changing threshold for hypertension during development. Such definitions are of heuristic value in identifying individuals on whom medical attention should be focused. But perhaps the real message of the different definitions is that they acknowledge an important feature of blood pressure during postnatal development: Blood pressure rises with age. Long ignored, the significance of the childhood, and indeed even prenatal, antecedents of hypertension are receiving increasing attention.[4,21]

The rise of blood pressure during childhood and adolescence follows a very stereotypical course, with a rapid increase during the first few weeks of life, a gradual increase throughout childhood, and a dramatic rise during puberty.[20] Blood pressure then remains relatively constant in most individuals throughout the remainder of the second and well into third decade, after which it again begins to rise.[4] It is during this period that most diastolic hypertension develops (i.e., blood pressures finally exceed 90 mm Hg diastolic). However, it has long been recognized that adult blood pressures are related to adolescent levels: Serial measures of blood pressure within individuals are correlated, and the coefficient of correlation becomes increasingly strong with aging.[21] As a consequence, adolescents with the highest relative rank of blood pressure have the highest risk of future hypertension. So where does hypertension begin? Is it when the blood pressure is established in the upper rank, as certainly can be determined during adolescence? Or alternatively, must we wait until middle age to diagnose hypertension? Because the pattern of high blood pressure is established early in life, hypertension may have its roots in early developmental events. Events contributing to high blood pressure in youth may result in pathophysiologic changes that cannot be subsequently reprogrammed or that set the stage so that events affecting blood pressure later in life have an enhanced hypertension-promoting effect.

Although the precise mechanisms affected early in development are unknown, several schema incorporating the general principle of early events conditioning later responses have been proposed:

1. *Vascular remodeling.* Observations by Folkow[22] and Sivertsson[23] that hypertensive vessels undergo adaptation by structural remodeling, which increases the wall:lumen ratio, identified an important mechanism that maintains chronically increased vascular resistance in established hypertension. Although partially reversible by long-term antihypertensive therapy, this structural adaptation persists to a degree even in effectively treated patients and progresses in uncontrolled hypertension.[24] Because structural changes are present even in borderline hypertension, it is likely that this adaptation begins early in the course of the blood pressure rise, probably before the hypertensive range is reached.[25,26]

2. *Hyperkinetic borderline hypertension.* Julius et al. described serial changes in cardiovascular function that result in a transition in the hemodynamics of blood pressure control from a state of increased cardiac output, largely sustained by the autonomic nervous system, to one of a sustained elevation of blood pressure dependent on increased vascular resistance and unrelated to increased autonomic tone.[27,28] The initiating factor for the early hyperkinetic circulatory state, increased sympathetic and decreased parasympathetic tone, is postulated to cause $\beta_1$-receptor down-regulation in the heart that, perhaps in concert with changes in myocardial function,[29] results in a regression of cardiac output to normal values. At the same time, structural enhancement of vascular resistance (increased wall:lumen ratio), induced by high blood pressure and sympathetic overactivity, results in a progressive increase in vascular tone even as sympathetic drive falls. The net effect of these adaptations is a transition from a state of increased cardiac output to one of increased vascular resistance.[30,31] Because the transition occurs over decades, serial longitudinal hemodynamic studies have been difficult to organize, but Lund-Johansen and Omvik documented the transition in a small group of subjects who presented with hyperkinetic borderline hypertension in youth and ended with typical high-resistance essential hypertension 20 years later.[32]

3. *Allometric dysfunction.* Weder and Schork proposed a schema in which the coordinated programs matching somatic and renal growth could be disrupted by an excessively vigorous growth pattern in youth and adolescence.[4] They postulated that the vigorous growth associated with modern childhood and adolescence, coupled with compression of the period of active growth by earlier puberty, might result in a fixed mismatch of some critical growth-related renal function and somatic metabolic demands. Such a mismatch might be compensated for by increased blood pressure, and since the fundamental defect could not be corrected after the cessation of growth at puberty, this fixed defect could promote hypertension throughout life. Although the precise nature of the renal defect leading to such a situation is unknown, underdevelopment of the medullary microcirculation or cortical afferent arterioles[33] appear to be important aspects of renal structure affecting sodium handling.[34] Aspects of this schema are pertinent to the subsequent discussion of how modernity causes hypertension.

4. *Synchronicity.* Schork et al. noted that in inbred animal strains, there is a temporal coupling of growth and blood pressure such that growth spurts regularly precede rises in blood pressure.[35] Similar findings have been reported for humans when serial changes in body size and blood pressure have been examined.[36] The vigor of the rise in blood pressure after a growth spurt appeared to be greater in genetically hypertensive rats compared with a genetically normotensive strain, suggesting that genetic programs controlling the coupling function could be responsible for initiating states of increasing blood pressure initially triggered by normal growth processes.

5. *Telomere shortening.* Aviv and Aviv proposed the interesting hypothesis that telomere shortening, a phenomenon accompanying normal aging, might contribute to hypertension.[37] There is considerable evidence that essential hypertension is closely linked to the growth, development, and aging of human beings. One biologic indicator of growth and aging that could provide a better understanding of the etiology of essential hypertension is the age-dependent telomere attrition rate in somatic cells, which registers the replicative history of somatic cells. Telomere attrition rate records the growth that results from the replication of somatic cells and their turnover—a process that is strongly linked to inflammation and oxidative stress, which are key factors in the biology of human aging.[38]

6. *Birth weight and hypertension.* Largely through the work of Barker, a relationship between low birth weight, increased placental weight, and increased risk of adult hypertension has been established.[39,40] These observations suggest that in utero events can condition, or in Barker's terminology, *program*, an infant to a phenotype characterized by insulin resistance and a tendency toward the development of hypertension and diabetes.[39] Barker argues that in utero growth retardation sets the stage for a thrifty phenotype that manifests itself as disease late in life.

The mechanism of such programming has been further investigated by Seckl, who has provided evidence that placental 11β-hydroxysteroid dehydrogenase activity may play a key role in such programming.[41] This enzyme converts physiologic glucocorticoids such as cortisol to inactive metabolites, thus decreasing the transfer of maternal steroids to the fetus. Experimental studies show that steroid exposure inhibits fetal growth but increases placental weight, the pattern identified by Barker as predisposing to hypertension.[39] Seckl demonstrated that in rats, in utero exposure to steroids increases the blood pressure of offspring,[42] suggesting that factors that control fetal steroid exposure, especially 11β-hydroxysteroid dehydrogenase activity, could play a role in promoting hypertension.

All these mechanisms share a common theme: Events at one point in development have consequences for the blood pressure level at a later stage. In searching for causal events, then, we would be well advised to look at the times at which such events are operative.

## HYPERTENSION: PROXIMATE AND ULTIMATE CAUSATION

Having stressed the importance to research in hypertension of the essential functions of the circulatory system, the integrated nature of cardiovascular-renal homeostasis and the importance of the temporal evolution of the level of blood pressure, let us turn to a consideration of why humans get hypertension.

No one can say with absolute certainty when hypertension first appeared in human history, but it is generally accepted to be a relatively modern disease of civilization. The emphasis on the importance of the acculturated environment somewhat undervalues the role of genes, and the term *syndrome of impaired genetic homeostasis* has been suggested as a better characterization of the problem.[43] The strongest support for the view that hypertension results from a fundamental mismatch between our ancient genes and our modern environment comes from observations of blood pressure in populations of modern-day hunter-gatherers.[44] Individuals in many of these societies pursue a lifestyle probably quite like that of the Neolithic period and do not develop hypertension or the progressive rise in systolic and mean blood pressure that is universally observed in individuals living in Westernized societies. Because adult hunter-gatherers have typical mammalian blood pressures (i.e., mean arterial blood pressures of about 100 mm Hg), elevated blood pressures in Westernized societies may reflect a response to some physiologic need imposed by our acculturation. Although we do not have an adaptive problem as obvious as the giraffe's long neck, modern environmental novelty apparently activates the flexible, powerful, highly evolutionarily preserved systems that alter the set-point of blood pressure control to a higher level in some individuals. Unlike the giraffe, we do not seem to "need" high blood pressure, for in general, there is no obvious physiologic dysfunction induced by lowering blood pressure through antihypertensive treatment. Furthermore, clinical trials show that the adverse consequences of sustained high blood pressure are ameliorated by such treatment.

Yet the indisputable fact that genes contribute to human hypertension implies an adaptive role for those genes.[45] We are unaware of any data suggesting an adaptive advantage or disadvantage for hypertension itself. Except for the relatively rare event of fatal malignant hypertension in youth, which could obviously affect reproductive potential, diseases arising from or aggravated by essential hypertension generally occur during postreproductive years. Thus, when considering high blood pressure in an evolutionary context, it is important to focus on issues other than high blood pressure, because that is not a trait likely to be related to reproductive success. It is reasonable to view hypertension as a pleiotropic effect of a genetic suite that subserves some important function other than blood pressure regulation.[1,35] The keys to hypertension are likely to reside in genetic-environmental interactions, with the genes involved those of our ancient hunter-gatherer–adapted genome and the environment that of our new human-created world: Hypertension is a response to environmental novelty.

What is it that Westernized society does to our bodies that causes high blood pressure? The increased dietary sodium intake of acculturated societies has been extensively studied, and the Intersalt trial has provided good evidence that in populations with minimal sodium intake, the prevalence of hypertension is very low.[46] However, other factors may also be important, as exemplified by the Kuna of Panama, some of whom follow a traditional lifestyle yet consume sodium at levels typical of Westernized societies and do not evidence hypertension.[47] Others have suggested that the ratio of sodium: potassium intake may be critical and have identified the weight gain associated with migration from rural to urban settings as a factor associated with the development of hypertension.[48] The most obvious features of Westernized lifestyle are calorie intake in excess of need and calorie expenditure far below that of our early ancestors. Hunting and gathering

involved nomadic foraging and persistent pursuit of game, both of which required vigorous physical exertion. Even as agriculture arose, life remained strenuous, and not until industrialization did humans begin to escape a lifestyle of obligatory physical activity. Such a lifestyle required considerable energy throughput, and the estimated daily energy expenditure of adult members of hunter-gatherer and traditional (nonmechanized) agricultural societies was on the order of 3000 kcal/day,[49,50] whereas individuals in our modern industrialized societies expend about 2000 kcal/day or less.

This shift is almost entirely the result of mechanization, as illustrated by estimates of the effect of mechanized farming in Japan, which reduced daily work expenditure for the average farmer by more than 50%.[51] The shift from a balanced energy throughput, characterized by high intake but equally high expenditure, to one of intake in excess of expenditure resulted in an altered body habitus with an increase in body fat and a loss of muscle mass.[52,53] Even recently studied hunter-gatherers, who have already been somewhat affected by the modern world, have skinfold thicknesses half those of Westernized North Americans.[52] The experience of the Inuit of the Northwestern Territories of Canada during the period when hunting by dog sled and kayak was superseded by travel on snowmobiles, all-terrain vehicles, and power boats is particularly powerful and instructive, as the effect of modernization occurred quickly and resulted in dramatic changes in body composition within a generation.[53] Eaton noted that for 20- to 29-year-old males, lean body mass declined 10.1% and body fat (estimated from skinfold thicknesses) increased 88.7% over one 20-year period; for women in the same age category, lean body mass fell 12.1% while body fat rose 40.1%.[43] Along with the observed changes in body habitus, which seem to inevitably follow Westernization, comes hypertension. It is reasonable to think that the effects on body habitus and blood pressure are related: The question is, how?

The most logical place to search for the causes of hypertension is in normal blood pressure regulatory systems, and the optimal time is before blood pressure rises to pathologic levels. In order to carry out such studies, we need to examine further how blood pressure changes during normal growth and development. Blood pressure rises in several reasonably stereotypical spurts, most notably during adolescence. This adolescent spurt is probably part of our fundamental human biology, as it appears in hunter-gatherer adolescents as well as in Westernized individuals.[54] However, hunter-gatherers do not go on to develop hypertension later in life, whereas we do. Most interest has traditionally focused on the period during which hypertension actually develops—adulthood. However, increasing attention is being paid to childhood and adolescence as evidence accumulates that the forces driving the blood pressure up may already be in play by that time. An alteration in the natural history of the adolescent growth spurt may be important in the pathophysiology of adult hypertension.

Schork et al. observed that the rise in blood pressure in young rats that corresponds to the adolescent blood pressure spurt in humans is coupled to a growth spurt: Rapid growth precedes a rise in blood pressure in a regular manner.[35] More recently, longitudinal observations in humans demonstrated the same sequence with the adolescent blood pressure spurt trailing the onset of the growth spurt by about 1 to 2 years.[36] The appearance of this sequence in both humans and rats suggests that blood pressure rises to serve some need imposed by growth, presumably as part of maintenance of overall homeostasis.[35] In humans, secular trends in growth and development suggest that the overall program of maturation may be greatly accelerated by modern life.[55] Interestingly, evidence suggests that human ancestors were quite tall, probably on average as tall as the upper 15% of the modern population,[56,57] so the amount of linear growth itself may not be the problem.

Historical data show a progressive compression of the period of active growth and development in children and adolescents,[58] such that the growth of contemporary adolescents is probably near its biologic limits for both the final height achieved and the rate at which linear growth proceeds.[59] Coupled with vigorous linear growth is a tendency to adiposity that results in a high average body mass index in the tallest adolescents. In addition, sexual maturity is now probably achieved almost as early as biologically possible,[55] and the relative obesity of adolescents may again play an important role. It has been suggested that a critical fat mass is a trigger of menarche (perhaps mediated by increasing leptin levels),[60] presumably because sufficient fat accumulation increases the potential for successful pregnancy and childbearing.[61] The earlier and greater accumulation of body fat by acculturated children may be part of the reason that sexual development is now much more rapid than in earlier times. We have previously proposed that this compression of growth and development has affected growth programs preserved during evolution and adapted for a more leisurely pace, resulting in mismatches between structure and function, perhaps at the level of the kidney.[4] If this hypothesis is correct, a rise in blood pressure to high levels in adolescents who grow rapidly to a large size and mature early is simply a mechanism by which the body maintains overall homeostasis. Because those adolescents who are driven by rapid and vigorous growth to develop high blood pressure are predisposed to adult hypertension, it may be that the effects of modern civilization are mediated in part by a disruption of normal (i.e., Paleolithic) growth patterns.

An important distinction between hunter-gatherers and us is lack of an adult rise in blood pressure in non-Westernized people. It is during this adult phase that hypertension actually develops. Hypertension has at least two developmental phases, an early phase (childhood and adolescence), during which the stage is set for future hypertension, and a later phase, during which progressively rising blood pressure finally achieves hypertensive levels. It seems likely that the later phase of hypertension development is a product of the same environmental influences that affected early growth and development, but in adulthood, where linear growth is no longer possible, the result of caloric excess is progressive adiposity, which ultimately promotes a rise in blood pressure and the development of hypertension. Some support for this view comes from an intriguing observation reported in the Framingham cohort that lean young hypertensives go on to develop obesity in adulthood, suggesting that factors that promote hypertension in youth may predispose to adiposity in adults.[62] As described previously, Barker et al. suggested that this tendency toward hypertension and obesity may actually be set during in utero development.[63] A pathophysiologic schema by which obesity may promote hypertension has been proposed by Landsberg.[64]

Our Paleolithic genes are affected by modern lifestyle factors with the result that we achieve less than optimal muscularity and a considerable excess of body fat, yet we grow linearly at an accelerated rate and achieve sexual maturity at a young age. These alterations in human natural history appear to provoke a rise in blood pressure through mechanisms not yet well described: Physiologists still have much to contribute to reveal the detailed mechanisms by which the set-point of blood pressure regulation is altered.

## GENETICS OF HYPERTENSION

Identifying genes predisposing to hypertension is a daunting challenge. Mutations have been described for several rare Mendelian hypertensive diseases with distinctive pathophysiologic features, and it is of interest that most relate to renal sodium handling, reinforcing the concept that the kidney has an overriding influence on blood pressure regulation.[65] These variants are not important causes of high blood pressure in the general population.

That genes contribute to hypertension is well established from twin and family studies. The diathesis for hypertension appears to be multigenic and to account for some 30% to 40% of total variation in blood pressure level. The number of "hypertension genes" transmitted to an at-risk individual is important: The relative risk of developing hypertension for offspring of hypertensive parents is higher if both parents are hypertensive and if the disease has had earlier onset in the parent(s).[66]

It is important to recognize that while estimates of heritability apportion part of the population variance of blood pressure to genetic factors, all blood pressure variance represents a gene-by-environment interaction. There are no "genes for hypertension," there are only genes predisposing to hypertension in our current environment. Most if not all the genetic component of hypertension is expressed only in a permissive environment, so-called context-dependency.[2,67] Defining what environmental factors promote and modify the expression of the genetic component hypertension is at least as difficult as identifying genes for hypertension, and most clues from cross-cultural or case-control studies are not carefully measured when population-based genetic epidemiologic studies are performed. Effects may be very subtle and in part be determined by an individual's life history. Even in a population of completely inbred animal models maintained under standardized conditions, blood pressure is normally distributed with a surprisingly large range.

Hypertension is a prototypical genetically complex disease; investigators seeking to identify individual genes for such diseases face many barriers (Figure 4–2):

1. *Diseases such as hypertension are not discrete.* Unlike Mendelian diseases with distinctive phenotypes, common diseases are often quantitative disorders, and definitions are based on arbitrary cut-points. Phenotypes employed for genetic studies are therefore somewhat poorly defined and probably etiologically heterogeneous. One of the clearest lessons from the secondary hypertensions is that there are many ways to sustain elevated blood pressure chronically. In addition, characterizing blood pressure is difficult; blood pressure itself is very labile, and there is no agreement as to what is the "right" blood pressure for analysis. Reducing variation by arbitrarily dichotomizing the population distribution into hypertensive and normotensive groups probably increases the problem of phenocopies.

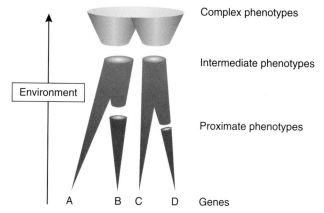

**Figure 4–2** Complex disease phenotypes arise from multiple genes. Proximate phenotypes (e.g., direct measurements of gene products) can identify discrete subtypes of complex diseases. Intermediate and complex phenotypes result from multiple gene-gene and gene-environment interactions, and identification of genes contributing to final phenotypes such as hypertension is increasingly difficult.

One promising approach accepts the premise that hypertension is not an isolated disorder of the regulation of the set-point of blood pressure control but rather reflects a complex disorder of multiple systems (e.g., those relating to the metabolic syndrome). Cluster analysis, a method for empirically in identifying phenotypic features that form distinctive phenotypes, may advance the identification of intermediate phenotypes more proximate to genetic disorders than blood pressure itself.[68] Other intermediate phenotypes based on physiologic (e.g., nonmodulation)[69] or biochemical (e.g., increased red blood cell sodium-lithium countertransport activity)[70,71] also hold promise.

2. *Hypertension is a disease of middle age.* Although as a group, offspring of hypertensives have higher blood pressures in youth than offspring of normotensives, the differences are modest, and subsequent tracking of blood pressure sufficiently variable to render reliable identification of normotensive individuals destined for future hypertension impossible. Families identified through hypertensive parental probands can therefore be studied only in populations for which hypertension status is known for at least two adult generations. Classical segregation analyses that track the vertical transmission of genetic markers in individuals with and without a disease are therefore of limited utility in hypertension except in studies of Mendelian hypertensions in which distinctive features can be identified early in life or by medical history.

Because of the great difficulties inherent in extended-family studies, alternative nonparametric approaches have recently been favored. Foremost among these is the affected sibling pair approach, in which genetic variants more common in hypertensive than nonhypertensive siblings are sought. Increasingly sophisticated analyses of the genetic transmission of such variants in nuclear families are slowly yielding clues to candidate genomic regions and genes. Such methods are less likely to be affected by problems of population stratification that can produce false positive findings in simple association studies.[72]

3. *Methodologic shortcomings constitute a third barrier to investigation of the genetics of hypertension.* While genetic linkage approaches have successfully identified genes causing Mendelian forms, application to essential hypertension has been less successful. By studying individuals with severe hypertension (defined either as a very high blood pressure level, early onset, or a requirement for multidrug therapy), the angiotensinogen gene was identified by linkage as a candidate for essential hypertension.[73,74] In truth, however, this gene would have been studied as a logical candidate anyway, and certainly its identification by linkage was greatly facilitated by prior knowledge of its physiologic role. More typically genomic regions identified by genetic linkage encompass broad chromosomal regions comprising a significant fraction of the genome and containing tens or hundreds of candidate genes, many with known or potential roles in cardiovascular function. It is not currently possible to sequence all such genes to look for functional variants, and prior characterization of hypertension-related physiologic or biochemical disorders potentially arising from differences in candidate genes is therefore still required to narrow the search. Unfortunately, relying upon what is already known probably risks missing new candidates, confounding the potential for gene discovery that is one of the appeals of the linkage approach.

Incorporating genomic structure via haplotype analysis may advance the understanding of which segments of genes harbor functional variants. Current efforts to build a genome-wide haplotype map will result in a framework that should facilitate gene discovery work in complex diseases, including hypertension. Haplotype analyses will still be complicated by the limitations noted above.

4. *Is hypertension the result of many relatively uncommon genetic variants or of common alleles?* Although still somewhat unsettled, the latter is favored.[75] In either case, in addition to phenotypic heterogeneity, genotypic heterogeneity is likely important in hypertension, complicating the search for genes. Furthermore, it is unlikely that most common single nucleotide polymorphisms are nonsynonymous, causing simple changes of the primary amino acid sequence of encoded proteins.[76] More likely, as is thought to be the case for the A(-6) allele of the angiotensinogen gene, common allelic variants will affect functions like gene expression or regulation or perhaps mRNA splicing. Single lesions may not be causal in themselves: Another of the lessons from animal models is that the genetic background upon which a variant is expressed may dramatically affect its phenotypic impact. Because such effects of gene-gene interactions are subtle, defining the functional consequences of genetic variation defined by linkage or association studies will be challenging. Here animal models, particularly those employing gene knockout or directed mutagenesis techniques, promise to be instructive.

5. *Race remains a vexing issue in the study of the genetics of hypertension.* There is a history of hypertension research on racial differences in physiologic and biochemical characteristics, which leads many to assume that there are unique genetic determinants of blood pressure in the races. At the same time, there is considerable debate as to whether genetic characterization of race is possible or desirable.[77,78] Given that there are certainly differences in allelic frequencies

between individuals whose ancestors spread from Africa to populate the world,[79] apparent genetic differences between hypertensives and normotensives may arise from population stratification or admixture. Because many differences in population-specific allelic frequencies arise from random genetic drift or other adaptively neutral processes, the conclusion that allelic frequency differences contribute to differences in the prevalence of hypertension in different populations must be viewed skeptically. We are all humans, and the mechanisms underlying blood pressure are likely to be quite similar in all of us.

Although challenging, identifying genes has proven not to be impossible. As noted previously, the angiotensinogen gene is thought to contribute to hypertension, although not all studies support the particular polymorphism originally described. A structural membrane protein, $\alpha$-adducin, first identified in the Milan Hypertensive Rat model, has been associated with blood pressure salt-sensitivity and diuretic responsiveness.[80] Several other polymorphisms including ones in the genes encoding the $\beta$ subunit of the G-protein complex[81] and the $\beta_2$-adrenergic receptor[82] are associated with hypertension. With genotyping becoming ever more efficient and increasingly affordable, more extensive surveys of candidate genes, including whole genome surveys using hundreds of thousands of single nucleotide polymorphisms will soon be feasible. Such intensive characterization should allow us to begin to define which genes are related to subtypes of essential hypertension as defined by intermediate phenotypes such as salt-sensitivity, nonmodulator status, or membrane transport abnormalities.

There are a huge number of additional issues to be addressed at every organizational level to answer the question of what causes hypertension. How we ask the question frames the answer we will get. Let us hope that we are clever enough to ask the right question.

# References

1. Strohman RC. Ancient genomes, wise bodies, unhealthy people: Limits of a genetic paradigm in biology and medicine. Perspect Biol Med 37:112-145, 1993.
2. Sing C, Havilland MB, Reilly SL. Genetic architecture of common multifactorial disease. *In* Chadwick D, Cardew G (eds). Variation in the Human Genome. Ciba Foundation Symposium 197. Chichester, UK, John Wiley & Sons, 1996; pp 211-232.
3. Schork NJ. Genetically complex cardiovascular traits: Origins, problems, and potential solutions. Hypertension 29:145-149, 1997.
4. Weder AB, Schork NJ. Adaptation, allometry, and hypertension. Hypertension 24:145-156, 1994.
5. Patterson JL, Goetz RH, Doyle JT, et al. Cardiorespiratory dynamics in the ox and giraffe, with comparative observations on man and other mammals. Ann NY Acad Sci 127:393-413, 1965.
6. Calder WA III. Scaling of physiological processes in homeothermic animals. Annu Rev Physiol 43:301-322, 1981.
7. Van Citters RL, Franklin DL, Vatner SF, et al. Cerebral hemodynamics in the giraffe. Trans Assoc Am Physicians 82:293-304, 1969.
8. Goetz RH, Warren JV, Gauer OH, et al. Circulation of the giraffe. Circ Res 8:1049, 1960.
9. Goetz RH. Preliminary observations on the circulation in the giraffe. Trans Am Coll Cardiol 5:239-248, 1955.
10. Dagg AI, Foster JB. The Giraffe. Its Biology, Behavior, and Ecology. New York, Van Nostrand Reinhold, 1976.
11. Starling EH. The Fluids of the Body. London, Constable, 1909; pp 104-133.
12. Guyton AC, Coleman TG, Cowley AV Jr, et al. Arterial pressure regulation: Overriding dominance of the kidneys in long-term regulation and in hypertension. Am J Med 52:584-594, 1972.
13. Guyton AC. Long-term arterial pressure control: An analysis from animal experiments and computer and graphic models. Am J Physiol 259:R865-877, 1990.
14. Kimura G, Brenner BM. Implications of the linear pressure-natriuresis relationship and importance of sodium sensitivity in hypertension. J Hypertens 15:1055-1061, 1997.
15. Johnson RJ, Herrera-Acosta J, Schreiner GF, et al. Subtle acquired renal injury as a mechanism of salt-sensitive hypertension. N Engl J Med 346:913-923, 2002.
16. Aviv A, Hollenberg NK, Weder A. Sodium glomerulopathy: Tubuloglomerular feedback and renal injury in African Americans. Kidney Int 65(2):361-368, 2004.
17. Schnermann J, Traynor T, Yang T, et al. Tubuloglomerular feedback: New concepts and developments. Kidney Int Suppl 67:S40-S45, 1998.
18. Wright JT, Bakris G, Greene T, et al. African American Study of Kidney Disease and Hypertension Study Group. Effect of blood pressure lowering and antihypertensive drug class on progression of hypertensive kidney disease: Results from the AASK trial. JAMA 288:2421-2431, 2002.
19. Pickering G. Normotension and hypertension: The mysterious viability of the false. Am J Med 65:561-563, 1978.
20. Task Force on Blood Pressure Control in Children. Report of the Second National Heart, Lung, and Blood Institute Task Force on Blood Pressure Control in Children—1987. Pediatrics 79:1-25, 1987.
21. Lever AF, Harrap SB. Essential hypertension: A disorder of growth with origins in childhood? J Hypertens 10:101-120, 1992.
22. Folkow B. Cardiovascular structural adaptation: Its role in the initiation and maintenance of primary hypertension. Clin Sci Mol Med 55:3, 1978.
23. Sivertsson R. The hemodynamic importance of structural vascular changes in essential hypertension. Acta Physiol Scand 343:1-56, 1970.
24. Schachter M. Drug-induced modification of vascular structure: Effects of antihypertensive drugs. Am Heart J 122:316-323, 1991.
25. Takeshita A, Mark AL. Decreased vasodilator capacity of forearm resistance vessels in borderline hypertension. Hypertension 2:610-616, 1980.
26. Zweifler AJ, Nicholls MG. Diminished finger volume pulse in borderline hypertension: Evidence for early structural vascular abnormality. Am Heart J 104:812-815, 1982.
27. Julius S, Quadir H, Gajendragadkar S. Hyperkinetic state: A precursor of hypertension? A longitudinal study of borderline hypertension. *In* Gross F, Strasser T (eds). Mild Hypertension: Natural History and Management. London, Pittman, 1979; pp 116-126.
28. Julius S, Schork NJ, Schork MA. Sympathetic hyperactivity in early stages of hypertension: The Ann Arbor data set. J Cardiovasc Pharmacol 12:S121-129, 1988.
29. Julius S, Randall OS, Esler MD, et al. Altered cardiac responsiveness and regulation in the normal cardiac output type of borderline hypertension. Circ Res 36-37(suppl I):I199-I207, 1975.
30. Julius S. Editorial review: The blood pressure seeking properties of the central nervous system. J Hypertens 6:177-185, 1988.
31. Julius S. Changing role of the autonomic nervous system in human hypertension. J Hypertens 8:S59-S65, 1990.
32. Lund-Johansen P, Omvik P. Hemodynamic patterns of untreated hypertensive disease. *In* Laragh JH, Brenner BM (eds). Hypertension: Pathophysiology, Diagnosis, and Management. New York, Raven, 1990; pp 305-327.

33. Norrelund H, Christensen KL, Samani NJ, et al. Early narrowed afferent arteriole is a contributor to the development of hypertension. Hypertension 24:301-308, 1994.

34. Majid DSA, Godfrey M, Navar LG. Pressure natriuresis and renal medullary blood flow in dogs. Hypertension 29: 1051-1057, 1997.

35. Schork NJ, Jokelainen P, Grant EJ, et al. Relationship of growth and blood pressure in inbred rats. Am J Physiol 266:R702-R708, 1994.

36. Akahoshi M, Soda M, Carter R, et al. Correlation between systolic blood pressure and physical development in adolescents. Am J Epidemiol 144:51-58, 1996.

37. Aviv A, Aviv H: Reflections on telomeres, growth, aging, and essential hypertension. Hypertension 29:1067-1072, 1997.

38. Aviv A. Chronology versus biology: Telomeres, essential hypertension, and vascular aging. Hypertension 40:229-232, 2002.

39. Barker DJP (ed). Fetal and Infant Origins of Adult Disease. London, BMJ, 1993.

40. Law CM, Shiell AW. Is blood pressure related to birth weight? The strength of evidence from a systematic review of the literature. J Hypertens 14:935-941, 1996.

41. Seckl JR: Glucocorticoids, feto-placental 11β-hydroxysteroid dehydrogenase type 2, and the early life origins of adult disease. Steroids 62:89-94, 1997.

42. Benediktsson R, Lindsay RS, Noble J, et al. Glucocorticoid exposure in utero: New model for adult hypertension. Lancet 341:339-341, 1993.

43. Neel JV, Weder AB, Julius S. Type II diabetes, essential hypertension, and obesity as "syndromes of impaired genetic homeostasis": The "thrifty genotype" hypothesis enters the 21st century. Perspect Biol Med 42:44-74, 1998.

44. James GD, Baker PT. Human population biology and blood pressure: Evolutionary and ecological considerations and interpretations of population studies. In Laragh JH, Brenner BM (eds). Hypertension: Pathophysiology, Diagnosis, and Management, 2nd ed. New York, Raven, 1995; pp 115-126.

45. Ward R. Familial aggregation and genetic epidemiology of blood pressure. In Laragh JH, Brenner BM (eds). Hypertension: Pathophysiology, Diagnosis, and Management, 2nd ed. New York, Raven, 1995; pp 67-88.

46. Intersalt Cooperative Research Group. Intersalt: An international study of electrolyte excretion and blood pressure. Results for 24 hour urinary sodium and potassium excretion. BMJ 297:319-328, 1988.

47. Hollenberg NK, Martinez G, McCullough M, et al. Aging, acculturation, salt intake, and hypertension in the Kuna of Panama. Hypertension 29:171-176, 1997.

48. Poulter NR, Khaw KT, Hopwood BE, et al. The Kenyan Luo migration study: Observations on the initiation of a rise in blood pressure. BMJ 300:967-972, 1990.

49. Hill K, Hawkes K, Hurtado M, et al. Seasonal variance in the diet of Ache hunter-gatherers in eastern Paraguay. Hum Ecol 12:101, 1984.

50. Heini AF, Minghelli AI, Diaz E, et al. Free-living energy expenditure assessed by two different methods in lean rural Gambian farmers. Eur J Clin Nutr 50(5):284-289, 1996.

51. Shimamoto T, Komachi Y, Inada H, et al. Trends for coronary heart disease and stroke and their risk factors in Japan. Circulation 79:503-515, 1989.

52. Eaton SB, Konner M, Shostak M. Stone agers in the fast lane: Chronic degenerative diseases in evolutionary perspective. Am J Med 84:739-749, 1988.

53. Rode A, Shepard RJ. Physiological consequences of acculturation: A 20-year study of fitness in an Inuit community. Eur J Appl Physiol 69:516-524, 1994.

54. Oliver WJ, Cohen EL, Neel JV. Blood pressure, sodium intake, and sodium related hormones in the Yanomamo Indians, a "no-salt" culture. Circulation 52:146-151, 1975.

55. Tanner JM. Earlier maturation in man. Sci Am 218:21-27, 1968.

56. Roberts MB, Stringer CB, Parfitt BP. A hominid tibia from middle Pleistocene sediments at Boxgrove, UK. Nature 369:311-313, 1994.

57. Walker A. Perspectives on the Nariokotome discovery. In Walker A, Leakey R (eds). The Nariokotome Homo erectus skeleton. Cambridge, MA, Harvard University Press, 1993; pp 411-430.

58. Tanner JM. Growth as a measure of the nutritional and hygienic status of a population. Horm Res 38:106–115, 1992.

59. Stini WA. Adaptive strategies of human populations under nutritional stress. In Watts ES, Johnston FE, Lasker GW (eds). Biosocial Interrelations in Population Adaptation. The Hague, The Netherlands, Mouton, pp 19-41, 1975.

60. Chehab FF, Mounzih K, Lu R, et al. Early onset reproductive function in normal female mice treated with leptin. Science 275:88-90, 1997.

61. Frisch RE. Body fat, puberty and fertility. Biol Rev 59:161-188, 1984.

62. Kannel WB, Brand N, Skinner JJ Jr, et al. The relation of adiposity to blood pressure and development of hypertension. Ann Intern Med 67:48-59, 1967.

63. Barker DJP, Bull AR, Osmond C, et al. Fetal and placental size and risk of hypertension in adult life. BMJ 301:259-262, 1990.

64. Kreiger DR, Landsberg L. Obesity and hypertension. In Laragh JH, Brenner BM (eds). Hypertension: Pathophysiology, Diagnosis, and Management, 2nd ed. New York, Raven, 1995; pp 2367-2388.

65. Lifton RP, Gharavi AG, Geller DS, et al. Molecular Mechanisms of Human Hypertension. Cell 104:545-565, 2001.

66. Hunt SC, Williams RR, Barlow GK. A comparison of positive family history definitions for defining risk of future disease. J Chron Dis 39:809-821, 1986.

67. Hunt SC, Cook NR, Oberman A, et al. Angiotensinogen genotype, sodium reduction, weight loss, and prevention of hypertension: Trials of hypertension prevention phase II. Hypertension 32:393-401, 1998.

68. Wu K-D, Hsiao C-F, Ho L-T, et al. Clustering and heritability of insulin resistance in Chinese and Japanese hypertensive families: A Stanford-Asian Pacific program in hypertension and insulin resistance sibling study. Hypertens Res 25:529-536, 2002.

69. Williams GH, Dluhy RG, Lifton RP, et al. Non-modulation as an intermediate phenotype in essential hypertension. Hypertension 20:788-796, 1992.

70. Canessa M, Adrangna N, Solomon HS, et al. Increased sodium-lithium countertransport in red cells of patients with essential hypertension. N Engl J Med 302:772-776, 1980.

71. Weder AB, Delgado MC, Zhu X, et al. Erythrocyte sodium-lithium countertransport and blood pressure: a genome-wide linkage study. Hypertension 41:842-846, 2003.

72. Cardon LR, Palmer LJ. Populations stratification and spurious allelic association. Lancet 361:598-604, 2003.

73. Inoue I, Nakajima T, Williams CS, et al. A nucleotide substitution in the promoter of human angiotensinogen is associated with essential hypertension and affects basal transcription in vitro. J Clin Invest 99:1786-1797, 1997.

74. Jeunemaitre X, Soubrier F, Kotelevtsev YV, et al. Molecular basis of human hypertension; role of angiotensinogen. Cell 71: 169-180, 1992.

75. Chakravarti A. Population genetics—making sense out of sequence. Nat Genet 22:56-60, 1999.

76. Halushka MK, Fan J-B, Bentley K, et al. Patterns of single-nucleotide polymorphisms in candidate genes for blood-pressure homeostasis. Nat Genet 22:239-247, 1999.

77. Cooper RS, Kaufman JS, Ward R. Race and genomics. New Engl J Med 348:1166-1170, 2003.

78. Burchard EG, Ziv E, Coyle N, et al. The importance of race and ethnic background in biomedical research and clinical practice. N Engl J Med 348:1170-1175, 2003.

79. Rosenberg NA, Pritchard JK, Weber JL, et al. Genetic structure of human populations. Science 298(5602):2381-2385, 2002.

80. Cusi D, Barlassina C, Azzani T, et al. Polymorphisms of alpha-adducin and salt sensitivity in patients with essential hypertension. Lancet 349:1353-1357, 1997.

81. Siffert W, Rosskopf D, Siffert G, et al. Association of human G-protein [beta]3 subunit variant with hypertension. Nat Genet 18:45-48, 1998.

82. Bray MS, Boerwinkle E. The role of beta(2)-adrenergic receptor variation in human hypertension. Curr Hyper Rep 2:39-43, 2000.

# Chapter 5

# Blood Pressure Genetics

## Stephen B. Harrap

Attempts to determine the genetic basis of blood pressure have encompassed a variety of approaches. These range from studies of blood pressure correlations between relatives,[1-3] to more direct analyses of associations between blood pressure and DNA variation. The potential of identifying the causative DNA variants has been reinforced by the release and refinement of the draft sequence of the human genome.[4-6] Beyond scientific curiosity, the impetus is a fundamental understanding of mechanisms to provide the basis for new means of detecting, preventing, and treating high blood pressure and allied cardiovascular disease.

The successful discovery of the molecular origins of rare familial Mendelian diseases that affect blood pressure[7] engendered optimism for genetic discovery in more common conditions such as clinical essential hypertension. However, the elucidation of genetic explanations of normal blood pressure variation and clinical hypertension are proving much more difficult.

## ASSUMPTIONS AND MODELS

Important to both the discovery and application of genetics of high blood pressure is a clear understanding of the epidemiologic characteristics of blood pressure and its relevance as a risk factor. In particular, the clinical concept of hypertension and the relationships with cardiovascular disease deserve scrutiny.

## Blood Pressure and Cardiovascular Disease

Much interest on the genetics of blood pressure has focused on hypertension, but the rationale owes more to clinical medicine than it does to the population burden of cardiovascular endpoints or the underlying biology of blood pressure.

### Hypertension Is an Arbitrarily Defined Risk Factor, Not a Disease

For individuals, the greatest relative cardiovascular risk is associated with the highest blood pressures.[8] This correlation justifies the medical approach of screening blood pressure and treating hypertensive subjects to reduce individual risk.

However, the population distribution of blood pressure is unimodal (Figure 5–1) and the definition of hypertension is operational.[9,10] Classifications such as hypertensive and normotensive are constantly changing[11,12] and do not necessarily differentiate individuals into meaningful biologic and, therefore, genetic groups.

### There Exists a Continuous Relationship between Blood Pressure and Cardiovascular Risk

Epidemiologic analyses indicate that the relationship between blood pressure and risk of cardiovascular disease is continuous.[8] In other words, across the entire population distribution an increment in pressure is associated with higher risk (Figure 5–2). However, such representations of individual risk reveal little of the impact of blood pressure in a population.

### Much Cardiovascular Disease Attributable to Blood Pressure Occurs in Normotensives

When the number of people exposed to a certain level of blood pressure is multiplied by the relevant relative risk, a different picture emerges.[13] For example, population attributable risk of blood pressure from the MRFIT study of 347,987 men (aged 35 to 57 years) is shown in Figure 5–3 as "excess deaths" from coronary heart disease (CHD) in relation to systolic blood pressure levels[14] after accounting for age, race, serum cholesterol, cigarettes per day, use of medication for diabetes, and income. Thirty-two percent of CHD deaths attributable to systolic blood pressure (SBP) occurred in men with a systolic pressure of less than 140 mm Hg, compared with 24% of excess CHD deaths attributable to SBP in subjects with pressures greater than 160 mm Hg.

### The Genetics of Higher Blood Pressure, Not Just Hypertension, Is Important

Although the individual burden rests with those with the highest pressures, the population burden is attributable to "average" pressures. Therefore, genetic explanations of the full range blood pressures are relevant to both individuals and to the entire community.

## THE RELATIVE IMPORTANCE OF GENES AND ENVIRONMENT

What is the evidence that human genes affect blood pressure and how can such effects be understood in relation to the influences of the environment?

## The Family Perspective

Biometric analyses are used to model blood pressure patterns within families and infer explanations based on genetic or environmental causation.[1-3,15]

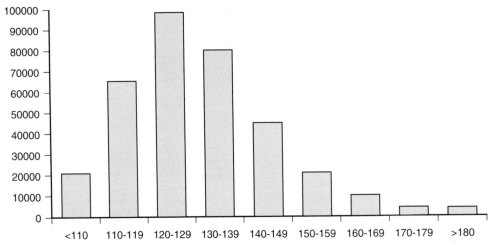

**Figure 5–1** Systolic blood pressure (SBP) distribution in 347,987 men aged 35 to 57 years screened for the Multiple Risk Factor Interventions Trial (MRFIT). These data have a unimodal distribution with a skew towards upper values. (Data from Stamler J, Stamler R, Neaton JD. Blood pressure, systolic and diastolic, and cardiovascular risks. US population data. Arch Intern Med 153:598-615, 1993.)

### Shared Genes

Genetic influence is suggested by the observation that the closer the genetic relatedness, the more similar the blood pressure. For example, the correlation coefficient for blood pressure between monozygotic twins (whose genetic similarity is 100%) is 0.78, while nontwin siblings (whose genetic similarity is 50% on average) show correlation coefficients of about 0.23.

### Shared Environment

The influence of shared environment is revealed by discrepancies in blood pressure correlations between relatives despite the same degree of genetic similarity. For example, with genetic relatedness of 50%, dizygotic twins, nontwin siblings, and parents and offspring show decreasing levels of blood pressure correlation.[15] Such differences can be ascribed only

to variation in the nature and extent of shared environmental factors such as diet and lifestyle.

Careful research design can provide interesting insights into such environmental effects. For example, the fact that the blood pressure correlation of adult offspring living apart exceeds that between those adult offspring and their parents suggests the persistent influence of environmental factors shared by offspring when they were living together in the family home.[3] It also suggests that the influence of such factors is more potent within a generation than it is across a generation, a manifestation of the generation gap. The importance of the shared family environment is also seen in the blood pressure correlations during childhood between genetically unrelated adopted siblings.[1] The higher blood pressure correlation between dizygotic twins than between nontwin siblings suggests possible additional environmental exposures.[3] In this respect the early life environment might be important.[16]

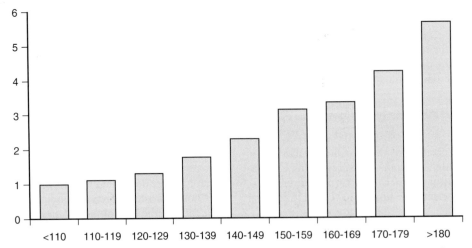

**Figure 5–2** Rate of deaths from coronary heart disease (CHD) (adjusted for age, race, serum cholesterol, cigarettes per day, diabetes, and income) relative to the group with the lowest SBP in 347,987 mean aged 35 to 57 years from Multiple Risk Factor Interventions Trial (MRFIT). These data show a stepwise increase in relative risk for each increment in SBP. (Data from Stamler J, Stamler R, Neaton JD. Blood pressure, systolic and diastolic, and cardiovascular risks. US population data. Arch Intern Med 153:598-615, 1993.)

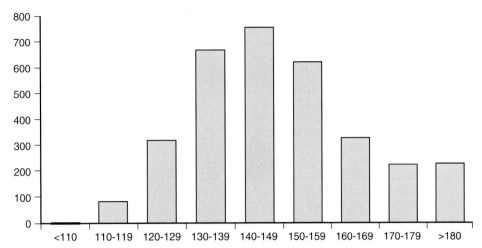

**Figure 5-3** Number of "excess deaths" from CHD attributable to SBP relative to the group with the lowest SBP in 347,987 mean aged 35 to 57 years from Multiple Risk Factor Interventions Trial (MRFIT). See text for details. These show a large number of people exposed to a modest risk (average blood pressure) account for many cases of cardiovascular death in a population. (Data from Stamler J, Stamler R, Neaton JD. Blood pressure, systolic and diastolic, and cardiovascular risks. US population data. Arch Intern Med 153:598-615, 1993.)

In adulthood the influence of shared environment is less apparent. The blood pressure correlation coefficient between parents is often of the order of 0.13[1-3] and does not increase significantly as the period of shared environment increases.[17]

### Defining the Balance between Genes and Environment

Sophisticated mathematical modelling and statistical analyses of family blood pressure patterns can partition variation of blood pressure into genetic and environmental compartments. The exact estimates depend on the research design and specific modelling parameters. Studies based on classical twin analyses tend to inflate the genetic component because the inherent assumption that the degree of shared environment is the same between monozygotic and dizygotic twins is usually violated.[18,19] Blood pressure heritability (the proportion of variance attributable to genes) estimates from twin-only studies can be as high as 80%.[20] Comprehensive familial analyses that include other relatives in addition to twins offer more reliable estimates. Such studies suggest that genetic factors account for 40% to 50% of blood pressure variance, while shared environment accounts for about 10% to 30% of variance.[1-3]

## The Population Perspective

Evidence of genetic and environmental effects from families is obtained from relatively stable groups over short time frames. A different perspective, particularly in terms of environmental effects, is obtained by the studies of populations subject to mass change over longer periods.

### Population Environment—Migration and Secular Trends

Blood pressures change significantly following migration.[21-24] Indeed, there appears to be a shift in the population mean blood pressures (Figure 5–4), such that there are changes at every level of the distribution.[25] These movements must be due to changes in the population environment because genes remain stable. In this context, "environment" encompasses economic, social, psychologic, and biologic elements. Furthermore, average blood pressures in geographically stable Western societies have been falling.[26-29] In the absence of major changes in the genetic constitution, such effects reflect the influence of subtle but cumulative transformation of the environment of the population as a whole.

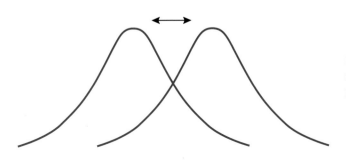

**Figure 5–4** Changes in the population environment with migration over time tend to shift the distribution of blood pressure as a whole.

Attempts to define the responsible environmental factors are very difficult indeed. Changes in blood pressure are often associated with increases in body weight, but there are inconsistencies. In migration, blood pressure and body weight tend to move in the same direction while recent secular declines in blood pressures in Western societies seem to be coinciding with increased levels of obesity.[30] Sometimes differences exist in simple comparisons between populations, as in urinary electrolyte excretion. However, attempts to define the causative nature of such differences are confounded by intercorrelated environmental characteristics, many of which are unmeasured.[31] Additionally, the influence of specific factors such as sodium is difficult to demonstrate between individuals within populations. Nevertheless, grouping of environmental exposures that are defined by socioeconomic status appear important correlations of blood pressure within populations.[32]

### Population Genetics

Within populations, individuals vary extensively across the genome, most commonly in the form of single nucleotide polymorphisms (see the section "Genetic Markers"). In general, the DNA sequence variation is greater within populations than it is between populations. Some estimates suggest that populations worldwide share 93% of the variation at individual genetic loci and 7% is unique to local populations.[33] Population-specific DNA variants tend to be younger and less frequent than the older, more frequent, global variants (Figure 5–5).[34] The unanswered question is to what extent population differences in blood pressure can be explained on population-specific differences.[35]

## The Individual Perspective

### Gene-Environment Combination

Individual blood pressure can be understood as the result of two underlying influences.[36] One, genotype, would determine an individual's rank within the population distribution (Figure 5–6). The other, population environment, would determine the mean for the population. Therefore, the final blood pressure would be the sum of these two influences and in this way depends on both genes and environment.

### Gene-Environment Interaction

It is possible that certain genotypes predispose to larger changes in blood pressure for a given change in the population environment. This phenomenon might explain the skewed distribution of blood pressure in Western societies. Migration studies have identified subgroups of individuals who appear to have exaggerated blood pressure responses to migration.[37] These clusters are often familial, although not explained by simple genetic inheritance.[37]

## MOLECULAR GENETICS

The limelight in genetic research has fallen on the molecular biologic laboratory and statistical genetic analysis. As it does so, something of the complex, underlying genetic architecture is revealed. The concept that specific variants in DNA

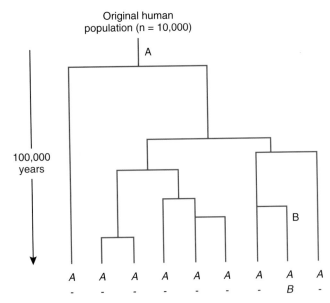

Original human population (n = 10,000)

100,000 years

Present day human population (n > 6,000,000,000)

**Figure 5–5** A schematic representation of the migration, expansion, and diversification of *Homo sapiens* from an ancient original population in West Africa to the present day. Allele **A** appeared over 100,000 years ago and is represented globally. Allele **B** appeared recently and is found in only one population. (From Harrap SB. Where are all the blood pressure genes? Lancet 361:2149-2151, 2003.)

sequence—known as alleles—in and around key genes might affect blood pressure has been proven by the discoveries relevant to monogenetic disease (discussed in the sections that follow). However, the number and nature of genetic variants that determine the physiologic variation in blood pressure and/or clinical hypertension remain largely mysterious. What seems certain is that the situation is not simple.

## Blood Pressure Polygenes

It is important to note that the similarity of blood pressure between blood relatives is not limited to high blood pressure. Low, middle, and high blood pressure levels are heritable. Herein lie clues to the genetic architecture underlying blood

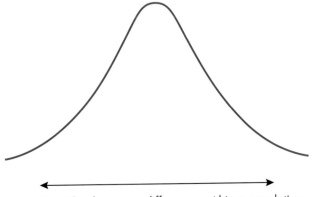

**Figure 5–6** Blood pressure differences within a population are likely to be explained by genetic differences between individuals.

pressure; as "hypertension genes" alone could not explain such patterns. Instead it is believed that a number of genes (polygenes) exist. Certain alleles at each polygene could exert incremental effects on blood pressure and in combination with other alleles at other polygenes could account for the quantitative variation and familial correlations of blood pressure (Figure 5–7). More direct evidence of polygenes has been obtained from molecular genome analyses (see "Genomic Discovery and Blood Pressure").

## Lessons from Mendelian Disease

The important question for both research and its application is how many blood pressure alleles might exist in a population. It has emerged that many "monogenic" diseases are in fact syndromes, comprising often hundreds of specific allelic forms. Similar clinical phenotypes can be caused by any one of several genes, for each of which one of many possible causative alleles is sufficient.[7]

If such genetic and allelic heterogeneity characterize "simple" monogenic disease, what are the prospects for complex conditions? Some theorists propose that the forces governing genetic architecture for rare and common conditions are different and as a result the allelic spectrum for conditions such as blood pressure might be simpler rather than more complex.[38] As things stand, two schools exist.

## Common Disease/Common Variants

According to the common disease/common variant (CD/CV) hypothesis,[39-41] there will exist a few key alleles in a population. Such alleles would be relatively common in genetic terms (population frequency >1%) and each would exert a moderate incremental effect on blood pressure. Related examples include the APOE4 allele in Alzheimer disease[42] or factor V[Leiden] in deep venous thrombosis.[43]

## Common Disease/Rare Alleles

In contrast, the common disease/rare allele (CD/RA) hypothesis postulates that allelic heterogeneity will be high with large numbers of uncommon alleles.[44,45] A large number of rare alleles would be difficult to detect in population-based studies[46] and because rare alleles tend to be younger and population-specific[34] they might be lost in studies of heterogeneous populations.[47]

For polygenic traits such as blood pressure both hypotheses might be relevant, with some polygenes fitting the CD/CV model and others fitting the CD/RA model.

# GENOMIC DISCOVERY AND BLOOD PRESSURE

## Genetic Markers

It has been estimated that one genome differs from another on average at 1 in every 1250 nucleotides. This allelic variation provides useful genetic markers. There are three major types of genetic markers: insertions and deletions of stretches of DNA (e.g., ACE I/D polymorphism[48,49]), variation in the number of times a characteristic DNA sequence is repeated (e.g., microsatellite short tandem nucleotide repeats[50]), and single nucleotide substitutions (known as single nucleotide polymorphisms [SNPs]).[51]

The most useful markers should be abundant and evenly distributed across the genome and they should be measurable easily and accurately. These criteria apply to microsatellites but especially to SNPs. Of the microsatellites, repeats of the dinucleotide CA(GT) are the most common and spread across the genome.[52] The number of repeats at any site is often highly variable (polymorphic), reducing the likelihood that they will be the same in any two individuals—a useful characteristic when tracing the inheritance of blood pressure in family linkage analyses (see "Linkage Studies").

### Single Nucleotide Polymorphisms

Of the estimated 15 million SNPs that dwell in the genomes of modern *Homo sapiens,* between 50,000 and 100,000 SNPs are in or around genes and are well placed to alter gene function and protein expression.[53] More than 1.4 million SNPs have been identified,[51] the most common being transitions between G⇔A and C⇔T.[54] For the typical gene one can expect to find 12 SNPs with a mean population frequency of 11% for the less common (i.e., the younger) allele at each SNP. About one half of SNPs are in coding sequences and one half of these alter protein sequence.[35] A survey of 75 genes of relevance to blood pressure homeostasis[35] found 874 SNPs, 209 of which changed the amino acid sequence. No association with blood pressure could be demonstrated in this relatively small analysis, but these protein-altering SNPs had the hallmarks of evolutionary youth, in that they each tended to be infrequent and in specific populations.

### Alleles, Markers, and Haplotypes

Both marker SNPs and SNPs that are functional alleles can be associated on stretches of DNA known as haplotypes. Consider an ancient chromosome in the original human population of 10,000 in West Africa 100,000 years ago.[55] On this chromosome exists an ancestral haplotype—a stretch of DNA with a series of nonfunctional specific SNP alleles (Figure 5–8). Within this haplotype a mutation appears and results in a new functional allele that causes an increment of blood pressure. At each subsequent generation, the process of recombination during meiosis (formation of eggs and

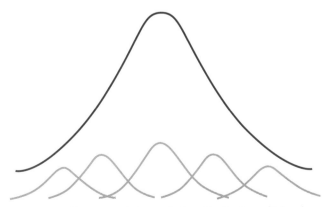

**Figure 5–7** The unimodal population distribution of blood pressure could be explained by many genetically distinct subpopulations defined by a number of polygenes.

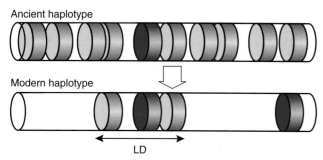

Ancient haplotype

Modern haplotype

LD

**Figure 5–8** Diagrammatic representation of a stretch of ancient chromosome and a haplotype comprising a group of specific markers (gray cylinders) around a new DNA variant (red cylinder) that causes an increment in blood pressure. Over the generations, recombination whittles away at markers surrounding the mutation so that those with high blood pressure as a result of the variant will have only close remnants of the ancient haplotype. The markers that have survived to the modern haplotype are said to be in linkage disequilibrium (LD) with the variant. Therefore, the specific markers would be associated with high blood pressure. The red marker more distant from the variant would be in linkage with the variant if the chance of recombination over a few generations were low.

sperm) tends to swap pieces of the chromosome with the equivalent region of its pair. In this way the association between the blood pressure and surrounding the marker alleles tends to be lost. The chance of such recombination depends on a variety of factors including the distance between the blood pressure and the marker alleles[56] (the farther away, the greater the likelihood of recombination) and the number of generations (i.e., opportunities to recombine).

### Linkage Disequilibrium

Specific SNP markers on remnants of the ancestral haplotype will lead by association to the blood pressure allele (see Figure 5–8). Such original marker alleles very close to the blood pressure allele will be preserved and are described as being in linkage disequilibrium (LD). The distance over which LD is preserved is typically less than 5000 nucleotides but varies in different parts of the genome from a few thousand nucleotides to more than 100,000 nucleotides.[57] Shorter distances of LD often occur in so-called recombination "hot spots."[56,58] Given the relative opportunities to recombine, ancient blood pressure alleles would be surrounded by shorter distances of LD than blood pressure alleles that emerged more recently.

### Linkage

Just outside the stretch of LD will be a variety of marker alleles that have been imported by recombination (see Figure 5–8). The precise nature of these new marker alleles might vary between families, but within families they will be coinherited with the blood pressure allele, provided they avoid being separated by recombination over a handful of generations. This situation is described as linkage between the blood pressure and marker alleles when they are inherited together. Linkage extends over much greater distances on either side of a blood pressure allele than LD.

## Discovery Strategies

From the starting point of the human genome, the first step is to focus on the likely or "candidate" region in which blood pressure alleles might exist. This focus is achieved either conceptually by simply nominating a candidate gene on the basis of physiologic plausibility or experimentally with a genome-wide scan. The former is potentially efficient, but blinkered. The latter is burdensome, but without prejudice and more likely to reveal novel causes.

A contemporary strategy for discovery involves the following steps:

Step 1. Genome-wide mapping to identify the candidate chromosomal region.
Step 2. Fine-mapping study to replicate and refine the localization.
Step 3. Allelic searches in and around genes within the candidate region, with priority given to those of known and relevant function.
Step 4. Identification of candidate alleles with likely functional implications.
Step 5. Testing of candidate alleles in living systems by physiologic genomic methods.
Step 6. Determination of the contribution by candidate alleles to population blood pressure variation.

## Linkage Studies

Studies based on linkage are used for genome-wide (step 1) and fine mapping (step 2). They necessarily involve families and test for coinheritance of blood pressure and adjacent marker alleles. The most informative linkage markers are highly polymorphic, so that the specific marker linked with a blood pressure allele in a particular family would be unlikely in other relatives by chance alone.

### Genome Maps

For genome scans, maps of 450 or so microsatellite markers, spaced on average 10,000 nucleotides apart, are generally used. For fine mapping, microsatellite markers more closely spaced across the candidate region are employed.

### Linkage Study Design

Linkage information is gathered family by family and the exact nature of the polymorphic marker linked with a certain blood pressure locus might vary between families. The minimum family unit for linkage studies comprises two relatives, often a pair of siblings.[59,60] Indeed, pairs of dizygotic twins can be especially useful because they have less environmental variability and a potentially sharper genetic signal.[61] Importantly, the sib-pair design is a pragmatic choice for conditions of middle age such as hypertension, in which parents might be dead and offspring difficult to classify. Both qualitative (hypertension, normotension, high, low) and quantitative (measured pressures) data can be used for sib-pair linkage studies.[62,63]

In linkage approaches, the selection of siblings with discordant phenotypes has been proposed.[64,65] Although there may be a theoretical argument for selecting from the extremes of the blood pressure distribution to increase statistical power[65,66] there are potential difficulties. The first is logistic. The more extreme the criteria, the fewer the eligible individuals and sibling pairs. Large screening phases are needed that can involve hundreds of thousands of individuals.[67] The second is etiologic. Pickering showed that familial correlation appeared to decline at very high levels of pressure and interpreted this as the result of inclusion of nonfamilial secondary forms of hypertension.[68] It can be difficult to effectively exclude nongenetic causes (sometimes transient) of very high or very low blood pressure in large scale screening programs. Finally doubt regarding the representativeness of individuals with extreme blood pressure will always remain, especially in relation to the genetic causes of middling levels of blood pressure around which most of the pressure-related complications occur.

## Association Studies

In association studies, the "family" is the population. Cases with high blood pressure who share common ancestors will also share the remains of the ancestral haplotype in which a blood pressure allele arose (see previous section "Alleles, Markers, and Haplotypes"). By inference, specific ancestral haplotype marker alleles in LD with a blood pressure allele will be found more frequently in cases (i.e., associated) with high blood pressure than in controls. Simple chi-square tests are used to determine the statistical significance of differences in proportion of marker alleles.

Association can be tested using individual SNPs one at a time. However, there might also be merit in testing association with combinations of SNPs in the region of interest. At each gene there are on average approximately 14 different SNP haplotypes.[54] One potential advantage of using SNP haplotypes is that the phenotypic effect might depend on the molecular interaction between a particular combination of SNPs. Examples exist of phenotypes that are associated with the whole SNP haplotype, but not with the individual SNP components.[69] Moreover, it might be possible to identify "tag SNPs" that distinguish certain haplotypes without the need for genotyping all SNPs in the haplotypes.[70]

### Association Study Design

The usual comparison in association studies is between hypertensive and normotensive subjects, who sit either side of an arbitrary line drawn in the population distribution (Figure 5–9). Theoretically, selecting from the top and bottom of the distribution should enhance genetic contrast and the power to detect association (Figure 5–10).[71,72] One practical example is the Four Corners Approach devised by Watt selects from the upper and lower ends of the blood pressure distribution using measured pressures from two generations.[73]

As LD extends over shorter distances than linkage (see previous section "Linkage Disequilibrium"), association studies have higher resolution especially when using closely spaced SNPs as markers for fine-mapping (step 2) and allelic searches (step 3). Indeed, SNPs might also be useful for LD mapping of the entire genome[46] (step 1). Although initial success in cardiovascular disease has been reported,[74] there is debate about the general utility of this approach[45,75,76] in which maps might require more than 1 million SNPs and high throughput methods to cope analytically.[77]

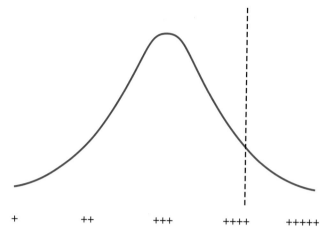

**Figure 5–9** Assuming that blood pressure rank is the result of the individual "dose" of polygenes, the genetic contrast between hypertensives (to the right of the dashed line) and normotensives (to the left of the dashed line) is not especially large.

### Single Nucleotide Polymorphism Discovery

Detailed allelic searches (step 3) demand a comprehensive catalog of SNPs in the region. This necessitates reference to global SNP databases combined with a phase of SNP discovery and verification in the relevant local population.[35,54] The gold standard is direct sequencing in and around candidate genes, at minimum covering the exons (coding regions, 5′ untranslated region, 3′ untranslated region), up to 100 nucleotides into the introns from the exon-intron boundaries and the 5′ upstream genomic region.[54]

### Potential Difficulties

SNP LD mapping should be successful if blood pressure is influenced by relatively old mutations that are at high frequency. However, should the CD/RA model pertain, the utility

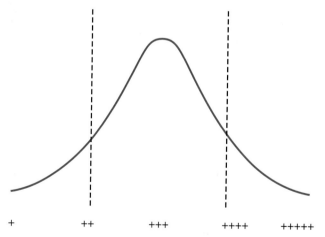

**Figure 5–10** Assuming that blood pressure rank is the result of the individual "dose" of polygenes, the genetic contrast between subjects with high (to the right of the upper dashed line) and low (to the left of the lower dashed line) blood pressure is greater than with the dichotomous strategy (see Figure 5–9).

of LD mapping will be limited with the existing statistical methods.[45,75] Indeed, any methods that depend on LD will struggle if high levels of allelic heterogeneity underpin blood pressure, simply because of the complexity imposed in detecting numerous and infrequent alleles. Under such circumstances, linkage methods that detect all blood pressure haplotypes in a chromosomal region might be better.

### Bias

For any discovery based on association studies, the possibility of false positives as a result of population stratification must be considered,[78] although the magnitude of the problem is debated.[79] Stratification arises when bias is introduced (often unwittingly) during the selection of cases and controls.[80] One important example is unrecognized racial or ethnic heterogeneity confounding analyses.[81] Where a racial or ethnic group is more prone to a disease (therefore, included more frequently as cases) any genetic variant characteristic of or more common in that group (even if not causative) will be mistakenly associated with the condition. Sometimes the causes of bias may be far more subtle and difficult to identify.

One approach has been to use independent markers at other loci to detect systemic genetic differences between cases and controls.[82] However, the preferred solution lies in combining approaches and performing association tests within families. Analyses such as the transmission disequilibrium test (TDT)[83] are not susceptible to population stratification and have an important role in confirming positive associations of putative causative DNA variants.

## GENETICS OF BLOOD PRESSURE DISEASES

Among the triumphs of molecular biology stand the definitions of genetic causes of rare Mendelian forms of blood pressure deviation.[7] Table 5–1 summarizes these discoveries.

One important lesson for essential hypertension from these Mendelian syndromes is that even blood pressure effects of major mutations are not guaranteed,[102] presumably as a result of interactions with other genes and the environment.

## GENETICS OF COMMON BLOOD PRESSURE VARIATION

### Candidate Genes

Before the advent of genomic maps, much of the early work analyzed associations between polymorphisms in candidate genes and clinical essential hypertension. The choice of candidates is directed by a variety of considerations.

### Candidates from Rare Mendelian Diseases

Although major mutations in genes responsible for Mendelian blood pressure diseases do not explain common hypertension,[103,104] other DNA variants in the same candidate genes with more subtle effects on gene expression or function might be relevant.

For example, the *SCNN1B* and *SCNN1G* genes encoding the β- and γ-subunits of the epithelial sodium channel that have been implicated in Liddle syndrome[86,87] make logical candidates and these genes have been linked with variation of SBP in the general population.[105] Causative DNA variation in these genes has yet to be identified for common hypertension, but these findings illustrate the potential relevance of rare syndromes to defining candidates for population genetic analyses. Other genetic loci from Table 5–1 are also worthy candidates.

### Candidates from Physiologic Plausibility

Careful physiologic study of blood pressure, and in particular the predisposition to high blood pressure, provides important clues to genes worthy of investigation. In contrast to the rare Mendelian syndromes, the pathophysiology is not predominantly renal and includes other neuronal and metabolic abnormalities.[106-110]

### Candidates with Functional Polymorphisms

Given the complex physiologic determination of blood pressure, the list of candidate genes is potentially enormous. However, those candidates for which functional DNA variation has been identified attract greater priority, especially if the variants are relatively common. For example, the simple I/D polymorphism of the ACE gene has been associated with differences in ACE enzyme activity[111,112] and variants of the angiotensinogen gene are associated with differences in plasma angiotensinogen levels.[118] A common polymorphism of the glucocorticoid receptor gene[108] has been related to tissue-specific differences in steroid sensitivity[113] and polymorphisms of the gene encoding the $\beta_2$-adrenergic receptor have been associated with changes in vascular reactivity.[114] SNPs of the natriuretic peptide A receptor also have functional effects on receptor mRNA levels.[115]

### Candidates from Linkage Mapping

The advent of genome-wide mapping offers an important means of selecting candidates that are located within chromosomal regions linked with blood pressure (see next paragraph). This approach will become increasingly important as linked loci are replicated to achieve confirmed status (see "Genome Scans" section).

### Candidate Association Analyses

Polymorphisms in and around a large range of candidates have been associated with blood pressure, including genes encoding ACE,[116,117] angiotensinogen,[118] glucocorticoid receptor,[108] insulin receptor,[119] complement C3F,[120] $\beta_2$-adrenergic receptor,[121,122] lipoprotein lipase,[123] type 1A dopamine receptor,[124] alpha-adducin,[125] $\alpha_{1B}$-adrenergic receptor,[124] endothelial nitric oxide synthase,[126] pancreatic phospholipase A2,[127] $\alpha_2$-adrenergic receptor,[128] SA gene,[129] angiotensin II type 1 receptor,[130] G-protein β3 subunit,[131] 6-phosphogluconate dehydrogenase,[132] prostacyclin synthase,[133] growth hormone,[134] Na,K,2Cl-cotransporter,[135] alpha(1)-Na,K-ATPase,[135] and GPR10.[136] However, almost every published positive result has been followed by a negative result.[137-149] Aspects of research design and analysis provide some possible

**Table 5-1** Rare Mendelian Forms of Blood Pressure Deviation

| Disease | Phenotype | Genetic Cause |
|---|---|---|
| Glucocorticoid remediable hyperaldosteronism[84] | Autosomal dominant, hypertension, variable hyperaldosteronism | Chimeric 11β-hydroxylase/aldosterone synthase gene |
| Syndrome of apparent mineralocorticoid excess[85] | Autosomal recessive, volume expansion, hypokalemia, low renin and aldosterone | Mutations in the 11β-hydroxysteroid dehydrogenase gene |
| Liddle syndrome[86,87] | Autosomal dominant, hypertension, volume expansion, hypokalemia, low renin and aldosterone | Mutation subunits of the epithelial sodium channel *SCNN1B* and *SCNN1G* genes |
| Pseudohypoaldosteronism type II (Gordon's syndrome)[88] | Autosomal dominant, hypertension, hyperkalemia, volume expansion, normal glomerular filtration rate | Linkage to chromosomes 1q31- q42 and 17p11- q21 |
| Gitelman's syndrome[89] | Autosomal recessive, low blood pressure, hypokalemic alkalosis, hypocalciuria | Mutations in the Na, Cl cotransporter *NCCT* gene |
| Bartter's syndrome[90,91] | Autosomal recessive, low blood pressure, hypokalemic alkalosis, hypercalciuria | Mutations in the Na, K, 2Cl cotransporter *NKCC2* gene or mutations in the K channel *ROMK* gene |
| Bartter's syndrome type III[92] | Autosomal recessive, low blood pressure, hypokalemic alkalosis, hypercalciuria without nephrocalcinosis | Mutations in the chloride channel *CLCNKB* gene |
| Pseudohypoaldosteronism type I—severe[93] | Autosomal recessive, low blood pressure, renal salt wasting, hyperkalemia and metabolic acidosis, elevated aldosterone levels | Mutation subunits of the epithelial sodium channel *SCNN1B* and *SCNN1G* genes |
| Pseudohypoaldosteronism type I—mild[94] | Autosomal dominant, low blood pressure, renal salt wasting, hyperkalemia and metabolic acidosis, elevated aldosterone levels that remit with age | Mutations in mineralocorticoid receptor gene |
| Polycystic kidney disease[95] | Autosomal dominant, renal cysts, hypertension and renal failure, liver cysts, cerebral aneurysms, valvular heart disease | Mutations in the *PKD1* and *PKD2* genes |
| Pheochromocytoma[96,97] | (a) Multiple endocrine neoplasia type 2A: autosomal dominant, medullary thyroid carcinoma, pheochromocytoma, hyperparathyroidism | (a) Mutations in the *RET* protooncogene |
| | (b) von Hippel-Lindau disease: autosomal dominant, retinal angiomas, hemangioblastomas of the cerebellum and spinal cord, renal cell carcinomas, adrenal pheochromocytomas[98] | (b) Mutations in the *VHL* tumour suppressor gene |
| | (c) Neurofibromatosis type 1: autosomal dominant, multiple neurofibromas, café au lait spots, Lisch nodules of the iris and pheochromocytomas[99] | (c) Mutations in the *NF1* tumour suppressor gene |
| | (d) Nonsyndromic pheochromocytomas | (d) Mutations in *RET, VHL, SDHB, SDHD* genes[100] |
| Hypertension exacerbated in pregnancy[101] | Autosomal dominant, early onset, severe hypertension with low aldosterone levels, exacerbated in pregnancy | Missense mutation resulting in substitution of leucine for serine at codon 810 ($MR_{L810}$) |

explanations for inconsistencies. However, the combination of chance and editorial bias[150] explains why certain positive results have not stood the test of time.

## Genome Scans

Figure 5–11 shows the results of a typical genome-wide scan, in this case a multipoint quantitative sib-pair analysis of SBP.[151] Each panel represents a probability plot (expressed as Z scores) along the length of each of the 22 autosomes and the

X chromosome. The Y chromosome is not included in linkage analyses because, other than at the very tips, the vast majority of the Y chromosome does not recombine and is, therefore, uninformative for linkage.

### *Genome-Wide Significance*

Evidence of linkage is derived from the magnitude of the probability and the likely location of the blood pressure locus is identified by the position along the chromosome

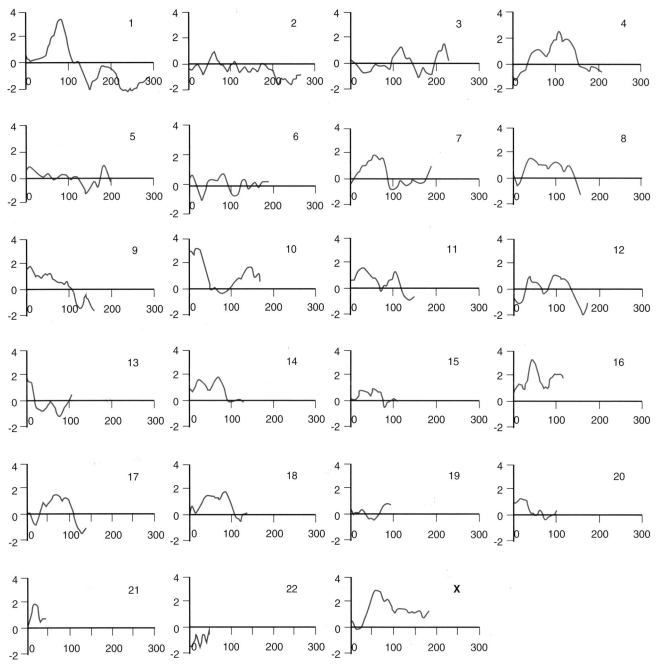

**Figure 5–11** Genome-wide probability plots for evidence of linkage with SBP. Each panel shows a chromosome (22 autosomes and X) with genetic distance in centiMorgans along the x-axis and probability (Z) along the y-axis. On chromosomes 1, 4, 16, and X, Z exceeds the evidence for suggestive linkage. (From Harrap SB, Wong ZY, Stebbing M, et al. Blood pressure QTLs identified by genome-wide linkage analysis and dependence on associated phenotypes. Physiol Genomics 8:99-105, 2002.)

(expressed for example as a genetic distance in centiMorgans from the p telomere) at which peak probability occurs. Because multiple markers (around 450 microsatellites per first pass scan) increase the likelihood of false positives, Lander and Kruglyak[152] proposed guidelines for accepting genome-wide significance with a series of gradings including "suggestive," "significant," and "highly significant." These correspond to the likelihoods of false positive being 1.00, 0.05, and 0.001, respectively, per genome-wide scan. These stringent guidelines have been questioned[153] as they may risk discarding important results in cases of inadequate statistical power. Many investigators use lower thresholds and the category of "promising" has been adopted with probabilities below "suggestive." Nevertheless, more important than arbitrary probability thresholds is the replication of linkage in independent populations. This essential step toward formal proof is central to the concept of a "confirmed" locus.[152]

Table 5–2 summarizes these results from genome-wide scans for blood pressure or hypertension that have reported chromosomal loci for which multipoint analyses reveal linkage evidence that exceeds the "promising" threshold. The summary has been restricted to multipoint analyses (using adjacent groups of markers simultaneously) as they increase the power to detect true linkages, they decrease the false-positive rate, and when linkage is detected, they provide localization and confidence intervals.[154]

### Mixed Success

One is struck immediately by the differences in the number, location, and statistical significance of blood pressure loci between the studies. Evidence of genome-wide suggestive linkage was reported for between 0 and 4 loci per study. Given that one suggestive locus is expected by chance, this leaves only nine studies with results that might be considered less likely to be false positives. This group includes six studies reporting more than one suggestive locus[67,158-161] and three others reporting a single locus at which linkage probability exceeded the "significant" threshold (log-of-the-odds [LOD] >3.6).[155-157]

### Where Are the Blood Pressure Polygenes?

The sparsity of linked loci might lead one to question the veracity of the polygenic model. But it is more likely that methodological problems impair the ability to detect the polygenes in linkage studies, especially if there are many of small individual effect.[174] If nothing else, the genome scans offer an attempt to define empirically the research designs that appear to provide the greatest success. This necessary process of trial and error will help chart the size and nature of further studies. The following identifies issues of potential relevance to both association and linkage analyses.

## Maximizing Success in Genetic Discovery
### Quantitative Versus Qualitative Phenotypes

Most of the nine "successful" genome-wide studies used quantitative methods (see Table 5–2). In qualitative analyses, clinical hypertension is most often used as the defining phenotype. However, the range of recorded pressures from any group of

hypertensives is very broad.[175] The qualitative assumption that all hypertensives are genetically similar is unlikely to be true and lumping together such genetic heterogeneity obscures valuable quantitative information that reflects to locus-specific effects that might be peculiar to certain families in linkage studies. Given the simple approaches for adjusting for the effects of antihypertensive treatments, quantitative analyses in treated subjects are feasible and worthwhile.[175]

### Different Pressure Phenotypes

Blood pressure can be measured as systolic, diastolic, mean, or pulse pressure in lying, sitting, standing, or ambulatory situations. Is any one better than another? From the genome scans, it appears that loci linked with SBP were reported more frequently than those with diastolic blood pressure (DBP) (see Table 5–2). However, this may simply be a function of the relatively high degree of individual-specific variation such as measurement error of DBP.[15]

The relationship between blood pressure and the underlying genotype might be complex or simple. If complex, a heterogeneous group of genes might influence blood pressure at any one of the numerous points of physiologic control (see Figure 5–7). By inference such alleles might be discovered when heterogeneity is minimized by subgrouping blood pressure according to underlying physiologic intermediate phenotypes.[176-181] Few genomic analyses have used this approach because detailed phenotypic characterizations in large numbers of subjects is very difficult. Nevertheless, simple dissection of blood pressure in large-scale studies is feasible. For example, analyses of postural changes[182,183] have the potential to reveal genetic factors related to the sympathetic nervous control of blood pressure. In hypertensive subjects the immediate blood pressure change on standing shows suggestive evidence of linkage to chromosome 18.[182] However this locus was not linked with the postural blood pressure change after 2 minutes standing,[182] suggesting genotypic heterogeneity even for the postural phenotypes.

If simple, there might exist DNA variants with pleiotropic effects (i.e., influencing all pressure phenotypes). Indeed, some evidence suggests that SBP and DBP,[15] lying and standing SBP,[183] and SBP and pulse pressure[184] share genetic determinants. For pleiotropic genes, the most appropriate phenotype would be 24-hour ambulatory recordings[185] with the added advantages of repeated measures and reduced measurement error. Ambulatory recordings would also allow analyses of blood pressures for genes whose effects are more obvious at one time of the day than another.[186]

Whether DNA variants are pleiotropic or highly specific in phenotypic effects, it is important that genetic analyses of blood pressure are precise and explicit in the selection of phenotypes. Furthermore, so that the measurements reflect the underlying genotype as reliably as possible,[187] measurement error must be minimized by careful standardization of techniques, training observers, and making repeated measures.

### Study Size

All other things being equal, the bigger the study size the greater the statistical power. However, meaningful power calculation for linkage is a difficult task without knowledge of the underlying genetic architecture and the potency of

**Table 5-2** Details of Genome-Wide Scans for Blood Pressure*

| Reference | Ethnicity/ Race | Study Design | Families/ Subjects | Significant Linkage Chr | cM | BP | Suggestive Linkage Chr | cM | BP | Promising Linkage Chr | cM | BP | Comments |
|---|---|---|---|---|---|---|---|---|---|---|---|---|---|
| Levy et al.[155] | W | F/QT | 332/1702 | 17 | 62 | SP | 18 | 7 | DP | | | | Longitudinal observations, adjustments for covariates and BP treatment effects |
| Hseuh et al.[156] | W | F/QT | 28/661 | 2 | 195 | DP | | | | | | | Amish, sitting BP, treated BPs excluded, identified through probands with type 2 diabetes |
| Kristjansson et al.[157] | W | F/QL | 120/490 | 18 | 89 | HT | | | | | | | Relatively isolated Icelandic families |
| Caulfield et al.[158] | W | SP/QL | 1599/2010 | 6 | qter | HT | 9 | 140 | HT | 2<br>5 | 155<br>80 | HT<br>HT | Severe and early-onset hypertension, excluding diabetics and subjects with BMI >30 kg/m² at diagnosis |
| Cooper et al.[159] | B | F/QT | 196/792 | | | | 3<br>10<br>19<br>19 | 22<br>76<br>42<br>78 | DP<br>DP<br>SP<br>SP | 1<br>2<br>2<br>2<br>5<br>7<br>7<br>8 | 148<br>24<br>104<br>128<br>102<br>81<br>109<br>117 | DP<br>DP<br>DP<br>SP<br>DP<br>DP<br>DP<br>DP | Nigerian farmers of the Yoruba group, adults and children sitting pressures, no treated BPs, wide pressure range |
| Rice et al.[160] | W | F/QT | 206/697 | | | | 2<br>5<br>7<br>8 | 114<br>45<br>135<br>87 | SP<br>SP<br>SP<br>SP | 1<br>19<br>22 | 120<br>4<br>45 | SP<br>SP<br>DP | Enriched with obese families, hypertensives excluded |
| Harrap et al.[151] | W | SP/QT | 274/548 | | | | 1<br>4<br>16<br>X | 86<br>108<br>49<br>67 | SP<br>SP<br>SP<br>SP | 5<br>10 | 203<br>17 | DP<br>SP | Population sample, young adults, supine BP, adjustments for BP treatment effects |
| Xu et al.[67] | C | SP/QL | 137/274 | | | | 16<br>15 | 64<br>105 | LCSP<br>LCDP | 3<br>11<br>17 | 6<br>58<br>24 | LCSP<br>EDSP<br>HCSP | Adults and children top and bottom age-adjusted deciles sitting BP, no treated BPs |
| Allayee et al.[161] | W | F/QT | 18/240 | | | | 4<br>6 | 26<br>89 | SP<br>DP | 8 | 45 | DP | Identified through hyperlipidemic probands; treated BPs—no adjustments or exclusion |

| Study | Race | Analysis | F/S | Chr | cM | Phenotype | Chr | cM | Phenotype | Comments |
|---|---|---|---|---|---|---|---|---|---|---|
| Rice et al.[162] | B,W | F/QT | 173/836 | 12 | 95 | BDP | 2<br>3<br>3<br>11<br>19 | 69<br>0<br>205<br>102<br>26 | BSP<br>WSP<br>WSP<br>WSP<br>BSP | Treated BPs excluded, adjustments for BP covariates |
| Hunt et al.[163] | W | F/QT/QL | 401/2959 | 6 | 89 | SP | 8<br>12<br>15 | 25<br>83<br>0 | DP<br>BT<br>DP | Adjustments for covariates and BP treatment effects, qualitative and quantitative approaches |
| Perola et al.[164] | W | SP/QL | 47/94 | 2 | 111 | MHT | 1<br>22 | 190<br>32 | MHT<br>HT | Obese and diabetics excluded, enriched with DZ twins divided by sex and parental region |
| Ranade et al.[165] | C,J | SP/QL | na/2462 | 10 | 30 | HT | 9<br>14 | 164<br>92 | LCBP<br>HT | High and low (bottom tertile) BP identified through hypertensive probands |
| Krushkal et al.[166] | W | SP/QL | 69/138 | 6 | 138 | SP | 15 | 90 | SP | Mean age 16 years, top vs. bottom quintiles |
| Theil et al.[167] | B,W | F/QT | 371/na | 1 | 170 | WDP | 11 | 76 | WSP | Identified through probands with BP in top quartile |
| Angius et al.[168] | W | F/QL | 35/77 | 2 | 27 | HT | | | | Isolated Sardinian village, hypertensive probands |
| Zhu et al.[169] | C | SP/QL | 79/232 | 2 | 161 | HT | | | | |
| Rao et al.[170] | B,W | SP/QL | 1076/1403 | | | | 2 | 61 | BHT | Selected for "severe" HT |
| Atwood et al.[171] | H | F/QL | 10/441 | | | | | | | Sitting BPs with random zero sphygmomanometer, adjustments for covariates and BP treatment effects |
| Sharma et al.[172] | W | SP/QL | 119/288 | | | | | | | |
| Kardia et al.[173] | B,W | SP/QL | 486/1457 | | | | | | | Random zero sphygmomanometer, no HT diagnostic criteria presented |

*Results are from multipoint linkage analyses only. Study samples comprise families (F) or sibling pairs (S) and analyses are either quantitative (QT) or qualitative (QL). Ethnicity and race of subjects were black (B), Chinese (C), Hispanic (H), Japanese (J), or white (W). After Lander and Krulyak[152] the following linkage probabilities were defined: for sibling pair studies, significant-log-of-the-odds (LOD) >3.6 (Z >4.07), suggestive-LOD >2.2 (Z >3.18) and promising-LOD >1.5 (Z >2.63); for family studies: significant-LOD >3.3 (Z >3.90), suggestive-LOD >1.9 (Z >2.96) and promising-LOD >1.5 (Z >2.63). The position of loci is quoted as centiMorgans (cM) from the p telomere. The following abbreviations apply for phenotypes: DP, diastolic pressure; SP, systolic pressure; LC, low concordant; ED, extreme discordant; HC, high concordant; B, Black; W, white; M, male; HT, hypertension; BMI, body mass index; DZ, dizygotic.

individual DNA variants. Variants of small effect will be difficult to detect by any means, but in general association studies are expected to be more powerful than linkage studies, unless the variants are rare in which case even association studies struggle.[188] The theoretical estimates of the required numbers of families for linkage studies range from several hundred to a few million.[46] A review of genome-wide scans, each comprising 20 to 1783 individuals (1 to 580 families) found that successful scans had on average twice as many subjects as unsuccessful scans.[189] Strangely, the same trend is not especially obvious for blood pressure (see Table 5–2) where some of the bigger searches were less successful. However, factors other than numerical size are relevant to study power.

### Population, Racial, and Ethnic Issues

The majority of genome-wide analyses have been based in outbred populations that have been sampled in a representative fashion[151,155,163,171] or with certain restrictions or selection criteria.* The nature of the selection criteria varied considerably and comprised enrichment or exclusion of obesity,[158,160,164] diabetes,[156,158,164] and hyperlipidemia.[161] The impact of ascertainment and selection on the genetic characteristics is unknown.

Four studies have been based in relatively isolated populations,[156,157,159,164,168] in which genetic heterogeneity and environmental variation are expected to be relatively low. However, the theoretical advantages of genetic isolates such as Finland[164] and Sardinia[168] for linkage mapping have been questioned.[190] For blood pressure, genetic isolates reported single loci, often at relatively high probability.[156,157] Nonetheless, these loci were not reproduced in other studies. Indeed, results were not found to be consistent between different genetic isolates within Finland itself,[164] raising questions (other things being equal) about the general inferences that might be obtained from genetically isolated populations.

The problem of population stratification (see previous section "Bias" ) is relevant not only for association studies but also for genome scans. If blood pressure alleles are ancient and predate the divergence of the human populations, they would be found globally and one might expect consistent findings between genomic analyses in different geographic, racial, and ethnic groups (see Figure 5–5).[47] However, little consistency exists for blood pressure genome scans (see Table 5–2).

One might infer, therefore, that in terms of its genetic causation, hypertension is a modern condition resulting from recently derived alleles that are population-specific. However, it is not possible to exclude the existence of ubiquitous ancient blood pressure alleles that are obscured in particular populations by environmental milieux that might constrain their expression.[191,192] Population differences, whether genetic or environmental will confound genetic studies that combine diverse populations.[193,194]

Nevertheless, not all evidence favors population-specific modern blood pressure alleles as some regions on chromosomes 2[158,159,164,169] and 16[67,151] have been identified in different populations. The locus at 16q13 was reported as suggestive in two quantitative analyses, one of the full range of SBPs in white subjects,[151] the other of low SBP in Chinese.[67] In addition, two other studies found evidence of promising linkage in this vicinity.[162,171] This locus is attractive because it encompasses a

number of plausible candidate genes including the *SCNN1B* and *SCNN1G* genes that encode the β- and γ-subunits, respectively, of the amiloride-sensitive epithelial sodium channel and *SLC12A3* that encodes the thiazide-sensitive NaCl cotransporter. These candidates have been proven relevant in genetic blood pressure diseases (see previous section "Candidates from Rare Mendelian Diseases") and it is conceivable that other DNA variants in and around these genes might have less dramatic but more common blood pressure effects.

### Dealing with Covariates

It is important to identify and, if necessary, control important sources of variation. However, in doing so, care must be taken not to jettison covariate effects that might share genetic origins with blood pressure. For example, blood pressures are often adjusted by regression methods for well-recognized sources of variation such as age and sex. However, removing the components of blood pressure variation associated with these covariates will obscure the phenotypic effects of genes whose effects might be age- or sex-dependent.[195,196]

### Age

In adulthood there is a positive correlation between age and blood pressure and many linkage studies* adjust pressure for age prior to analysis (see Table 5–2). However, some studies include adolescents[67,159,166] in whom the substantial effects of growth on blood pressure distort blood pressure ranking and correlations between blood pressure and age.[197] Indeed, genes for blood pressure found in growing adolescents might relate more to genes that determine the rate and timing of growth than to blood pressure per se.

### Sex

Sex is relevant to blood pressure genetics in a number of ways. First, blood pressure alleles might be on sex chromosomes. To date only one genome scan has included the X chromosome and reported suggestive evidence for a blood pressure locus.[151] Variation in the nonrecombining region of the Y chromosome has also been associated with significant blood pressure differences.[198,199] Second, the sexual phenotype and its hormonal milieu can influence gene expression. Dependence of expression on sex might explain why evidence of linkage[164] or association[196] with blood pressure is demonstrable in one but not the other sex.

Few studies make formal tests of the possible influence of sex, and simple mathematical adjustments will not necessarily help reveal loci whose phenotypic expression depends on the sexual phenotype. Unfortunately dividing studies into subgroups of single sexes reduces statistical power and novel statistical methods are needed for identifying sex-dependent genetic effects from entire data sets.

### Body Mass Index

Some analyses adjust blood pressures for variation in body mass index (BMI)[151,163] or exclude subjects with high BMI levels.[158,164] The rationale is to avoid the secondary nongenetic effects of BMI per se on blood pressure. However, there also appear to

---

*References 67, 160-162, 165-170, 172, 173.

*References 67, 151, 155, 162, 163, 171.

exist genetic factors that determine both blood pressure and BMI[15] that will be missed when adjustments for BMI are made. Genes that influence several related cardiovascular risk factors in such a way might be the most important to identify because of their multiplicative implications for coronary risk including conditions such as the metabolic syndrome. At least one genome scan has addressed this issue by comparing the linkage results for systolic pressure unadjusted and adjusted for BMI.[151] Three of the four suggestive loci were relatively unaffected by adjustment for BMI, but one locus showed a substantial reduction in linkage probability following adjustment of systolic pressure BMI.

### Antihypertensive Treatments

In quantitative analyses, problems can arise with pressures measured in subjects taking antihypertensive medication.[175] Measured pressures in treated subjects represent a biased distortion in a quantitative analysis because treatment lowers blood pressure and is usually applied to those with the highest values. For this reason, some studies have excluded treated individuals, but not only is important information lost from subjects most likely to have a genetic predisposition, but overall statistical power is weakened.[163] Relatively simple methods have been proposed to adjust for treatment in ways that maximize genetic information and statistical power.[175]

### Genotyping Errors

The benefits of reliable measures of appropriate phenotypes can be undermined if the same rigorous standards are not applied to genotyping itself. Small error rates of 1% to 2% can have serious repercussions for linkage results[200] and the rates of error are likely to increase with the use of extensive SNP maps and high-throughput technologies. It is possible to check for Mendelian transmission of marker alleles, but this method is not infallible, especially for small families and SNPs, and more comprehensive methods must be employed.[201] However, newer statistical methods are being developed to account for genotyping errors, even without actually correcting or deleting suspect genotypes.[202]

## THE FUTURE

There is still a long distance to travel before genetic mutations of significance to blood pressure are confirmed[203] and even further until they have an impact in everyday life. At the present stage we can claim to have made significant attempts at genome mapping (step 1 in the discovery strategy). However, there has been little reported evidence of the results of fine-mapping (step 2). As a result of thoughtful candidate gene selection there are well-documented alleles shown to be in linkage disequilibrium with functional variants (step 4) although their association with blood pressure is less certain.

In any case we can look ahead to the future where the genetics of blood pressure can be envisaged in terms of potential benefits for individuals and for populations.

### Individual Benefit

Genetic discovery might be utilized to predict our personal risks, to suggest the most appropriate antihypertensive treatments and even to design gene therapy.

### Genetic Diagnosis

Some hope that DNA analyses will identify genetic predisposition to high blood pressure and its complications. Such a possibility is predicated on reliable DNA tests that can be used to detect tangible and meaningful increases in risk. These possibilities will be hard to realize unless markers or variants conform to the CD/CV model. Vast numbers of infrequent alleles with small individual effects that typify the CD/RA paradigm will be difficult to locate and catalog in any comprehensive way. Even if discovered, they will not be useful individually for predictive screening because of their small effects.

In any case, genetic tests for complex human multifactorial disease might only ever provide an indication of predisposition and not predestination because of the modifying influence of other relevant genetic and environmental factors. Indeed, the true value of genetic markers of high blood pressure will not be known until large-scale epidemiologic studies demonstrate and quantify their predictive competency for major cardiovascular endpoints. Such evidence must not only achieve overall statistical significance but must also provide acceptably low rates of false positive and false negative results for individuals to avoid unnecessary anxiety or a false sense of security.

### Tailored Treatments

Pharmacogenomics is a growing discipline in which genomic information is used, amongst other things, to inform treatment choices.[204] DNA variants might be used to identify individuals who respond best to a certain class of antihypertensive drug treatment or to avoid certain treatments in particular patients in whom side effects are more likely to occur. Indeed, it might be that such DNA variants have no direct association with blood pressure but instead are relevant to drug pharmacokinetics or other physiologic control systems with which drugs might interact. Many large prospective clinical trials are incorporating genetic analyses in an attempt to identify variants that might be of use.[205]

### Gene Therapy

Beyond pharmacotherapy for hypertension, the possibility of gene therapy has been raised.[206-211] Some approaches are simply clever means of offering "symptomatic" treatment to achieve physiologic changes that can otherwise be achieved by pharmacologic treatment. Others might attempt to modulate a fundamental genetic defect. However, effective, safe, and cheap therapies exist to treat blood pressure and at this stage the difficulties and doubts about the long-term safety of gene therapy make it unattractive.

## Population Benefit: Common Disease/Common Mechanism

Genetics might never contribute to personalized diagnosis of common diseases simply because of the underlying complexities. But that does not diminish the far greater potential of genetics for prevention and treatment. It is not necessary to accumulate comprehensive catalogs of every blood pressure allele to discover novel and tractable biologic mechanisms of high blood pressure.

## Physiologic Convergence

We know from Mendelian cardiovascular diseases such as hypertrophic cardiomyopathy, that such phenotypes can be the common point upon which converge the effects of diverse alleles.[212] This physiologic distillation of molecular diversity provides unique targets for preventive and treatment strategies.[213] The CD/RA hypothesis does not sound the death knell for genetics if there is a common disease/common mechanism (CD/CM) paradigm toward which we can direct our attention.

Instead of genetic searches for the whereabouts of every blood pressure allele, we should search for molecular clues to the points of physiologic convergence. In theory a single allele could lead from a polygene to a subclinical phenotype for common hypertension in the way that such discoveries have been made in Mendelian hypertension. The physiologic intersection of a variety of genes provides an ideal target for developing methods to thwart the actions of several different genes simultaneously.

## Public Health Strategies

The identification of points of physiologic convergence facilitates tests of environmental variation on genetically determined mechanisms. Specific lifestyle or behavioral factors might be revealed as triggers of genetic predisposition and new strategies could be devised to minimize the impact of such mechanisms. If the behavioral or dietary modification is cheap and safe, then it could be (simply for consistency) implemented communitywide, even if the target genetic mechanism is not ubiquitous. Such an outcome might be the greatest contribution that genetics might make to blood pressure and cardiovascular disease.

# References

1. Mongeau JG, Biron P, Sing CF. The influence of genetics and household environment upon the variability of normal blood pressure: the Montreal Adoption Survey. Clin Exp Hypertens A. 8:653-660, 1986.
2. Longini IM, Jr., Higgins MW, Hinton PC, et al. Environmental and genetic sources of familial aggregation of blood pressure in Tecumseh, Michigan. Am J Epidemiol 120:131-144, 1984.
3. Harrap SB, Stebbing M, Hopper JL, et al. Familial patterns of covariation for cardiovascular risk factors in adults: The Victorian Family Heart Study. Am J Epidemiol 152:704-715, 2000.
4. International Human Genome Sequencing Consortium. Initial sequencing and analysis of the human genome. Nature 409: 860-921, 2001.
5. Venter JC, Adams MD, Myers EW, et al. The sequence of the human genome. Science 291:1304-1351, 2001.
6. Aach J, Bulyk ML, Church GM, et al. Computational comparison of two draft sequences of the human genome. Nature 409:856-859, 2001.
7. Lifton RP, Gharavi AG, Geller DS. Molecular mechanisms of human hypertension. Cell 104:545-556, 2001.
8. Lewington S, Clarke R, Qizilbash N, et al. Age-specific relevance of usual blood pressure to vascular mortality. Lancet 360:1903-1913, 2003.
9. Pickering G. Normotension and hypertension: The mysterious viability of the false. Am J Med 65:561-563, 1978.
10. Pickering G. Hypertension. Definitions, natural histories and consequences. Am J Med 52:570-583, 1973.
11. The seventh report of the Joint National Committee on prevention, detection, evaluation, and treatment of high blood pressure. JAMA 289:2560-2572, 2003.
12. Mancia G, Rosei A, DeBaker G, et al. 2003 European Society of Hypertension-European Society of Cardiology guidelines for the management of arterial hypertension. J Hypertens 21:1011-1053, 2003.
13. Rose G. Strategy of prevention: Lessons from cardiovascular disease. Br Med J Clin Res Ed 282:1847-1851, 1981.
14. Stamler J, Stamler R, Neaton JD. Blood pressure, systolic and diastolic, and cardiovascular risks. US population data. Arch Intern Med 153:598-615, 1993.
15. Cui J, Hopper JL, Harrap SB. Genes and family environment explain correlations between blood pressure and body mass index. Hypertension 40:7-12, 2002.
16. Lucas A, Fewtrell MS. Cole TJ. Fetal origins of adult disease-the hypothesis revisited. BMJ 319:245-249, 1999.
17. Knuiman MW, Divitini ML, Bartholomew HC, et al. Spouse correlations in cardiovascular risk factors and the effect of marriage duration. Am J Epidemiol 143:48-53, 1996.
18. Hopper JL. Why 'common environmental effects' are so uncommon in the literature. *In* Spector TD, Sneider H MacGregor AJ (eds). Advances in Twin and Sib-pair Analysis. London, Greenwich Medical Media Ltd, 2000; pp 151-165.
19. Phillips DI. Twin studies in medical research: can they tell us whether diseases are genetically determined? Lancet 341: 1008-1009, 1993.
20. Borhani NO, Feinleib M, Garrison RJ, et al. Genetic variance in blood pressure. Acta Geneticae Medicae et Gemellologiae 25:137-144, 1976.
21. Salmond CE, Prior IA, Wessen AF. Blood pressure patterns and migration: A 14-year cohort study of adult Tokelauans. Am J Epidemiol 130:37-52, 1989.
22. Sever PS, Poulter NR. A hypothesis for the pathogenesis of essential hypertension: the initiating factors. J Hypertens Suppl 7:S9-S12, 1989.
23. Ward RH, Chin PG, Prior IA. Tokelau Island Migrant Study: Effect of migration on the familial aggregation of blood pressure. Hypertension 2:I43-I54, 1980.
24. Winkelstein W Jr, Kagan A, Kato H, et al. Epidemiologic studies of coronary heart disease and stroke in Japanese men living in Japan, Hawaii and California: blood pressure distributions. Am J Epidemiol 102:502-513, 1975.
25. Rose G, Day S. The population mean predicts the number of deviant individuals. BMJ 301:1031-1034, 1990.
26. Wilhelmsen L. ESC Population Studies Lecture 1996: Cardiovascular monitoring of a city over 30 years. Eur Heart J 18:1220-1230, 1997.
27. Epstein FH. International trends in coronary heart disease epidemiology. Ann Clin Res 3:293-299, 1971.
28. Sarti C, Vartiainen E, Torppa J, et al. Trends in cerebrovascular mortality and in its risk factors in Finland during the last 20 years. Health Rep 6:196-206, 1994.
29. Wietlisbach V, Paccaud F, Rickenbach M, et al. Trends in cardiovascular risk factors (1984-1993) in a Swiss region: results of three population surveys. Prev Med 26:523-533, 1997.
30. James PT, Leach R, Kalamara E, et al. The worldwide obesity epidemic. Obes Res 9 Suppl 4:228S-233S, 2001.
31. Intersalt: An international study of electrolyte excretion and blood pressure. Results for 24 hour urinary sodium and potassium excretion. Intersalt Cooperative Research Group. BMJ 297:319-328, 1988.
32. Rose G, Marmot MG. Social class and coronary heart disease. Br Heart J 45:13-19, 1981.
33. Weiss KM, Clark AG. Linkage disequilibrium and the mapping of complex human traits. Trends Genet 18:19-24, 2002.

34. Thompson EA, Neel JV. Allelic disequilibrium and allele frequency distribution as a function of social and demographic history. Am J Hum Genet 60:197-204, 1997.

35. Halushka MK, Fan JB, Bentley K, et al. Patterns of single-nucleotide polymorphisms in candidate genes for blood-pressure homeostasis. Nat Genet 22:239-247, 1999.

36. Harrap SB. Hypertension: Genes versus environment. Lancet 344:169-171, 1994.

37. Ward RH. Genetic and sociocultural components of high blood pressure. Am J Phys Anthropol 62:91-105, 1983.

38. Reich DE, Lander ES. On the allelic spectrum of human disease. Trends Genet 17:502-510, 2001.

39. Cargill M, Altshuler D, Ireland J, et al. Characterization of single-nucleotide polymorphisms in coding regions of human genes. Nat Genet 22:231-238, 1999.

40. Chakravarti A. Population genetics—making sense out of sequence. Nat Genet 21:56-60, 1999.

41. Reich DE, Lander ES. On the allelic spectrum of human disease. Trends Genet 17:502-510, 2001.

42. Corder EH, Saunders AM, Strittmatter WJ, et al. Gene dose of apolipoprotein E type 4 allele and the risk of Alzheimer's disease in late onset families. Science 261: 921-923, 1993.

43. Bertina RM, Koeleman BP, Koster T, et al. Mutation in blood coagulation factor V associated with resistance to activated protein C. Nature 369:64-67, 1994.

44. Kaplan N, Morris R. Issues concerning association studies for fine mapping a susceptibility gene for a complex disease. Genet Epidemiol 20:432-457, 2001.

45. Pritchard JK. Are rare variants responsible for susceptibility to complex diseases? Am J Hum Genet 69:124-137, 2001.

46. Risch N, Merikangas K. The future of genetic studies of complex human diseases. Science 273:1516-1517, 1996.

47. Harrap SB. Where are all the blood pressure genes. Lancet 361:2149-2151, 2003.

48. Rigat B, Hubert C, Alhenc-Gelas F, et al. An insertion/deletion polymorphism in the angiotensin I-converting enzyme gene accounting for half the variance of serum enzyme levels. J Clin Invest 86:1343-1346, 1990.

49. Weber JL, David D, Heil J, et al.. Human diallelic insertion/deletion polymorphisms. Am J Hum Genet 71:854-862, 2002.

50. Weber JL, May PE. Abundant class of human DNA polymorphisms which can be typed using the polymerase chain reaction. Am J Hum Genet 44:388-396, 1989.

51. Sachidanandam R, Weissman D, Schmidt SC, et al. The International SNP Map Working Group. A map of human genome sequence variation containing 1.42 million single nucleotide polymorphisms. Nature 409:928-933, 2001.

52. Weber JL. Informativeness of human (dC-dA)n.(dG-dT)n polymorphisms. Genomics 7:524-530, 1990.

53. Botstein D, Risch N. Discovering genotypes underlying human phenotypes: past successes for Mendelian disease, future approaches for complex disease. Nat Genet 33:228-237, 2003.

54. Stephens JC, Schneider JA, Tanguay DA, et al. Haplotype variation and linkage disequilibrium in 313 human genes. Science 293:489-493, 2001.

55. Harpending HC, Batzer MA, Gurven M, et al. Genetic traces of ancient demography. Proc Nat Acad Sci (USA) 95:1961-1967, 1998.

56. Reich DE, Schaffner SF, Daly MJ, et al. Human genome sequence variation and the influence of gene history, mutation and recombination. Nat Genet 32:135-142, 2002.

57. Dunning AM, Durocher F, Healey CS. The extent of linkage disequilibrium in four populations with distinct demographic histories. Am J Hum Genet 67:1544-1554, 2000.

58. Jeffreys AJ, Neumann R. Reciprocal crossover asymmetry and meiotic drive in a human recombination hot spot. Nat Genet 31:267-271, 2002.

59. Wilson AF, Elston RC, Tran LD, et al. Use of the robust sib-pair method to screen for single-locus, multiple-locus, and pleiotropic effects: application to traits related to hypertension. Am J Hum Genet 48:862-872, 1991.

60. McCarthy MI, Kruglyak L, Lander ES. Sib-pair collection strategies for complex diseases. Genet Epidemiol 15:317-340, 1998.

61. MacGregor AJ, Snieder H, Schork NJ, et al. Twins: Novel uses to study complex traits and genetic diseases. Trends Genet 16: 131-134, 2000.

62. Kruglyak L, Lander ES. Complete multipoint sib-pair analysis of qualitative and quantitative traits Am J Hum Genet 57:439-454, 1995.

63. Zhang H, Risch N. Mapping quantitative-trait loci in humans by use of extreme concordant sib pairs: Selected sampling by parental phenotypes. Am J Hum Genet 59:951-957, 1996.

64. Risch NJ, Zhang H. Mapping quantitative trait loci with extreme discordant sib pairs: Sampling considerations. Am J Hum Genet 58:836-843, 1996.

65. Risch N, Zhang H. Extreme discordant sib pairs for mapping quantitative trait loci in humans. Science 268:1584-1589, 1995.

66. Zhang H, Risch N. Mapping quantitative-trait loci in humans by use of extreme concordant sib pairs: Selected sampling by parental phenotypes. Am J Hum Genet 59:951-957, 1996.

67. Xu X, Rogus JJ, Terwedow HA, et al. An extreme-sib-pair genome scan for genes regulating blood pressure. Am J Hum Genet 64:1694-1701, 1999.

68. Pickering GW. The nature of essential hypertension. Lancet i:1027-1028, 1959.

69. Drysdale CM, McGraw DW, Stack CB, et al. Complex promoter and coding region beta 2-adrenergic receptor haplotypes alter receptor expression and predict in vivo responsiveness. Proc Nat Acad Sci (USA) 97:10483-10488, 2000.

70. Zhang K, Calabrese P, Nordborg M, et al. Haplotype block structure and its applications to association studies: power and study designs. Am J Hum Genet 71:1386-1394, 2002.

71. Schork NJ, Nath SK, Fallin D, et al. Linkage disequilibrium analysis of biallelic DNA markers, human quantitative trait loci, and threshold-defined case and control subjects. Am J Hum Genet 67:1208-1218, 2000.

72. Abecasis GR, Cookson WOC, Cardon LR. The power to detect linkage disequilibrium with quantitative traits in selected samples. Am J Hum Genet 68:1463-1474, 2001.

73. Watt G. Design and interpretation of studies comparing individuals with and without a family history of high blood pressure. J Hypertens 4:1-7, 1986.

74. Ozaki K, Ohnishi Y, Iida A, et al. Functional SNPs in the lymphotoxin-alpha gene that are associated with susceptibility to myocardial infarction. Nat Genet 32:650-654, 2002.

75. Kruglyak L. Prospects for whole-genome linkage disequilibrium mapping of common disease genes. Nat Genet 22:139-144, 1999.

76. Weiss KM, Terwilliger JD. How many diseases does it take to map a gene with SNPs? Nat Genet 26:151-157, 2000.

77. Ohnishi Y, Tanaka T, Ozaki K, et al. A high-throughput SNP typing system for genome-wide association studies. J Hum Genet 46:471-477, 2001.

78. Thomas DC, Witte JS. Point: Population stratification: A problem for case-control studies of candidate-gene associations? Cancer Epidemiol Biomarkers Prev 11:505-512, 2002.

79. Wacholder S, Rothman N, Caporaso N. Counterpoint: Bias from population stratification is not a major threat to the validity of conclusions from epidemiological studies of common polymorphisms and cancer. Cancer Epidemiol Biomarkers Prev 11:513-520, 2002.

80. Little J, Bradley L, Bray MS, et al. Reporting, appraising, and integrating data on genotype prevalence and gene-disease associations. Am J Epidemiol 156:300-310, 2002.

81. Barley J, Carter ND, Cruickshank JK, et al. Renin and atrial natriuretic peptide restriction fragment length polymorphisms: association with ethnicity and blood pressure. J Hypertens 9:993-996, 1991.

82. Devlin B, Roeder K, Wasserman L. Genomic control, a new approach to genetic-based association studies. Theor Popul Biol 60:155-166, 2001.

83. Schulze TG, McMahon FJ. Genetic association mapping at the crossroads: Which test and why? Overview and practical guidelines. Am J Med Genet 114:1-11, 2002.

84. Lifton RP, Dluhy RG, Powers M, et al. A chimaeric 11 beta-hydroxylase/aldosterone synthase gene causes glucocorticoid-remediable aldosteronism and human hypertension. Nature 355:262-265, 1992.

85. Mune T, Rogerson FM, Nikkila H, et al. Human hypertension caused by mutations in the kidney isozyme of 11 beta-hydroxysteroid dehydrogenase. Nat Genet 10:394-399, 1995.

86. Shimkets RA, Warnock DG, Bositis CM, et al. Liddle's syndrome: heritable human hypertension caused by mutations in the beta subunit of the epithelial sodium channel. Cell 79:407-414, 1994.

87. Hansson JH, Nelson Williams C, Suzuki H, et al. Hypertension caused by a truncated epithelial sodium channel gamma subunit: genetic heterogeneity of Liddle syndrome. Nat Genet 11:76-82, 1995.

88. Mansfield TA, Simon DB, Farfel Z, et al. Multilocus linkage of familial hyperkalaemia and hypertension, pseudohypoaldosteronism type II, to chromosomes 1q31-42 and 17p11-q21. Nat Genet 16:202-205, 1997.

89. Simon DB, Nelson Williams C, Bia MJ, et al. Gitelman's variant of Bartter's syndrome, inherited hypokalaemic alkalosis, is caused by mutations in the thiazide-sensitive Na-Cl cotransporter. Nat Genet 12:24-30, 1996.

90. Simon DB, Karet FE, Hamdan JM, et al. Bartter's syndrome, hypokalaemic alkalosis with hypercalciuria, is caused by mutations in the Na-K-2Cl cotransporter NKCC2. Nat Genet 13:183-188, 1996.

91. Simon DB, Karet FE, Rodriguez Soriano J, et al. Genetic heterogeneity of Bartter's syndrome revealed by mutations in the K+ channel, ROMK. Nat Genet 14:152-156, 1996.

92. Simon DB, Bindra RS, Mansfield TA, et al. Mutations in the chloride channel gene, CLCNKB, cause Bartter's syndrome type III. Nat Genet 17:171-178, 1997.

93. Strautnieks SS, Thompson RJ, Gardiner RM, et al. A novel splice-site mutation in the gamma subunit of the epithelial sodium channel gene in three pseudohypoaldosteronism type 1 families. Nat Genet 13:248-250, 1996.

94. Geller DS, Rodriguez Soriano J, Vallo Boado A, et al. Mutations in the mineralocorticoid receptor gene cause autosomal dominant pseudohypoaldosteronism type I. Nat Genet 19:279-281, 1998.

95. Gallagher AR, Hidaka S, Gretz N, et al. Molecular basis of autosomal-dominant polycystic kidney disease. Cell Mol Life Sci 59:682-693, 2002.

96. Koch CA, Vortmeyer AO, Huang SC, et al. Genetic aspects of pheochromocytoma. Endocr Regul 35:43-52, 2001.

97. Woodward ER, Eng C, McMahon R, et al. Genetic predisposition to phaeochromocytoma: Analysis of candidate genes GDNF, RET and VHL. Hum Mol Genet 6:1051-1056, 1997.

98. Sims KB. Von Hippel-Lindau disease: Gene to bedside. Curr Opin Neurol 14:695-703, 2001.

99. Shen MH, Harper PS, Upadhyaya M. Molecular genetics of neurofibromatosis type 1 (NF1). J Med Genet 33:2-17, 1996.

100. Neumann HP, Bausch B, McWhinney SR, et al. The Freiburg-Warsaw-Columbus Pheochromocytoma Study Group. Germline mutations in nonsyndromic pheochromocytoma. N Engl J Med 346:1459-1466, 2002.

101. Geller DS. A mineralocorticoid receptor mutation causing human hypertension. Curr Opin Nephrol Hypertens 10:661-665, 2001.

102. Gates LJ, MacConnachie AA, Lifton RP, et al. Variation of phenotype in patients with glucocorticoid remediable aldosteronism. J Med Genet 33:25-28, 1996.

103. Chang H, Fujita T. Lack of mutations in epithelial sodium channel beta-subunit gene in human subjects with hypertension. J Hypertens 14:1417-1419, 1996.

104. Brand E, Kato N, Chatelain N, et al. Structural analysis and evaluation of the 11beta-hydroxysteroid dehydrogenase type 2 (11beta-HSD2) gene in human essential hypertension. J Hypertens 16:1627-1634, 1998.

105. Wong ZYH, Stebbing M, Ellis JA, et al. Genetic linkage of the beta and gamma subunits of the epithelial sodium channel with systolic blood pressure in the general population. Lancet 353:1222-1225, 1999.

106. Esler M, Jennings G, Lambert G. Noradrenaline release and the pathophysiology of primary human hypertension. Am J Hypertens 2:140S-146S, 1989.

107. Ferrannini E, Buzzigoli G, Bonadonna R, et al. Insulin resistance in essential hypertension. N Engl J Med 317:350-357, 1987.

108. Watt GCM, Harrap SB, Foy CJW, et al. Abnormalities of glucocorticoid metabolism and the renin-angiotensin system: A four corners approach to the identification of genetic determinants of blood pressure. J Hypertens 10:473-482, 1992.

109. Harrap SB, Fraser R, Inglis GC, et al. Abnormal epinephrine release in young adults with high personal and high parental blood pressures. Circulation 96:556-561, 1997.

110. Harrap SB, Cumming AD, Davies DL, et al. Glomerular hyperfiltration, high renin and low-extracellular volume in high blood pressure. Hypertension 35:952-957, 2000.

111. Rigat B, Hubert C, Alhenc Gelas F, et al. An insertion/deletion polymorphism in the angiotensin I-converting enzyme gene accounting for half the variance of serum enzyme levels. J Clin Invest 86:1343-1346, 1990.

112. Costerousse O, Allegrini J, Lopez M, et al. Angiotensin I-converting enzyme in human circulating mononuclear cells: genetic polymorphism of expression in T-lymphocytes. Biochem J 290:33-40, 1993.

113. Panarelli M, Holloway CD, Fraser R, et al. Glucocorticoid receptor polymorphism, skin vasoconstriction, and other metabolic intermediate phenotypes in normal human subjects. J Clin Endocrinol Metab 83:1846-18452, 1998.

114. Dishy V, Sofowora GG, Xie H, et al. The effect of common polymorphisms of the a2-adrenergic receptor on agonist-mediated vascular desensitization. N Engl J Med 345:1030-1035, 2001.

115. Knowles JW, Erickson LM, Guy VK, et al. Common variations in noncoding regions of the human natriuretic peptide receptor A gene have quantitative effects. Hum Genet 112:62-70, 2003.

116. Fornage M, Amos CI, Kardia S, et al. Variation in the region of the angiotensin-converting enzyme gene influences interindividual differences in blood pressure levels in young white males. Circulation 97:1773-1779, 1998.

117. O'Donnell CJ, Lindpaintner K, Larson MG, et al. Evidence for association and genetic linkage of the angiotensin-converting enzyme locus with hypertension and blood pressure in men but not women in the Framingham Heart Study. Circulation 97:1766-1772, 1998.

118. Jeunemaitre X, Soubrier F, Kotelevtsev YV, et al. Molecular basis of human hypertension: role of angiotensinogen. Cell 71:169-180, 1992.

119. Ying LH, Zee RY, Griffiths LR, et al. Association of a RFLP for the insulin receptor gene, but not insulin, with essential hypertension. Biochem Biophys Res Commun 181:486-492, 1991.

120. Schaadt O, Sorensen H, Krogsgaard AR. Association between the C3F-gene and essential hypertension. Clin Sci 61: 363S-365S, 1981.

121. Timmermann B, Mo R, Luft FC, et al. Beta-2 adrenoceptor genetic variation is associated with genetic predisposition to essential hypertension: The Bergen Blood Pressure Study. Kidney Int 53:1455-1460, 1998.

122. Kotanko P, Binder A, Tasker J, et al. Essential hypertension in African Caribbeans associates with a variant of the beta2-adrenoceptor. Hypertension 30:773-776, 1997.

123. Wu DA, Bu X, Warden CH, et al. Quantitative trait locus mapping of human blood pressure to a genetic region at or near the lipoprotein lipase gene locus on chromosome 8p22. J Clin Invest 97:2111-2118, 1996.

124. Krushkal J, Xiong M, Ferrell R, et al. Linkage and association of adrenergic and dopamine receptor genes in the distal portion of the long arm of chromosome 5 with systolic blood pressure variation. Hum Mol Gene 7:1379-1383, 1998.

125. Casari G, Barlassina C, Cusi D, et al. Association of the alpha-adducin locus with essential hypertension. Hypertension 25:320-326, 1995.

126. Miyamoto Y, Saito Y, Kajiyama N, et al. Endothelial nitric oxide synthase gene is positively associated with essential hypertension. Hypertension 32:3-8, 1998.

127. Frossard PM, Lestringant GG. Association between a dimorphic site on chromosome 12 and clinical diagnosis of hypertension in three independent populations. Clin Genet 48:284-287, 1995.

128. Lockette W, Ghosh S, Farrow S, et al. Alpha 2-adrenergic receptor gene polymorphism and hypertension in blacks. Am J Hypertens 8:390-394, 1995.

129. Iwai N, Ohmichi N, Hanai K, et al. Human SA gene locus as a candidate locus for essential hypertension. Hypertension 23:375-380, 1994.

130. Bonnardeaux A, Davies E, Jeunemaitre X, et al. Angiotensin II type 1 receptor gene polymorphisms in human essential hypertension. Hypertension 24:63-69, 1994.

131. Siffert W, Rosskopf D, Siffert G, et al. Association of a human G-protein beta3 subunit variant with hypertension. Nat Genet 18:45-48, 1998.

132. Wilson AF, Elston RC, Tran LD, et al. Use of the robust sib-pair method to screen for single-locus, multiple-locus, and pleiotropic effects: Application to traits related to hypertension. Am J Hum Genet 48:862-872, 1991.

133. Nakayama T, Soma M, Kanmatsuse K. Organization of the human prostacyclin synthase gene and association analysis of a novel CA repeat in essential hypertension. Adv Exp Med Biol 433:127-130, 1997.

134. Julier C, Delepine M, Keavney B, et al. Genetic susceptibility for human familial essential hypertension in a region of homology with blood pressure linkage on rat chromosome 10. Hum Mol Genet 6:2077-2085, 1997.

135. Glorioso N, Filigheddu F, Troffa C, et al. Interaction of alpha(1)-Na,K-ATPase and Na,K,2Cl-cotransporter genes in human essential hypertension. Hypertension 38:204-209, 2001.

136. Bhattacharyya S, Luan J, Challis B, et al. Association of polymorphisms in GPR10, the gene encoding the prolactin-releasing peptide receptor with blood pressure, but not obesity, in a U.K. Caucasian population. Diabetes 52:1296-1299, 2003.

137. Harrap SB, Davidson R, Connor JM, et al. The angiotensin I-converting enzyme gene and predisposition to high blood pressure in man. Hypertension 21:455-460, 1993.

138. Brand E, Chatelain N, Keavney B, et al. Evaluation of the angiotensinogen locus in human essential hypertension: A European study. Hypertension 31:725-729, 1998.

139. Harrap SB, Samani NJ, Lodwick D, et al. The SA gene: predisposition to hypertension and renal function in man. Clin Sci 88:665-670, 1995.

140. Jeunemaitre X, Lifton RP, Hunt SC, et al. Absence of linkage between the angiotensin converting enzyme locus and human essential hypertension. Nat Genet 1:72-75, 1992.

141. Nabika T, Bonnardeaux A, James M, et al. Evaluation of the SA locus in human hypertension. Hypertension 25:6-13, 1995.

142. Berge KE, Berg K. No effect of TaqI polymorphism at the human renal kallikrein (KLK1) locus on normal blood pressure level or variability. Clin Genet 44:196-202, 1993.

143. Kamitani A, Wong ZY, Fraser R, et al. Human alpha-adducin gene, blood pressure, and sodium metabolism. Hypertension 32:138-143, 1998.

144. Kreutz R, Hubner N, Ganten D, et al. Genetic linkage of the ACE gene to plasma angiotensin-converting enzyme activity but not to blood pressure. A quantitative trait locus confers identical complex phenotypes in human and rat hypertension. Circulation 92:2381-2384, 1995.

145. Bonnardeaux A, Nadaud S, Charru A, et al. Lack of evidence for linkage of the endothelial cell nitric oxide synthase gene to essential hypertension. Circulation 91:96-102, 1995.

146. Fornage M, Turner ST, Sing CF, et al. Variation at the M235T locus of the angiotensinogen gene and essential hypertension: a population-based case-control study from Rochester, Minnesota. Hum Genet 96:295-300, 1995.

147. Rotimi C, Morrison L, Cooper R, et al. Angiotensinogen gene in human hypertension. Lack of an association of the 235T allele among African Americans. Hypertension 24:591-594, 1994.

148. Takami S, Wong ZYH, Stebbing M, et al. Linkage analysis of endothelial nitric oxide synthase gene with human blood pressure. J Hypertens 17:1431-1436, 1999.

149. Takami S, Wong ZYH, Stebbing M, et al: Linkage analysis of the glucocorticoid and a2-adrenergic receptor genes with blood pressure and body mass index. Am J Physiol 276: H1379-H1384, 1999.

150. Dickersin K. The existence of publication bias and risk factors for its occurrence. JAMA 263:1385-1389, 1990.

151. Harrap SB, Wong ZY, Stebbing M, et al. Blood pressure QTLs identified by genome-wide linkage analysis and dependence on associated phenotypes. Physiol Genomics 8:99-105, 2002.

152. Lander E, Kruglyak L. Genetic dissection of complex traits: Guidelines for interpreting and reporting linkage results. Nat Genet 11:241-247, 1995.

153. Rao DC, Gu C. False positives and false negatives in genome scans. Adv Genet 42:487-498, 2001.

154. Almasy L, Blangero J. Multipoint quantitative-trait analysis in general pedigrees. Am J Hum Genet 62:1198-1211, 1998.

155. Levy D, DeStefano AL, Larson MG, et al. Evidence for a gene influencing blood pressure on chromosome 17: Genome scan linkage results for longitudinal blood pressure phenotypes in subjects from the Framingham heart study. Hypertension 36:477-483, 2000.

156. Hsueh WC, Mitchell BD, Schneider JL, et al. QTL influencing blood pressure maps to the region of PPH1 on chromosome 2q31-34 in Old Order Amish. Circulation 101:2810-2816, 2000.

157. Kristjansson K, Manolescu A, Kristinsson A, et al. Linkage of essential hypertension to chromosome 18q. Hypertension 39:1044-1049, 2002.

158. Caulfield M, Munroe P, Pembroke J, et al. Genome-wide mapping of human loci for essential hypertension. Lancet 361:2118-2123, 2003.

159. Cooper RS, Luke A, Zhu X, et al. Genome scan among Nigerians linking blood pressure to chromosomes 2, 3, and 19. Hypertension 40:629-633, 2002.

160. Rice T, Rankinen T, Province MA, et al. Genome-wide linkage analysis of systolic and diastolic blood pressure: the Quebec Family Study. Circulation 102:1956-1963, 2000.

161. Allayee H, de Bruin TW, Michelle Dominguez K, et al. Genome scan for blood pressure in Dutch dyslipidemic families reveals linkage to a locus on chromosome 4p. Hypertension 38:773-778, 2001.

162. Rice T, Rankinen T, Chagnon YC, et al. Genomewide linkage scan of resting blood pressure: HERITAGE Family Study. Health, Risk Factors, Exercise Training, and Genetics. Hypertension 39:1037-1043, 2002.

163. Hunt SC, Ellison RC, Atwood LD, et al. Genome scans for blood pressure and hypertension: The National Heart, Lung, and Blood Institute Family Heart Study. Hypertension 40:1-6, 2002.

164. Perola M, Kainulainen K, Pajukanta P, et al. Genome-wide scan of predisposing loci for increased diastolic blood pressure in Finnish siblings. J Hypertens 18:1579-1585, 2000.

165. Ranade K, Hinds D, Hsiung CA, et al. A genome scan for hypertension susceptibility loci in populations of Chinese and Japanese origins. Am J Hypertens 16:158-162, 2003.

166. Krushkal J, Ferrell R, Mockrin SC, et al. Genome-wide linkage analyses of systolic blood pressure using highly discordant siblings. Circulation 99:1407-1410, 1999.

167. Thiel BA, Chakravarti A, Cooper RS, et al. A genome-wide linkage analysis investigating the determinants of blood pressure in whites and African Americans. Am J Hypertens 16: 151-153, 2003.

168. Angius A, Petretto E, Maestrale GB, et al. A new essential hypertension susceptibility locus on chromosome 2p24-p25, detected by genomewide search. Am J Hum Genet 71:893-905, 2002.

169. Zhu DL, Wang HY, Xiong MM, et al. Linkage of hypertension to chromosome 2q14-q23 in Chinese families. J Hypertens 19:55-61, 2001.

170. Rao DC, Province MA, Leppert MF, et al. A genome-wide affected sibpair linkage analysis of hypertension: the HyperGEN network, Am J Hypertens 16:148-150, 2003.

171. Atwood LD, Samollow PB, Hixson JE, et al. Genome-wide linkage analysis of blood pressure in Mexican Americans. Genet Epidemiol 20:373-382, 2001.

172. Sharma P, Fatibene J, Ferraro F, et al. A genome-wide search for susceptibility loci to human essential hypertension. Hypertension 35:1291-1296, 2000.

173. Kardia SLR, Rozek LS, Krushkal J, et al. Genome-wide linkage analyses for hypertension genes in two ethnically and geographically diverse populations. Am J Hypertens 16:154-157, 2003.

174. Lander ES, Schork NJ. Genetic dissection of complex traits. Science 265:2037-2048, 1994.

175. Cui J, Hopper JL, Harrap SB. Antihypertensive treatments obscure familial contributions to blood pressure variation. Hypertension 41:207-210, 2003.

176. Williams RR, Hunt SC, Hasstedt SJ, et al. Multigenic human hypertension: Evidence for subtypes and hope for haplotypes. J Hypertens Suppl 8:S39-S46, 1990.

177. Drayer JI, Weber MA, Laragh JH, et al. Renin subgroups in essential hypertension. Clin Exp Hypertens A 4:1817-1834, 1982.

178. Hopkins PN, Hunt SC, Jeunemaitre X, et al. Angiotensinogen genotype affects renal and adrenal responses to angiotensin II in essential hypertension. Circulation 105:1921-1927, 2002.

179. Glorioso N, Filigheddu F, Cusi D, et al. Alpha-Adducin 460Trp allele is associated with erythrocyte Na transport rate in North Sardinian primary hypertensives. Hypertension 39:357-362, 2002.

180. Panarelli M, Holloway CD, Fraser R, et al. Glucocorticoid receptor polymorphism, skin vasoconstriction, and other metabolic intermediate phenotypes in normal human subjects. J Clin Endocrinol Metab 83:1846-1852, 1998.

181. Freeman K, Farrow S, Schmaier A, et al. Genetic polymorphism of the alpha 2-adrenergic receptor is associated with increased platelet aggregation, baroreceptor sensitivity, and salt excretion in normotensive humans. Am J Hypertens 8: 863-869, 1995.

182. Pankow JS, Rose KM, Oberman A, et al. Possible locus on chromosome 18q influencing postural systolic blood pressure changes. Hypertension 36:471-476, 2000.

183. Harrap SB, Cui JS, Wong ZY, et al. Familial and genomic analyses of postural changes in systolic and diastolic blood pressure. 243(3):586-591. 2004, [Epub 2004 Feb 09].

184. Camp NJ, Hopkins PN, Hasstedt SJ, et al. Genome-wide multi-point parametric linkage analysis of pulse pressure in large, extended Utah pedigrees. Hypertension 42:322-328, 2003.

185. Mancia G, Omboni S, Parati G. Lessons to be learned from 24-hour ambulatory blood pressure monitoring. Kidney Int Suppl 55:S63-S68, 1996.

186. Schwartz GL, Turner ST, Sing CF. Association of genetic variation with interindividual variation in ambulatory blood pressure. J Hypertens 14:251-258, 1996.

187. Terwilliger JD, Goring HH. Gene mapping in the 20th and 21st centuries: Statistical methods, data analysis, and experimental design. Human Biol 72:63-132, 2000.

188. Ardlie KG, Kruglyak L, Seielstad M. Patterns of linkage disequilibrium in the human genome. Nature Rev Genet 3:299-309, 2002.

189. Altmuller J, Palmer LJ, Fischer G, et al. Genomewide scans of complex human diseases: True linkage is hard to find. Am J Hum Genet 69:936-950, 2001.

190. Eaves IA, Merriman TR, Barber RA, et al. The genetically isolated populations of Finland and Sardinia may not be a panacea for linkage disequilibrium mapping of common disease genes. Nat Genet 25:320-323, 2000.

191. Weiss KM, Terwilliger JD. How many diseases does it take to map a gene with SNPs. Nat Genet 26:151-157, 2000.

192. Jaenisch R, Bird A. Epigenetic regulation of gene expression: how the genome integrates intrinsic and environmental signals. Nat Genet 33:245-254, 2003.

193. The FBPP Investigators. Multi-center genetic study of hypertension: The Family Blood Pressure Program (FBPP). Hypertension 39:3-9, 2002.

194. Province MA, Kardia SLR, Ranade K, et al. A meta-analysis of genome-wide linkage scans for hypertension: The National Heart, Lung and Blood Institute Family Blood Pressure Program. Am J Hypertens 16:144-147, 2003.

195. Perusse L, Moll PP, Sing CF. Evidence that a single gene with gender- and age-dependent effects influences systolic blood pressure determination in a population-based sample. Am J Hum Genet 49:94-105, 1991.

196. Ellis JA, Wong ZYH, Stebbing M, et al. Sex, genes and blood pressure. Clin Exp Pharmacol Physiol 28:1053-1055, 2001.

197. Lever AF, Harrap SB. Essential hypertension: A disorder of growth with origins in childhood? J Hypertension 10:101-120, 1992.

198. Ellis JA, Stebbing M, Harrap SB. Association of the human Y chromosome with high blood pressure in the general population. Hypertension 36:731-733, 2000.

199. Charchar FJ, Tomaszewski M, Padmanabhan S, et al. The Y chromosome effect on blood pressure in two European populations. Hypertension 39:353-356, 2002.

200. Abecasis GR, Cherny SS, Cardon LR. The impact of genotyping error on family-based analysis of quantitative traits. Eur J Hum Genet 9:130-134, 2002.

201. Douglas JA, Skol AD, Boehnke M. Probability of detection of genotyping errors and mutations as inheritance inconsistencies in nuclear-family data. Am J Hum Genet 70:487-495, 2002.

202. Sobel E, Papp JC, Lange K. Detection and integration of genotyping errors in statistical genetics. Am J Hum Genet 70: 496-508, 2002.

203. Page GP, George V, Go RC, et al. "Are we there yet?": deciding when one has demonstrated genetic causation in complex diseases and quantitative traits. Am J Hum Genet 73:711-719, 2003.

204. Bianchi G, Staessen JA, Patrizia F. Pharmacogenomics of primary hypertension—the lessons from the past to look toward the future. Pharmacogenomics 4:279-296, 2003.

205. Harrap SB, Tzourio C, Cambien F, et al. The ACE gene I/D polymorphism is not associated with the blood pressure and cardiovascular benefits of ACE inhibition. Hypertension 42:297-303, 2003.

206. Kurtz TW, Gardner DG. Transcription-modulating drugs: A new frontier in the treatment of essential hypertension. Hypertension 32:380-386, 1998.

207. Jin L, Zhang JJ, Chao L, et al. Gene therapy in hypertension: adenovirus-mediated kallikrein gene delivery in hypertensive rats. Hum Gene Ther 8:1753-1761, 1997.

208. Phillips MI. Antisense inhibition and adeno-associated viral vector delivery for reducing hypertension. Hypertension 29:177-187, 1997.

209. Lin KF, Chao J, Chao L. Human atrial natriuretic peptide gene delivery reduces blood pressure in hypertensive rats. Hypertension 26:847-853, 1995.

210. Lin KF, Chao L, Chao J. Prolonged reduction of high blood pressure with human nitric oxide synthase gene delivery. Hypertension 30:307-313, 1997.

211. Martens JR, Reaves PY, Lu D, et al. Prevention of renovascular and cardiac pathophysiological changes in hypertension by angiotensin II type 1 receptor antisense gene therapy. Proc Natl Acad Sci (USA) 95:2664-2669, 1998.

212. Bashyam MD, Savithri GR, Kumar MS, et al. Molecular genetics of familial hypertrophic cardiomyopathy (FHC). J Hum Genet 48:55-64, 2003.

213. Harrap SB, Petrou S. Utility of genetic approaches to common cardiovascular diseases. Am J Physiol 281:H1-H6, 2001.

# The Sympathetic Nervous System in Acute and Chronic Blood Pressure Elevation

## Joseph L. Izzo, Jr.

It has been almost 150 years since Claude Bernard proposed the concept of "sympathetic function," by which he meant an organized patterned response of an animal to its external environment. In his vision, vasomotor nerves helped preserve the "internal milieu" in an overall normative process later called homeostasis. We now know that there is a wide spectrum of responses of the sympathetic nervous system (SNS) that ranges from mild to massive and from acute to chronic. With respect to cardiovascular regulation, the SNS is the only system in the body capable of both momentary (seconds to minutes) and sustained (days to years) regulation of blood pressure (BP).[1,2] The SNS also plays a key role in extracellular volume regulation, metabolism, and thermoregulation. Because there is basal activity of the SNS at all times, it is logical to question whether hypertension and its associated metabolic abnormalities are related to SNS dysregulation. Such questions have been raised for more than a century but never satisfactorily resolved due to many factors, including the intrinsic complexity of the SNS; the cumbersome, expensive, and limited techniques required to study it; the complexity of the syndromes in which the SNS must be evaluated; the relative lack of direct clinical applications; and the failure of research agencies to fund investigations involving complex physiologic integrative science. Nevertheless, the conclusion that the SNS is intimately involved with all forms of hypertension is the inescapable theme of this chapter. Included are discussions of the organization of the SNS; links of sympathetic function with obesity, insulin resistance, and volume dysregulation; the complex effects of aging on SNS function; and the role of the SNS in secondary forms of hypertension.

## ORGANIZATION AND FUNCTION OF THE SYMPATHETIC NERVOUS SYSTEM

For the purposes of this discussion, the SNS will be considered to include the vasomotor control centers within the central nervous system (CNS), the peripheral afferent and efferent sympathetic nerves, and the adrenal medulla. The arborized, multilayered, cross-linked organizational pattern of the central and peripheral SNS provides numerous mechanisms by which the SNS can affect BP. A review of these mechanisms and selected animal studies provides an important backdrop for understanding the potential role of the SNS in human hypertension.

### Central Neuroanatomy and Sympathetic Nervous System Outflow Control

Much of our neuroanatomic understanding derives from the elegant studies of the late Donald Reis and others who identified the functional role of several CNS nuclei in acute and chronic BP regulation[3-6] (Figure 6–1). Reflex and behavioral control of arterial pressure is integrated in the rostral ventrolateral nucleus of the medulla oblongata (RVLM), which is sometimes called the vasomotor control center.[3,5] Cell bodies of efferent SNS cardiovascular stimulatory neurons lie in the $C_1$ subregion, which also receives and sends neural projections to and from many other CNS centers.[4,7] The most critical RVLM input comes from the adjacent nucleus tractus solitarius (NTS), which receives afferent fibers from stretch-sensitive mechanoreceptors in the carotid sinus and aortic arch (aorto-carotid baroreflexes), and the cardiac atria and ventricles (cardiopulmonary baroreflexes).[6-8] Signals from the NTS *inhibit* RVLM sympathetic outflow and tend to buffer acute BP changes.[6,9] In parallel, the NTS receives signals from *stimulatory* chemoreceptors in the kidneys and skeletal muscle.[6] The NTS integrates a variety of signals from stimulatory and inhibitory centers in the brain stem, basal ganglia, and cortex, including the overlying area postrema (AP) located in the floor of the fourth ventricle.[10] The NTS is also controlled by signals from the overlying AP, which does not have a blood-brain barrier.[11] The AP is exquisitely sensitive to circulating angiotensin II (Ang II), which acts to blunt the inhibitory effect of the NTS, thereby increasing RVLM-dependent SNS outflow.[11-14] The NTS-RVLM complex also receives sensory input from excitatory peripheral chemoreceptor afferent neurons in the kidneys and skeletal muscle that act to enhance or sustain RVLM-dependent SNS outflow.[6,7]

## The Brain Stem in Hypertensive Models

CNS centers that modulate or control SNS outflow clearly affect acute and chronic BP levels in animal models of hypertension. In spontaneously hypertensive rats (SHR), sympathectomy prevents the development of hypertension.[15] Brain stem regions in particular seem to participate in all forms of experimental hypertension. Ablation of the NTS in normal rats causes increased SNS outflow and either severe BP lability[9] or severe chronic hypertension with organ damage,[16] which can be abolished by simultaneous lesions of the RVLM.[17] Lesions in the AP lower BP in rats with genetic[17] and steroid-induced hypertension,[13,18] while stimulation of the AP by Ang II sustains genetic and steroid-induced hypertension.[11,13,14,18]

## Role of the Hypothalamus in Integration of Behavioral and Cardiovascular Responses

Stress, emotions, and drugs affect SNS function through a variety of CNS centers. Different patterns of stress responses are initiated by unique activation patterns of participating hypothalamic subregions, with each pattern driving a linked hemodynamic redistribution that optimizes the organisms' response to the environmental stimulus that is present. The

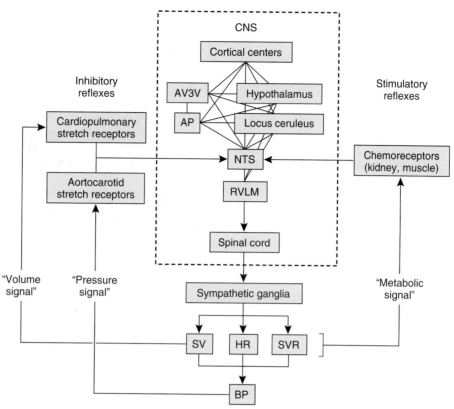

**Figure 6–1** CNS control of sympathetic outflow. Efferent SNS output is the result of integrated actions of several CNS centers, including many areas of the cortex as well as lower centers in the hypothalamus, basal ganglia (especially the locus ceruleus), and circumventricular regions, including the area postrema (AP) and the AV3V region. The critical integrator region is the nucleus tractus solitarius (NTS), which lies in the medulla oblongata. The NTS receives inhibitory afferent signals from the baroreflexes (volume and pressure signals) and stimulatory afferent signals from renal and muscular chemoreceptors (metabolic signals). SNS outflow is ultimately dependent on stimulation of the rostral ventrolateral medulla (the RVLM or vasomotor control center), which is tonically inhibited by the adjacent NTS. Circumventricular regions such as the AP are of particular interest because they have no blood-brain barrier; stimulation of the AP by circulating angiotensin II (Ang II) blunts the inhibitory effects of the NTS. Ultimately, RVLM stimulation sends signals via the spinal cord and sympathetic ganglia to regulate heart rate, cardiac stroke volume (SV), and systemic vascular resistance (SVR), which together determine momentary and chronic blood pressure (BP) levels.

posterolateral hypothalamus mediates defense reactions such as the global "fight or flight" response, which induces massive RVLM activation, with increased heart rate and BP and vasodilation in skeletal muscle.[19,20] Brody et al. identified the anteroventral third ventricular (AV3V) region as a region capable of modulating baroreflex function and SNS outflow in a complex pattern.[21-23] The median preoptic nucleus in this region serves to integrate water balance and thirst-sensing mechanisms with cardiovascular signals and may mediate organ-specific responses such as skeletal muscle vasodilation.[23] Thus, an interplay of CNS influences affects SNS outflow and these phenomena may also be involved in the heterogeneous syndrome of human essential hypertension.

Many other CNS nuclei have been found to modulate SNS outflow but a full discussion is beyond the limits of this work. For example, epinephrine release during exercise is blunted by benzodiazepine therapy.[24] The specificity of benzodiazepines for GABA-ergic neurons in the locus ceruleus strongly suggests a participatory role of that region of the basal ganglia in epinephrine-mediated hemodynamic responses.[25] Various other integrated hemodynamic response patterns are also necessary to meet different emotional and physiologic demands. For exam-

ple, an individual can experience different patterns of hemodynamic stimulation that are dependent on the individual's state-of-mind. Stimuli perceived as challenging or manageable are characterized by SNS-mediated increases in cardiac output, whereas stimuli perceived as threatening or outside the individual's range of control are associated with systemic vasoconstriction.[26,27] These differential hemodynamic responses are not genetically determined because they are not predicted by family history of hypertension and because both threat and challenge patterns can be seen in the same individual.[26] In extreme situations such as vagal syncope, bradycardia is the result of a general parasympathetic override of SNS outflow that involves the nucleus ambiguus and other hypothalamic centers.

## The Hypothalamus in Hypertensive Models

In addition to acute changes in BP, the hypothalamus may affect long-term BP control as well. Ablation of the posterior hypothalamus reduces BP in steroid-induced, genetic, and renal hypertension.[28] Lesions of the anterior hypothalamus dramatically increase BP via massive adrenomedullary stimulation in normotensive rats, whereas electrical stimulation of this region causes hypotension.[16,29] Ablation of the paraventricular nucleus prevents the development of hypertension in SHR.[30]

## The Spinal Cord and Peripheral Neurons

The SNS efferent impulses generated by cell bodies in the RVLM-C$_1$ region are conducted through efferent axons that run in the intermediolateral columns of the spinal cord and outward to the sympathetic ganglia. The pattern of neuronal arborization that is created allows an extremely small number of RVLM cell bodies to amplify the overall signal while allowing an extremely diverse system of linked organ-specific responses. Further amplification of the SNS signal occurs at the level of individual peripheral sympathetic neurons because each axon contains a series of norepinephrine (NE)-containing varicosities arranged like a string of beads that release NE in response to RVLM activation. Thus, the interlinked arborized organization of the SNS allows a spectrum of graded hemodynamic responses that range from subtle changes in regional blood flow to massive stimulation during fight or flight responses or in response to such major stimuli as severe hemorrhage, hypotension, hypoglycemia, or hypothermia.

## Peripheral Hyperinnervation in Hypertensive Models

A series of studies suggests that SHR are anatomically hyperinnervated, as reflected in the increased number,[31] axonal volume,[32] and granular NE content[33] of peripheral sympathetic nerves in these animals. In addition, the NE content[34] and expression of mRNA for nerve growth factor (NGF) in caudal and mesenteric arteries and kidney[35] are increased during development in these rats, and early treatment with antibody to NGF prevents this hyperinnervation and the accompanying vascular hypertrophy and lowers BP.[33] A pattern of accelerated growth of renal sympathetic innervation has also been described in SHR.[36]

## Adrenal Medulla

The adrenal medulla is a specialized postganglionic sympathetic organ that is responsible for the secretion of epinephrine and NE into the circulation in response to cardiovascular and metabolic stimuli. The adrenal medulla is dually controlled by the locus ceruleus and the RVLM area of the brain stem, as already noted.[24,37] Generally speaking, stimuli that cause substantial adrenomedullary responses are relatively major in magnitude, such as hypoglycemia, strenuous exercise beyond the anaerobic threshold, or hemorrhage. Whether the small increases in adrenal epinephrine secretion that occur during less intensive stimuli (postural change or mild mental stress) play a significant role in cardiovascular homeostasis is less clear.[37]

## Intrasynaptic Neuromodulation

The release of NE from storage granules in peripheral sympathetic varicosities is an exocytotic process dependent on intracellular calcium release.[38] Neuronally released NE faces one of three fates within the synapse: Reuptake (uptake 1) into the presynaptic noradrenergic varicosity removes about 80% of the NE released into the synapse; uptake and metabolism by postsynaptic cells (uptake 2) releases O-methylated metabolites in urine or plasma; diffusion (spillover) from the synaptic cleft releases NE into the extracellular fluid.[39] Speculation about reduced catecholamine uptake in states of SNS excess has not been clearly substantiated, however. A variety of substances act at specific receptors on postganglionic presynaptic membranes to modify local neurotransmission, either reducing or augmenting the amount of NE released with each electrical nerve impulse.[40-42] The most important of these presynaptic receptors is the $\alpha_2$ receptor, which is usually occupied by NE. $\alpha_2$ Receptors act as conservators of peripheral neurotransmission by signaling the noradrenergic neuron that NE is already present in the synaptic cleft and that subsequent nerve impulses need not release the same amount of NE as the immediately previous ones. This system thus provides a check and balance to excessive SNS discharge. Presynaptic $\alpha_2$ receptors are probably the main site of action of central sympatholytics such as clonidine, guanfacine, guanadrel, methyldopa, and rilmenidine, which compete with NE at $\alpha_2$ or imidazoline receptors to exert their effects. In direct opposition to these inhibitory presynaptic receptors are stimulatory presynaptic receptors such as $\beta_2$ receptors and Ang II receptors[42,43] that augment the amount of NE released per nerve impulse. Rand[42] first postulated that epinephrine facilitates SNS neurotransmission by functioning as a cotransmitter with NE. Under chronic stress, epinephrine initially released from the adrenal medulla is subsequently taken up into postganglionic neurons in parallel with NE. Subsequent SNS nerve impulses then cause the release of both epinephrine and NE from noradrenergic nerve terminals. If stress is protracted, the stimulatory effect of intrasynaptic epinephrine on presynaptic $\beta_2$ receptors counterbalances the inhibitory effects of intrasynaptic NE on $\alpha_2$ receptors. The clinical importance of this mechanism is not yet clear with respect to chronic hypertension, but studies suggest that the antihypertensive effect of nonselective $\beta$-blockers is related partly to blockade of intrasynaptic $\beta_2$ receptors.[40,44,45]

## Reinforcing Interactions of the Sympathetic Nervous System and Renin-Angiotensin-Aldosterone System

The body's two main BP defense mechanisms, the SNS and renin-angiotensin-aldosterone system (RAAS), have a unique set of mutually reinforcing actions that combine to raise BP acutely and chronically. A major impact of SNS activation is $\beta_1$ receptor–mediated release of renin from the kidney.[46] Renin in turn increases circulating Ang II, which acts at four or more levels to enhance further SNS outflow. First, circulating Ang II acts on CNS nuclei such as the AP, which does not have a blood-brain barrier, to enhance sympathetic outflow.[47,48] Second, Ang II acts on stimulatory presynaptic receptors in CNS and peripheral synapses to enhance the amount of NE (or epinephrine) released by each nerve impulse,[48] similar to the function of presynaptic $\beta$ receptors. Third, Ang II facilitates the effects of NE by virtue of its unique mechanism of inositide-dependent potentiation of calcium influx.[49] A fourth mechanism is the probable blunting of baroreflex suppression of SNS outflow.[11-14] In addition, Ang II has potent direct vasoconstrictive effects, principally via stimulation of AT$_1$ receptors, as well as stimulation of other physiologic responses that indirectly raise BP, including increased thirst, secretion of aldosterone from the adrenal cortex, and secretion of vasopressin (antidiuretic hormone) from the posterior pituitary.[49] Ang II acts together with catecholamines to promote structural changes such as hypertrophy of cardiac[50] and vascular smooth muscle.[51,52] Finally, Ang II promotes inappropriately high renal nerve activity, which directly promotes excessive salt and water retention and the phenotype of salt sensitivity.[53,54]

## Other Neuromodulators

A wide variety of other neurohormones, autacoids, and paracrine factors modify SNS activity centrally and peripherally. Nitric oxide (NO) has significant neuroinhibitory features, as demonstrated by increased SNS nerve traffic after NO synthase blockade.[55,56] Either neuronal NO deficiency or baroreflex desensitization[56] secondary to reduced NO availability has been postulated to contribute to chronic hypertension. Gamma amino butyric acid (GABA) is another neurodepressant, as evidenced by the ability of valproate or muscimol to lower BP in hypertensive rats.[25] Calcitonin gene-related peptide (CGRP) suppresses NE release from the brain stem in normotensive rats but not SHR.[57] The CNS effects of opiates,[58,59] atriopeptins,[60] and probably numerous other substances, are complex and dependent on the individual nuclei affected. Endogenous neurostimulatory substances also exist. SHR demonstrate augmented SNS responses due to activation of glutamate-sensitive neurons in the RVLM.[61] Ouabain also mediates increased RVLM-SNS outflow, but this effect depends to a degree on the presence of Ang II because the prohypertensive effects of ouabain are diminished by $AT_1$ receptor blockade.[62,63] Ouabain-Ang II interactions appear to exert their effects through altered cardiopulmonary baroreflex sensitivity.[63,64]

## Postsynaptic Adrenergic Receptors

$\alpha_1$-Adrenergic receptors tend to be found within adrenergic synapses, particularly on postsynaptic membranes on the adventitial side of the smooth muscle layer of blood vessels and their stimulation causes vasoconstriction, predominantly under the influence of NE. In addition to their intrasynaptic role, $\alpha_2$ receptors are found on endothelium, platelets, white blood cells, and fibroblasts. $\beta_1$ Receptors are found predominately in the heart and kidneys, whereas $\beta_2$ receptors are found in smooth muscle, endothelium, formed blood elements, and presynaptic neural membranes. Stimulation of $\beta_2$ receptors, which are preferentially occupied by epinephrine, tends to vasodilate directly and to increase cardiac output indirectly.

## Effects of Circulating Catecholamines

Contrary to their relatively weak effects on metabolic parameters,[65] physiologic-range elevations of circulating NE can increase plasma renin activity and diastolic blood pressure (DBP).[66,67] Thus, circulating NE should most properly be considered to be a cardiovascular hormone.[66,67] Other effects of physiologic increases in circulating NE include increased platelet and leukocyte number[68] and increased platelet aggregation.[69] Hypertensives have greater platelet aggregability than normotensives.[70]

## Cardiac Chromaffin Cells

The mammalian heart possesses unique perivascular catecholamine-producing cells that are not innervated by postganglionic sympathetic neurons and do not respond to SNS activation.[71] These cells have the potential to regulate a variety of physiologic processes, including growth and development,[72] but their clinical significance is unknown.

## INTEGRATED CARDIOVASCULAR, VOLUME, AND METABOLIC REGULATION

The richness and complexity of the physiologic responses mediated by the SNS is the basis for the complex patterns observed in physiologic and behavioral responses to environmental stimuli.

## Hemodynamic Regulation

The simplified physical equation describing BP (the product of cardiac output and systemic vascular resistance [SVR]) is shown in Figure 6–2, along with the proximal neurohumoral and receptor-mediated efferent factors that acutely control BP. It can be seen from Figure 6–2 that the SNS directly and indirectly affects many different parameters that directly control cardiac output (the product of heart rate and stroke volume) and SVR, which together determine the BP at the moment.

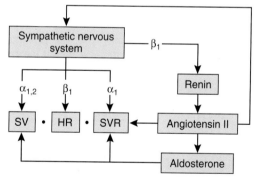

**Figure 6–2** Central position of the sympathetic nervous system (SNS) in blood pressure (BP) regulation. Changes in BP are directly effected by acute or chronic alterations in SNS activity. Hemodynamically, these changes depend on alterations of systemic vascular resistance *(SVR)* or cardiac output, which is the product of heart rate *(HR)* and stroke volume *(SV)*. Cardiac $\beta_1$ receptor stimulation directly increases HR and SV, while renal $\beta_1$ receptor stimulation indirectly increases extracellular fluid volume and cardiac filling pressure (preload). Preload is increased by stimulation of renal nerve–dependent renin release and subsequent production of Ang II and aldosterone. In addition, $\alpha_1$ receptor–mediated peripheral venoconstriction centralizes blood volume, while renal tubular $\alpha_2$ receptor stimulation enhances tubular sodium reabsorption. SVR is dependent on tonic arteriolar constriction that is affected by vascular $\alpha_1$ and Ang II receptors. Circulating Ang II exerts a *positive* feedback on CNS centers, increasing or sustaining SNS outflow.

Cardiac output is highly dependent on ventricular distension during diastole (preload); ventricular preload is in turn dependent on SNS-mediated peripheral venoconstriction and venous volume. Ventricular performance is diminished by factors that increase impedance to ventricular emptying, mainly increased systolic blood pressure (SBP) and central arterial stiffness. Under resting conditions, cardiac output and SVR counterregulate each other so that BP remains relatively constant. Maintenance of a relatively constant central BP in response to common physiologic stimuli is thus dependent on simultaneous matching of flow and resistance.[2,73,74] BP itself is only a loosely regulated physiologic variable that is directly influenced by the activity of the SNS. For example, during postural adaptation, venous return is limited by gravitational pooling of blood and cardiac output is about 20% to 25% less than that of the supine position. During dynamic exercise, cardiac output can increase by as much as fourfold and hypertensives exhibit a slightly greater increase in cardiac output with reduced exercise-induced systemic vasodilation.[75] Teleologically, it is probable that SNS-mediated central vasoregulation conferred adaptive advantages by allowing effective adjustments to upright posture but also aided in times of significant hemorrhage or dehydration.

The traditional view that hypertension is caused by an isolated increase in SVR is a gross oversimplification but the simplified hemodynamic model remains useful for instructional purposes. SVR measured under supine resting conditions in hypertensive subjects tends to be elevated, but the overlap with the normal range is extremely broad and the differences between normotensives and hypertensives are only modestly statistically significant. The dynamic physiologic variation in SVR is also extremely wide within and between individuals.[76-78] Accordingly, over the range of conditions experienced daily, hypertensives exhibit features of both inappropriately high cardiac output and inappropriately high SVR. The fact that hemodynamic differences between normotensives and hypertensives are both instantaneous and chronic provides a clue that the SNS participates in the pathogenesis of hypertension, at least in a permissive fashion; no other system in the body is capable of such rapid and dynamic responses.[2]

## High-Pressure (Aortocarotid) Baroreceptors and Pressure Regulation

Two distinct inhibitory baroreflex sensor systems exist: One responds to changes in arterial pressure (aortocarotid baroreflexes), the other to changes in cardiac volume and filling (cardiopulmonary baroreflexes). In general these two systems work in tandem to defend systemic perfusion pressure and blood flow. Arterial pressure increases are immediately counterregulated by the aortocarotid baroreflex arc, which begins with stretch receptors within the walls of large arteries (the pressure signal). Baroreceptor loading during acute increases in arterial pressure initiates negative afferent signals that act via the NTS to limit subsequent efferent RVLM-SNS outflow. Reductions in arterial pressure "unload" the aortocarotid baroreflexes, which send afferent signals via the NTS to activate efferent SNS outflow, thereby resulting in increased heart rate, enhanced myocardial contractility, and constriction of arteriolar and venous smooth muscle. The arterial baroreflex system can also respond to metabolic signals generated by the carotid sinus endothelium.[6] Aortocarotid baroreceptors are sensitized by

prostanoids[79] and respond to other factors that alter cellular ion transport.[80,81] Whether baroreflex feedback mechanisms continue to function appropriately in hypertension or whether they permit excessive BP variability[82] or inappropriately elevated SNS activity[83-89] remains a central issue in understanding the hemodynamic abnormalities in hypertension.

## Cardiopulmonary Baroreceptors and Volume Regulation

Operating in tandem with the arterial system are the low pressure stretch receptors in the heart and great veins (cardiopulmonary baroreflexes) that sense changes in cardiac stretch and central blood volume (cardiac preload). Decreases in preload, usually caused by loss of blood volume or severe salt depletion, lead to SNS activation; conversely, salt loading or extracellular volume expansion leads to suppression of SNS activity (the volume signal).[90,91] Thames et al. demonstrated that renal sympathetic nerve traffic was normally suppressed by volume loading even after ablation of afferent aortocarotid nerves,[92,93] demonstrating the intimate relationship between cardiac filling and renal nerve activity. In humans, cardiopulmonary baroreflexes can be stimulated separately by lower body negative pressure (LBNP), which increases muscle sympathetic nerve activity, renal vascular resistance, renal overflow of NE, glomerular filtration rate, plasma renin activity, and plasma Ang II, while reducing forearm and splanchnic blood flow.[94-97] Postural adaptation studies in humans also reveal the close relationship between cardiac filling and SNS activity; across both supine and upright postures, plasma NE correlates more strongly with reduced cardiac stroke volume and increased SVR than with central arterial pressure.[98] These integrated physiologic responses can occur independent of any changes in aortocarotid baroreflex activity,[97] although it is clear that the two baroreflex systems also have extensive interactions.[99,100] The net impact of cardiopulmonary baroreflex stimulation can thus supersede that of the aortocarotid system in controlling SNS and RAAS activity, especially during postural adaptation or other conditions that affect central blood volume in dogs[92,93,101] or humans.[98]

## Renal Nerves

Afferent and efferent renal sympathetic nerves are extremely important as direct controllers of renal hemodynamics and volume homeostasis. Renal nerve stimulation causes renal vasoconstriction[102,103] and also regulates renin release.[104-106] There are collateral synapses of RVLM-$C_1$ axons on noradrenergic cell bodies in the spinal cord that offer the opportunity for regional modulation of SNS responses.[4] The most relevant of these regional modulating influences is probably the reno-renal reflex that modifies contralateral renal hemodynamics in response to changes in ipsilateral flow and function.[107,108] Juxtaglomerular cells release renin primarily via activation of membrane $\beta_1$ adrenoceptors[109] but $\alpha_1$ adrenoceptors also stimulate renin release,[102,103] probably via altering tubular sodium content or macula densa function.[104] Given these interrelationships between the SNS and the RAAS, a permissive role of the SNS in renovascular hypertension could be anticipated. The physiologic importance of renal nerves is further demonstrated by experimental denervation of the kidney, which leads to a salt-wasting state.[110]

Relative salt wasting also occurs after pharmacologic sympathectomy with guanethidine in humans[111,112] and in autonomic insufficiency.[113] Renal salt wasting is a major reason why individuals with autonomic insufficiency have abnormally low blood volume and orthostatic hypotension. Renal nerves also mediate the hypertension caused by NO synthase inhibition in rats because renal denervation prevents the BP increases.[114]

## Baroreflex Abnormalities with Aging and Hypertension

Arterial baroreceptors exert an important permissive influence in chronic hypertension because they can never fully return BP or heart rate to normal if there is sufficient acute or chronic SNS stimulation. Two factors can be identified in the limitation of baroreflex activity, baroreflex resetting, and baroreflex blunting. Resetting of arterial baroreceptors is necessary in order for the baroreflex to continue to respond to acute changes in pressure, even when BP is mildly elevated.[115] Thus the SNS can never be completely suppressed by the baroreflex.[85,115-118] Although there remains an inverse correlation between resting plasma NE and arterial baroreflex sensitivity in chronic hypertension,[84] it can be argued that the apparent normal levels of SNS outflow are still inappropriately elevated. Chronic arterial baroreflex blunting also occurs with long-standing hypertension, where the relative ability of a given pressure increase to reduce SNS outflow is also diminished. Baroreflex blunting is associated with aging[116,118] and with conditions such as chronic hypertension[84] or renal failure,[119] in all of which there is increased arterial stiffness and presumably, reduced arterial mechanoreceptor distensibility.[118] Arterial baroreflex dysfunction in the setting of age-related arterial stiffness is an attractive explanation for the positive interrelationships among age, SNS activity, and BP.[87,88,120]

Altered sensitivity of cardiopulmonary baroreflexes may also play a significant role in permitting chronic increases in SNS activity with aging and hypertension. Hajduczok demonstrated that impaired cardiopulmonary baroreflexes contribute to the age-related increases in SNS activity.[86] When cardiac filling is reduced equally, borderline hypertensives exhibit augmented muscle sympathetic activation compared with normotensives.[97,121-123] In volume loading experiments in dogs with renal failure and hypertension, blunting of both cardiopulmonary and aortocarotid baroreflexes was found.[92,93] CNS ouabain and Ang II may play a role in cardiopulmonary baroreflex blunting because the slope of the curve in hypertensives is normalized by digitalis.[62,64]

## Metabolic Regulation and Thermoregulation

The SNS controls intermediary metabolism and body temperature by several interrelated mechanisms. Maintenance of peripheral metabolic homeostasis is generally blood flow dependent, and low-flow situations or conditions of high muscular energy expenditure decrease tissue pH and alter local redox potential, which stimulates peripheral chemoreceptors to enhance CNS sympathetic output in an effort to increase tissue blood flow (the metabolic signal).[6] The significance of these reflexes in hypertension has not been established. Thermoregulation is influenced by cutaneous blood flow reg-

ulation and sweating, which is mediated by acetylcholine rather than NE. Cold exposure creates the need for SNS activation to constrict blood flow to the extremities and the skin, reducing convective heat loss. Body temperature is also potentially influenced by the catabolic effects of catecholamines on adipose tissue, which can increase caloric availability and subsequent heat generation. In rodents, the metabolism of brown adipose tissue is regulated directly by catecholamines and adrenergic receptors.[124,125] Speculation exists that visceral fat in man is the rough equivalent of brown fat in rats.

The role of the SNS in the regulation of body temperature involves selective cutaneous vasoconstriction. A link exists to energy combustion because vascular sensitivity to NE is increased by free fatty acids, which are liberated by the action of catecholamines on adipose tissue.[125] Young and Landsberg demonstrated that sucrose overfeeding increases SNS activity, as manifested by increased cardiac NE turnover in rats.[126] In contrast, starvation decreases SNS activity in rats and humans.[126-128] The SNS also plays a major role in glucose homeostasis, providing an early line of defense against hypoglycemia.[126]

Both NE and epinephrine have diabetogenic properties and infusion of catecholamines causes a rise in blood glucose similar to that found in pheochromocytoma.[129] Increased SNS activity promotes hyperglycemia by a variety of mechanisms, including epinephrine-induced glucose biosynthesis from lactate and amino acids,[128,129] and β receptor–mediated decreases in glycogen synthase activity. The effects of NE in vivo on insulin and glucagon release are complicated by the influences of glucose, potassium, calcium, and growth hormone.[130] Stimulation of α-adrenergic receptors by catecholamines inhibits insulin secretion by pancreatic cells.[131] In contrast, pancreatic islet cells pretreated with NE show enhanced glucose-mediated secretion of insulin.[126]

## Microcirculatory Protective Effects of Sympathetic Nerves

Although excessive SNS activity may be globally harmful, catecholamines and sympathetic nerves may also have organ protective effects via reflex arteriolar constriction, which may protect the capillaries of the brain and kidney from surges in SBP. A baroprotective role of cerebral sympathetic nerves was uncovered by Heistad et al., who unilaterally denervated the cerebral vasculature in stroke-prone rats and found that fatal stroke occurred rapidly in the hemisphere ipsilateral to the sympathetic denervation.[132-134] In the syndrome of malignant hypertension, cerebral edema is worsened by sympathectomy, which causes increased cerebral blood flow.[134] In rats made acutely hypertensive by stellate ganglion stimulation, cerebral sympathetic nerve stimulation limits hyperemia.[135] In the kidney, afferent arteriolar constriction may slow the progression of glomerulosclerosis.[136] Presumably, sufficient lowering of systemic pressure in hypertensives reduces the need for precapillary arteriolar protection of the microcirculation.

## ENVIRONMENTAL STRESS AND BLOOD PRESSURE

The relatively loose regulation of BP is most apparent during times of physiologic stress, especially pain, exercise, and mental stress. The role of environmental and psychosocial stress in hypertensives is reviewed extensively in Chapter 7.

## Acute Mental Stress and Blood Pressure

The SNS stimulation that occurs repeatedly throughout the day as a result of mental stress and activity causes transitory increases in NE production and BP. Among the most important of these stimuli is physical activity. Although exercise raises BP, physical conditioning overrides this stimulatory effect and leads to effective reduction in basal and stimulated SNS activity and BP,[137,138] as well as cardiovascular risk.[139] Another important SNS stimulant is cigarette smoking.[140] Even though the effects of smoking are transient and BP is only increased for a short time, the repetitive nature of smoking causes an increase in average daily BP. Major stressors that cause acute hypertension are burns, brain injury, surgical interventions such as cardiopulmonary bypass, and general anesthesia, each of which results in marked SNS activation.[140] Exposure to cold and withdrawal from drugs such as opiates and central sympatholytics also acutely activate the SNS. Such episodes are transient, however, and are not associated with chronic hypertension.

## Chronic Stress, Personality Factors, and Blood Pressure

Among the most provocative simple observations about the effects of chronic stress on BP is that BPs are lower in primitive societies than complex societies. Lower socioeconomic groups within complex societies, who lead more stressful lives, have increased rates of hypertension.[141] Because of the difficulty in quantitating stress, however, large trials have generally ignored stress as a cardiovascular risk factor. When diary recordings have been combined with ambulatory BP monitoring, correlations have been found among stressful daily events, increased BP,[142-145] and increased left ventricular mass.[145,147] A major component of workplace BP elevation is stressful interpersonal relationships, particularly with one's immediate supervisor.[147] Specific personality subtypes also appear to predispose to hypertension and cardiovascular disease, but the original description that anxiety-prone individuals with "type A" personalities are at increased risk is no longer generally accepted. Rather, a personality pattern of suppressed hostility or "anger-in,"[148] with controlled, guilt-prone, and submissive characteristics has been found to be associated with hypertension. This personality pattern correlates with elevated plasma NE and increased plasma renin activity[149] and with increased cardiovascular morbidity and mortality.[150]

## Volume Regulation during Stress

Exaggerated stress-induced systemic and renal vasoconstriction contribute to increased SVR, reduced renal blood flow, and blunted natriuresis. Abnormally high renal sympathetic nerve tone thus is an important potential consideration in the pathogenesis of essential hypertension because excess salt and water retention during times of psychologic or physiologic stress contributes to high cardiac output. Delayed natriuresis due to renal vasoconstriction would also be important in sustaining the transient increase in extracellular volume and cardiac output for an extended period of time. If the frequency of significant stressors were sufficiently high, excessive volume retention would result.[107,151-154] Dibona et al. used an air jet stress paradigm to study renal nerves and salt and water excretion in SHR, which exhibited exaggerated renal vasoconstriction and excess salt and water retention during stress.[155] Other studies identified the importance of $\alpha_2$ receptors in CNS control centers in mediating this pattern.[151] In humans, Hollenberg et al. directly measured changes in renal blood flow during mental stress in normotensives with no parental history of hypertension, normotensives with a parental history of hypertension, and borderline hypertensives.[156] In borderline hypertensives there is decreased renal blood flow with mental stress.[156,157] Blunted natriuretic responses during stress would be further exacerbated by the blunting of cardiopulmonary baroreflex suppression of renal sympathetic nerve activity.[92] SNS activation also causes modifiable activation of the RAAS during mental stress,[158] an additional feature promoting impaired salt–water excretion.

## Circadian and Seasonal Variation in Sympathetic Nervous System Activity

The circadian rhythm of BP follows the circadian rhythm of the SNS, which decreases during sleep and then peaks in the morning hours in parallel with plasma renin activity, blood volume, cortisol secretion, cardiac output, body temperature, and other variables. Panza et al. used plethysmographic techniques to demonstrate that the basal vasomotor tone of the peripheral vasculature has a diurnal rhythm that is dependent on $\alpha$-receptor stimulation.[159] SNS activity decreases at night or during sleep along with BP, heart rate, cardiac output, and plasma catecholamines.[160] Superimposed on this circadian pattern are other daily SNS stimuli. Daytime BP is determined principally by daily activities rather than diurnal rhythms,[161,162] as shown most clearly in shift workers.[163] In addition to these high frequency and circadian patterns, seasonal and other ultradian variations in SNS activity have also been reported. During winter months, plasma and urinary catecholamine levels are increased[164-166] and there is increased systemic vasoconstriction, decreased blood volume and cardiac output, and in some cases, seasonal hypertension. Morbidity and mortality patterns also follow the patterns of SNS activation. The morning peaks of myocardial infarction and sudden cardiac death[167,168] and ischemic stroke[169] parallel the morning peak of SNS activity and platelet aggregability. This diurnal pattern is abolished by β-blockers.[167] A seasonal influence on coronary and cerebrovascular disease also exists with higher incidence of angina, heart failure, and mortality rates during winter months.[170-172]

# SYMPATHETIC NERVOUS SYSTEM HYPERACTIVITY IN ESSENTIAL HYPERTENSION

## General Considerations

The foregoing discussion has served to underscore the central position of the SNS in physiologic BP regulation and leads directly to the hypothesis that the SNS plays a major pathogenetic role in chronic human hypertension. At least five major questions arise in considering the role of the SNS in hypertension.

1. *Is the SNS only a trigger mechanism or a sustaining influence in hypertension?* The answer to this question is important for several reasons, including optimal therapy for the condition.
2. *What level of SNS activity is normal in the setting of chronic hypertension?* It can be argued that appropriate SNS outflow should be *low* in hypertension, not normal.
3. *What are the effects of aging or obesity on SNS outflow?* Age, weight, SNS activity, and BP all tend to increase together, so the question of causality or interaction is complex.
4. *If the SNS responds to so many cardiovascular and metabolic signals, can these influences be adequately controlled among individuals?* Assessment of SNS activation ideally requires control of time of day, body temperature, central blood volume, blood glucose, degree of emotional excitation, posture, and degree of physical activity to name several.
5. *Have appropriate study techniques been employed?* None of the current techniques is fully applicable to all forms of investigation.

## Genetic Markers

At present there are no genetic markers for increased SNS activity, but in SHR, the Y-chromosome confers higher BP and SNS activity but not increased pressor responses to physiologic or social stress.[173] The mechanism for this effect is not known but may be related to the stimulatory effects of testosterone on the rate-limiting catecholamine synthetic enzyme tyrosine hydroxylase.[174] Another catecholamine synthetic enzyme, dopamine beta hydroxylase (DBH) and its regulatory genes have been found to be deficient in certain patients with autonomic failure.[175]

## Family History Studies

Family history studies worldwide consistently reveal weak correlations between genetics and various indices of SNS overactivity. In a cross-sectional study of 557 Japanese, high plasma NE was found to predict future hypertension but was not closely related to family history of hypertension.[176-178] These investigators also found that family history of hypertension correlated with supranormal responses of NE and insulin to glucose loading.[176-178] In two smaller American studies, no relationship was found between family history of hypertension and plasma NE, urinary NE,[179] or plasma chromogranin A at rest or after mental stress.[180] A Swedish study, on the other hand, found that family history of hypertension predicted exaggerated responses of urinary catecholamines and heart rate to mental stress.[181] Similar findings, including an association with exaggerated BP responses were observed in an Italian study of children with hypertensive parents,[182] while an Australian study found that normotensives with a parental history of hypertension had elevated plasma NE and increased NE spillover.[183] In a small Swiss study[184] and in African Americans,[185] family history of hypertension was associated with exaggerated responses of muscle sympathetic activity to mental stress. A Canadian study demonstrated that the abnormal heart rate and forearm blood flow responses to mental stress in normotensives with a family history of hypertension could be abolished by α-β-blockade.[186] At the same time, arterial baroreflex sensitivity appears to be inherited separately from hypertension in humans.[187] In all these studies, the overlap between those with and without a family history of hypertension was substantial and the presence of a positive family history explained no more than 20% to 30% of the intergroup differences. Thus increased SNS activity and hypertension appear to be related more to environmental or acquired characteristics than to a strong genetic predetermination.

## Prehypertension and Early Hypertension

The first clinical evidence of SNS overactivity in prehypertensives was the observation that military recruits who later developed hypertension exhibited higher heart rates than those who remained normotensive.[188] Louis was the first to report elevated plasma catecholamines in hypertension, also observing that the abnormal catecholamines and hypertension could be proportionally reduced by the administration of ganglionic blockers.[189] Goldstein reviewed 78 studies published by 1982[190] and concluded that the majority of studies demonstrated elevated plasma NE values in young borderline hypertensives. Urinary catecholamines have been less consistently elevated in early hypertension.[191-193] In the Tecumseh study, 37% of borderline hypertensives were found to have elevated plasma NE along with increased heart rate, cardiac index, and forearm blood flow.[194] This pattern persisted from ages 5 to 23 and was also associated with a parental history of hypertension. More recently, a prospective 10-year follow-up study in initially normotensive Japanese found higher initial plasma NE values in those normotensives whose BPs subsequently increased than in those who remained normotensive,[177,178] clearly suggesting a role for the SNS in the initiation of hypertension. Elevated plasma epinephrine values have been reported to be elevated in early essential hypertensives,[195] who also have evidence of decreased β receptor responsiveness.[196] It has been suggested that increased circulating epinephrine could act as a cotransmitter with NE release that acts to "prime the pump" for sustained elevation of SNS outflow. Another SNS biochemical marker, plasma chromogranin A, is elevated in hypertension.[180]

In the hope of improving upon the relatively low sensitivity of plasma NE for detecting small changes in SNS activity, Esler et al. pioneered the use of steady-state radio-labeled NE infusion techniques to measure NE spillover and found increased whole-body NE spillover in early hypertension, corroborating the conclusions based on studies of plasma NE.[197-199] Kinetic techniques have also yielded data to suggest increased organ-specific NE spillover from the heart, kidney, and jugular vein of hypertensive subjects.[197,200] Despite the intuitive appeal of the kinetic approach, there are discrepancies with respect to data derived from direct muscle sympathetic nerve recordings. For example, kinetic techniques do not reveal increased skeletal muscle SNS traffic in hypertension, a finding consistently demonstrated by venous plasma NE values and by muscle sympathetic nerve recordings.[201,202] Curiously, muscle sympathetic activity has been reported to correlate with renal NE spillover.[203] Furthermore, obese individuals demonstrate reduced cardiac and increased renal NE spillover,[204] data that seem at odds with studies showing increased muscle sympathetic nervous activity in obesity.[205,206] These technical discrepancies should be interpreted in the context of the totality of evidence demonstrating increased SNS activity in early hypertension.

## The Metabolic Syndrome

Central obesity, hypertension, glucose intolerance, and dys-lipidemia compose the metabolic syndrome because they coexist in individuals at prevalence rates greater than would be predicted by chance alone[207,208] (see Chapter 13). The central feature of the metabolic syndrome is probably central adiposity, which is strongly and positively correlated with hypertension at all ages, regardless of gender or race.[209-211] In the Tecumseh study, obesity, insulin resistance, and sympathetic hyperactivity were highly correlated[194]; thus, increased SNS activity appears to be an under-recognized feature of the metabolic syndrome. Increased muscle sympathetic activity has been found in obese individuals[205,206] and there is growing realization of the potential role of the SNS in obesity-related hypertension.[212-214] There is thus a well-documented three-way association among increased SNS activity, obesity, and insulin resistance.[212-215] Not only does increased SNS activity cause insulin resistance but hyperinsulinemia clearly increases SNS activity[216] and probably favors weight gain. Thus, the vicious cycle of increased SNS activity; hyperinsulinemia may be a major pathophysiologic linkage between obesity and hypertension. Insulin-sensitizing drugs such as metformin[217] have been found to decrease SNS activity and BP. Given the diabetogenic actions of catecholamines, it is likely that increased SNS activity itself causes insulin resistance.[129] This hypothesis is consistent with studies showing that when the SNS is activated by lower body negative pressure, human forearm insulin resistance increases[218] and with the ability of the central sympatholytic drug clonidine to lower SNS output and plasma catecholamines while increasing insulin sensitivity in obese dogs.[219] Salt sensitivity is a lesser known association with the metabolic syndrome, as is "nondipping" status of overnight BP.[220]

## Sympathetic Nervous System-Renin-Angiotensin-Aldosterone System Interactions in Hypertension

Given the close relationship between SNS activity and RAAS activity, it would be logical to examine their interactions in essential hypertension. Esler found higher heart rates and cardiac indices among the high-renin hypertensives who also had isolated systolic hypertension.[221] In contrast, the normal-renin hypertensive group had normal heart rates and cardiac indices but elevated peripheral resistance. In addition, the degree of BP lowering following β-blockade was significant only in the high renin subgroup, suggesting that these individuals had neurogenic hypertension.[222] Other studies demonstrated a direct correlation between plasma renin activity and plasma NE in these younger individuals.[223,224] In essential hypertensives, Luft et al. found that mental stress caused exaggerated increases in glomerular filtration and plasma Ang II that were fully blocked by ACE inhibition.[225] Increased RAAS activity may play a role in insulin resistance as well, and insulin resistance may also stimulate Ang II production, because the insulin sensitizer troglitazone has been found to suppress Ang II along with insulin signaling in vascular smooth muscle cells.[226] Thus similar to the pattern observed for insulin resistance and SNS activity, bidirectional reinforcement may also exist for Ang II and insulin resistance.

## Sympathetic Nervous System Activity in Aging and Chronic Hypertension

The presence of multiple confounders in the assessment of appropriateness of SNS outflow has already been emphasized. The most important confounder of assessment of sympathetic activity in chronic hypertension is the close interrelationship among aging, increased SNS activity, and hypertension. Despite the prevalent view that SNS activation is present only in the early phases of hypertension, a more careful review of available information suggests that increased SNS activity remains a major pathogenetic component of essential hypertension at all stages of the disorder. Because body mass increases with age, it can at least be argued that a common thread linking aging, obesity, and hypertension is increased SNS activity. What remains to be identified are the precise mechanisms by which SNS activity increases with aging.

The prevalent view about the effects of aging on circulating catecholamines has been that age adjustment eliminates differences in SNS activity between hypertensives and normotensives. Upon closer scrutiny, however, this dogma appears to be incorrect. Messerli et al.[78] and Izzo et al.[120] found a significant positive correlation among age, plasma NE, and BP in hypertensives. After adjustment for age, a strong residual correlation between plasma NE and SVR remained.[120] Closely related to this pattern is the age-related decrease in β-adrenergic receptors that may explain in part the observed age-related decline in cardiac output.[227,228] In the Normative Aging Study,[229] one of the strongest residual relationships among the various parameters tested as determinants of BP was the age-independent relationship between urinary NE excretion and BP. Plasma epinephrine has also been reported to remain elevated in hypertensives beyond age 60, suggesting a continuing role in sustaining inappropriate SNS activity.[230] Although age-related increases in plasma NE were once believed to be reflections of reduced clearance rather than increased release,[231] this finding is probably explained by technical artifacts introduced by the use of tracer infusion techniques. Clear-cut age-related increases have been documented in muscular sympathetic nerve traffic in normotensives and hypertensives[232-234] and specifically in the resistance arterioles within these tissues.[233] In addition, positron imaging techniques have demonstrated increased cardiac sympathetic activity with advancing age.[235] On balance, it is highly likely that increased SNS activity is a central feature of the age-related increase in BP.

## Antihypertensive Therapy and Sympathetic Nervous System Activity in Sustained Hypertension

In the early twentieth century, the notion that vasomotor nerves contributed to vasoconstriction led to the variably successful practice of surgical sympathectomy of the lower extremities to treat hypertension. Pharmacologic studies were the first techniques used to corroborate increased SNS activity in hypertension. The fist class of oral antihypertensive drugs developed were the ganglionic blocking drugs, which lowered BP but caused significant postural hypotension.[236] These agents were found to cause proportional falls in BP and plasma NE in people with longstanding, severe hypertension.[189] Julius et al. concluded that because elevated cardiac outputs in borderline hypertensives were not normalized by β-blockade without atropine, there was a combination of sympathetic hyperactivity and parasympathetic dysfunction.[237,238] Goldstein found that hypertensive individuals with high resting plasma NE values exhibited a proportional fall in both BP and plasma NE after administration of the central $\alpha_2$-agonist clonidine,[239] confirming results with guanethidine.[189] Similar findings have been demonstrated in patients with kidney failure, another state of increased SNS activity.[240,241] Goldstein demonstrated that the $\alpha_2$ antagonist yohimbine increased SNS outflow and plasma NE to a greater degree in hypertensives than normals.[242] Similarly, Izzo et al. found that when BP was lowered by $\alpha_1$-blockade or nonspecific vasodilation, plasma NE doubled in hypertensive subjects,[243] while ACE inhibitors had no effect on plasma NE. The vasodilator studies of Goldstein and Izzo suggest that baroreflex suppression of SNS outflow masks the intrinsically increased SNS activity in chronic hypertension and, furthermore, that the RAAS plays a role in baroreflex blunting.[243] General clinical experience confirms the general utility of the central sympatholytic agents in hypertension, a finding that supports the concept of inappropriate SNS activity in all forms of chronic hypertension.

## α-Adrenergic Hyperresponsiveness

NE-induced vasoconstriction may be enhanced in hypertension.[244] Egan et al. found increased basal forearm vascular resistance in established hypertensives that could be normalized by α-blockade.[73] Philipp et al.[245] and Kiowski[246] examined the relative contributions of increased plasma NE and increased α-adrenergic vascular responsiveness in established hypertension. After stratification for BP, Phillip found a series of hyperbolic relationships between plasma NE concentration and α-adrenergic responsiveness; those with high plasma NE had low α-adrenergic responsiveness, whereas those with low plasma NE had high α-adrenergic responsiveness.[245] Thus, the impact of the SNS on BP is a combined effect of the amount of agonist and the tissue sensitivity to that agonist. Differential genetic expression of α-adrenergic receptors has been found in different vascular beds, and $\alpha_1$ gene expression increases with age, at least in the internal mammary artery.[248] Racial differences in α-adrenergic responsiveness have been described as well; Black children have higher BPs with lower urinary catecholamines.[248] Egan et al. have reported that α-adrenergic hyperresponsiveness is caused by increased endothelial fatty acid uptake, suggesting another link between metabolism and hypertension.[249] Vascular responses to SNS activation are generally attenuated by aging[250-252] and in diabetes.[250] The significance of this finding in age-related BP increases and hypertension has not been fully evaluated.

## SECONDARY HYPERTENSION

There is clear evidence that inappropriate SNS activity occurs in all forms of secondary hypertension.

## Steroid-induced Hypertension

A significant misconception exists that steroid-induced hypertension is simply volume-dependent hypertension. Substantial evidence in animals and humans suggests that steroid-induced hypertension is neurogenic in nature and is most clearly understood as a disturbance of the equilibrium between volume and SNS-mediated vasoconstriction. Normally, volume loading leads to a suppression of SNS outflow.[90,91] In steroid-induced hypertension, there is elevated or unsuppressable SNS outflow. Although rats implanted with deoxycorticosterone acetate (DOCA) develop hypertension with minimal elevations of catecholamines, their SNS outflow is accentuated by hemorrhage,[253] and pharmacologic interruption of neurotransmission results in BP normalization.[254] Zambraski et al. demonstrated that miniature swine implanted with DOCA, which do not require additional salt loading to manifest hypertension, exhibit increased plasma catecholamines that are normalized by pharmacologic sympathectomy.[255,256] In DOCA-salt rats, adrenalectomy significantly lowers BP and blunts NE release by a reduced cotransmitter effect on presynaptic $\beta_2$ receptors.[257] Although the mechanisms by which steroid excess engenders increased SNS outflow are not fully known, brain stem epinephrine synthesis increases during chronic steroid administration through induction of the epinephrine-synthesizing enzyme phenylethanolamine-N-methyl transferase (PNMT).[258,259] Local epinephrine exerts an excitatory effect on the RVLM to increase SNS outflow, which may interact with impaired cardiopulmonary baroreflexes[259] to sustain the hypertension.

## Renovascular Hypertension

Given the tight interrelationship between the SNS and the RAAS, a permissive role of the SNS in renovascular hypertension should be expected. Renal nerves participate in the maintenance of 2-kidney and 1-kidney renovascular hypertension in the rat because renal denervation substantially lowers BP in these animals.[260,261] In the 1-kidney renovascular model, Katholi et al. found that renal denervation reduced the abnormal hypothalamic NE metabolism that was found[262,263] and corrected the SNS overactivity.[263,264] In these animals, the development of hypertension could be prevented by posterior hypothalamic lesions, chemical sympathectomy, or thoracolumbar dorsal rhizotomy, which selectively ablates afferent renal nerves.[265-267] Thus, renal afferent nerves are important promoters of SNS overactivity, which contributes to the genesis and maintenance of renovascular hypertension.

## Renal Parenchymal Hypertension

Hypertension in renal failure may be simply an extension of essential hypertension, a subject that has recently been extensively reviewed.[268] Plasma catecholamines are elevated in chronic renal failure[240,269] in parallel with elevations in whole-body NE turnover[269] and BP. In uremic humans, hypertension is associated with increased muscle sympathetic nerve traffic.[270] Central sympatholytic drugs such as clonidine are extremely effective in uremic hypertension, causing proportional falls in plasma NE and BP.[240,241] Widespread clinical experience dictates that combined α-β-blockers are also extremely effective in treating hypertension in renal patients. The mechanisms for increased sympathetic discharge in uremia include cardiopulmonary baroreflex failure,[92,93] but it is also likely that abnormal afferent signals from renal nerves contribute to inappropriately high SNS outflow.[271]

## Pheochromocytoma

The paradigm of catecholamine hypertension is the naturally occurring model of pheochromocytoma. In this situation, excessive production of catecholamines directly causes hypertension and the removal of the autonomous catecholamine-secreting tissue cures the hypertension. In pheochromocytoma, plasma catecholamine levels are generally much higher than those observed in essential hypertension.[272] This argument has been used in the past to indicate that catecholamines play no role in essential hypertension. Because about 80% of NE released is immediately taken back up into that nerve terminal, however, the concentration of NE at the postsynaptic membrane in essential hypertension may be similar to that observed in pheochromocytoma.

## Preeclampsia

Microneurographic studies have demonstrated that the syndrome of preeclampsia is associated with marked increases in SNS activity, which was shown to return to normal as BP normalized after delivery.[273] Although this syndrome has features similar to profound volume depletion, the degree of SNS activation is higher than would be expected to occur from a compensatory response to hypovolemia.

## SUMMARY

The SNS is a diverse physiologic regulatory system that modulates normal cardiovascular, renal, and metabolic function in response to existing environmental conditions. Experimental evidence in animals and humans indicates that inappropriately high SNS activity is a feature of all stages and all forms of hypertension. Thus, the SNS participates at least as a facilitator of chronic hypertension and may be a primary etiologic factor in many situations.

## References

1. Izzo JL Jr. The sympathoadrenal system in the maintenance of elevated arterial pressure. J Cardiovasc Pharmacol 6:S514-S521, 1984.
2. Izzo JL Jr. Sympathoadrenal activity, catecholamines, and the pathogenesis of vasculopathic hypertensive target-organ damage. Am J Hypertens 2:305S-312S, 1989.
3. Reis DJ. The brain and hypertension: reflections on 35 years of inquiry into the neurobiology of the circulation. Circulation 70(Suppl III):31-45, 1984.
4. Reis DJ, Ruggiero DA, Morrison SF. The C1 area of the rostral ventrolateral medulla oblongata. Am J Hypertens 2:363S-374S, 1989.
5. Ross CA, Ruggiero DA, Park DH, et al. Tonic vasomotor control by the rostral ventrolateral medulla: effect of electrical or chemical stimulation of the area containing C1 adrenaline neurons on arterial pressure, heart rate and plasma catecholamines and vasopressin. J Neurosci 4:474-494, 1984.
6. Abboud FM. The sympathetic system in hypertension. Hypertension 4(Suppl II):208-225, 1982.
7. Walker JL, Abboud FM, Mark AL, et al. Interaction of cardiopulmonary and somatic reflexes in humans. J Clin Invest 65:1491-1497, 1980.
8. Ferrario CM, Barnes KL, Bohonek S. Neurogenic hypertension produced by lesions of the nucleus tractus solitarii alone or with sinoaortic denervation in the dog. Hypertension 3(Suppl 2): 112-118, 1981.
9. Nathan MA, Reis DJ. Chronic labile hypertension produced by lesions of the nucleus tractus solitarri in the cat. Circ Res 40: 72-80, 1977.
10. Ciriello J, Calaresu FR. Projections from buffer nerves to the nucleus of the solitary tract: an anatomical and electrophysiological study in the cat. J Auton Nerv Syst 3:299-310, 1981.
11. Fink GD, Haywood JR, Bryan WJ, et al. Central site for pressor action of blood-borne angiotensin in rat. Am J Physiol 239:R358-R361, 1980.
12. Lumbers ER, McCloskey DI, Potter EK. Inhibition by angiotensin II of baroreceptor-evoked activity in cardiac vagal efferent nerves in the dog. J Physiol 294:69-80, 1979.
13. Fink GD, Bruner CA, Mangiapane ML. Area postrema is critical for angiotensin-induced hypertension in rats. Hypertension 9:355-361, 1987.
14. Mangiapane ML, Skoog KM, Rittenhouse P, et al. Lesion of the area postrema region attenuates hypertension in spontaneously hypertensive rats. Circ Res. 64:129-135, 1989.
15. Lee RM, Borkowski KR, Leenen FH, et al. Interaction between sympathetic nervous system and adrenal medulla in the control of cardiovascular changes in hypertension. J Cardiovasc Pharmacol 17(Suppl 2):S114-S116, 1991.
16. Nathan MA, Reis DJ. Fulminating arterial hypertension with pulmonary edema from release of adrenomedullary catecholamines after lesions of the anterior hypothalamus in the rat. Circ Res 37: 226-235, 1975.
17. Granata AR, Ruggiero DA, Park DH, et al. Brain stem area with C1 epinephrine neurons mediates baroreflex vasodepressor responses. Am J Physiol 248:H547-H567, 1985.
18. Bruner CA, Mangiapane ML, Fink GD, et al. Area postrema ablation and vascular reactivity in deoxycorticosterone-salt-treated rats. Hypertension 11:668-673, 1988.
19. Juskevich JC, Robinson DS, Whitehorn D. Effect of hypothalamic stimulation in spontaneously hypertensive and Wistar-Kyoto rats. Eur J Pharmacol 51:429-439, 1978.
20. Takeda K, Bunag RD. Sympathetic hyperactivity during hypothalamic stimulation in spontaneously hypertensive rats. J Clin Invest 62:642-648, 1978.
21. Knuepfer MM, Johnson AK, Brody MJ. Identification of brain stem projections mediating hemodynamic responses to stimulation of the anteroventral third ventricle (AV3V) region. Brain Res 294:305-314, 1984.
22. Knuepfer MM, Johnson AK, Brody MJ. Vasomotor projections from the anteroventral third ventricle (AV3V). Am J Physiol 247:139-145, 1984.
23. Mangiapane ML, Brody MJ. Vasoconstrictor and vasodilator sites within anteroventral third ventricle region. Am J Physiol 253:827-831, 1987.
24. Stratton JR, Halter JB. Effect of a benzodiazepine (alprazolam) on plasma epinephrine and norepinephrine levels during exercise stress. Am J Cardiol 56:136-139, 1985.
25. Sasaki S, Nakata T, Kawasaki S, et al. Chronic central GABAergic stimulation attenuates hypothalamic hyperactivity and development of spontaneous hypertension in rats. J Cardiovasc Pharmacol 15(5):706-713, 1990.
26. Allen K, Shykoff BE, Izzo JL Jr. Cognitive appraisal of threat or challenge predicts hemodynamic responses to mental arithmetic and speech tasks. Am J Hypertens 11:134A, 1998.
27. Shykoff BE, Allen K, Izzo JL Jr. Interactions of social support and family history in blood pressure reactivity to psychological stressors. Am J Hypertens 11:134A, 1998.
28. Bunag RD, Eferakeya AD. Immediate hypotensive after effects of posterior hypothalamic lesions in awake rats with spontaneous, renal, or DOCA hypertension. Cardiovasc Res 10:663-671, 1976.
29. Folkow BB, Johansson, Oberg B. A hypothalamic structure with marked inhibitory effect on tonic sympathetic activity. Acta Physiol Scand 47:262-270, 1959.

30. Takeda K, Nakata T, Takesako T, et al. Sympathetic inhibition and attenuation of spontaneous hypertension by PVN lesions in rats. Brain Res 543(2):296-300, 1991.

31. Mangiarua EI, Lee RM. Increased sympathetic innervation in the cerebral and mesenteric arteries of hypertensive rats. Can J Physiol Pharmacol 68(4):492-499, 1990.

32. Albert V, Campbell GR. Relationship between the sympathetic nervous system and vascular smooth muscle: a morphometric study of adult and juvenile spontaneously hypertensive rat/Wistar-Kyoto rat caudal artery. Heart Vessels 5(3): 129-139, 1990.

33. Brock JA, Van Helden DF, Dosen P, et al. Prevention of high blood pressure by reducing sympathetic innervation in the spontaneously hypertensive rat. J Auton Nerv Syst 61(2): 97-102, 1996.

34. Antonaccio MJ, Robson RD, Burrell R. The effects of L-dopa and alpha-methyldopa on reflexes and sympathetic nerve function. Eur J Pharmacol 25:9-18, 1974.

35. Falckh PH, Harkin LA, Head RJ. Nerve growth factor mRNA content parallels altered sympathetic innervation in the spontaneously hypertensive rat. Clin Exp Pharmacol Physiol 19: 541-545, 1998.

36. Gattone VH 2nd, Evan AP, Overhage JM, et al. Developing renal innervation in the spontaneously hypertensive rat: Evidence for a role of the sympathetic nervous system in renal damage. J Hypertens 8(5):423-428, 1990.

37. Cryer PE. Physiology and Pathophysiology of the human sympathoadrenal neuroendocrine system. N Engl J Med 303:436-444, 1980.

38. Rubin RP. The role of calcium in the release of neurotransmitter substances and hormones. Pharmacol Rev 22:389-428, 1970.

39. Iverson LL. Catecholamine uptake process. Br Med Bull 29: 130-135, 1973.

40. Dixon WR, Mosimann WF, Weiner N. The role of presynaptic feedback mechanisms in regulation of norepinephrine release by nerve stimulation. J Pharmacol Exp Ther 209:196-204, 1979.

41. Langer SZ. Pre-synaptic regulation of the release of catecholamines. Pharmacol Rev 32:337-362, 1980.

42. Rand MJ, Majewski H. Adrenaline mediates a positive feedback loop in noradrenergic neurotransmission: its possible role in development of hypertension. Clin Exp Hypertens A6:347-370, 1984.

43. Floras JS, Aylward PE, Victor RG, et al. Epinephrine facilitates neurogenic vasoconstriction in humans. J Clin Invest 81: 1265-1274, 1988.

44. Chang PC, Kriek E, van Brummelen P. Sympathetic activity and presynaptic adrenoceptor function in patients with longstanding essential hypertension. J Hypertens 12(2):179-190, 1994.

45. Draper AJ, Meghji S, Redfern PH. Enhanced presynaptic facilitation of vascular adrenergic neurotransmission in spontaneously hypertensive rats. J Auton Pharmacol 9(2):103-111, 1989.

46. Bunag RD, Page IH, McCubbin JW. Neural stimulation of release of renin. Circ Res 19:851-858, 1966.

47. Zimmerman BG. Evaluation of peripheral and central components of action of angiotensin on the sympathetic nervous system. J Pharm Exp Ther, 158:1-10, 1967.

48. Zimmerman BG. Adrenergic facilitation by angiotensin: does it serve a physiological function? Clin Sci 60:343-348, 1981.

49. Marsden PA, Brenner BM, Ballerman BJ. Mechanisms of angiotensin action on vascular smooth muscle, the adrenal, and the kidney. In Laragh JH, Brenner BM, (eds). Hypertension: Pathophysiology, Diagnosis, and Treatment. New York, Raven Press, 1990; pp 1247-1272.

50. Waeber B, Brunner HR. Cardiovascular hypertrophy: Role of angiotensin II and bradykinin. J Cardiovasc Pharmacol 27(Suppl 2):S36-S40, 1996.

51. Dzau VJ, Gibbons GH. Cell biology of vascular hypertrophy in systemic hypertension. Am J Cardiol. 62:30G-35G, 1988.

52. Griffin SA, Brown WC, MacPherson F, et al. Angiotensin II causes vascular hypertrophy in part by a non-pressor mechanism. Hypertension 17:626-635, 1991.

53. Gavras I, Mulinari R, Gavras H. Renin-angiotensin and vasopressin in the development of salt-induced hypertension. J Hypertens 6:999-1002, 1988.

54. Ichihara A, Inscho EW, Imig JD, et al. Role of renal nerves in afferent arteriolar reactivity in angiotensin-induced hypertension. Hypertension 29(1 Pt 2):442-449, 1997.

55. Sander M, Hansen J, Victor RG. The sympathetic nervous system is involved in the maintenance but not initiation of the hypertension induced by N(omega)-nitro-L-arginine methyl ester. Hypertension 30(1):64-70, 1997.

56. Zanzinger J, Czachurski J, Seller H. Inhibition of sympathetic vasoconstriction is a major principle of vasodilation by nitric oxide in vivo. Circ Res 75(6):1073-1077, 1994.

57. Tsuda K, Tsuda S, Goldstein M, et al. Effects of calcitonin gene-related peptide on [3H]norepinephrine release in medulla oblongata of spontaneously hypertensive rats. Eur J Pharmacol 191(1):101-105, 1990.

58. May CN, Whitehead CJ, Heslop KE, et al. Evidence that intravenous morphine stimulates central opiate receptors to increase sympatho-adrenal outflow and cause hypertension in conscious rabbits. Clin Sci(Lond) 76(4):431-437, 1989.

59. Feuerstein G, et al. Effect of morphine on the hemodynamic and neuroendocrine responses to hemorrhage in conscious rats. Circ Shock 27:219-235, 1989.

60. Shirakami G, Nakao K, Yamada T, et al. Inhibitory effect of brain natriuretic peptide on central angiotensin II-stimulated pressor response in conscious rats. Neurosci Lett 91: 77-83, 1988.

61. Tsuchihashi T, Abe I, Fujishima M. Role of metabotropic glutamate receptors in ventrolateral medulla of hypertensive rats. Hypertension 24(6):648-652, 1994.

62. Budzikowski AS, Huang BS, Leenen FH. Brain "ouabain", a neurosteroid, mediates sympathetic hyperactivity in salt-sensitive hypertension. Clin Exp Hypertens 1998. 20(2):119-140, 1998.

63. Huang BS, Yuan B, Leenen FH. Chronic blockade of brain "ouabain" prevents sympathetic hyper-reactivity and impairment of acute baroreflex resetting in rats with congestive heart failure. Can J Physiol Pharmacol 78:45-53, 2000.

64. Lembo G, Rendina V, Iaccarino G, et al. Digitalis restores the forearm sympathetic response to cardiopulmonary receptor unloading in hypertensive patients with left ventricular hypertrophy. J Hypertens 11:1395-1402, 1993.

65. Silverberg AB, Shah SD, Haymond MW, et al. Norepinephrine: Hormone and neurotransmitter in man. Am J Physiol 234(3):E252-E256, 1978.

66. Izzo JL Jr. Cardiovascular hormonal effects of circulating norepinephrine. Hypertension, 5:787-789, 1983.

67. Licht MR, Izzo JL Jr. Humoral effect of norepinephrine on renin release in humans. Am J Hypertens 2:788-791, 1989.

68. Sloand JA, Hooper M, Izzo JL Jr. Effects of circulating norepinephrine on platelets, leukocytes, and RBC counts by alpha-1 adrenergic stimulation. Am J Cardiol 63:1140-1142, 1989.

69. Clayton S, Cross MJ. The aggregation of blood platelets by catecholamines and by thrombin. J Physiol(Lond), 169:82P-83P, 1963.

70. Vlachakis ND, Aledort L. Hypertension and propranolol therapy: Effect on blood pressure, plasma catecholamines and platelet aggregation. Am J Cardiol 45:321-325, 1980.

71. Huang MH, Friend DS, Sunday ME, et al. An intrinsic adrenergic system in mammalian heart. J Clin Invest 98(6):1298-1303, 1996.

72. Abboud FM. An intrinsic cardiac adrenergic system can regulate cardiac development and function. J Clin Invest 98(6):1275-1276, 1996.

73. Egan B, Panis R, Hinderliter A, et al. Mechanism of increased alpha adrenergic vasoconstriction in human essential hypertension. J Clin Invest 80:812-817, 1987.

74. Egan B, Schmouder R. The importance of hemodynamic considerations in essential hypertension. Am Heart J 116(2 Pt 2): 594-599, 1988.

75. Wilson MF, Sung BH, Pincomb GA, et al. Exaggerated pressure response to exercise in men at risk for systemic hypertension. Am J Cardiol 66:731-736, 1990.

76. Julius S, Conway J. Hemodynamic studies in patients with borderline blood pressure elevation. Circulation 38:282-288, 1968.

77. Safar ME, Weiss YA, Levenson JA, et al. Hemodynamic study of 85 patients with borderline hypertension. Am J Cardiol 31: 315-319, 1973.

78. Messerli FH, Frohlich ED, Suarez DH, et al. Borderline hypertension: Relationship between age, hemodynamics and circulating catecholamines. Circulation 64:760-764, 1981.

79. Chapleau MW, Hajduczok G, Abboud FM. Paracrine role of prostanoids in activation of arterial baroreceptors: An overview. Clin Exper Hypertens A 13(5):817-824, 1991.

80. Sharma RV, Chapleau MW, Hajduczok G, et al. Mechanical stimulation increases intracellular calcium concentration in nodose sensory neurons. Neuroscience 66(2):433-441, 1995.

81. Chapleau MW, Lu J, Hajduczok G, et al. Mechanism of baroreceptor adaptation in dogs: Attenuation of adaptation by the K+ channel blocker 4-aminopyridine. J Physiol 462: 291-306, 1993.

82. Mancia G, Parati G, Pomidossi G, et al. Arterial baroreflexes and blood pressure and heart rate variabilities in humans. Hypertension 8:147-153, 1986.

83. Izzo JL Jr, Taylor AA. The sympathetic nervous system and baroreflexes in hypertension and hypotension. Curr Hypertens Rep 1(3):254-263, 1999.

84. Goldstein DS. Arterial baroreflex sensitivity, plasma catecholamines, and pressor responsiveness in essential hypertension. Circulation 68(2):234-240, 1983.

85. Matsukawa T, Gotoh E, Hasegawa O, et al. Reduced baroreflex changes in muscle sympathetic nerve activity during blood pressure elevation in essential hypertension. J Hypertension 9(6):537-542, 1991.

86. Hajduczok C, Chapleau MW, Abboud FM. Increase in sympathetic activity with age. II. Role of impairment of cardiopulmonary baroreflexes. Am J Physiol 260:H1121-H1127, 1991.

87. Hajduczok G, Chapleau MW, Johnson SL, et al. Increase in sympathetic activity with age. I. Role of impairment of arterial baroreflexes. Am J Physiol 260(4 Pt 2):H1113-H120, 1991.

88. Hajduczok G, Chapleau MW, Abboud FM. Rapid adaptation of central pathways explains the suppressed baroreflex with aging. Neurobiol Aging 12(5):601-604, 1991.

89. Ebert TJ, Morgan BJ, Barney JA, et al. Effects of aging on baroreflex regulation of sympathetic activity in humans. Am J Physiol 263(3 Pt 2):H798-803, 1992.

90. Luft FC, Rankin LI, Henry DP, et al. Plasma and urinary norepinephrine at extremes of sodium intake in normal man. Hypertension 1:261-266, 1979.

91. Romoff MS, Keusch G, Campese VM, et al. Effect of sodium intake on plasma catecholamines in normal subjects. J Clin Endocrinol Metab 48:26-31, 1979.

92. Thames MD, Johnson LN. Impaired cardiopulmonary baroreflex control of renal nerves in renal hypertension. Circ Res 57:741-747, 1985.

93. Guo GB, Thames MD. Abnormal baroreflex control in renal hypertension is due to abnormal baroreceptors. Am J Physiol 245:420-428, 1983.

94. Tidgren B, Hjemdahl P, Theodorsson E, et al. Renal responses to lower body negative pressure in humans. Am J Physiol 259:F573-F579, 1990.

95. Schmedtje JF Jr, Varghese A, Gutkowska J, et al. Correlation of plasma norepinephrine and plasma atrial natriuretic factor during lower body negative pressure. Aviat Space Environ Med 61(6):555-558, 1990.

96. Joyner MJ, Shepherd JT, Seals DR. Sustained increases in sympathetic outflow during prolonged lower body negative pressure in humans. J Appl Physiol 68:1004-1009, 1990.

97. Westheim A, Os I, Kjeldsen SE, et al. Renal haemodynamic and sympathetic responses to head-up tilt in essential hypertension. Scand J Clin Lab Invest 50(8):815-822, 1990.

98. Izzo JL Jr, Sander E, Larrabee PS. Effect of postural stimulation on systemic hemodynamics and sympathetic nervous activity in systemic hypertension. Am J Cardiol 65:339-342, 1990.

99. Eckberg DL, Abboud FM, Mark AL. [AU6]Modulation of carotid baroreflex responsiveness in man: Effects of posture and propranolol labetalol in long-term treatment of hypertension. J Appl Physiol 41:383-387, 1976.

100. Thames MD, Schmid PG. Interaction between carotid and cardiopulmonary baroreflexes in control of plasma ADH. Am J Physiol 241:431-434, 1981.

101. Thames MD, Miller BD, Abboud FM. Baroreflex regulation of renal nerve activity during volume expansion. Am J Physiol 243:810-814, 1982.

102. Blair ML, Chen Y-H, Hisa H. Elevation of plasma renin activity by alpha-adrenoceptor agonists in conscious dogs. Am J Physiol 251(6 Pt 1):E695-E702, 1986.

103. Blair ML. Stimulation of renin secretion by alpha-adrenoceptor agonists. Am J Physiol 244(1):E37-E44, 1983.

104. Osborn JL, Thames MD, DiBona GF. Role of macula densa in renal nerve modulation of renin secretion. Am J Physiol 1982. 242:367-371.

105. Osborn JL, Roman RJ, Ewens JD. Renal nerves and the development of Dahl salt-sensitive hypertension. Hypertension 11(6 Pt 1):523-528, 1988.

106. Osborn JL, Plato CF, Gordin E, et al. Long-term increases in renal sympathetic nerve activity and hypertension. [Review] [30 refs]. Clin Exper Pharmacol & Physiol 24(1):72-76, 1997.

107. DiBona GF, Role of the renal nerves in hypertension. Sem Nephrol 11(5):503-511, 1991.

108. DiBona GF, Rios LL. Renal nerves in compensatory renal response to contralateral renal denervation. Am J Physiol 238:F26-F30, 1980.

109. Johnson JA, Davis JO, Gotshall RW, et al. Evidence for an intrarenal beta receptor in control of renin release. Am J Physiol 230(2):410-418, 1976.

110. Kamm DE, Levinsky NG. The mechanism of denervation natriuresis. J Clin Invest 44:93, 1965.

111. Gill JR Jr, Mason DT, Bartter FC. Adrenergic nervous system in sodium metabolism: Effects of guanethidine and sodium-retaining steroids in normal man. J Clin Invest 43:177, 1964.

112. Gill JR Jr, Bartter FC. Adrenergic nervous system in sodium metabolism. II. Effects of guanethidine on the renal response to sodium deprivation in normal man. N Engl J Med 275:1466-1471, 1966.

113. Wagner HN Jr. The influence of autonomic vasoregulatory reflexes on the rate of sodium and water excretion in man. J Clin Invest 36:1319-1327, 1957.

114. Matsuoka H, Nishida H, Nomura G, et al. Hypertension induced by nitric oxide synthesis inhibition is renal nerve dependent. Hypertension 23(6 Pt 2):971-975, 1994.

115. Xie PL, McDowell TS, Chapleau MW, et al. Rapid baroreceptor resetting in chronic hypertension. Implications for normalization of arterial pressure. Hypertension 17(1):72-79, 1991.

116. Gribbin B, Pickering TG, Sleight P, et al. Effect of age and high blood pressure on baroreflex sensitivity in man. Circulation Research 29(4):424-431, 1971.

117. Sleight P. Importance of cardiovascular reflexes in disease. Am J Med 84(suppl 3A):92-96, 1988.

118. Randall OS, Esler MD, Bulloch EG, et al. Relationship of age and blood pressure to baroreflex sensitivity and arterial compliance in man. Clin Sci Mol Med 51:357S-360S, 1976.

119. Pickering TG, Gribbin B, Oliver DO. Baroreflex sensitivity in patients on long-term hemodialysis. Clin Sci 43:645-647, 1972.

120. Izzo JL Jr, Smith RJ, Larrabee PS, et al. Plasma norepinephrine and age as determinants of systemic hemodynamics in men with established essential hypertension. Hypertension 9:415-419, 1987.

121. Simon AC, Safar ME, Weiss YA, et al. Baroreflex sensitivity and cardiopulmonary blood volume in normotensive and hypertensive patients. Br Heart J 39:799-805, 1977.

122. Mark AL, Kerber RE. Augmentation of cardiopulmonary baroreflex control of forearm vascular resistance in borderline hypertension. Hypertension 39-46, 1982.

123. Rea RF, Hamdan M. Baroreflex control of muscle sympathetic nerve activity in borderline hypertension. Circulation 82:856-862, 1990.

124. Saito M, Minokoshi Y, Shimazu T. Metabolic and sympathetic nerve activities of brown adipose tissue in tube-fed rats. Am J Physiol 257(3 Pt 1):E374-E378, 1989.

125. Rothwell NJ, Stock MJ. A role for brown adipose tissue in diet-induced thermogenesis. Obesity Res 5(6):650-656, 1997.

126. Landsberg L, Young JB. Catecholamines and the adrenal medulla. In Wilson JD, Foster DW (eds). Textbook of Endocrinology. Philadelphia, WB Saunders, 1985; pp 891-965.

127. Kushiro T, Kobayashi F, Osada H, et al. Role of sympathetic activity in blood pressure reduction with low calorie regimen. Hypertension 17(6 Pt 2):965-968, 1991.

128. Andersson B, Elam M, Wallin BG, et al. Effect of energy-restricted diet on sympathetic muscle nerve activity in obese women. Hypertension 18(6):783-789, 1991.

129. Izzo JL Jr, Swislocki ALM. Symposium on insulin and cardiovascular disease. Workshop III -Insulin resistance: Is it truly the link? Am J Med 90 (suppl 2A):26S-31S, 1991.

130. Bravo EL. The metabolic effects of catecholamines. Am J Hypertens 2:338S-343S, 1989.

131. Kjeldsen SE, Rostrup M, Moan A, et al. The sympathetic nervous system may modulate the metabolic cardiovascular syndrome in essential hypertension. J Cardiovasc Pharmacol, 20(Suppl 8):S32-S36, 1992.

132. MacKenzie ET, McCulloch J, O'Kean M, et al. Cerebral circulation and norepinephrine: relevance of the blood-brain barrier. Am J Physiol 231:483-488, 1976.

133. Sadoshima S, Busija D, Brody M, et al. Sympathetic nerves protect against stroke in stroke-prone hypertensive rats. Hypertension 3:I124-I127, 1981.

134. Sadoshima S, Thames M, Heistad DD. Cerebral blood flow during elevation of intracranial pressure: Role of sympathetic nerves. Am J Physiol 241:78-84, 1981.

135. Tuor UI. Acute hypertension and sympathetic stimulation: local heterogeneous changes in cerebral blood flow. Am J Physiol 263:H511-H518, 1992.

136. Beroniade VC, Lefebvre R, Falardeau P. Unilateral nodular diabetic glomerulosclerosis: Recurrence of an experiment of nature. Am J Nephrol 7:55-59, 1987.

137. Winder WW, Hagberg JM, Hickson RC, et al. Time course of sympathoadrenal adaptation to endurance exercise training in man. J Appl Physiol 45:370-374, 1978.

138. Winder WW, Hickson RC, Hagberg JM, et al. Training-induced changes in hormonal and metabolic responses to submaximal exercise. J Appl Physiol 46:766-771, 1979.

139. Paffenbarger RS Jr, Hyde RT, Wing AL, et al. Physical activity, all-cause mortality, and longevity of college alumni. N Engl J Med 314:605-613, 1986.

140. Cryer PE, Haymond MW, Santiago JV, et al. Norepinephrine and epinephrine release and adrenergic medication of smoking-associated hemodynamic and metabolic effects. N Engl J Med 295:573-577, 1976.

141. Harburg, E, et al. Socioecological stressor areas and black-white blood pressure: Detroit. J Chronic Dis 26:595-611, 1993.

142. Sokolow M, Werdegar D, Kain HK, et al. Relationship between level of blood pressure measured casually and by portable recorders and severity of complications in essential hypertension. Circulation 34(2):279-298, 1966.

143. Perloff D, Sokolow M, Cowan R. The prognostic value of ambulatory blood pressures. JAMA 249:2792-2798, 1983.

144. Pickering TG, Harshfield GA, Blank S, et al. Behavioral determinants of 24-hour blood pressure patterns in borderline hypertension. J Cardiovasc Pharmacol 8:S89-S92, 1986.

145. Clark LA, Denby L, Pregibon D, et al. A quantitative analysis of the effects of activity and time of day on the diurnal variations of blood pressure. J Chronic Dis 40:671-681, 1987.

146. Devereux RB, Pickering TG, Harshfield GA, et al. Left ventricular hypertrophy in patients with hypertension: importance of blood pressure response to regularly recurring stress. Circulation 3:470-476, 1983.

147. Schnall PL, Pieper C, Schwartz JE, et al. The relationship between 'job strain', workplace diastolic blood pressure, and left ventricular mass index. Results of a case-control study. JAMA 263:1929-1935, 1990. Erratum in: JAMA 267(9):1209, 1992.

148. Schneider RH, Egan BM, Johnson EH, et al. Anger and anxiety in borderline hypertension. Psychosomatic Med 48:242-248, 1986.

149. Julius S, Petrin J. Autonomic nervous and behavioral factors in hypertension. In Laragh JH, Brenner BM (eds). Hypertension: Pathophysiology, Diagnosis, and Management. New York, Raven Press, 1990; pp 2083-2090.

150. Alderman MH, Madhavan S, Ooi WL, et al. Association of the renin-sodium profile with the risk of myocardial infarction in patients with hypertension. N Engl J Med 324:1098-1104, 1991.

151. Kapusta DR, Knardahl S, Koepke JP, et al. Selective central alpha-2 adrenoceptor control of regional haemodynamic responses to air jet stress in conscious spontaneously hypertensive rats. J Hypertens 7:189-194, 1989.

152. DiBona GF. Stress and sodium intake in neural control of renal function in hypertension. Hypertension 17(4 Suppl):III2-I116, 1991.

153. DiBona, GF, Sawin LL. Role of renal nerves in sodium retention of cirrhosis and congestive heart failure. Am J Physiol 260(2 Pt 2):R298-R305, 1991.

154. DiBona GF, Jones SY. Acute environmental stress overrides cardiac volume receptor reflex in borderline hypertensive rats. J Hypertens 13(1):63-68, 1995.

155. DiBona GF, Jones SY, Sawin LL. Reflex effects on renal nerve activity characteristics in spontaneously hypertensive rats. Hypertension 30(5):1089-1096, 1997.

156. Hollenberg NK, Williams GH, Adams DF. Essential hypertension: Abnormal renal vascular and endocrine responses to a mild psychological stimulus. Hypertension 3:11-17, 1981.

157. Schmieder RE, Ruddel H, Schachinger H, et al. Renal hemodynamics and cardiovascular reactivity in the prehypertensive stage. Behav Med 19:5-12, 1993.

158. Allen K, Shykoff B-E, Izzo JL Jr. Pet ownership, but not ACE inhibitor therapy, blunts home blood pressure responses to mental stress. Hypertension 38(4):815-820, 2001.

159. Panza JA, Epstein SE, Quyyumi AA. Circadian variation in vascular tone and its relation to alpha-sympathetic vasoconstrictor activity. N Engl J Med 325:986-1039, 1991.

160. Watson RD, Hamilton CA, Reid JL, et al. Changes in plasma norepinephrine, blood pressure and heart rate during physical activity in hypertensive man. Hypertension 1(4):341-346, 1979.

161. Floras JS, Jones JV, Johnston JA, et al. Arousal and the circadian rhythm of blood pressure. Clin Sci Mol Med 55:395S-397S, 1978.

162. Floras JS, Hassan MO, Jones JV, et al. Factors influencing blood pressure and heart rate variability in hypertensive humans. Hypertension 11:273-281, 1988.

163. Sundberg S, Kohvakka A, Gordin A. Rapid reversal of circadian blood pressure rhythm in shift workers. J Hypertens 6(5):394-396, 1988.

164. Feller RP, Hale HB. Human sympatho-adrenal responsiveness in autumn, winter and spring. Technical document, Rep. SAM-TDR-63-46. Brooks Air Force Base, TX, USAF School of Aerospace Medicine, 1963.

165. Hata T, Ogihara T, Maruyama A, et al. The seasonal variation of blood pressure in patients with essential hypertension. Clin Exp Hypertens 3:341-354, 1982.

166. Izzo JL Jr, Larrabee PS, Sander E, et al. Hemodynamics of seasonal adaptation. Am J Hypertens 3:405-407, 1990.

167. Muller JE, Stone PH, Turi ZG, et al. Circadian variation in the frequency of onset of acute myocardial infarction. N Engl J Med 313:1315-1322, 1985.

168. Tofler GH, Brezinski D, Schafer AI, et al. Concurrent morning increase in platelet aggregability and the risk of myocardial infarction and sudden cardiac death. N Engl J Med 316: 1514-1518, 1987.

169. Argentino C, Toni D, Rasura M, et al. Circadian variation in the frequency of ischemic stroke. Stroke 21:387-389, 1990.

170. Bean WB, Mills CA. Coronary occlusion, heart failure and environmental temperatures. Am Heart J 16:701-713, 1938.

171. Anderson T, Le Riche W. Cold weather and myocardial infarction. Lancet i:291-296, 1970.

172. Protos A, Caracta A, Gross L. The seasonal susceptibility to myocardial infarction. J Am Geriatr Soc 19:526-535, 1971.

173. Ely D, Caplea A, Dunphy G, et al. Spontaneously hypertensive rat Y chromosome increases indexes of sympathetic nervous system activity. Hypertension 29(2):613-618, 1997.

174. Kumai T, Tanaka M, Watanabe M, et al. Possible involvement of androgen in increased norepinephrine synthesis in blood vessels of spontaneously hypertensive rats. Jpn J Pharmacol 66(4):439-444, 1994.

175. Robertson D, Goldberg MR, Onrot J, et al. Isolated failure of autonomic neurotransmission. Evidence for impaired beta-hydroxylation of dopamine. N Engl J Med 314:1494-1497, 1986.

176. Masuo K, Mikami H, Ogihara T, et al. Differences in insulin and sympathetic responses to glucose ingestion due to family history of hypertension. Am J Hypertens 9(8):739-745, 1996.

177. Masuo K, Mikami H, Ogihara T, et al. Sympathetic nerve hyperactivity precedes hyperinsulinemia and blood pressure elevation in young, nonobese Japanese population. Am J Hypertens 10(1):77-83, 1997.

178. Masuo K, Mikami H, Ogihara T, et al. Familial hypertension, insulin, sympathetic activity, and blood pressure elevation. Hypertension 32(1):96-100, 1998.

179. Manuck SB, Polefrone JM, Terrell DF, et al. Absence of enhanced sympathoadrenal activity and behaviorally evoked cardiovascular reactivity among offspring of hypertensives. Am J Hypertens 9(3):248-255, 1996.

180. Takiyyuddin MA, Cervenka JH, Hsiao RJ, et al. Chromogranin A. Storage and release in hypertension. Hypertension 15: 237-246, 1990.

181. Fredrickson M, Tuomisto M, Bergman-Losman B. Neuroendocrine and cardiovascular stress reactivity in middle-aged normotensive adults with parental history of cardiovascular disease. Psychophysiology 28(6):656-664, 1991.

182. Ferrara LA, Moscato TS, Pisanti N, et al. Is the sympathetic nervous system altered in children with familial history of arterial hypertension? Cardiology 75(3):200-205, 1988.

183. Ferrier C, Cox H, Esler M. Elevated total body noradrenaline spillover in normotensive members of hypertensive families. Clin Sci (Lond) 84(2):225-230, 1993.

184. Noll G, Wenzel RR, Schneider M, et al. Increased activation of sympathetic nervous system and endothelin by mental stress in normotensive offspring of hypertensive parents. Circulation 93(5):866-869, 1996.

185. Calhoun DA, Mutinga ML, Wyss JM, et al. Muscle sympathetic nervous system activity in black and Caucasian hypertensive subjects. J Hypertens 12(11):1291-1296, 1994.

186. Miller SB, Ditto B. Exaggerated sympathetic nervous system response to extended psychological stress in offspring of hypertensives. Psychophysiol 28(1):103-113, 1991.

187. Parmer RJ, Cervenka JH, Stone RA. Baroreflex sensitivity and heredity in essential hypertension. Circulation 85: 497-503, 1992.

188. Levy RL, et al. Transient tachycardia: Prognostic significance alone and in association with transient hypertension. JAMA 129(9):585-588, 1945.

189. Louis WJ, Doyle AE, Anavekar S. Plasma norepinephrine levels in essential hypertension. N Engl J Med 288:599-601, 1973.

190. Goldstein DS. Plasma catecholamines and essential hypertension: an analytical review. Hypertension 5:86-99, 1983.

191. Horky K, Kopecka J, Greogorova I, et al. Relationship between plasma renin activity and urinary catecholamines in various types of hypertension. Endokrinologie 67:331-342, 1976.

192. Januszewicz W, Wocial B. Urinary excretion of catecholamines and their metabolites in patients with renovascular hypertension. Jpn Heart J 19:468-478, 1978.

193. Saito I, Takeshita E, Hayashi S, et al. Comparison of clinic and home blood pressure levels and the role of the sympathetic nervous system in clinic-home differences. Am J Hypertens 3:219-224, 1990.

194. Julius S, Krause L, Schork NJ, et al. Hyperkinetic borderline hypertension in Tecumseh, Michigan. J Hypertens 9(1): 77-84, 1991.

195. Hofman A, Boomsma F, Schalekamp MA, et al. Raised blood pressure and plasma noradrenaline concentrations in teenagers and young adults selected from an open population. Br Med J 1:1536-1538, 1979.

196. Kjeldsen SE, Zweifler AJ, Petrin J, et al. Sympathetic nervous system involvement in essential hypertension: Increased platelet noradrenaline coincides with decreased beta-adrenoreceptor responsiveness. Blood Press 3(3):164-171, 1994.

197. Esler MD, Jennings GL, Johns J, et al. Estimation of 'total' renal, cardiac and splanchnic sympathetic nervous tone in essential hypertension from measurements of noradrenaline release. J Hypertens Suppl 2(3):S123-S125, 1984.

198. Esler M, Lambert, Jennings C. Increased regional sympathetic nervous activity in human hypertension: causes and consequences. J Hypertens Suppl 8:S53-S57, 1990.

199. Esler M, Ferrier C, Lambert G, et al. Biochemical evidence of sympathetic hyperactivity in human hypertension. Hypertension 17(4 suppl):III29-III35, 1991.

200. Ferrier C, Esler MD, Eisenhofer G, et al. Increased norepinephrine spillover into the jugular veins in essential hypertension. Hypertension 19(1):62-69, 1992.

201. Morlin C, Wallin BG, Eriksson BM. Muscle sympathetic activity and plasma noradrenaline in normotensive and hypertensive man. Acta Physiol Scand 119:117-121, 1983.

202. Wallin BG, Morlin, Hjemdahl P. Muscle sympathetic activity and venous plasma noradrenaline concentrations during static exercise in normotensive and hypertensive subjects. Acta Physiol Scand 129:489-497, 1987.

203. Wallin BG, Thompson JM, Jennings GL, et al. Renal noradrenaline spillover correlates with muscle sympathetic activity in humans. J Physiol 491(Pt 3):881-887, 1996.

204. Vaz M, Jennings G, Turner A, et al. Regional sympathetic nervous activity and oxygen consumption in obese normotensive human subjects. Circulation 96(10):3423-3429, 1997.

205. Grassi G, Seravalle G, Cattaneo BM, et al. Sympathetic activation in obese normotensive subjects. Hypertension 25(4 Pt 1): 560-563, 1995.

206. Gudbjornsdottir S, Lonnroth P, Sverrisdottir YB, et al. Sympathetic nerve activity and insulin in obese normotensive and hypertensive men. Hypertension 27(2):276-280, 1996.

207. Ferranini E, Haffner SM, Stern MP. Insulin sensitivity and hypertension. J Hypertens 8 (suppl 7):S169-S173, 1990.

208. DeFronzo RA, Ferrannini E. Insulin resistance: A multifaceted syndrome responsible for NIDDM, obesity, hypertension, dyslipidemia, and atherosclerotic cardiovascular disease. Diabetes Care 14(3):173-194, 1991.

209. Court JM, Hill GJ, Dunlop M, et al. Hypertension in childhood obesity. Aust Paediatr J 10:296-300, 1974.

210. Kannel WB, Brand N, Skinner JJ Jr, et al. The relation of adiposity to blood pressure and development of hypertension: The Framingham study. Ann Intern Med 67:48-49, 1976.

211. Stamler R, Stamler J, Riedlinger WF, et al. Weight and blood pressure findings in hypertension screening of 1 million Americans. JAMA 240:1607-1610, 1978.

212. Sowers JR, Whitfield LA, Catania RA, et al. Role of the sympathetic nervous system in blood pressure maintenance in obesity. J Clin Endocrinol Metab 54:1181-1186, 1982.

213. Daly PA, Landsberg L. Hypertension in obesity and NIDDM. Role of insulin and sympathetic nervous system. Diabetes Care 14(3):240-248, 1991.

214. Facchini FS, Stoohs RA, Reaven GM. Enhanced sympathetic nervous system activity. The linchpin between insulin resistance, hyperinsulinemia, and heart rate. Am J Hypertens 9(10 Pt 1):1013-1017, 1996.

215. Reaven GM, Lithell H, Landsberg L. Hypertension and associated metabolic abnormalities—The role of insulin resistance and the sympathoadrenal system. N Engl J Med 334(6):374-381, 1996.

216. Rowe JW, Young JB, Minaker KL, et al. Effect of insulin and glucose infusions on sympathetic nervous system activity in normal man. Diabetes 30:219-225, 1981.

217. Petersen JS, DiBona GF. Acute sympathoinhibitory actions of metformin in spontaneously hypertensive rats. Hypertension 27(3 Pt 2):619-625, 1996.

218. Jamerson K, Smith SD, Amerena JV, et al. Vasoconstriction with norepinephrine causes less forearm insulin resistance than a sympathetic reflex vasoconstriction. Hypertension 23:1006-1011, 1994.

219. Rocchini AP, Mao HZ, Babu K, et al. Clonidine prevents insulin resistance and hypertension in obese dogs. Hypertension 33(1 Pt 2):548-553, 1999.

220. Suzuki M, Kimura Y, Tsushima M, et al. Association of insulin resistance with salt sensitivity and nocturnal fall of blood pressure. Hypertension 35(4):864-868, 2000.

221. Esler MD, Julius S, Randall OS, et al. Relation of renin status to neurogenic vascular resistance in borderline hypertension. Am J Cardiol 36(5):708-715, 1975.

222. Esler MD, Nestel PJ. Renin and sympathetic nervous system responsiveness to adrenergic stimuli in essential hypertension. American J Cardiol 32(5):643-649, 1973.

223. DeQuattro V, Campese V, Miura Y, et al. Increased plasma catecholamines in high renin hypertension. Am J Cardiol 38:801-804, 1976.

224. Esler M, Julius S, Zweifler A, et al. Mild high-renin essential hypertension: neurogenic human hypertension? N Engl J Med 296:405-411, 1977.

225. Schmieder RE, Veelken R, Schobel H, et al. Glomerular hyperfiltration during sympathetic nervous system activation in early essential hypertension. J Am Soc Nephrol 8(6):893-900, 1997.

226. Fukuda N, Hu WY, Teng J, et al. Troglitazone inhibits growth and improves insulin signaling by suppression of angiotensin II action in vascular smooth muscle cells from spontaneously hypertensive rats. Atherosclerosis 163(2):229-39, 2002.

227. Izzo JL Jr. Hypertension in the elderly: A pathophysiologic approach to therapy. J Am Geriatrics Soc 30:352-359, 1982.

228. O'Malley K, Docherty JR, Kelly JG. Adrenoceptor status and cardiovascular function in aging. J Hypertens Suppl 6(1):S59-S62, 1988.

229. Ward KD, Sparrow D, Landsberg L, et al. Influence of insulin, sympathetic nervous system activity, and obesity on blood pressure: The Normative Aging Study. J Hypertens 14(3):301-308, 1996.

230. Cerasola G, Cottone S, D'Ignoto G, et al. Sympathetic activity in borderline and established hypertension in the elderly. J Hypertens Suppl 6(1):S55-S58, 1988.

231. Esler M, Skews H, Leonard P, et al. Age-dependence of noradrenaline kinetics in normal subjects. Clin Sci (Lond) 60:217-219, 1981.

232. Sverrisdottir YB, Johannsson G, Jungersten L, et al. Is the somatotropic axis related to sympathetic nerve activity in healthy ageing men? J Hypertens 19(11):2019-2024, 2001.

233. Dinenno FA, Jones PP, Seals DR, et al. Age-associated arterial wall thickening is related to elevations in sympathetic activity in healthy humans. Am J Physiol Heart Circ Physiol 278(4):H1205-H1210, 2000.

234. Grassi G, Seravalle G, Bertinieri G, et al. Sympathetic and reflex alterations in systo-diastolic and systolic hypertension of the elderly. J Hypertens 18(5):587-593, 2000.

235. Li ST, Holmes C, Kopin IJ, et al. Aging-related changes in cardiac sympathetic function in humans, assessed by 6-18F-fluorodopamine PET scanning. J Nucl Med 44(10): 1599-1603, 2003.

236. Freis ED. Origins and development of antihypertensive treatment. In Laragh JH, Brenner BM (eds). Hypertension: Pathophysiology, Diagnosis, and Management. New York, Raven Press, 1990; pp 2093-2105.

237. Simon G, Kiowski W, Julius S. Effect of beta adrenoceptor antagonists on baroreceptor reflex sensitivity in hypertension. Clin Pharmacol Ther 22:293-298, 1977.

238. Nicholls MG, Julius S, Zweifler AJ. Withdrawal of endogenous sympathetic drive lowers blood pressure in primary aldosteronism. Clin Endocrinol(Oxf) 15:253-258, 1981.

239. Goldstein DS, Levinson PD, Zimlichman R, et al. Clonidine suppression testing in essential hypertension. Ann Intern Med 102:42-49, 1985.

240. Campese VM, Romoff MS, Levitan D, et al. Mechanisms of autonomic nervous system dysfunction in uremia. Kidney Int 20:246-253, 1981.

241. Izzo JL Jr, Santarosa RP, Larrabee PS, et al. Increased plasma norepinephrine and sympathetic nervous activity in essential hypertensive and uremic humans: Effects of clonidine. J Cardiovasc Pharmacol 10(suppl. 12):S225-S229, 1987.

242. Goldstein DS, Keiser HR. Neural circulatory control in the hyperdynamic circulation syndrome. Am Heart J 109: 387-390, 1985.

243. Izzo JL Jr, Licht MR, Smith RJ, et al. Chronic effects of direct vasodilation (pinacidil), alpha-adrenergic blockade (prazosin) and angiotensin-converting enzyme inhibition (captopril) in systemic hypertension. Am J Cardiol 60:303-308, 1987.

244. Buhler FR, Amann FW, Bolli P, et al. Elevated adrenaline and increased alpha-adrenoceptor-mediated vasoconstriction in essential hypertension. J Cardiovasc Pharmacol 4(Suppl 1):S134-S138, 1982.

245. Philipp T, Distler A, Cordes U. Sympathetic nervous system and blood pressure control in essential hypertension. Lancet 2:959-963, 1978.

246. Kiowski W, van Brummelen P, Buhler FR. Plasma noradrenaline correlates with alpha-adrenoceptor-mediated vasoconstriction and blood pressure in patients with essential hypertension. Clin Sci (Lond) 57:177S-180S, 1979.

247. Rudner XL, Berkowitz DE, Booth JV, et al. Subtype specific regulation of human vascular alpha(1)-adrenergic receptors by vessel bed and age. Circulation 100(23):2336-2343, 1999.

248. Pratt JH, Manatunga AK, Bowsher RR, et al. The interaction of norepinephrine excretion with blood pressure and race in children. J Hypertens 10:93-96, 1992.

249. Stepniakowski KT, Lu G, Miller GD, et al. Fatty acids, not insulin, modulate alpha1-adrenergic reactivity in dorsal hand veins. Hypertension 30(5):1150-1155, 1997.

250. Stansberry KB, Hill MA, Shapiro SA, et al. Impairment of peripheral blood flow responses in diabetes resembles an enhanced aging effect. Diabetes Care 20(11):1711-1716, 1997.

251. Davy KP, Seals DR, Tanaka H. Augmented cardiopulmonary and integrative sympathetic baroreflexes but attenuated peripheral vasoconstriction with age. Hypertension 32(2): 298-304, 1998.

252. Dinenno FA, Dietz NM, Joyner MJ. Aging and forearm postjunctional alpha-adrenergic vasoconstriction in healthy men. Circulation 106:1349-1354, 2002.

253. Drolet G, Bouvier M, de Champlain J. Enhanced sympathoadrenal reactivity to haemorrhagic stress in DOCA-salt hypertensive rats. J Hypertens 7:237-242, 1989.

254. Chen, YF, Nagahama S, Winternitz SR, et al. Hyperresponsiveness of monoaminergic mechanisms in DOCA/NaCl hypertensive rats. Am J Physiol H71-H79, 1985.

255. Zambraski EJ, Ciccone CD, Izzo JL Jr. The role of the sympathetic nervous system in 2-kidney DOCA-hypertensive Yucatan miniature swine. Clin Exp Hypertens A8:411-424, 1986.

256. Thomas GD, O'Hagan KP, Zambraski EJ. Chemical sympathectomy alters the development of hypertension in miniature swine. Hypertension 17(3):357-362, 1991.

257. Moreau P, Drolet G, Yamaguchi N, et al. Role of presynaptic beta 2-adrenergic facilitation in the development and maintenance of DOCA-salt hypertension. Am J Hypertens 6: 1016-1024, 1993.

258. Saavedra JM. Brain catecholamines during development of DOCA-salt hypertension in rats. Brain Res 179:121-127, 1979.

259. Veelken R, Hilgers KF, Ditting T, et al. Impaired cardiovascular reflexes precede deoxycorticosterone acetate-salt hypertension. Hypertension 24(5):564-570, 1994.

260. Katholi RE, Winternitz SR, Oparil S. Role of the renal nerves in the pathogenesis of one-kidney renal hypertension in the rat. Hypertension 3:404-409, 1981.

261. Katholi RE, Whitlow PL, Winternitz SR, et al. Importance of the renal nerves in established two-kidney, one clip Goldblatt hypertension in the rat. Hypertension 4:166-174, 1982.

262. Eide I, Myers MR, DeQuattro V, et al. Increased hypothalamic noradrenergic activity in one-kidney one-clip renovascular hypertensive rats. J Cardiovasc Pharmacol 2:833-841, 1980.

263. Winternitz SR, Katholi RE, Oparil S. Decrease in hypothalamic norepinephrine content following renal denervation in the one-kidney one-clip Goldblatt hypertensive rat. Hypertension 4:369-373, 1982.

264. Katholi RE, Winternitz SR, Oparil S. Decrease in peripheral sympathetic nervous system activity following renal denervation or unclipping in the one-kidney one-clip Goldblatt hypertensive rat. J Clin Invest 69:55-62, 1982.

265. Dargie HL, Franklin SS, Reid JL. The sympathetic nervous system in renovascular hypertension in the rat. Br J Pharmacol 56:365-374, 1976.

266. Wyss JM, Aboukarsh N, Oparil S. Sensory denervation of the kidney attenuates renovascular hypertension in the rat. Am J Physiol 250:H82-H86, 1986.

267. Wyss JM, Aboukarsh N, Oparil S. Selective lesion of the renal afferents transiently lowers blood pressure in established 1 kidney, 1 clip Goldblatt hypertension. Circulation 70:429-435, 1984.

268. Izzo JL Jr, Campese VM. Hypertension and renal disease. *In* Brenner BM (ed). Brenner and Rector's The Kidney. Philadelphia, Saunders, 2004; pp 2109-2138.

269. Izzo JL Jr, Sterns RH. Abnormal norepinephrine release in uremia. Kidney Int 24(suppl.16):S221-S223, 1983.

270. Converse RL Jr, Jacobsen TN, Toto RD, et al. Sympathetic overactivity in patients with chronic renal failure. N Engl J Med 327:1912-1918, 1992.

271. Campese VM. Neurogenic factors and hypertension in chronic renal failure. J Nephrol 10(4):184-187, 1997.

272. Bravo EL, Tarazi RC, Fouad FM, et al. Clonidine-suppression test: A useful aid in the diagnosis of pheochromocytoma. N Engl J Med 305:623-626, 1981.

273. Schobel HP, Fischer T, Heuszer K, et al. Preeclampsia—a state of sympathetic overactivity. N Engl J Med 335:1480-1485, 1996.

# Chapter 7

# Environmental and Psychosocial Stress in Hypertension Onset and Progression

## Kathleen C. Light

Life events that evoke negative emotions such as anger, fear, and sadness have long been known to produce temporary elevations in blood pressure (BP).[1,2] Since the application of standardized laboratory experimental methods has become widely used to assess cardiovascular and neuroendocrine responses (psychophysiologic stress testing), a large body of evidence has shown that many other experiences also lead to short-term pressor responses. These experiences range from cognitive to physical challenges and from positive to negative emotional states. These laboratory studies have also shown that different adrenergic and hemodynamic patterns are involved during different types of stressors. Challenging tasks involving active coping and mental effort typically elicit a state involving increased β-adrenergic receptor activity characterized by increased heart rate, cardiac output, cardiac contractile force (frequently indicated by decreased pre-ejection period) and vasodilation in skeletal muscle.[3-5] This state is similar to the pattern originally identified through studies in animal models as "preparation for fight or flight" or the defense reaction, which is characterized by enhanced activity of the sympathetic adrenomedullary system.[6,7] Events that incorporate aspects of frustration, passive coping, loss of control, or helplessness tend to evoke less β-adrenergic activity and less cardiac activation but instead result in greater vasoconstriction, presumably owing to α-adrenergic activity.[3-5] This pattern resembles the "defeat reaction" of animal models, which is characterized by overactivity of the hypothalamic-pituitary-adrenocortical (HPAC) system.[6,7]

These psychophysiologic stress studies have also shown that even when the stressors themselves are highly standardized, individuals differ greatly in the magnitude that the BP increase evoked.[3] Those individuals who demonstrate BP increases that place them in the top 25% of those studied are often labeled *high stress reactors*. An active hypothesis guiding considerable research has focused on these hyperresponsive persons as a group that may be at increased risk of developing hypertension.[8] Studies have also shown that healthy normotensive men and women differ in their stress responses, with men showing greater systolic BP (SBP) increases, greater vasodilation during stressors evoking β-adrenergic activation, and greater vasoconstriction during stressors evoking α-adrenergic activation.[5,9] Men also show slower return of BP to prestress levels (slow recovery) after the stressful event has ended.[9] These gender differences are enhanced when women are tested in the phase of their menstrual cycle when female reproductive hormones, particularly estrogen and progesterone, are higher than when these are low. Estrogen has vasodilator effects, which may underlie both this observation and other findings suggesting that postmenopausal women have enhanced stress-induced BP increases compared with premenopausal women.[10,11] Ethnic differences in cardiovascular stress responses have also been shown in both normotensive and hypertensive adults, with African Americans demonstrating greater vasoconstriction during stress and sometimes greater BP increases than European Americans.[4,12,13] African Americans more frequently demonstrate another potentially maladaptive response to short-term stress exposure—increased sodium retention. This response, like exaggerated BP increases during stress, has been shown to occur more frequently in persons with risk factors for hypertension, including borderline hypertension and positive family history of hypertension.[14-16]

Laboratory stress studies in normotensive and hypertensive humans can be very informative about patterns of cardiovascular responses. They can also document the stability of high and low reactivity in a variety of cardiovascular measures. Stability at acceptable levels has been documented over periods ranging from weeks to months to as long as 10 years.[3,8,17] However, such studies cannot establish the long-term predictive significance of stress or of stress reactivity in the onset or progression of hypertension. This critical issue has been addressed in several other ways. This review summarizes recent findings in the following areas: (1) animal models involving stress showing progression to hypertension; (2) human studies showing relationship of environmental factors or personality or behavioral patterns to the development of hypertension; (3) prospective long-term follow-up studies of normotensive individuals characterized as high and low stress reactors; and (4) evidence that stress buffers and stress-management interventions are related to lower BP.

## ANIMAL MODELS OF STRESS-RELATED HYPERTENSION

One of the most influential leaders in the field of stress exposure, patterns of response, and health consequences was James P. Henry.[7] His model of stress-related hypertension in mice induced by social environments that increase territorial confrontations provided some of the strongest evidence to date that chronic stress exposure can indeed be a key precipitating factor in the pathogenesis of hypertension. The development of sustained hypertension was evident in dominant males (mean BP levels of 145 mm Hg) and was worsened in subdominant males (those just below the dominant ones in social status; mean levels of 160 mm Hg) but not in the truly subordinate males (mean levels of 125 mm Hg). The elevation was greater when the colony members were changed frequently versus when stable dominance hierarchies were allowed to remain intact. According to the interpretation of Henry and Stephens, dominant males showed a classic defense reaction with sympathetic activation as they exerted themselves but maintained control. Subdominant animals showed a more extreme defense reaction associated with striving but incomplete control. Subordinate animals showed a defeat reaction with enhanced corticosterone and HPAC activity.[18] In keeping with this as the era of genetic and molecular biology, it is important to emphasize that even in this model of social environmental hypertension, genetic influences are critical.

When Henry extended his work on social stress from mice to rats, he compared chronic social stress effects in rat strains that normally do not develop hypertension in standard laboratory environments.[7,19] Wistar-Kyoto hyperactive rats, classified as very peaceable, showed no BP rise with chronic unstable social environments, whereas the moderately peaceable Sprague-Dawley animals showed some rise in BP, and the aggressive Long-Evans rats showed much larger increases in BP, with rise in BP positively correlated with number of scars from aggressive encounters. This research was later expanded by Mormede, who reports that among six rat strains, both behavioral and adrenal and heart weight evidence can be used to identify those strains more vulnerable to social stress.[20] However, even strains showing high social stress sensitivity must also have related target organ vulnerability (renal, cardiac, or vascular) before the excess sympathetic adrenomedullary activity evoked by chronic social instability results in sustained BP increases.[20,21]

A second prominent model of stress-related hypertension is the borderline hypertensive rat (BHR) as developed and studied by Lawler et al.[22-26] This first-generation backcross of a spontaneously hypertensive rat (SHR) with a normotensive Wistar-Kyoto rat typically develops only high-normal or borderline hypertension in the usual laboratory environment. With daily exposure to a brief period of a shock avoidance conflict task for 16 weeks, the BHRs develop hypertension with target organ damage that persists even if the stress exposure is terminated. This stress-induced hypertension is blunted if the animals receive daily swimming exercise as well as the conflict task (Figure 7-1).[25] Hypertension also develops in BHRs if they are placed on a high intake of salt, and the combination of high salt and stress leads to greater adverse cardiovascular effects than either environmental factor individually.

A primary role for renal involvement in the hypertension resulting from either high stress or high salt is suggested by the observation that renal denervation delays onset of the rise in pressure. Work by DiBona et al. has shown that stress induces greater increases in sodium retention in SHRs and BHRs than in normotensive rat strains, and that this effect of stress can be prevented by renal denervation or reduction in central sympathetic outflow owing to administration of sympathetically active agents into the ventricles of the brain.[27-29] Lawler et al. have reported that in the early period of stress exposure plus high salt, norepinephrine content decreases in nuclei of the hypothalamus that are known to be involved in the classic defense reaction.[24]

A third animal model of stress-related hypertension described by Anderson et al. is the mongrel dog exposed to daily shock avoidance while on increased salt and low potassium intake.[30-32] This model requires both stress exposure and high salt intake to induce hypertension; neither factor alone is sufficient. The reversible hypertension that results involves retention of sodium, and either renal denervation or potassium supplementation is sufficient to prevent or reverse hypertension in this model. Thus, even in animals lacking clear genetic predisposition, a reversible form of hypertension may arise when three adverse environmental factors are present: excessive salt, potassium deficiency, and regular stress exposure.

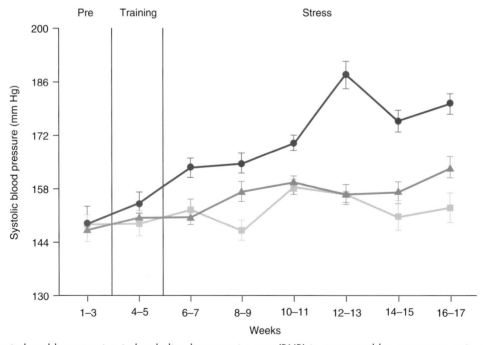

**Figure 7-1** Stress-induced hypertension in borderline hypertensive rats (BHR) is attenuated by concurrent swim training. Mean (±SEM) tail cuff systolic blood pressure (SBP) for each 2-week period before the stress manipulations *(Pre)*, during the 2 weeks when the stress was being progressively lengthened *(Training)*, and during the 12 weeks of daily swim or tail shock, or both *(Stress)*, in rats exposed to daily shock plus swim training *(triangles)*, shock only *(circles)*, or neither intervention *(squares)*. (From Cox RH, Hubbard JW, Lawler JE, et al. Exercise training attenuates stress-induced hypertension in the rat. Hypertension 7:747-751, 1985.)

In animal models, early life and even prenatal exposure to stress have also been shown to affect BP and stress responses throughout the life span.[33] In animals as well as humans, early loss of a parent or prolonged maternal separation has particularly profound effects including increased BP and corticosterone levels as an adult.[33-35] Conversely, early exposure to stress buffers such as enhanced maternal contact and stroking (known to increase central oxytocin activity), or multiday exogenous oxytocin administration, leads to decreased BP, corticosterone, and anxiety behavior into adolescence and adulthood.[36-37] Oxytocin, a mammalian neuropeptide/hormone linked to social bonding as well as maternal behavior, appears to decrease BP through alterations in central $\alpha$-adrenergic activity, as well as stimulating release of atrial natriuretic peptide and affecting cardiovascular function peripherally.[38]

These animal models provide the most definitive evidence to date that chronic life stress exposure can contribute to the development of hypertension in individuals with genetic susceptibility and/or when combined with other adverse environmental factors such as a high-salt/low-potassium diet. Also, the importance of early exposure to stress and/or stress buffers is highlighted. These observations lay the foundation for studies of environmental stress in humans, which cannot provide such direct and definitive evidence but do show important associations with parallels to the animal models.

## ENVIRONMENTAL STRESS EXPOSURE: CHRONIC JOB OR HOME LIFE STRESS AND ACUTE TRAUMATIC STRESS

Observations of people who move from stable, rural, traditional societies to unstable, urban, Westernized environments have indicated that contemporary urban conditions contribute to increases in BP over the life span.[39] For example, the nomadic Samburo warriors of Kenya show no BP increase with age in their traditional environment, yet when they join the Kenyan military, they show BP increases similar to those of recruits from more urban areas.[40,41] The principal factors that change with such a move and are believed to contribute to the pressure rise include (1) diet, (2) physical activity, (3) increased obesity, (4) reduction of supportive ties to the family and larger community, and (5) increased mental effort and active coping to perform work and home life activities under time pressure and competition. Waldron et al., after examining BP data from 84 different cultures and social groups, concluded that BP increases were independent of changes in salt intake and obesity (in men), and that the remaining factors, particularly economic competition and loss of family ties, appear to be the more universal contributing causes.[42]

Among Westernized societies, both urban and rural, people with less education, lower-status occupations, less total household income, and generally lower socioeconomic status (SES) have higher BP.[43] Although African Americans have on average fewer educational and economic resources and higher BP than age-matched European Americans, ethnic differences do not account for these differences in BP between lower and higher SES groups. Clear BP differences are seen between lower and higher SES African Americans, as between lower and higher SES whites and members of other ethnic minorities. Sources of these group differences have been reviewed by

Anderson et al.[44,45] All explanations involve multiple contributing factors, including *chronic stress,* defined as increased frequency of threats to the well-being of the individual and her or his close family and friends. This definition of chronic stress is so general that it leaves completely open which specific elements that differ between SES groups are most critical in their impact on BP. However, its generality is also one of its strengths in that it spans both the objective and the more individualized subjective perception of actual and anticipated life experiences as components of the stress exposure. Thus, it leaves room for individual differences in response to the same experience and for multiple models focusing on specific dimensions of low SES, such as economic insecurity or lack of control at work or at home.

One specific model that grew from the observed SES differences in BP is Dressler's model of lifestyle incongruity.[46] This model associates increased chronic stress and sympathetic nervous system (SNS) activity with the extent to which the individual's material acquisitions are higher than average for his or her occupation and income level (i.e., living beyond one's means). High lifestyle incongruity has been associated with increased BP levels. Dressler's current model also addresses incongruity in regard to noneconomic issues that are related to expectations about behavior and multiple roles or status within the family and community. Both economic and social incongruity appear to act, in part, through another important factor—reduction in social support from family and other sources.

Low occupational status and low control within the workplace are associated with lower SES, and both have been associated with increased job stress. Ever since early work by Rose et al. on air traffic controllers,[47] the hypothesis that daily stress exposure on the job may contribute to hypertension has been gaining support. Karasek et al.'s model of "job strain" was developed to formalize the study of stress on the job across a variety of occupations.[48] Job strain focuses on two dimensions of work stress: (1) psychological demands (i.e., how hard and how fast the worker perceives she or he must work) and (2) job decision latitude (i.e., the level of control over the nature and pace of the work). *Job strain* is defined as occurring when high psychological demand occurs together with low decision latitude.

Research on job strain as a contributing stress exposure factor in the onset and exacerbation of elevated BP has included more than 14 studies since the late 1980s. As summarized by Pickering, the method of BP assessment is critical.[39] Clinic assessments of BP are more time-efficient, but ambulatory BP obtained at intervals of every few minutes throughout a normal weekday spent at work and at home has distinct advantages for assessing response to daily work life demands at work and as they spill over to influence responses after work. Of seven studies using clinic assessments only, none has found a relationship between job strain and increased BP. Of another seven studies that employed ambulatory monitoring, all but one have observed a positive relationship for men. The most definitive work has come from Schnall et al., who have shown that job strain is related to higher BP at work and also at home and during sleep, to increased left ventricular mass, and to hypertensive status in a case-control study in 196 men.[49,50] They have also reported that job strain interacts with age such that the increase in BP with age is greater for high–job strain men, and that the combination of high job strain and increased alcohol use is related to greater increases in BP. Furthermore, in a 3-year follow-up study, this research team found that increases in pressure over time are greater for high–job strain than low–job strain men, controlling for BP at study entry.

High work demand and low control on the job have been related to increased urinary epinephrine but not cortisol,[51] suggesting that enhanced adrenergic receptor activity may contribute to the BP increase in high–job strain individuals. It is worth noting that research reported by Pickering[39] and another study by Light et al.[52] have observed no increase in work BP in women reporting job strain, although men in the same study showed the predicted relationship. This observation is consistent with recent work by Lundberg[53] and by Luecken et al.[54] suggesting that stress related to child care and other family duties is a greater influence than job-related stress on the mental and physical well-being of working women.

## PERSONALITY AND BEHAVIORAL PATTERNS ASSOCIATED WITH ELEVATED BLOOD PRESSURE

A number of psychological characteristics have been related to higher BP levels and/or increased prevalence of hypertension. Several of these traits are of relevance because they are presumed to act, in part, by increasing the individual's exposure to stress or perception of stress (e.g., cynical hostility) or because they themselves may be a consequence and thus a marker of excessive stress exposure (e.g., hopelessness and depressive symptoms).

Type A or the coronary-prone behavior pattern is associated with increased risk of atherosclerosis and coronary morbidity.[55] This pattern includes three semiindependent component traits: hostile outlook, competitiveness, and time urgency.[56] Of these traits, hostile outlook was the primary predictive factor in most studies that examined relationships of the individual factors. Additional research on hostility by Barefoot et al. has confirmed that this trait is stable over time and predicted both cardiovascular and all-cause mortality, in part through its relationship to increased BP.[56,59] Hostile outlook, described as a combination of angerability and cynical mistrust, leads to increased BP, vasoconstriction, and plasma cortisol and testosterone responses to laboratory stressors, as well as higher 24-hour urinary cortisol and ambulatory BP levels in normotensive and hypertensive individuals.[60-63] Some experts have interpreted such findings as evidence that hostile individuals demonstrate greater and more frequent stress reactions in daily life because they perceive more situations as threatening and because they provoke more conflicts and negative interpersonal interactions. Some studies have found no excessive BP responses to stress in high-hostility men and women during purely cognitive tasks such as mental arithmetic or the Stroop color-word task[64,65]; but other investigations in which the stressors involved interpersonal interactions, including efforts to control or dominate others or harassment and frustration by others, have consistently found greater pressor responses in high-hostility persons.[66] High-hostile young men reporting greater frequency and longer duration of angry episodes in their lives also demonstrate adrenergic receptor down-regulation, suggesting greater chronic SNS activity.[63]

Some studies have reported an apparently paradoxical association between low rather than high self-reports of hostility and higher BP. Work by Shapiro and Jamner et al. has suggested that these persons are not truly low in hostility, but instead they employ a defensive coping style, characterized by reluctance to admit to anger, anxiety, or other socially undesirable thoughts or feelings.[67,68] Defensive copers among paramedics and nurses showed higher ambulatory BP on the job, particularly under more stressful conditions. Defensive coping, like hostility, is more consistently related to high stress responsivity in men than in women, possibly because of differences in social expectations about expression of emotion between genders.[69,70] These observations indicate that it is not appropriate to conclude that there is a simple, unidirectional relationship between high scores on a hostility scale and risk of hypertension. Furthermore, several large-scale investigations have found that hostility scores decrease with increasing education and income.[71,72] Thus, it is important to separate the effects of social class from hostility by matching groups for education and economic resources or controlling statistically for group differences in these variables.

Anger-arousing experiences have long been known to raise BP and increase vasoconstriction.[1,2] One way in which hostile outlook may influence cardiovascular risk is through frequent bouts of anger. Three patterns of anger coping—high anger-out (hair trigger and explosive verbal and physical expression of anger), low anger-out (inability or unwillingness to show or express anger even when appropriate and justified), and high anger-in (denial of angry feelings toward others with unjustified self-blame)—have been hypothesized to lead to increased BP reactivity to stress and to hypertension.[73,74] The original research by Harburg et al. on African Americans living in high-crime areas of Detroit suggested that anger suppression or low anger-out was directly related to elevated BP in these stress-vulnerable people.[75] This pattern has been related to increased BP and heart rate during role play of conflicts and harassment in the laboratory, as well as to increased BP in wives after discussion of conflicts with their husbands.[59,76-80] Anger suppression, like hostility with its association of high-anger expression, has been related to down-regulation of β-adrenergic receptors, suggesting a stable pattern of sympathetic overactivity.[63,81,82] Engebretson et al. originally suggested that high cardiovascular reactivity was more frequent in both high–anger-in and high–anger-out persons if the stressor involved some provocation of angry feelings.[77] A recent prospective analysis of middle-aged men from the Kuopio, Finland study indicated that subjects who were at the extreme ends of the distribution for either anger-in or anger-out had a significantly higher risk of developing hypertension over the next 5 years.[83] These results confirm that extremes in either expressing or suppressing angry feelings are maladaptive and that moderation is the lowest-risk solution.

Another psychological factor related to increased BP is the desire to dominate and impress others, termed *power motivation*. McClelland found that inhibited power motivation in men predicted hypertension-related pathology in a 20-year study,[84] but few studies have confirmed an association between power motivation and either high reactivity or increased BP levels. Furthermore, a number of negative studies exist. The parallel of this pattern to Henry et al.'s psychosocial model of hypertension in rats and mice[7,18] is compelling and may provide a basis for integrating the contradictory results. Dominant and subdominant rats develop hypertension only if they are members of a strain that is vulnerable to stress-induced hypertension, and the BP increase occurs when aggressive contacts are high. In the truly dominant males, this occurs only when the social group members change, so that frequent bouts of aggression are required to assert dominance. In humans, the appropriate parallel might be that inhibited power motivation may lead to hypertension only when the individual's work and home environments are also unstable and the individual's social dominance is repeatedly threatened.

A related characteristic is the preference for active coping, or "John Henryism."[85-90] This trait is defined by the belief in individual control and that hard work and persistence despite obstacles will lead to future success. The theory regarding the active coping behavior pattern states specifically that it will not be related to increased sympathetic activity and BP if the environment is supportive and has adequate resources. Only if the individual's environment is deficient in some way, thus leading to excessive effort and sympathetic overactivity, will hypertension develop. James et al. showed that high John Henryism was associated with increased BP in lower–social class rural African Americans, whose environment offered little opportunity for success.[85,86] African American and white adolescents with the combination of high John Henryism and lower social class had increased BP and higher vascular resistance.[90] In another study in which the sample was limited to well-educated and employed African American and white adults, Light et al. observed that ambulatory BP at work was increased in women and African Americans with high-status professional and managerial jobs who scored high in this preference for active coping.[89] This effect was not seen among white male professionals and managers, and this was interpreted as evidence that this role is more threatening and less supportive for women and African Americans because of lack of peers in these jobs.

Attention has also focused on depressive symptoms and their relation to hypertension and cardiovascular risk.[91,92] Depression is different from previous psychological factors because it is assumed to be an impermanent mood state (characterized by sadness and loss of interest in work, hobbies, family, and friends) rather than a stable trait. However, longitudinal studies indicate that depressive states tend to recur and that past history of depression is a primary predictor of subsequent depressive states. Although fewer reports have supported a link between depression and hypertension versus a link between depression and cardiovascular or total mortality, the overall consistency of the pattern is compelling. Depression (as well as its correlated measure of distress, anxiety) is linked prospectively to onset of hypertension in both men and women, and in African American as well as white samples.[93] In elderly patients with established hypertension, men and women with higher depression scores show greater hypertension-related disease progression and increased incidence of stroke.[94,95] Depressive symptoms are predictive of more severe cardiac events. In patients with confirmed coronary heart disease (CHD), depressive symptoms are linked to increased myocardial infarction (MI), stroke, surgical intervention, and cardiac death; to decreased heart rate variability; and to increased cardiac activation and myocardial ischemia during Holter monitoring or mental stress in the laboratory.[91,96-100]

Depression can develop in susceptible persons as a reaction pattern to life stress, including stresses associated with health crises such as MI and other serious cardiovascular diagnoses.[96,97] In young healthy women, depressive symptoms were related to increased cardiac adrenergic tone and enhanced norepinephrine increases during a speech stressor.[101] In a larger subsequent study involving a biracial sample of both men and women, depressive symptoms were linked to increased ambulatory BP in persons with a genetic susceptibility to hypertension (i.e., those with hypertensive parents), but not in those with no susceptibility.[102] Stressful life events may contribute to worsening of depressive symptoms, and depression may in turn worsen sympathetic and cardiovascular responses to stress, producing a vicious circle effect. Frasure-Smith et al. have confirmed that in patients with a recent MI, depression predicts premature death due to recurrent MI, arrhythmic events, and congestive heart failure (CHF) at 6, 12, and 18 months' follow-up; risk was further increased in those whose post-MI depression was not their first depressive episode.[91,96,97] The effects of depression are strongest in the subgroup with premature ventricular complexes, a group especially vulnerable to arrhythmia and sudden death associated with alterations in cardiac autonomic activity, such as may be induced by severe acute life stress.

Hopelessness and pessimism are common among depressed and vitally exhausted individuals, but these can also occur without the severe sadness or loss of interest in life that are the true hallmarks of depression.[103] Unlike depression, which is more common in women than in men and less common in African Americans than in other ethnic groups, hopelessness is reported equally in both genders, and it may be equally or more common in minorities and those from lower social classes.[104] In the Kuopio Ischemic Heart Disease study, men with moderate to high hopelessness at baseline were 2.5 to 4 times more likely than men with lower levels of hopelessness to die of cardiovascular causes over a 6-year follow-up period, even after controlling for baseline BP, smoking, and other traditional cardiovascular risk factors.[105] Hopelessness also predicted all-cause mortality in this group of 2428 middle-aged men and carotid atherosclerotic lesion progression in the 942 men showing some carotid plaque at initial testing.[105,106] *The effect of persistent hopelessness was equivalent to that of smoking 2.5 packs of cigarettes daily.* Pessimism before coronary bypass surgery is also linked to increased likelihood of having a perioperative MI.[107,108] Less research has focused on the linkage of hopelessness and pessimism to hypertension, but the few studies reported to date support this relationship.[109] For example, in postmenopausal women, those who both had low SES and used a stable pessimistic attributional style (believing that bad events are permanent and cannot be controlled or improved) had increased ambulatory BP.[110] Helplessness and pessimism, like depression, are seen as both consequences of previous life stress and states that enhance the adverse cardiovascular effects of subsequent stress exposure.[111] Additional work on these important factors, which appear to parallel the defeat and helplessness state in animal models,[6,7] is currently in progress.

Altogether, there is substantial and growing evidence to support the association of hypertension and cardiac events with a number of psychological factors that involve stress as a causal factor in initiating the psychological condition or in contributing to its adverse cardiovascular consequences. Psychological states such as hostility, depression, anxiety, and hopelessness are thus ripe for serving as risk identifiers and as focal points for interventions to reduce risk. In two clinical trials, the Sadheart trial of pharmacotherapy for depression and the Enhanced Recovery in Coronary Heart Disease Patients (ENRICHD) trial of cognitive-behavioral therapy for clinical depression and/or social isolation, the addition of treatments for depression to standard medical care in patients with recent MI have alleviated psychological symptoms but did not further reduce cardiovascular morbidity and mortality.[112-114] Thus, it appears at this time that such psychological measures are best used as markers of additional risk that might be employed in an equation identifying persons for whom traditional medical interventions are even more vital to implement.[102]

## HIGH CARDIOVASCULAR RESPONSE TO STRESS IN PREDICTION OF LATER BLOOD PRESSURE ELEVATION

The hypothesis that those individuals who show exaggerated BP, heart rate, or other cardiovascular responses to behavioral stressors have increased risk of becoming hypertensive has generated considerable research and much debate since the late 1970s.[8,115] Indirect evidence supporting this hypothesis included observations that persons with borderline hypertension or those with hypertensive parents showed increased BP responses to stress in many studies, although not in all. Other evidence indicated that high response to stress was a stable characteristic of certain people, documented by highly correlated response levels when compared across stressors or on retesting after intervals as long as 1 to 10 years. Notably, response levels showed greater stability than did reactivity scores (calculated as increases from resting baseline levels).[3,17] More direct support for this hypothesis has been derived from several longitudinal studies. A number of these have employed a single stressor, often the cold pressor test, which elicits a BP increase via α-adrenergically mediated vasoconstriction. These investigations have not always yielded positive findings,[115] but the two largest investigations with the longest follow-up interval have supported the reactivity hypothesis by showing that individuals with the greatest BP increases to painful cold later developed hypertension at a higher rate than those with lesser BP increases.[116,117]

Several smaller-scale studies, particularly those focusing on young borderline-hypertensive individuals, have shown that high reactivity to active coping stressors like mental arithmetic that evoke BP increases through β-adrenergic activity and increased heart rate and cardiac output is predictive of later sustained hypertension.[118,119] Similar studies with active coping stressors using normotensive subjects have generated both positive and negative findings after partitioning out effects related to higher prestress BP, which is associated with high stress reactivity and later hypertension.[120-122] BP increases during *anticipation of upcoming physical or mental stress* and during *recovery after stress* are added effects of stress reactivity; increases in these measures are strongly predictive of later hypertension.[118,119,123]

Two prospective studies that included women as well as men in the sample have examined responses to multiple stressors. In the study by Matthews et al. involving parents and their children, high pressor reactivity to active coping stressors was related to increased BP after 6.5 years; the effects were more consistent for men and boys than for women and girls.[124] In the much larger Coronary Artery Risk Development in Young Adults (CARDIA) study involving more than 3300 African American and white young adults,[125] results after 5 years of follow-up indicated that high SBP reactivity to the active coping task, but not to the passive cold pressor test, was predictive of greater BP elevations and increased incidence of hypertension in African American and white men, even after controlling for baseline BP levels and other key covariates. In women regardless of race, neither task was effective in predicting later BP (Table 7–1).[125] The gender difference seen in the latter studies may have been related, in part, to the fact that women tend to develop hypertension at a later age, perhaps related to protective effects of female reproductive hormones during the ages under study. Another possibility is that video games may differentially engage higher active coping effort in men than in women.

Prior work by our group has supported the interpretation by the CARDIA investigators that individuals showing enhanced cardiac responses due to β-adrenergic activity during active coping stressors have a greater likelihood of demonstrating BP increases as young adults. In our investigation, the sample under study was small, but the follow-up testing involved more than 60 measures of BP from each subject obtained through ambulatory monitoring on a regular workday, providing greater confidence in the outcome measures.[120] Both high heart rate reactors and high BP responders to an active coping reaction time task demonstrated increased BP at work and at home as well as in the clinic 10 years later. The predictive effect of high heart rate reactivity most directly points to mediation via β-adrenergic activity, because our laboratory has confirmed through use of β-antagonists that heart rate and SBP elevations in response to active coping reaction time tasks primarily reflect such activity.[4,5]

More recently, our group has completed a second 10-year follow-up study using ambulatory BP monitoring.[126] This study reconfirmed that initially normotensive young men

**Table 7–1** Odds Ratios of Having Significant Blood Pressure Increase (8 mm Hg) Over 5-Year Follow-Up Function of Gender and Systolic Reactivity to Video Game: The CARDIA Study*

|  | Systolic Reactivity to Video Game (mm Hg)[†] | OR (95% CI) |
|---|---|---|
| Men | 5 | 0.8 (0.77, 0.92) |
|  | 10 | 1 |
|  | 20 | 1.4 (1.19, 1.69) |
|  | 30 | 2.0 (1.41, 2.86) |
| Women | 5 | 1.0 (0.89, 1.05) |
|  | 10 | 1 |
|  | 20 | 1.1 (0.91, 1.07) |
|  | 30 | 1.1 (0.83, 1.59) |

From Markovitz JH, Raczynski JM, Wallace D, et al. Cardiovascular reactivity to video game predicts subsequent blood pressure increases in young men: The CARDIA study. Psychosom Med 60:186-191, 1998.
OR, odds ratio; 95% CI, 95% confidence interval; BP, blood pressure.
*n = 889 with BP increase; n = 2722 without BP increase.
[†]Reference group = 10 mm Hg.

who were high heart rate and SBP responders to stress showed greater BP increases and a high incidence of borderline hypertension 10 years later. The results also showed that prediction of later development of borderline to stage 1 hypertension was strongest for the men who had hypertensive parents as well as high stress responsivity (Figure 7–2).[126] Finally, the study indicated that the stress exposure and stress buffers in the person's home and work environments could influence the predictive effect of high cardiovascular responsivity to stress. Clinic pressure was higher in high stress responders who reported high scores on the Daily Stress Inventory, but not for those reporting low daily stress. Similarly, ambulatory pressure at work was greater in high stress responders reporting low support from their work supervisor and greater during leisure at home from those reporting low overall social support, but not in high responders who had greater support in their lives. These findings encourage reconsideration of the reactivity hypothesis, expanding it to take into account genetic factors (e.g., parental hypertension); differences across individuals in chronic stress exposure, which affects expression of the predisposition to high heart rate and BP responses; and differences in exposure to stress buffers like social support.

In sum, these investigations provide cautious encouragement for continued research addressing high reactivity to stress as a potential risk factor for hypertension. Future research should avoid some of the oversimplified approaches of the past and utilize available opportunities to examine stress-response patterns in association with information about family history and factors relating to chronic stress level.

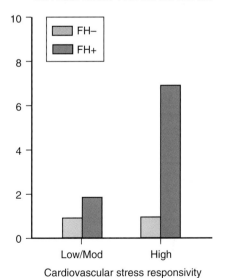

RELATIVE RISK OF HYPERTENSION
DEVELOPMENT TEN YEARS LATER

FH−
FH+

Cardiovascular stress responsivity

**Figure 7–2** High cardiovascular stress response predicts future hypertension in men with positive *(FH+)* but not negative family history of hypertension *(FH−* (Adapted from Light KC, Girdler SS, Sherwood A, et al. High stress responsivity predicts later blood pressure only in combination with positive family history and high life stress. Hypertension 33:1458-1464, 1999.)

## STRESS BUFFERS AND STRESS-REDUCTION INTERVENTIONS

As one of the spokesmen for models of stress and disease in humans, Cohen has incorporated a category of factors labeled *stress buffers* in his model.[127] Stress buffers include any factor that reduces perceived level of distress in individuals exposed to stress, that limits exposure to stressors, or that decreases adverse physiologic reactions to stress. The best-documented stress buffer is social support. Social isolation has been associated with high rates of premature death from cardiovascular disease and all causes combined.[128-131] In patients with MI, increased emotional social support was related to decreased mortality, even after controlling for age, Killip class, and other cardiovascular risk factors.[131] Laboratory studies have shown that BP and other cardiovascular responses to mental challenges are less when a supportive and nonevaluative person is present.[132-134] Similarly, even support from a pet dog or cat has been shown to reduce stress responses.[135] In contrast, when the supportive person may be evaluating the test subject based on her or his performance, or when support may increase the intensity of effort (such as arguing against racial discrimination in the presence of another person advocating the same position), cardiovascular responses can actually be increased rather than decreased when the supporter is present.[134-136] Support provided by a marital partner can be especially beneficial in reducing stress responses. In a recent study by Grewen et al., *BP and heart rate increases to a speech task were reduced by almost 50%* in 100 men and women tested immediately after a 10-minute period of warm contact with their partner (including hand-holding and a hug) versus 89 persons tested after solitary rest (Figure 7–3).[137]

In studies involving ambulatory BP monitoring, high perceived support is related to lower BP.[138-141] Again marital support is especially important. Persons reporting a more supportive relationship with their spouse/partner had lower ambulatory BP than those with no partner, but others who were married with a poor partner relationship had higher BP than those with no partner.[140] In a 3-year prospective study of hypertensive patients, more supportive marital relationships were prospectively associated with an 8% decrease, whereas poorer marital relationships were associated with a 6% increase in left ventricular mass.[141] In another study, Brownley et al. reported that high social support did not act by itself to lower BP in 129 healthy African American and white men and women, but it did interact with another factor that might increase stress and BP: a hostile outlook on life. In this sample, high-hostile persons lacking support had higher ambulatory BP, whereas high-hostile persons with social support showed no BP increase relative to low-hostile persons.[139] A similar interaction was seen in a prospective study of Swedish men, in which type A men lacking social support had increased mortality but other type A men reporting more support had no increase in risk relative to type B men.[142] Additional work addressing the potential stress-buffering effect of social support is needed, however. In particular, interactions of support with anger-coping styles and other psychological factors, with high stress reactivity, and with environmental stressors like job strain have clear potential to reveal important relationships.

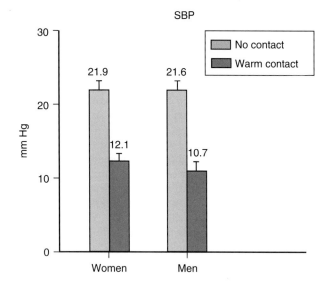

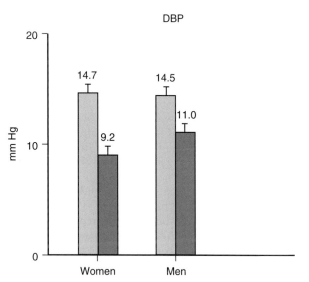

**Figure 7–3** Warm contact with spouse/partner prior to stress reduces systolic blood pressure (SBP) and diastolic blood pressure (DBP) increases to an anger-recall speech task. (Adapted from Grewen K, Anderson B, Girdler S, et al. Warm partner contact is related to lower cardiovascular reactivity. Behav Med 2003; 29:123-130.)

Another potential stress buffer is aerobic exercise. A number of studies have compared cardiovascular responses to stress after a period of exercise versus those following a control condition.[143-148] Some of these studies showed no differences, whereas others supported the hypothesis that stress responses are reduced after exercise.[148] Two factors that may influence the outcome of such studies are whether the subject is a high reactor to stress and whether his or her BP is elevated. Research in our laboratory has suggested that moderate aerobic exercise for only 20 to 30 minutes can evoke a reduction in vascular resistance in most individuals, but that BP will not decrease in all subjects.[144,147] BP responses during stress appear to be blunted after exercise in high stress reactors. This makes sense, because it is hard to reduce a response that is already minimal. Also, ambulatory BP levels have been shown to be reduced at work for up to 5 or more hours after exercise in borderline-hypertensive persons, whereas normotensive subjects typically show no reduction in BP, although they do show potentially beneficial decreases in total vascular resistance.[147,149] This appears to be related to homeostatic influences, such as baroreceptor activity, that elicit compensatory adjustments in circulatory control systems to prevent a fall in BP in normotensive individuals. Other research has indicated that reduced efferent SNS activity and lower circulating catecholamine levels contribute to the lower vascular resistance in the postexercise period.[150,151]

These studies addressed the effects of only a single bout of exercise on responses during the postexercise period. Other investigations have examined the effects of increased aerobic fitness level due to weeks of physical training on stress responses. These studies have similarly suggested that stress responses are reduced after aerobic training in some but not all persons, with hypertensive individuals being most likely to benefit. More rapid recovery of cardiovascular responses after stress has been observed as a more general benefit of training.[148] For this reason, regular exercise is strongly recommended both as adjunctive treatment and as a preventive intervention for hypertension.[109,151-153]

Stress-reduction interventions, including biofeedback, relaxation training, and cognitive behavioral therapies, have been extensively studied as potential ways to lower BP, with mixed success.[154-157] McGrady and Higgins attempted to develop a profile of hypertensive patients most likely to lower their BP through biofeedback. They found that young women with higher anxiety and tension levels and higher initial heart rates are the most successful in using this method.[155] Other studies have indicated that relaxation therapy is more effective with individuals whose daytime ambulatory BP is elevated versus those with lower daytime pressures.[154] Although some studies employing a "habituation control phase" have observed no changes with stress-reduction treatment,[157] falls in BP during both habituation and treatment have been seen in other well-designed investigations.[156]

There has been substantial rekindling of interest in stress-reduction interventions after the reports by Ornish et al.[158] and by Blumenthal et al.[159] that stress management can be part of a lifestyle intervention program that can reduce risk and even partially reverse vascular pathology in CHD patients. The former study employed stress management only in combination with other established methods, such as low-fat diet, exercise, and weight reduction, whereas the latter used stress management as a solitary intervention and compared its benefits with an exercise training group as well as to a usual care group. Patients given a combination of relaxation, biofeedback, and cognitive therapies to help them recognize and manage stress, anger, and depression demonstrated greater reduction in risk of subsequent cardiac events or interventions compared with patients given exercise training or usual care.[159] Although more studies are clearly needed, the overall pattern suggests that stress-management techniques are effective in reducing cardiovascular risks in some individuals. Benefits are more likely with interventions using cognitive therapy as well as simpler relaxation or biofeedback approaches and in patient groups with more cardiovascular and psychological risk factors. It is expected that more research on this topic will be forthcoming.

## SUMMARY

The preponderance of animal and human research shows that environmental and psychosocial stress have a clear impact on BP levels over the short term, and these may have a role in the onset and progression of hypertension in individuals with genetic or environmentally enhanced susceptibility (such as a high-salt, low-potassium diet). Increased SNS activity is a mediator of the effect of stress on BP, although other factors are also involved. Certain personality and behavioral patterns are associated with high stress responses and greater risk of hypertension and cardiovascular disease, and certain environmentally stressful conditions (ranging from the broadest, such as low SES, to the more specific, such as high job strain) are potential risk factors for hypertension. Buffers available to reduce the adverse effects of stress on BP include social support, exercise, and stress-management therapies. Since modern life in Western societies appears to make stress exposure unavoidable, more research on strategies to reduce the effects of stress exposure is needed.

## References

1. Schacter J. Pain, fear and anger in hypertensives and normotensives. Psychosom Med 19:17-29, 1957.
2. Sinha R, Lovallo WR, Parsons OA. Cardiovascular differentiation of emotions. Psychosom Med 54:422-435, 1992.
3. Sherwood A, Turner JR. A conceptual and methodological overview of cardiovascular reactivity research. In Turner JR, Sherwood A, Light KC (eds). Individual Differences in Cardiovascular Response to Stress. New York, Plenum, 1992; pp 3-32.
4. Light KC, Sherwood A. Race, borderline hypertension and hemodynamic responses to behavioral stress before and after beta-adrenergic blockade. Health Psychol 8:577-595, 1990.
5. Girdler SS, Hinderliter AL, Light KC. Peripheral adrenergic receptor contributions to cardiovascular reactivity: Influence of race and gender. J Psychosom Res 37:177-193, 1993.
6. Henry JP, Grim CE. Psychosocial mechanisms of primary hypertension. [Editorial review] J Hypertens 8:783-793, 1990.
7. Henry JP, Liu J, Meehan WP. Psychosocial stress and experimental hypertension. In Laragh JM, Brenner BM (eds). Hypertension. Pathophysiology, Diagnosis and Management. New York, Raven, 1995; pp 905-921.
8. Manuck SB. Cardiovascular reactivity in cardiovascular disease: "Once more unto the breach." Int J Behav Med 1:4-31, 1994.
9. Light KC, Girdler SS, West S, Brownley KA. Blood pressure responses to occupational challenges and laboratory stress in women. In Orth-Gomer K, Chesney MA, Wenger N (eds). Women, Stress and Heart Disease. Mahwah, NJ, Lawrence Erlbaum, 1998; pp 237-261.
10. Sudhir K, Jennings GL, Funder JW, et al. Estrogen enhances basal nitric oxide release in the forearm vasculature in perimenopausal women. Hypertension 28:330-334, 1996.
11. Owens JF, Stoney CM, Matthews KA. Menopausal status influences ambulatory blood pressure levels and blood pressure changes during mental stress. Circulation 88:2794-2802, 1993.
12. Light KC, Turner JR, Hinderliter AL, et al. Race and gender comparisons. I: Hemodynamic responses to a series of stressors. Health Psychol 12:354-365, 1993.
13. Sherwood A, May CW, Siegel WC, et al. Ethnic differences in hemodynamic responses to stress in hypertensive men and women. Am J Hypertens 8:552-557, 1995.
14. Light KC, Koepke JP, Obrist PA, et al. Psychological stress induces sodium and fluid retention in men at risk for hypertension. Science 220:429-431, 1983.
15. Light KC, Turner JR. Stress-induced changes in the rate of sodium excretion in healthy black and white men. J Psychosom Res 36:497-508, 1992.
16. Harshfield GA, Pulliam DA, Alpert BS. Patterns of sodium excretion during sympathetic nervous system arousal. Hypertension 17:1156-1170, 1992.
17. Sherwood A, Girdler SS, Bragdon EE, et al. Ten-year stability of cardiovascular responses to laboratory stressors. Psychophysiology 34:185-191, 1997.
18. Henry JP, Stephens PM. Stress, Health and the Social Environment: A Sociobiologic Approach to Medicine. New York, Springer-Verlag, 1977.
19. Folkow B. Physiological aspects of the "defense" and "defeat" reactions. Acta Physiol Scand 161(suppl 640):34-37, 1997.
20. Mormede P. Genetic influences on the responses to psychosocial challenges in rats. Acta Physiol Scand 161(suppl 640): 65-68, 1997.
21. Ely D, Caplea A, Dunphy G, et al. Physiological and neuroendocrine correlates of social position in normotensive and hypertensive rat colonies. Acta Physiol Scand 161(suppl 640):92-95, 1997.
22. Lawler JE, Barker GF, Hubbard JW, et al. Effect of stress on blood pressure and cardiac pathology in rats with borderline hypertension. Hypertension 3:496-501, 1981.
23. Sanders BJ, Cox RH, Lawler JE. Cardiovascular and renal responses to stress in borderline hypertensive rat. Am J Physiol 255:R431-R438, 1988.
24. Lawler JE, Zheng G, Li S, et al. Norepinephrine levels in discrete brain nuclei in borderline hypertensive rats exposed to compound stressors. Brain Res Bull 41:87-92, 1996.
25. Cox RH, Hubbard JW, Lawler JE, et al. Exercise training attenuates stress-induced hypertension in the rat. Hypertension 7: 747-751, 1985.
26. Sanders BJ, Lawler JE. The borderline hypertensive rat (BHR) as a model for environmentally induced hypertension: A review and update. Neurosci Biobeh Rev 16:207-217, 1992.
27. DiBona GF, Jones SY. Renal manifestations of NaCl sensitivity in borderline hypertensive rats. Hypertension 17:44-53, 1991.
28. Koepke JP, Jones SY, DiBona GF. Sodium responsiveness of central alpha-adrenergic receptors in spontaneously hypertensive rats. Hypertension 11:326-333, 1988.
29. Koepke JP, DiBona GF. Central adrenergic receptor control of renal function in conscious hypertensive rats. Hypertension 8:133-141, 1986.
30. Anderson DE, Kearns WD, Better WE. Progressive hypertension in dogs by avoidance conditioning and saline infusion. Hypertension 5:286-291, 1983.
31. Anderson DE, Kearns WD, Worden TJ. Potassium infusion attenuates avoidance-saline hypertension in dogs. Hypertension 5:415-420, 1983.
32. Anderson DA, Dietz JR, Murphy P. Behavioral hypertension in sodium-loaded dogs is accompanied by sustained sodium retention. J Hypertens 5:99-105, 1987.
33. Gutman D, Nemeroff CB. Neurobiology of early life stress: rodent studies. Semin Clin Neuropsychiatry 7:89-95, 2002.
34. Boccia ML, Pedersen CA. Brief vs. long maternal separations in infancy: contrasting relationships with adult maternal behavior and lactating levels of aggression and anxiety. Psychoneuroendocrinology 26:657-672, 2001.
35. Luecken LJ. Childhood attachment and loss experiences affect adult cardiovascular and cortisol function. Psychosom Med 60:765-772, 1998.
36. Holst S, Uvnas-Moberg K, Petersson M. Postnatal oxytocin treatment and postnatal stroking of rats reduce blood pressure in adulthood. Autonom Neurosci 99:85-90, 2002.
37. Pedersen CA, Boccia ML. Oxytocin links mothering received, mothering bestowed and adult stress responses. Stress 5: 259-267, 2002.

38. Petersson M. Cardiovascular effects of oxytocin. Prog Brain Res 139:281-288, 2002.

39. Pickering TG. The effects of environmental and lifestyle factors on blood pressure and the intermediary role of the sympathetic nervous system. J Hum Hypertens 11(suppl 1):S9-S18, 1997.

40. Shaper AG. Cardiovascular studies in the Samburo tribe of northern Kenya. Am Heart J 63:437-442, 1962.

41. Shaper AG, Leonard PJ, Jones KW, et al. Environmental effects on the body build, blood pressure and blood chemistry of nomadic warriors serving in the army in Kenya. East Afr Med J 46:282-289, 1969.

42. Waldron I, Nowotarski M, Freimer M, et al. Cross-cultural variation in blood pressure: A quantitative analysis of the relationship of blood pressure to cultural characteristics, salt consumption and body weight. Soc Sci Med 16:419-430, 1982.

43. Kaplan GA, Keil JE. Socioeconomic factors and coronary heart disease: A review of the literature. Circulation 88:1978-1998, 1993.

44. Anderson NB, Myers H, Pickering T, et al. Hypertension in blacks: Psychosocial and biological perspectives. J Hypertens 7:161-172, 1989.

45. Anderson NB, McNeilly M, Myers H. Toward understanding race difference in autonomic reactivity. *In* Turner JR, Sherwood A, Light KC (eds). Individual Differences in Cardiovascular Response to Stress. New York, Plenum, 1992; pp 125-145.

46. Dressler WW. Social support, lifestyle incongruity, and arterial blood pressure in a southern black community. Psychsom Med 53:608-620, 1991.

47. Rose RM, Jenkins CD, Hurst MW. Health change in air traffic controllers: A prospective study. I: Background and description. Psychosom Med 40:142-165, 1978.

48. Karasek RA, Baker D, Marxer F, et al. Job decision latitude, job demands and cardiovascular disease: A prospective study in Swedish men. Am J Pub Health 75:694-705, 1981.

49. Schnall PL, Pieper C, Schwartz JE, et al. The relationship between "job strain," workplace diastolic blood pressure and left ventricular mass index. JAMA 263:1929-1935, 1990; also see Correction, JAMA 267:1209, 1992.

50. Schnall PL, Schwartz JE, Landsbergis PA, et al. Relation between job strain, alcohol and ambulatory blood pressure. Hypertension 19:488-494, 1992.

51. Pollard TM, Ungpakorn G, Harrison GA, et al. Epinephrine and cortisol responses to work: A test of the models of Frankenhaeuser and Karasek. Ann Behav Med 18:229-237, 1996.

52. Light KC, Turner JR, Hinderliter AL. Job strain and ambulatory work blood pressure in healthy young men and women. Hypertension 20:214-218, 1992.

53. Lundberg U. Work and stress in women. *In:* Orth-Gomer K, Chesney MA, Wenger NK (eds): Women, Stress and Heart Disease. Mahwah, NJ, Lawrence Erlbaum, 1998; pp 41-56.

54. Luecken LJ, Suarez EC, Kuhn CM, et al. Stress in employed women: Impact of marital status and children at home on neurohormone output and home strain. Psychosom Med 59:352-359, 1997.

55. Rosenman RH, Brand RJ, Scholtz RI, et al. Multivariate prediction of coronary heart disease during the 8.5 year follow-up in the Western Collaborative Group Study. Am J Cardiol 37:903-912, 1976.

56. Houston BK, Chesney MA, Black GW, et al. Behavioral clusters and coronary heart disease risk. Psychosom Med 54:447-461, 1992.

57. Barefoot JC, Dahlstrom WG, Williams RB Jr. Hostility, CHD incidence and total mortality: A 25-year follow-up study of 255 physicians. Psychosom Med 45:59-63, 1983.

58. Dembroski TM, MacDougall JM, Costa PT, et al. Components of hostility as predictors of sudden death and myocardial infarction in the Multiple Risk Factor Intervention Trial. Psychosom Med 51:514-522, 1989.

59. Smith TW. Hostility and health: Current status of a psychosomatic hypothesis. Health Psychol 11:139-150, 1992.

60. Weidner G, Friend R, Ficarotto TJ, et al. Hostility and cardiovascular reactivity to stress in women and men. Psychosom Med 51:36-45, 1990.

61. Girdler SS, Jamner LD, Shapiro D. Hostility, testosterone and vascular reactivity to stress: Effects of gender. Int J Behav Med 4:242-263, 1998.

62. Jamner LD, Shapiro D, Hui KK, et al. Hostility and differences between clinic, self-determined and ambulatory blood pressure. Psychosom Med 55:203-211, 1993.

63. Suarez EC, Shiller AD, Kuhn CM, et al. The relationship between hostility and beta-adrenergic receptor physiology in healthy young males. Psychosom Med 59:481-487, 1997.

64. Sallis JF, Johnson CC, Trevorrow TR, et al. The relationship between cynical hostility and blood pressure reactivity. J Psychosom Res 31:111-116, 1987.

65. Smith MA, Houston BK. Hostility, anger expression, cardiovascular responsivity and social support. Biol Psychol 24:39-48, 1987.

66. Everson SA, McKey BS, Lovallo WR. Effect of trait hostility on cardiovascular responses to harassment in young men. Int J Behav Med 2:172-191, 1995.

67. Jamner LD, Shapiro D, Goldstein IB, et al. Ambulatory blood pressure and heart rate in paramedics: Effects of cynical hostility and defensiveness. Psychosom Med 53:393-406, 1992.

68. Shapiro D, Goldstein IB, Jamner LD. Effect of cynical hostility, anger out, anxiety and defensiveness on ambulatory blood pressure in black and white college students. Psychosom Med 58:354-364, 1996.

69. Helmers KF, Krantz DS. Defensive hostility, gender and cardiovascular levels and responses to stress. Ann Behav Med 18:246-254, 1996.

70. King AC, Taylor CB, Albright CA, et al. The relationship between repressive and defensive coping styles and blood pressure responses in healthy middle-aged men and women. J Psychosom Res 34:461-471, 1990.

71. Scherwitz L, Perkins L, Chesney M, et al. Cook-Medley Hostility Scale and subsets: Relationships to demographic and psychosocial characteristics in young adults in the CARDIA Study. Psychosom Med 53:36-49, 1991.

72. Barefoot JC, Peterson BL, Dahlstrom WG, et al. Hostility patterns and health implications: Correlates of Cook-Medley Hostility Scale scores in a national survey. Health Psychol 10:18-24, 1991.

73. Manuck SB, Morrison RL, Bellack AS, et al. Behavioral factors in hypertension: Cardiovascular responsivity, anger and social competence. *In* Chesney MA, Rosenman RM (eds). Anger and Hostility in Cardiovascular and Behavioral Disorders. Washington, DC, Hemisphere, 1985; pp 149-172.

74. Houston BK. Personality characteristics, reactivity, and cardiovascular disease. *In* Turner JR, Sherwood A, Light KC (eds). Individual Differences in Cardiovascular Response to Stress. New York, Plenum, 1992; pp 103-123.

75. Harburg E, Erfurt J, Hauenstein L, et al. Socio-ecological stress, suppressed hostility, skin color and Black-White male blood pressure: Detroit. Psychosom Med 35:276-296, 1973.

76. Durel LA, Carver CS, Spitzer SB, et al. Associations of blood pressure with self-report measures of anger and hostility among black and white men and women. Health Psychol 8:557-575, 1989.

77. Engebretson TO, Matthews KA, Scheier MF. Relations between anger expression and cardiovascular reactivity: Reconciling inconsistent findings through a matching hypothesis. J Pers Soc Psychol 58:844-854, 1989.

78. Powch IG, Houston BK. Hostility, anger-in and cardiovascular reactivity in white women. Health Psychol 15:200-208, 1996.

79. Houston BK. Anger, hostility and psychophysiological reactivity. *In* Siegman AW, Smith TW (eds). Anger, Hostility and the Heart. Hillsdale, NJ, Lawrence Erlbaum, 1996; pp 97-115.

80. Dimsdale JE, Pierce C, Schoenfeld D, et al. Suppressed anger and blood pressure: The effects of race, sex, social class, obesity and age. Psychosom Med 48:430-436, 1986.
81. Mills PJ, Dimsdale JE. Anger suppression: Its relationship to beta-adrenergic receptor sensitivity and stress-induced changes in blood pressure. Psychol Med 23:673-678, 1993.
82. Julius S, Amerena J, Smith S, et al. Autonomic and behavioral factors in hypertension. In Laragh JH, Brenner BM (eds). Hypertension: Pathophysiology, Diagnosis and Management. New York, Raven, 1995; pp 2557-2570.
83. Everson SA, Goldberg DE, Kaplan GA, et al. Anger expression and incident hypertension. Psychosom Med 60:730-735, 1998.
84. McClelland DC. Inhibited power motivation and high blood pressure in men. J Abnorm Psychol 8:182-190, 1979.
85. James SA, Harnett SA, Kalsbeek WD. John Henryism and blood pressure differences among black men. J Behav Med 6:259-278, 1983.
86. James SA, Keenan NL, Strogatz DS, et al. Socioeconomic status, John Henryism and blood pressure in black adults: The Pitt County Study. Am J Epidemiol 135:59-67, 1992.
87. Duijkers TJ, Drijver M, Kromhout D, et al. John Henryism and blood pressure in a Dutch population. Psychosom Med 50:353-359, 1988.
88. James SA. John Henryism and the health of African Americans. Cult Med Psychiatry 18:163-182, 1994.
89. Light KC, Brownley KA, Turner JR, et al. Job status and high-effort coping influence work blood pressure in women and blacks. Hypertension 25:554-559, 1995.
90. Wright LB, Treiber FA, Davis H, et al. Relationship of John Henryism to cardiovascular functioning at rest and during stress in youth. Ann Behav Med 18:146-150, 1996.
91. Frasure-Smith N, Lesperance F, Talajic M. Depression and 18-month prognosis after myocardial infarction. Circulation 91:999-1005, 1995.
92. Barefoot JC, Schroll M. Symptoms of depression, acute myocardial infarction and total mortality in a community sample. Circulation 93:1976-1980, 1996.
93. Jonas BS, Franks P, Ingram DD. Are symptoms of anxiety and depression risk factors for hypertension? Longitudinal evidence from the NHANES I Epidemiologic Follow-up Study. Arch Fam Med 6:43-49, 1997.
94. Wassertheil-Smoller S, Applegate WB, Berge K, et al. Change in depression as a precursor of cardiovascular events. SHEP Cooperative Research Group (Systolic Hypertension in the Elderly). Arch Intern Med 156:553-561, 1996.
95. Simonsick EM, Wallace RB, Balzer DG, et al. Depressive symptomatology and hypertension-associated morbidity and mortality in older adults. Psychosom Med 57:427-435, 1995.
96. Lesperance F, Frasure-Smith N, Talajic M. Major depression before and after myocardial infarction: Its nature and consequences. Psychosom Med 58:1-9, 1996.
97. Frasure-Smith N, Lesperance F, Talajic M. The impact of negative emotions on prognosis following myocardial infarction: Is it more than depression? Health Psychol 14:388-398, 1995.
98. Carney RM, Rich MW, Freedland KE, et al. Major depressive disorder predicts cardiac events in patients with coronary artery disease. Psychosom Med 50:627-633, 1988.
99. Carney RM, Saunders RD, Freedland KE, et al. Association of depression with reduced heart rate variability in patients with coronary artery disease. Am J Cardiol 76:562-564, 1995.
100. Krittayaphong R, Cascio WE, Light KC, et al. Heart rate variability in patients with coronary artery disease: Differences in patients with higher and lower depression scores. Psychom Med 59:231-235, 1997.
101. Light KC, Kothandapani RV, Allen MT. Enhanced cardiovascular and catecholamine responses in women with depressive symptoms. Int J Psychophysiol 28:157-166, 1998.
102. Grewen K, Girdler S, Hinderliter A, et al. Depressive symptoms are related to higher ambulatory blood pressure in persons with a family history of hypertension. Psychosom Med 2004 (in press).
103. Dua JK. Health, affect and attributional style. J Clin Psychol 51:507-518, 1995.
104. Greene SM. Levels of measured hopelessness in the general population. Br J Clin Psychol 20:11-14, 1981.
105. Everson SA, Goldberg DE, Kaplan GA, et al. Hopelessness and risk of mortality and incidence of myocardial infarction and cancer. Psychosom Med 58:113-121, 1996.
106. Everson SA, Kaplan GA, Goldberg DE, et al. Hopelessness and 4-year progression of carotid atherosclerosis. The Kuopio Ischemic Heart Disease Risk Factor Study. Arterioscler Thromb Vasc Biol 17:2-7, 1997.
107. Scheier MF, Matthews KA, Owens J, et al. Dispositional optimism and recovery from coronary artery bypass surgery: The beneficial effects on physical and psychological well-being. J Pers Soc Psychol 57:1024-1040, 1989.
108. Buchanan GM. Explanatory style and coronary heart disease. In Buchanon GM, Seligman MEP (eds). Explanatory Style. Hillsdale, NJ, Lawrence Erlbaum, 1995; pp 225-232.
109. Horan MJ, Lenfant C. Epidemiology of blood pressure and predictors of hypertension. Hypertension 15(suppl I):I20-I24, 1990.
110. Grewen K, Girdler SS, West SG, et al. Stable pessimistic attributions interact with socioeconomic status to influence blood pressure and vulnerability to hypertension. J Womens Health Gend Based Med 9:905-915, 2000.
111. Forest KB, Moen P, Dempster-McClain D. The effects of childhood family stress on women's depressive symptoms: A life course approach. Psychol Women Q 20:81-100, 1996.
112. Glassman AH, OConnor CM, Califf RM, et al. (Sadheart Group) Sertraline treatment of major depression in patients with acute myocardial infarction or unstable angina. JAMA 288:701-709, 2002.
113. Berkman LF, Blumenthal J, Burg M, et al. Effects of treating depression and low perceived social support on clinical events after myocardial infarction: The Enhancing Recovery in Coronary Heart Disease Patients (ENRICHD) Randomized Trial. JAMA 289:3171-3173, 2003.
114. Carney RM, Blumenthal JA, Catellier D, et al (ENRICHD Group). Depression as a risk factor for mortality after acute myocardial infarction. Am J Cardiol 92:1277-1281, 2003.
115. Pickering TG, Gerin W. Cardiovascular reactivity in the laboratory and the role of behavioral factors in hypertension: A critical review. Ann Behav Med 12:3-16, 1990.
116. Menkes MS, Matthews KA, Krantz DS, et al. Cardiovascular reactivity to the cold pressor as a predictor of hypertension. Hypertension 14:524-530, 1989.
117. Kasagi F, Akahoshi M, Shimaoki K. Relation between cold pressor test and development of hypertension based on 28-year follow-up. Hypertension 25:71-76, 1995.
118. Falkner B, Onesti G, Hamstra B. Stress response characteristics of adolescents with high genetic risk for essential hypertension. Clin Exp Hypertens 3:583-591, 1981.
119. Borghi C, Costa FV, Boschi S, et al. Predictors of stable hypertension in young borderline hypertensive subjects: A five-year follow-up study. J Cardiovasc Pharmacol 8(suppl 5):S138-S141, 1986.
120. Light KC, Dolan CA, Davis MR, et al. Cardiovascular responses to an active coping challenge as predictors of blood pressure patterns 10 to 15 years later. Psychosom Med 54:217-238, 1992.
121. Murphy JK, Alpert BS, Walker SS. Ethnicity, pressor reactivity and children's blood pressure: Five years of observations. Hypertension 20:327-332, 1992.
122. Carroll D, Smith GD, Sheffield D, et al. Pressor reactions to psychological stress and prediction of future blood pressure: Data from the Whitehall II Study. BMJ 310:771-776, 1995.

123. Everson SA, Kaplan GA, Goldberg DE, et al. Anticipatory blood pressure response to exercise predicts future high blood pressure in middle-aged men. Hypertension 27:1059-1064, 1996.

124. Matthews KA, Woodall KL, Allen MT. Cardiovascular reactivity to stress predicts future blood pressure status. Hypertension 22:479-485, 1993.

125. Markovitz JH, Raczynski JM, Wallace D, et al. Cardiovascular reactivity to video game predicts subsequent blood pressure increases in young men: The CARDIA Study. Psychosom Med 60:186-191, 1998.

126. Light KC, Girdler SS, Sherwood A, et al. High stress responsivity predicts later blood pressure only in combination with positive family history and high life stress. Hypertension 33:1458-1464, 1999.

127. Cohen S. Psychosocial models of the role of social support in the etiology of physical disease. Health Psychol 7:269-297, 1988.

128. House JS, Robbins C, Metzner HL. The association of social relationships and activities to mortality: Prospective evidence from Tecumseh Community Health Study. Am J Epidemiol 116:123-140, 1982.

129. Berkman L, Syme SL. Social networks, host resistance and mortality: A nine-year follow-up of Alameda County residents. Am J Epidemiol 109:186-204, 1979.

130. Williams RB, Barefoot JC, Califf RM, et al. Prognostic importance of social and economic resources among medically treated patients with angiographically documented coronary artery disease. JAMA 267:520-524, 1992.

131. Berkman LF, Leo-Summers L, Horwitz RI. Emotional support and survival after myocardial infarction. Ann Intern Med 117:1003-1009, 1992.

132. Gerin W, Milner D, Chawla S. Social support as a moderator of cardiovascular reactivity: A test of the direct and buffering hypotheses. Psychosom Med 57:16-22, 1995.

133. Lepore SJ, Allen KA, Evans GW. Social support lowers cardiovascular reactivity to an acute stressor. Psychosom Med 55:518-524, 1993.

134. Kamarck TW, Annunciato B, Amateau LM. Affiliation moderates the effects of social threat on stress-related cardiovascular responses: Boundary conditions for a laboratory model of social support. Psychosom Med 57:183-194, 1995.

135. Allen K, Blascovich J, Tomaka J, et al. Presence of human friends and pet dogs as moderators of autonomic responses to stress in women. J Pers Soc Psychol 61:582-589, 1991.

136. McNeilly MD, Robinson EL, Anderson NB, et al. Effects of racist provocation and social support on cardiovascular reactivity in African American women. Int J Behav Med 2:321-338, 1995.

137. Grewen K, Anderson B, Girdler S, et al. Warm partner contact is related to lower cardiovascular reactivity. Behav Med 2004 (in press).

138. Linden W, Chambers L, Maurice J, et al. Sex differences in social support, self-deception, hostility and ambulatory cardiovascular activity. Health Psychol 12:376-380, 1993.

139. Brownley KA, Light KC, Anderson NB. Social support and hostility interact to influence clinic, work and home blood pressure in black and white men and women. Psychophysiology 33:434-445, 1996.

140. Miller V, Grewen K, Light KC. Men and women in better partner relationships have better ambulatory blood pressure. Ann Behav Med 25 (Suppl 1): S143, 2003.

141. Baker B, Szalai JP, Paquette M, et al. Marital support, spousal contact and the course of mild hypertension. J Psychosom Res 55:229-233, 2003.

142. Orth-Gomer K, Unden A. Type A behavior, social support and coronary risk: Interaction and significance for mortality in cardiac patients. Psychosom Med 55:37-43, 1990.

143. Roskies E, Seraganian P, Oseasohn R, et al. The Montreal Type A Intervention Project: Major findings. Health Psychol 5:45-69, 1986.

144. Sherwood A, Light KC, Blumenthal JA. Effects of aerobic exercise on hemodynamic responses during psychosocial stress in normotensive and borderline hypertensive Type A men: A preliminary report. Psychosom Med 23:89-104, 1989.

145. Boone JB, Probst MM, Rogers MW, et al. Postexercise hypotension reduces cardiovascular responses to stress. J Hypertens 11:449-453, 1993.

146. Steptoe A, Kearsley N, Walters N. Cardiovascular activity during mental stress following vigorous exercise in sportsmen and inactive men. Psychophysiology 30:245-252, 1993.

147. West SG, Brownley KA, Light KC. Postexercise vasodilation reduces diastolic blood pressure responses to stress. Ann Behav Med 20:77-83, 1998.

148. Fillingim RB, Blumenthal JA. Does aerobic exercise reduce stress responses? In Turner JR, Sherwood A, Light KC (eds). Individual Differences in Cardiovascular Response to Stress. New York, Plenum, 1992; pp 203-217.

149. Brownley KA, West SG, Hinderliter AL, et al. Acute aerobic exercise reduces ambulatory blood pressure in borderline hypertensive men and women. Am J Hypertens 9:200-206, 1996.

150. Floras JS, Sinkey CA, Aylward PE, et al. Postexercise hypotension and sympathoinhibition in borderline hypertensive men. Hypertension 14:28-35, 1989.

151. Piepoli M, Coats AJS, Adamopoulos S, et al. Persistent peripheral vasodilation and sympathetic activity in hypotension after maximal exercise. J Appl Physiol 75:1807-1814, 1993.

152. World Hypertension League. Physical exercise in the management of hypertension: A consensus statement by the World Hypertension League. J Hypertens 9:283-287, 1991.

153. Gifford RW Jr, Committee Members. The Fifth Report of the Joint National Committee on Detection, Evaluation and Treatment of High Blood Pressure. Pub no. 93-1088. Bethesda, MD, National Institutes of Health, 1993; pp 11-15.

154. Van Montfrans GA, Karemaker JM, Weiling W, et al. Relaxation therapy and continuous ambulatory blood pressure in mild hypertension: A controlled study. BMJ 300:1368-1372, 1990.

155. McGrady A, Higgins JT Jr. Prediction of response to biofeedback-assisted relaxation in hypertensives: Development of a hypertensive predictor profile (HYPP). Psychosom Med 51:277-284, 1989.

156. Goebel M, Viol GW, Orebaugh C. An incremental model to isolate specific effects of behavioral treatments in essential hypertension. Biofeed Self-Regul 18:255-280, 1993.

157. Johnston DW, Gold A, Kentish J, et al. Effect of stress management on blood pressure in mild primary hypertension. BMJ 306:963-966, 1993.

158. Ornish D, Brown SE, Scherwitz LW, et al. Can lifestyle changes reverse coronary heart disease? Lancet 336:129-133, 1990.

159. Blumenthal JA, Jiang W, Babyak MA, et al. Stress management and exercise training in cardiac patients with myocardial ischemia: Effects on prognosis and evaluation of mechanisms. Arch Intern Med 157:2213-2223, 1997.

# Chapter 8

# Renin
## Timothy L. Reudelhuber

More than 100 years ago Tiegerstadt and Bergmann first noticed that extracts of rabbit kidney had the ability to raise blood pressure (BP). It eventually became clear that the active ingredient in this extract was a protease that would later be named *renin* (derived from *renal*), which plays a key role in the generation of the angiotensin vasoactive peptides (for a historical review see Hall[1]). Over the last century, the work of a host of laboratories across the world has led to our current understanding of the renin-angiotensin system (RAS; Figure 8–1). In humans, renin is coded for by a single gene located on chromosome 1. Although rats also have a single renin gene, most strains of laboratory and wild mice have two renin genes, both of which contribute to circulating renin.[2]

Renin is an aspartyl protease that is first synthesized as an enzymatically inactive precursor, prorenin. Although it is possible to activate prorenin by prolonged exposure to cold or acidic conditions in the laboratory, the primary mechanism for prorenin activation in vivo is the proteolytic removal of a 43 amino acid prosegment from its amino terminus. This proteolytic activation is not autocatalytic, and although several proteases have been shown to convert prorenin to renin in vitro, the most likely physiologically relevant proteases to date are cathepsin B, and the prohormone convertases 1 and 5 (PC1, PC5).[3-5]

The vast majority of the renin in the circulation originates in the juxtaglomerular (JG) cells surrounding the renal afferent arterioles (Figure 8–2, *A*). Removal of the prosegment occurs within the secretory pathway, after prorenin is targeted to immature secretory granules.[6] Once activated, renin is stored in these secretory granules until the cells receive a signal for its release. It has been estimated that JG cells divert roughly 20% of the prorenin they produce to secretory granules for activation,[7] while the remainder of the prorenin is secreted unmodified and constitutively. In humans, there is from 5 to 10 times more prorenin than renin in the plasma,[8,9] and there is no evidence to date that circulating prorenin contributes to the activity of the circulating RAS.

There have been some interesting variations proposed for the cell biology of renin, including the suggestion that active renin can be formed within the cytoplasm of cells (reviewed in Re[10]), and the finding of renin receptors,[11,12] at least one of which appears to generate an intracellular signal when bound to renin.[13] The importance of these phenomena to the biology of the RAS remains unclear, however.

## RENIN BIOLOGY AND ITS IMPORTANCE IN MEDICINE

### Tissue Origin and Activating Enzymes

The mechanism of activation of prorenin has received a lot of attention in recent years because organs other than the kidney, including the brain, pituitary, and adrenal glands; testes; uterus; and placenta, have been shown to express the renin gene (reviewed in Lavoie and Sigmund[14]). In fact, after nephrectomy renin virtually disappears from the circulation while prorenin persists,[15] demonstrating that nonrenal organs not only make prorenin but can also secrete it into the circulation. Other organs, such as the heart, are capable of taking up renin and prorenin from the circulation.[16,17] Because many of these tissues also make other components of the RAS, including angiotensinogen, angiotensin-converting enzyme (ACE), and angiotensin receptors, it has been suggested that *tissue* RAS could exist and be biologically important. The key question that remains is whether these tissues can activate prorenin to catalyze the first reaction in the RAS. Evidence supporting this possibility comes from three findings: First, enzymes are present in nonrenal tissues that can activate prorenin in the secretory pathway and lead to renin storage in secretory granules.[5] Second, prorenin with its prosegment still attached appears to display some enzymatic activity within tissues in transgenic mouse models.[18] Third, prorenin taken up from the circulation can be cleaved to active renin after uptake in certain cells.[19] Thus, while active renin in the circulation has been the primary focus for most physiologic studies and pharmacologic interventions, there is substantial experimental evidence suggesting that a tissue RAS could contribute to the local production and action of angiotensins.

## Control of Circulating Renin Levels

The primary mechanism by which the RAS contributes to acute changes in fluid and pressure homeostasis is by regulating renin levels in the circulation. This is accomplished in large part by modulating the release of renin-containing secretory granules from JG cells. The afferent arterioles contain baroreceptors and release renin in response to a perceived drop in BP or interstitial pressure. In addition, nerve terminals that make connections to the JG cells cause a release of renin in response to sympathetic nervous system activation. The JG cells also express angiotensin II type 1 (AT$_1$) receptors and decreases in circulating angiotensin II (Ang II) or inhibition of signaling through the AT$_1$ receptor (e.g., by pharmacologic blockade) stimulate renin release. In fact, chronic inhibition of the RAS actually causes the recruitment (or reactivation) of new JG cells (see Figure 8–2, *B*), leading to a further increase in renin secretion. Finally, the macula densa relays a signal to the JG cells to increase renin release when a drop in sodium is detected in the distal tubule. Renin secretion can also be inhibited by the converse of these same signals. For example, increases in BP, β-adrenergic blockade, increases in circulating Ang II, and a high urinary sodium concentration will all result in a decrease in renin secretion in an attempt to balance their effects on BP. These considerations are clinically important when tailoring therapy for hypertension, as the most common interventions (diuretics, β-blockers, ACE inhibitors, angiotensin receptor blockers [ARBs], low-sodium

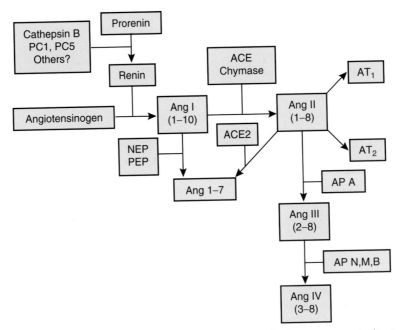

**Figure 8–1** Schematic representation of the renin-angiotensin system (RAS). The heavy arrows indicate the enzymes that catalyze the corresponding step. ACE, angiotensin-converting enzyme; Ang, angiotensin (Roman numerals refer to the nomenclature for the peptide; numbers in parentheses refer to the amino acid positions in the peptide relative to Ang I (10 amino acids)); NEP, neutral endopeptidase; $AT_1$, angiotensin II type 1; $AT_2$, angiotensin II type 2; PC1, prohormone convertase 1; PC 5, prohormone convertase 5; PEP, prolyl endopeptidase; AP, aminopeptidase.

diet) will cause a resetting in the activity of the circulating RAS that often requires a further adjustment in medication dosage.

## Renin as a Limiting Factor in the Renin-Angiotensin System

Laboratory measurements for renin are most commonly expressed as the capacity of plasma to generate angiotensin I (Ang I) when incubated either directly (plasma renin activity or PRA) or in the presence of excess angiotensinogen (plasma renin concentration or PRC). Thus, PRA reflects not only the amount of renin in the circulation, but also the amount of substrate angiotensinogen and is therefore the best measure of RAS activity in vivo. In most cases, PRC will parallel PRA, with the exception of patients with heart or liver failure, or other conditions that lead to increases in angiotensinogen.[20] The fact that PRA can be affected by changes in the levels of either angiotensinogen or renin is explained by the biochemistry of the RAS: In humans, the concentration of plasma angiotensinogen is close to the affinity constant (Km) of renin for angiotensinogen.[21] In practical terms, this means that the amount of angiotensin peptide generated in the plasma is a direct reflection of the concentrations of angiotensinogen and renin, because ACE is in over-abundance in the vascular wall. In general, this provides for rapid increases in activity of the RAS through the acute release of renin-containing granules from JG cells and more long-term regulation of the RAS by modulation of expression of the genes coding for both angiotensinogen and renin. Interestingly, in laboratory mice renin appears to be in excess and angiotensinogen is limiting for the activity of the RAS.[2]

## RENIN AS A RISK FACTOR AND DIAGNOSTIC TOOL

### Plasma Renin as a Predictor of Cardiovascular Complications

In a study involving 1717 hypertensive patients, Alderman et al. found that those with a high PRA (adjusted for urinary sodium content) were at significantly higher risk of suffering a myocardial infarction independent of other risk factors, including BP, race, sex, age, serum cholesterol, smoking, ECG evidence of left ventricular hypertrophy (LVH), history of cardiovascular disease, body mass index (BMI), and use of β-blockers.[22] This very striking result was the first indication that circulating renin might act via a mechanism other than by regulating BP and it provided a boost to those who championed the importance of tissue RAS. This association was later refuted in a study by Meade et al.,[23] who found that myocardial infarction correlated best with BP. Attempts to sort out the differences between these studies[24] have not been very fruitful, and the unfortunate conclusion has been that renin-sodium profiling may not be a good indicator of future cardiovascular complications.

### Renin Gene Mutations for Genetic Diagnosis and Prognosis

Because physiologic modulation of the activity of the RAS plays such a crucial role in fluid and pressure homeostasis, it is a natural extension to postulate that mutations in the genes coding for components of the RAS might result in activation of the system and therefore explain some forms of hypertension.

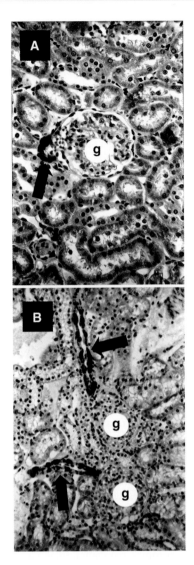

**Figure 8-2** Immunodetection of renin-producing cell in the juxtaglomerular (JG) apparatus (*dark arrows*) of rats either untreated **(A)** or after 2 weeks of treatment with the ACE inhibitor captopril **(B)**. g, glomeruli.

Early evidence suggesting a link between genetic variations in the angiotensinogen gene and hypertension[25] fueled an intense search for variations in the genes of the remaining components of the RAS, including renin. However, there have been many conflicting results over the years, with some suggesting a link between the renin gene and hypertension (see for example, Zhu et al.[26]), while others found no link (see for example, Jeunemaitre et al.[27]). This is a surprising result, because several rare forms of hypertension are associated with mutations in genes that code for downstream effectors of the RAS, including salt transport in the kidney.[28] The variable results in most association studies might be due to the small size of the patient populations or difficulty in defining the appropriate target group. Another possibility, suggested in a whole-genome scan study for hypertension-related genes, may be the fact that "BP regulation is most likely governed by multiple genetic loci, each with a relatively weak effect on BP in the population at large."[29]

Alternatively, the genes of the RAS may be "protected" from mutation because of their importance for some aspect of human survival. This possibility is supported by the finding that pharmacologic inhibition of the RAS during pregnancy in humans is fetotoxic, resulting in spontaneous abortion with severe defects of the fetus, including hypoplas-

tic organs and multiple defects of the kidney and urinary tract.[30] Hydronephrosis, defects in development of the urinary tract, and high neonatal mortality are also seen in laboratory mice in which the gene coding for renin,[31] as well as those coding for any of the other components of the RAS, including angiotensinogen, ACE, or the $AT_1$ receptor are inactivated (see Gurley et al.[32] for a review). These results probably explain why there has never been a report of a human mutation that completely inactivates the RAS because such a mutation would probably be lethal. Therefore, even though mutations in the renin gene have not been shown to cause hypertension to date, data on the consequences of blocking the RAS during development raise the possibility that such mutations may eventually explain some of the congenital abnormalities of the kidney and urinary tract (CAKUT).[33]

## Measurement of Renin to Tailor Therapy

The many physiologic, pharmacologic (discussed previously), and pathophysiologic (discussed in the following paragraphs) factors that can cause changes in circulating renin levels make the measurement of renin a capricious indicator of therapeutic potential. Studies have confirmed that PRA varies widely in hypertensives.[34,35] In a study involving more than 4000 hypertensive patients,[35] Alderman et al. divided their patient population into those with low renin (PRA <0.65 ng/ml/hr; 30% of the patients); medium renin, (PRA 0.66 to 4.5 ng/ml/hr; 60% of patients); or high renin, (PRA >4.5 ng/ml/hr; 10% of patients). They found that PRA varied according to sex, ethnicity, and age, but demographics alone could not predict the renin levels for any given patient group because of high interindividual variability. In spite of this complication, Laragh has proposed that hypertensive patients can be rationally subdivided into three groups to tailor therapy[36]: (1) "R" patients who have too much renin and who will respond best to interventions (β-blockers, ACE inhibitors, ARBs) that will block the RAS. (2) Hypertensive patients who have low renin levels and who will not respond well to this regimen. (3) "V" patients who have a predominantly volume and salt-dependent hypertension that will respond best to diuretics. Renin status as a guide for tailoring therapy remains hypothetical and the choice of drug class for the treatment of hypertension by most primary care physicians continues to be largely empirical.

## CONDITIONS OF RENIN EXCESS

With the key role that renin plays in the activity of the RAS in humans, it is not surprising that disorders of renin secretion would have deleterious effects on cardiovascular health. In fact, there are two clinical syndromes that are associated with renin-dependent hypertension. Diagnosis of these uncommon types of hypertension is made more difficult by the overwhelming prevalence of essential hypertension.

### Renovascular Hypertension

Obstruction of the renal artery leads to a drop in perfusion pressure in the JG apparatus, which reacts by increasing renin secretion. The relationship between renal artery stenosis and hypertension was elegantly demonstrated by the work of Goldblatt et al.,[37] who placed unilateral clips on the renal artery in rats and showed that the resulting increase in BP was initially due to a massive increase in renin production by the "clipped" kidney. Interestingly, as hypertension progresses in this model, it becomes less renin-dependent and may actually be fueled by a vicious cycle of secondary organ damage.[38]

The identification of patients with renovascular hypertension is important because they are more likely to progress to severe hypertension and to suffer from ischemic kidney injury. On the other hand, early diagnosis and treatment holds hope for reversal of the stenosis and resulting pathologies.

There are two major causes of renal artery stenosis, which are not seen with equal frequency in men and women. The most common cause of renovascular hypertension is atherosclerotic renal artery stenosis (ARAS; for a review see Safian[39] and Chapter 74). ARAS occurs more frequently in men than women, although gender differences tend to disappear in elderly individuals. Disease progression in these patients generally mirrors the development of atherosclerosis throughout the rest of the body and the vast majority of patients with ARAS have other clinical manifestations of atherosclerosis.

Fibromuscular dysplasia, in contrast, is restricted to the renal arteries. Although far less common overall that ARAS, fibromuscular dysplasia is the most common cause of renovascular hypertension in women younger than 50 years of age.[39,40]

The common clinical hallmarks of hypertension due to renal artery stenosis include the appearance of hypertension in young (<30 years) or old (>60 years) patients, the rapid progression of previously mild or controlled hypertension and/or the presence of an abdominal bruit. Associated clinical findings include unexplained acute or chronic azotemia. Although elevated renin is at the root of the problem, measurement of circulating renin either at rest, after ACE inhibitor "stimulation," or in the renal veins has not proven to be of great use because of the confounding effects of hypertension and antihypertensive medications on renin levels.[39,40]

Treatment of renovascular hypertension, particularly in the early phases, includes inhibition of the RAS including β-blockers, ACE inhibitors, and/or ARBs. In ARAS, aggressive risk reduction and use of lipid-lowering drugs are also recommended. In case of primary treatment failure, revascularization with angioplasty and/or stent placement is sometimes necessary. The diagnosis and treatment of renovascular hypertension are covered in more detail in Chapter 74.

### Renin-secreting Tumors

Renin-producing tumors represent the purest, albeit very rare, form of primary reninism resulting from unregulated secretion of renin, because the tumors have escaped the hemodynamic and hormonal control of the afferent arteriole. Two very thorough and informative reviews on renin-producing tumors have been published[41,42] and, because of the rarity of these cases, will likely remain excellent sources of information and reference for the interested reader for the foreseeable future. Renin-secreting tumors can be roughly divided into renal and nonrenal tumors, including lung cancers, hepatoblastomas, paragangliomas, pancreatic carcinomas, adenocarcinoma of the colon, adrenal carcinomas, and various types of ovarian and fallopian tube tumors. Production of renin by these tumor types is rare and unexpected and likely to be due to the particular chromosomal mutations or rearrangements undergone by the cancer cells. Treatment of hypertension in these cases has focused on the use of RAS inhibitors and tumor ablation, although hypertension is likely to reappear with new tumor growth or metastasis.

In the kidney, hypersecretion of renin is infrequently associated with renal carcinomas and quite frequently (>50% of cases) with Wilms' tumors. Although renal masses can cause compression-induced hypertrophy of the JG apparatus, leading to increased renin secretion, it is now clear that Wilms' tumor cells themselves secrete renin. Another exceedingly rare type of tumor associated with renin-dependent hypertension is the JG cell tumor, sometimes referred to as reninoma. These tumors are benign neoplasms that are most often clinically detected as causes of hypertension associated with severe hypokalemia in very young patients. The first report of such a tumor appeared in 1967, and to date the English literature contains less than 100 reports of such tumors.

Patients with renin-producing tumors are invariably hyperreninemic, resulting in hyperaldosteronemia and hypokalemia. Increased plasma renin activity (PRA) is not always apparent in these patients, however, and diagnosis by PRA is complicated in patients being treated for hypertension with medications that lead to increased renin secretion, such as ARBs and ACE inhibitors. Increased circulating renin is also seen in other conditions, including renovascular hypertension and renal failure, making the interpretation of increased PRA more equivocal. The best evidence in the diagnosis of a JG cell reninoma is the appearance of significant hypertension associated with hypokalemia in relatively young patients without other apparent risk factors.[41] In analyzing previously reported cases, Martin et al.[42] noted that the mean age at diagnosis was 26.8 years with less than one fourth of patients being diagnosed after 40 years of age. Many of these patients display hypertension that becomes increasingly difficult to control with standard therapy over time. If left untreated, patients may present with complaints commonly associated with severe hypertension, including headache, vomiting, polyuria, nocturia, and dizziness.

Three clinical tests have been used with limited success to provide support for the diagnosis of a reninoma. First, treatment with an ACE inhibitor or ARB, which normally results in a rise in renin secretion in patients with essential hypertension, will sometimes fail to elicit increased renin secretion in a patient with a reninoma, since the tumor cells may have escaped the normal feedback regulation of renin secretion. The hormonal response of these tumors is not uniform or entirely predictable, however.[41] It may also be impractical to administer such tests, as most suspect cases will already be dependent on RAS-targeted antihypertensive therapy to control their BP. Second, renal vein PRA measurements have been used to test for lateralization of renin secretion from the tumor-bearing kidney, because the healthy kidney suppresses renin secretion in response to the hypertension. Renin secretion from the tumor-bearing kidney is not always increased, however,[43,44] perhaps due to alternate vascularization of the tumor or to direct generation Ang II within some of the tumors. Patients with unilateral artery stenosis may lateralize renin secretion to the ischemic kidney, limiting the specificity of this diagnostic test. Finally, renal arteriograms may be used to detect larger tumors and in some cases to rule out stenosis as a cause of the hyperreninism. However, most reninomas are less than 4 cm in diameter[41,42] and may not appear on an arteriogram. A careful analysis of imaging studies of the kidneys will be the best adjunct when a reninoma is suspected, as it should have the necessary resolution to detect even small tumors, which can be clinically significant even at sizes under 1 cm in diameter. Importantly, there is no obvious correlation between the severity of hypertension and the size of the responsible reninoma.[42]

Treatment of hypertension associated with renin-secreting tumor of any sort consists of RAS-targeted antihypertensive therapy and may become more difficult with time as the tumor grows or metastasizes.[45] However, the ultimate correction of this problem is by ablation of the tumor. Patients harboring a JG cell reninoma have a particularly good prognosis. In greater than 90% of cases, reninoma-associated hypertension is smoothly and completely reversed by surgical resection of the tumor. In most of the remaining cases, only mild hypertension persists, perhaps due to secondary organ damage, and can be managed by standard therapy. As JG cell tumors are benign, there have been no reported cases of metastases or recurrence after surgery.

## PHARMACOLOGIC BLOCKADE

Several aspects make renin an ideal target for pharmacologic blockade. First, renin is limiting in the activity of the RAS, so its inhibition should be achievable and effective in blocking the generation of angiotensins. Second, although Ang I can be metabolized by alternate pathways (see Figure 8–1), renin is the only enzyme that can generate Ang I in vivo, as demonstrated by the inactivation of renin in mice,[31] making it the "gatekeeper" for activity of the RAS. Third, because renin has only one known substrate, angiotensinogen, a specific renin inhibitor would presumably only block the RAS and would thus have a low likelihood of side effects. Nevertheless, as of this writing there are no renin inhibitors approved for clinical use, presumably due to the high cost of synthesis, problems with bioavailability, and the obvious success of competitor classes of drugs. Would development of such an inhibitor be advantageous? Limited research has suggested that renin inhibitors might be more effective in lowering Ang II than ACE inhibition,[46] and there is the possibility that they could be used in combination with other RAS inhibitors to achieve more effective BP control. It therefore seems likely that the development of this new class of drugs will continue.

## SUMMARY

Renin modulates fluid balance and BP through its key role in controlling the activity of the RAS. Although measurement of renin activity and assessment of mutations in the genes encoding renin and other components of the RAS have not proven to be useful in the management of hypertension to date, understanding the factors that regulate the production and release of renin may be important in tailoring effective therapy. The future development of specific renin inhibitors may allow a more effective targeting and inhibition of the RAS in the treatment of cardiovascular disorders.

## References

1. Hall JE. Historical perspective of the renin-angiotensin system. Mol Biotechnol 24:27-39, 2003.
2. Lum C, Shesely EG, Potter DL, et al. Cardiovascular and renal phenotype in mice with one or two renin genes. Hypertension 43:79-86, 2004.
3. Wang PH, Do YS, Macaulay L, et al. Identification of renal cathepsin B as a human prorenin-processing enzyme. J Biol Chem 266:12633-12638, 1991.
4. Mercure C, Jutras I, Day R, et al. Prohormone convertase PC5 is a candidate processing enzyme for prorenin in the human adrenal cortex. Hypertension 28:840-846, 1996.
5. Reudelhuber TL, Ramla D, Chiu L, et al. Proteolytic processing of human prorenin in renal and non-renal tissues. Kidney Int 46:1522-1524, 1994.
6. Taugner R, Kim SJ, Murakami K, et al. The fate of prorenin during granulopoiesis in epithelioid cells. Immunocytochemical experiments with antisera against renin and different portions of the renin prosegment. Histochemistry 86:249-253, 1987.
7. Pratt RE, Carleton JE, Richie JP, et al. Human renin biosynthesis and secretion in normal and ischemic kidneys. Proc Natl Acad Sci USA 84:7837-7840, 1987.

8. Plouin PF, Chatellier G, Guyene TT, et al. Recent advances in the clinical study of the renin system. Reference values and conditions of validity. Presse Med 18:917-921, 1989.

9. Hsueh WA, Baxter JD. Human prorenin. Hypertension 17:469-477, 1991.

10. Re RN. Intracellular renin and the nature of intracrine enzymes. Hypertension 42, 117-122, 2003.

11. Sealey JE, Catanzaro DF, Lavin TN, et al. Specific prorenin/renin binding (ProBP). Identification and characterization of a novel membrane site. Am J Hypertens 9:491-502, 1996.

12. van den Eijnden MM, Saris JJ, de Bruin RJ, et al. Prorenin accumulation and activation in human endothelial cells: Importance of mannose 6-phosphate receptors. Arterioscler Thromb Vasc Biol 21:911-916, 2001.

13. Nguyen G, Delarue F, Burckle C, et al. Pivotal role of the renin/prorenin receptor in angiotensin II production and cellular responses to renin. J Clin Invest 109:1417-1427, 2002.

14. Lavoie JL, Sigmund CD. Minireview: Overview of the renin-angiotensin system–an endocrine and paracrine system. Endocrinology 144:2179-2183, 2003.

15. Sealey JE, White RP, Laragh JH, et al. Plasma prorenin and renin in anephric patients. Circ Res 41:17-21, 1977.

16. Prescott G, Silversides DW, Reudelhuber TL. Tissue activity of circulating prorenin. Am J Hypertens 15:280-285, 2002.

17. Prescott G, Silversides DW, Chiu SM, et al. Contribution of circulating renin to local synthesis of angiotensin peptides in the heart. Physiol Genomics 4:67-73, 2000.

18. Methot D, Silversides DW, Reudelhuber TL. In vivo enzymatic assay reveals catalytic activity of the human renin precursor in tissues. Circ Res 84:1067-1072, 1999.

19. Admiraal PJ, van Kesteren CA, Danser AH, et al. Uptake and proteolytic activation of prorenin by cultured human endothelial cells. J Hypertens 17:621-629, 1999.

20. Plouin PF, Cudek P, Arnal JF, et al. Immunoradiometric assay of active renin versus determination of plasma renin activity in the clinical investigation of hypertension, congestive heart failure, and liver cirrhosis. Horm Res 34:138-141, 1990.

21. Gould AB, Green D. Kinetics of the human renin and human substrate reaction. Cardiovasc Res 5:86-89, 1971.

22. Alderman MH, Madhavan S, Ooi WL, et al. Association of the renin-sodium profile with the risk of myocardial infarction in patients with hypertension. N Engl J Med 324: 1098-1104, 1991.

23. Meade TW, Cooper JA, Peart WS. Plasma renin activity and ischemic heart disease. N Engl J Med 329:616-619, 1993.

24. Alderman MH, Sealey JE, Laragh JH. Plasma renin activity and ischemic heart disease. N Engl J Med 330:506-507, 1994.

25. Jeunemaitre X, Soubrier F, Kotelevtsev YV, et al. Molecular basis of human hypertension: Role of angiotensinogen. Cell 71:169-180, 1992.

26. Zhu X, Chang YP, Yan D, et al. Associations between hypertension and genes in the renin-angiotensin system. Hypertension 41:1027-1034, 2003.

27. Jeunemaitre X, Rigat B, Charru A, et al. Sib pair linkage analysis of renin gene haplotypes in human essential hypertension. Hum Genet 88:301-306, 1992.

28. Lifton RP, Wilson FH, Choate KA, et al. Salt and blood pressure: New insight from human genetic studies. Cold Spring Harb Symp Quant Biol 67:445-450, 2002.

29. Thiel BA, Chakravarti A, Cooper RS, et al. A genome-wide linkage analysis investigating the determinants of blood pressure in whites and African Americans. Am J Hypertens 16:151-153, 2003.

30. Pryde PG, Sedman AB, Nugent CE, et al. Angiotensin-converting enzyme inhibitor fetopathy. J Am Soc Nephrol 3:1575-1582, 1993.

31. Yanai K, Saito T, Kakinuma Y, et al. Renin-dependent cardiovascular functions and renin-independent blood-brain barrier functions revealed by renin-deficient mice. J Biol Chem 275: 5-8, 2000.

32. Gurley SB, Le TH, Coffman TM. Gene-targeting studies of the renin-angiotensin system: Mechanisms of hypertension and cardiovascular disease. Cold Spring Harb Symp Quant Biol 67:451-457, 2002.

33. Nishimura H, Yerkes E, Hohenfellner K, et al. Role of the angiotensin type 2 receptor gene in congenital anomalies of the kidney and urinary tract, CAKUT, of mice and men. Mol Cell 3:1-10, 1999.

34. Meade TW, Imeson JD, Gordon D, et al. The epidemiology of plasma renin. Clin Sci (Lond) 64:273-280, 1983.

35. Alderman MH, Cohen HW, Sealey JE, et al. Plasma renin activity levels in hypertensive persons: Their wide range and lack of suppression in diabetic and in most elderly patients. Am J Hypertens 17:1-7, 2004.

36. Laragh JH. Abstract, closing summary, and table of contents for Laragh's 25 lessons in pathophysiology and 12 clinical pearls for treating hypertension. Am J Hypertens 14:1173-1177, 2001.

37. Goldblatt H, Lynch J, Hanzal RF, et al. Studies on experimental hypertension: Production of persistent elevation of systolic pressure by means of renal ischemia. J Exp Med 59:347-380, 1934.

38. Samani NJ, Godfrey NP, Major JS, et al. Kidney renin mRNA levels in the early and chronic phases of two-kidney, one clip hypertension in the rat. J Hypertens 7:105-112, 1989.

39. Safian RD. Atherosclerotic renal artery stenosis. Curr Treat Options Cardiovasc Med 5:91-101, 2003.

40. Bruni KR. Renovascular hypertension. J Cardiovasc Nurs 15: 78-90, 2001.

41. Corvol P, Pinet F, Plouin PF, et al. Renin-secreting tumors. Endocrinol Metab Clin North Am 23:255-270, 1994.

42. Martin SA, Mynderse LA, Lager DJ, et al. Juxtaglomerular cell tumor: A clinicopathologic study of four cases and review of the literature. Am J Clin Pathol 116:854-863, 2001.

43. Koriyama N, Kakei M, Yaekura K, et al. A case of renal juxtaglomerular cell tumor: Usefulness of segmental sampling to prove autonomic secretion of the tumor. Am J Med Sci 318:194-197, 1999.

44. Kashiwabara H, Inaba M, Itabashi A, et al. A case of renin-producing juxtaglomerular tumor: Effect of ACE inhibitor or angiotensin II receptor antagonist. Blood Press 6:147-153, 1997.

45. Arver S, Jacobsson H, Cedermark B, et al. Malignant human renin producing paraganglionoma-localization with 123I-MIBG and treatment with 131I-MIBG. Clin Endocrinol (Oxf) 51: 631-635, 1999.

46. Fisher ND, Hollenberg NK. Is there a future for renin inhibitors? Expert Opin Investig Drugs 10:417-426, 2001.

# Chapter 9

# Angiotensin-Converting Enzymes: Properties and Function

## Chris Tikellis, Colin I. Johnston

The renin-angiotensin system (RAS) is an important pathway that regulates blood pressure (BP)[1] and sodium/water homeostasis.[2] Angiotensin-converting enzyme (ACE) is a key component of the RAS. It is responsible for converting the inactive decapeptide, angiotensin I (Ang I), to the biologic active octapeptide angiotensin II (Ang II), as well as inactivating the vasodilator bradykinin.[3] Ang II is thought to be responsible for most of the physiologic and pathophysiologic effects of the RAS.

In mammals ACE occurs as two isoforms that are produced from a single gene with alternate splicing:

1. A somatic form (sACE), which is a type I integral membrane glycoprotein and which is widely distributed in many endothelial cells in variety of tissues, including the heart[4] and kidney and in the epithelial cells of proximal tubules,[5] small intestine[6] and a variety of neuronal cells in the brain.[7] This enzyme is anchored through the cell membrane and has a short intracellular extension with the major extracellular portion containing two duplicate domains, each containing a catalytic site.
2. A testicular form (germinal ACE or gACE) that is smaller as it only contains the C-terminal domain of somatic ACE and has only a single catalytic site. gACE is only expressed in differentiating male germinal cells,[8] and studies of ACE gene deletion in animal models have demonstrated a strong association with reduced fertility in males.[9]
3. A soluble form, which is formed in many body fluids, including the plasma and which arises from proteolytic cleavage, by a membrane "secretase"[10] at the membrane anchor of somatic ACE. Plasma ACE is catalytically active.

Gene deletion studies have shown that mice lacking endothelial ACE but having normal plasma ACE are unable to maintain normal BP, particularly when stressed by a low-salt diet, thus suggesting the functional primacy of the tissue RAS.[11,12] Twenty years after the introduction of specific inhibitors of ACE, the ACE inhibitors or "prills" have been established as preferred treatment for cardiovascular and renal disease (see Chapter 35). However, the classical view of the RAS has been challenged due to the discovery of other enzymes and angiotensin peptides that have been shown to have biologic activity and physiologic importance.

## ANGIOTENSIN-CONVERTING ENZYME 2

### Structure

Angiotensin-converting enzyme-related carboxypeptidase (ACE2), has been shown to cleave Ang I at different sites from ACE and to convert Ang II to angiotensin-(1-9) (Ang-[1-9]).[13,14] Analysis of the genomic sequence for ACE2 has shown that this gene contains 18 exons and maps to chromosomal location Xp22.[13] ACE2 is an 805 amino acid protein with a transmembrane domain (amino acids 740-763) and a single catalytic domain (amino acids 147-555) and has been classified as a metalloprotease due to its single HEXXH zinc-binding consensus (amino acids 374-378)[14] and its inhibition by EDTA.[13] Unlike ACE, ACE2 functions as a carboxypeptidase.[15] ACE2 has 60% homology with the testicular ACE isoform and 42% homology with somatic ACE at the metalloprotease catalytic domain[13,14] but differs from ACE in having only one enzymatic site.

In humans ACE2 transcripts have been identified in the heart, kidney, testis,[13,14] gastrointestinal tract, brain, and lung.[16] Preliminary data have also localized ACE2 to the retina (Tikellis C, Johnston CI, unpublished data), suggesting more ubiquitous expression than initially thought (Figure 9–1).

## Physiologic Function

The full physiologic functions of ACE2 are yet to be elucidated. To date it has been shown that recombinant ACE2 hydrolyses the carboxy terminal leucine from Ang I to generate Ang-(1-9)[13,14] and also cleaves the C-terminal residue of the peptides des-Arg[9]-bradykinin, neurotensin 1-13, and kinetensin.[14] Tipnis et al. showed that ACE2 was also able to cleave Ang II, resulting in its degradation to the vasodilator angiotensin-(1-7) (Ang-[1-7]).[13] In vitro studies showed that the catalytic efficiency of ACE2 is greater with Ang II as a substrate than with Ang I,[15] thus indicating that in the RAS the major role for ACE2 is probably the conversion of Ang II to Ang(1-7) (Figure 9–2). (See Chapter 10 for a more complete discussion of Ang-[1-7].)

Ang-(1-7) plays an important role in RAS as it counteracts most actions of Ang II (i.e., it has been shown to have vasodilator actions,[17-22] diuretic and natriuretic effects,[23] antiangiogenic action,[24] antithrombotic action,[25] and antiproliferative effects on vascular smooth muscle[26]). The biologic actions of Ang-(1-7) are not mediated via $AT_1$ or $AT_2$ receptors, and binding experiments have described specific Ang-(1-7) receptors.[18,27] With the use of knockout mouse technology, the *mas* protooncogene, a seven hydrophobic transmembrane domain protein that was previously described as an orphan G protein coupled receptor, was identified as a potential Ang-(1-7) receptor.[28] Furthermore, studies in *mas*-deficient mice confirmed that the Ang (1-7) receptor was expressed in the kidney and that Ang-(1-7) had an antidiuretic effect and a vasodilator effect on aortic rings. Ang-(1-7) undergoes further processing by ACE, which cleave two more amino acids at the C-terminal, resulting in Ang-(1-5)[14] and Ang-(3-5),[29] whose actions remain unknown.

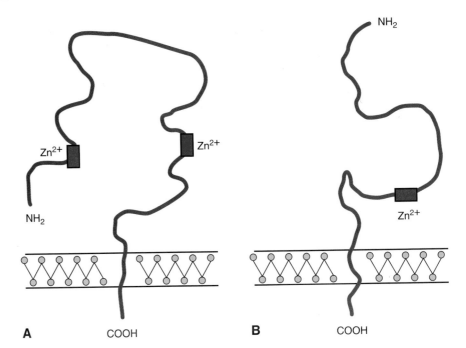

**Figure 9-1** Schematic representation of ACE **(A)** and ACE2 **(B)**, red box denotes active site.

ACE2 is not inhibited by classical ACE inhibitors such as captopril and lisinopril.[13,14] Potent (picomolar range) and selective inhibitors of ACE2 have been designed and synthesized,[30] which will greatly assist in elucidating the physiologic roles of ACE2 in vivo.

A preliminary insight into the physiologic roles of ACE2 was gained when Crackower et al. constructed ACE2 mutant mice.[31] They showed that deletion of ACE2 in these mice resulted in increases in the angiotensin peptides Ang I and Ang II in heart and kidney, implicating ACE2 as an important regulator of a number of angiotensins, including Ang I, Ang II, Ang-(1-9), and Ang-(1-7). Interestingly, BP was not altered in the ACE2 null mice even after the addition of the ACE inhibitor captopril. Most importantly, they demonstrated that ACE2 is essential for normal cardiac development, as deletion of the ACE2 gene in this mouse model resulted in cardiac contractile dysfunction. Furthermore, the loss of ACE2 induced the hypoxia-regulated genes, Bcl2/adenovirus EIB 19kD-interacting protein 3 (BNIP3) and plasminogen activator

inhibitor-1 (PAI-1), in the heart. Crackower et al. postulated that loss of ACE2 from the vascular endothelial cells resulted in constriction of the coronary vessels and thus reduced oxygen delivery to the myocytes.[31]

Other studies have provided further evidence implicating ACE2 in cardiovascular function. Ang-(1-7) formation has been reported to be increased in failing human hearts. A study by Zisman et al. examined Ang-(1-7) formation in human hearts and confirmed with the use of specific inhibitors that Ang-(1-7) formation was attributable to ACE2.[32] This is consistent with the hypothesis that ACE2 may have a cardioprotective role in damaged tissue, as in heart failure. In another study, ACE2 transgenic mice were generated that expressed a specific increase in cardiac ACE2.[33] These mice died from ventricular tachycardia and terminal ventricular fibrillation. They overexpressed ACE2 and had down-regulated gap junction proteins, connexin40 and connexin43, which are postulated to account for the electrophysiologic disturbances. The authors suggested that ACE2 may be important for certain aspects of ventricular remodeling. Additional evidence implicating ACE2 in cardiac function is provided by another study that showed increased Ang-(1-7) formation via increased cardiac expression of ACE2 in cardiac membranes from persons with various forms of heart failure.[32] Thus, a number of studies provide evidence to implicate ACE2 as an important component of the RAS, particularly in the heart. It is postulated that this enzyme may counterbalance the actions of ACE by converting Ang II, a potent vasoconstrictor, to Ang-(1-7), a vasodilator (see Figure 9-2).

ACE2 has been characterized in the kidney in a rodent model of type 1 diabetes mellitus. Previous studies in this model demonstrated that ACE is down-regulated in the tubules but up-regulated in the glomerulus of the diabetic kidney.[34] This redistribution has also been observed for ACE2. Treatment with an ACE inhibitor normalized the distribution of ACE and ACE2 protein,[35] suggesting that ACE2 may have a renoprotective role in diabetes.

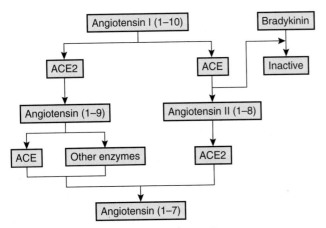

**Figure 9-2** The RAS pathway with ACE2.

Thus early studies provide evidence that implicates ACE2 as an important component of the RAS, as it counterbalances the actions of ACE by competing for and inactivating Ang II, a potent vasoconstrictor, generating Ang-(1-7), a vasodilator. Furthermore, the beneficial effect of ACE inhibitors may be due in part to the fact that these inhibitors do not inhibit ACE2.

## ACE POLYMORPHISMS

With the discovery of polymorphisms in the ACE gene there was great excitement about a possible association between ACE gene polymorphisms and some diseases. The most intensely studied of these polymorphisms was the biallelic ACE insertion/deletion (I/D) polymorphism, defined by the presence of an extra 287 base pair sequence inside intron 16 of the ACE gene (insertion or "I") or the absence of these extra base pairs (deletion or "D"). Inheritance of the I/D polymorphism follows Mendelian principles, with 25% of the population homozygous for the DD genotype, 25% homozygous for the II genotype, and 50% heterozygous for the DI genotype. Even though the ACE I/D polymorphism is in an intronic region of the ACE gene it is still responsible for at least half of the phenotypic variance observed in serum ACE levels.[36] The D genotype is strongly associated with increased plasma or serum ACE levels. Persons homozygous for deletion (DD) display the highest ACE values; those homozygous for insertion (II), the lowest ACE values; and those heterozygous (I/D), intermediate values.[37] Although persons with the ACE DD genotype have high ACE levels, their Ang I and Ang II levels are not elevated.[38,39]

Ethnic origin is also a determining factor in serum ACE activity. Caucasians with the ACE DD allele, have a greater vasodilator response to bradykinin than African Americans with ACE DD allele.[40] There are differences in serum ACE activity among ACE genotypes in Caucasians, but not in African Americans or African Caribbeans.[41-43]

The possible association between the ACE I/D polymorphism and cardiovascular disease remains controversial. Initially, small studies showed an association between the ACE DD genotype and cardiovascular disease. Later, larger and better-conducted trials showed no association. Some of the positive associations that have been identified appear only in certain ethnic groups and in subsets of patients. For example, a correlation was demonstrated between the ACE DD genotype and left ventricular hypertrophy (LVH) in a group of untreated hypertensive subjects, who had an increased risk of LVH .[44] In a meta-analysis, a positive association was demonstrated between the ACE DD genotype and common carotid artery intima-media thickness (IMT).[45] Initial studies also showed a positive correlation between the ACE DD genotype and myocardial infarction (MI).[46] However, more recent larger studies failed to confirm this association and did not demonstrate an increased risk of cardiovascular disease with the DD genotype.[47]

The relationship of the ACE DD genotype to other disorders such as diabetic nephropathy has also been closely examined. Meta-analyses of studies in type 1 and type 2 diabetic subjects demonstrated that the ACE DD genotype was significantly associated with diabetic nephropathy.[48,49] Similar studies have been carried out in many populations and in many ethnic groups, and a number of these have found no association between ACE genotype and nephropathy.[50,51] The mixed results may in part be explained by ethnic differences in the frequency of the D allele, although even within individual ethnic groups, the results of studies are conflicting.

Circulating levels of Ang II are different from levels found in tissues, and can make a pronounced contribution to vasoconstriction in tissue. Increased ACE activity has been observed in hearts of ACE DD persons,[52] and ACE mRNA levels were found to be increased in left ventricular tissue from heart failure patients with the ACE DD genotype.[53,54] It appears that the increased levels of ACE mRNA may be cell/tissue specific, as no association of ACE mRNA with ACE I/D genotype was observed in human atria.[55,56] Therefore, increased ACE mRNA expression may be tightly regulated and site specific, providing another possible reason for the conflicting nature of data from studies assessing ACE polymorphism in association with coronary heart disease (CHD) and LVH. Thus, the observation that tissue ACE mRNA levels are increased in association with the ACE DD allele warrants that future studies examining an association between the ACE DD allele and cardiovascular disease should measure tissue levels of ACE mRNA and activity as well as serum ACE activity.

The ACE I/D polymorphism may have a more important role as an indicator of patient responsiveness to standard ACE inhibitor therapy. In particular, the ACE I/D polymorphism may help identify patient groups who fail to respond to ACE inhibitor therapy. For example, patients with the DD genotype have been shown to be three times less likely to respond to ACE inhibitor therapy than patients with the II genotype.[57] For the moment there are insufficient data to make a firm conclusion about the role of the ACE I/D polymorphism as an accurate and reliable indicator of ACE inhibitor responsiveness in patients.

Genes encoding for other components of the RAS, such as the M235T polymorphism of the angiotensinogen gene and the A1166C polymorphism of the angiotensin II type I (AT$_1$) receptor gene, have also been implicated in cardiovascular and renal disease. Patients with the M235T polymorphism have been shown to have elevated ACE and angiotensinogen levels[58,59] and tend to exhibit hypertension[59] although no relationship with hypertension was seen in some studies.[60] However, data are conflicting on whether there is an association with cardiovascular and renal disease.[59,61-64] Among studies examining the association of the A1166C polymorphism of the AT$_1$ receptor with cardiovascular and renal disease, some have shown a positive correlation,[65,66] whereas others have not.[67,68]

## SUMMARY

The conflicting nature of the evidence to date emphasizes that any simple genetic variant is unlikely to have more than a minor impact in genetically complex conditions such as hypertension and cardiovascular or renal disease. In addition, the ACE I/D polymorphism is located in an intron, and the true loci that regulate ACE activity are still undefined. Thus it is highly likely that many interactions between genes and the environment all contribute to initiation and/or progression of cardiovascular and renal disease.

# References

1. Johnston CI. Franz Volhard Lecture. Renin-angiotensin system: a dual tissue and hormonal system for cardiovascular control. J Hypertens Suppl 10:S13-S26, 1992.
2. Dzau VJ, Bernstein K, Celermajer D, et al. The relevance of tissue angiotensin-converting enzyme: Manifestations in mechanistic and endpoint data. Am J Cardiol 88:1L-20L, 2001.
3. Erdos EG. Conversion of angiotensin I to angiotensin II. Am J Med 60:749-759, 1976.
4. Paul M, Stoll M, Kreutz R, et al. The cellular basis of angiotensin converting enzyme mRNA expression in rat heart. Basic Res Cardiol 91 Suppl 2:57-63, 1996.
5. Alhenc-Gelas F, Baussant T, Hubert C, et al. The angiotensin converting enzyme in the kidney. J Hypertens Suppl 7:S9-S13; discussion S14, 1989.
6. Erickson RH, Suzuki Y, Sedlmayer A, et al. Rat intestinal angiotensin-converting enzyme: purification, properties, expression, and function. Am J Physiol 263:G466-G473, 1992.
7. Whiting P, Nava S, Mozley L, et al. Expression of angiotensin converting enzyme mRNA in rat brain. Brain Res Mol Brain Res 11:93-96, 1991.
8. Sibony M, Segretain D, Gasc JM. Angiotensin-converting enzyme in murine testis: Step-specific expression of the germinal isoform during spermiogenesis. Biol Reprod 50:1015-1026, 1994.
9. Esther CR Jr, Howard TE, Marino EM, et al. Mice lacking angiotensin-converting enzyme have low blood pressure, renal pathology, and reduced male fertility. Lab Invest 74:953-965, 1996.
10. Turner AJ, Hooper NM. The angiotensin-converting enzyme gene family: Genomics and pharmacology. Trends Pharmacol Sci 23:177-183, 2002.
11. Cole JM, Khokhlova N, Sutliff RL, et al. Mice lacking endothelial ACE: normal blood pressure with elevated angiotensin II. Hypertension 41:313-321, 2003.
12. Cole J, Ertoy D, Bernstein KE. Insights derived from ACE knockout mice. J Renin Angiotensin Aldosterone Syst 1:137-141, 2000.
13. Tipnis SR, Hooper NM, Hyde R, et al. A human homolog of angiotensin-converting enzyme: Cloning and functional expression as a captopril-insensitive carboxypeptidase. J Biol Chem 275:33238-33243, 2000.
14. Donoghue M, Hsieh F, Baronas E, et al. A novel angiotensin-converting enzyme-related carboxypeptidase (ACE2) converts angiotensin I to angiotensin 1-9. Circ Res 87:E1-E9, 2000.
15. Vickers C, Hales P, Kaushik V, et al. Hydrolysis of biological peptides by human angiotensin-converting enzyme-related carboxypeptidase. J Biol Chem 277:14838-14843, 2002.
16. Harmer D, Gilbert M, Borman R, et al. Quantitative mRNA expression profiling of ACE 2, a novel homologue of angiotensin converting enzyme. FEBS Lett 532:107-110, 2002.
17. Haulica I, Bild W, Mihaila CN, et al. Biphasic effects of angiotensin (1-7) and its interactions with angiotensin II in rat aorta. J Renin Angiotensin Aldosterone Syst 4:124-8, 2003.
18. Brosnihan KB, Li P, Ferrario CM. Angiotensin-(1-7) dilates canine coronary arteries through kinins and nitric oxide. Hypertension 27:523-528, 1996.
19. Porsti I, Bara AT, Busse R, et al. Release of nitric oxide by angiotensin-(1-7) from porcine coronary endothelium: Implications for a novel angiotensin receptor. Br J Pharmacol 111:652-654, 1994.
20. Benter IF, Diz DI, Ferrario CM. Pressor and reflex sensitivity is altered in spontaneously hypertensive rats treated with angiotensin-(1-7). Hypertension 26:1138-1144, 1995.
21. Benter IF, Ferrario CM, Morris M, et al. Antihypertensive actions of angiotensin-(1-7) in spontaneously hypertensive rats. Am J Physiol 269:H313-H319, 1995.
22. Ferrario CM, Chappell MC, Tallant EA, et al. Counterregulatory actions of angiotensin-(1-7). Hypertension 30:535-541, 1997.
23. Hilchey SD, Bell-Quilley CP. Association between the natriuretic action of angiotensin-(1-7) and selective stimulation of renal prostaglandin I2 release. Hypertension 25:1238-1244, 1995.
24. Machado RD, Santos RA, Andrade SP. Opposing actions of angiotensins on angiogenesis. Life Sci 66:67-76, 2000.
25. Kucharewicz I, Chabielska E, Pawlak D, et al. The antithrombotic effect of angiotensin-(1-7) closely resembles that of losartan. J Renin Angiotensin Aldosterone Syst 1:268-272, 2000.
26. Freeman EJ, Chisolm GM, Ferrario CM, et al. Angiotensin-(1-7) inhibits vascular smooth muscle cell growth. Hypertension 28:104-8, 1996.
27. Tallant EA, Lu X, Weiss RB, et al. Bovine aortic endothelial cells contain an angiotensin-(1-7) receptor. Hypertension 29:388-393, 1997.
28. Santos RA, Simoes e Silva AC, Maric C, et al. Angiotensin-(1-7) is an endogenous ligand for the G protein-coupled receptor Mas. Proc Natl Acad Sci USA 100(14):8258-8263, 2003; Epub 2003 Jun 26.
29. Chappell MC, Pirro NT, Sykes A, et al. Metabolism of angiotensin-(1-7) by angiotensin-converting enzyme. Hypertension 31:362-367, 1998.
30. Dales NA, Gould AE, Brown JA, et al. Substrate-based design of the first class of angiotensin-converting enzyme-related carboxypeptidase (ACE2) inhibitors. J Am Chem Soc 124:11852-11853, 2002.
31. Crackower MA, Sarao R, Oudit GY, et al. Angiotensin-converting enzyme 2 is an essential regulator of heart function. Nature 417:822-828, 2002.
32. Zisman LS, Keller RS, Weaver B, et al. Increased angiotensin-(1-7)-forming activity in failing human heart ventricles: evidence for upregulation of the angiotensin-converting enzyme homologue ACE2. Circulation 108:1707-1712, 2003.
33. Donoghue M, Wakimoto H, Maguire CT, et al. Heart block, ventricular tachycardia, and sudden death in ACE2 transgenic mice with downregulated connexins. J Mol Cell Cardiol 35:1043-1053, 2003.
34. Anderson S, Jung FF, Ingelfinger JR. Renal renin-angiotensin system in diabetes: functional, immunohistochemical, and molecular biological correlations. Am J Physiol 265:F477-F486, 1993.
35. Tikellis C, Johnston CI, Forbes JM, et al. Characterization of renal angiotensin-converting enzyme 2 in diabetic nephropathy. Hypertension 41:392-397, 2003.
36. Rigat B, Hubert C, Alhenc-Gelas F, et al. An insertion/deletion polymorphism in the angiotensin I-converting enzyme gene accounting for half the variance of serum enzyme levels. J Clin Invest 86:1343-1346, 1990.
37. Huang W, Gallois Y, Bouby N, et al. Genetically increased angiotensin I-converting enzyme level and renal complications in the diabetic mouse. Proc Natl Acad Sci USA 98:13330-13334, 2001.
38. Danser AH, Deinum J, Osterop AP, et al. Angiotensin I to angiotensin II conversion in the human forearm and leg. Effect of the angiotensin converting enzyme gene insertion/deletion polymorphism. J Hypertens 17:1867-1872, 1999.
39. van Dijk MA, Kroon I, Kamper AM, et al. The angiotensin-converting enzyme gene polymorphism and responses to angiotensins and bradykinin in the human forearm. J Cardiovasc Pharmacol 35:484-490, 2000.
40. Gainer JV, Stein CM, Neal T, et al. Interactive effect of ethnicity and ACE insertion/deletion polymorphism on vascular reactivity. Hypertension 37:46-51, 2001.
41. Bloem LJ, Manatunga AK, Pratt JH. Racial difference in the relationship of an angiotensin I-converting enzyme gene polymorphism to serum angiotensin I-converting enzyme activity. Hypertension 27:62-66, 1996.
42. Chakravarti A. Population genetics—making sense out of sequence. Nat Genet 21:56-60, 1999.

43. Zhu X, McKenzie CA, Forrester T, et al. Localization of a small genomic region associated with elevated ACE. Am J Hum Genet 67:1144-1153, 2000.

44. van Berlo JH, Pinto YM. Polymorphisms in the RAS and cardiac function. Int J Biochem Cell Biol 35:932-943, 2003.

45. Sayed-Tabatabaei FA, Houwing-Duistermaat JJ, van Duijn CM, et al. Angiotensin-converting enzyme gene polymorphism and carotid artery wall thickness: A meta-analysis. Stroke 34:1634-1639, 2003.

46. Cambien F, Poirier O, Lecerf L, et al. Deletion polymorphism in the gene for angiotensin-converting enzyme is a potent risk factor for myocardial infarction. Nature 359:641-644, 1992.

47. Holmer SR, Hengstenberg C, Kraft HG, et al. Association of polymorphisms of the apolipoprotein(a) gene with lipoprotein(a) levels and myocardial infarction. Circulation 107:696-701, 2003.

48. Jeffers BW, Estacio RO, Raynolds MV, et al. Angiotensin-converting enzyme gene polymorphism in non-insulin dependent diabetes mellitus and its relationship with diabetic nephropathy. Kidney Int 52:473-477, 1997.

49. Marre M, Jeunemaitre X, Gallois Y, et al. Contribution of genetic polymorphism in the renin-angiotensin system to the development of renal complications in insulin-dependent diabetes: Genetique de la Nephropathie Diabetique (GENEDIAB) study group. J Clin Invest 99:1585-1595, 1997.

50. Schmidt S, Schone N, Ritz E. Association of ACE gene polymorphism and diabetic nephropathy? The Diabetic Nephropathy Study Group. Kidney Int 47:1176-1181, 1995.

51. Chowdhury TA, Dronsfield MJ, Kumar S, et al. Examination of two genetic polymorphisms within the renin-angiotensin system: No evidence for an association with nephropathy in IDDM. Diabetologia 39:1108-1114, 1996.

52. Danser AH, Schalekamp MA, Bax WA, et al. Angiotensin-converting enzyme in the human heart. Effect of the deletion/insertion polymorphism. Circulation 92:1387-1388, 1995.

53. Davis GK, Millner RW, Roberts DH. Angiotensin converting enzyme (ACE) gene expression in the human left ventricle: Effect of ACE gene insertion/deletion polymorphism and left ventricular function. Eur J Heart Fail 2:253-256, 2000.

54. Studer R, Reinecke H, Muller B, et al. Increased angiotensin-I converting enzyme gene expression in the failing human heart. Quantification by competitive RNA polymerase chain reaction. J Clin Invest 94:301-310, 1994.

55. Spruth E, Zurbrugg HR, Warnecke C, et al. Expression of ACE mRNA in the human atrial myocardium is not dependent on left ventricular function, ACE inhibitor therapy, or the ACE I/D genotype. J Mol Med 77:804-810, 1999.

56. Tamaki S, Iwai N, Ohmichi N, et al. Effect of genotype on the angiotensin-converting enzyme mRNA level in human atria. Clin Exp Pharmacol Physiol 24:305-308, 1997.

57. Jacobsen P, Rossing K, Rossing P, et al. Angiotensin converting enzyme gene polymorphism and ACE inhibition in diabetic nephropathy. Kidney Int 53:1002-1006, 1998.

58. Danser AH, Derkx FH, Hense HW, et al. Angiotensinogen (M235T) and angiotensin-converting enzyme (I/D) polymorphisms in association with plasma renin and prorenin levels. J Hypertens 16:1879-1883, 1998.

59. Sethi AA, Nordestgaard BG, Tybjaerg-Hansen A. Angiotensinogen gene polymorphism, plasma angiotensinogen, and risk of hypertension and ischemic heart disease: A meta-analysis. Arterioscler Thromb Vasc Biol 23:1269-1275, 2003.

60. Matsubara M, Metoki H, Katsuya T, et al. T+31C polymorphism (M235T) of the angiotensinogen gene and home blood pressure in the Japanese general population: The Ohasama Study. Hypertens Res 26:47-52, 2003.

61. Fogarty DG, Harron JC, Hughes AE, et al. A molecular variant of angiotensinogen is associated with diabetic nephropathy in IDDM. Diabetes 45:1204-1208, 1996.

62. Kinoshita JH, Nishimura C. The involvement of aldose reductase in diabetic complications. Diabetes Metab Rev 4:323-337, 1988.

63. Buraczynska M, Pijanowski Z, Spasiewicz D, et al. Renin-angiotensin system gene polymorphisms: Assessment of the risk of coronary heart disease. Kardiol Pol 58:1-9, 2003.

64. Nair KG, Shalia KK, Ashavaid TF, et al. Coronary heart disease, hypertension, and angiotensinogen gene variants in Indian population. J Clin Lab Anal 17:141-146, 2003.

65. Fradin S, Goulet-Salmon B, Chantepie M, et al. Relationship between polymorphisms in the renin-angiotensin system and nephropathy in type 2 diabetic patients. Diabetes Metab 28:27-32, 2002.

66. Dzida G, Sobstyl J, Puzniak A, et al. Polymorphisms of angiotensin-converting enzyme and angiotensin II receptor type 1 genes in essential hypertension in a Polish population. Med Sci Monit 7:1236-1241, 2001.

67. Tarnow L, Cambien F, Rossing P, et al. Angiotensin-II type 1 receptor gene polymorphism and diabetic microangiopathy. Nephrol Dial Transplant 11:1019-1023, 1996.

68. Ishanov A, Okamoto H, Watanabe M, et al. Angiotensin II type 1 receptor gene polymorphisms in patients with cardiac hypertrophy. Jpn Heart J 39:87-96, 1998.

# Chapter 10

# Angiotensin-(1-7)

## Debra I. Diz, Mark C. Chappell, E. Ann Tallant, Carlos M. Ferrario

Angiotensin-(1-7) (Ang-[1-7]) is the first amino-terminal angiotensin peptide product identified as possessing biologic actions. From this observation, new concepts regarding the regulation of cardiovascular function by the renin-angiotensin system (RAS) have evolved. The actions of Ang-(1-7) are as diverse as those of Ang II, including activation of a variety of vasodilator systems to oppose the actions of Ang II. There is strong evidence for a role of endogenous Ang-(1-7) in the control of blood pressure during states with prolonged activation of the RAS as a result of actions on at least one novel receptor [$AT_{(1-7)}$] as well other potential sites. In this chapter, we update the information available for the role of this peptide in the regulation of renal function.

In setting the stage for interpretation of the findings presented on the pleiotropic nature of the RAS, it is important to recognize that a variety of peptide systems express numerous biologically active C- and N-terminal metabolites. Responses to peptide fragments exhibit complex relationships with respect to the major actions of the parent peptides, with both similar and dissimilar actions noted for substance P, opioid, and vasopressin systems.[1-4] Indeed, extensive studies of the opiate and tachykinin systems reveal a family of receptors linked to different responses in different tissues.[5-10] For many of these peptide systems, the C-terminal metabolites retain the majority of the actions of the parent peptide, although they may have reduced affinity for binding at the receptor.[11-14] On the other hand, N-terminal metabolites for substance P (tachykinin), bradykinin, and vasopressin systems, which exist as peptides with a C-terminal proline,[3,12,15-18] may act as physiologic or pharmacologic antagonists. There is down-regulation/desensitization of the NK1 receptor by substance P-(1-7),[16,19] even though this peptide has low affinity for the NK1 receptor.[19] There are reports that weak agonists cause down-regulation of the serotonin,[20] parathyroid,[6] and endothelin[21] systems by a mechanism independent of receptor internalization. With these concepts in mind, there are striking parallels among other peptide systems and the RAS. Our initiation of the study of the N-terminal metabolite of Ang II nearly 15 years ago led to the recognition that many of the same features that are well accepted for other peptide systems may also be true for the angiotensin peptides and will be highlighted in this chapter.

## FORMATION AND METABOLISM OF ANG-(1-7) IN THE KIDNEY

Ang-(1-7) is present in the circulation and in various tissues including the kidney[22-24] at levels comparable to those of Ang II. Levels of the peptide in plasma, renal tissue, and urine are altered during physiologic or pathophysiologic conditions including those associated with changes in sodium and volume (hypertension, low- and high-salt diets). Emerging evidence also supports the concept of an intrarenal angiotensin system distinct from the circulating RAS,[25] with concentrations of Ang peptides in proximal tubular fluid,[26,27] isolated glomeruli,[28] interstitium,[29] and renal tissue[24,30-32] generally exceeding those of the circulation. Indeed, renin and angiotensinogen mRNA are present in JG cells, and proximal and distal tubules.[33-37] Ang-(1-7) exists within the tubular regions throughout the kidney as shown in Figure 10–1.[38]

The enzymes responsible for metabolism of the Ang peptides are distinct in pulmonary and renal tissues.[22] Processing pathways in the circulation, where Ang II is the predominant peptide by ~twofold, appear to employ the endopeptidase neprilysin as the major activity forming Ang-(1-7) from Ang I.[39] Ang-(1-7) is the primary product formed in preparations of isolated proximal tubules and exists in urine at ~fivefold higher levels than Ang II.[40] In the kidney, Ang-(1-7) can be formed directly from either Ang I or Ang II. Figure 10–2 illustrates schematically the pathways for formation and metabolism of Ang-(1-7) in this tissue. Several endopeptidases present within renal vascular and tubular tissue have the capacity to form and metabolize Ang-(1-7).[41] Neprilysin may contribute to the formation as well as the degradation of the peptide.[22,42,43] Neprilysin cleaves Ang I to Ang-(1-7) and Ang-(1-7) to Ang-(1-4). Neprilysin inhibitors augment the urinary levels of Ang-(1-7) in human and rat.[44-46] ACE also directly metabolizes Ang-(1-7) to Ang-(1-5). Significant urinary excretion of Ang-(1-7) occurs in both rats and humans,[24,44-46] and chronic ACE inhibitor treatment that lowers blood pressure and stimulates diuresis is associated with enhanced excretion of Ang-(1-7) in both normotensive and hypertensive rats.[45,46] The in vivo clearance of Ang-(1-7) is reduced sixfold with the ACE inhibitor lisinopril, which, depending upon the species (rat, dog, or human), may involve either the N-terminal or C-terminal catalytic domains of ACE.[47,48] Recent studies reveal that a homolog of ACE termed ACE2[49,50] (distinct from the ACE.2 knockout model developed by Bernstein and colleagues[51,52]) exhibits carboxypeptidase activity cleaving a single amino acid residue at the carboxy terminus. ACE2 is not inhibited by ACE inhibitors. ACE2 was originally reported to cleave Ang I to Ang-(1-9),[49,50] but recent kinetic studies suggest that the conversion of Ang II to Ang-(1-7) is preferred.[53] ACE2 expresses the highest efficiency ($k_{cat}/K_m$) among Ang-(1-7)–forming enzymes with a 500-fold greater $k_{cat}/K_m$ for Ang II as compared with Ang I. Ang II, apelin-(1-13), and dynorphin A share a $k_{cat}/K_m$ ranging from 1800 to 2900 $mM^{-1}sec^{-1}$, kinetics with at least an order of magnitude greater than for Ang I or [des-$Arg^9$]-bradykinin (BK 1-8). ACE2, like ACE, exists in both soluble and membrane-associated forms with the highest densities in the kidney, heart, gut, and testes.[49]

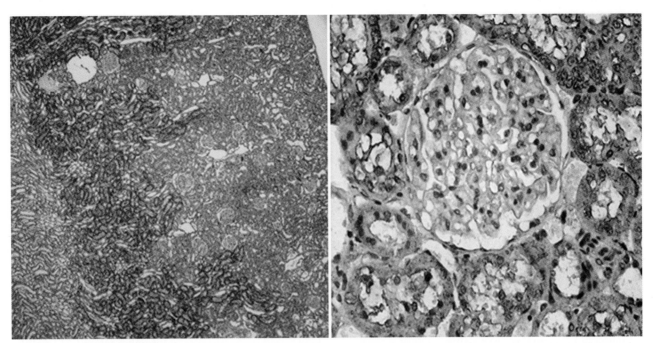

**Figure 10–1** Localization of Ang-(1-7) immunoreactivity in the kidney. Photomicrographs of SHR kidney sections showing immunostaining for Ang-(1-7) at 10× in the left panel and 100× in the right panel. Staining is densest in the tubules.

Differential and independent regulation of the formation of Ang-(1-7) and Ang II is reported in the kidney during ischemia and in hypertensive animals during changes in dietary sodium intake. In rats undergoing acute unilateral ischemia and subsequent reperfusion, increases in Ang II are not accompanied by

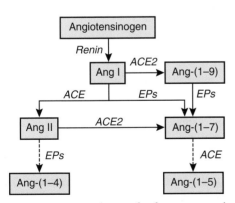

**Figure 10–2** Processing pathways for formation and metabolism of Ang-(1-7) in the kidney. Once formed from angiotensinogen by renin, angiotensin (Ang) I can be processed to Ang II or Ang-(1-7) by the pathways shown. The major endopeptidases (EPs) involved in formation of Ang-(1-7) from Ang I or Ang-(1-9) in the kidney include neprilysin, prolyl endopeptidase, and thimet oligopeptidase.[41] The critical positions of converting enzyme (ACE) and its recently identified homolog ACE2 with respect to reciprocal formation and metabolism of Ang II and Ang-(1-7) underscore the importance of studies aimed at determining the contribution of each enzyme during normal physiology and pathophysiology.

increases in Ang-(1-7).[24] In hypertensive animals maintained on low- and normal-salt diets differential changes in levels of the two peptides also occur.[30,46,54] In fact, Ang-(1-7) appears to contribute to maintenance of normal pressure during periods of salt restriction and the accompanying increase in Ang II levels in the circulation.[30] In salt-sensitive hypertension in the female mRen.2.Lewis congenics, there is increased ACE and a reduction in ACE2 in the kidney,[55] providing initial evidence that salt-sensitive hypertension may result from a deficit in formation of Ang-(1-7), as well as an increase in Ang II. In fact, during omapatrilat treatment of salt-sensitive hypertensive patients, this combined NEP and ACE inhibitor increases levels of Ang I and Ang-(1-7) dramatically.[45] In spontaneous hypertensive rats omapatrilat treatment is associated with sustained increases in Ang-(1-7) and a pronounced water diuresis, without increases in Ang II.[56] Furthermore, increased expression of ACE2 is seen in the proximal tubules of treated kidneys, which may contribute to the expression of Ang-(1-7) in this cortical area.[57] Studies in the ACE2 knockout mouse illustrate the importance of this enzyme in regulation of RAS, because higher circulating and tissue levels of Ang II occur.[58] Spontaneously hypertensive rats (SHR) and the Sabra salt-sensitive rats exhibit reduced mRNA levels and protein expression of ACE2.[58] Moreover, ACE2 maps to a QTL region on chromosome 10 known to be highly associated with the hypertensive phenotype.[58] Indeed, the results of these studies suggest that dysregulation of these two enzymatic systems (ACE and ACE2) may lead to altered levels of Ang II and Ang-(1-7). At the present time, little is known about the regulation of ACE2 and its role in hypertension and other cardiovascular pathologies. We would propose that the balance of ACE and ACE2 may serve to regulate the expression of Ang II and Ang-(1-7) in the kidney.

# INTRARENAL ACTIONS OF ANG-(1-7)

As illustrated previously, the presence and independent regulation of Ang II and Ang-(1-7) in kidney supports the concept of important and divergent actions for the two peptides within this organ. For Ang II, the actions include potent, but differential, constriction of diverse segments of the renal microvasculature as well as retention of sodium and water through stimulation of various transporters in the proximal epithelium. For Ang-(1-7), most actions are in opposition to those of Ang II. Ang-(1-7) infusions into the renal artery lead to diuresis and natriuresis accompanied by modest increases in glomerular filtration rate (GFR).[59-64] Ang-(1-7) induces dilation of preconstricted afferent arterioles.[65] Ang-(1-7) and Ang-(3-7) are potent inhibitors of $Na^+,K^+$-ATPase activity in isolated convoluted proximal tubules and the renal cortex.[60,66,67] Actions at the $Na^+/H^+$ exchanger may also occur.[68] Ang-(1-7) stimulates transcellular flux of sodium in renal tubular epithelial cells, which is associated with activation of phospholipase $A_2$.[69] Furthermore, inhibition of sodium transport by Ang I is markedly potentiated by captopril suggesting either a shift in processing pathways to Ang-(1-7) or reduced metabolism of the peptide in the proximal tubules of the kidney. The vasopeptidase inhibitor omapatrilat produces a chronic and pronounced diuresis associated with large increases in urinary excretion of Ang-(1-7) and enhanced immunocytochemical staining of the peptide as well as ACE2 in the kidney of the SHR.[55,56] That the diuresis consists of dilute urine is consistent with the localization of the Ang-(1-7) in all segments of the renal tubules.[56] The recent observations that the peptide may regulate aquaporin 1 in the proximal tubule[70] also reveal the potential of Ang-(1-7) as a key regulator in the control of water handling within the kidney.

Renal actions of Ang-(1-7) and Ang II are also comparable in several situations. In perfused straight proximal tubules, peritubular application of Ang-(1-7) displays biphasic effects on bicarbonate transport—a low concentration ($10^{-12}$ M) stimulates transport, whereas higher levels ($10^{-8}$ M) inhibit absorption—similar to what is seen with Ang II.[68] Intratubular application of Ang-(1-7) stimulates transport in the loop of Henle, but does not affect reabsorption in either the proximal or distal tubule.[71] The lack of an effect may result from the high luminal concentrations of Ang-(1-7) in the proximal or distal segments of the tubule. This would be similar to what occurs with Ang II where application of an $AT_1$ antagonist or ACE inhibitor attenuates basal reabsorption in the proximal tubule, but there is no additional effect of adding Ang II.[72] In fact, the natriuretic effects of high doses of Ang II may be due to the conversion of Ang II to Ang-(1-7) at the epithelial surface of the proximal tubule to functionally oppose the $AT_1$-dependent actions of Ang II. In water-loaded Wistar rats administration of Ang-(1-7) promotes an antidiuretic action.[73,74] Ang-(1-7) stimulates water transport in collecting duct tubules suggesting a site of action for Ang-(1-7), but the cellular mechanisms have not been defined.[75] Finally, Ang-(1-7) stimulates ouabain-insensitive $Na^+$-ATPase activity in the ovine renal cortex, but inhibits Ang II–dependent stimulation of this ATPase.[76,77] Burgelova et al.[78] showed that intrarenal administration of Ang-(1-7) produced natriuresis and blocked the antinatriuretic actions of Ang II. Ang-(1-7) did not attenuate the reduction in GFR or the increase in renal perfusion pressure associated with Ang II; however, it is simi-

lar to what was reported by Handa et al.[60] Finally, the renal actions of Ang-(1-7) also include an increase in oxidative stress markers such as thiobarbituric acid reactive species (TBARS), an indicator of lipid peroxidation, accompanied by a decrease in reduced glutathione as well as superoxide dismutase and glutathione peroxidase activities.[79] Together these studies emphasize the complexity of the actions and interactions of Ang-(1-7) and Ang II. Thus, the overall state of activity of the RAS and site(s) of the nephron exposed to the peptides clearly influence the ultimate physiologic action observed.

The cellular mechanisms responsible for actions of Ang-(1-7) in the kidney most likely involve mobilization of arachidonic acid and its subsequent processing through pathways yielding vasodilator and natriuretic products. The in vivo depressor response to Ang-(1-7) in the pithed rat was first shown to be dependent upon cyclooxygenase pathways.[80] Infusion of Ang-(1-7) into isolated rat kidneys causes an increase in prostacyclin in both the urine and the perfusate.[61] A renal source of circulating prostaglandins may in fact participate in the lowering of blood pressure produced by Ang-(1-7). Ang II infusions are associated with activation of prostanoid pathways within the kidney, and in the presence of thromboxane and $AT_1$ receptor antagonists, a blood pressure lowering effect is seen due to renal release of prostanoids.[81]

The natriuretic and diuretic actions of Ang-(1-7) in the perfused kidney are associated with increased levels of prostacyclin that are attenuated by the cyclooxygenase inhibitor indomethacin.[61] Ang-(1-7) infusion into SHR caused diuresis and natriuresis during the early days of infusion, concomitant with increases in urinary prostaglandins measured.[82] In hypertensive rats treated with lisinopril and losartan, indomethacin causes increases in blood pressure similar to those produced by an antibody to Ang-(1-7) or a neprilysin inhibitor and the treatments are not additive, suggesting that vasodilator prostaglandins mediate the effects of Ang-(1-7) in lisinopril/losartan-treated rats. Ang-(1-7) stimulates arachidonic acid release and inhibits transcellular sodium transport in renal tubular epithelial cells[69] and blocks the Ang II–stimulated $Na^+$-ATPase activity in the proximal tubule.[77] Low picomolar doses of Ang-(1-7) stimulate phosphatidylcholine incorporation in the renal cortex, providing a potential mechanism for supply of the arachidonic acid substrate[83]; however, there is no evidence for activation of phospholipase C by Ang-(1-7) in kidney.[84,85] Ang-(1-7)–dependent inhibition of ouabain-sensitive rubidium (Rb[86]) influx selectively activates the proximal epithelial cytochrome P450 (CYP450) system in isolated tubules to augment sodium excretion.[40,86] This contrasts with the stimulation of the vascular CYP450 system by Ang II to produce potent vasoconstrictors.[87-89] Cyclooxygenase products do not appear to play a role in this effect.[86]

An important concept generated by work over the past 5 years is that increased Ang-(1-7) levels may contribute to the actions of ACE inhibitors. On the basis of knowledge that ACE is a major factor in the clearance and metabolism of Ang-(1-7), early studies revealed that, in animals and patients, ~fivefold increases in circulating levels of Ang-(1-7) occur during chronic ACE inhibition. In agreement with these studies, patients chronically treated with the ACE inhibitor captopril have increases in plasma concentrations of prostacyclin with no significant effect on plasma concentrations of Ang II.[90] Blockade by the Ang-(1-7) receptor antagonist

D-[Ala⁷]-Ang-(1-7) or sequestration of the peptide with a specific monoclonal antibody reverses the blood pressure lowering actions of an ACE inhibitor alone or when combined with the AT₁ antagonist losartan.[54,91,92] Interestingly, the Ang-(1-7) receptor antagonist also reverses the blood pressure effects of treatment with losartan alone in the SHR; however, the Ang-(1-7) neutralizing antibody or the neprilysin inhibitor does not reverse the effects on blood pressure to the same extent.[92] These data suggest that the high levels of Ang II following chronic AT₁ receptor blockade due to disinhibition of renin release may spill over to an Ang-(1-7) receptor site to stimulate prostaglandin release.[92] Indeed, high resolution autoradiography revealed competition for Ang-(1-7) sites in the mesenteric artery or the aorta by [D-Ala⁷]-Ang-(1-7), Ang II and Ang-(1-7)—all assays were performed in the presence of AT₁(losartan) and AT₂ receptor (PD123319) antagonists.[91,92] Together these results suggest that Ang-(1-7) and prostacyclin may account for up to 30% of the antihypertensive actions of ACE inhibition and AT₁ receptor blockade.

## RECEPTORS RESPONSIBLE FOR ACTIONS OF ANG-(1-7) IN THE KIDNEY

Accumulated evidence, discussed subsequently, suggests that there are several mechanisms by which Ang-(1-7) produces its actions.[14,93] At least three potential mechanisms have been identified to account for these actions (Figure 10–3). These include (1) activation of antihypertensive systems (prostaglandins, nitric oxide) by actions at a novel non-AT₁/AT₂ receptor [AT₍₁₋₇₎] that are blocked by [D-Ala⁷]-Ang-(1-7); (2) actions of Ang-(1-7) that are blocked by AT₁ or AT₂ receptor antagonists in addition to [D-Ala⁷]-Ang-(1-7); and (3) Ang-(1-7)–induced homologous or heterologous down-regulation or desensitization of classic AT₁ receptors.

1. Activation of antihypertensive systems (prostaglandins, nitric oxide) by actions at a novel non-AT₁/AT₂ receptor [AT₍₁₋₇₎] that are blocked by [D-Ala⁷]-Ang-(1-7) (see Figure 10–3, First Panel). Many of the actions of Ang-(1-7) are blocked by the nonselective potent peptide antagonist,

[Sar¹-Thr⁸]-Ang II and sarcosine analogs of Ang II compete for Ang-(1-7) receptors in endothelial cells, whereas the AT₁ or AT₂ selective antagonists do not. [D-Ala⁷]-Ang-(1-7) selectively antagonizes several of the actions of Ang-(1-7), but not those of Ang II.[94] Non-AT₁/AT₂ receptor binding for Ang-(1-7) is reported in human skin fibroblasts,[95] canine coronary artery endothelium,[14] the mesenteric vasculature,[96,97] rat thoracic aorta,[98] and in rat thoracic aortic vascular smooth muscle cells (VSMC) in culture.[99] The response to an intravenous infusion of [Sar¹-Thr⁸]-Ang II was tested in SHR given the combination of lisinopril and losartan for 8 days, a treatment known to elevate Ang-(1-7) in plasma.[54,100] A pressor response was observed of magnitude and characteristics similar to that obtained by [D-Ala⁷]-Ang-(1-7), endogenous neutralization of Ang-(1-7) with a monoclonal antibody, or an inhibitor of Ang-(1-7) formation (neprilysin inhibitors). Thus, in the presence of both AT₁ (losartan) blockade and ACE inhibition, interference with the actions of Ang-(1-7) reverses the antihypertensive effect of the peptide, suggesting that the vasodepressor effects of Ang-(1-7) during the combined treatment are mediated by a non-AT₁/AT₂ angiotensin subtype receptor. This receptor is designated as AT₍₁₋₇₎.[101,102] The fact that these actions of Ang-(1-7) are manifest during ACE inhibition excludes interaction of the peptide with ACE[103,104] as the mechanism to account for these responses.

Ang-(1-7) infusion transiently decreases blood pressure in SHR and this effect is blocked by [D-Ala⁷]Ang-(1-7).[105] Ang-(1-7) also causes a depressor response in salt-sensitive Dahl rats that is blocked by [D-Ala⁷]Ang-(1-7).[106] Ang-(1-7) infusion increases release of prostacyclin and nitric oxide and reduces thromboxane A₂ levels, all of which are prevented by pretreatment with the [D-Ala⁷]Ang-(1-7). Other studies are consistent with the existence of an AT₍₁₋₇₎ receptor in renal tissue.[63,77,83] The in vivo actions of Ang-(1-7) are attenuated by the antagonist [D-Ala⁷]-Ang-(1-7), but not by the AT₁ antagonist losartan.[63,78] The natriuretic and diuretic effects of Ang-(1-7) and actions on the afferent arteriole are blocked by [D-Ala⁷]-Ang-(1-7), suggesting that the renal actions of Ang-(1-7) encompass both tubular

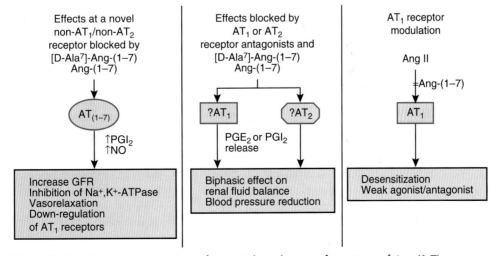

**Figure 10–3** Schematic presentation of potential mechanisms for actions of Ang-(1-7).

and vascular binding sites that are non-$AT_1/AT_2$ receptors. Intrarenal administration of D-[Ala[7]]-Ang-(1-7) to normotensive rats elicits a fall in GFR, urine volume, and sodium excretion, suggesting tonic activity of renal Ang-(1-7) in these animals.[78] In the afferent arteriole, Ang-(1-7) exhibits potent vasodilator effects that are blocked by D-[Ala[7]]-Ang-(1-7) and nitric oxide synthase inhibitors, but not $AT_1$ or $AT_2$ antagonists.[65] Actions of Ang-(1-7) to inhibit $Na^+,K^+$-ATPase activity ($^{86}Rb$ uptake) in isolated proximal tubules from normotensive rats,[40] consistent with natriuretic actions within the kidney, are blocked by D-[Ala[7]]-Ang-(1-7), but not $AT_1$ or $AT_2$ antagonists.

These data provide overwhelming evidence that the actions of Ang-(1-7) are mediated by a non-$AT_1/AT_2$ receptor. The unique $AT_{(1-7)}$ receptor is defined by its sensitivity to Ang-(1-7), its antagonism by [Sar[1]-Thr[8]]-Ang II and [D-Ala[7]]-Ang-(1-7), and its lack of response to losartan or PD123319, either functionally or in competition for binding. Importantly, data from Santos et al. reveal that the *mas* receptor gene codes for an Ang-(1-7) binding site.[107] Studies in *mas* receptor–deficient mice indicate the loss of $^{125}I$-Ang-(1-7) binding in the kidney of these animals. Functional assessments indicated the loss of vascular responses to Ang-(1-7) as well as effects of the heptapeptide in the collecting duct.[107] In addition, antisense oligonucleotides or small interfering RNAs to *mas* prevented responses to Ang-(1-7) (inhibition of mitogen-stimulated MAP kinase activity), in conjunction with a reduction in *mas* protein.[108] These findings further support the presence of a unique receptor in kidney responsible for the majority of actions of the peptide.

2. Actions of Ang-(1-7) that are blocked by $AT_1$ or $AT_2$ receptor antagonists in addition to [D-Ala[7]]-Ang-(1-7) (see Figure 10–3, Second Panel). As with most peptide systems, all of the actions of Ang-(1-7) cannot be attributed to activation of a single receptor. In fact, from the initial observation that Ang-(1-7)–released vasopressin from isolated hypothalamo-neurohypophysial explants,[109] many of the early actions of Ang-(1-7) appeared to be similar to Ang II. With identification of the Ang II receptor subtypes $AT_1$ and $AT_2$ by both pharmacologic and molecular approaches, subtype selective antagonists were used to attempt to characterize the actions of Ang-(1-7). The resulting pharmacologic data are far from clear. In addition to the actions of Ang-(1-7) at the novel $AT_{(1-7)}$ receptor highlighted previously, several actions of Ang-(1-7) are similar to those of Ang II or are blocked by $AT_1$ or $AT_2$ receptor antagonists. Examples of these responses, which occur at low doses or doses equivalent to Ang II, are found in several tissues, but especially brain and kidney. Moreover, in both binding and functional studies losartan and PD123319 compete for the same subpopulation of sites.[110-119]

In the kidney, Handa et al. reported that Ang-(1-7)–induced effects on oxygen consumption were due to actions blocked in part by losartan and completely by Sar[1]Thr[8]-Ang II.[60] Baracho and coworkers[120] reported that losartan and [D-Ala[7]]-Ang-(1-7) each caused 100% inhibition of the antidiuretic actions of Ang-(1-7) in isolated collecting tubules or in whole animals, but that neither $AT_2$ nor vasopressin antagonists had any effect. However, Ang-(1-7) has a poor ability to elicit vasoconstrictor or pressor responses or compete for Ang II binding. Infusion of Ang-(1-7) into the renal artery also does not antagonize the actions of Ang II on renal blood flow or GFR.[59-61] Thus, the actions of Ang-(1-7) contrast with the potent vasoconstriction elicited by Ang II through classic $AT_1$ sites.

To better understand the pharmacology of the receptors mediating the above responses, receptor-binding studies were carried out in membrane preparations from rat kidney. There was evidence for high affinity competition of $^{125}I$-[Sar[1]-Thr[8]]-Ang II binding by Ang-(1-7), which accounted for 10% to 20% of the total binding in the rat kidney (Figure 10–4). All of the binding was competed for by losartan, but both PD123319 and [D-Ala[7]]-Ang-(1-7) competed for 10% to 20% of the binding. Competition with [D-Ala[7]]-Ang-(1-7) was not additive with Ang-(1-7), suggesting that they compete for the same population of receptors. Alternatively, the biphasic nature of the losartan binding data suggest that losartan may discriminate between a classic $AT_1$ site and a second site that recognizes Ang-(1-7), [D-Ala[7]]-Ang-(1-7), and possibly PD123319, with high affinity. Further work by Garcia and Garvin[68] concluded that the biphasic effects of Ang-(1-7) in proximal tubules are inhibited primarily by losartan (80%); however, these effects of Ang-(1-7) are also inhibited significantly (40%) by the $AT_2$ antagonist PD123319. Other studies of low-dose Ang-(1-7) in proximal tubule preparations reveal that actions are blocked by [D-Ala[7]]-Ang-(1-7)[40,120]; thus, the binding data in kidney tissue strongly parallel the actions of Ang-(1-7) at a high affinity site.

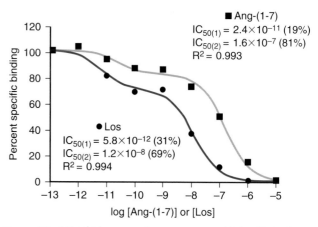

$^{125}I$-Sarthran Binding in Renal Medulla
Competition with Ang-(1–7) and Losartan

■ Ang-(1-7)
$IC_{50(1)} = 2.4 \times 10^{-11}$ (19%)
$IC_{50(2)} = 1.6 \times 10^{-7}$ (81%)
$R^2 = 0.993$

● Los
$IC_{50(1)} = 5.8 \times 10^{-12}$ (31%)
$IC_{50(2)} = 1.2 \times 10^{-8}$ (69%)
$R^2 = 0.994$

log [Ang-(1-7)] or [Los]

**Figure 10–4** Rat kidney membranes express high affinity for both losartan and Ang-(1-7). In membranes prepared from the renal medulla, as shown, or cortex of SD male rats (n = 3), binding to the antagonist $^{125}I$-[Sar[1],Thr[8]]-Ang II (0.2 nM) was competed for by Ang II with an $IC_{50}$ of 2 nM. Losartan (Los) competed for essentially all of the binding in a biphasic manner in the medulla. Competition by Ang-(1-7) also revealed two sites, one of high (<1 nM; 20%) and one of low affinity (0.2 μM; 80%). A similar percentage of binding was competed for by 1 μM [D-Ala[7]]-Ang-(1-7) and variably by 1 μM PD123319 (not shown). The competition by [D-Ala[7]]-Ang-(1-7) was not additive with 50 nM Ang-(1-7) suggesting that they both compete for the same high affinity site.

The aforementioned data are similar to what is reported for cultured mesangial cells.[115] In those studies, [125]I-[Sar[1]]-Ang II binding was displaced completely by losartan, a portion (~20%) was competed for by PD123319 but not CGP42112A, and a similar percentage of the binding (20%) showed a reasonably high affinity (20 nM) for Ang-(1-7). The relationship of the PD123319 component of the binding to the Ang-(1-7) component is not totally clear, because additive effects of the Ang-(1-7) and the AT$_2$ antagonists were not tested. Another report also found both a typical AT$_1$ receptor which accounted for 80% of the [125]I-Ang II binding in renal tissue as well as a PD123319-sensitive, losartan-sensitive component accounting for 20% of the total binding.[121] Ernsberger and colleagues[115] designated the novel binding site in the mesangial cells in culture an AT$_{1B}$ in earlier publications to distinguish it from the classic AT$_1$ receptor. This designation currently creates confusion with the molecular AT$_{1B}$ receptor. Whether the PD123319-sensitive effects represent a separate population of AT$_2$ receptors or overlap with the Ang-(1-7)– and [D-Ala[7]]-Ang-(1-7)–sensitive component is not clear and is the subject of ongoing investigations. However, a study in whole animals showed that PD123319 and [D-Ala[7]]-Ang-(1-7) each partially reverse the blood pressure lowering effects of AT$_1$ receptor blockade with losartan.[122] The effects of the two treatments were not additive, suggesting overlapping mechanisms if not receptors.

Therefore, available functional data support actions of Ang-(1-7) in the kidney through a losartan- and/or PD123319-sensitive site that is also inhibited by [D-Ala[7]]-Ang-(1-7). The receptor clearly does not fit the classical AT$_1$ receptor classification due to its recognition of Ang-(1-7) and [D-Ala[7]]-Ang-(1-7), because Ang-(1-7) does not activate phospholipase C.[123] The fact that only a subset (15%-20%) of the total losartan-sensitive receptors showed high affinity for Ang-(1-7) suggests that either these receptors are isoforms of the AT$_1$ or AT$_2$ receptors or the subtype selective antagonists are capable of interacting with AT$_{(1-7)}$ receptors. To begin to distinguish between these possibilities, we reported residual [125]I-[Sar[1]-Thr[8]]-Ang II binding sites in AT$_{1A}$ deficient mouse kidney that are losartan and/or PD123319 sensitive and also show high affinity for Ang-(1-7) and [D-Ala[7]]-Ang-(1-7).[124,125] That these sites contribute to less than 20% of the sites in wild-type mouse kidney, persist in the kidney of AT$_{1A}$ receptor knockout mice, and now account for the majority of residual binding reveals evidence for actions on a novel gene product. Data by Santos and colleagues[107] indicate the *mas* protein is a [D-Ala[7]]-Ang-(1-7)–sensitive receptor. However, this receptor does not recognize the presumed AT$_1$ or AT$_2$ selective antagonists. Alternately, we have evidence that expression of the AT$_{1B}$ receptor in VSMCs conveys an increase in a PD123319-sensitive site with high affinity for Ang-(1-7) and [D-Ala[7]]-Ang-(1-7).[126] Interestingly, the pattern of distribution of AT$_{1B}$ receptors in kidney parallels the distribution of the actions and binding of Ang-(1-7).[111-113,119,127]

3. Ang-(1-7)–induced homologous or heterologous down-regulation or desensitization of classic AT$_1$ receptors (see Figure 10–3, Third Panel). Regulation of receptors and receptor-mediated responses occurs at a number of different levels. These include regulation of the receptor by the ligand itself (homologous regulation) or by unrelated substances (heterologous regulation). Homologous regulation can be immediate and related to receptor internalization and rapid decreases in receptor numbers. It can be prolonged and include changes in number or affinity of the receptor through regulation at the mRNA and protein, or through alterations in the cellular signaling pathways. Desensitization or the functional uncoupling of the receptor from its effector system is typically a result of agonist-induced receptor phosphorylation.[128-130]

Reductions in AT$_1$ receptor density in the presence of elevated levels of Ang II may be due to receptor internalization.[131,132] Prior exposure to Ang II also may result in a rapid desensitization of cellular responses.[128,129-135] However, the reduction in the response to Ang II is not associated with changes in receptor number or affinity and inhibiting internalization does not prevent the desensitization. Acute and chronic exposure to elevated Ang-(1-7) decreases AT$_1$ receptors and AT$_1$ receptor–mediated responses in brain and kidney tissue and cells in culture. The mechanism for the Ang-(1-7) effects is not likely to be the result of direct pharmacologic antagonism (see next paragraph). Ang-(1-7) may act as a weak agonist at the AT$_1$ receptor to cause homologous receptor regulation, although the duration or magnitude may be less than that seen with a more potent agonist.[20,21] Indeed, studies in VSMC or CHO-AT$_{1A}$ cells indicate a direct effect of Ang-(1-7) at the AT$_1$ receptor, consistent with agonist-induced homologous down-regulation.[135,136] The response occurs rapidly, is present in cells containing only AT$_{1A}$ receptors without any evidence for Ang-(1-7) receptors, and may be accompanied by reduced activation of phospholipase C by Ang II.

In brain and peripheral tissues, the effects of ACE inhibitors on AT$_1$ receptors are variable, with decreases occurring in brain and increases occurring in the vasculature.[137,138-141] Because Ang II is decreased only acutely with ACE inhibition, the variety of responses indicates that factors other than Ang II contribute to the regulation of the AT$_1$ receptor. Termed heterologous regulation, this is known to occur in addition to the aforementioned ligand-mediated regulation.[132] Ang-(1-7) activates cellular mechanisms such as prostaglandin or nitric oxide release that may result in acute physiologic antagonism of the response to Ang II as indicated in the preceding sections. We propose that these mediators also participate in the regulation of AT$_1$ receptors based on a series of findings in cells in culture or kidney slices incubated with Ang-(1-7). Prostaglandins participate in heterologous down-regulation of opioid receptors[142] and substance P NK1 receptors.[19] Nitric oxide decreases AT$_1$ receptor mRNA.[143] Short-term incubation of isolated kidney slices with Ang-(1-7) results in a reduction in [125]I-Ang II–labeled receptors. This effect is reversed completely in the presence of meclofenamate and, at least in part, by [D-Ala[7]]-Ang-(1-7). Although Ang-(1-7) is associated with down-regulation of the AT$_1$ receptor following these relatively short-term treatments, Neves et al.[144] report that 24-hour treatment with Ang-(1-7) up-regulates AT$_1$ mRNA in VSMCs isolated from the Akron strain of WKY and SHR. This suggests that chronic exposure to Ang-(1-7) may alter the expression of the AT$_1$ receptor in a strain-specific manner. The physiologic relevance of these in vitro studies is underscored by the additional findings that WKY rats infused for 2 weeks with Ang-(1-7) have a reduction in Ang II–stimulated release of prostacyclin (Figure 10–5) as well as reduced pressor responses to exogenous Ang II.[145]

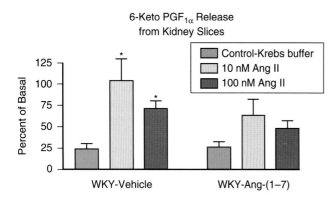

6-Keto PGF$_{1\alpha}$ Release
from Kidney Slices

* $p < 0.05$ compared with basal release

**Figure 10–5** Ang II–induced prostacyclin release from rat kidney slices is diminished in rats infused with Ang-(1-7). We tested whether basal or Ang II–stimulated PGI$_2$ release from kidney slices was altered after chronic treatment with Ang-(1-7) in WKY rats. *Ang-(1-7) (24 µg/kg/hr) or saline vehicle (V) was infused intravenously via osmotic minipumps for 2 weeks as described.[†] On day 2 or 12 of infusion, the kidneys were removed and slices prepared for incubation in oxygenated Krebs buffer at 37°C; data from both days were pooled for analysis. PGI$_2$ release was measured as 6-keto-PGF$_{1\alpha}$ in two consecutive 15-minute samples: before (basal) and during incubation with Krebs buffer (control) or 10 or 100 nM Ang II (n = 5-8 each). Ang II significantly increased 6-keto-PGF$_{1\alpha}$ release from kidney slices of vehicle-treated WKY rats threefold. The Ang II response was attenuated in rats that received prolonged infusion of Ang-(1-7). These findings suggest that increased Ang-(1-7) levels down-regulate the Ang II receptor or the receptor signaling pathways. (From *Diz DI, Benter IF, Bosch SM, Ferrario CM. Angiotensin-(1-7) infusion attenuates angiotensin II-induced prostacyclin release from kidney slices. Am J Hypertens 11:32A, 1998; [†]Benter IF, Ferrario CM, Morris M, Diz DI. Antihypertensive actions of angiotensin-(1-7) in spontaneously hypertensive rats. Am J Physiol Heart Circ Physiol 269:H313-H319, 1995, and Strawn WB, Ferrario CM, Tallant EA. Angiotensin-(1-7) reduces smooth muscle growth after vascular injury. Hypertension 33:207-211, 1999.)

At concentrations 1000-fold higher than that of Ang II, Ang-(1-7) does not antagonize Ang II–dependent vasoconstriction in the rat kidney.[60] However, high concentrations of Ang-(1-7) bind to the AT$_1$ receptor and either stimulate AT$_1$-like responses or antagonize Ang II responses. Ang-(1-7) prevents the Ang II–mediated increase in Ca$^{2+}$ in rat mesangial cells at micromolar concentrations and competes for the AT$_1$ receptor in these cells.[84] Micromolar concentrations of Ang-(1-7) constrict rat renal microvessels and reduce AT$_1$ receptor binding and Ang II–mediated phospholipase C activity in rat aortic VSMCs and CHO cells transfected with the AT$_{1A}$ receptor.[135,136,146] AT$_1$ receptor antagonists block down-regulation of the AT$_1$ receptor by Ang-(1-7), demonstrating that Ang-(1-7) interacts with the AT$_1$ receptor to reduce Ang II–mediated responses. Therefore, competition for the AT$_1$ receptor by pharmacologic concentrations of Ang-(1-7) may be responsible for blockade of contractile responses to Ang II by Ang-(1-7) in vascular studies that require micromolar amounts of Ang-(1-7).[147,148] However,

these supraphysiologic actions of the peptide do not explain the majority of actions attributed to Ang-(1-7) as illustrated in the preceding sections of this chapter.

## SUMMARY

The findings of many studies provide strong support for the premise that both exogenous administration and endogenous production of Ang-(1-7) elicit responses within tubular and vascular elements of the kidney. Most, but not all, actions oppose the effects of Ang II at least in part through prostaglandin production. The majority of actions of Ang-(1-7) are blocked by [D-Ala[7]]-Ang-(1-7). This argues strongly for involvement of novel receptors mediating the actions of the heptapeptide. However, as with many previously studied peptide systems, there is likely a family of receptors responsible for the myriad effects of Ang-(1-7). Pharmacologically, both actions and binding sites can be subdivided into those blocked solely by [D-Ala[7]]-Ang-(1-7) and those blocked by either or both presumed selective AT$_1$ and AT$_2$ antagonists in addition to the [D-Ala[7]]-Ang-(1-7). It is known that multiple protein isoforms exist within the AT$_1$ and AT$_2$ receptor categories based on glycosylation patterns or migration on isoelectric focusing gels. However, no one has yet determined whether these isoforms explain differences in the ability of these classic receptors to interact with Ang-(1-7). Finally, through its unique receptor or by direct interactions, the heptapeptide may play a role in down-regulation or desensitization of AT$_1$ receptors. Thus, Ang-(1-7) may influence Ang II–mediated responses in specific regions of the kidney by a variety of distinct mechanisms.

## References

1. Skilling SR, Smullin DH, Larson AA. Differential effects of C- and N-terminal substance P metabolites on the release of amino acid neurotransmitters from the spinal cord: potential role in nociception. J Neurosci 10:1309-1318, 1990.
2. Khan S, Grogan E, Whelpton R, Michael-Titus AT. N- and C-terminal substance P fragments modulate striatal dopamine outflow through a cholinergic link mediated by muscarinic receptors. Neurosci 73:919-927, 1996.
3. Kreeger JS, Larson AA. Substance P-(1-7), a substance P metabolite, inhibits withdrawal jumping in morphine-dependent mice. Eur J Pharmacol 238:111-115, 1993.
4. Strupp BJ, Bunsey M, Bertsche B, et al. Enhancement and impairment of memory retrieval by a vasopressin metabolite: an interaction with the accessibility of the memory. Behav Neurosci 104:268-276, 1990.
5. Helke CJ, Krause JE, Mantyh PW, et al. Diversity in mammalian tachykinin peptidergic neurons: Multiple peptides, receptors, and regulatory mechanisms. FASEB J 4:1606-1615, 1990.
6. Fukayama S, Tashjian AH Jr, et al. Signaling by N- and C-terminal sequences of parathyroid hormone-related protein in hippocampal neurons. Proc Natl Acad Sci USA 92:10182-10186, 1995.
7. Brinton RE, Gehlert DR, Wamsley JK, et al. Vasopressin metabolite, AVP4-9, binding sites in brain: distribution distinct from that of parent peptide. Life Sci 38:443-452, 1986.
8. Olson GA, Olson RD, Kastin AJ. Endogenous opiates: 1987. Peptides 10:205-236, 1989.
9. Hornfeldt CS, Sun X, Larson AA. The NH2-terminus of substance P modulates NMDA-induced activity in the mouse spinal cord. J Neuroscience 14:3364-3369, 1994.
10. Davis TP, Konings PN. Peptidases in the CNS: formation of biologically active, receptor-specific peptide fragments. [Review] [40 refs]. Crit Rev Neurobiol 7:163-174, 1993.

11. Krumins SA, Broomfield CA. C-terminal substance P fragments elicit histamine release from a murine mast cell line. Neuropeptides 24:5-10, 1993.

12. Khan S, Brooks N, Whelpton R, Michael-Titus AT. Substance P-(1-7) and substance P-(5-11) locally modulate dopamine release in rat striatum. Eur J Pharmacol 282:229-233, 1995.

13. Gardiner SM, Kemp PA, March JE, et al. Regional haemodynamic effects of angiotensin II (3-8) in conscious rats. Br J Pharmacol 110:159-162, 1993.

14. Ferrario CM, Chappell MC, Tallant EA, et al. Counter-regulatory actions of angiotensin-(1-7). Hypertension 30:535-541, 1997.

15. Stewart JM, Hall ME, Harkins J, et al. A fragment of substance P with specific central activity: SP(1-7). Peptides 3:851-857, 1982.

16. Herrera-Marschitz M, Terenius L, Sakurada T, et al. The substance P(1-7) fragment is a potent modulator of substance P actions in the brain. Brain Res 521:316-320, 1990.

17. Igwe OJ, Sun X, Larson AA. Correlation of substance P-induced desensitization with substance P amino terminal metabolites in the mouse spinal cord. Peptides 11:817-825, 1990.

18. Brattstrom A, de Jong W, Burbach JPH, et al. Vasopressin, vasopressin fragments and a C-terminal peptide of the vasopressin precursor share cardiovascular effects when microinjected into the nucleus tractus solitarii. Psychoneuroendocrinology 14:461-467, 1989.

19. Yukhananov RYu, Larson AA. An N-terminal fragment of substance P, substance P(1-7), down-regulates neurokinin-1 binding in the mouse spinal cord. Neurosci Lett 178:163-166, 1994.

20. VanHooft JA, Vijverberg HP. Full and partial agonists induce distinct desensitized states of the 5-HT3 receptor. J Recept Sign Transduct Res 17:267-277, 1998.

21. Cyr CR, Devi LA, Rudy B, et al. Heterologous desensitization of the human endothelin A and neurokinin A receptors in Xenopus laevis oocytes. Recept Signal Transduct 6:99-109, 1996.

22. Allred AJ, Diz DI, Ferrario CM, et al. Pathways for angiotensin-(1-7) metabolism in pulmonary and renal tissues. Am J Physiol Renal Physiol 279:F841-F850, 2000.

23. Kohara K, Brosnihan KB, Chappell MC, et al. Angiotensin-(1-7): A member of circulating angiotensin peptides. Hypertension 17:131-138, 1991.

24. Allred AJ, Chappell MC, Ferrario CM, et al. Differential actions of renal ischemic injury on the intrarenal angiotensin system. Am J Physiol Renal Physiol 279:F636-F645, 2000.

25. Navar LG, Harrison-Bernard LM, Nishiyama A, et al. Regulation of intrarenal angiotensin II in hypertension. Hypertension 39:316-322, 2002.

26. Braam B, Mitchell KD, Fox J, et al. Proximal tubular secretion of angiotensin II in rats. Am J Physiol Renal Physiol 264:F891-F898, 1993.

27. Navar LG, Lewis L, Hymel A, et al. Tubular fluid concentrations and kidney contents of angiotensins I and II in anesthetized rats. J Am Soc Nephrol 5:1153-1158, 1994.

28. Atiyeh BA, Arant BS Jr, Henrich WL, et al. In vitro production of angiotensin II by isolated glomeruli. Am J Physiol Renal Physiol 268:F266-F272, 1995.

29. Siragy HM, Howell NL, Ragsdale NV, et al. Renal interstitial fluid angiotensin. Hypertension. 25:1021-1024, 1995.

30. Iyer SN, Averill DB, Chappell MC, et al. Contribution of angiotensin-(1-7) to blood pressure regulation in salt-depleted hypertensive rats. Hypertension 36:417-422, 2000.

31. Fox J, Guan S, Hymel AA, et al. Dietary Na and ACE inhibition effects on renal tissue angiotensin I and II and ACE activity in rats. Am J Physiol Renal Physiol 262:F902-F909, 1992.

32. Campbell DJ, Anastasopoulos F, Duncan AM, et al. Effects of neutral endopeptidase inhibition and combined angiotensin converting enzyme and neutral endopeptidase inhibition on angiotensin and bradykinin peptides in rats. J Pharm Exp Ther 287:567-577, 1998.

33. Rohrwasser A, Morgan T, Dillon HF, et al. Elements of a paracrine tubular renin-angiotensin system along the entire nephron. Hypertension 34:1265-1274, 1999.

34. Zimpelmann J, Kumar D, Levine DZ, et al. Early diabetes mellitus stimulates proximal tubule renin mRNA expression in the rat. Kidney Int 58:2320-2330, 2000.

35. Kobori H, Nishiyama A, Abe Y, et al. Enhancement of intrarenal angiotensinogen in Dahl salt-sensitive rats on high salt diet. Hypertension 41:592-597, 2003.

36. Henrich WL, McAllister EA, Eskue A, et al. Renin regulation in cultured proximal tubular cells. Hypertension 27:1337-1340, 1996.

37. Ingelfinger JR, Zuo WM, Fon EA, et al. In situ hybridization evidence for angiotensinogen messenger RNA in the rat proximal tubule. J Clin Invest 85:417-423, 1990.

38. Ferrario CM, Averill DB, Brosnihan KB, et al. Vasopeptidase inhibition and Ang-(1-7) in the spontaneously hypertensive rat. Kidney Int 62:1349-1357, 2002.

39. Yamamoto K, Chappell MC, Brosnihan KB, et al. In vivo metabolism of angiotensin I by neutral endopeptidase (EC 3.4.24.11) in spontaneously hypertensive rats. Hypertension 19:692-696, 1992.

40. Chappell MC. Evidence for the formation of ang-(1-7) and the inhibitory actons of the peptide on $Na^+,K^+ATPase$ activity in rat proximal tubules. Hypertension 38:523, 2001.

41. Chappell MC, Allred AJ, Ferrario CM. Pathways of angiotensin-(1-7) metabolism in the kidney. Nephrol Dial Transplant 16:22-26, 2001.

42. Stephenson SL, Kenny AJ. Metabolism of neuropeptides. Biochem J 241:237-247, 1987.

43. Duncan AM, James GM, Anastasopoulos F, et al. Interaction between neutral endopeptidase and angiotensin converting enzyme inhibition in rats with myocardial infarction: Effects on cardiac hypertrophy and angiotensin and bradykinin peptide levels. Pharmacol Exp Ther 289:295-303, 1999.

44. Ferrario CM, Martell N, Yunis C, et al. Characterization of angiotensin-(1-7) in the urine of normal and essential hypertensive subjects. Am J Hypertens 11:137-146, 1998.

45. Ferrario CM, Smith RD, Brosnihan KB, et al. Effects of omapatrilat on the renin angiotensin system in salt sensitive hypertension. Am J Hypertens 15:557-564, 2002.

46. Yamada K, Iyer SN, Chappell MC, et al. Differential response of angiotensin peptides in the urine of hypertensive animals. Regul Pept 80:57-66, 1999.

47. Chappell MC, Pirro NT, Sykes A, et al. Metabolism of angiotensin-(1-7) by angiotensin converting enzyme. Hypertension 31:362-367, 1998.

48. Yamada K, Iyer SN, Chappell MC, et al. Converting enzyme determines the plasma clearance of angiotensin-(1-7). Hypertension 98:496-502, 1998.

49. Donoghue M, Hsieh F, Baronas E, et al. A novel angiotensin-converting enzyme-related carboxypeptidase (ACE2) converts angiotensin I to angiotensin 1-9. Circ Res 87:E1-E9, 2000.

50. Tipnis SR, Hooper NM, Hyde R, et al. A human homolog of angiotensin-converting enzyme. Cloning and functional expression as a captopril-insensitive carboxypeptidase. J Biol Chem 275:33238-33243, 2000.

51. Klein JD, Le Quach D, Cole JM, et al. Impaired urine concentration and absence of tissue ACE: involvement of medullary transport proteins. Am J Physiol Renal Physiol 283:F517-F524, 2002.

52. Esther CR, Marino EM, Howard TE, et al. The critical role of tissue angiotensin-converting enzyme as revealed by gene targeting in mice. J Clin Invest 99:2375-2385, 1997.

53. Vickers C, Hales P, Kaushik V, et al. Hydrolysis of biological peptides by human angiotensin-converting enzyme-related carboxypeptidase. J Biol Chem 277:14838-14843, 2002.

54. Iyer SN, Chappell MC, Averill DB, et al. Vasodepressor actions of angiotensin-(1-7) unmasked during combined treatment with lisinopril and losartan. Hypertension 31:699-705, 1998.

55. Chappell MC, Westwood BM, Averill DB, et al. Influence of gender on salt sensitivity in the mRen(2).Lewis rat. Hypertension 42:432, 2003.
56. Ferrario CM, Averill DB, Brosnihan KB, et al. Vasopeptidase inhibition and Ang-(1-7) in the spontaneously hypertensive rat. Kidney Int 62:1349-1357, 2002.
57. Chappell MC, Jung F, Gallagher PE, et al. Omapatrilat treatment is associated with increased ACE-2 and angiotensin-(1-7) in spontaneously hypertensive rats. Hypertension 40:409, 2002.
58. Crackower MA, Sarao R, Oudit GY, et al. Angiotensin-converting enzyme 2 is an essential regulator of heart function. Nature 417:822-828, 2002.
59. DelliPizzi A, Hilchey SD, Bell-Quilley CP. Natriuretic action of angiotensin (1-7). Br J Pharmacol 111:1-3, 1994.
60. Handa RK, Ferrario CM, Strandhoy JW. Renal actions of angiotensin-(1-7): In vivo and in vitro studies. Am J Physiol Renal Physiol 270:F141-F147, 1996.
61. Hilchey SD, Bell-Quilley CP. Association between the natriuretic action of angiotensin-(1-7) and selective stimulation of renal prostaglandin $I_2$ release. Hypertension 25:1238-1244, 1995.
62. Heyne N, Beer W, Muhlbauer B, et al. Renal response to angiotensin (1-7) in anesthetized rats. Kidney Int 47: 975-976, 1995.
63. Vallon V, Heyne N, Richter K, et al. [7-D-ALA]-Angiotensin 1-7 blocks renal actions of angiotensin 1-7 in the anesthetized rat. J Card Pharmacol 32:164-167, 1998.
64. Heller J, Kramer HJ, Maly J, et al. Effect of intrarenal infusion of angiotensin-(1-7) in the dog. Kidney Blood Press Res 23:89-94, 2000.
65. Ren Y, Garvin JL, Carretero OA. Vasodilator action of angiotensin-(1-7) on isolated rabbit afferent arterioles. Hypertension 39:799-802, 2002.
66. Handa RK. Angiotensin-(1-7) can interact with the rat proximal tubule AT(4) receptor system. Am J Physiol Renal Physiol 277:F75-F83, 1999.
67. Lopez O, Gironacci M, Rodriguez D, et al. Effect of angiotensin-(1-7) on ATPase activities in several tissues. Regul Pept 77:135-139, 1998.
68. Garcia NH, Garvin JL. Angiotensin 1-7 has a biphasic effect on fluid absorption in the proximal straight tubule. J Am Soc Nephrol 5:1133-1138, 1994.
69. Andreatta-Van Leyen S, Romero MF, Khosla MC, et al. Modulation of phospholipase A2 activity and sodium transport by angiotensin-(1-7). Kidney Int 44:932-936, 1993.
70. Jung F, Gupta M, Ferrario CM, Chappell MC. Angiotensin-(1-7) down-regulates aquaporin-1 expression in proximal tubule epithelial cells. Proceedings of the XVth InterAmerican Society of Hypertension. 2003; p 98.
71. Vallon V, Richter K, Heyne N, et al. Effect of intratubular application of Angiotensin 1-7 on nephron function. Kidney Blood Press Res 20:233-239, 1997.
72. Quan A, Baum M. Endogenous production of Angiotensin II modulates rat proximal tubule transport. J Clin Invest 97:2878-2882, 1996.
73. Santos RAS, Baracho NCV. Angiotensin-(1-7) is a potent antidiuretic peptide in rats. Braz J Med Biol Res 25:651-654, 1992.
74. Baracho NCV, Silva ACS, Khosla MC, et al. Characterization of the antidiuretic action of angiotensin-(1-7) in water-loaded rats. Hypertension 25:1408, 1995.
75. Santos RAS, Silva ACS, Magaldi AJ, et al. Evidence for a physiological role of angiotensin-(1-7) in the control of hydroelectrolyte balance. Hypertension 27:875-884, 1996.
76. Caruso-Neves C, Lara LS, Rangel LB, et al. Angiotensin-(1-7) modulates the ouabain-insensitive Na+-ATPase activity from basolateral membrane of the proximal tubule. Biochem Biophys Acta 1467:189-197, 2000.
77. Lara LS, Bica RB, Sena SL, et al. Angiotensin-(1-7) reverts the stimulatory effect of angiotensin II on the proximal tubule Na(+)-ATPase activity via a A779-sensitive receptor. Regul Pept 103:17-22, 2002.
78. Burgelova M, Kramer HJ, Teplan V, et al. Intrarenal infusion of angiotensin-(1-7) modulates renal functional responses to exogenous angiotensin II in the rat. Kidney Blood Press Res 25:202-210, 2002.
79. Gonzales S, Noriega GO, Tomaro ML, Pena C. Angiotensin-(1-7) stimulates oxidative stress in rat kidney. Regul Pept 106:67-70, 2002.
80. Benter IF, Diz DI, Ferrario CM. Cardiovascular actions of angiotensin-(1-7). Peptides 14:679-684, 1993.
81. Shebuski RJ, Aiken JW. Angiotensin II stimulation of renal prostaglandin synthesis elevates circulating prostacyclin in the dog. J Card Pharmacol 2:667-677, 1980.
82. Benter IF, Ferrario CM, Morris M, Diz DI. Antihypertensive actions of angiotensin-(I-7) in spontaneously hypertensive rats. Am J Physiol Heart Circ Physiol 269:H313-H319, 1995.
83. Gironacci MM, Fernandez-Tome MC, et al. Enhancement of phosphatidylcholine biosynthesis by angiotensin-(1-7) in the rat renal cortex. Biochem Pharmacol 63:507-514, 2002.
84. Chansel D, Vandermeersch S, Oko A, et al. Effects of angiotensin IV and angiotensin-(1-7) on basal and angiotensin II-stimulated cytosolic Ca2+ in mesangial cells. Eur J Pharmacol 414:165-175, 2002.
85. Heitsch H, Brovkovych S, Malinski T, et al. Angiotensin-(1-7)-stimulated nitric oxide and superoxide release from endothelial cells. Hypertension 37:72-76, 2001.
86. Chappell MC. Inhibition of $Na^+$, $K^+$-ATPase activity by angiotensin-(1-7) in rat proximal tubules is attenuated by cytochrome P450 blockade. FASEB J 16:A496, 2002.
87. Harder DR, Campbell WB, Roman RJ. Role of cytochrome P-450 enzymes and metabolites of arachidonic acid in the control of vascular tone. J Vasc Res 32:79-92, 1995.
88. McGiff JC, Quilley CP, Carroll MA. The contribution of cytochrome P450-dependent arachidonate metabolites to integrated renal function. Steroids 58:573-579, 1993.
89. Roman RJ, Alonso-Galicia M. P450-Eicosanoids: A novel signaling pathway regulating renal function. News Physiol Sci 14:238-242, 1999.
90. Luque M, Martin P, Martell N, et al. Effects of captopril related to increased levels of prostacyclin and angiotensin-(1-7) in essential hypertension. J Hypertens 14:799-805, 1996.
91. Chappell MC, Tallant EA, Diz DI, et al. The renin-angiotensin system and cardiovascular homeostasis. In Husain A, Graham R, (eds): Drugs, Enzymes and Receptors of the Renin Angiotensin System: Celebrating a Century of Discovery. Amsterdam, Harwood Academic Publishers, 2000; pp 3-21.
92. Iyer SN, Yamada K, Diz DI, et al. Evidence that prostaglandins mediate the antihypertensive actions of angiotensin-(1-7) during chronic blockade of the renin-angiotensin system. J Card Pharmacol 36:109-117, 2000.
93. Chappell MC, Iyer SN, Diz DI, et al. Antihypertensive effects of Ang-(1-7). Braz J Med Biol Res 31(9):1205-1212, 1998.
94. Santos RAS, Campagnole-Santos MJ, Baracho NCV, et al. Characterization of a new angiotensin antagonist selective for angiotensin-(1-7): Evidence that the actions of angiotensin-(1-7) are mediated by specific angiotensin receptors. Brain Res Bull 35:293-298, 1994.
95. Nickenig G, Geisen G, Vetter H, et al. Characterization of angiotensin receptors on human skin fibroblasts. J Mol Med 75:217-222, 1997.
96. Osei SY, Ahima RS, Minkes RK, et al. Differential responses to angiotensin-(1-7) in the feline mesenteric and hindquarters vascular beds. Eur J Pharmacol 234:35-42, 1993.
97. Oliveira MA, Fortes ZB, Santos RAS, et al. Synergistic effect of angiotensin-(1-7) on bradykinin-induced vasodilation on rat mesenteric microvessels in vivo, in situ. FASEB J 12:2270, 1998.

98. Tran Yl, Forster C. Angiotensin-(1-7) and the rat aorta: Modulation by the endothelium. J Card Pharmacol 30:676-682, 1997.

99. Freeman EJ, Chisolm GM, Ferrario CM, et al. Angiotensin-(1-7) [Ang.-(1-7)] inhibits vascular smooth muscle cell growth. Hypertension 28:104-108, 1996.

100. Iyer SN, Ferrario CM, Chappell MC. Angiotensin-(1-7) contributes to the antihypertensive effects of blockade of the renin-angiotensin system. Hypertension 31:356-361, 1998.

101. Bumpus FM, Catt KJ, Chiu AT, et al. Nomenclature for angiotensin receptors: A report of the Nomenclature Committee for the Council for High Blood Pressure Research. Hypertension 17:720-721, 1991.

102. de Gasparo M, Husain A, Alexander W, et al. Proposed update of angiotensin receptor nomenclature. Hypertension 25:924-927, 1995.

103. Deddish PA, Jackman HL, Wang HZ, et al. N-domain specific substrate and C-domain inhibitors of angiotensin converting enzyme: Angiotensin-(1-7) and keto-ACE. Hypertension 31:912-917, 1998.

104. Tom B, deVries R, Saxena PR, et al. Bradykinin potentiation by angiotensin-(1-7) and ACE inhibitors correlates with ACE C- and N-domain blockade. Hypertension 38:95-99, 2001.

105. Widdop RE, Sampey DB, Jarrott B. Cardiovascular effects of angiotensin-(1-7) in conscious spontaneously hypertensive rats. Hypertension 34:964-968, 1999.

106. Bayorh MA, Eatman D, Walton M, et al. A-779 attenuates angiotensin-(1-7) depressor response in salt-induced hypertensive rats. Peptides 23:57-64, 2002.

107. Santos RAS, Simoes e Silva AC, Maric C, et al. Angiotensin-(1-7) is an endogenous ligand for the G protein-coupled receptor Mas. Proc Natl Acad Sci USA 100:8258-8263, 2003.

108. Tallant EA, Chappell MC, Ferrario CM, et al. Inhibition of MAP kinase activity by angiotensin-(1-7) in vascular smooth muscle cells is mediated by the *mas* receptor. Hypertension 43:1348, 2004.

109. Schiavone MT, Santos RAS, Brosnihan KB, et al. Release of vasopressin from the rat hypothalamo-neurohypophysial system by angiotensin-(1-7) heptapeptide. Proc Natl Acad Sci USA 85:4095-4098, 1988.

110. Ernsberger P, Koletsky RJ, Collins LA, et al. Renal angiotensin receptor mapping in obese spontaneously hypertensive rats. Hypertension 21:1039-1045, 1993.

111. Ardaillou R, Chansel D, Chatziantoniou C, et al. Mesangial AT1 receptors: expression, signaling, and regulation. J Am Soc Nephrol 11:S40-S46, 1999.

112. Chansel D, LLorens-Cortes C, Vandermeersch S, et al. Regulation of angiotensin II receptor subtypes by dexamethasone in rat mesangial cells. Hypertension 27:867-874, 1996.

113. Ruan X, Purdy KE, Oliverio MI, et al. Effects of candesartan on angiotensin II-induced renal vasoconstriction in rats and mice. J Am Soc Nephrol 10:S202-S207, 1999.

114. Lorenzo O, Ruiz-Ortega M, Suzuki Y, et al. Angiotensin III activates nuclear transcription factor-kappaB in cultured mesangial cells mainly via AT(2) receptors: studies with AT(1) receptor-knockout mice. J Am Soc Nephrol 13:1162-1171, 2002.

115. Ernsberger P, Zhou J, Damon TH, et al. Angiotensin II receptor subtypes in cultured rat renal mesangial cells. Am J Physiol Renal Physiol 263:F411-F416, 1992.

116. Goto M, Mukoyama M, Suga S, et al. Growth-dependent induction of angiotensin II type 2 receptor in rat mesangial cells. Hypertension 30:358-362, 1997.

117. Dulin NO, Ernsberger P, Suciu DJ, et al. Rabbit renal epithelial angiotensin II receptors. Am J Physiol Renal Physiol 267:F776-F782, 1994.

118. Hedrick CC, Hassan K, Hough GP, et al. Short-term feeding of atherogenic diet to mice results in reduction of HDL and paraoxonase that may be mediated by an immune mechanism. Arterioscler Thromb Vasc Biol 20:1946-1952, 2000.

119. Zhou J, Ernsberger P, Douglas JG. A novel angiotensin receptor subtype in rat mesangium. Coupling to adenylyl cyclase. Hypertension 21:1035-1038, 1993.

120. Baracho NC, Simoes e Silva AC, Khosla MC, et al. Effect of selective angiotensin antagonists on the antidiuresis produced by angiotensin-(1-7) in water-loaded rats. Braz J Med Biol Res 31:1221-1227, 1998.

121. Chatziantoniou C, Dussaule J-C, Arendshorst WJ, et al. Angiotensin II receptors and renin release in rat glomerular afferent arterioles. Kidney Int 46:1570-1573, 1994.

122. Nakamura S, Averill DB, Chappell MC, et al. Contribution of angiotensin receptor subtypes to blood pressure regulation in salt depleted spontaneously hypertensive rats. FASEB J284:R164-R173, 2002.

123. Tallant EA, Higson JT. Angiotensin II activates distinct signal transduction pathways in astrocytes isolated from neonatal rat brain. Glia 19:333-342, 1997.

124. Chung CJ, Chappell MC, Callahan MF, et al. Angiotensin-(1-7) receptors defined by D-Ala$^7$-Ang-(1-7) are present in kidneys from AT$_{1A}$ deficient male and female mice. Hypertension 38:500, 2001.

125. Chung CJ, Chappell MC, Callahan MF, et al. Evidence for angiotensin-(1-7) receptors in murine kidney. FASEB J15:A778, 2001.

126. Diz DI, Chappell MC, Ferrario CM, et al. Vascular smooth muscle cells transfected with the AT$_{1b}$ receptor exhibit high affinity for Ang-(1-7) and [D-Ala$^7$]-Ang-(1-7). Hypertension 42:430, 2003.

127. Harrison-Bernard LM, Cook AK, Oliverio MI, et al. Renal segmental microvascular responses to AngII in AT1A receptor null mice. Am J Physiol Renal Physiol 284(3):F538-F545, 2002.

128. Bouscarel B, Wilson PB, Blackmore PF, et al. Agonist-induced down-regulation of the angiotensin II receptor in primary cultures of rat hepatocytes. J Biol Chem 263:14920-14924, 1988.

129. Oppermann M, Freedman NJ, Alexander RW, et al. Phosphorylation of the type 1A angiotensin II receptor by G protein-coupled receptor kinases and protein kinase C. J Biol Chem 271:13266-13272, 1996.

130. Yang H, Lu D, Raizada MK. Angiotensin II-induced phosphorylation of the AT1 receptor from rat brain neurons. Hypertension 30:351-357, 1997.

131. Conchon S, Monnot C, Teutsch B, et al. Internalization of the rat AT1a and AT1b receptors: pharmacological and functional requirements. FEBS Lett 349:365-370, 1994.

132. Lassegue B, Alexander RW, Nickenig G, et al. Angiotensin II down-regulates the vascular smooth muscle AT1 receptor by transcriptional and post-transcriptional mechanisms: Evidence for homologous and heterologous regulation. Mol Pharmacol 48:601-609, 1995.

133. Tang H, Shirai H, Inagami T. Inhibition of protein kinase C prevents rapid desensitization of type 1B angiotensin II receptor. Circ Res 77:239-248, 1995.

134. Thekkumkara TJ, Du J, Dostal DE, et al. Stable expression of a functional rat angiotensin II (AT1A) receptor in CHO-K1 cells: Rapid desensitization by angiotensin II. Mol Cell Biochem 146:79-89, 1995.

135. Clark MA, Tallant EA, Diz DI. Downregulation of the AT$_{1A}$ receptor by pharmacologic concentrations of angiotensin-(1-7). J Card Pharmacol 37:437-448, 2001.

136. Clark MA, Diz DI, Tallant EA. Angiotensin-(1-7) downregulates the angiotensin II type 1 receptor in vascular smooth muscle cells. Hypertension 37:1141-1146, 2001.

137. Wilson KM, Magargal W, Berecek KH. Long-term captopril treatment. Angiotensin II receptors and responses. Hypertension 11:I148-I152, 1988.

138. Berecek KH, Swords BH, Lo S, et al. Effect of angiotensin converting enzyme inhibitors upon brain angiotensin binding. J Hypertens 10:545-552, 1992.

139. Negoro N, Kanayama Y, Iwai J, et al. Angiotensin-converting enzyme inhibitor increases angiotensin type 1A receptor gene expression in aortic smooth muscle cells of spontaneously hypertensive rats. Biochem Biophys Acta 1226:19-24, 1994.

140. Diz DI, Bosch SM, Moriguchi A, et al. Converting enzyme inhibition lowers angiotensin II receptor density in medulla of transgenic (mREN2)27 rats. J Hypertension 12:S71, 1994.

141. Diz DI, Kohara K, Ferrario CM. Normalization of angiotensin (Ang) II receptors in the dorsal medulla oblongata of spontaneously hypertensive rats (SHR) follows converting enzyme inhibition and increases in plasma angiotensin-(1-7) concentrations. Am J Hypertens 5:16A, 1992.

142. Buzas B, Rosenberger J, Cox BM. Regulation of delta-opioid receptor mRNA levels by receptor-mediated and direct activation of the adenylyl cyclase-protein kinase A pathway. J Neurochem 68:610-615, 1997.

143. Ichiki T, Usui M, Kato M, et al. Downregulation of angiotensin II type 1 receptor gene transcription by nitric oxide. Hypertension 31:342-348, 1998.

144. Neves LA, Santos RA, Khosla MC, et al. Angiotensin-(1-7) regulates the levels of angiotensin II receptor subtype AT1 mRNA differentially in a strain-specific fashion. Regul Pept 95:99-107, 2000.

145. Benter IF, Diz DI, Ferrario CM. Pressor and reflex sensitivity is altered in spontaneously hypertensive rats treated with angiotensin-(1-7). Hypertension 26:1138-1144, 1995.

146. van Rodijnen WF, van Lambalgen TA, Tangelder GJ, et al. Reduced reactivity of renal microvessels to pressure and angiotensin II in fawn-hooded rats. Hypertension 39:111-115, 2002.

147. Mahon JM, Carr RD, Nicol AK, et al. Angiotensin-(1-7) is an antagonist at the type 1 angiotensin II receptor. J Hypertens 12:1377-1381, 1994.

148. Roks AJ, van Geel PP, Pinto YM, et al. Angiotensin-(1-7) is a modulator of the human renin-angiotensin system. Hypertension 34:296-301, 1999.

149. Diz DI, Benter IF, Bosch SM, et al. Angiotensin-(1-7) infusion attenuates angiotensin II-induced prostacyclin release from kidney slices. Am J Hypertens 11:32A, 1998.

150. Benter IF, Ferrario CM, Morris M, et al. Antihypertensive actions of angiotensin-(1-7) in spontaneously hypertensive rats. Am J Physiol Heart Circ Physiol 269:H313-H319, 1995.

151. Strawn WB, Ferrario CM, Tallant EA. Angiotensin-(1-7) reduces smooth muscle growth after vascular injury. Hypertension 33:207-211, 1999.

# The Angiotensin Receptors: AT$_1$ and AT$_2$

## Helmy M. Siragy, Robert M. Carey

Angiotensin II (Ang II), the principal effector hormone of the renin-angiotensin system (RAS), stimulates a variety of physiologic responses that control blood pressure (BP), renal function, and cellular growth (Figure 11–1). Ang II contributes to the pathogenesis of hypertension, cardiac hypertrophy, heart failure, diabetic renal disease, and myocardial infarction (MI). The biologic effects of Ang II are mediated through its interaction with its cell membrane receptors.[1-3] Most of the actions of Ang II are mediated by the Ang II type-1 (AT$_1$) receptor. In contrast to rodents that have two subtypes of the AT$_1$ receptor (AT$_{1A}$ and AT$_{1B}$), humans have only one form. The other angiotensin receptor isoform, the AT$_2$ receptor, has a less well-defined functional role in adult organisms.

## ANGIOTENSIN RECEPTORS

The development of highly selective Ang II receptor antagonists has allowed the characterization of at least two distinct Ang II receptor subtypes, AT$_1$ and AT$_2$.[4] Both receptors belong to the super-family of seven transmembrane-spanning region G-protein–coupled receptors[5,6] and bind Ang II with a similar affinity, but share only 34% sequence homology. The expression of these receptors is not static, and certain hormones, pharmacologic agents, and pathologic conditions can enhance or suppress their expression.[7,8]

## AT$_1$ RECEPTOR EXPRESSION AND REGULATION IN HUMANS

The AT$_1$ receptor gene is mapped to band 22 of chromosome 3 and has five exons.[9] Exon 1 enhances protein synthesis; exon 3 is responsible for amino-terminal extension of the AT$_1$ receptor; and exon 5 contains the coding region.[10-15] Multiple factors regulate AT$_1$ receptor expression. Glucocorticoids,[16] growth hormone,[17] and insulin[18] increase AT$_1$ receptor expression, whereas mineralocorticoids, estrogen,[19] and nitric oxide[20] reduce it. AT$_1$ receptor cDNA encodes a 39 amino acid protein with molecular weight of 41,000 Daltons.[21] The AT$_1$ receptor protein contains three potential sites for $N$-glycosylation on its putative extracellular domains. There are four extracellular domains that contain cysteine residues, which seem to be responsible for the sensitivity of Ang II binding to sulfhydryl reagents.

AT$_1$ receptor protein is widely distributed in the kidney.[22-26] It has been localized to the renal vasculature, mainly in vascular smooth muscle and endothelial cells. The AT$_2$ receptor is also found in the renal vasculature, glomeruli, and juxtaglomerular apparatus, as well as in the nephron, including proximal and distal tubules, particularly on proximal tubule brush border and basolateral membranes, thick ascending limb epithelia and collecting duct cells, glomerular podocytes, and macula densa cells.[22,26-31]

## AT$_1$ RECEPTOR SIGNALING

In humans the AT$_1$ receptor contains 359 amino acids and is coupled primarily to pertussis toxin-insensitive G-proteins that lead to activation of phospholipase C and calcium signaling. Once Ang II binds to the AT$_1$ receptor, it induces conformational changes in the receptor molecule that mediate signal transduction via several mechanisms. Interestingly the AT$_1$ receptor has a complex intracellular signaling system mediated by G-protein–coupled and G-protein–independent pathways. Ang II binding sites for the AT$_1$ receptor are in the N-terminal extracellular domain and the second extracellular loop, while the AT$_1$ receptor antagonist binding sites are located within the transmembrane regions of the receptor.[4] AT$_1$ receptor activation stimulates phospholipases C,[9,21] A$_2$, and D[32]; increases intracellular calcium and inositol 1,4,5-triphosphate; activates the mitogen-activated protein kinases, extracellular signal–regulated kinases (ERKs), and the JAK/STAT pathway; and enhances protein phosphorylation and stimulation of early growth response genes.[33-36] The AT$_1$ receptor has been shown to attenuate the production of cyclic adenosine 3′,5′-monophosphate (cAMP) via inhibition of adenylyl cyclase. AT$_1$ receptor activation enhances vasoconstriction through a reduction in cAMP and an increase in intracellular calcium. The signaling pathways for the AT$_1$ receptor clearly demonstrate its contribution to the development of hypertension, inflammation, cellular hypertrophy, and matrix formation (Box 11–1). Tyrosine phosphorylation appears to be the major signaling pathway for AT$_1$ receptor effects.[37]

## CHARACTERISTICS OF ANGIOTENSIN BINDING TO THE AT$_1$ RECEPTOR

Three dimensional structural analysis of the AT$_1$ receptor (Figure 11–2) has revealed that portions of the first and third extracellular loops are crucial for the Ang II binding, whereas the second and third intracellular loops are crucial for G-protein–coupling.[38-42]

## AT$_2$ RECEPTOR EXPRESSION AND DISTRIBUTION

The AT$_2$ receptor gene is encoded on chromosome Xq22-q2 in humans, and in the rat and mouse, on chromosome Xq3 and chromosome X.[43-45] It has three exons, but the entire AT$_2$ receptor coding sequence is contained in the third exon.[46,47] Absence

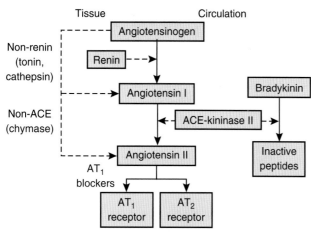

Figure 11–1 Schematic representation of different components of the renin-angiotensin system (RAS). There are circulating and local tissue paracrine components of this system. Also, multiple pathways can lead to angiotensin II (Ang II) formation. $AT_1$, angiotensin subtype $AT_1$ receptor; $AT_2$, angiotensin subtype $AT_2$ receptor.

Box 11–1 Effects of Angiotensin II via $AT_1$ Receptors

- Vasoconstriction
- Activate SNS
- Aldosterone, vasopressin, and endothelin secretion
- PAI-1 synthesis
- Platelet aggregation
- Thrombosis
- Cardiac contractility
- Super oxide production
- Vascular smooth muscle growth
- Myocyte growth
- Collagen formation

of an intron in the coding region indicates absence of isoforms for the $AT_2$ receptor. The regulation of the $AT_2$ receptor gene is not well elucidated. cAMP down-regulates the $AT_2$ receptor via destabilization of its mRNA. Expression of the $AT_2$ receptor is linked to growth states and growth factors. During embryogenesis and fetal development, the receptor is expressed in large quantities, and expression is decreased in the postnatal period. $AT_2$ receptor expression is significantly decreased in adults, but it is still detectable in multiple organs, including the heart, kidney, adrenal glands, brain, uterus, and ovaries.[48-52] $AT_2$ receptor expression is up-regulated in several pathologic conditions, such as vascular injury, sodium depletion, post-MI, and congestive heart failure (CHF).[48,51,53-58] In contrast, $AT_2$ receptor expression is down-regulated in diabetes mellitus.[59,60] Insulin, insulin-like growth factor-1, and interleukin-1β increase $AT_2$ receptor expression, whereas platelet-derived growth factor, basic fibroblast growth factor, exogenous Ang II, increased intracellular calcium, activation of protein kinase C, and norepinephrine administration down-regulate this receptor.[61-66]

## $AT_2$ RECEPTOR SIGNALING

The $AT_2$ receptor is considered a G-protein–coupled receptor, but its signaling mechanisms are different from those usually associated with this receptor family. Its receptor third intracellular loop domain is important for initiating cell signaling. The

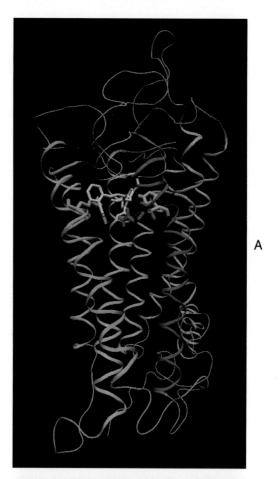

A

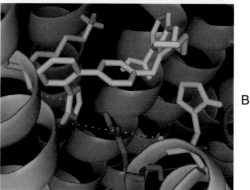

B

Figure 11–2 Molecular modeling of $AT_1$ receptor. **(A)** Model of rat $AT_{1A}$ receptor based on high-resolution structure of bovine rhodopsin. The Cα-trace of the entire receptor viewed from side color coded green except for TM-5 (pink) and TM6 (red). The ligand (yellow) bound to the receptor is candesartan, an insurmountable antagonist of the $AT_1$ receptor. **(B)** Candesartan (yellow) location in the pocket predicted by AutoDock Computer Program is shown. Residues are shown as Lys[199] (pink), His[256] (blue), and Glu[257] (red) that directly participate in candesartan binding. (From Takezako I, Gogonea C, Saad Y, et al. "Network leaning" as a mechanism of insurmountable antagonism of the angiotensin II type 1 receptor by non-peptide antagonists. J Biol Chem 279(15):15248-15257 2004; With permission.)

AT$_2$ receptor has low amino acid sequence homology (32%-34%) with the AT$_1$ receptor. The similarity between the AT$_1$ and AT$_2$ receptors is mainly confined to the transmembrane hydrophobic regions of the molecules, which allows for Ang II binding to these receptors.[67] The AT$_2$ receptor signaling region is located on the third intracellular loop is different from that of the AT$_1$ receptor, which allows for signaling mechanisms distinctive from those of the AT$_1$ receptor.[67] The differences between the third intracellular loops of these receptors, combined with the differences in their C-terminal domains, allow for unique binding to their respective agonists and antagonists.[67] The AT$_2$ receptor signaling mechanisms initiated by the third intracellular loop involve both G$_i$ and protein phosphotyrosine phosphatases.[68] The AT$_2$ receptor inhibits ERK activity via okadaic acid-sensitive serine/threonine phosphatase PP2A,[69] tyrosine/threonine phosphatase MKP-1,[70-72] and vanadate-sensitive tyrosine phosphatase (SHP-1),[73] leading to inhibition of cell growth. Inhibition of ERK contributes to initiation of MKP-1–mediated bcl-2-dephosphorylation.[72] The AT$_2$ receptor may activate phospholipase A$_2$ (PLA$_2$), leading to release of arachidonic acid and subsequent activation of MAP kinase and P21 *ras*.[73-75] The AT$_2$ receptor may influence renal tubular sodium reabsorption via this signaling pathway.

The AT$_2$ receptor induces sphingolipid and ceramide accumulation.[76,77] This effect may induce DNA fragmentation (apoptosis) via activation of capsase-3. The AT$_2$ receptor stimulates bradykinin[78,79] production with subsequent generation of nitric oxide (NO) and cyclic guanosine 3′,5′-monophosphate (cGMP).[80-82] Thus the AT$_2$ receptor can stimulate vasodilation through a bradykinin-NO-cGMP cascade.

## AT$_2$ RECEPTOR DISTRIBUTION

During fetal kidney development, the AT$_2$ receptor is highly expressed in mesenchymal cells of the mesonephros, immature glomeruli, cortical and medullary tubules, and interstitial cells.[48,83] Although AT$_2$ receptor expression rapidly declines in the postnatal period, the receptor can still be detected in the adult kidney. Sodium depletion increases AT$_2$ receptor expression in the kidney.[48] In the adult kidney, the AT$_2$ receptor is expressed in the renal vasculature, glomeruli, and tubules.[84] Autoradiography has revealed AT$_2$ receptor binding sites in the renal capsule[85] and juxtaglomerular apparatus.[86] In children, AT$_2$ receptors have been localized mainly in the interlobular arteries.[87] Immunohistochemistry of the adult rat and human kidneys revealed AT$_2$ receptor staining in glomerular epithelia, tubules, and large renal vessels.[22,48,83,84,88]

## RENAL EFFECTS OF THE AT$_2$ RECEPTOR

Chronic infusion of subpressor doses of Ang II reduced urinary sodium excretion in AT$_2$-null mice, but had no such effect in wild-type mice.[79] The lack of ability to enhance sodium excretion is attributed to inability of the AT$_2$-null mice to produce enough bradykinin, NO, and cGMP.[80-82] Similarly, under conditions of renal perfusion pressure, AT$_2$-null mice were unable to increase their sodium and water excretion as compared with wild-type mice.[89] These data strongly suggest a role for the AT$_2$ receptor in sodium excretion and pressure natriuresis (Box 11–2). The AT$_2$ receptor directly modulates

**Box 11–2** Effects of Angiotensin II via AT$_2$ Receptors

Tissue bradykinin production
Tissue NO production
Tissue cGMP production
Antiproliferation
Apoptosis
Cell differentiation
Tissue regeneration

blood vessel structure and function. Chronic treatment of wild-type mice or mice overexpressing the AT$_2$ receptor with Ang II produces a vasodepressor response.[90] In contrast, administration of subpressor dose of Ang II to AT$_2$-null mice produces a significant increase in BP.[79] These studies suggest a role for the AT$_2$ receptor in mediating vasodilation via the bradykinin-NO-cGMP cascade. Further studies have confirmed this hypothesis. Administration of Ang II to animals treated with losartan or valsartan caused a further reduction in BP,[91] and in animals treated with candesartan a sustained vasodilator response without desensitization.[92] This contrasts with responses via the AT$_1$ receptor, which internalizes and desensitizes in response to long-term agonist exposure. Similarly, administration of the selective AT$_2$ receptor agonist CGP-42112A decreases BP, an effect that is blocked by the AT$_2$ receptor antagonist PD123319 or the NO synthase inhibitor L-NAME.[91] The protective effect of the AT$_2$ receptor was demonstrated in a rat renal-wrap hypertension model.[78] In this study AT$_2$ receptor blockade reduced renal production of bradykinin, NO, and cGMP and reversed the BP-lowering effects of losartan.

The AT$_2$ receptor improves vascular remodeling by stimulating smooth muscle cell apoptosis. Study of vascular injury in AT$_2$-null mice demonstrates a reduction in the number of apoptotic cells.[93] Interestingly both AT$_1$ and AT$_2$ receptors can induce apoptosis of renal tubular cells.[94] AT$_2$ receptor blockade reduces tubular cell apoptosis in a rat model of unilateral ureteral obstruction.[95] In AT$_2$-null mice unilateral ureteral obstruction is associated with significantly fewer apoptotic cells, confirming the role of AT$_2$ receptors in stimulating apoptosis.[96] The most likely candidate signaling molecule that mediates AT$_2$ receptor-induced apoptosis is ceramide.[76,77] Consistent with these observations, AT$_2$ receptor blockade inhibits apoptosis in PC12W cells.[77]

The AT$_2$ receptor contributes to regulation of glomerular function. Afferent arteriole microperfusion studies demonstrate that the AT$_2$ receptor mediates vasodilation via release of epoxyeicosatrienoic acid (EET).[97] Reduction in glomerular AT$_2$ receptor expression has been seen in patients with glomerular disease.[98]

## AT$_1$ AND AT$_2$ RECEPTOR CROSS TALK

AT$_1$ and AT$_2$ receptors bind to Ang II with similar affinity, but have opposite functional effects (Box 11–3). Whereas the AT$_1$ receptor is responsible for vasoconstriction, natriuresis, cell hypertrophy, and matrix formation, the AT$_2$ receptor induces vasodilation, sodium excretion, and inhibition of cell growth and matrix formation. An increase in AT$_2$ receptor

**Box 11–3** Opposing Actions of Angiotensin II at $AT_1$ and $AT_2$ Receptors

| $AT_1$ | $AT_2$ |
|---|---|
| Vasoconstriction | Vasodilation |
| Antidiuresis/antinatriuresis | Diuresis/natriuresis |
| Cell growth and proliferation | Antiproliferation |
|     Aldosterone release |     Bradykinin production |
|     Vasopressin release |     NO release |

expression[99] and activity[100] may occur during $AT_1$ receptor blockade. The $AT_2$ receptor also regulates $AT_1$ receptor expression and activity, as $AT_2$-null mice have increased $AT_1$ receptors. Transfection of vascular smooth muscle cells with the $AT_2$ receptor gene decreased the expression of the $AT_1$ receptor.[101,102] At the cellular level, the $AT_1$ receptor promotes protein phosphorylation while the $AT_2$ receptor antagonizes this effect via stimulating protein dephosphorylation. While the $AT_1$ receptor increases intracellular $Ca^{2+}$ content to promote contraction, the $AT_2$ receptor produces the opposite effect. The $AT_2$ receptor had been shown to act as an $AT_1$ receptor antagonist.[103] This effect seems to be mediated via direct binding of the $AT_2$ receptor to the $AT_1$ receptor to for a heterodimer.

## SUMMARY

Although the RAS has been known for many years, only lately we began to understand the molecular and cellular mechanisms of action of Ang II. With the development of the nonpeptide antagonists and cloning of angiotensin receptors, we have begun to understand the pathophysiologic mechanisms that involve Ang II in development of renal and cardiovascular diseases. The discovery of opposing functions of $AT_1$ and $AT_2$ receptors will help develop new drugs and strategies to prevent and treat cardiovascular and renal diseases.

## References

1. Zitnay C, Siragy HM. Actions of angiotensin receptor subtypes on the renal tubules and vasculature: Implications for volume homeostasis and atherosclerosis. Miner Electrolyte Metab 24:362-370, 1998.
2. Siragy HM. $AT_1$ and $AT_2$ receptors in the kidney: Role in disease and treatment. Am J Kidney Dis 36:S4-S90, 2000.
3. Carson P, Giles T, Higginbotham M, et al. Angiotensin receptor blockers: Evidence for preserving target organs. Clin Cardiol 24:183-190, 2001.
4. de Gasparo M., Catt KJ, Inagami T, et al. International union of pharmacology. XXIII. The angiotensin II receptors. Pharmacol Rev 52:415-472, 2000.
5. Zou Y, Komuro I, Yamazaki T, et al. Cell type-specific angiotensin II-evoked signal transduction pathways: Critical roles of G-beta-gamma subunit, Src family and Ras in cardiac fibroblasts. Circ Res 82:337-345, 1998.
6. Kang J, Posner P, Sumners C. Angiotensin II type 2 receptor stimulation of neuronal K+ currents involves an inhibitory GTP binding protein. Am J Physio Cell Physiol 36:C1389-1397, 1994.
7. Kaschina E., Unger T. Angiotensin $AT_1/AT_2$ receptors: Regulation, signaling and function. Blood Press 12:70-88, 2003.
8. Carey RM, Siragy HM. Newly recognized components of the renin-angiotensin system: Potential roles in cardiovascular and renal regulation. Endocr Rev 24:261-271, 2003.
9. Murphy TJ, Alexander RW, Griendling KK, et al. Isolation of a cDNA encoding the vascular type-1 angiotensin II receptor. Nature 351:233-236, 1991.
10. Gaborik Z, Jagadeesh G, Zhang M, et al. The role of a conserved region of the second intracellular loop in $AT_1$ angiotensin receptor activation and signaling. Endocrinology 144:2220-2228, 2003.
11. Seta K, Sadoshirma J. Phosphorylation of tyrosine 319 of the angiotensin II type 1 receptor mediates angiotensin II-induced trans-activation of the epidermal growth factor receptor. J Biol Chem 278:9019-9026, 2003.
12. Leclerc PC, Auger-Messier M, Lanctot PM, et al. A polyaromatic caveolin-binding-like motif in the cytoplasmic tail of the type 1 receptor for angiotensin II plays an important role in receptor trafficking and signaling. Endocrinology 143:4702-4710, 2002.
13. Guo DF, Sun YL, Hamet P, et al. The angiotensin II type 1 receptor and receptor-associated proteins. Cell Res 11:165-180, 2001.
14. Luchtefeld M, Drexler H, Schieffer B. Role of G beta-subunit in angiotensin II-type 1 receptor signaling. Biochem Biophys Res Commun 280:756-760, 2001.
15. Saito Y, Berk BC. Transactivation: A novel signaling pathway from angiotensin II tyrosine kinase receptors. J Mol Cell Cardiol 33:3-7, 2001.
16. Della Bruna R, Ries S, Himmelstross C, et al. Expression of cardiac angiotensin II $AT_1$ receptor genes in rat hearts is regulated by steroids but not by angiotensin II. J Hypertens 13:763-769, 1995.
17. Wyse B, Sernia C. Growth hormone regulates AT-1a angiotensin receptors in astrocytes. Endocrinology 138:4176-4180, 1997.
18. Nickenig G, Roling J, Strehlow K, et al. Insulin induces upregulation of vascular $AT_1$ receptor gene expression by posttranscriptional mechanisms. Circulation 98:2453-2460, 1998.
19. Nickenig G, Baumer AT, Grohe C, et al. Estrogen modulates AT1 receptor gene expression in vitro and in vivo. Circulation 97:2197-2201, 1998.
20. Ichiki T, Usui M, Kato M, et al. Downregulation of angiotensin II type 1 receptor gene transcription by nitric oxide. Hypertension 31: 342-248, 1998.
21. Sasaki K, Yamano Y, Bardhan S, et al. Cloning and expression of a complementary DNA encoding a bovine adrenal angiotensin II type-1 receptor. Nature 351:230-233, 1991.
22. Miyata N, Park F, Li XF, et al. Distribution of angiotensin AT1 and AT2 receptor subtypes in the rat kidney. Am J Physiol 277:F437-446, 1999.
23. Pounarat, JS, Houillier P, Rismondo C, et al. The luminal membrane of rat thick limb expresses $AT_1$ receptor and aminopeptidase activities. Kidney Int 62:434-445, 2002.
24. Allen AM, Zhuo J, Mendelsohn FA. Localization and function of angiotensin AT1 receptors. Am J Hypertens 13:31S-38S, 2000.
25. Matsubara H, Sugaya T, Murasawa S, et al. Tissue-specific expression of human angiotensin II AT1 and AT2 receptors and cellular localization of subtype mRNAs in adult human renal cortex using in situ hybridization. Nephron 80:25-34, 1998.
26. Harrison-Bernard LM, Navar LG, Ho MM, et al. Immunohistochemical localization of Ang II $AT_1$ receptor in adult rat kidney using a monoclonal antibody. Am J Physiol 273:F170-F177, 1997.
27. Zhou J, Alcorn D, Allen AM, et al. High resolution localization of angiotensin II receptors in rat renal medulla. Kidney Int 42:1372-1380, 1992.
28. Zhuo J, Alcorn D, Harris PJ, et al. Localization and properties of angiotensin II receptors in rat kidney. Kidney Int 42:S40-S46, 1993.

29. Healy DP, Ye MQ, Troyanovskaya M. Localization of angiotensin II type 1 receptor subtype mRNA in rat kidney. Am J Physiol 268:F220-F226, 1995.

30. Kakinuma Y, Fogo A, Inagami T, et al. Intrarenal localization of angiotensin II type 1 receptor mRNA in the rat. Kidney Int 43:1129-1235, 1993.

31. Paxton WG, Runge M, Horaist C, et al. Immunohistochemical localization of rat angiotensin II AT₁ receptor. Am J Physiol 264:F989-F995, 1993.

32. de Gasparo M, Levens N. Does blockade of angiotensin II receptors offer clinical benefits over inhibition of angiotensin-converting enzyme? Pharmacol Toxicol 82:257-271, 1998.

33. Schmitz U, Berk BC. Angiotensin II signal transduction: Stimulation of multiple mitogen-activated protein kinase pathways. Trends Endocrinol Metab 8:261-266, 1997.

34. Schmitz U, Thommes K, Beier I, et al. Angiotensin II-induced stimulation of p21-activated kinase and c-Jun NH2-terminal kinase is mediated by Rac1 and Nck. J Biol Chem 276:22003-22010, 2001.

35. Ishida M, Ishida T, Thomas SM, et al. Activation of extracellular signal-regulated kinases (ERK1/2) by angiotensin II is dependent on c-Src in vascular smooth muscle cells. Circ Res 82:7-12, 1998.

36. Lijnen P, Petrov V. Renin-angiotensin system, hypertrophy and gene expression in cardiac myocytes. J Mol Cell Cardiol 31:949-970, 1999.

37. Giasson E, Servant MJ, Meloche S. Cyclic AMP-mediated inhibition of angiotensin II-induced protein synthesis is associated with suppression of tyrosine phosphorylation signaling in vascular smooth muscle cells. J Biol Chem 272:26879-26886, 1997.

38. Yamano Y, Ohyama K, Chaki S, et al. Identification of amino acid residues of rat angiotensin II receptor for ligand binding by site directed mutagenesis. Biochem Biophys Res Commun 87:1426-1431, 1992.

39. Hunyady L, Balla T, Catt KJ. The ligand binding site of the angiotensin AT₁ receptor. Trends Pharmacol Sci 17:135-140, 1996.

40. Karnik SS, Husain A, Graham RM. Molecular determinants of peptide and non-peptide binding to the AT1 receptor. Clin Exp Pharmacol Physiol Suppl 3:S58-S66, 1996.

41. Ji H, Leung M, Zhang Y, et al. Differential structural requirements for specific binding of nonpeptide and peptide antagonists to the AT1 angiotensin receptor. Identification of amino acid residues that determine binding of the antihypertensive drug losartan. J Biol Chem 269:16533-16536, 1994.

42. Schambye HT, von Wijk B, Hjorth SA, et al. Mutations in transmembrane segment VII of the AT1 receptor differentiate between closely related insurmountable and competitive angiotensin antagonists. Br J Pharmacol 113:331-333, 1994.

43. Koike G, Horiuchi M, Yamada T, et al. Human type 2 angiotensin II receptor gene: Cloned, mapped to the X chromosome, and its mRNA is expressed in the human lung. Biochem Biophys Res Commun 203:1842-1850, 1994.

44. Hein L, Dzau VJ, Barsh GS. Linkage mapping of the angiotensin AT2 receptor gene (Agtr2) to the mouse X chromosome. Genomics 30:369-371, 1995.

45. Tissir F, Riviere M, Guo DF, et al. Localization of the genes encoding the three rat angiotensin II receptors, Agtr1a, Agtr1b, Agtr2, and the human AGTR2 receptor respectively to rat chromosomes 17q12, 2q24 and Xq34, and the human Xq22. Cytogenet Cell Genet 71:77-80, 1995.

46. Ichiki T, Inagami T. Expression, genomic organization, and transcription of the mouse angiotensin II type 2 receptor gene. Circ Res 76:693-700, 1995.

47. Tsuzuki S, Ichiki T, Nakakubo H, et al. Molecular cloning and expression of the gene encoding human angiotensin II type 2 receptor. Biochem Biophys Res Commun 200:1449-1454, 1994.

48. Ozono R, Wang ZQ, Moore AF, et al. Expression of the subtype 2 angiotensin AT2 receptor protein in rat kidney. Hypertension 30:1238-1246, 1997.

49. Wang, ZQ, Moore AF, Ozono R, et al. Immunolocalization of subtype 2 angiotensin II AT2 receptor protein in rat heart. Hypertension 32:78-83, 1998.

50. Matsubara H, Sugaya T, Murasawa S, et al. Tissue-specific expression of human angiotensin II AT1 and AT2 receptors and cellular localization of subtype mRNAs in adult human renal cortex using in situ hybridization. Nephron 80:25-34, 1998.

51. Lopez JJ, Lorell BH, Ingelfinger JR, et al. Distribution and function of cardiac angiotensin AT1- and AT2-receptor subtypes in hypertrophied rat hearts. Am J Physiol 267:H 844-852, 1994.

52. de Gasparo M, Bottari S, Levens NR. Characteristics of angiotensin II receptors and their role in cell and organ physiology. In Laragh JH, Brenner BM (eds). Hypertension: Physiology, Diagnosis, and Management. New York, Raven, 1994; pp 100-110.

53. Ohkubo N, Matsubara H, Nozawa Y, et al. Angiotensin type 2 receptors are reexpressed by cardiac fibroblasts from failing myopathic hamster hearts and inhibit cell growth and fibrillar collagen metabolism. Circulation 96:3954-3962, 1997.

54. Nio Y, Matsubara H, Murasawa S, et al. Regulation of gene transcription of angiotensin II receptor subtypes in myocardial infarction. J Clin Invest 95:46-54, 1995.

55. Janiak P, Pillon A, Prost JF, et al. Role of angiotensin subtype 2 receptor in neointima formation after vascular injury. Hypertension 20:737-745, 1992.

56. Nakajima M, Hutchinson HG, Fujinaga M, et al. The angiotensin II type 2 (AT2) receptor antagonizes the growth effects of the AT1 receptor–Gain-of-function study using gene transfer. Proc Natl Acad Sci USA 92:10663-10667, 1995.

57. Viswanathan M, Saavedra JM. Expression of angiotensin II AT2 receptors in the rat skin during experimental wound healing. Peptides 13:783-786, 1992.

58. Tanaka M, Ohnishi J, Ozawa Y, et al. Characterization of angiotensin II receptor type 2 during differentiation and apoptosis of rat ovarian cultured granulosa cells. Biochem Biophys Res Commun 207:593-598, 1995.

59. Bonnet F, Candido R, Carey RM, et al. Renal expression of angiotensin receptors in long-term diabetes and the effects of angiotensin type 1 receptor blockade. J Hypertens 20: 1615-1624, 2002.

60. Wehbi GJ, Zimpelmann J, Carey RM, et al. Early streptozotocin-diabetes mellitus downregulates rat kidney AT2 receptors. Am J Physiol Renal Physiol 280:F254-265, 2001.

61. Kambayashi Y, Bardhan S, Inagami T. Peptide growth factors markedly decrease the ligand binding of angiotensin II type 2 receptor in rat cultured vascular smooth muscle cells. Biochem Biophys Res Commun 194:478-482, 1993.

62. Kambayashi Y, Nagata K, Ichiki T, et al. Insulin and insulin-like growth factors induce expression of angiotensin type-2 receptor in vascular-smooth-muscle cells. Eur J Biochem 239:558-565, 1996.

63. Ichiki T, Inagami T. Expression, genomic organization, and transcription of the mouse angiotensin II type 2 receptor gene. Circ Res 76:693-700, 1995.

64. Ichiki T, Inagami T. Transcriptional regulation of the mouse angiotensin II type 2 receptor gene. Hypertension 25:720-725, 1995.

65. de Gasparo M, Siragy HM. The AT2 receptor: Fact, fancy and fantasy. Regul Pept 81:11-24, 1999.

66. Kambayashi Y, Bardhan S, Takahashi K, et al. Molecular cloning of a novel angiotensin II receptor isoform involved in phospho-tyrosine phosphatase inhibition. J Biol Chem 268:24543-24546, 1993.

67. Hines J, Heerding JN, Fluharty SJ, et al. Identification of angiotensin II type 2 (AT2) receptor domains mediating high-affinity CGP 42112A binding and receptor activation. J Pharmacol Exp Ther 298:665-673, 2001.

68. Hayashida W, Horiuchi M, Dzau VJ. Intracellular third loop domain of angiotensin II type-2 receptor. Role in mediating signal transduction and cellular function. J Biol Chem 271:21985-21992, 1996.

69. Huang XC, Richards EM, Sumners C. Mitogen-activated protein kinases in rat brain neuronal cultures are activated by angiotensin II type 1 receptors and inhibited by angiotensin II type 2 receptors. J Biol Chem 271:15635-15641, 1996.

70. Tsuzuki S, Matoba T, Eguchi S, et al. Angiotensin II type 2 receptor inhibits cell proliferation and activates tyrosine phosphatase. Hypertension 28:916-918, 1996.

71. Yamada T, Horiuchi M, Dzau VJ. Angiotensin II type 2 receptor mediates programmed cell death. Proc Natl Acad Sci USA 93:56-160, 1996.

72. Horiuchi M, Hayashida W, Kambe T, et al. Angiotensin type 2 receptor dephosphorylates Bcl-2 by activating mitogen-activated protein kinase phosphatase-1 and induces apoptosis. J Biol Chem 272:19022-19026, 1997.

73. Bedecs K, Elbaz N, Sutren M, et al. Angiotensin II type 2 receptors mediate inhibition of mitogen-activated protein kinase cascade and functional activation of SHP-1 tyrosine phosphatase. Biochem J 325:449-454, 1997.

74. Dulin NO, Alexander LD, Harwalkar S, et al. Phospholipase A2-mediated activation of mitogen-activated protein kinase by angiotensin II. Proc Natl Acad Sci USA 95:8098-8102, 1998.

75. Jiao H, Cui XL, Torti M, et al. Arachidonic acid mediates angiotensin II effects on p21ras in renal proximal tubular cells via the tyrosine kinase-Shc-Grb2-Sos pathway. Proc Natl Acad Sci USA 95:7417-7421, 1998.

76. Gallinat S, Busche S, Schutze S, et al. AT2 receptor stimulation induces generation of ceramides in PC12W cells. FEBS Lett 443:75-79, 1999.

77. Lehtonen JY, Horiuchi M, Daviet L, et al. Activation of the de novo biosynthesis of sphingolipids mediates angiotensin II type 2 receptor-induced apoptosis. J Biol Chem 274:16901-16906, 1999.

78. Siragy HM, Carey RM. Protective role of the angiotensin AT2 receptor in a renal wrap hypertension model. Hypertension 33:1237-1242, 1999.

79. Siragy HM, Inagami T, Ichiki T, et al. Sustained hypersensitivity to angiotensin II and its mechanism in mice lacking the subtype-2 (AT2) angiotensin receptor. Proc Natl Acad Sci USA 96:6506-6510, 1999.

80. Siragy HM, Carey RM. The subtype-2 (AT2) angiotensin receptor regulates renal cyclic guanosine 3′, 5′-monophosphate and AT1 receptor-mediated prostaglandin E2 production in conscious rats. J Clin Invest 97:1978-1982, 1996.

81. Siragy HM, Carey RM. The subtype 2 (AT$_2$) angiotensin receptor mediates renal production of nitric oxide in conscious rats. J Clin Invest 100:264-269, 1997.

82. Siragy HM, de Gasparo M, Carey RM. Angiotensin type 2 receptor mediates valsartan-induced hypotension in conscious rats. Hypertension 2000; 35:1074-1077.

83. Kakucli J, Ichiki T, Kiyama S, et al. Developmental expression of renal angiotensin II receptor genes in the mouse. Kidney Int 47:140-147, 1995.

84. Carey RM, Wang ZQ, Siragy HM. Update: Role of the angiotensin type-2 (AT2) receptor in blood pressure regulation. Curr Hypertens Rep 2:198-201, 2000.

85. Herblin WF, Diamond SM, Timmermans PB. Localization of angiotensin II receptor subtypes in the rabbit adrenal and kidney. Peptides 12:581-584, 1991.

86. Gibson RE, Thorpe HH, Cartwright ME, et al. Angiotensin II receptor subtypes in renal cortex of rats and rhesus monkeys. Am J Physiol 261:F512-518, 1991.

87. Viswanathan M, Selby DM, Ray PE. Expression of renal and vascular angiotensin II receptor subtypes in children. Pediatr Nephrol 14:1030-1036, 2000.

88. Mifune M, Sasmura H, Nakazato Y, et al. Examination of angiotensin II type 1 and type 2 receptor expression in human kidney by immunohistochemistry. Clin Exp Hypertens 23:257-266, 2001.

89. Gross V, Schunck WH, Honeck H, et al. Inhibition of pressure natriuresis in mice lacking the AT2 receptor. Kidney Int 57:191-202, 2000.

90. Tsutsumi Y, Matsubara H, Masaki H, et al. Angiotensin II type 2 receptor overexpression activates the vascular kinin system and causes vasodilation. J Clin Invest 104:925-935, 1999.

91. Carey RM, Howell NL, Jin XH, et al. Angiotensin type 2 receptor-mediated hypotension in angiotensin type-1 receptor-blocked rats. Hypertension. 38:1272-1277, 2001.

92. Widdop RE, Matrougui K, Levy BI, et al. AT2 receptor-mediated relaxation is preserved after long-term AT1 receptor blockade. Hypertension 40:516-520, 2002.

93. Suzuki J, Iwai M, Nakagami H, et al. Role of angiotensin II-regulated apoptosis through distinct AT1 and AT2 receptors in neointimal formation. Circulation 106:847-853, 2002.

94. Thomas GL, Yang B, Wagner BE, et al. Cellular apoptosis and proliferation in experimental renal fibrosis. Nephrol Dial Transplan 13:2216-2226, 1998.

95. Morrissey JJ, Klahr S. Effect of AT2 receptor blockade on the pathogenesis of renal fibrosis. Am J Physiol 276:F39-45, 1999.

96. Ma J, Nishimura H, Fogo A, et al. Accelerated fibrosis and collagen deposition develop in the renal interstitium of angiotensin type 2 receptor null mutant mice during ureteral obstruction. Kidney Int 53:937-94, 1998.

97. Kohagura K, Endo Y, Ito O, et al. Endogenous nitric oxide and epoxyeicosatrienoic acids modulate angiotensin II-induced constriction in the rabbit afferent arteriole. Acta Physiol Scand 168:107-112, 2000.

98. Mifune M, Sasamura H, Nakazato Y, et al. Examination of angiotensin II type 1 and type 2 receptor expression in human kidneys by immunohistochemistry. Clin Exp Hypertens 23:257-266, 2001.

99. de Paolis P, Porcellini A, Gigante B, et al. Modulation of the AT2 subtype receptor gene activation and expression by the AT1 receptor in endothelial cells. J Hypertens 17:1873-1877, 1999.

100. Maeso R, Navarro-Cid J, Munoz-Garcia R, et al. Losartan reduces phenylephrine constrictor response in aortic rings from spontaneously hypertensive rats. Role of nitric oxide and angiotensin II type 2 receptors. Hypertension 28:967-972, 1996.

101. Jin XQ, Fukuda N, Su JZ, et al. Angiotensin II type 2 receptor gene transfer downregulates angiotensin II type 1a receptor in vascular smooth muscle cells. Hypertension 39:1021-1027, 2002.

102. Su JZ, Fukuda N, Jin XQ, et al. Effect of AT2 receptor on expression of AT1 and TGF-beta receptors in VSMCs from SHR. Hypertension 40:853-858, 2002.

103. AbdAlla S, Lother H, Abdel-tawab AM, et al. The angiotensin II AT2 receptor is an AT1 receptor antagonist. J Biol Chem 276(43):39721-39726, 2001.

# Chapter 12

# Aldosterone and Mineralocorticoids

## John W. Funder

## DEFINITIONS

### Aldosterone

Aldosterone is a steroid hormone produced primarily if not exclusively in the adrenal cortex. It is derived from cholesterol by sequential enzymatic reactions, including a final modification of the methyl ($CH_3$) group at carbon 18 (C18) to produce a unique aldehyde (CHO) group, whence the name aldosterone. Aldosterone is the physiologic mineralocorticoid hormone in terrestrial vertebrates; other steroids, most notably deoxycorticosterone (DOC), can also act as mineralocorticoids, but their secretion is not regulated in such a way that they are physiologic regulators of salt and water balance.

### Mineralocorticoid

Mineralocorticoid is defined in effector terms, as a hormone promoting unidirectional transepithelial sodium transport. Aldosterone was isolated from fractionated bovine adrenal glands half a century ago[1] on the basis of this mineralocorticoid activity, and not surprisingly its physiology has been almost exclusively described in epithelial terms. More recently, however, the definition of mineralocorticoid has had to be broadened, to accommodate physiologic actions of aldosterone on blood vessels and in the central nervous system, as detailed later in this chapter. The emerging pathophysiologic roles of mineralocorticoid receptors (MR), also dealt with toward the end of this chapter, similarly call for continuing refinement of their definition.

## ALDOSTERONE STRUCTURE AND SYNTHESIS

As noted in the preceding definition, aldosterone is characterized by an aldehyde group at C18. Aldehyde groups are chemically very reactive, and in solution the C18 aldehyde cyclizes with the hydroxyl (OH) group at C11 to form an 11,18 hemiacetal. In common with other adrenal steroids, aldosterone is produced by sequential enzymatic steps (side chain cleavage, 3β reduction, 21-hydroxylation) from cholesterol. Unlike other hormonal steroids, aldosterone synthesis in the adrenal gland is confined to its outermost layer, the zona glomerulosa. The final enzymatic step is catalyzed in most species by the enzyme aldosterone synthase (CYP11B2), by a multistep process with DOC as substrate; aldosterone synthase shares 11β hydroxylase activity with the closely related enzyme CYP11B1 (11β hydroxylase), responsible for the defining step in glucocorticoid (cortisol, corticosterone) synthesis. In some species (e.g., bovine) a single CYP11B enzyme appears responsible for both glucocorticoid and aldosterone synthesis, with the mechanism(s) determining zonal specificity yet to be determined.

## Regulation of Aldosterone Secretion

A number of positive (e.g., adrenocorticotropic hormone [ACTH]) and negative (e.g., nitric oxide [NO]) factors have been shown to affect aldosterone secretion in a variety of experimental situations, but there is consensus that angiotensin II (Ang II) and plasma potassium concentration ([$K^+$]) are the two major determinants of aldosterone secretion. The renin-angiotensin-aldosterone system (RAAS) has evolved to defend organ perfusion and blood pressure (BP), in response to reduced circulating volume monitored by the kidney, and to increased renal sympathetic drive. This level of integration provides a powerful counter-regulatory mechanism in situations of acute volume loss, such as major hemorrhage or massive gastrointestinal fluid and electrolyte loss. Although the primary role for aldosterone in the RAAS is usually considered to be that of volume expansion by epithelial sodium and water retention, it is now clear that aldosterone has additional sites of action. These include the amygdala, to stimulate salt appetite; the circumventricular region within the hypothalamus, to raise BP; and the vascular wall, acting as a vasoconstrictor.

Ang II is commonly considered the major determinant of aldosterone secretion, but this is not necessarily the case. Mice in which the gene for angiotensinogen has been knocked out are incapable of producing Ang II in response to physiologic stimuli such as salt restriction. In an elegant series of studies, however, angiotensinogen$^{-/-}$ mice were shown to respond indistinguishably from wild-type in terms of elevating aldosterone in response to a low-salt diet for 2 weeks.[2] When mice are placed on a low-[$Na^+$], low-[$K^+$] diet, two things are seen. First, even in wild-type mice the aldosterone response is less than to low [$Na^+$] alone. Second, for the first time, the angiotensinogen$^{-/-}$ mice no longer match the wild type in terms of aldosterone response, evidence for the importance of [$K^+$] in the process.

In the clinical context there are a number of factors that modify the evolutionary drives of catastrophic volume loss, restricted salt intake, or dietary potassium overload. Western diets are commonly sodium rich; increased sympathetic drive is similarly common, and manifests as essential hypertension. Although the dangers of diuretic-induced hypokalemia have been appropriately recognized, those of a modest and contained degree of hyperkalemia often appear exaggerated. The development of effective angiotensin-converting enzyme (ACE) inhibitors and Ang II receptor (AT$_1$) blockers has proven of immense clinical utility. The recent development of second-generation MR antagonists, and their side-effect–free therapeutic profile, promise to add an additional dimension to the treatment of cardiovascular disorders, including hypertension (see Chapter 70).

## Aldosterone Transport and Metabolism

Aldosterone can be secreted rapidly in response to elevation in Ang II or plasma [K$^+$], and circulates in the blood loosely bound to albumin (50%-60%) and free (40%-50%). This contrasts with most other adrenal steroids, which are commonly ≥95% bound, in considerable part (and with high affinity) to corticosteroid binding globulin (CBG, transcortin). Metabolism occurs both in the liver (glucuronidation) and in the kidney (reduction) to water soluble products that are largely excreted in urine, where free aldosterone represents only ~1% of the total product. The metabolic clearance rate for aldosterone in humans of the order of 1200 L/day, equivalent to the hepatic blood flow, and consistent with the albumin-bound fraction being extracted as equivalent to free in long transit time organs such as the liver.

## PHYSIOLOGIC ACTIONS OF ALDOSTERONE

Aldosterone was isolated on the basis of its effect on epithelial sodium transport, and this is commonly considered to be its principal physiologic role. Receptors for aldosterone were first identified in classical target tissues such as the kidney,[3] and subsequently in a variety of nonepithelial tissues. In some of the latter aldosterone appears to have physiologic actions,[4] whereas in others the effects are clearly pathophysiologic.[5]

Common to both epithelial and nonepithelial actions of aldosterone are MR and the enzyme 11β hydroxysteroid dehydrogenase type 2 (11βHSD2). Mineralocorticoid receptors are members of the steroid/thyroid/retinoid/orphan receptor family of nuclear transactivating factors, closely related to receptors for glucocorticoids (GR), androgens (AR), and progestins (PR).[6] MR are unusual in that they have equivalent high affinity for aldosterone and the physiologic glucocorticoid cortisol (and corticosterone, in mice and rats); in fact, cortisol and corticosterone have >30-fold higher affinity for MR than for GR. In addition, MR are found in fish, for example, which do not secrete aldosterone, suggesting the possibility of (patho)physiologic roles for MR occupied by glucocorticoids.[7]

Circulating plasma levels of glucocorticoids are commonly ~1000-fold higher than those of aldosterone, and plasma-free levels ~100-fold higher. Given their equivalent affinity for MR, a time-honored question is that of the mechanism allowing aldosterone to occupy and activate MR in its physiologic target tissues. Selectivity of the target-tissue response to aldosterone is vested in the enzyme 11βHSD2, which is coexpressed at very high levels (3.5–4 × 10$^6$ molecules per renal principal cell, for example) with MR in aldosterone target tissues. 11βHSD2 converts cortisol and corticosterone to their receptor-inactive 11-keto analogs cortisone and 11-dehydro-corticosterone; aldosterone is not similarly metabolized, as its 11-OH group is protected from enzymatic attack by its cyclization to the 11,18 hemiketal.[8,9]

Although from clinical studies the operation of 11BHSD2 is crucial to allow aldosterone to selectivity activate target tissue MR, conversion of cortisol to cortisone is only one part of the specificity-conferring mechanism. The other action of 11βHSD2 is to stoichometrically convert NAD to NADH. This action also appears crucial in preventing glucocorticoids from activating MR in aldosterone target tissues under normal circumstances. The NADH/redox state does play a role in inappropriate MR activation under pathophysiologic conditions, as will be discussed later.

The postreceptor events following MR activation have been relatively lightly explored. In common with other members of the superfamily, MR can act as transcription factor, binding to response elements in the promoter regions of particular genes, and binding an increasing array of coregulators serving to modulate the rate of gene transcription. A variety of candidate MR-regulated genes have been reported—Na$^+$,K$^+$-ATPase subunits, epithelial sodium channel (ENaC) subunits, CHIF (corticosteroid hormone induced factor), GILZ (glucocorticoid induced leucine zipper) protein—of which the most thoroughly explored has been SGK-1 (serum- and glucocorticoid-induced kinase-1). SGK-1 is constitutively expressed in glomeruli and in response to aldosterone in principal cells in the distal tubule.[10] SGK-1, when phosphorylated by insulin (probably inter alia), is ultimately responsible for the phosphorylation of ENaC subunits, thereby blocking ENaC internalization and thus increasing intracellular Na$^+$. Intracellular Na$^+$ is substrate for Na$^+$,K$^+$-ATPase on the basolateral surface of the cell membrane, which pumps Na$^+$ out of the cell into the interstitial space and ultimately the blood. These postreceptor studies have been largely done in kidney, renal cell lines, and to some extent distal colon; comparable studies in nonepithelial aldosterone target tissues are currently in progress.

Nonclassical aldosterone target tissues include the vasculature, the amygdala, and the A3V3 region of the hypothalamus. Vascular smooth muscle expresses both MR and 11βHSD2, and both rapid and prolonged effects of aldosterone at physiologic or near physiologic concentrations have been reported.[11-13] The amygdala similarly expresses both MR and 11βHSD2, but in terms of selectivity is at a disadvantage compared with peripheral tissues in that aldosterone has a very high reflection coefficient at the blood-brain barrier. The A3V3 region lies outside the blood-brain barrier, and expresses MR but not 11βHSD2. Experimental studies in rat and dog (but not sheep) show that aldosterone clearly can raise BP by acting on MR in the A3V3 region, though the extent to which this reflects a physiologic response in humans is yet to be determined.[14]

Finally, it is now clear that aldosterone has rapid nongenomic effects. Initially such effects were ascribed to interaction with a membrane receptor for aldosterone, distinct from the classical MR.[15] Subsequent studies in both vascular smooth muscle[12] and cardiomyocytes[16] have shown such rapid nongenomic effects to be mediated via classical MR; whether or not membrane-receptor mediated effects can be shown in these or other tissues remains to be systematically explored. Unlike the estrogen receptor (ER), MR do not have a myristoylation site in their sequence, and are thus unlikely to be plasma membrane located.

## CLINICAL SYNDROMES

There are various ways of categorizing clinical disorders, and for simplicity this section will begin with a consideration of disorders of aldosterone secretion, followed by disorders of mineralocorticoid receptor activation, with a final section on essential hypertension. Though some of the syndromes described are very rare, they have often been illustrative, with the pathophysiology providing insight into the normal physiology.

## Aldosterone Synthase Deficiency

Aldosterone deficiency may be part of a generalized hypoadrenal state, may follow deficiency in biosynthetic pathways shared with other adrenal steroids (e.g., 3βHSD, 21 hydroxylase), or may be "pure" aldosterone synthase deficiency. The condition commonly presents in infancy, and is characterized by the signs and symptoms of uncompensated sodium loss—failure to thrive, hyponatremia, hyperkalemia, hyperreninemia, and low or undetectable plasma and urinary aldosterone levels; the latter finding clearly distinguishes the syndrome from pseudohypoaldosteronism. The subject has been comprehensively reviewed.[17]

## Glucocorticoid Remediable Aldosteronism

Of more relevance to hypertension is the condition of glucocorticoid remediable aldosteronism (GRA), also known as glucocorticoid suppressible hypertension. GRA reflects the transcription of a chimeric gene, located at 8q24, which contains the 5′ end of CYP11B1 (11β hydroxylase) and the 3′ end of CYP11B2 (aldosterone synthase). Such a gene is not only transcriptionally activated by ACTH, but also is expressed throughout the adrenal cortex. The diagnosis should be suspected in patients with early onset familial hypertension, and can be confirmed or excluded by PCR for the chimeric gene. Treatment is optimally low dose (0.25-0.5 mg/day) dexamethasone. The occurrence of a chimeric CYP11B1/B2 gene reflects the two genes being located in tandem, and sharing 94% nucleotide identity, thus allowing the possibility of an unequal crossing over at meiosis.[18] The most common explanation for two highly homologous genes in tandem is a relatively recent gene duplication, consistent with the relatively recent appearance of aldosterone, in terrestrial vertebrates.

## Primary Aldosteronism

A year after the isolation and characterization of aldosterone in 1953, Jerome Conn reported resolution of hypertension and hypokalemia in a patient after removal of an aldosterone-producing adenoma.[19] For the next 40 years primary aldosteronism was considered to be a rare (<1%) cause of hypertension, despite Conn's estimate that up to 20% of patients with elevated BP may have primary aldosteronism. Over the past decade, thanks to the wider application of the aldosterone:renin ratio as a screening test, and adrenal venous catheterization to lateralize (or not) the source of the aldosterone, it has become clear that 8% to 15% of unselected hypertensives have autonomous aldosterone production; in a recent general practice population study, 30% of patients with moderate hypertension had elevated aldosterone:renin ratios.[20] In terms of diagnosis, patients increasingly are found to have bilateral adrenal hyperplasia rather than a discrete adenoma, and are commonly normokalemic, so that hypokalemia is no longer pathognomonic. Treatment is laparoscopic adrenalectomy, or mineralocorticoid receptor blockade in those with bilateral hyperplasia or who are unsuitable for surgery.

## Pseudohypoaldosteronism

Although more than 20 years ago defects in MR binding of aldosterone were postulated as the cause of pseudohypoaldosteronism (PHA) from studies on affected patients' leukocytes,[21] in subsequent studies no abnormalities in gene sequence were found.[22,23] This apparent conundrum has been resolved by the distinction between PHA type 1 and type 2, where one is caused by an epithelial sodium channel (ENaC) defect, and the other a defect in MR. The phenotype varies, but severe cases can be distinguished from aldosterone synthase deficiency by the often marked elevation in aldosterone as well as renin levels. Treatment is rigorous salt supplementation in infancy, with even severe cases appearing to improve with age, by mechanisms that remain poorly understood.

## Pregnancy-Associated Hypertension

In contrast to the inactivating MR mutations that may be found in PHA, a recently discovered point mutation[24] has been shown to result in a constitutively partially activated MR, in which both progesterone and spironolactone act as agonists, rather than as antagonists as is the case for the wild-type MR. The syndrome was discovered in a young male hypertensive, whose two sisters suffered severe exacerbations of hypertension in pregnancy, presumably reflecting the agonist effect of progesterone on the mutant MR. The syndrome is rare, and abnormal MR do not appear to underlie the relatively common finding of hypertension in pregnancy.

## Apparent Mineralocorticoid Excess

A more common, though still comparatively rare, condition of inappropriate MR activation is that of apparent mineralocorticoid excess (AME), first described by New and Ulick in 1977.[25] In this syndrome—of juvenile hypertension, sodium retention, and hypokalemia, in the presence of suppressed renin and aldosterone levels—epithelial MR are activated by cortisol, reflecting deficient activity of the specificity-conferring enzyme 11βHSD2. The finding of an elevated ratio of urinary free cortisol:cortisone is diagnostic, and patients are treated by MR blockade, on occasion with the suppression of cortisol by dexamethasone administration. Whereas previously it had been assumed that epithelial 11βHSD2 excluded glucocorticoids from MR, this has been shown not to be the case.[26] The enzyme acts to debulk intracellular glucocorticoid levels, from ~100-fold those of aldosterone to ~10-fold, consistent with a role for the forgotten cosubstrate (NAD, from which NADH is generated stoichiometrically) in activation of glucocorticoid-MR complexes, as briefly discussed subsequently and elsewhere in detail.[27,28]

## Essential Hypertension

Although an increasing number of patients with essential hypertension appear to have autonomous aldosterone secretion, the potential role of aldosterone, 11βHSD2, and MR in the majority of hypertensive patients remains unclear. A number of studies have linked allelic variation in 11βHSD2 or CYP11B2 with a higher incidence of elevated BP,[29,30] and there have similarly been sporadic reports of a subgroup of essential hypertensives with impaired conversion of cortisol to cortisone.

The selective MR antagonist eplerenone has been shown to be of equivalent potency to ACE inhibitors, $Ca^{2+}$ channel blockers, β-blockers, or angiotensin receptor blockers (ARBs) in terms of BP reduction.[31,32] In titration-to-effect studies, a wide (4- to 10-fold) dose range of eplerenone was needed in moderate hypertensives to reduce diastolic BP to <90 mm Hg, with comparable falls in BP (~16/12 mm Hg) at each dose level,[33] further evidence for a significant role for aldosterone in essential hypertension.

## Pathophysiology

Whereas the physiologic role of aldosterone in epithelia to retain $Na^+$ and water, and to excrete $K^+$, are well accepted, its other physiologic roles (as a vasoconstrictor, by a direct action on vascular smooth muscle cells (VSMCs), and in the brain to stimulate salt appetite) are less well explored. In other nonepithelial tissues it is unclear what, if any, are physiologic roles for aldosterone. What is clear, however, is that aldosterone may have direct pathophysiologic effects on blood vessels and cardiomyocytes, almost certainly inter alia, in the context of inappropriate salt status.

## Mineralocorticoid/Salt Imbalance

In physiologic terms, aldosterone and sodium have a reciprocal relationship; when salt status falls aldosterone rises, and vice versa. When, however, aldosterone secretion is no longer responsive to normal negative feedback—in primary aldosteronism, GRA or in animals infused with aldosterone and given only 0.9% NaCl solution to drink—this reciprocal nexus is broken, and aldosterone levels are inappropriate for salt status, and vice versa. Under these circumstances very marked cerebral, renal, and coronary vascular inflammation can be shown in experimental animals,[34,35,38] progressing to perivascular and interstitial cardiac fibrosis.[36,37] Importantly, if infused animals are on a low-salt diet with water as drinking fluid, these changes are not seen; in the human situation of prolonged $Na^+$ deficiency, very high levels of aldosterone coexist with no cardiac or vascular toxicity. The mechanisms involved in the deleterious synergy between aldosterone and inappropriate $Na^+$ status are currently unclear; their clarification would constitute a major advance in cardiovascular endocrinology.

## Vascular Inflammation and Cardiac Fibrosis

As noted previously, inappropriate aldosterone (or other mineralocorticoid) for salt status is followed by progressive vascular inflammation in a variety of organs. Animal models used include the stroke-prone spontaneously hypertensive rat (SHR-sp), where eplerenone has been shown to be very protective of both cerebral and renal vasculature, and tissue architecture[35]; the aldosterone infused rat on 0.9% NaCl solution to drink, in which eplerenone is similarly protective of renal and coronary vessels, and kidney/heart architecture[34,38]; and the AngII infused/0.9% NaCl drinking rat, in which BP is Ang II driven, and unaffected by eplerenone or adrenalectomy.[34,38] On the other hand, adrenalectomy or eplerenone administration completely reverses the vascular and perivascular inflammatory response produced by Ang II/salt, which is restored in adrenalectomized rats by aldosterone infusion. In all these models, markers of inflammation—ED-1, MCD-1, COX-2, IL-1β, IL-6, osteopontin—increase over the first 2 to 4 weeks of study, and their levels are returned toward or to baseline by MR blockade.

## MR Activation by Glucocorticoids

In tissues coexpressing MR and 11βHSD2, intracellular glucocorticoid levels are 10 times those of aldosterone, and in unprotected tissues (e.g., cardiomyocytes, most neurons) levels of glucocorticoids are ~100 times higher. Under normal circumstances these glucocorticoid-MR complexes appear inactive, and the glucocorticoid appears to act in tonic inhibitory mode.[5,39] In other circumstances, however, glucocorticoids act as MR agonists. The first of these is when 11βHSD2 is deficient or blocked, leading to the syndromes of AME or licorice intoxication. Under these circumstances intracellular cortisol levels rise from ~10 times those of aldosterone toward ~100 times; more importantly, however, levels of intracellular NADH fall precipitously. In other systems NADH has been shown to regulate transcription factor activity by activating corepressors.[40,41]

Secondly, when 11βHSD2 is blocked by administration of carbenoxolone, an identical pattern of vascular inflammation is seen as with mineralocorticoid/salt administration; importantly, these effects, presumably of glucocorticoids on MR occur when NADH levels fall as 11β hydroxysteroid dehydrogenase is blocked by carbenoxolone.[42] Third, experimental angioplasty in pigs is followed by a constriction in coronary luminal diameter, a constriction blocked by eplerenone treatment.[43] These animals were not receiving aldosterone or on a high-salt intake; our interpretation of these data is that under conditions of tissue damage and reactive oxygen species (ROS) generation, intracellular redox status changes—just as it does when 11βHSD2 is blocked—allowing normal levels of glucocorticoids to activate vascular MR and thus mimic the aldosterone/salt effects.

In this context it should be remembered that in both Randomized Aldactone Evaluation Study (RALES)[44] and Eplerenone Post-Acute Myocardial Infarction Heart Failure Efficacy and Survival Study (EPHESUS)[45] aldosterone levels were normal and salt status unremarkable. In the circumstances of heart failure—progressive or postmyocardial infarction—cardiomyocyte levels of ROS are known to be elevated. Under these circumstances, then, it would appear that spironolactone/eplerenone are not acting primarily as aldosterone blockers, but truly as MR antagonists blocking the effects of cortisol via MR in the context of tissue damage.

## FUTURE DIRECTIONS

Any prognostication is necessarily speculative, and thus these will be mentioned only briefly, and in no detail.

## Ectopic Aldosterone Synthesis

For the past decade there have been claims—commonly but not uniquely based on PCR of steroidogenic enzymes—that aldosterone can be synthesized in neurons, vascular wall and heart. Clinical data are conflicting—aldosterone is elaborated[46] or extracted[47] by the failing heart; in unpublished studies we were unable to find any consistent arteriovenous differences, in normal persons or those with severe heart failure. The Ang II/salt studies by Rocha et al.,[34,38] in which adrenalectomy totally reversed the vascular inflammation, argue powerfully against paracrine secretion of cardiac aldosterone of any consequence. Finally, the low levels of enzyme expression found by PCR, commonly between 0.01% and 1% of adrenal levels, means that each step of ectopic steroid synthesis becomes rate-limiting. Unless the enzymes are concentrated in merely a few cells, their contribution to even local aldosterone concentrations is likely to be negligible.

## MR-Independent Effects

Any molecule that circulates at subnanomolar concentrations can only act effectively by relatively high affinity binding. Many acute nongenomic effects of aldosterone have now been shown to be mediated via classical MR, in for example VSMC[12] and cardiomyocytes.[16] This does not exclude the possibility of another receptor for aldosterone, distinct from the classic MR, binding aldosterone and other mineralocorticoids with high affinity (and some degree of specificity, given their low circulating concentrations). It is unlikely that this is one of the 48 members of the steroid superfamily of nuclear transactivating factors identified in the human genome; it may, for example, be an analog of the membrane receptor for progesterone.[48]

## Therapeutic Implications

If aldosterone/salt imbalance is followed by inflammatory vascular and perivascular responses, and downstream tissue damage, then MR blockade assumes a particular therapeutic importance. If cortisol can activate MR in the context of tissue damage and ROS generation, leading to further ROS generation and exacerbation of tissue damage, MR blockade should prove of utility in breaking this potentially vicious cycle in conditions in addition to those characterized by mineralocorticoid/salt imbalance. MR blockade, therefore, may prove beneficial not only in the context of obvious cardiovascular disease (atherosclerosis/hypertension/myocarditis/heart failure), but also in conditions as diverse as diabetes, cerebrovascular protection and the prevention of premature labor. These possibilities need to be critically examined at the preclinical level, and if found of interest, transferred into the arena of clinical trials.

## References

1. Simpson S, Tait J, Wettstein A, et al. Isolierung eines neuen kristallierten Hormons aus Nebennieren mit besonders hoher Wirksamkeit auf den Mineralsoffwechsel. Experientia 9:333-335, 1953.
2. Okubo S, Niimura F, Nishimura H, et al. Angiotensin-independent mechanism for aldosterone synthesis during chronic extracellular fluid volume depletion. J Clin Invest 99:855-860, 1997.
3. Rousseau G, Baxter J, Funder J, et al. Glucocorticoid and mineralocorticoid receptors for aldosterone. J Steroid Biochem 3:219-227, 1972.
4. Funder JW, Pearce PT, Smith R, et al. Vascular type I aldosterone binding sites are physiological mineralocorticoid receptors. Endocrinology 125:2224-2226, 1989.
5. Qin, W, Rudolph A, Bond B, et al. A transgenic model of aldosterone-driven cardiac hypertrophy and heart failure. Circ Res 93:69-76, 2003.
6. Arriza JL, Weinberger C, Cerelli G, et al. Cloning of human mineralocorticoid receptor complementary DNA: structural and functional kinship with the glucocorticoid receptor. Science 237:268-275, 1987.
7. Greenwood A, Butler P, White R, et al. Multiple corticosteroid receptors in a teleost fish: Distinct sequences. Endocrinology 144:4226-4236, 2003.
8. Edwards CR, Stewart PM, Burt D, et al. Localisation of 11 beta-hydroxysteroid dehydrogenase—tissue specific protector of the mineralocorticoid receptor. Lancet 2:986-989, 1988.
9. Funder JW, Pearce P, Smith R, et al. Mineralocorticoid action: target-tissue specificity is enzyme, not receptor, mediated. Science 242:583-585, 1988.
10. Chen S, Bhargava A, Mastroberardino L, et al. Epithelial sodium channel regulated by aldosterone-induced protein SGK. Proc Natl Acad Sci USA 96:2514-2519, 1999.
11. Kornel L. Colocalization of 11 beta-hydroxysteroid dehydrogenase and mineralocorticoid receptors in cultured vascular smooth muscle cells. Am J Hypertens 7:100-103, (1994).
12. Alzamora R, Michea L, Marusic ET. Role of 11beta-hydroxysteroid dehydrogenase on nongenomic aldosterone effects in human arteries. Hypertension 35:1099-1104, 2000.
13. Romagni P, Rossie F, Guerrini L, et al. Aldosterone induces contraction of the resistance arteries in man. Atherosclerosis 166:345-349, 2003.
14. Gomez-Sanchez E, Funder J. Central mineralocorticoid receptors in the development of hypertension. Curr Opin Nephrol Hypertens in press, 2004.
15. Christ M, Douwes K, Eisen C, et al. Rapid effects of aldosterone on sodium transport in vascular smooth muscle cells. Hypertension 25:117-125, 1995.
16. Mihailidou A, Mardini M, Funder JW. Rapid, nongenomic effects of aldosterone in the heart mediated by epsilon protein kinase C. Endocrinology 145:773-780, 2004.
17. Dunlop F, Crock P, Montalto J, et al. A compound heterozygote case of type II aldosterone synthase deficiency. J Clin Endocrinol Metab 88:2518-2526, 2003.
18. Lifton R, Dluhy R, Powers M, et al. Hereditary hypertension caused by chimaeric gene duplications and ectopic expression of aldosterone synthase. Nat Genet 2:66-74, 1992.
19. Conn J. Primary aldosteronism: A new clinical syndrome. J Lab Clin Med 45:3-17, 1955.
20. Olivieri O, Ciacciarelli A, Signorelli D, et al. Aldosterone to renin ratio in a primary care setting: the Bussolengo study. J Clin Endocrinol Metab in press, 2004.
21. Armanini D, Kuhnle U, Strasser T, et al. Aldosterone-receptor deficiency in pseudohypoaldosteronism. New Engl J Med 313:1178-1181, 1985.
22. Komesaroff PA, Verity K, Fuller PJ. Pseudohypoaldosteronism: molecular characterization of the mineralocorticoid receptors. J Clin Endocrinol Metab 79:27-31, 1994.
23. Zennaro M-C, Borensztein P, Jeunemaitre X, et al. No alteration in the primary structure of the mineralocorticoid receptors in a family with pseudohypoaldosteronism. J Clin Endocrinol Metab 79:32-38, 1994.
24. Geller D, Farhi A, Pinkerton N, et al. Activating mineralocorticoid receptor mutation in hypertension exacerbated by pregnancy. Science 289:119-123, 2000.
25. New MI, Levine LS, Biglieri EG, et al. Evidence for an unidentified steroid in a child with apparent mineralocorticoid hypertension. J Clin Endocrinol Metab 44:924-933, 1977.
26. Funder JW, Myles K. Exclusion of corticosterone from epithelial mineralocorticoid receptors is insufficient for selectivity of aldosterone action: in vivo binding studies. Endocrinology 137:5264-5268, 1996.

27. Funder JW. The role of mineralocorticoid receptor antagonists in the treatment of cardiac failure. Expert Opin Investig Drugs 12:1963-1969, 2003.

28. Funder JW. Is aldosterone bad for the heart? Trends Endocrinol Metab 15:139-142, 2004.

29. Lim P, Macdonald T, Holloway C, et al. Variation at the aldosterone synthase (CYP11B2) locus contributes to hypertension in subjects with a raised aldosterone-to-renin ratio. J Clin Endocrinol Metab 87:4398-4402, 2002.

30. Connell JM, Fraser R, MacKenzie SM, et al. The impact of polymorphisms in the gene encoding aldosterone synthase (CYP11B2) on steroid synthesis and blood pressure regulation. Mol Cell Endocrinol 217:243-247, 2004.

31. Krum H, Nolly H, Workman D, et al. Efficacy of eplerenone added to renin-angiotensin blockade in hypertensive patients. Hypertension 40:117-123, 2002.

32. Weinberger M, Roniker B, Krause S, et al. Eplerenone, a selective aldosterone blocker, in mild-to-moderate hypertension. Am J Hypertens 15:709-716, 2002.

33. Levy D, Rocha R, Funder JW. Distinguishing the antihypertensive and electrolyte effects of eplerenone. J Clin Endocrinol Metab 89:2736-2740, 2004.

34. Rocha R, Rudolph A, Frierdich G, et al. Aldosterone induces a vascular inflammatory phenotype in the rat heart. Am J Physiol 283:H1802-H1810, 2002.

35. Chander P, Rocha R, Ranaudo J, et al. Aldosterone plays a pivotal role in the pathogenesis of thrombotic microangiopathy in SHRSP. J Am Soc Nephrol 14:1990-1997, 2003.

36. Brilla CG, Weber KT. Mineralocorticoid excess, dietary sodium, and myocardial fibrosis. J Lab Clin Med 120:893-901, 1992.

37. Young M, Fullerton M, Dilley R, et al. Mineralocorticoids, hypertension, and cardiac fibrosis. J Clin Invest 93:2578-2583, 1994.

38. Rocha R, Martin-Berger C, Yang P, et al. Selective aldosterone blockade prevents angiotensin II/salt-induced vascular inflammation in the rat heart. Endocrinology 143:4828-4836, 2002.

39. Sato A, Funder JW. High glucose stimulates aldosterone-induced hypertrophy via Type I mineralocorticoid receptors in neonatal rat cardiomyocytes. Endocrinology 137:4145-4153, 1996.

40. Zhang Q, Piston D, Goodman R. Regulation of corepressor function by nuclear NADH. Science 295:1895-1897, 2002.

41. Fjeld C, Birdsong W, Goodman R. Differential binding of NAD+ and NADH allows the transcriptional corepressor carboxyl-terminal binding protein to serve as a metabolic sensor. Proc Natl Acad Sci USA 100:9202-9207, 2003.

42. Young M, Moussa L, Dilley R, et al. Early inflammatory responses in experimental cardiac hypertrophy and fibrosis: Effects of 11 beta-hydroxysteroid dehydrogenase inactivation. Endocrinology 144:1121-1125, 2003.

43. Ward MR, Kanellakis P, Ramsey D, et al. Eplerenone suppresses constrictive remodeling and collagen accumulation after angioplasty in porcine coronary arteries. Circulation 104(4): 467-472, 2001.

44. Pitt B, Zannad F, Remme WJ, et al. The effect of spironolactone on morbidity and mortality in patients with severe heart failure. N Engl J Med 341:709-717, 1999.

45. Pitt B, Remme W, Zannad F, et al. Eplerenone, a selective aldosterone blocker, in patients with left ventricular dysfunction after myocardial infarction. N Engl J Med 348:1309-1321, 2003.

46. Mizuno Y, Yoshimura M, Yasue H, et al. Aldosterone production is activated in failing ventricle in humans. Circulation 103:72-77, 2001.

47. Tsutamoto T, Wada A, Maeda K, et al. Spironolactone inhibits the transcardiac extraction of aldosterone in patients with congestive heart failure. J Am Coll Cardiol 36:838-844, 2000.

48. Falkenstein E, Meyer C, Eisen C, et al. Full-length DNA sequence of a progesterone membrane-binding protein from porcine vascular smooth muscle cells. Biochem Biophys Res Commun 229:86-89, 1996.

# Chapter 13

# The Role of Insulin Resistance and Compensatory Hyperinsulinemia in Patients with Essential Hypertension

## Gerald M. Reaven

Essential hypertension is a multifactorial condition, and it should be obvious that one abnormality is not the "cause" of this syndrome. Rather, there are a number of physiologic changes that predispose individuals to develop high blood pressure. One of the goals of this chapter will be to review evidence that resistance to insulin-mediated glucose uptake and compensatory hyperinsulinemia may play such a role. In addition, there is a cluster of abnormalities associated with insulin resistance/hyperinsulinemia that contribute significantly to the risk of cardiovascular disease (CVD) in patients with essential hypertension. This chapter will address both of these issues by attempting to provide answers to the following three questions: (1) Do insulin resistance and/or compensatory hyperinsulinemia play a role in the pathogenesis of essential hypertension? (2) What are the mechanistic links between insulin resistance/hyperinsulinemia and essential hypertension? and (3) Is there a relationship between insulin resistance/hyperinsulinemia and CVD risk in patients with essential hypertension? Although there is considerable evidence from animal models of hypertension concerning these issues, as well as potentially relevant in vitro data, the evidence reviewed in this chapter will be limited to studies in human beings.

## DO INSULIN RESISTANCE AND/OR COMPENSATORY HYPERINSULINEMIA PLAY A ROLE IN THE PATHOGENESIS OF ESSENTIAL HYPERTENSION?

At the simplest level, there is substantial evidence that patients with essential hypertension are insulin resistant/hyperinsulinemic as compared with normotensive individuals.[1-8] Furthermore, it has been shown that insulin resistance/hyperinsulinemia exist in normotensive, first-degree relatives of patients with essential hypertension.[9-13] Despite this evidence of a strong link between insulin resistance/hyperinsulinemia and essential hypertension, the view that these changes in insulin metabolism play a role in blood pressure regulation continues to be debated. For example, the inability to detect a relationship between plasma insulin concentration and blood pressure in some cross-sectional studies has been interpreted to mean that insulin resistance/hyperinsulinemia is not involved in the pathogenesis of essential hypertension.[14-17] However, a very different view of the relationship between insulin resistance/compensatory hyperinsulinemia and blood pressure emerges from the results of the European Group for the Study of Insulin Resistance.[18] These investigators defined the relationship between a specific meas-

ure of insulin-mediated glucose disposal, fasting insulin concentration, and blood pressure in 333 normotensive individuals, studied in 20 different clinical research centers, and reported that blood pressure was directly related to both insulin resistance and insulin concentration. Furthermore, these relationships were independent of differences in age, gender, and degree of obesity.

The size of the European study, in addition to its use of a direct measure of insulin action, as contrasted to surrogate estimates, provides strong evidence that there is a relationship between insulin resistance, hyperinsulinemia, and blood pressure. In addition, results of prospective studies in which hyperinsulinemia has been used as a surrogate marker of insulin resistance support the view that insulin resistance/hyperinsulinemia are causally linked to the development of essential hypertension.[19-22] Perhaps the most compelling in this context is the study by Skarfors et al.,[19] who evaluated risk factors for the development of hypertension in 2130 men observed over a 10-year period. These investigators showed that the individuals with normal blood pressure at baseline who subsequently developed hypertension were more obese and higher plasma insulin (fasting and after intravenous glucose) and triglyceride (TG) concentrations. When baseline blood pressure was excluded from multivariate analysis, independent predictors of the progression to hypertension were obesity (as estimated by body mass index [BMI]), fasting and post-glucose challenge plasma insulin concentrations, and family history of hypertension.

Essentially similar results were reported by Lissner et al.,[20] who evaluated risk factors for the development of hypertension in 278 women followed over a 12-year period. In addition, they examined the relationship between blood pressure and risk factors in 219 women not receiving antihypertensive medication. Hypertension developed in approximately one third of the population in the 12-year period. In multiple logistic regression analysis, fasting hyperinsulinemia predicted the transition from normal to high blood pressure, independent of adjustments for initial BMI, waist:hip ratio, and weight gain. Individuals in the highest quartile in terms of fasting plasma insulin concentration were greater than threefold more likely to develop hypertension than those in the lowest quartile, and fasting insulin also predicted changes in blood pressure over the 12-year period.

The ability of insulin to predict changes in blood pressure over time in children and adolescents has also been shown on two occasions. One study[21] involved a population that ranged from 3 to 18 years at baseline, and was followed for 16 years. The results indicated that fasting insulin concentrations "seem to regulate actual blood pressure within the normal range and to predict future blood pressure"; conclusions that applied to both boys and girls, and were independent of differences in age and weight. In a somewhat more complicated study, 1865 children and adolescents were followed over a 6-year period, with essentially similar findings concerning the positive predictive power of baseline fasting insulin concentration.[22] Perhaps of greater interest was the finding that "high insulin levels seems to precede the development of a potentially atherogenic risk factor profile including low high-density lipoprotein cholesterol (HDL-C), high TG, and high systolic blood pressure."

More recent skepticism concerning the notion that insulin resistance/hyperinsulinemia plays a causal role in the genesis of essential hypertension stems from population-based studies in which the statistical technique of factor analysis is used to evaluate the relationship between insulin resistance and conditions thought to be related to it. The results of studies employing this approach have found that blood pressure appears to be a "factor" separate from the other cluster of abnormalities that associate with insulin resistance and/or hyperinsulinemia.[23] Although these findings are usually interpreted to signify the lack of an "independent" relationship between blood pressure and insulin resistance/hyperinsulinemia, the etiologic and clinical heterogeneity of patients with essential hypertension provides an obvious reason to question this conclusion. Resistance to insulin-mediated glucose disposal and compensatory hyperinsulinemia are continuous variables,[24] not dichotomous ones, and there is no simple way to classify a person as being insulin resistant or insulin sensitive.

An effort to estimate the number of persons with essential hypertension who are insulin resistant was made by measuring blood pressure and the plasma insulin response 120 minutes after a 75-g oral glucose challenge in an unselected population of 732 factory workers.[25] As a result of these

measurements, 41 individuals were identified as having essential hypertension.

Figure 13–1 illustrates the distribution of the plasma insulin responses to the glucose challenge of these individuals and those of 41 participants in the same survey with normal blood pressure. The two groups were matched for age, gender, degree of obesity, ethnic background, type of employment in the factory, and level of physical activity. Only 10% of the normotensive persons had plasma insulin concentrations that exceeded 80 mU/L when determined 120 minutes after the oral glucose challenge. In contrast, the plasma insulin concentration was >80 mU/L in 45% of the persons with essential hypertension. On the basis of these and other findings,[8] no more than half of the persons with essential hypertension can be considered to be insulin resistant/hyperinsulinemic.

If at most only half of the persons with high blood pressure are insulin resistant/hyperinsulinemic, it should not be surprising that population-based studies, in which surrogate markers of insulin resistance are applied to primarily normotensive individuals, do not always discern a relationship between insulin resistance and blood pressure. When the fact that at least half the persons with essential hypertension are not insulin resistant is added to these confounding variables, it is not difficult to understand why studies based on the use of factor analysis find that blood pressure does not segregate with whatever surrogate measures of insulin resistance are being used. It should also be emphasized that the results of population-based studies that conclude that insulin resistance is not related to the development of essential hypertension do not negate the observations that (1) the prevalence of insulin resistance/hyperinsulinemia is increased in patients with essential hypertension; (2) these changes can be seen in normotensive, first-degree relatives of patients with essential hypertension; and (3) insulin resistance/hyperinsulinemia have been shown in prospective studies to be independent predictors of the development of essential hypertension. The

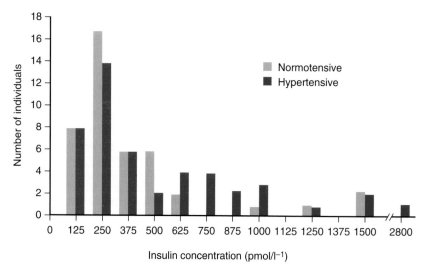

**Figure 13–1** Frequency distribution of the plasma insulin response 2 hours after a 75-g oral glucose challenge in normotensive and hypertensive volunteers. (Reprinted from Zavaroni I, Mazza S, Dall'Aglio E, et al. Prevalence of hyperinsulinaemia in patients with high blood pressure. J Intern Med 231:235-240, 1992, with permission of the authors and the journal.)

fact that insulin resistance/hyperinsulinemia does not contribute to the etiology of essential hypertension in some individuals should not obscure the conclusion, based on a large database, that it does in others.

Finally, the view that insulin resistance and compensatory hyperinsulinemia play a role in the pathogenesis of essential hypertension has been challenged by evidence that hyperinsulinemia, per se, does not necessarily result in an increase in blood pressure. Perhaps the evidence most often cited in this context is that the acute administration of insulin to normal volunteers causes vasodilation, and does not increase blood pressure.[26] On the other hand, there is no a priori reason to believe that the chronic effects of compensatory hyperinsulinemia on blood pressure regulation in insulin-resistant subjects should be the same as the acute effects of a primary increase in insulin concentration in healthy volunteers.

Turning to the association between chronic hyperinsulinemia and blood pressure regulation, it has been argued that the prevalence of hypertension is not increased in patients with insulin-secreting tumors of the pancreas. However, neither fasting nor postprandial plasma insulin concentrations in patients with an insulinoma are particularly elevated when the plasma concentration of proinsulin is considered, and the diagnosis of insulinoma is based upon the development of fasting hypoglycemia in the face of a plasma insulin concentration that does not decline as the plasma glucose level falls. At a more physiologic level, there is considerable evidence that chronic hyperinsulinemia plays a role in blood pressure regulation. For example, weight loss, which enhances insulin sensitivity and lowers plasma insulin concentrations in nondiabetic individuals,[27] can also decrease blood pressure in persons with essential hypertension.[28] This change seems to be correlated with the improvement in insulin resistance.[29] In a similar vein, there is evidence that blood pressure can be lowered in obese individuals by physical training without any change in weight, but only in those individuals who were hyperinsulinemic and/or hypertriglyceridemic before the training program was initiated.[30] Because there is also evidence that insulin sensitivity is directly related to level of habitual physical activity,[31] it is reasonable to conclude that the decrease in blood pressure in these individuals was associated with an improvement in insulin-stimulated glucose uptake. It is also worth noting that blood pressure falls when insulin dose is reduced in obese patients with type 2 diabetes and hypertension,[32] and that insulin treatment increases blood pressure in patients with type 2 diabetes.[33] Thus, evidence that the acute administration of insulin does not increase blood pressure in normal individuals, or that blood pressure is not elevated in patients with an insulinoma, appears to be, at the least, counterbalanced by evidence that modulation of insulin resistance and/or insulin level in insulin-resistant individuals leads to predictable changes in blood pressure.

## WHAT ARE THE POSSIBLE MECHANISTIC LINKS BETWEEN INSULIN RESISTANCE/HYPERINSULINEMIA AND ESSENTIAL HYPERTENSION?

Before discussing possible mechanisms by which insulin resistance/hyperinsulinemia increase the risk of developing hypertension, three fundamental issues must be emphasized. First, as

emphasized previously, not all persons with essential hypertension are insulin resistant, nor do all insulin-resistant individuals become hypertensive. Second, the relationship between insulin resistance and the development of hypertension is analogous to the role played by insulin resistance in the pathogenesis of type 2 diabetes.[34,35] Hyperglycemia develops in insulin-resistant individuals only when they no longer are able to secrete the large amount of insulin necessary to overcome the insulin resistance. In a similar fashion, it seems likely that hypertension develops only when some unknown compensatory response (or responses) is no longer able to overcome the metabolic changes associated with insulin resistance/hyperinsulinemia that favor an increase in blood pressure. Third, although insulin resistance is the fundamental defect, it is most likely that it is the compensatory hyperinsulinemia that increases the risk of an individual becoming hypertensive. This seeming paradox is because insulin action varies dramatically in a given individual as a function of the tissue in question. Resistance to insulin action at the level of the muscle (stimulation of glucose uptake) and the adipose tissue (inhibition of lipolysis) are highly correlated,[36] and the presence of these defects in insulin action can coexist in the same person with normal insulin action on the kidney and sympathetic nervous system.[37-40]

An example that may that best illustrate the general principles outlined previously is the relationship between insulin resistance/hyperinsulinemia, the kidney, and salt sensitivity. The fact that the infusion of insulin into normal individuals increases sodium retention has been known for some time,[41] and there is evidence that this is also true of persons with essential hypertension.[38] If the link between insulin resistance and hypertension is attributable to enhanced sodium retention, as a consequence of compensatory hyperinsulinemia, it might be predicted that such patients would also be salt sensitive. There is evidence in both normotensive and hypertensive individuals that this is the case.[42,43]

Perhaps the clearest example of the complex nature of the relationship between insulin resistance, compensatory hyperinsulinemia, the kidney and blood pressure regulation evolved from a study comparing changes in these variables in response with diets varying in sodium intake. Table 13–1 contains results of such measurements in 19 healthy volunteers who ingested alternating diets containing either low (25 mmol/day) or high (250 mmol/day) amounts of sodium, consumed in random order for 5 days each.[44] The high-sodium diet resulted in significant increases in body weight and 24-hour urinary sodium excretion, along with the expected decreases in concentrations of plasma renin activity (PRA) and aldosterone and increase in atrial natriuretic peptide (ANP) concentration. However, the average mean arterial pressure (MAP) of the 19 individuals in this study did not change. Insulin-mediated glucose disposal, as quantified by determining the steady-state plasma glucose (SSPG) concentration at the end of a 180-minute infusion of octreotide, insulin, and glucose, was similar when measured at the end of each dietary sodium intake. Because the steady-state plasma insulin concentrations were the same on both occasions, insulin-mediated glucose disposal rates were not affected by the 10-fold difference in sodium intake. Furthermore, plasma insulin concentrations 120 minutes after a 75-g oral glucose challenge were also similar when measured at the end of each period of sodium intake. Finally, there was an increase in 24-hour urinary nitrate and nitrite (NOx) excretion of borderline statistical significance.

**Table 13-1** Experimental Variables at the End of the Low- and High-Sodium Diets (Mean + SEM)

| Variable | Low | High | p |
|---|---|---|---|
| Weight (kg) | 78.8 + 3.1 | 79.4 + 3.0 | .005 |
| Urinary Na (mmol/day) | 12.7 + 2.8 | 174 + 14 | .0001 |
| MAP (mm Hg) | 82.7 + 2.6 | 82.9 + 2 | NS |
| SSPI (pmol/L) | 306 + 42 | 330 + 49 | NS |
| SSPG (mmol/L) | 8.25 + 1.01 | 7.83 + 1.00 | NS |
| Insulin (pmol/L) | 270 + 33 | 258 + 32 | NS |
| ANP (pmol/L) | 4.6 + 0.7 | 10.3 + 1.3 | .009 |
| PRA (ng/ml/hr) | 2.8 + 0.4 | 0.41 + 0.1 | .0001 |
| Aldosterone (pmol/L) | 674 + 75 | 92 + 11 | .0001 |
| Urinary NOx (umol/day) | 1119 + 94 | 1353 + 136 | .06 |

Adapted from Facchini FS, DoNascimento C, Reaven GM, et al. Blood pressure, sodium intake, insulin resistance, and urinary nitrate excretion. Hypertension 33:1008-1012, 1999. Na, sodium; SSPI, steady-state plasma insulin; SSPG, steady-state plasma glucose; ANP, atrial natriuretic peptide; PRA, plasma renin activity.

The salt-induced increase in body weight was directly related to baseline degree of insulin resistance (SSPG, $p = .03$) and plasma insulin concentration 120 minutes after an oral glucose challenge ($p = .07$), and inversely related to the ability to increase urinary sodium excretion ($p = .01$). The inability to increase sodium excretion was also significantly related to both SSPG ($p = .04$) and the postglucose challenge insulin concentration ($p = .11$). In contrast, changes in ANP, PRA, and aldosterone concentrations and urinary NOx excretion were unrelated to the changes in body weight and sodium excretion in response to the high-salt diet.

Although the data in Table 13-1 indicated that MAP did not change significantly with the high-salt diet, there was considerable individual variability, and multiple regression analysis in the whole population showed that the greater the weight gain in response to the high-salt diet, the greater the increase in MAP ($r = 0.51$, $p < .05$). The only other significant variable associated with a salt-induced increase in MAP was the 24-hour urinary NOx excretion, and the results in Figure 13-2 demonstrate a highly significant inverse relationship ($r = -0.77$, $p < .001$) between these two variables. These results suggest that only those individuals who were insulin resistant/hyperinsulinemic retained a significant amount of salt and gained weight in response to a high-salt diet. However, as seen in Figure 13-2, if insulin-resistant individuals increased their urinary NOx excretion, their blood pressure did not increase. Obviously, 24-hour urinary NOx excretion is only a surrogate measure of nitric oxide production, but it can be speculated that the daylong increase in circulating insulin concentrations that is characteristic of insulin-resistant individuals acts on a insulin-sensitive kidney to retain-salt and water in response to a high-salt diet. Unless this can be compensated for by an increase in nitric oxide production, blood pressure is likely to increase. Whether or not this ultimately proves to be a correct formulation remains to be seen, but these results help explain why the prevalence of salt sensitivity is increased in insulin-resistant/ hyperinsulinemic individuals.[42,43]

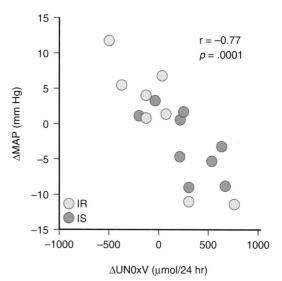

**Figure 13-2** Relationship between the change in mean arterial blood pressure (ΔMAP) in response to the high-salt diet and the concomitant change in the 24-hour urinary excretion of nitrites and nitrates (ΔUNOxV) in insulin-resistant (IR) and insulin-sensitive (IS) individuals. (Reprinted from Facchini FS, DoNascimento C, Reaven GM, et al. Blood pressure, sodium intake, insulin-resistance, and urinary nitrate excretion. Hypertension 33:1008-1012, 1999, with permission of the authors and the journal.)

Insulin activation of the sympathetic nervous system (SNS) provides a somewhat broader approach to understanding why insulin-resistant and hyperinsulinemic individuals are at increased risk to develop hypertension. An increase in heart rate is recognized as not only a manifestation of enhanced SNS activity, but also as a significant predictor of the development of hypertension.[45,46] The fact that heart rate is also related to both insulin resistance and hyperinsulinemia[39] is consistent with the view that these abnormalities of insulin metabolism predispose individuals to develop hypertension via activation of the SNS. Results of the population-based Normative Aging Study provide further support for this point of view in that SNS activity, as estimated by 24-hour urinary excretion of norepinephrine, was elevated in hyperinsulinemic, and presumably insulin-resistant subjects.[47] Furthermore, results of that study identified a significant relationship between plasma insulin concentration and urinary norepinephrine excretion, independent of differences in other relevant variables, including BMI and regional fat distribution.

Finally, the possibility that stimulation of the SNS by compensatory hyperinsulinemia in insulin-resistant individuals plays a role in the development of essential hypertension is another example of differential insulin sensitivity. Specifically, both heart rate and plasma norepinephrine concentrations appear to increase normally in response to hyperinsulinemia in individuals who demonstrate a defect in insulin-mediated glucose disposal by muscle.[48]

This discussion of the possible causal relationship between insulin resistance/hyperinsulinemia and the development of essential hypertension has focused on two, somewhat related, potential mechanisms. These are not the only possibilities, but they seem to be the explanations for which there is the most evidence at this time. At the least, they provide a testable hypothesis as to the nature of these relationships.

## INSULIN RESISTANCE, COMPENSATORY HYPERINSULINEMIA, AND CARDIOVASCULAR DISEASE IN PATIENTS WITH ESSENTIAL HYPERTENSION

The advent of more effective antihypertensive drugs has greatly decreased morbidity and mortality in patients with high blood pressure. However, the beneficial effects of lowering blood pressure have been more obvious in decreasing risk of stroke as compared with CVD.[49] Because CVD is the major cause of morbidity and mortality in patients with hypertension, this apparent paradox has received a great deal of attention. Not surprisingly, many different explanations have been proposed to account for this finding, but the simplest explanation is that approximately half of the patients with essential hypertension are insulin resistant/hyperinsulinemic, and exhibit the cluster of CVD risk factors common to such individuals.[25] Thus the subset of patients with essential hypertension that are also insulin resistant are likely to have some degree of glucose intolerance, as well as the atherogenic lipoprotein phenotype characteristic of insulin-resistant/hyperinsulinemic individuals: high TG and low HDL-C concentrations, smaller and denser low-density lipoprotein particles, and an exaggerated degree of postprandial lipemia.[50]

Furthermore, there is evidence that patients in whom essential hypertension is associated with insulin resistance are at the greatest CVD risk.[51-53] For example, Figure 13–3 compares the plasma glucose and insulin concentrations in response to a 75-g oral glucose challenge in untreated patients with essential hypertension, without clinical evidence of CVD, who have ischemic heart disease by Minnesota

Code criteria, with those of healthy volunteers, as well as a matched group of equally hypertensive individuals with normal electrocardiograms.[51] It is apparent that patients with essential hypertension *and* electrocardiographic evidence of CVD were somewhat glucose intolerant and hyperinsulinemic as compared with either the normotensive control group or those with normal electrocardiograms. Not surprisingly, measurement of insulin-mediated glucose disposal demonstrated that patients with essential hypertension and ischemic electrocardiographic changes were insulin resistant. In addition, the data in Table 13–2 show that patients with high blood pressure and abnormal electrocardiograms were also significantly more dyslipidemic (higher plasma TG and lower HDL-C concentrations) as compared with normotensive individuals or hypertensive patients with normal electrocardiograms. The existence of these CVD risk factors in the hypertensive patients with abnormal electrocardiograms was seen in the absence of pharmacologic treatment of their high blood pressure. Furthermore, the magnitude of the abnormalities in insulin, glucose, and lipid metabolism in patients with high blood pressure is much greater than the adverse effects of any antihypertensive treatment.[54] Finally, lowering blood pressure with antihypertensive treatment does not return these metabolic abnormalities to normal.[5,6]

The importance of the link between dyslipidemia and CVD in insulin-resistant/hyperinsulinemic patients with essential hypertension and CVD has received additional support from two reports from the Copenhagen Male Study. In the first publication,[52] Jeppesen et al. evaluated the hypothesis that blood pressure is less predictive of CVD in individuals with the dyslipidemia characteristic of insulin-resistant/hyperinsulinemic individuals—a high TG and a low HDL-C concentration—than in those without these changes in lipid metabolism. Their results were consistent with the proposed hypothesis in that the development of CVD in individuals with a high TG and low HDL-C concentration was independent of differences in baseline systolic or diastolic blood pressure. In contrast, the

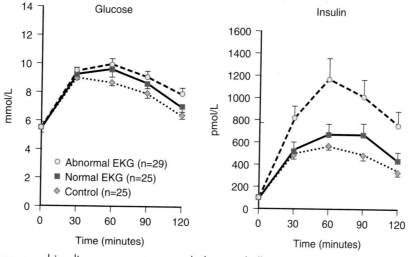

**Figure 13–3** Plasma glucose and insulin responses to an oral glucose challenge in control and hypertensive patients with either a normal or an abnormal electrocardiogram as defined by Minnesota Code Criteria. (Reprinted from Sheuh WH-H, Jeng C-Y, Shieh S-M, et al. Insulin resistance and abnormal electrocardiograms in patients with high blood pressure. Am J Hypertens 5:444-448, copyright 1992, with permission from the American Journal of Hypertension, Ltd.)

**Table 13–2** Lipid and Lipoprotein Concentrations (Mean ± SEM)

| Group | Cholesterol (mmol/L) | LDL Cholesterol (mmol/L) | HDL Cholesterol (mmol/L) | Cholesterol:HDL Cholesterol (ratio) | Triglyceride (mmol/L) |
|---|---|---|---|---|---|
| Control (n =25) | 5.05 ± 0.24 | 3.11 ± 0.22 | 1.36 ± 0.08 | 3.95 ± 0.31 | 1.16 ± 0.12 |
| Normal ECG (n = 24) | 4.79 ± 0.19 | 3.03 ± 0.18 | 1.28 ± 0.07 | 4.00 ± 0.25 | 1.21 ± 0.14 |
| Abnormal ECG (n = 29) | 5.36 ± 0.18 | 3.39 ± 0.17 | 1.10 ± 0.06* | 5.04 ± 0.23** | 1.81 ± 0.13** |

From Sheuh WH-H, Jeng C-Y, Shieh S-M, et al. Insulin resistance and abnormal electrocardiograms in patients with high blood pressure. Am J Hypertens 5:444-448, 1992.
*Different from control ($p < .01$).
**Different from control and normal ECG ($p < .02$).

higher the systolic ($p < .001$) or diastolic ($p < .03$) blood pressure at the beginning of the study, the greater the incidence of CVD in those without the dyslipidemia associated with insulin resistance/hyperinsulinemia.

In a second study,[53] the 2906 participants enrolled in the Copenhagen Male Study were divided into three groups on the basis of their fasting plasma TG and HDL-C concentrations. Individuals whose plasma TG and HDL-C concentrations were in the upper third or lower third, respectively, of the whole population, were assigned to the high TG/low HDL-C group. At the other extreme, a low TG/high HDL-C group was composed of those individuals whose plasma TG and HDL-C concentrations were in the lower third and upper third, respectively, of the study population for these two lipid measurements. The intermediate group consisted of those participants whose lipid values did not qualify them for either of the two extreme groups. The investigators then defined the interaction between TG/HDL-C groups and four conventional CVD risk factors: smoking, sedentary lifestyle, hypercholesterolemia, and essential hypertension. Irrespective of which of the four conventional CVD risk factors were considered, there was a two to three times higher risk of CVD in the high TG/low HDL-C group. The incidence of CVD in the face of any of the four conventional CVD risk factors was less than 5% during the 8-year period of observation as long as the individual with one of the conventional risk factors was also in the lowest TG/highest HDL-C group.

It should be emphasized that Jeppesen et al. used a high plasma TG and low HDL-C concentration as a surrogate marker of insulin resistance/hyperinsulinemia, without necessarily suggesting that these specific changes in lipoprotein metabolism were the total explanation of why CVD risk was increased in this subset of the population with essential hypertension. There is no reason to suspect that the hyperinsulinemia, glucose intolerance, dyslipidemia, and procoagulant state associated with the insulin-resistance syndrome will not contribute to the increased CVD risk in those patients with essential hypertension that are also insulin resistant.[50] In addition, changes in endothelial function that might contribute to increased CVD risk also vary as a function of differences in insulin-mediated glucose disposal in patients with essential hypertension. For example, the first step in the process of atherogenesis is the binding of circulating mononuclear cells to the endothelium,[55] and the data in the right panel of Figure 13–4 indicate that the binding of mononuclear cells isolated from patients with hypertension to endothelial cells in vitro is directly related to their degree of insulin resistance as quantified by the SSPG concentration at the end of a 180-minute infusion of octreotide, insulin, and glucose.[56] However, it can also be seen by comparing the two panels of Figure 13–4 that the relationship between SSPG concentration and binding of isolated mononuclear cells to endothelium was similar in normotensive and hypertensive volunteers in that the more insulin resistant an individual (the higher the SSPG concentration), the greater the adherence of his or her isolated mononuclear cells to endothelium.

Essentially identical findings were observed when the relationship between plasma asymmetric dimethylarginine (ADMA) concentration and insulin-mediated glucose disposal was evaluated.[57] Plasma concentrations of ADMA, an endogenous inhibitor of nitric oxide synthase, have been shown to be predictive of CVD in several clinical syndromes,[58] and Figure 13–5 depicts the relationship between SSPG concentration (the specific measurement of insulin resistance) and plasma ADMA concentrations in normal volunteers (*left panel*) and patients with essential hypertension (*right panel*). While plasma ADMA and SSPG concentrations vary widely in both experimental groups, the elevations in plasma ADMA concentrations are associated with higher SSPG concentrations (greater degrees of insulin resistance) irrespective of blood pressure. Thus plasma ADMA concentrations are increased to a similar degree in insulin-resistant individuals, whether normotensive or hypertensive.

## SUMMARY

There is a large body of experimental evidence that insulin resistance and compensatory hyperinsulinemia are more prevalent in patients with essential hypertension than in their first-degree relatives. Insulin resistance and/or compensatory hyperinsulinemia have also been shown in several large prospective, population-based studies to predict the development of essential hypertension. However, not all patients with essential hypertension are insulin resistant/hyperinsulinemic, and the

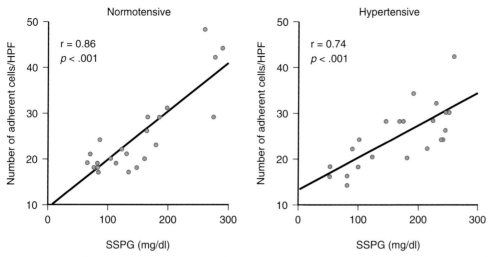

**Figure 13–4** Relationship between the steady-state plasma glucose (SSPG) concentration and the adherence of mononuclear cells isolated from the plasma of volunteers (*left panel*) who are normotensive and patients with essential hypertension (*right panel*) to cultured endothelial cells. The SSPG concentration is the average of four measurements of plasma glucose concentration obtained during the last 30 minutes of a 180-minute infusion of somatostatin, glucose, and insulin; the higher the SSPG concentration the more insulin resistant the individual. (Adapted from Chen N-G, Abbasi F, Lamendola, C, et al. Mononuclear cell adherence to cultured endothelium is enhanced by hypertension and insulin resistance in healthy nondiabetic volunteers. Circulation 100:940-943, 1999, with permission of the authors and the journal.)

increase in blood pressure in these individuals is unrelated to any change in insulin action. This heterogeneity in the multiple factors that increase the likelihood of a person developing hypertension almost certainly accounts for the continuing argument as to whether insulin resistance/hyperinsulinemia play a role in the etiology of essential hypertension. The fact that insulin resistance/compensatory hyperinsulinemia does not provide a single unifying hypothesis to account for the etiology of essential hypertension should not obscure the important role played by the defect in insulin-mediated glucose disposal in increasing the likelihood that blood pressure will increase. Of greater clinical relevance is the compelling evidence that it is the subset of patients with essential hypertension that are also insulin resistant, with the well-known cluster of associated CVD risk factors, that are at greatest CVD risk. Consequently, effective treatment of patients with essential hypertension should not be limited to simply lowering blood pressure, but must also address the multiple CVD risk factors often present in these patients.

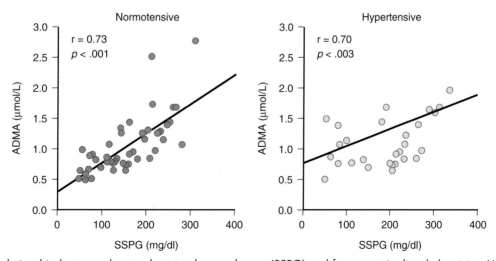

**Figure 13–5** Relationship between the steady-state plasma glucose (SSPG) and f asymmetric dimethylarginine (ADMA) concentrations in normotensive (*left panel*) and hypertensive (*right panel*) individuals. The SSPG concentration providers a measure of insulin resistance as described in the legend to Figure 13–4. (Adapted from Stuhlinger MC, Abbasi F, Chu JW, et al. Relationship between insulin resistance and an endogenous nitric oxide synthase inhibitor. JAMA 287:1420-1426, 2002, with permission of the authors and the journal.)

# References

1. Welborn TA, Breckenridge A, Rubinstein AH, et al. Serum-insulin in essential hypertension and in peripheral vascular disease. Lancet 1:1136-1137, 1966.
2. Lucas CP, Estigarribia JA, Darga LL, et al. Insulin and blood pressure in obesity. Hypertension 7:702-706, 1985.
3. Modan M, Halkin H, Almog S, et al. Hyperinsulinemia: A link between hypertension, obesity and glucose intolerance. J Clin Invest 75:809-817, 1985.
4. Ferrannini E, Buzzigoli G, Bonadona R. Insulin resistance in essential hypertension. N Engl Journal of Med 317:350-357, 1987.
5. Shen D-C, Shieh S-M, Fuh M, et al. Resistance to insulin-stimulated glucose uptake in patients with hypertension. J Clin Endocrinol Metab 66:580-583, 1988.
6. Swislocki ALM, Hoffman BB, Reaven GM. Insulin resistance, glucose intolerance and hyperinsulinemia in patients with hypertension. Am J Hypertens 2:419-423, 1989.
7. Pollare T, Lithell H, Berne C. Insulin resistance is a characteristic feature of primary hypertension independent of obesity. Metabolism 39:167-174, 1990.
8. Marigliano A, Tedde R, Sechi LA, et al. Insulinemia and blood pressure: Relationships in patients with primary and secondary hypertension, and with or without glucose metabolism impairment. Am J Hypertens 3:521-526, 1990.
9. Ferrari P, Weidmann P, Shaw S, et al. Altered insulin sensitivity, hyperinsulinemia and dyslipidemia in individuals with a hypertensive parent. Am J Med 91:589-596, 1991.
10. Allemann Y, Horber FF, Colombo M, et al. Insulin sensitivity and body fat distribution in normotensive offspring of hypertensive parents. Lancet 341:327-331, 1993.
11. Facchini F, Chen Y-DI, Clinkingbeard C, et al. Insulin resistance, hyperinsulinemia, and dyslipidemia in nonobese individuals with a family history of hypertension. Am J Hypertens 5:694-699, 1992.
12. Ohno Y, Suzuki H, Yamakawa H, et al. Impaired insulin sensitivity in young, lean normotensive offspring of essential hypertensive: Possible role of disturbed calcium metabolism. J Hypertens 11:421-426, 1993.
13. Beatty OL, Harper R, Sheridan B, et al. Insulin resistance in offspring of hypertensive parents. BMJ 307:92-96, 1993.
14. Mbanya J-C, Wilkinson R, Thomas T, et al. Hypertension and hyperinsulinemia: A relation in diabetes but not in essential hypertension. Lancet I:733-734, 1988.
15. Donhaue RP, Skyler JS, Sneiderman N, et al. Hyperinsulinemia and elevated blood pressure: Cause, confounder, or coincidence? Am J Epidemiol 132:827-836, 1990.
16. Collins VR, Dowse GK, Finch CF, et al. An inconsistent relationship between insulin and blood pressure in three Pacific Island populations. J Clin Epidemiol 43:1369-1378, 1990.
17. Saad MF, Lillioja S, Nyomba BL, et al. Racial differences in the relation between blood pressure and insulin resistance. N Eng J Med 324:733-739, 1991.
18. European Group for the Study of Insulin Resistance (EGIR). Insulin resistance, hyperinsulinemia, and blood pressure. Role of age and obesity. Hypertension 30:1144-1149, 1992.
19. Skarfors ET, Lithell HO, Selinus I. Risk factors for the development of hypertension: A 10-year longitudinal study in middle-aged men. J Hypertens 9:217-223, 1991.
20. Lissner L, Bengtsson C, Lapidus L, et al. Fasting insulin in relation to subsequent blood pressure changes and hypertension in women. Hypertension 20:797-801, 1992.
21. Taittonen L, Uhari M, Nuutinen M, et al. Insulin and blood pressure among healthy children. Am J Hypertens 9:193-199, 1996.
22. Raitakari OT, Porkka KVK, Rönnemaa T, et al. The role of insulin in clustering of serum lipids and blood pressure in children and adolescents. Diabetologia 38:1042-1050, 1995.
23. Meigs JB. Invited commentary: Insulin resistance syndrome? Syndrome X? A syndrome at all? Factor analysis reveals patterns in the fabric of correlated metabolic risk factors. Am J Epidemiol 152:908-911, 2000.
24. Yeni-Komshian H, Carantoni M, Abbasi F, et al. Relationship between several surrogate estimates of insulin resistance and quantification of insulin-mediated glucose disposal in 490 healthy, nondiabetic volunteers. Diabetes Care 23:171-175, 2000.
25. Zavaroni I, Mazza S, Dall'Aglio E, et al. Prevalence of hyperinsulinaemia in patients with high blood pressure. J Intern Med 231:235-240, 1992.
26. Anderson AE, Mark AL. The vasodilator action of insulin: Implications for the insulin hypothesis of hypertension. Hypertension 21:136-141, 1993.
27. Olefsky JM, Reaven GM, Farquhar JW. Effects of weight reduction on obesity: Studies or carbohydrate and lipid metabolism. J Clin Invest 53:64-76, 1974.
28. Reisin E, Abel R, Modan M, et al. Effect of weight loss without salt restriction on the reduction of blood pressure in overweight hypertensive patients. N Engl J Med 298:1-6, 1978.
29. Su H-Y, Sheu WH-H, Chin H-ML, et al. Effect of weight loss on blood pressure and insulin resistance in normotensive and hypertensive obese individuals. Am J Hypertens 8:1016-1071, 1995.
30. Krotkiewski M, Mandroukas K, Sjostrom L, et al. Effects of long-term physical training on body fat metabolism, and blood pressure in obesity. Metabolism 28:650-658, 1979.
31. Rosenthal M, Haskell WL, Solomon R, et al. Demonstration of a relationship between level of physical training and insulin-stimulated glucose utilization in normal humans. Diabetes 32:408-411, 1983.
32. Tedde R, Sechi LA, Marigliano A, et al. Antihypertensive effect of insulin reduction in diabetic-hypertensive patients. Am J Hypertens 2:163-170, 1989.
33. Randeree HA, Omar MAK, Motala AA, et al. Effect of insulin therapy on blood pressure in NIDDM patients with secondary failure. Diabetes Care 15:1258-1263, 1992.
34. Reaven GM. Role of insulin resistance in human disease. Diabetes 37:1595-1607, 1988.
35. Reaven GM. The insulin resistance syndrome. Curr Atheroscler Rep 5:364-371, 2003.
36. Abbasi F, McLaughlin T, Lamendola C, et al. The relationship between glucose disposal in response to physiological hyperinsulinemia and basal glucose and free fatty acid concentrations in healthy volunteers. J Clin Endocrinol Metab 85:1251-1254, 2000.
37. Skott P, Vaag A, Bruum NE, et al. Effect of insulin on renal sodium handling in hyperinsulinemic type 2 (non-insulin-dependent) diabetic patients with peripheral insulin resistance. Diabetologia 34:275-281, 1991.
38. Muscelli E, Natali A, Bianchi S, et al. Effect of insulin on renal sodium and uric acid handling in essential hypertension. Am J Hypertens 9:746-752, 1996.
39. Facchini FS, Riccardo A, Stoohs A, et al. Enhanced sympathetic nervous system activity-the linchpin between insulin resistance, hyperinsulinemia, and heart rate. Am J Hypertens 9:1013-1017, 1996.
40. Reaven GM. The kidney: An unwilling accomplice in Syndrome X. Am J Kidney Dis 30:928-931, 1997.
41. DeFronzo RA, Cooke C, Andres R, et al. The effect of insulin in renal handling of sodium, potassium, calcium and phosphate in man. J Clin Invest 55:845-855, 1975.
42. Sharma AM, Schorr U, Distler A. Insulin resistance in young salt-sensitive normotensive subjects. Hypertension 21:273-279, 1993.
43. Zavaroni I, Coruzzi P, Bonini L, et al. Association between salt sensitivity and insulin concentrations in patients with hypertension. Am J Hypertens 8:855-858, 1995.
44. Facchini FS, DoNascimento C, Reaven GM, et al. Blood pressure, sodium intake, insulin resistance, and urinary nitrate excretion. Hypertension 33:1008-1012, 1999.

45. Paffenbarger RS, Thorne MC, Wing AL. Chronic disease in former college students: VIII. Characteristics in youth predisposing to hypertension in later years. Am J Epidemiol 88:25-32, 1968.

46. Selby JV, Friedman GD, Quesenberry CP. Precursors of essential hypertension: Pulmonary function, heart rate, uric acid, serum cholesterol and other serum chemistries. Am J Epidemiol 131:1017-1027, 1990.

47. Troisi RJ, Weiss ST, Parker DR, et al. Relation of obesity, insulin, and sympathetic nervous system activity. Hypertension 17:669-677, 1991.

48. O'Hare JA, Minaker KL, Meneilly GS, et al. Effect of insulin on plasma norepinephrine and 3,4 dihydroxyphenylalanine in obese men. Metabolism 38:322-329, 1989.

49. Collins R, Peto R, MacMahon S, et al. Blood pressure, stroke and coronary heart disease. Pt. 2. Short-term reductions in blood pressure: Overview of randomized drug trials in their epidemiological context. Lancet 335:827-838, 1990.

50. Reaven GM. Insulin resistance, compensatory hyperinsulinemia, and coronary heart disease: Syndrome X. *In* Sobell BE, Schneider DJ, (eds): Medical Management of Diabetes and Heart Disease. Marcel Dekker, New York, 2002; pp 117-136.

51. Sheuh WH-H, Jeng C-Y, Shieh S-M, et al. Insulin resistance and abnormal electrocardiograms in patients with high blood pressure. Am J Hypertens 5:444-448, 1992.

52. Jeppesen J, Hein HO, Suadicani P, et al. High triglycerides and low HDL cholesterol and blood pressure and risk of ischemic heart disease. Hypertension 36:226-239, 2000.

53. Jeppesen J, Hein HO, Suadicani P, et al. Low triglycerides-high high-density lipoprotein cholesterol and risk of ischemic heart disease. Arch Intern Med 161:361-366, 2001.

54. Reaven GM. Treatment of hypertension; focus on prevention of coronary heart disease. J Clin Endocrinol Metab 76:537-540, 1993.

55. Ross R. The pathogenesis of atherosclerosis. N Engl J Med 314:488-500, 1986.

56. Chen N-G, Abbasi F, Lamendola C, et al. Mononuclear cell adherence to cultured endothelium is enhanced by hypertension and insulin resistance in healthy nondiabetic volunteers. Circulation 100:940-943, 1999.

57. Stuhlinger MC, Abbasi F, Chu JW, et al. Relationship between insulin resistance and an endogenous nitric oxide synthase inhibitor. JAMA 287:1420-1426, 2002.

58. Vallance P. Importance of asymmetrical dimethylarginine in cardiovascular risk. Lancet 358:2096-2097, 2001.

# Chapter 14

# Remodeling of Resistance Arteries in Hypertension

## Ernesto L. Schiffrin, Hope Intengan

Essential hypertension is characterized by the presence of increased peripheral vascular resistance to blood flow.[1] This results from increased energy dissipation which occurs mainly at the level of small arteries and arterioles, vessels with a lumen diameter measuring less than 400 µm and usually more than 50 µm, the major site of generation of vascular resistance.[2] These vessels include small arteries with a lumen of 400 to 100 µm and arterioles that have smaller diameters. Resistance arteries may play an important role in the development of hypertension and its complications.[3,4] Resistance to flow varies inversely with the fourth power of the blood vessel radius according to Poiseuille's Law. Thus, small decreases in lumen size will significantly increase resistance. The vascular changes that result in a decreased lumen size in resistance arteries in hypertension may be structural, mechanical, or functional. We do not know whether they are a primary abnormalities or the consequences of hemodynamic or endocrine, paracrine, or autocrine effects triggered by blood pressure elevation or other unknown mechanisms, which could be genetic, metabolic, or humoral.

## STRUCTURAL CHANGES IN RESISTANCE ARTERIES IN HYPERTENSION

### Small Arteries

Structural changes of small, resistance arteries in hypertension may occur as eutrophic or hypertrophic remodeling (Figure 14–1).[5] Eutrophic remodeling is usually found in mild to moderate (stage 1) hypertension.[6,7] It is characterized by a reduced outer diameter and lumen, whereas the cross-sectional area of the media is normal, resulting in a greater media:lumen ratio. In this type of remodeling there is no true vascular hypertrophy, but rather a rearrangement of smooth muscle cells around a smaller lumen, associated with an increased extracellular matrix deposition (mainly collagen fibers and fibronectin).[8] In experimental hypertensive models, this type of remodeling is generally found when the renin-angiotensin system plays an important role, such as in spontaneously hypertensive rats (SHR)[9] and 2-kidney 1 clip Goldblatt hypertensive rats.[10] In humans, eutrophic remodeling is found in patients with essential hypertension and modest blood pressure elevations.[5-8,11] The mechanism that leads to eutrophic remodeling is unclear. Maintenance of media volume may involve a combination of growth and apoptosis, the latter localized peripherally in the vessel. Inward cell growth decreases lumen diameter. Enhanced apoptosis occurs indeed in various models of hypertension, including deoxycorticosterone (DOCA)-salt hypertensive rats[12] and angiotensin-induced hypertensive rats.[13] Eutrophic remodeling may also be the result of chronic vasoconstriction.[14]

In hypertrophic remodeling there is true vascular hypertrophy, with thickening of the media that encroaches on the lumen, associated with increased media:lumen ratio and media cross-sectional area (see Figure 14–1). Hypertrophic remodeling predominates in rat models of severe hypertension in which the endothelin system is activated, such as DOCA-salt hypertensive rats,[15] 1-kidney 1 clip Goldblatt hypertensive rats,[16] and Dahl-salt sensitive hypertensive rats.[17] In humans, hypertrophic remodeling has been reported in renovascular hypertension and pheochromocytoma.[18] Both types of remodeling may be present to varying degrees, and "remodeling" and "growth" indices[11] are used to approximate their relative contributions. In hypertrophic remodeling there may be increased smooth muscle cell number and/or size[19] as well as augmented deposition of extracellular proteins such as collagen and fibronectin. In small arteries from SHR[20] and from essential hypertensive patients,[8] collagen deposition is significantly enhanced, which may play an important role modulating cell growth (Figure 14–2).

Diminished activity of matrix metalloproteinases (MMP), which degrade extracellular matrix proteins,[21] may play a role in the accumulation of extracellular matrix in resistance arteries. Serum concentrations of MMP-1 were diminished in hypertensive patients in whom vascular type I collagen was augmented.[22] In the mesenteric arterial bed, MMP-1 and MMP-3 activity were decreased in young SHR before established hypertension developed, whereas pro-MMP2 and activated MMP-2 were diminished in mesenteric arteries from adult SHR.[23] These changes may favor accumulation of types IV and V collagen, fibronectin, and proteoglycans.[24,25]

The stiffness of the wall of small arteries is altered in experimental and essential hypertension.[23] Distensibility and compliance of the vessel wall are determined by the stiffness of wall components, the geometry of the vessel and intraluminal pressure. Second-order cerebral small arteries from stroke-prone SHR (SHR-sp) are less distensible than those of their normotensive counterparts, which may account in part for the reduction in their external diameter.[26] In contrast, third-order small arteries of less than 200 µm in diameter have normal wall mechanics, and therefore present true remodeling rather than changes attributable to altered wall mechanics.[26] In genetic and experimental rat models of salt-sensitive hypertension, mesenteric resistance artery stiffness not different from that in normotensive controls.[27,28] However, in SHR the stiffness of mesenteric small arteries may be initially reduced,[29] followed later by increases in the stiffness of wall components, with reduced compliance and distensibility, in part a consequence of collagen deposition.[20] This underlines the heterogeneity of remodeling and mechanical changes in resistance vessels along the vascular tree, in different vascular beds and in different experimental models. Wall stiffness of subcutaneous small arteries from hypertensive patients either

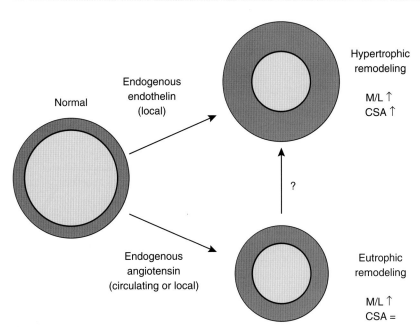

Normal

Endogenous
endothelin
(local)

Endogenous
angiotensin
(circulating or local)

Hypertrophic
remodeling

M/L ↑
CSA ↑

?

Eutrophic
remodeling

M/L ↑
CSA =

**Figure 14–1** Eutrophic and hypertrophic remodeling of resistance arteries in hypertension and potential agents that play a role in inducing the different types of remodeling of small arteries. As hypertension progresses, eutrophic remodeling may evolve toward hypertrophic remodeling under the influence of angiotensin II and/or endothelin-1, other growth factors, and high blood pressure. (Reproduced with permission from Intengan HD, Schiffrin EL. Structure and mechanical properties of resistance arteries in hypertension: Review. Hypertension 36:312-318, 2000.)

was not increased compared with that of normotensive subjects[30] or was slightly decreased.[8] Different mechanisms may account for changes in stiffness. As a consequence of the closer alignment of cellular and fibrillar components resulting from changes in cell-extracellular attachment, collagen fibers may be recruited at higher distending pressures in small arteries from mild hypertensive patients early in the disease. Later, because of the smaller lumen and greater collagen:elastin ratio, compliance of resistance arteries may be progressively reduced in vessels from hypertensive subjects as a result of tensing of the collagen jacket at earlier portions of the pressure curve. Decreased wall stiffness in cerebral arterioles from SHR-sp, has been attributed to increased elastin content.[31] In contrast, in peripheral resistance arteries, small artery stiffness was increased in SHR in association with increased volume density of collagen and/or increased collagen:elastin ratio.[20] Extracellular constituents other than collagen and elastin, such as proteoglycans may also modulate vascular stiffness. Removal of chondroitin-dermatan sulfate–containing glycosaminoglycans from mesenteric resistance arteries may increase their stiffness.[32]

## Arterioles

Large arterioles (lumen diameter <100 μm) also undergo remodeling as described for small arteries. Rarefaction, with reduction of arteriolar density, occurs at the level of smaller arterioles (lumen diameter <40 μm) and may increase vascular resistance. It may initially be functional and later anatomic and permanent. Rarefaction has been reported in different experimental rat models of hypertension.[33]

## FUNCTIONAL ABNORMALITIES OF RESISTANCE ARTERIES IN HYPERTENSION

Enhanced constriction of resistance arteries in hypertension may increase peripheral resistance by reducing lumen diameter.

Increased responsiveness to norepinephrine and enhanced myogenic tone have been reported in experimental hypertension.[34,35] Impaired endothelium-dependent relaxation has been repeatedly reported[36] and may also contribute to increased constriction. However, most vasoconstrictor agents, including endothelin-1, vasopressin, and norepinephrine elicit normal or diminished constrictor responses,[34,37] suggesting that augmented vasoconstriction in hypertension may result from amplification of vasoconstrictor responses by the structural or mechanical reduction of lumen diameter, according to Laplace's law.[38] Whether this actually occurs has been challenged.[39] Enhanced constriction in response to angiotensin II may be present as a consequence of post-receptor signaling changes, either in the coupling of the receptor to G proteins or in other events in the cascade that lead to increased calcium release and entry into the smooth muscle cell in hypertension.[40]

Extracellular matrix components may contribute to abnormal function of resistance arteries in hypertension (see Figure 14–2). Peptides with the integrin-binding sequence arginine-glycine-aspartate (RGD) induced endothelium-dependent relaxation of rat skeletal muscle arterioles by binding to $\alpha_v\beta_3$ integrins.[41] Because $\alpha_v\beta_3$ integrins are more abundant in arteries from adult SHR,[20] $\alpha_v\beta_3$-mediated relaxation could be enhanced. However, in hypertension, $\alpha_v\beta_3$ integrins may be unavailable for ligand binding or occupied, and may therefore not induce vascular relaxation. Another RGD-containing peptide, glycine-arginine-glycine-aspartate-serine-proline (GRGDSP), induced endothelium-independent afferent arteriole constriction with increased intracellular calcium concentration.[42] In hypertension and with aging, fibronectin and $\alpha_5\beta_1$ integrins are increased,[20] and accordingly $\alpha_5\beta_1$-integrin occupancy could contribute to increased contractility and vascular resistance. Modulation of MMPs may also play a role in changes in vasoactive behavior. Inhibition of vascular MMP-2 in rat mesenteric arteries reduced the vasoconstrictor effects of big endothelin-1. The mechanism for this effect was cleavage of big endothelin-1 and release of the new vasoconstrictor peptide ET-1[1-32].[43]

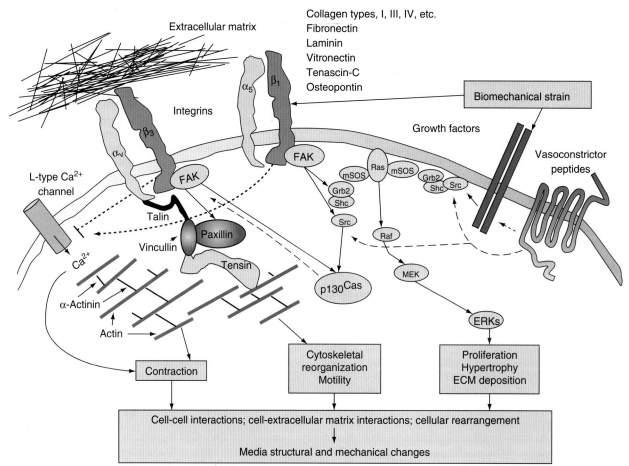

**Figure 14–2** Associations between extracellular matrix proteins and integrins on the smooth muscle cell surface, and intracellular signaling pathways leading to cytoskeletal reorganization and to cell motility, migration, and growth. These processes contribute to rearrangement of smooth muscle cells, increased deposition of extracellular matrix components and changes in cell-cell and cell-matrix interactions, processes that are at the origin of mechanical alterations and structural remodeling in hypertension. G-protein–coupled receptors (angiotensin, endothelin, and others), acting directly or via transactivation of growth factor receptors, as well as biomechanical strain, activate MAP kinases via membrane-associated c-Src that induces association with the adaptor protein complex Shc-Grb-Sos and downstream activation of the Ras:Raf:MAP kinase cascade. MAP kinase acts on nuclear and cytoplasmic targets to initiate cell growth. G-protein–coupled receptors interact with integrins via p130^Cas. Extracellular matrix components directly activate integrins, and via focal adhesion kinase (FAK)-dependent pathways, phosphorylate cytoskeletal proteins (paxillin, talin, actin) that regulate cytoskeletal organization and motility. Integrin-activated FAK also influences cell growth by activating MAP kinases. By mechanisms that remain unclear, integrin activation triggers opening of various channels, including L-type $Ca^{2+}$ channels, modifying $Ca^{2+}$ transport and vascular smooth muscle cell contraction. Functional and structural interactions between extracellular matrix proteins and smooth muscle cells through adhesion molecules may be important in maintaining vascular wall integrity. Alterations in these interactions, possibly by modifications in cell attachment sites, could contribute to changes in vascular media stiffness. ECM, extracellular matrix; FAK, p125 focal adhesion kinase; ERKs; extracellular signal-regulated kinases, also known as mitogen-activated protein (MAP) kinases; MEK, mitogen-activated ERK-activating kinase, also known as MAP kinase kinase (MAPKK). (Reproduced with permission from Intengan HD, Schiffrin EL. Structure and mechanical properties of resistance arteries in hypertension: Review. Hypertension 36:312-318, 2000.)

## SUMMARY

Abnormalities of endothelial cells, smooth muscle cells, adhesion molecules, and the extracellular matrix in the vasculature may contribute to structural, mechanical, or functional changes that reduce the lumen diameter of small arteries and arterioles and contribute to increases in vascular resistance in hypertension. A deeper understanding of these

vascular alterations and the mechanisms that produce them may lead to the development of new therapeutic approaches to prevent target organ damage in cardiovascular disease.

## Acknowledgments

The authors' work was supported by grant 13570 and by a group grant to the Multidisciplinary Research Group on

Hypertension both from the Canadian Institutes of Health Research (CIHR).

# References

1. Lund-Johanson P. Haemodynamics in early essential hypertension—still an area of controversy. J Hypertens 1:209-213, 1983.
2. Bohlen HG. Localization of vascular resistance changes during hypertension. Hypertension 8:181-183, 1986.
3. Schiffrin EL. Reactivity of small blood vessels in hypertension: Relation with structural changes. Hypertension 19(Suppl II): II1-II9, 1992.
4. Schiffrin EL. Resistance arteries as endpoints in hypertension. Blood Pressure 6(Suppl 2):24-30, 1997.
5. Mulvany MJ, Baumbach GL, Aalkjaer C, et al. Vascular remodeling. Letter to the Editor. Hypertension 28:505-506, 1996.
6. Schiffrin EL, Deng LY, Larochelle P. Morphology of resistance arteries and comparison of effects of vasoconstrictors in mild essential hypertensive patients. Clin Invest Med 16:177-186, 1993.
7. Schiffrin EL, Deng LY, Larochelle P. Effects of a beta blocker or a converting enzyme inhibitor on resistance arteries in essential hypertension. Hypertension 23:83-91, 1994.
8. Intengan HD, Deng LY, Li JS, Schiffrin EL. Mechanics and composition of human subcutaneous resistance arteries in essential hypertension. Hypertension 33:569-574, 1999.
9. Deng LY, Schiffrin EL. Effects of endothelin-1 and vasopressin on resistance arteries of spontaneously hypertensive rats. Am J Hypertens 5:817-822, 1992.
10. Li JS, Knafo L, Turgeon A, et al. Effect of endothelin antagonism on blood pressure and vascular structure in renovascular hypertensive rats. Am J Physiol Heart Circ Physiol 40:H88-H93, 1996.
11. Heagerty AM, Aalkjaer C, Bund SJ, et al. Small artery structure in hypertension: Dual processes of remodeling and growth. Hypertension 21:391-397, 1993.
12. Heagerty AM, Aalkjaer C, Bund SJ, et al. Small artery structure in hypertension: Dual processes of remodeling and growth. Hypertension 21:391-397, 1993.
13. Diep QN, Li JS, Schiffrin EL. In vivo study of AT(1) and AT(2) angiotensin receptors in apoptosis in rat blood vessels. Hypertension 34:617-624, 1999.
14. Bakker ENTP, Van der Meulen ET, Van den Berg BM, et al. Inward remodeling follows chronic vasoconstriction in isolated resistance arteries. J Vasc Res 39:12-20, 2002.
15. Deng LY, Schiffrin EL. Effects of endothelin on resistance arteries of DOCA-salt hypertensive rats. Am J Physiol 262:H1782-787, 1992.
16. Deng LY, Schiffrin EL. Morphologic and functional alterations of mesenteric small resistance arteries in early renal hypertension in the rat. Am J Physiol 261:H1171-1177, 1991.
17. D'Uscio LV, Barton M, Shaw S, et al. Structure and function of small arteries in salt-induced hypertension—effects of chronic endothelin-subtype-a-receptor blockade. Hypertension 30:905-911, 1997.
18. Rizzoni D, Porteri E, Castellano M, et al. Vascular hypertrophy and remodeling in secondary hypertension. Hypertension 28:785-790, 1996.
19. Lee RM. Vascular changes at the prehypertensive phase in the mesenteric arteries from spontaneously hypertensive rats. Blood Vessels 22:105-126, 1985.
20. Intengan HD, Thibault G, Li JS, et al. Resistance artery mechanics, structure, and extracellular components in spontaneously hypertensive rats. Effects of angiotensin receptor antagonism and converting enzyme inhibition. Circulation 100:2267-2275, 1999.
21. Galis ZS, Sukhova GK, Lark MW, et al. Increased expression of matrix metalloproteinases and matrix degrading activity in vulnerable regions of human atherosclerotic plaques. J Clin Invest 94:2494-2503, 1994.
22. Laviades C, Varo N, Fernandez J, et al. Abnormalities of the extracellular degradation of collagen type I in essential hypertension. Circulation 98:535-540, 1998.
23. Intengan HD, Schiffrin EL. Structure and mechanical properties of resistance arteries in hypertension: Review. Hypertension 36:312-318, 2000.
24. Hein M, Fisher J, Kim DK, et al. Vascular smooth muscle phenotype influences glycosaminoglycan composition and growth effects of extracellular matrix. J Vasc Res 33:433-441, 1996.
25. Castro CM, Cruzado MC, Miatello RM, et al. Proteoglycan production by vascular smooth muscle cells from resistance arteries of hypertensive rats. Hypertension 34:893-896, 1999.
26. Hadju MA, Baumbach GL. Mechanics of large and small cerebral arteries in chronic hypertension. Am J Physiol 266:H1027-H1033, 1994.
27. Intengan HD, Schiffrin EL. Mechanical properties of mesenteric resistance arteries from Dahl salt-resistant and salt-sensitive rats: role of endothelin-1. J Hypertens 16:1907-1912, 1998.
28. Intengan HD, He G, Schiffrin EL. Effect of vasopressin antagonism on structure and mechanics of small arteries and vascular expression of endothelin-1 in deoxycorticosterone acetate salt hypertensive rats. Hypertension 32:770-777, 1998.
29. Laurant PM, Touyz RM, Schiffrin EL. Effect of pressurization on mechanical properties of mesenteric small arteries from spontaneously hypertensive rats. J Vasc Res 34:117-125, 1997.
30. Thybo NK, Mulvany MJ, Jastrup B, et al. Some pharmacological and elastic characteristics of isolated subcutaneous small arteries from patients with essential hypertension. J Hypertens 14:993-998, 1996.
31. Baumbach GL, Dobrin PB, Hart MN, et al. Mechanics of cerebral arterioles in hypertensive rats. Circ Res 62:56-64, 1988.
32. Gandley RE, McLaughlin MK, Koob TJ, et al. Contribution of chondroitin-dermatan sulfate-containing proteoglycans to the function of rat mesenteric arteries. Am J Physiol 273: H952-H960, 1997.
33. Hashimoto H, Prewitt RL, Efaw CW. Alterations in the microvasculature of one-kidney, one-clip hypertensive rats. Am J Physiol 253:H933-940, 1987.
34. Aalkjaer C, Heagerty AM, Petersen KK, et al. Evidence for increased media thickness, increased neuronal amine uptake, and depressed excitation-contraction coupling in isolated resistance vessels from essential hypertensives. Circ Res 61:181-186, 1987.
35. Izzard AS, Heagerty AM. Impaired flow-dependent dilatation in distal mesenteric arteries from the spontaneously hypertensive rat. J Physiol 518:239-245, 1999.
36. Deng LY, Li JS, Schiffrin EL. Endothelium-dependent relaxation of small arteries from essential hypertensive patients: Mechanisms and comparison with normotensive subjects and with responses of vessels from spontaneously hypertensive rats. Clin Sci 88:611-622, 1995.
37. Schiffrin EL, Deng LY, Larochelle P. Blunted effects of endothelin upon small subcutaneous resistance arteries of mild essential hypertensive patients. J Hypertens 10:437-444, 1992.
38. Folkow B. Physiological aspects of primary hypertension. Physiol Rev 62:347-504, 1982.
39. Izzard AS, Bund SJ, Heagerty AM. Increased wall-lumen ratio of mesenteric vessels from the spontaneously hypertensive rat is not associated with increased contractility under isobaric conditions. Hypertension 28:604-608, 1996.
40. Touyz RM, Schiffrin EL. Signal transduction mechanisms mediating the physiological and pathophysiological actions of angiotensin II in vascular smooth muscle cells. Pharmacol Rev 52:639-672, 2000.
41. Mogford JE, Davis GE, Platts SH, et al. Vascular smooth muscle $\alpha_v\beta_3$ integrin mediates arteriolar vasodilation in response to RGD peptides. Circ Res 79:821-826, 1996.

42. Mogford JE, Davis GE, Meininger GA. RGDN peptide interaction with endothelial $\alpha_5\beta_1$ integrin causes sustained endothelin-dependent vasoconstriction of rat skeletal muscle arterioles. J Clin Invest 100:1647-1653, 1997.

43. Fernandez-Patron C, Radomski MW, Davidge ST. Vascular matrix metalloproteinase-2 cleaves big endothelin-1 yielding a novel vasoconstrictor. Circ Res 85:906-911, 1999.

# Chapter 15

# Clinical Applications of Arterial Stiffness in Hypertension

## Roland Asmar

Epidemiologic studies have shown that cardiovascular disease related to arterial lesions is the leading cause of morbidity and mortality in the Western countries. Arterial abnormalities have been observed at early stages of cardiovascular diseases, particularly in the presence of risk factors, principally hypertension. The arteries are the site of hypertension-induced organ damage that compromises the function of various organs: the kidney (nephrosclerosis), the brain (stroke), the heart (angina-myocardial infarction), and the aorta (aneurysm). Therapeutic trials have shown that arterial lesions appear in some treated hypertensive patients and that the effect of cardiovascular drugs on the arterial wall may differ among compounds. Accordingly, assessment of arterial wall properties has been embraced by the world of hypertension research as an important activity.

During the last decade we have had an extraordinary advance in the methodologic aspects of noninvasive determination of the mechanical properties of the large arteries, principally arterial stiffness, related to the development of new ultrasound techniques and computer processing. A consequence of this remarkable development is the availability of devices that allow not only the evaluation of arterial stiffness but also its estimation at different sites in the arterial tree and assessment of other hemodynamic parameters of the arterial wall such as pulse pressure, pulse contour analysis, arterial diameter, wall thickness, and distal compliance.

The growing interest in arterial stiffness is reflected by an increasing number of publications, by the number of ongoing studies, and by development of drugs that act specifically on the arterial wall. Despite this increasing interest, there remains a profusion of methodology and terminology in the literature that can cause confusion and make it impossible to compare results between studies and between research groups.[1] This review is focused on the clinical applications of arterial stiffness measurements in patients at high cardiovascular risk, principally those with hypertension.

## DEFINITIONS AND REFERENCE VALUES

In clinical research, *arterial stiffness* is the most simple and common term used to describe the mechanical properties of the large arteries.[2-5] The terms *compliance* and *distensibility* are also widely used, although they imply a more quantitative approach. Some fundamental hemodynamic principles should be recalled to understand the different definitions used to describe arterial stiffness in clinical practice, to note their limitations, and to provide some normal values.

### Hemodynamic Basis

The most widely accepted model of the arterial system is a simple tube with one end representing the peripheral resist-ance and the other receiving blood from the heart.[5] A wave generated by cardiac contraction travels along the tube toward the periphery and is reflected back from the periphery. Thus the pressure wave at any point along the tube is the resultant of both the incident and the reflected waves (Figure 15–1). The incident wave is influenced by the left ventricular ejection and the arterial stiffness (pulse wave velocity [PWV]); the reflected wave is related to arterial stiffness and the characteristics of the reflected waves. *Local* arterial stiffness refers to measurements performed locally on a cross-sectional area of straight artery. *Regional* (segmental) stiffness refers to measurements performed over a segment of the arterial tree or on a regional arterial circulation. *Systemic* (global) stiffness refers to the compliance of the whole arterial tree. In clinic, arterial stiffness should be investigated either locally to explore vascular damage or in the regional and/or systemic circulations to explore the interactions between the heart and vessels (Table 15–1).

## Indices of Local Arterial Stiffness

In most cases, measurements are done locally on superficial and straight arteries. The vessel is considered a portion of a cylindrical tube in which the relationship between blood pressure and volume (or lumen diameter or cross-sectional area) is established, and its slope represents an index of stiffness. From these measurements, stiffness changes were described as universally accepted indices called *distensibility*, *compliance*, *elastic modulus* (Peterson), and *incremental elastic modulus* (Young) (see Table 15–1). Because of the curvilinearity of the pressure-diameter relationship, all of these parameters are highly pressure dependent. Thus, to evaluate the degree of stiffness of the arterial wall material, blood pressure should be considered and isobaric measurements should be performed according to the local arterial pressure.

Local determinations of arterial stiffness are performed by using ultrasound techniques in which several aspects have to be considered. First, the stiffness indices represent dynamic and not static measurements.[5,6] Therefore, changes in pressure (pulse pressure) and changes in volume (or lumen diameter or cross-sectional area) are measured locally at the same arterial location (e.g., the carotid). Second, because the measurements are exclusively cross-sectional, it is assumed that the length of the artery remains constant over time. Third, because the arterial tree is heterogeneous, it is important to investigate both proximal (elastic) and distal arteries (muscular).[7]

## Indices of Regional and Systemic Arterial Stiffness

The most common measure of regional (segmental) arterial stiffness is PWV.[8] The principle of PWV is based on the fact that left ventricular ejection volume of blood into the

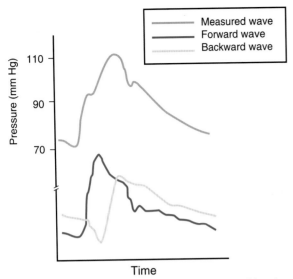

**Figure 15–1** Decomposition of the measured ( – ) blood pressure into a forward (— incident) wave and a backward (.... reflected) wave.

ascending aorta dilates the aortic wall and generates a pulse wave that is propagated throughout the arterial tree at a finite speed determined by the elastic and geometric properties of the arterial wall and the characteristics (density) of the contained fluid (blood). Higher velocity corresponds to higher arterial stiffness. PWV is related to the Young's modulus (E) of a thin-walled homogenous elastic tube by the formula PWV = $\sqrt{E.h/2r\rho}$, where $\rho$ is the density of blood (1.05), $E$ the

incremental elastic modulus, and *h/2r* the wall thickness divided by diameter. PWV velocity is calculated by using the formula PWV = D/T, where *D* represents the distance traveled by the pulse between two recording sites and *T* represents the transit time needed by the front wave (which is not influenced by wave reflection) to travel from one site to the other (Figure 15–2).

Characteristic impedance is another valuable index of arterial stiffness and relates absolute arterial pressure to absolute velocity of flow at the same site in the absence of wave reflections.[5] Characteristic impedance (Zc) is related to PWV by the formula Zc = PWV/$\rho$ ($\rho$ = blood density).

It is important to note that the mechanical properties of arteries and wave reflections are constantly interacting. When the arterial wall is stiff, wave travel is rapid, and the reflected wave merges with the systolic part of the incident wave, causing a supplementary increase in pressure in systole (called augmentation index) and a low pressure in diastole, resulting in an increase in pulse pressure.[5,9] This is a manifestation rather than a measure or index of arterial stiffness.

Systemic or total (called also "capacitive") arterial compliance (C) is an estimate of the compliance of the whole arterial tree via simple models of the arterial circulation by using analysis of the arterial pressure wave. During diastole, the general shape of the diastolic pressure curve commonly assumes a simple monoexponential form, enabling an analogy with the electrical RC model. The limitation of this classical model is that pressure oscillations are considered to be instantaneous and occurring simultaneously in all parts of the arterial tree.[10] Moreover, methods for calculating total arterial compliance likewise require noninvasive estimation of cardiac output and assumption of a Windkessel model in which no wave reflection

**Table 15–1** Definition and Units of the Various Indices of Arterial Stiffness

| | |
|---|---|
| Arterial distensibility | Relative diameter (or area) change for a pressure increment; the inverse of elastic modulus<br>$\Delta D/(\Delta P.D)$ (mm Hg$^{-1}$) |
| Arterial compliance | Absolute diameter (or area) change for a given pressure step at fixed vessel length<br>$\Delta D/\Delta P$ (cm/mm Hg) (or cm$^2$/mm Hg) |
| Volume elastic modulus | Pressure step required for (theoretical) 100% increase in volume<br>$\Delta P/(\Delta V/V)$ (mm Hg) = $\Delta P/(\Delta A/A)$ (mm Hg) where there is no change in length |
| Elastic modulus | The pressure step required for (theoretical) 100% stretch from resting diameter at fixed vessel length<br>$(\Delta P.D)/\Delta D$ (mm Hg) |
| Young's modulus | Elastic modulus per unit area; the pressure step per square centimeter required for (theoretical) 100% stretch from resting length<br>$\Delta P.D/(\Delta D.h)$ (mm Hg/cm) |
| Pulse wave velocity | Speed of travel of the pulse along an arterial segment<br>Distance/$\Delta t$ (cm/s) |
| Characteristic impedance | Relationship between pressure change and flow velocity in the absence of wave reflections<br>$\Delta P/\Delta V$ [(mm Hg/cm)/s] |
| Stiffness index | Ratio of logarithm (systolic/diastolic pressures) to (relative change in diameter)<br>$\beta$ Index = (Ps/Pd)/[(Ds – Dd)/Dd] (nondimensional) |
| "Capacitive compliance" | Relationship between pressure fall and volume fall in the arterial tree during the exponential component of diastolic pressure decay<br>$\Delta V/\Delta P$ (cm$^3$/mm Hg) |
| "Oscillatory compliance" | Relationship between oscillating pressure change and oscillating volume change around the exponential pressure decay during diastole<br>$\Delta V/\Delta P$ (cm$^3$/mm Hg) |

Note that mm Hg were used (100 mm Hg = 13.33 KPa) and that the ratio between stroke volume and pulse pressure or the beta index, a semi-logarithmic transformation of the volume elastic modulus, are not considered as true indices of arterial stiffness.
Abbreviations: P, pressure; D, diameter; V, volume; h, wall thickness; t, time; s, systolic; d, diastolic; A, cross-sectional area.

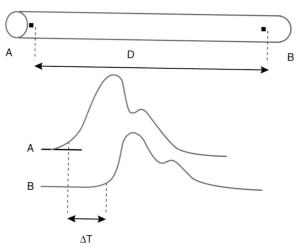

**Figure 15–2** Pulse wave velocity measurement. A = Wave recorded by the proximal transducer; B = wave recorded by the distal transducer; ΔT = time delay between the foot waves; D = distance travelled by the wave.

exits. Nevertheless, methods of pulse wave analysis concentrated exclusively on diastolic decay and using a modified Windkessel model have been proposed.[11]

## METHODS, DEVICES, AND PROCEDURES

This chapter will not give an exhaustive analysis of all the available methods and their reproducibility but will focus on some of those commonly used (Table 15–2).

### Assessment of Systemic and Segmental Arterial Stiffness and Wave Reflections

Most of these devices use measurements of pulse transit time or pulse contour analysis.

### Automated Doppler Recording for Pulse Wave Velocity Measurement

This system gives an automated measurement of PWV by using continuous Doppler.[12]

### Cardiovision System

The Cardiovision System (IMDP, Las Vegas, NV) uses computerized oscillometry (obtained from a brachial pressure cuff) to measure blood pressure and to derive an index of unloaded brachial arterial stiffness.[13]

### Complior System

The Complior System (Artech-Medical, Pantin, France) gives an automated measurement of PWV based on dedicated pressure transducers directly applied on the skin.[14] Two arterial segments, mainly the aortic trunk, the upper or the lower limbs, can be evaluated simultaneously. The system allows an indirect estimation of the central pulse pressure according to the classical water-hammer formula.

### HDI/Pulse Wave CR 2000

This technique (Hypertension Diagnosis Inc., Minnesota) is based on the radial pulse recording with a piezoelectric sensor strapped on the wrist and calibrated with a brachial oscillometric blood pressure recording.[11,15] The modified Windkessel model, on which this method is based, allows determination of proximal "capacitive" compliance (C1, which normally approximates 1.71-2.2 $cm^3/mm$ Hg) and distal "oscillatory" compliance (C2, which normally approximates 0.054-0.075 $cm^3/mm$ Hg).

### Magnetic Resonance Imaging

Magnetic resonance imaging (MRI) has been proposed as a non-invasive means of obtaining local distensibility or arterial PWV.[16]

### QKd System

The method is developed as an add-on device of the ambulatory blood pressure monitoring (ABPM) recording device Diasys (Novacor, Rueil-Malmaison, France).[17]

### Second Derivative of the Finger Plethysmogram (SDPTG)

This method (Fukuda Electric Co., Tokyo, Japan) is based on the analysis of the information contained in the derivatives of

**Table 15–2** Methods and Devices to Assess Arterial Stiffness

| Method/Device | Global Stiffness | Local Stiffness |
|---|---|---|
| Applanation Tonometry | PCA | |
| Automated Ultrasound recording | PWV | |
| Cine MRI | PWV | Aorta |
| Complior | PWV | |
| CR-2000 | PCA | |
| QKD System | Assimilated to transit time | |
| Second derivative of the finger plethysmograph | PCA | |
| SphygmoCor | PCA/PWV | |
| Subclavian pulse tracing-Doppler echocardiography | PCA | |
| Transesophageal echocardiography | | Aorta |
| Vascular echography-Frame Grabler processing | | Carotid |
| Wall Track System | PWV | Superficial arteries |

Cine MRI, cine magnetic resonance imaging; PCA, pulse contour analysis; PWV, pulse wave velocity.

the peripheral blood pressure pulse waveform obtained by finger plethysmography.[18]

### SphygmoCor System

The SphygmoCor device (PWV Medical, Sydney, Australia) is based on a peripheral pressure pulse recording with the applanation tonometer (Millar).[9,19] From the radial or carotid artery recording, this system calculates an index of wave reflection, the augmentation index, and the carotid and aortic pulse pressure. It also allows the measurements of transit time to calculate PWV between two arterial pressure waves recorded successively with the R wave of the electrocardiogram (ECG).

### Subclavian Pulse Tracing and Doppler Echocardiography Method

Measurements of arterial pressure at the level of the subclavian artery with a strain gauge transducer and measurement of aortic flow velocity with Doppler echocardiography are computerized to calculate arterial compliance with an electrical model.[20]

## Assessment of Local Arterial Stiffness

### Transesophageal Echocardiography

Transesophageal echocardiography enables measurement of the ascending aorta wall thickness and changes in diameter. Combination with the subclavian blood pressure enables calculation of the elastic modulus.[21]

### Vascular Echography Coupled with Frame Grabber Processing

Simultaneous measurement of blood pressure, carotid arterial diameter, and intima media thickness allows calculation of Peterson's elastic modulus, Young's elastic modulus, and beta index, which requires a semi-logarithmic transformation of the pressure measurements.[22]

### Wall Track System

The Wall Track System (WTS) (Pie Medical, Maastricht, The Netherlands) includes a vascular echo tracking device for the measurement of internal diameter at diastole, its pulsatile changes, and the intima media wall thickness.[23] The WTS also allows measurements of transit time to calculate PWV between two arterial sites recorded successively with the R wave of the ECG. The combination of WTS and local blood pressure recordings allows the calculation of local compliance and wall distensibility coefficients. Use of an additional pressure-adjusted water-filled cuff allows the calculation at the level of the radial artery of the elastic modulus over a large range of distension pressures.

## User Procedures: Standardization of the Examination Conditions

The patient conditions and the examination procedure are very similar to those used for blood pressure measurements and are summarized in Box 15–1.[24-29]

# DIAGNOSTIC VALUE OF ARTERIAL STIFFNESS MEASUREMENTS

## Age and Gender

Numerous studies have shown that arterial stiffness is closely related to age, the major factor influencing the mechanical properties of arteries. Various mechanisms, including the role of the endothelium, and media have been invoked to explain the observed changes with age.

An age-dependent increase in arterial stiffness and pulse pressure (both accompanied by an increase in systolic blood pressure [SBP] and a decrease in diastolic blood pressure [DBP] with age) in both healthy populations and populations with cardiovascular disease has been described independently of mean blood pressure or presence of other risk factors.[5,30] Aging has a different effect on central (elastic) arteries than on peripheral (muscular) arteries and arterioles. Central arteries stiffen progressively, whereas the stiffness of muscular arteries changes little with age.[7,31] These results have been reported in both sexes, although arterial diameter and length are smaller in women than in men. The extent of the increase in arterial stiffness with age may depend on several environmental or genetic factors.

## Blood Pressure

Relationships between arterial stiffness and blood pressure level vary widely among studies, depending on whether we consider the central or peripheral arterial pulse wave and the systolic, diastolic, mean, or pulse pressure. Population studies

---

**Box 15–1** Standardization of the Examination Procedure

- Rest period for at least 10 minutes at stable room temperature.
- Supine position is preferred. Patients may neither speak nor sleep during assessments.
- Patients have to refrain from smoking, eating, and drinking caffeine or alcohol for at least 3 hours before the examination.
- Repeated measurements should be performed under the same conditions, by the same observer, and using validated automated procedures where possible.
- The time of drug intake should be mentioned.
- A quality control of the obtained data has to be performed.
- If appropriate, correction for important confounding factors is possible. Absolute unadjusted values must always be given.
- Investigators have to be trained to avoid observer bias errors.

performed in untreated normotensives and hypertensives with large ranges of age and without any cardiovascular disease analyzed the determinants of PWV by using adequate statistical methods. Their results are in agreement and show that the major determinants of PWV are, independently, age and SBP. These findings are predictable, because the major determinant of SBP is the stiffness of large arteries. The influence of age and SBP differs in central arteries (carotid-femoral PWV), in which age is the major determinant, and in peripheral arteries (arm PWV), in which blood pressure is the major determinant. Table 15–3 shows the normal values of PWV measured in different arterial segments.

## Hypertension

Increased PWVs have been reported in hypertensives as compared with normotensives. However, these results have varied according to the arterial segment, blood pressure, and age adjustment.

It is well established that arterial abnormalities appear at an early stage of hypertension. These cannot be attributed solely to the stretching effect of elevated blood pressure but also reflect intrinsic alterations of the arterial wall that could represent either adaptive changes to the increase in arterial pressure or primary abnormalities of the vessel wall.

### Borderline and White-Coat Hypertension

Comparison of aortic (carotid-femoral) and arm (brachial-radial) PWVs, between young borderline hypertensives and age-matched normotensives showed higher PWVs in the borderline hypertensives at any mean blood pressure level.[32] These results suggested that the increased arterial stiffness noticed in borderline hypertensive patients is not solely due to the elevated pressure but also reflects intrinsic arterial wall changes (Figure 15–3). Similar results were observed in patients with white-coat hypertension as compared with normotensive controls.

### Persistent Hypertension

Numerous studies have reported stiffer arteries in patients with established hypertension as compared with normoten-

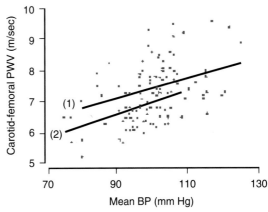

**Figure 15–3** Correlation between PWV and mean BP in borderline hypertensives (1,●) and normotensives (2▲). At any BP level, PWV is higher in age-matched hypertensives. (Adapted from Girerd X, Chanudet X, Larroque P, et al. Early arterial modifications in young patients with borderline hypertension. J Hypertens 7(Suppl):S45-S47, 1989.)

sive controls. Comparison of aortic (carotid-femoral) and arm (brachial-radial) PWVs between patients with essential hypertension and age-matched normotensive controls showed higher PWVs in hypertensives at any age. A population study of aortic pulse wave velocity (carotid-femoral) in normotensive and hypertensive patients showed higher PWV in hypertensives as compared with normotensives (11.8 ± 2.7 versus 8.5 ± 1.5 m/sec) (Figure 15–4).

Taken together, these findings showed (1) in borderline hypertension, higher carotid-femoral and brachial-radial PWV than in age-matched normotensives; (2) in white-coat hypertension, higher carotid-femoral PWV than in age-matched normotensives; (3) in sustained hypertension, higher pulse wave velocity than in normotensives at any given age. The elevated PWV and increased arterial stiffness cannot be attributed solely to the stretching effect of elevated blood pressure. Early hypertension-related abnormalities in the arterial wall also contribute.

In normotensives, there is a continuous decrease in compliance and distensibility from central to peripheral arteries.[5,33]

**Table 15–3** Normal Values of Pulse Wave Velocity

| Velocity | Normal Values |
|---|---|
| Thoracic aorta | 400–530 cm/sec |
| Abdominal aorta | 500–570 cm/sec |
| Aortic arch-femoral | 5.1 age (years) + 533 cm/sec |
| | 9.2 age (years) + 615 cm/sec |
| Carotid-femoral (site to site) | 775–980 cm/sec |
| | 0.06 systolic BP (mm Hg) + 0.09 age (years)-2.3 × $10^2$ m/sec |
| Carotid-femoral (distance substraction) | 620–930 cm/sec |
| Brachial-radial | 880 cm/sec |
| | 0.61 age (years) + 817 cm/sec |
| | 4.8 age (years) + 998 cm/sec |
| Femoral-foot artery | 830 cm/sec |
| | 4.43 age (years) + 718 cm/sec |
| | 5.6 age (years) + 791 cm/sec |

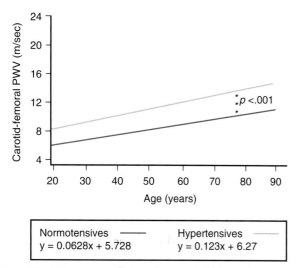

| Normotensives | Hypertensives |
|---|---|
| y = 0.0628x + 5.728 | y = 0.123x + 6.27 |

**Figure 15–4** Linear correlations between PWV and age in established hypertensive patients (–) and in normotensive persons (—). PWV is higher in hypertensives than in normotensives. (Adapted from Asmar et al.)[30]

This physiologic stiffness gradient is significantly attenuated in hypertensives whether they are young or old. The reduced stiffness gradient in hypertensives is mainly due to a significant decrease in distensibility of central arteries, whereas minimal changes in distensibility of the peripheral muscular arteries are usually observed.[33,34]

## Hypertension and Other Cardiovascular Risk Factors

### Diabetes

Most authors have reported stiffer arteries in diabetic than in nondiabetic (both type 1 and 2) patients with or without hypertension, even at early stages of the disease.[30,35] The stiffness changes occurred predominantely in the central aorta and the lower limb. Moreover, some authors found a relationship between arterial stiffness and glycemia control or duration of disease, a finding that is disputed by others. Several mechanisms have been proposed to explain the stiffer arteries: hemostatic abnormalities, hyperinsulinemia, nonenzymatic glycosylation, changes in the autonomic nervous system, and clustering of other risk factors. Specific studies of the relationship between insulin or insulin resistance and arterial stiffness are emerging.

### Dyslipidemia

Based on experimental and clinical studies, it has been reported that cholesterol excess alters endothelial function, leading to a decreased ability of arterial vessels to relax. Whether this abnormality is associated with increased stiffness of the arterial wall in humans remains controversial.[30] At present, there is limited evidence for an association between cholesterol levels or dyslipidemia and large artery stiffness.[36] Longitudinal studies relating arterial stiffness to cholesterol metabolism and to endothelial function are lacking.

### Smoking

Cigarette smoking increases stiffness of both medium and large arteries. Whether the arterial effect of smoking is related to concomitant blood pressure changes or is pressure independent is still debated. Longitudinal studies involving smoking and arterial stiffness as a primary goal are lacking.[37]

## Hypertension and Organ Damage

### Congestive Heart Failure

Arterial compliance measured at the aortic, carotid, iliac, or brachial artery levels is significantly impaired in patients with congestive heart failure (CHF).[5,11,30,38] Further studies are needed to evaluate the role of arterial stiffness in the prognosis of CHF and its improvement with treatment.

### End-Stage Renal Disease

Patients with end-stage renal disease (ESRD) have a high prevalence of systolic hypertension caused by increased arterial stiffness. In comparison with nonuremic patients, aortic PWV is increased in ESRD, especially in younger persons. The arterial stiffening is more pronounced in the aorta than in the peripheral arteries, in association with arterial calcification, low high-density lipoprotein cholesterol levels, and altered mechanisms of endothelium-dependent flow dilation.[39]

## ARTERIAL STIFFNESS AND PROGNOSIS

Prospective epidemiologic studies have directed attention to SBP and pulse pressure PP as a better predictor of cardiovascular and all-cause mortality than DBP. These studies highlighted the role of pulse pressure and arterial stiffness in the pathophysiology of cardiovascular disease and emphasized that these parameters give more information than blood pressure determination alone.[40-44]

## Aortic Pulse Wave Velocity as an Independent Predictor of Cardiovascular Risk

Because left ventricular ejection remains stable or even decreases with age, arterial stiffness is probably the principal factor responsible for increased SBP and pulse pressure during aging. Thus the question has arisen whether the aortic PWV might be a risk factor for cardiovascular or overall mortality. Blacher et al.[45] showed three significant predictors of cardiovascular mortality in patients with ESRD: aortic PWV, age, and duration of hemodialysis. After adjustment for all confounding factors, the odds ratio for PWV (>1270 cm/sec) was 4.4 (confidence interval [CI]: 2.3-8.5) for all-cause mortality and 5.0 (CI: 2.3-10.9) for cardiovascular mortality.

In patients with essential hypertension, a study based on calculation of cardiovascular risk with the Framingham equations[46] showed an increased risk of cardiovascular complications in parallel with the increase in aortic PWV, with aortic PWV being the strongest predictor of cardiovascular mortality. Elsewhere, Laurent et al.[47] analyzed the prognostic value of PWV in a longitudinal study in hypertensive patients and

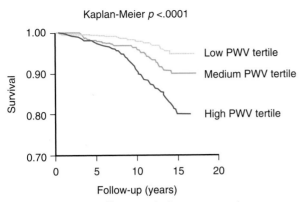

**Figure 15–5** Aortic stiffness and all-cause mortality in hypertensive patients. Mortality is higher in the high PWV tertile. Similar results were observed for cardiovascular mortality. (Adapted from Laurent et al.)[47]

clearly demonstrated that aortic stiffness, as evaluated by carotid-femoral PWV, is an independent predictor of all-cause and cardiovascular mortality. The same authors showed that aortic stiffness is also an independent predictor of primary coronary events and of fatal stroke in hypertensive patients.[48,49] These findings suggest that increased arterial stiffness, as evaluated by aortic PWV, should be considered an independent predictor of all-cause and cardiovascular mortality, primary coronary events, and fatal stroke in patients at high cardiovascular risk with hypertension.

## ARTERIAL STIFFNESS: PHARMACOLOGY AND THERAPEUTICS

### Hypertension

There is a need for pharmacologic studies focusing on arterial wall properties at both proximal and distal levels. This has been investigated with nitrates and nitrite donors,[50] which have been shown to decrease arterial stiffness at doses not affecting resistance vessels, and to a lesser extent, with angiotension-converting enzyme inhibitors and calcium antagonists.

In principle, the demonstrated ability of antihypertensive agents to reduce arterial stiffness is not surprising, because blood pressure reduction unloads the stiffer components of the arterial wall. Whether classes of antihypertensive agents vary in their ability to affect arterial structure and thus influence arterial stiffness via a pressure-independent mechanism is more difficult to demonstrate, because the demonstration requires large-scale trials. In long-term studies it is generally accepted that angiotensin-converting enzyme inhibitors, calcium antagonists, and some β-blocking agents share a similar ability to decrease arterial stiffness in hypertensive patients. Results with diuretics may differ according to the patient's age and the arterial site.[51-53]

In the short term, a pressure-independent decrease in arterial stiffness is generally mediated by smooth muscle relaxation caused either by a direct drug effect or by a resultant change in endothelial function. In the long term, the occurrence of a pressure-independent decrease in arterial stiffness implies a pharmacologic remodeling of the arterial wall.

Various pressure-independent changes in arterial structure have been described in response to long-term drug treatment, including angiotensin-converting enzyme inhibitors (with or without diuretics), aldosterone antagonists, or even amino-guanidine derivatives.[54,55] Reduction in pulsatile mechanical stress through the decrease in arterial stiffness is a desirable goal of drug treatment to reduce arterial wall hypertrophy and lumen enlargement.

Guérin et al.[45,59] analyzed the impact of PWV reduction (improvement in arterial stiffness) in terms of mortality in patients at high cardiovascular risk caused by ESRD. Their results showed that the degree of PWV reduction is an independent predictor of mortality (Figure 15–6). These important findings showed that improvement of PWV has a direct benefit in terms of mortality.

Clinical trials including the study of polymorphisms of candidate genes should consider not only the renin-angiotensin system but also the various systems involved in arterial structure, vasomotor tone, and remodeling. A pressure-independent decrease in arterial stiffness was observed in hypertensive persons with a polymorphism in the angiotension II type 1 ($AT_1$) receptor gene.[56]

## Other Arterial Diseases

Studies of the effects of drugs on arterial stiffness in persons with cardiovascular risk factors are scarce. In patients with familial hypercholesterolemia, radial artery compliance was largely increased after a 2-year treatment with simvastatin, whereas no significant change was observed after 6 months of treatment.[57] Systemic compliance is higher, and aortic-femoral PWV and central pulse pressure lower in women receiving menopausal hormonal therapy, suggesting that such therapy may decrease stiffness of the aorta and large arteries in postmenopausal women. Removing women from their hormonal therapy for 4 weeks reduced arterial compliance, and reinstating therapy for a further 4 weeks restored compliance to prestudy levels, independent of blood pressure changes.[58]

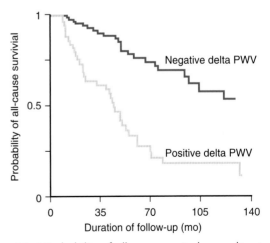

**Figure 15–6** Probability of all-cause survival according to delta PWV under antihypertensive therapy. Comparison between PWV responders (negative delta PWV) and nonresponders (positive delta PWV) was highly significant ($p < .00001$). (Adapted from Guérin et al.)[59]

## Nonpharmacologic Treatment

Most studies of nonpharmacologic therapies have involved relatively small numbers of persons. Aerobically trained athletes have greater large arterial compliance than matched sedentary controls. A single, 30-minute cycling exercise at 65% of maximal oxygen consumption induced a small increase in aortic compliance and reduction in PWV and central SBP. Furthermore, 4 weeks of moderate-intensity exercise (65% max) performed for 30 minutes, three times per week in previously sedentary persons increased resting arterial compliance. A pressure-independent decrease in arterial stiffness may be observed through changes in several environmental factors such as sodium intake. Weight loss in healthy obese men induced a significant fall in mean blood pressure, associated with a tendency toward a blood pressure–dependent decrease in large artery stiffness. Six-week fish oil therapy improved systemic arterial compliance in non–insulin-dependent diabetes mellitus, whereas no change occurred in blood pressure, cardiac output, and systemic vascular resistance. PWV increased less in healthy adults who were taking more than 300 mg/day of standardized garlic powder for more than 2 years than in age- and sex-matched control subjects. Finally, isoflavones derived from either soy products or red clover increased large artery compliance in postmenopausal women.

## References

1. Lehmann ED. Terminology for the definition of arterial elastic properties. Path Biol 47(6):656-664, 1999.
2. Glagov S. Microarchitecture of arteries and veins. *In* Abramson D, Dobrin P (eds). Blood Vessels and Lymphatics. Orlando, FL, Academic Press, 1984; pp 3-16.
3. Dobrin PB. Mechanical properties of arteries. Physiol Rev 58:397-460, 1978.
4. Milnor WR. Hemodynamics, 2nd ed. Baltimore, Williams & Wilkins, 1989; pp 56-243.
5. Nichols WW, O'Rourke M. McDonald's Blood Flow in Arteries: Theoretical, Experimental and Clinical Principles, 4th ed. London, Edward Arnold, 1998; pp 54-113, 201-222, 284-292, 347-401.
6. Bergel DH. The dynamic elastic properties of the arterial wall. J Physiol 156:458-69, 1961.
7. Boutouyrie P, Laurent S, Benetos A, et al. Opposing effects of ageing on distal and proximal large arteries in hypertensives. J Hypertens 10(6):S87-S91, 1992.
8. Bramwell JC, Hill AV. Velocity of transmission of the pulse wave and elasticity of arteries. Lancet 1:891-892, 1922.
9. Kelly R, Hayward C, Avolio A, et al. Non-invasive determination of age-related changes in the human arterial pulse. Circulation 80:1652-9, 1989.
10. O'Rourke MF. Mechanical principles in arterial disease. Hypertension 26:2-9, 1995.
11. Cohn JN, Finkelstein S, McVeigh G, et al. Noninvasive pulse wave analysis for the early detection of vascular disease. Hypertension 26:503-508, 1995.
12. Lehmann E, Hopkins KD, Rawesh A, et al. Relation between number of cardiovascular risk factors/events and noninvasive Doppler ultrasound assessments of aortic compliance. Hypertension 32:565-569, 1998.
13. Shimazu H, Kawarada A, Ito H, et al. Electric impedance cuff for the indirect measurement of blood pressure and volume elastic modulus in human limb and finger arteries. Med Biol Eng Comput 27:477-483, 1989.
14. Asmar R, Benetos A, Topouchian J, et al. Assessment of arterial distensibility by automatic pulse wave velocity measurement. Validation and clinical application studies. Hypertension 26:485-490, 1995.
15. Watt TB, Burrus CS. Arterial pressure contour analysis for estimating human vascular properties. J Appl Physiol 40:171-176, 1976.
16. Resnick LM, Militianu D, Cunnings AJ, et al. Direct magnetic resonance determination of aortic distensibility in essential hypertension: Relation to age, abdominal visceral fat, and in situ intracellular free magnesium. Hypertension 30(3 Pt 2): 654-659, 1997.
17. Gosse P, Guillo P, Ascher G, et al. Assessment of arterial distensibility by monitoring the timing of Korotkoff sounds. Am J Hypertens 7:228-233, 1994.
18. Takazawa K, Tanaka N, Fujita M, et al. Assessment of vasoactive agents and vascular aging by the second derivative of photoplethysmogram waveform. Hypertension 32:365-70, 1998.
19. Chen C-H, Ting C-T, Nussbacher A, et al. Validation of carotid artery tonometry as a means of estimating augmentation index of ascending aortic pressure. Hypertension 27:168-175, 1996.
20. Marcus RH, Korcarz C, McCray G, et al. Noninvasive method for determination of arterial compliance using Doppler echocardiography and subclavian pulse tracings. Validation and clinical application of a physiological model of the circulation. Circulation 89:2688-2699, 1994.
21. Lang RM, Cholley BP, Korcarz C, et al. Measurement of regional elastic properties of the human aorta: A new application of transesophageal echocardiography with automated border detection and calibrated subclavian pulse tracings. Circulation 90:1875-1882, 1994.
22. Roman ML, Saba PS, Pini R, et al. Parallel cardiac and vascular adaptation in hypertension. Circulation 86:1909-1918, 1992.
23. Hoeks APG, Brands PJ, Smeets FAM, et al. Assessment of the distensibility of superficial arteries. Ultrasound Med Biol 16:121-128, 1990.
24. van der Heijden-Spek JJ, Staessen JA, Fagard RH, et al. Effect of age on brachial artery wall properties differs from the aorta and is gender dependent. A population study. Hypertension 35:637-642, 2000.
25. Kool MJ, Wijnen JA, Hoeks AP, et al. Diurnal pattern of vessel-wall properties of large arteries in healthy men. J Hypertens 9(Suppl 6):S108-S109, 1991.
26. Failla M, Grappiolo A, Carugo S, et al. Effects of cigarette smoking on carotid and radial artery distensibility. J Hypertens 15:1659-1664, 1997.
27. Kool MJF, Hoeks APG, Struijker Boudier HAJ, et al. Short- and long-term effects of smoking on arterial wall properties in habitual smokers. J Am Coll Cardiol 22:1881-1886, 1993.
28. Kelbaek H, Munck O, Christensen NJ, et al. Central haemodynamic changes after a meal. Br Heart J 61:506-509, 1989.
29. Hayoz D, Tardy Y, Rutschmann B, et al. Spontaneous diameter oscillations of the radial artery in humans. Am J Physiol 264:H2080-H2084, 1993.
30. Asmar R. Arterial Stiffness and Pulse Wave Velocity: Clinical Applications. Amsterdam, Elsevier, 1999; pp 30-33.
31. Benetos A, Laurent S, Hoeks AP, et al. Arterial alterations with aging and high blood pressure: A noninvasive study of carotid and femoral arteries. Arterioscler Thromb 13:90-97, 1993.
32. Girerd X, Chanudet X, Larroque P, et al. Early arterial modifications in young patients with borderline hypertension. J Hypertens 7:S45-S47, 1989.
33. Safar ME, London GM. The arterial system in human hypertension. *In* Swales JD (ed). Textbook of Hypertension. London, Blackwell Scientific, 1994; pp 85-102.
34. Laurent S, Girerd X, Mourad JJ, et al. Elastic modulus of arterial artery wall material is not increased hypertension. Arterioscler Thromb 14:1233-1231, 1994.

35. van Dijk R, Nijpels G, Twisk JWR. Change in common carotid artery diameter, distensibility and compliance in subjects with a recent history of impaired glucose tolerance: A 3-year follow-up study. J Hypertens 18:293-300, 2000.

36. Cameron JD, Jennings GL, Dart AM. The relationship between arterial compliance, age, blood pressure and serum lipid levels. J Hypertens 13:1718-1723, 1995.

37. Stefanadis C, Tsiamis E, Vlachopoulos C, et al. Unfavorable effect of smoking on the elastic properties of the aorta. Circulation 95:31-38, 1997.

38. Giannattasio C, Failla M, Stella ML, et al. Alterations of radial artery compliance in patients with congestive heart failure. Am J Cardiol 76:381-5, 1995.

39. London GM, Marchais SJ, Safar ME, et al. Aortic and large artery compliance in end-stage renal failure. Kidney Int 37:137-142, 1990.

40. Darne B, Girerd X, Safar M, et al. Pulsatile versus steady component of blood pressure: A cross-sectional and a prospective analysis on cardiovascular mortality. Hypertension 13:392-400, 1989.

41. Madhavan S, Ooi WL, Cohen H, et al. Relation of pulse pressure and blood pressure reduction to the incidence of myocardial infarction. Hypertension 23:395-401, 1994.

42. Safar M, London G. Therapeutic studies and arterial stiffness in hypertension: Recommendations of the European Society of Hypertension. J Hypertens 18:1527-1535, 2000.

43. Benetos A, Rudnichi A, Safar M, et al. Pulse pressure and cardiovascular mortality in normotensive and hypertensive subjects. Hypertension 35:560-564, 1998.

44. Mitchell GF, Moye LM, Braunwald E, et al. Sphygmomanometrically determined pulse pressure is a powerful independent predictor of recurrent events after myocardial infarction in patients with impaired left ventricular function. Circulation 96:4254-4260, 1997.

45. Blacher J, Guérin AP, Pannier B, et al. Impact of aortic stiffness on survival in end-stage renal disease. Circulation 99:2434-2439, 1999.

46. Blacher J, Asmar S, Djane S, et al. Aortic pulse wave velocity as a marker of cardiovascular risk in hypertensive patients. Hypertension 33:1111-1117, 1999.

47. Laurent S, Boutouyrie P, Asmar R, et al. Aortic stiffness is an independent predictor of all-cause and cardiovascular mortality in hypertensive patients. Hypertension 37:1236-1241, 2001.

48. Boutouyrie P, Tropeano AI, Asmar R, et al. Aortic stiffness is an independent predictor of primary coronary events in hypertensive patients: A longitudinal study. Hypertension 39:10-15, 2002.

49. Laurent S, Katsahian S, Fassot C, et al. Aortic stiffness is an independent predictor of fatal stroke in essential hypertension. Stroke 34:1203-1206, 2003.

50. Laurent S, Arcaro G, Benetos A, et al. Mechanism of nitrate-induced improvement on arterial compliance depends on vascular territory. J Cardiovasc Pharmacol 19:641-649, 1992.

51. Van Merode T, Van Bortel LM, Smeets FA, et al. Verapamil and nebivolol improve carotid artery distensibility in hypertensive patients. J Hypertens 7(Suppl 6):262-263, 1989.

52. Boutouyrie P, Bussy C, Lacolley P, et al. Local steady and pulse pressure and arterial remodeling. Circulation 100:1387-1393, 1999.

53. Topouchian J, Asmar R, Sayegh F, et al. Changes in arterial structure and function under trandolapril-verapamil combination in hypertension. Stroke 30:1056-1064, 1999.

54. Asmar R, Topouchian J, Pannier B, et al. Pulse wave velocity as endpoint in large-scale intervention trial: The Complior study. J Hypertens 19:813-818, 2001.

55. Asmar R, London G, O'Rourke M, et al. Improvement in blood pressure, arterial stiffness and wave reflections with a very low dose perindopril-indapamide combination in hypertensive patient. Hypertension 38:922-926, 2001.

56. Benetos A, Cambien F, Gautier S, et al. Influence of the angiotensin II type 1 receptor gene polymorphism on the effects of perindopril and nitrendipine on arterial stiffness in hypertensive individuals. Hypertension 28:1081-1084, 1996.

57. Giannattasio C, Mangoni AA, Faila M, et al. Impaired radial artery compliance in normotensive subjects with familial hypercholesterolemia. Atherosclerosis 124:249-260, 1996.

58. Waddell TK, Rajkumar C, Cameron JD, et al. Withdrawal of hormonal therapy for 4 weeks decreases arterial compliance in postmenopausal women. J Hypertens 17:413-418, 1999.

59. Guérin A, Blacher J, Pannier B, et al. Impact of arterial stiffness attenuation on survival of patients in end-stage renal failure. Circulation 103:987-992, 2001.

# Chapter 16

# Endothelium in Hypertension: Nitric Oxide

## Lukas E. Spieker, Thomas F. Lüscher

The vascular endothelium synthesizes and releases a spectrum of vasoactive substances and therefore plays a fundamental role in the basal and dynamic regulation of the circulation.[1] Due to its strategic anatomic position, the endothelium is constantly exposed to the different risk factors for atherosclerosis.

## NITRIC OXIDE

Nitric oxide (NO)—originally described as endothelium-derived relaxing factor (EDRF)—is released from endothelial cells in response to shear stress produced by blood flow, and in response to activation of a variety of receptors (Figure 16–1).[2-4] NO is a free radical gas with an in vivo half-life of a few seconds, which is readily able to cross biologic membranes.[2,5,6] After diffusion from endothelial to vascular smooth muscle cells, NO increases intracellular cyclic guanosine monophosphate (cGMP) concentrations by activation of the enzyme guanylate cyclase leading to relaxation of the smooth muscle cells.[7]

NO is synthesized by NO synthase (NOS) from L-arginine.[7] The conversion from L-arginine to NO can be inhibited by false substrates for the NOS, for example, by $N^G$-monomethyl-arginine (L-NMMA).[8] Because there is a continuous basal release of NO that determines the tone of peripheral blood vessels, systemic inhibition of NO synthesis causes an increase in arterial blood pressure.[9-13] There are two major types of NOS in the vasculature: a constitutive and an inducible isoform. The former, which is present in endothelial cells, is called endothelial NOS (eNOS), the latter is an important inflammatory mediator released by macrophages in response to immunologic stimuli.[9] NO has also antithrombogenic, antiproliferative, leukocyte-adhesion inhibiting effects, and influences myocardial contractility.[10,13,15,16] The hemodynamic effects of pharmacologic NO inhibition include an increase in systemic and pulmonary arterial blood pressure, and a decrease in cardiac output (Table 16–1).

### Nitric Oxide in Experimental Hypertension

Endothelium-derived NO-mediated vascular relaxation is impaired in spontaneously hypertensive animals.[10-13] Thus, the bioavailability of NO is reduced. Surprisingly, the NO pathway is paradoxically up-regulated in the resistance circulation and the heart of spontaneously hypertensive rats (SHR).[14,15] Adult SHR possess a higher activity of eNOS than their normotensive counterparts.[16] Very young prehypertensive SHR have, in contrast, lower eNOS activity than young normotensive rats without a genetic background for hypertension, indicating that the increased activity of eNOS in adult SHR is indeed related to hypertension (Figure 16–2).

Moreover, the plasma concentrations of the oxidative product of NO metabolism, nitrate, are higher in hypertensive rats than in normotensive controls.[14] These results indicate that the basal release of NO is increased in hypertensive rats.

Thus, it appears that in SHR, there must be a factor blunting the hemodynamic effect of NO.[17] Indeed, NO production is increased in stroke-prone SHR (SHR-sp), but bioavailability is reduced.[18] Direct in situ measurement of NO release by a porphyrinic microsensor in SHR-sp confirmed that hypertension is associated with increased NO decomposition by superoxide anions, (i.e., free oxygen radicals) (Figure 16–3).[19]

In other models of hypertension (i.e., in Dahl salt-sensitive rats; in two-kidney, one clip experimental hypertension; and in deoxycorticosterone [DOCA]-salt hypertensive rats) endothelium-dependent relaxation is also impaired.[20-24] However, NO production by eNOS is reduced rather than up-regulated in Dahl salt-sensitive rats (see Figure 16–3).[22,25,26] L-Arginine, the substrate of NO production by eNOS, normalizes blood pressure and simultaneously increases urinary excretion of nitrate, the degradation product of nitric oxide, in Dahl salt-sensitive rats.[27-30] Further mechanisms contribute to the pathogenesis of salt-sensitive hypertension, for example, decreased expression of endothelial endothelin B receptors, which mediate NO release,[23,25,31] and altered expression of the constitutive brain NOS as well as the inducible NOS isoform, possibly leading to alterations in renal sympathetic nervous activity and sodium handling.[32-35]

### Nitric Oxide in Human Hypertension

There are several techniques for the assessment of NO bioavailability in humans. Most often, flow-mediated vasodilation of the brachial artery, a marker of endothelial function, is assessed by high-resolution ultrasonography (Figure 16–4). Alternatively, endothelium-dependent and endothelium-independent vasomotion in reaction to intraarterially infused vasoactive substances are assessed using venous occlusion plethysmography (Figure 16–5). Among the most often used endothelium-dependent vasodilators are acetylcholine and serotonin. Sodium nitroprusside or nitroglycerine serve as endothelium-independent vasodilators.

Endothelium-dependent vasodilation in response to acetylcholine is impaired in patients with arterial hypertension, in forearm circulation (see Figure 16–5),[36-46] as well as in the coronary vascular bed.[47,48] Endothelium-dependent vasodilation in the human forearm and coronary vascular beds are strongly correlated.[49,50]

Basal NO activity is decreased in hypertensive patients.[51] Furthermore, urinary excretion of the metabolic oxidation product of nitric oxide, $^{15}N$ nitrate, after administration of $^{15}N$-labeled arginine (i.e., the substrate for the generation of NO) is reduced in hypertensive patients compared with

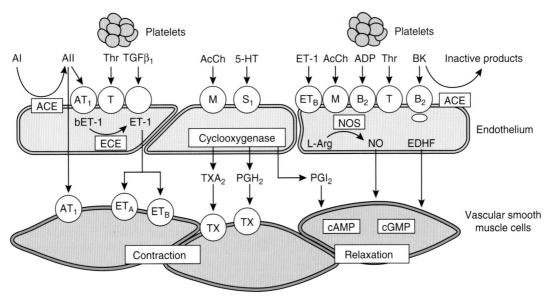

**Figure 16-1** Endothelium-derived vasoactive substances. Nitric oxide (NO) is released from endothelial cells in response to shear stress and to activation of a variety of receptors. NO exerts vasodilating and antiproliferative effects on smooth muscle cells and inhibits thrombocyte-aggregation and leukocyte-adhesion. Endothelin-1 (ET-1) exerts its major vascular effects—vasoconstriction and cell proliferation—through activation of specific $ET_A$ receptors on vascular smooth muscle cells. In contrast, endothelial $ET_B$ receptors mediate vasodilation via release of NO and prostacyclin. Additionally, $ET_B$ receptors in the lung were shown to be a major pathway for the clearance of ET-1 from plasma. ACE, angiotensin-converting enzyme; ACh, acetylcholine; AII, angiotensin II; $AT_1$, angiotensin 1 receptor; BK, bradykinin; COX, cyclooxygenase; ECE, endothelin-converting enzyme; EDHF, endothelium-derived hyperpolarizing factor; $ET_A$ and $ET_B$, endothelin A and B receptor; ET-1, endothelin-1; $PGH_2$, prostaglandin $H_2$; $PGI_2$, prostacyclin; S, serotoninergic receptor; Thr, thrombin; T, thromboxane receptor; $TXA_2$, thromboxane; 5-HT, 5-hydroxytryptamine (serotonin). (Modified from Lüscher TF, Noll G. Endothelium-derived vasoactive substances. In Braunwald E (ed). Heart Disease, 5th ed. Philadelphia, WB Saunders, 1997; p 1165.)

**Table 16-1** Hemodynamic Effects of NOS Inhibition in Healthy Volunteers

|  | **Baseline** | **L-NMMA (mg/kg/min)** | |
| --- | --- | --- | --- |
|  |  | **0.3** | **1.0** |
| **SBP** | 134 ± 7 | 152 ± 5 | 150 ± 3* |
| **DBP** | 73 ± 4 | 87 ± 5 | 85 ± 5† |
| **SVR** | 1114 ± 124 | 1413 ± 145* | 1973 ± 203‡ |
| **HR** | 67 ± 4 | 70 ± 6 | 63 ± 6 |
| **CI** | 3.5 ± 0.3 | 3.1 ± 0.2* | 2.3 ± 0.2§ |
| **SVI** | 53 ± 6 | 48 ± 6 | 38 ± 5† |
| **CVP** | 4 ± 0.7 | 3.6 ± 0.4 | 4.3 ± 0.05 |
| **B/min** | 23.1 ± 3.5 | 14 ± 4.5 | 18.6 ± 5.5 |

Modified after Spieker LE, Corti R, Binggeli C, et al. Baroreceptor dysfunction induced by nitric oxide synthase inhibition in humans. J Am Coll Cardiol 36:213-218, 2000.
*$p < .05$, †$p < .01$, ‡$p < .001$, §$p < .0001$, for each data point compared with baseline values.
L-NMMA, NG-monomethyl-L-arginine; SBP, systolic blood pressure (mm Hg); DBP, diastolic blood pressure (mm Hg); SVR, systemic vascular resistance (dyne·s⁻¹·cm⁻⁵); HR, heart rate (beats/min); CI, cardiac index (L·min⁻¹·m⁻²); SVI, stroke volume index (ml·min⁻¹·m⁻²); CVP, central venous pressure (mm Hg); B/min, sympathetic bursts per minute.

normotensive controls (see Figure 16-5).[52] Thus whole-body NO production in patients with essential hypertension is diminished under basal conditions. In line with these findings, the vasoconstrictor response to L-NMMA, an inhibitor of NO synthesis, was significantly less in hypertensive patients compared with normotensives, whereas there was no difference in the response to norepinephrine, an endothelium-independent vasoconstrictor, between hypertensives and normotensives.[51,53]

Normotensive offspring of hypertensive parents exhibit impaired endothelium-dependent vasodilation to acetylcholine.[54] In parallel to manifest hypertension, in normotensive offspring, vasoconstriction resulting from inhibition of NO synthesis is decreased.[55] Thus derangement of endothelial function in hypertension is likely to be caused in part by genetic factors, and not just a consequence of elevated blood pressure (although the hemodynamic factor importantly contributes).[56]

## NITRIC OXIDE AND OXIDATIVE STRESS IN HYPERTENSION

Oxidative stress plays an important role in the pathogenesis of hypertension (Figure 16–6). Superoxide anion ($O_2^-$), an oxygen radical, can scavenge NO to form peroxynitrite ($ONOO^-$), effectively reducing the bioavailability of endothelium-derived NO.[19,57] In addition, $O_2^-$ can act as a vasoconstrictor.[58-61] Nicotinamide adenine dinucleotide (NADH) dehydrogenase,

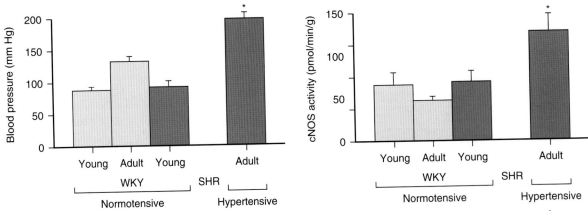

**Figure 16–2** Increased activity of constitutive nitric oxide synthase (NOS) in cardiac endothelium of spontaneously hypertensive rats (SHR; *black bars*). Adult SHR possess a higher activity of constitutive NOS than their normotensive counterparts (Wystar-Kyoto rats, WKY; *open bars*). Very young prehypertensive SHR have, in contrast, lower constitutive NOS activity than the normotensive, indicating that the increased activity of NOS in adult SHR is indeed related to hypertension. (Modified from Nava E, Noll G, Lüscher TF. Increased activity of constitutive nitric oxide synthase in cardiac endothelium in spontaneous hypertension. Circulation 91:2310-2313, 1995.)

a mitochondrial enzyme of the respiratory chain, seems to be a major source of $O_2^-$.[62] Expression of NAD(P)H oxidase in human coronary artery smooth muscle cells is up-regulated by pulsatile stretch, generating increased oxidative stress.[63] Another source of $O_2^-$ is cyclooxygenase (COX).[64] In contrast, xanthine oxidase, another generator of superoxide anions, does not appear to play a significant role in essential hypertension.[63,65]

Paradoxically, NOS (i.e., the NO-generating enzyme) can also produce $O_2^-$.[66-68] Production of $O_2^-$ in SHR-sp, an experimental model of genetic hypertension, can be prevented by NOS inhibition.[68] Administration of exogenous tetrahydro-biop-terin ($BH_4$), an essential cofactor for NOS, can reduce excess $O_2^-$ in the aorta of SHR-sp (see Figure 16–6).[68] In prehypertensive SHR, the calcium ionophore A23187-stimulated -

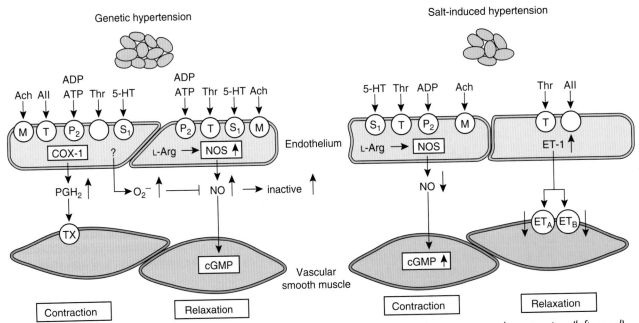

**Figure 16–3** Heterogeneity of endothelial dysfunction in experimental hypertension. In spontaneous hypertension *(left panel)* nitric oxide synthase (NOS) is up-regulated and nitric oxide (NO) is inactivated by superoxide anions ($O_2^{-1}$). In addition, the production of thromboxane ($TXA_2$) and prostaglandin H2 ($PGH_2$) is increased. In salt-related hypertension *(right panel)* NO production is reduced and the endothelin (ET) system is up-regulated. ACE, angiotensin-converting enzyme; ACh, acetylcholine; AII, angiotensin II; $AT_1$, angiotensin 1 receptor; cGMP, cyclic guanosine monophosphate; COX, cyclooxygenase; $ET_A$ and $ET_B$, endothelin A and B receptor; ET-1, endothelin-1; L-Arg, L-arginine; M, muscarinergic receptor; $\cdot O_2^-$, superoxide anion; $PGI_2$, prostacyclin; S, serotoninergic receptor; T, thrombin receptor; Thr, thrombin; TX, thromboxane receptor; 5-HT, 5-hydroxytryptamine (serotonin). (Modified from Spieker LE, Noll G, Ruschitzka FT, et al. Working under pressure: The vascular endothelium in arterial hypertension. J Hum Hypertens 14:617-630, 2000.)

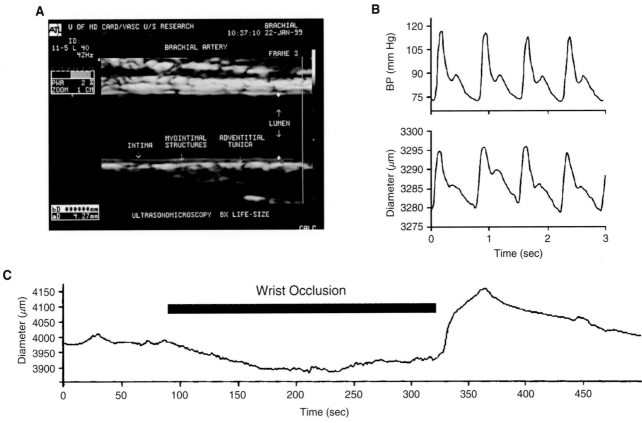

**Figure 16-4** Flow-mediated vasodilation of the brachial artery is measured by high-resolution ultrasonography **(A)**. With the use of echo-tracking, arterial diameter can be measured on a beat-to-beat base **(B)**. After establishing stable baseline conditions, flow-mediated vasodilation is measured after release of a blood pressure cuff placed around the wrist and inflated to suprasystolic pressure for 5 minutes **(C)**. The resulting hyperemic blood flow to the hand after release of the wrist cuff leads to a more or less pronounced vasodilation of the brachial artery, which is mediated by endothelium-derived nitric oxide (NO).

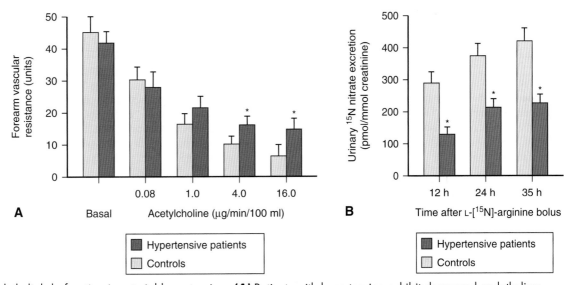

**Figure 16-5** Endothelial dysfunction in arterial hypertension. **(A)** Patients with hypertension exhibit decreased endothelium-dependent vasodilation in response to acetylcholine compared with normotensive controls. **(B)** Cumulative urinary excretion of $^{15}N$ nitrate after administration of $^{15}N$-labeled arginine (i.e., the substrate for enzymatic production of nitric oxide [NO]). Urinary excretion of the metabolic oxidation product of NO, nitrate, is reduced in hypertensive patients compared with normotensive controls. These data show that whole-body NO production in patients with essential hypertension is diminished under basal conditions. (A modified from Linder L, Kiowski W, Bühler FR, et al. Indirect evidence for release of endothelium-derived relaxing factor in human forearm circulation in vivo: Blunted response in essential hypertension. Circulation 81:1762-1767, 1990. B modified from Forte P, Copland M, Smith LM, et al. Basal nitric oxide synthesis in essential hypertension. Lancet 349:837-842, 1997.)

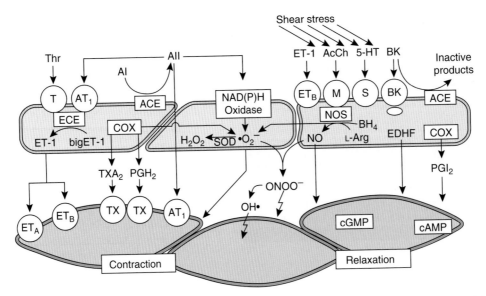

**Figure 16-6** Role of oxidative stress in the pathogenesis of endothelial dysfunction in hypertension. Superoxide anion ($\cdot O_2^-$), generated by angiotensin II–activated NAD(P)H oxidase, by dysfunctional nitric oxide synthase (NOS), and by cyclooxygenase (COX), can scavenge the vasodilator NO to form the highly reactive peroxynitrite. Peroxynitrite can damage cell membranes and oxidize lipids. In addition, $\cdot O_2^-$ can act as a vasoconstrictor. ACE, angiotensin-converting enzyme; ACh, acetylcholine; AII, angiotensin II; $AT_1$, angiotensin 1 receptor; $BH_4$, tetrahydrobiopterin; BK, bradykinin; COX, cyclooxygenase; ECE, endothelin-converting enzyme; EDHF, endothelium-derived hyperpolarizing factor; $ET_A$ and $ET_B$, endothelin A and B receptor; ET-1, endothelin-1; $H_2O_2$, hydrogen peroxide; L-Arg, L-arginine; NAD(P)H oxidase, nicotinamide adenine dinucleotide oxidase; $\cdot O_2^-$ superoxide anion; OH$\cdot$, hydroxyl radical; ONOO$^-$, peroxynitrite; $PGH_2$, prostaglandin $H_2$; $PGI_2$, prostacyclin; S, serotoninergic receptor; SOD, superoxide dismutase; Thr, thrombin; TXA, thromboxane receptor; $TXA_2$, thromboxane; 5-HT, 5-hydroxytryptamine (serotonin). (Modified from Spieker LE, Noll G, Ruschitzka FT, et al. Working under pressure: The vascular endothelium in arterial hypertension. J Hum Hypertens 14:617-630, 2000.)

(i.e., a receptor-independent activator of NOS) production of $O_2^-$ was significantly higher than in control rats. NO release was reduced in SHR aortas, with opposite results in the presence of exogenous $BH_4$. Thus, dysfunctional eNOS may be a source of $O_2^-$ in prehypertensive SHR and contribute to the development of hypertension and its vascular complications.[66,69]

$O_2^-$ is finally detoxified by superoxide dismutase (SOD), forming $H_2O_2$, which is further metabolized by catalase.[70] However, the reaction between the two radicals $O_2^-$ and NO is three times faster than the detoxification of $O_2^-$ by SOD.[71] Depending on the relative concentrations of NO and SOD, there may be a propensity for $O_2^-$ to preferentially react with NO, resulting in decreased bioavailability of NO.

The gene for cytosolic SOD (i.e., SOD1) is located on the 21q22.1 region of chromosome 21.[72] Therefore, patients with Down syndrome (trisomy 21) have an extra copy of the SOD gene. Because of gene dosage excess, their SOD activity is 50% greater than in the diploid population, leading to reduced $O_2^-$ levels.[73] Indeed, patients with Down syndrome have lower blood pressure levels, indicating a major role for $O_2^-$ in the regulation of arterial blood pressure. Furthermore, the normal age-associated increase of blood pressure is absent in patients with Down syndrome.[74]

### Interactions between Nitric Oxide, Angiotensin II, and Superoxide Anions

The renin-angiotensin system plays a major role in hypertension (see Figure 16–1).[75] Apart from direct vasoconstrictor effects of angiotensin II (Ang II), there are important interactions between Ang II, oxygen radicals, and NO.

Ang II stimulates generation of $O_2^-$ by increasing the expression of the NAD(P)H oxidase gene (p22phox) and increasing the activity of NAD(P)H oxidase.[76-79] The vasoconstrictor effect of Ang II is enhanced in the absence of NO, and diminished during coinfusion of the antioxidant vitamin C.[80] Thus, the vasoconstrictive effect of Ang II is modulated by reactive oxygen species, mainly $O_2^-$, and their interaction with endothelium-derived NO (see Figure 16–6). Furthermore, Ang II increases the production of endothelin (ET) in the blood vessel wall, which exerts vasoconstriction and induces proliferation of the vascular smooth muscle cells.[81]

## NITRIC OXIDE AND PROSTAGLANDINS

Prostacyclin ($PGI_2$) is an endothelium-derived relaxing factor, which is released in response to shear stress (see Figure 16–1).[3,82-84] $PGI_2$ is synthesized by COX from arachidonic acid.[85] $PGI_2$ increases intracellular cyclic adenosine monophosphate (cAMP) in smooth muscle cells and platelets. In contrast to NO, $PGI_2$ does not contribute to the maintenance of basal vascular tone of large conduit arteries.[86] Instead, its platelet inhibitory effects are most important. The synergistic effect of both $PGI_2$ and NO enhances their antiplatelet activity.[87] A novel interesting concept in atherosclerosis is selective inhibition of COX-2, which lowers CRP levels and improves endothelial function.[88]

Depending on the animal model of hypertension and the vascular bed, endothelium-dependent contractions to acetylcholine, a muscarinic receptor-dependent stimulator of NO synthesis, have been documented (see Figure 16–3). Because this response is inhibited by COX inhibitors and thromboxane receptor antagonists, the most likely contractile factors are thromboxane $A_2$ and prostaglandin $H_2$.[89,90]

Interactions between COX products and NO have been demonstrated.[91] In hypertensive patients, indomethacin, a COX inhibitor, significantly increased the response to acetylcholine, an effect that could be blocked by coinfusion of L-NMMA, an inhibitor of NO synthesis.[92] Therefore, COX inhibition restores NO-mediated vasodilation in essential hypertension, suggesting that COX-dependent substances can impair NO bioavailability. COX is indeed a source of the NO-scavenger $O_2^-$.[64]

## NITRIC OXIDE AND ENDOTHELIUM-DERIVED HYPERPOLARIZING FACTOR

Inhibitors of the L-arginine pathway do not prevent all endothelium-dependent relaxations.[93] Because vascular smooth muscle cells become hyperpolarized under these conditions, an endothelium-dependent hyperpolarizing factor (EDHF) of unknown chemical structure has been proposed (see Figure 16–1).[94,95] There is evidence that a calcium-dependent potassium channel on endothelial or smooth muscle cells is important in mediating endothelium-dependent hyperpolarization, a mechanism that is impaired in arterial hypertension.[96-98] Endothelium-dependent hyperpolarization may also be involved in the compensation for the impaired NO-system in patients with essential hypertension.[99,100]

## INTERACTIONS BETWEEN NITRIC OXIDE AND ENDOTHELIN

More than a decade ago, a novel vasoconstrictor peptide synthesized by vascular endothelial cells was identified.[101,102] The family of ETs consists of three closely related peptides—ET-1, ET-2, and ET-3—which are converted by endothelin-converting enzymes (ECE) from "big endothelins" originating from large preproendothelin peptides cleaved by endopeptidases.[103-107] The ET peptides are synthesized not only in vascular endothelial and smooth muscle cells, but also in neural, renal, and pulmonary cells, and some leukocytes.[108,109] The chemical structure of the endothelins is closely related to neurotoxins (sarafotoxins) produced by scorpions and snakes.[110-112] Factors modulating the expression of ET-1 include shear-stress, epinephrine, Ang II, thrombin, inflammatory cytokines (tumor necrosis factor α, interleukin-1, and interleukin-2), transforming growth factor β, and hypoxia.[113-125] ET-1 is metabolized by a neutral endopeptidase, which also cleaves natriuretic peptides.[126,127]

Imbalance of endothelium-derived relaxing and contracting substances disturbs the normal function of the vascular endothelium.[1,128] Endothelin acts as the natural counterpart to endothelium-derived NO, which exerts vasodilating, antithrombotic, and antiproliferative effects, and inhibits leukocyte-adhesion to the vascular wall.[113] In addition to its pressor effect in humans,[129,130] ET-1 induces vascular and myocardial hypertrophy,[131-133] independent risk factors for cardiovascular morbidity and mortality.[134-136] In patients with essential hypertension, carotid wall thickening and left ventricular mass correlate with reduced endothelium-dependent vasodilation.[137,138]

ET-1 has a paracrine rather than an endocrine mode of action, which is reflected by plasma levels of ET-1 in the picomolar range.[139,140] Infusion of an ET receptor antagonist into the brachial artery or systemically in healthy humans leads to vasodilation, indicating a role of ET-1 in the maintenance of basal vascular tone.[141,142] When ET-1 is infused, vasoconstriction follows a brief phase of vasodilation, which may be explained by relaxation of smooth muscle cells caused by $ET_B$ receptor-mediated release of the vasodilators NO and $PGI_2$ (see Figure 16–1). Additionally, ET-1 may also exert effects on the central and autonomic nervous systems and alter baroreflex function.[143-154] In the kidney, sodium reabsorption is modulated.[155]

The ET system is activated in several but not all animal models of arterial hypertension.[132,156-165] ET plasma levels have been reported to be elevated in certain patients with essential hypertension,[166] but this is a subject of controversy.[53,167] The causal role of ET-1 in the pathogenesis of hypertension thus remains unclear.[168]

Because most ET-1 synthesized in endothelial cells is secreted abluminally, it might attain a higher concentration in the vessel wall than in plasma. Indeed, significant correlations between the amount of immunoreactive ET-1 in the tunica media and blood pressure, total serum cholesterol, and number of atherosclerotic sites have been found.[169] In blood vessels of healthy controls, ET-1 was detectable almost exclusively in endothelial cells, whereas in patients with coronary artery disease and/or arterial hypertension, sizable amounts of ET-1 were detectable in the tunica media of different types of arteries.[169] Furthermore, there is evidence that certain gene polymorphisms of ET-1 and ET receptors can be associated with blood pressure.[170-173] Moreover, in hypertensive patients, TAK-044, a mixed $ET_{A/B}$ receptor antagonist, caused a significantly greater vasodilation than in normotensive subjects.[53] Because in this study, plasma levels of ET-1 were similar in normotensive and hypertensive patients, increased sensitivity to endogenous ET-1 in hypertension has to be postulated. Decreased bioavailability of NO may be involved in this phenomenon, because NO antagonizes some of the effects of ET-1.

## EFFECTS OF ANTIHYPERTENSIVE THERAPY ON NO BIOAVAILABILITY IN HYPERTENSIVE PATIENTS

In hypertensive animals, most classes of antihypertensive drugs (e.g., calcium-channel blockers, ACE inhibitors, $AT_1$ receptor antagonists) improve endothelium-dependent vasodilation.[99,174-180] Surprisingly and in contrast to animal experiments, antihypertensive therapy cannot consistently restore impaired endothelium-dependent vasodilation in patients with arterial hypertension.[36-46,181] However, depending on the antihypertensive drug and its pharmacologic profile, improvements in endothelium-dependent vasodilation can be achieved (Table 16–2).[38,40,42,182-192] The multifactorial etiology of essential hypertension as well as the duration of blood pressure elevation may explain certain inconsistent results of different investigators.[193,194]

**Table 16–2** Effect of Antihypertensive Therapy on Endothelial Function in Patients with Arterial Hypertension

| Author | Antihypertensive Therapy | Duration of Treatment | NO-Release Agonist/ Antagonist | Improvement in Endothelium-Dependent Vasomotion |
|---|---|---|---|---|
| | **ACE-inhibitors** | | | |
| Hirooka et al.[38] | Captopril | Acute | ACh | Yes |
| Creager et al.[43] | Captopril | 7-8 weeks | MCh | No |
| | Enalapril | 7-8 weeks | MCh | No |
| Taddei et al.[191] | Lisinopril | Acute | ACh | No |
| | | | Bk | Yes |
| | | 1 and 12 months | ACh | No |
| | | | Bk | Yes |
| Lyons et al.[184] | Enalapril | 6 weeks | L-NMMA | Yes |
| Millgard et al.[185] | Captopril | Acute | MCh | Yes |
| | | 3 months | MCh | Yes |
| Schiffrin et al. | Cilazapril | 1 and 2 years | ACh | Yes |
| | **Ang II antagonist** | | | |
| Ghiadoni et al. | Candesartan | 2 months | ACh | No |
| | | 12 months | ACh | (Yes)* |
| | **β-Blocker** | | | |
| Schiffrin et al. | Atenolol | 2 years | ACh | No |
| Dawes et al.[188] | Nebivolol | Acute | L-NMMA | Yes |
| | **Ca antagonists** | | | |
| Hirooka et al.[38] | Nifedipine | Acute | ACh | No |
| Millgard et al.[85] | Nifedipine | Acute | MCh | No |
| Sudano et al.[189] | Nifedipine | 6 months | ACh | Yes |
| Schiffrin et al. | Nifedipine | Chronic | ACh | Yes |
| Taddei et al.[191] | Lacidipine | 2 and 8 months | ACh and Bk | Yes |
| Lyons et al.[184] | Amlodipine | 6 weeks | L-NMMA | Yes |
| Perticone et al.[192] | Isradipine | 2 and 6 months | ACh | Yes |
| | **Other** | | | |
| Panza et al. | Various (diuretics, verapamil, β-blockers, clonidine, α-methyldopa) | Chronic vs. 2 weeks withdrawal | ACh ACh | No No |
| Taddei et al.[42] | Potassium | Acute | ACh | Yes |

Modified from Spieker LE, Noll G, Ruschitzka FT, et al. Working under pressure: The vascular endothelium in arterial hypertension. J Hum Hypertens14:617-630, 2000.
*This effect was paralleled by an enhanced endothelium-independent vasodilation to dosium nitroprusside.
Ang II, angiotensin II; ACE, angiotensin-converting enzyme; ACh, acetylcholine; Bk, bradykinin; Ca, calcium; L-NMMA, N$^G$-monomethyl-L-arginine; MCh, methacholine; NO, nitric oxide.

In addition to certain ACE inhibitors, several calcium channel blocking agents were successful in improving endothelial function in human hypertension (see Table 16–2). Antioxidant properties of an antihypertensive drug are important, because oxidative stress plays a central role in the pathophysiology of human hypertension. Endothelial function of patients with hypertension is improved by ascorbic acid, an antioxidant vitamin, which restores the imbalance of increased NO decomposition by superoxide.[195] Scavenging of reactive oxygen species by antioxidants may become an important therapeutic strategy,[19,196] because chronic treat-

ment with vitamin C is in fact able to lower blood pressure in patients with hypertension.[197]

Treatment with candesartan, an AT$_1$-receptor antagonist, reduced the vasodilator response to the mixed ET$_{A/B}$-receptor antagonist TAK-044 that was initially more pronounced in hypertensive patients than in normotensive controls.[187] This was paralleled by a reduction in circulating plasma ET-1 levels. Furthermore, the impaired vasoconstrictor response to L-NMMA, an inhibitor of NO synthesis, was augmented by antihypertensive treatment in hypertensives. Thus, the Ang II receptor blocker candesartan improves tonic NO release and reduces vasoconstriction to endogenous ET-1 in the forearm of hypertensive patients.

Interestingly, infusion of nebivolol, but not other β-blockers, intraarterially in the forearm of healthy subjects is associated with an increase in forearm blood flow.[198] The increase in forearm blood flow achieved by nebivolol can be prevented by coinfusion of the NO synthesis inhibitor L-NMMA. Similar results have been obtained in the human venous circulation.[199] This strongly suggests that nebivolol stimulates the formation of NO in the vasculature and may therefore have an interesting hemodynamic profile, which leads—unlike other β-blockers—to peripheral vasodilation in addition to the classical β-blocking effects on the sympathetic nervous system, heart rate, and cardiac contractility.[200,201] Nebivolol also causes NO-dependent vasodilation in hypertensive patients.[188] It is currently not known if this favorable effect persists during chronic treatment with this new type of $\beta_1$-blocker.

The effects of newer antihypertensive agents (e.g., ET receptor antagonists, ECE inhibitors, and inhibitors of neutral endopeptidases cleaving natriuretic peptides) on endothelial function in hypertension remain to be elucidated.

## SUMMARY

The vascular endothelium, by synthesizing and releasing vasoactive substances, plays a crucial role in the pathogenesis of hypertension. Because of its position between intraarterial pressure and smooth muscle cells responsible for peripheral resistance, the endothelium is thought to be both victim and offender in arterial hypertension. The delicate balance of endothelium-derived factors, which is disturbed in hypertension, can be restored by specific antihypertensive and antioxidant treatment.

## References

1. Lüscher TF, Vanhoutte PM. The Endothelium: Modulator of Cardiovascular Function. Boca Raton, CRC Press, 1990.
2. Furchgott RF, Zawadzki JV. The obligatory role of endothelial cells in the relaxation of arterial smooth muscle by acetylcholine. Nature 288:373-376, 1980.
3. Rubanyi GM, Romero JC, Vanhoutte PM. Flow-induced release of endothelium-derived relaxing factor. Am J Physiol 250:H1145-H149, 1986.
4. Anderson EA, Mark AL. Flow-mediated and reflex changes in large peripheral artery tone in humans. Circulation 79:93-100, 1989.
5. Palmer RM, Ferrige AG, Moncada S. Nitric oxide release accounts for the biological activity of endothelium-derived relaxing factor. Nature 327:524-526, 1987.
6. Stamler JS, Singel DJ, Loscalzo J. Biochemistry of nitric oxide and its redox-activated forms. Science 258:1898-1902, 1992.
7. Palmer RM, Ashton DS, Moncada S. Vascular endothelial cells synthesize nitric oxide from L-arginine. Nature 333:664-666, 1988.
8. Palmer RMJ, Rees DD, Ashton DS, Moncada S. L-arginine is the physiological precursor for the formation of nitric oxide in endothelium-dependent relaxation. Biochem Biophys Res Commun 153:1251-1256, 1988.
9. Palmer RM, Bridge L, Foxwell NA, et al. The role of nitric oxide in endothelial cell damage and its inhibition by glucocorticoids. Br J Pharmacol 105:11-12, 1992.
10. Lüscher TF, Vanhoutte PM. Endothelium-dependent contractions to acetylcholine in the aorta of the spontaneously hypertensive rat. Hypertension 8:344-348, 1986.
11. Lüscher TF, Romero JC, Vanhoutte PM. Bioassay of endothelium-derived substances in the aorta of normotensive and spontaneously hypertensive rats. J Hypertension 4 (Suppl 6):81, 1986.
12. Dohi Y, Thiel MA, Bühler FR, Lüscher TF. Activation of endothelial L-arginine pathway in resistance arteries. Effect of age and hypertension. Hypertension 16:170-179, 1990.
13. Diederich D, Yang ZH, Bühler FR, et al. Impaired endothelium-dependent relaxations in hypertensive resistance arteries involve cyclooxygenase pathway. Am J Physiol 258:H445-H451, 1990.
14. Nava E, Farre AL, Moreno C, et al. Alterations to the nitric oxide pathway in the spontaneously hypertensive rat. J Hypertens 16:609-615, 1998.
15. Kelm M, Feelisch M, Krebber T, et al. The role of nitric oxide in the regulation of coronary vascular resistance in arterial hypertension: Comparison of normotensive and spontaneously hypertensive rats. J Cardiovasc Pharmacol 20:S183-S186, 1992.
16. Nava E, Noll G, Lüscher TF. Increased activity of constitutive nitric oxide synthase in cardiac endothelium in spontaneous hypertension. Circulation 91:2310-2313, 1995.
17. Grunfeld S, Hamilton CA, Mesaros S, et al. Role of superoxide in the depressed nitric oxide production by the endothelium of genetically hypertensive rats. Hypertension 26:854-857, 1995.
18. McIntyre M, Hamilton CA, Rees DD, et al. Sex differences in the abundance of endothelial nitric oxide in a model of genetic hypertension. Hypertension 30:1517-1524, 1997.
19. Tschudi MR, Mesaros S, Luscher TF, et al. Direct in situ measurement of nitric oxide in mesenteric resistance arteries. Increased decomposition by superoxide in hypertension. Hypertension 27:32-35, 1996.
20. Lüscher TF, Raij L, Vanhoutte PM. Endothelium-dependent vascular responses in normotensive and hypertensive Dahl rats. Hypertension 9:157-163, 1987.
21. Lee J, Choi KC, Yeum CH, et al. Impairment of endothelium-dependent vasorelaxation in chronic two-kidney, one clip hypertensive rats. Nephrol Dial Transplant 10:619-623, 1995.
22. Hayakawa H, Hirata Y, Suzuki E, et al. Mechanisms for altered endothelium-dependent vasorelaxation in isolated kidneys from experimental hypertensive rats. Am J Physiol 264:H1535-H1541, 1993.
23. Hirata Y, Hayakawa H, Suzuki E, et al. Direct measurements of endothelium-derived nitric oxide release by stimulation of endothelin receptors in rat kidney and its alteration in salt-induced hypertension. Circulation 91:1229-1235, 1995.
24. Dohi Y, Criscione L, Lüscher TF. Renovascular hypertension impairs formation of endothelium-derived relaxing factors and sensitivity to endothelin-1 in resistance arteries. Br J Pharmacol 104:349-354, 1991.
25. Kakoki M, Hirata Y, Hayakawa H, et al. Effects of hypertension, diabetes mellitus, and hypercholesterolemia on endothelin type B receptor-mediated nitric oxide release from rat kidney. Circulation 99:1242-1248, 1999.
26. Ni Z, Oveisi F, Vaziri ND. Nitric oxide synthase isotype expression in salt-sensitive and salt-resistant Dahl rats. Hypertension 34:552-557, 1999.
27. Chen PY, Sanders PW. L-arginine abrogates salt-sensitive hypertension in Dahl/Rapp rats. J Clin Invest 88:1559-1567, 1991.
28. Chen PY, St. John PL, Kirk KA, et al. Hypertensive nephrosclerosis in the Dahl/Rapp rat. Initial sites of injury and effect of dietary L-arginine supplementation. Lab Invest 68:174-184, 1993.
29. Chen PY, Sanders PW. Role of nitric oxide synthesis in salt-sensitive hypertension in Dahl/Rapp rats. Hypertension 22:812-818, 1993.
30. Hu L, Manning RD, Jr. Role of nitric oxide in regulation of long-term pressure-natriuresis relationship in Dahl rats. Am J Physiol 268:H2375-H2383, 1995.
31. Matsuoka H, Itoh S, Kimoto M, et al. Asymmetrical dimethylarginine, an endogenous nitric oxide synthase inhibitor, in experimental hypertension. Hypertension 29:242-247, 1997.

32. Deng AY, Rapp JP. Locus for the inducible, but not a constitutive, nitric oxide synthase cosegregates with blood pressure in the Dahl salt-sensitive rat. J Clin Invest 95:2170-2177, 1995.

33. Ikeda Y, Saito K, Kim JI, et al. Nitric oxide synthase isoform activities in kidney of Dahl salt-sensitive rats. Hypertension 26:1030-1034, 1995.

34. Simchon S, Manger W, Blumberg G, et al. Impaired renal vasodilation and urinary cGMP excretion in Dahl salt-sensitive rats. Hypertension 27:653-657, 1996.

35. Rudd MA, Trolliet M, Hope S, et al. Salt-induced hypertension in Dahl salt-resistant and salt-sensitive rats with NOS II inhibition. Am J Physiol 277:H732-H739, 1999.

36. Linder L, Kiowski W, Bühler FR, et al. Indirect evidence for release of endothelium-derived relaxing factor in human forearm circulation in vivo: Blunted response in essential hypertension. Circulation 81:1762-1767, 1990.

37. Panza JA, Quyyumi AA, Brush JJ, et al. Abnormal endothelium-dependent vascular relaxation in patients with essential hypertension. N Engl J Med 323:22-27, 1990.

38. Hirooka Y, Imaizumi T, Masaki H et al. Captopril improves impaired endothelium-dependent vasodilation in hypertensive patients. Hypertension 20:175-180, 1992.

39. Panza JA, Casino PR, Kilcoyne CM, et al. Role of endothelium-derived nitric oxide in the abnormal endothelium-dependent vascular relaxation of patients with essential hypertension. Circulation 87:1468-1474, 1993.

40. Panza JA, Quyyumi AA, Callahan TS, et al. Effect of antihypertensive treatment on endothelium-dependent vascular relaxation in patients with essential hypertension. J Am Coll Cardiol 21:1145-1151, 1993.

41. Panza JA, Casino PR, Badar DM, Quyyumi AA. Effect of increased availability of endothelium-derived nitric oxide precursor on endothelium-dependent vascular relaxation in normal subjects and in patients with essential hypertension. Circulation 87:1475-1481, 1993.

42. Taddei S, Mattei P, Virdis A, et al. Effect of potassium on vasodilation to acetylcholine in essential hypertension. Hypertension 23:485-490, 1994.

43. Creager MA, Roddy MA. Effect of captopril and enalapril on endothelial function in hypertensive patients. Hypertension 24:499-505, 1994.

44. Panza JA, Casino PR, Kilcoyne CM, et al. Impaired endothelium-dependent vasodilation in patients with essential hypertension: Evidence that the abnormality is not at the muscarinic receptor level. J Am Coll Cardiol 23:1610-1616, 1994.

45. Taddei S, Virdis A, Mattei P, et al. Aging and endothelial function in normotensive subjects and patients with essential hypertension. Circulation 91:1981-1987, 1995.

46. Taddei S, Virdis A, Mattei P, et al. Hypertension causes premature aging of endothelial function in humans. Hypertension 29:736-743, 1997.

47. Treasure CB, Klein JL, Vita JA, et al. Hypertension and left ventricular hypertrophy are associated with impaired endothelium-mediated relaxation in human coronary resistance vessels. Circulation 87:86-93, 1993.

48. Egashira K, Suzuki S, Hirooka Y, et al. Impaired endothelium-dependent vasodilation of large epicardial and resistance coronary arteries in patients with essential hypertension: Different responses to acetylcholine and substance P. Hypertension 25:201-206, 1995.

49. Anderson TJ, Uehata A, Gerhard MD, et al. Close relation of endothelial function in the human coronary and peripheral circulation. J Am Coll Cardiol 26:1235-1241, 1995.

50. Takase B, Uehata A, Akima T, et al. Endothelium-dependent flow-mediated vasodilation in coronary and brachial arteries in suspected coronary artery disease. Am J Cardiol 82:1535-1539, A7-A8, 1998.

51. Calver A, Collier J, Moncada S, Vallance P. Effect of local intra-arterial NG-monomethyl-L-arginine in patients with hypertension: The nitric oxide dilator mechanism appears abnormal. J Hypertens 10:1025-1031, 1992.

52. Forte P, Copland M, Smith LM, Milne E, Sutherland J, Benjamin N. Basal nitric oxide synthesis in essential hypertension. Lancet 349:837-842, 1997.

53. Taddei S, Virdis A, Ghiadoni L, et al. Vasoconstriction to endogenous endothelin-1 is increased in the peripheral circulation of patients with essential hypertension. Circulation 100:1680-1683, 1999.

54. Taddei S, Virdis A, Mattei P, et al. Endothelium-dependent forearm vasodilation is reduced in normotensive subjects with familial history of hypertension. J Cardiovasc Pharmacol 20:S193-S195, 1992.

55. McAllister AS, Atkinson AB, Johnston GD, et al. Basal nitric oxide production is impaired in offspring of patients with essential hypertension. Clin Sci (Colch) 97:141-147, 1999.

56. Millgard J, Lind L. Acute hypertension impairs endothelium-dependent vasodilation. Clin Sci (Colch) 94:601-607, 1998.

57. Rubanyi GM, Vanhoutte PM. Superoxide anions and hyperoxia inactivate endothelium-derived relaxing factor. Am J Physiol 250:H822-H827, 1986.

58. Katusic ZS, Vanhoutte PM. Superoxide anion is an endothelium-derived contracting factor. Am J Physiol 257:H33-H37, 1989.

59. Auch-Schwelk W, Katusic ZS, Vanhoutte PM. Contractions to oxygen-derived free radicals are augmented in aorta of the spontaneously hypertensive rat. Hypertension 13:859-864, 1989.

60. Cosentino F, Sill JC, Katusic ZS. Role of superoxide anions in the mediation of endothelium-dependent contractions. Hypertension 23:223-235, 1994.

61. Katusic ZS, Schugel J, Cosentino F, et al. Endothelium-dependent contractions to oxygen-derived free radicals in the canine basilar artery. Am J Physiol 264:H859-H864, 1993.

62. Turrens JF, Boveris A. Generation of superoxide anion by the NADH dehydrogenase of bovine heart mitochondria. Biochem J 191:421-427, 1980.

63. Hishikawa K, Oemar BS, Yang Z, et al. Pulsatile stretch stimulates superoxide production and activates nuclear factor-kappa B in human coronary smooth muscle. Circ Res 81:797-803, 1997.

64. Kontos HA, Wei EP, Ellis EF, et al. Appearance of superoxide anion radical in cerebral extracellular space during increased prostaglandin synthesis in cats. Circ Res 57:142-151, 1985.

65. Cardillo C, Kilcoyne CM, Cannon RO, 3rd, et al. Xanthine oxidase inhibition with oxypurinol improves endothelial vasodilator function in hypercholesterolemic but not in hypertensive patients. Hypertension 30:57-63, 1997.

66. Cosentino F, Patton S, d'Uscio LV, et al. Tetrahydrobiopterin alters superoxide and nitric oxide release in prehypertensive rats. J Clin Invest 101:1530-1537, 1998.

67. Stroes E, Hijmering M, van Zandvoort M, et al. Origin of superoxide production by endothelial nitric oxide synthase. FEBS Lett 438:161-164, 1998.

68. Kerr S, Brosnan MJ, McIntyre M, et al. Superoxide anion production is increased in a model of genetic hypertension: Role of the endothelium. Hypertension 33:1353-1358, 1999.

69. Jameson M, Dai FX, Luscher T, et al. Endothelium-derived contracting factors in resistance arteries of young spontaneously hypertensive rats before development of overt hypertension. Hypertension 21:280-288, 1993.

70. Fridovich I, Freeman B. Antioxidant defenses in the lung. Annu Rev Physiol 48:693-702, 1986.

71. Thomson L, Trujillo M, Telleri R, et al. Kinetics of cytochrome c2+ oxidation by peroxynitrite: Implications for superoxide measurements in nitric oxide-producing biological systems. Arch Biochem Biophys 319:491-497, 1995.

72. Levanon D, Lieman-Hurwitz J, Dafni N, et al. Architecture and anatomy of the chromosomal locus in human chromosome 21 encoding the Cu/Zn superoxide dismutase. EMBO J 4:77-84, 1985.

73. De La Torre R, Casado A, Lopez-Fernandez E, et al. Overexpression of copper-zinc superoxide dismutase in trisomy 21. Experientia 52:871-873, 1996.

74. Morrison RA, McGrath A, Davidson G, et al. Low blood pressure in Down's syndrome: A link with Alzheimer's disease? Hypertension 28:569-575, 1996.

75. Goldblatt H, Lynch J, Hanzal RF, et al. Studies on experimental hypertension, I: The production of persistent elevation of systolic blood pressure by means of renal ischemia. J Exp Med 59:347-379, 1934.

76. Fukui T, Ishizaka N, Rajagopalan S, et al. p22phox mRNA expression and NADPH oxidase activity are increased in aortas from hypertensive rats. Circ Res 80:45-51, 1997.

77. Rajagopalan S, Kurz S, Munzel T, et al. Angiotensin II-mediated hypertension in the rat increases vascular superoxide production via membrane NADH/NADPH oxidase activation. Contribution to alterations of vasomotor tone. J Clin Invest 97:1916-1923, 1996.

78. Laursen JB, Rajagopalan S, Galis Z, et al. Role of superoxide in angiotensin II-induced but not catecholamine-induced hypertension. Circulation 95:588-593, 1997.

79. Zafari AM, Ushio-Fukai M, Akers M, et al. Role of NADH/NADPH oxidase-derived H2O2 in angiotensin II-induced vascular hypertrophy. Hypertension 32:488-495, 1998.

80. Dijkhorst-Oei LT, Stroes ES, Koomans HA, et al. Acute simultaneous stimulation of nitric oxide and oxygen radicals by angiotensin II in humans in vivo. J Cardiovasc Pharmacol 33:420-424, 1999.

81. Moreau P, d'Uscio LV, Shaw S, et al. Angiotensin II increases tissue endothelin and induces vascular hypertrophy: Reversal by ET(A)-receptor antagonist. Circulation 96:1593-1597, 1997.

82. Pohl U, Holtz J, Busse R, et al. Crucial role of endothelium in the vasodilator response to increased flow in vivo. Hypertension 8:37-44, 1986.

83. Koller A, Kaley G. Prostaglandins mediate arteriolar dilation to increased blood flow velocity in skeletal muscle microcirculation. Circ Res 67:529-534, 1990.

84. Okahara K, Sun B, Kambayashi J. Upregulation of prostacyclin synthesis-related gene expression by shear stress in vascular endothelial cells. Arterioscler Thromb Vasc Biol 18:1922-1926, 1998.

85. Moncada S, Gryglewski R, Bunting S, Vane JR. An enzyme isolated from arteries transforms prostaglandin endoperoxides to an unstable substance that inhibits platelet aggregation. Nature 263:663-665, 1976.

86. Joannides R, Haefeli WE, Linder L, et al. Nitric oxide is responsible for flow-dependent dilatation of human peripheral conduit arteries in vivo. Circulation 91:1314-1319, 1995.

87. Radomski MW, Palmer RM, Moncada S. Comparative pharmacology of endothelium-derived relaxing factor, nitric oxide and prostacyclin in platelets. Br J Pharmacol 92:181-187, 1987.

88. Chenevard R, Hurlimann D, Bechir M, et al. Selective COX-2 inhibition improves endothelial function in coronary artery disease. Circulation 107:405-409, 2003.

89. Küng CF, Lüscher TF. Different mechanisms of endothelial dysfunction with aging and hypertension in rat aorta. Hypertension 25:194-200, 1995.

90. Noll G, Lang MG, Tschudi MR, et al. Endothelial vasoconstrictor prostanoids modulate contractions to acetylcholine and ANG II in Ren-2 rats. Am J Physiol 272:H493-H500, 1997.

91. Yang ZH, von Segesser L, Bauer E, et al. Different activation of the endothelial L-arginine and cyclooxygenase pathway in the human internal mammary artery and saphenous vein. Circ Res 68:52-60, 1991.

92. Taddei S, Virdis A, Ghiadoni L, et al. Cyclooxygenase inhibition restores nitric oxide activity in essential hypertension. Hypertension 29:274-279, 1997.

93. Richard V, Tanner FC, Tschudi M, et al. Different activation of L-arginine pathway by bradykinin, serotonin, and clonidine in coronary arteries. Am J Physiol 259:H1433-H1439, 1990.

94. Vanhoutte PM. Vascular physiology: The end of the quest? [news]. Nature 327:459-460, 1987.

95. Taylor SG, Weston AH. Endothelium-derived hyperpolarizing factor: A new endogenous inhibitor from the vascular endothelium. Trends Pharmacol Sci 9:272-274, 1988.

96. Van de Voorde J, Vanheel B, Leusen I. Endothelium-dependent relaxation and hyperpolarization in aorta from control and renal hypertensive rats. Circ Res 70:1-8, 1992.

97. Fujii K, Tominaga M, Ohmori S, et al. Decreased endothelium-dependent hyperpolarization to acetylcholine in smooth muscle of the mesenteric artery of spontaneously hypertensive rats. Circ Res 70:660-669, 1992.

98. Edwards G, Dora KA, Gardener MJ, Garland CJ, Weston AH. K+ is an endothelium-derived hyperpolarizing factor in rat arteries. Nature 396:269-272, 1998.

99. Takase H, Moreau P, Kung CF, et al. Antihypertensive therapy prevents endothelial dysfunction in chronic nitric oxide deficiency. Effect of verapamil and trandolapril. Hypertension 27:25-31, 1996.

100. Taddei S, Ghiadoni L, Virdis A, et al. Vasodilation to bradykinin is mediated by an ouabain-sensitive pathway as a compensatory mechanism for impaired nitric oxide availability in essential hypertensive patients. Circulation 100:1400-1405, 1999.

101. Yanagisawa M, Kurihara H, Kimura S, et al. A novel potent vasoconstrictor peptide produced by vascular endothelial cells. Nature 332:411-415, 1988.

102. Hickey KA, Rubanyi G, Paul RJ, et al. Characterization of a coronary vasoconstrictor produced by cultured endothelial cells. Am J Physiol 248:C550-C556, 1985.

103. Ikegawa R, Matsumura Y, Tsukahara Y, et al. Phosphoramidon, a metalloproteinase inhibitor, suppresses the secretion of endothelin-1 from cultured endothelial cells by inhibiting a big endothelin-1 converting enzyme. Biochem Biophys Res Commun 171:669-675, 1990.

104. Takahashi M, Matsushita Y, Iijima Y, et al. Purification and characterization of endothelin-converting enzyme from rat lung. J Biol Chem 268:21394-21398, 1993.

105. Ohnaka K, Takayanagi R, Nishikawa M, et al. Purification and characterization of a phosphoramidon-sensitive endothelin-converting enzyme in porcine aortic endothelium. J Biol Chem 268:26759-26766, 1993.

106. Shimada K, Takahashi M, Tanzawa K. Cloning and functional expression of endothelin-converting enzyme from rat endothelial cells. J Biol Chem 269:18275-18278, 1994.

107. Rossi GP, Albertin G, Franchin E, et al. Expression of the endothelin-converting enzyme gene in human tissues. Biochem Biophys Res Commun 211:249-253, 1995.

108. Inoue A, Yanagisawa M, Takuwa Y, et al. The human preproendothelin-1 gene. Complete nucleotide sequence and regulation of expression. J Biol Chem 264:14954-14959, 1989.

109. Inoue A, Yanagisawa M, Kimura S, et al. The human endothelin family: Three structurally and pharmacologically distinct isopeptides predicted by three separate genes. Proc Natl Acad Sci USA 86:2863-2867, 1989.

110. Fleminger G, Bousso-Mittler D, Bdolah A, et al. Immunological and structural characterization of sarafotoxin/endothelin family of peptides. Biochem Biophys Res Commun 162:1317-1323, 1989.

111. Kloog Y, Bousso-Mittler D, Bdolah A, et al. Three apparent receptor subtypes for the endothelin/sarafotoxin family. FEBS Lett 253:199-202, 1989.

112. Kloog Y, Ambar I, Sokolovsky M, et al. Sarafotoxin, a novel vasoconstrictor peptide: Phosphoinositide hydrolysis in rat heart and brain. Science 242:268-270, 1988.

113. Boulanger C, Lüscher TF. Release of endothelin from the porcine aorta. Inhibition of endothelium-derived nitric oxide. J Clin Invest 85:587-590, 1990.

114. Boulanger CM, Tanner FC, Bea ML, et al. Oxidized low density lipoproteins induce mRNA expression and release of endothelin from human and porcine endothelium. Circ Res 70: 1191-1197, 1992.

115. Yoshizumi M, Kurihara H, Sugiyama T, et al. Hemodynamic shear stress stimulates endothelin production by cultured endothelial cells. Biochem Biophys Res Commun 161:859-864, 1989.

116. Kourembanas S, Marsden PA, McQuillan LP, et al. Hypoxia induces endothelin gene expression and secretion in cultured human endothelium. J Clin Invest 88:1054-1057, 1991.

117. Shirakami G, Nakao K, Saito Y, et al. Acute pulmonary alveolar hypoxia increases lung and plasma endothelin-1 levels in conscious rats. Life Sci 48:969-976, 1991.

118. Hieda HS, Gomez-Sanchez CE. Hypoxia increases endothelin release in bovine endothelial cells in culture, but epinephrine, norepinephrine, serotonin, histamine and angiotensin II do not. Life Sci 47:247-251, 1990.

119. Kohno M, Murakawa K, Yokokawa K, et al. Production of endothelin by cultured porcine endothelial cells: Modulation by adrenaline. J Hypertens Suppl 7:S130-S131, 1989.

120. Ohta K, Hirata Y, Imai T, et al. Cytokine-induced release of endothelin-1 from porcine renal epithelial cell line. Biochem Biophys Res Commun 169: 578-584, 1990.

121. Kanse SM, Takahashi K, Lam HC, et al. Cytokine stimulated endothelin release from endothelial cells. Life Sci 48:1379-1384, 1991.

122. Miyamori I, Takeda Y, Yoneda T, et al. Interleukin-2 enhances the release of endothelin-1 from the rat mesenteric artery. Life Sci 49:1295-1300, 1991.

123. Woods M, Bishop-Bailey D, Pepper JR, et al. Cytokine and lipopolysaccharide stimulation of endothelin-1 release from human internal mammary artery and saphenous vein smooth-muscle cells. J Cardiovasc Pharmacol 31:S348-S350, 1998.

124. Dohi Y, Hahn AW, Boulanger CM, et al. Endothelin stimulated by angiotensin II augments contractility of spontaneously hypertensive rat resistance arteries. Hypertension 19:131-137, 1992.

125. Barton M, Shaw S, d'Uscio LV, et al. Angiotensin II increases vascular and renal endothelin-1 and functional endothelin converting enzyme activity in vivo: Role of ETA receptors for endothelin regulation. Biochem Biophys Res Commun 238:861-865, 1997.

126. Abassi ZA, Tate JE, Golomb E, et al. Role of neutral endopeptidase in the metabolism of endothelin. Hypertension 20:89-95, 1992.

127. Abassi ZA, Golomb E, Bridenbaugh R, et al. Metabolism of endothelin-1 and big endothelin-1 by recombinant neutral endopeptidase EC.3.4.24.11. Br J Pharmacol 109:1024-1028, 1993.

128. Lüscher TF. Imbalance of endothelium-derived relaxing and contracting factors: A new concept in hypertension? Am J Hypertens 317:317-330, 1990.

129. Vierhapper H, Wagner O, Nowotny P, et al. Effect of endothelin-1 in man. Circulation 81:1415-1418, 1990.

130. Kiely DG, Cargill RI, Struthers AD, Lipworth BJ. Cardiopulmonary effects of endothelin-1 in man. Cardiovasc Res 33:378-386, 1997.

131. Ito H, Hirata Y, Hiroe M, et al. ET-1 induces hypertrophy with enhanced expression of muscle specific genes in cultured neonatal rat cardiomyocytes. Circ Res 69:209-215, 1991.

132. Barton M, d'Uscio LV, Shaw S, et al. ET(A) receptor blockade prevents increased tissue endothelin-1, vascular hypertrophy, and endothelial dysfunction in salt-sensitive hypertension. Hypertension 31:499-504, 1998.

133. Yang Z, Krasnici N, Lüscher TF. Endothelin-1 potentiates smooth muscle cell growth to PDGF: Role of ETA and ETB receptor blockade. Circulation 100:5-8, 1999.

134. Kannel WB, Gordon T, Offutt D. Left ventricular hypertrophy by electrocardiogram. Prevalence, incidence, and mortality in the Framingham study. Ann Intern Med 71:89-105, 1969.

135. Bots ML, Hoes AW, Koudstaal PJ, et al. Common carotid intima-media thickness and risk of stroke and myocardial infarction: The Rotterdam Study. Circulation 96:1432-1437, 1997.

136. O'Leary DH, Polak JF, Kronmal RA, et al. Carotid-artery intima and media thickness as a risk factor for myocardial infarction and stroke in older adults. Cardiovascular Health Study Collaborative Research Group. N Engl J Med 340:14-22, 1999.

137. Ghiadoni L, Taddei S, Virdis A, et al. Endothelial function and common carotid artery wall thickening in patients with essential hypertension. Hypertension 32:25-32, 1998.

138. Perticone F, Maio R, Ceravolo R, et al. Relationship between left ventricular mass and endothelium-dependent vasodilation in never-treated hypertensive patients. Circulation 99: 1991-1996, 1999.

139. Wagner OF, Christ G, Wojta J, et al. Polar secretion of endothelin-1 by cultured endothelial cells. J Biol Chem 267:16066-16068, 1992.

140. Sorensen SS. Radio-immunoassay of endothelin in human plasma. Scand J Clin Lab Invest 51:615-623, 1991.

141. Haynes WG, Webb DJ. Contribution of endogenous generation of endothelin-1 to basal vascular tone. Lancet 344:852-854, 1994.

142. Haynes WG, Ferro CJ, O'Kane KP, et al. Systemic endothelin receptor blockade decreases peripheral vascular resistance and blood pressure in humans. Circulation 93:1860-1870, 1996.

143. Yang Z, Bauer E, von Segesser L, et al. Different mobilization of calcium in endothelin-1-induced contractions in human arteries and veins: Effects of calcium antagonists. J Cardiovasc Pharmacol 16:654-660, 1990.

144. Yang ZH, Richard V, von Segesser L, et al. Threshold concentrations of endothelin-1 potentiate contractions to norepinephrine and serotonin in human arteries. A new mechanism of vasospasm? Circulation 82:188-195, 1990.

145. Lysko PG, Feuerstein G, Pullen M, et al. Identification of endothelin receptors in cultured cerebellar neurons. Neuropeptides 18:83-86, 1991.

146. Nambi P, Pullen M, Feuerstein G. Identification of endothelin receptors in various regions of rat brain. Neuropeptides 16:195-199, 1990.

147. Knuepfer MM, Han SP, Trapani AJ, et al. Regional hemodynamic and baroreflex effects of endothelin in rats. Am J Physiol 257:H918-H926, 1989.

148. Gardiner SM, Compton AM, Kemp PA, et al. Regional and cardiac haemodynamic responses to glyceryl trinitrate, acetylcholine, bradykinin and endothelin-1 in conscious rats: Effects of NG-nitro-L-arginine methyl ester. Br J Pharmacol 101: 632-639, 1990.

149. Nakamoto H, Suzuki H, Murakami M, et al. Different effects of low and high doses of endothelin on haemodynamics and hormones in the normotensive conscious dog. J Hypertens 9:337-344, 1991.

150. Donckier JE, Hanet C, Berbinschi A, et al. Cardiovascular and endocrine effects of endothelin-1 at pathophysiological and pharmacological plasma concentrations in conscious dogs. Circulation 84:2476-2484, 1991.

151. van den Buuse M, Itoh S. Central effects of endothelin on baroreflex of spontaneously hypertensive rats. J Hypertens 11:379-387, 1993.

152. Kannan H, Tanaka H, Ueta Y, et al. Effects of centrally administered endothelin-3 on renal sympathetic nerve activity and renal blood flow in conscious rats. J Auton Nerv Syst 49: 105-113, 1994.

153. Chapleau MW, Hajduczok G, Abboud FM. Suppression of baroreceptor discharge by endothelin at high carotid sinus pressure. Am J Physiol 263:R103-R108, 1992.

154. Mosqueda-Garcia R, Appalsamy M, Fernandez-Violante R, et al. Modulatory effects of endothelin on baroreflex activation in the nucleus of the solitary tract. Eur J Pharmacol 351: 203-207, 1998.

155. Sorensen SS, Madsen JK, Pedersen EB. Systemic and renal effect of intravenous infusion of endothelin-1 in healthy human volunteers. Am J Physiol 266:F411-F418, 1994.

156. Miyauchi T, Ishikawa T, Tomobe Y, et al. Characteristics of pressor response to endothelin in spontaneously hypertensive and Wistar-Kyoto rats. Hypertension 14:427-434, 1989.

157. Lariviere R, Day R, Schiffrin EL. Increased expression of endothelin-1 gene in blood vessels of deoxycorticosterone acetate-salt hypertensive rats. Hypertension 21:916-920, 1993.

158. Lariviere R, Thibault G, Schiffrin EL. Increased endothelin-1 content in blood vessels of deoxycorticosterone acetate-salt hypertensive but not in spontaneously hypertensive rats. Hypertension 21:294-300, 1993.

159. Li JS, Lariviere R, Schiffrin EL. Effect of a nonselective endothelin antagonist on vascular remodeling in deoxycorticosterone acetate-salt hypertensive rats. Evidence for a role of endothelin in vascular hypertrophy. Hypertension 24:183-188, 1994.

160. Schiffrin EL, Lariviere R, Li JS, et al. Deoxycorticosterone acetate plus salt induces overexpression of vascular endothelin-1 and severe vascular hypertrophy in spontaneously hypertensive rats. Hypertension 25:769-773, 1995.

161. Doucet J, Gonzalez W, Michel JB. Endothelin antagonists in salt-dependent hypertension associated with renal insufficiency. J Cardiovasc Pharmacol 27:643-651, 1996.

162. Lariviere R, Sventek P, Schiffrin EL. Expression of endothelin-1 gene in blood vessels of adult spontaneously hypertensive rats. Life Sci 56:1889-1896, 1995.

163. Hocher B, Rohmeiss P, Zart R, et al. Significance of endothelin receptor subtypes in the kidneys of spontaneously hypertensive rats: Renal and hemodynamic effects of endothelin receptor antagonists. J Cardiovasc Pharmacol 26:S470-S472, 1995.

164. Hocher B, Rohmeiss P, Zart R, et al. Function and expression of endothelin receptor subtypes in the kidneys of spontaneously hypertensive rats. Cardiovasc Res 31:499-510, 1996.

165. Hocher B, George I, Rebstock J, et al. Endothelin system-dependent cardiac remodeling in renovascular hypertension. Hypertension 33:816-22, 1999.

166. Saito Y, Nakao K, Mukoyama M, et al. Increased plasma endothelin level in patients with essential hypertension [letter]. N Engl J Med 322:205, 1990.

167. Miyauchi T, Yanagisawa M, Iida K, et al. Age- and sex-related variation of plasma endothelin-1 concentration in normal and hypertensive subjects. Am Heart J 123:1092-1093, 1992.

168. Haynes WG, Ferro CJ, Webb DJ. Bosentan in essential hypertension [letter; comment]. N Engl J Med 339:346; discussion 347, 1998.

169. Rossi GP, Colonna S, Pavan E, et al. Endothelin-1 and its mRNA in the wall layers of human arteries ex vivo. Circulation 99:1147-1155, 1999.

170. Stevens PA, Brown MJ. Genetic variability of the ET-1 and the ETA receptor genes in essential hypertension. J Cardiovasc Pharmacol 26:S9-S12, 1995.

171. Tiret L, Poirier O, Hallet V, et al. The Lys198Asn polymorphism in the endothelin-1 gene is associated with blood pressure in overweight people. Hypertension 33:1169-1174, 1999.

172. Nicaud V, Poirier O, Behague I, et al. Polymorphisms of the endothelin-A and -B receptor genes in relation to blood pressure and myocardial infarction: The Etude Cas-Temoins sur l'Infarctus du Myocarde (ECTIM) Study. Am J Hypertens 12:304-310, 1999.

173. Sharma P, Hingorani A, Jia H, et al. Quantitative association between a newly identified molecular variant in the endothelin-2 gene and human essential hypertension. J Hypertens 17:1281-1287, 1999.

174. Lüscher TF, Vanhoutte PM, Raij L. Antihypertensive treatment normalizes decreased endothelium-dependent relaxations in rats with salt-induced hypertension. Hypertension 9:193-197, 1987.

175. Tschudi MR, Criscione L, Novosel D, et al. Antihypertensive therapy augments endothelium-dependent relaxations in coronary arteries of spontaneously hypertensive rats. Circulation 89:2212-2218, 1994.

176. d'Uscio LV, Shaw S, Barton M, et al. Losartan but not verapamil inhibits angiotensin II-induced tissue endothelin-1 increase: Role of blood pressure and endothelial function. Hypertension 31:1305-1310, 1998.

177. Maeso R, Rodrigo E, Munoz-Garcia R, et al. Chronic treatment with losartan ameliorates vascular dysfunction induced by aging in spontaneously hypertensive rats. J Hypertens 16:665-672, 1998.

178. Rodrigo E, Maeso R, Munoz-Garcia R, et al. Endothelial dysfunction in spontaneously hypertensive rats: Consequences of chronic treatment with losartan or captopril. J Hypertens 15:613-618, 1997.

179. Boulanger CM, Desta B, Clozel JP, Vanhoutte PM. Chronic treatment with the CA2+ channel inhibitor RO 40-5967 potentiates endothelium-dependent relaxations in the aorta of the hypertensive salt sensitive Dahl rat. Blood Press 3:193-196, 1994.

180. Dohi Y, Criscione L, Pfeiffer K, et al. Angiotensin blockade or calcium antagonists improve endothelial dysfunction in hypertension: Studies in perfused mesenteric resistance arteries. J Cardiovasc Pharmacol 24:372-379, 1994.

181. Panza JA, Garcia CE, Kilcoyne CM, et al. Impaired endothelium-dependent vasodilation in patients with essential hypertension. Evidence that nitric oxide abnormality is not localized to a single signal transduction pathway. Circulation 91: 1732-1738, 1995.

182. Creager MA, Roddy M-A, Coleman SM, et al. The effect of ACE inhibition on endothelium-dependent vasodilation in hypertension. J Vasc Res 29:97, 1992.

183. Taddei S, Virdis A, Ghiadoni L, et al. Effects of angiotensin converting enzyme inhibition on endothelium-dependent vasodilatation in essential hypertensive patients. J Hypertens 16:447-456, 1998.

184. Lyons D, Webster J, Benjamin N. The effect of antihypertensive therapy on responsiveness to local intra-arterial NG-monomethyl-L-arginine in patients with essential hypertension. J Hypertens 12:1047-1052, 1994.

185. Millgard J, Hagg A, Sarabi M, et al. Captopril, but not nifedipine, improves endothelium-dependent vasodilation in hypertensive patients. J Hum Hypertens 12:511-516, 1998.

186. Schiffrin EL, Deng LY, Larochelle P. Progressive improvement in the structure of resistance arteries of hypertensive patients after 2 years of treatment with an angiotensin I-converting enzyme inhibitor. Comparison with effects of a beta-blocker. Am J Hypertens 8:229-236, 1995.

187. Ghiadoni L, Virdis A, Magagna A, et al. Effect of the angiotensin II type 1 receptor blocker candesartan on endothelial function in patients with essential hypertension. Hypertension 35:501-506, 2000.

188. Dawes M, Brett SE, Chowienczyk PJ, et al. The vasodilator action of nebivolol in forearm vasculature of subjects with essential hypertension. Br J Clin Pharmacol 48:460-463, 1999.

189. Sudano I, Taddei S, Virdis A, et al. Nifedipine enhances endothelium-dependent relaxation and inhibits contractions

to endothelin-1 and phenylephrine in hypertension. J Hypertens 16:1115(abstract), 1998.

190. Schiffrin EL, Deng LY. Structure and function of resistance arteries of hypertensive patients treated with a beta-blocker or a calcium channel antagonist. J Hypertens 14:1247-1255, 1996.

191. Taddei S, Virdis A, Ghiadoni L, et al. Lacidipine restores endothelium-dependent vasodilation in essential hypertensive patients. Hypertension 30:1606-1612, 1997.

192. Perticone F, Ceravolo R, Maio R, et al. Calcium antagonist isradipine improves abnormal endothelium-dependent vasodilation in never treated hypertensive patients. Cardiovasc Res 41:299-306, 1999.

193. Cockcroft JR, Chowienczyk PJ, Benjamin N, et al. Preserved endothelium-dependent vasodilatation in patients with essential hypertension. N Engl J Med 330:1036-1040, 1994.

194. Perticone F, Ceravolo R, Maio R, et al. Angiotensin-converting enzyme gene polymorphism is associated with endothelium-dependent vasodilation in never treated hypertensive patients. Hypertension 31:900-905, 1998.

195. Taddei S, Virdis A, Ghiadoni L, et al. Vitamin C improves endothelium-dependent vasodilation by restoring nitric oxide activity in essential hypertension. Circulation 97:2222-2229, 1998.

196. Nakazono K, Watanabe N, Matsuno K, et al. Does superoxide underlie the pathogenesis of hypertension? Proc Natl Acad Sci USA 88:10045-10048, 1991.

197. Duffy SJ, Gokce N, Holbrook M, et al. Treatment of hypertension with ascorbic acid. Lancet 354, 1999.

198. Cockcroft JR, Chowienczyk PJ, Brett SE, et al. Nebivolol vasodilates human forearm vasculature: Evidence for an L-arginine/NO-dependent mechanism. J Pharmacol Exp Ther 274:1067-1071, 1995.

199. Bowman AJ, Chen CP, Ford GA. Nitric oxide mediated venodilator effects of nebivolol. Br J Clin Pharmacol 38:199-204, 1994.

200. Van Nueten L, De Cree J. Nebivolol: Comparison of the effects of dl-nebivolol, d-nebivolol, l-nebivolol, atenolol, and placebo on exercise-induced increases in heart rate and systolic blood pressure. Cardiovasc Drugs Ther 12:339-344, 1998.

201. Wallin BG, Sundlof G, Stromgren E, et al. Sympathetic outflow to muscles during treatment of hypertension with metoprolol. Hypertension 6:557-662, 1984.

202. Spieker LE, Corti R, Binggeli C, et al. Baroreceptor dysfunction induced by nitric oxide synthase inhibition in humans. J Am Coll Cardiol 36:213-218, 2000.

203. Spieker LE, Noll G, Ruschitzka FT, et al. Working under pressure: The vascular endothelium in arterial hypertension. J Hum Hypertens 14:617-630, 2000.

204. Lüscher TF, Noll G. Endothelium-derived vasoactive substances. *In* Braunwald E (ed). Heart Disease. 5th ed. Philadelphia, WB Saunders, 1997; p 1165.

# Chapter 17

# Endothelin in Hypertension

## John A. Schirger, Guido Boerrigter, and John C. Burnett, Jr.

The endothelin (ET) system has been the focus of much attention in recent years, and excellent reviews are available.[1-4] In this chapter we provide an overview of the ET system before focusing on it in hypertension and its major complication, heart failure. We also provide a special emphasis on clinical trials.

The vascular endothelium is an important source of vasodilating and vasoconstricting factors (Figure 17–1). One of these vasoconstricting factors is ET-1, the most-potent human vasoconstrictor identified so far,[5] which opposes, for example, the vasodilating actions of nitric oxide (NO) and the C-type (vascular) natriuretic peptide CNP. The ET system includes three 21-amino acid peptide hormones—ET-1, ET-2, and ET-3—with ET-1 playing the prominent role in the cardiovascular system. ET is not stored in vesicles, and its secretion is primarily regulated at the level of synthesis. The final step in the biosynthesis is cleavage of ET from its precursor big-ET by an endothelin-converting enzyme (ECE). Stimuli for ET secretion include intraarterial pressure, low shear stress, angiotensin II (Ang II), vasopressin, catecholamines, and transforming growth factor β. There are two ET receptor subtypes, ET-A and ET-B, which belong to the superfamily of transmembrane receptors linked with guanine-nucleotide binding (G) proteins. In the vasculature, ET vasoconstricts via ET-A and ET-B receptors on vascular smooth muscle cells (VSMCs), while activation of ET-B receptors on endothelial cells leads to vasodilation. Under physiologic conditions, ET-1 appears to act as an autocrine and paracrine factor rather than an endocrine hormone, with about 80% of ET secreted via the basal membrane. The ET system contributes to basal vascular tone, as pharmacologic ET receptor blockade lowers the mean arterial pressure (MAP) by about 10 mm Hg. Apart from its vasomotor actions, ET promotes VSMC proliferation and has been implicated in the pathogenesis of atherosclerosis.[6] In addition to their presence in the vasculature, ETs and their receptors are present and function in various tissues (Figure 17–2).

Physiologic actions of ET include participation in the redistribution of tissue blood flow that occurs during physical exercise. In a rat model, ET-A receptor blockade attenuated the physiologic blood flow reduction to the internal organs, thus decreasing blood flow to active muscles during exercise.[7] In addition, exercise training in rats led not only to improved cardiac function with physiologic hypertrophy but also to an increase in ET messenger ribonucleic acid (mRNA) expression.[8] However, the same authors report that pathologic hypertrophy in spontaneously hypertensive rats is associated with an increase in ET mRNA expression, whereas exercise-induced physiologic hypertrophy in Wistar-Kyoto rats is not associated with alterations in ET mRNA.[9] Subsequently we discuss in more depth the vascular, renal, myocardial, and humoral actions of ET.

## BIOLOGIC ACTIONS OF ENDOTHELIN

### Vascular Actions

Vasoconstriction, with an increase in arterial pressure, is the most central action of ET. In the key study by Yanagisawa, bolus administration of ET in the rat produced a marked sustained hypertensive response.[5] In isolated porcine coronary arteries, ET produced a dose-dependent and sustained vasoconstriction. In other animal preparations, exogenous ET produced marked increases in systemic and regional vascular resistances, with decreases in cardiac output—the latter thought to be related, in part, to myocardial ischemia secondary to intense coronary vasoconstriction.[6,10] ET was even more constricting in isolated veins as compared with arteries, in part secondary to the reduced presence of NO in veins.[11]

The role of ET as a vasoconstrictor and regulator of arterial pressure has been demonstrated in studies in which the ET gene was transferred by adenoviral gene delivery into normal rats.[12] ET gene transfer resulted in an increase in arterial pressure that could be reversed by ET receptor blockade. These vasoconstrictor responses have not been limited to animal models or tissues. Administration of ET or big ET to normal humans has produced potent and reversible vasoconstrictor responses.[13] Infusion of exogenous ET has been reported to produce significant coronary vasoconstriction in humans, supporting a role for ET as an important potential mediator of myocardial ischemia in states of ET activation. Such vasoconstricting actions may be most important in the presence of a deficiency of counter regulatory humoral factors such as NO and CNP, as in some forms of hypertension. Thus the vasoconstricting action of ET in vivo probably reflects not simply a direct action of ET but rather an imbalance between ET, NO, and CNP. This concept has been underscored by the report that inhibition of NO in vivo markedly potentiates the coronary, renal, pulmonary, and systemic vasoconstricting and hypertensive responses to exogenous ET administered at pathophysiologic concentrations.[14]

Growth of the vascular wall in states such as hypertension has been thought to be due in part to ET.[15] This effect on vascular remodeling is most evident in isolated VSMCs and can be reversed by ET receptor blockade or by counterregulatory humoral factors such as atrial natriuretic peptide (ANP) or CNP.

### Renal Actions

The kidney has emerged as central in the biology of ET. Studies have clearly demonstrated that the renal circulation may be more sensitive than others in vasoconstrictor responsiveness to ET. Administration of ET at concentrations that mimic those observed in pathophysiologic states results in renal vasoconstriction in association with a decrease in

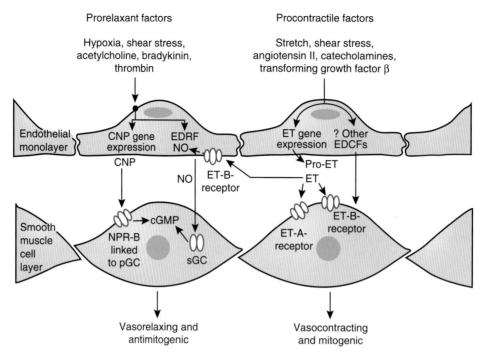

**Figure 17-1** Schematic diagram of endothelial and vascular smooth muscle cells with vasorelaxing (left) and vasoconstricting (right) factors. CNP, C-type natriuretic peptide; NO, nitric oxide; ET, endothelin; NPR-B, natriuretic peptide B-receptor; pGC, particulate guanylate cyclase; sGC, soluble guanylate cyclase; cGMP, cyclic guanosine monophosphate; EDRF, endothelium-derived relaxing factor; EDCF, endothelium-derived constricting factors. (From Boerrigter G, Burnett JC. Endothelin in neurohormonal activation in heart failure. Coronary Artery Disease 14:495-500, 2003.)

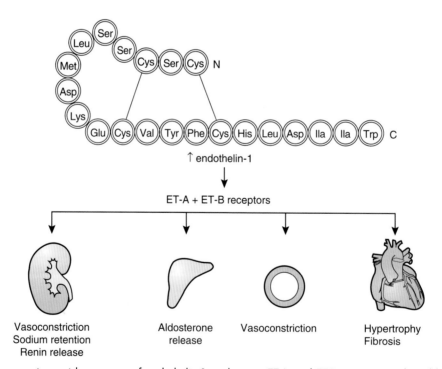

**Figure 17-2** Twenty-one amino acid sequence of endothelin-1 and major ET-A and ET-B receptor-mediated biologic actions.

sodium excretion.[16] These studies are complemented by evidence that ET administration to normal humans produces renal vasoconstriction and sodium retention.[17] It is important to note, however, that although the renal actions of exogenously administered ET in dogs and humans appear to be mediated by the ET-A receptor (see section Endothelin Receptors), and ET-A receptor antagonism may attenuate decreases in urinary sodium excretion and glomerular filtration rate (GFR) in the normal dog,[18] administration of an ET-A receptor antagonist in a model of canine congestive heart failure (CHF) results in sustained sodium retention without changing GFR (see discussion of congestive heart failure).[19]

These important renal actions of ET in humans and experimental animals have prompted studies to determine whether ET has a role in renal disease. Such a role is supported by increased renal production of ET in disease models such as acute and chronic renal failure (CRF), as well as by reports of increased urinary ET in models of renal transplant rejection and contrast nephropathy.[20,21] Thus ET is an important modulator of renal function and may participate in the pathophysiology of renal diseases that are associated with elevations in arterial pressure.

## Myocardial Actions

Another important target for ET is the heart. ET has been reported to have positive inotropic actions in isolated cardiomyocytes and in the intact heart.[22] Although this effect may be offset by coronary vasoconstriction and myocardial ischemia, the autocrine/paracrine action of endogenous ET may augment myocardial contractility. In an animal model of CHF with increased expression of ET, ET-A receptor blockade results in improved cardiac relaxation.[10,23]

ET may also have growth-promoting effects on ventricular myocytes and cardiac fibroblasts. In an animal model of ventricular hypertrophy produced by pressure overload of the left ventricle, blockade of ET attenuated ventricular hypertrophy independent of any reduction in cardiac afterload.[24] In isolated cardiac fibroblasts, ET receptors are expressed and may be activated by other humoral factors such as Ang II. Once activated, ET may serve as a mediator for production of collagen and thus induce cardiac fibrosis and impair myocardial relaxation.[25]

It is well established that ET is synthesized in cardiac myocytes and fibroblasts as well as endothelial cells, and it has been reported that ET mediates Ang II–induced myocyte hypertrophy and fibroblast proliferation.[26,27] Also, ET directly stimulates collagen synthesis through the ET-A receptor in adult rat cardiac fibroblasts.[28] ET is reported to reduce matrix metalloproteinase (MMP)-1 (interstitial collagenase) in skin fibroblasts and in adult rat cardiac fibroblasts[29] and to decrease MMP-2 in rat mesangial cells and in adult canine cardiac fibroblasts.[30] Similar to data for Ang II, these data suggest that ET stimulates myocardial fibrosis, not only by enhancing collagen synthesis, but also by diminishing MMP activity. Interestingly, Fernandez-Patron et al.[31] reported that MMP-2 cleaved big ET-1 to produce mature ET, suggesting an interaction between the MMP system and ET in the regulation of vascular reactivity.

We have investigated the crosstalk between cardiotrophin 1 (CT-1) and the ET system. CT-1 is a potent hypertrophic factor in cardiomyocytes and signals through the glycoprotein 130/leukemia inhibitory factor (gp130/LIF) receptor complex.[32,33] We have elucidated in canine cardiac fibroblasts an interaction between the CT-1/gp130/LIF receptor complex and the ET/ET-A receptor axis in regulatory DNA synthesis.[25] ET, derived from cardiac fibroblasts, has been known to mediate a hypertrophic response via the ET-A receptor in cardiomyocytes.[26] In addition, CT-1 and ET share a common signal transduction system, which includes mitogen-activated protein kinase activation.[32] Saito et al. have reported that ANP- and β-major histocompatibility complex–luciferase activation by ET was inhibited when cardiomyocytes were transfected with a dominant negative mutant of gp130.[34] We hypothesized that CT-1 activation of DNA synthesis in the cardiac fibroblast

would be modulated by ET via the ET-A receptor. This was confirmed by the findings that the specific ET-A receptor antagonist, BQ-123, inhibited not only ET-stimulated but also CT-1–stimulated DNA synthesis. Conversely, pretreatment with antibodies for the gp130/LIF receptor abolished the action of ET. We also demonstrated that ET stimulates the translocation of the LIF receptor from the cytosol to the cell surface. Our data suggest that an interaction between the CT-1/gp130/LIF receptor and ET/ET-A receptor occurs in cardiac fibroblasts and that crosstalk between these two systems may be of importance in cardiac fibroblast activation and cardiac remodeling.

## Humoral Actions

ET has key interactions with other neurohumoral systems. ET interacts importantly with NO via activation of the ET-B receptor (see later section), which is expressed primarily in vascular endothelium. ET thus releases NO, underscoring the unique balance between these two humoral pathways that mediate divergent actions on underlying vascular smooth muscle. ET also releases other vasodilating humoral factors of endothelial cell origin, such as CNP and adrenomedullin.[35,36] In addition, the production and release of ANP are linked to ET.

An important synergism exists between Ang II and ET. Ang II may enhance the vascular responsiveness to a given concentration of ET. Studies have also demonstrated that many of the myocardial actions of Ang II may occur via ET.[37] Ang II–mediated myocardial hypertrophy may involve activation of an ET receptor subtype, activation of myocardial ET production, or both. Furthermore, Ang II is a potent stimulus for ET gene expression in isolated cultured cardiac fibroblasts,[38] and inhibition of Ang II generation may therefore inhibit the tissue activation of ET. We have reported that activation of circulating and tissue ET in a model of heart failure could be markedly attenuated by chronic angiotensin-converting enzyme (ACE) inhibition.[39] The latter observation supports the view that some of the actions of ACE inhibition occur through inhibition of ET synthesis.

An additional key action of ET involves stimulation of the synthesis and release of aldosterone.[40] Studies in isolated zona glomerulosa cells have reported that ET is a potent activator of aldosterone synthesis.[41] Both ET-A and ET-B receptors appear to be involved.[42] The report that the aldosterone system coexists with ET in the heart, along with the known promoting effect of aldosterone on myocardial fibrosis, underscores the importance of exploring the emerging relationship between the ET system and aldosterone.

## ENDOTHELIN RECEPTORS

The multiple biologic actions of ET are mediated by at least two receptor subtypes, ET-A and ET-B (Figure 17–3). The ET-A receptor is widely expressed and is the principal receptor for the ET system in vascular smooth muscle. The ET-A receptor has higher affinity for ET-1 than for ET-3. ET-A receptor activation results in vasoconstriction via activation of phospholipase C and an increase in intracellular calcium.[43] The ET-B receptor was initially thought to be expressed only in vascular endothelial cells and to release vasodilating substances such as NO and prostacyclin, as well as the newly identified vasodilating peptide adrenomedullin. More-recent studies have

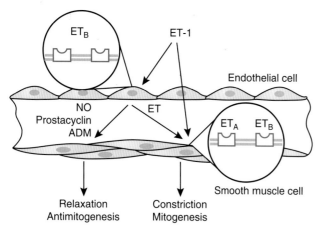

**Figure 17–3** ET receptor subtypes. ET-B receptors on endothelial cells stimulate secretion of the vasorelaxing and antimitogenic factors nitric oxide (NO), prostacyclin, and adrenomedullin (ADM), as well as the vasoconstrictor endothelin. Both ET-A and ET-B receptors on vascular smooth muscle cells promote vasoconstriction and mitogenesis.

demonstrated expression of the ET-B receptor in other vascular tissues such as the aorta, pulmonary vasculature, and coronary circulation and that its expression may be upregulated in pathophysiologic states in which the endothelium is damaged.[44-47] ET-B expression may be regulated by other humoral factors, such as Ang II.[48]

In addition to mediating vasorelaxation through the release of endogenous vasodilators, a vasoconstricting role for ET-B receptor activation has been reported in vitro, and studies suggest that ET-B receptor blockade may be necessary to reverse all of the vasoconstricting actions of ET. ET-A receptor antagonism with the selective ET-A receptor antagonist BQ-123 has been shown in vitro to incompletely inhibit the actions of ET. Furthermore, Fukuroda et al. demonstrated that the combination of a selective ET-B antagonist, BQ-788, with BQ-123 produced a synergistic inhibition of ET-mediated vasoconstriction in vitro.[49] Leadly et al. demonstrated in normal dogs a vasoconstrictor response to low doses of the selective ET-B receptor agonist sarafotoxin S6c in vivo, with increases in peripheral but not renal vascular resistance.[50] In addition, Haynes et al. reported that selective ET-B receptor activation with sarafotoxin S6c resulted in significant vasoconstriction in the human forearm.[51]

ET-B receptor activation has both direct and indirect vasoconstricting actions, the latter by increasing endogenous ET secretion, resulting in ET-A receptor activation. In vitro studies demonstrate that activation of the ET-B receptor upregulates the preproET-1 gene, with increased ET secretion from cultured endothelial and mesangial cells and cardiac myocytes.[52] This mechanism could account for ET-B receptor-mediated vasoconstriction via local activation of the ET-A receptor. Rasmussen et al. demonstrated that ET-B receptor activation with sarafotoxin S6c mediates systemic and pulmonary vasoconstriction, with decreases in cardiac output and SvO$_2$.[53] Selective ET-A receptor blockade attenuated the systemic vasoconstrictor action of high-dose sarafotoxin S6c. In addition, dual ET-A and ET-B receptor antagonism attenuated the increases in systemic and pulmonary vascular resist-

ance and the decreases in cardiac output seen with S6c. These studies suggest a role for the ET-B receptor in promoting vasoconstriction, at least to some extent via the ET-A receptor, probably through increased endogenous ET production. However, although the potential cardiopulmonary protective properties of dual ET-A/ET-B receptor blockade may represent an important therapeutic strategy in states of ET activation, there remains concern that blockade of ET-B, which can also serve as a clearance receptor, could enhance circulating concentrations of ET during dual receptor inhibition.[54]

## ACTIVATION AND BLOCKADE OF THE ENDOTHELIN SYSTEM IN HYPERTENSION

Given the success of antagonizing vasoconstricting neurohormonal systems that are activated in cardiovascular disease, it seems reasonable to try to antagonize the ET system in hypertension and heart failure. Consequently, a multitude of ET blockers have been developed and tested (Table 17–1). From a theoretical perspective, three ways to antagonize ET actions appear promising: (1) combined/dual ET-A/ET-B receptor blockade, (2) selective ET-A receptor blockade, or (3) inhibition of the ECE.

The potent vasoconstricting and growth-promoting properties of ET have suggested a potential role for ET in the pathogenesis of systemic hypertension. Circulating ET is not usually increased in hypertension, and any observed elevations are small and usually related to renal dysfunction.[55] In contrast, circulating ET is markedly increased in humans with hemangioendothelioma or severe forms of transplant-related hypertension.[56,57] Plasma ET is also increased in several models of experimental hypertension, including mineralocorticoid hypertension, the spontaneously hypertensive rat, and renovascular hypertension.[58,59] The lack of increase of plasma ET in human essential hypertension could be explained by the paracrine/autocrine function of ET; that is, ET secretion from the endothelial cell is albuminally directed, thus increasing tissue and not circulating concentrations of ET.[60]

Overexpression of ET-1 by gene transfer techniques has resulted in transient increases in plasma ET with associated hypertension.[12] Furthermore, ET synthesis has been shown to be increased in the vascular wall of the mineralocorticoid hypertensive rat.[61] A correlation has been reported between the magnitude of vascular wall hypertrophy and ET gene expression in this model of hypertension. However, this positive correlation is offset by an attenuated vascular responsiveness to exogenous ET, suggesting receptor down-regulation.

In human hypertension, however, the vasoconstricting responsiveness to ET has been reported to be enhanced.[62] ET infusion has been shown to result in an enhanced vasoconstrictor response in the hand veins of human hypertensives.[63] In contrast, no difference in the response to α receptor stimulation or in basal plasma ET concentration was observed between hypertensive and normotensive individuals in this study. Although some studies support a predominant role for the ET-A receptor in mediating the vasoconstrictor effects of ET-1 in hypertension, others report vasoconstriction mediated through the ET-B receptor in hypertension as well.[64] This may be due to a modification in the relative distribution of ET-B receptors on the endothelium and vascular smooth muscle in hypertension. Although the effect of ET-A activation appears straightforward,

**Table 17-1** Endothelin Inhibitors

| Drug Type | Peptide | Nonpeptide |
|---|---|---|
| ET-A receptor antagonist | BQ123 FR139317 | ABT627, BMS182874 BMS193884, LU135252, PD156707, PD176856, TTA78Ro611790, S0139, SB234551, T0201, TBC11251, ZD1611 |
| ET-A/ET-B receptor antagonist | PD142893 TAK044 | A182086, CGS27830, L754142, LU224332, PD160672, PD160874, Ro462005, Ro470203, SB209670, SB217242, J104121 |
| ET-B receptor antagonist | BQ788 IRL2500 RES7011 | A192621, K8794, RES11491, Ro468443, TBC10894 |
| ECE inhibitor | FR901533 WS75624A, B | CGS26303, PD069185, SA7060 |
| ECE/NEP inhibitor | | CGS26303, SLV-306 |

Peptide and nonpeptide inhibitors of the endothelin system. ET, endothelin; ECE, endothelin-converting enzyme; NEP, neutral endopeptidase.

the effect of ET-B receptor activation is more complex and quite controversial. As mentioned previously, some studies have shown that ET-B blockade in addition to ET-A blockade enhances vasodilation, whereas other studies have shown the opposite. Just et al. used different experimental strategies to elucidate the role of the ET-B receptor in the rat renal microcirculation and concluded that ET-B receptors when stimulated alone exert a net vasoconstrictor response but cause a net dilator influence when costimulated with ET-A receptors.[65] These findings suggest a complex interaction between the two receptor subtypes. The effect of ET-B activation/ET-B antagonism appears to be complex and to depend on factors such as species, vascular bed, pathophysiologic status, and experimental strategy. For that reason, absent large clinical trials comparing nonselective ET antagonists with selective ET-A antagonists, the controversy regarding which strategy would be more beneficial in hypertension will likely continue.

Hypertension in association with chronic kidney disease is common and may contribute to further renal damage, as well as to acceleration of atherosclerosis and ventricular dysfunction. ET concentration in blood vessels and glomeruli have been reported to be increased in experimental models of CRF.[66] Furthermore, ET receptor antagonists lower arterial pressure and reduce renal glomerular sclerosis and proteinuria in these models.[67]

Goddard and colleagues have addressed the pathophysiologic significance of ET in the pathophysiology of CRF.[68] These investigators studied the systemic and renal hemodynamic effects of ET receptor antagonists in CRF, examining differences between ET-A versus selective ET-B and combined ET-A and ET-B receptor blockade. In this key randomized placebo-controlled crossover study, ET-A blockade alone and in combination with ET-B blockade reduced blood pressure in patients with CRF. This effect was greater with ET-A blockade alone (Figure 17-4). ET-A blockade significantly increased renal blood flow and reduced renal vascular resistance when administered alone but not when combined with ET-B blockade. These changes in renal hemodynamics were associated with a reduction in effective filtration fraction. In healthy controls, ET-A blockade alone or in combination with ET-B blockade had minimal effects

on renal hemodynamics. Furthermore, ET-B blockade alone produced systemic and renal vasoconstriction both in patients with CRF and in healthy controls. Thus, this study demonstrated that ET-A receptor antagonism was highly effective in decreasing blood pressure in CRF—findings also consistent with renal protection. Importantly, because ET-B appears to play a key role in the maintenance of renal blood flow, combined ET-A and ET-B receptor antagonism, although it results in a lowering of blood pressure, does not confer these renal protective actions.

Nonselective and selective ET receptor blockade have been evaluated in clinical trials in patients with systemic hypertension. The nonselective ET-A/ET-B antagonist bosentan (500 and 2000 mg daily) reduced diastolic and systolic blood pressure significantly as compared with placebo and to a similar degree as enalapril (20 mg once daily).[69] Bosentan, which has been approved for the treatment of pulmonary hypertension, is associated with considerable risk of liver toxicity, making it an unlikely first-line drug in systemic hypertension, for which many alternatives are available. The selective ET-A antagonist darusentan significantly reduced diastolic and systolic pressure as compared with placebo.[70] No increase in hepatic transaminases was observed. Importantly, both clinical trials had, as their primary endpoint, change in blood pressure, and the treatment periods were 4 and 6 weeks, respectively. Given the known effects of ET-1 on VSMC hypertrophy and proliferation, it would be important to see how long-term selective or nonselective ET antagonism compares with established antihypertensive drug treatment in preventing hypertension-related target organ damage. Important endpoints in addition to mortality include cardiac hypertrophy and heart failure, as well as stroke and myocardial infarction.

## ENDOTHELIN IN CONGESTIVE HEART FAILURE

The ET system is clearly activated in both experimental and human CHF.[71] Plasma ET correlates with the severity of CHF,[72] and ET is known to promote vasoconstriction, as well as myocardial remodeling and fibrosis in CHF. These findings

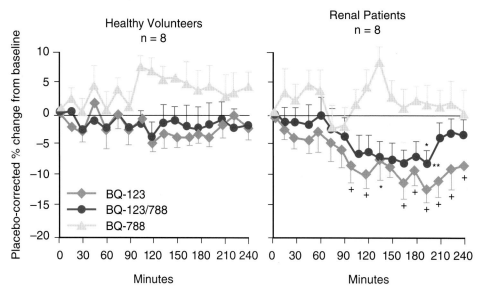

**Figure 17–4** Mean systemic arterial pressure after endothelin receptor antagonism in healthy humans and patients with chronic renal failure. Values are given as mean placebo-corrected % change from baseline ± standard error of measurement. Infusion of low-dose antagonist/placebo was done from 0-15 minutes; infusion of high-dose antagonist (10x low-dose)/placebo was done from 90-105 minutes. BQ-123, selective endothelin-A receptor antagonist, diamonds; BQ-788, selective endothelin-B receptor antagonist, triangle; BQ-123/BQ-788, circles. (From Goddard J, Johnston NR, Hand MF, et al. Endothelin-A receptor antagonism reduces blood pressure and increases renal blood flow in hypertensive patients with chronic renal failure. Circulation 109:1186-1193, 2004.)

have led to studies in experimental models of CHF that established hemodynamic improvements with ET receptor antagonism.[73,74] Initial clinical studies also showed improved hemodynamic function with administration of ET receptor antagonists.[75,76] The issue of whether nonselective or selective ET-A receptor antagonism is the best strategy to pursue is controversial. Although the ET-B receptor serves a clearance function and promotes vasorelaxation under physiologic conditions, under pathophysiologic conditions such as CHF, it promotes vasoconstriction and may activate other growth-promoting and vasoconstrictive factors. Nevertheless, studies with both selective and nonselective ET receptor antagonism showed hemodynamic improvement.

Disappointingly, clinical trials with both selective and nonselective ET receptor antagonism failed to show improvements in myocardial remodeling and, indeed, in one case showed an increase in congestive symptoms (see later). The reasons for this are not entirely clear, but a previous animal study showed that ET-A receptor antagonism in normal dogs results in increased sodium retention.[18] We have carried out a series of studies that suggest mechanisms for these clinical findings.[19] We first established that the ET system is activated early in the course of CHF. Specifically, at the transition to overt CHF as defined by the onset of sodium retention, the ET system is activated in both tissue and plasma in the absence of activation of Ang II or aldosterone (the renin-angiotensin-aldosterone system, RAAS). In a model of severe pacing-induced canine CHF, we defined the effects of chronic ET-A receptor antagonism initiated early in the progression of CHF on cardiac hemodynamics, neurohumoral function, and sodium homeostasis. We found that in addition to improving cardiac function and decreasing MAP, ET-A receptor blockade

resulted in sustained sodium retention and further activation of the RAAS (Figure 17–5). These findings suggest a mechanism for the increase in congestive symptoms noted in clinical trials with ET receptor antagonism. Carefully designed clinical trials that use dosing regimens different from those in the original studies may be warranted given the clear pathophysiologic role of ET in CHF.

Following are short summaries of studies with ET antagonists in experimental or human CHF. Several of these studies are available only as summaries from scientific meetings or as abstracts, because it is not uncommon that the results of negative trials are not published in full form.

Bosentan (RO 470203) is the best-developed ET-A/ET-B blocker and the only one to have been tested in a large clinical trial. Bosentan improved survival in a rat model of CHF when started 7 days after coronary artery ligation.[77] However, in a randomized placebo-controlled trial in 1613 patients with CHF (Endothelin Antagonist Bosentan for Lowering Cardiac Events in Heart Failure), bosentan did not improve mortality.[78] Bosentan was not different from placebo in the primary endpoints but was associated with worsening CHF caused by fluid retention, perhaps related to the renal mechanisms discussed in the preceding paragraph.

Tezosentan (RO 610612) was developed as an intravenous dual ET receptor antagonist for use in acute heart failure. Compared with placebo, tezosentan dose dependently increases cardiac index (CI) and decreases pulmonary capillary wedge pressure (PCWP) and pulmonary and systemic vascular resistance (PVR and SVR).[79] In the Randomized Intravenous TeZosentan (RITZ)-2 trial with 184 patients, tezosentan increased CI, decreased PCWP, and improved dyspnea score as compared with placebo.[80] In the symptom-

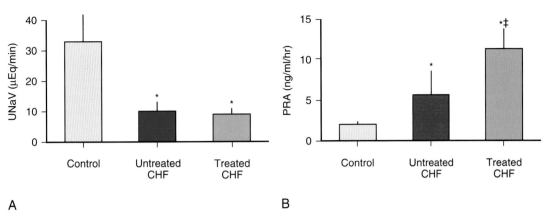

**Figure 17–5** Urinary sodium excretion (UNaV) (left) and plasma renin activity (PRA) in control (open bar), untreated congestive heart failure (black bar), and congestive heart failure treated with LU 135252 (hatched bar). *p <.05 vs. control; ‡p <.05 vs. untreated. (From Schirger JA, Chen HH, Jougasaki M, et al. Endothelin A receptor antagonism in experimental congestive heart failure results in augmentation of the renin-angiotensin system and sustained sodium retention. Circulation 109:249-254, 2004.)

based RITZ-1 trial with 675 patients, tezosentan did not improve the primary endpoint (the patient's assessment of dyspnea after 24 hours). Furthermore, tezosentan did not change the combined secondary endpoint, time to death, or worsening symptoms of CHF. Likewise, mortality at 6 months was unchanged.

In the Enrasentan Cooperative Randomized Evaluation (ENCORE) trial, patients taking standard medication were randomized to enrasentan or placebo.[80] Enrasentan (SB 217242) treatment was associated with trends to worsening CHF, increased rate of withdrawal for adverse events, and excess mortality. Patients taking enrasentan were almost three times as likely to be hospitalized. In another randomized controlled trial, 72 patients with asymptomatic left ventricular dysfunction were randomized to enrasentan or the ACE inhibitor enalapril. Compared with enalapril, enrasentan increased CI signficantly after 6 months of treatment; however, the primary endpoint, left ventricular end-diastolic volume index, was significantly increased, suggesting an adverse remodeling effect of enrasentan.[81]

Sakai et al. demonstrated that ET-A blockade with the peptide BQ-123 could improve long-term survival in a rat model of CHF.[24] In contrast, orally available darusentan (LU 135252) in a similar rat model did not improve survival. When given in combination with the ACE inhibitor trandolapril, there was no additional survival benefit as compared with trandolapril alone.[82] There have been several human trials with selective ET-A blockers. Darusentan in addition to standard therapy was evaluated in 157 patients in the Heart Failure ET(A) Receptor Blockade Trial (HEAT).[83] ET-A blockade with darusentan for 3 weeks increased CI and decreased SVR without changes in MAP or PCWP. However, there was a worrisome trend for higher mortality and a higher percentage of patients with worsening CHF in the treatment group. This might be attributed in part to the fact that patients were immediately assigned to either 30, 100, or 300 mg of darusentan without careful up-titration. The Endothelin-A Receptor Antagonist Trial in Heart Failure (EARTH) evaluated the effect of darusentan in addition to standard medication over a 6-month period. Although darusentan administration was safe, no benefit was apparent

for the treatment group (European Society of Cardiology Meeting, 2002, Berlin, Anand IS and Luescher TF).

Givertz et al. studied the effect of acute intravenous administration of the selective ET-A receptor antagonist sitaxsentan (TBC 11251) in a randomized placebo-controlled trial in 48 patients with New York Heart Association classes III and IV CHF.[84] Sitaxsentan decreased PVR, mean and systolic pulmonary artery pressure, and right atrial pressure. Interestingly, heart rate, MAP, PCWP, CI, and SVR remained unchanged. As expected, sitaxsentan administration was associated with a decrease in circulating ET.

In summary, ET receptor antagonism in CHF has not been demonstrated to be widely safe or efficacious to date. A novel molecule has recently been introduced that inhibits both ECE and neutral endopeptidase 24.11 (NEP). NEP is an enzyme that degrades the natriuretic peptides as well as other vasoactive compounds such as ET. Selective NEP inhibitors were tested in the past to enhance the beneficial vasodilating and natriuretic actions of the natriuretic peptides, but in CHF trials NEP inhibitors were not superior to standard therapy, perhaps because of the simultaneous inhibition of ET degradation. As mentioned previously, ET antagonism in clinical trials appears to be associated with fluid retention. Therefore, combined NEP/ECE inhibition could combine the beneficial actions of both strategies while attenuating the negative effects. Mulder et al. reported that ECE-NEP inhibition in a rat model of CHF was associated with beneficial effects as compared with placebo and NEP inhibition alone,[85] whereas Dickstein et al. reported the beneficial hemodynamic effects of combined ECE-NEP inhibition with SLV306 in patients with CHF.[86] Further studies appear warranted to pursue the strategy of dual ECE-NEP inhibition in cardiovascular diseases.

## SUMMARY

The lack of adequate antihypertensive treatment strategies underscores our lack of understanding of the mechanisms responsible for blood pressure elevation and its complications, including stroke, myocardial infarction, and heart failure. A neurohumoral basis for hypertension is supported by studies of humans with hypertension, of their offspring, and of experimental models.

ET, a peptide primarily of endothelial origin, may play a role in the pathogenesis of hypertension. ET possesses many of the properties that result in increased arterial pressure as well as its multiorgan complications. The elevation of blood pressure with genetic overexpression of ET by gene transfer and the lowering of blood pressure with ET receptor antagonism in humans with essential hypertension and hypertension associated with CRF provide the rationale for examining the contribution of this peptide to these disease processes.

## References

1. Miyauchi T, Masaki T. Pathophysiology of endothelin in the cardiovascular system. Annu Rev Physiol 61:391-415, 1999.
2. Kedzierski RM, Yanagisawa M. Endothelin system: The double-edged sword in health and disease. Annu Rev Pharmacol Toxicol 41:851-876, 2001.
3. Boerrigter G, Burnett JC. Endothelin in neurohormonal activation in heart failure. Coron Artery Dis 14:495-500, 2003.
4. Rich S, McLaughlin VV. Endothelin receptor blockers in cardiovascular disease. Circulation 108:2184-2190, 2003.
5. Yanagisawa M, Kurihara H, Kimura S, et al. A novel potent vasoconstrictor peptide produced by vascular endothelial cells. Nature 332:411-415, 1988.
6. Lerman A, Edwards BS, Hallett JW, et al. Circulating and tissue endothelin immunoreactivity in advanced atherosclerosis. N Engl J Med 325:997-1001, 1991.
7. Maeda S, Miyauchi T, Iemitsu M, et al. Involvement of endogenous endothelin-1 in exercise-induced redistribution of tissue blood flow: An endothelin receptor antagonist reduces the redistribution. Circulation 106:2188-2193, 2002.
8. Iemitsu M, Miyauchi T, Maeda S, et al. Effects of aging and subsequent exercise training on gene expression of endothelin-1 in rat heart. Clin Sci 103(Suppl 48):152S-157S, 2002.
9. Iemitsu M, Miyauchi T, Maeda S, et al. Physiological and pathological cardiac hypertrophy induce different molecular phenotypes in the rat. Am J Physiol Regul Integr Comp Physiol 281:R2029-R2036, 2001.
10. Miller WL, Redfield MM, Burnett JC, Jr. Integrated cardiac, renal, and endocrine actions of endothelin. J Clin Invest 83:317-320, 1989.
11. Moreland S, McMullen DM, Delaney CL, et al. Venous smooth muscle contains vasoconstrictor ET-Blike receptors. Biochem Biophys Res Commun 184:100-106, 1992.
12. Niranjan V, Telemaque S, deWit D, et al. Systemic hypertension induced by hepatic overexpression of human preproendothelin-1 in rats. J Clin Invest 98:2364-2372, 1996.
13. Pernow J, Kaijser J, Lennart L, et al. Comparable potent coronary constrictor effects of endothelin-1 and big endothelin-1 in humans. Circulation 94:2077-2082, 1996.
14. Lerman A, Sandok EK, Hildebrand FL, Jr., et al. Inhibition of endothelium-derived relaxing factor enhances endothelin-mediated vasoconstriction. Circulation 85:1894-1898, 1992.
15. Alberts GF, Peifley KA, Johns A, et al. Constitutive endothelin-1 overexpression promotes smooth muscle cell proliferation via an external autocrine loop. J Biol Chem 269:10112-10118, 1994.
16. Clavell AL, Stingo AJ, Margulies KB, et al. Role of endothelin receptor subtypes in the in vivo regulation of renal function. Am J Physiol 268:F455-F460, 1995.
17. Rabelink TJ, Kaassjager KAH, Boer P, et al. Effects of endothelin-1 on renal function in humans: Implications for physiology and pathophysiology. Kidney Int 46:376-378, 1994.
18. Syed N, Gulmi FA, Chou SY, et al. Renal actions of endothelin-1 under endothelin receptor blockade by BE-18257B. J Urol 159(2):563-566, 1998.
19. Schirger JA, Chen HH, Jougasaki M, et al. Endothelin A receptor antagonism in experimental congestive heart failure results in augmentation of the renin-angiotensin system and sustained sodium retention. Circulation 109:249-254, 2004.
20. Benigni A, Zola C, Corna D, et al. Blocking both type A and B endothelin receptors in the kidney attenuates renal injury and prolongs survival in rats with remanant kidney. Am J Kidney Dis 27:416-423, 1996.
21. Margulies KB, Hildebrand FL, Heublein DM, et al. Radio contrast increases plasma and urinary endothelin. J Am Soc Nephrol 2:1041-1045, 1991.
22. Ishikawa T, Yanagisawa M, Kimura S, et al. Positive inotropic actions of novel vasoconstrictor peptide on guinea pig atria. Am J Physiol 255:H970-H973, 1988.
23. Sakai S, Miyauchi T, Saruta T, et al. Endogenous endothelin-1 participates in the maintenance of cardiac function in rats with congestive heart failure. Circulation 93, 1214-1222, 1996.
24. Sakai S, Miyauchi T, Kobayashi M, et al. Inhibition of myocardial endothelin pathway improves long-term survival in heart failure. Nature 384:353-355, 1996.
25. Tsuruda T, Jougasaki M, Boerrigter G, et al. Cardiotrophin-1 stimulation of cardiac fibroblast growth: Roles for glycoprotein 130/leukemia inhibitory factor receptor and the endothelin type A receptor. Circ Res 90:128-134, 2002.
26. Gray MO, Long CS, Kalinyak JE, et al. Angiotensin II stimulates cardiac myocyte hypertrophy via paracrine release of TGF-β1 and endothelin-1 from fibroblasts. Cardiovasc Res 40:352-363, 1998.
27. Fujisaki H, Ito H, Hirata Y, et al. Natriuretic peptides inhibit angiotensin II-induced proliferation of rat cardiac fibroblasts by blocking endothelin-1 gene expression. J Clin Invest 96:1059-1065, 1995.
28. Guarda E, Katwa LC, Myers PR, et al. Effects of endothelins on collagen turnover in cardiac fibroblasts. Cardiovasc Res 27:2130-2134, 1993.
29. Xu S, Denton CP, Holmes A, et al. Endothelins: Effect on matrix biosynthesis and proliferation in normal and scleroderma fibroblasts. J Cardiovasc Pharmacol 31:S360-S363, 1998.
30. Yao J, Morioka T, Li B, et al. Endothelin is a potent inhibitor of matrix metalloproteinase-2 secretion and activation in rat mesangial cells. Am J Physiol Renal Physiol 280:F628-F635, 2001.
31. Fernandez-Patron C, Radomski MW, Davidge ST. Vascular matrix metalloproteinase-2 cleaves big endothelin-1 yielding a novel vasoconstrictor. Circ Res 85:906-911, 1999.
32. Heinrich PC, Behrmann I, Müller-Newen G, et al. Interleukin-6–type cytokine signalling through the gp130/Jak/STAT pathway. Biochem J 334:297-314, 1998.
33. Pennica D, Shaw KJ, Swanson TA, et al. Cardiotrophin-1: Biological activities and binding to the leukemia inhibitory factor receptor/gp130 signaling complex. J Biol Chem 270:10915-10922, 1995.
34. Saito S, Aikawa R, Shiojima I, et al. Endothelin-1 induces expression of fetal genes through the interleukin-6 family of cytokines in cardiac myocytes. FEBS Lett 456:103-107, 1999.
35. Kullo IJ, Burnett JC, Jr. C-type natriuretic peptide: The vascular component of the natriuretic peptide system. In Sowers JR (ed). Contemporary Endocrinology: Endocrinology of the Vasculature. Totowa, NJ, Humana, 1996; pp 79-93.
36. Jougasaki M, Schirger JA, Simari RD, et al. Autocrine role for the endothelin-B receptor in the secretion of endothelial-derived adrenomedullin. Hypertension 32:917-922, 1998.
37. Ito H, Hirata Y, Adachi S, et al. Endothelin-1 is an autocrine/paracrine factor in the mechanism of angiotensin II-induced hypertrophy in cultured rat cardiomyocytes. J Clin Invest 92:398-403, 1993.

38. Farch J, Touyz RM, Schiffrin EL, et al. Endothelin-1 and angiotensin II receptors in cells from rat hypertrophied heart, receptor regulation and intracellular $Ca^{2+}$ modulation. Circ Res 78:302-311, 1996.

39. Clavell A, Mattingly M, Nir A, et al. Angiotensin-converting enzyme inhibition modulates endogenous endothelin in chronic canine thoracic inferior vena cava constriction. J Clin Invest 97:1286-1292, 1996.

40. Cozza EN, Gomez-Sanchez CE, Foecking MF, et al. Endothelin binding to cultured calf adrenal glomerulosa cells and stimulation of aldosterone secretion. J Clin Invest 84:1032-1035, 1989.

41. Andreis PG, Neri G, Tortorella C, et al. Mechanisms transducing the aldosterone secretagogue signal of endothelins in the human adrenal cortex. Peptides 23:561-566, 2002.

42. Silvestre J-S, Robert V, Heymes C, et al. Myocardial production of aldosterone and corticosterone in the rat. J Biol Chem 273:4883-4891, 1998.

43. Xuan YT, Wang OL, Whorton AR. Regulation of endothelin-induced $Ca^{2+}$ mobilization in smooth muscle cells by protein kinase C. Am J Physiol 266(6 Pt 1):C1560-C1567, 1994.

44. Gray GA, Mickley EJ, Webb DJ, et al. Localization and function of ET-1 and ET receptors in small arteries post-myocardial infarction: Upregulation of smooth muscle ET-B receptors that modulate contraction. Br J Pharmacol 130:1735-1744, 2000.

45. Sumner MJ, Cannon TR, Mundin JW, et al. Endothelin ET-A and ET-B receptors mediate vascular smooth muscle contraction. Br J Pharmacol 107:858-860, 1992.

46. Kobayashi T, Miyauchi T, Iwasa S, et al. Corresponding distributions of increased endothelin-B receptor expression and increased endothelin-1 expression in the aorta of apolipoprotein E-deficient mice with advanced atherosclerosis. Pathol Int 50:929-936, 2000.

47. Bauer M, Wilkens H, Langer F, et al. Selective upregulation of endothelin B receptor gene expression in severe pulmonary hypertension. Circulation 105:1034-1036, 2002.

48. Wong NL, Tsui JK. Angiotensin regulates endothelin-B receptor in rat inner medullary collecting duct. Metabolism 50(6):661-666, 2001.

49. Fukuroda T, Ozaki S, Ihara M, et al. Synergistic inhibition by BQ-123 and BQ-788 of endothelin-1-induced contractions of the rabbit pulmonary artery. Br J Pharmacol 113:336-338, 1994.

50. Leadly RJ, Jr., Zhu JL, Goetz KL. Effects of endothelin-1 and sarafotoxin S6b on regional hemodynamics in the conscious dog. Am J Physiol 260:R1210-R1217, 1991.

51. Haynes WG, Webb DJ. Endothelium-dependent modulation of responses to endothelin-1 in human veins. Clin Sci 84:427-433, 1993.

52. Iwasaki S, Homma T, Matsuda Y, et al. Endothelin receptor subtype-B mediates autoinduction of endothelin-1 in rat mesangial cells. J Biol Chem 270:6997-7003, 1995.

53. Rasmussen TE, Jougasaki M, Supaporn T, et al. Cardiovascular actions of ET-B activation in vivo and modulation by receptor antagonism. Am J Physiol 274:R131-R138, 1998.

54. Fukuroda T, Fujikawa T, Ozaki S, et al. Clearance of circulating endothelin-1 by ET-B receptors in rats. Biochem Biophys Res Commun 199:1461-1465, 1994.

55. Kohno M, Yasunari K, Murakawa K, et al. Plasma immunoreactive endothelin in essential hypertension. Am J Med 88:614-618, 1990.

56. Yokokawa K, Tahara H, Kohno M, et al. Hypertension associated with endothelin-secreting malignant-hemangioendothelioma. Ann Intern Med 114:213-215, 1991.

57. Lerman A, Click RL, Narr BJ, et al. Elevation of plasma endothelin associated with systemic hypertension in humans following orthotopic liver transplantation. Transplantation 51:646-650, 1991.

58. Moreau P, Schiffrin EL. Role of endothelins in animal models of hypertension: Focus on cardiovascular protection. Can J Physiol Pharmacol 81:511-521, 2003.

59. Kohno M, Murakawa K, Horio T, et al. Plasma immunoreactive endothelin-1 in experimental malignant hypertension. Hypertension 18:93-100, 1991.

60. Wagner OF, Christ G, Wojta J, et al. Polar secretion of endothelin-1 by cultured endothelial cells. J Biol Chem 267:16066-16068, 1992.

61. Lariviere R, Thibault G, Schiffrin EL. Increased endothelin-1 content in blood vessels of deoxycorticosterone acetate-salt hypertensive but not spontaneously hypertensive rats. Hypertension 21:294-300, 1993.

62. Taddei S, Virdis A, Ghiadoni I, et al. Vasoconstriction to endogenous endothelin-1 is increased in the peripheral circulation of patients with essential hypertension. Circulation 100:1680-1683, 1999.

63. Haynes WG, Hand MF, Johnstone HA, et al. Direct and sympathetically mediated venoconstriction in essential hypertension. Enhanced responses to endothelin-1. J Clin Invest 94:1359-1364, 1994.

64. Cardillo C, Kilcoyne CM, Waclawiw M, et al. Role of endothelin in the increased vascular tone of patients with essential hypertension. Hypertension 33:753-758, 1999.

65. Just A, Olson AJ, Arendshorst WJ. Dual constrictor and dilator actions of ET(B) receptors in the rat renal microcirculation: Interactions with ET(A) receptors. Am J Physiol Renal Physiol 286:F660-F668, 2004.

66. Lariviere R, Lebel M, Kingma I, et al. Effects of losartan and captopril on endothelin-1 production in blood vessels and glomeruli of rats with reduced renal mass. Am J Hypertens 11:989-997, 1998.

67. Ding SS, Qiu C, Hess P, et al. Chronic endothelin receptor blockade prevents both early hyperfiltration and late overt diabetic nephropathy in the rat. J Cardiovasc Pharmacol 42:48-54, 2003.

68. Goddard J, Johnston NR, Hand MF, et al. Endothelin-A receptor antagonism reduces blood pressure and increases renal blood flow in hypertensive patients with chronic renal failure. Circulation 109:1186-1193, 2004.

69. Krum H, Viskoper RJ, Lacourciere Y, et al. The effect of an endothelin-receptor antagonist, bosentan, on blood pressure in patients with essential hypertension. Bosentan Hypertension Investigators. N Engl J Med 338:784-790, 1998.

70. Nakov R, Pfarr E, Eberle S, HEAT Investigators. Darusentan: An effective endothelinA receptor antagonist for treatment of hypertension. Am J Hypertens 15(7 Pt 1):583-589, 2002.

71. Wei C, Lerman A, Rodeheffer R, et al. Endothelin in human congestive heart failure. Circulation 89:1580-1586, 1994.

72. Galatius-Jensen S, Wroblewski H, Emmeluth C, et al. Plasma endothelin levels in congestive heart failure: A predictor of cardiac death? J Card Fail 2:71-76, 1996.

73. Borgeson DD, Grantham JA, Williamson EE, et al. Chronic oral endothelin type A receptor antagonism in experimental heart failure. Hypertension 31:766-770, 1998.

74. Spinale FG, Walker JD, Mukherjee R, et al. Concomitant endothelin receptor subtype-A blockade during progression of pacing induced congestive heart failure in rabbits. Circulation 95:1918-1929, 1997.

75. Sutsch G, Kiowski W, Yan X, et al. Short-term oral endothelin-receptor antagonist therapy in conventionally treated patients with symptomatic severe chronic heart failure. Circulation 98:2262-2268, 1998.

76. Love MP, Haynes WG, Gray GA, et al. Vasodilator effects of endothelin-converting enzyme inhibition and endothelin ETA receptor blockade in chronic heart failure patients treated with ACE inhibitors. Circulation 94:2131-2137, 1996.

77. Mulder P, Richard V, Derumeaux G, et al. Role of endogenous endothelin in chronic heart failure: Effect of long-term treatment with an endothelin antagonist on survival, hemodynamics, and cardiac remodeling. Circulation 96:1976-1982, 1997.

78. Kalra PR, Moon JC, Coats AJ. Do results of the ENABLE (Endothelin Antagonist Bosentan for Lowering Cardiac Events in Heart Failure) study spell the end for non-selective endothelin antagonism in heart failure? Int J Cardiol 85:195-197, 2002.

79. Torre-Amione G, Young JB, Durand J, et al. Hemodynamic effects of tezosentan, an intravenous dual endothelin receptor antagonist, in patients with class III to IV congestive heart failure. Circulation 103:973-980, 2001.

80. Louis A, Cleland JG, Crabbe S, et al. Clinical Trials Update: CAPRICORN, COPERNICUS, MIRACLE, STAF, RITZ-2, RECOVER and RENAISSANCE and cachexia and cholesterol in heart failure. Highlights of the Scientific Sessions of the American College of Cardiology, 2001. Eur J Heart Fail 3:381-387, 2001.

81. Prasad S, Smith G, Dargie H, et al. Enrasentan compared with enalapril in patients with asymptomatic left ventricular dysfunction. Circulation 106:II-470, 2002.

82. Mulder P, Boujedaini H, Richard V, et al. Long-term survival and hemodynamics after endothelin-A receptor antagonism and angiotensin-converting enzyme inhibition in rats with chronic heart failure: Monotherapy versus combination therapy. Circulation 106:1159-1164, 2002.

83. Luscher TF, Enseleit F, Pacher R, et al. Hemodynamic and neurohumoral effects of selective endothelin A (ET(A)) receptor blockade in chronic heart failure: The Heart Failure ET(A) Receptor Blockade Trial (HEAT). Circulation 106:2666-2672, 2002.

84. Givertz MM, Colucci WS, LeJemtel TH, et al. Acute endothelin A receptor blockade causes selective pulmonary vasodilation in patients with chronic heart failure. Circulation 101:2922-2927, 2000.

85. Mulder P, Barbier S, Monteil C, et al. Sustained improvement of cardiac function and prevention of cardiac remodeling after long-term dual ECE-NEP inhibition in rats with congestive heart failure. J Cardiovasc Pharmacol 43:489-494, 2004.

86. Dickstein K, De Voogd HJ, Miric MP, et al. Effect of single doses of SLV306, an inhibitor of both neutral endopeptidase and endothelin-converting enzyme, on pulmonary pressures in congestive heart failure. Am J Cardiol 94:237-239, 2004.

# Chapter 18

# Natriuretic Peptides

## Vito M. Campese, Mitra K. Nadim

Since the discovery by DeBold et al.[1] in 1981 that atrial extracts have potent natriuretic and vasodepressor activity, the natriuretic system has become known as a functionally important endocrine system of cardiovascular and renal origin that participates in the integrative control of their function. This led to the discovery of the atrial natriuretic peptide (ANP) and to the recognition of its importance in the regulation of sodium balance and blood pressure. Subsequently, four other natriuretic peptides, brain natriuretic peptide (BNP), C-type natriuretic peptide (CNP), dendroaspis natriuretic peptide (DNP), and urodilatin were discovered. Elevated plasma ANP levels have been reported in a variety of disease states associated with pathologic volume expansion such as congestive heart failure (CHF), chronic renal failure, and cirrhosis. It has been proposed that elevated ANP levels may represent a compensatory homeostatic response to chronic volume overload. The term *natriuretic peptides* has remained even though these peptides perform a multitude of functions besides natriuresis, including vasodilation, antiproliferative effects, vascular remodeling, and modulation of noradrenergic and the renin-angiotensin-aldosterone systems.

## CHEMISTRY OF NATRIURETIC PEPTIDES

Five distinct natriuretic peptides have been recognized, and at least three are the products of separate genes and subject to independent regulation. The first to be identified was ANP, a 28-amino acid (AA) peptide synthesized and secreted by the atria.[1] ANP contains a 17-AA ring closed by a disulfide bond between two cysteine residues. The ANP gene in humans is located on the short arm of chromosome 1 and is composed of three exons separated by two introns with regulatory elements upstream of the coding sequence.[2] ANP is synthesized as a 151-AA preprohormone (preproANP) and is stored in atrial myocytes as a 126-AA prohormone (proANP). When secreted, proANP is cleaved between AA 98 and 99 yielding an N-terminal moiety of 98-AA (N-ANP) and the biologically active C-terminal hormone (ANP) in equimolar amounts.[3] ANP has a very short half-life (2.5 minutes), whereas N-ANP has a much longer half-life (approximately 21 minutes) in plasma. Thus the plasma concentration of N-ANP is approximately 50 times greater than that of ANP. The AA sequence of ANP is identical in most mammals studied, with the exception of rodents and rabbits, in which isoleucine replaces methionine at position 110.

BNP is a 32-AA peptide, structurally similar to ANP that retains the 17-AA ring structure. A single copy gene consisting of three exons and two introns, which is also located on chromosome 1, encodes human BNP. The gene regulation of BNP is completely different from that of ANP: ANP is stored largely as proANP, whereas BNP is stored as the mature hormone in human and rat heart, and as proBNP in pig and sheep heart.[4] In contrast to ANP, the structure of BNP shows marked interspecies variability. In humans, the mature circulating form consists of a 32-AA residue peptide and a higher-molecular-weight component, probably proBNP. Two precursor forms of relatively high molecular mass, preproBNP (134-AAs) and proBNP (108-AAs) have been identified in human cardiac tissue[5] and plasma.[6] In rats, the circulating mature form is a 45-AA residue peptide, whereas in pigs, two circulating forms have been identified. Because of interspecies variability in structure, it is not surprising that species-specific antisera are required for measurements of BNP in plasma, and actions of BNP differ among species.

The third peptide to be discovered was CNP.[7] Human CNP consists of a precursor preproCNP of 126-AAs and a proCNP of 103-AAs, which is then processed to form two peptides, CNP-53 and CNP-22. CNP-22 is the only form that possesses substantial biologic activity.[8] Among the natriuretic peptides, CNP has the highest AA identity between species. Human CNP-53 has two AA substitutions as compared with the porcine and rat CNP-53, whereas human CNP-22 is identical to the porcine and rat CNP-22.[8] Structures of CNP-22 and proCNP appear to be identical in all mammalian species studied. CNP shares the 17-AA ring configuration, which is essential for biologic activity, with ANP and BNP, but lacks the carboxy terminal extension. The CNP gene is located on human chromosome 2.[9] It also has three exons, although the coding region of preproCNP is encoded within the first two. The regulatory mechanisms for the transcription of the CNP gene appear to differ from those that regulate ANP and BNP.[10]

Recently a new member of the natriuretic peptide family, DNP, a 38-AA natriuretic peptide, was isolated from the venom of the green mamba snake, *Dendroaspis angusticeps*.[11] DNP contains a 17-AA disulfide ring structure similar to ANP, BNP, and CNP with a 15-residue carboxy terminal extension. In addition, it has 12-and 14-AA residues in common with ANP and BNP-respectively. The gene encoding the peptide has yet to be cloned.

A nonglycosylated 32-AA natriuretic peptide was isolated from human urine and termed *urodilatin*.[12] Initially, this compound was thought to be ANP excreted in the urine. Subsequent studies demonstrated that urodilatin and ANP are different. The AA sequence of urodilatin is identical to that of ANP except for the presence of four additional AAs (Thr-Ala-Pro-Arg) in the amino terminal.[13] Urodilatin and ANP are derived from the same gene and a common precursor peptide, proANP.[13] In contrast to ANP, urodilatin is not detected in plasma and appears to be restricted to kidney.

## TISSUE DISTRIBUTION OF NATRIURETIC PEPTIDES

ANP gene expression is highest in normal adult atria and much lower in ventricles. However, in pathologic states, such as heart failure and ventricular hypertrophy, ANP gene expression in the ventricles may increase markedly. ANP mRNA is present in several areas of the brain, particularly in areas involved with blood pressure regulation, such as hypothalamus and brain stem. ANP mRNA has also been found in the anterior pituitary; kidney; vascular tissue; and particularly, the great cardiac veins, inferior vena cava, adrenal medulla, eye, lung, and gastrointestinal tract.[14]

BNP was initially isolated from the brain of pigs[15] and dogs.[16] Shortly thereafter, its name became a misnomer when it was discovered that the highest expression level of BNP was in the ventricular myocardium. Whereas ANP mRNA is largely present in atria, BNP mRNA is expressed in ventricles. BNP mRNA has also been found in extracardiac tissues, including porcine and human brain, bovine adrenal medulla, and human amnion tissue. In rats, extracardiac expression of this peptide is scant. Two types of secretory granules have been identified in human and porcine myocytes: One contains only ANP and the other contains both ANP and BNP.[17] Cosecretion of ANP and BNP has been demonstrated in porcine cardiocytes.[18]

CNP was also initially isolated from porcine brain,[7] and subsequently from rat and human brain extracts,[19] in which it occurs in greater concentration than either ANP or BNP. CNP is the only hormone in the heart and brain of the primitive cartilaginous fish and is believed to be an ancestral peptide of the natriuretic peptide family.[20] Immunoreactive CNP and CNP gene transcripts are found in abundance in the cerebral cortex, brain stem, cerebellum, basal ganglia, hypothalamus, and spinal cord of most species. In cerebrospinal fluid, CNP is about 10-fold higher in concentration than ANP or BNP. The concentration of CNP in plasma, however, is at the lower limit of detection and it has been proposed to act in a paracrine or autocrine manner to regulate local vascular tone.[21] CNP is detectable in a variety of peripheral tissues including endothelium, kidney, adrenal glands, heart, small and large bowel, thymus, uterus, and testis.[22-28] CNP in the atrial and ventricular myocardium may have important local actions. Some have suggested that CNP in the myocardium derives from the endothelium of coronary arteries.[29] CNP has been localized in the endothelium in humans, primarily as the CNP-53 AA precursor, which may be a storage form to be transformed into the active CNP-22 when needed. CNP-53 has also been detected in human plasma, suggesting a possible physiologic role.[30] It is not clear, however, whether plasma concentrations of CNP provide a sensitive index of local production in the vasculature or in other tissues. Using in situ hybridization, Cataliotti et al. have demonstrated CNP mRNA expression in tubular epithelium and in the visceral and parietal layer of glomeruli in human kidneys.[31] CNP immunoreactivity was positive in the proximal, distal, and medullary collecting ducts.

DNP-like immunoreactivity has been detected in canine and human plasma and atrial myocardium.[32, 33] Urodilatin is synthesized exclusively in kidney tubules and secreted into the tubular lumen.[34] Immunohistochemical studies have shown urodilatin-like immunoreactivity in the distal and collecting tubules, especially in the cortical collecting duct. Urodilatin is not detectable in plasma and is presumed to be processed in the distal tubule from the same precursor as ANP.[35] However, urodilatin gene expression has not been detected in kidney.

## NATRIURETIC PEPTIDE RECEPTORS

All natriuretic peptides exert their biologic effects by interacting with specific receptors. Molecular cloning techniques have identified three different subtypes of natriuretic peptide receptors (NPRs), NPR-A, NPR-B and NPR-C, which have been localized to three human chromosomes; however, the designations do not correspond to the relative affinities for ANP, BNP, and CNP.[36] NPR-A and NPR-B mediate the biologic actions of the hormones, whereas NPR-C mainly acts as a clearance receptor.[37] The NPRs are transmembrane proteins that are members of the receptor guanylyl cyclase family found in target tissues of the natriuretic peptides. Each receptor contains an extracellular binding domain to which a natriuretic peptide can bind. NPR-A and NPR-B have an extracellular ligand-binding domain, an intracellular guanylate cyclase domain, and a protein kinase-like domain that catalyzes the formation of cyclic guanosine monophosphate (cGMP) from guanosine triphosphate (GTP).[38] Intracellular cGMP targets include cGMP-dependent protein kinases, cGMP-gated ion channels, and cGMP-regulated cyclic nucleotide phosphodiesterases.[39] ANP, BNP, and urodilatin selectively activate NPR-A. In canines, synthetic DNP increases urinary cGMP excretion, suggesting that DNP may function through the NPR-A receptor, which is linked to particulate guanylyl cyclase and cGMP generation.[33] However, the existence of a new, yet to be discovered natriuretic peptide receptor cannot be excluded. ANP has greater affinity for the NPR-A than does BNP,[40] whereas CNP has very low affinity for this receptor. By contrast, CNP binds more selectively with NPR-B, with an affinity three orders of magnitude greater than that of either ANP or BNP.[41] This raises the possibility of developing specific antagonists for these receptors.

ANP, BNP, and CNP all bind to the NPR-C receptor, which functions mainly as a clearance receptor.[42,43] NPR-C contains an extracellular ligand binding domain and a short (37-AA) intracellular domain, but unlike NPR-A and NPR-B, lacks the intracellular protein kinase-like and guanylyl cyclase regions. NPR-C is thought to act through internalization and lysosomal hydrolysis of the natriuretic peptide-receptor complex, followed by return to the cell surface. Some studies suggest that NPR-C acts by activating the phosphoinositol pathway[44] or by inhibiting cyclic adenosine monophosphate (cAMP) production;[45] others have suggested that this receptor may mediate antiproliferative effects of ANP, as well as the inhibitory effects of ANP on adrenergic neurotransmission in peripheral tissues and cells.[46] The neuromodulatory effects of ANP via NPR-C involves suppression of adenylyl cyclase activity via a pertussis-toxin–sensitive G protein.[47]

The number and distribution of NPRs vary widely among tissues. NPR-A is expressed in heart, lungs, kidney, adrenal glands, adipose tissue, eye, pregnant uterus, and placenta.[48,49] In the kidney, NPR-A is expressed in renal vessels, glomeruli, inner medullary collecting duct, and papillae, consistent with the predominant role of ANP at these sites.[50] The distribution of NPR-B overlaps somewhat with that of NPR-A, but this receptor is present in lower density than NPR-A in large vessels and kidney and in higher density in brain. The distribution of NPR-B in kidneys of Sprague-Dawley rats was studied by reverse transcriptase polymerase chain reaction (RT-PCR) techniques: NPR-B receptors were present in glomeruli, distal convoluted tubules, and cortical and outer medullary and inner medullary tubules, but not in proximal convoluted tubules or in thin or thick ascending limbs.[51] Using RT-PCR, expression of NPR-A has been shown to be four times more abundant in human arteries than in veins, whereas expression of NPR-B was approximately the same.[52] NPR-C is the most abundant NPR in most tissues, and is expressed in the heart, kidney, brain, endothelium, smooth muscle cells, and adrenal glands.[4,37] More than 90% of all ANP receptors in kidney are NPR-C. These receptors are mainly localized in the vascular and glomerular structures of the cortex, particularly in the podocytes of glomerular cells.[50,53] Genes for all three NPR subtypes are expressed in the rat heart.[54] cGMP generation in purified myocytes was stimulated only by ANP and BNP, which bind specifically to NPR-A, whereas CNP, which binds to NPR-B, was ineffective. Therefore, rat ventricular myocytes appear to express predominantly NPR-A. The mRNAs for all three NPRs were also found in cultures of fibroblasts from the rat heart.[54] In contrast to myocytes, large increases in cGMP were observed in response to both ANP and CNP in cardiac fibroblasts.

The number and distribution of NPRs may vary in response to a variety of hormones, intracellular mediators, and metabolic and pathologic conditions. In sheep kidney, sodium depletion enhances expression of NPR-B mRNA twofold.[55] In cultured bovine carotid artery endothelial cells, high-salt medium induced a marked reduction in the number of NPR-C, whereas NPR-A density was not affected.[56] Chronic oral salt supplementation in mice resulted in selective downregulation of NPR-C gene expression in the kidney independent of changes of ANP levels and expression of NPR-A.[57] NPR-C gene expression is also reduced in the kidney of Dahl salt-sensitive and salt-resistant rats after chronic salt loading, whereas expression of NPR-A and NPR-B is not altered.[53] These studies support the notion that NPR-C plays an important role in the regulation of salt balance and in the pathophysiology of salt-sensitive hypertension. After induction of myocardial infarction (MI) in rats, NPR-C expression increased in the infarcted and noninfarcted regions of the left ventricular wall, while it decreased in the kidneys and lungs. BNP and ANP mRNA levels, as well as circulating ANP and BNP also increased, suggesting that the increase in circulating ANP and BNP levels in this condition may be due, at least in part, to reduced peripheral clearance by NPR-C.[58]

Recently, the mechanisms involved in the regulation of NPR-C have received considerable attention. Downregulation of NPR-C in tissues has typically been attributed to increased ANP levels in the circulation, which result in increased cGMP production through the activation of NPR-A and guanylate cyclase.[59,60] However, in vitro, NPR-C gene expression in pulmonary arterial smooth muscle cells was not reduced by high concentrations of ANP or cGMP.[61] In addition, studies in ANP knockout mice (-/-) subjected to hypoxia or dietary salt supplementation indicate selective reduction in NPR-C in the absence of circulating ANP.[57,62,63] This downregulation may contribute to the increase in circulating ANP levels seen under hypoxic conditions and may enhance the vasodilator effects of ANP in lung, thus regulating hypoxic pulmonary vasoconstriction and hypertension. A variety of growth factors, including fibroblast growth factor (FGF), protein kinase A and C, platelet-derived growth factor (PDGF), and β-adrenergic agonists have recently been shown to regulate ANP receptors in tissues.[62,64,65] In pulmonary arterial smooth muscle cells, rapid reduction in NPR-C mRNA levels have been demonstrated in response to very low concentrations of FGF and PDGF.[61] This observation was found to be mediated by overexpression of tyrosine kinase-activating growth factors. This study suggests that, in vivo, these growth factors could also potentially be physiologic regulators of NPR-C gene expression.

# REGULATION OF NATRIURETIC PEPTIDE SECRETION

ANP and BNP are continuously released from the heart, but certain mechanical and neuroendocrine stimuli also increase their rate of synthesis and/or secretion. Atrial stretch is the principal stimulus for ANP release. In response to acute stretching of the atria, ANP secretion from atrial cardiocytes is increased, leading to an immediate rise in plasma levels of the hormone. Release of ANP is not $Ca^{2+}$ dependent and derives from an acutely releasable pool that is exhausted within minutes after the initial stretch stimulus. Stretch over a 4-hour period does not alter ANP gene expression in atria but does stimulate it after 24 hours. Studies in isolated atrial tissues and myocytes have revealed an increase in ANP release after resting tension is increased, suggesting that atrial stretch-induced ANP release acts independently of central nervous system (CNS) effects and heart beat.[14] The transplanted heart resembles the normal heart in its response to exercise by increasing secretion of ANP.[66]

Stretch of myocardial cells affects the secretion of natriuretic peptides only transiently, suggesting that chronic stimulation of ANP secretion may be under the influence of other factors, such as endothelin-1 (ET-1),[67,68] catecholamines,[69] acetylcholine, glucocorticoids, angiotensin II (Ang II),[70] thyroid hormones, prostaglandins,[71] Na, K-ATPase inhibitors,[72] vasopressin, and adrenomedullin.[73] Of these factors, ET-1 appears to be the most powerful stimulator of ANP, although this action is transient, probably as a result of desensitization of ET-1 receptor binding, and down-regulation of phospholipase C activity.[74] Administration of BQ123, an ET-1 subtype A ($ET_A$) receptor antagonist, reduces stretch-induced ANP release, suggesting that ET-1 acts as a modulator of ANP secretion in a paracrine fashion. In a study by Leskinen et al., the release of ANP in response to atrial stretch in rats was shown to be mediated by endothelin (ET) as opposed to a direct mechanical effect.[68] However, ET receptor blockers had no significant effect on baseline plasma concentrations of ANP in the absence of stretch. ET-1 also stimulates BNP gene expression in cultured neonatal atrial cardiocytes as well as in adult atrial tissue.[75] Using isolated rabbit hearts, Focaccio et al. showed that Ang II causes release of ANP in the absence of hemodynamic changes.[70] How much of this effect is due to atrial stretch as a result of change in hemodynamics versus direct action of the vasoconstrictor remains to be determined.

The neuroendocrine component of ANP release from the atria is mediated by oxytocin.[76] Baroreceptors in the brain respond to blood volume expansion by releasing oxytocin.[77]

Specific oxytocin receptors in the heart mediate the action of oxytocin to release ANP, which then exerts negative inotropic and chronotropic effects via activation of guanylyl cyclase and elevation of cGMP. BNP release is not affected by oxytocin.

Transcriptional control of natriuretic peptide production is not the same in atria as in ventricles.[78-81] Whereas natriuretic peptide expression in the atria appears to be governed by mechanical stimuli, in the ventricles, the expression of ANP and BNP appear to be mainly dependent on the endocrine environment. Following aortic banding in rats, Ogawa et al. reported down-regulation of ventricular expression of natriuretic peptides following treatment with a low dose of the angiotensin-converting enzyme (ACE) inhibitor ramipril, whereas ANP production did not change with either a low or high dose of the ACE inhibitor.[80] In rats with deoxycorticosterone acetate (DOCA)-salt hypertension and renovascular hypertension, ventricular ANP and BNP gene expression, blood pressure and the development of left ventricular hypertrophy (LVH) were reduced after chronic blockade of $ET_A$.[78,79] However, natriuretic peptide stores and mRNA levels in the atria were not modified by $ET_A$ blockade, suggesting that, in vivo, modulation of ANP production is independent of endocrine factors and is mainly determined by atrial wall stretch. In contrast, in DOCA-salt hypertension, blockade of ET receptor type B ($ET_B$) worsened hypertension and increased LVH without an increase in ventricular natriuretic peptide (VNP) transcript levels in comparison with animals treated with DOCA-salt alone.[81] This study supports the hypothesis that mechanical stimuli per se are not the only determinant of ventricular natriuretic peptide gene expression and that the increase in blood pressure does not correlate with the enhancement of natriuretic peptide expression in the ventricles.

BNP secretion and gene expression are affected by acute stretch in some, but not all experimental models.[82] Because BNP is predominantly secreted from the ventricles, the main stimulus for BNP release appears to be ventricular stretch. With chronic stimulation, as seen in DOCA-salt treated rats, both ANP and BNP mRNAs increase in atria and ventricles.[83] ANP and BNP mRNA levels are also increased in the hearts of spontaneously hypertensive rats (SHR),[84] of dogs subjected to rapid ventricular pacing,[85] and of humans with CHF.[86]

ANP and BNP are cosecreted, but seem to respond differently to the same stimuli. For example, unlike ANP, the plasma concentration of BNP does not change when normal subjects assume the supine position. BNP release is stimulated by increases in left ventricular end-diastolic pressure, pulmonary artery pressure, and pulmonary artery wedge pressure.[87,88] In patients with chronic renal failure, removal of fluids reduced blood levels of BNP.[89] In isolated perfused heart, BNP and ANP release is stimulated by ventricular stretch.[90]

The transcription of the CNP gene is regulated by many factors, such as tumor necrosis factor (TNF), interleukin-1, and transforming growth factor (TGF). These cytokines influence vascular cell proliferation, migration, and contraction, effects that can be modulated by CNP. In conditions characterized by widespread damage to endothelium, such as sepsis, hypoxia, and chronic renal failure, blood levels of CNP are elevated.[91] The markedly elevated plasma levels of CNP in chronic renal failure could be related in part to endothelial damage and in part to reduced clearance of the peptide. Plasma concentrations of CNP are not increased in chronic

CHF, a condition associated with very high levels of ANP and BNP. Whether this reflects no increase in myocardial production or whether plasma concentrations are not necessarily a marker of tissue activation of CNP remains to be established.

## METABOLISM OF NATRIURETIC PEPTIDES

The metabolism of natriuretic peptides involves two main pathways: enzymatic degradation by neutral endopeptidase 24.11 (NEP) and receptor-mediated clearance via the NPR-C clearance receptor.[49] NEP 24.11 is a membrane-bound metalloprotease that cleaves ANP between AA 105 and 106, thus, opening the ring structure and inactivating the peptide.[92] It is widely distributed throughout the body and is expressed in high concentrations in the brush border membranes of the renal proximal tubules.[93] NEP degrades the peptides in the following order of CNP < ANP < BNP.[94] The second mechanism involved in elimination of natriuretic peptides is via clearance receptors. NPR-C serves a clearance function for natriuretic peptides in tissues. NPR-C binds to natriuretic peptides in the order of ANP < CNP < BNP.[40] Urodilatin is also inactivated by NPR-C and by enzymatic degradation through NEP, but is more resistant to enzymatic degradation than ANP, which may explain the greater natriuretic effects of urodilatin than ANP.[95] Recently, natriuretic and renal hemodynamic actions of synthetic DNP were shown to be attenuated by HS-142, a natriuretic peptide receptor antagonist, while NEP inhibition had no effect.[96] These findings suggest that the actions of DNP are mediated partly via the natriuretic peptide guanylyl cyclase receptors and that DNP either is resistant to degradation by NEP due to its long C-terminus or is not a substrate at all.

Inhibition of NEP and occupation of NPR-C produce increases in plasma ANP concentration, urine sodium and volume excretion, and a decrease in blood pressure.[97,98] Coadministration of these agents produces greater effects than those achieved when either of these agents is administered alone.[97] At physiologic plasma concentrations of ANP, NPR-C may play a dominant role over NEP. In rats with heart failure, inhibition of NEP and NPR-C induces a significant rise in plasma ANP with vasodilation, natriuresis, and diuresis.[84] Under these circumstances, the clearance receptor appears to play a lesser role than that of NEP in the metabolism of the peptide because of receptor occupancy, receptor down-regulation, or decreased internalization of the receptor-ligand complex.[99]

## OTHER NATRIURETIC PEPTIDES

The cardiac ventricle of rainbow trout contains a VNP structurally more similar to ANP than to BNP.[100] Only VNP has been isolated from rainbow trout or from a related species, the chum salmon, *Oncorhynchus keta*. In these species, attempts to isolate ANP from atria using immunoreactivity to mammalian ANP as an assay system have been unsuccessful. A new natriuretic peptide isolated from trout atria exhibits low relaxant activity in the chick rectum and extremely low vasorelaxant activity in the rat aortic strip (only 1/400 that of human ANP). This peptide was equipotent with trout VNP and human ANP in relaxing trout epibranchial arteries.[101]

Two related peptides are guanylin and uroguanylin, 15-AA and 16-AA peptides produced primarily in the gastrointestinal mucosa. These peptides act through the cGMP pathway to regulate sodium and water transport across the intestinal mucosa and may also coordinate intestinal absorption with subsequent renal excretion of sodium.[102]

# PHYSIOLOGIC ACTIONS OF NATRIURETIC PEPTIDES

## Renal Effects

In low doses, sufficient to achieve a doubling of basal plasma levels, ANP causes natriuresis but no change in blood pressure, unless the infusion is prolonged.[103,104] ANP causes intravascular volume contraction, as documented by increases in serum albumin and hematocrit, due in part to diuresis and in part to a shift of fluids from the capillary beds into the interstitium,[105] resulting in decreased preload and blood pressure.[106]

Qualitatively, the effects of BNP are similar to those of ANP. BNP is natriuretic in both animals and human subjects, even at doses that produce plasma levels comparable with those in heart failure. Equimolar infusions of ANP and BNP achieve similar increments in plasma concentrations, but the increase in cGMP during ANP infusion is fourfold that observed during BNP infusion. The natriuresis and contraction in plasma volume caused by the two peptides are comparable.

The mechanisms of the natriuretic action of BNP and ANP are complex. ANP raises glomerular filtration rate (GFR) in the isolated perfused rat kidney in spite of decreased systemic arterial pressure and renal blood flow,[107] and increased single nephron GFR, measured by the micropuncture technique.[108] ANP also increases GFR in normal subjects[109] and in patients with essential hypertension.[110] These findings suggest that the renal hemodynamic effects of ANP account, at least in part, for its natriuretic action. The increase in GFR has been ascribed to constriction of the efferent glomerular arterioles, accompanied by dilation of the afferent glomerular arterioles.[107] Unlike ANP, despite similar natriuretic effects, BNP does not alter GFR in humans,[111] suggesting that at least some of the natriuretic effects of natriuretic peptides must be due to mechanisms other than changes in GFR. ANP inhibits sodium transport in the proximal tubule[112] and in the inner medullary collecting duct.[113] ANP causes diuresis and natriuresis, at least in part by inhibiting the V2 receptor-mediated action of vasopressin in the collecting duct. The site of interaction of ANP and vasopressin is post cAMP synthesis.[114]

Shin et al. demonstrated increases in ANP mRNA expression in the kidneys of streptozotocin-induced diabetic rats; urinary ANP excretion correlated with urinary sodium excretion in these animals.[115] In a subsequent study, the authors were able to demonstrate an increase in renal cortical and medullary CNP mRNA levels in the diabetic rats with an accompanying elevation of urinary CNP excretion rate that improved with salt restriction and insulin treatment, implying that CNP synthesized in kidney is responsive to the alteration of water and electrolyte homeostasis in diabetic rats.[116]

DNP is similar to ANP and BNP in that it has potent natriuretic and diuretic properties.[33] In dogs, infusion of DNP was associated with increases in plasma cGMP and urinary cGMP excretion independent of increases in plasma ANP, BNP, or CNP suggesting that the renal actions of DNP are direct and not mediated by the other natriuretic peptides.[33] In addition, administration of exogenous DNP led to decreases in distal tubular reabsorption of sodium and arterial pressure in the absence of any change in GFR or renal blood flow.

The discovery of selective antagonists of natriuretic peptides has allowed further clarification of their physiologic roles. A selective NPR antagonist, HS-142-1, was isolated from a fungal culture broth of *Aureobasidium* species.[117] HS-142-1 selectively and reversibly blocks guanylyl cyclase-linked NPR-A and NPR-B receptors and interferes with cGMP production.[118] Studies with HS-142-1 have confirmed a role for the endogenous natriuretic peptides in the control of renal sodium excretion and in the natriuretic response to volume expansion. This drug blocks the natriuretic and diuretic actions of the ANPs in control animals as well as in animals with experimentally induced heart failure. HS-142-1 increases renal vascular resistance, renin, aldosterone, and catecholamines secretion, but does not affect basal renal blood flow.[118,119]

Using NPR-A knockout mice, the contribution of NPR-A signaling to acute renal salt handling has been studied.[120] Following intravenous administration of ANP, wild-type mice responded with elevated urine and sodium excretion, whereas NPR-A–null mice were unresponsive to ANP. This suggests that ANP regulation of diuresis and natriuresis is solely through NPR-A and that no other receptor can compensate. In order to determine whether natriuretic factors other than ANP are released by the heart in response to elevated blood pressure, NPR-A knockout and wild-type mice were volume expanded.[120] Plasma ANP concentrations were elevated in animals of both genotypes, but urine flow, sodium excretion and urinary cGMP were increased only in the wild type. These results imply that for acute sodium and volume handling, NPR-A is most likely the sole mediator of renal response to cardiac peptides. Because basal urine and sodium excretory rates did not differ between wild-type and null mice, it seems likely that a mechanism other than natriuretic peptide signaling through NPR-A regulates chronic salt and water handling by the kidney.

Transgenic mice overexpressing an ANP fusion gene have low blood pressure regardless of their dietary salt composition but are not different from wild-type mice in their urinary salt output.[121] These mice adequately compensate for the renal effects but not the hemodynamic effects of ANP.[122] This suggests the presence of a compensatory mechanism, which prevents renal salt and water loss in the face of high natriuretic peptide levels. This compensatory mechanism can be overridden by acute volume expansion, and thus ANP-induced natriuresis is observed.[121]

Urodilatin, by means of its renal paracrine interaction, exerts essential physiologic regulation of sodium and water excretion. Urodilatin excretion correlates directly with urinary sodium excretion.[13] High dietary sodium intake or saline infusion results in increased urodilatin excretion, whereas no such correlation is evident between urine sodium excretion and ANP excretion.[13] In addition, circadian rhythm of urinary sodium excretion is correlated with urinary urodilatin excretion. Intravenous administration of urodilatin in normal volunteers results in greater natriuresis than administration of ANP with fewer hypotensive effects.[123] When injected into healthy men in doses >20 ng/kg/min, urodilatin induces diuresis and natriuresis and inhibits renin secretion; higher doses lower blood pressure.[123] The natriuretic action of urodilatin is due in part to an increase in GFR and in part to direct effects on distal tubules. Urinary excretion of urodilatin increases in concert with renal sodium excretion, being higher during salt ingestion or after an acute saline infusion.[124] The natriuretic effect of urodilatin is stronger than that of ANP in healthy men and in experimental models of CHF.[95,125] This has led to the suggestion that urodilatin may be more important than ANP in the regulation of sodium excretion. The mechanisms underlying the greater potency of urodilatin over ANP are not clear, but its relative resistance to NEP degradation may be a contributory factor.

## Hemodynamic Effects

Homozygous ANP-null mice develop hypertension and cardiac hypertrophy. Following a high-salt diet, ANP-deficient mice had significantly higher blood pressures than those maintained on a standard diet, suggesting a salt-sensitive form of hypertension.[126] Sustained low-dose infusions of ANP reduce peripheral vascular resistance and blood pressure in animals and in humans, whereas infusions of higher doses cause a decrease in blood pressure accompanied by a rise in peripheral vascular resistance, probably as a result of activation of counterregulatory hormones. In this instance, the hypotensive action of ANP is largely related to a shift of intravascular fluid into the interstitium, thus decreasing preload. Infusion of BNP in high doses into hypertensive rats also causes a profound and sustained fall in blood pressure.[127] However, when administered to hypertensive or normotensive human subjects in doses sufficient to raise plasma concentrations to levels comparable with those seen in heart failure, BNP causes no significant change in blood pressure or heart rate.[128] When administered in higher doses to normal subjects, BNP causes decreases in systemic vascular resistance and in blood pressure, a rise in cardiac index, and significant reductions in pulmonary capillary wedge pressure, pulmonary vascular resistance, and right atrial pressure.[129] When administered in high doses to patients with CHF, BNP causes similar hemodynamic changes, but systemic blood pressure and pulmonary vascular resistance do not change. The vasorelaxation caused by BNP is associated with and, probably dependent on, the release of cGMP.

ANP and BNP may attenuate the vasoconstriction caused by infusion of norepinephrine and angiotensin II. Thus ANP and BNP may modulate changes in blood pressure caused by other neuroendocrine homeostatic mechanisms and local endothelial factors. Studies of the role of natriuretic peptides in the control of basal cardiovascular tone have been made possible by the discovery of selective antagonists. HS-142-1 causes constriction of the coronary circulation in anesthetized mongrel dogs without any significant change in systemic hemodynamics, including arterial pressure, heart rate, or cardiac filling pressure.[130] These actions were associated with a decrease in plasma cGMP; circulating ANP levels did not change. This observation suggests that ANP is an important regulator of basal coronary vascular tone.

CNP is produced in blood vessels and in cultured vascular endothelial cells and acts as an endothelium-derived relaxing peptide.[131] CNP can induce relaxation and inhibit growth of vascular smooth muscle cells and has powerful venodilator effects.[132-134] Using a NPR-B specific monoclonal antibody that inhibited CNP-stimulated cGMP accumulation, Drewett et al. demonstrated that CNP relaxes vascular smooth muscle by virtue of its binding to NPR-B.[132] In vitro studies have shown that CNP dilates saphenous, femoral, and renal veins, both in the presence and in the absence of the endothelium, but the venous relaxation is more potent in the absence of the endothelium.[135] In addition, CNP may be an important regulator of basal coronary vascular tone. This effect may be due to receptor-mediated clearance of CNP by endothelial NPR-C, CNP-mediated release of endothelium-dependent vasoconstrictors, or metabolism by endothelial NEP. In isolated human blood vessels in vitro, CNP causes venous relaxation and, to a lesser degree, arterial relaxation. Arterial relaxation is less pronounced with CNP than with ANP.[136] In human gastroepiploic artery, Ikeda et al.[52] found that ANP raised cGMP production by one order of magnitude more than in veins. CNP stimulated cGMP production weakly and equally in these vessels. Analyzed by RT-PCR, expression of NPR-A receptor was four times more abundant in arteries than in veins. Expression of NPR-B was approximately the same in arteries and veins. In cardiac myocytes, CNP reduces contractility and induces accumulation of cGMP, effects opposite of those induced by ET-1.[137]

Intravenous administration of CNP to normal rats (5-50 μg/kg) induces hypotension, a fall in right atrial pressure, and a small diuresis and natriuresis.[30] These responses are attenuated in SHR.[138] In dogs, intravenous infusions of CNP cause hemodynamic effects similar to those in rats, but the natriuretic effect is less evident.[139] Intravenous injection of CNP in normal humans elicits limited biologic actions. When infused intravenously in doses sufficient to achieve plasma concentrations of approximately 60 fmol/ml (circulating levels of CNP in humans are <10 fmol/ml), CNP has no significant biologic actions.[140] When infused in doses sufficient to achieve plasma concentrations of 770 fmol/ml, CNP exerts significant natriuretic, kaliuretic, and hypotensive actions.[141] However, the natriuretic action of CNP appears to be less than that of ANP or BNP. The hemodynamic actions of CNP are more pronounced than those of ANP despite lesser increase in plasma cGMP, raising the possibility that some of the actions of CNP are not mediated by cGMP. Wei et al. showed that the vasorelaxant effects of CNP are inhibited by potassium chloride, but not by blockade of adrenoreceptors, nitric oxide synthase, prostaglandin synthesis, or by methylene blue, an inhibitor of guanylate cyclase.[142] CNP causes potassium channel activation and membrane hyperpolarization in porcine coronary artery smooth muscle cells.[142]

DNP has been shown to relax isolated rodent aorta and canine coronary arteries[11,143] with a potency comparable with ANP. In addition, DNP augments the formation of cGMP in aortic endothelial and smooth muscle cells and displaces ANP binding from the NPRs.[11] Relaxation of an isolated canine coronary artery by DNP was reduced by HS-142, an inhibitor of guanylate cyclase.[143] In vitro, DNP has been shown to cause a dose-dependent relaxation of human blood vessels with a greater effect on the arteries than the veins.[144] DNP resulted in less arterial relaxation than ANP or CNP and similar relaxation to BNP, while in veins, DNP caused the greatest relaxation of the natriuretic peptides.

Mice with genetically altered natriuretic peptide expression have been used to investigate the contribution of natriuretic peptides to blood pressure regulation. Overexpression of the ANP gene lowers systemic blood pressure.[145] On the other hand, ANP knockout mice have higher blood pressures than wild-type controls, independent of salt intake.[146] ANP-deficient mice on a high-salt diet have significantly higher blood pressures than those maintained on a standard diet, suggesting a salt-sensitive form of hypertension. In response to acute intravascular volume expansion, wild-type mice show a greater natriuresis than ANP-null mice while on a low-salt diet. However, animals fed a high-salt diet exhibit enhanced natriuresis irrespective of genotype. These studies demonstrated that ANP lowers blood pressure independently of renal salt excretion.[126] Given that both ANP knockout and transgenic mice can maintain salt balance regardless of dietary salt intake, ANP may be more important for blood pressure regulation than for renal salt handling.

NPR-A knockout mice have been used to investigate the contribution of natriuretic peptides to blood pressure regulation via NPR-A.[147,148] Disruption of the NPR-A gene has been shown to result in chronic elevations of blood pressure in mice on normal and high-salt diets.[147] Aldosterone and ANP concentrations are not affected by genotype, suggesting that mutations in the NPR-A gene could explain some salt-resistant forms of essential hypertension and that the NPR-A signaling pathway could potentially operate independently of ANP. In a study by Lopez et al., both ANP and BNP caused dose-dependent relaxation of precontracted aortic rings from wild-type but not NPR-A–null mice. In wild-type animals, ANP was much more potent than CNP in lowering blood pressure; however, in NPR-A–null animals, ANP had no effect on blood pressure even at very high levels, whereas CNP was as effective as in wild-type animals.[147] This study demonstrates that ANP and BNP act through NPR-A, whereas CNP acts through another receptor to regulate blood pressure.

## Antiproliferative Effect

Vascular remodeling is central to the pathophysiology of hypertension and atherosclerosis. The pivotal role of vasoactive substances present in the blood vessel in the control of vascular growth is well known. Whereas vasoconstricting peptides such as Ang II promote vascular growth, vasodilating substances such as natriuretic peptides inhibit vascular growth. ANP has been shown to be antimitogenic in endothelial and vascular smooth muscle cells[133,149,150] and to attenuate the growth response to adrenergic stimuli[151] and induce apoptosis in neonatal rat cardiomyocytes.[152] Moreover, ANP-induced apoptosis occurs through the induction of p53 and inhibition of Bcl2 proteins.[153] The apoptotic effect of ANP can be inhibited by specific blockade of NPR-A or modulated by ET (an antiapoptotic factor). Similar effects have been noted in neonatal rat cardiac myocytes.[152]

In cultured vascular smooth muscle cells, CNP exerts a growth-inhibitory action and antagonizes the growth-promoting action of Ang II, which is mediated through the Ang II subtype 1 receptor.[154] CNP, like the other natriuretic factors, blunts stimulated ET-1 production in vitro,[155] apparently via cGMP. As ET-1 causes vascular smooth muscle cell proliferation, CNP could locally inhibit vascular smooth muscle cell proliferation via this mechanism. CNP exerts growth inhibitory effects in human vascular smooth muscle cells and can reduce the response of these cells to growth factors.[133,156,157]

Endothelial secretion of CNP is stimulated by various cytokines and growth factors, such as TGF-β and TNF-α, that are produced and activated in proliferative vascular lesions.[131,158] In vivo, CNP infusion reduces the extent of the vascular injury response in rats with carotid artery injury.[159]

Overexpression of CNP via local adenovirus-mediated gene transfer has been shown to suppress vascular remodeling and thus prevent restenosis in porcine coronary arteries in vivo following balloon injury.[160] This strategy may prevent restenosis after angioplasty in humans. In the rat mesangio-proliferative anti-Thy 1.1 model, CNP was involved in the regulation of mesangial cell proliferation and matrix production, suggesting that it may regulate tissue homeostasis and contribute to resolution of mesangioproliferative diseases.[161]

## Modulation of Sympathetic Nervous System Activity

The effects of ANP on blood pressure and fluid and electrolyte balance are largely mediated via the kidney and the vasculature. However, evidence indicates that the effects of ANP on the CNS also contribute to fluid and electrolyte balance and hemodynamic regulation. Although natriuretic peptides are unable to cross the blood-brain barrier, they are capable of reaching sites in the CNS outside this barrier such as the subfornical organ, hypothalamic median eminence, and area postrema. ANP decreases sympathetic tone via an action on the brain stem.[162] Dampening of baroreceptors, suppression of the release of catecholamines from autonomic nerve endings and suppression of sympathetic outflow from the CNS are some of the mechanisms that are responsible for this reduction in sympathetic tone.[162,163] Injection of BNP into the ventrolateral medulla, an area of the brain important in the noradrenergic control of blood pressure, causes a decrease in blood pressure and heart rate in rats.[164] Microinjection of a monoclonal anti-ANP antibody into the anterior hypothalamus decreases blood pressure in SHR, but not in normotensive control Wistar-Kyoto (WKY) rats.[165,166] This suggests that the activity of ANP is enhanced in the hypothalamus of SHR as a result of either increased production of ANP in the brain or increased receptor sensitivity.[167] On the other hand, inhibition of the action of endogenous ANP in the nucleus tractus solitarius raises blood pressure, suggesting a role in the tonic regulation of cardiovascular baroreceptor signal to this area of the brain.[163] ANP synthesis in key brain nuclei that regulate the cardiovascular system is affected by changes in blood volume.[168] ANP inhibits salt appetite, water drinking, and vasopressin secretion from the pituitary, and this central action of the peptide contributes to controlling fluid and electrolyte homeostasis.[169,170] Patients with advanced CHF manifest activation of the sympathetic nervous system (SNS), decreased heart rate variability, and loss of modulation of muscle SNS activity in the low-frequency range. Infusion of ANP augments the variability of SNS activity, suggesting a beneficial effect on neurogenic circulatory control.[171]

ANP and BNP are present in Purkinje fibers of several mammals, including humans.[172-174] ANP has also been shown in the nodose ganglia of the heart, pathways that carry afferent stimuli from the cardiopulmonary area.[175] Furthermore, ANP interferes with α$_1$-adrenergic receptor activation in the rat heart[176] and the human kidney.[177] The physiologic relevance of these observations is not fully understood.

CNP was initially considered to act principally as a neuropeptide. However, the functional significance of CNP within the CNS remains largely unknown. In neuronal cell lines, CNP increases cGMP production.[178] Studies in rats and sheep indicate that CNP may stimulate water drinking and reduce blood pressure and adrenocortical activity.[179] CNP may exert prejunctional inhibition of norepinephrine release.[180] The highest concentration of CNP in the body is present in the pituitary, where it may inhibit the release of luteinizing hormone (LH) via NPR-A activation.[181] CNP increases catecholamine synthesis in the adrenal medulla via cGMP-mediated activation of tyrosine hydroxylase, a rate-limiting enzyme in the synthesis of these amines.[182] By contrast, in incubated rat hypothalamic slices, CNP inhibits spontaneous release of norepinephrine and increases its neuronal uptake and storage.[183] These studies suggest that CNP may be involved in the regulation of noradrenergic neurotransmission at the presynaptic level.

## Antiinflammatory Effects

A link between natriuretic peptides, specifically ANP, and the immune system has recently been demonstrated.[184-188] ANP mediates macrophage function by influencing the production of proinflammatory factors. ANP has recently been reported to inhibit the production of TNF-α in macrophages,[185,186] reperfused liver,[187] and whole human blood[185] and to attenuate changes in endothelial morphology and permeability induced by TNF-α,[189] thus influencing important pathophysiologic features of inflammation. More recently, several studies have demonstrated that ANP[184,187,188] and CNP[188] specifically suppress TNF-α–induced expression of adhesion molecules via cGMP-mediated inhibition of nuclear factor (NF)-κB expression.[187,188,190]

## Effects on the Renin-Angiotensin-Aldosterone System (RAAS)

Secretion of renin and aldosterone are markedly inhibited following ANP infusion.[191] ANP decreased renin secretion from isolated renin-secreting cells, but failed to inhibit renin secretion in nonfiltering kidneys, or to alter furosemide-induced renin release from isolated afferent arterioles.[191] However, NEP inhibition blunted the rise in renin secretion in bumetanide-treated rats, suggesting that ANP may influence, directly or indirectly, intracellular signaling in the macula densa.[192] In human subjects, BNP causes a fall or no change in plasma renin activity.[129,193] ANP, but not BNP, inhibits the plasma aldosterone response to Ang II.[194] The decrease in plasma aldosterone is due to the decrease in plasma renin activity and to a direct effect of ANP on the adrenal zonal glomerulosa to inhibit aldosterone synthesis. The increase in sodium load delivered to the macula densa following ANP infusion may be responsible for the decrease in renin secretion.

Infusion of small doses of ANP and BNP inhibits the RAAS, but CNP does not appear to affect this system when infused in doses that do not alter blood pressure. Only when infused in very high doses does CNP decrease plasma aldosterone and increase plasma and urinary concentrations of cGMP. CNP modulates adrenocorticotropic hormone–induced aldosterone secretion[195] and inhibits vascular ACE activity and thus may serve as an endogenous regulator of the RAAS.[196]

Following Ang II inhibition via an ACE inhibitor or Ang II receptor blocker, renal CNP mRNA expression increased in streptozocin-diabetic (STZ) rats and controls; this effect was more pronounced in the controls. These results demonstrate a direct stimulatory effect of the RAAS on renal CNP mRNA levels.[197] In patients with essential hypertension, plasma ANP levels increased by 15.7% despite the drop in blood pressure and the slight decrease of atrial and ventricular diameters following treatment with irbesartan, an Ang II receptor blocker.[198]

Infusion of Ang II in isolated rat kidney leads to decreased renal excretion of urodilatin. The alterations in urodilatin excretion cannot be explained by vasoconstriction per se, because ET-1 infusion does not alter urodilatin excretion.[199]

In addition to renin and aldosterone suppression, ANP also antagonizes all of the known effects of Ang II, including peripheral vasoconstriction, stimulation of proximal sodium fluid reabsorption, central dipsogenic actions, and growth-promoting activities in vascular smooth muscle cells. These effects have been attributed to ANP-induced decreases in cytosolic calcium due to cGMP-dependent stimulation of sarcolemmal $Ca^{2+}$ ATPase activity.[200]

## Other Actions of Natriuretic Peptides

CNP has been isolated from the small and large intestine of rats,[183] and administration of CNP to dogs reduced jejunal electrolyte and fluid secretion.[201] This suggests that CNP may contribute to fluid homeostasis by modulating intestinal excretion of electrolytes. CNP relaxes pulmonary arteries and bronchial smooth muscle cells of guinea pigs.[202] In vitro, CNP causes dose-dependent relaxation of bronchial smooth muscle and stimulates cGMP release from human respiratory epithelial cells.[203] The significance of these observations in pulmonary diseases remains to be ascertained.

Negative,[204,205] positive,[206-208] biphasic (initially inotropic then negative inotropic),[209] and no inotropic[210] effect have been reported for CNP in different species. These discrepancies could be due to differential effects of CNP on various cell types (i.e., endothelial cells or fibroblasts versus cardiac myocytes) or to species differences.

Transgenic mice overexpressing BNP exhibit skeletal abnormalities due to endochondral ossification, such as elongated limbs and crooked tails, the severity of which correlated with the elevation in plasma BNP concentration.[211] In vitro, CNP was more potent than BNP in promoting growth of embryonic mouse tibias, whereas ANP overexpressing mice had no skeletal defects.[211] Mice deficient in cGMP-dependent protein kinase II, an intracellular mediator of guanylyl cyclase signaling, have defects in endochondral ossification that lead to dwarfism.[212] These studies support a role for natriuretic peptide modulation of bone and cartilage growth via guanylyl cyclase-coupled receptors.

## INTERACTIONS AMONG NATRIURETIC PEPTIDES

Potentially important interactions among natriuretic peptides occur in vivo. Very high infusion rates (0.1 μg/kg/min) of BNP increase plasma levels of ANP in humans; much lower infusion rates of CNP (5 pmol/kg/min) increase plasma concentrations of ANP but not BNP.[213] CNP production and release by bovine aortic endothelial cells is enhanced by ANP or BNP.[214] In the presence of background low-dose ANP infusions, coinfusion of BNP abruptly and reversibly increases plasma ANP levels by 50% and has additive physiologic effects. Similarly, in the presence of background BNP infusion, coinfusion of ANP causes a reversible increase in plasma BNP concentration and results in additive physiologic effects. These studies support the notion that natriuretic peptides compete for clearance in shared degradative pathways, rather than affecting each other's production rates.[213]

## PATHOPHYSIOLOGY OF NATRIURETIC PEPTIDES

### Hypertension

ANP is involved in the pathogenesis of salt-sensitive hypertension. Molecular genetic studies show that disruption of the proANP gene in mice causes a form of salt-sensitive hypertension and cardiac hypertrophy.[146] By contrast, transgenic mice overexpressing the genes for ANP or BNP have lower blood pressure than normal littermates and do not develop pulmonary hypertension when exposed to chronic hypoxia.[145,215] Chronic blockade of endogenous ANP with a monoclonal antibody has been shown to accelerate the development and exacerbate the severity of hypertension in stroke-prone SHR (SHR-sp) and DOCA-salt hypertensive rats.[216] In contrast, administration of an NEP inhibitor, SCH 34826, which protects endogenous ANP from hydrolysis, prevents salt-sensitive hypertension in SHR.[217]

ANP levels are increased in response to salt loading in WKY rats but not in salt-sensitive SHR.[218] ANP infusion in doses that achieved plasma ANP levels well within the physiologic range abolished the salt-induced exacerbation of hypertension in salt-sensitive SHR.[219] ANP secretion in response to increased atrial pressure was impaired in prehypertensive Dahl salt-sensitive rats but exaggerated in more advanced phases when hypertension was complicated by LVH.[220] In normotensive salt-resistant rats, dietary salt supplementation is associated with increased plasma ANP levels.[221] In contrast, salt-sensitive SHR fail to increase plasma ANP levels appropriately in response to dietary salt supplementation, resulting in an inability to mount a natriuretic response and normalize blood pressure in the presence of dietary salt.[221, 222] In hypertension caused by excess mineralocorticoid, the concentration of ANP increases in concert with the phenomenon of "escape." Administration of HS-142-1 exacerbates hypertension in this model.[223]

Measurements of plasma ANP levels in patients with essential hypertension have provided conflicting results. Some studies have shown low to normal plasma ANP levels,[224-226] whereas others have shown increased levels.[227-229] Sagnella et al. showed an increase in plasma ANP levels during high salt intake in patients with essential hypertension.[230] Kohno et al.[231] showed that sodium loading increased plasma ANP more in salt-sensitive than in salt-resistant patients. Nimura, on the other hand, showed a blunted increase in plasma ANP in response to high dietary salt intake in salt-sensitive compared with salt-resistant patients.[232] We have demonstrated that salt-sensitive hypertensive African Americans manifest abnormal ANP secretion in response to increased dietary sodium intake.[233]

Salt-resistant patients fail to manifest the expected rise in ANP, whereas salt-sensitive patients show a paradoxical decrease in ANP. In these patients, reduced atrial secretion of ANP could be, at least in part, responsible for the reduced ability to excrete sodium and for the sodium-induced rise in blood pressure. In whites, we noticed a similar tendency for ANP to decrease during high salt intake, but the decrease did not reach statistical significance. The discrepancies in the literature could be due partly to methodologic differences in ANP measurement and to differences in age, dietary salt intake, left ventricular function, and genetics among populations studied.

Ferrari et al.[234] and Weidmann et al.[235] observed markedly reduced plasma ANP during high sodium intake in offspring of hypertensive parents compared with offspring of normotensive parents. They suggested that a relative ANP deficiency might predispose individuals to develop essential hypertension. Male and female offspring of hypertensive individuals manifest lower BNP levels than offspring of normotensive individuals.[236]

Using the candidate gene approach, Rutledge et al.[237] have shown that an Hpa II variant within a polymorphic region in intron 2 of the ANP gene is more common among hypertensive African Americans (25%) than among normotensive controls (3.4%). Although subjects were not characterized according to their salt-sensitivity status, this study supports the hypothesis that a deficit of ANP secretion or augmented metabolism may be genetically determined and contribute to salt-sensitivity and hypertension in African Americans. Frequency of the Hpa II allelic variant was also higher among a cohort of white hypertensive Germans compared with normotensive individuals.[238] In a case control study of a Japanese population, an association was found between a polymorphic marker located within the 5' region of the ANP gene and hypertension.[239] By contrast, no difference in the prevalence of the ANP-Hpa II wild-type allele was found between salt-sensitive and salt-resistant normotensive Caucasians.[240] Other investigators have also failed to find an association between the ANP gene and high blood pressure.[241] One possible explanation for these differences is that the pathogenetic role of ANP may vary among populations of different ethnic backgrounds, or that appropriate size populations were not used in some of these studies. In aldosterone-producing adenoma, a secondary form of hypertension, a significant association between allelic variants of the ANP gene and aldosterone responsiveness to Ang II has been demonstrated.[242] A second polymorphic marker (Sca I) for ANP has been identified at position 2238 (T and C), but the prevalence of this marker did not differ between hypertensive and normotensive Blacks. In a Japanese study of 233 individuals with essential hypertension and 213 age-matched normotensive controls, neither the G1837A nor the T2238C polymorphism of the ANP gene was associated with hypertension.[243]

A pathophysiologic role of natriuretic peptides and their receptors in the development of obesity-related hypertension has been suggested by several investigators.[244-247] High levels of NPR-A and NPR-C have been detected in animal and human adipose tissue.[247-249] Suppression of NPR-C gene expression in adipose tissue, accompanied by increased ANP activity, resulting in natriuresis and diuresis was demonstrated in rats following fasting.[247] In obese hypertensive subjects, NPR-A:NPR-C ratio and ANP levels were significantly lower than in nonobese hypertensive subjects, suggesting that overexpression of NPR-C may lead to increased peripheral clearance of natriuretic peptides such as ANP and thus lower its biologic activity. Lower biologic activity of ANP is further suggested by the presence of higher plasma renin and aldosterone levels, which are physiologically inhibited by ANP, in obese hypertensives in comparison to obese normotensives.[247]

Elevated plasma ANP levels have been demonstrated in pregnant women compared with nonpregnant controls.[250-252] ANP levels were even higher in pregnant women suffering from both gestational hypertension and preeclampsia.[250-254] The increase in plasma ANP levels seen in preeclampsia does not appear to reflect underlying volume status, because preeclampsia is usually associated with normal or reduced blood volume[255] and low right atrial pressures.[256] The increase in ANP levels may be due to ET, because ET has been shown to stimulate ANP release in vivo and in vitro[257] and maternal plasma levels of ET-1 are elevated in preeclampsia.[258]

Taken together, experimental and clinical studies suggest a role for ANP in the regulation of blood pressure and in the pathogenesis of some forms of hypertension.

## Congestive Heart Failure

In acute congestive heart failure (CHF), secretion of ANP increases in response to an acute rise in atrial filling pressure and atrial stretch. By contrast, controversy remains with regard to the acute response of BNP. In vitro studies have indicated that when isolated myocytes are subjected to acute stretch, BNP gene expression may be more immediately responsive than ANP gene expression.[259] In vivo studies, however, have indicated that acute changes in cardiac filling pressures caused by volume expansion,[260] mitral stenosis repair in humans,[261] or rapid left ventricular pacing in anesthetized dogs do not increase circulating BNP levels.[262] This is consistent with the observation that BNP concentrations in the normal heart are markedly lower than those of ANP. In anesthetized dogs with acute CHF, an infusion of exogenous BNP sufficient to achieve circulating concentrations similar to those observed in chronic CHF resulted in markedly increased plasma and urine cGMP, reduced cardiac filling pressure, diuresis, natriuresis, attenuated release of renin, and inhibition of distal tubular sodium reabsorption.[262] This provides a rationale for the use of BNP in the management of acute CHF. In anesthetized dogs with acute CHF induced by rapid ventricular pacing, administration of HS-142-1 caused a decrease in GFR and an increase in distal fractional sodium reabsorption, supporting a functional role for the endogenous natriuretic peptide system in preserving sodium homeostasis and GFR in acute CHF.[263]

Increased levels of DNP have been detected in the atrial and ventricular myocardium of dogs with CHF[264] and in the blood of patients with New York Heart Association (NYHA) class III or IV heart failure,[32] suggesting that DNP increase may be part of a compensatory neurohumoral response of the failing heart to maintain cardiovascular homeostasis.

In CHF, ANP secretion increases in proportion to the severity of heart failure. Ventricular production of ANP increases, but remains lower than atrial production.[265] Plasma levels of BNP also increase and may exceed levels of ANP. Plasma BNP correlates more closely than ANP with severity of heart failure and outcome.[266] Plasma BNP levels correlate with left ventric-

ular wall thickness and left ventricular mass.[267] BNP is considered to be a backup hormone that, in chronic CHF, is synthesized and released into the plasma to complement the actions of ANP. In contrast, plasma CNP does not change, even though cardiac tissue content may be increased.[136]

Natriuretic peptides secreted in CHF inhibit the production of Ang II, aldosterone, catecholamines, and ETs, defending the patient against sodium and water retention. The vasodilator and volume contracting properties of the natriuretic peptides reduce systemic vascular resistance, decrease ventricular filling pressure, and improve myocardial performance. Blocking the actions of these peptides with specific receptor antagonists results in accelerated progression of heart failure and stimulation of renin, aldosterone, catecholamines, and ET-1.[119,268] Furthermore, these peptides inhibit the growth of cardiac fibroblasts, thus reducing cardiac remodeling and collagen accumulation. Calderone et al. reported the ability of ANP to attenuate the growth-promoting effects of noradrenaline on myocardial cells, thus, protecting the heart from the adverse effects of enhanced sympathetic activity such as interstitial fibrosis and myocardial hypertrophy.[269] Similar effects have been shown for BNP and CNP.

The cGMP response to ANP in heart failure is diminished compared with that in normal subjects, probably due to down-regulation of specific receptors caused by chronic exposure to high levels of the peptide. This results in further deterioration of heart failure. In contrast, the cGMP response to CNP is enhanced in patients with CHF compared with normal subjects, suggesting receptor up-regulation.[270] The significance of these changes remains obscure.

## Ischemic Heart Disease

After acute myocardial infarction (AMI), levels of BNP rise during the first 24 hours.[271-275] AMI is associated with stimulation of the RAAS and SNS. Elevation of natriuretic peptides may be a counterregulatory attempt to control the extent of vasoconstriction. BNP levels are higher in patients with unstable angina than in those with stable angina or healthy controls.[276] BNP gene expression and tissue BNP stores increased in an experimental model of transmural infarction.[277] These studies suggest that myocardial ischemia augments the synthesis and release of BNP. Marumoto et al. measured levels of ANP and BNP during exercise in patients with stable angina and normal resting left ventricular function and in normal control subjects.[278] Despite similar rate-pressure products, the levels of both ANP and BNP during exercise were significantly elevated in patients with angina compared with normal controls.

Some evidence suggests that natriuretic peptides may themselves contribute to myocardial injury. Infarct size after ischemia-reperfusion is smaller in genetically engineered mice lacking NPR-A and mice pretreated with HS-142-1, an NPR-A antagonist, than in wild-type or untreated controls. This reduction in infarct size was accompanied by decreases in neutrophil infiltration, P-selectin expression, and activation of NF-κB. ANP directly induced P-selectin expression and $H_2O_2$-induced activation of NF-κB.[279] These results suggest that blockade of NPR-A may alleviate ischemia-reperfusion injury and provide the basis for future clinical interventions. By contrast, other evidence suggests that administration of natriuretic peptide may alleviate ischemia-induced myocardial damage. Administration of low-dose urodilatin at the time of reperfusion results in a dose-dependent increase in myocardial cGMP and limits necrosis.[280] The reason for these apparently conflicting data is not clear and more studies are necessary.

## Arrhythmia

ANP and BNP levels are reportedly increased in patients with supraventricular and ventricular tachyarrhythmias.[281-288] Successful treatment with chemical or electrical cardioversion was followed by a decrease in plasma ANP levels in these patients. In patients with atrial fibrillation, elevated ANP levels were unrelated to echocardiographic dimensions, ventricular rate, and blood pressure.[281] Increased plasma ANP concentration in atrial arrhythmias has been attributed to elevation of atrial pressure,[287] and the reduction in ANP levels following cardioversion has been explained by the decrease in atrial pressure resulting from restoration of sinus rhythm.[283] BNP levels have been shown to be beneficial in detecting patients with nonvalvular atrial fibrillation who are at high risk for thromboembolic complications.[289]

## Atherosclerosis

CNP, which is expressed in the vascular endothelium, has antiatherosclerotic effects. The migration of medial smooth muscle cells (SMCs) into the intima is proposed to be an important contributor to intimal thickening in atherosclerotic lesions. Natriuretic peptides, particularly CNP, inhibit oxidized-low-density lipoprotein–mediated SMC migration through a cGMP-dependent process, suggesting that they may act as antimigration factors during the process of intimal thickening in hypercholesterolemia-induced coronary atherosclerosis.[290-292] In cultured vascular SMC, CNP has been shown to antagonize the mitogenic activity of Ang II.[154] Furthermore, NPR-B is up-regulated in vivo in SMCs in the intimal layer of atherosclerotic arteries. This finding could support a regulatory role of natriuretic peptides in atherogenesis.[293] In addition, the vasodilator effects of ANP and cGMP are reduced in atherosclerotic rabbit aortas.[294]

Increased NEP activity has been demonstrated in atherosclerotic arteries and plasma of cholesterol-fed rabbits.[295] Treatment with an NEP inhibitor (UK73967) decreased plasma cholesterol, preserved the arterial concentration of CNP by suppressing local degradation, and inhibited atheroma formation in these animals. The precise mechanism for inhibition of atheroma formation by the NEP inhibitor and whether these findings are reproducible in humans with hypercholesterolemia remain to be determined.

## Nephrotic Syndrome

Most,[296] although not all,[297,298] studies have demonstrated slightly elevated ANP levels in nephrotic patients, particularly in those with low plasma renin activity, suggesting that the increase in ANP may be the result of volume expansion. Increased plasma CNP concentrations and urinary CNP excretion have also been reported in patients with nephrotic syndrome.[31] Some have attempted to treat edema in nephrotic patients with ANP infusion, but the natriuretic response was less than that seen in control subjects.[299]

## Chronic Kidney Disease

Patients with end-stage renal disease have been shown to have markedly elevated ANP and BNP levels that decline somewhat after dialysis.[300-303] The main factors responsible for the high plasma concentrations of ANP and BNP are extracellular volume expansion, decreased metabolism and clearance of the peptides and concomitant heart disease. In studies on dialysis patients without heart failure, both BNP and ANP were strong independent predictors of left ventricular mass, ejection fraction, and risk of death.[304-306] A positive correlation between ANP and left ventricular mass and severity of hypertension was observed in 21 pediatric patients on chronic peritoneal dialysis.[307]

CNP gene expression has been detected in human kidneys, and increased plasma concentrations of CNP have been reported in patients with chronic kidney disease.[141] The renal actions of CNP remain unclear, however.

## Respiratory Diseases

Animal studies have shown that ANP and BNP reduce elevated pulmonary vascular tone and attenuate hypoxia-induced pulmonary hypertension.[308-311] Plasma ANP levels are elevated in chronic respiratory failure and do not change with short-term oxygen therapy.[312] BNP levels are also elevated in patients with chronic obstructive pulmonary disease (COPD) and acute hypoxia and are positively correlated with the degree of hypoxia.[313] In one study, plasma levels of ANP and BNP were elevated in patients with COPD and $PaO_2$ <60 mm Hg and correlated significantly with the degree of hypoxemia. Plasma CNP was not detectable in these patients. Plasma levels of ANP and BNP were significantly decreased by long-term oxygen therapy. Moreover, plasma ANP and BNP levels were elevated in COPD patients with right ventricular hypertrophy compared with patients without right ventricular hypertrophy.[314] These data suggest that in COPD patients, the major stimulus for ANP and BNP secretion may be hypoxemia, but a rise in right ventricular pressure may also play a role.

Plasma ANP concentrations have been reported to be markedly elevated in patients with acute lung injury and to correlate well with the severity of the injury.[315,316] In patients with chronic thromboembolic pulmonary hypertension, BNP levels were strongly associated with the severity of pulmonary hypertension and decreased significantly following pulmonary thromboendarterectomy.[317] Sustained elevation of postoperative BNP indicated the presence of residual pulmonary hypertension, suggesting a role for BNP measurement in the evaluation of the efficacy of pulmonary thromboendarterectomy in this condition. In patients with acute pulmonary embolism, BNP levels were also significantly higher in those who had concomitant right ventricular dysfunction.[318] Thus plasma BNP levels may be of clinical importance as a tool for assessment of right ventricular function in patients with acute pulmonary embolism.

## Stroke

Stroke susceptibility loci in SHR-sp have been mapped close to a marker derived from the ANP gene, and structural and functional differences in the ANP gene have been reported in SHR-sp versus stroke-resistant SHR.[319] Molecular variants, including a polymorphism within exon 1 (G664A) that encodes a valine-to-methionine substitution in the biologically active proANP, have been identified in humans.[320] Studies looking at whether G664A is a risk factor in stroke patients and whether there is an association with any particular ischemic stroke subtype have provided conflicting results.[320,321] Hassan et al. studied 436 patients who presented with ischemic stroke or transient ischemic attack and compared them with 295 community control subjects.[321] Their results indicated that the ANP gene G664A polymorphism was unlikely to be a major risk factor for ischemic stroke. In contrast, in a study by Rubattu et al., this marker was associated with a twofold increase in the incidence of stroke in human subjects.[320] In the latter study, patients with hemorrhagic stroke were included and an ethnically mixed population was tested, possibly accounting for the differences between the two studies. The prevalence of this polymorphic marker in African Americans remains to be established.

Increased levels of ANP have been found in patients with stroke.[322] ANP has been shown to act directly on the nervous system to inhibit water and sodium accumulation in ischemic brain edema, and thus may be protective through both its vascular and antiedema effects.

## Alzheimer's Disease

Accumulation of the neurotoxic peptide amyloid beta-protein Abeta in the cerebrum is thought to play a central role in the pathogenesis of Alzheimer's disease.[323] Interestingly, Abeta is degraded by a protease which is indistinguishable from insulin-degrading enzyme, a thiol metalloendopeptidase related to NEP that also metabolizes insulin, glucagon, and ANP.[324] Insulin and ANP inhibit the metabolism of Abeta by competing for the insulin-degrading enzyme.[324] The role of ANP in the prevention or treatment of Alzheimer's disease remains to be determined.

## Cirrhosis

The mechanisms of sodium retention in cirrhosis are complex and include activation of vasoconstrictors, such as Ang II and norepinephrine.[325] Increased secretion of prostaglandins and ANP compensates, at least in part, for the sodium-retaining actions of these vasoconstrictors. Plasma levels of ANP and BNP are usually elevated in patients with cirrhosis,[326, 327] with the exception of patients with hyponatremia, in whom the levels may actually be decreased.[328] By contrast, urinary excretion of urodilatin is unchanged in patients with cirrhosis even in the presence of increased plasma levels of ANP,[329] suggesting that ANP and urodilatin in cirrhosis are regulated independently. Patients with well-compensated cirrhosis remain in sodium balance, presumably as a result of the natriuretic effects of these elevated levels of ANP. When cirrhosis decompensates, ANP becomes unable to offset the sodium-retaining actions of Ang II and aldosterone and of increased activation of the SNS.[330] With the development of refractory ascites, cirrhotic patients become unresponsive to the natriuretic effects of ANP. This may be in part mediated by further increased activity of the SNS.[331] In a rat model of cirrhosis, the ANP response could be entirely restored by renal denervation, suggesting a key role for the SNS in the mediation of unresponsiveness to ANP.[332] Increased circulating DNP levels have been demonstrated in patients with cirrhosis and ascites when compared with both cirrhotic patients without ascites and healthy subjects. In addition, circulating levels of DNP increased in relation to the severity of cirrhosis.[333] Unlike ANP, BNP, and DNP, CNP levels are decreased in patients with cirrhosis.[334]

Administration of HS-142-1 reduces renal plasma flow and GFR in cirrhotic rats with ascites, suggesting that natriuretic peptides may play a role in preservation of renal function and urine sodium excretion in this condition.[335]

# CLINICAL USES OF NATRIURETIC PEPTIDES

## Diagnostic Use

During the past several years there as been interest in the use of natriuretic peptides as tools for emergent diagnosis and screening of the population for left ventricular systolic and diastolic dysfunction, particularly targeting high-risk groups.[336-341] Plasma BNP levels have a higher sensitivity and specificity for identification of left ventricular systolic dysfunction than ANP, are capable of differentiating between chronic heart failure patients with moderately and severely impaired exercise capacity and provide a useful indication of which patients are more likely to have heart failure and require further clinical assessment.[342-344]

Plasma BNP concentration has been suggested as a surrogate therapeutic end-point for patients with heart failure.[345-347] In a double blind study in patients with NYHA class III or IV heart failure, Troughton et al.[345] demonstrated that pharmacotherapy guided by BNP levels reduces cardiovascular events and delays time to first cardiovascular event compared with intensive clinically guided therapy.

In patients with type 1 diabetes without evidence of microalbuminuria, ANP infusion has been shown to increase albumin excretion.[348-350] Thus, ANP infusion may unmask underlying alterations in glomerular permselectivity and predict diabetic nephropathy. Longitudinal studies are needed to determine whether measurement of ANP-induced microalbuminuria might allow the early detection of at risk patients with diabetes.

## Prognostic Use

Plasma concentrations of BNP and ANP are increased in patients with chronic heart failure and accurately predict left ventricular ejection fraction, morbidity and mortality in these patients.[273,274,346,351-353] In patients admitted with decompensated CHF, changes in BNP levels during treatment were strong predictors for mortality and early readmission.[346,354] Plasma N-ANP and BNP levels also predict severity of AMI, including infarct size, likelihood of ventricular remodeling and lower ejection fraction and associated mortality independent of ventricular function.[271,355-361] In the Cooperative New Scandinavian Enalapril Survival Study (CONSENSUS) II trial[362] and the Survival and Ventricular Enlargement (SAVE) trial,[363] levels of ANP, measured post-MI, were related to survival. However, when left ventricular ejection fraction was added to the analysis, the independent prognostic value of ANP was diminished. N-ANP was an independent predictor of death, cardiovascular mortality, and heart failure in a subgroup of patients with AMI from the CONSENSUS II trial,[364] Thrombolysis in Myocardial Infarction (TIMI) II trial,[358] and SAVE trial.[365]

## Therapeutic Use

Natriuretic peptides, particularly BNP, have been shown to have therapeutic potential for various pathologic conditions. Nesiritide, a recombinant human BNP, recently gained FDA approval as the first new parenteral agent approved for heart failure therapy. In patients with decompensated CHF, nesiritide, in addition to standard therapy resulted in improvement in hemodynamics, including a prompt fall in systemic vascular resistance and pulmonary capillary wedge pressure, associated with rapid clinical improvement and a reduction in self-reported symptoms.[366-369] Nesiritide also caused fewer arrhythmias in patients with decompensated CHF compared with dobutamine.[370] This therapy represents a novel approach to the management of CHF, enhancing naturally occurring protective mechanisms.

Infusion of ANP into patients with AMI improved left ventricular ejection fraction and appeared to be more beneficial in its effects on autonomic nervous activity, plasma renin activity, and myocardial oxygen consumption than nitroglycerin.[371,372] Infusion of ANP during exercise thallium stress testing in patients with stable angina and normal left ventricular function decreased the extent and severity of the myocardial perfusion defect and prevented ischemia ST-segment depression.[373] In patients with angina pectoris induced by hyperventilation, both ANP[374] and BNP[375] have been shown to suppress chest pain and electrocardiographic changes by preventing vasospasm via cGMP amplification. In patients with compensated cirrhosis, infusion of ANP in doses that increase plasma concentrations to levels comparable with those observed in patients with ascites, decreases left ventricular end-diastolic volume, stroke volume, cardiac output, and blood pressure, and increases GFR and urinary sodium excretion.[376] However, the use of ANP in cirrhosis is generally limited by intolerable drug-induced hypotension, in part because the hypotensive action of ANP in these patients is not associated with an appropriate increase in plasma norepinephrine.[377] When combined with terlipressin (a vasopressor analog), increased systemic vascular resistance prevented ANP-induced vasodilation and enhanced the natriuretic effect of ANP in patients with cirrhosis and refractory ascites.[378]

Use of ANP in patients with renal failure has not been promising. In patients with renal insufficiency receiving ANP or mannitol infusion prior to cardiac catheterization, acute renal failure occurred to a similar extent in both groups.[379] In a multicenter, randomized, double-blind, placebo-controlled study, administration of anaritide, a synthetic form of ANP, in critically ill patients with acute tubular necrosis did not improve the overall rate of dialysis-free survival.[380] Anaritide improved dialysis-free survival in patients with oliguria, but worsened it in those with nonoliguric acute renal failure. A more recent study showed no significant beneficial effect of ANP in dialysis-free survival or reduction in dialysis in subjects with oliguric acute renal failure.[381]

In a study by Mitaka et al.,[382] infusion of ANP-induced diuresis and improved pulmonary gas exchange in patients with acute lung injury during mechanical ventilation. Bindels et al.[383] studied the effects of infusion of ANP versus inhalation of nitric oxide in patients with an early acute respiratory distress syndrome. ANP did not alter mean pulmonary artery pressure, pulmonary artery resistance index, extravascular lung water index, or pulmonary gas exchange. In contrast, nitric oxide inhalation improved all these indices.

Although the role of ANP as a pharmacotherapeutic agent is limited due to its low oral bioavailability, its narrow therapeutic range, and short half-life, ANP gene therapy may potentially be useful for some conditions. ANP gene delivery has been shown to reduce mortality due to cerebrovascular disorders and stroke in Dahl salt-sensitive rats.[384] A single injection of an adenovirus harboring the human ANP gene (Ad.RSV-cANP) caused a significant reduction of blood pressure that lasted for more than 3 weeks. The stroke mortality rate of Dahl salt-sensitive rats decreased significantly from 54% to 17% at 3 weeks after ANP gene delivery compared with rats injected with control virus. A significant reduction in salt-induced aortic hypertrophy as evidenced by decreased thickness of the aortic wall was evident following ANP gene delivery. This technology may have potential value in treating individuals at high risk of stroke.

Administration of synthetic DNP to dogs with severe CHF has beneficial cardiovascular, renal, and humoral effects.[264] DNP decreased right atrial and pulmonary capillary wedge pressure, increased GFR in association with natriuresis and diuresis despite a reduction in mean arterial pressure, increased plasma and urinary cGMP, and suppressed plasma renin activity. Thus DNP may have potential as a new intravenous agent for the treatment of decompensated CHF.

Agents that interfere with the receptor binding or metabolism of natriuretic peptides are potential therapeutic targets. Selective antagonists of NPRs have helped define the functions of these natriuretic peptides, but have not yet proved useful in the clinical arena. More promising are the NEP inhibitors. Potent inhibitors of NEP provided useful tools to test the role of NEP in the inactivation of natriuretic peptides, as well as in probing the functions of these peptides. These drugs potentiate the natriuretic and hypotensive responses to intravenous infusions of ANP, as well as the natriuretic response to volume expansion.[385] NEP inhibition results in diuresis and natriuresis in rats with CHF[386,387] and chronic kidney disease.[388] In rats with chronic heart failure, ONO-9902, a NEP inhibitor, reduced left ventricular end-diastolic pressure and increased cardiac output. These changes were associated with decreased plasma levels of ANP, BNP, and ET-1.[389] In salt-sensitive models of hypertension, such as the DOCA-salt rat model, NEP inhibitors reduce blood pressure.[390] These actions occur despite minimal increases in plasma ANP levels and are associated with increased urinary excretion of cGMP, suggesting that the antihypertensive response to NEP inhibition cannot be attributed exclusively to changes in plasma concentration of ANP and that NEP inhibitors may raise local tissue levels of ANP without increasing plasma levels. The actions of NEP inhibitors have also been attributed to reduced inactivation of other vasoactive peptides, such as bradykinin.[391] This hypothesis is unlikely because SCH 34826, an oral NEP inhibitor, failed to affect the depressor response to bradykinin.[390] Moreover, administration of a bradykinin antagonist failed to alter the hypotensive response to the oral administration of SCH 34826 in the DOCA-salt rat. NEP inhibitors can also potentiate the renal effects of ANP, and this response is partially inhibited by bradykinin antagonists.[392]

Studies with NEP inhibitors in humans have been promising. In patients with heart failure caused by left ventricular systolic dysfunction, administration of candoxatril, a specific NEP inhibitor, increased sodium excretion, reduced right and left atrial pressures without any increase in renin activity and improved exercise capacity.[393-396] NEP inhibitors such as phosphoramidion and UK 73967 have been shown to potentiate the myocardial protective action of ANP and BNP against neutrophil-induced endothelial cytotoxicity, which is known to play a role in ischemia-reperfusion myocardial injury.[397]

Vasopeptidase inhibitors are a new class of drugs that inhibit both NEP and ACE, augmenting any beneficial effect of the elevation of natriuretic peptides.[398,399] Simultaneous inhibition of NEP and ACE results in increases in natriuretic peptides (ANP, BNP, and CNP) and vasodilatory peptides (bradykinin and adrenomedullin), thereby enhancing vasodilation, decreasing vascular tone, and lowering blood pressure. None of these drugs has been approved for human use due to a high frequency of angioedema.

Since the discovery of the natriuretic peptides in 1981, extensive research has revealed many potential therapeutic uses of these peptides. Future efforts in this in this area may allow fulfillment of their therapeutic potential.

## References

1. de Bold AJ, Borenstein HB, Veress AT, et al. A rapid and potent natriuretic response to intravenous injection of atrial myocardial extract in rats. Life Sci 28:89-94, 1981.
2. Yandle TG. Biochemistry of natriuretic peptides. J Intern Med 235:561-576, 1994.
3. Mathisen P, Hall C, Simonsen S. Comparative study of atrial peptides ANF (1-98) and ANF (99-126) as diagnostic markers of atrial distension in patients with cardiac disease. Scand J Clin Lab Invest 53:41-49, 1993.
4. Espiner EA, Richards AM, Yandle TG, et al. Natriuretic hormones. Endocrinol Metab Clin North Am 24:481-509, 1995.
5. Sudoh T, Maekawa K, Kojima M, et al. Cloning and sequence analysis of cDNA encoding a precursor for human brain natriuretic peptide. Biochem Biophys Res Commun 159:1427-1434, 1989.
6. Yandle TG, Richards AM, Gilbert A, et al. Assay of brain natriuretic peptide (BNP) in human plasma: Evidence for high molecular weight BNP as a major plasma component in heart failure. J Clin Endocrinol Metab 76:832-838, 1993.
7. Sudoh T, Minamino N, Kangawa K, et al. C-type natriuretic peptide (CNP): A new member of natriuretic peptide family identified in porcine brain. Biochem Biophys Res Commun 168:863-870, 1990.
8. Tawaragi Y, Fuchimura K, Tanaka S, et al. Gene and precursor structures of human C-type natriuretic peptide. Biochem Biophys Res Commun 175:645-651, 1991.
9. Ogawa Y, Nakao K, Nakagawa O, et al. Human C-type natriuretic peptide. Characterization of the gene and peptide. Hypertension 19:809-813, 1992.
10. Tawaragi Y, Fuchimura K, Nakazato H, et al. Gene and precursor structure of porcine C-type natriuretic peptide. Biochem Biophys Res Commun 172:627-632, 1990.
11. Schweitz H, Vigne P, Moinier D, et al. A new member of the natriuretic peptide family is present in the venom of the Green Mamba (Dendroaspis angusticeps). J Biol Chem 267:13928-13932, 1992.
12. Schulz-Knappe P, Forssmann K, Herbst F, et al. Isolation and structural analysis of "urodilatin," a new peptide of the cardiodilatin-(ANP)-family, extracted from human urine. Klin Wochenschr 66:752-759, 1988.
13. Forssmann WG, Richter R, Meyer M. The endocrine heart and natriuretic peptides: Histochemistry, cell biology, and functional aspects of the renal urodilatin system. Histochem Cell Biol 110:335-357, 1998.
14. Ruskoaho H. Atrial natriuretic peptide: Synthesis, release, and metabolism. Pharmacol Rev 44:479-602, 1992.
15. Sudoh T, Kangawa K, Minamino N, et al. A new natriuretic peptide in porcine brain. Nature 332:78-81, 1988.
16. Itoh H, Nakao K, Saito Y, et al. Radioimmunoassay for brain natriuretic peptide (BNP) detection of BNP in canine brain. Biochem Biophys Res Commun 158:120-128, 1989.
17. Hasegawa K, Fujiwara H, Itoh H, et al. Light and electron microscopic localization of brain natriuretic peptide in relation to atrial natriuretic peptide in porcine atrium. Immunohistocytochemical study using specific monoclonal antibodies. Circulation 84:1203-1209, 1991.
18. Iida T, Hirata Y, Takemura N, et al. Brain natriuretic peptide is cosecreted with atrial natriuretic peptide from porcine cardiocytes. FEBS Lett 260:98-100, 1990.
19. Komatsu Y, Nakao K, Suga S, et al. C-type natriuretic peptide (CNP) in rats and humans. Endocrinology 129:1104-1106, 1991.
20. Suzuki R, Togashi K, Ando K, et al. Distribution and molecular forms of C-type natriuretic peptide in plasma and tissue of a dogfish, Triakis scyllia. Gen Comp Endocrinol 96:378-384, 1994.
21. Kaneko T, Shirakami G, Nakao K, et al. C-type natriuretic peptide (CNP) is the major natriuretic peptide in human cerebrospinal fluid. Brain Res 612:104-109, 1993.
22. Chen HH, Burnett JC Jr. C-type natriuretic peptide: The endothelial component of the natriuretic peptide system. J Cardiovasc Pharmacol 32:S22-S28, 1998.
23. Mattingly MT, Brandt RR, Heublein DM, et al. Presence of C-type natriuretic peptide in human kidney and urine. Kidney Int 46:744-747, 1994.
24. Stingo AJ, Clavell AL, Heublein DM, et al. Presence of C-type natriuretic peptide in cultured human endothelial cells and plasma. Am J Physiol 263:H1318-H1321, 1992.
25. Vollmar AM, Wolf R, Schulz R. Co-expression of the natriuretic peptides (ANP, BNP, CNP) and their receptors in normal and acutely involuted rat thymus. J Neuroimmunol 57:117-127, 1995.
26. Stepan H, Faber R, Stegemann S, et al. Expression of C-type natriuretic peptide in human placenta and myometrium in normal pregnancies and pregnancies complicated by intrauterine growth retardation. Preliminary results. Fetal Diagn Ther 17:37-41, 2002.
27. Middendorff R, Muller D, Paust HJ, et al. Natriuretic peptides in the human testis: Evidence for a potential role of C-type natriuretic peptide in Leydig cells. J Clin Endocrinol Metab 81:4324-4328, 1996.
28. Vollmar AM, Gerbes AL, Nemer M, et al. Detection of C-type natriuretic peptide (CNP) transcript in the rat heart and immune organs. Endocrinology 132:1872-1874, 1993.
29. Heublein DM, Clavell AL, Stingo AJ, et al. C-type natriuretic peptide immunoreactivity in human breast vascular endothelial cells. Peptides 13:1017-1019, 1992.
30. Totsune K, Takahashi K, Murakami O, et al. Elevated plasma C-type natriuretic peptide concentrations in patients with chronic renal failure. Clin Sci (Lond) 87:319-322, 1994.
31. Cataliotti A, Giordano M, De Pascale E, et al. CNP production in the kidney and effects of protein intake restriction in nephrotic syndrome. Am J Physiol Renal Physiol 283:F464-F472, 2002.

32. Schirger JA, Heublein DM, Chen HH, et al. Presence of Dendroaspis natriuretic peptide-like immunoreactivity in human plasma and its increase during human heart failure. Mayo Clin Proc 74:126-130, 1999.

33. Lisy O, Jougasaki M, Heublein DM, et al. Renal actions of synthetic dendroaspis natriuretic peptide. Kidney Int 56:502-508, 1999.

34. Feller SM, Gagelmann M, Forssmann WG. Urodilatin: A newly described member of the ANP family. Trends Pharmacol Sci 10:93-94, 1989.

35. Greenwald JE, Needleman P, Wilkins MR, et al. Renal synthesis of atriopeptin-like protein in physiology and pathophysiology. Am J Physiol 260:F602-F607, 1991.

36. Lowe DG, Klisak I, Sparkes RS, et al. Chromosomal distribution of three members of the human natriuretic peptide receptor/guanylyl cyclase gene family. Genomics 8:304-312, 1990.

37. Maack T, Okolicany J, Koh GY, et al. Functional properties of atrial natriuretic factor receptors. Semin Nephrol 13:50-60, 1993.

38. Koller KJ, Goeddel DV. Molecular biology of the natriuretic peptides and their receptors. Circulation 86:1081-1088, 1992.

39. Lincoln TM, Cornwell TL. Intracellular cyclic GMP receptor proteins. FASEB J 7:328-338, 1993.

40. Suga S, Nakao K, Hosoda K, et al. Receptor selectivity of natriuretic peptide family, atrial natriuretic peptide, brain natriuretic peptide, and C-type natriuretic peptide. Endocrinology 130:229-339, 1992.

41. Koller KJ, Lowe DG, Bennett GL, et al. Selective activation of the B natriuretic peptide receptor by C-type natriuretic peptide (CNP). Science 252:120-123, 1991.

42. Nussenzveig DR, Lewicki JA, Maack T. Cellular mechanisms of the clearance function of type C receptors of atrial natriuretic factor. J Biol Chem 265:20952-20958, 1990.

43. Fuller F, Porter JG, Arfsten AE, et al. Atrial natriuretic peptide clearance receptor. Complete sequence and functional expression of cDNA clones. J Biol Chem 263:9395-9401, 1988.

44. Hirata M, Chang CH, Murad F. Stimulatory effects of atrial natriuretic factor on phosphoinositide hydrolysis in cultured bovine aortic smooth muscle cells. Biochim Biophys Acta 1010:346-351, 1989.

45. Anand-Srivastava MB, Sairam MR, Cantin M. Ring-deleted analogs of atrial natriuretic factor inhibit adenylate cyclase/cAMP system. Possible coupling of clearance atrial natriuretic factor receptors to adenylate cyclase/cAMP signal transduction system. J Biol Chem 265:8566-8572, 1990.

46. Drewett JG, Ziegler RJ, Trachte GJ. Neuromodulatory effects of atrial natriuretic peptides correlate with an inhibition of adenylate cyclase but not an activation of guanylate cyclase. J Pharmacol Exp Ther 260:689-696, 1992.

47. Levin ER. Natriuretic peptide C-receptor: More than a clearance receptor. Am J Physiol 264:E483-E489, 1993.

48. Itoh H, Sagawa N, Hasegawa M, et al. Expression of biologically active receptors for natriuretic peptides in the human uterus during pregnancy. Biochem Biophys Res Commun 203:602-607, 1994.

49. Nakao K, Ogawa Y, Suga S, et al. Molecular biology and biochemistry of the natriuretic peptide system. II: Natriuretic peptide receptors. J Hypertens 10:1111-1114, 1992.

50. Martin ER, Lewicki J, Scarborough RM, et al. Expression and regulation of ANP receptor subtypes in rat renal glomeruli and papillae. Am J Physiol Renal Fluid Electrolyte Physiol 257:F649-F657, 1989.

51. Lohe A, Yeh I, Hyver T, et al. Natriuretic peptide B receptor and C-type natriuretic peptide in the rat kidney. J Am Soc Nephrol 6:1552-1558, 1995.

52. Ikeda T, Itoh H, Komatsu Y, et al. Natriuretic peptide receptors in human artery and vein and rabbit vein graft. Hypertension 27:833-8337, 1996.

53. Nagase M, Ando K, Katafuchi T, et al. Role of natriuretic peptide receptor type C in Dahl salt-sensitive hypertensive rats. Hypertension 30:177-183, 1997.

54. Lin X, Hanze J, Heese F, et al. Gene expression of natriuretic peptide receptors in myocardial cells. Circ Res 77:750-758, 1995.

55. Fraenkel MB, Aldred GP, McDougall JG. Sodium status affects GC-B natriuretic peptide receptor mRNA levels, but not GC-A or C receptor mRNA levels, in the sheep kidney. Clin Sci (Lond) 86:517-522, 1994.

56. Katafuchi T, Mizuno T, Hagiwara H, et al. Modulation by NaCl of atrial natriuretic peptide receptor levels and cyclic GMP responsiveness to atrial natriuretic peptide of cultured vascular endothelial cells. J Biol Chem 267:7624-7629, 1992.

57. Sun JZ, Chen SJ, Majid-Hasan E, et al. Dietary salt supplementation selectively downregulates NPR-C receptor expression in kidney independently of ANP. Am J Physiol Renal Physiol 282:F220-F227, 2002.

58. Hystad ME, Oie E, Grogaard HK, et al. Gene expression of natriuretic peptides and their receptors type-A and -C after myocardial infarction in rats. Scand J Clin Lab Invest 61:139-150, 2001.

59. Cohen D, Koh GY, Nikonova LN, et al. Molecular determinants of the clearance function of type C receptors of natriuretic peptides. J Biol Chem 271:9863-9869, 1996.

60. Lewicki J, Protter A. Molecular determinants of natriuretic peptide clearance receptor function. In Samson WK, Levin ER, (eds). Contemporary Endocrinology: Natriuretic Peptides in Health and Disease. Totowa, NJ, Humana Press, 1997; pp 51-70.

61. Sun JZ, Oparil S, Lucchesi P, et al. Tyrosine kinase receptor activation inhibits NPR-C in lung arterial smooth muscle cells. Am J Physiol Lung Cell Mol Physiol 281:L155-L163, 2001.

62. Sun JZ, Chen SJ, Li G, et al. Hypoxia reduces atrial natriuretic peptide clearance receptor gene expression in ANP knockout mice. Am J Physiol Lung Cell Mol Physiol 279:L511-L519, 2000.

63. Li H, Oparil S, Meng QC, et al. Selective downregulation of ANP-clearance-receptor gene expression in lung of rats adapted to hypoxia. Am J Physiol 268:L328-L335, 1995.

64. Itoh H, Zheng J, Bird IM, et al. Basic FGF decreases clearance receptor of natriuretic peptides in fetoplacental artery endothelium. Am J Physiol 277:R541-R547, 1999.

65. Paul RV, Wackym PS, Budisavljevic M, et al. Regulation of atrial natriuretic peptide clearance receptors in mesangial cells by growth factors. J Biol Chem 268:18205-18212, 1993.

66. Weston MW, Cintron GB, Giordano AT, et al. Normalization of circulating atrial natriuretic peptides in cardiac transplant recipients. Am Heart J 127:129-142, 1994.

67. Schiebinger RJ, Gomez-Sanchez CE. Endothelin: A potent stimulus of atrial natriuretic peptide secretion by superfused rat atria and its dependency on calcium. Endocrinology 127:119-125, 1990.

68. Leskinen H, Vuolteenaho O, Ruskoaho H. Combined inhibition of endothelin and angiotensin II receptors blocks volume load-induced cardiac hormone release. Circ Res 126:587-595, 1997.

69. Schiebinger RJ, Baker MZ, Linden J. Effect of adrenergic and muscarinic cholinergic agonists on atrial natriuretic peptide secretion by isolated rat atria. Potential role of the autonomic nervous system in modulating atrial natriuretic peptide secretion. J Clin Invest 80:1687-1691, 1987.

70. Focaccio A, Volpe M, Ambrosio G, et al. Angiotensin II directly stimulates release of atrial natriuretic factor in isolated rabbit hearts. Circulation 87:192-198, 1993.

71. Gardner DG, Schultz HD. Prostaglandins regulate the synthesis and secretion of the atrial natriuretic peptide. J Clin Invest 86:52-59, 1990.

72. Bloch KD, Zamir N, Lichtstein D, et al. Ouabain induces secretion of proatrial natriuretic factor by rat atrial cardiocytes. Am J Physiol 255:E383-E387, 1988.

73. Kaufman S, Deng Y. Adrenomedullin suppresses atrial natriuretic factor (ANF) secretion from isolated atrium. Life Sci 63:1017-1022, 1998.

74. Leite MF, Page E, Ambler SK. Regulation of ANP secretion by endothelin-1 in cultured atrial myocytes: Desensitization and receptor subtype. Am J Physiol 267:H2193-H2203, 1994.

75. Suzuki E, Hirata Y, Kohmoto O, et al. Cellular mechanisms for synthesis and secretion of atrial natriuretic peptide and brain natriuretic peptide in cultured rat atrial cells. Circ Res 71:1039-1048, 1992.

76. Favaretto AL, Ballejo GO, Albuquerque-Araujo WI, et al. Oxytocin releases atrial natriuretic peptide from rat atria in vitro that exerts negative inotropic and chronotropic action. Peptides 18:1377-1381, 1997.

77. Gutkowska J, Jankowski M, Lambert C, et al. Oxytocin releases atrial natriuretic peptide by combining with oxytocin receptors in the heart. Proc Natl Acad Sci USA 94:11704-11709, 1997.

78. Bianciotti LG, de Bold AJ. Effect of selective ET(A) receptor blockade on natriuretic peptide gene expression in DOCA-salt hypertension. Am J Physiol Heart Circ Physiol 279:H93-H101, 2000.

79. Bianciotti LG, de Bold AJ. Modulation of cardiac natriuretic peptide gene expression following endothelin type A receptor blockade in renovascular hypertension. Cardiovasc Res 49:806-816, 2001.

80. Ogawa T, Linz W, Stevenson M, et al. Evidence for load-dependent and load-independent determinants of cardiac natriuretic peptide production. Circulation 93:2059-2067, 1996.

81. Bianciotti LG, de Bold AJ. Natriuretic peptide gene expression in DOCA-salt hypertension after blockade of type B endothelin receptor. Am J Physiol Heart Circ Physiol 282:H1127-34.

82. Mantymaa P, Vuolteenaho O, Marttila M, et al. Atrial stretch induces rapid increase in brain natriuretic peptide but not in atrial natriuretic peptide gene expression in vitro. Endocrinology 133:1470-1473, 2002.

83. de Bold AJ, Bruneau BG, Kuroski de Bold ML. Mechanical and neuroendocrine regulation of the endocrine heart. Cardiovasc Res 31:7-18, 1996.

84. Chiu PJ, Tetzloff G, Romano MT, et al. Influence of C-ANF receptor and neutral endopeptidase on pharmacokinetics of ANF in rats. Am J Physiol 260:R208-R216, 1991.

85. Perrella MA, Schwab TR, O'Murchu B, et al. Cardiac atrial natriuretic factor during evolution of congestive heart failure. Am J Physiol 262:H1248-55, 1992.

86. Mukoyama M, Nakao K, Hosoda K, et al. Brain natriuretic peptide as a novel cardiac hormone in humans. Evidence for an exquisite dual natriuretic peptide system, atrial natriuretic peptide and brain natriuretic peptide. J Clin Invest 87:1402-1412, 1991.

87. Richards AM, Crozier IG, Espiner EA, et al. Plasma brain natriuretic peptide and endopeptidase 24.11 inhibition in hypertension. Hypertension 22:231-236, 1993.

88. Kohno M, Horio T, Yokokawa K, et al. Pulmonary arterial brain natriuretic peptide concentration and cardiopulmonary hemodynamics during exercise in patients with essential hypertension. Metabolism 41:1273-1275, 1992.

89. Lang CC, Choy AM, Henderson IS, et al. Effect of haemodialysis on plasma levels of brain natriuretic peptide in patients with chronic renal failure. Clin Sci (Lond) 82:127-131, 1992.

90. Kinnunen P, Vuolteenaho O, Ruskoaho H. Mechanisms of atrial and brain natriuretic peptide release from rat ventricular myocardium: Effect of stretching. Endocrinology 132:1961-1970, 1993.

91. Hama N, Itoh H, Shirakami G, et al. Detection of C-type natriuretic peptide in human circulation and marked increase of plasma CNP level in septic shock patients. Biochem Biophys Res Commun 198:1177-1182, 1994.

92. Soleihac JM, Lucan E, Beaumont A, et al. A 94-kDa protein identified as neutral endopeptidase 24.11, can inactivate atrial natriuretic peptide in the vascular endothelium. Mol Pharmacol 41:609-614, 1992.

93. Seymour AA, Abboa-Offei BE, Smith PL, et al. Potentiation of natriuretic peptides by neutral endopeptidase inhibitors. Clin Exp Pharmacol Physiol 22:63-69, 1995.

94. Dussaule JC, Stefanski A, Bea ML, et al. Characterization of neutral endopeptidase in vascular smooth muscle cells of rabbit renal cortex. Am J Physiol 264:F45-F52, 1993.

95. Saxenhofer H, Raselli A, Weidmann P, et al. Urodilatin, a natriuretic factor from kidneys, can modify renal and cardiovascular function in men. Am J Physiol 259:F832-F838, 1990.

96. Chen HH, Lainchbury JG, Burnett JC. Natriuretic peptide receptors and neutral endopeptidase in mediating the renal actions of a new therapeutic synthetic natriuretic peptide dendroaspsis natriuretic peptide. J Am Coll Cardiol 40:1186-1191, 2002.

97. Sybertz EJ Jr, Chiu PJ, Watkins RW, et al. Neutral metalloendopeptidase inhibitors as ANF potentiators: Sites and mechanisms of action. Can J Physiol Pharmacol 69:1628-1635. 1991.

98. Seymour AA, Fennell SA, Swerdel JN. Potentiation of renal effects of atrial natriuretic factor-(99-126) by SQ 29,072. Hypertension 14:87-97, 1989.

99. Kishimoto I, Nakao K, Suga S, et al. Downregulation of C-receptor by natriuretic peptides via ANP-B receptor in vascular smooth muscle cells. Am J Physiol 265:H1373-H1379, 1993.

100. Takei Y, Takano M, Itahara Y, et al. Rainbow trout ventricular natriuretic peptide: Isolation, sequencing, and determination of biological activity. Gen Comp Endocrinol 96:420-426, 1994.

101. Takei Y, Fukuzawa A, Itahara Y, et al. A new natriuretic peptide isolated from cardiac atria of trout, *Oncorhynchus mykiss.* FEBS Lett 414:377-380, 1997.

102. Greenberg RN, Hill M, Crytzer J, et al. Comparison of effects of uroguanylin, guanylin, and *Escherichia coli* heat-stable enterotoxin STa in mouse intestine and kidney: Evidence that uroguanylin is an intestinal natriuretic hormone. J Investig Med 45:276-282, 1997.

103. Richards AM, Crozier IG. Physiological role of atrial natriuretic peptide. Int J Cardiol 25:141-143, 1989.

104. Janssen WM, de Zeeuw D, van der Hem GK, et al. Antihypertensive effect of a 5-day infusion of atrial natriuretic factor in humans. Hypertension 13:640-646, 1989.

105. Weidmann P, Hasler L, Gnadinger MP, et al. Blood levels and renal effects of atrial natriuretic peptide in normal man. J Clin Invest 77:734-742, 1986.

106. Charles CJ, Espiner EA, Richards AM. Cardiovascular actions of ANF: Contributions of renal, neurohumoral, and hemodynamic factors in sheep. Am J Physiol 264:R533-538, 1993.

107. Camargo MJ, Kleinert HD, Atlas SA, et al. Ca-dependent hemodynamic and natriuretic effects of atrial extract in isolated rat kidney. Am J Physiol 246:F447-F456, 1984.

108. Briggs JP, Steipe B, Schubert G, et al. Micropuncture studies of the renal effects of atrial natriuretic substance. Pflugers Arch 395:271-276, 1982.

109. Weidmann P, Gnadinger MP, Ziswiler HR, et al. Cardiovascular, endocrine and renal effects of atrial natriuretic peptide in essential hypertension. J Hypertens Suppl 4:S71-S83, 1986.

110. Weder AB, Sekkarie MA, Takiyyuddin M, et al. Antihypertensive and hypotensive effects of atrial natriuretic factor in men. Hypertension 10:582-589, 1987.

111. Holmes SJ, Espiner EA, Richards AM, et al. Renal, endocrine, and hemodynamic effects of human brain natriuretic peptide in normal man. J Clin Endocrinol Metab 76:91-96, 1993.

112. Seymour AA, Blaine EH, Mazack EK, et al. Renal and systemic effects of synthetic atrial natriuretic factor. Life Sci 36:33-44, 1985.

113. Gunning M, Ballermann BJ, Silva P, et al. Brain natriuretic peptide: Interaction with renal ANP system. Am J Physiol 258:F467-F472, 1990.

114. Inoue T, Nonoguchi H, Tomita K. Physiological effects of vasopressin and atrial natriuretic peptide in the collecting duct. Cardiovasc Res 51:470-480, 2001.

115. Shin SJ, Lee YJ, Tan MS, et al. Increased atrial natriuretic peptide mRNA expression in the kidney of diabetic rats. Kidney Int 51:1100-1105, 1997.

116. Shin SJ, Wen JD, Lee YJ, et al. Increased C-type natriuretic peptide mRNA expression in the kidney of diabetic rats. J Endocrinol 158:35-42, 1998.

117. Morishita Y, Sano T, Ando K, et al. Microbial polysaccharide, HS-142-1, competitively and selectively inhibits ANP binding to its guanylyl cyclase-containing receptor. Biochem Biophys Res Commun 176:949-957, 1991.

118. Stevens TL, Wei CM, Aahrus LL, et al. Modulation of exogenous and endogenous atrial natriuretic peptide by a receptor inhibitor. Hypertension 23:613-618, 1994.

119. Wada A, Tsutamoto T, Matsuda Y, et al. Cardiorenal and neurohumoral effects of endogenous atrial natriuretic peptide in dogs with severe congestive heart failure using a specific antagonist for guanylate cyclase-coupled receptors. Circulation 89:2232-2240, 1994.

120. Kishimoto I, Dubois SK, Garbers DL. The heart communicates with the kidney exclusively through the guanylyl cyclase-A receptor: Acute handling of sodium and water in response to volume expansion. Proc Natl Acad Sci USA 93:6215-6219, 1996.

121. Veress AT, Chong CK, Field LJ, et al. Blood pressure and fluid-electrolyte balance in ANF-transgenic mice on high- and low-salt diets. Am J Physiol 269:R186-R192, 1995.

122. Koh GY, Klug MG, Field LJ. Atrial natriuretic factor and transgenic mice. Hypertension 22:634-639, 1993.

123. Carstens J, Jensen KT, Pedersen EB. Effect of urodilatin infusion on renal haemodynamics, tubular function and vasoactive hormones. Clin Sci (Lond) 92:397-407, 1997.

124. Drummer C, Fiedler F, Konig A, et al. Urodilatin, a kidney-derived natriuretic factor, is excreted with a circadian rhythm and is stimulated by saline infusion in man. J Am Soc Nephrol 1:1109-1113, 1991.

125. Villarreal D, Freeman RH, Johnson RA. Renal effects of ANF (95-126), a new atrial peptide analogue, in dogs with experimental heart failure. Am J Hypertens 4:508-515, 1991.

126. John SW, Veress AT, Honrath U, et al. Blood pressure and fluid-electrolyte balance in mice with reduced or absent ANP. Am J Physiol 271:R109-R114, 1996.

127. Kita T, Kida O, Yokota N, et al. Effects of brain natriuretic peptide-45, a circulating form of rat brain natriuretic peptide, in spontaneously hypertensive rats. Eur J Pharmacol 202:73-79, 1991.

128. Stephenson SL, Kenny AJ. The hydrolysis of alpha-human atrial natriuretic peptide by pig kidney microvillar membranes is initiated by endopeptidase-24.11. Biochem J 243:183-187, 1987.

129. Yoshimura M, Yasue H, Morita E, et al. Hemodynamic, renal, and hormonal responses to brain natriuretic peptide infusion in patients with congestive heart failure. Circulation 84: 1581-1588, 1991.

130. Supaporn T, Wennberg PW, Wei CM, et al. Role for the endogenous natriuretic peptide system in the control of basal coronary vascular tone in dogs. Clin Sci (Lond) 90:357-362, 1996.

131. Suga S, Nakao K, Itoh H, et al. Endothelial production of C-type natriuretic peptide and its marked augmentation by transforming growth factor-beta. Possible existence of "vascular natriuretic peptide system." J Clin Invest 90:1145-1149, 1992.

132. Drewett JG, Fendly BM, Garbers DL, et al. Natriuretic peptide receptor-B (guanylyl cyclase-B) mediates C-type natriuretic peptide relaxation of precontracted rat aorta. J Biol Chem 270:4668-4674, 1995.

133. Itoh H, Pratt RE, Dzau VJ. Atrial natriuretic polypeptide inhibits hypertrophy of vascular smooth muscle cells. J Clin Invest 86:1690-1697, 1990.

134. Doi K, Itoh H, Ikeda T, et al. Adenovirus-mediated gene transfer of C-type natriuretic peptide causes G1 growth inhibition of cultured vascular smooth muscle cells. Biochem Biophys Res Commun 239:889-894, 1997.

135. Wei CM, Aarhus LL, Miller VM, et al. Action of C-type natriuretic peptide in isolated canine arteries and veins. Am J Physiol 264:H71-H73, 1993.

136. Wei CM, Heublein DM, Perrella MA, et al. Natriuretic peptide system in human heart failure. Circulation 88:1004-1009, 1993.

137. Fixler R, Hasin Y, Eilam Y, et al. Opposing effects of endothelin-1 on C-type natriuretic peptide actions in rat cardiomyocytes. Eur J Pharmacol 423:95-98, 2001.

138. Wei CM, Kim CH, Khraibi AA, et al. Atrial natriuretic peptide and C-type natriuretic peptide in spontaneously hypertensive rats and their vasorelaxing actions in vitro. Hypertension 1994; 23:903-907.

139. Clavell AL, Stingo AJ, Wei CM, et al. C-type natriuretic peptide: A selective cardiovascular peptide. Am J Physiol 264:R290-R295, 1993.

140. Hunt PJ, Richards AM, Espiner EA, et al. Bioactivity and metabolism of C-type natriuretic peptide in normal man. J Clin Endocrinol Metab 78:1428-1435, 1994.

141. Igaki T, Itoh H, Suga S, et al. C-type natriuretic peptide in chronic renal failure and its action in humans. Kidney Int Suppl 55:S144-S147, 1996.

142. Wei CM, Hu S, Miller VM, et al. Vascular actions of C-type natriuretic peptide in isolated porcine coronary arteries and coronary vascular smooth muscle cells. Biochem Biophys Res Commun 205:765-771, 1994.

143. Collins E, Bracamonte MP, Burnett JC Jr, et al. Mechanism of relaxations to dendroaspis natriuretic peptide in canine coronary arteries. J Cardiovasc Pharmacol 35:614-618, 2000.

144. Best PJ, Burnett JC, Wilson SH, et al. Dendroaspis natriuretic peptide relaxes isolated human arteries and veins. Cardiovasc Res 55:375-384, 2002.

145. Steinhelper ME, Cochrane KL, Field LJ. Hypotension in transgenic mice expressing atrial natriuretic factor fusion genes. Hypertension 16:301-307, 1990.

146. John SW, Krege JH, Oliver PM, et al. Genetic decreases in atrial natriuretic peptide and salt-sensitive hypertension. Science 267:679-681, 1995.

147. Lopez MJ, Wong SK, Kishimoto I, et al. Salt-resistant hypertension in mice lacking the guanylyl cyclase-A receptor for atrial natriuretic peptide. Nature 378:65-68, 1995.

148. Lopez MJ, Garbers DL, Kuhn M. The guanylyl cyclase-deficient mouse defines differential pathways of natriuretic peptide signaling. J Biol Chem 272:23064-23068, 1997.

149. Hutchinson HG, Trindade PT, Cunanan DB, et al. Mechanisms of natriuretic-peptide-induced growth inhibition of vascular smooth muscle cells. Cardiovasc Res 35:158-167, 1997.

150. Itoh H, Pratt RE, Ohno M, et al. Atrial natriuretic polypeptide as a novel antigrowth factor of endothelial cells. Hypertension 19:758-761, 1992.

151. Horio T, Nishikimi T, Yoshihara F, et al. Inhibitory regulation of hypertrophy by endogenous atrial natriuretic peptide in cultured cardiac myocytes. Hypertension 35:19-24, 2000.

152. Wu CF, Bishopric NH, Pratt RE. Atrial natriuretic peptide induces apoptosis in neonatal rat cardiac myocytes. J Biol Chem 272:14860-14866, 1997.

153. Suenobu N, Shichiri M, Iwashina M, et al. Natriuretic peptides and nitric oxide induce endothelial apoptosis via a cGMP-dependent mechanism. Arterioscler Thromb Vasc Biol 19:140-46, 1999.

154. Itoh H, Nakao K. Antagonism between the vascular renin-angiotensin and natriuretic peptide systems in vascular remodelling. Blood Press Suppl 5:49-53, 1994.

155. Kohno M, Yasunari K, Yokokawa K, et al. Inhibition by atrial and brain natriuretic peptides of endothelin-1 secretion after stimulation with angiotensin II and thrombin of cultured human endothelial cells. J Clin Invest 87:1999-2004, 1991.

156. Furuya M, Aisaka K, Miyazaki T, et al. C-type natriuretic peptide inhibits intimal thickening after vascular injury. Biochem Biophys Res Commun 193:248-253, 1993.

157. Morishita R, Gibbons GH, Pratt RE, et al. Autocrine and paracrine effects of atrial natriuretic peptide gene transfer on vascular smooth muscle and endothelial cellular growth. J Clin Invest 94:824-829, 1994.

158. Suga S, Itoh H, Komatsu Y, et al. Cytokine-induced C-type natriuretic peptide (CNP) secretion from vascular endothelial cells—evidence for CNP as a novel autocrine/paracrine regulator from endothelial cells. Endocrinology 133:3038-3041, 1993.

159. Tsutsui M, Yanagihara N, Minami K, et al. C-type natriuretic peptide stimulates catecholamine synthesis through the accumulation of cyclic GMP in cultured bovine adrenal medullary cells. J Pharmacol Exp Ther 268:584-589, 1994.

160. Morishige K, Shimokawa H, Yamawaki T, et al. Local adenovirus-mediated transfer of C-type natriuretic peptide suppresses vascular remodeling in porcine coronary arteries in vivo. J Am Coll Cardiol 35:1040-1047, 2000.

161. Canaan-Kuhl S, Ostendorf T, Zander K, et al. C-type natriuretic peptide inhibits mesangial cell proliferation and matrix accumulation in vivo. Kidney Int 53:1143-1151, 1998.

162. Schultz HD, Gardner DG, Deschepper CF, et al. Vagal C-fiber blockade abolishes sympathetic inhibition by atrial natriuretic factor. Am J Physiol 255:R6-R13, 1988.

163. Yang RH, Jin HK, Wyss JM, et al. Pressor effect of blocking atrial natriuretic peptide in nucleus tractus solitarii. Hypertension 19:198-205, 1992.

164. Ermirio R, Avanzino GL, Ruggeri P, et al. Cardiovascular effects of microinjection of ANF and brain natriuretic peptide into ventrolateral medulla. Am J Physiol 259:R32-R37, 1990.

165. Yang RH, Jin HK, Chen YF, et al. Blockade of endogenous anterior hypothalamic atrial natriuretic peptide with monoclonal antibody lowers blood pressure in spontaneously hypertensive rats. J Clin Invest 86:1985-1990, 1990.

166. Oparil S, Chen YF, Peng N, et al. Anterior hypothalamic norepinephrine, atrial natriuretic peptide, and hypertension. Front Neuroendocrinol 17:212-246, 1996.

167. Grove KL, Goncalves J, Picard S, et al. Comparison of ANP binding and sensitivity in brains from hypertensive and normotensive rats. Am J Physiol 272:R1344-R1353, 1997.

168. Imura H, Nakao K, Itoh H. The natriuretic peptide system in the brain: Implications in the central control of cardiovascular and neuroendocrine functions. Front Neuroendocrinol 13:217-249, 1992.

169. Burrell LM, Lambert HJ, Baylis PH. Effect of atrial natriuretic peptide on thirst and arginine vasopressin release in humans. Am J Physiol 260:R475-R479, 1991.

170. Blackburn RE, Samson WK, Fulton RJ, et al. Central oxytocin and ANP receptors mediate osmotic inhibition of salt appetite in rats. Am J Physiol 269:R245-R251, 1995.

171. Kubo T, Ando S, Picton P, et al. Atrial natriuretic peptide augments the variability of sympathetic nerve activity in human heart failure. J Hypertens 19:619-626, 2001.

172. Back H, Stumpf WE, Ando E, et al. Immunocytochemical evidence for CDD/ANP-like peptides in strands of myoendocrine cells associated with the ventricular conduction system of the rat heart. Anat Embryol (Berl) 175:223-226, 1986.

173. Wharton J, Anderson RH, Springall D, et al. Localisation of atrial natriuretic peptide immunoreactivity in the ventricular myocardium and conduction system of the human fetal and adult heart. Br Heart J 60:267-274, 1988.

174. Hansson M, Eriksson A, Forsgren S. Natriuretic peptide immunoreactivity in nerve structures and Purkinje fibres of human, pig and sheep hearts. Histochem J 29:329-336, 1997.

175. Debinski W, Gutkowska J, Kuchel O, et al. ANF-like peptide(s) in the peripheral autonomic nervous system. Biochem Biophys Res Commun 1986; 134:279-284.

176. Atchison DJ, Ackermann U. The interaction between atrial natriuretic peptide and cardiac parasympathetic function. J Auton Nerv Syst 42:81-88, 1993.

177. Lang CC, Choy AM, Balfour DJ, et al. Prazosin attenuates the natriuretic response to atrial natriuretic factor in man. Kidney Int 42:433-441, 1992.

178. Toki S, Morishita Y, Sano T, et al. HS-142-1, a novel non-peptide ANP antagonist, blocks the cyclic GMP production elicited by natriuretic peptides in PC12 and NG108-15 cells. Neurosci Lett 135:117-120, 1992.

179. Samson WK, Skala KD, Huang FL. CNP-22 stimulates, rather than inhibits, water drinking in the rat: Evidence for a unique biological action of the C-type natriuretic peptides. Brain Res 568:285-258, 1991.

180. Trachte GJ, Drewett JG. C-type natriuretic peptide neuromodulates independently of guanylyl cyclase activation. Hypertension 23:38-43, 1994.

181. Samson WK, Huang FL, Fulton RJ. C-type natriuretic peptide mediates the hypothalamic actions of the natriuretic peptides to inhibit luteinizing hormone secretion. Endocrinology 132:504-509, 1993.

182. Vatta MS, Presas M, Bianciotti LG, et al. B and C types natriuretic peptides modulate norepinephrine uptake and release in the rat hypothalamus. Regul Pept 65:175-184, 1996.

183. Wilcox JN, Augustine A, Goeddel DV, et al. Differential regional expression of three natriuretic peptide receptor genes within primate tissues. Mol Cell Biol 11:3454-3462, 1991.

184. Tsukagoshi H, Shimizu Y, Kawata T, et al. Atrial natriuretic peptide inhibits tumor necrosis factor-alpha production by interferon-gamma-activated macrophages via suppression of p38 mitogen-activated protein kinase and nuclear factor-kappa B activation. Regul Pept 99:21-29, 2001.

185. Kiemer AK, Hartung T, Vollmar AM. cGMP-mediated inhibition of TNF-alpha production by the atrial natriuretic peptide in murine macrophages. J Immunol 165:175-181, 2000.

186. Kiemer AK, Baron A, Gerbes AL, et al. The atrial natriuretic peptide as a regulator of Kupffer cell functions. Shock 17:365-371, 2002.

187. Kiemer AK, Vollmar AM, Bilzer M, et al. Atrial natriuretic peptide reduces expression of TNF-alpha mRNA during reperfusion of the rat liver upon decreased activation of NF-kappaB and AP-1. J Hepatol 33:236-246, 2000.

188. Kiemer AK, Weber NC, Vollmar AM. Induction of IkappaB: Atrial natriuretic peptide as a regulator of the NF-kappaB pathway. Biochem Biophys Res Commun 295:1068-1076, 2002.

189. Kiemer AK, Weber NC, Furst R, et al. Inhibition of p38 MAPK activation via induction of MKP-1: Atrial natriuretic peptide reduces TNF-alpha-induced actin polymerization and endothelial permeability. Circ Res 90:874-881, 2002.

190. Collard CD, Agah A, Reenstra W, et al. Endothelial nuclear factor-kappaB translocation and vascular cell adhesion molecule-1 induction by complement: Inhibition with anti-human C5 therapy or cGMP analogues. Arterioscler Thromb Vasc Biol 19:2623-2629, 1999.

191. Burnett JC Jr, Granger JP, Opgenorth TJ. Effects of synthetic atrial natriuretic factor on renal function and renin release. Am J Physiol 247:F863-F866, 1984.

192. Haloui M, Messika-Zeitoun D, Louedec L, et al. Potentiation of urinary atrial natriuretic peptide interferes with macula densa function. Cardiovasc Res 51:542-552, 2001.

193. McGregor A, Richards M, Espiner E, et al. Brain natriuretic peptide administered to man Actions and metabolism. J Clin Endocrinol Metab 70:1103-1107, 1990.

194. Hunt PJ, Espiner EA, Nicholls MG, et al. Differing biological effects of equimolar atrial and brain natriuretic peptide infusions in normal man. J Clin Endocrinol Metab 81:3871-3876, 1996.

195. Totsune K, Takahashi K, Murakami O, et al. Natriuretic peptides in the human kidney. Hypertension 24:758-762, 1994.

196. Davidson NC, Barr CS, Struthers AD. C-type natriuretic peptide. An endogenous inhibitor of vascular angiotensin-converting enzyme activity. Circulation 93:1155-1159, 1996.

197. Walther T, Schuitheiss HP, Tschope C. Impaired angiotensin II regulation of renal C-type natriuretic peptide mRNA expression in experimental diabetes mellitus. Cardiovasc Res 51: 562-566, 2001.

198. Kotridis P, Kokkas B, Karamouzis M, et al. Plasma atrial natriuretic peptide in essential hypertension after treatment with irbesartan. Blood Press 11:91-94, 2002.

199. Heringlake M, Bahlmann L, Klaus S, et al. Effects of angiotensin II and the AT(1) receptor antagonist losartan on the renal excretion of urodilatin. Kidney Blood Press Res 24:79-83, 2001.

200. Maack T. Role of atrial natriuretic factor in volume control. Kidney Int 49:1732-1737, 1996.

201. Morita H, Hagiike M, Horiba T, et al. Effects of brain natriuretic peptide and C-type natriuretic peptide infusion on urine flow and jejunal absorption in anesthetized dogs. Jpn J Physiol 42:349-353. 1992.

202. Takagi K, Araki N, Suzuki K. Relaxant effect of C-type natriuretic peptide on guinea-pig tracheal smooth muscle. Arzneimittelforschung 42:1329-1331, 1992.

203. Geary CA, Goy MF, Boucher RC. Synthesis and vectorial export of cGMP in airway epithelium: Expression of soluble and CNP-specific guanylate cyclases. Am J Physiol 265:L598-L605, 1993.

204. Brusq JM, Mayoux E, Guigui L, et al. Effects of C-type natriuretic peptide on rat cardiac contractility. Br J Pharmacol 128:206-212, 1999.

205. Nir A, Zhang DF, Fixler R, et al. C-type natriuretic peptide has a negative inotropic effect on cardiac myocytes. Eur J Pharmacol 412:195-201 2001.

206. Beaulieu P, Cardinal R, Page P, et al. Positive chronotropic and inotropic effects of C-type natriuretic peptide in dogs. Am J Physiol 273:H1933-H1940, 1997.

207. Beaulieu P, Cardinal R, De Lean A, et al. Direct chronotropic effects of atrial and C-type natriuretic peptides in anaesthetized dogs. Br J Pharmacol 118:1790-1796, 1996.

208. Hirose M, Furukawa Y, Kurogouchi F, et al. C-type natriuretic peptide increases myocardial contractility and sinus rate mediated by guanylyl cyclase-linked natriuretic peptide receptors in isolated, blood-perfused dog heart preparations. J Pharmacol Exp Ther 286:70-76, 1998.

209. Pierkes M, Gambaryan S, Boknik P, et al. Increased effects of C-type natriuretic peptide on cardiac ventricular contractility and relaxation in guanylyl cyclase A-deficient mice. Cardiovasc Res 53:852-861, 2002.

210. Shah AM, Mebazaa A, Wetzel RC, et al. Novel cardiac myofilament desensitizing factor released by endocardial and vascular endothelial cells. Circulation 89:2492-2497, 1994.

211. Suda M, Ogawa Y, Tanaka K, et al. Skeletal overgrowth in transgenic mice that overexpress brain natriuretic peptide. Proc Natl Acad Sci USA 95:2337-2342, 1998.

212. Pfeifer A, Aszodi A, Seidler U, et al. Intestinal secretory defects and dwarfism in mice lacking cGMP-dependent protein kinase II. Science 274:2082-2086, 1996.

213. Hunt PJ, Espiner EA, Richards AM, et al. Interactions of atrial and brain natriuretic peptides at pathophysiological levels in normal men. Am J Physiol 269:R1397-R1403, 1995.

214. Hu RM, Levin ER, Pedram A, et al. Atrial natriuretic peptide inhibits the production and secretion of endothelin from cultured endothelial cells. Mediation through the C receptor. J Biol Chem 267:17384-17389, 1992.

215. Ogawa Y, Itoh H, Tamura N, et al. Molecular cloning of the complementary DNA and gene that encode mouse brain natriuretic peptide and generation of transgenic mice that overexpress the brain natriuretic peptide gene. J Clin Invest 93:1911-1921, 1994.

216. Itoh H, Nakao K, Mukoyama M, et al. Chronic blockade of endogenous atrial natriuretic polypeptide (ANP) by monoclonal antibody against ANP accelerates the development of hypertension in spontaneously hypertensive and deoxycorticosterone acetate-salt-hypertensive rats. J Clin Invest 84:145-154, 1989.

217. Jin H, Mathews C, Chen YF, et al. Effects of acute and chronic blockade of neutral endopeptidase with Sch 34826 on NaCl-sensitive hypertension in spontaneously hypertensive rats. Am J Hypertens 5:210-218, 1992.

218. Jin HK, Chen YF, Yang RH, et al. Impaired release of atrial natriuretic factor in NaCl-loaded spontaneously hypertensive rats. Hypertension 11:739-744, 1988.

219. Jin HK, Yang RH, Chen YF, et al. Atrial natriuretic factor prevents NaCl-sensitive hypertension in spontaneously hypertensive rats. Hypertension 15:170-176, 1990.

220. Onwochei MO, Rapp JP. Hyposecretion of atrial natriuretic factor by prehypertensive Dahl salt-sensitive rat. Hypertension 13:440-448, 1989.

221. Jin H, Chen YF, Yang RH, et al. Atrial natriuretic factor in NaCl-sensitive and NaCl-resistant spontaneously hypertensive rats. Hypertension 14:404-412, 1989.

222. Jin HK, Yang RH, Chen YF, et al. Altered stores of atrial natriuretic peptide in specific brain nuclei of NaCl-sensitive spontaneously hypertensive rats. Am J Hypertens 4:449-455, 1991.

223. Yokota N, Bruneau BG, Kuroski de Bold ML, et al. Atrial natriuretic factor significantly contributes to the mineralocorticoid escape phenomenon. Evidence for a guanylate cyclase-mediated pathway. J Clin Invest 94:1938-1946, 1994.

224. Schiffrin EL, St-Louis J, Essiambre R. Platelet binding sites and plasma concentration of atrial natriuretic peptide in patients with essential hypertension. J Hypertens 1988; 6:565-572.

225. Nakaoka H, Kitahara Y, Amano M, et al. Effect of beta-adrenergic receptor blockade on atrial natriuretic peptide in essential hypertension. Hypertension 1987; 10:221-225.

226. Talartschik J, Eisenhauer T, Schrader J, et al. Low atrial natriuretic peptide plasma concentrations in 100 patients with essential hypertension. Am J Hypertens 3:45-47, 1990.

227. Montorsi P, Tonolo G, Polonia J, et al. Correlates of plasma atrial natriuretic factor in health and hypertension. Hypertension 10:570-576, 1987.

228. Dessi-Fulgheri P, Palermo R, Di Noto G, et al. Plasma levels of atrial natriuretic factor in mild to moderate hypertensives without signs of left ventricular hypertrophy: Correlation with the known duration of hypertension. J Hum Hypertens 2: 177-182, 1988.

229. Kohno M, Yasunari K, Matsuura T, et al. Circulating atrial natriuretic polypeptide in essential hypertension. Am Heart J 113:1160-1163 1987.

230. Sagnella GA, Markandu ND, Buckley MG, et al. Atrial natriuretic peptides in essential hypertension: Basal plasma levels and relationship to sodium balance. Can J Physiol Pharmacol 69:1592-1600, 1991.

231. Kohno M, Yasunari K, Murakawa K, et al. Effects of high-sodium and low-sodium intake on circulating atrial natriuretic peptides in salt-sensitive patients with systemic hypertension. Am J Cardiol 59:1212-1213, 1987.

232. Nimura S. Attenuated release of atrial natriuretic factor due to sodium loading in salt-sensitive essential hypertension. Jap Heart J 32:167-178, 1991.

233. Campese VM, Tawadrous M, Bigazzi R, et al. Salt intake and plasma atrial natriuretic peptide and nitric oxide in hypertension. Hypertension 28:335-340, 1996.

234. Ferrari P, Weidmann P, Ferrier C, et al. Dysregulation of atrial natriuretic factor in hypertension-prone man. J Clin Endocrinol Metab 71:944-951, 1990.

235. Weidmann P, Ferrari P, Allemann Y, Ferrier C, Shaw SG. Developing essential hypertension: A syndrome involving ANF deficiency? Can J Physiol Pharmacol 69:1582-1591, 1991.

236. Pitzalis MV, Iacoviello M, Massari F, et al. Influence of gender and family history of hypertension on autonomic control of heart rate, diastolic function and brain natriuretic peptide. J Hypertens 19:143-148, 2001.

237. Rutledge DR, Sun Y, Ross EA. Polymorphisms within the atrial natriuretic peptide gene in essential hypertension. J Hypertens 13:953-955, 1995.

238. Beige J, Ringel J, Hohenbleicher H, et al. HpaII-polymorphism of the atrial-natriuretic-peptide gene and essential hypertension in whites. Am J Hypertens 10:1316-1318, 1997.

239. Kato N, Sugiyama T, Morita H, et al. Genetic analysis of the atrial natriuretic peptide gene in essential hypertension. Clin Sci (Lond) 98:251-258, 2000.

240. Schorr U, Beige J, Ringel J, et al. Hpa II polymorphism of the atrial natriuretic peptide gene and the blood pressure response to salt intake in normotensive men. J Hypertens 15:715-718, 1997.

241. Berge KE, Berg K. No effect on blood pressure level or variability of polymorphisms in DNA at the locus for atrial natriuretic factor (ANF). Clin Genet 46:433-435, 1994.

242. Tunny TJ, Jonsson JR, Klemm SA, et al. Association of restriction fragment length polymorphism at the atrial natriuretic peptide gene locus with aldosterone responsiveness to angiotensin in aldosterone-producing adenoma. Biochem Biophys Res Commun 204:1312-1317, 1994.

243. Rahmutula D, Nakayama T, Soma M, et al. Association study between the variants of the human ANP gene and essential hypertension. Hypertens Res 24:291-294, 2001.

244. Maoz E, Shamiss A, Peleg E, et al. The role of atrial natriuretic peptide in natriuresis of fasting. J Hypertens 10:1041-1044, 1992.

245. Maoz E, Shamiss A, Peleg E, et al. The effect of weight reduction on the levels of atrial natriuretic peptide (ANP) in obese hypertensive and normotensive subjects. Metabolism 40:110-111, 1991.

246. Dessi-Fulgheri P, Sarzani R, Tamburrini P, et al. Plasma atrial natriuretic peptide and natriuretic peptide receptor gene expression in adipose tissue of normotensive and hypertensive obese patients. J Hypertens 15:1695-1699, 1997.

247. Dessi-Fulgheri P, Sarzani R, Rappelli A. The natriuretic peptide system in obesity-related hypertension: New pathophysiological aspects. J Nephrol 11:296-299, 1998.

248. Sarzani R, Paci VM, Dessi-Fulgheri P, et al. Comparative analysis of atrial natriuretic peptide receptor expression in rat tissues. J Hypertens Suppl 11:S214-S215, 1993.

249. Sarzani R, Dessi-Fulgheri P, Paci VM, et al. Expression of natriuretic peptide receptors in human adipose and other tissues. J Endocrinol Invest 19:581-585, 1996.

250. Castro LC, Hobel CJ, Gornbein J. Plasma levels of atrial natriuretic peptide in normal and hypertensive pregnancies: A meta-analysis. Am J Obstet Gynecol 171:1642-1651, 1994.

251. Spaanderman M, Ekhart T, van Eyck J, et al. Preeclampsia and maladaptation to pregnancy: A role for atrial natriuretic peptide? Kidney Int 60:1397-406, 2001.

252. Minegishi T, Nakamura M, Abe K, et al. Adrenomedullin and atrial natriuretic peptide concentrations in normal pregnancy and pre-eclampsia. Mol Hum Reprod 5:767-770, 1999.

253. Pouta AM, Vuolteenaho OJ, Laatikainen TJ. An increase of the plasma N-terminal peptide of proatrial natriuretic peptide in preeclampsia. Obstet Gynecol 89:747-753, 1997.

254. Senoz S, Sahin N, Ozcan T, et al. The concentration of plasma atrial natriuretic peptide in normotensive and preeclamptic pregnancies. Eur J Obstet Gynecol Reprod Biol 62:173-177, 1995.

255. Soffronoff EC, Kaufmann BM, Connaughton JF. Intravascular volume determinations and fetal outcome in hypertensive diseases of pregnancy. Am J Obstet Gynecol 127:4-9, 1977.

256. Visser W, Wallenburg HC. Central hemodynamic observations in untreated preeclamptic patients. Hypertension 17:1072-1077, 1991.

257. Stasch JP, Hirth-Dietrich C, Kazda S, et al. Endothelin stimulates release of atrial natriuretic peptides in vitro and in vivo. Life Sci 45:869-875, 1989.

258. Florijn KW, Derkx FH, Visser W, et al. Elevated plasma levels of endothelin in pre-eclampsia. J Hypertens Suppl 9:S166-S167, 1991.

259. Nakagawa O, Ogawa Y, Itoh H, et al. Rapid transcriptional activation and early mRNA turnover of brain natriuretic peptide in cardiocyte hypertrophy. Evidence for brain natriuretic peptide as an "emergency" cardiac hormone against ventricular overload. J Clin Invest 96:1280-1287, 1995.

260. Wambach G, Koch J. BNP plasma levels during acute volume expansion and chronic sodium loading in normal men. Clin Exp Hypertens 17:619-629, 1995.

261. Tharaux PL, Dussaule JC, Hubert-Brierre J, et al. Plasma atrial and brain natriuretic peptides in mitral stenosis treated by valvulotomy. Clin Sci (Lond) 87:671-677, 1994.

262. Grantham JA, Borgeson DD, Burnett JC Jr. BNP: Pathophysiological and potential therapeutic roles in acute congestive heart failure. Am J Physiol 272:R1077-R1083, 1997.

263. Stevens TL, Rasmussen TE, Wei CM, et al. Renal role of the endogenous natriuretic peptide system in acute congestive heart failure. J Card Fail 2:119-125, 1996.

264. Lisy O, Lainchbury JG, Leskinen H, et al. Therapeutic actions of a new synthetic vasoactive and natriuretic peptide, dendroaspis natriuretic peptide, in experimental severe congestive heart failure. Hypertension 37:1089-1094, 2001.

265. Hosoda K, Nakao K, Mukoyama M, et al. Expression of brain natriuretic peptide gene in human heart. Production in the ventricle. Hypertension 17:1152-1155, 1991.

266. Motwani JG, McAlpine H, Kennedy N, et al. Plasma brain natriuretic peptide as an indicator for angiotensin-converting-enzyme inhibition after myocardial infarction. Lancet 341:1109-1113, 1993.

267. Hirata Y, Matsumoto A, Aoyagi T, et al. Measurement of plasma brain natriuretic peptide level as a guide for cardiac overload. Cardiovasc Res 51:585-591, 2001.

268. Stevens TL, Burnett JC Jr., Kinoshita M, et al. A functional role for endogenous atrial natriuretic peptide in a canine model of early left ventricular dysfunction. J Clin Invest 95:1101-1108, 1995.

269. Calderone A, Thaik CM, Takahashi N, et al. Nitric oxide, atrial natriuretic peptide and cGMP inhibit the growth-promoting effects of norepinephrine in cardiac myocytes and fibroblasts. J Clin Invest 101:812-818, 1998.

270. Nakamura M, Arakawa N, Yoshida H, et al. Vasodilatory effects of C-type natriuretic peptide on forearm resistance vessels are distinct from those of atrial natriuretic peptide in chronic heart failure. Circulation 90:1210-1214, 1994.

271. Darbar D, Davidson NC, Gillespie N, et al. Diagnostic value of B-type natriuretic peptide concentrations in patients with acute myocardial infarction. Am J Cardiol 78:284-287, 1996.

272. Morita E, Yasue H, Yoshimura M, et al. Increased plasma levels of brain natriuretic peptide in patients with acute myocardial infarction. Circulation 88:82-91, 1993.

273. Omland T, Aakvaag A, Bonarjee VV, et al. Plasma brain natriuretic peptide as an indicator of left ventricular systolic function and long-term survival after acute myocardial infarction. Comparison with plasma atrial natriuretic peptide and N-terminal proatrial natriuretic peptide. Circulation 93:1963-1969, 1996.

274. Richards AM, Doughty R, Nicholls MG, et al. Plasma N-terminal pro-brain natriuretic peptide and adrenomedullin: Prognostic utility and prediction of benefit from carvedilol in chronic ischemic left ventricular dysfunction. Australia-New Zealand Heart Failure Group. J Am Coll Cardiol 37:1781-1787, 2001.

275. Tan AC, van Loenhout TT, Lamfers EJ, et al. Atrial natriuretic peptide after myocardial infarction. Am Heart J 118:490-494, 1989.

276. Kikuta K, Yasue H, Yoshimura M, et al. Increased plasma levels of B-type natriuretic peptide in patients with unstable angina. Am Heart J 132:101-107, 1996.

277. Hama N, Itoh H, Shirakami G, et al. Rapid ventricular induction of brain natriuretic peptide gene expression in experimental acute myocardial infarction. Circulation 92:1558-1564, 1995.

278. Marumoto K, Hamada M, Hiwada K. Increased secretion of atrial and brain natriuretic peptides during acute myocardial ischaemia induced by dynamic exercise in patients with angina pectoris. Clin Sci (Lond) 88:551-556, 1995.

279. Izumi T, Saito Y, Kishimoto I, et al. Blockade of the natriuretic peptide receptor guanylyl cyclase-A inhibits NF-kappaB activation and alleviates myocardial ischemia/reperfusion injury. J Clin Invest 108:203-213, 2001.

280. Padilla F, Garcia-Dorado D, Agullo L, et al. Intravenous administration of the natriuretic peptide urodilatin at low doses during coronary reperfusion limits infarct size in anesthetized pigs. Cardiovasc Res 51:592-600, 2001.

281. Wozakowska-Kaplon B, Opolski G. Atrial natriuretic peptide level after cardioversion of chronic atrial fibrillation. Int J Cardiol 83:159-165 2002.

282. Rossi A, Enriquez-Sarano M, Burnett JC Jr., et al. Natriuretic peptide levels in atrial fibrillation: A prospective hormonal and Doppler-echocardiographic study. J Am Coll Cardiol 35:1256-1262, 2000.

283. Ellenbogen KA, Rogers R, Walsh M, et al. Increased circulating atrial natriuretic factor (ANF) release during induced ventricular tachycardia. Am Heart J 116:1233-1238, 1988.

284. Mookherjee S, Anderson G Jr, Smulyan H, et al. Atrial natriuretic peptide response to cardioversion of atrial flutter and fibrillation and role of associated heart failure. Am J Cardiol 67:377-380, 1991.

285. Petersen P, Kastrup J, Vilhelmsen R, et al. Atrial natriuretic peptide in atrial fibrillation before and after electrical cardioversion therapy. Eur Heart J 9:639-641, 1988.

286. Arakawa M, Miwa H, Kambara K, et al. Changes in plasma concentrations of atrial natriuretic peptides after cardioversion of chronic atrial fibrillation. Am J Cardiol 70:550-552, 1992.

287. Roy D, Paillard F, Cassidy D, et al. Atrial natriuretic factor during atrial fibrillation and supraventricular tachycardia. J Am Coll Cardiol 1987; 9:509-514, 1987.

288. Inoue S, Murakami Y, Sano K, et al. Atrium as a source of brain natriuretic polypeptide in patients with atrial fibrillation. J Card Fail 6:92-96, 2000.

289. Shimizu H, Murakami O, Inoue S, et al. High plasma brain natriuretic polypeptide level as a marker of risk for thromboembolism in patients with nonvalvular atrial fibrillation. Stroke 33:1005-1010, 2002.

290. Kohno M, Yokokawa K, Yasunari K, et al. Effect of the endothelin family of peptides on human coronary artery smooth-muscle cell migration. J Cardiovasc Pharmacol 31:S84-S89, 1998.

291. Ikeda M, Kohno M, Yasunari K, et al. Natriuretic peptide family as a novel antimigration factor of vascular smooth muscle cells. Arterioscler Thromb Vasc Biol 17:731-736, 1997.

292. Kohno M, Yokokawa K, Yasunari K, et al. Effect of natriuretic peptide family on the oxidized LDL-induced migration of human coronary artery smooth muscle cells. Circ Res 81:585-590, 1997.

293. Suga S, Nakao K, Mukoyama M, et al. Characterization of natriuretic peptide receptors in cultured cells. Hypertension 19:762-765, 1992.

294. Hirata K, Akita H, Yokoyama M, et al. Impaired vasodilatory response to atrial natriuretic peptide during atherosclerosis progression. Arterioscler Thromb 12:99-105, 1992.

295. Kugiyama K, Sugiyama S, Matsumura T, et al. Suppression of atherosclerotic changes in cholesterol-fed rabbits treated with an oral inhibitor of neutral endopeptidase 24.11 (EC 3.4.24.11). Arterioscler Thromb Vasc Biol 16:1080-1087, 1996.

296. Pedersen EB, Danielsen H, Eiskjaer H, et al. Increased atrial natriuretic peptide in the nephrotic syndrome. Relationship to the renal function and the renin-angiotensin-aldosterone system. Scand J Clin Lab Invest 48:141-147, 1988.

297. Rodriguez-Iturbe B, Colic D, Parra G, et al. Atrial natriuretic factor in the acute nephritic and nephrotic syndromes. Kidney Int 38:512-517, 1990.

298. Tulassay T, Rascher W, Lang RE, et al. Atrial natriuretic peptide and other vasoactive hormones in nephrotic syndrome. Kidney Int 31:1391-1395, 1987.

299. Jespersen B, Eiskjaer H, Mogensen CE, et al. Reduced natriuretic effect of atrial natriuretic peptide in nephrotic syndrome: A possible role of decreased cyclic guanosine monophosphate. Nephron 71:44-153, 1995.

300. Mair J, Friedl W, Thomas S, et al. Natriuretic peptides in assessment of left-ventricular dysfunction. Scand J Clin Lab Invest Suppl 230:132-142, 1999.

301. Jensen KT, Carstens J, Ivarsen P, et al. A new, fast and reliable radioimmunoassay of brain natriuretic peptide in human plasma. Reference values in healthy subjects and in patients with different diseases. Scand J Clin Lab Invest 57:529-540, 1997.

302. Buckley MG, Sethi D, Markandu ND, et al. Plasma concentrations and comparisons of brain natriuretic peptide and atrial natriuretic peptide in normal subjects, cardiac transplant recipients and patients with dialysis-independent or dialysis-dependent chronic renal failure. Clin Sci (Lond) 83:437-444, 1992.

303. Tonolo G, McMillan M, Polonia J, et al. Plasma clearance and effects of alpha-hANP infused in patients with end-stage renal failure. Am J Physiol 254:F895-F899, 1988.

304. Zoccali C, Mallamaci F, Benedetto FA, et al. Cardiac natriuretic peptides are related to left ventricular mass and function and predict mortality in dialysis patients. J Am Soc Nephrol 12:1508-1515, 2001.

305. Mallamaci F, Zoccali C, Tripepi G, et al. Diagnostic potential of cardiac natriuretic peptides in dialysis patients. Kidney Int 59:1559-1566, 2001.

306. Nitta K, Kawashima A, Yumura W, et al. Plasma concentration of brain natriuretic peptide as an indicator of cardiac ventricular function in patients on hemodialysis. Am J Nephrol 18:411-415, 1998.

307. Holtta T, Happonen JM, Ronnholm K, et al. Hypertension, cardiac state, and the role of volume overload during peritoneal dialysis. Pediatr Nephrol 16:324-331, 2001.

308. Jin H, Yang RH, Chen YF, et al. Atrial natriuretic peptide in acute hypoxia-induced pulmonary hypertension in rats. J Appl Physiol 71:807-814, 1991.

309. Jin H, Yang RH, Chen YF, et al. Atrial natriuretic peptide attenuates the development of pulmonary hypertension in rats adapted to chronic hypoxia. J Clin Invest 85:115-120, 1990.

310. Klinger JR, Petit RD, Curtin LA, et al. Cardiopulmonary responses to chronic hypoxia in transgenic mice that overexpress ANP. J Appl Physiol 75:198-205, 1993.

311. Zhao L, Long L, Morrell NW, et al. NPR-A-Deficient mice show increased susceptibility to hypoxia-induced pulmonary hypertension. Circulation 99:605-607, 1999.

312. Winter RJ, Davidson AC, Treacher D, et al. Atrial natriuretic peptide concentrations in hypoxic secondary pulmonary hypertension: Relation to haemodynamic and blood gas variables and response to supplemental oxygen. Thorax 44:58-62, 1989.

313. Lang CC, Coutie WJ, Struthers AD, et al. Elevated levels of brain natriuretic peptide in acute hypoxaemic chronic obstructive pulmonary disease. Clin Sci (Lond) 83:529-533, 1992.

314. Ando T, Ogawa K, Yamaki K, et al. Plasma concentrations of atrial, brain, and C-type natriuretic peptides and endothelin-1 in patients with chronic respiratory diseases. Chest 110:462-468, 1996.

315. Tanabe M, Ueda M, Endo M, et al. Effect of acute lung injury and coexisting disorders on plasma concentrations of atrial natriuretic peptide. Crit Care Med 22:1762-1768, 1994.

316. Mitaka C, Hirata Y, Nagura T, et al. Plasma alpha-human atrial natriuretic peptide concentration in patients with acute lung injury. Am Rev Respir Dis 146:43-46, 1992.

317. Nagaya N, Ando M, Oya H, et al. Plasma brain natriuretic peptide as a noninvasive marker for efficacy of pulmonary thromboendarterectomy. Ann Thorac Surg 74:180-184; discussion 184, 2002.

318. Tulevski, II, Hirsch A, Sanson BJ, et al. Increased brain natriuretic peptide as a marker for right ventricular dysfunction in acute pulmonary embolism. Thromb Haemost 86:1193-1196, 2001.

319. Rubattu S, Lee-Kirsch MA, DePaolis P, et al. Altered structure, regulation, and function of the gene encoding the atrial natriuretic peptide in the stroke-prone spontaneously hypertensive rat. Circ Res 85:900-905, 1999.

320. Rubattu S, Ridker P, Stampfer MJ, et al. The gene encoding atrial natriuretic peptide and the risk of human stroke. Circulation 100:1722-1726, 1999.

321. Hassan A, Ali N, Dong Y, et al. Atrial natriuretic peptide gene G664A polymorphism and the risk of ischemic cerebrovascular disease. Neurology 57:1726-1728, 2001.

322. Estrada V, Tellez MJ, Moya J, et al. High plasma levels of endothelin-1 and atrial natriuretic peptide in patients with acute ischemic stroke. Am J Hypertens 7:1085-1089, 1994.

323. Yan SD, Fu J, Soto C, et al. An intracellular protein that binds amyloid-beta peptide and mediates neurotoxicity in Alzheimer's disease. Nature 389:689-695, 1997.

324. Qiu WQ, Walsh DM, Ye Z, et al. Insulin-degrading enzyme regulates extracellular levels of amyloid beta-protein by degradation. J Biol Chem 273:32730-32738, 1998.

325. Valdivieso A. The kidney in chronic liver disease: Circulatory abnormalities, renal sodium handling and role of natriuretic peptides. Biol Res 31:291-304, 1998.

326. Bernardi M, Fornale L, Di Marco C, et al. Hyperdynamic circulation of advanced cirrhosis: A re-appraisal based on posture-induced changes in hemodynamics. J Hepatol 22:309-318, 1995.

327. La Villa G, Romanelli RG, Casini Raggi V, et al. Plasma levels of brain natriuretic peptide in patients with cirrhosis. Hepatology 16:156-161, 1992.

328. Akriviadis EA, Ervin MG, Cominelli F, et al. Hyponatremia of cirrhosis: Role of vasopressin and decreased 'effective' plasma volume. Scand J Gastroenterol 32:829-834, 1997.

329. Salo J, Jimenez W, Kuhn M, et al. Urinary excretion of urodilatin in patients with cirrhosis. Hepatology 24:1428-1432, 1996.

330. Wong F, Blendis L. Pathophysiology of sodium retention and ascites formation in cirrhosis: Role of atrial natriuretic factor. Semin Liver Dis 14:59-70, 1994.

331. Morali GA, Floras JS, Legault L, et al. Muscle sympathetic nerve activity and renal responsiveness to atrial natriuretic factor during the development of hepatic ascites. Am J Med 91:383-392, 1991.

332. Koepke JP, Jones S, DiBona GF. Renal nerves mediate blunted natriuresis to atrial natriuretic peptide in cirrhotic rats. Am J Physiol 252:R1019-R1023, 1987.

333. Fabrega E, Crespo J, Rivero M, et al. Dendroaspis natriuretic peptide in hepatic cirrhosis. Am J Gastroenterol 96:2724-2729, 2001.

334. Gulberg V, Moller S, Henriksen JH, et al. Increased renal production of C-type natriuretic peptide (CNP) in patients with cirrhosis and functional renal failure. Gut 47:852-857, 2000.

335. Angeli P, Jimenez W, Arroyo V, et al. Renal effects of natriuretic peptide receptor blockade in cirrhotic rats with ascites. Hepatology 20:948-954, 1994.

336. Lubien E, DeMaria A, Krishnaswamy P, et al. Utility of B-natriuretic peptide in detecting diastolic dysfunction: Comparison with Doppler velocity recordings. Circulation 105:595-601, 2002.

337. Krishnaswamy P, Lubien E, Clopton P, et al. Utility of B-natriuretic peptide levels in identifying patients with left ventricular systolic or diastolic dysfunction. Am J Med 111:274-279, 2001.

338. Maisel AS, Koon J, Krishnaswamy P, et al. Utility of B-natriuretic peptide as a rapid, point-of-care test for screening patients undergoing echocardiography to determine left ventricular dysfunction. Am Heart J 141:367-374, 2001.

339. McCullough PA, Nowak RM, McCord J, et al. B-type natriuretic peptide and clinical judgment in emergency diagnosis of heart failure: Analysis from Breathing Not Properly (BNP) Multinational Study. Circulation 106:416-422, 2002.

340. Maisel AS, Krishnaswamy P, Nowak RM, et al. Rapid measurement of B-type natriuretic peptide in the emergency diagnosis of heart failure. N Engl J Med 347:161-167, 2002.

341. Dao Q, Krishnaswamy P, Kazanegra R, et al. Utility of B-type natriuretic peptide in the diagnosis of congestive heart failure in an urgent-care setting. J Am Coll Cardiol 37:379-385, 2001.

342. Kruger S, Graf J, Kunz D, et al. brain natriuretic peptide levels predict functional capacity in patients with chronic heart failure. J Am Coll Cardiol 40:718-722, 2002.

343. Cowie MR, Struthers AD, Wood DA, et al. Value of natriuretic peptides in assessment of patients with possible new heart failure in primary care. Lancet 350:1349-1353, 1997.

344. McDonagh TA, Robb SD, Murdoch DR, et al. Biochemical detection of left-ventricular systolic dysfunction. Lancet 351:9-13, 1998.

345. Troughton RW, Frampton CM, Yandle TG, et al. Treatment of heart failure guided by plasma aminoterminal brain natriuretic peptide (N-BNP) concentrations. Lancet 355:1126-1130, 2000.

346. Cheng V, Kazanagra R, Garcia A, et al. A rapid bedside test for B-type peptide predicts treatment outcomes in patients admitted for decompensated heart failure: A pilot study. J Am Coll Cardiol 37:386-391, 2001.

347. Kawai K, Hata K, Takaoka H, et al. Plasma brain natriuretic peptide as a novel therapeutic indicator in idiopathic dilated cardiomyopathy during beta-blocker therapy: A potential of hormone-guided treatment. Am Heart J 141:925-932, 2001.

348. Vervoort G, Wetzels JF, Lutterman JA, et al. Atrial natriuretic peptide-induced microalbuminuria is associated with endothelial dysfunction in noncomplicated type 1 diabetes patients. Am J Kidney Dis 40:9-15, 2002.

349. Prasad N, Clarkson PB, MacDonald TM, et al. Atrial natriuretic peptide increases urinary albumin excretion in men

with type 1 diabetes mellitus and established microalbuminuria. Diabet Med 15:678-682, 1998.

350. Zietse R, Derkx FH, Weimar W, et al. Effect of atrial natriuretic peptide on renal and vascular permeability in diabetes mellitus. J Am Soc Nephrol 5:2057-2066, 1995.

351. Lerman A, Gibbons RJ, Rodeheffer RJ, et al. Circulating N-terminal atrial natriuretic peptide as a marker for symptomless left-ventricular dysfunction. Lancet 341:1105-1109, 1993.

352. Tsutamoto T, Wada A, Maeda K, et al. Plasma brain natriuretic peptide level as a biochemical marker of morbidity and mortality in patients with asymptomatic or minimally symptomatic left ventricular dysfunction. Comparison with plasma angiotensin II and endothelin-1. Eur Heart J 20:1799-1807, 1999.

353. Tsutamoto T, Wada A, Maeda K, et al. Attenuation of compensation of endogenous cardiac natriuretic peptide system in chronic heart failure: Prognostic role of plasma brain natriuretic peptide concentration in patients with chronic symptomatic left ventricular dysfunction. Circulation 96:509-516, 1997.

354. Bettencourt P, Ferreira S, Azevedo A, et al. Preliminary data on the potential usefulness of B-type natriuretic peptide levels in predicting outcome after hospital discharge in patients with heart failure. Am J Med 113:215-219, 2002.

355. Jernberg T, Stridsberg M, Lindahl B. Usefulness of plasma N-terminal proatrial natriuretic peptide (proANP) as an early predictor of outcome in unstable angina pectoris or non-ST-elevation acute myocardial infarction. Am J Cardiol 89:64-66, 2002.

356. Richards AM, Nicholls MG, Yandle TG, et al. Plasma N-terminal pro-brain natriuretic peptide and adrenomedullin: New neurohormonal predictors of left ventricular function and prognosis after myocardial infarction. Circulation 97:1921-1929, 1998.

357. Omland T, de Lemos JA, Morrow DA, et al. Prognostic value of N-terminal pro-atrial and pro-brain natriuretic peptide in patients with acute coronary syndromes. Am J Cardiol 89:463-465, 2002.

358. Hall C, Cannon CP, Forman S, et al. Prognostic value of N-terminal proatrial natriuretic factor plasma levels measured within the first 12 hours after myocardial infarction. Thrombolysis in Myocardial Infarction (TIMI) II Investigators. J Am Coll Cardiol 26:1452-1456 1995.

359. Arakawa N, Nakamura M, Aoki H, et al. Plasma brain natriuretic peptide concentrations predict survival after acute myocardial infarction. J Am Coll Cardiol 27:1656-1661, 1996.

360. Nagaya N, Nishikimi T, Goto Y, et al. Plasma brain natriuretic peptide is a biochemical marker for the prediction of progressive ventricular remodeling after acute myocardial infarction. Am Heart J 135:21-28, 1998.

361. de Lemos JA, Morrow DA, Bentley JH, et al. The prognostic value of B-type natriuretic peptide in patients with acute coronary syndromes. N Engl J Med 345:1014-1021, 2001.

362. Omland T, Aarsland T, Aakvaag A, et al. Prognostic value of plasma atrial natriuretic factor, norepinephrine and epinephrine in acute myocardial infarction. Am J Cardiol 72:255-259, 1993.

363. Rouleau JL, Packer M, Moye L, et al. Prognostic value of neurohumoral activation in patients with an acute myocardial infarction: Effect of captopril. J Am Coll Cardiol 24:583-591, 1994.

364. Omland T, Bonarjee VV, Nilsen DW, et al. Prognostic significance of N-terminal pro-atrial natriuretic factor (1-98) in acute myocardial infarction: Comparison with atrial natriuretic factor (99-126) and clinical evaluation. Br Heart J 70:409-414, 1993.

365. Hall C, Rouleau JL, Moye L, et al. N-terminal proatrial natriuretic factor. An independent predictor of long-term prognosis after myocardial infarction. Circulation 89:1934-1942, 1994.

366. Mills RM, LeJemtel TH, Horton DP, et al. Sustained hemodynamic effects of an infusion of nesiritide (human b-type natriuretic peptide) in heart failure: A randomized, double-blind, placebo-controlled clinical trial. Natrecor Study Group. J Am Coll Cardiol 34:155-162, 1999.

367. Colucci WS. Nesiritide for the treatment of decompensated heart failure. J Card Fail 7:92-100, 2001.

368. Colucci WS, Elkayam U, Horton DP, et al. Intravenous nesiritide, a natriuretic peptide, in the treatment of decompensated congestive heart failure. Nesiritide Study Group. N Engl J Med 343:246-253, 2000.

369. Publication Committee for the VMAC Investigators (Vasodilatation in the Management of Acute CHF). Intravenous nesiritide vs nitroglycerin for treatment of decompensated congestive heart failure: A randomized controlled trial. JAMA 287:1531-1540, 2002.

370. Burger AJ, Horton DP, LeJemtel T, et al. Effect of nesiritide (B-type natriuretic peptide) and dobutamine on ventricular arrhythmias in the treatment of patients with acutely decompensated congestive heart failure: The PRECEDENT study. Am Heart J 144:1102-1108, 2002.

371. Hayashi M, Tsutamoto T, Wada A, et al. Intravenous atrial natriuretic peptide prevents left ventricular remodeling in patients with first anterior acute myocardial infarction. J Am Coll Cardiol 37:1820-1826, 2001.

372. Kosuge M, Miyajima E, Kimura K, et al. Comparison of atrial natriuretic peptide versus nitroglycerin for reducing blood pressure in acute myocardial infarction. Am J Cardiol 81: 781-784, 1998.

373. Lai CP, Egashira K, Tashiro H, et al. Beneficial effects of atrial natriuretic peptide on exercise-induced myocardial ischemia in patients with stable effort angina pectoris. Circulation 87:144-151, 1993.

374. Tanaka H, Yasue H, Yoshimura M, et al. Suppression of hyperventilation-induced attacks with infusion of atrial natriuretic peptide in patients with variant angina pectoris. Am J Cardiol 72:128-133, 1993.

375. Kato H, Yasue H, Yoshimura M, et al. Suppression of hyperventilation-induced attacks with infusion of B-type (brain) natriuretic peptide in patients with variant angina. Am Heart J 128:1098-1104, 1994.

376. La Villa G, Lazzeri C, Pascale A, et al. Cardiovascular and renal effects of low-dose atrial natriuretic peptide in compensated cirrhosis. Am J Gastroenterol 92:852-857, 1997.

377. Brenard R, Moreau R, Pussard E, et al. Hemodynamic and sympathetic responses to human atrial natriuretic peptide infusion in patients with cirrhosis. J Hepatol 14:347-356, 1992.

378. Gadano A, Moreau R, Vachiery F, et al. Natriuretic response to the combination of atrial natriuretic peptide and terlipressin in patients with cirrhosis and refractory ascites. J Hepatol 26:1229-1234, 1997.

379. Kurnik BR, Weisberg LS, Cuttler IM, et al. Effects of atrial natriuretic peptide versus mannitol on renal blood flow during radiocontrast infusion in chronic renal failure. J Lab Clin Med 116:27-36, 1990.

380. Allgren RL, Marbury TC, Rahman SN, et al. Anaritide in acute tubular necrosis. Auriculin Anaritide Acute Renal Failure Study Group. N Engl J Med 336:828-834, 1997.

381. Lewis J, Salem MM, Chertow GM, et al. Atrial natriuretic factor in oliguric acute renal failure. Anaritide Acute Renal Failure Study Group. Am J Kidney Dis 36:767-774, 2000.

382. Mitaka C, Hirata Y, Nagura T, et al. Beneficial effect of atrial natriuretic peptide on pulmonary gas exchange in patients with acute lung injury. Chest 114:223-228, 1998.

383. Bindels AJ, van der Hoeven JG, Groeneveld PH, et al. Atrial natriuretic peptide infusion and nitric oxide inhalation in patients with acute respiratory distress syndrome. Crit Care 5:151-157, 2001.

384. Lin KF, Chao J, Chao L. Atrial natriuretic peptide gene delivery reduces stroke-induced mortality rate in Dahl salt-sensitive rats. Hypertension 33:219-224, 1999.

385. Danilewicz JC, Barclay PL, Barnish IT, et al. UK-69,578, a novel inhibitor of EC 3.4.24.11 which increases endogenous ANF levels and is natriuretic and diuretic. Biochem Biophys Res Commun 164:58-65, 1989.

386. Tikkanen I, Helin K, Tikkanen T, et al. Elevation of plasma atrial natriuretic peptide in rats with chronic heart failure by SCH 39370, a neutral metalloendopeptidase inhibitor. J Pharmacol Exp Ther 254:641-645, 1990.

387. Northridge DB, Jardine AG, Alabaster CT, et al. Effects of UK 69 578: A novel atriopeptidase inhibitor. Lancet 2:591-593, 1989.

388. Lafferty HM, Gunning M, Silva P, et al. Enkephalinase inhibition increases plasma atrial natriuretic peptide levels, glomerular filtration rate, and urinary sodium excretion in rats with reduced renal mass. Circ Res 65:640-646, 1989.

389. Maki T, Nasa Y, Yamaguchi F, et al. Long-term treatment with neutral endopeptidase inhibitor improves cardiac function and reduces natriuretic peptides in rats with chronic heart failure. Cardiovasc Res 51:608-617, 2001.

390. Sybertz EJ, Chiu PJ, Vemulapalli S, et al. SCH 39370, a neutral metalloendopeptidase inhibitor, potentiates biological responses to atrial natriuretic factor and lowers blood pressure in desoxycorticosterone acetate-sodium hypertensive rats. J Pharmacol Exp Ther 250:624-631, 1989.

391. Gafford JT, Skidgel RA, Erdos EG, et al. Human kidney "enkephalinase", a neutral metalloendopeptidase that cleaves active peptides. Biochemistry 22:3265-3271, 1983.

392. Smits GJ, McGraw DE, Trapani AJ. Interaction of ANP and bradykinin during endopeptidase 24.11 inhibition: Renal effects. Am J Physiol 258:F1417-F1424, 1990.

393. Northridge DB, Currie PF, Newby DE, et al. Placebo-controlled comparison of candoxatril, an orally active neutral endopeptidase inhibitor, and captopril in patients with chronic heart failure. Eur J Heart Fail 1:67-72, 1999.

394. Northridge DB, Newby DE, Rooney E, et al. Comparison of the short-term effects of candoxatril, an orally active neutral endopeptidase inhibitor, and frusemide in the treatment of patients with chronic heart failure. Am Heart J 138:1149-1157, 1999.

395. Newby DE, McDonagh T, Currie PF, et al. Candoxatril improves exercise capacity in patients with chronic heart failure receiving angiotensin converting enzyme inhibition. Eur Heart J 19:1808-1813, 1998.

396. Westheim AS, Bostrom P, Christensen CC, et al. Hemodynamic and neuroendocrine effects for candoxatril and frusemide in mild stable chronic heart failure. J Am Coll Cardiol 34:1794-1801, 1999.

397. Matsumura T, Kugiyama K, Sugiyama S, et al. Neutral endopeptidase 24.11 in neutrophils modulates protective effects of natriuretic peptides against neutrophils-induced endothelial cytotoxity. J Clin Invest 97:2192-2203, 1996.

398. Corti R, Burnett JC Jr., Rouleau JL, et al. Vasopeptidase inhibitors: A new therapeutic concept in cardiovascular disease? Circulation 104:1856-1862, 2001.

399. Burnett JC. Vasopeptidase inhibition. Curr Opin Nephrol Hypertens 9:465-468, 2000.

# Vasodilator Peptides: CGRP, Substance P, and Adrenomedullin

## Ralph E. Watson, Donald J. DiPette, Scott C. Supowit, Khurshed. A Katki, Huawei Zhao

There is mounting evidence that the potent vasodilator peptides calcitonin gene-related peptide (CGRP), substance P (SP), and adrenomedullin (ADM) regulate cardiovascular function both in the normal state and in hypertension. Evidence from human studies and experiments in rat and mouse models of hypertension has shed more light on the possible roles of these neuropeptides in human hypertension.

## CALCITONIN GENE-RELATED PEPTIDE

CGRP is a 37-amino acid neuropeptide derived from the tissue-specific splicing of the primary RNA transcript of the calcitonin/CGRP gene,[1,2] which will be referred to as the α-CGRP gene. Calcitonin is produced mainly in the parafollicular cells of the thyroid, but CGRP synthesis occurs almost exclusively in regions of the central and peripheral nervous systems.[3] β-CGRP is a second CGRP gene that does not produce calcitonin, but also produces CGRP, primarily in central neuronal tissues.[3,4] The two CGRP genes, α-CGRP and β-CGRP in the rat and I and II in humans, differ in their protein sequences by one and three amino acids respectively, and the biologic activities of the two peptides are quite similar in most vascular beds.[5]

### Distribution and Localization of CGRP

Immunoreactive CGRP and its receptors are widely distributed in the nervous and cardiovascular systems.[5,6] In the peripheral nervous system, common sites of CGRP synthesis are in the spinal nerve dorsal root ganglia (DRG). These structures contain the cell bodies of sensory nerves that terminate centrally in laminae I/II of the dorsal horn of the spinal cord and peripherally in blood vessels and all other tissues innervated by the sensory nervous system.[7] Blood vessels in all vascular beds are surrounded by a dense perivascular CGRP neural network.[3] Circulating CGRP is thought to be a spillover phenomenon from the perivascular nerve terminals caused by release of CGRP to promote vasodilation and other functions.[3] Receptors for CGRP have been identified in the media and intima of resistance vessels.

### Cardiovascular Actions of CGRP

CGRP is the most potent vasodilator discovered to date, and it has positive chronotropic and inotropic effects.[8,9] CGRP selectively dilates many vascular beds, especially the coronary vasculature.[3,8,10] Systemic administration of CGRP decreases blood pressure (BP) in a dose-dependent manner in nor-motensive animals and humans.[3,6] The primary mechanism is peripheral arterial dilation.[3,6,9] The CGRP receptors are coupled to G proteins. G proteins are located in the intracellular portion of the plasma membrane, and they bind activated receptor complexes. Through conformational changes and cyclic binding and hydrolysis of guanosine triphosphate, G proteins, directly or indirectly, affect alterations in channel gating, thus coupling cell surface receptors to intracellular responses. In a number of tissues, including vascular smooth muscle, CGRP increases intracellular cyclic adenosine monophosphate (cAMP). CGRP may also activate adenosine triphosphate–activated potassium channels of vascular smooth muscle.[3] The vasodilator response evoked by CGRP may, in part, be mediated by nitric oxide (NO) release.[3] Various vascular beds may differ in their dependence on the endothelium for the dilator response to CGRP.[3] The NO-mediated vasodilator response is endothelium dependent, whereas the other mechanisms directly affect the vascular smooth muscle. Thus CGRP can dilate blood vessels through endothelium-dependent and endothelium-independent mechanisms.

### Role of CGRP in Human Hypertension

CGRP administration can significantly decrease BP in humans,[3,6] but it is not clear what role CGRP plays in human hypertension. The levels of circulating immunoreactive CGRP in hypertensive humans reported in different studies have been inconsistent.[3,6] Several factors are probably responsible, including the assay itself, heterogeneity of essential hypertension, severity and duration of the BP elevation, the degree of target organ damage, and the variety of treatment regimens used in the patients.[3]

### Role of CGRP in Rat Models of Experimental Hypertension

In contrast to human hypertension, a direct role for CGRP in experimental hypertension has now been established. We have previously reported that CGRP plays a compensatory vasodilator role to attenuate the BP increase in three rat models of acquired hypertension: (1) deoxycorticosterone-salt (DOC-salt),[11,12] (2) subtotal nephrectomy-salt (SN-salt),[13] and (3) N-nitro-L-arginine methyl ester (L-NAME)-induced hypertension during pregnancy.[14] Considerable progress has been made in elucidating the mechanism of the antihypertensive effects of CGRP in these settings. In the DOC-salt model, the depressor activity of CGRP appears to be mediated by a significant increase in the neuronal synthesis and release of the peptide, whereas in the SN-salt and L-NAME models, the BP lowering effect of CGRP is mediated by a marked increase in vascular reactivity to the dilator actions of the neuropeptide. In contrast, the spontaneously hypertensive rat (SHR), a genetic model of hypertension,[15] displays a significant age-related decrease in CGRP production, which may contribute to the increased BP through the loss of a potent vasodilator system.[16] These and related studies have been the subject of several reviews.[7,17] Therefore, we will focus on recent reports that use α-CGRP null mice.

## Characterization of the α-CGRP Knockout Mouse

To assess the long-term role of CGRP in the regulation of cardiovascular function, permanent deletion of this gene was achieved by targeted disruption of the calcitonin/α-CGRP gene locus.[18] The β-CGRP gene is intact in these knockout (KO) mice; however, α-CGRP is by far the predominant CGRP species produced in DRG neurons.[3] The mice used in these studies were genotyped using standard polymerase chain reaction techniques. In our initial studies, systolic blood pressure, determined by tail-cuff BP, was significantly ($p < .01$) higher in the KO mice (160 ± 6.1 mm Hg) compared with controls (125 ± 5 mm Hg).[19] To confirm this finding, previously instrumented KO and wild-type (WT) mice (25- to 30-g males) were studied fully awake and unrestrained. As shown in Figure 19–1, the mean arterial pressure (MAP) was significantly elevated in the KO mice compared with the controls. The mice were sacrificed and the DRG were removed and frozen for later quantification of α-CGRP, β-CGRP, and SP mRNA and peptide levels. Figure 19–2 shows the absence of the α-CGRP mRNA in the KO mice following Northern blot analysis. Experiments were also performed to determine whether β-CGRP and SP mRNA levels were altered in KO mice. As expected, the mRNA species for β-CGRP and SP were present in both groups, and normalization of the hybridization signals (β-CGRP and SP) to 18S rRNA levels indicated that there was no significant difference in the synthesis of these mRNAs between genotypes.

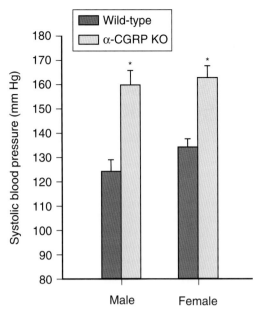

**Figure 19–1** Systolic BP measurements in α-CGRP KO and WT mice of either sex, with the tail-cuff method. BP values were obtained for each animal by taking four to six readings daily for 5 days. Mean ± SEM for each group (n = 7) are presented for both male and female mice. Asterisk indicates significant differences from WT (p <.05). (From Gangula PR, Zhao H, Supowit SC, et al. Increased blood pressure in alpha-calcitonin gene-related peptide/calcitonin gene knockout mice. Hypertension 35:470-475, 2000.) BP, blood pressure; KO, knockout; WT, wild-type; SEM, standard error of measure.

Immunostaining for immunoreactive CGRP (iCGRP) was performed in the spinal cords of both KO and control mice. We observed intense staining of CGRP in laminae I/II of the dorsal horn of the spinal cord in the WT mice. Even though the antibody used in these studies recognizes both α- and β-CGRP, no staining of iCGRP was observed in the KO mice.

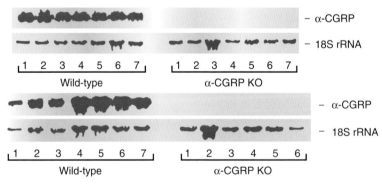

**Figure 19–2** Northern blot analysis of mRNA from DRG from WT and α-CGRP KO male **(A)** and female **(B)** mice. Total cellular RNA samples isolated from DRG taken from WT and α-CGRP KO mice were fractionated on a denaturing formaldehyde-agarose gel and transferred to a nylon membrane. The membrane was hybridized with the [32]P-labeled α-CGRP genomic DNA insert. The α-CGRP was removed from the membrane, which was subsequently hybridized with [32]P-labeled 18S rDNA probe (bottom). After hybridization with each probe, the membrane was washed and placed on a phosphor screen, and the image was generated from PhosphorImager analyses of the exposed screen. Note the lack of α-CGRP mRNA in the α-CGRP KO group. (From Gangula PR, Zhao H, Supowit SC, et al. Increased blood pressure in alpha-calcitonin gene-related peptide/calcitonin gene knockout mice. Hypertension 35:470-475, 2000.) mRNA, messenger ribonucleic acid; DRG, dorsal root ganglion; WT, wild-type; KO, knockout; rDNA, ribosomal deoxyribonucleic acid.

In later studies the BP phenotype of the mutant mice was confirmed by radiotelemetric recording. Both α-CGRP KO and WT controls underwent probe implantation and recording was begun 1 week after the surgery to allow for recovery. The telemetric analyses were based on data for 7 consecutive days. Comparisons were made of harmonic patterns, rhythm-adjusted mean (MESOR = average 24-hour arterial pressure), amplitude, and acrophase (clock time of peak amplitude).[20] As anticipated, both the α-CGRP KO and WT mice displayed a 24-hour rhythm characterized by several nighttime peaks. As shown in Figure 19–3, the average 24-hour MAP was approximately 12 to 20 mm Hg higher in the KO mice compared with the controls, consistent with our previous data. These mice were then placed on a high-salt (3.2% Na) diet for 2 weeks and BP and heart rate were recorded by telemetry. No increase in MAP or heart rate was observed in either strain. These findings are in agreement with our previous studies showing that a chronic high-salt diet does not increase the MAP (measured acutely) in either the α-CGRP KO or WT mice.

It should be noted that, to delete the α-CGRP gene, it was also necessary to inactivate the calcitonin gene, as well as katacalcin, that is derived from the processing of the calcitonin peptide precursor.[3] It is important to note that it has been clearly demonstrated that neither endogenous calcitonin nor katacalcin plays a role in cardiovascular regulation.[3,21] A second KO mouse, specific for α-CGRP, has been generated, but on a different genetic background, by Lu et al.[22] Interestingly these KO mice do not appear to display an increased baseline MAP. Another α-CGRP–specific KO strain that has the same genetic background as the mice used in our study has been generated and shown to display a significantly elevated BP and heart rate compared with controls.[23] Although differences in genetic background or experimental approach may account for the discrepancy between the findings of Lu et al.[22] and the results reported by us and Oh-hashi et al.,[23] these data indicate that α-CGRP plays a significant role in the regulation of basal BP.

## DOC-Salt–Induced Hypertension in the α-CGRP KO Mouse

Hypertension was induced in 8- to 10-week-old male α-CGRP KO mice and their WT counterparts by uninephrectomy, DOC administration, and 0.9% saline drinking water. Control KO and WT mice were sham operated and given tap water to drink. Three weeks after initiation of the protocol, all mice had arterial catheters surgically placed for continuous MAP recording and were studied in a conscious and unrestrained state. The DOC-salt protocol produced a significant increase in MAP in the α-CGRP KO and WT animals. When normalized to baseline BP, the MAP was 15% and 30% higher in the WT and CGRP KO mice, respectively. This MAP increase in the DOC-salt KO mice compared with untreated KO mice was significantly greater than that observed in the WT groups. Cardiac hypertrophy (heart/body weight) was present in the control CGRP KO (0.51 ± 0.02) compared with control WT (0.45 ± 0.01) mice. As expected, there was a significant increase in heart to body weight ratios in the two DOC groups (DOC-salt KO, 0.68 ± 0.02 vs. DOC-salt WT, 0.68 ± 0.02) when compared with their matching control group. These data indicate that deletion of the α-CGRP gene not only increases baseline BP and cardiac weight, but also enhances the BP response to DOC-salt treatment.[24]

## Blood Pressure Response to Capsaicin Administration in α-CGRP KO and WT Mice

Several lines of evidence indicate that the efferent vasodilator activity of the sensory nervous system is mediated primarily by capsaicin (the active ingredient in pepper)-sensitive C-fiber and Aδ-fiber classes of sensory nerves. To study the hypotensive role of CGRP following stimulation of capsaicin-sensitive sensory nerves, we used α-CGRP KO mice and WT controls in conjunction with the CGRP antagonist (CGRP$_{8-37}$).[25] In the anesthetized state the MAP of the KO mice was still approximately 15 mm Hg higher than that of the WT controls. Intravenous administration of capsaicin to WT mice produced a rapid but transient (~30 seconds) bradycardia accompanied by a 40% decrease in MAP. This response was followed by a sustained (4-6 minutes) hypotensive effect that reduced the MAP by 20%. Pretreatment of the WT mice with atropine abolished the transient bradycardia and hypotension, but was without effect on the prolonged hypotensive response. In contrast, the prolonged hypotensive response was blocked by administration of CGRP$_{8-37}$. In the CGRP KO mice, capsaicin again produced a transient, atropine-sensitive bradycardia and reduction in MAP (40%), but the sustained hypotensive response was absent. Pretreatment of both mouse strains with

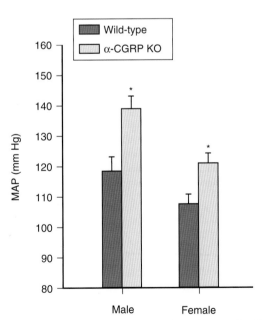

**Figure 19–3** MAP determinations made with an indwelling carotid arterial catheter in α-CGRP KO and WT mice of either sex in a fully awake and unrestrained state. Mean ± SEM for each group (n = 7) are presented for both male and female mice. Asterisk indicates significant differences from WT (p <.05). (From Gangula PR, Zhao H, Supowit SC, et al. Increased blood pressure in alpha-calcitonin gene-related peptide/calcitonin gene knockout mice. Hypertension 35:470-475, 2000.) MAP, mean arterial pressure; KO, knockout; WT, wild-type; SEM, standard error of measure.

the capsaicin antagonist, capsazepine, blocked all of the actions of capsaicin. These data indicate that although the initial hemodynamic effects of capsaicin treatment result from transient vagal stimulation, the sensory nerve component of the sustained capsaicin-mediated hypotensive response is primarily dependent on α-CGRP.

## Coronary Flows in the α-CGRP KO Mouse

Studies performed in the rat suggest that capsaicin-sensitive sensory nerves participate in the regulation of basal coronary blood flow. To test the hypothesis that α-CGRP plays a critical role in the regulation of coronary blood flow, Langendorff-perfused heart preparations were used to compare coronary flow rates between α-CGRP KO and WT control mice under various pressure-loading conditions.[26] Deletion of the α-CGRP gene in both sexes resulted in a significant 20% to 30% reduction in coronary flow at all pressures tested. In addition, coronary flow for both strains of mice was consistently lower in females than in males. These data suggest that CGRP is responsible for up to 30% of basal coronary blood flow. Histopathologic analysis showed no obvious structural or pathologic alterations in the myocardium or coronary vasculature between genotypes. Because blood vessel diameter is directly related to coronary flow, studies were performed to determine the range of blood vessel diameters (optical micrometer) in heart sections from the KO and WT mice. No detectable differences were observed between strains. Thus, the mechanism of this reduction in coronary flow is likely to be decreased coronary vasodilation resulting from ablation of α-CGRP from perivascular sensory nerve terminals.

## Summary

CGRP and its receptors are widely distributed in the nervous and cardiovascular systems. CGRP is the most potent vasodilator discovered to date and has positive chronotropic and inotropic effects. CGRP selectively dilates many vascular beds, especially the coronary vasculature. Systemic administration of CGRP decreases BP in a dose-dependent manner in normotensive animals and humans, primarily by peripheral arterial dilation. It can dilate blood vessels through endothelium-dependent and endothelium-independent mechanisms. Although CGRP administration can significantly decrease high BP in humans, it is not clear what role CGRP plays in human hypertension. However, a direct role for CGRP in experimental hypertension has now been established in several models of hypertension. In acquired rat models, CGRP plays a compensatory vasodilator role to attenuate the BP increase. In the DOC-salt model, the depressor activity of CGRP appears to be mediated by a significant increase in the neuronal synthesis and release of the peptide. In the SN-salt and L-NAME models, the BP lowering effect of CGRP is mediated by a marked increase in vascular reactivity to CGRP. By contrast, the SHR, a genetic model of hypertension, displays a significant age-related decrease in CGRP production, which may contribute to the increased BP through the loss of a potent vasodilator system.

MAPs in mice with a permanent deletion of the α-CGRP gene are significantly elevated compared with controls. This deletion also increases cardiac weight and enhances the BP response to DOC-salt hypertension. In addition, whereas the initial hemodynamic effects of capsaicin treatment in mice result from transient vagal stimulation, the sensory nerve component of the sustained capsaicin-mediated hypotensive response is primarily dependent on α-CGRP. Studies of CGRP KO mice suggest that CGRP is responsible for up to 30% of basal coronary blood flow.

# SUBSTANCE P

SP is an 11-amino acid peptide sensory neurotransmitter that mediates pain, touch, and temperature. It is involved in many physiologic activities including smooth muscle contraction and vasodilation.[5,6,17,27-29] SP was first described in 1931 as "an atropine-resistant factor, which stimulates smooth muscle and lowers blood pressure."[30] Its structure was first identified in 1971.[31] SP is a member of the tachykinin family. The five major mammalian tachykinins are SP, neurokinin A (NKA), neurokinin B (NKB), neuropeptide K, and neuropeptide-γ (NP-γ).[32-34] SP is derived from tissue-specific alternative splicing of the preprotachykinin I gene and is produced almost exclusively in neuronal tissues.[32] An important site of SP synthesis is the DRG, which contain the cell bodies of sensory neurons that extend centrally to the spinal cord and peripherally to blood vessels.[7] SP and its receptor (NK-1 receptor) are present throughout the central and peripheral nervous systems.[35-37] SP receptors are also found in endothelial cells.[35] SP is often located in and released from the same sensory nerve endings as CGRP.[36] SP has been shown to regulate blood flow of various organs.

## Cardiovascular Actions of Substance P

SP is a potent vasodilator, but has little effect on heart rate and cardiac contractility.[35] Of the three tachykinin receptor subtypes NK-1, NK-2, and NK-3, SP is the preferred ligand (binding-molecule) for NK-1 receptors, NKA for NK-2, and NKB for NK-3, but all three tachykinins have some affinity for all three NK receptors if a high enough dose is given.[35] The three receptors all belong to the superfamily of G-protein–coupled receptors. SP induces vasodilation by an endothelium-dependent mechanism involving the release of both NO and a hyperpolarizing/vasodilator factor different from NO.[6,35,38]

## Release of Substance P from Sensory Nerve Terminals

Sensory nerve fibers are classified as capsaicin-sensitive and capsaicin-insensitive. The capsaicin-sensitive nerves have the receptor for capsaicin. When capsaicin-sensitive sensory nerve fibers are exposed to capsaicin, they release SP. SP-rich nerve fibers are part of the sensory nervous system, comprising mostly capsaicin-sensitive C-fiber and Aδ-fiber nerves that respond to chemical, thermal, and mechanical stimuli.[27,28,39] These stimuli cause SP release. If the stimulus is powerful enough, it also causes propagation of sensory information back to the central nervous system. Although these nerves have traditionally been thought to "sense" stimuli in the periphery and transmit the information centrally, there is evidence that they also have an efferent function. It is clear that DRG-neuron–derived peptides are released at peripheral sensory nerve terminals in the absence of afferent nerve stimulation.[40] The continuous release of peptides from DRG neurons may reflect a paracrine function, with the released peptides binding to nearby receptors. This implies that these neurons participate in the continuous regulation of blood flow and other tissue activities. It has been postulated that some DRG neurons are specialized in controlling peripheral effector mechanisms, but have no role in sensation.[40]

## Role of Substance P in Hypertension

Decreased levels of SP have been found in stroke-prone spontaneously hypertensive rats (SHR-sp) and in human essential hypertension.[41] Therefore, SP could contribute to elevated BP by the decreased activity of a counterregulatory mechanism. A nonpeptide SP receptor (NK-1) antagonist has been used to study the hemodynamic role of the peptide in five experimental models of hypertension, including the DOC-salt; SN-salt; SHR; two-kidney, one-clip rats; and one-kidney, one-clip rats.[15,41-43] In conscious unrestrained rats, the SP antagonist induced significant increases in MAP in the three salt-dependent models, DOC-salt, SN-salt, and one-kidney, one-clip rats. However, the antagonist caused no significant effect on the MAP in the salt-independent models, SHR and two-kidney, one-clip. This suggests that SP may act as a partial compensatory mechanism to counteract the BP increase in salt-dependent hypertension.

Studies performed in our laboratory, confirmed the depressor effects of SP using a peripherally acting NK-1 receptor antagonist (spantide-II) and determined the neuronal expression and release of SP in both the SN-salt and DOC-salt models.[42,43] In addition, we studied the Dahl salt-sensitive and Dahl salt-resistant rats, a model of hypertension that has both genetic and salt-dependent components.[44]

To determine the role and mechanism of action of SP in SN-salt hypertension, we induced hypertension in 4- to 6-week-old male Sprague-Dawley rats by subtotal nephrectomy and 1% saline drinking water. Sham-operated rats were given either tap water or 1% saline to drink.[42] Eleven to 13 days later, all rats had intravenous (for drug administration) and arterial (for continuous monitoring of MAP) catheters surgically implanted and were studied in the conscious and unrestrained state. Baseline MAP was significantly elevated in the SN-salt rats (157 ± 6 mm Hg) compared with tap water–fed (128 ± 3 mm Hg) and 1% saline–fed controls (132 ± 5 mm Hg). As shown in Figure 19–4, intravenous vehicle administration did not significantly alter the MAP in any of the groups. In contrast, intravenous administration of spantide-II resulted in a rapid increase of the already elevated MAP in the SN-salt rats compared with both control groups.[42] To determine whether neuronal expression of SP is altered in this model, we quantified SP mRNA and peptide levels in DRG from all the study groups. As shown in Figure 19–5, the SP mRNA and peptide levels were not elevated in the SN-salt rats compared with controls.[42] To determine whether the mechanism of the antihypertensive effect of SP in the SN-salt model is due to increased vascular reactivity to the dilator activity of this neuropeptide, similar to our findings with CGRP, we administered exogenous SP to these three groups.[42] As shown in Figure 19–6, this resulted in a significantly greater decrease in MAP in the SN-salt rats compared with both control groups. This suggests that, in SN-salt hypertension, SP plays a counterregulatory role in the absence of an increase in production

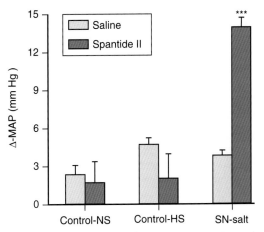

**Figure 19–4** Span-II increases the MAP in SN-salt rats but not in control rats. Rats were instrumented for continuous MAP recording and span-II administration as described in the text. With the rats fully awake and unrestrained, bolus doses of the vehicle (0.1 ml of saline) and span-II (0.2 μmol/L in 0.1 ml) were administered intravenously. Values reported are change in MAP ± SEM (mm Hg) from baseline MAP. ***$p$ <.001 SN-salt versus control-NS (tap water) and control-HS (1% saline). (From Katki KA, Supowit SC, DiPette DJ. Substance P in subtotal nephrectomy-salt hypertension. Hypertension 39[part 2]:389-393, 2002.) Span-II, spantide-II; MAP, mean arterial pressure; SN, subtotal nephrectomy; SEM, standard error of measure.

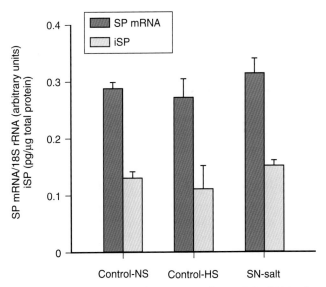

**Figure 19–5** SP mRNA and iSP content from DRG of SN-salt and control-NS (tap water) and control-HS (1% saline). The SP mRNA:18S rRNA ratios were determined by scanning densitometry. Values reported are mean ± SEM arbitrary units. Immunoreactive SP was quantified using a commercially available rabbit antirat SP RIA kit. Values are reported in pg iSP/μg total protein. (From Katki KA, Supowit SC, DiPette DJ. Substance P in subtotal nephrectomy-salt hypertension. Hypertension 2002; 39[part 2]:389-393.) SP, substance P; mRNA, messenger ribonucleic acid; iSP, immunoreactive substance P; DRG, dorsal root ganglion; SN, subtotal nephrectomy; rRNA, ribosomal ribonucleic acid; SEM, standard error of measure; RIA, radioimmunoassay.

of SP. One possible mechanism of this compensatory vasodilator response is enhanced vascular reactivity to SP.[42]

## Summary

Taken together, various lines of research suggest a potential dual role of SP in essential hypertension and regulation of regional organ blood flow:

1. A deficiency of SP could result in hypertension and decreased organ blood flow.
2. Enhanced vascular reactivity to SP could be a compensatory vasodilator response to hypertension or decreased organ blood flow.

All of these experiments were performed acutely, so the long-term participation of SP in hypertension is unknown. Studies in humans are also needed. Nevertheless, these studies point to the SP-containing sensory afferent neurons having an important efferent cardiovascular function.

## ADRENOMEDULLIN

Adrenomedullin (ADM) was discovered in 1993, when peptide extracts from human pheochromocytoma were studied.[45] The name comes from its abundance in normal adrenal medulla, as well as in pheochromocytoma tissue arising from adrenal medulla.[45] It is a 52-amino acid peptide with a unique 6-amino acid ring structure formed by an intramolecular disulfide bond between residues 16 and 21. It also has a C-terminal amide structure. Both of these features are similar to structures found in CGRP and amylin (a 37-amino acid peptide packaged with insulin in pancreatic β-cell secretory granules that inhibits glycogen synthesis and glucose utilization).[46] Thus ADM is considered a member of the CGRP/amylin/calcitonin superfamily of peptides. ADM has a potent and long-lasting hypotensive effect.[45] The ADM gene is situated in a single locus of chromosome 11.[47] ADM antagonists such as ADM-(22-52) and ADM-(40-52) do not contain the ring and lack agonist activity.[46]

### Distribution of Adrenomedullin

ADM immunoreactivity in the rat and pig is found in the adrenal gland, heart, lung, and kidney.[48,49] Since the discovery that the ADM gene is more highly expressed in endothelial cells than even the adrenal medulla,[50] ADM is now regarded as a secretory product of the vascular endothelium, like NO and endothelin, and ADM expression has been found in all tissues of the body.[51]

### Adrenomedullin in Human Hypertension

Plasma ADM levels are increased in hypertensive patients compared with normotensive controls, especially if there is an increase in serum creatinine or renin levels.[52-57] There is a progressive rise in ADM proportionate to the severity of the hypertension and the target organ damage.[55-57] This suggests that ADM is released to compensate for the elevated BP.[51] After control of BP with antihypertensive medication, plasma ADM levels do not come down.[52] Plasma ADM levels are directly proportional to serum creatinine levels and inversely related to

glomerular filtration rates (GFRs) in hypertensive patients.[52] Neither acute nor chronic salt-loading changes plasma ADM levels in normotensives or essential hypertensives.[58]

### Adrenomedullin in Experimental Models of Hypertension

In Dahl salt-sensitive rats, plasma ADM and cardiac ventricle ADM concentration and mRNA levels were higher in rats with high-salt than low-salt intake.[59] Plasma ADM correlated well with the weight of the left ventricle, suggesting that ADM participates in the pathophysiology of salt-dependent hypertension and cardiac hypertrophy.[59] In DOCA-treated SHR that developed malignant hypertension, plasma and renal tissue ADM were significantly higher than in control rats.[60] Chronic ADM infusion in Dahl salt-sensitive rats significantly improved renal function (serum creatinine, creatinine clearance, and urinary protein excretion) and histologic findings (glomerular injury score) without changing MAP compared with untreated controls, suggesting that ADM has renoprotective effects in this experimental model of hypertension.[61] Chronic infusion of ADM significantly prolonged life in this model.[62] Human ADM gene delivery delays BP rise and protects against cardiovascular remodeling and renal injury in several rat models of hypertension.[63-65]

### Circulating Adrenomedullin in Other Disease States

ADM levels are also increased in patients with congestive heart failure (CHF),[66] renal disease,[53] and acute myocardial infarction (MI).[67] In CHF, there is a progressive increase in plasma ADM level from New York Heart Association classification I to IV.[66] Among acute MI patients, plasma ADM levels were higher in those who developed CHF than those without CHF. ADM may be increased to compensate for the increase in vasoconstrictors seen in acute MI.[67]

In hepatic cirrhosis, a progressive increase in ADM levels has been observed with increasing disease severity.[68] There is an inverse relationship between ADM levels and GFR,[69] creatinine clearance, and sodium excretion,[70] suggesting that ADM might play a role in the hemodynamic changes that lead to ascites and edema in cirrhosis.[51,70]

Of all the conditions studied, the greatest increase in ADM is seen in septic shock.[71,72] ADM likely plays a key role in its pathophysiology. Because a correlation between ADM levels and the relaxation of vascular tone has been demonstrated,[73] it is likely that ADM is directly responsible for the hypotension characteristic of septic shock.[51]

### Biologic Actions of Adrenomedullin

Intravenous infusion of ADM into many animals and humans causes a potent and sustained hypotension, mainly through NO production in blood vessels.[51] The effects are comparable with CGRP.[51] Interestingly, injection of ADM directly into the corpus cavernosum of the cat penis causes a significant, dose-dependent increase in penile length and increased intracavernous pressure.[74] The mechanism is unclear but is not NO dependent, because the NO inhibitor (Nω-nitro-L-arginine methyl ester) does not block the effect. ADM has antiproliferative effects and inhibits coronary artery smooth muscle migration, and so may inhibit vascular remodeling.[75] It also may have a role in uterine growth and revascularization.[76] There is still considerable debate about the exact role of ADM in cell and tumor growth.[51]

ADM inhibits adrenocorticotropic hormone (ACTH) release from the pituitary and aldosterone production, but may increase renal blood flow, urine output, and urinary sodium excretion.[51] It may also play a paracrine regulatory role in skeletal growth. It causes pulmonary vasodilation and inhibits bronchoconstriction. ADM is expressed in most key mucosal surfaces and has antimicrobial properties against both gram-positive and gram-negative bacteria.

## Adrenomedullin Receptors

Are there separate ADM receptors or do CGRP receptors mediate the effects of ADM? ADM receptors have always been linked to the CGRP receptors.[3,51] There are two subtypes of CGRP receptors, based on the potency of the CGRP receptor antagonist fragment $CGRP_{8-37}$.[77] $CGRP_1$ receptors require much lower concentrations of $CGRP_{8-37}$ than $CGRP_2$ receptors for antagonism. The vasodilating effects of ADM on the rat mesenteric vessels (a prototypic $CGRP_1$ receptor) are blocked by $CGRP_{8-37}$.[78] Many subsequent studies have documented the blocking of some ADM effects by $CGRP_{8-37}$. In addition, ADM binds with high affinity to and activates CGRP receptors in neuroblastoma cells, a model of $CGRP_1$ receptors.[79] Several later studies supported the high-affinity binding of ADM to almost all CGRP receptors, with an affinity of one tenth to one hundredth that of CGRP itself.[51]

ADM has a low affinity for the CGRP receptors in guinea pig vas deferens, a model of $CGRP_2$ receptors, suggesting that ADM has lower affinity for $CGRP_2$ than $CGRP_1$ receptors.[80] However studies of the inhibitory effects of $CGRP_{8-37}$ on ADM actions must be interpreted with caution.[51] In some studies, very high concentrations of $CGRP_{8-37}$ were used, which may bind to specific ADM receptors and make interpretation difficult.[51,81] In vivo studies demonstrating that $CGRP_{8-37}$ blocks CGRP effects but not ADM effects at the same concentrations provide strong evidence for specific ADM effects.[51,82-84]

Are there specific ADM receptors? It is clear that CGRP receptors mediate at least *some* of the effects of ADM, but receptors in cultured rat vascular smooth muscle cells were found to have 23 times greater affinity for ADM than for CGRP, which is unlike any known CGRP receptor.[85] This suggests that a specific ADM receptor exists. Surprisingly, the effects of ADM on these cells were inhibited by high doses of $CGRP_{8-37}$.[85] In another study, $CGRP_{8-37}$ blocked the effects of ADM in cultured rat vascular smooth muscle cells, but the binding of ADM in these cells was not inhibited by CGRP or high doses of $CGRP_{8-37}$.[86] These two studies clearly indicate the existence of receptors with higher affinity for ADM than for CGRP, which make these very different from any known CGRP receptors.[51,85,86] Specific ADM binding sites have been found in rat heart, lung, spleen, liver, skeletal muscle, and spinal cord.[87]

The human ADM fragment $ADM_{22-52}$ is a specific ADM receptor antagonist.[88] In rabbit endothelial cells and rat cerebral blood vessels, it is an effective antagonist,[89,90] but in rat mesangial (glomerular support) cells and human neuroblas-

toma cells, it was no more potent an antagonist of ADM than $CGRP_{8-37}$.[88] In rat vascular smooth muscle cells, $ADM_{22-52}$ is a very weak antagonist.[91] In rat cardiac cells and cat hindlimb vascular bed, $ADM_{22-52}$ not only is inactive against ADM, but inhibits CGRP effects.[92,93] Therefore, a much better antagonist needs to be developed.

The identification and characterization of the functional CGRP and ADM receptor(s) has been very controversial, especially since the publication of the "RAMP" (receptor activity modifying protein) hypothesis.[94] This hypothesis states that both ADM and CGRP signal through a common receptor, calcitonin receptor-like receptor (CRLR). Ligand specificity is determined by coexpression of either of two chaperone proteins RAMP1 (CGRP) or RAMP2 (ADM). Another RAMP (RAMP3) has also been postulated to confer ADM specificity to CRLR. So far, three biologic functions for RAMPs have been defined: They transport CRLR to the cell surface, define its pharmacology, and determine its glycosylation state. It now appears that a functional CGRP (or ADM) receptor must include three proteins in a complex: the ligand-binding, membrane-spanning protein (CRLR); a chaperone (RAMP1 or 2); and a third peptide, the receptor component protein, that couples the receptor to the cellular signal transduction pathway.[95]

## Summary

ADM may play a significant role in human hypertension as a compensatory vasodilator. Studies in several rat models of hypertension suggest that ADM delays BP rise and protects against cardiovascular remodeling and renal injury. ADM levels are increased in several other disease states, usually as a compensatory response to vascular changes. But the greatest increase in plasma ADM levels is seen in septic shock, where ADM is probably directly responsible for the characteristic hypotension.

The effects of ADM are probably the result of binding to both CGRP and specific ADM binding sites. These effects can be blocked by both a $CGRP_1$ receptor antagonist ($CGRP_{8-37}$) and an ADM receptor antagonist ($ADM_{22-52}$). However, neither of these antagonists is very potent, and their specificities are doubtful. We need small, nonpeptide, potent, specific antagonists to definitively study the physiology of ADM receptors.

In addition to vasodilation, ADM has many other actions, including the following:

1. Antiproliferative inhibition of smooth muscle cell migration, and thus inhibition of vascular remodeling
2. A role in uterine growth and revascularization
3. Possibly a role in cell and tumor growth
4. Inhibition of ACTH release from the pituitary and of aldosterone production
5. Increases in renal blood flow, GFR, and urinary sodium excretion and decreases in distal tubular sodium reabsorption
6. Regulation of skeletal growth
7. Pulmonary vasodilation and inhibition of bronchoconstriction
8. Antimicrobial properties against both gram-positive and gram-negative bacteria

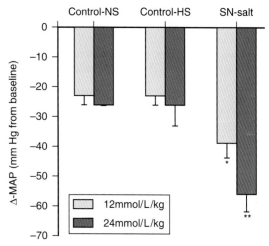

**Figure 19-6** SP decreases MAP in SN-salt rats in a dose-dependent manner. The three groups of animals (n = 6/group) were instrumented for continuous MAP recording and intravenous drug administration as described previously. With the rats fully awake and unrestrained, the vehicle (0.1 ml of saline) was administered followed by a single dose of 12 nmol • $L^{-1}$ • $kg^{-1}$ SP, and the change in MAP was recorded. In another experiment, the same three groups of animals were used, and a dose of 24 nmol • $L^{-1}$ • $kg^{-1}$ of SP was injected intravenously. Values reported are decrease in MAP ± SEM (mm Hg). *$p < .05$ SN-salt versus control-NS (tap water) and control-HS (1% saline) at the indicated dose. **$p < .01$ SN-salt versus control-NS (tap water) and control-HS (1% saline) at the indicated dose. (From Katki KA, Supowit SC, DiPette DJ. Substance P in subtotal nephrectomy-salt hypertension. Hypertension 39[part 2]:389-393, 2002.) SP, substance P; MAP, mean arterial pressure; SN, subtotal nephrectomy; SEM, standard error of measure.

The mechanisms of action of ADM are still not clear. cAMP is often a second messenger for ADM, but other processes are probably involved. The role of NO is also unclear.

## SUMMARY

Several lines of evidence suggest that the vasodilator peptides CGRP, SP, and ADM may play important roles in human hypertension. These exact roles still need to be elucidated.

## Acknowledgments

The authors thank Becky McMahon for her excellent clerical service. We also thank Dr. George Abela and Dr. Hongbao Ma for their invaluable contributions to this work.

## References

1. Amara SG, Jonas V, Rosenfeld MG, et al. Alternative RNA processing in calcitonin gene expression generates mRNA encoding different polypeptide products. Nature 298:240-244, 1982.
2. Rosenfeld MG, Mermod JJ, Amara SG, et al. Production of a novel neuropeptide encoded by the calcitonin gene via tissue-specific RNA processing. Nature 304:129-133, 1983.
3. Wimalawansa SJ. Calcitonin gene-related peptide and its receptors: Molecular genetics, physiology, pathophysiology, and therapeutic potentials. Endocrine Rev 17:533-585, 1996.
4. Breimer LH, MacIntyre I, Zaidi M. Peptides from the calcitonin genes: Molecular genetics, structure, and function. Biochem J 255:377-390, 1988.
5. Dockray GJ. Physiology of enteric neuropeptides. *In* Johnson LR (ed). Physiology of the Gastrointestinal Tract. New York, Raven Press, 1994; p 169.
6. Yaksh TL, Bailey SB, Roddy DR. Peripheral release of substance P from primary afferents. *In* Dubner R, Gebhart GF, Bond MR (eds). Proceedings of the Vth World Congress on Pain. Amsterdam, Elsevier, 1988; p 51.
7. DiPette DJ, Supowit SC. Calcitonin gene-related peptide and hypertension. *In* Oparil S, Weber MA (eds). Hypertension: A Companion to Brenner and Rector's The Kidney. Philadelphia, WB Saunders, 2000; pp 182-189.
8. Asimakis GK, DiPette DJ, Conti VR, et al. Hemodynamic action of calcitonin gene-related peptide in the isolated rat heart. Life Sci 41:597-603, 1987.
9. DiPette DJ, Schwarzenberger K, Kerr N, et al. Dose dependent systemic and regional hemodynamic effects of calcitonin gene-related peptide. Am J Med Sci 297:65-70, 1989.
10. Brain SD, Williams TJ, Tippins JR, et al. Calcitonin gene-related peptide is a potent vasodilator. Nature 313:54-56, 1985.
11. Supowit SC, Guraraj A, Ramana CV, et al. Enhanced neuronal expression of calcitonin gene-related peptide in mineralocorticoid-salt hypertension. Hypertension 25:1333-1338, 1995.
12. Supowit SC, Zhao H, Hallman DM, et al. Calcitonin gene-related peptide is a depressor of deoxycorticosterone-salt hypertension in the rat. Hypertension 29:945-950, 1997.
13. Supowit SC, Zhao H, Hallman DM, et al. Calcitonin gene-related peptide is a depressor in subtotal nephrectomy hypertension. Hypertension 31:391-396, 1998.
14. Gangula PR, Supowit SC, Wimalawansa SJ, et al. Calcitonin gene-related peptide is a depressor in NG-nitro-L-arginine methyl ester (L-NAME)-induced preeclampsia. Hypertension 29:248-253, 1997.
15. Watson RE, DiPette DJ. Experimental models of hypertension. *In* Izzo JL, Black HR (eds). Hypertension Primer: The Essentials of High Blood Pressure, 3rd ed. Baltimore, Lippincott Williams & Wilkins, 2002.
16. Supowit SC, Zhao H, DiPette DJ. Nerve growth factor enhances calcitonin gene-related peptide expression in the spontaneously hypertensive rat. Hypertension 37:728-732, 2001.
17. Watson RE, Supowit SC, Zhao H, et al. Role of sensory nervous system vasoactive peptides in hypertension. Braz J Med Biol Res 35:1033-1045, 2002.
18. Hoff AO, Thomas PM, Cote GJ, et al. Generation of a calcitonin knockout mouse model [Abstract]. Bone 23:S64, 1998.
19. Gangula PR, Zhao H, Supowit SC, et al. Increased blood pressure in alpha-calcitonin gene-related peptide/calcitonin gene knockout mice. Hypertension 35:470-475, 2000.
20. Carlson SH, Wyss MJ. Long-term telemetric recording of arterial pressure and heart rate in mice fed nasal and high NaCl diets. Hypertension 35:1-11, 2000.
21. DiPette DJ, Wimalawansa SJ. Cardiovascular actions of calcitonin gene-related peptide. *In* Crass J, Avioli LV (eds). Calcium Regulating Hormones and Cardiovascular Function. Ann Arbor, MI, CRC Press, 1994; p 239.
22. Lu JT, Son YT, Lee J, et al. Mice lacking alpha-calcitonin gene-related peptide exhibit normal cardiovascular regulation and neuromuscular development. Mol Cell Neurosci 14:99-120, 1999.
23. Oh-hashi Y, Shindo T, Kurihara Y, et al. Elevated sympathetic nervous activity in mice deficient in alpha-CGRP. Circ Res 89:983-990, 2001.
24. Supowit SC, Zhao H, Watson RE, et al. The blood pressure increase in deoxycorticosterone-salt-induced hypertension is

enhanced in alpha-calcitonin gene-related peptide null mice [Abstract]. Am J Hypertens 15:183A, 2002.

25. Zhao H, Supowit SC, Li J, et al. Capsaicin-induced hypotension: Role of calcitonin gene-related peptide [Abstract]. FACEB J 16:A831, 2002.

26. Ma H, Huang R, Abela GS, et al. Coronary flow is decreased in the alpha-calcitonin gene-related peptide knockout mouse [Abstract]. Hypertension 40:384, 2002.

27. Lembeck F, Holzer P. Substance P as a neurogenic mediator of antidromic vasodilation and neurogenic plasma extravasation. Naunyn Schmiedebergs Arch Pharmacol 310:175-183, 1979.

28. Holzer P. Local effector functions of capsaicin-sensitive sensory nerve endings: Involvement of tachykinins, calcitonin gene-related peptide, and other neuropeptides. Neuroscience 45: 739-768, 1988.

29. Stewart-Lee A, Burnstock G. Actions of tachykinins in the rabbit mesenteric artery: Substance P and [Glp6,L-Pro9]SP6-11 are potent agonists for endothelial neurokinin-1 receptors. Br J Pharmacol 97:1218-1224, 1989.

30. von Euler US, Gaddum JH. An unidentified depressor substance in certain tissue extracts. J Physiol (Lond) 72:74-87, 1931.

31. Chang MM, Leeman SE, Nial HD. Amino acid sequence of substance P. Nature New Biol 232:86-87, 1971.

32. Hokfelt T, Broberger C, Xu ZQ, et al. Neuropeptides: An overview. Neuropharmacology 39:1337-1356, 2000.

33. MacDonald MR, Takeda J, Rice CM, et al. Multiple tachykinins are produced and secreted upon post-translational processing of the three substance P precursor proteins, alpha-, beta-, and gamma-preprotachykinin. Expression of the preprotachykinins in AtT-20 cells infected with vaccinia virus recombinants. J Biol Chem 264:15578-15592, 1989.

34. Hokfelt T, Pernow B, Wahren J. Substance P: A pioneer amongst neuropeptides. J Intern Med 249:27-40, 2001.

35. Maggi CA. The mammalian tachykinin receptors. Gen Pharmacol 26:911-944, 1995.

36. Mau SE. Effects of substance P on cellular signaling systems in the rat anterior pituitary. Danish Med Bull 46:35-56, 1999.

37. Ribeiro da Silva A, Hokfelt T. Neuroanatomical localisation of substance P in the CNS and sensory neurons. Neuropeptides 34:256-271, 2000.

38. Marti E, Gibson SJ, Polak JM, et al. Ontogeny of peptide-and-amine-containing neurones in motor, sensory and autonomic regions of rat and human spinal cord, dorsal root ganglia and rat skin. J Comp Neurol 226:332-359, 1987.

39. Rang HP, Bevan SJ, Dray A. Nociceptive peripheral neurones: Cellular properties. In Wall PD, Melzak R (eds): Textbook of Pain. Edinburgh, Churchill-Livingstone, 1994; pp 57-78.

40. Holzer P, Maggi CA. Dissociation of dorsal root ganglion neurons into afferent and efferent-like neurons. Neuroscience 86:389-398, 1998.

41. Kohlmann O, Cesaretti ML, Ginoza M, et al. Role of substance P in blood pressure regulation in salt-dependent experimental hypertension. Hypertension 29:506-509, 1997.

42. Katki KA, Supowit SC, DiPette DJ. Substance P in subtotal nephrectomy-salt hypertension. Hypertension 39(part 2): 389-393, 2002.

43. Katki KA, Supowit SC, DiPette DJ. Enhanced expression of substance P in deoxycorticosterone acetate-induced hypertension [Abstract]. Circulation 102(Suppl II):II348-II349, 2000.

44. Katki KA, Supowit SC, DiPette DJ. Role of calcitonin gene-related peptide and substance P in Dahl-salt hypertension. Hypertension 38(part 2):679-682, 2001.

45. Kitamura K, Kangawa K, Kawamoto M, et al. Adrenomedullin: A novel hypotensive peptide isolated from human pheochromocytoma. Biochem Biophys Res Commun 192:553-560, 1993.

46. Champion HC, Nussdorfer GG, Kadowitz PJ. Structure-activity relationships of adrenomedullin in the circulation and adrenal gland. Regul Pept 85:1-8, 1999.

47. Jougasaki M, Burnett JC. Adrenomedullin: Potential in physiology and pathophysiology. Life Sci 66:855-872, 2000.

48. Sakata J, Shimokubo T, Kitamura K, et al. Distribution and characterization of immunoreactive rat adrenomedullin in tissue and plasma. FEBS Lett 352:105-108, 1994.

49. Ichiki Y, Kitamura K, Kangawa K, et al. Distribution and characterization of immunoreactive adrenomedullin in porcine tissue, and isolation of adrenomedullin [26-52] and adrenomedullin [34-52] from porcine duodenum. J Biochem (Tokyo) 118:765-770, 1995.

50. Sugo S, Minamino N, Kangawa K, et al. Endothelial cells actively synthesize and secrete adrenomedullin. Biochem Biophys Res Commun 201:1160-1166, 1994.

51. Hinson JP, Kapas S, Smith DM. Adrenomedullin, a multifunctional regulatory peptide. Endocrine Rev 21:138-167, 2000.

52. Kohno M, Hanehira T, Kano H, et al. Plasma adrenomedullin concentrations in essential hypertension. Hypertension 27: 102-107, 1996.

53. Tanaka M, Kitamura K, Ishizaka Y, et al. Plasma adrenomedullin in various diseases and exercise-induced change in adrenomedullin in healthy subjects. Intern Med (Tokyo) 34:728-733, 1995.

54. Letizia C, Subioli S, Cerci S, et al. High plasma adrenomedullin concentrations in patients with high-renin essential hypertension. J Renin Angiotensin Aldosterone Syst 3:126-129, 2002.

55. Kitamura K, Ichiki Y, Tanaka M, et al. Immunoreactive adrenomedullin in human plasma. FEBS Lett 341:288-290, 1994.

56. Cheung B, Leung R. Elevated plasma levels of human adrenomedullin in cardiovascular, respiratory, hepatic and renal disorders. Clin Sci (Lond) 92:59-62, 1997.

57. Ishimitsu T, Nishikimi T, Saito Y, et al. Plasma levels of adrenomedullin, a newly identified hypotensive peptide, in patients with hypertension and renal failure. J Clin Invest 94:2158-2161, 1994.

58. Ishimitsu T, Nishikimi T, Matsuoka H, et al. Behavior of adrenomedullin during acute and chronic salt loading in normotensive and hypertensive subjects. Clin Sci (Lond) 91: 293-298, 1996.

59. Shimokubo T, Sakata J, Kitamura K, et al. Adrenomedullin changes in circulating and cardiac tissue concentration in Dahl salt-sensitive rats on a high salt diet. Clin Exp Hypertens 18:949-961, 1996.

60. Nishikimi T, Yoshihara F, Kanazawa A, et al. Role of increased circulating and renal adrenomedullin in rats with malignant hypertension. Am J Physiol Regul Integr Comp Physiol 281:R2079-R2087, 2001.

61. Nishikimi T, Mori Y, Kobayashi N, et al. Renoprotective effect of chronic adrenomedullin infusion in Dahl salt-sensitive rats. Hypertension 39:1077-1082, 2002.

62. Mori Y, Nishikimi T, Kobayashi N, et al. Long-term adrenomedullin infusion improves survival in malignant hypertensive rats. Hypertension 40:107-113, 2002.

63. Chao J, Kato K, Zhang JJ, et al. Human adrenomedullin gene delivery protects against cardiovascular remodeling and renal injury. Peptides 22:1731-1737, 2001.

64. Dobrzynski E, Wang C, Chao J, et al. Adrenomedullin gene delivery attenuates hypertension, cardiac remodeling, and renal injury in deoxycorticosterone acetate-salt hypertensive rats. Hypertension 36:995-1001, 2000.

65. Chao J, Jin L, Lin KF, et al. Adrenomedullin gene delivery reduces blood pressure in spontaneously hypertensive rats. Hypertens Res 20:269-277, 1997.

66. Nishikimi T, Saito Y, Kitamura K, et al. Increased plasma levels of adrenomedullin in patients with heart failure. J Am Coll Cardiol 26:1424-1431, 1995.

67. Kobayashi K, Kitamura K, Hirayama N, et al. Increased plasma adrenomedullin in acute myocardial infarction. Am Heart J 131:676-680, 1996.

68. Fabrega E, Casafont F, Crespo J, et al. Plasma adrenomedullin levels in patients with hepatic cirrhosis. Am J Gastroenterol 92:1901-1904, 1997.
69. Guevara M, Gines P, Jimemez W, et al. Increased adrenomedullin levels in cirrhosis: Relationship with hemodynamic abnormalities and vasoconstrictor systems. Gastroenterology 114:336-343, 1998.
70. Kojima G, Tsujimoto T, Uemura M, et al. Significance of increased plasma adrenomedullin concentration in patients with cirrhosis. J Hepatol 28:840-846, 1998.
71. Ehlenz K, Koch B, Preuss P, et al. High levels of circulating adrenomedullin in severe illness: Correlation with C-reactive protein and evidence against the adrenal medulla as site of origin. Exp Clin Endocrinol Diabetes 105:156-162, 1997.
72. Hirata Y, Mitaka C, Sato K, et al. Increased circulating adrenomedullin, a novel vasodilatory peptide, in sepsis. J Clin Endocrinol Metab 81:1449-1453, 1996.
73. Nishio K, Akai Y, Murao Y, et al. Increased plasma concentrations of adrenomedullin correlate with relaxation of vascular tone in patients with septic shock. Crit Care Med 25:953-957, 1997.
74. Champion HC, Wang R, Shenassa BB, et al. Adrenomedullin induces penile erection in the cat. Eur J Pharmacol 319:71-75, 1997.
75. Kohno M, Yokokawa K, Kano H, et al. Adrenomedullin is a potent inhibitor of angiotensin II-induced migration of human coronary artery smooth muscle cells. Hypertension 29: 1309-1313, 1997.
76. Zhao Y, Hague S, Manek S, et al. PCR display identifies tamoxifen induction of the novel angiogenic factor adrenomedullin by a non estrogenic mechanism in the human endothelium. Oncogene 16:409-415, 1998.
77. Dennis T, Fournier A, Cadieux A, et al. hCGRP8-37, a calcitonin gene-related peptide antagonist revealing calcitonin gene-related peptide receptor heterogeneity in the brain and periphery. J Pharmacol Exp Ther 254:123-128, 1990.
78. Nuki C, Kawasaki H, Kitamura K, et al. Vasodilator effect of adrenomedullin and calcitonin gene-related peptide receptors in rat mesenteric vascular beds. Biochem Biophys Res Commun 196:245-251, 1993.
79. Entzeroth M, Doods HN, Wieland HA, et al. Adrenomedullin mediates vasodilation via CGRP1 receptors. Life Sci 56:L19-L25, 1995.
80. Poyner DR, Taylor GM, Tomlinson AE, et al. Characterization of receptors for calcitonin gene-related peptide and adrenomedullin on the guinea pig vas deferens. Br J Pharmacol 126:1276-1282, 1999.
81. Coppock HA, Owji AA, Austin C, et al. Rat-2 fibroblasts express specific adrenomedullin receptors, but not calcitonin gene-related peptide receptors, which mediate increased intracelluar cAMP and inhibit mitogen-activated protein kinase activity. Biochem J 338:15-22, 1999.
82. Nandha KA, Taylor GM, Smith DM, et al. Specific adrenomedullin binding sites and hypotension in the rat systemic vascular bed. Regul Pept 62:145-151, 1996.
83. Pinto A, Sekizawa K, Yamaya M, et al. Effects of adrenomedullin and calcitonin gene-related peptide on airway and pulmonary vascular smooth muscle in guinea pigs. Br J Pharmacol 119:1477-1483, 1996.
84. Hjelmqvist H, Keil R, Mathai M, et al. Vasodilation and glomerular binding of adrenomedullin in rabbit kidney are not CGRP receptor mediated. Am J Physiol 273:R716-R724, 1997.
85. Eguchi S, Hirata Y, Kano H, et al. Specific receptors for adrenomedullin in cultured rat vascular smooth muscle cells. FEBS Lett 340:226-230, 1994.
86. Ishizaka Y, Tanaka M, Kitamura K, et al. Adrenomedullin stimulates cyclic AMP formation in rat vascular smooth muscle cells. Biochem Biophys Res Commun 200:642-646, 1994.
87. Owji AA, Smith DM, Coppock HA, et al. An abundant and specific binding site for he novel vasodilator adrenomedullin in the rat. Endocrinology 136:2127-2134, 1995.
88. Disa J, Dang K, Tan KB, et al. Interaction of adrenomedullin with calcitonin receptor in cultured human breast cancer cells, T 47D. Peptides 19:247-251, 1998.
89. Muff R, Leuthauser K, Buhlmann N, et al. Receptor activity modifying proteins regulate the activity of a calcitonin gene-related peptide receptor in rabbit aortic endothelial cells. FEBS Lett 441:366-368, 1998.
90. Dogan A, Suzuki Y, Koketsu N, et al. Intravenous infusion of adrenomedullin and increase in regional cerebral blood flow and prevention of ischemic brain injury after middle cerebral artery occlusion in rats. J Cereb Blood Flow Metab 17:19-25, 1997.
91. Eguchi S, Hirata Y, Iwasaki H, et al. Structure-activity relationship of adrenomedullin, a novel vasodilatory peptide, in cultured rat vascular smooth muscle cells. Endocrinology 135:2454-2458, 1994.
92. Nishikimi T, Horio T, Yoshihara F, et al. Effect of adrenomedullin on cAMP and cGMP levels in rat cardiac myocytes and nonmyocytes. Eur J Pharmacol 353:337-344, 1998.
93. Champion HC, Santiago JA, Murphy WA, et al. Adrenomedullin-(22-52) antagonizes vasodilator responses to CGRP but not adrenomedullin in the cat. Am J Physiol 272:R234-R242, 1997.
94. Foord SM, Marshall FH. RAMPs: Accessory proteins for seven transmembrane domain receptors. Trends Pharmacol Sci 20:184-187, 1999.
95. Evans BN, Rosenblatt MI, Mnayer LO, et al. CGRP-RCP, a novel protein required for signal transduction at calcitonin gene-related peptide and adrenomedullin receptors. J Biol Chem 275:31438-31443, 2000.

# The Kallikrein-Kinin System as a Regulator of Cardiovascular and Renal Function

## Oscar A. Carretero, Xiao-Ping Yang, Nour-Eddine Rhaleb

Both genetic and environmental factors acting via intermediate phenotypes participate in the regulation of blood pressure, the etiology of hypertension, and the development of target organ damage. Vasoactive systems are important components of these intermediate phenotypes. They can act as local hormones (intracrine, autocrine, and paracrine) or as endocrine and neuroendocrine systems. We use the term *intracrine* to indicate hormones that act within the cells that synthesize them, such as reactive oxygen species ($O_2^-$) and products of protooncogenes. The term *autocrine* is used to indicate hormones that act on the cell membrane receptors where they are produced, such as growth factors. The term *paracrine* denotes hormones that act near the site where they are produced, such as kinins, eicosanoids, nitric oxide (NO), and endothelium-derived hyperpolarizing factor (EDHF). *Endocrine* refers to hormones such as aldosterone that are released into the extracellular fluid and act on distant target tissues, although they can also act in an autocrine and paracrine faction. Finally, *neuroendocrine* hormones such as catecholamines are released by neurons and act near or distant from the site of release.

Blood pressure is the result of a balance between vasopressor and vasodepressor systems. Alteration of this equilibrium may result in (1) hypertension, (2) target organ damage, (3) effective antihypertensive treatment, or (4) hypotension and shock. Changes in this balance could be caused by (1) genetic factors such as mutations in one of the genes of the vasoactive system and/or (2) environmental factors that alter the activity of vasoactive systems. Endocrine and neuroendocrine vasopressor systems, such as the renin-angiotensin-aldosterone system and catecholamines, play a well-established and important role in the regulation of blood pressure, the pathogenesis of some forms of hypertension, and target organ damage. The role of vasodepressor systems is less well established; however, evidence suggests that they play an important role in the regulation of blood flow, renal function, the pathogenesis of salt-induced hypertension and target organ damage, and the cardioprotective effects of angiotensin-converting enzyme (ACE) inhibitors and angiotensin receptor blockers (ARBs).[1-5] Vasodepressor hormones such as kinins, eicosanoids, NO, and EDHF act as local hormonal systems, opposing the effects of vasopressor systems. Some vasodepressor systems such as atrial (ANP), brain (BNP), and C-type (CNP) natriuretic peptides may act as both endocrine and local hormones. Here we will review the kinin-generating system and the role of kinins in (1) the regulation of local blood flow, (2) water and sodium excretion, (3) the regulation of blood pressure and the pathogenesis of hypertension, and (4) the therapeutic effects of ACE inhibitors and ARBs.

## THE KININ-GENERATING SYSTEM

Kininogenases such as glandular and plasma kallikreins are enzymes that generate kinins by hydrolyzing substrates known as *kininogens*, which circulate at high concentrations in plasma. Kinins are rapidly destroyed by a group of peptidases known as kininases (Figure 20–1). Plasma and glandular (tissue) kallikrein are potent kininogenases and both are serine proteases. A single gene encodes for plasma kallikrein, and there is a large family of glandular kallikrein genes; however, KLK1 is the only glandular kallikrein that generates kinins (hereafter referred to as *glandular kallikrein*, or simply *kallikrein*). Plasma kallikrein, also known as *Fletcher factor*, is expressed mainly in the liver; in plasma it is found in the zymogen form (prekallikrein) and differs from glandular kallikrein in its biochemical, immunologic, and functional characteristics. It preferentially releases bradykinin from high-molecular-weight kininogen (HMWK), also known as *Fitzgerald factor*. Together with HMWK and Hageman factor, it is involved in coagulation, fibrinolysis, and possibly, activation of the complement system. The plasma kallikrein-HMWK system, acting through the release of bradykinin, could be involved in the local regulation of blood flow and in some of the effects of ACE inhibitors. On the other hand, patients with congenital deficiency of plasma HMWK (Fitzgerald trait) have normal amounts of kinins in their blood.[6] (For a review of the plasma kallikrein-HMWK system, see references 7-9.)

Glandular kallikrein belongs to a family of serine proteases with very high homology; the genes encoding for these enzymes are tightly clustered and arranged in tandem on the same chromosome. The number of family members varies widely among mammals; it is estimated that the kallikrein family contains at least three genes in humans, 20 in the rat, and 23 to 30 in the mouse, many of them pseudogenes.[10] Despite the highly homologous amino acid composition of the serine proteases encoded by the glandular kallikrein gene family, most are not kininogenases and act on entirely different substrates. For example, tonin, a rat enzyme of the kallikrein family, hydrolyzes angiotensinogen and generates angiotensin II; prostate-specific antigen, a human enzyme of the kallikrein family, hydrolyzes semenogelin, a high-molecular-weight seminal vesicle protein.[11,12] We have isolated a new member of the kallikrein family from the submandibular gland.[13,14] This protease produces contraction of isolated aortic rings and (like tonin) also generates angiotensin II, suggesting that localized regions of variability are important in determining substrate specificity and possibly function of all enzymes of the kallikrein family. (For a review of the

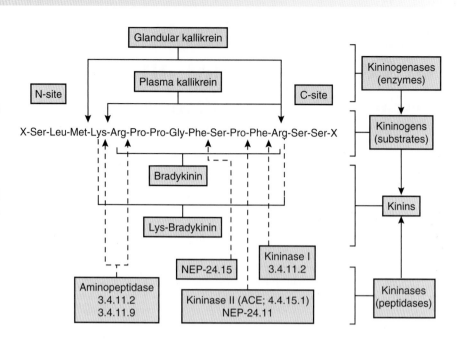

**Figure 20–1** Site of kininogen cleavage *(solid arrows)* by the main kininogenases (glandular and plasma kallikrein). The *broken arrows* indicate sites of kinin cleavage by kininases (kininase I, kininase II, neutral endopeptidases 24.11 and 24.15, and aminopeptidases). (From Carretero OA, Scicil AG. Kinins paracrine hormone. 34(Suppl 26):S-52-S-59, 1988.)

molecular biology of the glandular kallikrein-kininogen system see references 15-17.)

True glandular kallikrein or KLK1 is encoded by a single gene having five exons and four introns. Other members of the kallikrein gene family have a similar exonic and intronic structure, with the splice junctions completely conserved. The 5′ and 3′ flanking regions have a high homology among the various genes; however, gene regulation and site of expression are different, suggesting that small variations in the nucleotide sequence of the 5′ region are important in the regulation of expression. The glandular kallikrein gene is expressed mainly in the submandibular gland, pancreas, and kidney; however, using the polymerase chain reaction, we have demonstrated its mRNA in vascular tissue, heart, and adrenal glands, although in smaller amounts.[18,19] Glandular kallikrein and kallikrein-like enzymes have also been found in the arteries and veins,[20] heart,[21] brain,[22] pituitary gland,[23,24] pancreas,[25] intestine,[26,27] salivary and sweat glands,[28] spleen,[29] adrenal glands,[30] blood cells,[19] and the exocrine secretions of these structures. Some of these are probably true glandular kallikrein, whereas others may be separate members of the kallikrein family.

There is immunoreactive glandular kallikrein in plasma, primarily the inactive form; however, a small portion is in the active form.[31-35] In humans[36] and rabbits,[37] 50% or more of urinary kallikrein is the inactive or zymogen form, whereas in rats most is in the active form.[38] Glandular kallikrein can release kinins from low-molecular-weight kininogen (LMWK) and HMWK. In humans, glandular kallikrein releases lys-bradykinin (kallidin), whereas in rodents it releases bradykinin.[39,40]

Kininogens (kallikrein substrates) are the precursors of kinins. In plasma there are two main forms, characterized as LMWK and HMWK.[41,42] Both are potent inhibitors of cysteine proteinases such as calpain and cathepsins H, L, and B.[43-45] In the rat there is a third kininogen known as t-kininogen, because it releases kinins when incubated with trypsin but not with tissue or plasma kallikrein. It is one of the main acute phase reactants of inflammation in the rat. All kininogens inhibit thiol proteases such as cathepsin M, H, and calpains.[46-49] HMWK is involved in the early stages of surface-activated coagulation (intrinsic coagulation pathway).[7,9,50]

Kininases are peptidases found in blood and other tissues that hydrolyze kinins and other peptidic hormones.[51] The best known is ACE or kininase II, which converts angiotensin I to II and inactivates kinin substance P and other peptides.[51,52] Another important kininase is neutral endopeptidase 24.11 (NEP-24.11), also known as enkephalinase, which not only hydrolyzes kinins and enkephalins but also destroys ANP, BNP, and endothelin.[53,54] Research performed in our laboratory suggests that it may be an important renal kininase, at least in the rat.[55] Other kininases include MEP-24.15, aminopeptidases, and carboxypeptidases; however, it is not known whether they play an important role in the degradation of kinins in vivo. After inhibition of most of these enzymes in vivo, plasma concentrations of endogenous kinins do not increase significantly, and their half-life remains less than 20 seconds, suggesting that other peptidases are also important in kinin metabolism.[56]

Kinins are oligopeptides containing the sequence of bradykinin in their structure. They act mainly as local hormones, because they circulate at very low concentrations (1- 50 fmol/ml) and are rapidly hydrolyzed by kininases. In tissues such as the kidney, heart, and aorta, kinin concentrations are higher (100-350 fmol/g).[57] Eicosanoids, NO, EDHF, tissue plasminogen activator (tPA), and cytokines mediate at least some of the effects of exogenously administered kinins[58-62] (Figure 20–2). At least two subtypes of kinin receptors have been well characterized by using analogs of bradykinin, $B_1$ and $B_2$.[63,64] These receptors have been cloned and belong to the family of seven transmembrane receptors linked to G proteins.[65] $B_1$ receptors are not present or are present only at very low density in normal tissues but are expressed and synthesized de novo during tissue injury, inflammation, and administration of lipopolysaccharides such as endotoxin. In some species, including rabbits, they mediate contraction of the isolated aorta and relaxation of mesenteric arteries. The

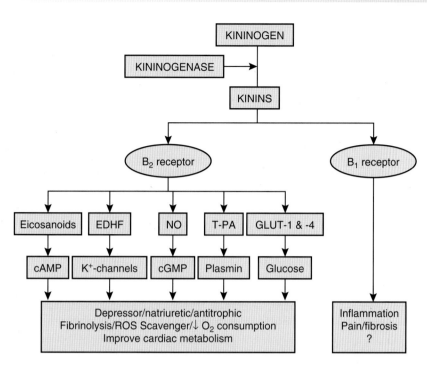

**Figure 20-2** Kinins act via the $B_2$ and $B_1$ receptors. Most of the known effects of kinins are mediated by the $B_2$ receptor, which acts by stimulating the release of various intermediaries: eicosanoids, endothelial-derived hyperpolarizing factor (EDHF), nitric oxide (NO), tissue plasminogen activator (tPA), and glucose transporter (GLU-1 and -2. (Modified from Carretero OA. Kinins: Local hormones in regulation of blood pressure and renal function. Choices Cardiol 7(Suppl 1): 10-14, 1993.)

main agonists for this receptor are des-Arg⁹-bradykinin and des-Arg⁹-kallidin. $B_2$ receptors mediate most of the effects of bradykinin and are the main receptors for the agonists bradykinin and kallidin (lys-bradykinin). Studies using kinin analogs with agonistic and antagonistic properties in various tissues suggest the existence of other subtypes of receptors.[66-69] Stewart and Vavrek[70] discovered that substitution of D-phenylalanine for proline at position 7 of bradykinin converts it into a specific antagonist for $B_2$ receptors, while the substitution of Phe8 in des-Arg⁹-BK by a residue with aliphatic (Ala, Ile, Leu, D-Leu, norleucine) or saturated cyclic hydrocarbon chains (cyclohexyalanine) produced antagonists for $B_1$ receptors.[71,72] Further modifications have resulted in a very potent $B_2$ receptor antagonist with long-lasting effects in vivo, DArg⁰-Hyp³-Thi⁵-DThi⁷-Oic⁸-bradykinin or icatibant (Hoe-140),[73] which has become an important tool for studying the role of kinins. Orally active kinin antagonists have been developed for the possible treatment of inflammation, hyperalgesia, and perhaps cancer.[74-78]

In humans, it has been reported that the $B_2$ receptor is activated by kallikreins and other serine proteases and that this effect is blocked by the kinin antagonist icatibant.[79] Some ACE inhibitors potentiate the effect of bradykinin not only by inhibiting its hydrolysis but also by cross-talk between ACE and the $B_2$ receptor.[80] The $B_2$ receptor forms heterodimers with the angiotensin type 1 receptor ($AT_1$), causing increased activation of the angiotensin receptor. The stability of this heterodimer is not affected by bradykinin, angiotensin, or their antagonists.[81] The $B_2$ receptor also forms a complex with endothelial NO synthase (eNOS), inhibiting the generation of NO, and this effect is reversed by bradykinin.[82] The pathophysiologic role of these interactions of the $B_2$ receptor is not known; however, it has been reported that in preeclampsia there is an increase in $AT_1$ and $B_2$ heterodimers that could mediate an enhanced response to angiotensin II. Thus, in some situations these interactions of the $B_2$ receptor could play a physiopathologic role.

## THE KALLIKREIN-KININ SYSTEM IN THE VASCULATURE AND IN THE REGULATION OF LOCAL BLOOD FLOW

Arteries and veins contain a kallikrein-like enzyme, and both vascular tissue and smooth muscle cells in culture contain mRNA for glandular kallikrein.[18,20] Vascular smooth muscle cells in culture release both glandular kallikrein and kininogen[83]. Thus the components of the kallikrein-kinin system are present in vascular tissue, where they could play an important role in the regulation of vascular resistance. Blood flow-induced dilation of isolated arteries from mice with deletion of the gene expressing glandular kallikrein was found to be significantly reduced as compared with controls, suggesting that the kallikrein-kinin system in the arterial wall participates in this process.[84,85] The action of ACE inhibitors on local potentiation of the vasodilator effect of kinins appears to be partly attributable to their prevention of bradykinin degradation and subsequent increases in the production of endothelium-derived relaxing factors (EDRFs) such as NO. In spontaneously hypertensive rats (SHR) and in the canine coronary artery, ACE inhibitors potentiate the endothelium-dependent relaxation evoked by bradykinin.[86,87] This vasorelaxation appears to be associated primarily with increased release of NO.

When the arterial endothelium is removed, the smooth muscle cells begin to proliferate in the medium; they then migrate across the internal elastic lamina into the intima, where they cause neointimal hyperplasia, mimicking some of the vascular changes that occur in atherosclerosis. ACE inhibitors have been shown to inhibit neointima formation.[88,89] Blocking kinins or inhibiting NO synthesis lessens the protective effect of the ACE inhibitor, suggesting that it may be mediated by a local increase in kinins, which stimulates the release of NO.[90,91]

Kinins play an important role in the local regulation of blood flow in organs rich in glandular kallikrein such as the submandibular gland, uteroplacental complex, and kidney.[92-95] In rats nephrectomized 48 hours earlier to exclude the renal renin-angiotensin system, use of an ACE (kininase II) inhibitor significantly increased blood flow in the submandibular gland but did not affect blood pressure. In contrast, 10 minutes after sympathetic stimulation of the gland to increase kallikrein secretion in the vascular compartment, the ACE inhibitor markedly decreased blood pressure and increased kinin concentrations in arterial blood.[35,96] Changes in both blood flow and blood pressure were blocked by antibodies to kinins and glandular kallikrein. The effect of the ACE inhibitor on basal glandular blood flow was also blocked by a kinin antagonist.[92] At low doses, the antagonist caused no significant change in blood flow when the ACE inhibitor was not administered, whereas at high doses, basal blood flow decreased significantly. These data suggest that in organs rich in glandular kallikrein, kinins play a role in the regulation of basal blood flow. Studies using kinin antibodies and antagonists clearly indicate that kinins act as paracrine hormones, regulating blood flow within the gland. These studies also indicate that the effect of ACE inhibitors on blood flow is mediated by kinins.[92] In nephrectomized pregnant rabbits infused with an angiotensin antagonist to block the uterine renin-angiotensin system, ACE inhibitors increased both uterine and placental blood flow and immunoreactive prostaglandin $E_2$ ($PGE_2$), whereas these effects were blocked by a kinin antibody.[93] This suggests that endogenously generated kinins play a role in the regulation of uterine blood flow, either directly or through the release of prostaglandins.

In organs rich in glandular kallikrein, such as the submandibular gland and uteroplacental complex, kinins appear to play an important role in the regulation of blood flow, especially when ACE is inhibited. In addition, the local arterial kallikrein-kinin system also participates in the regulation of blood flow and in the vascular protective effect of ACE inhibitors.

## KININS IN THE REGULATION OF RENAL BLOOD FLOW

Kinins may play an important role in the regulation of renal blood flow. Blocking renal kinins by infusing low doses of a kinin antagonist into the renal artery of sodium-depleted dogs decreased renal blood flow and autoregulation of the glomerular filtration rate (GFR) without changing blood pressure.[97] The changes in renal blood flow were blocked by prior inhibition of ACE, suggesting that either they were mediated by renin release caused by an agonistic effect of the antagonist or else renal kinins may have increased when ACE was inhibited, thereby competing more effectively with the antagonist. The changes in GFR autoregulation were not altered by the ACE inhibitor and may have been due to a change in either the relationship between afferent and efferent glomerular arteriolar resistance or the coefficient of filtration.[97] We have shown that the vasodilator effect of bradykinin in the renal efferent arteriole is mediated by cytochrome P450 metabolites

of arachidonic acid called *epoxyeicosatrienoic acids* (EETs) and that bradykinin stimulates the glomeruli to release another cytochrome P450 metabolite, the vasoconstrictor eicosanoid 20-hydroxyeicosatetraenoic acid (20-HETE), and also an unidentified vasodilator prostaglandin, which together participate in regulation of the downstream glomerular circulation and perhaps in the regulation of GFR.[98,99]

We examined the role of kinins in the regulation of renal blood flow distribution by using a laser-Doppler flowmeter.[94] The kinin antagonist lowered papillary blood flow without altering outer cortical blood flow, suggesting that intrarenally formed kinins are important in regulating blood flow in the inner medulla. This study also showed that renin plays an important role in the regulation of papillary blood flow, because after kinins were blocked, enalaprilat increased flow significantly. When we inhibited both ACE and neutral endopeptidase-24.11 (NEP-24.11), papillary blood flow increased by 50%, as compared with 25% when they were inhibited separately. These increases were blocked by the kinin antagonist, indicating that the augmented papillary blood flow induced by both ACE and NEP-24.11 inhibitors is mediated by increased kinin concentrations in the interstitial space. We observed no consistent effect on water or sodium excretion; however, water excretion tends to decrease in animals treated with a kinin antagonist.

In anesthetized rats, blocking kinins decreased renal blood flow.[95] In dogs, when kallikrein excretion was stimulated by sodium deprivation, a kinin antagonist (given intrarenally) partially blocked the effect of enalaprilat on renal blood flow.[100] This suggests that although blockade of the renin-angiotensin system accounted for a significant portion of the increase in renal blood flow caused by the ACE inhibitor, a substantial component was contributed by endogenous kinins. Similar results were reported in rats in which the kallikrein-kinin system was stimulated by deoxycorticosterone.[101]

In the kidney, kinins normally play a minor role in the regulation of blood flow. However, when the kallikrein-kinin system is stimulated by low-sodium intake or mineralocorticoids, or when endogenous kinin degradation is inhibited, kinins appear to participate in the regulation of renal blood flow. In addition, the data suggest that kinins play an important role in the regulation of papillary blood flow and that during reduction of renal perfusion pressure, kinins may aid in regulation of the GFR.

## KININS IN THE REGULATION OF WATER AND ELECTROLYTE EXCRETION

Renal kallikrein is located in the connecting cells of the connecting tubule; it is released in significant amounts in this segment of the nephron and excreted in the urine (Figure 20–3).[37,102,103] Kallikrein releases kinins into the lumen of the distal nephron, either from filtered kininogen or kininogen produced in the principal cells of the distal nephron.[104,105] Kinin receptors are also present in the collecting duct.[106] In addition, kallikrein is released on the basolateral side of the nephron, where it may liberate kinins from plasma kininogens.[107] The renal interstitial fluid contains a high concentration of kinins.[108] The role of kinins in the regulation of water and sodium excretion has been studied by

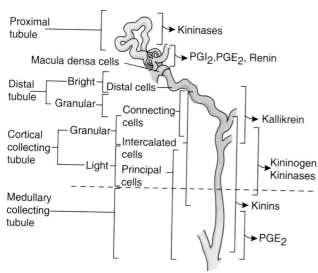

**Figure 20–3** Localization of the kallikrein-kinin system, renin, and prostaglandin in the nephron (*right brackets*); anatomical subdivisions of the nephron (*outer left brackets*); and type of cells found in the distal nephron (*inner left brackets*). $PGE_2$, prostaglandin $E_2$; $PGI_2$, prostacyclin.

either increasing intrarenal kinins or blocking kinins. Infusion of kinins into the late proximal nephron doubled excretion of simultaneously administered[22] Na,[109] and that part of this effect was mediated by prostaglandins,[110] whereas infusion of a kinin antagonist into the late proximal nephron reduced[22] Na recovery significantly.[111] After systemic administration of phosphoramidon, an inhibitor of NEP-24.11 (a major kininase in the nephron), urinary excretion of kinins doubled; diuresis increased by 15%, and natriuresis increased by 37%.[55] These data support the hypothesis that increased kinins in the nephron participate in intrarenal control of water and electrolyte excretion, but it is also possible that the effect of this peptidase inhibitor is mediated by blocking hydrolysis of other peptides such as atrial natriuretic factor (ANF).[112]

The infusion of aprotinin inhibited the enzymatic activity of urinary kallikrein but did not affect acute water or electrolyte excretion in euvolemic and sodium- or water-expanded rats.[113] A transient decrease in sodium excretion has been observed during aprotinin administration in mineralocorticoid-treated rats.[114] Infusion of kinin antibodies into saline-expanded rats decreased sodium excretion.[115] Caution should be used in interpreting this finding, because antibodies may stimulate release of histamine, cause an anaphylactoid reaction, or form a high-molecular-weight complex with kininogen that is then deposited in the nephron, any of which might alter water and sodium excretion. To avoid these problems, we use Fab fragments of kinin antibodies, which are rapidly distributed in the extracellular fluid and excreted by the kidney; moreover, they do not form high-molecular-weight complexes or activate complement and other proteolytic systems in plasma, thus reducing the risk of anaphylactoid reactions. In unanesthetized rats, the Fab fragments blocked 70% of the effect of an injection of 100 ng bradykinin on blood pressure and appeared rapidly in the urine, suggesting that they block the effect of kinins not only in the vascular and interstitial spaces but also in the lumen of the distal nephron. Using these Fab fragments and a kinin antagonist, we studied a model in which the renal kallikrein-kinin system is stimulated—namely, DOCA-salt-treated rats.[116] Both the Fab fragments and kinin antagonist significantly decreased urine volume and increased urinary osmolarity; however, only the Fab fragments significantly lessened urinary sodium excretion. Neither altered blood pressure, renal blood flow, or GFR. The antidiuretic effect of the Fab fragments and kinin antagonist may be due to blockade of kinins in the vascular interstitial space of the kidney, since the antagonist is likely hydrolyzed in the proximal tubule and does not reach the lumen of the distal nephron. On the other hand, the antinatriuretic effect of Fab fragments of kinin antibodies on sodium excretion may be due to blockade of kinins in both the vascular/interstitial and urinary compartments or only in the latter compartment, because the antibody appeared in the urine and the antidiuretic effect was not observed with the antagonist. Thus kinins may aid in the regulation of water and sodium excretion when the kallikrein-kinin system is stimulated. In normal nonanesthetized rats, inhibition of kinin release in the lumen of the nephron by Fab fragments of monoclonal antibodies to kallikrein causes urinary $PGE_2$, UV, and $U_{Na}V$ to decrease. The changes in UV and $U_{Na}V$ mimic those of $PGE_2$, suggesting that the natriuretic and diuretic effects of kinins are mediated in part by $PGE_2$.[117]

In vitro, stimulation of the release of EDRF from endothelial cells by bradykinin or acetylcholine increases cGMP content and inhibits $Na^+$ transport by cortical collecting duct cells.[118] In vivo, stimulation of EDRF release by bradykinin results in natriuresis and diuresis without affecting the GFR.[119] In conclusion, kinins acting as local hormones play a role in the regulation of renal hemodynamic and excretory function, either directly or via the release of $PGE_2$ and EDRF.

## KININS AS REGULATORS OF BLOOD PRESSURE AND THE PATHOGENESIS OF HYPERTENSION

The development of antibodies to kinins and kallikrein, kinin antagonists, and kininase inhibitors—as well as gene knockout (KO) models of the kallikrein-kinin system and the discovery of kininogen-deficient rats and humans with various spontaneous mutations of the system—has allowed us to study the role of kinins in various physiologic and pathologic conditions. The role of the kallikrein-kinin system in the pathogenesis of hypertension has been studied by (1) measurements of the various components of the system, (2) the use of bradykinin $B_2$ receptor antagonists, (3) the use of mice in which the $B_2$ receptor has been deleted by homologous recombination, (4) deletion of the kallikrein gene, and (5) use of rats deficient in kininogen. Decreased activity of the kallikrein-kinin system may play a role in hypertension. Low urinary kallikrein excretion in children is one of the major genetic markers associated with a family history of essential hypertension, and children with high urinary kallikrein excretion have less probability of a genetic background of hypertension.[120-123] A restriction fragment length polymorphism for the kallikrein gene family in spontaneously hypertensive rats has been linked to high blood pressure,[124] and urinary kallikrein excretion is decreased in several models of genetic hypertension. Urinary and/or arterial tissue kallikrein are also decreased in renovascular hypertension and genetically hypertensive rats.[125-128] Although these reductions may be secondary to increases in blood pressure, urinary kallikrein is decreased in normotensive children of patients with essential hypertension and in genetically hypertensive and Dahl salt-sensitive rats before the development of hypertension,[129-133] suggesting that these decreases may be primary abnormalities.

Kinins circulate in concentrations of approximately 5 to 50 pg/ml of blood.[6] These concentrations need to be increased to at least 100 pg in humans[134] and 1000 pg in rats[135] to cause acute decreases in blood pressure. Although blood kinin concentrations may increase in some physiologic and pathologic situations, they seldom reach levels that could explain changes in blood pressure, save for exceptional experimental conditions such as stimulation of the sympathetic nerve of the submandibular gland in animals treated with ACE inhibitors (see section on blood flow regulation). Thus kinins must act as paracrine hormones, regulating local vascular resistance and organ function.

In early studies, acute administration of a kinin antagonist at high doses increased blood pressure in most rats tested, while a vasodepressor effect was observed in some.[136] Using a more potent antagonist,[137] also at high doses, we found that it produced a transient biphasic response: first a small pressor effect, followed by a depressor effect.[138] At lower doses, although still sufficient to block exogenous bradykinin, the same antagonists did not alter normal blood pressure. These studies are compatible with the hypothesis that kinins play a role in the regulation of blood pressure. However, to demonstrate the pressor effect, the kinin antagonist has to be used at much higher doses than those needed to block the vasodepressor effect of exogenous bradykinin. High doses may be needed to displace kinins bound to tissue receptors. We must be cautious in interpreting these data, because we cannot rule out the possibility that these kinin antagonists have a vasopressor effect that is unrelated to kinin-blocking activity. Studies by our group using kinin antibodies or their Fab frag-ments showed that although they partially block the vasodepressor effect of kinins, they do not cause acute changes in blood pressure.

Chronic blockade of $B_2$ kinin receptors with a potent and selective $B_2$ antagonist, icatibant, did not increase blood pressure under normal conditions or under conditions that favor the development of hypertension in rats such as (1) chronic infusion of a subpressor or pressor dose of angiotension II, (2) a high-salt diet, or (3) mineralocorticoids and salt.[139,140] However, these results are not universal.[141-144]

Mice with the bradykinin $B_2$ receptor deleted by homologous recombination (gene knockout) have normal blood pressure (Figure 20–4). However, they develop hypertension when fed a high-sodium diet (8%) for at least 2 months.[145,146] Thus, low kinin activity may be involved in the development and maintenance of salt-sensitive high blood pressure. However, in these mice, mineralocorticoid hypertension was not exacerbated.[147] It has been reported that as these mice grow older, they also develop hypertension and left ventricular hypertrophy (LVH) even on a normal sodium diet.[148] However, we were unable to demonstrate that ablation of $B_2$ kinin receptors renders mice spontaneously hypertensive.[149] Others were also unable to confirm the hypothesis that $B_2$ kinin receptors are major components in the maintenance of normal blood pressure and cardiac structure.[146,147,150,151] Mice deficient in kinin $B_2$ receptors or tissue kallikrein had blood pressure similar to wild-type controls, confirming that kinins are not an important determinant of blood pressure.[151]

In kininogen-deficient Brown Norway Katholiek rats (BNK), administration of mineralocorticoids and salt or angiotensin II reportedly causes blood pressure to increase similarly to rats with a normal kallikrein-kinin system.[139] This contradicts other reports.[141-143]

These studies suggest that kinins do not play an important role in the regulation of normal blood pressure or in the pathogenesis of hypertension, although they may be involved in the pathogenesis of salt-induced hypertension. Overall, chronic blockade of the kallikrein-kinin system does not appear to cause hypertension or potentiate hypertensinogenic stimuli, although the data are inconsistent.

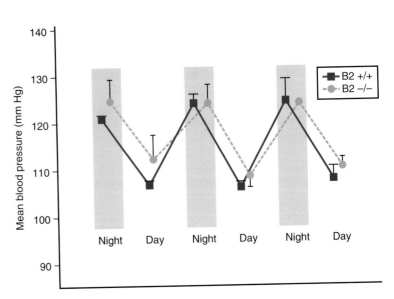

**Figure 20–4** Diurnal and nocturnal mean blood pressure of bradykinin $B_2$ receptor knockout (–/–) and wild-type (+/+) mice. Blood pressure was measured over 24 hours by a telemetric system. (Rhaleb N-E and Carretero OA, unpublished data.)

# ROLE OF KININS IN THE ANTIHYPERTENSIVE EFFECT OF ACE INHIBITORS

Inhibition of kinin and degradation of other oligopeptides may contribute to the antihypertensive effect of ACE inhibitors. Although blockade of angiotensin II formation appears to be important in this regard, the role of kinins is less well established. Orally active ACE inhibitors are effective antihypertensive agents, not only in high-renin hypertension but also in clinical and experimental models in which the renin-angiotensin system has not been pathogenetically implicated.[152,153] Thus, some effects of ACE inhibitors may be mediated by a local renin-angiotensin system, kinins, or some other undetermined mechanism, because ACE can hydrolyze other peptides (Figure 20–5). ACE inhibitors may also potentiate the effect of kinins by a direct interaction with the kinin $B_2$ receptor.[80]

Blood kinins are unchanged or moderately increased after administration of ACE inhibitors.[1,154,155] (For review, see references 156-157.) Kinins in the urine reportedly increase more consistently after administration of ACE inhibitors, indicating that their concentration in renal tissue likewise increases.[55,158-161] This may contribute to the antihypertensive effect of ACE inhibitors by altering renovascular resistance and increasing sodium and water excretion.

Many studies have assessed the role of kinins in the acute antihypertensive effect of ACE inhibitors. In various experimental models of hypertension, the acute antihypertensive effect of ACE inhibitors is attenuated by blocking kinins with either high titers of kinin antibodies[162-165] or with a $B_2$ kinin receptor antagonist.[154,155,166] Kinin antagonists also partially reverse the antihypertensive effect of ACE inhibition in rats with renovascular hypertension.[165] We assessed the influence of kinins on the acute antihypertensive effect of enalaprilat in rats with severe hypertension induced by aortic ligation between the renal arteries.[155] In this model, renin plays an important role in the pathogenesis of hypertension.[152] Acute and severe hypertension can produce endothelial damage that may lead to activation of plasma kallikrein and increased kinin formation. We found that enalaprilat lowered mean blood pressure by 48 ± 6 mm Hg in the controls and 21 ± 4

mm Hg in the kinin antagonist group ($p$ <.01). However, kinin concentrations in arterial plasma were not significantly altered by the ACE inhibitor (41 ± 10 vs. 68 ± 20 pg/ml) (Figure 20–6). As indicated earlier, if mean arterial pressure in the unanesthetized rat is to be decreased, kinins in arterial blood must reach at least 1000 pg/ml.[135] Thus the effect of the ACE inhibitor may be due to an increase in tissue kinins, which could act as a paracrine hormonal system regulating vascular resistance. Cachofeiro et al.[154] demonstrated that pretreatment with either a bradykinin antagonist or an NO synthesis inhibitor attenuated the acute antihypertensive effects of both captopril and ramipril in SHR, but pretreatment with a prostaglandin synthesis inhibitor failed to alter the effects of ACE inhibitors, suggesting that this acute antihypertensive effect is due to bradykinin acting via the release of NO. However, in the dog, kinins may play a role in the acute hypotensive effect of ACE inhibitors through the release of prostaglandins.[167]

In humans, an ACE insertion (I)/deletion (D) polymorphism in intron 16 of the ACE gene could be an important determinant of bradykinin metabolism[168]; ACE activity is higher in subjects with ACE D and is associated with a high rate of bradykinin degradation. In normotensive persons and hypertensive persons with low and normal renin, aprotinin (an inhibitor of kallikrein and other proteases) blocked part of the acute blood pressure–lowering effect of captopril.[169] The influence of aprotinin could be due to inhibition of kinin formation or other effects. However, when using a specific $B_2$ kinin receptor antagonist (icatibant), the short-term blood pressure effects of ACE inhibitors were attenuated in both normotensive and hypertensive persons.[170] These studies suggest that part of the acute effect of ACE inhibitors on blood pressure is mediated by kinins, which affect local and peripheral vascular resistance either directly or through release of prostaglandins and NO.

The contribution of kinins to the chronic antihypertensive effects of ACE inhibitors is more controversial. In renovascular hypertension (2K1C), chronic blockade of kinin receptors interferes with the blood pressure–lowering activity of ramipril.[171] In mineralocorticoid hypertension, in which kallikrein-kinin and ACE activity are reportedly increased,[172] chronic ACE inhibition has a small but significant antihypertensive effect; blocking the $B_2$ receptor with icatibant blunted

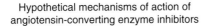

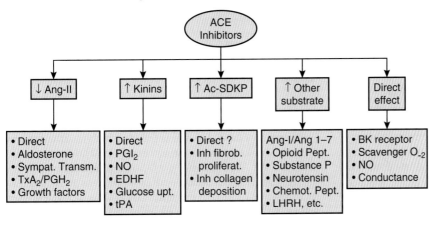

**Figure 20–5** ACE has multiple substrates, and inhibition of their hydrolysis may explain the cardioprotective effect of ACE inhibitors.

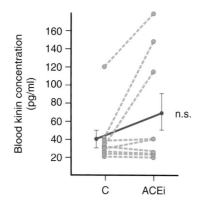

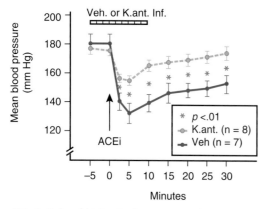

**Figure 20-6** Role of kinins in the acute antihypertensive effects of an ACE inhibitor (enalaprilat) in rats with severe hypertension. *Top,* Blood kinin concentrations before (C) and after administration of the ACE inhibitor. *Bottom,* Mean blood pressure before and after ACE inhibition; *open* and *closed circles* represent rats pretreated with a kinin antagonist or vehicle, respectively. Values are mean ± standard error of measure (bottom). (Reprinted from Carbonell LF, Carretero OA, Stewart JM, Scicli AG. Effect of a kinin antagonist on the acute antihypertensive activity of enalaprilat in severe hypertension. Hypertension 11:239-243, 1988.)

this chronic antihypertensive action,[139,173] suggesting that in this model, kinins may play a role in the antihypertensive effect of ACE inhibitors. However, they do not appear to contribute to the chronic antihypertensive effect of ACE inhibitors in SHR[171] or in hypertension induced by aortic coarctation.[154,174,175] Therefore the role of kinins in the long-term antihypertensive effect of ACE inhibitors depends on the model. To our knowledge, no studies of chronic blockade of the kallikrein-kinin system have been conducted in humans.

## ROLE OF KININS IN THE CARDIAC ANTIHYPERTROPHIC EFFECT OF ACE INHIBITORS

ACE inhibitors have been shown to reverse LVH in essential hypertension and in various experimental models. This decrease is partly due to reduced afterload, but it has been postulated that it may be partially independent of the decrease in blood pressure. A decrease in angiotensin II, which stimu-

lates various protooncogenes and growth factors, may participate in the antihypertrophic effect of ACE inhibitors acting independently of their effect on blood pressure. The cardiac kallikrein-kinin system may also participate in the effect of ACE inhibitors on the heart. Doses of ACE inhibitors that do not decrease blood pressure reverse LVH in rats with hypertension caused by aortic coarctation.[176] To be certain that blood pressure does not decrease, direct 24-hour measurements are needed. The antihypertrophic effects of ACE inhibitors have been reported to be reversed by a kinin antagonist.[177] However, using a very similar protocol, we have not been able to confirm this.[175] Further studies are needed to determine whether doses of ACE inhibitors that do not decrease blood pressure (24-hour blood pressure monitoring) reverse cardiac hypertrophy and whether kinins participate in this process.

Capillary length and density increase in hearts of SHR treated with an ACE inhibitor at both "antihypertensive" and "nonantihypertensive" doses. There is strong evidence that angiotensin II also has significant angiogenic effects.[178] However, the effect of an ACE inhibitor on capillary growth cannot be attributed to inhibition of angiotensin production alone, because it is blocked by concomitant treatment with the selective $B_2$ receptor antagonist, icatibant, suggesting that it may be due to kinins.[179]

## ROLE OF KININS IN MYOCARDIAL ISCHEMIA AND IN THE PROTECTIVE EFFECT OF ISCHEMIC PRECONDITIONING AND ACE INHIBITORS

Both human and animal studies have demonstrated that kinins are released from the heart and that their release is increased during ischemia. This release of kinins could have a cardioprotective effect.[180-182] Indeed, experimental studies have shown that intracoronary infusion of bradykinin significantly limited infarct size, reduced the incidence of ventricular arrhythmias, improved cardiac performance and normalized myocardial metabolism.[183-185] It has also been suggested that kinins are important mediators of ischemic preconditioning, in which repeated brief coronary occlusions render the myocardium more resistant to injury from subsequent prolonged ischemia. In patients undergoing angioplasty, balloon inflation for 1 minute (which mimics ischemic preconditioning) increased kinin concentrations in the coronary sinus 50-fold as compared with preinflation values.[2] Preconditioning almost doubled cardiac interstitial kinin concentrations as compared with nonpreconditioned hearts subjected to ischemia.[182] The role of kinins in ischemic preconditioning was further demonstrated in our laboratory with animals genetically lacking $B_2$ kinin receptors or deficient in kinins. We found that in $B_2$ kinin receptor KO mice, as well as in rats deficient in HMWK, the cardioprotective effect of preconditioning was abolished or significantly blunted.[3]

During myocardial ischemia followed by sympathetic nerve stimulation, kinins in coronary sinus blood increase significantly.[186] An ACE inhibitor was shown to reduce myocardial infarct size after ischemia/reperfusion, whereas an angiotensin II antagonist (losartan) did not.[187] In nephrectomized dogs in which infarction was induced by occlusion of the coronary artery for 90 minutes, blockade of local angiotensin II formation with protease inhibitors had no significant effect on myocardial infarct size despite decreased angiotensin II release. Captopril did not alter local angiotensin II formation but did increase bradykinin and reduce infarct size, suggesting that kinins were responsible for the effect of the ACE inhibitor on infarct size.[181] Similarly, when low doses of the ACE inhibitor ramiprilat (which had no systemic effect) were infused into the left coronary artery in dogs, they reduced the size of the infarction caused by ligation of the descending branch of the left coronary artery.[183] This cardioprotective effect of ramiprilat was mimicked by bradykinin and abolished by coadministration of a kinin antagonist.

ACE inhibitors have been shown to reduce ischemia/reperfusion injury, including infarct size and reperfusion arrhythmias. The cardioprotective effect of ACE inhibitors is due to inhibition of both angiotensin II formation and kinin degradation.[4,5,187-190] In animal models of ischemia/reperfusion injury, we and others have shown that ACE inhibitors reduced infarct size and ventricular arrhythmias and that these effects of ACE inhibitors were abolished or attenuated by coadministration of a $B_2$ kinin antagonist.[183,187,191] We further showed that the infarct-limiting and antiarrhythmic effects of ACE inhibitors were blocked by inhibition of NO or prostaglandin synthesis[191] and diminished in eNOS gene KO mice.[192]

The cardioprotective effect of kinins may be mediated in several ways. Release of NO from the endothelium may be stimulated either directly or via prostaglandins. It has been shown that myocardial ischemia increases kinin release, accompanied by increased release of cGMP (an indicator of NO production) and 6-keto-$PGF_1$ (a metabolite of prostacyclin),[193,194] whereas inhibiting NO or prostaglandin synthesis diminishes or blocks the cardioprotective effect of kinins.[195,196] Kinins improve cardiac metabolism by increasing high-energy phosphate production and glucogen content in the heart, which could be mediated by facilitating translocation of intracellular glucose transporters (GLUT1 and GLUT4), thereby increasing glucose uptake.[197,198] This is important because during ischemia, the source of energy production is shifted from oxidation of fatty acids to glycolysis. Also, activation of protein kinase C (PKC) has been shown to be involved in the protective mechanism of preconditioning.[199-201] Activation of kinins causes further phosphorylation of a secondary effector, presumably the adenosine triphosphate (ATP)-sensitive potassium channels ($K_{ATP}$). Kinins have been shown to activate PKC, thereby stimulating the opening of $K_{ATP}$ and leading to cardioprotection.[202,203] Such responses may favorably influence functional and metabolic events during ischemic episodes and protect against ischemia/reperfusion injury.

## ROLE OF KININS IN THE CARDIOPROTECTIVE EFFECT OF ACE INHIBITORS IN HEART FAILURE AFTER MYOCARDIAL INFARCTION

ACE inhibitors reduce morbidity and mortality, improve cardiac function, regress left ventricular remodeling, and prolong life in patients with heart failure. We showed that in a rat model of heart failure caused by surgically induced myocardial infarction (MI), ACE inhibitors improved cardiac function and attenuated remodeling, as evidenced by increased

ejection fraction and decreased left ventricular dilation, myocyte hypertrophy, and interstitial fibrosis. These beneficial cardiac effects of ACE inhibitors were diminished by blockade of kinins.[190] The role of kinins in the cardioprotective effect of ACE inhibitors was confirmed by the fact that in $B_2$ kinin receptor KO mice and kininogen-deficient rats after MI, the effect of ACE inhibitors was significantly diminished or absent.[5,189] Although the precise mechanism by which kinins protect the heart is not yet well defined, accumulated evidence suggests that kinin-stimulated release of NO and/or prostaglandins may be largely responsible. Bradykinin stimulates release of NO from the mouse myocardium and decreases myocardial oxygen consumption; these effects are blocked by a $B_2$ kinin antagonist and absent in $B_2$ receptor KO mice.[204] We have shown that in eNOS KO mice with heart failure after MI, the effect of the ACE inhibitor was almost abolished.[205] Considered together, these findings may suggest that kinins acting on the $B_2$ receptor play an important role in the cardioprotective action of ACE inhibitors via the release of NO.

In patients with heart failure, ACE inhibitors have been shown not only to improve cardiac function and increase survival but also to decrease the rate of myocardial reinfarction.[206] The mechanism of this decrease is not known, but because ACE inhibitors may block kinin degradation in the coronary circulation, one hypothesis is that kinins stimulate the release of EDRF and $PGI_2$, important inhibitors of platelet aggregation. Because kinins are potent stimulators of the release of tPA,[62,207] it is also possible that this potentiation of tPA release may activate plasmin and fibrinolysis. Although the exact mechanism of action of ACE inhibitors in reinfarction is not known, these hypotheses open up an exciting new area of cardiovascular research.

## ROLE OF KININS IN THE CARDIOPROTECTIVE EFFECT OF ANGIOTENSIN RECEPTOR BLOCKERS

Two subtypes of angiotensin II receptors, $AT_1$ and $AT_2$, have been identified. Most biologic actions of angiotensin II are mediated by the $AT_1$ receptor, whereas little is known about the function of $AT_2$ receptors. In cultured endothelial cells, angiotensin II stimulates the release of NO. This effect is blocked by either an $AT_2$ or $B_2$ receptor antagonist, indicating that angiotensin II–stimulated NO release is mediated via activation of the $AT_2$ receptor and a kinin-dependent mechanism.[208] Mice overexpressing the $AT_2$ receptor were reported to have increased kininogenase activity in the vasculature.[209] Because blockade of the $AT_1$ receptor increases angiotensin II levels, which in turn may activate the $AT_2$ receptor, it is rational to hypothesize that the cardioprotective effect of ARBs is mediated in part by kinins via activation of the $AT_2$ receptor. In fact, we found that ARBs improved cardiac function and ameliorated remodeling in rats with congestive heart failure after MI and that these effects were significantly attenuated by an $AT_2$ or $B_2$ receptor antagonist[190] or in mice lacking the $AT_2$ receptor.[210] Using $B_2$ kinin receptor KO mice and kininogen-deficient rats, as well as eNOS KO mice, we confirmed that a lack of kinins or endothelium-derived NO diminished the cardioprotective effect of ARBs,[4,5,205] indicating that increased release of kinins and NO cause by activation of the $AT_2$

receptor is an important mediator of the cardioprotective effect of ARBs.

Because angiotensin II also plays a critical role in the regulation of blood pressure and in the pathogenesis of many models of hypertension, the interaction of the renin-angiotensin-aldosterone system and the kallikrein-kinin system and their contribution of these two systems to the effects of ACE inhibitors and ARBs should not be underestimated. Figure 20–7 illustrates some of these interactions. The $AT_1$ receptor and the bradykinin $B_2$ receptor form stable heterodimers, causing increased activation of G[alpha]$_q$ and G[alpha]$_i$ (the two major signaling proteins triggered by $AT_1$). Also, the endocytotic pathways of both receptors change with heterodimerization. This appears to be the first reported example of signal enhancement triggered by heterodimerization of two different vasoactive hormone receptors.[81] Interaction of the $AT_1$ and $B_2$ receptors potentiates the pressor effect of angiotensin II. On the other hand, angiotensin-(1-7) interacting with bradykinin has emerged as an endogenous antihypertensive/antitrophic mechanism, opposing many of the actions of angiotensin II that are mediated by the $AT_1$ receptor.[211-213] It has been demonstrated that angiotensin-(1-7), acting via receptors other than $AT_1$ or $AT_2$, induced bradykinin-mediated hypotension in SHR and normotensive rats[214] and dilation of porcine coronary arteries.[215,216] Angiotensin I and II are cleaved to angiotensin-(1-7) by various endopeptidases.[217,218] This constitutes another mecha-

nism by which kinins could contribute to the beneficial effects of ACE inhibitors or ARBs. Bradykinin also appears to play an important role in mediating the counterregulatory protective effect of $AT_2$ receptors, which oppose the effect of the $AT_1$ receptor.[190,210,219] Thus there is a close interaction between kinins and angiotensins in the regulation of cardiovascular and renal function.

Kinins appear not to play a fundamental role in the pathogenesis of hypertension, because humans, rats, and mice with a deficiency of one component of the kallikrein-kinin system or with chronic blockade of the kallikrein-kinin system do not have hypertension. In the kidney, kinins participate in the regulation of papillary blood flow and water and sodium excretion. $B_2$-KO mice appear to be hypersensitive to the hypertensinogenic effect of salt. Kinins participate in the acute antihypertensive effect of ACE inhibitors but in general are not involved in their chronic antihypertensive effects, save for mineralocorticoid-salt–induced hypertension. Kinins acting via NO participate in the vascular protective effect of ACE inhibitors during neointima formation. In MI produced by ischemia/reperfusion, kinins play an important role in the reduction of infarct size induced by preconditioning or ACE inhibitors. In heart failure secondary to infarction, the therapeutic effects of ACE inhibitors are partially mediated by kinins via the release of NO. The therapeutic effect of ARB in heart failure is partly due to activation of $AT_2$ receptors that act via kinins and NO. Thus kinins play an important role in

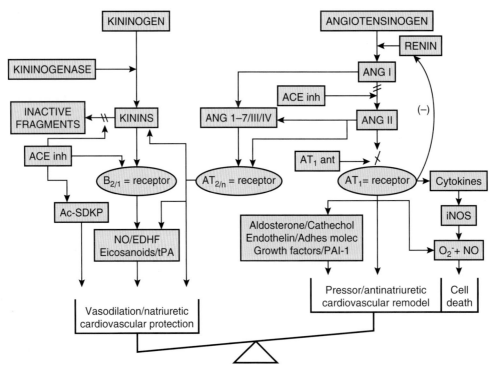

**Figure 20–7** The renin-angiotensin and kallikrein-kinin systems. In both systems, a substrate is cleaved by an enzyme of restricted specificity, releasing a peptide that is either already active (lys-bradykinin, bradykinin) or inactive (angiotensin I). On further processing by a specific peptidase, angiotensin I is converted to a vasoactive peptide (angiotensin II). In turn, vasoactive peptides are inactivated by peptidases. Angiotensin-converting enzyme is common to both systems but has different roles: it processes angiotensin I to angiotensin II and is the main kinin-inactivating peptidase. From Liu Y, Yang X, Sharov VG, et al. Effects of Angiotensin-converting enzyme inhibitors and Angiotensin II Type I receptor antagonists in rats with heart failure. J Clin Invest 99:1926-1935, 1997.

the regulation of cardiovascular and renal function as well as in many of the beneficial effects of ACE inhibitors and ARBs.

## SUMMARY

Autocrine, endocrine, and neuroendocrine hormonal systems are important factors that regulate cardiovascular and renal function. Alteration of the balance among these systems may result in hypertension and target-organ damage. Changes in this balance could be due to (1) genetic factors and/or (2) environmental factors. Endocrine and neuroendocrine vasopressor hormonal systems—such as the renin-angiotensin system, aldosterone, and catecholamines—play a well-established and important role in the regulation of blood pressure and the pathogenesis of some forms of hypertension and target-organ damage. The role of vasodepressor autacoids such as kinins is less well established. However, there is increasing evidence that vasodepressor hormones not only play an important role in the regulation of blood pressure and renal function but may also oppose remodeling of the cardiovascular system. This chapter reviews the role of kinins, oligopeptides containing the sequence of bradykinin. They are generated from precursors known as *kininogens* by enzymes such as glandular (tissue) enzymes and plasma kallikrein. Some of the effects of kinins are mediated via autacoids such as eicosanoids, NO, EDHF, and/or tPA. Acting via these mediators, kinins play an important role in the regulation of cardiovascular and renal function as well as some of the cardiovascular and renal effects of ACE and ARBs. A study of Utah families revealed that a dominant kallikrein gene expressed as high urinary kallikrein excretion was associated with a decreased risk of essential hypertension. Also, a restriction fragment length polymorphism (RFLP) that distinguishes the kallikrein gene family in one strain of SHR from normotensive Brown Norway rats has been identified; in recombinant inbred substrains derived from these SHR and Brown Norway strains, the RFLP marking the kallikrein gene family of the SHR cosegregated with an increase in blood pressure. However, humans, rats, and mice with a deficiency of one component of the kallikrein-kinin system or chronic blockade of the kallikrein-kinin system do not have hypertension. In the kidney, kinins participate in the regulation of papillary blood flow and water and sodium excretion. Mice with homologous deletion of the gene for the $B_2$ receptor for bradykinin appear to be more sensitive to the hypertensinogenic effect of salt.

Kinins participate in the acute antihypertensive effect of ACE inhibitors; however, in general they are not involved in the chronic antihypertensive effects of ACE inhibitors save for mineralocorticoid-salt–induced hypertension. Kinins acting via nitric oxide NO participate in the vascular protective effect of ACE inhibitors during neointima formation. In MI produced by ischemia/reperfusion, kinins play an important role in the reduction of infarct size induced by preconditioning or ACE inhibitors. In heart failure secondary to infarction, the therapeutic effects of ACE inhibitors are partially mediated by kinins via the release of NO. The therapeutic effect of ARB in heart failure is partly due to activation of angiotensin type 2 receptors via kinins and NO. Thus kinins could play an important role in the regulation of cardiovascular and renal function as well as in many of the beneficial effects of ACE inhibitors and ARB.

## References

1. Carretero OA, Scicli AG. Kinins paracrine hormone. Kidney Int 34(Suppl 26):S-52-S-59, 1988.
2. Parratt JR, Vegh A, Papp JG. Bradykinin as an endogenous myocardial protective substance with particular reference to ischemic preconditioning: A brief review of the evidence. Can J Physiol Pharmacol 73:837-842, 1995.
3. Yang X-P, Liu Y-H, Scicli GM, et al. Role of kinins in the cardioprotective effect of preconditioning. Study of myocardial ischemia/reperfusion injury in $B_2$ kinin receptor knockout mice and kininogen-deficient rats. Hypertension 30:735-740, 1997.
4. Liu Y-H, Yang X-P, Shesely EG, et al. Role of angiotensin II type 2 receptors and kinins in the cardioprotective effect of angiotensin II type 1 receptor antagonists in rats with heart failure. J Am Coll Cardiol 43:1473-1480, 2004.
5. Yang X-P, Liu Y-H, Mehta D, et al. Diminished cardioprotective response to inhibition of angiotensin-converting enzyme and angiotensin II type 1 receptor in $B_2$ kinin receptor gene knockout mice. Circ Res 88:1072-1079, 2001.
6. Scicli AG, Mindroiu T, Scicli G, et al. Blood kinins, their concentration in normal subjects and in patients with congenital deficiency in plasma prekallikrein and kininogen. J Lab Clin Med 100:81-93, 1982.
7. Colman RW. Patho-physiology of kallikrein system. Ann Clin Lab Sci 10:220-226, 1980.
8. Kaplan AP, Silverberg M. The coagulation-kinin pathway of human plasma. Blood 70:1-15, 1987.
9. Sundsmo JS, Fair DS. Relationships among the complement, kinin, coagulation and fibrinolytic systems in the inflammatory reaction. Clin Physiol Biochem 1:225-284, 1983.
10. Clements JA. The glandular kallikrein family of enzymes: Tissue-specific expression and hormonal regulation. Endocr Rev 10:393-419, 1989.
11. Boucher R, Demassieux S, Garcia R, et al. Tonin, angiotensin II system. Circ Res 41:26-29, 1977.
12. Lilja H. A kallikrein-like serine protease in prostatic fluid cleaves the predominant seminal vesicle protein. J Clin Invest 76:1899-1903, 1985.
13. Yamaguchi T, Carretero OA, Scicli AG. A novel serine protease with vasoconstrictor activity coded by the kallikrein gene S3. J Biol Chem 266:5011-5017, 1991.
14. Yamaguchi T, Carretero OA, Scicli AG. A potent vasoconstrictor in the rat submandibular gland. Hypertension 17:101-106, 1991.
15. Carretero OA, Carbini LA, Scicli AG. The molecular biology of the kallikrein-kinin system: I. General description, nomenclature and the mouse gene family. J Hypertens 11:693-697, 1993.
16. Scicli AG, Carbini LA, Carretero OA. The molecular biology of the kallikrein-kinin system: II. The rat gene family. J Hypertens 11:775-780, 1993.
17. Carbini LA, Scicli AG, Carretero OA. The molecular biology of the kallikrein-kinin system: III. The human kallikrein gene family and kallikrein substrate. J Hypertens 11:893-898, 1993.
18. Saed GM, Carretero OA, MacDonald RJ, et al. Kallikrein messenger RNA in rat arteries and veins. Circ Res 67:510-516, 1990.
19. Nolly H, Saed G, Carretero OA, et al. Adrenal kallikrein. Hypertension 21:911-915, 1993.
20. Nolly H, Scicli AG, Scicli G, et al. Characterization of a kininogenase from rat vascular tissue resembling tissue kallikrein. Circ Res 56:816-821, 1985.
21. Nolly H, Carbini LA, Scicli G, et al. A local kallikrein-kinin system is present in rat hearts. Hypertension 23:919-923, 1994.
22. Chao J, Chao L, Swain CC, et al. Tissue kallikrein in rat brain and pituitary: Regional distribution and estrogen induction in the anterior pituitary. Endocrinology 120:475-482, 1987.

23. Clements JA, Matheson BA, MacDonald RJ, et al. The expression of the kallikrein gene family in the rat pituitary: Oestrogen effects and the expression of an additional family member in the neurointermediate lobe. J Neuroendocrinol 1:199-203, 1989.

24. Powers CA, Nasjletti A. A major sex difference in kallikrein-like activity in the rat anterior pituitary. Endocrinology 114:1841-1844, 1984.

25. Frey EK, Kraut H, Werle E. Kallikrein padutin [English transl. (1977) ed by R Vogel]. Stuttgart, Ferdinand Enke Verlag, 1950.

26. Zimmermann A, Geiger R, Kortmann H. Similarity between a kininogenase (kallikrein) from human large intestine and human urinary kallikrein. Hoppe-Seylers Z Physiol Chem 360:1767-1773, 1979.

27. Schachter M, Longridge DJ, Wheeler GD, et al. Immunocytochemical and enzyme histochemical localization of kallikrein-like enzymes in colon, intestine, and stomach of rat and cat. J Histochem Cytochem 34:927-934, 1986.

28. Hilton SM. The physiological role of glandular kallikreins. *In* Erdös EG (ed). Handbook of Experimental Pharmacology, Vol 25: Bradykinin, Kallidin and Kallikrein. 2nd ed. New York: Springer-Verlag, 1970;389-399.

29. Chao J, Chao L, Margolius HS. Isolation of tissue kallikrein in rat spleen by monoclonal antibody-affinity chromatography. Biochim Biophys Acta 801:244-249, 1984.

30. Scicli G, Nolly H, Carretero OA, et al. Glandular kallikrein-like enzyme in adrenal glands. Adv Exp Med Biol 247B:217-222, 1989.

31. Rabito SF, Scicli AG, Carretero OA. Immunoreactive glandular kallikrein in plasma. *In* Gross F, Vogel G (eds). Enzymatic Release of Vasoactive Peptides. New York, Raven Press, 1980;247-256.

32. Rabito SF, Scicli AG, Kher V, et al. Immunoreactive glandular kallikrein in rat plasma: A radioimmunoassay for its determination. Am J Physiol 242:H602-H610, 1982.

33. Geiger R, Clausnitzer B, Fink E, et al. Isolation of an enzymatically active glandular kallikrein from human plasma by immunoaffinity chromatography. Hoppe Seylers Z Physiol Chem 361:1795-1803, 1980.

34. Lawton WJ, Proud D, Frech ME, et al. Characterization and origin of immunoreactive glandular kallikrein in rat plasma. Biochem Pharmacol 30:1731-1737, 1981.

35. Scicli AG, θrstavik TB, Rabito SF, et al. Blood kinins after sympathetic nerve stimulation of the rat submandibular gland. Hypertension 5(Suppl I):I-101-I-106, 1983.

36. Pisano JJ, Corthorn J, Yates K, et al. The kallikrein-kinin system in the kidney. Contrib Nephrol 12:116-125, 1978.

37. Omata K, Carretero OA, Itoh S, et al. Active and inactive kallikrein in rabbit connecting tubules and urine during low and normal sodium intake. Kidney Int 24:714-718, 1983.

38. Noda Y, Yamada K, Igic R, et al. Regulation of rat urinary and renal kallikrein and prekallikrein by corticosteroids. Proc Natl Acad Sci USA 80:3059-3063, 1983.

39. Alhenc-Gelas F, Marchetti J, Allegrini J, et al. Measurement of urinary kallikrein activity: Species differences in kinin production. Biochim Biophys Acta 677:477-488, 1981.

40. Mindroiu T, Scicli G, Perini F, et al. Identification of a new kinin in human urine. J Biol Chem 261:7407-7411, 1986.

41. Jacobsen S. Substrates for plasma kinin-forming enzymes in human, dog and rabbit plasmas. Br J Pharmacol 26:403-411, 1966.

42. Jacobsen S. Separation of two different substrates for plasma kinin-forming enzymes. Nature 210:98-99, 1966.

43. Müller-Esterl W, Fritz H, Machleidt W, et al. Human plasma kininogens are identical with α-cysteine proteinase inhibitors: Evidence from immunological, enzymological and sequence data. FEBS Lett 182:310-314, 1985.

44. Ohkubo I, Kurachi K, Takasawa T, et al. Isolation of a human cDNA for $\alpha_2$-thiol proteinase inhibitor and its identity with low molecular weight kininogen. Biochemistry 23:5691-5697, 1984.

45. Sueyoshi T, Enjyoji K, Shimada T, et al. A new function of kininogens as thiol-proteinase inhibitors: Inhibition of papain and cathepsins B, H and L by bovine, rat and human plasma kininogens. FEBS Lett 182:193-195, 1985.

46. Barlas A, Okamoto H, Greenbaum LM. T-kininogen: The major plasma kininogen in rat adjuvant arthritis. Biochem Biophys Res Commun 129:280-286, 1985.

47. Furuto-Kato S, Matsumoto A, Kitamura N, et al. Primary structures of the mRNAs encoding the rat precursors for bradykinin and T-kinin: Structural relationship of kininogens with major acute phase protein and α1-cysteine proteinase inhibitor. J Biol Chem 260:12054-12059, 1985.

48. Okamoto H, Greenbaum LM. Kininogen substrates for trypsin and cathepsin D in human, rabbit and rat plasmas. Life Sci 32:2007-2013, 1983.

49. Okamoto H, Greenbaum LM. Pharmacological properties of T-kinin (isoleucyl-seryl-bradykinin) from rat plasma. Biochem Pharmacol 32:2637-2638, 1983.

50. Kaplan AP, Silverberg M, Ghebrehiwet B, et al. The kallikrein-kinin system in inflammation. Adv Exp Med Biol 247:125-136, 1989.

51. Erdös EG. Kininases. *In* Erdös EG (ed). Handbook of Experimental Pharmacology, Vol XXV, Suppl: Bradykinin, Kallidin and Kallikrein. Berlin, Springer-Verlag, 1979;427-487.

52. Erdös EG. Angiotensin I converting enzyme. Circ Res 36:247-255, 1975.

53. Skidgel RA, Schulz WW, Tam L-T, et al. Human renal angiotensin I converting enzyme and neutral endopeptidase. Kidney Int 31 (Suppl 20):S-45-S-48, 1987.

54. Vijayaraghavan J, Scicli AG, Carretero OA, et al. The hydrolysis of endothelins by neutral endopeptidase 24.11 (enkephalinase). J Biol Chem 265:14150-14155, 1990.

55. Ura N, Carretero OA, Erdös EG. Role of renal endopeptidase 24.11 in kinin metabolism in vitro and in vivo. Kidney Int 32:507-513, 1987.

56. Ishida H, Scicli AG, Carretero OA. Role of angiotensin converting enzyme and other peptidases in in vivo metabolism of kinins. Hypertension 14:322-327, 1989.

57. Campbell DJ, Kladis A, Duncan A-M. Bradykinin peptides in kidney, blood, and other tissues of the rat. Hypertension 21:155-165, 1993.

58. Cherry PD, Furchgott RF, Zawadzki JV, et al. Role of endothelial cells in relaxation of isolated arteries by bradykinin. Proc Natl Acad Sci USA 79:2106-2110, 1982.

59. Vane JR, Änggård EE, Botting RM. Regulatory functions of the vascular endothelium. N Engl J Med 323:27-36, 1990.

60. Vanhoutte PM. Endothelium and control of vascular function: State of the art lecture. Hypertension 13:658-667, 1989.

61. Tiffany CW, Burch RM. Bradykinin stimulates tumor necrosis factor and interleukin-1 release from macrophages. FEBS Lett 247:189-192, 1989.

62. Smith D, Gilbert M, Owen WG. Tissue plasminogen activator release in vivo in response to vasoactive agents. Blood 66:835-839, 1985.

63. Regoli D. Pharmacology of bradykinin and related kinins. Adv Exp Med Biol 156:569-584, 1983.

64. Regoli D, Rhaleb NE, Drapeau G, et al. Basic pharmacology of kinins: pharmacologic receptors and other mechanisms. Adv Exp Med Biol 247:399-407, 1989.

65. McEachern AE, Shelton ER, Bhakta S, et al. Expression cloning of a rat B$_2$ bradykinin receptor. Proc Natl Acad Sci USA 88:7724-7728, 1991.

66. Regoli D, Rhaleb N-E, Dion S, et al. New selective bradykinin receptor antagonists and bradykinin $B_2$ receptor characterization. Trends Pharmacol Sci 11:156-161, 1990.

67. Burch RM, Farmer SG, Steranka LR. Bradykinin receptor antagonists. Med Res Rev 10:237-269, 1990.

68. Regoli D, Rhaleb N-E, Drapeau G, et al. Kinin receptor subtypes. J Cardiovasc Pharmacol 15(Suppl 6):S30-S38, 1990.

69. Saha JK, Sengupta JN, Goyal RK. Effect of bradykinin on opossum esophageal longitudinal smooth muscle: evidence for novel bradykinin receptors. J Pharmacol Exp Ther 252:1012-1020, 1990.

70. Stewart JM, Vavrek RJ. Bradykinin competitive antagonists for classical kinin systems. In Greenbaum LM, Margolius HS (eds). Kinins IV, Part A. New York, Plenum Press, 1986; 537-542.

71. Regoli D, Barabe J. Pharmacology of bradykinin and related kinins. Pharmacol Rev 32:1-46,1980.

72. Marceau F, Hess JF, Bachvarov DR. The $B_1$ receptors for kinins. Pharmacol Rev 50:357-386, 1998.

73. Wirth K, Hock FJ, Albus U, et al. Hoe 140 a new potent and long acting bradykinin-antagonist: In vivo studies. Br J Pharmacol 102:774-777, 1991.

74. Stewart JM, Gera L, York EJ, et al. Metabolism-resistant bradykinin antagonists: Development and applications. Biol Chem 382:37-41, 2001.

75. Burgess GM, Perkins MN, Rang HP, et al. Bradyzide, a potent non-peptide B(2) bradykinin receptor antagonist with long-lasting oral activity in animal models of inflammatory hyperalgesia. Br J Pharmacol 129:77-86, 2000.

76. Whalley ET, Hanson WL, Stewart JM, et al. Oral activity of peptide bradykinin antagonists following intragastric administration in the rat. Can J Physiol Pharmacol 75:629-632, 1997.

77. Stewart JM. Bradykinin antagonists as anti-cancer agents. Curr Pharm Des 9:2036-2042, 2003.

78. Bock MG, Longmore J. Bradykinin antagonists: New opportunities. Curr Opin Chem Biol 4:401-406, 2000.

79. Hecquet C, Tan F, Marcic BM, et al. Human bradykinin $B_2$ receptor is activated by kallikrein and other serine proteases. Mol Pharmacol 58:828-836, 2000.

80. Marcic BM, Erdös EG. Protein kinase C and phosphatase inhibitors block the ability of angiotensin I-converting enzyme inhibitors to resensitize the receptor to bradykinin without altering the primary effects of bradykinin. J Pharmacol Exp Ther 294:605-612, 2000.

81. AbdAlla S, Lother H, Quitterer U. $AT_1$-receptor heterodimers show enhanced G-protein activation and altered receptor sequestration. Nature 407:94-98, 2000.

82. Ju H, Venema VJ, Marrero MB, et al. Inhibitory interactions of the bradykinin $B_2$ receptor with endothelial nitric-oxide synthase. J Biol Chem 273:24025-24029, 1998.

83. Oza NB, Schwartz JH, Goud HD, et al. Rat aortic smooth muscle cells in culture express kallikrein, kininogen, and bradykininase activity. J Clin Invest 85:597-600, 1990.

84. Bergaya S, Meneton P, Bloch-Faure M, et al. Decreased flow-dependent dilation in carotid arteries of tissue kallikrein-knockout mice. Circ Res 88:593-599, 2001.

85. Meneton P, Bloch-Faure M, Hagege AA, et al. Cardiovascular abnormalities with normal blood pressure in tissue kallikrein-deficient mice. Proc Natl Acad Sci USA 98:2634-2639, 2001.

86. Mombouli J-V, Illiano S, Nagao T, et al. Potentiation of endothelium-dependent relaxations to bradykinin by angiotensin I converting enzyme inhibitors in canine coronary artery involves both endothelium-derived relaxing and hyperpolarizing factors. Circ Res 71:137-144, 1992.

87. Clozel M. Mechanism of action of angiotensin converting enzyme inhibitors on endothelial function in hypertension. Hypertension 18(Suppl II):II-37-II-42, 1991.

88. Powell JS, Müller RKM, Rouge M, et al. The proliferative response to vascular injury is suppressed by angiotensin-converting enzyme inhibition. J Cardiovasc Pharmacol 16(Suppl 4): S42-S49, 1990.

89. Osterrieder W, Müller RKM, Powell JS, et al. Role of angiotensin II in injury-induced neointima formation in rats. Hypertension 18(Suppl II):II-60-II-64, 1991.

90. Farhy R, Ho K-L, Carretero OA, et al. Kinins mediate the antiproliferative effect of ramipril in rat carotid artery. Biochem Biophys Res Commun 182:283-288, 1992.

91. Farhy RD, Carretero OA, Ho K-L, et al. Role of kinins and nitric oxide in the effects of angiotensin converting enzyme inhibitors on neointima formation. Circ Res 72:1202-1210, 1993.

92. Berg T, Carretero OA, Scicli AG, et al. Role of kinin in regulation of rat submandibular gland blood flow. Hypertension 14:73-80, 1989.

93. Seino M, Carretero OA, Albertini R, et al. Kinins in regulation of uteroplacental blood flow in the pregnant rabbit. Am J Physiol 242:H142-H147, 1982.

94. Roman RJ, Kaldunski ML, Scicli AG, et al. Influence of kinins and angiotensin II on the regulation of papillary blood flow. Am J Physiol 255:F690-F698, 1988.

95. Seino M, Abe K, Nushiro N, et al. Effects of a competitive antagonist of bradykinin on blood pressure and renal blood flow in anesthetized rats. J Hypertens 6:867-871, 1988.

96. Ørstavik TB, Carretero OA, Johansen L, et al. Role of kallikrein in the hypotensive effect of captopril after sympathetic stimulation of the rat submandibular gland. Circ Res 51:385-390, 1982.

97. Beierwaltes WH, Carretero OA, Scicli AG. Renal hemodynamics in response to a kinin analogue antagonist. Am J Physiol 255:F408-F414, 1988.

98. Ren Y, Garvin J, Carretero OA. Mechanism involved in bradykinin-induced efferent arteriole dilation. Kidney Int 62:544-549, 2002.

99. Wang H, Carretero OA, Garvin JL. Inhibition of apical $Na^+/H^+$ exchangers on the macula densa cells augments tubuloglomerular feedback. Hypertension 41:688-691, 2003.

100. Zimmerman BG, Raich PC, Vavrek RJ, et al. Bradykinin contribution to renal blood flow effect of angiotensin converting enzyme inhibitor in the conscious sodium-restricted dog. Circ Res 66:234-240, 1990.

101. Nakagawa M, Nasjletti A. Renal function as affected by inhibitors of kininase II and of neutral endopeptidase 24.11 in rats with and without desoxycorticosterone pretreatment. Adv Exp Med Biol 247:495-499, 1989.

102. Omata K, Carretero OA, Scicli AG, et al. Localization of active and inactive kallikrein (kininogenase activity) in the microdissected rabbit nephron. Kidney Int 22:602-607, 1982.

103. Scicli AG, Carretero OA, Hampton A, et al. Site of kininogenase secretion in the dog nephron. Am J Physiol 230:533-536, 1976.

104. Scicli AG, Gandolfi R, Carretero OA. Site of formation of kinins in the dog nephron. Am J Physiol 234:F36-F40, 1978.

105. Figueroa CD, MacIver AG, Mackenzie JC, et al. Localisation of immunoreactive kininogen and tissue kallikrein in the human nephron. Histochemistry 89:437-442, 1988.

106. Tomita K, Pisano JJ. Binding of [$^3$H]bradykinin in isolated nephron segments of the rabbit. Am J Physiol 246:F732-F737, 1984.

107. Vio CP, Churchill L, Rabito SF, et al. Renal kallikrein in venous effluent of filtering and non-filtering isolated kidneys. Adv Exp Med Biol 156B:897-905, 1983.

108. Siragy HM, Jaffa AA, Margolius HS. Stimulation of renal interstitial bradykinin by sodium depletion. Am J Hypertens 6: 863-866, 1993.

109. Kauker ML. Bradykinin action on the efflux of luminal $^{22}$Na in the rat nephron. J Pharmacol Exp Ther 214:119-123, 1980.

110. Kauker ML. Kallidin effect on renal tubular function in meclofenamate- and vehicle-pretreated rats. Proc Soc Exp Biol Med 193:60-64, 1990.

111. Kauker ML, Gisi PJ, Zawada ET. Renal kinins and sodium transport: Influence of a bradykinin receptor antagonist (BKRA) [abstract]. FASEB J 4:A990, 1990.

112. Sybertz EJ, Chiu PJS, Vemulapalli S, et al. Atrial natriuretic factor-potentiating and antihypertensive activity of SCH 34826: An orally active neutral metalloendopeptidase inhibitor. Hypertension 15:152-161, 1990.

113. Pollock DM, Butterfield MI, Ader JL, et al. Dissociation of urinary kallikrein activity and salt and water excretion in the rat. Am J Physiol 250:F1082-F1089, 1986.

114. Nasjletti A, McGiff JC, Colina-Chourio J. Interrelations of the renal kallikrein-kinin system and renal prostaglandins in the conscious rat. Influence of mineralocorticoids. Circ Res 43:799-807, 1978.

115. Marin Grez M. The influence of antibodies against bradykinin on isotonic saline diuresis in the rat. Evidence for kinin involvement in renal function. Pflugers Arch 350:231-239, 1974.

116. Düsing R, Struck A, Göbel BO, et al. Effects of n-3 fatty acids on renal function and renal prostaglandin E metabolism. Kidney Int 38:315-319, 1990.

117. Saitoh S, Scicli AG, Peterson E, et al. Effect of inhibiting renal kallikrein on prostaglandin E$_2$, water, and sodium excretion. Hypertension 25:1008-1013, 1995.

118. Stoos BA, Carretero OA, Farhy RD, et al. Endothelium-derived relaxing factor inhibits transport and increases cGMP content in cultured mouse cortical collecting duct cells. J Clin Invest 89:761-765, 1992.

119. Lahera V, Salom MG, Fiksen-Olsen MJ, et al. Mediatory role of endothelium-derived nitric oxide in renal vasodilatory and excretory effects of bradykinin. Am J Hypertens 4:260-262, 1991.

120. Sinaiko AR, Glasser RJ, Gillum RF, et al. Urinary kallikrein excretion in grade school children with high and low blood pressure. J Pediatr 100:938-940, 1982.

121. Uchiyama M, Otsuka T, Sakai K. Urinary kallikrein excretion in children of parents with essential hypertension. Arch Dis Child 60:974-975, 1985.

122. Wollheim E, Peterknecht S, Dees C, et al. Defect in the excretion of a vasoactive polypeptide fraction A possible genetic marker of primary hypertension. Hypertension 3:574-579, 1981.

123. Zinner SH, Margolius HS, Rosner B, et al. Familial aggregation of urinary kallikrein concentration in childhood: Relation to blood pressure, race and urinary electrolytes. Am J Epidemiol 104:124-132, 1976.

124. Pravenec M, Kren V, Kunes J, et al. Cosegregation of blood pressure with a kallikrein gene family polymorphism. Hypertension 17:242-246, 1991.

125. Carretero OA, Amin VM, Ocholik T, et al. Urinary kallikrein in rats bred for their susceptibility and resistance to the hypertensive effect of salt. A new radioimmunoassay for its direct determination. Circ Res 42:727-731, 1978.

126. Carretero OA, Polomski C, Hampton A, et al. Urinary kallikrein, plasma renin and aldosterone in New Zealand genetically hypertensive (GH) rats. Clin Exp Pharmacol Physiol 3(Suppl):55-59, 1976.

127. Carretero OA, Scicli AG, Piwonska A, et al. Urinary kallikrein in rats bred for susceptibility and resistance to the hypertensive effect of salt and in New Zealand genetically hypertensive rats. Mayo Clin Proc 52:465-467, 1977.

128. Keiser HR, Geller RG, Margolius HS, et al. Urinary kallikrein in hypertensive animal models. Fed Proc 35:199-202, 1976.

129. Carretero OA, Scicli AG. The renal kallikrein-kinin system in human and in experimental hypertension. Klin Wochenschr 56(Suppl I):113-125, 1978.

130. Holland OB, Chud JM, Braunstein H. Urinary kallikrein excretion in essential and mineralocorticoid hypertension. J Clin Invest 65:347-356, 1980.

131. Margolius HS, Horwitz D, Pisano JJ, et al. Urinary kallikrein excretion in hypertensive man. Relationships to sodium intake and sodium-retaining steroids. Circ Res 35:820-825, 1974.

132. Seino M, Abe K, Otsuka Y, et al. Urinary kallikrein excretion and sodium metabolism in hypertensive patients. Tohoku J Exp Med 116:359-367, 1975.

133. Sustarsic DL, McPartland RP, Rapp JP, et al. Urinary kallikrein and urinary prostaglandin E$_2$ in genetically hypertensive mice. Proc Soc Exp Biol Med 163:193-199, 1980.

134. Bönner G, Preis S, Schunk U, et al. Hemodynamic effects of bradykinin on systemic and pulmonary circulation in healthy and hypertensive humans. J Cardiovasc Pharmacol 15(Suppl 6): S46-S56, 1990.

135. Salgado MCO, Rabito SF, Carretero OA. Blood kinin in one-kidney, one clip hypertensive rats. Hypertension 8(Suppl I): I-110-I-113, 1986.

136. Benetos A, Gavras I, Gavras H. Hypertensive effect of a bradykinin antagonist in normotensive rats. Hypertension 8:1089-1092, 1986.

137. Beierwaltes WH, Carretero OA, Scicli AG, et al. Competitive analog antagonists of bradykinin in the canine hindlimb. Proc Soc Exp Biol Med 186:79-83, 1987.

138. Carbonell LF, Carretero OA, Madeddu P, et al. Effects of a kinin antagonist on mean blood pressure. Hypertension 11(Suppl I):I-84-I-88, 1988.

139. Rhaleb N-E, Yang X-P, Nanba M, et al. Effect of chronic blockade of the kallikrein-kinin system on the development of hypertension in rats. Hypertension 37:121-128, 2001.

140. Madeddu P, Parpaglia PP, Demontis MP, et al. Bradykinin B$_2$-receptor blockade facilitates deoxycorticosterone-salt hypertension. Hypertension 21:980-984, 1993.

141. Majima M, Katori M, Hanazuka M, et al. Suppression of rat deoxycorticosterone-salt hypertension by kallikrein-kinin system. Hypertension 17:806-813, 1991.

142. Majima M, Yoshida O, Mihara H, et al. High sensitivity to salt in kininogen-deficient Brown Norway Katholiek rats. Hypertension 22:705-714, 1993.

143. Majima M, Mizogami S, Kuribayashi Y, et al. Hypertension induced by a nonpressor dose of angiotensin II in kininogen-deficient rats. Hypertension 24:111-119, 1994.

144. Madeddu P, Parpaglia PP, Demontis MP, et al. Chronic inhibition of bradykinin B$_2$-receptors enhances the slow vasopressor response to angiotensin II. Hypertension 23:646-652, 1994.

145. Alfie ME, Yang X-P, Hess F, et al. Salt-sensitive hypertension in bradykinin B$_2$ receptor knockout mice. Biochem Biophys Res Commun 224:625-630, 1996.

146. Cervenka L, Harrison-Bernard LM, Dipp S, et al. Early onset salt-sensitive hypertension in bradykinin B$_2$ receptor null mice. Hypertension 34:176-180, 1999.

147. Rhaleb N-E, Peng H, Alfie M, et al. Effect of ACE inhibitor on DOCA-salt- and aortic coarctation-induced hypertension in mice. Do kinin B$_2$ receptors play a role? Hypertension 33:329-334, 1999.

148. Emanueli C, Maestri R, Corradi D, et al. Dilated and failing cardiomyopathy in bradykinin B$_2$ receptor knockout mice. Circulation 100:2359-2365, 1999.

149. Rhaleb N-E, Yang X-P, Peng H, et al. Cardiovascular phenotype of male 129/SvEvTac, 129/SvJ and B$_2$-KO mice [abstract]. FASEB J 15:A101, 2001.

150. Milia AF, Gross V, Plehm R, et al. Normal blood pressure and renal function in mice lacking the bradykinin B$_2$ receptor. Hypertension 37:1473-1479, 2001.

151. Trabold F, Pons S, Hagege AA, et al. Cardiovascular phenotypes of kinin B$_2$ receptor- and tissue kallikrein-deficient mice. Hypertension 40:90-95, 2002.
152. Carretero OA, Kuk P, Piwonska SS, et al. Role of the renin-angiotensin system in the pathogenesis of severe hypertension in rats. Circ Res 29:654-663, 1971.
153. Marks ES, Bing RF, Thurston H, et al. Vasodepressor property of the converting enzyme inhibitor captopril (SQ 14 225): The role of factors other than renin-angiotensin blockade in the rat. Clin Sci 58:1-6, 1980.
154. Cachofeiro V, Sakakibara T, Nasjletti A. Kinins, nitric oxide, and the hypotensive effect of captopril and ramiprilat in hypertension. Hypertension 19:138-145, 1992.
155. Carbonell LF, Carretero OA, Stewart JM, et al. Effect of a kinin antagonist on the acute antihypertensive activity of enalaprilat in severe hypertension. Hypertension 11:239-243, 1988.
156. Carretero OA Scicli AG. The kallikrein-kinin system as a regulator of cardiovascular and renal function. In Laragh JH, Brenner BM (eds). Hypertension: Physiology, Diagnosis, and Management. 2nd ed. New York, Raven Press, 1995;983-999.
157. Campbell DJ. The kallikrein-kinin system in humans. Clin Exp Pharmacol Physiol 28:1060-1065, 2001.
158. Clappison BH, Anderson WP, Johnston CI. Role of the kallikrein-kinin system in the renal effects of angiotensin-converting enzyme inhibition in anaesthetized dogs. Clin Exp Pharmacol Physiol 8:509-513, 1981.
159. McCaa RE. Studies in vivo with angiotensin I converting enzyme (kininase II) inhibitors. Fed Proc 38:2783-2787, 1979.
160. Nasjletti A, Colina-Chourio J, McGiff JC. Disappearance of bradykinin in the renal circulation of dogs. Effects of kininase inhibition. Circ Res 37:59-65, 1975.
161. Vinci JM, Horwitz D, Zusman RM, et al. The effect of converting enzyme inhibition with SQ20,881 on plasma and urinary kinins, prostaglandin E and angiotensin II in hypertensive man. Hypertension 1:416-426, 1979.
162. Carretero OA, Miyazaki S, Scicli AG. Role of kinins in the acute antihypertensive effect of the converting enzyme inhibitor, captopril. Hypertension 3:18-22, 1981.
163. Carretero OA, Ørstavik TB, Rabito SF, et al. Interference of converting enzyme inhibitors with the kallikrein-kinin system. Clin Exp Hypertens [A] 5:1277-1285, 1983.
164. Carretero OA, Scicli AG, Maitra SR. Role of kinins in the pharmacological effects of converting enzyme inhibitors. In Horovitz ZP (ed). Angiotensin Converting Enzyme Inhibitors: Mechanisms of Action and Clinical Implications. Baltimore, Urban & Schwarzenberg, 1981;105-121.
165. Benetos A, Gavras H, Stewart JM, et al. Vasodepressor role of endogenous bradykinin assessed by a bradykinin antagonist. Hypertension 8:971-974, 1986.
166. Danckwardt L, Shimizu I, Bönner G, et al. Converting enzyme inhibition in kinin-deficient Brown Norway rats. Hypertension 16:429-435, 1990.
167. Pontieri V, Lopes OU, Ferreira SH. Hypotensive effect of captopril. Role of bradykinin and prostaglandinlike substances. Hypertension 15(Suppl I):I-55-I-58, 1990.
168. Murphey LJ, Gainer JV, Vaughan DE, et al. Angiotensin-converting enzyme insertion/deletion polymorphism modulates the human in vivo metabolism of bradykinin. Circulation 102:829-832, 2000.
169. Overlack A, Stumpe KO, Heck I, et al. Identification of angiotensin II- and kinin-dependent mechanisms in essential hypertension. In Philipp T, Distler A (eds). Hypertension: Mechanisms and Management. Berlin, Springer-Verlag, 1980;183-191.
170. Gainer JV, Morrow JD, King DJ, et al. Effect of bradykinin receptor blockade on response to angiotensin converting enzyme inhibition in salt-deplete normotensive subjects. N Engl J Med (submitted).
171. Bao G, Gohlke P, Qadri F, et al. Chronic kinin receptor blockade attenuates the antihypertensive effect of ramipril. Hypertension 20:74-79, 1992.
172. Nakagawa M, Nasjletti A. Plasma kinin concentration in deoxycorticosterone-salt hypertension. Hypertension 11:411-415, 1988.
173. Carretero OA. High-mineralocorticoid conditions: Kinins (paracrine hormones) in the regulation of renal function and blood pressure. In, Mornex R, Jaffiol C, Leclère J (eds). Progress in Endocrinology: The Proceedings of the Ninth International Congress of Endocrinology, Nice, 1992. Carnforth, Lancashershire, UK, Parthenon Publications Group, 1993;536-540.
174. Gohlke P, Linz W, Schölkens BA, et al. Angiotensin-converting enzyme inhibition improves cardiac function. Role of bradykinin. Hypertension 23:411-418, 1994.
175. Rhaleb N-E, Yang X-P, Scicli AG, et al. Role of kinins and nitric oxide in the antihypertrophic effect of ramipril. Hypertension 23:865-868, 1994.
176. Schölkens BA, Linz W, Martorana PA. Experimental cardiovascular benefits of angiotensin-converting enzyme inhibitors: Beyond blood pressure reduction. J Cardiovasc Pharmacol 18(Suppl 2):S26-S30, 1991.
177. Linz W, Schölkens BA. A specific B$_2$-bradykinin receptor antagonist HOE 140 abolishes the antihypertrophic effect of ramipril. Br J Pharmacol 105:771-772, 1992.
178. Fernandez LA, Twickler J, Mead A. Neovascularization produced by angiotensin II. J Lab Clin Med 105:141-145, 1985.
179. Unger T, Mattfeldt T, Lamberty V, et al. Effect of early onset angiotensin converting enzyme inhibition on myocardial capillaries. Hypertension 20:478-482, 1992.
180. Hashimoto K, Hamamoto H, Honda Y, et al. Changes in components of kinin system and hemodynamics in acute myocardial infarction. Am Heart J 95:619-626, 1978.
181. Noda K, Sasaguri M, Ideishi M, et al. Role of locally formed angiotensin II and bradykinin in the reduction of myocardial infarct size in dogs. Cardiovasc Res 27:334-340, 1993.
182. Pan H-L, Chen S-R, Scicli GM, et al. Cardiac interstitial bradykinin release during ischemia is enhanced by ischemic preconditioning. Am J Physiol Heart Circ Physiol 279:H116-H121, 2000.
183. Martorana PA, Kettenbach B, Breipohl G, et al. Reduction of infarct size by local angiotensin-converting enzyme inhibition is abolished by a bradykinin antagonist. Eur J Pharmacol 182:395-396, 1990.
184. Linz W, Wiemer G, Schölkens BA. ACE-inhibition induces NO-formation in cultured bovine endothelial cells and protects isolated ischemic rat hearts. J Mol Cell Cardiol 24:909-919, 1992.
185. Linz W, Martorana PA, Schölkens BA. Local inhibition of bradykinin degradation in ischemic hearts. J Cardiovasc Pharmacol 15 (Suppl 6):S99-S109, 1990.
186. Shimamoto K, Miura T, Miki T, et al. Activation of kinins on myocardial ischemia. Agents Actions 38:90-97, 1992.
187. Hartman JC, Wall TM, Hullinger TG, et al. Reduction of myocardial infarct size in rabbits by ramiprilat: Reversal by the bradykinin antagonist HOE 140. J Cardiovasc Pharmacol 21:996-1003, 1993.
188. Witherow FN, Helmy A, Webb DJ, et al. Bradykinin contributes to the vasodilator effects of chronic angiotensin-converting enzyme inhibition in patients with heart failure. Circulation 104:2177-2181, 2001.
189. Liu Y-H, Yang X-P, Mehta D, et al. Role of kinins in chronic heart failure and in the therapeutic effect of ACE inhibitors in kininogen-deficient rats. Am J Physiol Heart Circ Physiol 278:H507-H514, 2000.
190. Liu Y-H, Yang X-P, Sharov VG, et al. Effects of angiotensin-converting enzyme inhibitors and angiotensin II type 1

receptor antagonists in rats with heart failure: Role of kinins and angiotensin II type 2 receptors. J Clin Invest 99:1926-1935, 1997.

191. Liu Y-H, Yang X-P, Sharov VG, et al. Role of kinins, nitric oxide and prostaglandins in the protective effect of ACE inhibitors on ischemia/reperfusion myocardial infarction in rats [abstract]. Hypertension 24:380, 1994.

192. Yang X-P, Liu Y-H, Shesely EG, et al. Endothelial nitric oxide gene knockout mice. Cardiac phenotypes and the effect of angiotensin-converting enzyme inhibitor on myocardial ischemia/reperfusion injury. Hypertension 34:24-30, 1999.

193. Linz W, Wiemer G, Schölkens BA. Role of kinins in the pathophysiology of myocardial ischemia: In vitro and in vivo studies. Diabetes 45 (Suppl 1):S51-S58, 1996.

194. Rubin LE, Levi R. Protective role of bradykinin in cardiac anaphylaxis. Coronary- vasodilating and antiarrhythmic activities mediated by autocrine/paracrine mechanisms. Circ Res 76: 434-440, 1995.

195. Goto M, Liu Y, Yang X-M, et al. Role of bradykinin in protection of ischemic preconditioning in rabbit hearts. Circ Res 77:611-621, 1995.

196. Vegh A, Szekeres L, Parratt JR. Protective effects of preconditioning of the ischaemic myocardium involve cyclo-oxygenase products. Cardiovasc Res 24:1020-1023, 1990.

197. Schoelkens BA, Linz W. Bradykinin-mediated metabolic effects in isolated perfused rat hearts. Agents Actions 38(Suppl): 36-42, 1992.

198. Rett K, Wicklmayr M, Dietze GJ, et al. Insulin-induced glucose transporter (GLUT1 and GLUT4) translocation in cardiac muscle tissue is mimicked by bradykinin. Diabetes 45(Suppl 1):S66-S69, 1996.

199. Ytrehus K, Liu Y, Downey JM. Preconditioning protects ischemic rabbit heart by protein kinase C activation. Am J Physiol 266:H1145-H1152, 1994.

200. Speechly-Dick ME, Mocanu MM, Yellon DM. Protein kinase C. Its role in ischemic preconditioning in the rat. Circ Res 75:586-590, 1994.

201. Wolfrum S, Schneider K, Heidbreder M, et al. Remote preconditioning protects the heart by activating myocardial PKCe-isoform. Cardiovasc Res 55:583-589, 2002.

202. Menasché P, Kevelaitis E, Mouas C, et al. Preconditioning with potassium channel openers. A new concept for enhancing cardioplegic protection? J Thorac Cardiovasc Surg 110:1606-1613, 1995.

203. Brew EC, Mitchell MB, Rehring TF, et al. Role of bradykinin in cardiac functional protection after global ischemia-reperfusion in rat heart. Am J Physiol 269:H1370-H1378, 1995.

204. Loke KE, Curran CML, Messina EJ, et al. Role of nitric oxide in the control of cardiac oxygen consumption in $B_2$-kinin receptor knockout mice. Hypertension 34:563-567, 1999.

205. Liu Y-H, Xu J, Yang X-P, et al. Effect of ACE inhibitors and angiotensin II type 1 receptor antagonists on endothelial NO synthase knockout mice with heart failure. Hypertension 39:375-381, 2002.

206. Pfeffer MA, Braunwald E, Moyé LA, et al. Effect of captopril on mortality and morbidity in patients with left ventricular dysfunction after myocardial infarction. Results of the Survival and Ventricular Enlargement trial. N Engl J Med 327:669-677, 1992.

207. Gertz SD, Kurgan A. Tissue plasminogen activator and selective coronary vasodilation [letter]. Am J Cardiol 62:173, 1988.

208. Seyedi N, Xu X, Nasjletti A, et al. Coronary kinin generation mediates nitric oxide release after angiotensin receptor stimulation. Hypertension 26:164-170, 1995.

209. Tsutsumi Y, Matsubara H, Masaki H, et al. Angiotensin II type 2 receptor overexpression activates the vascular kinin system and causes vasodilation. J Clin Invest 104:925-935, 1999.

210. Xu J, Carretero OA, Liu Y-H, et al. Role of $AT_2$ receptors in the cardioprotective effect of $AT_1$ antagonists in mice. Hypertension 40:244-250, 2002.

211. Ferrario CM. Angiotensin-(1-7) and antihypertensive mechanisms. J Nephrol 11:278-283, 1998.

212. Freeman EJ, Chisolm GM, Ferrario CM, et al. Angiotensin-(1-7) inhibits vascular smooth muscle cell growth. Hypertension 28:104-108, 1996.

213. Ferrario CM, Averill DB, Brosnihan KB, et al. Vasopeptidase inhibition and Ang-(1-7) in the spontaneously hypertensive rat. Kidney Int 62:1349-1357, 2002.

214. Gorelik G, Carbini LA, Scicli AG. Angiotensin 1-7 induces bradykinin-mediated relaxation in porcine coronary artery. J Pharmacol Exp Ther 286:403-410, 1998.

215. Abbas A, Gorelik G, Carbini LA, et al. Angiotensin-(1-7) induces bradykinin-mediated hypotensive responses in anesthetized rats. Hypertension 30:217-221, 1997.

216. Brosnihan KB, Li P, Ferrario CM. Angiotensin-(1-7) dilates canine coronary arteries through kinins and nitric oxide. Hypertension 27:523-528, 1996.

217. Chappell MC, Gomez MN, Pirro NT, et al. Release of angiotensin-(1-7) from the rat hindlimb: influence of angiotensin-converting enzyme inhibition. Hypertension 35:348-352, 2000.

218. Chappell MC, Allred AJ, Ferrario CM. Pathways of angiotensin-(1-7) metabolism in the kidney. Nephrol Dial Transplant 16(Suppl 1):22-26, 2001.

219. Siragy HM, Inagami T, Ichiki T, et al. Sustained hypersensitivity to angiotensin II and its mechanism in mice lacking the subtype-2 ($AT_2$) angiotensin receptor. Proc Natl Acad Sci USA 96:6506-6510, 1999.

220. Carretero OA. Kinins: Local hormones in regulation of blood pressure and renal function. Choices Cardiol 7 (Suppl 1): 10-14, 1993.

# SECTION 3

# Target Organ Damage/ Cardiovascular Events

## Chapter 21

## The Concept of Total Risk

### William J. Elliott, Henry R. Black

## RISK—DEFINITIONS AND TYPES

*Webster's New Pocket Dictionary* defines *risk* as "the chance of harm, injury, etc." Risk, however, has many different meanings, depending on the context and the background and training of the user or audience. In the discipline of surgery, a person who is a "poor surgical risk" is an individual whose likelihood of death or other adverse outcome during the perioperative period is high, compared with the chance of a desirable outcome. In commerce, risk comes in at least three varieties: "Business risk" can be loosely defined as the chance that something will go wrong with an individual company, resulting in a loss. "Systemic risk" includes potential threats to an area's financial structure, which could make the entire region suffer economically. "Market risk" quantitates the probability that when one wishes to sell an asset, the proceeds will be less than expected. When the term *risk factor* was first added to the medical vocabulary by the Framingham Heart Study, its heritage, in fact, came from the financial world.

In medicine (and epidemiology, the basic science that forms the foundation for evidence-based medicine), risk is most easily defined as the proportion of previously unaffected individuals who, on average, will acquire the disease of interest during a defined period of time. Because risk is given as a proportion, it typically has no specific units, although the time period of interest is usually given in academic discussions. For short-term changes in health status (e.g., intensive-care unit medicine), the time period of interest is usually minutes, hours, or days. For longer-term evaluations of disease emergence, the time period of interest is often measured in years or decades.

Risk comes in two basic types: *absolute risk*—the definition of which is essentially the same as risk, as given previously, except that the time frame is *always* included; and *relative risk*, which is essentially a ratio of the risks for a group of interest, compared with another "control" group. A variant of relative risk is *attributable risk*, which is the amount or proportion of disease that can be said to be associated with exposure to a particular factor; its use is more common if there are "competing risks" (more than one factor being evaluated, to be discussed shortly).

Perhaps the easiest way to illustrate the difference between absolute and relative risk is in the context of a clinical trial. In the 1980s, there was still debate as to whether older people with "isolated systolic hypertension" (defined, at that time as systolic blood pressure [SBP] ≥160 mm Hg, but a normal diastolic blood pressure [DBP], <90 mm Hg) should be given antihypertensive medications. There was concern not only that there would be few, if any, benefits, but also that the side effects of the drugs would be more troublesome to older people, in whom the typical elevation in SBP may be only a result of "stiffer" arteries. The Systolic Hypertension in the Elderly Program (SHEP) therefore enrolled 4736 people aged 60 years or older, in normal sinus rhythm, with blood pressures (BPs) in the range of 160 to 209/<90 mm Hg, and randomly allocated 2365 of them to treatment, beginning with 12.5 mg/day of chlorthalidone.[1] The other 2371 people received placebo tablets, but were allowed to begin open-label treatment during follow-up if one of several prespecified criteria was met. The primary outcome measure was fatal or nonfatal stroke, but other cardiovascular endpoints, including coronary heart disease (CHD) and heart failure, were also collected. The study, on average, lasted 4.5 years. At the completion of the study, there were 106 fatal or nonfatal strokes in the treatment group, as compared with 159 in the group originally assigned placebo.[1] The absolute risk of fatal or nonfatal stroke, therefore, in the placebo-treated group was 159 strokes/2371 people allocated to placebo treatment/4.5 years of follow-up, or approximately 1.5% per year. The absolute risk of fatal or nonfatal stroke in the actively treated group was, analogously 106 strokes/2365 people allocated to active treatment/4.5 years of follow-up, or approximately 1.0% per year. The relative risk of fatal or nonfatal stroke for the actively treated group, compared with those who were initially given placebo, can be estimated as the ratio of these two absolute risks: 106/2365:159/2371, or 0.668. The relative risk reduction in fatal or nonfatal stroke, calculated by this method, would therefore be 0.332, or 33.2%. This simple estimate compares rather favorably with the 36% calculated by the more complex proportional hazards model (which takes into account the incidence of stroke over the entire time of follow-up that is ignored in the simple risk ratio calculated previously).[1]

It is interesting and important to contrast estimates of absolute and relative risk reduction. In the previous example, the relative risk reduction in stroke, for actively treated versus placebo-treated people in SHEP, was about 33% to 36% (depending on the method used for its calculation). The *absolute risk reduction*, however, was the difference between the two groups' absolute risk estimates: 1.490% to 0.996% per year, or about 0.494% per year. Headline writers and many physicians are much more easily impressed with relative risk reduction estimates, because these are somewhat better understood by most lay people, and are often easier to remember.[2] However, there are good reasons to consider, and perhaps even to prefer, absolute risk reduction estimates. Because relative risk estimates always require reference to a specific "con-

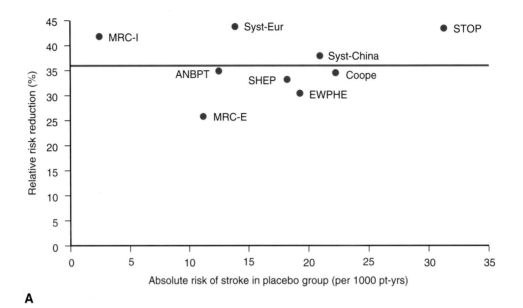

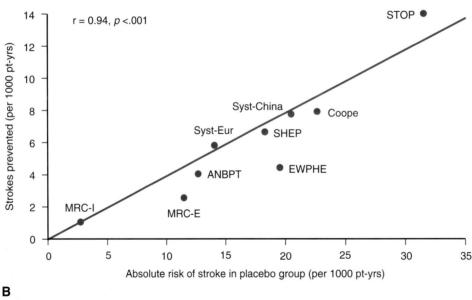

**Figure 21–1** Relationships between absolute risk of stroke (calculated as the stroke rate per 1000 patient-years in the control group, either placebo or no treatment) and **(A)** the relative risk reduction of stroke with active treatment compared with control; and **(B)** the absolute risk difference between active treatment and control (equivalent to the number of strokes prevented per 1000 patient-years by antihypertensive drug therapy). Each circle represents a single clinical trial. Abbreviations: MRC-I, Medical Research Council Trial in Mild Hypertension[8]; MRC-E, Medical Research Council Trial in Older Adults[72]; ANBPT, Australian National Blood Pressure Trial[73]; Syst-Eur, Systolic Hypertension Trial in Europe[74]; SHEP, Systolic Hypertension in the Elderly Program[1]; EWPHE, European Working Party on Hypertension in the Elderly[75]; Syst-China, Systolic Hypertension Trial in China[76]; Coope, Coope and Warrender[77]; STOP, Swedish Trial in Old Patients with Hypertension.[7] (Updated from The sixth report of the Joint National Committee on Prevention, Detection, Evaluation, and Treatment of High Blood Pressure (JNC VI). Arch Intern Med 157:2413-2446, 1997 and Lever AF, Ramsay LE. Treatment of hypertension in the elderly. J Hypertens 13:571-579, 1995).

trol group," such estimates tend to be somewhat less useful across time, particularly as the science of medicine evolves. For example, the relative risk estimate for drug treatment of "isolated systolic hypertension" is not of great interest today, because most physicians, an important meta-analysis,[3] and all guidelines since 1993 agree that such treatment is desirable and should be routine. Additionally, neither group in SHEP received intensive drug treatment for dyslipidemia, despite the fact that most eligible people with isolated systolic hypertension today would be recommended to receive it. Such treatment would likely decrease the relative risk reduction for stroke that could be attributed to antihypertensive drug treatment, because a meta-analysis of 3-hydroxy-3-methyl-glutaryl-coenzyme A reductase treatment suggests a relative risk reduction of about 24% in primary stroke prevention.[4]

A further positive attribute of absolute risk is that it can be easily compared across studies; this is particularly easy and appropriate when all studies are placebo-controlled. Figure 21–1, *A*, shows a plot of the relative risk reduction for stroke (on the y-axis) across many clinical trials in hypertension, indexed to the absolute risk of stroke (on the x-axis) for the population studied.

These data show that the relative risk reduction for stroke for nearly all trials was typically about 36% ± 6% (mean ± standard deviation). Although this is perhaps useful and interesting, a meta-analysis would probably provide a more precise assessment of the pooled point estimate. Alternatively, focusing on the absolute risk difference, Figure 21–1, *B*, shows the number of strokes prevented (on the y-axis), indexed as before to the absolute risk of stroke (on the x-axis). This graph illustrates the very powerful effect of "risk stratification" for individual patients,[5] and also shows why estimates of risk are very important to decisions regarding therapy.[6] For example, giving antihypertensive drug therapy to the much older patients in the Swedish Trial of Old Patients with Hypertension (STOP-Hypertension)[7] prevents approximately 14 strokes per 1000 patient-years of treatment. This would be a much more cost-effective use of medications than giving similar antihypertensive drug therapy to the much younger patients (age 35-64 years old) in the first Medical Research Council (MRC-I)[8] trial, which observed approximately one stroke saved for every 1000 patient-years of therapy. This observation is also consistent with the adage, "One cannot prevent a stroke that isn't likely to occur."

Another major advantage of the absolute risk estimate (over relative risk) is that it can easily be tied to the "NNT" (number needed to treat), which provides an overall estimate of the effectiveness of an intervention.[5] Simply put, the NNT is an estimate of the number of people who would need to be treated with the studied regimen to prevent a *single* outcome of interest. The NNT is simply the reciprocal of the absolute risk difference: For SHEP, the 1-year NNT is 1/0.494 or about 202. This suggests that one fatal or nonfatal stroke would be prevented by the antihypertensive drug treatment regimen used in SHEP for each 202 individuals treated for 1 year. Because most antihypertensive drug studies (and indeed SHEP) gathered data for nearly 5 years, it is more traditional to present the 5-year NNT data; for SHEP, the 5-year NNT shrinks to 40.

Another variant of risk that is most useful in large populations where there are competing risk factors is *attributable risk*. For example, many conditions influence the future risk of stroke, including the presence or absence of atrial fibrillation, hypertension, smoking habit, dyslipidemia, and possibly over-weight/obesity. The relative importance of each of these factors can be most easily apportioned using a completely untreated population (e.g., the Framingham Heart Study). Discerning a significant risk reduction can be difficult in treated populations, because the overall risk for the event of interest can be reduced by therapy, leading to an incorrect estimate of the risk attributable to one or more other risk factors. Perhaps the best recent example of this was the Anglo-Scandinavian Cardiac Outcomes Trial (ASCOT), in which (in a 2 × 2 factorial design) two active antihypertensive treatment regimens were compared, while simultaneously atorvastatin was compared with placebo, in the prevention of fatal or nonfatal myocardial infarction (MI).[9] Fortunately, the degree of BP lowering was not significantly different across the two randomized groups (atorvastatin vs. placebo). This allowed the investigators to estimate the relative risk reduction for fatal or nonfatal MI attributable to atorvastatin at 36% (95% confidence interval: 17%-50%, $p = .0005$), without interference from the effect of BP lowering.[10] Most studies are not as fortunate, and therefore most estimates of attributable risk must be understood in the context of the degree of treatment of other risk factors, and the potential interaction of the two or more risk factors and their treatment. Within a given large population, the population-attributable risk (PAR) takes into account not only the relative risk for an endpoint, but also the prevalence of the potential risk factor within the population (or proportion of cases with the endpoint exposed to the factor). For example, a recent publication from the Framingham Heart Study suggested that the PAR for overweight, as a possible risk factor for stroke, in men was significant, at about 15%.[11]

## TOTAL RISK

Statistical evaluations of risk factors must necessarily consider *only* clearly defined endpoints, for example, stroke, CHD, end-stage renal disease (ESRD), or "cardiovascular events" (which has been variably defined). As a result, what constitutes "total risk" depends somewhat on one's perspective. Because medicine tends to be fragmented, with specialists usually focusing on one specific organ or disease, little attention is routinely given to statistical evaluations that encompass *all* diseases commonly associated with common interdisciplinary conditions, such as hypertension. Thus, hypertension is a well-known risk factor for stroke, CHD, heart failure, and ESRD. Because stroke tends to be the province of neurologists, CHD is studied most intensively by cardiologists, and ESRD is of greatest interest to nephrologists, these hypertension-associated endpoints tend to be segmented when statistical evaluations of risk factors and risk assessments are performed.

As with attributable risk, population-based data often help define total risk. Projections were that, in the United States in 2003, a first diagnosis of CHD would be made in more than 650,000, stroke in more than 500,000, and ESRD in nearly 100,000 people.[12] Preliminary national vital statistics data (derived from death certificates) from 2001 show that heart disease accounted for 28.9%, stroke for 6.7%, and nephritis (a category that includes many types of renal disease) for about 1.6% of the 2,4017,798 deaths,[13] but these data probably underestimate mortality resulting from renal disease, because dialysis patients most often die from heart disease.[12] In the Framingham Heart Study, in participants younger than 75 years, CHD consistently accounted for more than half of the cardiovascular events from 1948 to 1998, whereas stroke incidence markedly decreased during this time period. Framingham cannot provide meaningful information about ESRD, because their original population included only 5209 people. Even using the 1999 nationwide incidence of ESRD, fewer than two of their original participants should have required dialysis or renal transplantation.

There is increasing interest in the use of risk equations to guide public policy, which depends not only on the rates of disease emergence, but the cost of each episode. U.S. national data estimate the per-patient cost of therapy for ESRD ($54,917/year for dialysis, $51,096/year for renal transplantation)[14] much higher than for heart disease ($11,273 per hospitalization for MI, and $5501 per hospitalization for heart failure) or stroke ($5955 per hospitalization for stroke).[12] Because the incidence of ESRD has grown steadily while the rates for heart disease and stroke have declined since 1980, there is much interest from federal and other authorities to find quantitative methods for estimating the risk for combined cardiovascular and renal disease. Some authors have concluded that, on an economic basis, risk assessment is too labor- and laboratory-intensive for application to the entire population, and should be limited to demographic groups with an inherently higher risk (e.g., older people).[15] The National Institutes of Health is currently exploring ways to combine other longitudinal data (from sources such as the Cardiovascular Health Study[16] and the Atherosclerosis Risk in Communities study[17]) with those from the Framingham Heart Study (which included no minority participants) to provide a more universally accepted risk equation for the U.S. population.

Rather than generating a single risk equation that encompasses both cardiovascular and renal endpoints, most recent efforts have focused on risk prediction scores for cardiovascular events (which include MI, heart failure, stroke, and other cardiovascular disease–related deaths).[18] There are many reasons for this, including the fact that many risk factors other than hypertension impact the risk of both cardiovascular and renal endpoints, but with different weights. Probably the two best examples are the degree of microalbuminuria and/or proteinuria,[19,20] and serum creatinine concentration, which is probably the best single predictor of ESRD, but a relatively insensitive and nonspecific predictor of cardiovascular events.[21] Estimated glomerular filtration rate (which incorporates serum creatinine concentration[22]), however, has been shown to be a powerful predictor of both renal and cardiovascular endpoints.[23]

## COMPETING RISKS

One of the basic tenets of modern statistical methods is the strict minimization of bias. In general, individuals who have already suffered an endpoint (e.g., a first MI) are at significantly higher risk for a second endpoint of a similar nature (e.g., a second MI, which is about 2 to 4 times more likely than in individuals without such a prior history). The best and most widely accepted way to avoid this sort of bias in risk assessment is to simply use the time-to-first event methodology (e.g., Kaplan-Meier life-table analyses) and "censor" (or ignore) all events that occur subsequent to the first one. Although this has a major advantage in statistical modeling, it leads to underestimates of the incidence of major adverse events, especially

cardiovascular events. Whereas ESRD is typically encountered only once in any given person's lifetime, MIs, strokes, and hospitalizations for heart failure can (and do) recur.

The issue of "competing risks" is particularly important when attempting to integrate cardiovascular and renal event data into a single risk equation. As noted previously, there are multiple risk factors that are shared by the two types of events, including age, gender, and BP. Serum creatinine concentration, probably the best predictor of the need for renal replacement therapy, has been associated with a significantly higher risk of cardiovascular events in several datasets.[21,24-27] Some of this association can be attributed to the elevated creatinine being a result of poorly controlled hypertension, which itself increases cardiovascular risk.[28] In addition, ESRD itself is an independent risk factor for cardiovascular events and cardiovascular death: ESRD patients have an 80% 1-year mortality after MI, compared with about 10% in the non-ESRD population.[29] People on dialysis or who have had a kidney transplant have an increased propensity to infection, a predisposition to cancer inherent to immunosuppressants, and a continued risk of the disease that brought them to renal replacement therapy (most commonly diabetes in the United States). Despite these risks, nearly half of the Americans with ESRD disease die of cardiovascular disease (CVD). In the 2001 death registry maintained by the U.S. Renal Data Systems (which includes all individuals in the United States whose ESRD treatment is funded through Medicare or Medicaid), 43.7% died from a cardiac cause, and another 5.2% succumbed to a stroke.[14]

A further confounder of any attempt to integrate both cardiovascular and renal risk into a single equation is potential differential effects of treatment. Theoretically, any treatment that delays a fatal MI or stroke is likely to increase the chance that the patient will live long enough to develop ESRD. Similarly, a therapy that delays the time to ESRD may lengthen life sufficiently so that an MI or stroke may occur. Another potential concern is the possibility of a treatment that may significantly decrease the risk of ESRD, but increase the risk of cardiovascular events. This phenomenon may have been observed in the Irbesartan Diabetic Nephropathy Trial (IDNT), in which the angiotensin II receptor antagonist irbesartan significantly reduced the primary renal endpoint (doubling of serum creatinine, ESRD, or death) compared with amlodipine, by 23% ($p = .006$).[30] There were no significant differences between these two randomized treatment groups in the composite secondary outcome that included cardiovascular events, but the nonsignificant trends favored amlodipine over irbesartan for cardiovascular death (relative risk reduction of 26%), MI (35%), and stroke (35%).[31]

## INTERRELATION OF TYPES OF CARDIOVASCULAR RISK

Probably the simplest type of quantitative risk assessment should be based on cardiovascular death as the endpoint, because this would preclude some of the issues related to competing risks discussed previously. A method for calculating the 5-year risk of cardiovascular death has been derived from eight clinical trials involving 47,088 patients followed for a mean of 5.2 years, and resulting in 1639 deaths.[32] The small proportion of people who die (which limits statistical power) can be overcome by longer follow-up.[33] Although cardiovascular death is gaining favor as the preferred endpoint among European epidemiologists, health economists and policymakers (especially in the United States) object, because it would ignore any and all expensive and debilitating events that precede death.

A second logical endpoint is all cardiovascular events, which include CHD events and stroke. Some authors prefer to include heart failure among the CHD events, but others restrict it to fatal and nonfatal MI. This endpoint is particularly favored (over CHD alone) by many groups interested in hypertension treatment, because BP lowering reduces stroke more (in terms of relative risk, about 36%) than CHD (about 18%-21%) in nearly all clinical trials. In most Western hypertension clinical trials, CHD events account for about 75% of the cardiovascular events; in most studies performed in China and older studies in Japan, stroke comprises a higher proportion of the total events. Several recent comparisons of various risk estimators suggest that a cutoff of CVD risk ≥20% over 10 years is roughly equivalent to a CHD risk ≥15% over 10 years.[34,35]

The most common endpoint for Western risk assessment has become CHD events. Although this endpoint ignores stroke, it lends itself readily to a discussion not only of the potential benefits of antihypertensive drug therapy, but also aspirin and lipid-lowering agents. An obvious disadvantage of using this method is the fact that CHD displays wide (but predictable) variability across regions and countries that is not easily explained by differences in the prevalence of the usual CHD risk factors.[36] Thus a person with the same set of risk factors will typically have markedly different risk for CHD in Italy compared with Finland[37]; this has proven to be a major challenge for groups trying to develop a single overall risk estimator for all of Europe.[6,38-40]

## CURRENT CARDIOVASCULAR RISK ASSESSMENT TOOLS

Perhaps because of the difficulty in integrating both cardiovascular and renal risk in a single risk equation, most recent authors have focused on developing, testing, and comparing risk assessment algorithms for cardiovascular (most especially cardiac) events. The algorithms that have been used vary in complexity from simply counting the existing risk factors[41] to complex equations (derived from a Weibull accelerated failure

**Table 21-1** Some Methods of Estimating Risk

| Model | Population Studied | Risk Factors Included | Validated? |
|---|---|---|---|
| Framingham Heart Study* | About 11,332 residents of Framingham, MA | Age, gender, SBP and DBP; total, LDL and HDL cholesterol; diabetes; smoking | Widely |
| Cardiovascular Disease Life Expectancy Model | 3700 men and women from USA and Canada, aged 35-74 (from Lipid Research Clinics follow-up cohort) | Age, gender, mean BP, total and HDL cholesterol, diabetes, smoking, cardiovascular disease | Yes |
| Munster Heart Study | 4400 German men and women, aged 40-65 (workplace-based) | Age, SBP, total and HDL cholesterol, diabetes, smoking, family history, angina symptoms | Not in women |
| British Regional Heart Study Risk Function | 7735 men aged 40-59 (general practitioner-based) | Mean BP, total cholesterol, diabetes, smoking, family history, angina symptoms | No |
| Dundee Coronary Risk Disk | 5203 men aged 40-59 (UK Heart Disease Prevention Project) | Total cholesterol, SBP, smoking | Not in women |
| New Zealand Guidelines* | Based on Framingham equation | Age, gender, diabetes, smoking, SBP, DBP, total:HDL cholesterol ratio | No |
| Joint British Societies Risk Tables* | Based on Framingham equation, modified with epidemiologic data from Britain | Age, gender, diabetes, smoking, SBP, total:HDL cholesterol ratio, family history | Yes |
| European Society of Cardiology Tables* | Based on Framingham equation, modified with epidemiologic data from Europe | Age, gender | Yes |
| Sheffield Tables* | Based on Framingham equation, modified with epidemiologic data from Scotland | Age, gender, total:HDL cholesterol ratio, hypertension, smoking, diabetes, LVH on ECG, family history of CHD | Yes |

*Denotes models that are discussed more fully in text. SBP, systolic blood pressure; DBP, diastolic blood pressure; BP, blood pressure; LDL, low-density lipoprotein; HDL, high-density lipoprotein; LVH, left ventricular hypertrophy; ECG, electrocardiogram; CHD, coronary heart disease.

regression model).[42] Some of these, and the populations from which they have been derived, are summarized in Table 21–1.

## Counting Risk Factors

The simplest type of risk assessment is probably the one recommended by the sixth Report of the Joint National Committee on Prevention, Detection, Evaluation, and Treatment of High Blood Pressure (JNC VI).[41] In this scheme, people were divided into three broad categories of risk (A, B, or C). Risk Group A, which is defined without mention of any threshold of absolute risk, are those without any of the traditional cardiovascular risk factors, target organ damage related to hypertension, or concomitant CVD. These very-low-risk individuals include only premenopausal women and comprised only 9% of the hypertensive population in the National Health and Nutrition Examination Survey (NHANES) I Epidemiological Follow-up Study.[43] The majority (nearly 72%) of the hypertensive population had one or more risk factors for CVD, but no diabetes, target organ damage, or concomitant CVD, and were placed in Risk Group B. The highest-risk group (Risk Group C) with either diabetes, evidence of target organ damage, or concomitant CVD, accounted for 19.2% of the NHANES sample. After correcting for regression-dilution bias, Ogden et al. calculated that the number of people needed to be treated for 10 years to prevent a CVD death ranged from 34 to 486 (Risk Group A) to 11 to 21 (Risk Group C), with the higher numbers associated with the lower levels of BP.

JNC VI recommended using this simple system to decide on the intensity and type of initial treatment for high-normal and high BP. Unless the initial BP exceeded 180/110 mm Hg, only lifestyle modifications were recommended for people in Risk Groups A and B; the latter were to receive them for a shorter time before drugs should be started. Both antihypertensive drug therapy and lifestyle modifications were initially recommended for people in Risk Group C.

The obvious advantage of this simple system was that it is easy to use. It did not require a computer or access to complex figures or tables. The authors of JNC VI were not concerned with making precise estimates of cardiovascular risk, but instead focusing attention on hypertensive individuals whose overall risk was very low or very high, independent of the BP level. However, the specificity of the JNC VI risk stratification system, when compared with the most recent Framingham risk equation, in a group of 202 people representative of a Scottish population, was only 9%.[35] This would presumably lead to drug treatment for a high number of people, many of whom are unlikely to benefit from it (in terms of cardiovascular event protection). Another potential disadvantage of the JNC VI risk stratification system was the inclusion of age (the most important risk factor for cardiovascular events) only as a dichotomous variable (older or younger than 60 years); this probably accounted for much of the low specificity. The JNC VI scheme is still the only risk stratification system that includes postmenopausal status as a cardiovascular risk factor for women. As with the World Health Organization/International Society of Hypertension (WHO/ISH) guidelines discussed next, JNC VI counted a family history of premature CVD (first-degree female relatives younger than age 65, or men younger than age 55); this is mentioned only as a footnote in other risk estimators.

The risk stratification scheme published in 1999 as part of the WHO/ISH guidelines included more detail than, but was similar to, the JNC VI risk stratification method.[44] One major difference was that there were four categories of risk: low, medium, high, or very high. These corresponded rather generally to categories of absolute risk of CVD over 10 years: <15%, 15% to 20%, 20% to 30%, and >30%, respectively. Low-risk people included men younger than 55 years of age and women younger than 65 years of age with grade 1 hypertension (140-159/90-99 mm Hg) and no other cardiovascular risk factors, target organ damage, diabetes, or associated clinical conditions (existing CVD). Medium-risk individuals included grade 1 hypertensives with one or two other risk factors, or grade 2 hypertensives (160-179/100-109 mm Hg) with zero to two other risk factors, but again no target organ damage, diabetes, or associated clinical conditions. High-risk people had either grade 3 hypertension (≥180/≥110 mm Hg) and no other risk factors, or grade 1 or 2 hypertension and three or more risk factors, or target organ damage or diabetes. People with associated clinical conditions were all very high risk, as were grade 3 hypertensives with one or more risk factors, target organ damage, or diabetes. The WHO/ISH risk stratification system therefore went somewhat beyond a simple counting of risk factors, but relied heavily on the counted number to categorize hypertensive people according to their need for therapy. Not surprisingly, this slightly more complex method was superior to the simple JNC VI stratification scheme, especially in correctly estimating risk for low-risk hypertensives.[35] Two potential disadvantages of the WHO/ISH risk stratification system were its complexity and unclear relationship to treatment; even today, most practicing doctors do not take the time to count the risk factors and classify individual patients, before starting antihypertensive drug therapy.

The seventh report of the Joint National Committee on Prevention, Detection, Evaluation, and Treatment of High Blood Pressure (JNC 7) does not provide much information about formal risk assessment of hypertensive patients.[45,46] It does recommend a thiazide-type diuretic for most patients with stage 1 hypertension, and a two-drug combination for most patients with stage 2 hypertension, but it omits a discussion of examining a patient's BP in the context of other risk factors and the global cardiovascular risk. Perhaps the most important reason for this was previous recommendation of the National Cholesterol Education Panel's III Adult Treatment Panel for physicians to use, in everyday clinical practice, a modified Framingham equation to estimate absolute risk of CHD.[47] The Executive Committee also wished to focus attention on hypertension per se and to avoid potential differences of opinion with other guidelines committees for the United States, including a proposal to consolidate recommendations across many healthcare advocacy groups (including the National Heart, Lung, and Blood Institute; National High Blood Pressure Education Program; National Cholesterol Education Program; American Diabetes Association; and National Kidney Foundation). A second important reason for omitting a discussion of risk stratification was that only when stratification leads to differential treatment strategies does it really impact on clinical practice. Because JNC 7 recommends antihypertensive drug treatment for all hypertensives (≥140/≥90 mm Hg) and all those with "compelling indications" for a specific drug or drug class, there was little to be gained by refocusing attention on global cardiovascular risk assessment that would not change the existing treatment plan.

The 1999 risk stratification system of the WHO/ISH has been updated by the European Society of Hypertension (ESH) and European Society of Cardiology (ESC).[48] This extensive document now provides five levels of risk, based on an interaction of the untreated BP level and the presence or absence of risk factors, target organ damage, or associated clinical conditions. The "average risk" individual has either "normal" (120-129/80-84 mm Hg) or "high-normal" (130-139/85-89 mm Hg) BPs and no other risk factors (which now include both abdominal waist circumference and C-reactive protein[49]). "Low added risk" includes individuals with no other risk factors and grade 1 hypertension (140-159/90-99 mm Hg) or one to two risk factors and either normal or high-normal BPs. "Moderate added risk" includes people with grade 2 hypertension (160-179/100-109 mm Hg) and no other risk factors; grade 1 or 2 hypertension with one to two risk factors; or normal BPs and three or more risk factors, tar-

get organ damage, or diabetes. Individuals with "high added risk" include grade 3 hypertension (≥180/≥110 mm Hg) and no other risk factors; three or more risk factors, target organ damage, or diabetes and either high-normal BP or grade 1 or 2 hypertension; and normal BP and established CVD. Everyone with established CVD with a BP >130/85 mm Hg is at "very high added risk," according to the new ESH/ESC guidelines. The need for immediate drug treatment of hypertension is tied loosely to the risk category. Individuals at high or very high added risk begin drug treatment promptly; those at moderate added risk are to be monitored closely for at least 3 months and treated if the individual so desires or remains persistently hypertensive. Interestingly, and perhaps uniquely, the new ESH/ESC guidelines recommend withholding antihypertensive drug therapy for at least 3 months from a 64-year-old female smoker with dyslipidemia (or any other individual with two risk factors) and a BP of up to 179/109 mm Hg. Because the ESH/ESC risk stratification system is so new, formal evaluations of its predictive value have not yet been undertaken.

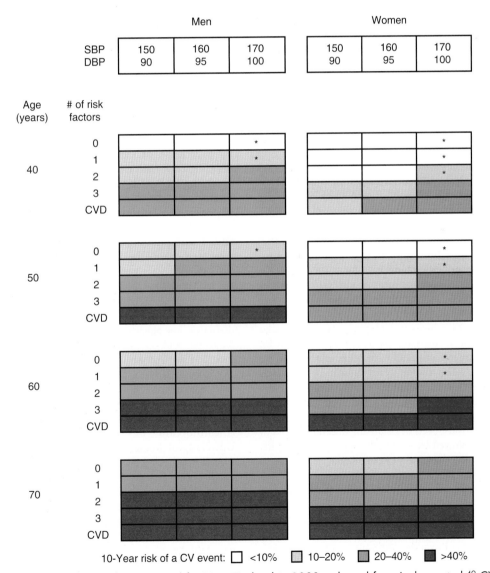

**Figure 21-2** Risk stratification algorithm proposed for New Zealand in 1993, adapted from Jackson et al.[49] CV, cardiovascular; CVD, (existing) cardiovascular disease. The asterisk (*) indicates groups with low absolute risk for whom treatment is nonetheless recommended.

## Counting Risk Factors and Stratification by Age

In 1993, a group of physicians in New Zealand broke new ground in considering risk for hypertensive patients and recommended that treatment generally be initiated only for hypertensive individuals (defined then as BP ≥150/90 mm Hg) whose absolute cardiovascular risk exceeded 20% in 10 years (Figure 21–2).[50] They suggested that the threshold for hypertension treatment should not be based only on the level of BP, but instead on absolute risk of CVD. These novel proposals, as intended, have been debated widely, but have resulted in several refinements (discussed in the following paragraphs) that have been generally widely accepted in Europe, and to a lesser extent in the United States; they have been updated in 2000.[51]

The original New Zealand treatment guidelines departed somewhat from their intended goal, in that they recommended antihypertensive drug therapy for all with initial BPs higher than 170/100 mm Hg. According to their calculations, 40- to 59-year-old men with zero to one risk factor(s) and 40- to 60-year-old women with zero to two risk factor(s) have an absolute risk lower than the recommended threshold (>20% risk of CVD in 10 years), yet these individuals should still receive drug therapy (see asterisks in Figure 21–2). The New Zealand authors chose cutpoints for BP that were different from other guidelines: 150/90, 160/95, and 170/100 mm Hg. Epidemiologic data indicate that cardiovascular risk increases continuously, from a BP <115/75 mm Hg,[52] but the New Zealand guidelines ignore these lower levels of BP. Like the Framingham group, the New Zealand authors prepared separate risk tables for each gender, a practice that has become common. Unlike American guidelines, the New Zealand group included obesity (body mass index >30 kg/m$^2$) and the ratio of total:high-density lipoprotein (HDL) cholesterol (>6:1) as risk factors. Their definition of a positive family history is somewhat more conservative than that used in JNC VI, because both male and female relatives must have had a CVD event before age 55.

Despite these differences from simpler risk estimators, the New Zealand guidelines still merely *count* cardiovascular risk factors, without giving each one a specific weight. For example, diabetes and a family history of premature cardiovascular events are equivalent in this strategy, which may account for its poorer performance compared with other, more complex risk estimators.[35,53] The major contribution of the New Zealand group was to stratify the risk calculation by age and gender and to recommend treatment only for those whose absolute CVD risk exceeded a given threshold. Their approach of displaying the various levels of risk using different colors or patterns has been followed by many other groups, to simplify the results of sometimes complex calculations.

There is some reluctance, particularly in the United States, to rely on these (more complex) estimates of cardiovascular risk as a guide to treatment. First, it takes time and effort to compile the required data for each patient and to perform the calculation, even with web-based resources or personal digital assistants. Unless it was linked to reimbursement, busy practitioners would likely find this exercise to be an inconvenience and a waste of time for patients' return office visits. A second challenge derives from biologic variability and medicolegal risk. Although today's risk estimators can provide a reason-able "guess" of an individual's absolute risk of a CVD or CHD event, there is sufficient variability in the estimate that even complex equations may result in an inexact and incorrect prediction.[54] There is a finite possibility that an individual with a calculated "low-risk" of a cardiovascular event, who avoids treatment, will suffer such an event. If the decision not to treat is based solely or primarily on the risk score, it will be difficult to mount a successful defense about the withholding of antihypertensive treatment, if the prevailing local standard is to treat every hypertensive person with drug therapy.

## Tables Using Weighted Coefficients for Risk Factors

Several different groups have issued tables that are similar to those of the New Zealand guidelines. The most important and most heavily studied of these are from the ESC, the Joint British Societies (JBS), and Sheffield, England.

The ESC has published a set of guidelines for prevention of CHD.[55] These guidelines include a risk estimator that is based on prior work of the Framingham Heart Study, but which uses weightings for each of the risk factors that are derived from epidemiologic data from Europe (especially Northern Europe). The ESC risk estimator uses total serum cholesterol and assumes a constant HDL cholesterol of 1.0 mm/L (39 mg/dl). As might be expected, this model gives overall results that are similar to those provided by the Framingham risk equation, with perhaps slightly less specificity for American patients.[56]

In 1998, the JBS (Cardiac, Hyperlipidaemia, Hypertension, and Diabetes) met and agreed on a set of recommendations for prevention of CHD.[57] Their risk estimator, a modified Framingham risk equation that weighs each risk factor according to British national data, has several forms, which originated at the University of Manchester. For the practicing physician, the equations are "simplified" into a set of colored tables. Unlike other similar tables, in which every box in the table (corresponding to a set of risk factors) has a single risk level (and color), the JBS tables often have boxes that contain two colors. This is presumably useful in identifying individuals with risk that is intermediate between the cutoff levels (<15%, 15%-30%, or >30% risk of CHD over 10 years). There are two separate tables, one for diabetics and another for nondiabetics. The age groups are categorized as 35 to 44, 45 to 54, 55 to 64, and 65 to 74 years. The other major risk factors included are smoking habit ("which should reflect lifetime exposure to tobacco and not simply tobacco at the time of risk assessment"[57]), SBP, and total:HDL cholesterol ratio. A somewhat more complex "Cardiac Risk Assessor" (which includes DBP and left ventricular hypertrophy [LVH] by electrocardiogram [ECG]) has also been developed at the University of Manchester and is available on the Internet.[58] The JBS tables[35] and computer program[59] have been tested against other risk estimators, with reasonably good results.

Investigators from Sheffield, England have published and been very active in testing a series of tables, the most recent of which is based on the Framingham equations, supplemented by data from the 1995 Scottish health survey.[60] Their new tables (one for men, another for women) use age and total:HDL cholesterol ratio (with 22 choices for men, 18 for women), and dichotomize hypertension (defined as ≥140/90 mm Hg, or taking treatment), smoking, and diabetes. With a few modifications (e.g., doubling of risk with LVH on ECG, increasing age by 6 years if family history of premature CHD), these tables have been reasonably well validated.[34,35] Some physicians and nurses have found the Sheffield tables difficult to use,[61] and they do not address levels of risk different from the 15% and 30% risk of CHD over 10 years.[59] Surprisingly, the Sheffield investigators indicated that the actual level of BP (treated or untreated) affected overall risk of CHD only slightly; this is why their tables dichotomize hypertension as being present or not. This approach differs, in this respect, from many others, and from the data on more than 1 million people in 61 observational studies indicating that the risk for coronary and cerebrovascular mortality doubles for each 20/10–mm Hg increase in BP over 115/75 mm Hg.[52]

## Framingham Risk Equations

The Framingham Heart Study has published several equations that are useful in risk estimation, but are, of their very nature, quite complex.[42,62] Although derived from 5541 men and 5791 women, mostly white, who lived in Framingham, Massachusetts (the original Framingham cohort who survived until 1971, and their spouses or offspring, aged 35 to 74 years), the Framingham equations have been found to be useful in other populations, including minorities and people from other countries.[17,56,63-65] The Framingham risk score has also been used to standardize cardiovascular risk (as a single baseline covariate) across randomized treatment groups in the LIFE (Losartan Intervention for Endpoint reduction) study.[66]

The Framingham risk equations have been greatly simplified by means of a scoring system that allows each risk factor to be rated and a composite score to be calculated, which is proportional to the 10-year risk of CHD.[42] This was the approach chosen by the National Cholesterol Education Program's Adult Treatment Panel III, which included an even more simplified version of this scoring system as the final page of its Executive Summary.[47]

**Box 21–1** Tests That May Improve Prediction of Risk for Cardiovascular Disease

**Serum Markers**
High-sensitivity C-reactive protein, homocysteine, fibrinogen, lipoprotein(a)

**Imaging Studies**
Electron-beam computed tomography of the coronary arteries; magnetic resonance imaging of heart, brain, and major blood vessels; B-mode ultrasound of carotid arteries

**Physiologic Studies**
Pulse-wave velocity in radial artery, treadmill and other types of exercise testing, ankle-brachial index

**Blood Pressure Specific**
Ambulatory blood pressure (BP) monitoring data; nocturnal versus daytime BPs, urinary albumin:creatinine ratio

## FUTURE METHODS FOR RISK ESTIMATION

As epidemiologists continue to identify new risk factors for CVD, these may be incorporated into newer equations that improve the accuracy of (and maybe even simplify) such calculations.[67] Box 21–1 is a partial list of these, some of which (e.g., high-sensitivity C-reactive protein[48,49]) have already been incorporated into risk stratification systems. It is likely, however, that new equations will not ignore the "classical" risk factors, including hypertension.[68] Two papers have reexamined the decades-old allegation that less than half the people hospitalized with an acute coronary syndrome have even one established risk factor; both studies have shown that the true prevalence of "risk factor–free" individuals who develop coronary events (including coronary death) is probably 5% to 15%.[69,70]

## SUMMARY

Although the concept of "total risk" is attractive, there are few well-validated methods of estimating a composite of both cardiovascular and renal risk in hypertensive patients. Many methods exist for computing short-term (e.g., 10-year) risk for CHD (typically defined as fatal or nonfatal MI and new-onset angina pectoris). The most well-known of these is the Framingham risk score. Whether any of these risk estimators (with all their complexity), novel genetic markers, and/or risk equations based on genomic techniques will lead to more cost-effective risk stratification and better use of limited healthcare resources remains to be seen.

## References

1. Prevention of stroke by antihypertensive drug treatment in older persons with isolated systolic hypertension. Final results of the Systolic Hypertension in the Elderly Program (SHEP). SHEP Cooperative Research Group. JAMA 265:3255-3264, 1991.
2. Bucher HC, Weinbacher M, Gyr K. Influence of method of reporting study results on decisions of physicians to prescribe drugs to lower cholesterol concentration. BMJ 309:761-764, 1994.
3. Staessen JA, Gasowski J, Wang JG, et al. Risks of untreated and treated isolated systolic hypertension in the elderly: Meta-analysis of outcome trials. Lancet 355:865-872, 2000.
4. Sirol M, Bouzamondo A, Sanchez P, et al. [Does statin therapy reduce the risk of stroke? A meta-analysis] (in French). Ann Med Intern 152:188-193, 2001.
5. Pignone M, Mulrow CD. Using cardiovascular risk profiles to individualise hypertensive treatment. BMJ 322:1165-1166, 2001.
6. Wallis EJ, Ramsay LE, Jackson PR. Cardiovascular and coronary risk estimation in hypertension management. Heart 88: 306-312, 2002.
7. Dahlöf B, Lindholm LH, Hansson L, et al. Morbidity and mortality in the Swedish Trial in Old Patients with Hypertension (STOP-Hypertension). Lancet 338:1281-1285, 1991.
8. MRC Trial of treatment of mild hypertension: Principal results. Medical Research Council Working Party. Brit Med J (Clin Res) 291:97-104, 1985.
9. Sever PS, Dahlöf B, Poulter NR, et al. Rationale, design, methods and baseline demography of participants of the Anglo-Scandinavian Cardiac Outcomes Trial. J Hypertens 16:1139-1147, 2001.

10. Sever PS, Dahlöf B, Poulter NR, et al. Prevention of coronary and stroke events with atorvastatin in hypertensive patients who have average or lower-than-average cholesterol concentrations, in the Anglo-Scandinavian Cardiac Outcomes Trial—Lipid Lowering Arm (ASCOT-LLA): A multicentre randomised controlled trial. Lancet 361:1149-1158, 2003.

11. Wilson PWF, D'Agostino RB, Sullivan L, et al. Overweight and obesity as determinants of cardiovascular risk: The Framingham experience. Arch Intern Med 162:1867-1872, 2002.

12. American Heart Association. 2003 Heart and Stroke Statistical Update. Dallas, TX, American Heart Association. 2002.

13. Arias E, Smith BL. Deaths: Preliminary Data for 2001. Hyattsville, MD, National Center for Health Statistics, 2003; pp 1-48.

14. United States Renal Data System. USRDS 2002 Annual Data Report. Bethesda, MD, National Institutes of Health, National Institute of Diabetes and Digestive and Kidney Disease, 2002.

15. Marshall T, Rouse A. Resource implications and health benefits or primary prevention strategies for cardiovascular disease in people aged 30 to 74: Mathematical modelling study. BMJ 325:197, 2002.

16. Lumley T, Kronmal RA, Cushman M, et al. A stroke prediction score in the elderly: Validation and Web-based application. J Clin Epidemiol 55:129-136, 2002.

17. D'Agostino RB Sr, Grundy S, Sullivan LM, et al. Validation of the Framingham coronary heart disease prediction scores: Results of multiple ethnic groups investigation. CHD Risk Prediction Group. JAMA 286:180-187, 2001.

18. Padwal R, Straus SE, McAlister FA. Cardiovascular risk factors and their effects on the decision to treat hypertension: Evidence based review. BMJ 322:977-980, 2001.

19. Dinneen S, Gerstein HC. The association of microalbuminuria and mortality in non-insulin-dependent diabetes mellitus. A systemic overview of the literature. Arch Intern Med 157:1413-1418, 1997.

20. Gerstein HC, Mann JF, Yi Q, et al. Albuminuria and risk of cardiovascular events, death, and heart failure in diabetic and non-diabetic individuals. HOPE Study Investigators. JAMA 286:421-426, 2001.

21. Scillaci G, Reboldi G, Verdecchia P. High-normal serum creatinine concentration is a predictor of cardiovascular risk in essential hypertension. Arch Intern Med 161:886-891, 2001.

22. Levey AS, Bosch JP, Lewis JB, et al. A more accurate method to estimate glomerular filtration rate from serum creatinine: A new prediction equation. Ann Intern Med 130:461-470, 1999.

23. Muntner P, He J, Hamm L, et al. Renal insufficiency and subsequent death resulting from cardiovascular disease in the United States. J Am Soc Nephrol 13:745-753, 2002.

24. Holland DC, Lam M. Predictors of hospitalization and death among pre-dialysis patients: A retrospective cohort study. Nephrol Dialy Transplant 15:650-658, 2000.

25. Wang JG, Staessen JA, Fagard RH, et al. Prognostic significance of serum creatinine and uric acid in older Chinese patients with isolated systolic hypertension. Hypertension 37:1068-1074, 2001.

26. Mann JF, Gerstein HC, Pogue J, et al. Renal insufficiency as a predictor of cardiovascular outcomes and the impact of ramipril: The HOPE randomized trial. Ann Intern Med 134:629-636, 2001.

27. Shlipak MG, Simon JA, Grady D, et al. Renal insufficiency and cardiovascular events in postmenopausal women with coronary heart disease. Heart and Estrogen/progestin Replacement Study (HERS) Investigators. J Am Coll Cardiol 38:705-711, 2001.

28. Hall WD. Abnormalities of kidney function as a cause and a consequence of cardiovascular disease. Am J Med Sci 317:176-182, 1999.

29. Herzog CA, Ma JZ, Collins AJ. Poor long-term survival after acute myocardial infarction among patients on long-term dialysis. N Engl J Med 339:799-805, 1998.

30. Lewis EJ, Hunsicker LG, Clarke WR, et al. Renoprotective effect of the angiotensin-receptor antagonist irbesartan in patients with nephropathy due to Type 2 diabetes. Collaborative Study Group. N Engl J Med 345:841-860, 2001.

31. Berl T, Hunsicker LG, Lewis JB, et al. Cardiovascular outcomes in the Irbesartan Diabetic Nephropathy Trial of patients with type 2 diabetes and overt nephropathy. Irbesartan Diabetic Nephropathy Trial Collaborative Study Group. Ann Intern Med 138:542-549, 2003.

32. Pocock S, McCormack V, Gueyffier F, et al. A score for predicting risk of death from cardiovascular disease in adults with raised blood pressure, based on individual patient data from randomised controlled trials. INDANA Project Steering Committee. BMJ 323:75-81, 2001.

33. Miura K, Daviglus ML, Dyer AR, et al. Relationship of blood pressure to 25-year mortality due to coronary heart disease, cardiovascular diseases, and all causes in young adult men: The Chicago Heart Association Detection Project in Industry. Arch Intern Med 161:1501-1508, 2001.

34. Wallis EJ, Ramsay LE, Haq IU, et al. Is coronary risk an accurate surrogate for cardiovascular risk for treatment decisions in hypertension? A population validation. J Hypertension 19:691-696, 2001.

35. Yikona JINM, Wallis EJ, Ramsay LE, et al. Coronary and cardiovascular risk estimation in uncomplicated mild hypertension. A comparison of risk assessment methods. J Hypertension 20:2173-2182, 2002.

36. van den Hoogen PCW, Feskens EJM, Nagelkerke NJD, et al. The relation between blood pressure and mortality due to coronary heart disease among men in different parts of the world. N Engl J Med 342:1-8, 2000.

37. Menotti A, Puddu PE, Lanti M. Comparison of the Framingham risk function-based coronary chart with risk function from an Italian population study. Eur Heart J 21:365-370, 2000.

38. Haq IU, Ramsay LE, Yeo WW, et al. Is the Framingham risk function valid for northern European populations? A comparison of methods for estimating absolute coronary risk in high risk men. Heart 81:40-46, 1999.

39. Diverse Populations Collaborative Group. Prediction of mortality from coronary heart disease among diverse populations: Is there a common predictive function? Heart 88:222-228, 2002.

40. Conroy RM, Ryörälä K, Fitzgerald AP, et al. Prediction of ten-year risk of fatal cardiovascular disease in Europe: The SCORE Project. The SCORE Project Group. Eur Heart J 24:987-1003, 2003.

41. The sixth report of the Joint National Committee on Prevention, Detection, Evaluation, and Treatment of High Blood Pressure (JNC VI). Arch Intern Med 157:2413-2446, 1997.

42. D'Agostino RB, Russel MW, Huse DM, et al. Primary and subsequent coronary risk appraisal: New results from the Framingham Study. Am Heart J 139:272-281, 2000.

43. Ogden LG, He J, Lydick E, et al. Long-term absolute benefit of lowering blood pressure in hypertensive patients according to the JNC VI Risk Stratification. Hypertension 34:539-543, 2000.

44. 1999 World Health Organisation-International Society of Hypertension Guidelines for the Management of Hypertension. Guidelines Subcommittee. J Hypertension 17:151-183, 1999.

45. Chobanian AV, Bakris GL, Black HR, et al. The seventh report of the Joint National Committee on The Prevention, Detection, Evaluation, and Treatment of High Blood Pressure (JNC 7)—EXPRESS. JAMA 289:2560-2672, 2003.

46. Chobanian AV, Bakris GL, Black HR, et al. Seventh report of the Joint National Committee on The Prevention, Detection, Evaluation, and Treatment of High Blood Pressure (JNC 7)—COMPLETE VERSION. Hypertension 42:1206-1252, 2003.

47. Executive Summary of the Third Report of the National Cholesterol Education Program (NCEP) Expert Panel on Detection, Evaluation, and Treatment of High Blood

Cholesterol in Adults (Adult Treatment Panel III). JAMA 285:2486-2497, 2001.

48. 2003 European Society of Hypertension—European Cardiology guidelines for the management of arterial hypertension. Guidelines Committee. J Hypertension 21:1011-1053, 2003.

49. Ridker PM, Rifai N, Rose L, et al. Comparison of C-reactive protein and low-density lipoprotein cholesterol levels in the prediction of first cardiovascular events. N Engl J Med 347:1557-1565, 2002.

50. Jackson R, Barham P, Bils J, et al. Management of raised blood pressure in New Zealand: A discussion document. BMJ 307:107-110, 1993.

51. Jackson R. Updated New Zealand cardiovascular disease risk-benefit prediction guide. BMJ 320:709-710, 2000.

52. Lewington S, Clarke R, Qizillbash N, et al. Age-specific relevance of usual blood pressure to vascular mortality. Lancet 360:1903-1913, 2002.

53. McManus RJ, Mant J, Meulendijks CF, et al. Comparison of estimates and calculations of risk of coronary heart disease by doctors and nurses using different calculation tools in general practice: Cross sectional study. BMJ 324:459-464, 2002.

54. Franklin SS, Wong ND. Cardiovascular risk evaluation: An inexact science. J Hypertension 20:2127-2130, 2002.

55. Prevention of coronary heart disease in clinical practice: Recommendations of the Second Joint Task Force of European and other Societies on coronary prevention. Eur Heart J 19:1434-1503, 1998.

56. Orford JL, Sesso HD, Stedman M, et al. A comparison of the Framingham and European Society of Cardiology coronary heart disease risk prediction models in the normative aging study. Am Heart J 144:95-100, 2002.

57. Wood D, Durrington P, Poulter N, et al. on behalf of the British Cardiac Society, British Hyperlipidaemia Association, British Hypertension Society and endorsed by the British Diabetic Association. Joint British recommendations on prevention of coronary heart disease in clinical practice. Heart 80:S1-S29, 1998.

58. Cardiac risk assessor. University of Manchester, UK. Available at: www.hyp.ac.uk/bhs/risk.xls a3D0.

59. Durrington PN. Risk in cardiovascular disease: Joint British societies recommend their computer program for risk calculations. BMJ 321:174, 2000.

60. Wallis EJ, Ramsay LE, Haq IU, et al. Coronary and cardiovascular risk estimation for primary prevention: Validation of a new Sheffield table in the 1995 Scottish health survey population. BMJ 320:671-676, 2000.

61. Isles CG, Ritchie LD, Murchie P, et al. Risk assessment in primary prevention of coronary heart disease: Randomised comparison of three scoring methods. BMJ 320:690-691, 2000.

62. Lloyd-Jones DM, Larson MG, Leip EP, et al. Lifetime risk for developing congestive heart failure: The Framingham Heart Study. Circulation 106:3068-3072, 2002.

63. Ramachandran S, French JM, Vanderpump MPJ, et al. Using the Framingham model to predict heart disease in the United Kingdom: Retrospective study. BMJ 320:676-677, 2000.

64. Cappuccio FP, Oakeshott P, Strazzullo P, et al. Application of Framingham risk estimates to ethnic minorities in United Kingdom and implications for primary prevention of heart disease in general practice: cross sectional population based study. BMJ 325:1271, 2002.

65. Nanchahal K, Duncan JR, Durrington PN, et al. Analysis of predicted coronary heart disease risk in England based on Framingham study risk appraisal models published in 1991 and 2000. BMJ 325:194-195, 2002.

66. Dahlöf B, Devereux RB, Kjeldsen SE, et al. for the LIFE study group. Cardiovascular morbidity and mortality in the Losartan Intervention for Endpoint reduction in hypertension study (LIFE): A randomised trial against atenolol. Lancet 359:995-1003, 2002.

67. Pearson TA. New tools for coronary risk assessment: What are their advantages and limitations? Circulation 105:886-892, 2002.

68. Magnus PMB, Beaglehole R. The real contribution of the major risk factors to the coronary epidemics: Time to end the "Only-50%" myth. Arch Intern Med 161:2657-2660, 2001.

69. Greenland P, Knoll MD, Stamler J, et al. Major risk factors as antecedents of fatal and nonfatal coronary heart disease events. JAMA 290:891-897, 2003.

70. Khot UN, Knot MB, Bajzer CT, et al. Prevalence of conventional risk factors in patients with coronary heart disease. JAMA 290:898-904, 2003.

71. Lever AF, Ramsay LE. Treatment of hypertension in the elderly. J Hypertens 13:571-579, 1995.

72. MRC Working Party. Medical Research Council trial of treatment of hypertension in older adults. Principal results. BMJ 304:405-412, 1992.

73. Management Committee. The Australian therapeutic trial in mild hypertension. Lancet 1:1261-1267, 1980.

74. Staessen JA, Fagard R, Thijs L, et al. for the Systolic Hypertension—Europe (Syst-EUR) Trial Investigators. Morbidity and mortality in the placebo-controlled European Trial on Isolated Systolic Hypertension in the Elderly. Lancet 360:757-764, 1997.

75. Amery A, Brixko P, Clement D, et al. Mortality and morbidity results from the European Working Party on High Blood Pressure in the Elderly Trial. Lancet 1:1349-1354, 1985.

76. Liu L, Wang J, Gong L, et al. for the Systolic Hypertension in China (Syst-China) Collaborative Group. Comparison of active treatment and placebo in older Chinese patients with isolated systolic hypertension. J Hypertension 16:1823-1829, 1998.

77. Coope J, Warrender TS. Randomised trial of treatment of hypertension in the elderly in primary care. Br Med J 293:1145-1151, 1986.

# Chapter 22

# New Interpretations of Blood Pressure: The Importance of Pulse Pressure

## Stanley S. Franklin

The traditional epidemiologic definition of hypertension as a cardiovascular risk factor is based on two components of the arterial pulse wave—the peak systolic blood pressure (SBP) and end-diastolic blood pressure (DBP)—as measured from the brachial artery by means of the sphygmomanometer. More recently, attention has been directed toward the pulse pressure (PP) as a pulsatile component of cardiovascular risk. PP, the difference between SBP and DBP, is due to the force imparted to the arterial blood column by left ventricular contraction, which produces a pressure increment over and above the existing DBP. There is abundant evidence that the increase in PP after the sixth decade of life is a surrogate risk marker for central artery stiffness.[1-3] There is also evidence that central artery stiffness is an independent risk factor for cardiovascular disease.[1-3] Still unsettled, however, is whether PP is superior to SBP or to mean arterial pressure (MAP = ⅓ SBP + ⅔ DBP) as a predictor of cardiovascular risk. The objective of this chapter is to review the clinical usefulness of PP as a predictor of cardiovascular risk.

## HISTORICAL PERSPECTIVE

Our understanding of the relationship between the various blood pressure (BP) indices and cardiovascular risk has undergone considerable change since the introduction of the sphygmomanometer at the beginning of the twentieth century. Initially, elevated DBP was thought the best measure of cardiovascular risk because it was equated to the resistance that the heart had to overcome, whereas elevation in SBP was largely ignored because it was equated with the maximum force of the heart.[4] Indeed, interventional studies between the 1960s and 1980s invariably defined the severity of hypertension solely on the basis of DBP. However, since publication of data from the Framingham Heart Study in 1971, more weight has been given to SBP in defining hypertensive cardiovascular risk.[5-7] Nevertheless, it was only after the benefits of antihypertensive therapy in isolated systolic hypertension (ISH) were clearly demonstrated in the 1990s that national and international guidelines first recommended therapy for elevated SBP in the absence of associated diastolic hypertension. Although the current guidelines acknowledge that both SBP and DBP define hypertensive cardiovascular risk,[8,9] they contain a number of limitations. SBP and DBP represent only the two extremes of the propagated arterial pulse wave that is measured by sphygmomanometry at the brachial artery. Since the late 1980s, new evidence suggests that the relationship of BP components to cardiovascular risk is surprisingly more complex than initially thought. Part of this complexity involves the effect of ageing on BP indices and the possible role of PP in predicting cardiovascular risk.

## AGE-RELATED CHANGES IN BLOOD PRESSURE

Population studies,[10,11] including those from Framingham,[12] demonstrate that SBP rises from adolescence, whereas DBP, although initially increasing with age, levels off at ages 50 to 55 and decreases after ages 60 to 65 years. Thus PP increases after ages 50 to 55: a change that is accelerated from the ages of 60 to 65 and beyond. The rise in SBP and DBP up to ages 50 to 55 can best be explained by the dominance of peripheral vascular resistance (Table 22–1). In contrast, after the fifth decade of life (1) increasing PP and decreasing DBP are surrogate measurements for central elastic artery stiffening. Indeed, the fall in DBP with increasing aortic stiffness is explained by a diminished hydraulic buffering system, leading to greater peripheral run-off of stroke volume during systole. Thus, with less blood remaining in the aorta at the beginning of diastole, and with diminished elastic recoil, DBP decreases with increased steepness of diastolic decay. (2) After age 60, central arterial stiffness overrides increased systemic vascular resistance and becomes the dominant hemodynamic factor in both normotensive and hypertensive individuals, as manifested by an increase in SBP, a decrease in DBP and hence a rise in PP. (3) Hypertension, left untreated, may accelerate stiffening of elastic arteries, which, in turn, may set up a vicious cycle of worsening hypertension and further increases in elastic artery stiffness.[12]

The Third National Health and Nutrition Examination Survey[13] (NHANES III) showed that three of four adult persons with hypertension are 50 years of age or older. Moreover, 80% of untreated or inadequately treated persons with hypertension in this age group have ISH, which by definition consists of elevated PP. In addition to ISH being the predominant form of geriatric hypertension, there is evidence that widened PP may complement SBP as a predictor of cardiovascular risk.

## USEFULNESS OF PULSE PRESSURE IN PREDICTING CORONARY HEART DISEASE RISK

Using almost the same Framingham cohort as in the previous study, 1924 men and women between 50 and 79 years of age at baseline with no clinical evidence of coronary heart disease (CHD) and free from antihypertensive drug therapy, were followed for up to 20 years (Figure 22–1).[14] In this population, CHD risk was inversely correlated with DBP at any level of SBP greater than 120 mm Hg, suggesting that PP was an important component of risk. There was a far greater increase in CHD risk with increments in PP for a given SBP than with increments in SBP with a constant PP. The Framingham study

**Table 22-1** Hemodynamic Patterns of Age-Related Changes in Blood Pressure

| Age (years) | DBP (mm Hg) | SBP (mm Hg) | MAP (mm Hg) | PP (mm Hg) | Hemodynamics |
|---|---|---|---|---|---|
| 30-39 | ↑ | ↑ | ↑ | →↑ | R > S |
| ↑ | → | ↑ | → | ↑↑ | R = S |
| ≥60 | ↓ | ↑ | →↑ | ↑↑↑↑ | S > R |

Adapted from Franklin SS, Gustin W, Wong ND, et al. Hemodynamic patterns of age-related changes in blood pressure. The Framingham Heart Study. Circulation 96:308-315, 1997; with permission.
DBP, diastolic blood pressure; SBP, systolic blood pressure; MAP, mean arterial pressure; PP, pulse pressure; ↑, increase; ↓, decrease; →, no change; R, small-vessel resistance; S, large-vessel stiffness.

supports the findings of earlier workers[15-17] that PP may be useful as an adjunct to SBP in predicting risk and that CHD events are more related to the pulsatile stress of elastic artery stiffness during systole (as reflected in a rise in PP) than the steady-state stress of resistance during diastole (as reflected in a parallel rise in SBP and DBP). Seven additional publications, including a total of 12 different databases from around the world, have clearly shown an inverse relation of risk with DBP, so that PP becomes superior to the reference SBP in predicting total and cardiovascular mortality[18-24]; three additional studies have shown the same relation for predicting CHD risk.[25-27] Furthermore, the value of PP in predicting risk in the elderly has been confirmed by 24-hour conventional[28] and intraarterial[24] ambulatory BP monitoring.

PP may predict cardiovascular risk when SBP is normal or low as a result of ventricular dysfunction. This has been described in postmyocardial infarction,[29] end-stage renal disease

(ESRD) on hemodialysis,[30] and frank heart failure[31] and is consistent with "reverse causation," expressed as an increased cardiac mortality in association with a falling SBP. In the presence of compromised myocardial function, DBP decreases at a more rapid rate than SBP, so that the rise in PP rather than the fall in SBP becomes the stronger predictor of future cardiac events, including cardiac death.

## USEFULNESS OF PULSE PRESSURE IN PREDICTING BENEFIT OF THERAPY

The benefit of effective antihypertensive therapy may be related to the extent of increased PP. There is evidence from a meta-analysis of eight intervention trials involving elderly individuals with ISH (defined by a SBP ≥160 and DBP <95 mm Hg) that fewer patients had to be treated to prevent one cardiovascular death if the PP at baseline was 90 mm Hg or greater.[23] The importance of a wide PP in ensuring a robust therapeutic outcome was confirmed in the Losartan Intervention for Endpoint Reduction (LIFE) trial of patients with hypertension and left ventricular hypertrophy (LVH). The therapeutic benefit of losartan was compared with that of atenolol in persons with ISH (SBP ≥160 and DBP <90 mm Hg) enrolled in LIFE, and that benefit was compared with the benefit achieved in LIFE participants with combined systolic-diastolic hypertension (SDH, defined as a SBP ≥160 and DBP ≥90 mm Hg). There was a 46% decrease in cardiovascular mortality from losartan over atenolol therapy in the ISH group as compared with no difference between treatments in the SDH group, although SBP was reduced almost equally in both arms of the study.[32] The most logical interpretation of this analysis is that effective therapy with an angiotensin II antagonist resulted in a significant benefit over atenolol in reducing cardiovascular mortality in the group with the highest PP and hence the greatest risk.

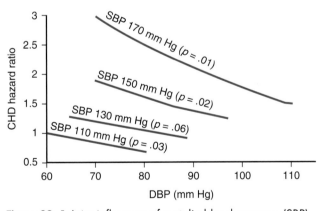

**Figure 22-1** Joint influences of systolic blood pressure (SBP) and diastolic blood pressure (DBP) risk. Coronary heart disease (CHD) hazard ratios were determined from the level of DBP within SBP groups. Hazard ratios were set to a reference value of 1.0 for SBP of 130 mm Hg and DBP of 80 mm Hg and plotted for SBP values of 110, 130, 150, 170 mm Hg, respectively. The p-values were for the β coefficients for model. All estimates were adjusted for age, sex, body mass index, cigarettes smoked per day, glucose intolerance, and total cholesterol:high-density lipoprotein. (Adapted with permission from Franklin SS, Khan SA, Wong ND, et al. Is pulse pressure useful in predicting risk for coronary heart disease? The Framingham Heart Study. Circulation 100:354-360, 1999.)

## PULSE PRESSURE AS A MARKER FOR CENTRAL ARTERY STIFFNESS: PATHOLOGIC CONSEQUENCES

Increased PP may be a surrogate marker for several possible pathologic mechanisms, all originating from the underlying increased central arterial stiffness and contributing to disorders of the myocardium.[33] Increased aortic pulsatile load elevates left ventricular wall stress, decreases coronary flow reserve, impairs left ventricular relaxation, and may lead to diastolic dysfunction. Increased aortic pulsatile load is the major factor in the development of LVH with increased coronary blood flow requirements. Simultaneously, the decrease in DBP that characterizes ISH further compromises the oxygen supply:demand ratio by reducing coronary blood flow. In addition, increased pulsatile stress leads to endothelial dysfunction with a greater propensity for coronary atherosclerosis and for rupture of unstable atherosclerotic plaques.

## HOW DOES AGE INFLUENCE THE CUFF PRESSURE ASSESSMENT OF CHD RISK?

The Framingham Heart Study examined the relationship between BP and CHD risk as a function of age (Figure 22–2).[34] From the ages of 20 to 79 years there was a continuous, graded shift from DBP to SBP and eventually to PP as predictors of CHD risk. From age 60 onward, when considered with SBP, DBP was negatively related to CHD risk, so that PP emerged as the best predictor.[34] All three BP indices in the Framingham study[34] were equally predictive of CHD risk in the transitional ages of 50 to 59 years, whereas in the younger group (<50 years of age), DBP was a more powerful predictor of CHD risk than SBP; PP itself was not predictive. Evidence favoring DBP over SBP in predicting CHD risk in young adults was also noted in a number of earlier large observational studies[35-37] and in a later study utilizing intraarterial BP measurements.[24] These findings are consistent with the NHANES III study, which showed that there were twice as many hypertensive persons younger than age 50 up-staged by DBP as compared with SBP.[13] The bias toward DBP over SBP by earlier generations of physicians may be, in part, due to the emphasis on hypertension as a young person's condition. However, with the ageing of the population over the past half-century, hypertension has become largely a condition affecting older persons with ISH.

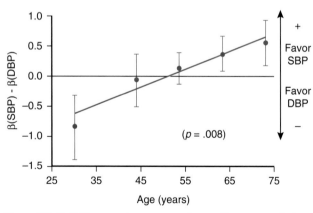

**Figure 22–2** Difference in coronary heart disease prediction between systolic blood pressure (SBP) and diastolic blood pressure (DBP) as function of age. Difference in β coefficients (from Cox proportional-hazards regression) between SBP and DBP is plotted as function of age, obtaining this regression line: β(SBP)–β(DBP) = −1.49848 + 0.0290 ¥ age (p = .008). (From Franklin SS, Larson MG, Khan SA, et al. Does the relation of blood pressure to coronary heart disease risk change with aging? The Framingham Heart Study. Circulation 103:1245-1249, 2001; with permission.)

Curiously, the underlying hemodynamics that favor DBP as the predominant predictor of CHD risk in young hypertensive subjects are poorly understood.

## THE IMPORTANCE OF PULSE WAVE REFLECTION

Conventional hemodynamic mechanisms do not explain why cuff DBP is superior to cuff SBP and PP in predicting CHD risk in young adults. The studies of Elzinga and Westerhof[38] showed that increased peripheral resistance was associated with a nearly parallel rise in aortic SBP and aortic DBP (or a greater rise in SBP than DBP in conjunction with some increase in arterial stiffness), whereas increased arterial stiffness alone was associated with a rise in aortic SBP and a fall in aortic DBP.[39] Thus the concept that increased peripheral vascular resistance alone is responsible for a greater rise in cuff DBP than SBP is a myth; an additional hemodynamic factor—wave reflection—must be present to explain these findings (Figure 22–3).

In young subjects the reflected pressure waves return to the ascending aorta in diastole and serve to elevate mean DBP, thus boosting coronary artery perfusion.[40] In addition, the summation of the incident pressure wave with the reflected wave in young adults produces a normal phenomenon of pressure amplification of PP and SBP from the aorta to the brachial artery.[40] In contrast, as arteries stiffen with advancing age, a larger reflected pressure wave returns to the ascending aorta earlier during late systole and increases or "augments" the central SBP and PP, thus decreasing pressure amplification and simultaneously contributing to increase cardiac afterload.[41]

Studies by Wilkinson et al.,[42] using radial artery waveforms recorded noninvasively by applanation tonometry, have shown that peripheral amplification of PP and SBP decreases significantly as peripheral DBP increases in persons younger than 50 years of age; however, only a small, nonsignificant further decrease in amplification occurs in older subjects, largely because there is already increased early wave reflection within a stiffened arterial tree. In contrast, peripheral and central DBP and MAP track in a near parallel manner at all ages. Thus as peripheral vascular resistance rises in younger subjects, there is less change in peripheral SBP because of reduced pressure amplification. This explains why DBP is a better predictor of CHD risk in younger subjects. Further support for this concept comes for the studies of Millasseau et al.,[43] who showed that pulse wave velocity, as a surrogate measurement for aortic stiffness, was more closely correlated with peripheral DBP than SBP in subjects older than age 50 but not in those age 50 or younger.

## SPURIOUS SYSTOLIC HYPERTENSION

Peripheral amplification, when exaggerated in tall, fit young men with highly elastic central arteries, may produce spurious upper limb systolic hypertension.[44,45] This normal variant represents extreme pressure amplification of the brachial and radial systolic cuff pressures. Characteristically, these young men have normal central SBP and DBP and normal peripheral DBP and heart rates. The frequency of this form of pseudosystolic hypertension is unknown. This exaggerated

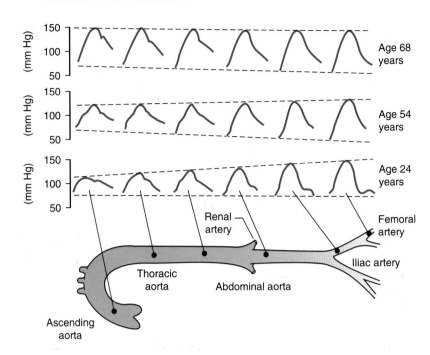

**Figure 22–3** Pressure wave recorded along the arterial tree from the proximal ascending aorta to the femoral artery in three subjects aged 24, 54, and 68 years. (From Nichols WW, et al. In O'Rourke MF, Safar ME, Dzau V (eds). Arterial Vasodilation: Mechanisms and Therapy. London, Edward Arnold, 1993; with permission.)

peripheral amplification in some young, tall individuals with highly elastic central arteries represents a second example of why DBP is superior to SBP in predicting cardiovascular risk.

## PARADIGM SHIFT IN THE INTERPRETATION OF BLOOD PRESSURE MEASUREMENTS

Paradoxically, the heart only "sees" SBP in the ascending aorta, and pressure wave amplification distorts the relationship between central and peripheral systolic pressure, as measured at the brachial artery by the sphygmomanometer. Therefore, central and not peripheral SBP, regardless of age, determines cardiac afterload and hence CHD risk. The changing pattern of age-related brachial artery BP components that predict CHD risk results from altered peripheral resistance, aortic stiffness, and early wave reflection, all acting in concert to raise SBP, decrease DBP, and abolish pressure amplification; this leads to an age-related shift from sphygmomanometric-determined DBP to SBP and ultimately to PP in the prediction of CHD risk. Overall, these findings validate the hemodynamic factors associated with aging and hypertension that were described more than 20 years ago by O'Rourke and Nichols.[46,47] In addition, these findings represent a significant paradigm shift in our understanding of how we use brachial artery cuff BP components to predict CHD risk.

## CLINICAL IMPLICATIONS

The reliance on DBP in the young and on SBP in the middle-aged to predict CHD risk appears straightforward, but there are questions regarding the best clinical approach for using PP as a predictor of CHD risk in the older patient. Cuff PP cannot replace SBP as a single measure of CHD risk, because it significantly underestimates peripheral vascular resistance.[48]

Furthermore, MAP or DBP consistently underestimates peripheral resistance, central artery stiffness, and early wave reflection in this older age group.[48] In contrast, elevation in cuff SBP fully represents increased peripheral vascular resistance and partially represents increased central elastic artery stiffness and early wave reflection. Of the four BP indices, SBP is usually the single best predictor for middle-aged and older persons with systolic-diastolic hypertension (SBP ≥140 and DBP ≥90 mm Hg). However, evaluation of SBP and DBP jointly allows the assessment of the total cardiac load (i.e., the full influence of resistance, stiffness, and reflection) and therefore provides the best estimation of cardiovascular risk. Thus, the best strategy for assessing risk in this age group is to determine the level of SBP elevation, and then adjust risk upward in the presence of discordantly low DBP and hence high PP ISH.[48]

The greatest prognostic value of a wide PP in this older age group may be in the categories of high-normal (higher half of the prehypertensive classification) SBP and stage 1 systolic hypertension (i.e., from SBP of 130 to 159 mm Hg), a BP span that encompasses almost two thirds of all adult CHD events.[49] The concurrent presence of wide PP in either of these two BP groups could shift an individual into a higher risk category and therefore possibly dictate a change in therapy. In addition, a wide PP could be helpful in identifying high-risk persons who may profit from more aggressive therapy for control of their BP.

## CAVEATS IN EQUATING PULSE PRESSURE WITH CARDIOVASCULAR RISK

If PP is a surrogate for central artery stiffness, it is the stiffness that is the cardiovascular risk factor; strictly speaking, PP is a risk marker of stiffness. There are certain caveats to consider when using PP as a predictor of cardiovascular risk.

First, in middle-aged, healthy populations or older individuals with both systolic and diastolic hypertension, SBP and

MAP may be equal or superior to PP as predictors of cardiovascular risk[50-52]; in this population, there is such high colinearity between SBP and PP that it often becomes impossible to show an advantage of one index over another in predicting risk. Only when SBP increases and DBP decreases, as described in most observational studies, does the superiority of PP over SBP as a predictor of cardiovascular risk become apparent in uncomplicated hypertension.

Second, with advanced age and after adjustment for cardinal risk factors, PP becomes an independent predictor of CHD risk. Therefore, despite the high colinearity between SBP with PP, the latter predominates as the single best predictor of CHD risk because of the contribution of pulsatile stress in a minority of subjects with discordantly low DBP values. It should be noted that the MAP equation ($\frac{1}{3}$ SBP + $\frac{2}{3}$ DBP) grossly underestimates vascular resistance after ages 50 to 60 as DBP levels off and even falls.[12] Hence, beyond middle-age, PP becomes a better predictor and the MAP a poorer predictor of cardiovascular risk. Paradoxically, the value or MAP has been highlighted with the recent publication of meta-analyses by the Prospective Studies Collaboration (PSC)[53] and the Asian Pacific Cohort Studies Collaboration (APCSC),[54] using 61 and 37 cohort studies, respectively. These investigators concluded that MAP, in both the young and old, was a far superior predictor of CHD risk than was PP. Their conclusions are in total disregard of the proven importance of arterial stiffness and early wave reflection as important risk factors in middle-aged and elderly individuals with ISH. A meta-analysis of a smaller number of well-performed, observational studies, rather than the multiple diverse studies included in the PSC and APCSC, might have provided a different picture of the importance of PP in predicting cardiovascular risk.

PP becomes an even stronger predictor of cardiovascular risk (1) when combined with a cluster of risk factors[55]; (2) in the presence of target organ damage, such as LVH[56] or albuminuria[57]; (3) in association with diabetes[58]; and (4) in the presence of prior cardiovascular complications that lead to ventricular dysfunction.[29-31]

The totality of evidence supports PP as a surrogate risk marker for arterial stiffness, although at times an imperfect one. Despite high colinearity of PP with SBP, PP can be a more useful predictor of cardiovascular risk above and beyond the predictive power of MAP, SBP, or DBP. Clearly, these findings call into question the prevailing belief that elevation of SBP and DBP contribute equally to cardiovascular risk. However, there is as yet scanty evidence supporting the reduction of PP instead of SBP as a therapeutic goal. In addition, we have little information on the utility of using PP and SBP together, rather than SBP alone, to classify hypertensive risk. Furthermore, a public health recommendation that focuses on PP may detract from the importance of SBP in the diagnosis and treatment of hypertension. At present, it would be premature to modify current guidelines on the basis of prevailing data.

## FUTURE FRONTIERS OF NONINVASIVE ASSESSMENT OF CENTRAL BLOOD PRESSURE

Although the use of cuff PP as a prognostic guide to cardiovascular risk may have some utility in older persons, this may not hold true under all circumstances. Aortic PP is the result of integration of three principal factors (i.e., stroke volume, arterial stiffness, and the intensity and timing of wave reflections). Each of these factors can influence PP independently, but usually they act in concert. However, individual changes in pressure amplification, heart rate, stroke-volume and cardiac contractility may distort the relation between PP and arterial stiffness. Because central artery stiffness is established early, noninvasive assessment of arterial stiffness may allow better assessment of cardiovascular risk before hypertension develops, and long before the onset of cardiovascular complications.[59-64] In addition, assessment of aortic stiffness may allow targeted primary prevention of cardiovascular disease and may be a useful tool for monitoring the success or failure of antihypertensive therapy. Thus noninvasive assessment of arterial stiffness and central BP appears to be a promising area for further investigation. There is hope that physicians of the twenty-first century will have a simple office method of measuring central pulse waveforms that will supplement or possibly replace the sphygmomanometer.

## References

1. Dart AM, Kingwell BA. Pulse pressure—a review of mechanisms and clinical relevance. J Am Coll Cardiol 37:975-984, 2001.
2. Van Bortel LMAB, Struijker-Boudier HAJ, et al. Pulse pressure, arterial stiffness, and drug treatment of hypertension. Hypertension 38:914-921, 2001.
3. Safar ME, Levy BL, Struijker-Boudier HAJ. Current perspectives on arterial stiffness and pulse pressure in hypertension and cardiovascular diseases. Circulation 107:2864-2869, 2003.
4. Mackenzie J. Principles of Diagnosis and Treatment of Heart Affections, 3rd ed. London, Oxford University Press, 1926.
5. Kannel WB, Gordon T, Schwartz MJ. Systolic versus diastolic blood pressure and the risk of coronary heart disease. Am J Cardiol 27:335-346, 1971.
6. Stamler J, Neaton JD, Wentworth DN. Blood pressure (systolic and diastolic) and risk of fatal coronary heart disease. Hypertension 13:I2-I12, 1989.
7. Rutan GH, McDonald RH, Chula LH. A historical perspective of elevated systolic vs diastolic blood pressure from an epidemiological and clinical trial viewpoint. J Clin Epidemiol 42:663-673, 1989.
8. Chobanian AV, Bakris GL, Black HR, et al. The seventh report of the Joint National Committee on Prevention, Detection, Evaluation, and Treatment of High Blood Pressure (JNC 7). JAMA 289:2560-2572, 2003.
9. Mancia G, Rosei A, DeBaker G, et al. 2003 European Society of Hypertension-European Society of Cardiology Guidelines for the Management of Arterial Hypertension. J Hypertens 21:1011-1053, 2003.
10. Whelton PK, He J, Klag MJ. Blood pressure in westernized populations. In Swales JD (ed). Textbook of Hypertension. Oxford, UK, Blackwell Scientific Publications. 1994.
11. Burt VL, Whelton P, Roccella EJ, et al. Prevalence of hypertension in the US adult population: Results from the Third National Health and Nutrition Examination Survey, 1988-1991. Hypertension 25:305-313, 1995.
12. Franklin SS, Gustin W, Wong ND, et al. Hemodynamic patterns of age-related changes in blood pressure. The Framingham Heart Study. Circulation 96:308-315, 1997.
13. Franklin SS, Jacobs MJ, Wong ND, et al. Predominance of isolated systolic hypertension among middle-aged and elderly US hypertensives. Hypertension 37:869-874, 2001.
14. Franklin SS, Khan SA, Wong ND, et al. Is pulse pressure useful in predicting risk for coronary heart disease? The Framingham Heart Study. Circulation 100:354-360, 1999.
15. Darne B, Girerd X, Safar M, et al. Pulsatile versus steady component of blood pressure: A cross-sectional analysis and a

prospective analysis on cardiovascular mortality. Hypertension 13:392-400, 1989.

16. Fang J, Madhavan S, Cohen H, et al. Measures of blood pressure and myocardial infarction in treated hypertensive patients. J Hypertens 13:413-419, 1995.

17. Benetos A, Safar M, Rudnichi A, et al. Pulse Pressure. A predictor of long-term cardiovascular mortality in a French male population. Hypertension 30:1410-1415, 1997.

18. Lee MT, Rosner BA, Weiss CT. Relationship of blood pressure to cardiovascular death: The effect of pulse pressure in the elderly. Ann Epidemiol 9:101-107, 1999.

19. Domanski MJ, Davis BR, Pfeffer MA, et al. Isolated systolic hypertension. Prognostic information provided by pulse pressure. Hypertension 34:375-380, 1999.

20. Glynn RG, Chae CU, Guralnik JM, et al. Pulse pressure and mortality in older people. Arch Intern Med 160:2765-2772, 2000.

21. Blacher J, Staessen JA, Girerd X, et al. Pulse pressure not mean pressure determines cardiovascular risk in older hypertensive patients. Arch Intern Med 160:1085-1089, 2000.

22. Benetos A, Zureik M, Morcet J, et al. A decrease in diastolic blood pressure combined with an increase in systolic blood pressure is associated with a higher cardiovascular mortality in men. J Am Coll Cardiol 35:673-680, 2000.

23. Staessen JA, Gasowski, Wang JG, et al. Risks of untreated and treated isolated systolic hypertension in the elderly: Meta-analysis of outcome trials. Lancet 104:865-872, 2000.

24. Khattar RS, Swales JD, Dore C, et al. Effect of aging on the prognostic significance of ambulatory systolic, diastolic, and pulse pressure in essential hypertension. Circulation 104: 783-789, 2001.

25. Millar JA, Lever AF, Burke V. Pulse pressure as a risk factor for cardiovascular events in the MRC mild hypertension trial. J Hypertens 17:1065-1072, 1999.

26. Sesso HD, Stampfer MJ, Rosner B, et al. Systolic and diastolic blood pressure, pulse pressure, and mean arterial pressure as predictors of cardiovascular disease risk in men. Hypertension 36:801-807, 2000.

27. Vaccarino V, Holford TR, Krumholz HM. Pulse pressure and risk for myocardial infarction and heart failure in the elderly. J Am Coll Cardiol 36:130-138, 2000.

28. Verdecchia P, Schillaci G, Borgione C, et al. Ambulatory pulse pressure: A potent predictor of total cardiovascular risk in hypertension. Hypertension 32:983-988, 1998.

29. Mitchell GF, Moye LA, Braunwald E, et al. Sphygmomanometrically determined pulse pressure is a powerful independent predictor of recurrent events after myocardial infarction in patients with impaired left ventricular function. Circulation 96:4254-4260, 1997.

30. Klassen PS, Lowrie EG, Reddan DN, et al. Association between pulse pressure and mortality in patients undergoing maintenance hemodialysis. JAMA 287:1548-1555, 2002.

31. Chae CU, Pfeffer MA, Glynn RJ, et al. Increased pulse pressure and risk of heart failure in the elderly. JAMA 281:634-639, 1999.

32. Kjeldsen SE, Dahlof B, Devereux RB, et al. Effects of losartan on cardiovascular morbidity and mortality in patients with isolated systolic hypertension and left ventricular hypertrophy. JAMA 288:1491-1498, 2002.

33. Franklin SS, Izzo JL. Aging, hypertension, and arterial stiffness. In Izzo JL, Black HR (eds). Hypertension Primer. Philadelphia, Lippincott, Williams & Wilkins, 2003; pp 170-175.

34. Franklin SS, Larson MG, Khan SA, et al. Does the relation of blood pressure to coronary heart disease risk change with aging? The Framingham Heart Study. Circulation 103: 1245-1249, 2001.

35. Lichtenstein MJ, Shipley MJ, Rose G. Systolic and diastolic blood pressure as predictors of coronary heart disease mortality in the Whitehall study. Br Med J 291:243-245, 1985.

36. Tverdal A. Systolic and diastolic blood pressures as predictors of coronary heart disease in middle-aged Norwegian men. Br Med J 294:671-673, 1987.

37. Neaton JD, Kuller L, Stamler J, et al. Impact of systolic and diastolic blood pressure on cardiovascular mortality. In Laragh JH, Brenner BM (eds). Hypertension: Pathophysiology, Diagnosis, and Management, 2nd ed. New York, Raven Press, 1995; pp 127-144.

38. Elzinga G, Westerhof N. Pressure and flow generated by the left ventricle against different impedances. Circ Res 32:178-186, 1973.

39. Berne RM, Levy MN. Cardiovascular Physiology. St Louis, Mosby, 1992; pp 135-151.

40. O'Rourke MF, Kelly RP. Wave reflection in the systemic circulation and its implications in ventricular function. J Hypertens 11:327-337, 1993.

41. Murgo JP, Westerhof N, Giolma JP, et al. Aortic input impedance in normal man: Relationship to pressure waveforms. Circulation 62:105-116, 1980.

42. Wilkinson IB, Franklin SS, Hall IR, et al. Pressure amplification explains why pulse pressure is unrelated to risk in young subjects. Hypertension 38:1461-1466, 2001.

43. Millasseau S, Ritter JM, Chowienczyk P. Relationship between blood pressure and aortic pulse wave velocity in young and old subjects with essential hypertension. J Hypertens 21:S253, 2003.

44. O'Rourke MF, Viachopoulos C, Graham RM. Spurious systolic hypertension in youth. Vasc Med 5:141-145, 2000.

45. Mahmud A, Feely J. Spurious systolic hypertension of youth: Fit young men with elastic arteries. Am J Hypertens 16:229-232, 2003.

46. O'Rourke MF. Arterial hemodynamics in hypertension. Circ Res 26/27(Suppl II):123-133, 1970.

47. Nichols WW, O'Rourke MF. McDonald's Blood Flow in Arteries, 4th ed. London, Arnold, Hodder Headline Group, 1998.

48. Franklin SS. Ageing and hypertension: The assessment of blood pressure indices in predicting coronary heart disease. J Hypertens 17:S29-S36, 1999.

49. Stamler J, Stamler R, Neaton JD. Blood pressure, systolic and diastolic, and cardiovascular risks. US population data. Arch Intern Med 153:598-615, 1993.

50. Antikainen RL, Jousiliahti P, Vanhanen H, et al. Excess mortality associated with increased pulse pressure among middle-aged men and women is explained by high systolic blood pressure. J Hypertens 18:417-23, 2000.

51. Miura K, Daviglus, Dyer AR, et al. Relationship of blood pressure to 25-year mortality due to coronary heart disease, cardiovascular diseases, and all causes in young adult men: The Chicago Heart Association Detection Project in Industry. Arch Intern Med 161:1501-1508, 2001.

52. Domanski M, Mitchell G, Pfeffer M, et al. Pulse pressure and cardiovascular disease-related mortality. JAMA 287:2677-2683, 2002.

53. Prospective Studies Collaboration. Age-specific relevance of usual blood pressure to vascular mortality: A meta-analysis of individual data for one million adults in 61 prospective studies. Lancet 360:1903-1913, 2002.

54. Asia Pacific Cohort Studies Collaboration. Blood pressure indices and cardiovascular disease in the Asia Pacific Region. A pooled analysis. Hypertension 42:69-75, 2003.

55. Glynn RJ, L'Italien GJ, Season HD, et al. Development of prediction for long-term cardiovascular risk associated with systolic and diastolic blood pressure. Hypertension 39:105-110, 2002.

56. Gardin JM, Arnold A, Gottdiener JS, et al. Left ventricular mass in the elderly. The Cardiovascular Health Study. Hypertension 29:1095-1103, 1997.

57. Pedrinelli R, Dell'Omo G, Penno G, et al. Microalbuminuria and pulse pressure in hypertensive and atherosclerotic men. Hypertension 35:48-54, 2000.

58. Schram MT, Kostense PJ, van Dijk RAJM, et al. Diabetes, pulse pressure and cardiovascular mortality: The Hoorn Study. J Hypertens 20:1743-1752, 2002.

59. Blacher J, Asmar R, Djane S, et al. Aortic pulse wave velocity as a marker of cardiovascular risk in hypertensive patients. Hypertension 33:1111-1117, 1999.

60. Boutouyrie P, Bussy C, Lacolley P, et al. Association between local pulse pressure, mean blood pressure, and large-artery remodeling. Circulation 100:1387-1393, 1999.

61. Wilkinson IB, MacCallum H, Rooijmans DF, et al. Increased augmentation index and systolic stress in type 1 diabetes mellitus. QJM 93:441-448, 2000.

62. Laurent S, Boutouyrie P, Asmar R, et al. Aortic stiffness is an independent predictor of all-cause and cardiovascular mortality in hypertensive patients. Hypertension 37:1236-1241, 2001.

63. Nishijima T, Nakayama Y, Tsumura K, et al. Pulsatility of ascending aortic blood pressure waveform is associated with an increased risk of coronary heart disease. Am J Hypertens 14(5 Pt 1):469-473, 2001.

64. Waddell TK, Dart AM, Medley TL, et al. Carotid pressure is a better predictor of coronary artery disease severity than brachial pressure. Hypertension 38:927-931, 2001.

# Chapter 23

# Coronary Atherosclerotic Sequelae of Hypertension

## William B. Kannel

Hypertension is a highly prevalent predisposing condition for the development of cardiovascular disease (CVD) in the United States, and one of the major contributors to coronary heart disease (CHD) the leading cause of cardiovascular death from this cause. Hypertension affects about 50 million persons in the United States and is destined to increase further as the population ages.[1] Framingham Study data indicate that 90% of 50-year-old normotensive persons can expect to develop hypertension in their lifetime.[2] Persistent elevation of blood pressure (BP) is a critical element in the evolution of atherosclerotic cardiovascular morbidity and mortality. Animal experiments indicate that hypertension accelerates lipid-induced atherosclerosis and that lowering the BP retards the pathology.[3] Also, low-pressure segments of the human circulation such as the pulmonary arteries or veins are virtually immune to atherosclerosis, despite exposure to the same lipid-laden blood as the systemic arteries supplying the heart, brain, and limbs. Atherosclerotic vascular pathology has now replaced the fibrinoid necrosis of malignant hypertension as the chief outcome of poorly controlled hypertension. However, the relation of hypertension to atherosclerosis is complex, interacting with other major risk factors that greatly influence its potential to enhance atherogenesis in the coronary arteries and elsewhere. The continuing high prevalence of hypertension in the general population, its great impact on cardiovascular morbidity and mortality rates and our ability to treat and control it, give it a high priority among measures to prevent CVD in general and CHD in particular. Treatment of hypertension and the CVD it promotes, account for a large portion of our health care expenditures.

## PREVALENCE AND INCIDENCE

Hypertension (BP >140/90 mm Hg) is a dangerously prevalent condition afflicting one in four American adults. About 4% of persons younger than age 30 years have this condition and it increases in prevalence with age, reaching 65% in persons age 80 years and older.[4] Each year about 2 million individuals are added to the pool of hypertensive persons requiring evaluation and treatment. The seventh Report of the Joint National Committee on Detection, Evaluation, and Treatment of High Blood Pressure (JNC 7) has designated systolic blood pressures (SBPs) of 120 to 139 mm Hg or diastolic blood pressures (DBPs) of 80 to 89 mm Hg as *prehypertension*.[1] These patients are at twice the risk for developing *hypertension* as those with lower values.[5]

Over 26 years of follow-up, 25% to 50% of the normotensive segment of the Framingham Study cohort developed hypertension.[6] Those with high-normal pressures developed "hypertension" at a twofold to threefold higher rate than those with strictly normal pressures.[5-7] The incidence of new onset of hypertension increased threefold and eightfold from the third to the fifth decade of age in men and women, respectively.[6]

## OPTIMAL BLOOD PRESSURE

It is difficult to specify at what BP a significant excess risk of hypertensive atherosclerotic cardiovascular sequelae *begins* to occur. Epidemiologic investigations report an excess risk of such events at BPs well below those often designated to define hypertension.[1,8,9] To assess accurately the incremental risk of CVD at BPs in the nonhypertensive range, it is necessary to have huge population samples. A reasonably precise assessment of the risk of mortality at relatively low BPs can be obtained from the more than 350,000 men screened for eligibility in the Multiple Risk Factor Intervention Trial (MRFIT).[9] Ten-year mortality rates in relation to baseline BP in that study increased stepwise from the lowest SBP (<110 mm Hg) on up. Compared with this lowest pressure, those with SBPs of only 120 to 129 mm Hg had an 18% higher overall and 35% higher cardiovascular mortality.[9] Thus the optimal SBP appears to be less than 110 mm Hg because 40% of all deaths and 35% of cardiovascular deaths occurred in the "normotensive" range of 110 to 139 mm Hg. Based on these data, it appears that the majority of the population have higher than optimal SBPs, because only 6% of MRFIT screenees had pressures less than 110 mm Hg. A report based on another large population sample also shows a continuous relationship between CVD and BP in 40- to 70-year-old persons. Each 20-mm Hg increment in SBP or 10–mm Hg increase in DBP confers a doubling of the risk of CVD across the range of BPs from 115/75 to 185/115 mm Hg.[10] Framingham Study data also suggest a continuous graded influence of BP on myocardial infarction (MI) occurrence in particular, beginning below 120 mm Hg systolic and 75 mm Hg diastolic, in men younger than age 65 years. For men older than age 65 years, an even steeper gradient of risk is noted throughout the SBP range. For DBP, incremental risk is noted as pressures increase above 75 mm Hg (Figure 23–1).

The population-attributable risk statistic provides the best indication of the population impact of hypertension because it takes into account both the prevalence of designated stages of hypertension and their risk ratios. Based on Framingham Study data, this indicates that, together, all grades of hypertension account for 28.5% of atherosclerotic cardiovascular events in men ages 35 to 64 years; 18.1% is attributed to JNC VI stages I and II hypertension. In women, the corresponding

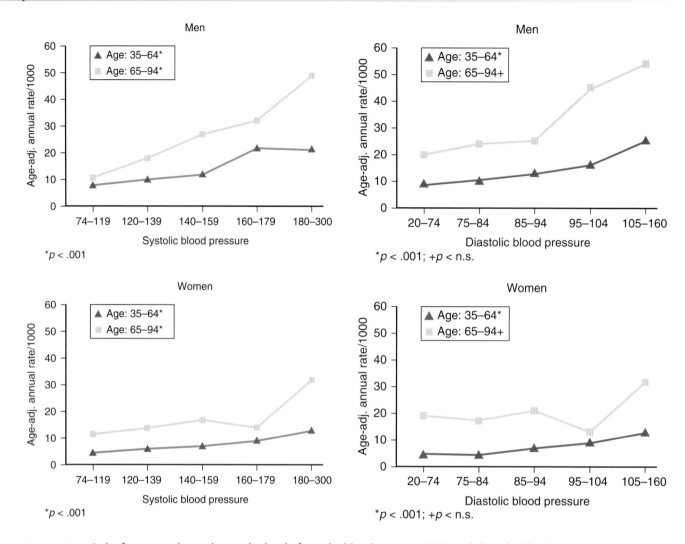

**Figure 23–1** Risk of coronary heart disease by level of systolic blood pressure (SBP) and diastolic blood pressure (DBP) in each sex at specified ages. Framingham Study: 30-year follow-up. (From Vokonas PS, Kannel WB. Epidemiology of coronary heart disease in the elderly. In DD Tresh, WS Aronow (eds). Cardiovascular Disease in the Elderly, 2nd ed. New York, Marcel Dekker, 1999; pp 139-164.

attributable risk figures are 29.6% and 14.2%. Similar proportions of cardiovascular events are attributable to hypertension in the elderly. The relative and absolute risk of CHD to the individual increases sharply with the degree of BP elevation, but the population impact, signified by the population-attributable risk, is greatest for JNC VI stages I and II hypertension.

Control of existing hypertension remains far from complete and the incidence of newly acquired hypertension has not declined, indicating a need for primary prevention by weight control, salt restriction, and exercise, targeted at persons with a strong family history of hypertension, Blacks, and the obese.[11] Because there is a high prevalence in the population of persons with high-normal prehypertensive pressures who are at increased risk of developing more severe grades of hypertension, these nonpharmacologic approaches to control the discretionary environmental determinants of elevated BP need greater attention. The goal for hypertension control in the general population is to shift the BP distribution down to a more acceptable average value by hygienic measures, as well as treating those with already elevated pressures.

For physicians using medication to control BP, somewhat higher pressures are recommended as thresholds for treatment. However, it is important to recognize that the average pressure at which atherosclerotic cardiovascular events occur is not extremely elevated. The average BP at which men aged 30 to 62 years in the Framingham Study developed CHD was only 146/91 mm Hg; and for women, 161/94 mm Hg (Table 23–1). The median BP at which cardiovascular events occurred tended to increase with age, and has declined over succeeding calendar decades, both in those untreated and those under treatment. By the 1980s, half the cardiovascular events in Framingham Study men not on treatment occurred at pressures below 135/81 mm Hg, and in women, at pressures below 136/80 mm Hg.

## ATHEROSCLEROTIC SEQUELAE

Hypertension is clearly a major contributor to the occurrence of atherosclerotic CVD in the general population, imposing a twofold to fourfold increased risk of a major atherosclerotic cardiovascular event in persons ages 35 to 64 years and about a twofold risk in the elderly (Table 23–2). Thus it contributes to the risk of such events at all ages in either sex. The risk ratios are largest for heart failure and stroke, but CHD is the most common and lethal sequela for individuals younger than age 65 years, equaling in incidence all the other adverse outcomes combined. Although the absolute and excess risk of atherosclerotic CVD imposed by hypertension in women is less than in men, the relative risk is just as high for women as for men older than and younger than age 65 years (see Table 23–2).

## Coronary Hazards

The less-than-expected efficacy of antihypertensive therapy to reduce the risk of coronary morbidity and mortality in early trials led to some unjustified questioning of the importance of BP in the development of CHD. Prospective epidemiologic investigation has in fact shown that hypertension is a powerful independent risk factor for the occurrence of coronary events.[12] In the Framingham Study, risk of every clinical manifestation of CHD was increased in persons with antecedent hypertension (Table 23–3). Although the CHD incidence rates of hypertensive women are substantially lower than those of men, the risk ratios comparing rates in hypertensives

with nonhypertensives are higher in women than men. Hypertension increases the risk of an MI almost twofold in men younger than age 65 years and threefold in such women (see Table 23–3).

For reasons that are unclear, hypertension predisposes disproportionately to MIs that go unrecognized, and the more severe the hypertension, the greater the proportion unrecognized (Table 23–4). This association persists even after excluding persons on therapy that might mask symptoms, persons with electrocardiogram (ECG) evidence of left ventricular hypertrophy (LVH) that might be confused with anterior MIs, and persons with coexistent diabetes who are known to be more prone to silent MIs. Unrecognized MIs are surprisingly common in general and particularly so in hypertensive persons. In hypertensive men, 35% of MIs go unrecognized, and in hypertensive women, 48%. This propensity to silent or unrecognized MIs makes periodic ECG surveillance of hypertensive patients for evidence of an MI mandatory.

As for CVD in general, risk of coronary events increases with the BP in a continuous graded fashion with no indication of a critical value where normal pressure leaves off and abnormal ensues (see Figure 23–1). It has been suggested that there is an excess risk of CHD at very low DBPs. However, in the Framingham Study of healthy persons taken as a whole, there was no indication of a J-curve relation of DBP to the occurrence

**Table 23–1** Mean Initial Blood Pressure of Those Developing Coronary Heart Disease (CHD) Versus Those Remaining Disease Free for 14 Years in the Framingham Study

| | Systolic Blood Pressure (mm Hg) | | | | Diastolic Blood Pressure (mm Hg) | | | |
|---|---|---|---|---|---|---|---|---|
| | Men | | Women | | Men | | Women | |
| Ages | CHD (323) | Controls (1959) | CHD (169) | Controls (2676) | CHD | Controls | CHD | Controls |
| 30-39 | 138* | 132* | 126† | 124 | 90* | 83 | 83† | 79 |
| 40-49 | 143* | 135* | 149* | 136 | 92* | 86 | 91* | 85 |
| 50-62 | 150* | 141* | 168* | 150 | 91* | 87 | 97* | 90 |
| Total | 146‡ | 135* | 161‡ | 135 | 91‡ | 85 | 94‡ | 84 |

*p <.05.
†Not significant.
‡p <.01.
CHD, coronary heart disease.

**Table 23–2** Relation of Hypertension to Atherosclerotic Cardiovascular Outcomes: 36-Year Follow-up in the Framingham Study

| | Ages 35-64 Years | | | | Ages 65-94 Years | | | |
|---|---|---|---|---|---|---|---|---|
| Cardiovascular Sequelae | Biennial Age-Adjusted Rate/1000 | | Age-Adjusted Risk Ratio | | Biennial Age-Adjusted Rate/1000 | | Age-Adjusted Risk Ratio | |
| | Men | Women | Men | Women | Men | Women | Men | Women |
| Coronary Disease | 45 | 21 | 2.0* | 2.2* | 73 | 44 | 1.6* | 1.9* |
| Stroke | 12 | 6 | 3.8* | 2.6* | 36 | 39 | 1.9† | 2.3* |
| Peripheral Artery Disease | 10 | 7 | 2.0* | 3.7* | 17 | 10 | 1.6‡ | 2.0* |
| Heart Failure | 14 | 6 | 4.0* | 3.0* | 33 | 24 | 1.9* | 1.9* |

From Kannel WB. Hypertension in the elderly. Cardiol Elderly 1:359-363, 1993.
*p <.001.
†p <.01.
‡p <.05.

**Table 23-3** Clinical Manifestations of Coronary Heart Disease by Hypertensive Status: 40-Year Follow-up in the Framingham Study*

| Clinical Manifestation | Ages 35-64 Years Annual Age-Adjusted Rate/1000 | | | | Ages 65-94 Years Annual Age-Adjusted Rate/1000 | | | |
|---|---|---|---|---|---|---|---|---|
| | HBP Absent | | HBP Present | | HBP Absent | | HBP Present | |
| | Men | Women | Men | Women | Men | Women | Men | Women |
| Myocardial infarction | 4.8 | 0.9 | 9.3 | 2.9 | 11.7 | 3.8 | 20.8 | 8.8 |
| Angina pectoris | 4.6 | 2.2 | 9.4 | 5.9 | 6.7 | 4.1 | 9.4 | 7.8 |
| Sudden death | 0.74 | 0.20 | 1.95 | 0.55 | 2.6 | 1.1 | 4.8 | 1.8 |

*HBP = 140/90 mm Hg or taking medication.
HBP, high blood pressure.

**Table 23-4** Percent of Myocardial Infarctions Unrecognized by Hypertensive Status

| Hypertensive Status | Excluding Diabetics* | | Excluding Anti-HBP Rx* | | Excluding LVH* | |
|---|---|---|---|---|---|---|
| | Men | Women | Men | Women | Men | Women |
| Normal | 18.5 | 30.7 | 17.8 | 26.6 | 19.6 | 29.0 |
| Mild | 28.3 | 36.1 | 30.2 | 35.5 | 30.1 | 35.3 |
| Definite | 33.2 | 48.1 | 34.8 | 48.5 | 32.7 | 50.5 |

*Also excludes persons with coronary heart disease at examination immediately preceding MI.
HBP, high blood pressure; Rx, medication; LVH, left ventricular hypertrophy.

of coronary mortality.[13] Only in persons with elevated SBP and those who already had an MI was an upturn in coronary mortality seen at DBPs below 75 mm Hg. The reason for this excess of mortality at low DBPs is at present unclear, but it is likely that it is confined to those with an increased pulse pressure.

It has been suggested that increased coronary mortality at low DBPs is a reflection of ill health, poor left ventricular function, or overtreatment.[14-16] Overtreatment does not appear to be a likely explanation, because the J-curve BP relationship has been observed in both treated and untreated persons who have sustained an MI in the Framingham Study and elsewhere.[13,17] Because low DBP appears to be associated with a poor outcome in patients with overt CHD and not in those free of such disease, it is possible that the presence of a low pressure, whether induced by treatment or not, is potentially lethal in the presence of a severely compromised coronary circulation. Although the Framingham Study took into account the fall in pressure that may result from an extensive MI and excluded persons with heart failure, it remains possible that the low DBP following MI is a manifestation of the extent of myocardial damage sustained.

## Reinfarction and Death

A wide range of clinical, demographic, and biochemical risk factors have been investigated for prognostic value following an MI, but only a few studies have assessed the outlook beyond 5 years, as the Framingham Study has done. Assessment of the influence of BP on the outlook following MI is complicated because the BP can fall *as a result of* the infarction, so its association with the prognosis may depend on when the BP was measured with respect to the time of

occurrence of the infarction.[13,14] Hypertension appears to confer a poor prognosis after an MI only when the BP is assessed after it has stabilized from the drop in pressure that often occurs postinfarction.[15,16] Patients whose BPs fall as a result of an MI have a worse outlook than those whose pressures remain stable.[13,14,17] Framingham Study data indicate that after excluding those who had a significant (i.e., 10 mm Hg) fall in BP immediately post-MI, there is a distinct relationship of the post-MI BP to mortality (Figure 23-2).

In the Framingham Study, where BPs were measured about 1 year after surviving the MI, and patients were followed for reinfarction or coronary death up to 30 years, both SBP and DBP were found to be important risk factors.[18] Mean SBP

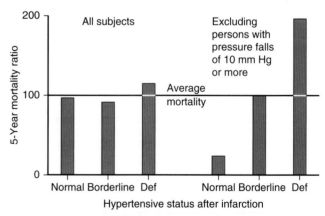

**Figure 23-2** Mortality following myocardial infarction (MI) according to blood pressure status after interim MI. Framingham Study.

and DBP were higher in persons who experienced a reinfarction or coronary fatality. Each 25–mm Hg increase in SBP conferred a 53% increase in propensity to reinfarction and a 42% increased likelihood of coronary mortality adjusted for age and other risk factors for CHD.[18] This strong association of postinfarction SBP with reinfarction and coronary mortality is in agreement with the findings of others.[19,20]

## COMPONENTS OF BLOOD PRESSURE

For most of the past century arterial hypertension was regarded as an arteriolar disease leading to increased resistance and hence increased mean arterial pressure (MAP). Because MAP is closer to the DBP than SBP, elevation of the diastolic component of the BP was considered the hallmark of arterial hypertension.[21] DBP was considered a clinical measure of arteriolar tone and SBP, a measure of cardiac strength.

The increase in BP with age was regarded as a natural phenomenon. Although challenged by Framingham Study investigators in relation to risk of both stroke and heart attack many decades before,[22] the idea that the increase in SBP with age is innocuous persisted until the Systolic Hypertension in the Elderly Program (SHEP) trial.[23]

Clinical decisions and trials concerned with the efficacy of treating hypertension emphasized the diastolic component of the BP for too long because high DBPs were believed to be more pathologic than SBP elevations. However, epidemiologic data from the Framingham Study[22,24] and elsewhere[9] do not suggest that the DBP has a greater impact than the SBP on the occurrence of CVD in general or CHD in particular. SBP has a significantly greater impact than DBP on the rate of development of cardiovascular sequelae of hypertension, including CHD.[9,22]

Current staging of hypertension is based on the levels of both SBP and DBP. Franklin et al. have examined whether the pulse pressure adds useful information for estimating the risk of initial coronary events in the population-based Framingham Study[25] (see Chapter 22). They found that when SBPs and DBPs were jointly entered into multivariable analysis, CHD risk was positively associated with SBP and inversely for DBP. Cross-classification examination of CHD risk by SBP and DBP confirmed this result (Table 23–5). These findings suggested that the pulse pressure is an important determinant of the BP-related risk of CHD. For any level of SBP, persons with higher pulse pressure (i.e., lower DBP) had a substantial increase in risk (Figure 23–3). Risk of CHD increased in a continuous graded fashion with the pulse pressure at all levels of SBP.

These results support the prior Framingham Study data indicating that in persons whose DBPs had not exceeded 90 mm Hg, the risk of cardiovascular events increased steeply with the SBP (and hence pulse pressure) at all ages in both sexes.[24] In the Framingham Study, the age-adjusted incidence of CHD was substantially greater for isolated systolic than isolated diastolic hypertension in both sexes. Age-specific analysis of Framingham Study data indicates that this conclusion may need to be modified because of an observed variable impact of the BP components according to age. An examination of the relative importance of systolic, diastolic, and pulse pressure as CHD predictors in different age groups suggests that there is a gradual shift with advancing age from diastolic to systolic and finally to pulse pressure as dominant predictors of CHD. In younger (<50 years) persons, DBP and to a lesser extent SBP, predict CHD, whereas in older individuals SBP and pulse pressure are superior predictors of the risk.[26]

## RISK FACTOR CLUSTERING

A tendency for hypertension to cluster with other major coronary risk factors has long been noted in the Framingham

**Table 23–5** Risk of Coronary Heart Disease According to Systolic and Diastolic Blood Pressure: 20-Year Follow-up in the Framingham Study of Persons Ages 50-79 Years

| | Relative Risks | | | |
| | Systolic Blood Pressure | | | |
| Diastolic Blood Pressure | <120 | 120-139 | 140-159 | ≥160 |
|---|---|---|---|---|
| ≥90 | — | 1.7 | 2.3† | 2.8‡ |
| 80-89 | 1.4 | 1.9* | 1.9* | 4.0‡ |
| 70-79 | 1.1 | 2.1† | 3.4‡ | 6.8‡ |
| <70 | 1.0 | 2.4* | 4.2† | — |

From Franklin SS, Khan BS, Wong ND, et al. Is pulse pressure useful in predicting coronary heart disease? Circulation 100:354-360, 1999.
*p <.05.
†p <.0.
‡p <.001.
Adjusted for age, sex, body mass index, cigarette smoking, glucose tolerance, and total:high-density lipoprotein cholesterol ratio.

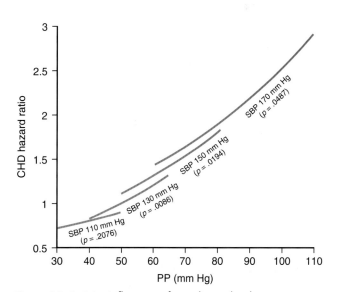

**Figure 23–3** Joint influences of systolic and pulse pressure on risk of coronary heart disease. (From Franklin SS, Khan SA, Wong ND, et al. Is pulse pressure useful in predicting coronary heart disease? The Framingham heart study. Circulation 100:354-360, 1999.)

Study and elsewhere, and many of the risk factors with which it tends to cluster also predict the occurrence of the hypertension.[1,27] It has become increasingly apparent that the magnitude of the risk of CHD associated with any degree of BP elevation is markedly influenced by the associated burden of other risk factors (Figure 23–4).[27] Only 20% to 24% of the elevated (upper quintile) BP (>138 mm Hg in men and >130 mm Hg in women) that occurred in the Framingham Study was accompanied by other risk factors (upper quintiles of total cholesterol, body mass index [BMI], triglycerides, glucose,

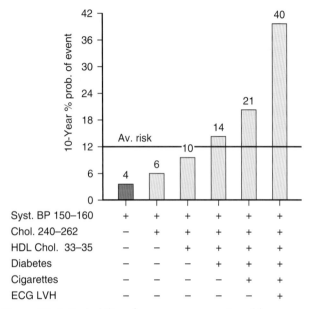

**Figure 23–4** Probability of a coronary event in mild hypertension by intensity of associated risk factors. Men aged 45 years. (From Kannel WB, Wilson PWF. Hypertension as a cardiovascular risk factor. *In* CJ Bulpitt, (ed). Handbook of Hypertension, Vol. 20: Epidemiology of Hypertension. Amsterdam, Elsevier Science BV, 2000; pp 19-42.

or lower-quintile high-density lipoprotein [HDL] cholesterol). Clusters of two or more of these additional risk factors occurred in 49% of men and 54% of women, a rate greatly exceeding that expected by chance. The bulk of CHD events—63% in men and 78% in women—occurred in those hypertensives with two or more additional risk factors (Table 23–6).

The tendency for elevated BP to cluster with other risk factors suggests that hypertension may be a reflection of some more fundamental process that accelerates atherogenesis[28] (see Chapter 13). Abdominal obesity promotes insulin resistance and abnormal sympathoadrenal activity and has been postulated as an underlying mechanism.[29] Abnormalities of lipoprotein metabolism, insulin resistance, and glucose tolerance are commonly encountered in persons with essential hypertension and their close relatives.[30] These abnormalities do not cluster with secondary hypertension. Hyperinsulinemia, signifying insulin resistance, is found in both obese and nonobese persons with hypertension and may persist despite antihypertensive therapy.[28] However, insulin resistance and hyperinsulinemia are more severe and more closely associated with hypertension in obese than nonobese persons. Also, weight gain worsens all the elements of the insulin resistance syndrome and weight loss improves them. In the Framingham Study the extent of risk factor clustering increased stepwise with the degree of obesity: A 5-pound increase in weight imposed a 30% increase in the extent of risk factor clustering with hypertension. Persons with elevated BP characteristically have elevated triglycerides and reduced HDL cholesterol. Such persons also tend to have atherogenic small-dense low-density lipoprotein particles.[31] It is uncertain what percentage of hypertensive persons have the insulin resistance syndrome; it has been estimated that about half may have it.

In the Framingham Study, BP-related risk of developing CHD increased stepwise with the extent of risk factor clustering (see Table 23–6). Among persons with elevated BP it is estimated that about 40% of coronary events in men and 68% in women are attributable to clusters of two or more additional risk factors.

**Table 23–6** 16-Year CHD Incidence by Number of Other Risk Factors: Framingham Heart Study Offspring with Elevated Blood Pressure (Persons Ages 30-65 Years at Baseline)

| Number of Other Risk Factors | Relative Risk (95% CI) | Prevalence | Number of CHD Events (%) | Population-Attributable Risk (Multivariate) |
|---|---|---|---|---|
| **Men** | | | | |
| 0 | 1.0 (referent) | 22% | 10 (14%) | — |
| 1 | 1.33 (0.57, 3.06) | 29% | 17 (24%) | 0.09 |
| ≥2 | 2.28 (1.09, 4.78) | 49% | 45 (63%) | 0.39 |
| *Total* | | | 72 (100%) | |
| Women | | | | |
| 0 | 1.0 (referent) | 18% | 2 (5%) | — |
| 1 | 2.05 (0.41, 10.18) | 28% | 7 (18%) | 0.23 |
| ≥2 | 4.93 (1.14, 21.27) | 54% | 31 (78%) | 0.68 |
| *Total* | | | 40 (100%) | |

High blood pressure defined as SPB ≥138 mm Hg (men) and ≥130 mm Hg (women). Other risk factors included the top quintiles of other factors (total cholesterol, BMI, triglycerides, glucose) and bottom quintile for HDL cholesterol.
CI, confidence interval; CHD, coronary heart disease; BMI, body mass index; SBP, systolic blood pressure; HDL, high-density lipoprotein.

Whatever the cause of the risk factor clustering in persons with elevated BP, it is clear that it should be anticipated and routinely screened for. Also, when three or more of the specified risk factors—increased waist girth, elevated triglycerides, reduced HDL cholesterol, elevated blood sugar, and BP—are found, it seems reasonable to suspect the presence of the insulin resistance or metabolic syndrome.[1]

## GLOBAL RISK ASSESSMENT

Because of the tendency of risk factors to cluster with hypertension and the variable risk depending on the amount of clustering that accompanies the hypertension, it is advisable to undertake a global coronary risk assessment in all hypertensive patients. To facilitate this, CHD risk factor prediction charts were developed based on Framingham Study multivariate risk formulations (Table 23–7). Using this scoring system it is possible to conveniently estimate the global CHD risk of hypertensive patients, taking the associated burden of other risk factors into account. To an extent, designation by the JNC 7 guidelines of the *metabolic syndrome* as one of the "special situations" to consider in evaluation and treatment of hypertension invokes multivariable risk assessment. However, most of the ingredients of the syndrome are components of the Framingham Study risk profile; the value of detecting persons with the syndrome has greater implications for the choices of therapy than risk assessment.

### Renin

Hypertension is heterogeneous in its pathophysiology and clinical sequelae. Much research has been directed at determining and understanding the pathophysiology of the factors that increase the risk of CHD in hypertension. In this connection, the role of the renin-angiotensin system (RAS) has been the focus of attention for some time.[32] An activated RAS has been postulated to be another risk factor for CHD in hypertension.[33] In addition to causing vasoconstriction and sodium retention, angiotensin II increases vascular smooth muscle cell growth and promotes neointima formation after vascular injury.[32] Experimentally, angiotensin-converting enzyme (ACE) inhibitors reduce myocardial ischemia, decrease atherosclerosis, prevent restenosis after arterial injury, and prevent ventricular dilation.[32] However, it is not yet clear whether high renin plays a causal role in the risk of an MI in hypertension or is only a marker for an activated sympathetic or neurohormonal state.[32] High renin with respect to the level of sodium excretion has been reported in a case-control comparison and a prospective epidemiologic investigation to be another predictor of MI in patients with hypertension.[33,34] A retrospective study similar to the earlier retrospective study that claimed to show a relationship of renin to heart attacks and strokes failed to confirm this claim.[34,35] It is possible that hypertensive patients with high renin profiles could benefit more than those with low renin from treatment with β-blockers or ACE inhibitors to prevent CHD, but this remains to be demonstrated.

### Left Ventricular Hypertrophy

LVH, whether manifested by ECG, chest radiograph, or echocardiogram, is an ominous feature of hypertension. ECG LVH, particularly when accompanied by repolarization abnormality, is a harbinger of impending clinical CHD in the hypertensive patient. It further escalates the risk of all the major sequelae of elevated BP; most commonly CHD (Table 23–8). Framingham Study participants with higher baseline voltages and more severe repolarization abnormalities had higher BPs, and serial changes in these ECG parameters were accompanied by corresponding changes in BP. The risk of CVD increases over a threefold range in relation to the size of the R-wave on the ECG and, compared with normal, severe repolarization abnormality increases the risk almost sixfold for men and 2.5-fold for women.[36] Framingham Study participants observed to have a decrease in voltage over time had only one half the risk of cardiovascular events of those with no change.[36] Because ECG LVH carries as serious a prognosis as an MI detected by routine ECG examination, it is appropriate to regard hypertensive persons with this condition as seriously as if they have diagnosed CHD.[8] LVH on radiograph is not as ominous as the ECG version, but adds to risk when it accompanies ECG hypertrophy.[8] Echocardiography is a more sensitive and more easily quantifiable detector of hypertensive LVH, and hypertrophy detected by echocardiogram has also been shown to be associated with an increased risk of developing CHD.[37] Risk of coronary events is related to the left ventricular mass observed in hypertensive persons in a continuous graded fashion, with no critical value that separates compensatory from pathologic hypertrophy (Figure 23–5).[37]

### Heart Rate

Hypertensive persons tend to have higher heart rates than normotensive people, and persons with more rapid heart rates tend to develop hypertension at a greater rate.[38,39] Hypertension with a rapid heart rate is also more dangerous. The Framingham Study observed an independent effect of the heart rate that accompanies hypertension on the rate of subsequent mortality from CHD (Table 23–9). The observed effect was stronger for the occurrence of fatal than nonfatal coronary events, and particularly for acutely fatal attacks, consistent with a direct effect of heart rate, mediated through the autonomic nervous system. Apparently as hypertension exacts its toll on the myocardium, the heart rate must increase to compensate for a decreased stroke output.[39]

### The Elderly

The impact of hypertension on the development of CHD is perceived to weaken in advanced age.[11,40] In the very old, it has been claimed that hypertension may actually protect against mortality.[40] This has resulted in a reluctance to treat hypertension aggressively in the aged.[11] The risk ratio for clinical CHD in hypertensive participants in the Framingham Study decreases slightly with advance in age, but this is offset by a distinctly higher absolute, excess, and attributable risk, owing to the high incidence of CHD in the elderly, the high prevalence of hypertension in this age group, and the significant risk ratio in older persons (Table 23–10). Because there is a disproportionate rise in SBP compared with DBP with advancing age, isolated systolic hypertension (ISH) is the predominant type of hypertension in the elderly. ISH is clearly a risk factor for the development of CHD in

**Table 23-7** Coronary Heart Disease Risk Factor Prediction Chart*

### 1. Find Points For Each Risk Factor

| Age (If Female) | | Age (If Male) | | HDL Cholesterol | | Total Cholesterol | | Systolic Blood Pressure | | Other | |
|---|---|---|---|---|---|---|---|---|---|---|---|
| *Age | Pts. | Age | Pts. | HDLC | Pts. | Total C | Pts. | SBP | Pts. | | Pts. |
| 30 | -12 | 30 | -2 | 25-26 | 7 | 139-151 | -3 | 98-104 | -2 | Cigarettes | 4 |
| 31 | -11 | 31 | -1 | 27-29 | 6 | 152-166 | -2 | 105-112 | -1 | Diabetic—male | 3 |
| 32 | -9 | 32-33 | 0 | 30-32 | 5 | 167-182 | -1 | 113-120 | 0 | Diabetic—female | 6 |
| 33 | -8 | 34 | 1 | 33-35 | 4 | 183-199 | 0 | 121-129 | 1 | ECG LVH | 9 |
| 34 | -6 | 35-36 | 2 | 36-38 | 3 | 200-219 | 1 | 130-139 | 2 | | |
| 35 | -5 | 37-38 | 3 | 39-42 | 2 | 220-239 | 2 | 140-149 | 3 | 0 pts for each | NO |
| 36 | -4 | 39 | 4 | 43-46 | 1 | 240-262 | 3 | 150-160 | 4 | | |
| 37 | -3 | 40-41 | 5 | 47-50 | 0 | 263-288 | 4 | 161-172 | 5 | | |
| 38 | -2 | 42-43 | 6 | 51-55 | -1 | 289-315 | 5 | 173-185 | 6 | | |
| 39 | -1 | 44-45 | 7 | 56-60 | -2 | 316-330 | 6 | | | | |
| 40 | 0 | 46-47 | 8 | 61-66 | -3 | | | | | | |
| 41 | 1 | 48-49 | 9 | 67-73 | -4 | | | | | | |
| 42-43 | 2 | 50-51 | 10 | 74-80 | -5 | | | | | | |
| 44 | 3 | 52-54 | 11 | 81-87 | -6 | | | | | | |
| 45-46 | 4 | 55-56 | 12 | 88-96 | -7 | | | | | | |
| 47-48 | 5 | 57-59 | 13 | | | | | | | | |
| 49-50 | 6 | 60-61 | 14 | | | | | | | | |
| 51-52 | 7 | 62-64 | 15 | | | | | | | | |
| 53-55 | 8 | 65-67 | 16 | | | | | | | | |
| 56-60 | 9 | 68-70 | 17 | | | | | | | | |
| 61-67 | 10 | 71-73 | 18 | | | | | | | | |
| 68-74 | 11 | 74 | 19 | | | | | | | | |

### 2. Sum Points For All Risk Factors

| Age | + | HDLC | + | Total C | + | SBP | + | Smoker | + | Diabetes | + | ECG LVH | = | Point Total |

NOTE: *Subtract Minus Points From Total.*

### 3. Look Up Risk Corresponding To Point Total

| Pts. | Probability 5 Yr | Probability 10 Yr | Pts. | Probability 5 Yr | Probability 10 Yr | Pts. | Probability 5 Yr | Probability 10 Yr | Pts. | Probability 5 Yr | Probability 10 Yr |
|---|---|---|---|---|---|---|---|---|---|---|---|
| ≤1 | <1% | <2% | 10 | 2% | 6% | 19 | 8% | 16% | 28 | 19% | 33% |
| 2 | 1% | 2% | 11 | 3% | 6% | 20 | 8% | 18% | 29 | 20% | 36% |
| 3 | 1% | 2% | 12 | 3% | 7% | 21 | 9% | 19% | 30 | 22% | 38% |
| 4 | 1% | 2% | 13 | 3% | 8% | 22 | 11% | 21% | 31 | 24% | 40% |
| 5 | 1% | 3% | 14 | 4% | 9% | 23 | 12% | 23% | 32 | 25% | 42% |
| 6 | 1% | 3% | 15 | 5% | 10% | 24 | 13% | 25% | | | |
| 7 | 1% | 4% | 16 | 5% | 12% | 25 | 14% | 27% | | | |
| 8 | 2% | 4% | 17 | 6% | 13% | 26 | 16% | 29% | | | |
| 9 | 2% | 5% | 18 | 7% | 14% | 27 | 17% | 31% | | | |

### 4. Compare With Average 10-Year Risk

| Age | Probability Women | Probability Men |
|---|---|---|
| 30-34 | <1% | 3% |
| 35-39 | <1% | 5% |
| 40-44 | 2% | 6% |
| 45-49 | 5% | 10% |
| 50-54 | 8% | 14% |
| 55-59 | 12% | 16% |
| 60-64 | 13% | 21% |
| 65-69 | 9% | 30% |
| 70-74 | 12% | 24% |

*These charts were prepared with the help of William B. Kannel, M.D., Professor of Medicine and Public Health, and Ralph D'Agostino, Ph.D., Head, Department of Mathematics, both at Boston University; Keaven Anderson, Ph.D., Statistician; NHLBI, Framingham Study; Daniel McGee, Ph.D., Associate Professor, University of Arizona. From American Heart Association.

**Table 23-8** Risk of Coronary Heart Disease by Hypertensive and ECG LVH Status: 32-Year Follow-up in the Framingham Study

| | Biennial Age-Adjusted Rate/1000 | | | | | |
| | Ages 35-64 Years* | | | Ages 65-94 Years* | | |
| | ECG LVH | | | ECG LVH | | |
| Hypertension* | None | Voltage | Voltage + Repolarization | None | Voltage | Voltage + Repolarization |
|---|---|---|---|---|---|---|
| Men | | | | | | |
| Absent | 22 | 35 | 54 | 43 | 75 | 117 |
| Present | 44 | 35 | 110 | 69 | 111 | 168 |
| Women | | | | | | |
| Absent | 9 | 19 | — | 23 | 83 | 90 |
| Present | 19 | 17 | 85 | 41 | 53 | 136 |

*Hypertension includes all receiving treatment.
ECG, electrocardiogram; LVH, left ventricular hypertrophy.

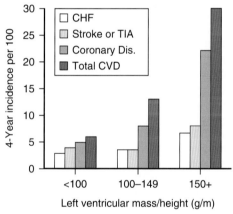

**Figure 23-5** Four-year incidence of cardiovascular events according to left ventricular mass. Men ages 65-90 years. (Framingham Study.)

**Table 23-9** Risk of Fatal and Nonfatal Coronary Events per 40 BPM. Increase in Heart Rate: Hypertensive Individuals. 30-Year Follow-up in the Framingham Study.

| | Odds Ratio for 40 BPM Increment (BP Age-Adjusted) | |
| Coronary Event | Men | Women |
|---|---|---|
| All fatal CHD events | 1.80* | 1.59[†] |
| Fatal within 30 days | 2.37[‡] | 2.46[§] |
| Nonfatal within 30 days | 1.14[†] | 0.82[†] |
| All fatal and nonfatal | 1.33[§] | 0.98[†] |

*$p < .01$.
[†]NS.
[‡]$p < .05$.
[§]$p < .001$.
BPM, beats per minute; BP, blood pressure; CHD, coronary heart disease.

**Table 23-10** Risk of Coronary Heart Disease Associated with Hypertension by Age in Each Sex: 40-Year Follow-up in the Framingham Study

| | Age-Adjusted Rate/1000 | | Age-Adjusted Risk Ratio | | Excess Rate/1000 | |
| Age (years) | Men | Women | Men | Women | Men | Women |
|---|---|---|---|---|---|---|
| 35-64 | 1.95 | 0.55 | 2.6 | 2.8 | 1.20 | 0.35 |
| 65-94 | 4.75 | 0.80 | 1.9 | 1.7 | 2.20 | 0.75 |

the elderly, possibly more so than in the middle aged (Figure 23–6). The high SBP and pulse pressure in the hypertensive elderly appears to be a direct cause of the excess CHD rather than only a sign of a diseased rigid artery, because the systolic hypertension persists as a risk factor when the associated arterial rigidity is taken into account.[41] The chief determinant of ISH in the elderly appears to be an elevated BP in middle age.[42]

Whether predominantly systolic, diastolic, or combined, hypertension is a hazard for CHD in the elderly. However, SBP elevation is a more reliable predictor of CHD in the elderly than the DBP, and reliance on the DBP to assess risk can be misleading in the aged with systolic hypertension.[6] Although their absolute risk of developing clinical CHD is lower than in men, the relative risks are higher in women than men for all clinical events other than sudden death.

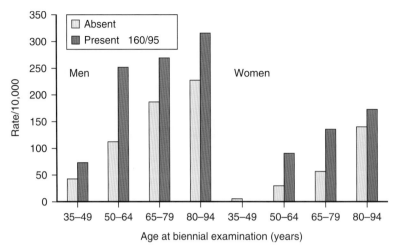

**Figure 23–6** Average annual incidence of myocardial infarction associated with isolated systolic hypertension by age and sex. (Framingham Study.)

**Table 23–11** Percent Prevalence of Associated Cardiovascular Conditions in Hypertensive Elderly: Framingham Study (1970-1982), Persons Aged 65-94 Years

| Associated Cardiovascular Conditions | Men | Women |
|---|---|---|
| Angina | 12 | 16 |
| Myocardial infarction | 12 | 5 |
| Cardiac failure | 3 | 5 |
| Stroke | 10 | 5 |
| Peripheral artery disease | 9 | 6 |
| Any cardiovascular disease | 31 | 27 |

Hypertension in the elderly is likely to be accompanied by overt CHD. In the Framingham Study, 24% of hypertensive elderly men also had angina or an MI. In elderly hypertensive women, 21% had these manifestations of CHD (Table 23–11). Stroke, heart failure, and peripheral artery disease are also commonly present. Some 31% of men and 27% of women in this age group will have one or more of these cardiovascular conditions. These greatly increase the hazard of the hypertension and must be taken into account in treatment decisions.

## PREVENTIVE IMPLICATIONS

In the 1950s there was limited knowledge about the long-term outlook of what was called "essential hypertension," and the condition was considered benign. Physicians were unimpressed with the hazards of such hypertension and, even if they were concerned, could do little about it. Over the past four decades we have come to recognize that idiopathic hypertension is an insidious and long-term promoter of accelerated atherogenesis and lethal cardiovascular events. Also, during this period effective, tolerable, and safe antihypertensive medications were produced that made it possible to control elevated BP and determine the effects of BP control on CVD outcomes.

BPs obtained routinely in the office predict the rate of development of CVD in general and CHD in particular.

Although there is some evidence that home BPs and 24-hour monitoring of BP may be useful refinements (see Chapters 27 and 28), risk assessment and treatment can be based on the average of several office BPs. Treatment should not be initiated on the basis a single casual office BP elevation, nor should the efficacy of treatment be judged from less than the average of multiple BP measurements. The lowest of a series of BPs should not be used to determine either the need for, or efficacy of, antihypertensive therapy.

In evaluating the hazard of hypertension and the need to treat it, more attention needs to be given to the SBP. For too long there has been an overemphasis on the diastolic component of the BP. Risk of CHD has been consistently shown to be more strongly related to the SBP than the DBP. ISH is not an innocuous accompaniment of advanced age. Treatment based on the SBP in patients with ISH has been shown to be at least as effective as that based on the DBP in preventing cardiovascular morbidity and mortality.[23,43]

Coexistent risk factors that cluster with hypertension exert a greater influence on the cardiovascular and coronary hazards of hypertension than the character of the BP elevation. Hypertension seldom occurs in isolation of other major risk factors to which it is metabolically linked. This makes it mandatory to test for the other risk factors and to conceptualize hypertension as a component of a cardiovascular risk profile. This avoids the possibility of either overreacting to an isolated moderate BP elevation or being falsely reassured by a return of BP to high-normal levels. Accompanied by multiple abnormalities of other risk factors, a seemingly innocuous degree of hypertension can be dangerous. When hypertension is accompanied by elevated triglycerides, reduced HDL cholesterol, and abdominal obesity, insulin resistance is likely and treatment should be modified accordingly. Prevention of CHD is more likely to be effective if in addition to lowering the BP, a more favorable coronary risk profile is achieved. Not uncommonly, elderly hypertensive patients when first encountered may already have overt angina, an MI, peripheral artery disease, or cardiac failure. These associated conditions must be taken into account in judging the urgency for treatment and in choosing the optimal therapeutic agents.

Antihypertensive therapy has been shown to regress LVH in hypertensive patients.[44] Although it is not yet established by controlled trials whether this regression consistently reduces the formidable increase in CVD risk imposed by LVH, Framingham Study data indicate that when improvement in the ECG evidence of hypertrophy is observed, there is a substantially lower risk of cardiovascular sequelae compared with those in whom there is no change or progression (Table 23–12).[36] Thus, therapy that eliminates or slows progression of LVH may improve the outlook of the hypertensive patient with this dangerous condition. When LVH accompanies hypertension, there should be a greater urgency for aggressive antihypertensive therapy.

Because heart rate appears to directly influence the coronary mortality rate associated with hypertension, antihypertensive medications that lower the heart rate may have an advantage over those that accelerate it. In an analysis of β-blocker trials, a strong relationship between the reduction in heart rate achieved and the reduction in mortality was found.[45] Analysis of the Norwegian Multicenter Timolol Trial found that the postinfarction resting heart rate predicts later cardiac mortality and that the benefit of treatment was a result of the achieved reduction in heart rate.[46] Treatment with β-blockers has been reported to reduce silent ischemic events in relation to the reduction in heart rate achieved.[46]

Because hypertension predisposes to the occurrence of silent or unrecognized MI, hypertensive persons should be periodically monitored by ECG for such an occurrence. These unrecognized MIs must be detected and dealt with aggressively because they impose a long-term outlook that is little different from that of overtly manifest MIs.[47]

The greatest burden of hypertension-related CHD occurs in the elderly, in whom ISH predominates. In contrast to earlier reports, meta-analysis of the efficacy of antihypertensive therapy in the elderly indicates a significant 25% decrease in coronary mortality.[48,49] Practitioners caring for elderly ambulatory hypertensive patients should attempt to control elevated BP of any variety. Reduction of SBP in the elderly with ISH resulted in substantial decreases in coronary events.[39,46] In the

very oldest and most ill and frail, further trials are needed before well-founded recommendations can be made (see Chapter 55).

The elderly with a favorable risk profile and only mild hypertension can be managed with weight control, a moderate exercise program, salt and alcohol restriction, and advice against smoking. These measures help reduce the dosage of antihypertensive medication required to control hypertension and also help to control other often-associated risk factors. Polypharmacy may be a significant problem in managing hypertension in the elderly, who often take nonsteroidal antiinflammatory drugs for arthritis. There is much to be gained in treating hypertension in the elderly because their risk of disabling cardiovascular events is so high. However, despite convincing evidence of the benefit of treating ISH, the third National Health and Nutrition Examination Survey found that only about half of hypertensive patients receive therapy and only 27% of those under treatment are adequately controlled.[1]

ISH is the least likely form of hypertension to be treated, and even when treated, it is seldom controlled. Examination of the rates of control to goal SBPs and DBPs in the Framingham Study indicates that among those receiving antihypertensive therapy, only 49.0% are controlled to the systolic goal of <140 mm Hg compared with 89.7% to the diastolic goal of <90 mm Hg, and only 47.8% to both goals.[49] Older age, LVH, and higher BMI are associated with poor SBP control. Because ACE inhibitors both lower BP and improve arterial distensibility, they seem a logical choice for treating ISH. However, diuretics and calcium antagonists have been shown to reduce coronary events in ISH.[39,46]

Prevention of CHD requires more than reduction of the BP. Excess risk is concentrated in those who have other risk factors or evidence of target organ involvement, such as proteinuria, cardiomegaly, vascular bruits, or ECG abnormalities. Optimal preventive management should include reduced saturated fat, cholesterol, and salt intake; increased physical activity; smoking cessation; and avoidance of excessive alcohol intake. Inducing the hypertensive cigarette smoker to quit can promptly reduce the risk of CHD to half that of those who continue to smoke, a risk reduction greater than that expected from reduction in the BP per se.

The benefits of treating hypertension, particularly for ISH in the elderly, are now better appreciated.[23,43] Low-dose combination therapy using antihypertensive agents with different modes of action can substantially reduce the BP, virtually eliminate unpleasant side effects, and maintain a good quality of life in those under treatment.

**Table 23–12** Risk of Cardiovascular Events as a Function of Serial ECG Changes in Persons with Left Ventricular Hypertrophy: Framingham Study

|  | Odds Ratio | |
| --- | --- | --- |
|  | **Men** | **Women** |
| **Voltage Change** | | |
| Decrease | 0.46 | 0.56* |
| No change | 1.00 | 1.00 |
| Increase | 1.86 | 1.61 |
| **Repolarization Change** | | |
| Improved | 0.45 | 1.19* |
| No change | 1.00 | 1.00 |
| Worsened | 1.89 | 2.02 |

From Levy D, Salomon M, D'Agostino RB, et al. Prognostic implications of baseline electrocardiographic features and their serial changes in subjects with left ventricular hypertrophy. Circulation 90(4):1786-1793, 1994.
*Not significant.

## SUMMARY

Over the past two decades the percentage of hypertensive persons who have become aware of their problem and have come under treatment has improved substantially. Concomitant with these improvements, major declines in coronary and stroke mortality have occurred. Because of the large population-attributable risk for hypertension as a risk factor for CHD and stroke, it is inferred that the improved detection and control of hypertension in the general population contributed substantially to these declines.

Epidemiologic investigation has shown the importance of elevated BP as a contributor to cardiovascular morbidity and mortality in general and CHD in particular. It has demonstrated that BP exerts a continuous graded influence, so the concept of an acceptable BP has changed from that which is usual in an apparently healthy population to that which confers the greatest freedom from its cardiovascular sequelae. Risk of developing the cardiovascular consequences of hypertension increases linearly over a sixfold range with each increment of BP, even within the range of pressures usually considered high-normal. The bulk of cardiovascular events, including coronary events, occur in persons with stage 1 and stage 2 hypertension. Three times as many cardiovascular events are attributable to this less severe hypertension than stage 3 hypertension. The odds of developing CVD in stages 1 and 2 hypertension is double that of persons with normal BPs.

Epidemiologic investigation has also shown that the adverse consequences of hypertension are more closely related to elevation of SBP than DBP. It is now evident that hypertension seldom occurs in isolation and that high-risk hypertension is concentrated in those with a cluster of other metabolically linked risk factors. Hypertension is often one component of an insulin resistance syndrome.

Epidemiologic investigation has established the importance of hypertension as a risk factor for CHD in the elderly and clinical trials have shown the efficacy of treating both systolic and diastolic hypertension at all ages. The ominous significance of LVH is now well documented and the potential benefit of causing it to regress shown.

Physicians now have a good deal more information to guide them in their efforts to delay or prevent the sequelae of hypertension than was available only a decade ago. However, this increase in information has made clinical decisions and therapeutic choices in managing hypertension more complex. Evaluation and management of hypertension is no longer based solely on determining the height of the BP, and lowering it to a more acceptable level. New classification schemes place more emphasis on SBP, lesser BP elevations, and the presence of other associated risk factors.[1] The number of available antihypertensive agents, with different modes of action, suitable for monotherapy and combined therapy, has grown. There is controversy about first-choice agents and whether therapy should necessarily be tailored to take into account the associated dyslipidemia, glucose intolerance, LVH, and insulin resistance commonly present.

The goal of antihypertensive therapy is to prevent cardiovascular morbidity and mortality rather than simply to bring the BP under control. BP control must be achieved in the least intrusive way, and use of low dose combinations of agents is preferred over resorting to high doses of single drugs to achieve goal BPs. Trials have clearly shown that treatment reduces stroke and heart failure events, but some question the efficacy of antihypertensive treatment, without concomitantly improving the multivariate risk profile in reducing CHD. There is some interest in cautious step-down therapy for patients whose BPs have been well controlled over time.

Maintaining long-term compliance with treatment remains a problem. There is continuing concern about the safety of drastic lowering of the BP in hypertensive persons with concomitant CHD. For those with stage 1 hypertension, optimal treatment requires improvement in the patient's global risk by serious attention to the often-associated cluster of atherogenic risk factors. Only in this way can we target mildly hypertensive persons for cost-effective treatment without needlessly alarming or falsely reassuring them.

Despite potent antihypertensive therapies and clinical trial evidence that treatment reduces cardiovascular and renal sequelae, more than one fourth of the 50 million hypertensive persons in the United States remain unaware that they have the condition, and three fourths of those known to have it are poorly controlled.[1] Most cases of uncontrolled hypertension are in persons with elevated SBP.[50,51] This is regrettable because it is in these persons that antihypertensive therapy has been shown to be most effective in reducing the incidence of MI, overall mortality, stroke, and heart failure.[23,43] Poor control of hypertension is attributable to adverse effects of drugs, medication costs, patients' knowledge and beliefs, and physicians' knowledge and attitudes.[52] Approximately one half of patients prescribed medication discontinue it by the end of 1 year (see Chapter 37). Physicians are often reluctant to treat systolic hypertension for fear of doing harm by lowering the DBP too much. The validity of the J-curve phenomenon and fear of impairing cognitive function by excessive reduction in BP are not supported by clinical trial data.[53] Dementia incidence in the Syst-Eur trial was actually 50% lower in the treated than in the control group.[53] Intensified efforts to modify BP and its often-associated risk factors must become a national priority if we are to continue to decrease death and disability from CHD.

# References

1. Chobanian AV, Bakris GL, Black HR, et al. The Seventh Report of the Joint National Committee on Detection, Evaluation and Treatment of High Blood Pressure. The JNC 7 Report. JAMA 289:2560-2572, 2003.
2. Vasan RS, Beiser A, Seshardi S, et al. Residual lifetime risk for developing hypertension in middle-aged women and men: The Framingham Heart Study. JAMA 287:1003-1010, 2002.
3. Chobanian A. 1989 Corcoran Lecture: Adaptive and maladaptive responses of the arterial wall to hypertension. Hypertension 15:666-674, 1990.
4. Morbidity & Mortality: Chartbook on Cardiovascular, Lung, and Blood Diseases. Bethesda, MD, National Heart, Lung, and Blood Institute (NHLBI), National Institutes of Health (NIH); pp 43-45
5. Vasan RS, Larson MG, Leip EP, et al. Assessment of frequency of progression to hypertension in non-hypertensive participants in the Framingham Heart Study. Lancet 358:1682-1686, 2001.
6. Garrison RJ, Kannel WB, Stokes J III, et al. Incidence and precursors of hypertension in young adults: The Framingham Offspring Study. Prev Med 16:234-251, 1987.
7. Leitschuh L, Cupples LA, Kannel WB, et al. High-normal blood pressure progression to hypertension in the Framingham Heart Study. Hypertension 17:22-27, 1991.
8. Wilson PWF, Kannel WB. Hypertension, other risk factors and the risk of cardiovascular disease. In JH Laragh, BM Brenner (eds). Hypertension: Pathophysiology, Diagnosis, and Management, 2nd ed. New York, Raven, 1995; pp 99-114.
9. Neaton JD, Kuller L, Stamler J, et al. Impact of systolic and diastolic blood pressure on cardiovascular mortality. In Laragh JH, Brenner BM (eds). Hypertension: Pathophysiology, Diagnosis, and Management, 2nd ed. New York, Raven, 1995; pp 1903-1913.
10. Lewington S, Clark R, Qislbash N, et al. Age-specific relevance of usual blood pressure to vascular mortality. Lancet 360:1903-1913, 2002.
11. Whelton PK, He J, Appel LJ, et al. Primary prevention of hypertension: Clinical and public health advisory from the National

High Blood Pressure Education Program. JAMA 288:1882-1888, 2002.

12. Kannel WB. Framingham Study insights into hypertensive risk of cardiovascular disease. Hypertens Res 18:181-196, 1995.

13. D'Agostino RB, Belanger AJ, Kannel WB, et al. Relation of low diastolic blood pressure to coronary heart disease in the presence of myocardial infarction: The Framingham Study. BMJ 303:385-389, 1991.

14. Stewart IM. Relation of reduction in pressure to first myocardial infarction in patients receiving treatment for severe hypertension. Lancet 1:861-865, 1979.

15. Coope J. Hypertension: The cause of the J-curve. J Hum Hypertens 4:1-4, 1990.

16. Fletcher A, Bulpitt J. How far should blood pressure be lowered? N Engl J Med 326:251-254, 1992.

17. Staessen J, Bulpitt C, Clement D, et al. Relation between mortality and treated blood pressure in elderly patients with hypertension: Report of the European Working Party on High Blood Pressure in the Elderly. BMJ 298:1552-1556, 1989.

18. Kannel WB, Sorley P, Castelli WP, et al. Blood pressure and survival after myocardial infarction. The Framingham Study. Am J Cardiol 45:326-330, 1980.

19. The Coronary Drug Project Research Group. Blood pressure in survivors of myocardial infarction. J Am Coll Cardiol 4:1135-1147, 1984.

20. Khaw K-T, Barrett-Conner E. Prognostic factors for mortality in a population-based study of men and women with a history of heart disease. J Cardiopulm Rehabil 6:474-480, 1986.

21. O'Rourke MF. Isolated systolic hypertension, pulse pressure and arterial stiffness as risk factors for cardiovascular disease. Curr Hypertens Rep 3:204-211, 1999.

22. Kannel WB, Gordon T, Schwartz MJ. Systolic versus diastolic blood pressure and risk of coronary heart disease: The Framingham Study. Am J Cardiol 27:335-345, 1971.

23. SHEP Cooperative Research Group. Prevention of stroke by antihypertensive drug treatment in older persons with isolated systolic hypertension: Final results of the Systolic Hypertension in the Elderly Program (SHEP). JAMA 265:3255-3264, 1991.

24. Kannel WB. Epidemiology of essential hypertension: The Framingham Study experience. Proc R Coll Phys Edinb 21:273-287, 1991.

25. Franklin SS, Khan BS, Wong ND, et al. Is pulse pressure useful in predicting coronary heart disease? Circulation 100(4):354-360, 1999.

27. Franklin SS, Larson MG, Shehzad A, et al. Does the relation of blood pressure to coronary heart disease risk change with aging? The Framingham Heart Study. Circulation 103:1245-1249, 2001.

28. Kannel WB. Potency of vascular risk factors as the basis for antihypertensive therapy. Eur Heart J 13(suppl G):34-42, 1992.

29. Reaven GM, Chen YD. Insulin resistance, its consequences and coronary heart disease [editorial comment]. Circulation 93:1780-1783, 1996.

30. Despres JP. Abdominal obesity as an important component of the insulin resistance syndrome. Nutrition 9:452-459, 1993.

31. Reaven GM. Insulin resistance, hyperinsulinemia, and hypertriglyceridemia in the etiology and clinical course of hypertension. Am J Med 90:7S-12S, 1991.

32. Siegal RD, Cupples LA, Schaefer EJ, et al. Lipoproteins, apolipoproteins and low-density lipoprotein size among diabetics in the Framingham Offspring Study. Metabolism 45:1267-1272, 1996.

33. Dzau VJ. Renin and myocardial infarction in hypertension. N Engl J Med 324:1128-1130, 1991.

34. Alderman MH, Madhavan S, Ooi WL, et al. Association of the renin-sodium profile with the risk of myocardial infarction in patients with hypertension. N Engl J Med 324:1098-1104, 1991.

35. Brunner HR, Sealey JE, Laragh JH. Renin as a risk factor in essential hypertension: More evidence. Am J Med 55:295-302, 1973.

36. Meade TW, Imeson JD, Gordon D, et al. The epidemiology of plasma renin. Clin Sci (Lond) 64:273-289, 1983.

37. Levy D, Salomon M, D'Agostino RB, et al. Prognostic implications of baseline electrocardiographic features and their serial changes in subjects with left ventricular hypertrophy. Circulation 90:1780-1793, 1994.

38. Levy D, Garrison RJ, Savage DD, et al. Prognostic implications of echocardiographically determined left ventricular mass in the Framingham Heart Study. Ann Intern Med 322:1561-1566, 1990.

39. Gillman MW, Kannel WB, Belanger AJ, et al. Influence of heart rate on mortality among persons with hypertension. The Framingham Study. Am Heart J 125:1148-1154, 1993.

40. Kannel WB. Risk factors in hypertension. J Cardiovasc Pharmacol 13(Suppl 1):4-10, 1989.

41. Langer RD, Ganiats TG, Barrett-Conner E. Paradoxical survival in elderly men with high blood pressure. Br Med J 29:1356-1358, 1989.

42. Kannel WB, Wolf PA, McGee DL, et al. Systolic blood pressure, arterial rigidity and stroke. The Framingham Study. JAMA 245:1225-1228, 1981.

43. Wilking SVP, Belanger A, Kannel WB, et al. Determinants of isolated systolic hypertension. JAMA 260:3451-3455, 1988.

44. Staessen JA, Fagard R, Thijs L, et al. Randomized double blind comparison of placebo and active treatment for older patients with isolated systolic hypertension. Lancet 350:757-764,1997.

45. Dahlof B, Pennert K, Hansson L. Reversal of left ventricular hypertrophy in hypertensive patients: A meta-analysis of 109 treatment studies. Am J Hypertens 5:95-110, 1992.

46. Kjekshus JK. Comments: Beta blockers—heart rate reduction: A mechanism of action. Eur Heart J 6(suppl):29, 1985.

47. Gunderson T, Grottum P, Pederson T, et al. Effect of timolol and reinfarction after acute myocardial infarction: Prognostic importance of heart rate at rest. Am J Cardiol 58:20, 1986.

48. Kannel WB, Abbott RD. Incidence and prognosis of unrecognized myocardial infarction: An update on the Framingham Study. N Engl J Med 311:1144-1147, 1984.

49. Insua JT, Sacks HS, Lau T-S, et al. Drug treatment of hypertension in the elderly. Ann Intern Med 121:355-362, 1994.

50. Collins R, Peto R, MacMahon S, et al. Blood pressure, stroke and coronary heart disease. Part 2. Short term reductions in blood pressure: Overview of randomized drug trials in their epidemiological context. Lancet 335:827-838, 1990.

51. Lloyd-Jones DM, Evans JC, Larson MG, et al. Differential control of systolic and diastolic blood pressure. Factors associated with lack of blood pressure control in the community. Hypertension 36:594-599, 2000.

52. Hyman DJ, Pavlik VN. Characteristics of patients with uncontrolled hypertension in the United States. N Engl J Med 345:479-486, 2001.

53. Chobabian AV. Control of hypertension—An important national priority. N Engl J Med 345:534-535, 2001.

54. Forrette F, Seux MI, Staessen JA, et al. Prevention of dementia in randomized double blind placebo-controlled systolic hypertension in Europe (Syst-Eur) trial. Lancet 352:1347-1351, 1998.

# Chapter 24

# Left Ventricular Hypertrophy, Congestive Heart Failure, and Coronary Flow Reserve Abnormalities in Hypertension

## Joseph A. Diamond, Robert A. Phillips

Hypertensive heart disease is a result of a complex interaction of genetic and hemodynamic factors inducing structural and functional adaptations that lead to increased left ventricular (LV) mass, diastolic dysfunction, congestive heart failure (CHF), arrhythmias, and abnormalities of blood flow due to microvascular disease. These changes increase the risk of coronary heart disease, CHF, stroke, and sudden death. Echocardiographically determined left ventricular hypertrophy (LVH) is defined as LV mass in the upper 2.5% to 5% of the adult population. It occurs in 15% to 20% of hypertensive patients.[1] Considered as a discrete, categorical variable, LVH significantly increases the risk of coronary artery disease, CHF, cerebrovascular accidents, ventricular arrhythmia, and sudden death.[2-4] LVH increases the relative risk of mortality by twofold in persons with coronary artery disease and by fourfold in those with normal epicardial coronary arteries.[5,6] In addition, when LV mass is considered as a continuous variable, a direct and progressive relationship exists between cardiovascular risk and absolute LV mass[3] (Figure 24–1). This chapter covers the following areas:

- Causes of LVH and CHF
- Myocardial and structural alterations in LVH
- Identification and treatment of LVH in clinical practice
- LV mass regression—does the choice of antihypertensive matter?
- Diastolic dysfunction and CHF: mechanisms and treatments
- Coronary microcirculation in patients with hypertension

## CAUSES OF LEFT VENTRICULAR HYPERTROPHY AND CONGESTIVE HEART FAILURE IN PATIENTS WITH HYPERTENSION

### Genetic Factors in the Development of Left Ventricular Hypertrophy and Congestive Heart Failure

It is estimated that up to 60% of the variance of LV mass may be due to genetic factors independent of blood pressure (BP).[7] Epidemiologic evidence for genetic influence on LV mass includes offspring studies that generally, but not uniformly, demonstrate that LV mass in children of hypertensive parents is elevated independently of BP and other known determinants of LVH.[8,9] In the Framingham Heart Study, there are significant parent-child and sibling correlations of LV mass after adjustments for age, height, weight, and systolic blood pressure (SBP). However, the overall contribution of heredity to LV mass is small.[9,10] Furthermore, one twin study, in which monozygotic twins had only minimally less intertwine variation in wall thickness than dizygotic twins or sibling pairs, indicates that genetic influences on LV mass can be modified by environmental factors.[11]

Additional evidence for a genetic influence on LV mass is that race appears to be a determinant of ventricular structure. Studies over the past three decades suggest that for equal levels of BP, Blacks have increased relative wall thickness and LV mass compared with whites. In the Evans County, Georgia Study, conducted between 1960 and 1962, electrocardiographic evidence of LVH was twofold to threefold higher in Blacks at any given level of BP.[12] In the early 1980s, Dunn et al., using M-mode echocardiography, showed that for the same level of BP, Blacks had greater LV mass.[13] Hammond et al. showed that for the same BP and LV mass, relative wall thickness (concentric remodeling) was greater in Blacks.[14] Similarly, in the Treatment of Mild Hypertension Study (TOMHS), even though BP and LV mass were the same, Blacks had greater wall thickness than whites.[15] Similarly, a study from London showed that for equal levels of previously untreated BP, Blacks had greater LV mass and relative wall thickness than whites.[16] Hinderliter et al. showed that even in the absence of hypertension, young adult Blacks tend to have greater relative wall thickness than whites, suggesting that differences in ventricular structure may be independent of hemodynamic factors.[17] The increase in LV mass and relative wall thickness observed in Blacks may in part be due to a greater total hemodynamic burden as compared with whites, due to a more blunted fall in nocturnal BP.[18] This altered BP pattern begins in adolescence.

One of the first and most studied genetic factors in the development of LVH in hypertensive humans is an insertion/deletion polymorphism of a 287 base-pair marker in intron 16 (noncoding region) of the gene for the angiotensin-converting enzyme (ACE). It is estimated from population studies that the ACE gene contributes 3% to 4% to the variation of BP in the general population. The homozygous genotype for the deletion (DD) is associated with electrocardiographic evidence of LVH.[19] The association was strongest in men who were normotensive, supporting the concept that this association is independent of hemodynamic factors. However, the Framingham study did not find a relation between echocardiographically measured LV mass and ACE genotype.[19,20] An Italian study showed that the DD genotype was a risk factor for increased echocardiographically determined LV mass.[21] Furthermore, a study in an ethnically diverse New York City population found that the DD genotype was associated with

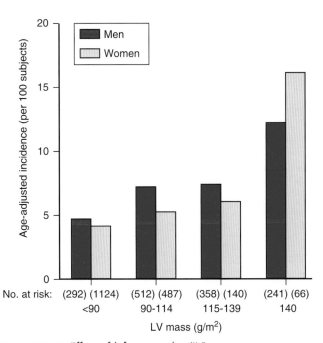

**Figure 24-1** Effect of left ventricular (LV) mass on age-adjusted incidence of cardiovascular disease over a 4-year period in the Framingham Heart Study. (Adapted with permission from Levy D, Garrison RJ, Savage DD, et al. Prognostic implications of echocardiographically determined left ventricular mass in the Framingham Heart Study. N Engl J Med 322:1561-1566, 1990. Copyright © 1990 Massachusetts Medical Society.)

concentric remodeling of the LV, a geometric pattern associated with increased cardiovascular risk.[22]

In addition to the ACE gene, there is strong evidence that other genes affecting the renin-angiotensin system are influential in the development of LVH. A polymorphism (344C/T) in the promoter region of the aldosterone synthase gene on chromosome 8, resulting in increased intracardiac aldosterone production (independent of adrenal synthesis) has been associated with increased LV mass in individuals with mild to moderate hypertension.[23,24] The angiotensinogen gene (on chromosome 1) also contributes to the development of LVH in hypertensive individuals. In the Hypertension Genetic Epidemiology Network (HyperGEN) study, two polymorphisms of the angiotensinogen gene have been associated with LVH. The M235T polymorphism on exon 2 of the angiotensinogen gene appears to be a marker for a functional variant, the G-6A polymorphism, which is tightly linked to the marker (6 base pairs away) and affects the transcriptional rate of the gene.[25] Additional studies applying the principles of physiologic genomics are assessing the effect of the ACE and angiotensinogen genes on hypertensive heart disease. This is accomplished by altering expression levels via transgenics, knockouts, and gene targeting in animal models.[26] In spontaneously hypertensive rats (SHR), antisense targeted to angiotensinogen mRNA delivered by an adeno-associated virus produced sustained reduction in BP and reduction in LVH.[27] This suggests a potential future gene therapy approach for the treatment of hypertension and regression of LVH.

In addition to the renin-angiotensin system, other studies are focusing on genes with different physiologic mechanisms that

could contribute to hypertensive heart disease. For example, Nakayama et al. identified an insertion/deletion mutation in the human type A natriuretic peptide receptor gene (hNPRA) on chromosome 1 that appears to result in LVH in a population of Japanese hypertensive subjects.[28] Another gene under study is the G-protein $\beta_3$-subunit gene (CNB3) on chromosome 12 that encodes the $\beta_3$ subunit of G proteins. A single base substitution (C → T) at position 825 of the gene results in a change in the splicing of exon 9, resulting in the loss of 41 amino acids in the resulting altered, but functioning, protein. Enhanced G-protein activation has been demonstrated and is thought to be the cause of the phenotypic observation of enhanced $Na^+,H^+$ exchanger activity, which has been associated with hypertension and LVH. Poch et al. showed increased LV mass by echocardiography in Spanish individuals with the 825T allele.[29] However, this was not confirmed in other population studies.[30] Table 24–1 summarizes the genes that appear to contribute to LVH.

In addition to genes that contribute to the development of LVH, studies have also identified genes that affect LV contractility in individuals with hypertensive heart disease. One study implicates a gene on the short arm of chromosome 11. This gene is likely involved in the production of myosin-binding protein C (MyBP-C), a protein with several important structural and regulatory functions in the contractility of myocytes.[31] It may play a particularly important role in LV contractility in Blacks. Another gene on chromosome 22 may play a less important though significant role in regulating LV contractility. This gene may regulate the production of $\beta$-adrenergic receptor kinase ($\beta$ARK), which with elevated expression, attenuates $\beta$-adrenergic signaling and contributes to contractile dysfunction.[32,33]

## Hemodynamic Factors and Left Ventricular Hypertrophy

The effect of BP, as well as virtually every factor known to influence BP, has been investigated for its independent effect on LV mass (Table 24–2). There is very strong evidence for a causal relationship between BP and absolute LV mass. This was first reported 70 years ago[34] and led to the view that myocardial hypertrophy is an adaptive cardiac response that reduces wall stress and allows the ventricle to maintain mechanical efficiency.[35,36] In the Framingham Heart Study, 10% of the variation in LV mass among persons was accounted for by differences in SBP averaged over 30 years.[37] Similarly, average BP obtained during awake hours in hypertensive subjects accounts for 10% to 25% of LV mass variation,[38-40] whereas a blunted nocturnal fall in BP is associated with increased LV mass.[41] Ambulatory BP monitoring (ABPM) correlates more closely than clinic BP with LV mass and carotid artery intimal-medial thickness, and may more accurately predict the risk for cardiovascular disease than clinic BP measurements[39,42-46] (see Chapters 27 and 28).

In hypertensive persons, approximately 40% (r = 0.66, p <.001) of the variance in LV mass is accounted for by total LV load or peak meridional wall stress.[47] In normotensive persons, enhanced augmentation of SBP by reflected waves, a process associated with aging of the arterial tree, elevates wall stress and is associated with increased LV mass.[48] Other hemodynamic factors associated with increased mass are volume, which obviously directly increases LV mass, and intrinsic contractility of the ventricle. An intrinsically hypercontractile

**Table 24–1** Genes Implicated in the Development of Left Ventricular Hypertrophy in Essential Hypertension

| Gene | Location | Physiologic role |
|------|----------|------------------|
| ACE gene[19,22,374] | Insertion/deletion polymorphism of 287 base pair marker in intron 16 on chromosome 17 | Production of angiotensin II |
| X-linked angiotensin II type 2 receptor gene[375] | Intronic polymorphism (-1332 G/A) on the X-chromosome | Oppose the effects of $AT_1$ receptor |
| Angiotensinogen gene[376] | G-6A polymorphism in exon 2 on chromosome 1 | Production of angiotensinogen |
| Aldosterone synthase gene[24] | –344C/T polymorphism in the promoter region of the aldosterone synthase gene on chromosome 8 | Production of intracardiac aldosterone |
| G-protein $\beta_3$-subunit gene[29,377] | Single base substitution at position 825 of exon 9 on the short arm of chromosome 12 | Enhanced $Na^+,H^+$ exchange due to enhanced G-protein activation |
| Type A human natriuretic peptide receptor gene[28] | Deletion mutation of the 5′ flanking region on chromosome 1 | Elevated BNP due to decrease in natriuretic peptide receptors |

ACE, angiotensin-converting enzyme; $AT_1$, angiotension II type1; BNP, brain natriuretic peptide.

**Table 24–2** Association Between Left Ventricular Mass, Hemodynamic Factors, and Nonhemodynamic Factors

| Factor | Strength of Evidence Supporting a Causal Role in LV Mass |
|--------|----------------------------------------------------------|
| Blood pressure/ wall stress | Very strong[34,37-41,47,378] |
| Stroke volume | Very strong[47,379] |
| Obesity | Very strong[62,70,71,73,74] |
| Growth hormone and IGF-1 | Strong[89,90] |
| Gender | Strong[65,69,380,381] |
| Race | Strong[12,15-17,382] |
| Age | Strong (women only?)[60-64] |
| Intracellular [$Ca^{2+}$] | Strong[51,75] |
| Insulin resistance | Strong[70,92,93] |
| Angiotensin II | Strong[80,383] |
| Alcohol | Needs confirmation[384] |
| Intrinsic myocardial contractility | Needs confirmation[47] |
| Blood viscosity | Needs confirmation[385] |
| Parathyroid hormone | Needs confirmation[78] |
| Aldosterone (collagen synthesis) | Needs confirmation[82,383,386] |
| Sodium intake | Needs confirmation[387] |
| $Na^+,H^+$ exchanger and $Na^+,K^+,Cl^-$ cotransport system | Needs confirmation[388] |
| Polymorphism of the ACE gene | Controversial[19,21] |
| Plasma renin activity | Controversial[77-79] |
| Norepinephrine | Controversial[11,77,85,86,88] |
| $Na^+,Li^+$ exchanger | Controversial[388,389] |
| βARK | Controversial[32,33] |

ACE, angiotensin-converting enzyme; βARK, β-adrenergic receptor kinase; IGF-1, insulin-like growth factor-1; LV, left ventricular.

ventricle requires less wall thickening to overcome wall stress. Thus, an inverse relation exists between degree of LV mass and intrinsic myocardial contractility.[47]

The sequence of events that leads from increased wall stress to cellular hypertrophy is only beginning to be elucidated.[49] Because failure to hypertrophy in response to increased wall stress would result in a mechanical disadvantage and decreased LV function, it is likely that there are redundant systems that translate wall stress into cardiac myocyte hypertrophy. Increased wall stress may activate a stretch receptor, which, through a series of cellular and subcellular events, activates fetal cardiac and growth genes, such as c-*myc* and c-*jun*, to up-regulate myocardial cell protein synthesis. Shear stress has been shown to activate these growth genes in endothelial cells by stimulating the production of several mitogen-activated protein kinases (Figure 24–2).[50] The molecular mechanisms that couple hypertrophic signals at the cell membrane to the reprogramming of cardiomyocyte gene expression are beginning to be elucidated. Intracellular calcium release may be an early response to myocyte stretch and other humoral stimuli, including angiotensin II (Ang II), phenylephrine, and endothelin. The increase in intracellular calcium results in activation of the phosphatase calcineurin, which then dephosphorylates transcription factor NF-AT3, resulting in its translocation to the nucleus. In the nucleus, AT3 interacts with another transcription factor, GATA4, to initiate transcription of genes that lead to myocyte hypertrophy,[51] such as β-myosin heavy chain and β-skeletal actin (Figure 24–3). In the hypertrophic response, other genes, such as those for atrial natriuretic peptide and phospholamban, are also up-regulated.[52]

Calcineurin appears to be both necessary and sufficient to induce hypertrophy. Pharmacologic inhibition of calcineurin activity with cyclosporine blocks development of hypertrophy in several circumstances: (1) mice prone to LVH because they are genetically engineered to produce high levels of calcineurin,[51] (2) mice genetically predisposed to develop hypertrophic cardiomyopathy,[53] and (3) rats whose aorta was banded to produce a pressure stimulus for hypertrophy.[53] Although cyclosporine is not clinically useful in the nontransplant population, it is likely that new classes of calcineurin inhibitors

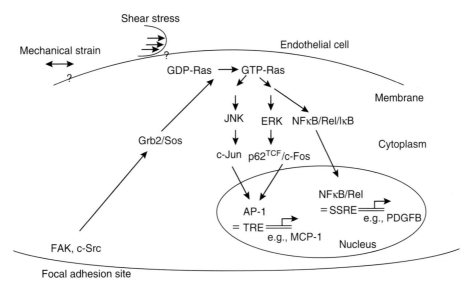

**Figure 24–2** The sequential events of signaling and gene expression in endothelial cells in response to shear stress or mechanical strain. Tyrosine kinases in the focal adhesion site of endothelial cells such as FAK and c-SRC are involved in the mechanochemical transduction. Through the Src homology 2–containing adaptor Grbe, the small GTPase Ras is activated by Sos, a guanine nucleotide exchange factor that converts the inactive GDP-Ras to the activated GTP-Ras. As a result, JNK and ERK in the cytoplasm are activated to phosphorylate, respectively c-Jun and p62$^{TCF}$/c-Fos, which are components of the transcription factor AP-1. In the nucleus, the action of the activated AP-1 on its target sequence (e.g., the TRE site in the promoter of the MCP-1 gene) causes an up-regulation of gene expression. Concurrently, NFκB/Rel is activated by eliminating its inhibitor IκB so that genes with a shear stress–responsive element or κB site (e.g., PDGF-B can be activated). (Reproduced with permission from Chien S, Li S, Shyy YJ. Effects of mechanical forces on signal transduction and gene expression in endothelial cells. Hypertension 31:162-169, 1998.)

(e.g., tacrolimus [FK506]) that regulate transcription will become available to modulate responses such as hypertrophy.[54] It is likely that the ACE inhibitors and angiotensin receptor blockers (ARBs) also attenuate the development of cardiac hypertrophy by preventing angiotensin from up-regulating the production of factors that stimulate fetal-type genes, particularly calcineurin. Nonantihypertensive doses of the ARB candesartan suppress calcineurin production and subsequent LVH and fibrosis in salt-sensitive hypertensive Dahl (DS) rats.[54]

Two large community-based studies indicate that hypertension is the most common risk factor for CHF, both with and without systolic dysfunction.[55,56] In the Framingham study, after adjusting for age and other risk factors in proportional hazards regression models, the risk for developing CHF due to systolic dysfunction (CHF-S) in hypertensive compared with normotensive persons was nearly twofold in men and threefold in women. Hypertension was the highest risk factor for CHF-S by multivariate analysis, accounting for 39% of cases in men and 59% in women.[55] Another population-based study of CHF in Olmsted County, Minnesota showed similar findings. Of 216 persons studied, 52% presented with hypertension. Of these patients, 137 underwent evaluation of LV systolic function. Hypertension was the underlying risk factor in 53% of persons with LV ejection fraction (LVEF) <50% and was present in 58% of those with LVEF ≥50%. Of note, long-term survival was not significantly different between persons with normal or low LVEF.[56] The prognosis for hypertensive patients with newly diagnosed CHF-S was poor in both studies (≤35% survival by 5 years).

BP control effectively prevents the development of CHF. In the Systolic Hypertension in the Elderly Program (SHEP) study, patients with isolated systolic hypertension (ISH) and a prior history of myocardial infarction (MI) (by electrocardiogram [ECG]) who were treated with diuretic-based therapy with BP lowering to <150 mm Hg systolic had only a 2% to 3% chance of developing CHF over a 4-year period. By contrast, those patients treated with placebo had an 8% to 10% chance of developing CHF.[57] Meta-analysis of randomized placebo-controlled antihypertensive therapy trials demonstrated that adequate BP control decreases the incidence of CHF by half.[58]

## Nonhemodynamic Factors and Left Ventricular Hypertrophy

LV mass is not significantly different in boys and girls during infancy and childhood, but a difference becomes evident at puberty, when sex-specific hormonal influences occur.[59] With aging, LV mass increases in both genders, but this effect may be more pronounced in women than men.[60-64] Women have less LV mass for the same level of office-determined BP,[65] but whether this difference is biologic or an artifact of the method of BP measurement or indexation of LV mass is controversial. For similar levels of clinic BP, women often have lower ambulatory BPs than men. This results in less hypertrophy in women for the same level of clinic pressure.[66-68] Additionally, some of the gender difference is accounted for by less lean muscle mass in women than in men.[69] When LV mass is indexed by the lean body mass (obtained by bioelectrical impedance), the gender difference in LV mass disappears.

Determinants of LV mass may also differ between men and women. In the Tecumseh study of normotensive adults, LVH

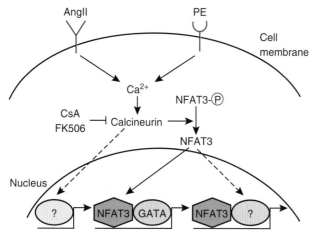

**Figure 24–3** A model for the calcineurin-dependent transcriptional pathway in cardiac hypertrophy. Angiotensin II (Ang II), PE, and possibly other hypertrophic stimuli acting at the cell membrane lead to elevation of intracellular $Ca^{2+}$ and activation of calcineurin in the cytoplasm. Calcineurin dephosphorylates NFAT3, resulting in its translocation to the nucleus, where it interacts with GATA4 to synergistically activate transcription. Whether all actions of NFAT3 are mediated by its interaction with GATA4 or whether there are GATA4- independent pathways for activation of certain hypertrophic responses remains to be determined. *Solid arrows* denote pathways that are known. *Dotted lines* denote possible pathways that have not been demonstrated. (reproduced with permission from Molkentin JD, Lu JR, Antos CL, et al. A calcineurin-dependent transcriptional pathway for cardiac hypertrophy. Cell 93:215-228, 1998.)

in men was associated with evidence of increased sympathetic nervous system activity and hyperinsulinemia, whereas in women, obesity was the major determinant of LVH.[70] In a study by De Simone et al., obesity was the predominant factor determining LV mass in women, whereas in men, hemodynamic factors, age, and degree of obesity all contributed.[71] The association of obesity with LVH may account for the increased risk of morbidity and mortality associated with LVH in Black women. In one study of 163 Black men and 273 Black women, after adjusting for age, BP, and ejection fraction, the relative risk for total mortality in individuals with LVH versus those without LVH was 2.0 (0.8-5.0, 95% confidence interval [CI]) for men and 4.3 (1.6-11.7, 95% CI) for women.[72]

In the Framingham study, obesity was associated with increased LV mass in elderly men and women.[62] The greater incidence of LVH in obese persons is accounted for by increased wall thickness and often by increased LV internal dimension.[71,73,74] These changes are reversible with weight loss.[74]

Several hormones have been related to the hypertrophic process.[49,75,76] The role of the renin-angiotensin-aldosterone axis in hypertensive target organ pathophysiology has been extensively explored (see Chapters 8, 9, 10, and 72). Experimental and human studies[77,78] have linked plasma renin activity to degree of LVH, but this is not universally accepted.[79] The product of renin activity, angiotensin I (Ang I), is the substrate for ACE. Expression and regulation of the ACE gene and thus

Ang II levels, may modulate development of LVH. This is supported by in vitro studies in which local release of Ang II in response to the mechanical stretch is a necessary permissive factor for induction of the hypertrophic growth response.[80] Although there is ample evidence that Ang II is involved in the hypertrophic response, it is apparently not necessary. This was shown in a study in which LVH developed in mice in response to pressure overload despite homologous deletion of the Ang II type 1 ($AT_1$) receptor.[81] Aldosterone, the synthesis of which is partially controlled by Ang II levels, appears to regulate cardiac fibroblast metabolism and growth.[82] These observations may explain why elevated plasma renin levels confer a greater risk for MI in patients with hypertension.[83]

Several lines of evidence suggest that norepinephrine may influence LV mass. Regression of LVH in SHR is enhanced by drugs that inhibit adrenergic stimuli.[77] Elevated plasma norepinephrine levels in the absence of hypertension cause LVH in dogs[84] and significant increases in LV mass are induced by several weeks of diet-induced elevated endogenous catecholamine levels in normotensive offspring of hypertensive parents.[85] These observations may be explained by the stimulatory effect of norepinephrine on the renin-angiotensin-aldosterone axis, and by evidence in cell culture that, through $\alpha_1$ receptors, norepinephrine can activate growth promoting oncogenes.[86] However, the importance of adrenergic stimuli in development of LVH has been questioned.[79] Cardiac and vascular structural changes, seen in renovascular hypertension and hyperaldosteronism, are not observed in patients with essential hypertension or pheochromocytoma.[87] Furthermore, only a minority of patients with pheochromocytoma have LVH despite extraordinarily high levels of norepinephrine.[88]

Hormones and growth factors that regulate general growth may also be involved in myocardial hypertrophy. For example, marked increases in LV mass may occur in persons with acromegaly as a result of elevated growth hormone and insulin-like growth factor 1 (IGF-1).[89] IGF-1 levels are higher in hypertensive patients with LVH.[90] In utero, insulin is a trophic factor that causes macrosomia.[91] Insulin levels and the degree of insulin resistance may independently modulate LV mass in normotensive and borderline hypertensive subjects.[70,92,93] This may be because insulin resistance leads to increased levels of intracellular calcium, possibly as a result of decreased $Na^+,K^+$-ATPase activity.[94] Elevated intracellular calcium, which appears to be caused by calcineurin, may be an important stimulus for myocardial actin and myosin synthesis.[75] This ionic hypothesis[95] may also explain the association between parathyroid hormone levels and LV mass in hypertensive persons.[78]

## MYOCARDIAL COMPOSITION IN LEFT VENTRICULAR HYPERTENSION AND CORONARY HEART FAILURE

Increases in myocyte and interstitial mass that occur as the heart hypertrophies adversely alter ventricular and vascular performance, creating a substrate for increased cardiovascular morbidity and mortality. The heart is composed of several different cell types and an extracellular matrix. Myocytes constitute approximately 75% of the heart mass (Figure 24–4); the remaining 25% is cardiac interstitium that is composed of the coronary vasculature, fibroblasts, macrophages, and mast cells. In hypertensive heart disease, myocytes hypertrophy and

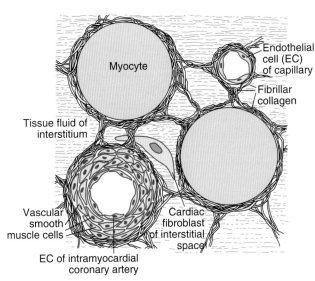

**Figure 24–4** Schematic representation of the cellular composition of the myocardium. The heart is composed of several different cell types and an extracellular matrix. Monocytes constitute approximately 75% of the heart mass. The remaining 25% is the cardiac interstitium, which is composed of the coronary vasculature, fibroblasts, macrophages, and mast cells. (Reproduced with permission from Weber KT, Brilla CG. Pathological hypertrophy and cardiac interstitium. Fibrosis and renin-angiotensin-aldosterone system. Circulation 83:1849-1865, 1991.)

interstitial components undergo hyperplasia, hypertrophy, and remodeling.[34,82] Excess collagen production by fibroblasts increases total interstitial and periarteriolar fibrosis. This reduces ventricular compliance. Echocardiographically derived parameters (pixel intensity, skewness, kurtosis, and the broad band of echoes about the distribution) have been shown to correlate with histologically assessed collagen volume in patients with hypertension and LVH.[96] Vascular smooth muscle cells undergo hyperplasia and hypertrophy, resulting in medial hypertrophy, coronary artery wall remodeling, and increased coronary wall:lumen ratio.[97] These structural changes decrease vasodilator capacity.

Although the precise structural changes that lead to decompensated systolic and diastolic function from compensated LVH are not currently known, myocardial fibrosis likely plays an important role. As part of the hypertrophic response, cardiac fibroblasts undergo a phenotypic change, assuming a myofibroblast configuration. Stimulated myofibroblasts proliferate and increase production of extracellular matrix proteins, including fibronectin, laminin, and collagen I and III. This results in progressive fibrosis. Many of these processes are controlled by integrins, which are cell surface receptors that mediate the cell's ability to interact with its environment.[52]

Progressive fibrosis of the heart is a major component of the remodeling process in hypertensive heart disease and leads to LV systolic dysfunction (CHF-S) through impaired myocyte contractility, oxygenation, and metabolism. Several studies, including a study of hypertensive patients that showed that $AT_1$ receptor blockade with losartan results in decreased plasma levels of growth factors including endothelin-1, basic fibroblast growth factor, and platelet-derived growth factor, suggest that this process may be reversed.[98] This may help explain the pos-

itive survival impact of ACE inhibitors and may suggest positive benefits of ARBs in patients with CHF-S.[99,100]

Myocyte hypertrophy may decrease the efficiency of excitation-contraction coupling, leading to decreased efficiency of contraction and development of CHF.[101] Normally, depolarization triggers influx of calcium through dihydropyridine receptors (L-type $Ca^{2+}$ channels), leading to local cytoplasmic increases in $Ca^{2+}$ concentration. This local increase "sparks" the release of $Ca^{2+}$ from the sarcoplasmic reticulum (SR) through activation of ryanodine receptors (RyRs). The efflux of $Ca^{2+}$ from the SR causes myocyte contraction by activating the troponin-actin-myosin complex. Physical alteration of the hypertrophied myocyte in LVH increases the distance between the voltage-dependent $Ca^{2+}$ channels and the RyRs on the SR, resulting in failure of the local $Ca^{2+}$ to trigger sarcoplasmic $Ca^{2+}$ release.

## MEASUREMENT OF LEFT VENTRICULAR HYPERTROPHY AND USE IN CLINICAL TRIALS AND PRACTICE

### M-Mode Echocardiography

M-mode echocardiography is the most widely used, anatomically validated method for determining LV mass.[102] Most laboratories acquire M-mode tracings with two-dimensional (2D) directed imaging.[103] To obtain a technically adequate study, the patient is imaged in the parasternal short-axis view from the highest possible interspace. This increases the likelihood of achieving an image plane orthogonal to the LV anatomic long axis, yielding a "round" LV image in the parasternal view. The M-mode cursor is then directed through the center of the 2D parasternal short axis, just distal to the mitral valve leaflets, and the M-mode gains are adjusted to optimize endocardial and epicardial interfaces. To measure walls and prevent inclusion of right- and left-sided chordal echoes in the septal and posterior wall, several guidelines are helpful. The M-mode tracing should be recorded with simultaneous viewing of the 2D image, measuring interfaces that show continuous motion throughout the cardiac cycle and discarding tracings that show abrupt posterior motion of the septum in midsystole. The latter finding reflects an incorrect angle beam from a low parasternal window. In research studies, interfaces are usually measured using the Penn convention, which excludes endocardial and epicardial surfaces in measurement of wall thickness and includes endocardial surfaces in the LV dimension measurement.[102] Measurements are made in diastole on the R wave of the QRS complex. LV mass is calculated according to the following formula:*

$$1.04[(ivs + pwd + lvid)^3 - lvid^3] - 13.6$$

Comparable LV mass values can be obtained with measurements made according to the American Society of Echocardiography (ASE) convention using the following formula[104]:

$$0.8 \text{ (ASE mass)} + 0.6 \text{ g}$$

ASE measurements are made at the onset of the QRS and are based on the leading-edge method.[105] It is important to note that many large multicenter epidemiologic studies are now

---

*ivs, interventricular septum; pwd, posterior wall dimensions; lvid, left ventricular internal dimension (diastole).

measuring wall thickness from still-frame 2D images when the M-mode is inadequate. This is in recognition of the fact that many clinical echocardiographic laboratories where these studies are performed are not sufficiently expert at obtaining research-quality M-mode images.

No uniform method is available for indexing LV mass measurements by body size or composition. The method of indexing may be irrelevant; a study comparing different methods of indexing LV mass suggested that prediction of mortality is similar for various indices, including those based on height or body surface area.[106] Most published studies index mass by body surface area, expressed as g/m².[69] De Simone et al. suggested that indexing LV mass by height to the 2.7 power avoids underestimation of LVH in obese subjects.[107] Until late 1994, most publications from the Framingham Heart Study indexed LV mass by the person's height in meters,[1] but Framingham now recommends indexing mass by the person's height to the second power.[108] Partition values for LVH based on different indexing methods are listed in Table 24–3.

Despite careful attention to the technical points noted previously, several studies indicate considerable variability in an individual measurement of LV mass.[109,110] In TOMHS, the width of the 95% confidence interval for a single replicate measurement of LV mass was 60 g, or approximately 35 g/m².[111]

This raises the issue of whether 2D-directed M-mode echocardiography should be used to guide decisions about initiation or intensity of antihypertensive therapy in the patient with borderline or stage 1 hypertension. Most of the data on reduction of cardiovascular events have been derived from trials that focused on treatment of a single risk factor. If the only risk for cardiovascular disease is diastolic BP >110 mm Hg, then more than 100 patients must be treated with antihypertensive therapy to prevent one event in 5 years.[112,113] However, patients present to the physician with varying degrees of risk based on absence or presence of multiple risk factors. Because of this variability, the concept is emerging that deciding whether to treat, or determining intensity of treatment, should be based on the aggregate of risk factors, that is, "absolute" risk[112,114] (see Chapter 21). LVH is a major risk factor for future cardiovascular events, but it is unclear how to integrate information from echocardiography into a treatment algorithm when the echocardiographic measurement has such great intrinsic variability.

A statistically based resolution of the problem of inherent variability in the measurement of LV mass is needed. We derived an estimate of the probability that LVH is present for any given value of LV mass (Figure 24–5). This calculation is based on the Z-statistic, using methodology similar to that employed to determine the probability that hypertension is present for any given level of ambulatory BP.[115] If the cutoff for LVH is 125 g/m² (95th percentile for LV mass), then a person with an LV mass index ≥110 g/m² has least a 20% chance of having LVH. Because of the prognostic implications of LVH, we propose that intensive treatment for LV mass reduction begin when there is at least a 20% probability that LVH is present. Similarly, if LV mass is <110 g/m², the risk of a cardiovascular event in a patient with stage 1 hypertension is low; therefore, initiation or intensity of treatment would be determined by presence or absence of other risk factors.

## Role of 2D Echocardiography, Magnetic Resonance Imaging, Computed Tomography, and 3D Imaging

Two-dimensional measurements of LV mass using Simpson's rule and the area-length method have been have been standardized and may be reproducible.[116,117] However, acceptance of these measurements is limited by several factors. These include lack of anatomic validation of the technique, which may be a result of incorrect assumptions about ventricular geometry in unusually shaped ventricles, and technical difficulties in obtaining endocardial and epicardial interfaces, especially of the lateral wall.[104]

Newer techniques focus on more accurate visualization of the LV. Many of these are less dependent on calculations based on geometric assumptions about the shape of the ventricle.[118] Magnetic resonance imaging (MRI), for example, may give highly reliable and anatomically validated LV mass measurements.[119-121] Transverse slices are obtained and the endocardial and epicardial contours are determined. Computer summation of all the pixels in the circumscribed muscle area of each slice may then be determined. The multiple of slice thickness and number of slices, and the specific gravity of 1.06 g/ml, is then calculated to obtain LV mass. There are no assumptions regarding the shape of the ventricle in this method.

A similar technique may be used in ultrafast computed tomography (CT) images.[122] Although significantly more costly than echocardiography, MRI may be an effective tool

**Table 24–3** Partition Value for Defining Left Ventricular Hypertrophy (LVH) Based on Various Indexing Methods

| | LVM/Height²·⁷ (g/m²·⁷)[108] | LVM/BSA (g/m²)[2,69] | LVM/Height (g/m)[108,390] | LVM/Height² (g/m²)[108] |
|---|---|---|---|---|
| | | **95th percentile** | | |
| Men | 52 | 125 | 138 | 78 |
| Women | 41 | 100 | 95 | 58 |
| | | **97th percentile** | | |
| Men | | 134 | | |
| Women | | 110 | | |
| Mean + 2 SD | | | | |
| Men | | | 143 | |
| Women | | | 102 | |

LVM, left ventricular mass, Penn convention; BSA, body surface area; SD, standard deviation.

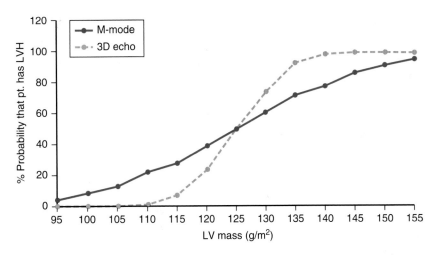

**Figure 24–5** Estimated probability that an observed left ventricular (LV) mass index (LV mass/body surface area) obtained by either M-mode or three-dimensional (3D) echocardiography is >125 g/m². This is based on a standard deviation for M-mode 17.4 g/m² and for 3D = 6.8 g/m² (assumption that body surface area = 1.7).

for monitoring changes in LV mass for an individual patient or for groups of patients in a research protocol.[118,121] Less expensive and technically less demanding methods of assessing LV mass have used computer-automated algorithms with technetium-99m-sestamibi single-photon emission CT myocardial perfusion imaging.[123,124] These techniques rely on determining counts per pixel of myocardium and thus do not depend on assumptions about the shape of the ventricle. Early studies are promising; however, this technique is still in development.[125]

New techniques in echocardiography are allowing noninvasive, accurate assessments of LV mass. Three-dimensional echocardiography eliminates problems of the geometric assumptions used in M-mode and 2D echocardiographic techniques, allowing for more accurate assessment of LV mass. In vitro correlation of 3D-determined LV mass and weight of fixed animal hearts is high, and in vivo correlation with MRI measurement in humans is also very good over a wide range of weights.[126-130] A new generation of intravenously administered ultrasound contrast agents (microbubbles) capable of consistent and persistent detection within the LV cavity and myocardium now allows easier visualization of the endocardial and epicardial edges, permitting more accurate measurements for conventional M-mode– and 2D-determined LV mass. In experimental studies, 3D echocardiography performed with new echocardiographic contrast agents has been used to display myocardial mass and the mass of infarcted myocardium.[131]

## LEFT VENTRICULAR MASS REGRESSION

Regression of LV mass with effective BP reduction has been demonstrated in more than 400 clinical studies, but fewer than 10% have been double-blind and placebo-controlled.[132] Data indicate that LV mass regression improves survival in hypertensive patients. In one small trial that followed hypertensive patients for more than 10 years, the cumulative incidence of nonfatal cardiovascular events was significantly higher among patients without regression of LVH as compared with those with significant reduction of LV mass.[133] Verdecchia et al. showed decreased risk of cardiac events with LV mass regression independent of the baseline LV mass, baseline clinic and ambulatory BP, and the degree of BP

reduction.[134] Similar findings were reported in a prospective study of 172 patients with essential hypertension, in whom the absence or presence of LVH on follow-up echocardiogram was the strongest predictor of subsequent morbid events.[135] Total cardiovascular events were also reduced in TOMHS, in which there was LV mass regression.[136] A mechanism that might explain these findings is that midwall fractional shortening, a sensitive measure of intrinsic myocardial systolic performance, appears to improve with LV mass regression, as does Doppler assessed stroke volume.[137,138]

BP reduction with all classes of antihypertensive agents reduces LV mass, with the possible exception of pure vasodilators such as minoxidil and hydralazine.[77] A meta-analysis of more than 100 studies yielded a moderately strong relationship between BP reduction and LV mass regression.[139] This confirms the hemodynamic contribution to LV mass.

It is not clear, however, whether antihypertensive agents can regress LV mass independent of their effect on BP. In animal studies, low-dose ACE inhibitors can reduce LV mass without lowering BP.[140] The Losartan Intervention for Endpoint Reduction (LIFE) study showed a significant and progressive decrease in LV mass over a 3-year treatment period, despite only a small reduction in BP after the first year of blinded therapy with atenolol or losartan.[142,143] However, one meta-analysis suggested that for equal levels of BP reduction, β-blockers, ACE inhibitors, and calcium channel blockers (CCBs) cause the same degree of LVH regression, whereas diuretics reduce chamber dimension but do not lead to regression of hypertrophied muscle.[132] This conclusion has been challenged in two randomized trials that suggest that diuretics are as effective if not more effective than other drug classes for reducing LV mass. In TOMHS, BP was reduced by a combination of weight loss plus either placebo or one of five antihypertensive drug classes (β-blocker, α-blocker, CCB, ACE inhibitor, or diuretic).[136] At 1 and 4 years, all groups showed LV mass regression, confirming that weight loss in conjunction with BP reduction reduces LV mass. Surprisingly, only participants receiving chlorthalidone had greater LV mass regression than those undergoing weight loss and receiving placebo. Reduced internal dimension as well as reduced wall thickness accounted for this finding. The Veterans Administration (VA) Cooperative Study Group reported similar results: For equal levels of BP reduction, hydrochlorothiazide had a greater effect on LV mass regression than other antihypertensive agents.[141] In this trial of 493 patients who completed 1 year of maintenance antihypertensive therapy, LV mass was not reduced despite hemodynamic improvement in patients taking prazosin, clonidine, or diltiazem, but ACE inhibition was nearly as beneficial as diuretic-based therapy. In the LIFE trial, LV mass regression (by Cornell ECG voltage criteria) occurred with both atenolol and the ARB losartan, but the reduction was significantly more pronounced with losartan.[142] Additional data (not analyzed by drug assignment) from a subset of patients who underwent serial echocardiograms (n = 754) showed significant regression in LV mass after 1 year of treatment (despite small overall reduction in BP) and continued regression of LV mass by 2 years with sustained BP reduction.[143] (See Chapter 31 for a more complete discussion of the LIFE trial.)

Although the patient with hypertension and LVH is typically treated with more than one agent, few studies have evaluated the effect of combination therapy on LV mass regression. However, the 4E-LVH study (Effects of Eplerenone, Enalapril, and Eplerenone/Enalapril) reported that the combination of eplerenone (an aldosterone antagonist) with the ACE inhibitor enalapril was more effective in reducing LV mass than either treatment alone.[144]

## NEW PHARMACOLOGIC APPROACHES FOR LEFT VENTRICULAR MASS REGRESSION

### Targeting Structural, Functional, and Genetic Adaptations That Lead to Increased Left Ventricular Mass

The factors that predict why some patients respond to antihypertensive treatment with LV mass regression and others do not, have not been identified. It is likely that genetically based differences may account for heterogeneity of response.

"Nonantihypertensive" medications may interfere with the pathways that lead to cellular (and therefore cardiac) hypertrophy. In addition to providing cardiovascular benefit by their cholesterol-lowering actions, hydroxymethylglutaryl coenzyme A (HMG-CoA) reductase inhibitors may also reduce cardiac morbidity and mortality by preventing cardiac hypertrophy. The activation of fetal cardiac and growth genes such as c-*myc* and c-*jun* to up-regulate myocardial cell protein synthesis is accomplished by stimulating the production of several mitogen-activated protein kinases (e.g., the *Ras-Raf1-ERK1* kinase cascade). HMG-CoA reductase inhibitors disrupt the proper plasma membrane localization of GTP-binding proteins such as Ras. Thus in animal models of LVH (aortic-banded Wistar rats), simvastatin has been shown to limit the development of cardiac hypertrophy by inhibiting Ras signaling.[145] In aortic banded mice, rapamycin attenuated the development of hypertrophy.[146] Rapamycin inhibits the mammalian target of rapamycin (mTOR), a component of the phosphoinositide 3-kinase pathway, which is also thought to be an important determinant of cell size. Rapamycin also appears to affect the mitogen-activated protein kinase pathways by inhibiting JNK1.

## DIASTOLIC FUNCTION IN HYPERTENSION

### Clinical Presentation and Etiology

The clinical presentation of diastolic dysfunction in hypertensive heart disease is variable, ranging from asymptomatic findings on noninvasive testing to overt CHF despite normal systolic function.[147-152] The prevalence of asymptomatic LV filling abnormalities in adults without hypertrophy and with ambulatory awake BP >130/85 mm Hg may be as high as 33%.[40] Once LVH or ischemia develops, these asymptomatic abnormalities may cause decreased exercise ejection fraction and blunt the expected rise in exercise cardiac output.[153] An estimated 30% to 45 % of patients with CHF have normal systolic function but abnormal diastolic function (CHF-D).[152] In the Olmsted County study, the prognosis for patients with CHF-D was poor. Survival at 3 months, 1 year, and 5 years was 86%, 76%, and 48%, respectively (Figure 24–6).[56] In a cohort of patients with CHF-D and underlying coronary artery disease, 7-year cardiovascular mortality approached 50%. Many

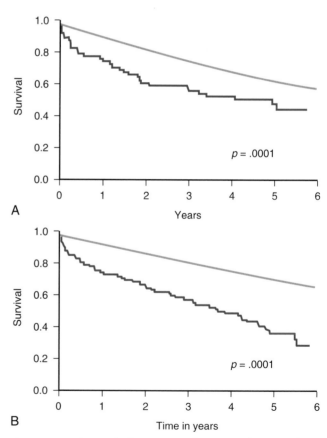

**Figure 24–6** Survival of patients with ejection fraction of ≥50% **(A)** and <50% **(B)** compared with that for age- and sex-matched population. (Reproduced with permission from Senni M, Tribouilloy CM, Rodeheffer RJ, et al. Congestive heart failure in the community: A study of all incident cases in Olmsted County, Minnesota, in 1991. Circulation 98:2282-2289, 1998.)

of these patients were also hypertensive.[154] Symptoms in CHF-D are accounted for by prolonged LV relaxation or decreased compliance, which causes shifts in the diastolic LV pressure-volume relation that result in elevated left atrial and LV filling pressures.[155]

## Factors Affecting Diastolic Function

Genetic,[156] structural, metabolic, and hemodynamic factors can affect diastolic function under resting conditions and during states of increased demand or ischemia (Figure 24–7).

### Genetic Factors

Using E and A Doppler mitral inflow velocities as a phenotype for diastolic filling, the Hypertension Genetic Epidemiology Network study performed linkage analyses that identified two potentially significant genes on chromosome 5 that contribute to diastolic dysfunction in hypertension.[157] One is a calcium-modulating cyclophilin ligand (CAMLG), an integral membrane protein involved in the regulation of $Ca^{2+}$ ion signaling. This protein is expressed in multiple tissues, and may play a role in $Ca^{2+}$ transport in myocardial contraction/relaxation. The other is the α-1B adrenergic receptor (ADRA1B) gene, which is expressed in myocardium and may indirectly stimulate intracellular $Ca^{2+}$ release and protein kinase C activation. Other genes likely involved in diastolic dysfunction include the SR-$Ca^{2+}$ ATPase pump, which is up-regulated in CHF, and phospholamban, which is overexpressed in rats with prolonged isovolumic relaxation and increased LV end-diastolic pressure. In addition, abnormal diastolic filling parameters have been associated with ACE I/D and G-protein $\beta_3$-subunit C825T gene polymorphisms.

### Structural Factors

Reports in the late 1980s and early 1990s suggested that diastolic abnormalities occur early in the course of hypertension and precede detectable hypertrophy.[40,148,158-160] Later studies challenged the notion that diastolic abnormalities are the first sign of hypertensive heart disease; they suggest that diastolic abnormalities do not precede structural changes, but rather occur simultaneously. In general, diastolic function is inversely related to LV mass in patients with hypertension[148,149,161-163]

and regression of LV mass with CCBs, β-blockers, and ACE inhibitors is often,[164-169] but not always,[170] associated with improved LV diastolic function. In the Hypertension and Ambulatory Recording Venetia Study (HARVEST), an Italian study comparing young (age 18-45 years) patients with stage 1 hypertension with matched normotensive controls, the former had significantly greater LV mass and more concentric remodeling.[171] However, there was no significant difference in Doppler mitral inflow velocity (E/A) ratio, a marker of diastolic dysfunction. Experimental data suggest that a diastolic abnormality in the absence of frank hypertrophy indicates that the heart is beginning to hypertrophy in response to hemodynamic or nonhemodynamic stimuli. For example, dogs with aortic banding simultaneously develop abnormalities of LV filling and increased LV mass.[172] This early change appears to be dependent on increased myocyte size rather than increased fibrosis.[173] However, there is also strong evidence that abnormal filling is partially accounted for by interstitial collagen deposition that occurs with LVH and aging, leading to passive structural changes that result in increased chamber stiffness.[82,174,175]

### Ischemia

Ischemia has pronounced effects on diastolic function, and these are exacerbated in even the minimally hypertrophied heart.[176] Several metabolic/biochemical factors, which are not fully elucidated, help slow inactivation of the actin-myosin complex and delay relaxation. Baseline adenosine triphosphate (ATP) levels in the pressure-overload hypertrophied heart are similar to or slightly lower than those in control hearts.[177,178] Although it may be normal in the resting state,[179] the rate of sarcoplasmic uptake of $Ca^{2+}$, an energy-dependent and ATP-requiring step, is markedly reduced by hypoxia.[180] However, diastolic dysfunction in the hypertrophied ventricle may not be fully explained by depletion of high-energy phosphates. In one study, when the isolated buffer-perfused rat heart was subjected to hypoxia, significantly more ischemia developed in hypertrophied hearts than in control hearts at equivalent rates of coronary flow and with similar rates of ATP depletion.[177] This led the authors to conclude that hypertrophy-induced alterations in $Ca^{2+}$ handling, such as changes in the calcium transient that are abnormal even at rest,[181] might contribute to ischemia-induced diastolic dysfunction in LVH. In the intact

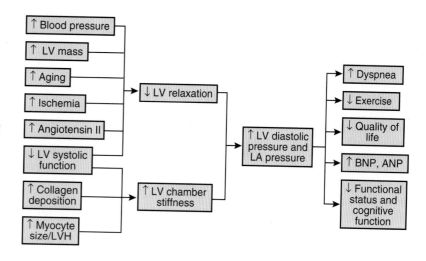

**Figure 24–7** Causes of left ventricular (LV) diastolic dysfunction and its clinical consequences. ANP, atrial natriuretic peptide; BNP, brain natriuretic peptide; LA, left atrial; LVH, LV hypertrophy.

dog, however, under conditions of increased oxygen demand, there was decreased conversion of phosphocreatinine to ATP in the hypertrophied heart,[178] suggesting that high-energy phosphate metabolism is impaired by hypertrophy. Differences in results between the isolated heart and the intact heart may be due to failure of the intact heart to deliver adequate blood flow because of decreased coronary flow reserve.

### Hemodynamic Load

Increased hemodynamic load affects diastolic performance. In isolated hearts, increases in afterload early in systole impair relaxation.[182] Wall stress in untreated hypertensive persons is inversely related to diastolic function.[163] When studied with ABPM, previously untreated borderline and mild hypertensive patients demonstrate a linear relation between BP and abnormal LV filling.[40,183] The degree to which an acute reduction in BP per se improves LV diastolic performance is not known, and studies are difficult to interpret becauce the agents used can themselves affect performance.[184,185]

CHF-D may be characterized by a higher pressure/volume ratio at end-diastole in comparison with normal individuals, but no difference in the ratio at end of systole. This appears on the pressure-volume loop curve as a shift upward and to the left, thus indicating an abnormality of passive diastolic relaxation with decreased capacitance (a decrease in filling volume at any specified filling pressure). Kawaguchi et al.[186] invasively compared LV pressure-volume relationships in patients with CHF-D versus age-matched and young controls. They showed an elevation of end-diastolic pressure:volume ratio (EDPVR) in patients with CHF-D. However, they also showed changes in systolic-ventricular and arterial stiffening and suggested that CHF-D may be due to an adverse coupling of diastolic relaxation abnormality with systolic-ventricular and arterial stiffness.[186] Some investigators have even proposed that CHF-D is not a disease of abnormal LV relaxation, but is a complex of different pathophysiologic processes that produce the clinical scenario of CHF-D.[187]

### Systolic Function

Systolic function, as measured by ejection fraction, does not appear to decrease during episodes of severe hypertension with pulmonary edema.[188] However, systolic and diastolic dysfunction are closely linked. Midwall fractional shortening, a more sensitive measure of intrinsic myocardial systolic function than endocardial fractional shortening, is abnormal in a substantial portion of asymptomatic hypertensive persons.[189,190] Schussheim et al. found that depressed midwall fractional shortening and diastolic dysfunction occur simultaneously in asymptomatic hypertensive persons with normal endocardial fractional shortening.[191] Conversely, those with normal midwall fractional shortening tend to have normal Doppler indices of mitral inflow. In the Hypertension Genetic Epidemiology Network Study, impaired LV relaxation, measured by prolonged isovolumic relaxation time, was associated with lower midwall fractional shortening, but not with lower fractional shortening.[157] The prognostic implications of these findings were illustrated in the Cardiovascular Health Study, a population-based study of 5201 men and women ≥65 years. Those at highest risk for CHF were those with the highest LV mass index and lowest stress-corrected midwall fractional shortening.[192]

### Aging

Aging has profound effects on diastolic function, reflected in a reduced rate of LV relaxation and increased diastolic stiffness. This effect has been confirmed by various noninvasive measurements of diastolic function.[40,61,193-198] Among normal persons in the Framingham Heart Study, age was the predominant factor affecting Doppler indices of diastolic function, with a Pearson correlation coefficient of −0.80 between age and the E/A ratio.[199] Hypertension, including ISH, further depresses diastolic function in older subjects,[159,200,201] but this finding has been questioned.[202]

The effect of exercise on age-related changes in diastolic function is also controversial. A prospectively designed exercise program in men between the ages of 60 and 82 demonstrated reversal of depressed LV diastolic function with aging.[203] However, a cross-sectional study of younger (52-76 years) male athletes demonstrated similar impairment of diastolic LV filling similar to sedentary peers.[204] In contrast, a study of healthy persons in all age ranges showed that diastolic function improved with regular modest use of alcohol or regular aerobic exercise.[205]

### Hormones and Paracrine Factors

Catecholamines are believed to favorably affect diastolic performance by improving systolic performance.[206,207] Other studies suggest that Ang II adversely affects diastolic function by impairing LV relaxation and stimulating aldosterone-mediated myocardial fibrosis.[82] In an echocardiographic study of 84 nonhypertensive Finnish men and women age 36 to 37 years, polymorphism in the gene encoding aldosterone synthase (CYP11B2), an enzyme catalyzing critical steps in aldosterone synthesis, was linked to diastolic dysfunction and LV mass. Persons with the −344TT polymorphism in the promoter region of this gene had mean early:late peak velocity (A/E) ratios and LV mass significantly greater than individuals with −344CT and −344CC genotypes.[23] In contrast, a later study of hypertensive persons showed the opposite finding, with higher LV mass in individuals with the −344CC variant.[24] Clinical studies of aldosterone antagonists appear to demonstrate improvement of echocardiographic parameters of diastolic dysfunction and LV mass independent of the degree of BP lowering.[144,208]

## Noninvasive Measurement of Diastolic Function

Diastolic function can be evaluated by several methods. The rate of isovolumic pressure decay, early and late LV filling, and pressure-volume relations can be derived from cardiac catheterization.[209-211] Although these measurements are the most accurate indices of diastolic function, they require an invasive procedure. Inferences regarding the diastolic properties of the ventricle can be obtained noninvasively with radionuclide angiography[212] and M-mode[213] or Doppler echocardiography[214] and acoustic quantification.[215] These techniques yield information on all phases of diastole, including isovolumetric relaxation, early and late LV filling,[40,159,216] and temporal differences in regional filling (regional nonuniformity).[217]

Radionuclide angiography was one of the first noninvasive techniques for assessment of LV filling properties. It is based on analysis of the LV time-activity curve. The time-activity curve represents relative volume changes throughout the cardiac cycle. Several parameters of diastolic function can be computed from the time-activity curve, including the peak rate of rapid diastolic filling, time to peak filling rate and the relative contributions of the rapid filling period and of atrial systole to total LV stroke volume. In addition, the duration of the isovolumetric relaxation period may be computed in approximately 80% of patients. Decreased peak filling rate, increased time to peak filling rate, and decreased third and one-half filling fractions are reported.

Hypertensive patients with LVH and impaired diastolic filling at rest also have decreased exercise-induced augmentation in end-diastolic volume, leading to reduced stroke volume and impaired exercise ejection fraction.[148] Attention must be given to technical details of data acquisition and analysis for evaluation of diastolic events using radionuclide angiography. In particular, the effects of cycle length variability (in gated studies), temporal resolution, temporal smoothing, and normalization parameters must be considered. For diastolic studies, high-count double-buffered, left anterior oblique 32-frame images are used.

Doppler echocardiographic evaluation of LV inflow is the most widely used noninvasive measure of diastolic function.[218] The LV diastolic flow velocity profile obtained with Doppler echocardiography correlates well with radionuclide angiographic variables in the evaluation of LV diastolic function.[212] However, Doppler echocardiographic assessment is easy and convenient and does not add much time to data acquisition. Furthermore, significant prognostic information may be obtained from Doppler determined mitral inflow. The Strong Heart Study evaluated the prognostic significance of abnormal mitral inflow as a measure of diastolic dysfunction in a population-based sample of middle-aged and elderly American Indians. In this population, a restrictive pattern of inflow with mitral E/A ratio >1.5 was associated with a three-fold increase in cardiac mortality independent of other covariates.[219] A low E/A ratio (i.e., <0.6), indicative of delayed LV relaxation, was also associated with increased cardiovascular mortality, but not as an independent variable. A younger Italian population was evaluated in the Progretto Ipertensione Umbria Monitoraggio Ambulatoriale (PIUMA) study. They did not observe a J-shaped pattern as noted in the Strong Heart Study. There was, however, significantly increased cardiovascular mortality associated with a low E/A ratio, with a 21% higher risk of cardiovascular events for each 0.3 decrease in age-adjusted E/A ratio below the median value for the group (0.98).[220]

In the setting of normal ventricular relaxation, immediately after mitral valve opening LV pressure is significantly lower than left atrial pressure, and therefore the gradient between the left atrium and LV is relatively high. This results in a high peak velocity of early filling (E) and significant emptying of the blood in the left atrium in early diastole. As a result, the peak velocity of the late filling wave (A) is low. If LV relaxation is prolonged, the LV pressure decline after mitral valve opening is delayed, so the gradient between the left atrium and LV in early diastole is reduced, and equilibration of pressure between the two chambers may be delayed. In the setting

of normal LV function, this is reflected on the Doppler recording as a reduced E and higher A/E ratio and/or a prolonged deceleration time of the early filling wave[221-223] (Figures 24–8 and 24–9). The enhanced A wave may be a result of two factors: (1) LV pressure is lower than normal just before the atrial contraction due to decreased LV filling, and (2) the delayed atrial emptying causes a rise in atrial pressure. These two factors lead to a higher gradient between the left atrium and LV at atrial systole and, hence, an enhanced peak A wave.

Using Doppler echocardiography, one group studied normal persons between the ages of 20 and 50 years (mean 35 ± 9 years), with heart rates ≤90 beats/min and no evidence of coronary artery disease. The average value peak A/E ratio was 0.67 ± 0.16; an A/E ratio of 0.99 was 2 standard deviations (SDs) above this mean value.[40] These data have been corroborated by others, who have shown that an A/E ratio ≥1 in persons younger than 50 years of age is significantly higher than the range for normal subjects.[196] Framingham Heart Study data, however, suggest that an A/E ratio of 1 may be in the upper range of normal for a for a 40- to 50-year-old, and is clearly abnormal only in persons younger than age 40 years (Figure 24–10).[224] Studies using Doppler echocardiography show that approximately 20% of untreated prehypertensive or stage 1 hypertensive persons have diastolic filling abnormalities in the absence of LVH.[40,225] In addition, there may be a threshold of average awake ambulatory BP, 130/85 mm Hg, below which neither diastolic abnormalities nor LVH is detected (Figure 24–11).[40]

### Pitfalls in Interpretation of Noninvasive Measurements

Information derived from Doppler echocardiography should be interpreted in the context of the many dynamic factors that can affect Doppler variables. These include changes in afterload, systolic performance, heart rate, and cardiac filling pressures.[221,226] For example, the peak velocity of late LV filling (peak A) is directly related to heart rate.[227] Therefore, a pharmacologic intervention that simultaneously increases heart rate and the height of the A wave could be incorrectly interpreted as adversely affecting diastolic function. Conversely, a pharmacologic intervention that raises LV end-diastolic pressure could be misinterpreted as beneficial if it simultaneously lowers the A wave and raises the E wave (i.e., "pseudonormalization" of the Doppler profile). This was demonstrated in a study in which verapamil was given to patients with coronary artery disease.[228] This intervention resulted in an increased early filling velocity (E wave) and a shortening of isovolumetric relaxation. Invasive studies, however, showed that these seemingly beneficial changes were in fact associated with a prolongation of the time constant of relaxation and an increase in LV end-diastolic pressure. Thus, increased LV end-diastolic pressure and left atrial filling pressures—not improved LV relaxation—caused a pattern of Doppler "pseudonormalization" characterized by a higher E wave, lower A wave, and shortened isovolumetric relaxation time.

### Emerging Techniques to Measure Diastolic Function

A challenge in noninvasive evaluation of diastolic function is to devise methods by which LV end-diastolic pressure can be serially evaluated. One group suggested that plasma atrial

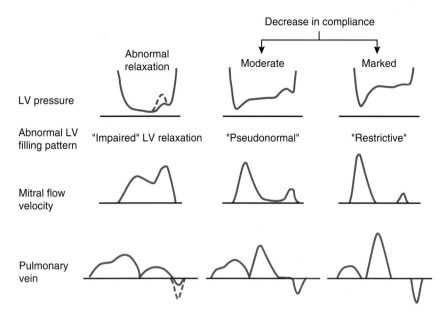

**Figure 24–8** The three basic abnormal left ventricular (LV) (mitral flow velocity) filling patterns together with representative LV pressure recordings and pulmonary venous flow velocity recordings. (Reproduced with permission from Appleton CP. Left ventricular diastolic function. *In* Murphy JG, (ed). Mayo Clinic Cardiology Review. Armonk, NY, Futura, 1997; pp 43-56.)

natriuretic peptide, a measure of LV filling pressures, be used to interpret changes in noninvasively derived LV filling parameters. Plasma atrial natriuretic peptide levels increase when the atria are stretched as a result of increased filling pressures[229-231] and fall as LV end-diastolic pressure decreases. This knowledge was exploited to interpret a Doppler evaluation of diastolic function in severely hypertensive persons treated for 1 year with nifedipine.[169] Over the year, the Doppler early filling (E wave) increased while the A wave decreased. Atrial natriuretic peptide levels fell, suggesting that LV end-diastolic pressure had decreased. The investigators concluded that it was likely that the increased velocity of early filling and decreased A wave were due to improved LV relaxation.

Several merging Doppler techniques may allow for serial noninvasive interpretation of LV end-diastolic pressure. Among these is measurement of pulmonary venous inflow.[232-234] During atrial contraction, flow into the pulmonary veins reverses as the pulmonary veins become a "low-pressure sink" for the contracting atrium. Increased LV end-diastolic pressures create more "afterload" for the atrium, leading to increased height and duration of the "reverse flow" wave. Furthermore, the difference in pulmonary venous and mitral flow velocity duration during atrial contraction is related to the increase in LV end-diastolic pressure.[233] Therefore, prolonged pulmonary venous velocity duration during atrial contraction, coupled with a shortened duration of the mitral A wave, suggests increasing LV end-diastolic pressure.

Conversely, a shorter pulmonary venous velocity duration coupled with a lengthened transmitral A wave during atrial contraction suggests decreasing LV end-diastolic pressure (see Figure 24–8).

Another promising Doppler technique to assess LV end-diastolic pressure rests on the observation that diastolic flow is initially directed toward the ventricular apex (transmitral A wave) and then wraps around and enters the LV outflow tract just before ejection.[235,236] This "preejection wave," termed the *Ar wave,* can be identified on recordings of the LV outflow tract. The time from peak of the transmitral A wave to peak of the Ar wave (A-Ar interval) is inversely related to LV chamber stiffness and LV end-diastolic pressure[235] (i.e., the stiffer the ventricle or the higher the LV end-diastolic pressure, the shorter the A-Ar interval).

Color M-mode assessment of LV filling expands on this concept. It is based on the interval from color M-mode peak velocity at the mitral leaflet tips to peak velocity in the apical region of the LV. A first wave propagates from the left atrium to the LV apex, corresponding to early filling, and a second wave follows atrial contraction. The magnitude of these velocities is highest above the mitral tips and decreases as flow approaches the apex. The velocity at which flow propagates within the ventricle ($V_p$) is given by the slope of the color wavefront. The time delay of the first wave of early filling from its appearance at the mitral leaflets to its appearance in the LV apex (TD) is also measured and is directly related to the time constant of isovolumetric relaxation.

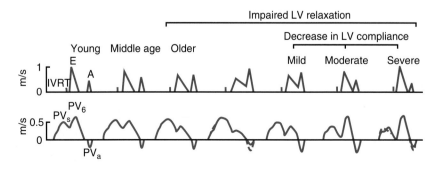

**Figure 24–9** Natural history of left ventricular (LV) filling patterns. A, mitral flow velocity at atrial contraction; E, mitral flow velocity in early diastole; PVs, pulmonary venous flow velocity in systole. (Reproduced with permission from Appleton CP. Left ventricular diastolic function. *In* Murphy JG, (ed). Mayo Clinic Cardiology Review. Armonk, NY, Futura, 1997; pp 43-56.)

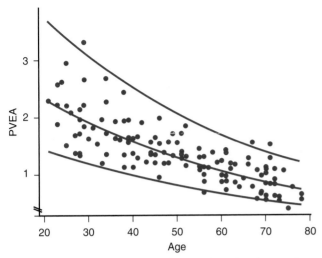

**Figure 24–10** Predicted value of ratio of peak velocity of early filling/late filling (PVEA) ratio in normal subjects studied in the Framingham Heart Study. *Solid outer lines* represent the 95% confidence intervals. At approximately age 40, a PVEA ratio below 1 is outside of the 95% confidence interval. (From Benjamin EJ, Levy D, Anderson KM, et al. Determinants of Doppler indexes of left ventricular diastolic function in normal subjects (the Framingham Heart Study). Am J Cardiol 70:508-515, 1992, with permission from Excerpta Medica.)

In hypertensive patients with abnormal relaxation, and in patients with restrictive heart disease, there is reduced $V_p$ and prolonged TD.[237] These variables may be independent of heart rate and LV end-diastolic pressure. Thus, this technique may become extremely useful in serial assessment of LV relaxation.

Tissue Doppler imaging (TDI) is an ultrasound technique based on color Doppler imaging principles. It allows quantification of intramural myocardial velocities by detection of consecutive phase shifts of the ultrasound signal reflected from contracting myocardium. Large Doppler signals obtained from the ventricular wall can be selectively displayed as a color or pulsed Doppler images by eliminating small Doppler signals produced by the blood flow.[238,239] There are significant correlations between early and late myocardial velocities obtained by TDI and the invasively determined time constant of LV pressure decay during an isovolumetric diastole (tau).[240] This suggests that TDI variables are load and heart rate independent reflections of intrinsic diastolic function. As a result, and because of the availability of TDI on most new commercially available ultrasound equipment, TDI will probably emerge as the measure of choice for assessing diastolic function.

Ultrasonic backscatter is an echocardiographic technique in which quantitative characterization of myocardial texture is obtained by analysis of ultrasonic reflectivity. The amount of backscatter produced when ultrasound interacts with components of tissue appears to correlate with the degree of myocardial fibrillar collagens type I and type III. An association between myocardial ultrasonic reflexivity and extent of diastolic dysfunction defined by traditional ultrasound Doppler methods has been demonstrated.[241]

## Effect of Treatment on CHF-D

Although CHF-D has been recognized for nearly two decades, treatment of hypertensive patients with symptoms of CHF-D is guided by relatively few studies. Topol et al., in a landmark study, analyzed the effect of treatment on morbidity and mortality in 21 elderly hypertensive patients with marked concentric hypertrophy, supernormal LV systolic function, and depressed LV diastolic function. These patients were treated with a variety of antihypertensive and cardioactive agents because of CHF, angina, stroke, or syncope.[151] Of the 12 patients who received vasodilators (nitrates, hydralazine, prazosin, or captopril), 6 had a severe hypotensive reaction and 1 died. In contrast, all 9 patients who received β-blockers or calcium antagonists improved, and 4 had less dyspnea after discontinuation of digoxin and furosemide. In a study of 144 patients with CHF and Doppler evidence of restrictive LV diastolic filling as measured by a shortened deceleration time of early mitral filling, cardiac mortality was assessed after 2 years of unblinded oral therapy. Various combinations of digoxin, diuretics, ACE inhibitors, nitrates, and β-blockers were used. Survival was significantly better in patients with prolongation of the deceleration time over the treatment period compared with patients with no change in deceleration time.[242] The latter group used more digoxin. No other significant difference in medication use was noted. Thus, although reversing diastolic dysfunction may relieve symptoms and prolong survival, the optimal regimen is still not clear.

Systematic studies of various agents on CHF-D are few, and the paucity of the resulting data have formed the basis for conflicting recommendations by authorities on the optimal treatment of CHF-D. This suggests a need for a randomized controlled trial utilizing drug classes whose efficacy in treatment of CHF-D has not been proved.

### ACE Inhibitors and Angiotensin Receptor Blockers in the Treatment of CHF-D

Three studies have evaluated the efficacy of ACE inhibitors in CHF-D. In one study, 10 persons with hypertension, LVH, and CHF-D were treated in a nonrandomized, uncontrolled study with the ACE inhibitor enalapril and a low-sodium diet.[168] After an average of 9 months of treatment, CHF symptoms resolved in all subjects, without use of diuretics. Diastolic function as measured by Doppler echocardiography did not change after the initial decrease in BP, but improved significantly (decreased A/E ratio and deceleration time) after LV mass regression. Another study compared treatment with an ACE inhibitor to standard therapy without enalapril in 21 elderly patients with CHF-D, prior non–Q-wave MI, and normal ejection fraction.[243] In the enalapril group, BP and LV mass were significantly reduced with treatment, and this was accompanied by a significant improvement in New York Heart Association functional score (decrease from 3.0 to 2.4, *p* <.01), increased exercise time on a treadmill, and an improvement in diastolic function as measured by Doppler echocardiography. In the third study, 35 patients with hypertension and LVH underwent endocardial biopsy after 6 months of treatment with lisinopril.[244] There was evidence of significant regression of myocardial fibrosis as evidenced by collagen volume fraction and myocardial hydroxyproline concentration, irrespective of the degree of LVH regression. This was accompanied by echocardiographic signs of improved LV

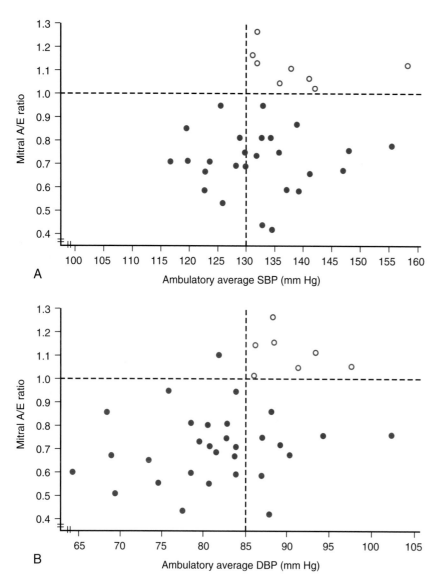

**Figure 24-11** Ratio of late (A) to early (E) left ventricular inflow velocity (A/E ratio) in 37 persons (<50 years old) plotted against *(panel **A**)* average ambulatory awake systolic blood pressure (SBP) and *(panel **B**)* average awake ambulatory diastolic blood pressure (DBP). All subjects were untreated and had no evidence of coronary disease and were referred for evaluation borderline hypertension. *Horizontal hatched lines* indicate A/E ratio ≥1 is abnormal in this population; vertical hatched lines indicate BP above which abnormal A/E ratio was detected. All subjects (eight, *open circles* in upper right quadrant of panel **A**) had SBP >130 mm Hg. In upper left quadrant of panel **B,** only 1 of 22 subjects *(closed circles)* with diastolic pressure <85 mm Hg had abnormal A/E ratio, and this subject had SBP >130; all other subjects with abnormal A/E ratio (seven, *open circles* in upper right quadrant of panel **B**) had DBP >85. (From Phillips RA, Goldman ME, Ardeljan M, et al. Determinants of abnormal left ventricular filling in early hypertension. J Am Coll Cardiol 14: 979-985, 1989, with permission from the American College of Cardiology Foundation.)

diastolic function, including increased E/A and decreased isovolumic relaxation time.

In the Candesartan in Heart Failure Assessment of Reduction in Mortality and Morbidity (CHARM)-preserved study, an ARB was assessed in comparison with placebo in 3023 patients with history of classes II-IV CHF, but LVEF >40%. This study showed a significant benefit of the ARB over placebo preventing further hospitalizations for CHF.[245] However, these results might be explained by a significantly greater reduction in BP in the candesartan group compared with the placebo group (6.9 mm Hg systolic and 2.9 mm diastolic, *p* <.0001).

### Calcium Channel Blockers in the Treatment of CHF-D

Two small, short-term studies have been reported in which CCBs were the mainstays of therapy for CHF. In a prospective study of 20 patients (15 of whom had hypertension), verapamil and placebo were compared in a 5-week crossover design. Compared with baseline, verapamil significantly improved LV filling, decreased symptoms and improved exercise time,[246] whereas placebo had no significant effect.

However, possibly because of a "carryover" effect of verapamil-induced improvement into the placebo phase of the crossover design, there was no difference between verapamil and placebo in LV filling. In six severely hypertensive patients followed for 4 months, of whom four received a concomitant diuretic, treatment with nifedipine was associated with symptomatic improvement.[247]

### β-Blockers in the Treatment of CHF-D

There is very limited data regarding the role of β-blockers in isolated CHF-D. A study in patients with idiopathic dilated cardiomyopathy (ejection fraction <25%) evaluated the effect of metoprolol, up to 50 mg three times daily, on diastolic dysfunction.[248] Diastolic function improved within 3 months of treatment, and the investigators suggested that better diastolic performance might have allowed for the subsequent observed boost in systolic function. Another study compared atenolol with nebivolol in hypertensive patients with history of CHF-D. After 6 months of treatment, they found significant improvement in E/A ratio with all patients, though somewhat more pronounced with the latter treatment group.[249]

### Diuretics in the Treatment of CHF-D

Although no clinical trial data are available, some investigators recommend cautious use of diuretics to reduce the congested state in CHF-D.[150,250] Diuretics reduce congestion by lowering LV preload and reducing right ventricular filling pressure, thereby relieving pericardial restraint on the LV.[251] However, use of diuretics remains controversial because of the lack of clinical trial evaluation of this strategy and the concern that preload may be inappropriately reduced with "overdiuresis." In fact, the Fifth Report of the Joint National Committee on the Detection, Evaluation, and Treatment of Hypertension (JNC V) considers diuretic therapy in diastolic dysfunction as "relatively or absolutely contraindicated" in patients with hypertensive hypertrophic cardiomyopathy with diastolic dysfunction.[252] On the other hand, diuretic-based therapy very effectively prevents development of CHF in patients with hypertension.

### Digoxin and Inotropes in the Treatment of CHF-D

Although digoxin may improve LV filling by decreasing heart rate, its ability to increase intracellular calcium may increase LV stiffness.[253] In the National Institutes of Health–sponsored Digitalis Investigation Group trial, with nearly 8000 patients,[254] digoxin did not appear to be deleterious in those with abnormal systolic function (CHF-S) and might have improved functional status.

### Summary of Treatment of CHF-D

Although 2 million Americans have CHF-D, few have been enrolled in published studies that specifically evaluated the effect of drug therapy on this syndrome. Some authorities recommend that first-line treatment include β-blockers or calcium antagonists.[250,252] However, until recently, β-blockers were contraindicated in patients with CHF. Others recognize that management of symptoms in these patients often requires use of diuretics,[150] but physicians should prescribe diuretics cautiously in this setting. Still others advocate improvement of diastolic dysfunction by inhibition of the renin-angiotensin system with ACE inhibitors, ARBs, and/or aldosterone antagonists, with the aim of reversing of interstitial cardiac fibrosis.[255] The Seventh Report of the Joint National Committee on Prevention, Detection, Evaluation, and Treatment of High Blood Pressure (JNC 7) recommends ACE inhibitors, β-blockers, ARBs, and aldosterone blockers along with diuretics for patients with symptomatic CHF with either systolic or diastolic ventricular dysfunction. Evaluation for ischemic heart disease is also recommended in these patients.[256]

## Effect of Antihypertensive Treatment on Asymptomatic Diastolic Dysfunction

The effect of antihypertensive treatment on noninvasively derived LV filling abnormalities in asymptomatic subjects has been studied with a variety of agents. No study has reported conversion from asymptomatic to symptomatic status with treatment. Thus, analysis of therapy relies on serial measurements of noninvasively derived measures of LV filling. These studies are difficult to evaluate without data on filling pressures, which are rarely provided. For example, one 8-week study comparing verapamil with lisinopril suggested that verapamil was superior because treatment resulted in shorter time to peak LV filling, reduced isovolumetric relaxation time, and greater first-half filling. In that study, lisinopril prolonged resting isovolumetric relaxation time.[257] An equally compelling alternative explanation is that the effect of verapamil was a result of increased filling pressures[228] and the effect lisinopril was due to decreased filling pressures.

### Calcium Channel Blockers in the Treatment of Asymptomatic Diastolic Dysfunction

Many studies suggest that the CCBs verapamil and dihydropyridine improve diastolic function.[164,167,169,257-259] Some of these salubrious effects are likely pharmacologic, but some studies also suggest that improved filling is dependent on coincident LV mass regression.[164,167,169] Studies with diltiazem showed no significant benefit, but these were flawed by short duration of treatment[149] or by inclusion of patients whose LV diastolic function was nearly normal at baseline.[260]

### β-Blockers in the Treatment of Asymptomatic Diastolic Dysfunction

β-Blockers are routinely advocated as first-line agents in treatment of CHF-D.[250,261] However, the effects of β-blocker therapy on diastolic function have been variable. Some studies show improved filling (in association with, but possibly independent of, LV mass regression).[164-166] Two studies, including one in elderly hypertensive patients, failed to demonstrate LV mass regression or improvement in diastolic function.[167,262] Because β-blockade antagonizes catecholamine-mediated LV relaxation, it has been suggested that β-blockers can improve diastolic function only if accompanied by BP reduction, relief of ischemia, and prolongation of the time for LV filling.[150,262]

### ACE Inhibitors in the Treatment of Asymptomatic Diastolic Dysfunction

Studies of the effects of ACE inhibitors on asymptomatic diastolic function in hypertensive patients have revealed variable effects. Because Ang II has a direct negative effect on myocardial relaxation,[264] inhibition of Ang II would be expected to improve LV filling. In one study in which captopril induced significant LV mass regression, Doppler indices of LV filling did not change.[170] However, LV filling was normal at baseline; thus, LV filling would not be expected to improve. Both lisinopril[265] and enalapril have been shown to improve Doppler or M-mode derived indices of diastolic function.[266]

## CORONARY MICROCIRCULATION ABNORMALITIES IN THE PATIENT WITH HYPERTENSION

In hypertensive patients with LVH, structural and functional alterations in the small coronary vessels, increasing ventricular wall stress and alterations in the rheologic properties of blood (e.g., increased viscosity) inhibit the ability of the coronary microcirculation to regulate overall coronary blood flow.[267] These abnormalities result in diminished coronary flow reserve, the increase in total coronary blood flow that occurs with maximal vasodilation (Figure 24–12). A better (though less frequently used) term may be *myocardial perfusion reserve*, because this reflects the total circulation of the myocardium rather than just the epicardial coronary arteries. Abnormal coronary flow reserve may predispose the hypertensive patient to ischemic syndromes, which lead to CHF, MI, and sudden death.

## Coronary Vessel Pathology in Left Ventricular Hypertrophy

Various vascular abnormalities result in a reduction in the total maximal cross-sectional area of the coronary microvasculature. These include inadequate vascular growth in response to increasing muscle mass, changes in vessel wall composition, vascular remodeling, and vascular endothelial dysfunction.

### Rarefaction of Arterioles

Morphometric studies in various animal models suggest that inadequate growth of the coronary microvascular bed is one factor limiting myocardial perfusion in the presence of pressure-overload myocardial hypertrophy.[268-275] The capacity for coronary angiogenesis decreases over time. Between the ages of 9 to 14 years, heart weight increases fourfold, while capillary density decreases by 28%. Capillary density in the hypertrophied heart is also age dependent. Adults with acquired aortic stenosis have decreased capillary density, whereas children with congenital aortic stenosis maintain capillary density by increasing capillary supply in proportion to myocyte volume.[273,276,277] As hypertrophy progresses in the adult with hypertension, there is insufficient angiogenesis to compensate for the increasing myocardial mass.

Defective angiogenesis may be a mechanism in the inheritance of hypertension. Higher vascular resistance and lower

capillary density (in the dorsum of the finger) were demonstrated in mildly hypertensive young men with hypertensive parents but not in mildly hypertensive men without hypertensive parents.[278] The mechanisms of angiogenesis are complex. Factors released with increased vascular wall tension that influence cell to cell interactions, extracellular matrix molecules, and the inhibition and stimulation of endothelial growth factors may be important.[279,280] Vascular endothelial growth factor (VEGF) is one such factor that has received much attention in the developing field of cardiac molecular therapy. VEGF promotes the sprouting of new vessels via its effects on angiopoietin. ACE inhibition has in part been thought to promote angiogenesis and thus augment coronary flow reserve by up-regulation of VEGF, as well as other related factors.[281] Another factor, hepatocyte growth factor (HGF), is a mesenchyme-derived pleiotropic factor that regulates cell growth, cell motility, and morphogenesis of vascular tissue (among other types of cells). Myocardial HGF concentrations are low in SHR and are inversely proportional to LV weight. Concentrations of cardiac and vascular Ang II, a suppressor of HGF, are increased in SHR. In addition, administration of an ACE inhibitor or an ARB results in a significant increase in cardiac HGF concentration.[282]

### Medial Wall Thickening

Pressure overload with coronary arterial hypertension causes vascular medial hypertrophy with decreased lumen diameter and increased ratio of media thickness to lumen diameter (media:lumen ratio).[283-285] Comparisons of coronary vascular morphology and coronary resistance in normotensive Wistar-Kyoto (WKY) and SHR showed a nearly twofold increase in medial thickness in the coronary arterioles of the hypertensive rats.[267] There was also a significantly increased ratio of medial thickness to vessel radius and increased minimal coronary resistance in the hypertensive

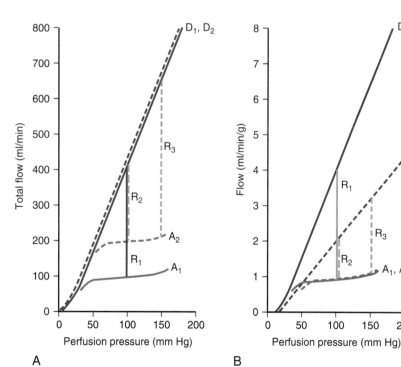

**Figure 24–12** Diagram of coronary flow reserve in the presence of hypertrophy. In panel **A,** absolute flow is measured (ml/min). In panel **B,** flow per unit mass (ml/min/g) is measured. A, autoregulated flows; D, pressure flow line during maximal vasodilation; R, flow reserve. Normal are A1, D1, R1, and solid lines. Hypertrophied are A2, D2, R2, R3, and *dashed lines*. In both scenarios, coronary flow reserve is diminished. R3 represents coronary flow reserve when perfusion pressures are elevated. (Reproduced with permission from Hoffman JI. A critical view of coronary reserve. Circulation 75:16-11, 1987.)

A                                    B

animals. The cellular basis for this increase in medial thickness is predominantly rearrangement of smooth muscle cells within the medial layers of the arterial wall, not increases in individual myocyte cell size.[286] The factors responsible for this rearrangement are slowly becoming understood.

Endothelin plays a significant role, because blockade of endothelin subtype A ($ET_A$) receptors inhibits hypertrophic vascular remodeling in salt-sensitive forms of hypertension.[287] This factor, as well as other agents important for control of smooth muscle cell hypertrophy and proliferation (endothelial growth factor [EGF], platelet-derived growth factor [PDGF], Ang II, mechanical stretch, and fluid shear stress), induce a series of cellular kinase cascades, known collectively as the mitogen-activated protein (MAP) kinase cascades, which have been implicated in vascular smooth muscle cell proliferation and hypertrophy.[288] These kinases lead to activation of the protooncogenes c-*fos* and c-*jun*, which are components of the nuclear transcription factor AP-1. Activation of this transcription factor results in increased gene expression for processes that initiate vascular growth and hypertrophy[289] (see Figure 24–2). The magnitude of vascular structural alteration, however, may be independent of the extent of endothelial dysfunction in hypertension.[290]

### Perivascular and Interstitial Fibrosis

In addition to medial hypertrophy, pressure-overloaded cardiac hypertrophy with hypertension causes increased vascular and perivascular deposition of collagen.[291] Inhibition of collagen deposition in vascular and extravascular myocardial tissue in the Wistar rat shows that coronary flow reserve is mainly determined by medial thickening, independent of collagen deposition. Nevertheless, collagen deposition does affect coronary blood flow, since there is more reversal of coronary flow abnormalities after removing the pressure load on the heart (aortic banding) in the rats with less collagen deposition.[291]

### Increased Vascular Water Content

A 10% to 15% increase in the water content of arterial walls occurs in hypertensive patients. A high concentration of vascular water produces thickening of the vascular walls (even in the absence of hypertrophy) and may also cause a reduction in coronary flow reserve.[267]

### Endothelial Dysfunction

In the heart and systemic vessels, nitric oxide (NO) appears to reverse smooth muscle cell hypertrophy and hyperplasia.[292] Thus, expression of NO in hypertension may help protect from target end-organ damage. Impairment of endothelial function is an early vascular abnormality resulting in abnormal myocardial blood flow in patients with coronary artery disease, angina pectoris with normal coronary arteriograms, and hypertension with LVH. Although hypertensive patients have appropriate responses to the endothelial-independent vasodilators, most studies demonstrate a blunted response to acetylcholine-stimulated endothelial-dependent vasodilation.[293-297] Imbalance between endothelial-mediated vasodilation and vasoconstriction may be an early lesion in hypertension. In SHR, impaired endothelial-dependent relaxation occurs before the development of overt hypertension.[298]

Attention has focused on substance P and bradykinin, native peptides of the coronary endothelium that are extremely potent in triggering endothelium-dependent dilation of small coronary arteries. They contribute to the resting level of coronary blood flow and partially mediate flow-dependent dilation in response to increased myocardial demand.[299,300] A cytochrome P450 product, not NO, may regulate production of these vasodilators.[300]

## Myocardial Hypertrophy and Wall Stress

Increased wall stress (one factor initiating the development of LVH in hypertensive patients) may directly modulate coronary flow reserve by causing physical compression of blood vessels. Elevated wall stress may stimulate the release of vasoactive substances that alter vascular function and growth.[267] Patients with nonhypertensive LVH, without ventricular dilation and increased wall tension (i.e., some cases of aortic stenosis, hypertrophic obstructive and hypertrophic nonobstructive cardiomyopathy with no ventricular dilation) do not have decreased coronary flow reserve. Those with hypertension with similar degrees of LVH, or aortic stenosis with ventricular dilation and increased LV end-diastolic pressures, however, show abnormally decreased flow reserve.[301,302] This effect is also seen in patients with dilated cardiomyopathy[303] and dilated ventricles due to aortic regurgitation.[304,305]

## Alterations of Coronary Autoregulation and Flow Reserve with Left Ventricular Hypertrophy

The coronary circulation is able to maintain a relatively stable blood supply over a wide range of perfusion pressures.[306-309] This range varies in different experiments but is generally between 70 and 130 mm Hg in humans.[310] Coronary flow decreases markedly when perfusion pressure drops below the lower limit of autoregulation.

### Proposed Mechanisms of Autoregulation

Both metabolic and myogenic mechanisms may produce autoregulation of coronary flow. Different sites in the microvasculature may have different dominant mechanisms of control.[311] The smallest coronary arterioles are predominantly sensitive to metabolic factors, whereas larger arterioles are more reactive to myogenic stimuli. According to the metabolic theory, a decrease in coronary artery perfusion pressure results in decreased blood flow. Subsequent decreases in myocardial substrate availability, or increases in production of metabolites, produce vasodilation.[312] Potential mediators include oxygen (myocardial oxygen tension), $K^+$ and $Ca^{2+}$ ion concentrations (transmembrane potentials), osmolality, adenosine, prostaglandins, and carbon dioxide ($CO_2$) and $H^+$ concentrations.[313-315] The endogenous vasodilator NO has been shown to inhibit coronary autoregulation.[316]

Myogenic regulation is an intrinsic mechanism: Application of force to vascular smooth muscle results in contraction.[317-319] In the coronary circulation, there are difficulties in demonstrating myogenic responses, because these are closely integrated with metabolic factors.[320] These mechanisms result in both microvascular dilation and increased recruitment of arterioles,[321] thus resulting in changes in intramyocardial blood volume. Myocardial contrast echocardiography can quantify autoregulatory increases in intramyocardial blood volume, and thus may provide a noninvasive method for studying coronary autoregulation.[322]

### Relationship Between Autoregulated Coronary Flow and Maximal Coronary Flow

Coronary flow reserve is, for any given perfusion pressure, the decrease in coronary resistance over the resting state that occurs after maximal coronary vasodilation. A normal human heart can increase coronary flow by a factor of 4 to 5 times over the resting state.[301] Coronary flow increases above resting autoregulated levels after transient coronary arterial occlusion (reactive hyperemia), exercise, pacing, or injection of agents such as dipyridamole, adenosine, papaverine, or hyperosmolar iodinated contrast media.[323] Loss of autoregulation occurs during these events. Coronary flow reserve is a dynamic value that is dependent on coronary perfusion pressure. Because there is no autoregulation during states that produce maximal coronary flow, the relationship between coronary flow and coronary perfusion pressure is linear. Relatively small changes in perfusion pressure produce large changes in coronary flow reserve.

## Factors that Confound the Measurement of Coronary Flow Reserve

Increased heart rate, contractility, and afterload all decrease coronary flow reserve and therefore confound its measurement. It is not clear if these factors increase baseline flow, decrease maximal flow, or both.[324,325] In humans, Doppler measurements of coronary blood flow during pacemaker-induced tachycardia show increases in resting flow velocity, but not in peak velocity with papaverine administration.[325] The use of potent vasodilators to quantify coronary flow reserve may result in a blunted measurement if there is any significant increase in heart rate. Body size may also influence absolute values of maximal coronary blood flow.[326]

Elevations in aortic pressure increase myocardial oxygen consumption and blood flow. Consequently, shifts in mean aortic pressure produce alterations in autoregulated (resting) blood flow. By using the relationship between mean aortic pressure, coronary flow reserve, and coronary vascular resistance (coronary flow = mean aortic pressure/coronary resistance), one may calculate a coronary resistance ratio.[327] The resistance ratio may be less sensitive than a flow ratio to changes in arterial pressure.[323]

In addition to external confounding factors, there are intrinsic factors in the definition and measurement of coronary flow reserve that produce confusion. Coronary flow reserve can be measured as either the difference of maximal and resting flow (absolute coronary flow reserve) or the ratio of maximal flow to resting flow (relative coronary flow reserve). It is not clear which measurement is clinically more relevant. In hypertensive patients with LVH, it is possible to have a normal or mildly increased absolute coronary flow reserve with a reduced relative coronary flow reserve.[323]

Many current methods of measuring coronary flow reserve are not sensitive to changes in coronary flow reserve over different layers of myocardium. Coronary flow reserve is lower in subendocardial muscle for all perfusion pressures. Some of the newer noninvasive techniques such as cine-CT and nuclear magnetic resonance may be able to measure coronary flow reserve in the different layers of myocardium, but data are still very preliminary.

## Effect of Hypertension and Left Ventricular Hypertrophy on Coronary Flow Reserve

Coronary flow reserve can be measured as absolute flow (ml/min) or flow per unit muscle mass (ml/min/g) (see Figure 24–12).[310] Although resting absolute coronary blood flow in the entire LV increases with LVH, resting coronary blood flow per gram of myocardium is unchanged. Total maximal ventricular flow does not significantly change with acquired LVH, whereas total flow per gram of myocardium decreases. This is due to the lack of vascular growth in response to increasing muscle mass. Thus, when absolute flow is measured, resting flow is high and maximal flow is normal (see Figure 24–12, A). If flow per gram is measured, resting flow per gram myocardium is normal but maximal flow per gram myocardium is reduced (see Figure 24–12, B). Consequently, coronary flow reserve is less than normal whether measured as absolute flow (ml/min) or flow per gram (ml/min/gm) of myocardium.

In the presence of hypertension, absolute coronary flow reserve may theoretically be normal or increased, despite higher resting absolute coronary blood flow. This is due to the higher coronary perfusion pressure (shift to the right side of the curve), as shown by R3 in Figure 24–12, A. Nevertheless, in most cases of hypertensive heart disease, vascular abnormalities and increased LV end-diastolic pressure result in reduced maximal flow and thus a decrease in coronary flow reserve.[302,328-330] Most,[304,329,331] but not all[332,333] studies show an inverse linear relationship between the extent of LVH and vascular endothelial function as noted by either forearm blood flow or coronary flow reserve (Figure 24–13).

Other factors (e.g., race, gender, diabetes, cigarette smoking, and prior therapies) also influence coronary flow reserve.[334-338] Evaluation of endothelial-dependent dilation of the brachial artery has shown that reduced flow-mediated dilation is related to age. Noticeable decline begins in men after age 40 years but is preserved in women until their 50s.[339] This delay in women may be due to protective effects of estrogen, because their decline appears to correlate with the onset of menopause. Estrogen treatment of postmenopausal women improves endothelial-dependent vasodilation.[340] This may be a direct effect of estrogen on vascular function or an indirect effect through altered lipid metabolism, because increased high-density lipoprotein appears to improve NO bioavailability.[341] Tamoxifen acts as a selective estrogen receptor modulator (SERM) in women and has estrogen-like activities on some cardiovascular risk factors (e.g., lipids). In one study, tamoxifen was shown to augment endothelium-dependent forearm flow-mediated vasodilation in men with coronary artery disease.[342] In a study of the coronary circulation, age and total serum cholesterol were found to be independent predictors of a blunted vasodilator response to acetylcholine.[342] Analysis of SHR and normotensive rats showed that hypertension and aging independently result in structural alterations in coronary resistance vasculature, with a decrease in the ratio of lumen diameter to wall thickness. Aging did not decrease arteriolar density.[344] Racial differences were demonstrated in a study showing that Blacks have decreased coronary flow reserve compared with whites, independent of LVH.[334]

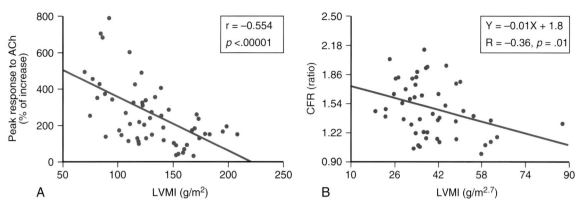

**Figure 24-13** Inverse relationship between LV mass and vascular endothelial function. **(A),** increase in left ventricular mass index (LVMI) is associated with a decrease in the increase in forearm blood flow in response to acetylcholine (ACh) infusion. **(B),** the same relationship is shown when comparing LVMI with coronary flow reserve (CFR) as determined by "split-dose" Tl-201 single photon emission tomography in subjects with moderate to severe hypertension. (Part A from Perticone F, Maio R, Ceravolo R, et al. Relationship between left ventricular mass and endothelium-dependent vasodilation in never-treated hypertensive patients. Circulation 99:1991-1996, 1999. Part B from Diamond JA, Krakoff LR, Goldman A, et al. Comparison of two calcium blockers on hemodynamics, left ventricular mass, and coronary vasodilatory in advanced hypertension. Am J Hypertens 14:231-240, 2001, with permission from the American Journal of Hypertension, Ltd.)

Hypertension may alter coronary flow reserve prior to the development of LVH. This was suggested by a cross-sectional analysis of hypertensive and nonhypertensive patients. Although coronary flow reserve was lowest in untreated hypertensive patients with increased LV mass, patients with hypertension and normal LV mass had lower coronary flow reserve than normotensive patients.[345] This must be viewed with caution, however, because cross-sectional studies do not allow one to analyze other factors that may influence coronary blood flow, such as duration of hypertension and prior antihypertensive therapies. Whether or not linearly related, most studies suggest that LVH is strongly associated with reduced coronary flow reserve. Thus, abnormalities of coronary flow reserve may partially explain why patients with hypertension and LVH are at increased risk for myocardial ischemia and infarction.[3]

## Effect of Blood Pressure Reduction on Autoregulated Blood Flow and Coronary Flow Reserve

Experimental and clinical studies demonstrate that BP reduction in hypertensive patients with LVH may increase myocardial ischemia. Resting absolute coronary flow is high in these patients, and loss of autoregulated flow occurs at higher perfusion pressures (the autoregulatory curve is shifted upward and to the right). In experimentally induced LVH, although marked reductions in coronary perfusion pressure from 100 to 40 mm Hg have minimal effect on autoregulation in the subepicardium, the ability of the subendocardium to autoregulate is reduced by >50%.[346] This may account for the increased size of MI associated with experimentally induced coronary ligation in hypertrophied hearts.[347,348] Recovery of stunned myocardium (systolic thickening and regional myocardial blood flow) in the period immediately following transient coronary occlusion is delayed in the presence of LVH, and even more so when BP is lowered during this early reperfusion period.[349]

BP reduction in hypertensive humans without LVH does not significantly change resting coronary blood flow when perfusion pressure is acutely lowered with nitroprusside from 120 to 70 mm Hg. However, LVH accompanies hypertension, there is a marked decline in flow as perfusion pressure decreases from 90 to 70 mm Hg (Figure 24–14).[350] This suggests that a reduction of BP to <90 mm Hg in patients with LVH could cause ischemia. This observation may in part explain the limited impact of BP reduction on mortality from coronary artery disease compared with nonfatal and fatal stroke in patients with both systolic and diastolic hypertension. Analysis of several large prospective observational studies suggests that a 5– to 6–mm Hg decrease in diastolic blood pressure (DBP) would cause a 20% to 25% reduction in coronary events. However, this degree of reduction in BP has resulted in only a 14% decrease in coronary events.[112,351] This finding was confirmed by the Blood Pressure Lowering Treatment Trialists' Collaboration review of 29 major trials, which assessed major cardiovascular outcomes based on class of antihypertensive medication and degree of BP lowering. Overall, larger reductions in BP resulted in the larger reductions in overall cardiovascular risk. The largest impact of BP reduction was on stroke.[352]

A J-curve may describe the relation between mortality rate from MI and treated DBP.[353] Traditionally the J-curve does not specifically address hypertensive patients with no coronary artery disease. These patients may benefit from decreasing BP as much as possible. However, those with ischemic disease and a treated DBP of <85 to 95 mm Hg may have an upturn in coronary events. This is presumably a result of inadequate pe fusion of coronary arteries. Support for and against this relation is based on differing interpretations and results of retrospective analyses of several large treatment trials or programs.[354-358] For example, in one retrospective analysis, men with LVH or ischemic patterns on ECG had an increased incidence of MI when treated DBPs were below 95 mm Hg.[359] By contrast, in the Systolic Hypertension in the Elderly Program (SHEP) trial, coronary events were decreased in patients with

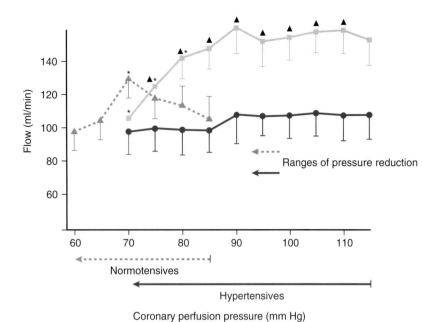

**Figure 24-14** Effect of acute reduction in coronary perfusion pressure on coronary autoregulation in controls with normotension, patients with hypertension without left ventricular hypertrophy (LVH), and patients with hypertension and LVH. The autoregulatory curve for hypertension with LVH is shifted upward and to the right. At coronary perfusion pressure <90 mm Hg, patients with hypertension and LVH have marked loss of coronary autoregulation. (Reproduced with permission from Polese A, DeCesare N, Montorsi P, et al. Upward shift of the lower range of coronary flow autoregulation in hypertensive patients with hypertrophy of the left ventricle. Circulation 83:845-853, 1991.)

evidence of LVH by ECG criteria and low treatment DBP.[360] Although this may argue against a J-curve, it is important to realize that these patients had low DBPs prior to treatment, and hence their autoregulatory curve was already adjusted to lower pressure. Systolic hypertension in older patients with decreased arterial compliance (increased stiffness) is associated with higher cardiac morbidity and mortality and may explain the association of increased cardiac death in patients with low DBP or increased pulse pressure[361-363] (see Chapters 15 and 22).

Recommendations for the safest level of BP reduction in patients with LVH can be only speculative at this point. In patients with isolated systolic hypertension, in whom the pretreatment DBP is already low, SHEP trial data indicate that further reduction to a DBP of 65 mm Hg is safe.[364] JNC recommends lowering BP to <130/80 mm Hg in patients with target organ damage, including chronic kidney disease and diabetes, but this is not based on a wealth of data.[256,365]

## Effect of Antihypertensive Treatment on Coronary Flow Reserve

### ACE Inhibitors and Angiotensin Receptor Blockers in the Treatment of Coronary Flow Reserve

Few human studies have examined the effects of antihypertensive therapy on coronary flow reserve. Data using the gas chromatographic argon method of quantifying coronary flow reserve showed improvement in hypertensive patients after 12 months of therapy with enalapril.[366] By blocking the production of Ang II, ACE inhibitors may be effective in improving coronary flow reserve. This may be due to reduction in perivascular and interstitial fibrosis.[367] Akinboboye et al. used [15]O-water positron emission tomography (PET) to quantify myocardial perfusion reserve in a small population (n = 17) of predominantly African Americans with hypertension. This study demonstrated improved myocardial perfusion reserve after treatment with lisinopril for a mean of 11 months,[368] but no significant change in myocardial flow reserve after treat-

ment with losartan. Using a modification of traditional Tl-201 myocardial perfusion imaging for quantification of myocardial perfusion reserve, Diamond et al. showed modest improvement after 6 months of antihypertensive treatment with the ARB eprosartan.[369] However, there was no significant change in myocardial perfusion reserve with the ACE inhibitor enalapril. This may have been due to the short follow-up period in the study.

### Calcium Channel Blockers in the Treatment of Coronary Flow Reserve

The effect of CCBs on coronary flow reserve is even less clear. Although they produce favorable hemodynamic effects, with reversal of pressure-overload and regression of LVH, several studies suggest that certain CCBs do not significantly change or may even reduce coronary flow reserve. Theoretically, CCBs may reduce coronary flow reserve by blocking the effect of endogenous vasodilators such as adenosine.[370]

### β-Blockers in the Treatment of Coronary Flow Reserve

Using PET quantification of myocardial perfusion, β-blockers have been shown to augment coronary flow reserve in healthy volunteers. Billinger et al. showed in patients with coronary artery disease that postischemic coronary flow reserve (hyperemic flow) is significantly augmented in patients taking the β-blocker metoprolol.[371] By augmenting coronary flow reserve, oxygen supply to the heart is enhanced. This may in part explain the benefit of β-blockers in patients with coronary artery disease.

## References

1. Levy D, Anderson KM, Savage D, et al. Echocardiographically detected left ventricular hypertrophy: Prevalence and risk factors. The Framingham Heart Study. Ann Intern Med 108:7-13, 1988.

2. Casale PN, Devereux RB, Milner M, et al. Value of echocardiographic measurement of left ventricular mass in predicting cardiovascular morbid events in hypertensive men. Ann Intern Med 105:173-178, 1986.

3. Levy D, Garrison RJ, Savage DD, et al. Prognostic implications of echocardiographically determined left ventricular mass in the Framingham Heart Study. N Engl J Med 322:1561-1566, 1990.

4. Bikkina M, Larson MG, Levy D. Asymptomatic ventricular arrhythmias and mortality risk in subjects with left ventricular hypertrophy. J Am Coll Cardiol 22:1111-1116, 1993.

5. Cooper RS, Simmons BE, Castaner A, et al. Left ventricular hypertrophy is associated with worse survival independent of ventricular function and number of coronary arteries severely narrowed. Am J Cardiol 65:441-445, 1990.

6. Ghali JK, Liao Y, Simmons B, et al. The prognostic role of left ventricular hypertrophy in patients with or without coronary artery disease. Ann Intern Med 117:831-836, 1992.

7. Deschepper CF, Boutin-Ganache I, Zahabi A, et al. In search of cardiovascular candidate genes: Interactions between phenotypes and genotypes. Hypertension 39:332-336, 2002.

8. Himmelmann A, Svensson A, Hansson L. Blood pressure and left ventricular mass in children with different maternal histories of hypertension: The Hypertension in Pregnancy Offspring Study. J Hypertens 11:263-268, 1993.

9. van Hooft IMS, Grobbee DE, Waal-Manning HJ, et al. Hemodynamic characteristics of the early phase of primary hypertension: The Dutch Hypertension and Offspring study. Circulation 87:1100-1106, 1993.

10. Post WS, Larson MG, Myers RH, et al. Heritability of left ventricular mass: The Framingham Heart Study. Hypertension 30:1025-1028, 1997.

11. Adams TD, Yanowitz FG, Fisher AG, et al. Heritability of cardiac size: An echocardiographic and electrocardiographic study of monozygotic and dizygotic twins. Circulation 71:39-44, 1985.

12. Beaglehole R, Tyroler HA, Cassel JC, et al. An epidemiological study of left ventricular hypertrophy in the biracial population of Evans County, Georgia. J Chronic Dis 28:549-559, 1974.

13. Dunn FG, Oigman W, Sungard-Rise K, et al. Racial differences in cardiac adaptation to essential hypertension determined by echocardiographic indexes. J Am Coll Cardiol 5:1348-1351, 1983.

14. Hammond IW, Alderman MH, Devereux RB, et al. Contrast in cardiac anatomy and function between black and white patients with hypertension. J Natl Med Assoc 76:247-255, 1984.

15. Liebson PR, Grandits G, Prineas R, et al. Echocardiographic correlates of left ventricular structure among 844 mildly hypertensive men and women in the treatment of mild hypertension study (TOMHS). Circulation 87:476-486, 1993.

16. Mayet J, Shahi M, Foale RA, et al. Racial differences in cardiac structure and function in essential hypertension. BMJ 308:1011-1014, 1994.

17. Hinderliter AL, Light KC, Willis PW. Racial differences in left ventricular structure in healthy young adults. Am J Cardiol 69:1196-1199, 1992.

18. Harshfield GA, Alpert BS, Willey ES, et al. Race and gender influence ambulatory blood pressure patterns of adolescents. Hypertension 14:598-603, 1989.

19. Schunkert H, Hense H-W, Holmer SR, et al. Association between a deletion polymorphism of the angiotensin converting-enzyme gene and left ventricular hypertrophy. N Engl J Med 330:1634-1638, 1994.

20. Lindpaintner K, Lee M, Larson MG, et al. Absence of association or genetic linkage between the angiotensin-converting-enzyme gene and left ventricular mass [see comments]. N Engl J Med 334:1023-1028, 1996.

21. Perticone F, Ceravolo R, Cosco C, P et al. Deletion polymorphism of angiotensin-converting enzyme gene and left ventricular hypertrophy in southern Italian patients. J Am Coll Cardiol 29:365-369, 1997.

22. Gharavi AG, Lipkowitz MS, Diamond JA, et al. Deletion Polymorphism of the angiotensin-converting enzyme gene is independently associated with left ventricular mass and geometric remodeling in systemic hypertension. Am J Cardiol 77:1315-1319, 1996.

23. Kupari M, Hautanen A, Lankinen L, et al. Associations between human aldosterone synthase (CYP11B2) gene polymorphisms and left ventricular size, mass, and function. Circulation 97(6):569-575, 1998.

24. Stella P, Bigatti G, Tizzoni L, et al. Association between aldosterone synthase (CYP11B2) polymorphism and left ventricular mass in human essential hypertension. J Am Coll Cardiol 43:265-270, 2004.

25. Lifton RP, Gharavi AG, Geller DS. Molecular mechanisms of human hypertension. Cell 104:545-556, 2001.

26. Glueck SB, Dzau VJ. Physiological genomics: Implications in hypertension research. Hypertension 39:310-315, 2002.

27. Kimura B, Mohuczy D, Tang X, Phillips MI. Attenuation of hypertension and heart hypertrophy by adeno-associated virus delivering angiotensinogen antisense. Hypertension 37:376-380, 2001.

28. Nakayama T, Soma M, Takahashi Y, et al. Functional deletion mutation of the 5'-flanking region of type A human natriuretic peptide receptor gene and its association with essential hypertension and left ventricular hypertrophy in the Japanese. Circ Res 86:841-845, 2000.

29. Poch E, Gonzalez D, Gomez-Angelats E, et al. G- Protein beta(3) subunit gene variant and left ventricular hypertrophy in essential hypertension. Hypertension 35(1 Pt 2):214-218, 2000.

30. Sedlacek K, Fischer M, Erdmann J, S et al. Relation of the G protein beta3-subunit polymorphism with left ventricle structure and function. Hypertension 40:162-167, 2002.

31. Arnett DK, Devereux RB, Kitzman D, et al. Linkage of left ventricular contractility to chromosome 11 in humans: The HyperGEN Study. Hypertension 38:767-772, 2001.

32. Akhter SA, Milano CA, Shotwell KF, et al. Transgenic mice with cardiac overexpression of alpha1B-adrenergic receptors. In vivo alpha1-adrenergic receptor-mediated regulation of beta-adrenergic signaling. J Biol Chem 272:21253- 21259, 1997.

33. Choi DJ, Koch WJ, Hunter JJ, et al. Mechanism of beta-adrenergic receptor desensitization in cardiac hypertrophy is increased beta-adrenergic receptor kinase. J Biol Chem 272(27):17223-17229, 1997.

34. Chanutin A, Barksdale EE. Experimental renal insufficiency produced by partial nephrectomy. II. Relationship of left ventricular hypertrophy, the width of the cardiac muscle fiber and hypertension in the rat. Arch Intern Med 52:739-744, 1933.

35. Grossman W, Jones D, McLaurin LP. Wall stress and patterns of hypertrophy in the human left ventricle. J Clin Invest 56:56-64, 1975.

36. Badeer HS. Biological significance of cardiac hypertrophy. Am J Cardiol 14:133-137, 1964.

37. Lauer MS, Anderson KM, Levy D. Influence of contemporary versus 30-year blood pressure levels on left ventricular mass and geometry: The Framingham Heart Study. J Am Coll Cardiol 18:1287-1294, 1991.

38. Rowlands DB, Glover DR, Ireland MA, et al. Assessment of left-ventricular mass and its response to antihypertensive treatment. Lancet 1:467-470, 1982.

39. Devereux RB, Pickering TG, Harshfield GA. Left ventricular hypertrophy in patients with hypertension: Importance of blood pressure response to regular recurring stress. Circulation 68:470-476, 1983.

40. Phillips RA, Goldman ME, Ardeljan M, et al. Determinants of abnormal left ventricular filling in early hypertension. J Am Coll Cardiol 14:979-985, 1989.

41. Guerrier M, Schillaci G, Verdecchia P, et al. Circadian blood pressure changes and left ventricular hypertrophy in essential hypertension. Circulation 81:528-536, 1990.

42. Stanford JL, Weiss NS, Voigt LF, et al. Combined estrogen and progestin hormone replacement therapy in relation to risk of breast cancer in middle-aged women. JAMA 274:137-142, 1995.

43. Cavallini MC, Roman MJ, Pickering TG, et al. Is white coat hypertension associated with arterial disease or left ventricular hypertrophy? Hypertension 26:413-419, 1995.

44. Perloff D, Sokolow M, Cowan R. The prognostic value of ambulatory blood pressures. JAMA 249:2792-2798, 1983.

45. Hoegholm A, Kristensen KS, Bang LE, et al. Left ventricular mass and geometry in patients with established hypertension and white coat hypertension. Am J Hypertens 6:282-286, 1993.

46. White WB, Schulman P, McCabe EJ, et al. Average daily blood pressure, not office blood pressure determines cardiac function in patients with hypertension. JAMA 261:873-877, 1989.

47. Ganau A, Devereux RB, Pickering TG, et al. Relation of left ventricular hemodynamic load and contractile performance to left ventricular mass in hypertension. Circulation 81:25-36, 1990.

48. Saba PS, Roman MJ, Pini R, et al. Relation of carotid pressure waveform to left ventricular anatomy in normotensive subjects. J Am Coll Cardiol 22:1873-1880, 1993.

49. Morgan HE, Baker KM. Cardiac hypertrophy. Mechanical, neural and endocrine dependence. Circulation 83:13-25, 1991.

50. Schunkert H, Jahn L, Izumo S, et al. Localization and regulation of c-fos and c-jun protooncogene induction by systolic wall stress in normal and hypertrophied rat hearts. Proc Natl Acad Sci USA 88:11480-11484, 1991.

51. Molkentin JD, Lu JR, Antos CL, et al. A calcineurin-dependent transcriptional pathway for cardiac hypertrophy. Cell 93:215-228, 1998.

52. Hsueh WA, Law RE, Do YS. Integrins, adhesion, and cardiac remodeling. Hypertension 1998; 31(1 Pt 2):176-180.

53. Sussman MA, Lim HW, Gude N, et al. Prevention of cardiac hypertrophy in mice by calcineurin inhibition. Science 281:1690-1693, 1998.

54. Nagata K, Somura F, Obata K, et al. AT1 receptor blockade reduces cardiac calcineurin activity in hypertensive rats. Hypertension 40:168-174, 2002.

55. Levy D, Larson MG, Vasan RS, et al. The progression from hypertension to congestive heart failure [see comments]. JAMA 1996; 275:1557-1562.

56. Senni M, Tribouilloy CM, Rodeheffer RJ, et al. Congestive heart failure in the community: A study of all incident cases in Olmsted County, Minnesota, in 1991. Circulation 98:2282-2289, 1998.

57. Kostis JB, Davis BR, Cutler J, et al. Prevention of heart failure by antihypertensive drug treatment in older persons with isolated systolic hypertension. JAMA 278:212-216, 1997.

58. Moser M, Hebert PR. Prevention of disease progression, left ventricular hypertrophy and congestive heart failure in hypertension treatment trials. J Am Coll Cardiol 27:1214-1218, 1996.

59. De Simone G, Devereux RB, Daniels SR, et al. Gender differences in left ventricular growth. Hypertension 26(6 Pt 1):979-983, 1995.

60. Savage DD, Drayer JIM, Henry WL, et al. Echocardiographic assessment of cardiac anatomy and function in hypertensive patients. Circulation 1979; 59:623-632.

61. Gerstenblith G, Frederiksen J, Yin FCP, et al. Echocardiographic assessment of a normal adult aging population. Circulation 56:273-278, 1977.

62. Levy D, Garrison RJ, Savage DD, et al. Left ventricular mass and incidence of coronary heart disease in an elderly cohort: The Framingham Heart Study. Ann Intern Med 110:101-107, 1989.

63. Shub C, Klein AL, Zachariah PK, et al. Determination of left ventricular mass by echocardiography in a normal population: Effect of age and sex in addition to body size. Mayo Clin Proc 69:205-211, 1994.

64. De Simone G, Devereux RB, Roman MJ, et al. Gender differences in left ventricular anatomy, blood viscosity and volume regulatory hormones in normal adults. Am J Cardiol 68:1704-1708, 1991.

65. Hinderliter AL, Light KC, Park WW 4th. Gender differences in left ventricular structure and function in young adults with normal or marginally elevated blood pressure. Am J Hypertens 5:33-36, 1992.

66. Eison H, Phillips RA, Ardeljan M, et al. Differences in ambulatory blood pressure between men and women with mild hypertension. J Hum Hypertens 4:400-404, 1990.

67. Diamond JA, Krakoff LR, Martin K, et al. Comparison of ambulatory blood pressure and amounts of left ventricular hypertrophy in men versus women with similar levels of hypertensive clinic blood pressures. Am J Cardiol 79:505-508, 1997.

68. Verdecchia P, Porcellati C, Schillaci G, et al. Ambulatory blood pressure: An independent predictor of prognosis in essential hypertension. Hypertension 24:793-801, 1994.

69. Devereux RB, Lutas EM, Casale PN, et al. Standardization of M-mode echocardiographic left ventricular anatomic measurements. J Am Coll Cardiol 4:1222-1230, 1984.

70. Marcus R, Krause L, Weder AB, et al. Sex-specific determinants of increased left ventricular mass in the Tecumseh blood pressure study. Circulation 90:928-936, 1994.

71. De Simone G, Devereux RB, Roman MJ, et al. Relation of obesity and gender to left ventricular hypertrophy in normotensive and hypertensive adults. Hypertension 23:600-606, 1994.

72. Liao Y, Cooper RS, Mensah GA, et al. Left ventricular hypertrophy has a greater impact on survival in women than in men. Circulation 92:805-810, 1995.

73. Lauer MS, Anderson KM, Levy D. Separate and joint influences of obesity and mild hypertension on left ventricular mass and geometry: The Framingham Heart Study. J Am Coll Cardiol 19:130-134, 1992.

74. MacMahon SW, Wilcken DEL, MacDonald GJ. The effect of weight reduction on left ventricular mass. N Engl J Med 314:334-339, 1986.

75. Marban E, Koretsune Y. Cell calcium, oncogenes, and hypertrophy. Hypertension 15:652-658, 1990.

76. Dubus I. Origin and mechanisms of heart failure in hypertensive patients: Left ventricular remodelling in hypertensives heart disease. Eur Heart J 14(Suppl J):76-81, 1993.

77. Sen S, Tarazi RC, Khairallah PA, et al. Cardiac hypertrophy in spontaneously hypertensive rats. Circ Res 35:775-781, 1974.

78. Bauwens FR, Duprez DA, De Buyzere ML, et al. Influence of the arterial blood pressure and nonhemodynamic factors on left ventricular hypertrophy in moderate essential hypertension. Am J Cardiol 68:925-929, 1991.

79. Devereux RB, Pickering TG, Cody RJ, et al. Relation of renin-angiotensin system activity to left ventricular hypertrophy and function in experimental and human hypertension. J Clin Hypertens 3:87-103, 1987.

80. Sadoshima J, Xu Y, Slayter HS, et al. Autocrine release of angiotensin II mediates stretch-induced hypertrophy of cardiac myocytes in vitro. Cell 75:977-984, 1993.

81. Harada K, Komuro I, Shiojima I, et al. Pressure overload induces cardiac hypertrophy in angiotensin II type 1A receptor knockout mice [see comments]. Circulation 97:1952-1959, 1998.

82. Weber KT, Brilla CG. Pathological hypertrophy and cardiac interstitium. Fibrosis and renin-angiotensin-aldosterone system Pathological hypertrophy and cardiac interstitium. Fibrosis and renin-angiotensin-aldosterone system. Circulation 83:1849-1865, 1991.

83. Alderman MH, Madhavan S, Ooi WL, et al. Association of the renin-sodium profile with the risk of myocardial infarction in patients with hypertension. N Engl J Med 324:1098-1104, 1991.

84. Laks MM, Morady F, Swan HJC. Myocardial hypertrophy produced by chronic infusion of subhypertensive doses of norepinephrine in the dog. Chest 64:75-78, 1973.

85. Trimarco B, Ricciardelli B, De Luca N, et al. Participation of endogenous catecholamines in the regulation of left ventricular mass in progeny of hypertensive parents. Circulation 72:38-46, 1985.

86. Simpson P. Role of proto-oncogenes in myocardial hypertrophy. Am J Cardiol 62:13G-19G, 1988.

87. Rizzoni D, Lorenza M, Porteri E, et al. Relations between cardiac and vascular structure in patients with primary and secondary hypertension. J Am Coll Cardiol 32:985-992, 1998.

88. Shub C, Cueto-Garcia L, Sheps S, et al. Echocardiographic findings in pheochromocytoma. Am J Cardiol 57:971-975, 1986.

89. Lim MJ, Barkan AL, Buda AJ. Rapid reduction of left ventricular hypertrophy in acromegaly after suppression of growth hormone hypersecretion. Ann Intern Med 117:719-726, 1992.

90. Andronico G, Mangano M-T, Nardi E, et al. Insulin-like growth factor 1 and sodium-lithium countertransport in essential hypertension and in hypertensive left ventricular hypertrophy. J Hypertens 11:1097-1101, 1993.

91. Geffner ME, Golde DW. Selective insulin action on skin, ovary and heart in insulin-resistant states. Diabetes Care 11:500-505, 1988.

92. Phillips RA, Krakoff LR, Ardeljan M, et al. Relation of left ventricular mass to insulin resistance and blood pressure in nonobese subjects. J Am Coll Cardiol 23:48A, 1994. [Abstract]

93. Phillips RA, Krakoff LR, Dunaif A, et al. Relation among left ventricular mass, insulin resistance, and blood pressure in nonobese subjects. J Clin Endocrinol Metab 83:4284-4288, 1998.

94. Prakash TR, MacKenzie SJ, Ram JL, et al. Insulin stimulates gene transcription and activity of Na+K+ATPase in vascular smooth muscle cells. Hypertension 20:443, 1992. [Abstract]

95. Resnick LM. Ionic basis of hypertension, insulin resistance, vascular disease, and related disorders: The mechanism of "syndrome X". Am J Hypertens 6:123S-134S, 1993.

96. Ciulla M, Paliotti R, Hess DB, et al. Echocardiographic patterns of myocardial fibrosis in hypertensive patients: Endomyocardial biopsy versus ultrasonic tissue characterization. J Am Soc Echocardiogr 10:657-664, 1997.

97. Schwartzkopff B, Motz W, Frenzel H, et al. Structural and functional alterations of the intramyocardial coronary arterioles in patients with arterial hypertension. Circulation 88:993-1003, 1993.

98. Cottone S, Vadala A, Vella MC, et al. Changes of plasma endothelin and growth factor levels, and of left ventricular mass, after chronic AT1-receptor blockade in human hypertension. Am J Hypertens 11:548-553, 1998.

99. Moye LA, Pfeffer MA, Wun CC, et al. Uniformity of captopril benefit in the SAVE Study: Subgroup analysis. Survival and Ventricular Enlargement Study. Eur Heart J 15(Suppl B):2-8, 1994.

100. Dahlof B, Devereux R, de-Faire U, et al. The Losartan Intervention For Endpoint reduction (LIFE) in Hypertension study: Rationale, design, and methods. The LIFE Study Group. Am -J-Hypertens 10:705-713, 1997.

101. Gomez AM, Valdivia HH, Cheng H, et al. Defective excitation-contraction coupling in experimental cardiac hypertrophy and heart failure [see comments]. Science 276:800-806, 1997.

102. Devereux RB, Reichek N. Echocardiographic determination of left ventricular mass in man: Anatomic validation of the method. Circulation 55:613-618, 1977.

103. Feigenbaum H. The echocardiographic examination. In: Feigenbaum H (ed). Echocardiography, 4e. Philadelphia, Lea & Febiger, 1986; pp 50-187.

104. Devereux RB, Alonso DR, Lutas EM, et al. Echocardiographic assessment of left ventricular hypertrophy: Comparison to necropsy findings. Am J Cardiol 57:450-458, 1986.

105. Sahn DJ, DeMaria A, Kisslo J, et al. The Committee on M-mode Standardization of Echocardiography: Recommendations regarding quantitation in M-mode echocardiography: Results of a survey of echocardiographic measurements. Circulation 58:1073-1078, 1978.

106. Liao Y, Cooper RS, Durazo-Arvizu R, et al. Prediction of mortality risk by different methods of indexation for left ventricular mass. J Am Coll Cardiol 29:641-647, 1998.

107. De Simone G, Daniels SR, Devereux RB, et al. Left ventricular mass and body size in normotensive children and adults: Assessment of allometric relations and impact of overweight. J Am Coll Cardiol 20:1251-1260, 1992.

108. Lauer MS, Anderson KM, Larson M, et al. A new method for indexing left ventricular mass for differences in body size. Am J Cardiol 74:487-491, 1994.

109. Devereux RB. Detection of left ventricular hypertrophy by M-mode echocardiography. Anatomic validation, standardization, and comparison to other methods. Hypertension ≈ 9(Suppl II):II19-II26.

110. Gottdiener JS, Livengood SV, Meyer PS, et al. Should echocardiography be performed to assess effects of antihypertensive therapy? Test-retest reliability of echocardiography for assessment of left ventricular mass and function. J Am Coll Cardiol 25:424-430, 1995.

111. Grandits GA, Liebson PR, Dianzumba S, et al. Echocardiography in multicenter clinical trials: Experience from the Treatment of the Mild Hypertension Study. Control Clinic Trials. 15:395-410, 1995.

112. Collins R, Peto R, MacMahon S, et al. Blood pressure, stroke, and coronary heart disease. Part 2, short-term reductions in blood pressure: Overview of randomized drug trials in their epidemiological context. Lancet 335:827-838, 1990.

113. Cook RJ, Sackett DL. The number needed to treat: A clinically useful measure of treatment effect [published erratum appears in BMJ 1995 310:1056] [see comments]. BMJ 310:452-454, 1995.

114. Alderman MH. Blood pressure management: Individualized treatment based on absolute risk and the potential for benefit [see comments]. Ann Intern Med 119:329-335, 1993.

115. Moore CR, Krakoff LR, Phillips RA. Confirmation or exclusion of stage I hypertension by ambulatory blood pressure monitoring. Hypertension 29:1109-1113, 1997.

116. Schiller NB, Shah PM, Crawford M, et al. Recommendations for quantitation of the left ventricle by two-dimensional echocardiography. American Society of Echocardiography Committee on Standards, Subcommittee on Quantitation of Two-Dimensional Echocardiograms. J Am Soc Echocardiogr 2:358-367, 1989.

117. Collins HW, Kronenberg MW, Byrd BF. Reproducibility of left ventricular mass measurements by two-dimensional and M-mode echocardiography. J Am Coll Cardiol 14:672-676, 1989.

118. Myerson SG, Bellenger NG, Pennell DJ. Assessment of left ventricular mass by cardiovascular magnetic resonance. Hypertension 39:750-755, 2002.

119. Keller AM, Peschock RM, Malloy CR, et al. In vivo measurement of myocardial mass using nuclear magnetic resonance imaging. J Am Coll Cardiol 8:113-117, 1986.

120. Riley-Hagan M, Peshock RM, Stray-Gundersen J, et al. Left ventricular dimensions and mass using magnetic resonance imaging in female endurance athletes. Am J Cardiol 69:1067-1074, 1992.

121. Bottini PB, Carr AA, Prisant LM, et al. Magnetic resonance imaging compared to echocardiography to assess left ventricular mass in the hypertensive patient. Am J Hypertens 8:221-228, 1995.

122. Yamaoka O, Yabe T, Okada M, et al. Evaluation of left ventricular mass: Comparison of ultrafast computed tomography, magnetic resonance imaging, and contrast left ventriculography. Am Heart J 126:1372-1379, 1993.

123. Wolfe CL, O'Connell JW, Sievers RE, et al. Assessment of perfused left ventricular mass in normal, ischemic, and reperfused myocardium by means of single-photon emission computed tomography of technetium-99m isonitrile. Am Heart J 126:1275-1286, 1993.

124. Williams KA, Lang RM, Reba RC, et al. Comparison of technetium-99m sestamibi-gated tomographic perfusion imaging with echocardiography and electrocardiography for determination of left ventricular mass. Am J Cardiol 77:750-755, 1996.

125. Faber TL, Folks RD, Cooke JP, et al. Left ventricular mass from ungated perfusion images: Comparison to MRI. J Nucl Med 38:20P, 1997. [Abstract]

126. Gopal AS, Keller AM, Shen Z, et al. Three-dimensional echocardiography: In vitro and in vivo validation of left ventricular mass and comparison with conventional echocardiographic methods. J Am Coll Cardiol 24:504-513, 1994.

127. Gopal AS, Shen Z, Sapin PM, et al. Assessment of cardiac function by three-dimensional echocardiography compared with conventional noninvasive methods. Circulation 92: 842-853, 1995.

128. Jiang L, Vazquez de Prada A, et al. Three-dimensional echocardiography: In vivo validation for right ventricular free wall mass as an index of hypertrophy. J Am Coll Cardiol 23:1715-1722, 1994.

129. Keller AM, Gopal AS, Sapin PM, et al. Three-dimensional echocardiography: An advance in quantitative assessment of the left ventricle. Coron Artery Dis 6:42-48, 1995.

130. Rodevand O, Bjornerheim R, Kolbjornsen O, et al. Left ventricular mass assessed by three-dimensional echocardiography using rotational acquisition. Clin Cardiol 20:957-962, 1997.

131. Kaul S. New developments in ultrasound systems for contrast echocardiography. Clin Cardiol 20(10 Suppl 1):I27-I30, 1997.

132. Schmieder RE, Martus P, Klingbeil A. Reversal of left ventricular hypertrophy in essential hypertension. A meta-analysis of randomized double-blind studies [see comments]. JAMA 275:1507-1513, 1996.

133. Muiesan ML, Salvetti M, Rizzoni D, et al. Association of change in left ventricular mass with prognosis during long-term antihypertensive treatment. J Hypertens 13:1091-1095, 1995.

134. Verdecchia P, Schillaci G, Borgioni C, et al. Prognostic significance of serial changes in left ventricular mass in essential hypertension. Circulation 97: 48-54, 1998.

135. Koren MJ, Ulin RJ, Koren AT, et al. Left ventricular mass change during treatment and outcome in patients with essential hypertension. Am J Hypertens 15:1021-1028, 2002.

136. Neaton JD, Grimm RH Jr, Prineas RJ, et al. Treatment of mild hypertension study: Final results. JAMA 270:713-724, 1993.

137. Schussheim AE, Diamond JA, Phillips RA. Left ventricular midwall function improves with antihypertensive therapy and regression of left ventricular hypertrophy in patients with asymptomatic hypertension. Am J Cardiol 87:61-65, 2001.

138. Wachtel K, Palmieri V, Olsen MH, et al. Change in systolic left ventricular performance after 3 years of antihypertensive treatment: The Losartan Intervention for Endpoint (LIFE) Study. Circulation 106:227-232, 2002.

139. Dahlof B, Pennert K, Hansson L. Reversal of left ventricular hypertrophy in hypertensive patients. A metaanalysis of 109 treatment studies. Am J Hypertens 5:95-110, 1992.

140. Linz W, Schaper J, Wiemer G, et al. Ramipril prevents left ventricular hypertrophy with myocardial fibrosis without blood pressure reduction: A one year study in rats. Br J Pharmacol 107:970-975, 1992.

141. Gottdiener JS, Reda DJ, Massie BM, et al. Effect of single-drug therapy on reduction of left ventricular mass in mild to moderate hypertension: Comparison of six antihypertensive agents. The Department of Veterans Affairs Cooperative Study Group on Antihypertensive Agents [see comments]. Circulation 95:2007-2014, 1997.

142. Okin PM, Devereux RB, Jern S, et al. Regression of electrocardiographic left ventricular hypertrophy by losartan versus atenolol: The Losartan Intervention for Endpoint reduction in Hypertension (LIFE) Study. Circulation 108:684-690, 2003.

143. Devereux RB, Palmieri V, Liu JE, et al. Progressive hypertrophy regression with sustained pressure reduction in hypertension: The Losartan Intervention For Endpoint Reduction study. J Hypertens 20:1445-1450, 2002.

144. Pitt B, Reichek N, Willenbrock R, et al. Effects of eplerenone, enalapril, and eplerenone/enalapril in patients with essential hypertension and left ventricular hypertrophy: The 4E-left ventricular hypertrophy study. Circulation 108(:1831-1838, 2003.

145. Indolfi C, Di Lorenzo E, Perrino C, et al. Hydroxymethylglutaryl coenzyme A reductase inhibitor simvastatin prevents cardiac hypertrophy induced by pressure overload and inhibits p21ras activation. Circulation 106:2118-2124, 2002.

146. Shioi T, McMullen JR, Tarnavski O, et al. Rapamycin attenuates load-induced cardiac hypertrophy in mice. Circulation 107:1664-1670, 2003.

147. Fouad FM, Slominiski JM, Tarazi RC. Left ventricular diastolic function in hypertension: Relation to left ventricular mass and systolic function. J Am Coll Cardiol 3:1500-1506, 1984.

148. Smith VE, Schulman P, Karimeddini M, et al. Rapid ventricular filling in left ventricular hypertrophy II. Pathological hypertrophy. J Am Coll Cardiol 5:869-874, 1985.

149. Inouye I, Massie B, Loge D, et al. Abnormal left ventricular filling: An early finding in mild to moderate systemic hypertension. Am J Cardiol 53:120-126, 1984.

150. Bonow RO, Udelson JE. Left ventricular diastolic dysfunction as a cause of congestive heart failure: Mechanisms and management. Ann Intern Med 117:502-510, 1992.

151. Topol EJ, Traill GV, Fortuin NJ. Hypertensive cardiomyopathy of the elderly. N Engl J Med 312:277-282, 1985.

152. Soufer R, Wohlgelernter D, Vita N, et al. Intact systolic left ventricular function in clinical congestive heart failure. Am J Cardiol 55:1032-1036, 1985.

153. Cuocolo A, Sax FL, Brush JE, et al. Left ventricular hypertrophy and impaired diastolic filling in essential hypertension. Diastolic mechanisms for systolic dysfunction during exercise. Circulation 81:978-986, 1990.

154. Setaro JF, Soufer R, Remetz MS, et al. Long- term outcome in patients with congestive heart failure and intact systolic left ventricular performance. Am J Cardiol 69:1212-1216, 1992.

155. Carroll JD, Lang RM, Neumann AL, et al. The differential effects of positive inotropic and vasodilator therapy on diastolic properties in patients with congestive cardiomyopathy. Circulation 74:815-825, 1986.

156. Graettinger WF, Neutel JM, Smith DHG, et al. Left ventricular diastolic filling alterations in normotensive young adults with a family history of systemic hypertension. Am J Cardiol 68: 51-56, 1991.

157. Tang W, Arnett DK, Devereux RB, et al. Linkage of left ventricular early diastolic peak filling velocity to chromosome 5 in hypertensive African Americans: The HyperGEN echocardiography study. Am J Hypertens 15:621-627, 2002.

158. Snider AR, Gidding SS, Rocchini AP, et al. Doppler evaluation of left ventricular diastolic filling in children with systemic hypertension. Am J Cardiol 56:921-926, 1985.

159. Phillips RA, Coplan NL, Krakoff LR, et al. Doppler echocardiographic analysis of left ventricular filling in treated hypertensive patients. J Am Coll Cardiol 9:317-322, 1987.

160. Dianzumba SB, DiPette DJ, Cornman C, et al. Left ventricular filling characteristics in mild untreated hypertension. Hypertension 1986; 8(Suppl I):I156-I160.

161. Shapiro LM, McKenna WJ. Left ventricular hypertrophy: Relationship of structure to diastolic function in hypertension. Br Heart J 51:637-642, 1984.

162. Hartford M, Wikstrand J, Wallentin I, et al. Diastolic function of the heart in untreated primary hypertension. Hypertension 6:329-338, 1984.

163. Fouad FM, Slominski JM, Tarazi RC. Left ventricular diastolic function in hypertension: Relation to left ventricular mass and systolic function. J Am Coll Cardiol 3:1500-1506, 1984.

164. Smith VE, White WB, Meeran MK, et al. Improved left ventricular filling accompanies reduced left ventricular mass during therapy of essential hypertension. J Am Coll Cardiol 8:1449-1454, 1986.

165. White WB, Schulman P, Karimeddini MK, et al. Regression of left ventricular mass is accompanied by improvement in rapid left ventricular filling following antihypertensive therapy with metoprolol. Am Heart J 117:145-150, 1989.

166. Trimarco B, DeLuca N, Rosiello G. Improvement of diastolic function after reversal of left ventricular hypertrophy induced long-term antihypertensive treatment with tertatolol. Am J Cardiol 64:745-751, 1989.

167. Schulman SP, Weiss JL, Becher LC, et al. The effects of antihypertensive therapy on left ventricular mass in elderly patients. N Engl J Med 322:1350-1356, 1990.

168. Gonzalez-Fernandez RB, Altieri PI, Diaz LM, et al. Effects of enalapril on heart failure in hypertensive patients with diastolic dysfunction. Am J Hypertens 5:480-483., 1992.

169. Phillips RA, Ardeljan M, Shimabukuro S, et al. Normalization of left ventricular mass and associated changes in neurohormones and atrial natriuretic peptide after one year of sustained nifedipine therapy for severe hypertension. J Am Coll Cardiol 17:1595-1602, 1991.

170. Shahi M, Thorn S, Poulter N, et al. Regression of hypertensive left ventricular hypertrophy and left ventricular diastolic dysfunction. Lancet 336:458-461, 1990.

171. Palatini P, Visentin P, Mormino P, et al. Structural abnormalities and not diastolic dysfunction are the earliest left ventricular changes in hypertension. HARVEST Study Group. Am J Hypertens 11:147-154, 1998.

172. Douglas PS, Berko B, Lesh M, et al. Alterations in diastolic function in response to progressive left ventricular hypertrophy. J Am Coll Cardiol 13:461-467, 1989.

173. Douglas PS, Tallant B. Hypertrophy, fibrosis and diastolic dysfunction in early canine experimental hypertension. J Am Coll Cardiol 17:530-536, 1991.

174. Brilla CG, Janicki JS, Weber KT. Cardioreparative effects of lisinopril in rats with genetic hypertension and left ventricular hypertrophy. Circulation 83:1771-1779, 1991.

175. Villari B, Campbell SE, Hess OM, et al. Influence of collagen network on left ventricular systolic and diastolic function in aortic valve disease. J Am Coll Cardiol 22:1477-1484, 1993.

176. Lorell BH, Grice WN, Apstein CS. Influence of hypertension with minimal hypertrophy on diastolic function during demand ischemia. Hypertension 13:361-370, 1989.

177. Wexler LF, Lorell BH, Momomura S, et al. Enhanced sensitivity to hypoxia-induced diastolic dysfunction in pressure-overload left ventricular hypertrophy in the rat: Role of high-energy phosphate depletion. Circ Res 62:766-775, 1988.

178. Osbakken M, Douglas PS, Ivanics T, et al. Creatinine kinase kinetics studied by phosphorus-31 nuclear magnetic resonance in a canine model of chronic hypertension-induced cardiac hypertrophy. J Am Coll Cardiol 19:223-228, 1992.

179. Ito Y, Suko J, Chidsey CA. Intracalcium and myocardial contractility. V. Calcium uptake of sarcoplasmic reticulum fractions in hypertrophied and failing rabbit hearts. J Mol Cell Cardiol 6:237-247, 1974.

180. Harding DP, Poole-Wilson PA. Calcium exchange in rabbit myocardium during and after hypoxia: Effect of temperature and substrate. Cardiovasc Res 14:435-445, 1980.

181. Gwathmey JK, Morgan JP. Altered calcium handling in experimental pressure-overload hypertrophy in the ferret. Circ Res 57:836-843, 1985.

182. Brutsaert DL, Rademakers FE, Sys SU, et al. Analysis of relaxation in the evaluation of ventricular function of the heart. Prog Cardiovasc Dis 28:143-163, 1985.

183. White WB, Schulman P, Dey HM, et al. Effects of age and 24-hour ambulatory blood pressure on rapid left ventricular filling. Am J Cardiol 63:13431-1347, 1989.

184. Franchi F, Fabbri G, Monopoli A, et al. Left ventricular diastolic filling improvement obtained by intravenous verapamil in mild to moderate essential hypertension: A complex effect. Cardiology 76:32-41, 1989.

185. Betocchi S, Cuocolo A, Pace L, et al. Effect of intravenous verapamil administration on left ventricular diastolic function in systemic hypertension. Am J Cardiol 59:624-629, 1987.

186. Kawaguchi M, Hay I, Fetics B, et al. Combined ventricular systolic and arterial stiffening in patients with heart failure and preserved ejection fraction: Implications for systolic and diastolic reserve limitations. Circulation 107:714- 720, 2003.

187. Burkhoff D, Maurer MS, Packer M. Heart failure with a normal ejection fraction: Is it really a disorder of diastolic function? Circulation 107:656-658, 2003.

188. Gandhi SK, Powers JC, Nomeir AM, et al. The pathogenesis of acute pulmonary edema associated with hypertension. N Engl J Med 344:17-22, 2001.

189. De Simone G, Devereux RB, Koren MJ, et al. Midwall left ventricular mechanics. An independent predictor of cardiovascular risk in arterial hypertension. Circulation 93:259- 265, 1996.

190. De Simone G, Devereux RB, Roman MJ, et al. Assessment of left ventricular function by the midwall fractional shortening/end-systolic stress relation in human hypertension [published erratum appears in J Am Coll Cardiol 24:844, 1994]. J Am Coll Cardiol 23:1444-1451, 1994.

191. Schussheim AE, Diamond JA, Jhang JS, et al. Midwall fractional shortening is an independent predictor of left ventricular diastolic dysfunction in asymptomatic patients with systemic hypertension. Am J Cardiol 82:1056-1059, 1998.

192. Aurigemma GP, Gottdiener JS, Shemanski L, et al. Predictive value of systolic and diastolic function for incident congestive heart failure in the elderly: The cardiovascular health study. J Am Coll Cardiol 37:1042-1048, 2001.

193. Harrison TR, Dixon K, Russell RO, et al. The relation of age to the duration of contraction, ejection, and relaxation of the normal human heart. Am Heart J 67:189-199, 1964.

194. Miyatake K, Okamoto M, Kinoshita N, et al. Augmentation of atrial contribution to left ventricular inflow with aging as assessed by intracardiac Doppler flowmetry. Am J Cardiol 64:315-323, 1984.

195. Phillips RA, Krakoff LR, Coplin NL, et al. Normal aging produces left ventricular diastolic abnormalities detectable by Doppler echocardiography. Clin Res 34:336A, 1986. [Abstract]

196. Van Dam I, Fast T, DeBoo J, et al. Normal diastolic filling patterns of the left ventricle. Eur Heart J 9:165-171, 1988.

197. Spirito P, Maron BJ. Influence of aging on Doppler echocardiographic indices of left ventricular diastolic function. Br Heart J 59:672-679, 1988.

198. Arora RR, Machac J, Goldman ME, et al. Atrial kinetics and left ventricular diastolic filling in the healthy elderly. J Am Coll Cardiol 9:1255-1260, 1987.

199. Benjamin EJ, Plehn JF, D'Agostino RB, et al. Mitral annular calcification and the risk of stroke in an elderly cohort. N Engl J Med 327:374-379, 1992.

200. Psaty BM, Furberg CD, Kuller LH, et al. Isolated systolic hypertension and subclinical cardiovascular disease in the elderly: Initial findings from the Cardiovascular Health Study. JAMA 268:1287-1291, 1992.

201. Sagie A, Benjamin EJ, Galderisi M, et al. Echocardiographic assessment of left ventricular structure and diastolic filling in elderly subjects with borderline isolated systolic hypertension (the Framingham Heart Study). Am J Cardiol 72:662-665, 1993.

202. Nicolino A, Ferrara N, Longobardi G, et al. Left ventricular diastolic filling in elderly hypertensive patients. J Am Geriatr Soc 41:217-222, 1993.

203. Levy WC, Cerqueira MD, Abrass IB, et al. Endurance exercise training augments diastolic filling at rest and during exercise in healthy young and older men. Circulation 88:116-126, 1993.

204. Fleg JL, Shapiro EP, O'Connor F, et al. Left ventricular diastolic filling performance in older male athletes. JAMA 273(17):1371-1375, 1995.

205. Voutilainen S, Kupari M, Hippelainen M, et al. Factors influencing Doppler indexes of left ventricular filling in healthy persons. Am J Cardiol 68:653-659, 1991.

206. Nixdorff U, de Mey C, Belz GG, et al. Beta- adrenergic stimulation enhances left ventricular diastolic performance in normal subjects. J Cardiovasc Pharmacol 29:476-484, 1997.

207. Tanaka M, Hashimoto Y, Numano F. Decreased left ventricular contractility reserve in patients with never-treated essential hypertension. Clin Exp Pharmacol Physiol 27:871-875, 2000.

208. Grandi AM, Imperiale D, Santillo R, et al. Aldosterone antagonist improves diastolic function in essential hypertension. Hypertension 40:647-652, 2002.

209. Weiss JL, Frederiksen JW, Weisfeldt ML. Hemodynamic determinants of the time-course of fall in canine left ventricular pressure. J Clin Invest 58:751-760, 1976.

210. Grossman W, McLaurin LP. Diastolic properties of the left ventricle. Ann Intern Med 84:316-326, 1976.

211. Hess OM, Ritter M, Schneider J, et al. Diastolic stiffness and myocardial structure in aortic valve disease before and after valve replacement. Circulation 69:855-865, 1984.

212. Spirito P, Maron BJ, Bonow RO. Noninvasive assessment of left ventricular diastolic function: Comparative analysis of Doppler echocardiographic and radionuclide angiographic techniques. J Am Coll Cardiol 7:518-526, 1986.

213. Shapiro LM, Mackinnon J, Beevers DG. Echocardiographic features of malignant hypertension. Br Heart J 46:374-379, 1981.

214. Kitabatake A, Inoue M, Asao M, et al. Transmitral blood flow reflecting diastolic behavior of the left ventricle in health and disease: A study by pulsed Doppler technique. Jpn Circ J 46:92-102, 1982.

215. Chenzbraun A, Pinto FJ, Popylisen S, et al. Filling patterns in left ventricular hypertrophy: A combined acoustic quantification and Doppler study. J Am Coll Cardiol 23:1179-1185, 1994.

216. Hanrath P, Mathey DG, Siegert R, Bleifeld W. Left ventricular relaxation and filling pattern in different forms of left ventricular hypertrophy: An echocardiographic study. Am J Cardiol 45:15-23, 1980.

217. Nakashima Y, Nii T, Ikeda M, et al. Role of left ventricular regional nonuniformity in hypertensive diastolic dysfunction. J Am Coll Cardiol 22:790-795, 1993.

218. Spirito P, Maron BJ. Doppler echocardiography for assessing left ventricular diastolic function. Ann Intern Med 109:122-126, 1988.

219. Bella JN, Palmieri V, Roman MJ, et al. Mitral ratio of peak early to late diastolic filling velocity as a predictor of mortality in middle-aged and elderly adults: The Strong Heart Study. Circulation 105(16):1928-1933, 2002.

220. Schillaci G, Pasqualini L, Verdecchia P, et al. Prognostic significance of left ventricular diastolic dysfunction in essential hypertension. J Am Coll Cardiol 39:2005-2011, 2002.

221. Choong CY, Abascal VM, Thomas JD, et al. Combined influence of ventricular loading and relaxation on the transmitral flow velocity profile in dogs measured by Doppler echocardiography. Circulation 78:672-683, 1988.

222. Himura Y, Kumada T, Kambayashi M, et al. Importance of left ventricular systolic function in the assessment of left ventricular diastolic function with Doppler transmitral flow velocity recording. J Am Coll Cardiol 18:753-760, 1991.

223. Appleton CP. Left ventricular diastolic function. In: Murphy JG, (ed). Mayo Clinic Cardiology Review. Armonk, NY, Futura, 1997; pp 43-56.

224. Benjamin EJ, Levy D, Anderson KM, et al. Determinants of Doppler indexes of left ventricular diastolic function in normal subjects (the Framingham Heart Study). Am J Cardiol 70:508-515, 1992.

225. Laufer E, Jennings GL, Dewar E. Prevalence of cardiac structural and functional abnormalities in untreated primary hypertension. Hypertension 13:151-162, 1989.

226. Ishida Y, Meisner JS, Tsujioka K, et al. Left ventricular filling dynamics: Influence of left ventricular relaxation and left atrial pressure. Circulation 74:187-196, 1986.

227. Appleton CP, Carucci MJ, Henry CP, et al. Influence of incremental changes in heart rate on mitral flow velocity: Assessment in lightly sedated, conscious dogs. J Am Coll Cardiol 17:227-236, 1991.

228. Nishimura RA, Schwartz RS, Holmes DR, et al. Failure of calcium channel blockers to improve ventricular relaxation in humans. J Am Coll Cardiol 21:182-188, 1993.

229. Raine AEG, Erne P, Burgisser E, et al. Atrial natriuretic peptide and atrial pressure in patients with congestive heart failure. N Engl J Med 315:533-537, 1986.

230. Eison HB, Rosen MJ, Phillips RA, Krakoff LR. Determinants of atrial natriuretic factor in the adult respiratory distress syndrome. Chest 95:1040-1045, 1988.

231. Rodeheffer RJ, Tanaka I, Imada T, et al. Atrial pressure and secretion of atrial natriuretic factor into the human central circulation. J Am Coll Cardiol 8:18-26, 1986.

232. Matsuda Y, Toma Y, Matsuzaki M, et al. Change of left atrial systolic pressure waveform in relation to left ventricular end-diastolic pressure. Circulation 82:1659-1667, 1990.

233. Rossvoll O, Hatle LK. Pulmonary venous flow velocities recorded by transthoracic Doppler ultrasound: Relation to left ventricular diastolic pressures. J Am Coll Cardiol 21:1687-1696, 1993.

234. Appleton CP, Galloway JM, Gonzales MS, et al. Estimation of left ventricular filling pressures using two- dimensional and Doppler echocardiography in adult patients with cardiac disease. Additional value of analyzing left atrial size, left atrial ejection fraction and the difference in duration of pulmonary venous and mitral flow velocity at atrial contraction. J Am Coll Cardiol 22:1972-1982, 1993.

235. Pai RG, Suzuki M, Heywood JT, et al. Mitral A wave velocity transit time to the outflow tract as a measure of left ventricular diastolic stiffness: Hemodynamic correlations in patients with coronary artery disease. Circulation 89:553-557, 1994.

236. Pai RG, Shakudo M, Yoganathan AP, et al. Clinical correlates of the rate of transmission of transmitral "A" wave to the left ventricular outflow tract in left ventricular hypertrophy secondary to systemic hypertension, hypertrophic cardiomyopathy or aortic valve stenosis. Am J Cardiol 73:831-834, 1994.

237. Garcia MJ, Thomas JD, Klein AL. New Doppler echocardiographic applications for the study of diastolic function. J Am Coll Cardiol 32:865-875, 1998.

238. Derumeaux G, Ovize M, Loufoua J, et al. Doppler tissue imaging quantitates regional wall motion during myocardial ischemia and reperfusion. Circulation 97(19):1970-1977, 1998.

239. Galiuto L, Ignone G, DeMaria AN. Contraction and relaxation velocities of the normal left ventricle using pulsed-wave tissue Doppler echocardiography. Am J Cardiol 81:609-614, 1998.

240. Oki T, Tabata T, Yamada H, et al. Clinical application of pulsed Doppler tissue imaging for assessing abnormal left ventricular relaxation. Am J Cardiol 79:921-928, 1997.

241. Maceira AM, Barba J, Beloqui O, et al. Ultrasonic backscatter and diastolic function in hypertensive patients. Hypertension 40:239-243, 2002.

242. Temporelli PL, Corra U, Imparato A, et al. Reversible restrictive left ventricular diastolic filling with optimized oral therapy predicts a more favorable prognosis in patients with chronic heart failure. J Am Coll Cardiol 31:1591-1597, 1998.

243. Aronow WS, Kronzon I. Effect of enalapril on congestive heart failure treated with diuretics in elderly patients with prior myocardial infarction and normal left ventricular ejection fraction. Am J Cardiol 71:602-604, 1993.

244. Brilla CG, Funck RC, Rupp H. Lisinopril-mediated regression of myocardial fibrosis in patients with hypertensive heart disease [see comments]. Circulation 102:1388-1393, 2000.

245. Yusuf S, Pfeffer MA, Swedberg K, et al. Effects of candesartan in patients with chronic heart failure and preserved left-ventricular ejection fraction: The CHARM-Preserved Trial. Lancet 362:777-781, 2003.

246. Setaro JF, Zaret BL, Schulman DS, et al. Usefulness of verapamil for congestive heart failure associated with abnormal left ventricular diastolic filling and normal left ventricular systolic performance. Am J Cardiol 66:981-986, 1990.

247. Given BD, Lee TH, Stone PH, et al. Nifedipine in severely hypertensive patients with congestive heart failure and preserved ventricular systolic function. Arch Intern Med 145: 281-285, 1985.

248. Andersson B, Caidahl K, di Lenarda A, et al. Changes in early and late diastolic filling patterns induced by long-term adrenergic beta-blockade in patients with idiopathic dilated cardiomyopathy. Circulation 94:673-682, 1996.

249. Nodari S, Metra M, Dei CL. Beta-blocker treatment of patients with diastolic heart failure and arterial hypertension. A prospective, randomized, comparison of the long- term effects of atenolol vs. nebivolol. Eur J Heart Fail 5:621-627, 2003.

250. Gaasch WH. Diagnosis and treatment of heart failure based on left ventricular systolic or diastolic dysfunction [see comments]. JAMA 271(16):1276-1280, 1994.

251. Packer M. Abnormalities of diastolic function as a potential cause of exercise intolerance in chronic heart failure. Circulation 81(2 Suppl):III78-III86, 1990.

252. The Fifth Report of the Joint National Committee on Detection, Evaluation, and Treatment of High Blood Pressure (JNC V). Arch Intern Med 153:154-183, 1993.

253. Lorell BH, Isoyama S, Grice WN, et al. Effects of ouabain and isoproterenol on left ventricular diastolic function during low-flow ischemia in isolated, blood- perfused rabbit hearts. Circ Res 63:457-467, 1988.

254. The effect of digoxin on mortality and morbidity in patients with heart failure. The Digitalis Investigation Group [see comments]. N Engl J Med 336:525-533, 1997.

255. Brutsaert DL, Sys SU, Gillebert TC. Diastolic failure: Pathophysiology and therapeutic implications [published erratum appears in J Am Coll Cardiol 22:1272, 1993]. J Am Coll Cardiol 22:318-325, 1993.

256. Chobanian AV, Bakris GL, Black HR, et al. The Seventh Report of the Joint National Committee on Prevention, Detection, Evaluation, and Treatment of High Blood Pressure: The JNC 7 Report. JAMA 289:2560-2571, 2003.

257. Clements IP, Bailey KR, Zachariah PK. Effects of exercise and therapy on ventricular emptying and filling in mildly hypertensive patients. Am J Hypertens 7:695-702, 1994.

258. Zusman RM, Christensen DM, Higgins J, et al. Nifedipine improves left ventricular function in patients with hypertension. J Cardiovasc Pharmacol 18:843-848, 1991.

259. Hung MJ, Cherng WJ, Wang CH, et al. Effects of verapamil in normal elderly individuals with left ventricular diastolic dysfunction. Echocardiography 18:123-129, 2001.

260. Szlachcic J, Tubau JF, Vollmer C, et al. Effects of diltiazem on left ventricular mass and diastolic filling in mild to moderate hypertension. Am J Cardiol 63:198-201, 1989.

261. Topol EJ, Traill TA, Fortuin NJ. Hypertensive hypertrophic cardiomyopathy of the elderly. N Engl J Med 312:277-283, 1985.

262. Zusman RM, Christensen DM, Federman EB, et al. Nifedipine, but not propranolol, improves left ventricular systolic and diastolic function in patients with hypertension. Am J Cardiol 64:51F-61F, 1989.

263. Fouad FM, Slominski MJ, Tarazi RC, et al. Alterations in left ventricular filling with beta-adrenergic blockade. Am J Cardiol 51:161-164, 1983.

264. Schunkert H, Dzau VJ, Tang SS, et al. Increased rat cardiac angiotensin converting enzyme activity and mRNA expression in pressure overload left ventricular hypertrophy. J Clin Invest 86:1913-1920, 1990.

265. Esper RJ, Burrieza OH, Cacharrón JL, et al. Left ventricular mass regression and diastolic function improvement in mild and moderate hypertensive patients treated with lisinopril. Cardiology 83:76-81, 1993.

266. Grandi AM, Venco A, Barzizza F, et al. Effect of enalapril on left ventricular mass and performance in essential hypertension. Am J Cardiol 63:1093-1097, 1989.

267. Strauer BE. The concept of coronary flow reserve. J Cardiovasc Pharmacol 19 Suppl. 5:S67-S80, 1992.

268. Bache RJ. Effects of hypertrophy on the coronary circulation. Prog Cardiovasc Dis 31:403-440, 1988.

269. Anversa P, Sonnenblick EH. Ischemic cardiomyopathy: Pathophysiologic mechanisms. Prog Cardiovasc Dis 32: 1-22, 1990.

270. Greene AS, Tonellato PJ, Lui J, et al. Microvascular rarefaction and tissue vascular resistance in hypertension. Am J Physiol 256:H126-H131, 1989.

271. Rakusan K. Microcirculation in the stressed heart. In: Legato MJ, (ed). The Stressed Heart. Boston/Norwell, MA, Martinus Nijhoff Publishing, 1987; pp 107-123.

272. Marcus ML, Harrison DG, Chilian WM, et al. Alterations in the coronary circulation in hypertrophied ventricles. Circulation 75 (Suppl I):I19-I25, 1987.

273. Breisch EA, White FC, Nimmo LE, et al. Cardiac vasculature and flow during pressure-overload hypertrophy. Am J Physiol 251:H1031-H1037, 1986.

274. Rakusan K, Wicker P, Abdul-Samad M, et al. Failure of swimming exercise to improve capillarization in cardiac hypertrophy of renal hypertensive rats. Circ Res 61:641-647, 1987.

275. Smolich JJ, Walker AM, Campbell GR, et al. Left and right ventricular myocardial morphometry in fetal, neonatal, and adult sheep. Am J Physiol 257:H1-H9, 1989.

276. Rakusan K, Flanagan MF, Geva T, et al. Morphometry of human coronary capillaries during normal growth and the effect of age in left ventricular pressure-overload hypertrophy. Circulation 86:38-46, 1992.

277. Tomanek RJ. Effects of age and exercise on the extent of the myocardial capillary bed. Anat Rec 167:55-62, 1970.

278. Noon JP, Walker BR, Webb DJ, et al. Impaired microvascular dilatation and capillary rarefaction in young adults with a predisposition to high blood pressure. J Clin Invest 99:1873-1879, 1997.

279. D'Amore PA, Thompson RW. Mechanisms of angiogenesis. Annu Rev Physiol 49:453-464, 1987.

280. Hudlicka O. What makes blood vessels grow? J Physiol 444: 1-24, 1991.

281. Britz-Cunningham SH, Adelstein SJ. Molecular targeting with radionuclides: State of the science. J Nucl Med 44: 1945-1961, 2003.

282. Nakano N, Moriguchi A, Morishita R, et al. Role of angiotensin II in the regulation of a novel vascular modulator,

hepatocyte growth factor (HGF), in experimental hypertensive rats. Hypertension 30(6):1448-1454, 1997.

283. James TN. Morphologic characteristics and functional significance of focal fibromuscular dysplasia of small coronary arteries. Am J Cardiol 65:126-136, 1990.

284. Tomanek RJ, Plamer PY, Pfeiffer GL, et al. Morphologic characteristics and functional significance of focal fibromuscular dysplasia of small coronary arteries, arterioles and capillaries during hypertension and left ventricular hypertrophy. Circ Res 58:38-46, 1986.

285. Schwartzkopff B, Motz W, Knauer S, et al. Morphometric investigation of intramyocardial arterioles in right septal endomyocardial biopsy of patients with arterial hypertension and left ventricular hypertrophy. J Cardiovasc Pharmacol 20: 2-7, 1992.

286. Korsgaard N, Aalkjaer C, Heagerty AM, et al. Histology of subcutaneous small arteries from patients with essential hypertension Hypertension 22:523-526, 1993.

287. Barton M, d'Uscio LV, Shaw S, et al. ET(A) receptor blockade prevents increased tissue endothelin-1, vascular hypertrophy, and endothelial dysfunction in salt-sensitive hypertension. Hypertension 31:499-504, 1998.

288. Force T, Bonventre JV. Growth factors and mitogen-activated protein kinases. Hypertension 31:152-161, 1998.

289. Chien S, Li S, Shyy YJ. Effects of mechanical forces on signal transduction and gene expression in endothelial cells. Hypertension 31:162-169, 1998.

290. Rizzoni D, Porteri E, Castellano M, et al. Endothelial dysfunction in hypertension is independent from the etiology and from vascular structure. Hypertension 31:335-341, 1998.

291. Isoyama S, Ito J, Sato K, et al. Collagen deposition and the reversal of coronary reserve in cardiac hypertrophy. Hypertension 20:491-500, 1992.

292. Raij L. relationship with renal injury and left ventricular hypertrophy. Hypertension 31:189-193, 1998.

293. Brush JE, Faxon DP, Salmon S, et al. Abnormal endothelium-dependent coronary vasomotion in hypertensive patients. J Am Coll Cardiol 19:809-815, 1992.

294. Motz W, Vogt M, Rabenau O, et al. Evidence of endothelial dysfunction in coronary resistance vessels in patients with angina pectoris and normal coronary angiograms. Am J Cardiol 68:996-1003, 1991.

295. Panza JA, Quyyumi AA, Brush JE, et al. Abnormal endothelium-dependent vascular relaxation in patients with essential hypertension. N Engl J Med 323:22-27, 1990.

296. Treasure CB, Klein JL, Vita JA, et al. Hypertension and left ventricular hypertrophy are associated with impaired endothelium-mediated relaxation in human coronary resistance vessels. Circulation 87:86-93, 1993.

297. Vrints CJ, Bult H, Hilter E, et al. Impaired endothelium-dependent cholinergic coronary vasodilation in patients with angina and normal coronary arteriograms. J Am Coll Cardiol 19:21-31, 1992.

298. Jameson M, Dai F-X, Lüscher T, et al. Endothelium-derived contracting factors in resistance arteries of young spontaneously hypertensive rats before development of overt hypertension. Hypertension 21:280-288, 1993.

299. Groves P, Kurz S, Just H, et al. Role of endogenous bradykinin in human coronary vasomotor control. Circulation 92: 424-430, 1995.

300. Gauthier-Rein KM, Rusch NJ. Distinct endothelial impairment in coronary microvessels from hypertensive Dahl rats. Hypertension 31:328-334, 1998.

301. Strauer BE. Coronary hemodynamics in hypertensive heart disease. Basic concepts, clinical consequences, and experimental analysis of regression of hypertensive microangiopathy. Am J Med 84 (Suppl 3A):45-54, 1988.

302. Strauer BE. Ventricular function and coronary hemodynamics in hypertensive heart disease. Am J Cardiol 44:999-1006, 1979.

303. Cannon RO, Cunnion RE, Parrillo JE, et al. Dynamic limitation of coronary vasodilator reserve in patients with dilated cardiomyopathy and chest pain. J Am Coll Cardiol 10:1190-1200, 1987.

304. Prichard AD, Smith H, Holt J, et al. Coronary vascular reserve in left ventricular hypertrophy secondary to chronic aortic regurgitation. Am J Cardiol 51:315-320, 1983.

305. Villari B, Hess OM, Moccetti D, et al. Effect of progression of left ventricular hypertrophy on coronary artery dimensions in aortic valve disease. J Am Coll Cardiol 20:1073-1079, 1992.

306. Rouleau J, Boerboom LE, Surjadhana A, et al. The role of autoregulation and tissue diastolic pressures in the transmural distribution of left ventricular blood flow in anesthetized dogs. Circ Res 45:804-815, 1979.

307. Guyton RA, McClenathan JH, Michaelis LL. Evolution of regional ischemia distal to a proximal coronary stenosis: Self propagation of ischemia. Am J Cardiol 40:381-392, 1977.

308. Mosher P, Ross J, McFate PA, et al. Control of coronary blood flow by an autoregulatory mechanism. Circ Res 14: 250-259, 1964.

309. Driscol TE, Moir TW, Eckstein RW. Autoregulation of coronary blood flow: Effect of intraarterial pressure gradients. Circ Res 15:103-111, 1964.

310. Hoffman JI. A critical view of coronary reserve. Circulation 75(Suppl I):I6-I11, 1987.

311. DeFily DV, Chilian WM. Regulation of myocardial blood flow. Coordination of the responses of vascular microdomains in the coronary circulation. In: Cardiology in Review. Baltimore, Williams & Wilkins, 1994; pp 67-76.

312. Berne RM, Rubio R. Cardiac nucleotides in hypoxia: Possible role in regulation of coronary blood flow. Am J Physiol 204:317-322, 1963.

313. Marcus ML. Metabolic regulation of coronary blood flow. In: Marcus ML. The Coronary Circulation in Health and Disease. New York, McGraw-Hill, 1983; pp 84-85.

314. Dole WP, Nuno DW. Myocardial oxygen tension determines the degree and pressure range of coronary autoregulation. Circ Res 59:202-215, 1986.

315. Samaha FF, Heineman C, Ince J, et al. ATP-sensitive potassium channel is essential to maintain basal coronary vascular tone in vivo. Am J Physiol 262:C1220-C1227, 1992.

316. Avontuur JA, Bruining HA, Ince C. Nitric oxide causes dysfunction of coronary autoregulation in endotoxemic rats. Cardiovasc Res 35:368-376, 1997.

317. Bayliss WM. On the local reaction of the arterial wall to changes in internal pressure. J Physiol 28:220-231, 1902.

318. Folkow B. Intravascular pressure as a factor regulating the tone of the small vessels. Acta Physiol Scand 17:289-310, 1949.

319. Marcus ML. Myogenic regulation of coronary blood flow. In: Marcus ML: The Coronary Circulation in Health and Disease. New York: McGraw-Hill, 1983; pp 147-154.

320. Johnson PC. The myogenic response. In: Borh DF, Somlyo AP, Sparks HV, (eds). The Cardiovascular System. Handbook of Physiology, Vol 2, 1980; pp 409-442.

321. Chilian WM. Coronary microcirculation in health and disease. Summary of an NHLBI workshop. Circulation 95: 522-528, 1997.

322. Wu CC, Feldman MD, Mills JD, et al. Myocardial contrast echocardiography can be used to quantify intramyocardial blood volume: New insights into structural mechanisms of coronary autoregulation [see comments]. Circulation 96: 1004-1011, 1997.

323. Hoffman JIE. Maximal coronary flow and the concept of coronary vascular reserve. Circulation 70:153-159, 1984.

324. Cleary RM, Ayon D, Moore NB, et al. Tachycardia, contractility and volume loading alter conventional indexes of

coronary flow reserve, but not the instantaneous hyperemic flow versus pressure slope index. J Am Coll Cardiol 20:1261-1269, 1992.

325. Rossen JD, Winniford MD. Effect of increases in heart rate and arterial pressure on coronary flow reserve in humans. J Am Coll Cardiol 21:343-348, 1993.

326. O'Keefe DD, Hoffman JIE, Cheitlin R, et al. Coronary blood flow in experimental canine left ventricular hypertrophy. Circ Res 43:43-51, 1978.

327. Bretschneider HJ. Parmakotherapie coronarer durchblutungsstorungen mit kreislaufwirksamen subtanzen. Deutsch Ges Med 69:583, 1963.

328. Opherk D, Mall G, Zebe H, et al. Reduction of coronary reserve: A mechanism for angina pectoris in patients with arterial hypertension and normal coronary arteries. Circulation 69:1-7, 1984.

329. Prichard AD, Gorlin R, Smith H, det al. Coronary flow studies in patients with left ventricular hypertrophy of the hypertensive type: Evidence for an impaired coronary vascular reserve. Am J Cardiol 47:547-554, 1981.

330. Goldstein RA, Haynie M. Limited myocardial perfusion reserve in patients with left ventricular hypertrophy. J Nucl Med 31:255-258, 1990.

331. Diamond JA, Machac J, Henzlova MJ, et al. Quantitative adenosine-thallium perfusion imaging for assessing coronary flow reserve in arterial hypertension. J Am Coll Cardiol 21(Suppl A):288A. 1993.[Abstract]

332. Houghton JL, Frank MJ, Carr AA, et al. Relations among impaired coronary flow reserve, left ventricular hypertrophy and thallium perfusion defects in hypertensive patients without obstructive coronary artery disease. J Am Coll Cardiol 15:43-51, 1990.

333. Marcus ML, White CW. Coronary flow reserve in patients with normal coronary angiograms. J Am Coll Cardiol 6:1254-1256, 1985.

334. Houghton JL, Prisant M, Carr AA, et al. Racial differences in myocardial ischemia and coronary flow reserve in hypertension. J Am Coll Cardiol 23:1123-1129, 1994.

335. Gould KL, Martucci JP, Goldberg DI, et al. Short-term cholesterol lowering decreases size and severity of perfusion abnormalities by positron emission tomography after dipyridamole in patients with coronary artery disease. A potential noninvasive marker of healing coronary endothelium. Circulation 89:1530-1538, 1994.

336. Quillen JE, Rossen JD, Oskarsson HJ, et al. Acute effects of cigarette smoking on the coronary circulation: Constriction of epicardial and resistance vessels. J Am Coll Cardiol 22:642-647, 1993.

337. Celermajer DS, Sorensen KE, Georgakopoulos D, et al. Cigarette smoking is associated with dose-related and potentially reversible impairment of endothelium-dependent dilation in healthy young adults. Circulation 88:2149-2155, 1993.

338. Nasher PJ, Brown RE, Oskarsson H, et al. Maximal coronary flow reserve and metabolic coronary vasodilation in patients with diabetes mellitus. Circulation 91:635-640, 1995.

339. Celermajer DS, Sorensen KE, Spiegelhalter DJ, et al. Aging is associated with endothelial dysfunction in healthy mean years before the age-related decline in women. J Am Coll Cardiol 24:471-476, 1994.

340. Leiberman EH, Gerhard MD, Uehata A, et al. Estrogen improves endothelium-dependent, flow-mediated vasodilation in postmenopausal women. Ann Intern Med 121:936-941, 1994.

341. O'Connell BJ, Genest JJ. High-density lipoproteins and endothelial function. Circulation 104(16):1978-1983, 2001.

342. Clarke SC, Schofield PM, Grace AA, et al. Tamoxifen effects on endothelial function and cardiovascular risk factors in men with advanced atherosclerosis. Circulation 103:1497-1502, 2001.

343. Zeiher AM, Drexler H, Saurbier B, et al. Endothelium-mediated coronary blood flow modulation in humans. Effects of age, atherosclerosis, hypercholesterolemia, and hypertension. J Clin Invest 92:652-662, 1993.

344. Vitullo JC, Penn MS, Rakusan K, et al. Effects of hypertension and aging on coronary arteriolar density. Hypertension 21:406-414, 1993.

345. Antony I, Nitenberg A, Foult J-M, et al. Coronary vasodilator reserve in untreated and treated hypertensive patients with and without left ventricular hypertrophy. J Am Coll Cardiol 22:514-520, 1993.

346. Harrison DG, Florentine MS, Brooks LA, et al. The effect of hypertension and left ventricular hypertrophy on the lower range of coronary autoregulation. Circulation 77:1108-1115, 1988.

347. Koyanagi S, Eastham CL, Harrison DG, et al. Increased size of myocardial infarction in dogs with chronic hypertension and left ventricular hypertrophy. Circ Res 50:55-62, 1982.

348. Dellsperger KC, Clothier JL, Hartnett JA, et al. Acceleration of the wavefront of myocardial necrosis by chronic hypertension and left ventricular hypertrophy in dogs. Circ Res 63:87-96, 1988.

349. Taylor AL, Murphree S, Buja LM, et al. Segmental systolic responses to brief ischemia and reperfusion in the hypertrophied canine left ventricle. J Am Coll Cardiol 20:994-1002, 1992.

350. Polese A, DeCesare N, Montorsi P, et al. Upward shift of the lower range of coronary flow autoregulation in hypertensive patients with hypertrophy of the left ventricle. Circulation 83:845-853. 1991.

351. MacMahon S, Peto R, Cutler J, et al. Blood pressure, stroke, and coronary heart disease. Part 1, prolonged differences in blood pressure: Prospective observational studies corrected for the regression dilution bias. Lancet 335:765-774, 1990.

352. Turnbull F. Effects of different blood-pressure- lowering regimens on major cardiovascular events: Results of prospectively-designed overviews of randomised trials. Lancet 362:1527-1535, 2003.

353. Cruickshank JM, Thorp JM, Zacharias FJ. Benefits and potential harm of lowering high blood pressure. Lancet 1:581-584, 1987.

354. Alderman MH, Ooi WL, Madhavan S, Cohen H. Treatment-induced blood pressure reduction and the risk of myocardial infarction. JAMA 262:920-924, 1989.

355. Farnett L, Mulrow CD, Linn WD, et al. The J-curve phenomenon and the treatment of hypertension. Is there a point beyond which pressure reduction is dangerous? JAMA 265:489-495, 1991.

356. Fletcher AE, Bulpitt CJ. How far should blood pressure be lowered? N Engl J Med 326:251-254, 1992.

357. McCloskey LW, Psaty BM, Koepsell TD, et al. Level of blood pressure and risk of myocardial infarction among treated hypertensive patients. Arch Intern Med 152:513-520, 1992.

358. Weinberger MH. Do no harm. Antihypertensive therapy and the "J" curve. Arch Intern Med 152:473-476, 1992.

359. Lindblad U, Rastam L, Ryden L, et al. Control of blood pressure and risk of first acute myocardial infarction: Skaraborg hypertension project. BMJ 308:681-686, 1994.

360. Hansson L. Future goals for the treatment of hypertension in the elderly with reference to STOP-hypertension, SHEP, and the MRC trial in older adults. Am J Hypertens 6 Suppl..40S-43S, 1993.

361. Benetos A, Zureik M, Morcet J, et al. A decrease in diastolic blood pressure combined with an increase in systolic blood pressure is associated with a higher cardiovascular mortality in men. J Am Coll Cardiol 35:673-680, 2000.

362. Franklin SS, Khan SA, Wong ND, et al. Is pulse pressure useful in predicting risk for coronary heart disease? The Framingham Heart Study. Circulation 100:354-360, 1999.

363. Khattar RS, Swales JD, Dore C, et al. Effect of aging on the prognostic significance of ambulatory systolic, diastolic, and pulse pressure in essential hypertension. Circulation 104: 783-789, 2001.

364. Prevention of stroke by antihypertensive drug treatment in older persons with isolated systolic hypertension. Final results of the Systolic Hypertension in the Elderly Program (SHEP). SHEP Cooperative Research Group. JAMA 265(24):3255-3264, 1991.

365. Lenfant C, Chobanian AV, Jones DW, et al. Seventh Report of the Joint National Committee on the Prevention, Detection, Evaluation, and Treatment of High Blood Pressure (JNC 7): Resetting the hypertension sails. Hypertension 41:1178-1179. 2003. [Epub 2003 May 19.]

366. Vogt M, Motz WH, Schwartzkopf B, et al. Pathophysiology and clinical aspects of hypertensive hypertrophy. Eur Heart J 14(Suppl D):2-7, 1993.

367. Yamada H, Fabris B, Allen AM, et al. Localization of angiotensin converting enzyme in the rat heart. Circ Res 68:141-149, 1991.

368. Akinboboye OO, Chou RL, Bergmann SR. Augmentation of myocardial blood flow in hypertensive heart disease by angiotensin antagonists: A comparison of lisinopril and losartan. J Am Coll Cardiol 40:703-709, 2002.

369. Diamond JA, Gharavi AG, Roychoudhury D, et al. Effect of long-term eprosartan versus enalapril antihypertensive therapy on left ventricular mass and coronary flow reserve in stage I-II hypertension. Curr Med Res & Opin 15:1-8, 1999.

370. Merrill G, Young M, Dorell S, et al. Coronary interactions between nifedipine and adenosine in the intact dog heart. Eur J Pharmacol 81:543-550, 1982.

371. Billinger M, Seiler C, Fleisch M, et al. Do beta-adrenergic blocking agents increase coronary flow reserve? J Am Coll Cardiol 38:1866-1871, 2001.

372. Perticone F, Maio R, Ceravolo R, et al. Relationship between left ventricular mass and endothelium-dependent vasodilation in never-treated hypertensive patients. Circulation 99(15):1991-1996, 1999.

373. Diamond JA, Krakoff LR, Goldman A, et al. Comparison of two calcium blockers on hemodynamics, left ventricular mass, and coronary vasodilatory in advanced hypertension. Am J Hypertens 14:231-240, 2001.

374. Perticone F, Ceravolo R, Cosco C, et al. Deletion polymorphism of angiotensin-converting enzyme gene and left ventricular hypertrophy in southern Italian patients. J Am Coll Cardiol 29:365-369, 1997.

375. Alfakih K, Maqbool A, Sivananthan M, et al. Left ventricle mass index and the common, functional, X-linked angiotensin II type-2 receptor gene polymorphism (-1332 G/A) in patients with systemic hypertension. Hypertension 43:1189-1194. 2004. [Epub 2004 May 03.]

376. Tang W, Devereux RB, Rao DC, et al. Associations between angiotensinogen gene variants and left ventricular mass and function in the HyperGEN study. Am Heart J 143:854-860, 2002.

377. Obineche EN, Frossard PM, Bokhari AM. An association study of five genetic loci and left ventricular hypertrophy amongst Gulf Arabs. Hypertens Res 24(6):635-639, 2001.

378. Fagard R, Staessen J, Thijs L, et al. Relation of left ventricular mass and filling to exercise blood pressure and rest blood pressure. Am J Cardiol 75:53-57, 1995.

379. Jones EC, Devereux RB, O'Grady MJ, et al. Relation of hemodynamic volume load to arterial and cardiac size. J Am Coll Cardiol 29:1303-1310, 1997.

380. Cabral AM, Vasquez EC, Moyses MR, et al. Sex hormone modulation of ventricular hypertrophy in sino-aortic denervated rats. Hypertension 11(Suppl 1):93-97, 1988.

381. Douglas PS, Katz SE, Weinberg EO, et al. Hypertrophic remodeling: Gender differences in the early response to left ventricular pressure overload. J Am Coll Cardiol 32:1118-1125, 1998.

382. Cubeddu LX, Aranda J, Bingh B, et al. Comparison of verapamil and propranolol for the initial treatment of hypertension: Racial differences in response. JAMA 256:2214-2221, 1986.

383. Schmieder RE, Langenfeld MR, Friedrich A, et al. Angiotensin II related to sodium excretion modulates left ventricular structure in human essential hypertension. Circulation 94(6):1304-1309, 1996.

384. Manolio TA, Levy D, Garrison RJ, et al. Relation of alcohol intake to left ventricular mass: The Framingham study. J Am Coll Cardiol 17,3:717-721, 1991.

385. Devereux RB, Drayer JIM, Chien S, et al. Whole blood viscosity as a determinant of cardiac hypertrophy in systemic hypertension. Am J Cardiol 54:592-595, 1986.

386. Rossi GP, Sacchetto A, Visentin P, et al. Changes in left ventricular anatomy and function in hypertension and primary aldosteronism. Hypertension 27:1039-1045, 1996.

387. Schmieder RE, Messerli FH, Garavaglia GE, et al. Dietary salt intake: Adeterminant of cardiac involvement in essential hypertension. Circulation 78:951-956, 1988.

388. De la Sierra A, Coca A, Paré JC, et al. Erythrocyte ion fluxes in essential hypertensive patients with left ventricular hypertrophy. Circulation 88:1628-1633, 1993.

389. Nosadini R, Semplicini A, Fioretto P, et al. Sodium-lithium countertransport and cardiorenal abnormalities in essential hypertension. Hypertension 18:191-198, 1991.

390. Levy D, Savage DD, Garrison RJ, et al. Echocardiographic criteria for left ventricular hypertrophy: The Framingham Heart Study. Am J Cardiol 59:956-960, 1987.

# Renal Protection in Chronic Kidney Disease

## Donna S. Hanes, Matthew R. Weir

Chronic kidney disease (CKD) has become a major public health problem in the United States and threatens to escalate over the next few decades. In the Third National Health and Nutrition Examination Survey (NHANES III), an estimated 3% of the adult population, or 5.6 million people, were found to have abnormal renal function, as defined by a serum creatinine greater than 1.6 mg/dl.[1] Even more concerning, the number of patients predicted to develop kidney failure by the year 2010 is twofold to threefold higher than the number today and will likely exceed 650,000.[2] However, even this approximation grossly underestimates the prevalence of kidney disease, because many people have significant proteinuria or other abnormalities that will certainly progress to end-stage renal disease (ESRD) in the face of a normal serum creatinine and normal to reduced glomerular filtration rate (GFR). Extrapolating the estimated number of patients with all stages of kidney failure indicates that more than 11% of the population has kidney disease.

It is commonly accepted that once there is a decline in the GFR, progressive loss of renal function is inevitable. This final common pathway occurs despite the lack of persistent disease activity. Moreover, a heterogeneous variety of insults including diabetes, glomerulonephritis, and hypertension all result in a similar pattern of renal injury. The histologic hallmarks of CKD include glomerulosclerosis, interstitial fibrosis, and renal cell apoptosis. Other morphologic features may include monocytic or macrophage infiltration.

The rate of loss of renal function is determined by the underlying disease process and other factors. The main determinants of renal progression include (1) activity of the primary disease process, (2) intrarenal adaptations, and (3) local and systemic mediators.[3] The latter include systemic and glomerular hypertension, proteinuria, metabolic derangements of glucose and lipids, smoking, dietary protein, anemia, race, and gender, many of which cluster together in the same patient[4] (Figure 25–1).

Therefore intensive efforts are underway to modify the rate of loss of renal function. Over the last few decades, much has been learned about the specific factors that can slow renal disease progression, affording the clinician both a means to treat specific patients and a better understanding of the underlying pathophysiology of renal injury. Currently the most important renoprotective interventions include reduction of blood pressure, inhibition of the renin-angiotensin-aldosterone system (RAAS), and reduction of proteinuria. Many trials have provided insight into the importance of each of these modifiers. By carefully following currently recommended guidelines, the rate of loss of renal function can be slowed and the need for renal replacement therapy can be significantly delayed. Ultimately this will improve patient outcomes, reduce cardio-vascular morbidity and mortality, and improve quality of life while simultaneously saving millions of Medicare dollars.

This chapter highlights the importance of the known risk factors for renal injury and outlines methods to intervene in these pathways. Emphasis is placed on the interrelationship between kidney and cardiac disease, the importance of blood pressure reduction and RAAS inhibition, and the recently recognized concept of proteinuria reduction independent of changes in blood pressure.

## ASSOCIATION BETWEEN NEPHROPATHY AND CARDIOVASCULAR RISK

The link between cardiovascular risk and nephropathy has been well described. In an analysis of the United Kingdom Prospective Diabetes Study (UKPDS), the annual cardiovascular death rate for patients with normoalbuminuria (<30 mg/dl) was 0.7%; in patients who progressed to microalbuminuria (30-299 mg/dl) and macroalbuminuria (>300 mg/dl), the annual death rates rose to 2.0% and 3.5%, respectively. Once a patient developed an increase in serum creatinine or required renal replacement therapy, the annual death rate more than tripled, to 12.1% (Table 25–1).[5]

In 1998, the National Kidney Foundation (NKF) Task Force on Cardiovascular Disease in Chronic Renal Disease issued a report emphasizing the high risk of cardiovascular disease (CVD) in CKD.[6] In this report it was demonstrated that death caused by CVD was 10 to 30 times higher in dialysis patients as compared with the general population. The task force further recommended that patients with CKD be treated aggressively as the highest risk group for CVD events. In keeping with this strategy, the Joint National Committee on Prevention, Detection, Evaluation, and Treatment of High Blood Pressure (JNC 7) classified patients with kidney disease in the same high-risk category as those with diabetes.[7] These guidelines recommend a blood pressure goal of <130/80 mm Hg in such patients.

The extent to which traditional risk factors contribute to increased CVD in CKD patients is uncertain. Certainly many patients with CKD have diabetes, older age, and left ventricular hypertrophy. However, the Framingham risk equation appears to be insufficient to capture the extent of CVD risk in patients with CKD.[8] It has been proposed that the "missing link" that explains the astounding burden of CVD in CKD may be related to nontraditional risk factors.[9] Patients with kidney failure have an inordinate amount of oxidant stress, dyslipidemia, elevated inflammatory markers, hyperhomocysteinemia, anemia, and other factors that promote atherogenesis[10] (Table 25–2). Although no direct cause-and-effect relationship

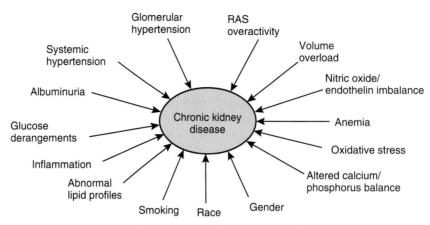

**Figure 25-1** Factors contributing to the pathophysiology of CKD.

**Table 25-1** Annual Cardiovascular Death Rates in Diabetic Patients with Various Stages of Chronic Kidney Disease

| Urinary Albumin Excretion (mg/day) | Annual Death Rate (%) |
|---|---|
| <150 mg | 0.7 |
| 150-300 mg | 2.0 |
| >300 mg | 3.5 |
| >300 mg and requiring renal replacement therapy | 12.1 |

Adapted from Adler AI, Stevens RJ, Manley SE, et al. Development and progression of nephropathy in type 2 diabetes: The United Kingdom Prospective Diabetes Study (UKPDS 64). Kidney Int 63:225-232, 2003.

**Table 25-2** Traditional and Nontraditional Cardiovascular Risk Factors in CKD

| Traditional Risk Factors | Nontraditional Risk Factors |
|---|---|
| Age | Albuminuria |
| Male sex | Homocysteine |
| Hypertension | Lipoprotein (a) |
| High LDL cholesterol | Anemia |
| Low HDL cholesterol | Abnormal calcium/phosphate |
| Diabetes | Volume overload |
| Smoking | Electrolyte imbalance |
| Physical inactivity | Oxidative stress |
| Menopause | Malnutrition |
| Family history of CVD | Inflammation |
| LVH | Sleep disturbances |
|  | Altered nitric oxide/endothelin balance |

Modified from Oberg BP, McMenamin E, Lucas FL, et al. Increased prevalence of oxidant stress and inflammation in patients with moderate to severe chronic kidney disease. Kidney Int 65:1009-1016, 2004.
LDL, low-density lipoprotein; HDL, high-density lipoprotein; CVD, cardiovascular disease; LVH, left ventricular hypertrophy.

has been established between these nontraditional risk factors and CVD events in CKD patients, ongoing clinical trials to reduce the burden of these factors will assess their importance in this patient population.

## STAGES OF CHRONIC KIDNEY DISEASE

As shown in Table 25–3, the current classification of CKD is based on the estimated glomerular filtration rate (eGFR). In the Clinical Practice Guidelines published by the NKF, CKD is defined as either kidney damage for ≥3 months (defined by structural or functional abnormalities of the kidney) or GFR <60 ml/min/1.73 m² for ≥3 months (with or without kidney damage).[11] A GFR of <60 ml/min/1.73 m² was chosen because it represents (1) the level at which mortality increases significantly, (2) loss of greater than 50% of normal renal function, and (3) the level below which laboratory abnormalities associated with CKD become manifest. Therefore there is a strong impetus to preserve the GFR above the critical threshold of 60 ml/min/1.73 m² from the perspective of both the heart and kidney.

## PROTEINURIA AS A MARKER FOR CARDIOVASCULAR DISEASE

Microalbuminuria (defined as a random urine albumin: creatinine ratio [ACR] of 30-300 mg/g) and macroalbuminuria (ACR >300 mg/g) are increasingly being recognized as independent risk factors for CVD. Large clinical trials have demonstrated that proteinuria is more predictive of a cardiovascular event than any of the traditional risk factors.[12] Microalbuminuria, the hallmark of diabetic nephropathy, is strongly associated with increased cardiovascular risk and strongly predicts renal disease progression. The greater the amount of protein excreted, the greater is the risk for renal disease progression and CVD.[13]

### Pathophysiology of Progressive Renal Failure

It is generally accepted that renal injury and loss of glomerular volume result in hyperfiltration and overcompensation by the

**Table 25-3** Classification of Chronic Kidney Disease According to the National Kidney Foundation

| GFR Stage | Description | ml/min/1.73 m² | Action |
|---|---|---|---|
| 1 | Kidney with normal or increased GFR | >90 | Diagnosis and treatment<br>Treat comorbid conditions<br>Slow progression CVD risk reduction |
| 2 | Kidney damage with mild decrease in GFR | 60-89 | Estimating progression |
| 3 | Moderately decreased GFR | 30-59 | Evaluate and treat complications |
| 4 | Severely decreased GFR | 15-29 | Preparation for renal replacement therapy |
| 5 | Kidney failure | <15 | Renal replacement |

Increased rates of adverse cardiovascular events occur when patients approach stage 3 CKD.
Adapted from Kidney Disease Outcomes Quality Initiative (K/DOQI). Clinical practice guidelines on hypertension and antihypertensive agents in chronic kidney disease. Am J Kidney Dis 43:S1-290, 2004.

remainder of the kidney. Brenner's "remnant nephron" theory postulates that it is this hyperfiltration, or overload, that causes progressive loss of the remaining glomeruli. Once the GFR is <60 ml/min/1.73 m², the remaining nephrons assume the entire filtration load. Consequently, they acquire greater oxygen demands and are then more susceptible to hypoxia and oxidative injury. Other pathophysiologic processes have also been proposed to promote progressive renal injury. In a simplified form, early insult can lead to sodium retention and angiotensin II (Ang II) production, which promote systemic and glomerular hypertension. The result is an increase in glomerulosclerosis and progressive decline in GFR.

Albuminuria has been known for many years to be a marker for kidney disease, but the pathogenic role of proteinuria has been appreciated only recently. Proteinuria frequently precedes the development of glomerulosclerosis even in the absence of glomerular hypertension.[14] Proteinuria has also been shown to have tubulotoxic effects. Remuzzi and Bertani suggest that the first step in renal deterioration is disruption of glomerular permselectivity, which may be mediated by mechanical injury to the capillary wall, or in the absence of increased glomerular capillary pressure, toxins, or immune reactants.[15] Once the permselectivity has been disrupted, the progression to kidney failure is triggered by the exposure of glomerular, mesangial, and tubulointerstitial cells to an abnormal protein load.[16] In keeping with this finding, numerous clinical trials in very diverse kidney diseases have demonstrated that the severity of proteinuria correlated best with the rate of renal function decline.[17]

However, some patients do progress to renal failure in the absence of significant proteinuria. Thus, although proteinuria is a key factor in the downward spiral that is CKD progression, it is not critical. Interestingly, Wright et al. have reported that the differences in the rate of progression of kidney disease between the different renal disorders were no longer apparent after correction for proteinuria.[18]

Several other factors contribute to progressive decline in renal function. The most important of these include hypertension and the effects of Ang II. Systemic hypertension is the second most common cause of ESRD (the most common being diabetes). For many years, the causal role of hypertension in renal disease progression was not well defined. It was clear that malignant hypertension leads to a rapid loss of renal function, but this is the cause in only about 6% of patients.[19] Milder forms of hypertension have been recognized to be associated with ESRD more recently. One of the first trials to demonstrate the association was the Multiple Risk Factor Intervention Trial (MRFIT).[20] In this large epidemiologic study with more than 332,544 middle-aged men, high blood pressure was a strong predictor of increased renal risk (Figure 25-2). The risk of renal injury was seen even at very modest elevations in blood pressure, such as a diastolic and systolic blood pressure of

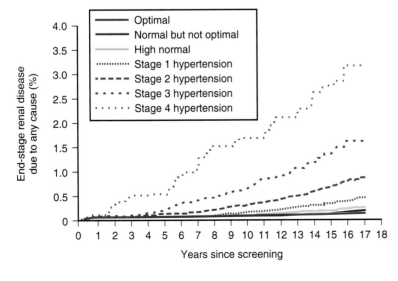

**Figure 25-2** High blood pressure and the cumulative risk of end-stage renal disease in men. (From Klag MJ, Whelton PK, Randall BL, et al. Blood pressure and end-stage renal disease in men. N Engl J Med 334:13-18, 1996.)

82 mm Hg and 127 mm Hg, respectively. Other studies have confirmed this finding in the general population.[21,22] Among African Americans, the severity of glomerulosclerosis has been shown to correlate with the level of blood pressure.[23] Perhaps the most striking data come from type 2 diabetics. In a multivariate model of diabetic kidney disease, every 10–mm Hg rise in baseline systolic blood pressure increased the risk of ESRD or death by 6.7%.[24] Moreover, patients with the highest pulse pressure, indicating a significant loss of vascular elasticity, had the highest risk for disease progression.

The difficulty with these data is that they do not explain the tremendous variability in the rate of decline of renal function among hypertensive patients. Not all patients with hypertension develop renal disease, and those who do progress toward ESRD at very different rates. Even among normotensives, there is a linear increase in the risk of renal disease as blood pressure rises from optimal to high-normal levels (Figure 25–2). Therefore, other concomitant conditions and individual renal susceptibility to hypertensive renal damage must contribute to the long-term effects of blood pressure on nephron integrity. Nonetheless, as will be discussed, strict control of blood pressure remains the cornerstone of cardiorenal protection.

## Role of Angiotensin II

The progression of renal disease is also mediated by Ang II. Ang II raises systemic blood pressure by causing direct vasoconstriction, activation of the sympathetic nervous system, and aldosterone release. This, in turn, causes salt and water retention, further contributing to elevated blood pressure. The increased blood pressure may be transmitted to the glomerulus, promoting intraglomerular hypertension and glomerular capillary damage. This is particularly concerning in the face of diseases that damage renal autoregulatory capacity. For example, in diabetics, the ability of the afferent arteriole to constrict and protect the glomerulus in the setting of systemic hypertension is blunted. This may explain why hypertension in these patients causes an accelerated decline in renal function.

Ang II also contributes to renal injury because of its differential effects on the vasculature of the nephron. It preferentially constricts the efferent arteriole, causing an increase in intraglomerular pressure and perpetuating renal injury.[25] Ang II has other detrimental effects on the nephron that are unrelated to elevated blood pressure. Importantly, it stimulates the growth of vascular smooth muscle and mesangial cells, leading to further renal impairment.[26,27] In diabetics, the tissue RAAS is also a mediator of vascular injury induced by transforming growth factor-β (TGF-β). Uncontrolled and persistent activation of the tissue RAAS with elevated levels of Ang II increases TGF-β, which causes progressive fibrosis. The local production of Ang II directly stimulates TFG-β expression, leading to increased matrix production, decreased degradation, and transformation of cell-surface integrin proteins that facilitate matrix assembly.[28,29]

## Impact of Hyperlipidemia

Hyperlipidemia, either primary or secondary to renal disease, is thought to aggravate renal damage in a number of diverse diseases.[3] Dyslipidemia is common in renal disease, particularly in patients with proteinuria. Proteinuria is associated with a distinct form of dyslipidemia, and under experimental conditions, the glomerular leakage of lipoproteins initiates a sequence of pathophysiologic responses in the kidney, promoting glomerulosclerosis and interstitial sclerosis.[30-32] The potential of lipids to cause toxic injury to the kidneys is well established. Histologic examination of kidney tissue has demonstrated glomerular deposition of lipids and lipid-laden macro-phages.[33] Apolipoprotein (apo) B and apo E often accumulate in mesangial tissue, particularly in association with proteinuria and hyperlipidemia. When hyperlipidemia is present, it is commonly associated with more-severe mesangial hypercellularity and glomerulosclerosis.

Clinical evidence suggests that hyperlipidemia modifies the rate of renal deterioration, at least in some diseases.[34] In nondiabetic kidney disease, patients with hyperlipidemia progressed to ESRD more quickly than those without it.[35] Specifically, it has been suggested that a high ratio of low-density lipoprotein (LDL):high-density lipoprotein (HDL), elevated levels of apo B or triglyceride-rich apo B, and low HDL levels all contribute to more-rapid renal deterioration.[36] However, this relationship has not been demonstrated consistently in all studies, and the effects do not appear to be substantial.

## STRATEGIES TO PRESERVE KIDNEY FUNCTION AND DELAY PROGRESSION OF KIDNEY DISEASE

Because the majority of patients with kidney disease are in the early stages of injury, the opportunity to preserve renal function and hence cardiovascular health is of primary importance. In general, the cornerstone of long-term cardiorenal protection involves three major strategies: (1) control of blood pressure, (2) inhibition of the RAAS, and (3) lifestyle modification. It is critically important to emphasize that although angiotensin-converting enzyme (ACE) inhibitors and angiotensin receptor blockers (ARB) are uniquely protective, they must be used in conjunction with other agents such as diuretics, calcium antagonists (CAs), and β-blockers to achieve the recommended blood pressure levels. Currently there is no evidence to suggest that treatment should be determined by race, age, or gender.

### Nonpharmacologic Strategies

Lifestyle interventions such as dietary salt reduction, limitation of dietary protein, regular exercise, weight loss, and smoking cessation should be encouraged in all patients with CKD.[7,37] Reducing dietary salt enhances the blood pressure–lowering effect of virtually all antihypertensive medications and also augments the reduction of proteinuria. Similarly, weight loss to a target body mass index <25 kg/m$^2$ can help lower blood pressure and reduce urinary protein excretion independent of blood pressure changes. Exercise for 30 minutes per day, most days a week, should be stressed. Smoking cessation, particularly in diabetics, should always be reinforced, because smoking can independently promote deterioration of renal function and enhance urinary protein excretion in addition to its myriad detrimental effects on overall health. It is imperative to keep in mind that the various lifestyle modifications have more impact in some ethnic groups. For example, dietary salt reduction may be more important in African Americans, who tend to be more salt sensitive. Women, particularly African Americans, carry the burden of the greatest prevalence of obesity and may benefit the most from weight reduction. Thus the efficacy of lifestyle interventions varies considerably depending on the individual patient. This is not the case with pharmacologic intervention, in that recommendations are much more uniform and effects are much more consistent.

## Achieving Target Blood Pressure Pharmacologically

Whether hypertension is the cause or consequence of CKD, numerous clinical trials have demonstrated that achievement of an optimal blood pressure is one of the most important strategies to preserve renal function (Figure 25–3).[38-40] Optimal blood pressure can be defined as systolic blood pressure <120 mm Hg. This has been demonstrated in all ethnic groups. It is also clear that most patients will require three or more medications to achieve that goal. Furthermore, the higher the baseline systolic blood pressure, the greater will be the relative benefit with drugs that inhibit the RAAS. JNC 7 recommends a goal blood pressure of <130/80 mm Hg in patients with CKD. We are far from reaching that goal. In the NHANES III subgroup that included patients with CKD, only 75% of the patients with hypertension received pharmacologic treatment. Even more alarming is the fact that only 11% of these patients reached the target blood pressure of <130/85 mm Hg and only 27% reached the target of <140/90 mm Hg.[1] Treated hypertensive individuals with elevated serum creatinine levels had a mean blood pressure of 147/77 mm Hg; an astounding 48% of these patients were prescribed only one antihypertensive medication.

Most patients require two or more antihypertensives to achieve these blood pressure goals. If the blood pressure is >20/10 mm Hg above the target, a combination of drugs should be started at the outset.[7] Because the average number of agents needed to control blood pressure in patients with CKD is 2.6 to 4.3, and the likelihood of these patients having a cardiovascular event is high, therapy should be designed with both diseases in mind.

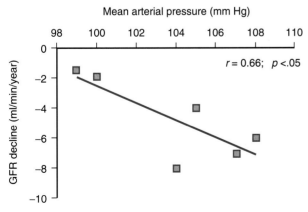

**Figure 25–3** Slower decline in renal function with lower blood pressure goals. Results of studies ≥3 years in patients with type 2 diabetic nephropathy. (From Bakris GL. Diabetes Res Clin Pract 39(suppl):S35-42, 1998.)

# DRUG CLASS EFFECTS ON THE KIDNEY

## Inhibitors of the Renin-Angiotensin-Aldosterone System: The ACE Inhibitors

There has been considerable interest in the ability of the ACE inhibitors to protect the kidney from the unrelenting deterioration that occurs with hypertension and renal insufficiency. The ACE inhibitors have a number of hemodynamic and nonhemodynamic effects that afford such protection (Box 25–1). In patients with hypertension, ACE inhibitors have the ability to restore the pressure-natriuresis relationship to normal, allowing sodium balance to be maintained at a lower arterial pressure.[41] The mechanism responsible for this effect is direct inhibition of proximal, and possibly distal, tubular sodium reabsorption.[42] This increase in renal excretory capacity plays a major role in the long-term antihypertensive efficacy of the drugs. Clinically, the increase in sodium excretion is transitory because the reduction in arterial pressure returns sodium excretion to normal. However, the maintenance of normal sodium excretion at lower arterial pressures correlates with increased excretion in the setting of hypertension.[42] After several days, inhibition of Ang II and aldosterone contribute to the natriuresis.[43-45]

The long-term effects of ACE inhibitors on water excretion are less certain. ACE inhibitors induce an initial increase in free water clearance, but there are no long-term changes in total body weight, plasma, or extracellular fluid volume.[46] The decrease in aldosterone caused by ACE inhibition also correlates with decreased potassium excretion,[45] particularly in patients with impaired renal function. The antikaliuretic effect appears to be transient but can be exacerbated by concomitant administration of potassium-sparing diuretics, supplements, and nonsteroidal antiinflammatory drugs and should be monitored rigorously.

Potential renoprotective effects noted in experimental models include attenuation of oxidative stress,[47] scavenging free radicals, and attenuating lipid peroxidation.[48] ACE inhibitors also ameliorate the deranged lipid profile in patients with nephrotic-range proteinuria, which may impact the rate of progression of renal failure.[49,50] The clinical importance of these effects is under investigation.

Insofar as the degree of proteinuria correlates best with the rate of decline of renal function, and a decrease in proteinuria correlates better with renal function outcome than a reduction in blood pressure, reduction of proteinuria has a substantial

**Box 25–1** Potential Renoprotective Effects of ACE Inhibitors

Restore pressure/natriuresis relationship to normal
Inhibit tubular sodium resorption
Decrease arterial pressure
Decrease aldosterone production
Decrease proteinuria
Improve altered lipid profiles
Decrease renal blood flow
Decrease filtration fraction
Decrease renal vascular resistance
Reduce scarring and fibrosis
Attenuate oxidative stress and free radicals

impact.[51] All ACE inhibitors decrease urinary protein excretion[52] in normotensive and hypertensive patients with renal disease of various origins.[53-55] Individual response rates vary from a rise of 31% to a fall of 100% and are strongly influenced by drug dose and changes in dietary sodium. There is a clear dose-response relationship between increasing doses and reduction of proteinuria that is not dependent on changes in blood pressure, renal plasma flow (RPF), or GFR. Furthermore, the effect of ACE inhibitors on reduction of proteinuria is abolished with high salt intake.[56] In normotensive diabetics, studies demonstrate that ACE inhibitors can normalize GFR, markedly attenuate the progression of renal disease, and normalize microalbuminuria.[57] The effect is noted in the first month of therapy and is maximal at 14 months.

Several mechanisms account for the reduction in urinary protein excretion seen with ACE inhibitors: a decrease in glomerular capillary hydrostatic pressure, a decrease in mesangial uptake and clearance of macromolecules, and improved glomerular basement membrane permselectivity.[58] ACE inhibitors have superior antiproteinuric efficacy when compared with other classes of antihypertensive agents, with the exception of ARBs. The antiproteinuric effect is additive with the ARBs and does not depend on changes in creatinine clearance, GRF, or blood pressure.[59,60] Clinical trials also demonstrate a superior renoprotective effect of ACE inhibitor treatment in African Americans, once thought not to benefit from this class. In the African American Study of Kidney Disease and Hypertension (AASK) trial, hypertensive patients with proteinuria >300 mg/day had a much slower rate of progression of kidney disease when treated with an ACE inhibitor when compared with a dihydropyridine CA or β-blocker.[61]

Evidence suggests that the majority of vasoconstrictor action of Ang II is confined to the efferent arteriole. ACE inhibitors preferentially dilate the efferent arteriole by reducing the systemic and intrarenal levels of Ang II. The result is a reduction in intraglomerular capillary pressure. ACE inhibitors uniformly increase renal blood flow, decrease filtration fraction, have variable to no effect on GFR, decrease renal vascular resistance, reduce urinary protein excretion, and impair microvascular autoregulation in patients with hypertension. Long-term administration is associated with a decrease in renal perfusion, with a tendency to higher filtration fraction and lower afferent resistances. Marked improvement in GFR occurs and is sustained for up to 3 years.[62,63]

Many patients with impaired renal function exhibit a reversible fall in GFR with ACE inhibitor therapy that is not detrimental. Numerous studies demonstrate that the GFR declines initially because of the hemodynamic changes, but the long-term reduction in perfusion pressure is renoprotective. In fact, patients with the greatest initial decline in GFR have the slowest rate of loss of renal function over time.[64] It should be emphasized that ACE inhibitors should not be withdrawn immediately if an increase in serum creatinine is noted; a 20% to 30% decline in GFR can be expected, and close monitoring is warranted. Inappropriate, early withdraw of ACE inhibitors for reductions in GFR is one of the most common mistakes made when treating patients with renal disease.

In patients with an activated RAAS, ACE inhibitors cause a decrease in GFR and can precipitate acute renal failure. Patients with severe bilateral renal artery stenosis, unilateral renal artery stenosis of a solitary kidney, severe hypertensive nephrosclerosis, volume depletion, congestive heart failure, cirrhosis, or a transplanted kidney are at high risk for renal deterioration with ACE inhibitors.[65,66] These patients typically have a precipitous drop in blood pressure and deterioration of renal function when treated with ACE inhibitors. In these states of reduced renal perfusion caused by low effective arterial circulating volume or reduced flow through an obstructed artery, the maintenance of renal blood flow and GFR is highly dependent on increased efferent arteriolar vasoconstriction mediated by Ang II. Interruption of the increased tone causes a critical reduction in perfusion pressure and can lead to dramatic reductions in GFR and urinary flow, as well as worsening of renal ischemia, and in select cases, anuria.[67] Therefore a reduction of GFR greater than 30% should prompt an evaluation for renal artery stenosis.

## Renoprotective Effects of Angiotensin II Type 1 Receptor Antagonists

Intrarenal Ang II receptors are widely distributed in the afferent and efferent arterioles, glomerular mesangial cells, inner stripe of the outer medulla, and medullary interstitial cells and on the luminal and basolateral membranes of the proximal and distal tubular cells, collecting ducts, podocytes, and macula densa cells.[68] The majority of receptors are of the $AT_1$ subclass. Ang II, predominantly produced locally but also delivered in the systemic circulation, interacts with its receptors to exert its effects. Ang II may work at the cell surface through a second messenger pathway or the receptor ligand complex in the intracellular compartment following internalization of and release of Ang II into the intracellular fluid. Studies suggest that the majority of renal interstitial Ang II is formed at sites not readily accessible to ACE inhibition or is formed via non-ACE pathways.[69] ARBs antagonize the binding of Ang II to the $AT_1$ receptor and cause a number of intrarenal changes. The renal hemodynamic responses to $AT_1$ receptor blockade are variable depending on the counteracting influences of the decrease in arterial pressure.[70] Decreases in systemic arterial pressure caused by ARBs may be associated with compensatory activation of the intrarenal sympathetic nervous system, resulting in decreased renal function.[71] This effect is more pronounced in sodium-depleted states in which activation of the RAAS helps maintain arterial and renal pressure.[72]

In contrast, direct intrarenal infusions of ARBs cause an increase in sodium excretion.[73] This has been shown to be by direct inhibition of sodium reabsorption in the proximal tubules but may also be due to hemodynamic changes in medullary blood flow and tubular absorption in distal nephron segments.[74] Because Ang II blockade enhances the ability of the kidneys to excrete sodium, sodium balance can be maintained at lower arterial pressures. Ang II blockade also reduces tubuloglomerular feedback sensitivity by decreasing macula densa transport of sodium chloride to the afferent arteriole.[75] This leads to an increased delivery of sodium chloride to the distal segments for excretion without compensatory changes in GFR.

A unique property of the ARB losartan is its ability to lower serum uric acid in a dose-dependent manner. It appears to inhibit urate reabsorption in the proximal tubule, resulting in a reduction of serum urate by approximately 0.4 mg/dl.[76] The clinical implications of this effect are unknown, but it may be beneficial, because it has been suggested that hyperuricemia is a risk factor for renal disease progression and coronary artery disease.[3] It has been suggested that some of the cardiovascular and renal benefits of losartan are a direct result of its uricosuric effect.[77]

ARB treatment of hypertensive patients with normal or impaired renal function elicits renal responses similar to or slightly greater than those elicited by ACE inhibitor treatment.[78,79] In addition to decreases in systolic and diastolic blood pressure, patients demonstrate increases in renal blood flow, decreases in filtration fraction and renal vascular resistance, and no substantial changes in GFR.[80] These effects are likely a result of combined decreases in both preglomerular and postglomerular resistances. It has been suggested that elevated intrarenal Ang II levels in the face of $AT_1$ receptor blockade stimulate $AT_2$ receptors, which can increase preglomerular vasodilator actions of bradykinin, cyclic guanosine monophosphate, and nitric oxide.[81,82] ACE inhibitors can potentiate this effect.[80] The clinical importance of this finding has yet to be established.

Ang II blockade may significantly reduce GFR in underperfused kidneys, and patients with low perfusion pressures, dehydration, or renal artery stenosis may experience severe decreases in GFR but less severe than with ACE inhibitors.[83,84]

Under conditions of overperfusion, such as hypertension associated with glomerulosclerosis and nephron loss or diabetes, Ang II blockade is protective. Such patients often have a suboptimal suppression of the RAAS. The lowering of efferent arteriole resistance reduces intraglomerular hydrostatic pressure, attenuating the progression of renal injury, and increases renal sodium excretory capacity. In concert with the reduction in systemic arterial pressure, these actions provide more renal protection with the ARBs than with other classes of antihypertensive agents in the presence of equivalent reductions of blood pressure.[13,85-87]

Urinary protein excretion is significantly decreased with ARBs and parallels findings with ACE inhibitors. Antiproteinuric effects have been described in diabetic and nondiabetic patients and those with renal transplants.[88] Interestingly, in individual patients, the course of long-term renal function correlates with the antiproteinuric response to therapy.[89] The antiproteinuric effect has a slow onset. The dose-response curves for the antiproteinuric effects differ from those of the antihypertensive effects. The maximal effect occurs at 3 to 4 weeks, and the peak of the dose-response curve has not been determined.[90] Whether

the antiproteinuric effects of the ARBs are equivalent to, or better than, those of ACE inhibitors remains to be determined. ARBs and ACE inhibitors appear to have additive and similar hemodynamic and antiproteinuric effects.[51] In a number of trials, ACE inhibitor or ARB therapy reduced proteinuria by up to 40%, whereas combined therapy resulted in a 70% reduction of proteinuria with no further changes in blood pressure.[91,92] Such findings suggest that the mechanism of antiproteinuric effect may differ between the two classes. Although evidence in support of this approach is limited,[11] some authorities recommend that patients on ACE inhibitor therapy with persistent hypertension or proteinuria be treated with additional ARB therapy.[93] This combination appears to reduce intrarenal Ang II and TGF-β levels more than high doses of either agent alone.[94,95] Furthermore, combined ACE inhibitor–ARB treatment has been shown to be more effective than monotherapy with either class of agent in retarding the progression of nondiabetic renal disease (Figure 25–4).[60]

Clinical trials demonstrate superior antiproteinuric effects of the ARBs when compared with conventional antihypertensive treatment. In patients with diabetic nephropathy, ARBs reduce macroproteinuria up to 28% and can revert microproteinuria to normal in 33% of patients (Figure 25–5).[13,86,87] Long-term renoprotection with these agents substantially retards the progression of renal disease. Patients with diabetic nephropathy and >900 mg/dl protein per day receiving ARBs had a 20% reduction in the risk of composite endpoints (doubling of serum creatinine, developing ESRD, or death).[13,86] The risk of doubling of the serum creatinine was 33% lower in the ARB arm than in the placebo group and 37% lower than in the amlodipine arm. These effects were independent of changes in blood pressure. Thus, strong clinical trial evidence indicates that ARBs are more effective than other drug classes in slowing the progression of kidney disease.[11,96] Studies currently underway will assess whether very-high-dose ARBs and/or ARB/ACE inhibitor combinations will provide even more protection. Remarkably, analyses of the results of currently available trials have demonstrated for the first time that the reduction in proteinuria with ARBs correlates with a reduction in cardiovascular morbidity and mortality (Figure 25–6).[97,98]

Like the ACE inhibitors, ARBs have multiple nonhemodynamic effects that may contribute to renoprotection. These include antiproliferative actions on the vasculature and

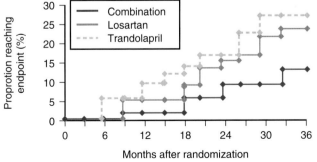

| No. at risk | | | | | | | |
|---|---|---|---|---|---|---|---|
| Losartan | 89 | 88 | 84 | 79 | 65 | 59 | 47 |
| Trandolapril | 86 | 85 | 83 | 75 | 72 | 63 | 58 |
| Combination | 88 | 87 | 86 | 83 | 76 | 73 | 67 |

**Figure 25–4** Proportion of patients reaching renal endpoints treated with a single ACE inhibitor versus an ARB versus both. (From Nakao N, Yoshimura A, Morita H, et al. Combination treatment of angiotensin-II receptor blocker and angiotensin-converting-enzyme inhibitor in non-diabetic renal disease [COOPERATE]: A randomized controlled trial. Lancet 361:117-124, 2003.)

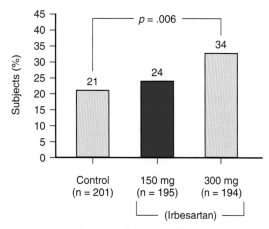

**Figure 25–5** Normalization of urinary albumin excretion rate in patients with diabetic nephropathy treated with irbesartan versus standard care. (Adapted from Parving HH, Lehnert H, Brochner-Mortensen J, et al. The effect of irbesartan on the development of diabetic nephropathy in patients with type 2 diabetes. N Engl J Med 345:870-878, 2001.)

mesangium, inhibition of TGF-$\beta$,[95,99] inhibition of atherogenesis[100,101] and vascular deterioration,[102] reduced superoxide production and increased nitric oxide bioavailability,[103,104] reduced collagen formation, reduced mesangial matrix production, improved vascular wall remodeling, decreased vasoconstrictor effects of endothelin-1, improved endothelial function,[103] reduced oxidative stress, and protection from calcineurin inhibitor injury. The clinical importance of these effects is currently under investigation.

An important consideration when using ACE inhibitors or ARBs is the potential for the development of hyperkalemia. This complication occurs in up to 10% of patients and is more common in diabetics and those with impaired renal function.[105] Serious hyperkalemia is found in only 1% to 2% of patients. Hyperkalemia often results from one or more of three disturbances that impair the excretion of potassium: decreased delivery of sodium to the distal nephron, aldosterone deficien-

cy, and abnormal functioning of the collecting duct.[106] These abnormalities can result from the effects of other drugs, from underlying disease, or from both. Management of hyperkalemia is outlined in Box 25–2.

## β-Blockers

β-Adrenergic receptors in the kidney mediate vasodilation and increase renin secretion. β-Adrenergic blockers might be expected to influence renal blood flow and GFR through their effects on cardiac output and blood pressure in addition to their direct effects on intrarenal adrenergic receptors. $\beta_2$ Receptors predominate in the kidney; thus the specificity of a β-blocker will influence its effect on the kidney. Acute administration of β-blockers usually results in a reduction in GFR and effective RPF.[107] Chronic administration is associated with a 10% to 20% decrement in RPF and GFR.[108] This modest reduction in GFR is probably not of great clinical importance. In contrast to the effect with RAAS inhibitors, the reduction in GFR with β-blockers does not seem to correlate with the stabilization of renal function.[108]

## Renoprotective Effects of Calcium Antagonists

The potential benefits of CAs in acute and chronic kidney disease have been well described. There are multiple mechanisms whereby they alter or protect renal function, notably as natriuretics, vasodilators, and antiproteinuric agents. All CAs exert natriuretic and diuretic effects. Experimental and clinical studies in hypertension indicate that the increase in sodium excretion is, in part, independent of vasodilation or changes in GFR, renal blood flow, or filtration fraction.[110,111] This effect likely is the result of changes in renal sodium handling that can potentiate the antihypertensive effects of CA on the vasculature. In normotensive subjects, CAs increase sodium excretion from 10% to 240%, often in the absence of changes in blood pressure.[112]

The natriuretic effect appears to persist long term. Chronic administration of CAs to hypertensive patients results in a

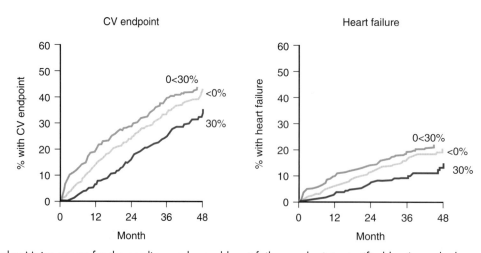

**Figure 25–6** Kaplan-Meier curves for the cardiovascular and heart failure endpoints stratified by 6-month changes in albuminuria. Percent represents change from baseline proteinuria. (Adapted from de Zeeuw D, Remuzzi G, Parving HH, et al. Proteinuria, a target for renoprotection in patients with type 2 diabetic nephropathy: Lessons from RENAAL. Kidney Int 65:2309-2320, 2004.)

**Box 25–2** Approach to Patients at Risk for Hyperkalemia Caused by Inhibitors of the Renin-Angiotensin System

Discontinue drugs that interfere with renal potassium excretion, such as nonsteroidal antiinflammatory drugs, cyclooxygenase-2 inhibitors, and trimethoprim-sulfamethoxazole.
Inquire about the use of herbal preparations.
Prescribe low-potassium diet; inquire about the use of potassium-containing salt substitutes.
Prescribe thiazide or loop diuretics (loop diuretics are necessary when the creatinine clearance in less than 30 ml/min).
Consider prescribing sodium bicarbonate to correct metabolic acidosis.
Initiate therapy with low-dose ACE inhibitor or ARB.
Measure potassium 1 week after initiating therapy or changing doses.
If potassium increases to >5.5 mmol/L, decrease the dose of the drug; if the patient is taking a combination of ACE inhibitor and ARB, and/or aldosterone-receptor blocker, discontinue one and recheck potassium.
The dose of spironolactone should not exceed 25 mg when used in combination with ACE inhibitors or ARBs and should not be given at all when the creatinine clearance is less than 30 ml/min.
If potassium is consistently >5.5 mmol/L despite these steps, discontinue drugs.

Adapted from Palmer BF. Managing hyperkalemia caused by inhibitors of the renin-angiotensin-aldosterone system. N Engl J Med 351:585-592, 2004.

cumulative sodium deficit that is abruptly reversed with discontinuation of the drug.[113] Natriuresis commonly occurs 3 to 6 hours after the morning dose[114,115]; the net negative sodium balance plateaus after the first 2 to 3 days but persists throughout the duration of therapy. There are no significant changes in long-term body weight, potassium, urea nitrogen, catecholamines, or GFR.

## Renal Hemodynamic Effects of Calcium Antagonists

The renal hemodynamic effects of CAs are variable and depend primarily on which vasoconstrictors modulate renal vascular tone.[111] Experimentally, CAs improve GFR in the presence of the vasoconstrictors norepinephrine, Ang II, and others by preferentially attenuating afferent arteriolar resistance.[116] The efferent arteriole appears to be refractory to this vasodilatory effect. Patients with primary hypertension appear to be more sensitive to the renal hemodynamic effects of CAs than are normotensives, and these effects are more pronounced with advancing kidney disease.[117,118] Acute administration of CAs results in little change, or augmentation of the GFR and RPF, no change in the filtration fraction, and reduction of renal vascular resistance. Chronic administration is not associated with significant changes in renal hemodynamics. The response is maximal in the presence of Ang II, which selectively causes postglomerular vasoconstriction. Clinically significant changes are counteracted by the reduction in renal perfusion pressure coincident with the reduction in blood pressure.

The long-term effects of CAs on renal function are controversial and variable. In hypertensive patients, the effects on renal hemodynamics vary. Some patients exhibit no change in GFR, whereas others have an exaggerated increase in GFR and RPF. Normotensive patients with a family history of hypertension also have exaggerated hemodynamic responses.[119]

## Antiproteinuric Effects of Calcium Antagonists

The antiproteinuric effects of CAs are also controversial and variable with respect to the class of drug and the level of blood pressure reduction achieved.[120,121] Some dihydropyridines may increase protein excretion by up to 40%. It is not clear whether this is a result of vasodilation of the afferent arteriole, resulting in increased glomerular capillary pressure, because CAs directly impair renal autoregulation. Changes in glomerular basement membrane permeability or increased intrarenal Ang II may also play a role in the increased proteinuria associated with CAs.[122,123] In contrast, felodipine, diltiazem, and verapamil do not appear to have a proteinuric effect and may lower protein excretion, possibly by decreasing efferent arteriolar tone and glomerular pressure. The clinical implications remain to be determined.

Large clinical trials underscore the controversy. In African Americans with hypertension and mild to moderate renal insufficiency and proteinuria >1 g/day, ACE inhibitor therapy was associated with a renoprotective effect, whereas the dihydropyridine CA amlodipine was associated with deteriorating renal function.[124] This effect was independent of blood pressure reduction and was more evident in proteinuric patients; it also occurred in patients with baseline proteinuria <300 mg/day. Hypertensive patients with diabetic nephropathy also fare worse with amlodipine therapy as compared with therapy with an ARB.[86] In one study, patients experienced higher rates of progression of renal disease in the amlodipine and placebo groups as compared with the ARB group. This effect was also independent of blood pressure levels achieved. There were no significant differences in cardiovascular death, myocardial infarction, or stroke between the treatment groups.[125] Coadministration of amlodipine with an ARB does not abrogate the renoprotective effect of the ARB.[13] It is postulated that selective dilation of the afferent arteriole induced by CAs favors an increase in glomerular capillary pressure that accelerates renal disease progression.

## Additional Renoprotective Effects

CAs possess many nonhemodynamic effects that may afford renoprotection. In addition to lowering blood pressure, they act as free radical scavengers; retard renal growth and kidney weight[126,127]; reduce the entrapment of macromolecules in the mesangium[128]; attenuate the mitogenic actions of platelet-derived growth factor and platelet-activating factor[127]; block mitochondrial overload of calcium[129]; decrease lipid peroxidation; decrease glomerular basement membrane thickness; augment the antioxidant activities of superoxide dismutase, catalase, and glutathione peroxidase; inhibit metalloproteinase-1 and collagenolytic activity; suppress the expression of the angiogenic growth factors, vascular endothelial growth factor, β-fibrogenic growth factor, TGF-β, and endothelial nitric oxide synthetase[130]; and prevent renal cortical remodeling and scarring[131,132] (Box 25–3). The clinical implications of these findings remain speculative at present.

## Diuretics

Although diuretics have a mechanism of action centered in the kidney, they have no specific renoprotective effect beyond blood pressure lowering. Moreover, thiazides, the recommended first-line agents in the treatment of uncomplicated hypertension, lose their efficacy in patients with CKD and an estimated GFR of <30 ml/min.[133] Thus thiazides are a much less important class of drugs for CKD patients. A loop diuretic is often needed to help control extracellular fluid volume and blood pressure in such patients, but no data suggest that loop diuretics improve cardiovascular or renal survival.

## ADDITIONAL STRATEGIES TO DELAY RENAL DISEASE PROGRESSION

### Treatment of Hyperlipidemia

Pharmacologic reduction of elevated lipids attenuates the progression of renal disease in experimental animals.[134] In humans the data are very limited but suggest that the reduction of lipids with drugs can slow the rate of progression of renal disease. For example, Bianchi et al. conducted a prospective, randomized, controlled trial to evaluate the effects of 1 year of treatment with atorvastatin versus no treatment on proteinuria and progression of renal disease in patients with CKD.[135] The authors concluded that treatment with atorvastatin, added to standard therapy with a regimen of ACE inhibitors or ARBs, may reduce proteinuria and the rate of decline of renal function in patients with proteinuria, CKD, and hypercholesterolemia. Multiple small trials with agents that inhibit hydroxymethylglutaryl-coenzyme A (HMG-CoA) reductase have demonstrated similar findings. These agents reduce total cholesterol, LDL cholesterol, and apo B.[136-138] In these trials, a reduction in proteinuria was achieved but no significant changes in the course of renal disease were noted. It has been suggested that the time course of the trials was not sufficient to detect such changes, because the antiproteinuric effects may not be manifest for up to a year.[139] A meta-analysis of the results of 13 clinical trials of antihyperlipidemic drugs on renal function showed a tendency toward renal preservation with lipid reduction.[140]

Because CKD is considered a coronary heart disease equivalent, the NKF Task Force on Cardiovascular Disease recommends aggressive management of all risk factors in patients with CKD. The Kidney Foundation Kidney Disease Outcomes Quality Initiative developed guidelines for the management of dyslipidemias in CKD patients. The Working Group recommended that LDL cholesterol levels should be targeted to <100 mg/dl in patients with CKD.[11]

### Management of Anemia

Interstitial fibrosis plays a critical role in the progression of renal disease by reducing the ability of the kidney to synthesize erythropoietin. Consequently, anemia is perpetuated and the remaining functioning tissue, with a higher metabolic demand than normal, becomes more susceptible to ischemic injury and further fibrosis. Analyses of the biologic effects of erythropoietin and the pathophysiology of interstitial fibrosis suggest that treatment with recombinant human erythropoietin (epoetin) may slow the progression of CKD.[141] Exogenous epoetin both decreases interstitial fibrosis and protects against its consequences (Figure 25–7). Clinical trial evidence supports this theory. In one trial, the investigators compared 20 patients with CKD who were treated with epoetin with 43 patients who had a similar degree of renal failure but who were less anemic and thus did not receive epoetin. The rate of decline of creatinine clearance did not change over time in the control group, whereas in the treated group, it was significantly slower after epoetin therapy had been started.[142]

## SUMMARY

The importance of recognizing early kidney disease is now becoming evident in clinical practice. Major advances have allowed us to better understand renal disease progression, and the last decade has been marked by important discoveries that can slow the rate of decline in renal function. Although several dietary and lifestyle changes may help, by far the most important strategies to delay renal disease progression include strict blood pressure control and inhibition of the RAAS.

Because the reduction of proteinuria predicts long-term renal and cardiovascular protection, proteinuria cannot be overlooked. Proteinuria is not only a determinant of renal risk but also of the benefit that can be attained by pharmacologic intervention. Promising trials are now underway to assess the effects of high-dose RAAS inhibition. In the future we may be

---

**Box 25–3** Renal Protective Mechanisms of CAs

↓ Blood pressure
↓ Proteinuria
Scavenge free radicals
↓ Kidney growth
↓ Mesangial molecule entrapment
Attenuate antigenic PDGF and PAF
Block mitochondrial calcium overload
↓ Lipid peroxidation
↓ Glomerular basement membrane thickness
Augment antioxidant effects of superoxide
　　dismutase/catalase and glutathione peroxidase
Inhibit collagenolytic activity
Suppress angiogenic growth factors
Prevent renal cortical remodeling
Ameliorate cyclosporine A toxicity
Block thromboxane- and endothelin-induced
　　vasoconstriction

PDGF, platelet-derived growth factor; PAF, platelet-activated factor.

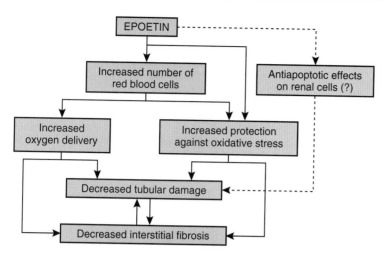

**Figure 25-7** Schematic representation of the potential beneficial effects of epoetin treatment. (Adapted from Rossert J, Fouqueray B, Boffa JJ. Anemia management and the delay of chronic renal failure progression. J Am Soc Nephrol 14:S173-S177, 2003.)

titrating the dose of RAAS inhibitors to the degree of proteinuria rather than to blood pressure. For the present, any potential intervention that may benefit a patient with early nephropathy should be started.

## References

1. Coresh J, Wei GL, McQuillan G, et al. Prevalence of high blood pressure and elevated serum creatinine level in the United States: Findings from the third National Health and Nutrition Examination Survey (1988-1994). Arch Intern Med 161:1207-1216, 2001.
2. U.S. Renal Data System. USRDS 2003 Annual Data Report: Atlas of End-Stage Renal Disease in the United States. National Institutes of Health. National Institute of Diabetes and Digestive and Kidney Diseases. Bethesda, MD, NIH, 2003.
3. Navis G, de Jong PE, de Zeeuw D. Specific Pharmacologic Approaches to Clinical Renoprotection, Ch. 56. In Brenner B (ed). Brenner & Rector's The Kidney, 7th ed. Philadelphia, Saunders, 2004; pp 2453-2490.
4. Ejerblad E, Fored CM, Lindblad P, et al. Association between smoking and chronic renal failure in a nationwide population-based case-control study. J Am Soc Nephrol 15:2178-2185, 2004.
5. Adler AI, Stevens RJ, Manley SE, et al. Development and progression of nephropathy in type 2 diabetes: The United Kingdom Prospective Diabetes Study (UKPDS 64). Kidney Int 63:225-232, 2003.
6. Levey AS, Beto JA, Coronado BE, et al. Controlling the epidemic of cardiovascular disease in chronic renal disease: What do we know? What do we need to learn? Where do we go from here? National Kidney Foundation Task Force on Cardiovascular Disease. Am J Kidney Dis 32:853-906, 1998.
7. Chobanian AV, Bakris GL, Black HR, et al. The seventh Report of the Joint National Committee on Prevention, Detection, Evaluation, and Treatment of High Blood Pressure: The JNC 7 report. JAMA 289:2560-2572, 2003.
8. Sarnak MJ, Levey AS, Schoolwerth AC, et al. Kidney disease as a risk factor for development of cardiovascular disease: A statement from the American Heart Association Councils on Kidney in Cardiovascular Disease, High Blood Pressure Research, Clinical Cardiology, and Epidemiology and Prevention. Hypertension 42:1050-1065, 2003.
9. Muntner P, Hamm LL, Kusek JW, et al. The prevalence of non-traditional risk factors for coronary heart disease in patients with chronic kidney disease. Ann Intern Med 140:9-17, 2004.
10. Oberg BP, McMenamin E, Lucas FL, et al. Increased prevalence of oxidant stress and inflammation in patients with moderate to severe chronic kidney disease. Kidney Int 65:1009-1016, 2004.
11. K/DOQI clinical practice guidelines on hypertension and anti-hypertensive agents in chronic kidney disease. Am J Kidney Dis 43:S1-S290, 2004.
12. Heart Outcomes Prevention Evaluation Study Investigators. Effects of ramipril on cardiovascular and microvascular outcomes in people with diabetes mellitus: Results of the HOPE study and MICRO-HOPE substudy. Lancet 355:253-259, 2000.
13. Brenner BM, Cooper ME, de Zeeuw D, et al. Effects of losartan on renal and cardiovascular outcomes in patients with type 2 diabetes and nephropathy. N Engl J Med 345:861-869, 2001.
14. Fogo A, Yoshida Y, Glick AD, et al. Serial micropuncture analysis of glomerular function in two rat models of glomerular sclerosis. J Clin Invest 82:322-330, 1988.
15. Remuzzi G, Bertani T. Is glomerulosclerosis a consequence of altered glomerular permeability to macromolecules? Kidney Int 38:384-394, 1990.
16. Gansevoort RT, Mimran A, de Zeeuw D, et al. AT1 receptor antagonists and the kidney. In Epstein M, Brunner H (eds). Angiotensin II Receptor Antagonists. Philadelphia, Hanley & Belfus, 2001; pp 295-316.
17. Gansevoort RT, Navis GJ, Wapstra FH, et al. Proteinuria and progression of renal disease: Therapeutic implications. Curr Opin Nephrol Hypertens 6:133-140, 1997.
18. Wright JP, Salzano S, Brown CB, et al. Natural history of chronic renal failure: A reappraisal. Nephrol Dial Transplant 7:379-383, 1992.
19. Agodoa LY, Jones CA, Held PJ. End-stage renal disease in the USA: Data from the United States Renal Data System. Am J Nephrol 16:7-16, 1996.
20. Klag MJ, Whelton PK, Randall BL, et al. Blood pressure and end-stage renal disease in men. N Engl J Med 334:13-18, 1996.
21. Iseki K, Iseki C, Ikemiya Y, et al. Risk of developing end-stage renal disease in a cohort of mass screening. Kidney Int 49:800-805, 1996.
22. Bakris GL, Williams M, Dworkin L, et al. Preserving renal function in adults with hypertension and diabetes: A consensus approach. National Kidney Foundation Hypertension and Diabetes Executive Committees Working Group. Am J Kidney Dis 36:646-661, 2000.
23. Fogo A, Breyer JA, Smith MC, et al. Accuracy of the diagnosis of hypertensive nephrosclerosis in African Americans: A report from the African American Study of Kidney Disease (AASK) Trial. AASK Pilot Study Investigators. Kidney Int 51:244-252, 1997.
24. Bakris GL, Weir MR, Shanifar S, et al. Effects of blood pressure level on progression of diabetic nephropathy: Results from the RENAAL study. Arch Intern Med 163:1555-1565, 2003.
25. Eiskjaer H, Sorensen SS, Danielsen H, et al. Glomerular and tubular antinatriuretic actions of low-dose angiotensin II infusion in man. J Hypertens 10:1033-1040, 1992.

26. Dubey RK, Jackson EK, Rupprecht HD, et al. Factors controlling growth and matrix production in vascular smooth muscle and glomerular mesangial cells. Curr Opin Nephrol Hypertens 6:88-105, 1997.

27. Wolf G, Ziyadeh FN. The role of angiotensin II in diabetic nephropathy: Emphasis on nonhemodynamic mechanisms. Am J Kidney Dis 29:153-163, 1997.

28. Hanes DS, Nahar A, Weir MR. The tissue renin-angiotensin-aldosterone system in diabetes mellitus. Curr Hypertens Rep 6:98-105, 2004.

29. Houlihan CA, Akdeniz A, Tsalamandris C, et al. Urinary transforming growth factor-beta excretion in patients with hypertension, type 2 diabetes, and elevated albumin excretion rate: Effects of angiotensin receptor blockade and sodium restriction. Diabetes Care 25:1072-1077, 2002.

30. Keane WF, Kasiske BL, O'Donnell MP, et al. The role of altered lipid metabolism in the progression of renal disease: Experimental evidence. Am J Kidney Dis 17:38-42, 1991.

31. Moorhead JF. Lipids and the pathogenesis of kidney disease. Am J Kidney Dis 17:65-70, 1991.

32. Joven J, Villabona C, Vilella E, et al. Abnormalities of lipoprotein metabolism in patients with the nephrotic syndrome. N Engl J Med 323:579-584, 1990.

33. Lee HS, Lee JS, Koh HI, et al. Intraglomerular lipid deposition in routine biopsies. Clin Nephrol 36:67-75, 1991.

34. Manttari M, Tiula E, Alikoski T, et al. Effects of hypertension and dyslipidemia on the decline in renal function. Hypertension 26:670-675, 1995.

35. Maschio G, Oldrizzi L, Rugiu C, et al. Factors affecting progression of renal failure in patients on long-term dietary protein restriction. Kidney Int Suppl 22:S49-S52, 1987.

36. Levey AS, Gassman JJ, Hall PM, et al. Assessing the progression of renal disease in clinical studies: Effects of duration of follow-up and regression to the mean. Modification of Diet in Renal Disease (MDRD) Study Group. J Am Soc Nephrol 1:1087-1094, 1991.

37. Lakkis J, Weir MR. Pharmacological strategies for kidney function preservation: Are there differences by ethnicity? Adv Ren Replace Ther 11:24-40, 2004.

38. Peterson JC, Adler S, Burkart JM, et al. Blood pressure control, proteinuria, and the progression of renal disease. The Modification of Diet in Renal Disease Study. Ann Intern Med 123:754-762, 1995.

39. Ruilope LM, Salvetti A, Jamerson K, et al. Renal function and intensive lowering of blood pressure in hypertensive participants of the hypertension optimal treatment (HOT) study. J Am Soc Nephrol 12:218-225, 2001.

40. Hebert LA, Kusek JW, Greene T, et al. Effects of blood pressure control on progressive renal disease in blacks and whites. Modification of Diet in Renal Disease Study Group. Hypertension 30:428-435, 1997.

41. Hall JE. Angiotensin converting enzyme inhibition: Renal effects and their role in reducing arterial pressure. *In* MacGregor GA, Sever PS (eds). Current Advances in ACE Inhibition. London, Churchill Livingstone, 1989.

42. Atlas SA, Case DB, Sealey JE, et al. Interruption of the renin-angiotensin system in hypertensive patients by captopril induces sustained reduction in aldosterone secretion, potassium retention and natruiresis. Hypertension 1:274-280, 1979.

43. Hollenberg NK, Swartz SL, Passan DR, et al. Increased glomerular filtration rate after converting-enzyme inhibition in essential hypertension. N Engl J Med 301:9-12, 1979.

44. Hollenberg NK, Meggs LG, Williams GH, et al. Sodium intake and renal responses to captopril in normal man and in essential hypertension. Kidney Int 20:240-245, 1981.

45. Larochelle P, Gutkowska J, Schiffrin E, et al. Effect of enalapril on renin, angiotensin converting enzyme activity, aldosterone and prostaglandins in patients with hypertension. Clin Invest Med 8:197-201, 1985.

46. Reams GP, Bauer JH, Gaddy P. Use of the converting enzyme inhibitor enalapril in renovascular hypertension. Effect on blood pressure, renal function, and the renin-angiotensin-aldosterone system. Hypertension 8:290-297, 1986.

47. de Cavanagh EM, Inserra F, Toblli J, et al. Enalapril attenuates oxidative stress in diabetic rats. Hypertension 38:1130-1136, 2001.

48. Liu X, Engelman RM, Rousou JA, et al. Attenuation of myocardial reperfusion injury by sulfhydryl-containing angiotensin converting enzyme inhibitors. Cardiovasc Drugs Ther 6:437-443, 1992.

49. Sakemi T, Baba N. Effects of antihypertensive drugs on the progress of renal failure in hyperlipidemic Imai rats. Nephron 63:323-329, 1993.

50. Keilani T, Schlueter WA, Levin ML, et al. Improvement of lipid abnormalities associated with proteinuria using fosinopril, an angiotensin-converting enzyme inhibitor. Ann Intern Med 118:246-254, 1993.

51. Kasiske BL, Kalil RS, Ma JZ, et al. Effect of antihypertensive therapy on the kidney in patients with diabetes: A meta-regression analysis. Ann Intern Med 118:129-138, 1993.

52. Heeg JE, de Jong PE, van der Hem GK, et al. Reduction of proteinuria by angiotensin converting enzyme inhibition. Kidney Int 32:78-83, 1987.

53. Herlitz H, Edeno C, Mulec H, et al. Captopril treatment of hypertension and renal failure in systemic lupus erythematosus. Nephron 38:253-256, 1984.

54. Hommel E, Parving HH, Mathiesen E, et al. Effect of captopril on kidney function in insulin-dependent diabetic patients with nephropathy. Br Med J (Clin Res Ed) 293:467-470, 1986.

55. Reams GP, Bauer JH. Effect of enalapril in subjects with hypertension associated with moderate to severe renal dysfunction. Arch Intern Med 146:2145-2148, 1986.

56. Navis G, de Jong PE, Donker AJ, et al. Moderate sodium restriction in hypertensive subjects: Renal effects of ACE-inhibition. Kidney Int 31:815-819, 1987.

57. Apperloo AJ, de Zeeuw D, de Jong PE. A short-term antihypertensive treatment-induced fall in glomerular filtration rate predicts long-term stability of renal function. Kidney Int 51:793-797, 1997.

58. de Zeeuw D, Heeg JE, Stelwagen T, et al. Mechanism of the antiproteinuric effect of angiotensin-converting enzyme inhibition. Contrib Nephrol 83:160-165, 1990.

59. Ferrari P, Marti HP, Pfister M, et al. Additive antiproteinuric effect of combined ACE inhibition and angiotensin II receptor blockade. J Hypertens 20:125-130, 2002

60. Nakao N, Yoshimura A, Morita H, et al. Combination treatment of angiotensin-II receptor blocker and angiotensin-converting-enzyme inhibitor in non-diabetic renal disease (COOPERATE): A randomised controlled trial. Lancet 361:117-124, 2003.

61. Wright JT Jr, Bakris G, Greene T, et al. Effect of blood pressure lowering and antihypertensive drug class on progression of hypertensive kidney disease: Results from the AASK trial. JAMA 288:2421-2431, 2002.

62. Simon G, Morioka S, Snyder DK, et al. Increased renal plasma flow in long-term enalapril treatment of hypertension. Clin Pharmacol Ther 34:459-465, 1983.

63. Reams GP, Bauer JH. Long-term effects of enalapril monotherapy and enalapril/hydrochlorothiazide combination therapy on blood pressure, renal function, and body fluid composition. J Clin Hypertens 2:55-63, 1986.

64. Lewis EJ, Hunsicker LG, Bain RP, et al. The effect of angiotensin-converting-enzyme inhibition on diabetic nephropathy. The Collaborative Study Group. N Engl J Med 329:1456-1462, 1993.

65. Hricik DE. Captopril-induced renal insufficiency and the role of sodium balance. Ann Intern Med 103:222-223, 1985.

66. Murphy BF, Whitworth JA, Kincaid-Smith P. Renal insufficiency with combinations of angiotensin converting enzyme inhibitors and diuretics. Br Med J (Clin Res Ed) 288:844-845, 1984.

67. Levenson DJ, Dzau VJ. Effects on angiotensin-converting enzyme inhibition on renal hemodynamics in renal artery stenosis. Kidney Int Suppl 20:S173-S179, 1987.

68. Mendelsohn FA, Dunbar M, Allen A, et al. Angiotensin II receptors in the kidney. Fed Proc 45:1420-1425, 1986.

69. Nishiyama A, Seth DM, Navar LG. Renal interstitial fluid angiotensin I and angiotensin II concentrations during local angiotensin-converting enzyme inhibition. J Am Soc Nephrol 13:2207-2212, 2002.

70. Cervenka L, Navar LG. Renal responses of the nonclipped kidney of two-kidney/one-clip Goldblatt hypertensive rats to type 1 angiotensin II receptor blockade with candesartan. J Am Soc Nephrol 10(Suppl 11):S197-S201, 1999.

71. Takishita S, Muratani H, Sesoko S, et al. Short-term effects of angiotensin II blockade on renal blood flow and sympathetic activity in awake rats. Hypertension 24:445-450, 1994.

72. Jover B, Saladini D, Nafrialdi N, et al. Effect of losartan and enalapril on renal adaptation sodium restriction in rat. Am J Physiol 267:F281-F288, 1994.

73. Peng Y, Knox FG. Comparison of systemic and direct intrarenal angiotensin II blockade on sodium excretion in rats. Am J Physiol 269:F40-F46, 1995.

74. Knox FG, Burnett JC Jr, Kohan DE, et al. Escape from the sodium-retaining effects of mineralocorticoids. Kidney Int 17:263-276, 1980.

75. Navar LG, Inscho EW, Majid SA, et al. Paracrine regulation of the renal microcirculation. Physiol Rev 76:425-536, 1996.

76. Schaefer KL, Porter JA. Angiotensin II receptor antagonists: The prototype losartan. Ann Pharmacother 30:625-636, 1996.

77. Hoieggen A, Alderman MH, Kjeldsen SE, et al. The impact of serum uric acid on cardiovascular outcomes in the LIFE study. Kidney Int 65:1041-1049, 2004.

78. Shaw W. Safety and efficacy of losartan in hypertensive patients with renal impairment. J Am Soc Nephrol 567, 1994.

79. Doig JK, MacFadyen RJ, Sweet CS, et al. Dose-ranging study of the angiotensin type I receptor antagonist losartan (DuP753/MK954) in salt-depleted normal man. J Cardiovasc Pharmacol 21:732-738, 1993.

80. Buter H, Navis G, de Zeeuw D, et al. Renal hemodynamic effects of candesartan in normal and impaired renal function in humans. Kidney Int Suppl 63:S185-S187, 1997.

81. Siragy HM, Carey RM. Protective role of the angiotensin AT2 receptor in a renal wrap hypertension model. Hypertension 33:1237-1242, 1999.

82. Delles C, Jacobi J, John S, et al. Effects of enalapril and eprosartan on the renal vascular nitric oxide system in human essential hypertension. Kidney Int 61:1462-1468, 2002.

83. Textor SC, Tarazi RC, Novick AC, et al. Regulation of renal hemodynamics and glomerular filtration in patients with renovascular hypertension during converting enzyme inhibition with captopril. Am J Med 76:29-37, 1984.

84. Cooper ME, Webb RL, de Gasparo M. Angiotensin receptor blockers and the kidney: Possible advantages over ACE inhibition? Cardiovasc Drug Rev 19:75-86, 2001.

85. Bohlen L, de Courten M, Weidmann P. Comparative study of the effect of ACE-inhibitors and other antihypertensive agents on proteinuria in diabetic patients. Am J Hypertens 7:84S-92S, 1994.

86. Lewis EJ, Hunsicker LG, Clarke WR, et al. Renoprotective effect of the angiotensin-receptor antagonist irbesartan in patients with nephropathy due to type 2 diabetes. N Engl J Med 345:851-860, 2001.

87. Parving HH, Lehnert H, Brochner-Mortensen J, et al. The effect of irbesartan on the development of diabetic nephropathy in patients with type 2 diabetes. N Engl J Med 345:870-878, 2001.

88. Ersoy A, Dilek K, Usta M, et al. Angiotensin-II receptor antagonist losartan reduces microalbuminuria in hypertensive renal transplant recipients. Clin Transplant 16:202-205, 2002.

89. Wapstra FH, Navis G, de Jong PE, et al. Prognostic value of the short-term antiproteinuric response to ACE inhibition for prediction of GFR decline in patients with nondiabetic renal disease. Exp Nephrol 4(Suppl 1):47-52, 1996.

90. Gansevoort RT, de Zeeuw D, de Jong PE. Dissociation between the course of the hemodynamic and antiproteinuric effects of angiotensin I converting enzyme inhibition. Kidney Int 44:579-584, 1993.

91. Russo D, Pisani A, Balletta MM, et al. Additive antiproteinuric effect of converting enzyme inhibitor and losartan in normotensive patients with IgA nephropathy. Am J Kidney Dis 33:851-856, 1999.

92. Kuriyama S, Tomonari H, Abe A, et al. Augmentation of antiproteinuric effect by combined therapy with angiotensin II receptor blocker plus calcium channel blocker in a hypertensive patient with IgA glomerulonephritis. J Hum Hypertens 16:371-373, 2002.

93. Taal MW, Brenner BM. Combination ACEI and ARB therapy: Additional benefit in renoprotection? Curr Opin Nephrol Hypertens 11:377-381, 2002.

94. Komine N, Khang S, Wead LM, et al. Effect of combining an ACE inhibitor and an angiotensin II receptor blocker on plasma and kidney tissue angiotensin II levels. Am J Kidney Dis 39:159-164, 2002.

95. Agarwal R, Siva S, Dunn SR, et al. Add-on angiotensin II receptor blockade lowers urinary transforming growth factor-beta levels. Am J Kidney Dis 39:486-492, 2002.

96. Sica DA, Bakris GL. Type 2 diabetes: RENAAL and IDNT: The emergence of new treatment options. J Clin Hypertens (Greenwich) 4:52-57, 2002.

97. de Zeeuw D, Remuzzi G, Parving HH, et al. Proteinuria, a target for renoprotection in patients with type 2 diabetic nephropathy: Lessons from RENAAL. Kidney Int 65:2309-2320, 2004.

98. Isben H, Wachtell K, Olsen MH, et al. Does albuminuria predict cardiovascular outcome on treatment with losartan versus atenolol in hypertension with left ventricular hypertrophy? A LIFE substudy. J Hypertens 22:1805-1811, 2004.

99. Inigo P, Campistol JM, Lario S, et al. Effects of losartan and amlodipine on intrarenal hemodynamics and TGF-beta(1) plasma levels in a crossover trial in renal transplant recipients. J Am Soc Nephrol 12:822-827, 2001.

100. Ferrario CM, Smith R, Levy P, et al. The hypertension-lipid connection: Insights into the relation between angiotensin II and cholesterol in atherogenesis. Am J Med Sci 323:17-24, 2002.

101. Ferrario CM. Use of angiotensin II receptor blockers in animal models of atherosclerosis. Am J Hypertens 15:9S-13S, 2002.

102. Schiffrin EL. Vascular changes in hypertension in response to drug treatment: Effects of angiotensin receptor blockers. Can J Cardiol 18(Suppl A):15A-18A, 2002.

103. Brosnan MJ, Hamilton CA, Graham D, et al. Irbesartan lowers superoxide levels and increases nitric oxide bioavailability in blood vessels from spontaneously hypertensive stroke-prone rats. J Hypertens 20:281-286, 2002.

104. Taddei S, Virdis A, Ghiadoni L, et al. Effects of antihypertensive drugs on endothelial dysfunction: Clinical implications. Drugs 62:265-284, 2002.

105. Reardon LC, Macpherson DS. Hyperkalemia in outpatients using angiotensin-converting enzyme inhibitors. How much should we worry? Arch Intern Med 158:26-32, 1998.

106. Palmer BF. Managing hyperkalemia caused by inhibitors of the renin-angiotensin-aldosterone system. N Engl J Med 351:585-592, 2004.

107. Zech P, Pozet N, Labeeuw M, et al. Acute renal effects of beta-blockers. Am J Nephrol 6(Suppl 2):15-19, 1986.

108. Valvo E, Gammaro L, Bedogna V, et al. Effects of nadolol on systemic and renal hemodynamics in patients with reno-parenchymal hypertension and various degrees of renal function. Int J Clin Pharmacol Ther Toxicol 24:202-206, 1986.

109. Epstein M, Oster JR. Beta blockers and renal function: A reappraisal. J Clin Hypertens 1:85-99, 1985.

110. Weir MR, Hanes DS, Klassen DK. Antihypertensive Drugs, Ch 55. In Brenner B (ed). Brenner & Rector's The Kidney, 7th ed. Philadelphia, Saunders, 2004; pp 2381-2451.

111. Epstein M. Calcium antagonists and the kidney. Implications for renal protection. Am J Hypertens 4:482S-486S, 1991.

112. Wallia R, Greenberg A, Puschett JB. Renal hemodynamic and tubular transport effects of nitrendipine. J Lab Clin Med 105:498-503, 1985.

113. MacGregor GA, Pevahouse JB, Cappuccio FP, et al. Nifedipine, diuretics and sodium balance. J Hypertens Suppl 5:S127-S131, 1987.

114. Hulthen UL, Katzman PL. Renal effects of acute and long-term treatment with felodipine in essential hypertension. J Hypertens 6:231-237, 1988.

115. Krusell LR, Jespersen LT, Schmitz A, et al. Repetitive natriuresis and blood pressure. Long-term calcium entry blockade with isradipine. Hypertension 10:577-581, 1987.

116. Loutzenhiser R, Epstein M. Effects of calcium antagonists on renal hemodynamics. Am J Physiol 249:F619-F629, 1985.

117. Sunderrajan S, Reams G, Bauer JH. Long-term renal effects of diltiazem in essential hypertension. Am Heart J 114:383-388, 1987.

118. Reams GP, Lau A, Hamory A, et al. Amlodipine therapy corrects renal abnormalities encountered in the hypertensive state. Am J Kidney Dis 10:446-451, 1987.

119. Blackshear JL, Garnic D, Williams GH, et al. Exaggerated renal vasodilator response to calcium entry blockade in first-degree relatives of essential hypertensive subjects. Hypertension 9:384-389, 1987.

120. Demarie BK, Bakris GL. Effects of different calcium antagonists on proteinuria associated with diabetes mellitus. Ann Intern Med 113:987-988, 1990.

121. Bakris GL. Effects of diltiazem or lisinopril on massive proteinuria associated with diabetes mellitus. Ann Intern Med 112:707-708, 1990.

122. Isshiki T, Amodeo C, Messerli FH, et al. Diltiazem maintains renal vasodilation without hyperfiltration in hypertension: Studies in essential hypertension in man and the spontaneously hypertensive rat. Cardiovasc Drugs Ther 1:359-366, 1987.

123. Brunner FP, Hermle M, Theil G. Verapamil in contrast to enalapril aggravates hyperfiltration despite lowered blood pressure in rats with reduced renal mass [abstract]. Proceedings of the Tenth International Congress of Nephrology 497, 1987.

124. Sica DA, Douglas JG. The African American Study of Kidney Disease and Hypertension (AASK): New findings. J Clin Hypertens (Greenwich) 3:244-251, 2001.

125. Berl T, Hunsicker LG, Lewis JB, et al. Cardiovascular outcomes in the Irbesartan Diabetic Nephropathy Trial of patients with type 2 diabetes and overt nephropathy. Ann Intern Med 138:542-549, 2003.

126. Dworkin LD. Impact of calcium entry blockers on glomerular injury in experimental hypertension. Cardiovasc Drugs Ther 4:1325-1330, 1990.

127. Sweeney C, Shultz P, Raij L. Interactions of the endothelium and mesangium in glomerular injury [abstract]. J Am Soc Nephrol 1:S13, 1990.

128. Keane WF, Raij L. Relationship among altered glomerular barrier permselectivity, angiotensin II, and mesangial uptake of macromolecules. Lab Invest 52:599-604, 1985.

129. Schwertschlag U, Schrier RW, Wilson P. Beneficial effects of calcium channel blockers and calmodulin binding drugs on in vitro renal cell anoxia. J Pharmacol Exp Ther 238:119-124, 1986.

130. Jesmin S, Sakuma I, Hattori Y, et al. Long-acting calcium channel blocker benidipine suppresses expression of angiogenic growth factors and prevents cardiac remodelling in a type II diabetic rat model. Diabetologia 45:402-415, 2002.

131. Mandarim-de-Lacerda CA, Pereira LM. Renal cortical remodelling by NO-synthesis blockers in rats is prevented by angiotensin-converting enzyme inhibitor and calcium channel blocker. J Cell Mol Med 5:276-283, 2001.

132. Wada Y, Kato S, Okamoto K, et al. Diltiazem, a calcium antagonist, inhibits matrix metalloproteinase-1 (tissue collagenase) production and collagenolytic activity in human vascular smooth muscle cells. Int J Mol Med 8:561-566, 2001.

133. Niemeyer C, Hasenfuss G, Wais U, et al. Pharmacokinetics of hydrochlorothiazide in relation to renal function. Eur J Clin Pharmacol 24:661-665, 1983.

134. Diamond JR, Hanchak NA, McCarter MD, et al. Cholestyramine resin ameliorates chronic aminonucleoside nephrosis. Am J Clin Nutr 51:606-611, 1990.

135. Bianchi S, Bigazzi R, Caiazza A, et al. A controlled, prospective study of the effects of atorvastatin on proteinuria and progression of kidney disease. Am J Kidney Dis 41:565-570, 2003.

136. Rabelink AJ, Hene RJ, Erkelens DW, et al. Partial remission of nephrotic syndrome in patient on long-term simvastatin. Lancet 335:1045-1046, 1990.

137. Prata MM, Nogueira AC, Pinto JR, et al. Long-term effect of lovastatin on lipoprotein profile in patients with primary nephrotic syndrome. Clin Nephrol 41:277-283, 1994.

138. Kasiske BL, Velosa JA, Halstenson CE, et al. The effects of lovastatin in hyperlipidemic patients with the nephrotic syndrome. Am J Kidney Dis 15:8-15, 1990.

139. Rayner BL, Byrne MJ, van Zyl SR. A prospective clinical trial comparing the treatment of idiopathic membranous nephropathy and nephrotic syndrome with simvastatin and diet, versus diet alone. Clin Nephrol 46:219-224, 1996.

140. Fried LF, Orchard TJ, Kasiske BL. Effect of lipid reduction on the progression of renal disease: A meta-analysis. Kidney Int 59:260-269, 2001.

141. Rossert J, Fouqueray B, Boffa JJ. Anemia management and the delay of chronic renal failure progression. J Am Soc Nephrol 14:S173-S177, 2003.

142. Jungers P, Choukroun G, Oualim Z, et al. Beneficial influence of recombinant human erythropoietin therapy on the rate of progression of chronic renal failure in predialysis patients. Nephrol Dial Transplant 16:307-312, 2001.

# SECTION 4

# Diagnosis

## Chapter 26

# Initial Evaluation and Follow-Up Assessment

## Lawrence R. Krakoff

High arterial pressure, hypertension, is a highly prevalent disorder of the adult population in the United States and other nations with "Western" cultures. Hypertension is one of the most common reasons for a patient to visit a physician's office or clinic. The initial evaluation or work-up for hypertension and its follow-up assessment is quite different from that for acute disease processes. For those disorders with sudden onset, the initial evaluation or work-up is often considered as a definitive assessment that reveals the likely cause, needed diagnostic tests, and appropriate treatment. After the acute disease is successfully treated, follow-up in the clinics may not be needed or may be limited to a few visits.

The initial assessment of hypertensive patients differs from the evaluation for acute illnesses in large part because the diagnostic focus is less on finding a cause (secondary hypertension) than on determining the overall risk status of the patient. Staging comes first, and cause a distant second. Furthermore, the management of hypertensive patients takes place over an extended period of time, many years or decades. During this long interval, many changes can be anticipated as the patient's status becomes the result of treatment, evolution of related or unrelated disease states, and aging. Hence, periodic reevaluation of hypertensive patients is a necessary part of their management.

In the past few years there has been increasing recognition that in adults, and to some extent in adolescents and children as well, high blood pressure (BP) occurs in many individuals who have other predictors and risk factors for future cardiovascular disease. Smoking, overweight, abnormal serum lipid patterns, and diabetes mellitus (usually type 2) in varying combinations, often accompany hypertension. In addition, hypertensive individuals often have target organ damage (TOD) that has already led to symptoms or impairment, but also predicts likelihood of additional disease in the future. The absolute risk of future cardiovascular disease is then a composite of reversible risk factors and target organ pathology involving the heart, brain, kidneys, and arteries. Aging adds irreversibly and inexorably to the absolute risk of cardiovascular disease. Figure 26–1 is a schematic to summarize these complex relationships. The diagnostic process must combine reasonable completeness, efficiency, and practicality for the limited time and resources available to busy clinicians. This will be the guiding approach summarized in this chapter.

## WHEN IS HYPERTENSION PRESENT?

### Arterial Pressure and Risk

The risk of future cardiovascular disease increases in a direct and somewhat linear relationship to systolic and diastolic arterial pressure.[1] For systolic blood pressure (SBP), this relationship continues into older age groups.[2,3] The relationship between diastolic blood pressure (DBP) and risk of cardiovascular disease in older groups is more complex because the pulse pressure (systolic-diastolic pressure) assumes more importance.[4] In those older than 50 years of age, for equally high SBPs, a lower DBP (wider pulse pressure) confers a worse prognosis.[5,6] In a similar manner, the risk of future end-stage renal disease (ESRD) increases significantly when BP is only minimally elevated above the normal range, but increases steeply when the pressure is very high.[7]

For practical diagnostic purposes, ranges of BP were grouped into "high-normal pressure" and stages 1 to 3, in the Sixth Report of the Joint National Committee on Detection, Prevention, and Treatment of Hypertension (JNC VI)[8] and generally accepted by international guidelines.[9] The most recent guideline from the United States, the Seventh Report of the Joint National Committee on Prevention, Detection, and Treatment of High Blood Pressure (JNC 7) adds a new term, "prehypertension," referring to those who have BPs above 120/80 mm Hg and below 140/90 mm Hg.[10] The rationale for this classification is based on the very high lifetime risk of hypertension found in the Framingham Heart Study for those with pressures above the ideal level for minimum risk.[11] Whether prehypertension, as a diagnosis, is a helpful tool for getting those younger patients to adopt a better lifestyle and prevent hypertension[12] is uncertain. A modified version of the BP classification is given in Table 26–1 as a basis for considering levels of BP in relation to diagnosis and treatment.

Some have suggested that the minute-to-minute *variability* in arterial BP also contributes to disease, in addition to average levels. A cross-sectional study of intraarterial pressures suggested that excessive variation in pressure is correlated with TOD.[13] However, as a predictor of future disease in prospective studies and a basis for treatment, variability per se, has yet to be shown as an independent risk factor when adjusted for other factors.[14]

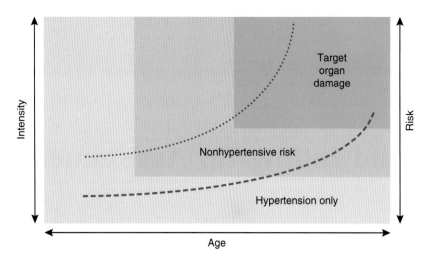

**Figure 26-1** A schematic representation for assessing absolute risk of future cardiovascular disease in hypertensive patients. Likelihood of a fatal or nonfatal stroke or myocardial infarction is related to age, the "intensity" of each risk factor (e.g., level of BP or of low-density lipoprotein cholesterol), and absence or presence of target organ damage (TOD) (e.g., left ventricular hypertrophy). The *dashed lines* indicate that for any combination of risk factors and TOD, age will increase the risk.

## Accurate Measurement, Errors, and Bias

Accurate measurement of BP is clearly needed for correct diagnostic classification. When arterial pressure is either well in the normal range (SBP <130 mm Hg and DBP <80 mm Hg) or markedly elevated (SBP >180 mm Hg and DBP >110 mm Hg), even a somewhat inaccurate method of BP measurement will approximate the true average, so the likelihood of a false-positive or false-negative diagnosis of hypertension is very small.[15] However, many have average or usual pressures that fall in the ranges of 130 to 160 mm Hg for SBP and 80 to 105 mm Hg for DBP. BPs measured by the ordinary clinical method (stethoscope and cuff with either a mercury or aneroid manometer) may be inaccurate or misrepresentative. This can lead to a misclassification that is even more likely when the average pressures are close to one of the dividing points for diagnosis (i.e., high-normal pressure versus JNC VI stage 1).[15,16] Attention needs to be paid to (1) correct cuff size for the patient, (2) accuracy of the manometer, (3) training and reliability of the observer,[17] and (4) sufficient number of measurements for a reasonable approximation of the average pressure.[15]

## Supplemental Pressures

BP measurements obtained outside of the clinic may be helpful to arriving at average pressure and have important prognostic value. The use of either ambulatory BP monitoring[18] or home BPs[19] has gained recognition in this regard. Such measurements may reveal "white-coat hypertension" in which BP elevation is limited to the clinic or office, or its opposite state, in which clinic pressures are lower than average daily pressures.[20,21] These topics are discussed in Chapters 27 and 28.

**Table 26-1** Recommended Evaluation and Initial Management for Various Blood Pressure (BP) Levels Found at Initial Clinic Measurement of Asymptomatic Adult Subjects*

| BP Levels | Recommended Treatment |
| --- | --- |
| Systolic ≥220 mm Hg or Diastolic ≥115 mm Hg | Rapid evaluation by comprehensive history, physical examination and laboratory tests. Start treatment within 24 hours. |
| Systolic ≥180 mm Hg or Diastolic ≥105 mm Hg | Comprehensive evaluation within 1 week. Begin treatment if BP remains at this level. |
| Systolic ≥160 mm Hg or Diastolic ≥100 mm Hg | Comprehensive evaluation within 2-4 weeks. Treatment decision depends on overall status. |
| Systolic 140-159 mm Hg or Diastolic 90-99 mm Hg | Comprehensive evaluation within 1 month. Initiate lifestyle changes. Ordinarily withhold drug treatment for 1-6 months. Supplemental pressure, ambulatory monitoring, or self-measurement may be helpful. |
| Systolic >120 mm Hg or Diastolic >80 mm Hg | Prehypertension suggesting that hypertension may develop in the future (years). Provide advice regarding diet, exercise, salt intake. Reassess yearly. |

*For symptoms or abnormal findings on physical examination, individual decisions are more appropriate. The BP levels approximately correspond to stages 1 to 3 of the JNC VI report,[8] with the additional classification of "prehypertension" added in the JNC 7 report.[10]

## NONHYPERTENSIVE RISK FACTORS

### Definitions

Hypertension is an unequivocal risk factor for cardiovascular mortality and morbidity. Before clinical trials established the benefit of lowering BP, the term *risk factor* was limited to mean a measurable trait that predicts future disease and is presumed to play a causal role for future pathology. Now that clinical trials have established the effectiveness of antihypertensive therapy, the term *risk factor* includes the implication that reduction of pressure confers benefit. Thus, a cardiovascular risk factor predicts disease, is a cause of pathology, and can be reduced by a treatment that prevents disease.

Some hypertensive patients have no other risk factors to worsen their prognosis. Many, however, have the combination of high BP and other, independent predictors and causes of stroke, coronary heart disease (CHD), and/or renal insuffi-

**Table 26–2** Nonhypertensive Risk Factors to be Assessed in the Work-up of Hypertensive Patients

| Major Risk Factors | Comment |
|---|---|
| Smoking status | Cessation of smoking reduces risk of CHD within 2 years by 50%. Stroke and peripheral vascular disease can be prevented. |
| Diabetes mellitus | More likely in hypertensive groups. Invariably increases risk. Can be treated. |
| Serum lipid–lipoprotein levels | The benefit of reducing high LDL concentrations is firmly established. Correction of high triglyceride level and low HDL status is likely to be beneficial. |
| Overweight and increased waist:hip ratio | Overweight and obesity are clearly related to cardiovascular disease. Weight reduction lowers BP and other risk factors. |
| Excess alcohol use | Clearly associated with increased pressure and likelihood of disease. Low alcohol use may be beneficial. |
| Reduced aerobic exercise | Evidence supports the value of regular exercise for preventing cardiovascular disease. |

CHD, coronary heart disease; LDL, low-density lipoprotein.

ciency. Table 26–2 lists those risk factors that are have strong epidemiologic association with cardiovascular disease. These risk factors are reversible and should be taken into consideration during the initial and continuing evaluation and management of *every* hypertensive patient. A brief review of each of these risk factors now follows.

## Smoking

A history of current or recent cigarette smoking nearly doubles risk of stroke and CHD and is well correlated with likelihood of peripheral arterial disease. Furthermore, smoking is related to the occurrence of malignant hypertension.[22,23] Those who stop smoking can rapidly reduce risk of CHD within a few years.[24] Ongoing counseling during follow-up visits may reduce smoking behavior, as demonstrated in the Multiple Risk Factor Invention Trial (MRFIT).[25] More recently, pharmacologic options have become available (e.g., nicotine chewing gum, nicotine transcutaneous patches, clonidine, and bupropion). These strategies, together with aggressive public education programs, may achieve a sustained elimination of smoking behavior and thus reduce long-term risk of stroke, CHD, and peripheral vascular disease.

## Lipids and Lipoproteins

Many serum lipoprotein patterns have been associated with altered cardiovascular risk and the list of possible candidates is increasing. Increased low-density lipoprotein (LDL) cholesterol or reduced high-density lipoprotein (HDL) cholesterol are well-accepted predictors. The metabolic syndrome, associated with insulin resistance, low HDL cholesterol, and elevated serum triglyceride concentration, appears to be a predictor of CHD.

Randomized placebo-controlled clinical trials carried out in persons with a high risk of future CHD have demonstrated that reduction of serum cholesterol by statin therapy is effective in the presence or absence of hypertension.[26-28] Statin therapy is effective in preventing coronary events even when baseline cholesterol levels are "normal" (i.e., LDL cholesterol ≤100 mg/dl [or ≤2.7 mM/L] or total cholesterol ≤207 mg/dl [or ≤5.6 mM/L]). For those at high risk due to low HDL levels, fibrate therapy

with gemfibrozil may be effective, at least for those with prior CHD.[29] Other fibrates have not been studied in outcome trials.

## Diabetes, Glucose, and Insulin Resistance

Every hypertensive patient should be assessed for diabetes when first seen and during follow-up. Hypertensives are twice as likely to develop new type 2 diabetes compared with normotensives.[30] The importance of overt diabetes, high-normal fasting glucose, or glucose intolerance as adding to potentially reversible risk within the hypertensive population and even in those with high-normal pressure cannot be overemphasized.[31]

Within the hypertensive population, a fraction have normal fasting glucose and glucose tolerance, but the syndrome of insulin resistance (the metabolic syndrome).[32,33] It is not yet certain that this syndrome, apart from its frequent correlates of obesity and altered serum lipoprotein pattern, confers independent risk. Furthermore, insulin resistance is not easily defined outside of research settings. For a more extensive discussion of insulin resistance in essential hypertension, see Chapter 13.

For ordinary clinical purposes, the fasting serum glucose is all that is needed to define the metabolic state of most patients. However, new definitions of both diabetes and the borderline state of impaired fasting glucose have been reached through an evidence-based process and the consensus of experts and should be used to classify hypertensive patients.[34] The diagnosis of diabetes is based on an *average fasting glucose* (two or more separate measurements) of >125 mg/dl (or ≥7 mM/L). When the average falls between 100 and 126 mg/dl, impaired fasting glucose is the correct label; such patients should be reevaluated at 1- to 2-year intervals for possible conversion to type 2 diabetes.

If a patient is known to have had either insulin-dependent or non–insulin-dependent diabetes for several years, additional evaluation for complications of the diabetic state including the presence of retinopathy, neuropathy, nephropathy, and evidence of peripheral macrovascular and microvascular disease (i.e., foot ulcers) needs to be undertaken.

## Weight, Build, and Overweight

Measurement of weight and height are, or should be, part of the initial assessment of all patients. At a glance, one can tell if the body build is slim, muscular, mildly overweight, obese, or morbidly obese. It is useful, however, to have a single and simple calculation that gives a numerical counterpart to the clinical impression. The calculated body mass index (BMI) is widely used in clinical studies to convey body build that relates weight to height. The calculation for BMI is weight (kg)/height in meters squared ($m^2$) or $kg/m^2$. For those measuring height in inches and weight in pounds, the formula for BMI, equivalent to using metric units, with a correction factor is $705 \times$ weight (lbs)/height in inches$^2$. Generally, desirable BMI is $\leq 25$, mild overweight is 25 to 29, and definite overweight is $\geq 30$ or $\geq 20\%$ above desirable weight.

Weight distribution may also predict future cardiovascular disease and the likelihood of hypertension or the tendency to non–insulin-dependent diabetes mellitus (NIDDM). The "apple" shape is relatively incriminated, while the "pear" shape is less so. These adjectives are reflected in a simple measurement, the waist:hip ratio, normally well below 0.9. As the ratio increases in overweight patients, the body build is more of the "apple" or high-risk type.[35]

Overweight hypertensives may be considered to have a reversible disorder, whose correction (i.e., weight loss) may not only lower their BP, but improve overall risk status (elevated serum LDL cholesterol, impaired glucose metabolism, or NIDDM) as well. National trends suggest that overweight is relentlessly increasing in the United States.[36]

## Exercise Pattern—Fitness

A pattern of regular exercise may lower BP by 4 to 5 mm Hg,[37] even reduce left ventricular hypertrophy (LVH)[38] and contribute to prevention of future cardiovascular disease.[39-41] As part of the initial evaluation, assessment of exercise is advisable along with encouragement to maintain or increase daily physical activity for its benefit.

## Alcohol Use or Over Use

Appraisal of day-to-day ingestion of alcoholic beverages should be part of the initial and recurring assessment of hypertensive patients for several reasons. Low-level alcohol intake may be a preventive measure for future cardiovascular disease[42] and can be encouraged if there is no evidence of harm.[43] However, sustained high alcohol intake may contribute to both hypertension and cardiovascular disease,[44] whereas reduction of high alcohol ingestion may lower BP and even prevent the onset of hypertension.[45-47] Those hypertensive patients who continue high alcohol use may be difficult to control because of poor compliance with antihypertensive therapy.

## Other Potential Risk Factors

### Renin as a Risk Factor and Renin Profiling

The renin-angiotensin-aldosterone system participates in control of arterial pressure and fluid-volume balance. This system can be assessed with widely available clinical measurements. Classification of hypertensive patients into low, normal, and high renin subgroups has prognostic significance in that the low renin subgroup tends to have less CHD, both in an observational study[48] and a prospective cohort analysis,[49] in contrast to higher rates of CHD in normal and high renin groups. Renin profiling may predict response to antihypertensive drug treatment and add useful information for detection of secondary hypertension, especially renal artery stenosis and primary aldosteronism.

As an indirect assessment, an unusually good response to treatment with either an angiotension-converting enzyme inhibitor or angiotensin type 1 receptor blocker (drugs that specifically block the renin-angiotensin system) implies an overactive renin system. In contrast, the lack of any BP response to either of these drug classes suggests a low renin state, as occurs in primary aldosteronism. The sensitivity and specificity of clinical responses to these drugs are, however, not defined.

The use of renin profiling has not become a widespread approach for initial assessment, unless secondary hypertension is suspected. However, renin profiling may have a role for those patients who are resistant to treatment with two to three drugs. Recent studies report high detection rates of primary aldosteronism in patients with refractory hypertension,[50,51] and the addition of spironolactone or other mineralocorticoid receptor antagonists may be effective in this setting.[52,53]

### Homocysteine and C-Reactive Protein

New candidates as predictors or possible participating causes of cardiovascular disease are often reported. The level of serum homocysteine has been correlated with stroke[54] and CHD.[55] Homocysteine levels are partly related to the availability and normal metabolism of folic acid and vitamin $B_{12}$ via methylation pathways.[56] An adequate dietary supply of folic acid is needed to minimize homocysteine concentration. Supplementing the diet with folic acid may reduce homocysteine and is potentially beneficial for prevention of cardiovascular disease.[57]

The plasma level of C-reactive protein (CRP), a manifestation of inflammation, is another candidate risk factor for stroke, CHD, and peripheral arterial disease.[58] It has been suggested that the atherosclerotic process includes a low-grade inflammation, which can elevate CRP.[59,60] Thus an elevated CRP might be viewed as reflecting TOD, rather than being a candidate risk factor. The overall effect of aspirin in reducing risk of CHD[61] might then include an antiinflammatory effect (on atherogenesis) in addition to an antithrombotic action. It has also been suggested the benefit of statin therapy in preventing CHD is partly mediated by an antiinflammatory effect related to CRP levels. Whether measurement of CRP levels adds enough information to be useful as a screening procedure remains contoversial.[62]

## TARGET ORGAN DAMAGE

Treatment of hypertension prevents the development of cardiac, renal, and vascular pathology, (i.e., TOD). Nonetheless, many patients have evidence for TOD when seen initially or during follow-up. Detection of TOD in hypertensive patients is a crucial and necessary diagnostic requirement for initial evaluation and subsequent interval reassessments. Presence of TOD adds to risk of future cardiovascular disease and mortality. Furthermore, treatment may reverse TOD (e.g., regress LVH) or delay progression (e.g., reduce decline in renal function). Both the medical history and pertinent physical examination are clearly useful to detect some forms of TOD. Relevant and cost-effective testing is needed for improving precision in many instances.

Table 26–3 lists the major sites of TOD to be surveyed, how these are to be assessed in the initial medical history and physical examination, and the most often used tests or imaging procedures for confirmation.

## INITIAL ASSESSMENT OF HYPERTENSIVE PATIENTS

Hypertension is usually first considered during periodic check-up visits or as part of ordinary screening when patients are seen for unrelated minor illnesses. Hypertension, presenting as an emergency, is rare and will require hospitalization and immediate treatment (see Chapter 78).

Most hypertensives will be managed at clinic or office visits. The initial evaluation should consist of a careful medical history, appropriately comprehensive physical examination, and *necessary* tests. For adult hypertensive patients, the tests that I include, as a minimum, are as follows:

1. Electrocardiogram: Is there evidence for left ventricular enlargement or ischemic disease?
2. Fasting glucose, serum creatinine, and electrolytes ($Na^+$, $K^+$ $Cl^-$, $HCO_3^-$) to assess for diabetes, hypokalemia, and renal function.
3. Serum lipid profile: HDL and LDL cholesterol fractions and triglyceride concentration.
4. Urinalysis: Is proteinuria or an abnormal sediment present?

Once this information is available, the issues addressed in Table 26–4 should be dealt with. The first row of Table 26–4 indicates that the initial assessment should provide the overall absolute cardiovascular risk of each patient, as portrayed in Figure 26–2. Additional tests may be needed to define TOD (see Table 26–3). The second row of Table 26–4 places emphasis on those features derived from the medical history that are often overlooked in overviews and guidelines for patient management and yet are crucial in establishing strategy for long-term management of hypertensive patients. The individual patient's ordinary activities, socioeconomic status, ability to understand his or her risk, comprehension of what may be a complex medical regimen, and support systems are pertinent to management. Will this patient be compliant with medication, and reliable about follow-up visits and reporting symptoms? What financial burdens can he or she deal with for tests and medications? Accurate assessment of these issues may determine whether a patient can be expected to change lifestyle or take medication regularly. The third row of Table 26–4 states that the initial work-up will lead to a plan that will include recommendations for treatment and for appropriate follow-up evaluations, which will be covered in the upcoming sections.

The fourth row in Table 26–4 indicates that an estimate of the likelihood of secondary hypertension should be made. Many forms of secondary hypertension can be detected through a careful history and physical examination. Table 26–5 provides a guide to these disorders and also indicates the

**Table 26–3** Assessment of Target Organ Damage (TOD) to be Suspected in Hypertensive Patients with or without Other Risk Factors

| Site/Pathology | Detection by History and Examination | Pertinent Additional Tests |
|---|---|---|
| Retina: arteriolar thickening, hemorrhage, exudates, papilledema | Ophthalmoscopy | Fluorescein angiography, *rarely needed* |
| Carotid artery stenosis | Auscultation for bruits | Carotid ultrasound assessment* |
| LVH; diastolic and systolic dysfunction | History of dyspnea, fatigue; examination for $S_4$, increased $S_2$, cardiac enlargement–left ventricular heave | ECG; echocardiogram for selected cases |
| Coronary artery disease | History of angina, or previous myocardial infarction | ECG, stress tests* |
| Cerebrovascular disease | History of stroke or transient ischemic attack, screening neurologic examination | Carotid ultrasound assessment*; additional imaging with CT scan or MRI sometimes appropriate |
| Renal pathology | History of renal disease or diabetes >5 years, unexplained edema | Urinalysis for protein, abnormal sediment; spot urine for microalbumin; albumin: creatinine ratio; calculated creatinine clearance as estimate of glomerular filtration rate |
| Abdominal aortic aneurysm | History of abdominal mass or discomfort, detection of pulsatile mass on physical examination | Ultrasound of abdomen,* CT scan, MRI, MRA |
| Peripheral arterial stenosis | History of claudication, reduced pulses on physical examination | Measurement of arm and calf pressures for ankle/arm index* |

*Indicated as initial test when history or physical examination reveals positive findings.
LVH, left ventricular hypertrophy; $S_4$, fourth heart sound; $S_2$, second heart sound; ECG, electrocardiogram; CT, computed tomography; MRI, magnetic resonance imaging; MRA, magnetic resonance angiography.

**Table 26–4** Information to be Derived from Initial Assessment of Hypertensive Patients

| Assessment | Information Derived |
|---|---|
| Overall risk status of future cardiovascular disease | Composite of: Average blood pressure level Nonhypertensive risk factors Target organ damage |
| Assessment for management strategy | Potential for education, change in lifestyle, compliance with medication |
| Plan for treatment and follow-up | Choice of lifestyle change and/or medication; schedule for follow-up, rescreening |
| Likelihood of secondary hypertension | Clues provided by history, physical examination, and initial laboratory tests |

need for appropriate laboratory assessment as initial screening strategy. Characteristics of many diagnostic tests frequently used to detect secondary hypertension have been calculated with regard to sensitivity, specificity, and predictive value.[63] When secondary hypertension is considered likely, on clinical grounds, combinations of tests used judiciously may provide the greatest accuracy.[63,64]

## INITIAL MANAGEMENT

After evaluating hypertensive patients, decisions will be made regarding goals for treatment and strategies for achieving these goals. In general, some combination of lifestyle change and drug therapy will be recommended. When the pressure is higher, drug treatment will be started immediately. For those

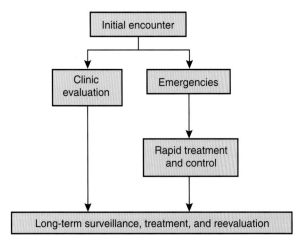

**Figure 26–2** A simplified flow diagram for management of hypertensive patients, after their initial detection. The few hypertensive emergencies will be rapidly evaluated and treated. Most patients will be evaluated entirely in clinic or office settings. All should be kept under observation with reevaluation, adjustment in treatment, and appropriate diagnostic assessment for as long as possible.

with pressures in the range of 140 to 150 mm Hg/90 to 100 mm Hg, without TOD, initial nonpharmacologic choices, particularly weight reduction, with or without reduced salt intake may be appropriate. Diets that have high fruit, vegetable, and low-fat dairy product content with low-salt intake such as the Dietary Approaches to Stop Hypertension (DASH)-sodium diet can be recommended as an effective lifestyle change.[65,66] When smoking, increased LDL cholesterol, or diabetes is found, attention to these may be as important as BP reduction.

Apart from the general advice given in guidelines or consensus documents, there is surprisingly little information in the medical literature about specific strategies for getting each patient to the goal of a reduced overall risk of future cardiovascular disease. The patient's ability to understand and comply with treatment needs attention, as well as his or her various personal, social, and economic characteristics. In setting a plan for management, the time frame for achieving specific goals needs to be discussed with the patient. Trying to do too much in too short a time often leads to frustration and less optimal compliance, compared with a gradual introduction of one intervention at a time over several visits, spaced out over several months.

## REEVALUATION AND FOLLOW-UP

After the initial work-up, management of hypertension and cardiovascular risk ought to become a long-term partnership between doctor and patient so that periodic surveillance and reassessment are coupled with continuing motivation and education. The success of randomized clinical trials in demonstrating the efficacy of antihypertensive drug therapy and cholesterol reduction has depended on recruiting and maintaining a high fraction of patients on treatment who are willing to remain enrolled under observation. Whether the same degree of compliance and adherence can be achieved in ordinary clinical settings remains a challenge.

Most patients with well-controlled BP after 6 to 9 months of treatment remain stable for long periods and, in my view can be seen every 6 months thereafter. Even this frequency may be too demanding for many patients who work or have family responsibilities and are free of symptoms, unless a highly convenient medical care system is available. Adjunct resources such as work-site clinics may be helpful.[67] Self-measurement of BPs at home has the potential for reducing need for office or clinic visits[68] and may improve control of hypertension.[69]

When hypertension remains uncontrolled despite appropriate multidrug treatment, the terms *refractory hypertension* or *resistant hypertension* apply. Some of these patients have normal pressures by ambulatory BP monitoring[70-72] or home monitoring[19] because of a large white-coat effect. Many of those with refractory hypertension probably have reduced adherence to medication and need additional education and counseling to improve use of medication.[73] Other considerations should include underdosing of partially effective medications (especially in very obese patients), ineffective drug combinations, use of steroids or nonsteroidal antiinflammatory drugs that may raise pressure, and secondary hypertension (see following paragraphs).

My own suggestions for follow-up evaluations are given in Table 26–6. There are, however, many exceptions or intercurrent changes that warrant highly individual choices. Even when

**Table 26-5** Initial Assessment for Secondary Hypertension—Some Examples of More Well-known Forms

| Specific Disease | Findings by History and Physical Examination | Usual Screening or Initial Tests |
|---|---|---|
| Coarctation of the aorta | Decreased pulsation and pressure in legs, interscapular bruit | Chest radiograph for abnormal aortic contour, chest CT or MRI |
| Cushing's syndrome | Obesity, "moon" face, "buffalo hump" of cervical fat pad, acne, bruises, purple abdominal striae | 24-hour free cortisol and overnight dexamethasone suppression test |
| Primary aldosteronism, other forms of mineralocorticoid excess | Normal appearance, vague symptoms, fatigue, weakness, rarely tetany | Serum electrolytes, plasma renin, serum or urine aldosterone; measure other mineralocorticoids for rare conditions |
| Renal artery stenosis | Subcostal bruit, signs of widespread atherosclerotic arterial disease | High renin profile, positive captopril test, duplex Doppler study of renal arteries, MRA of renal arteries |
| Polycystic kidney disease | History of familial hypertension and renal disease, palpable flank masses | Ultrasound of kidneys |
| Chronic renal disease | History of abnormal urinalysis, known connective tissues disease (e.g., lupus erythematosus), edema, hematuria, recurrent urinary tract infections or stones | Complete urinalysis; creatinine clearance, urinary protein, appropriate serologic studies |
| Pheochromocytoma | Highly variable pressure, symptoms of paroxysmal palpitations, anxiety, sweating, headache, constipation or diarrhea, weight loss, family history of endocrine disease or "birthmark" diseases | 24-hour urine metanephrine excretion or serum metanephrines; CT scan for detection of tumor |
| Drug reactions: diet pill overdose, cocaine use, ephedra, other drugs, or alcohol withdrawal | Often abrupt increase in blood pressure with headaches, *accurate history is crucial,* including *recent use* of any drugs | Chemical screens for amphetamines, cocaine, alcohol, other drugs |
| Obstructive sleep apnea | History of snoring or abnormal breathing during sleep, daytime somnolence | Overnight sleep study with $O_2$ saturation (somnography) |
| Hyperthyroidism* | Typical symptoms, tachycardia or atrial fibrillation, wide pulse pressure with normal-low diastolic pressure | Serum TSH with "reflex" test for free thyroxine level |
| Hypothyroidism* | Typical symptoms, bradycardia, increase in systolic pressure | Serum TSH with "reflex" test for free thyroxine level |
| Hyperparathyroidism* | Compatable symptoms: renal stones, osteoporosis, intestinal disorders | Serum calcium level, followed by appropriate studies for parathyroid hormone excess |

CT, computed tomography; MRI, magnetic resonance imaging; MRA, magnetic resonance angiography; TSH, thyroid-stimulating hormone.
*Whether disorders of thyroid or parathyroid function are specific causes of hypertension remains uncertain. Because hypertension is highly prevalent, these disorders may appear by chance, but patients should be fully evaluated when these disorders are suspected.

hypertension and other risk factors are well controlled over long periods of observation, hypertensive patients remain likely to have cerebrovascular and cardiovascular disease.[74] Thus clinicians should be aware that the syndromes of cerebrovascular disease or CHD are ever in the background despite effective therapy. This implies that screening tests for arterial disease, particularly cardiac stress tests and ultrasound interrogations of the carotid artery and the abdominal aorta may have value for hypertensives treated for many years, espe-

cially if they are older (>55 years) or have wide pulse pressures or any prior cardiovascular disease. Men older than age 65 may benefit from screening by ultrasound for abdominal aortic aneurysms.[75] This strategy is not cost-effective for women.[76]

Secondary hypertension may occur, on occasion, in those with essential hypertension during their course of prolonged management. Atherosclerotic renal artery stenosis may develop when there are multiple risk factors for atherosclerosis or carotid or peripheral artery disease. Development of renal

**Table 26-6** Suggested Follow-up Assessment for Hypertensive Patients, Based on Level of Absolute Risk and Response to Treatment*

| Measurement or Procedure | Comment |
| --- | --- |
| Weight | Every visit |
| Sitting BP | Every visit |
| Standing BP | Initial visit, if patient dizzy, if tendency to orthostatic hypotension known or suspected; older patients |
| Listen for carotid bruit, cardiac examination, peripheral vascular assessment | 1-2 years, unless new symptoms or abnormalities present in past |
| For nondiabetic patients: fasting glucose, lipid profile | For stable patients without abnormalities at baseline, every 2 years For overweight patients, or unusual change in weight, recheck glucose and lipids more often |
| Patients with drug-treated hyperlipidemia | Monitor serum lipids every 6-12 months |
| Diabetic patients | Glucose, HgbA$_1$C, serum lipids initially as often as necessary for optimal management; once stable, every 6-12 months; check for microalbuminuria annually after 5 years |
| ECG | Every 2 years unless new symptoms or known abnormalities at baseline |
| Renal function: creatinine, urine for microalbumin, electrolytes | Every 1-2 years, unless abnormal at baseline or high-dose diuretics prescribed |
| Echocardiography, cardiac stress test, creatinine clearance | Only for change in status from baseline suspected by new symptoms |
| Work-up for secondary hypertension | New symptoms, hypokalemia, impaired renal function; consider for some patients with refractory hypertension |

*The suggestions are based on several current guidelines and clinical experience, but individual patients may require different kinds of ongoing assessment.
BP, blood pressure; ECG, electrocardiogram.

insufficiency in elderly patients who used to be hypertensive, but now have congestive heart failure with lower arterial pressure, should raise the suspicion of renal arterial disease and ischemic nephropathy.[77,78]

Refractory hypertension might also raise the question of underlying disease. In addition to renal artery stenosis, hypothyroidism should be considered and is easily detected by measuring thyroid-stimulating hormone (TSH). Primary aldosteronism has recently been reported as a more common cause of drug-resistant hypertension.[50,51]

Each follow-up visit of a hypertensive patient is not only a reevaluation of medical status, but can be viewed as an opportunity to maintain or enhance the goals of optimal preventive care. Brief and focused emphasis on reinforcing positive changes in lifestyle, education about risk and value of compliance with treatment may contribute to the patient's overall commitment to staying on treatment. The message to be conveyed is that such periodic evaluations are part of the long-range plan for reducing the odds of cardiovascular disease through an effective partnership between doctor and patient.

## SUMMARY

The initial and follow-up evaluations of hypertensive patients are, taken together, a complex scheme for preventing or reversing cardiovascular and renal disease over time intervals from years to decades. The tools available to clinicians for work-up now include a wide spectrum from the most basic skills (the medical history and physical examination) to sophisticated imaging techniques and biochemical assays. It is now possible with reasonable cost and efficiency to predict absolute risk of future cardiovascular disease with far greater precision when many risk factors are taken together, and not rely on BP alone. Such a strategy then can lead to more rational therapy focused on reversible risk factors and pathology, as revealed from clinical trials. Secondary hypertension, although rare, can now be detected with more precise, but less invasive methods because of progress in diagnostic technology. Nonetheless, for most hypertensive patients, it is sustained surveillance and reassessment, coupled with strategies for education and motivation to achieve their active participation in optimal treatment that will be the crucial determinants in reducing the likelihood of stroke, CHD, congestive heart failure, and progression to ESRD.

## References

1. Prospective Studies Collaboration. Age-specific relevance of usual blood pressure to vascular mortality: a meta-analysis of individual data for one million adults in 61 prospective studies. Lancet 1903-1913, 2002.
2. Glynn RJ, Field TS, Rosner B, et al. Evidence for a positive linear relation between blood pressure and mortality in elderly people. Lancet 345:825-829, 1995.

3. Vasan RS, Larson MG, Leip E, et al. Impact of high-normal blood pressure on the risk of cardiovascular disease. N Engl J Med 345:1291-1297, 2001.

4. Franklin SS, Khan SA, Wong ND, et al. Is pulse pressure useful in predicting risk for coronary heart disease? The Framingham Heart Study. Circulation 100:354-360, 1999.

5. Staessen J, Gasowski J, Wang JG, et al. Risks of untreated and treated isolated systolic hypertension in the elderly: meta-analysis of outcome trials. Lancet 355:865-872, 2000.

6. Franklin SS, Larson M, Kahn S, et al. Does the relation of blood pressure to coronary heart disease risk change with aging? The Framingham Heart Study. Circulation 103: 1245-1249, 2001.

7. Klag MJ, Whelton PK, Randall BL, et al. Blood pressure and end-stage renal disease in men. N Engl J Med 334:13-18, 1996.

8. The Sixth Report of the Joint National Committee on Prevention, Detection, Evaluation, and Treatment of High Blood Pressure. Arch Intern Med 157:2413-2445, 1997.

9. Guidelines Subcommittee. 1999 World Health Organization-International Society of Hypertension Guidelines for the Management of Hypertension. J Hypertens 17:151-183, 1999.

10. Chobanian AV, Bakris GL, Black HR, et al. The seventh report of the Joint National Committee on Prevention, Detection, Evaluation and Treatment of High Blood Pressure: The JNC 7 Report. EXPRESS VERSION: JAMA 2003; 289:2560-2572; COMPLETE VERSION: Hypertension 42:1206-1252, 2003.

11. Vasan RS, Beiser A, Seshadri S, et al. Residual lifetime risk for developing hypertension in middle-aged women and men: The Framingham Heart Study. JAMA 287:1003-1010, 2002.

12. He J, Whelton PK, Appel LJ, et al. Long-term effects of weight loss and dietary sodium reduction on incidence of hypertension. Hypertension 35:544-549, 2000.

13. Parati G, Pomidossi G, Albini F, et al. Relationship of 24-hour blood pressure mean and variability to severity of target-organ damage in hypertension. J Hypertens 5:93-98, 1987.

14. Verdecchia P, Borgioni C, Ciucci A, et al. Prognostic significance of blood pressure variability in essential hypertension. Blood Pressure Monitoring 1:3-11, 1996.

15. Perry HM Jr, Miller JP. Difficulties in diagnosing hypertension: implications and alternatives. J Hypertens 10:887-896, 1992.

16. Schechter CB, Adler RS. Bayesian analysis of diastolic blood pressure measurement. Med Decis Making 8:182-190, 1991.

17. Bruce NG, Shaper AG, Walker M, et al. Observer bias in blood pressure studies. J Hypertens 6:375-380, 1988.

18. Clement D, De Buyzere M, De Bacqer DA et al. Prognostic value of ambulatory blood-pressure recordings in patients with treated hypertension. N Engl J Med 348:2407-2415, 2003.

19. Bobrie G, Genes N, Vaur L, et al. Is "isolated home" hypertension as opposed to "isolated office" hypertension a sign of greater cardiovascular risk? Arch Intern Med 161(18): 2205-2211, 2001.

20. Liu JE, Roman MJ, Pini R, et al. Cardiac and arterial target organ damage in adults with elevated ambulatory and normal office blood pressure. Ann Intern Med 131:564-572, 1999.

21. Jain A, Krakoff LR. Effect of recorded home blood pressure measurements on staging of hypertensive patients. Blood Pressure Monitoring 7(3):157-161, 2002.

22. Isles C, Brown JJ, Cumming AMM, et al. Excess smoking in malignant-phase hypertension. BMJ 1:579-581, 1979.

23. Bloxham CA, Beevers DG, Walker JM. Malignant hypertension and cigarette smoking. BMJ 1:581-583, 1979.

24. Rosenberg L, Kaufman DW, Helmrich SP, et al. The risk of myocardial infarction after quitting smoking in men under 55 years of age. N Engl J Med 313:1511-1514, 1985.

25. Multiple Risk Factor Intervention Trial Research Group. Multiple risk factor intervention trial: Risk factor changes and mortality results. JAMA 248:1465-1477, 1982.

26. Shepard J, Cobbe SM, Ford I, et al. Prevention of coronary heart disease with pravastatin in men with hypercholesterolemia. N Engl J Med 333:1301-1307, 1995.

27. Heart Protection Study Collaborative Group. MRC/BHF heart protection study of cholesterol lowering with simvastatin in 20536 high-risk individuals: a randomised placebo-controlled trial. Lancet 360:7-22, 2002.

28. Sever PS, Dahlöf B, Poulter NR, et al. Prevention of coronary and stroke events with atorvastatin in hypertensive patients who have average or lower-than-average cholesterol concentrations, in the Anglo-Scandavanavian Cardiac Outcomes Trial-Lipid Lowering Arm (ASCOT-LLA): A multicentre randomised controlled trial. Lancet 361:1149-1158, 2003.

29. Rubins HB, Robins SJ, Collins D, et al. Gemfibrozil for the secondary prevention of coronary heart disease in men with low levels of high-density lipoprotein cholesterol. Veterans Affairs High-Density Lipoprotein Cholesterol Intervention Trial Study Group. N Engl J Med 341(6):410-418, 1999.

30. Gress TW, Nieto J, Shahar E, et al. Hypertension and antihypertensive therapy as risk factors for type 2 diabetes. N Engl J Med 342:905-912, 2000.

31. Gerstein HC, Yusuf S. Dysglycemia and risk of cardiovascular disease. Lancet 347:949-950, 1996.

32. Saad MF, Knowler WC, Pettitt DJ, et al. Insulin and hypertension—Relationship to obesity and glucose intolerance in Pima Indians. Diabetes 39:1430-1435, 1990.

33. Shen DC, Sheih SM, Chen YD, et al. Resistance to insulin-stimulated glucose uptake in patients with hypertension. J Clin Endocrinol Metab 66:580-583, 1988.

34. American Diabetes Association. Standards of medical care in diabetes. Diabetes Care 27:S15-S35, 2004.

35. Haffner SM, Miettinen H, Gaskill SP, et al. Metabolic precursors of hypertension. The San Antonio heart study. Arch Intern Med 156:1994-2000, 1996.

36. Flegel KM, Carroll MD, Ogden CL, et al. Prevalence and trends in obesity among US adults, 1999-2000. JAMA 288:1723-1727, 2002.

37. Whelton SP, Chin A, Xin X, et al. Effect of aerobic exercise on blood pressure: a meta-analysis of randomized, controlled trials. Ann Intern Med 136:493-503, 2002.

38. Kokkinos PF, Narayan P, Colleran JA, et al. Effects of regular exercise on blood pressure and left ventricular hypertrophy in African-American men with severe hypertension. N Engl J Med 333:1462-1467, 1995.

39. Ekelund L-G, Haskell WL, Johnson JL, et al. Physical fitness as a predictor of cardiovascular mortality in asymptomatic North American Men. N Engl J Med 319:1379-1384, 1988.

40. Fries JF, Singh G, Morfield D. Running and the development of disability with age. Ann Int Med 121:502-509, 1994.

41. Paffenbarger RS Jr, Hyde RT, Wing AL, et al. The association of changes in physical-activity level and among other lifestyle characteristics with mortality among men. N Engl J Med 328:538-545, 1993.

42. Gill JS, Zezulka AV, Shipley MJ, et al. Stroke and alcohol consumption. N Engl J Med 315:1041-1046, 1986.

43. Stampfer MJ, Colditz GA, Willett WC, et al. A prospective study of moderate alcohol consumption and the risk of coronary disease and stroke in women. N Engl J Med 319:267-273, 1988.

44. Beilin LJ. The fifth Sir George Pickering memorial lecture: Epitaph to essential hypertension-a preventable disorder of known aetiology? J Hypertens 6:85-94, 1988.

45. Whelton PK, He J, Appel LJ, et al. Primary prevention of hypertension: clinical and public health advisory from the National High Blood Pressure Education Program. JAMA 288: 1882-1888, 2002.

46. Puddey IB, Parker M, Beilin LJ, et al. Effects of alcohol and caloric restrictions on blood pressure and serum lipids in overweight men. Hypertension 20:533-541, 1992.

47. Marmot MG, Elliott P, Shipley MJ, et al. Alcohol and blood pressure: the INTERSALT Study. BMJ 308:1263-1267, 1994.

48. Brunner HR, Laragh JH, Baer L, et al. Essential hypertension: renin, and aldosterone, heart attack and stroke. N Engl J Med 286:441-449, 1972.

49. Alderman MH, Madhavan S, Ooi WL, et al. Association of the renin-sodium profile with the risk of myocardial infarction in patients with hypertension. N Engl J Med 324:1098-1104, 1991.

50. Calhoun DA, Nishizaka MK, Zaman MA, et al. Hyperaldosteronism among Black and White subjects with resistant hypertension. Hypertension 40:892-896, 2002.

51. Lim PO, Jung RT, MacDonald TM. Is aldosterone the missing link in refractory hypertension?: aldosterone-to-renin ratio as a marker of inappropriate aldosterone activity. J Hum Hypertens 16(3):153-158, 2002.

52. Ouzan J, Perault C, Lincoff AM, et al. The role of spironolactone in the treatment of patients with refractory hypertension. Am J Hypertens 15(4 Pt 1):333-339, 2002.

53. Nishizaka MK, Zaman MA, Calhoun DA. Efficacy of low-dose spironolactone in subjects with resistant hypertension. Am J Hypertens 16:925-930, 2003.

54. Perry IJ, Refsum H, Morris RW, et al. Prospective study of serum total homocysteine concentration and risk of stroke in middle-aged British men. Lancet 346:1995-1398, 1995.

55. Nygard O, Nordrehaug JE, Refsum H, et al. Plasma homocysteine levels and mortality in patients with coronary artery disease. N Engl J Med 337:230-236, 1998.

56. Mayer EL, Jacobsen DW, Robinson K. Homocysteine and coronary atherosclerosis. J Am Coll Cardiol 27:517-527, 1996.

57. Jacques PF, Selhyb J, Bostom AG, et al. The effect of folic acid fortification on plasma folate and total homocysteine. N Engl J Med 340:1449-1454, 1999.

58. Ridker PM, Cushman M, Stampfer MJ, et al. Plasma concentration of C-reactive protein and risk of developing peripheral vascular disease. Circulation 97:425-428, 1998.

59. Grau AJ, Buggle F, Becher H, et al. The association of leukocyte count, fibrinogen, and C-reactive protein with vascular risk factors and ischemic vascular disease. Thromb Res 82:245-255, 1996.

60. Danesh J, Collins R, Appleby P, et al. Association of fibrinogen, C-reactive protein, albumin, or leukocyte count with coronary heart disease: meta-analyses of prospective studies. JAMA 279:1477-1482, 1998.

61. Steering Committee of the Physician's Health Study Research Group. Final report on the aspirin component of the ongoing physicians health study. N Engl J Med 321:129-135, 1989.

62. Mosca L. C-reactive proteins–to screen or not to screen? N Engl J Med 347:1615-1617, 2002.

63. Krakoff LR. Secondary or curable hypertension. *In* Krakoff LR. Management of the Hypertensive Patient. New York, Churchill Livingstone, 1995; pp 75-86.

64. Pauker SG, Kopelman RI. Interpreting hoofbeats: Can Bayes help clear the haze? N Engl J Med 327:1009-1013, 1992.

65. Sacks FM, Svetkey LP, Vollmer WM, et al. Effects on blood pressure of reduced dietary sodium and the dietary approaches to stop hypertension (DASH) study. N Engl J Med 344:3-10, 2001.

66. John JH, Ziebland S, Yudkin P, et al. Effects of fruit and vegetable consumption on plasma antioxidant concentrations and blood pressure: A randomised controlled trial. Lancet 359:1969-1974, 2002.

67. Foote A, Efurt JC. Hypertension control at the work site: Comparison of screening alone, referral and follow-up, and on-site treatment. N Engl J Med 308:809-813, 1983.

68. Soghikian K, Casper SM, Fireman BH, et al. Home blood pressure monitoring: Effect on use of medical services and medical care costs. Med Care 30:855-865, 1992.

69. Rogers MAM, Small D, Buchan DA, et al. Home monitoring service improves mean arterial pressure in patients with essential hypertension. Ann Intern Med 134:1024-1032, 2001.

70. Mezzetti A, Pierdomenico SD, Costantini F, et al. White-coat resistant hypertension. Am J Hypertens 10:1302-1307, 1997.

71. Redon J, Campos C, Rodicio JL, et al. Prognostic value of ambulatory blood pressure monitoring in refractory hypertension: a prospective study. Hypertension 31:712-718, 2001.

72. Brown MA, Buddle ML, Martin A. Is resistant hypertension really resistant? Am J Hypertens 14:1263-1269, 2003.

73. Burnier M, Schneider MP, Chiolero A, et al. Electronic compliance monitoring in resistant hypertension: the basis for rational therapeutic decisions. J Hypertens 19(2):335-341, 2001.

74. Alderman MH, Cohen H, Madhavan S. Distribution and determinants of cardiovascular events during 20 years of successful antihypertensive treatment. J Hypertens 16:761-769, 1998.

75. The Multicentre Aneurysm Screening Study Group. The Multicentre Aneurysm Screening Study (MASS) into the effect of abdominal aortic aneurysm screening on mortality in men: a randomised controlled trial. Lancet 360:1531-1539, 2002.

76. Scott RA, Bridgewater SG, Ashton HA. Randomized clinical trial of screening for abdominal aortic aneurysm in women. Br J Surg 89(3):283-285, 2002.

77. Rimmer JM, Gennari FJ. Atherosclerotic renovascular disease and progressive renal failure. Ann Int Med 118:712-719, 1993.

78. MacDowell P, Kalra PA, O'Donoghue DJ, et al. Risk of morbidity from renovascular disease in elderly patients with congestive cardiac failure. Lancet 352:13-16, 1998.

# Prognostic and Diagnostic Value of Ambulatory Blood Pressure Monitoring

## Gianfranco Parati, Grzegorz Bilo, Giuseppe Mancia

The currently employed method for blood pressure (BP) measurement in physicians' offices is still based on the auscultatory sphygmomanometric technique, developed by Riva-Rocci[1] and Korotkoff more than a century ago, which has remained the usual approach for the diagnosis and management of hypertension in clinical practice. This technique has provided us with most of the available information on the prognostic consequences of a high BP, and on the protective effect of BP reduction obtained by antihypertensive treatment.

However, over the years a considerable number of problems associated with this time-honored method have been acknowledged. The main limitations of office BP measurements are related to the following:

1. Their inability to provide a large number of BP values (necessary to account for the physiologic variability typical of this parameter).
2. The fact that measurements are usually taken in a health care facility setting, which may cause an alerting reaction in the patient, followed by a BP rise that is frequently of a relevant magnitude (even 30 mm Hg or more), known as the "white-coat effect" (WCE).
3. The often improper application of the auscultatory sphygmomanometric technique (inappropriate conditions of measurement, error in positioning or selecting the arm cuff, wrong arm position, observer's bias and digit preference).
4. The inherent inaccuracy of auscultatory BP readings, mainly for diastolic BP (DBP) measurements, in a number of clinical conditions.
5. The incoming banning of mercury from diagnostic applications and devices, until now routinely used in the clinical setting. The safety issues related to this highly toxic metal may be expected to lead to the disappearance of mercury sphygmomanometers, which have already been banned in some European countries.[2,3]

The first four issues can be considered responsible for the high degree of between-measurement variability that can be observed both within and between physician's visits, this phenomenon can be explained only in part by physiologic mechanisms.

In the attempt to overcome these limitations, a number of different approaches to BP measurement have been proposed, aimed at obtaining a more precise definition of patients' "true" BP level. Two of them are now widely used in clinical practice, namely self–BP measurement (SBPM) at home and 24-hour ambulatory BP monitoring (ABPM). This chapter focuses on the clinical value of the information obtained by performing ABPM in the management of hypertensive patients.

## TECHNIQUE OF AMBULATORY BLOOD PRESSURE MONITORING—ITS HISTORY AND CURRENT ACHIEVEMENTS

The occurrence of pronounced BP fluctuations over time was first observed by Stephen Hales in 1733, when performing his famous experiments on "the arterial pulse" by inserting a glass pipe into the crural artery of mares (Figure 27–1). In the following years, additional information on the occurrence of BP variations with time was obtained in humans, although only through indirect methods aimed at quantifying the arterial pulse, in most cases at the level of the radial artery (Figure 27–2). Further insights into the variations of BP in humans under the effects of exercise, stress, and emotions were later made possible by the introduction of the sphygmomanometric technique by Riva-Rocci[1] and Korotkoff.

A major breakthrough occurred in the last decades of the twentieth century, when a portable intraarterial ABPM system was developed by the Oxford group. This technique, using a catheter placed in the radial or brachial artery and connected with an electronic transducer and a perfusion unit positioned at heart level, was able to yield a detailed recording of beat-by-beat BP changes, stored on an analog tape recorder. The application of this system to ABPM in humans has provided us with the first demonstration that BP is characterized by pronounced oscillations over the entire 24 hours (Figure 27–3).[4] These include both long-term fluctuations, such as those between wakefulness and sleep, and rapid changes over a time scale of seconds and minutes, due to the cardiovascular effects of emotion, exercise, and behavioral challenges.[5,6] Application of this technique to subjects characterized by different BP levels has led to the demonstration that BP variability (as quantified by the standard deviation [SD] of average 24-hour BP levels) increases progressively with the increase in 24-hour mean BP levels. It has also allowed a dynamic observation of BP and heart rate changes during the physician's visit, at the time when a sphygmomanometric measurement is performed. Through the application of this technique, we provided the first direct assessment of the magnitude and time course of the WCE and quantification of the differential impact on BP and heart rate exerted by BP measurements performed by a doctor and a nurse, respectively.[7,8]

The invasive nature of this method has prevented its widespread use in a clinical setting, for which noninvasive approaches are required. This need has been met by progress in technology that led to the development of two alternative approaches to noninvasive BP monitoring. The first consists of a noninvasive system able to yield beat-by-beat BP recordings similar to those offered by the intraarterial technique, but without need of intraarterial catheters. This was achieved

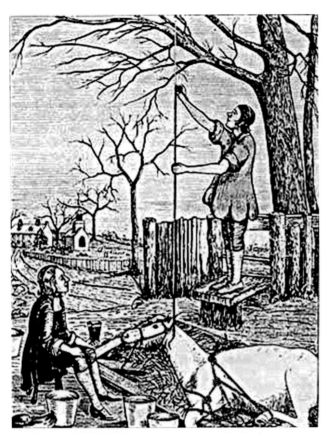

**Figure 27–1** The first blood pressure measurement, by Hales, 1733. (Illustration by Elizabeth Cuzzort. From Medical Times, Volume 72, 1944.)

through the photo-plethysmographic arterial clamping technique described by Penaz and further improved by Wesseling, based on the application of small cuffs on the middle or ring fingers of the patient's hand.[9,10] This technique was first applied to the development of a stationary device (Finapres, Ohmeda Inc., Ohmeda, Colorado, USA) now improved, refurbished, and made commercially available with the new name of Finometer (FMS, Arnhem, The Netherlands).

Subsequently, the same technology was implemented in a portable device (Portapres, FMS, Arnhem, The Netherlands), which until now remains the only available approach to non-invasive 24-hour, beat-by-beat ABPM. These devices have been shown to be accurate for tracking of BP changes, but the absolute BP values they yield do not always precisely reflect sphygmomanometric BP obtained at the arm level.[11] The accuracy of this system has been improved by implementing a hydrostatic height correction system, able to correct the recorded BP values for the hydrostatic height difference between the finger cuff and heart level, and by applying a mathematical transformation to finger BP waveforms aimed at reconstructing brachial BP waveforms and at approaching arm BP levels[12] (Figure 27–4).

Techniques for continuous BP monitoring have provided us with a large amount of interesting data on the physiologic mechanisms regulating the cardiovascular system and on their derangement in pathologic conditions.[13] This has been obtained through computer analysis of spontaneous BP and heart rate variations. This approach has yielded new information not only on the magnitude but also on the rapidity of spontaneous BP fluctuations, the latter found to be steeper in hypertensive than in normotensive persons.[14] In spite of their great potential, techniques for continuous BP monitoring have been largely confined to a research setting, mainly because of their high cost and complexity.

The other approach to ABPM is based on the use of portable, noninvasive, discontinuous BP monitoring devices, which have become widely used tools to assess BP changes over the 24 hours in the clinical setting.[15] The first ABPM devices, known as *Remler devices,*[16,17] were based on semiautomatic techniques. The measurement was started manually by the patient, who was asked to inflate the arm cuff, while the cuff deflation and the BP readings (based on microphonic detection of the Korotkoff sounds) were done automatically. Despite its limitations, including inability to yield information on nighttime BP and the need of an interactive, time-consuming procedure by a technician to individually derive the recorded BP values, this technique made it possible for the first time to obtain evidence on the prognostic relevance of ABPM.[18]

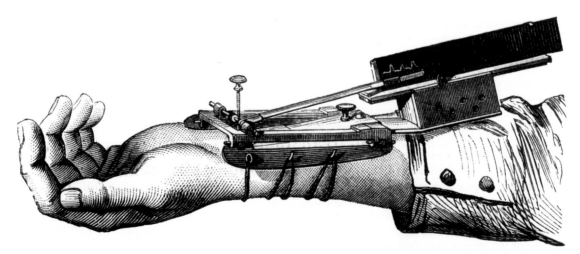

**Figure 27–2** The "direct" sphygmograph, by Etienne Jules Marey, 1860. (From Marey EJ. La circulation du sang. Paris, Masson, 1881; p 214. Courtesy of The Wellcome Library, London.)

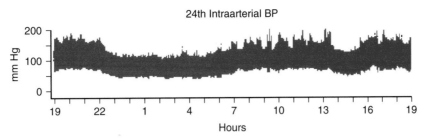

**Figure 27-3** An example of 24-hour beat-by-beat intraarterial ambulatory blood pressure (BP) recording documenting the pronounced variability that characterizes BP over day and night periods. (From Mancia G, Parati G, Di Rienzo M, et al. Blood pressure variability. *In* Zanchetti A, Mancia G (eds). Handbook of Hypertension, Vol. 17: Pathophysiology of Hypertension. London, Elsevier Science BV 1997; pp 117-169: by permission.)

Further technologic development in this field has led to the introduction of fully automated ABPM devices in which BP measurement by the microphonic technique (rather susceptible to interference, especially by external noise) has been progressively replaced by the oscillometric approach. Currently, fully automated oscillometric devices, if validated according to internationally accepted protocols,[19-21] are the method of choice for performing ABPM.[22] The need to focus on validated devices is related to the fact that oscillometric monitors do not directly measure systolic BP (SBP) and DBP, but just mean BP, whereas systolic and diastolic values are derived from mean values through use of proprietary device-specific algorithms. A list of devices validated for clinical application according to the aforementioned protocols is published[23] and is available and regularly updated on a dedicated website (*www.dableducational.com*).

## PROGNOSTIC IMPORTANCE OF AMBULATORY BLOOD PRESSURE

Although most of the available data on the prognostic importance of an elevated BP and on the benefits obtainable by its reduction through effective antihypertensive treatment are based on office readings,[24] an increasing number of studies have indicated that ABPM may provide diagnostic and prognostic information that is not only equivalent but probably superior to that yielded by traditional office measurements.[25]

A number of these studies have focused on the relationship of office and ambulatory BP with target organ damage. They have almost invariably demonstrated the superiority of ambulatory values in this regard. This was the case in terms of cardiac, renal, cerebral, and vascular changes (both in large and small arteries), as well as in terms of a general organ damage score, in studies specifically focusing on this issue[26-30] (Figure 27–5),[27] and also in analysis of the baseline data of large prospective outcome studies such as the European Lacidipine Study on Atherosclerosis (ELSA—data on macrovascular changes)[31] (Figure 27–6).

A few longitudinal studies showing that ABPM provides data that are prognostically superior to those obtained by means of office measurement are also available. The first longitudinal data were those of Perloff et al.,[18] followed by data on target organ progression such as those obtained over a 6- to 7-year follow-up of the patients included in our study using intraarterial ABPM[32] and those obtained when prospectively focusing on target organ damage reduction by treatment in the Study on Ambulatory Monitoring of Pressure and Lisinopril Evaluation (SAMPLE)[33] (Figure 27–7).

Longitudinal data on the ability of ABPM to provide important prognostic information on the occurrence of cardiovascular events are also available. Such data were provided by the uncontrolled observations by Verdecchia et al. obtained in the cohort of subjects included in the PIUMA (Progetto Ipertensione Umbria Monitoraggio Ambulatoriale) database[34] and by Redon et al.[35] in patients with resistant hypertension. An important contribution to the demonstration of the prognostic value of ABPM was also provided by analysis of data obtained from the adult population of Ohasama in Japan.

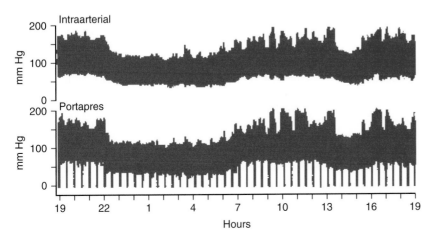

**Figure 27-4** Comparison of blood pressure values obtained with invasive technique and with Portapres device.

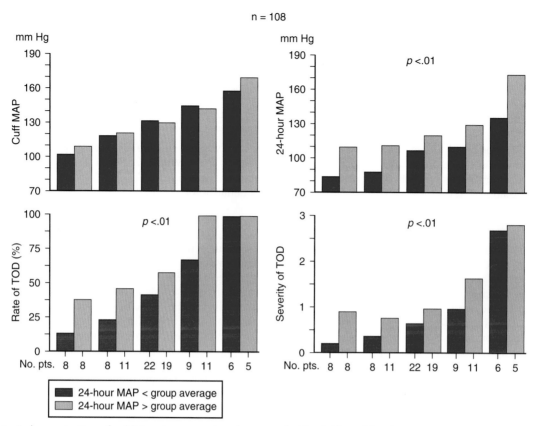

n = 108

**Figure 27-5** A demonstration of additional prognostic value provided by 24-hour blood pressure (BP) in terms of target organ damage (TOD). For every quintile of office BP, the presence of a higher 24-hour mean arterial pressure (MAP) was associated with more severe target organ changes. (From Parati G, Pomidossi G, Albini F, et al. Relationship of 24-hour blood pressure mean and variability to severity of target organ damage. J Hypertens 5:93-98, 1987; by permission.)

After 5 years of follow-up, it was evident that having ambulatory SBP in the highest quintile of the population data distribution was associated with an elevated risk of death from cardiovascular causes, whereas no such close association was found for casual BP values.[36] Similarly, in the analysis of data from the Syst-Eur study (Systolic Hypertension in Europe Trial),[37] in the group of elderly hypertensives receiving placebo, a 10–mm Hg higher ambulatory SBP (but not office BP) at baseline was an independent predictor of both cardiovascular and total mortality over the follow-up period. The predictive power was stronger for nighttime mean BP (Figure 27–8).[37]

The prognostic value of ABPM was further confirmed in treated antihypertensive patients in the OvA study (Office versus Ambulatory Blood Pressure Study).[38] In this study baseline ambulatory BP (more SBP than DBP) was a powerful significant predictor of risk of cardiovascular events over 5.5 years of follow-up even after correction for differences in office BP had been made (Figure 27–9).

It has to be considered, however, that the superior prognostic value of ambulatory BP and of its reduction by treatment (as shown in the SAMPLE study[33]) compared with office BP readings is particularly evident in case of reproducible ambulatory BP data[39] compared with "casual" office BP measurements. The difference in predictive power between office and ambulatory BP becomes less pronounced when repeated and carefully performed office BP measures are considered or when, on the other hand, poorly reproducible ambulatory BP

data are taken into account. This has been emphasized in a few studies, including a paper by Fagard et al.,[40] although another study from this group has demonstrated that even when changes in office BP are significantly predictive of left ventricular mass reduction with treatment, changes in ambulatory BP provide additional prognostic information.[41]

Several advantages of ABPM over office readings might explain its greater predictive power[25,42,43] (Box 27–1). The two most important advantages are (1) the large number of BP readings obtainable with ABPM, which makes the resulting mean values much more stable and reproducible (an observation in line with the previously mentioned demonstration by Fagard et al.[40] that repeated office BP measurements obtained under standardized conditions may have similar prognostic value to 24-hour ABPM) and (2) the fact that ABPM is devoid of a major confounder in the assessment of BP-related cardiovascular risk (i.e., the WCE[45]; see Chapter 28). Additional factors responsible for the superiority of ABPM over office readings may be the noise introduced in the latter approach by an insufficient quality of office measurements (use of devices in poor technical condition, inappropriate conditions of measurement, observer bias and end-digit preference) and, for the assessment of the effects of antihypertensive treatment, the fact that ABPM is virtually devoid of any placebo effect.[46]

A further advantage of ABPM is related to its ability to provide information not only on average BP values over the 24-hour period, but also on different patterns of BP variation

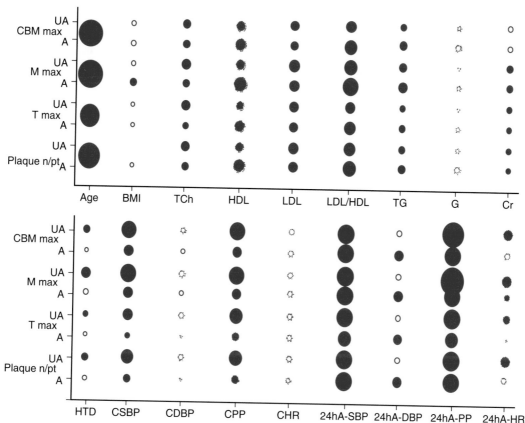

**Figure 27–6** The data from ELSA study. The circles represent Spearman correlation coefficients of baseline ultrasonographic variables with a number of possible determinants, including baseline blood pressure (BP) and heart rate. The size of each circle is proportional to the correlation: *full circle,* positive correlation; *dashed circle,* negative correlation; *gray circle,* significant correlation. *Abbreviations:* UA, unadjusted coefficients, A, adjusted coefficients; BMI, body mass index; HDL, high-density lipoprotein; LDL, low-density lipoprotein; HTD, hypertension duration; CSBP, clinic systolic blood pressure; CDBP, clinic diastolic blood pressure; CPP, clinic pulse pressure; CHR, clinic heart rate; 24hA-SBP, 24-hr mean ambulatory systolic blood pressure; 24hA-DBP, 24-hr mean ambulatory diastolic blood pressure; 24hA-PP, 24-hr mean ambulatory pulse pressure; 24hA-HR, 24-hr mean ambulatory heart rate; CBM max, mean of the maximum of intima-media thickness (IMT) of the four far walls of the carotid bifurcations and distal common carotid arteries; M max, changes in the mean thickness of up to 12 different sites (right and left, near and far walls, distal common, bifurcation and proximal internal carotid); T max, overall mean maximum IMT. From 1444 patients in whom complete baseline data were available. (From Zanchetti A, Bond MG, Hennig M, et al. Risk factors associated with alterations in carotid intima-media thickness in hypertension: Baseline data from the European Lacidipine Study on Atherosclerosis. J Hypertens 16:949-961, 1998; by permission.)

during the 24 hours. Although the evidence supporting the prognostic value of average 24-hour, daytime or nighttime BP values is extensive and convincing, the prognostic significance of BP variability is still a research issue, even if already supported by several studies.[27,32,47-52] This is the case for overall BP variability, as quantified by the SD of the average BP values of the 24-hours, the daytime or the nighttime. This is also the case for its different components during 24 hours. The patterns of BP variability that have most commonly been considered to bear a prognostic value are the following.

1. *Nocturnal BP fall (dipping).* The absence of this physiologic phenomenon in groups of persons at high cardiovascular risk (e.g., patients with diabetes, chronic renal failure, obstructive sleep apnea syndrome, and some forms of secondary hypertension) has raised a question whether it should be considered an independent cardiovascular risk factor. A number of studies have demonstrated that nondipping is associated with more target

organ damage and an increased risk of cardiovascular events,[53] but it remains unclear whether this additional risk depends on impaired cardiovascular regulation (as is the case in diabetic neuropathy) or if it is simply the result of an increased BP load at night. In the latter case, the absolute level of BP at night should be prognostically more important than the magnitude of the difference in BP between daytime and nighttime. These possibilities are not mutually exclusive and each may explain the additional risk associated with an alteration of the sleep-wakefulness cycle in BP to a different degree in different patients. The situation is made even more complex by the observations of Kario et al., that in elderly persons also an excessive BP fall at night results in an increased risk of ischemic cerebral damage and stroke.[54] The issue of the clinical relevance of nocturnal BP dipping needs to be addressed with caution because of the demonstration that this phenomenon is poorly reproducible.[55] Thus the

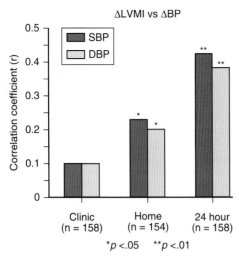

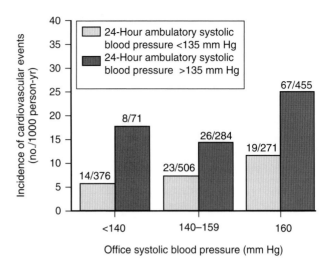

**Figure 27-7** SAMPLE study data. Average correlation coefficients between treatment—induced changes in blood pressures (BPs) measured in study and treatment-induced change in left ventricular mass index (LVMI) after 12 months of treatment. Numbers in parentheses refer to subjects used for correlations. (From Mancia G, Zanchetti A, Agabiti-Rosei E, et al. Ambulatory BP is superior to clinic BP in predicting treatment-induced regression of left ventricular hypertrophy. SAMPLE Study Group. Study on Ambulatory Monitoring of Blood Pressure and Lisinopril Evaluation. Circulation 95:1464-1470, 1997; by permission.)

**Figure 27-9** Incidence of cardiovascular events in the OvA study according to category of office systolic blood pressure. (From Clement DL, De Buyzere ML, De Bacquer DA, et al. Prognostic value of ambulatory blood-pressure recordings in patients with treated hypertension. N Engl J Med 348:2407-2415, 2003. Copyright 2003 Massachusetts Medical Society.)

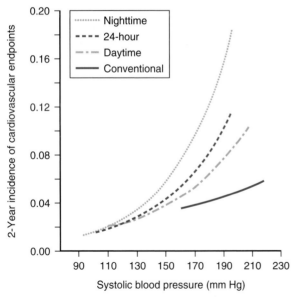

**Figure 27-8** Systolic blood pressures on conventional, 24-hour, daytime, and nighttime measurement at entry as predictors of the 2-year incidence of cardiovascular endpoints in the placebo group in the Syst-Eur Study. Incidence is given as a fraction (i.e., 0.02 is an incidence of 2 events per 100 people). Using multiple Cox regression, the event rate was standardized to female sex, 69.6 years (mean age), no previous cardiovascular complications, nonsmoking status, and residence in western Europe. (From Staessen JA, Thijs L, Fagard R, et al. Hypertension in Europe Trial Investigators. Predicting cardiovascular risk using conventional vs ambulatory blood pressure in older patients with hypertension. JAMA 282:539-546, 1999; by permission.)

isolated finding of lack of nocturnal BP fall on ABPM should be carefully considered, to avoid the erroneous classification of subjects as "nondippers," a label that might carry an adverse prognostic meaning, while they might have simply been "nonsleepers."

2. *Morning surge of BP.* The rate of cardiovascular events (ischemic cardiac events, sudden death, stroke) is higher in the morning hours,[56] at a time when increases in BP, heart rate, sympathetic activity, and platelet aggregability occur in association with awakening. It is not clear, however, whether the morning BP surge and the associated increase in event rate are both the result of a common cause (i.e., an increased sympathetic nervous system activity, leading to an increased risk of arrhythmias and BP peaks) or whether there is a causal link between morning BP surge and a higher event rate (a steeper morning BP rise might increase cardiac and vascular stress and thus contribute to the occurrence of events).[57] Only one study has investigated this relationship directly and has demonstrated that, in fact, an increased morning BP surge is associated with a higher incidence of stroke in the follow-up period.[58] Importantly, given on one side the aforementioned demonstration that an increased rate of cerebrovascular events may be related to the presence of extreme dipping,[54] and on the other side the observation that this phenomenon is often associated with a more pronounced morning BP rise, it is not clear which of these two patterns is prognostically more important. In other words, it is not clear whether the adverse prognostic significance of extreme dipping depends on its postulated risk of organ underperfusion or on its association with a resulting steeper morning BP surge.[58]

3. *Overall BP variability,* including its "erratic," noncircadian components, which are usually quantified as the SD of average 24-hour, daytime, or nighttime ambulatory BP

**Box 27–1** Advantages and Limitations of Ambulatory Blood Pressure Monitoring (ABPM)

**Advantages**
- No observer bias and digit preference
- Large number of BP values available over 24 hours in daily life
- No alerting reaction to blood pressure (BP) automated measurements (no "white-coat effect")
- Higher reproducibility of 24-hour average BP
- No placebo effect
- Assessment of 24-hour, daytime, nighttime, and hourly BP values
- Assessment of BP variability (although limited with discontinuous BP monitoring)
- Assessment of day-night BP changes (dippers, nondippers, extreme dippers); better if performed over repeated recordings
- 24-hour average BP more closely related to target organ damage of hypertension
- Superior prognostic value of 24-hour, daytime, or nighttime average BP
- Assessment of effectiveness and time distribution of BP control by treatment over 24 hours, also through mathematical indices (trough/peak ratio and smoothness index)

**Limitations**
- Possible inaccuracy of automated BP readings, particularly in true ambulatory conditions
- Interference with patient's daily activities
- Quality of sleep more or less affected
- Limited reproducibility of hourly BP values
- Reference "normal" ambulatory BP values still under debate
- Need of more evidence on prognostic value of ABPM
- High cost

From Parati G, de Leeuw P, Illyes M, et al. Blood pressure measurement in research. Blood Press Monit 7:83-87, 2002; by permission.)

values. There are convincing data demonstrating that elevated BP variability is related to target organ damage, as well as to cardiovascular events[27,32,48,49] (Figures 27–10 and 27–11). The impact of elevated BP variability on cardiovascular mortality has been clearly demonstrated in population studies. In the Ohasama study,[49] this was particularly evident in case of daytime BP SD values: An increase in daytime SBP variability was associated with increased risk of cardiovascular mortality in this Japanese population. In terms of target organ damage, the predictive value of increased BP variability has been confirmed by data coming from the PAMELA (Pressioni Arteriose Monitorate E Loro Associazioni) study.[59] In this northern Italian population, the focus was on the so-called erratic component of BP variability, that is, the 24-hour BP variability "purified" from the influence of nocturnal BP fall and of the BP fall associated with siesta (i.e., from its most important cyclic components), identified by means of spectral analysis (Fourier transform). The results showed that in this population only the erratic component of 24 BP SD was significantly correlated with left ventricular mass. All of the aforementioned results differ from those obtained by Verdecchia et al. in the PIUMA study,[60] where the influence of BP variability on cardiovascular mortality, evident in univariate analysis, became marginally significant after adjustment for confounders. Differences in study design, quality of ambulatory BP recordings, and characteristics of the populations considered might however partly explain this discrepancy. The prognostic value of BP variability has been further supported by additional data from the Syst-Eur study, showing that how SBP variability (only during nighttime in this case) was a significant and independent predictor of stroke in elderly hypertensive patients with isolated systolic hypertension (ISH).[51]

It has to be emphasized that, while the first papers demonstrating clinical relevance of BP variability were based on the analysis of continuous intraarterial ambulatory BP recordings, yielding a very accurate assessment of BP variability,[27,32]

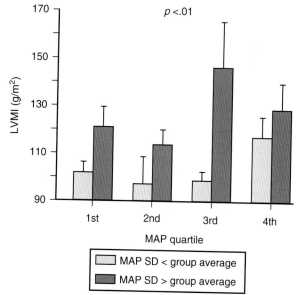

**Figure 27–10** A demonstration of additional prognostic value provided by 24-hour blood pressure (BP) variability in terms of target organ damage. For every quartile of baseline 24-hour mean arterial pressure (MAP), the presence of a greater MAP variability (MAP SD) was associated with a higher left ventricular mass index over the follow-up period. (From Frattola A, Parati G, Cuspidi C, et al. Prognostic value of 24-hour blood pressure variability. J Hypertens 11:1133-1137, 1993; by permission.)

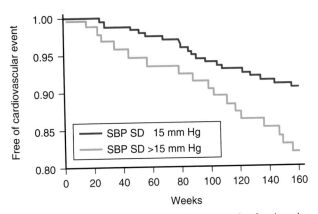

**Figure 27-11** Kaplan-Meier survival analysis for fatal and nonfatal cardiovascular morbid events in patients with increased (>15 mm Hg) and normal (≤15 mm Hg) daytime systolic blood pressure (SBP) variability. (From Parati G, Bilo G, Vettorello M, et al. Assessment of overall blood pressure variability and its different components. Blood Press Monit 8:155-9, 2003; by permission.)

all subsequent studies were based on discontinuous noninvasive ABPM, which cannot offer the same accuracy in assessing the magnitude and the frequency of BP variations over time due to loss of information on rapid BP changes.[61]

Although the prognostic importance of BP variability over the 24 hours is unquestionable, a number of aspects of the association between different patterns of BP variation and target organ damage/cardiovascular events remain unclear. This is related to a number of yet unsolved problems, such as the definition of "normal" reference values for BP variability; the difficulties in providing a reproducible estimate of this phenomenon; the inaccuracies in estimating BP variability from discontinuous BP samples obtained at a relatively low frequency; and the important interactions between some components of 24-hour BP variability that may raise difficult mathematical and pathophysiologic issues, as exemplified by the reported relation between nocturnal dip and morning BP surge or by the relation between either of these and 24-hour BP SD.

Further evidence is thus needed to evaluate the extent to which alterations in different components of BP variability might cause cardiovascular damage or, on the contrary, to what extent these alterations only constitute a marker of an impairment in cardiovascular control mechanisms associated with a preexisting pathology.

## AMBULATORY BLOOD PRESSURE MONITORING IN THE DIFFERENTIAL DIAGNOSIS OF "SUSTAINED HYPERTENSION" AND "WHITE-COAT HYPERTENSION"

Office BP measurements remain the method recommended for the diagnosis of hypertension in daily practice. However, measurements performed in the physician's office are commonly associated with an alerting reaction induced in the patient by the procedure. This alerting reaction is responsible

for a BP elevation of variable magnitude, often exceeding 20 to 30 mm Hg[7] (Figure 27-12), which might overestimate the patient's actual BP levels and/or underestimate the efficacy of antihypertensive treatment. This phenomenon, termed *white-coat effect* (WCE), cannot be easily quantified in clinical practice, because its precise assessment would require continuous BP recordings to be performed before and during the physician's visit. Because of this difficulty, surrogate measures of WCE are commonly used. The most popular of these is based on the calculation of the difference between office BP and mean daytime ambulatory BP. Based on this approach, *white-coat hypertension* (WCH,[62] also termed *isolated office hypertension* [IOH]) is defined as the coexistence of elevated office BP values and normal BP levels outside of the physician's office. Differences in terminology and methodology applied in this context, however, have caused confusion and some discrepancy in the assessment of the clinical relevance of WCH among studies (Box 27-2).[63]

For this reason, although ABPM is recommended for patients affected by either a pronounced WCE or by WCH (in the United States a suspicion of WCH is the clinical situation in which ABPM is reimbursed by Centers for Medicare and Medicaid Services [CMS][64]), no standard procedure has yet been defined to identify these patients. In particular, there is still discussion on whether out-of-office BP should be measured by self–BP monitoring at home or by ABPM. There is no general agreement whether ABPM should be performed only in patients with a discrepancy between office and home BP values, or whether ABPM should be adopted anytime a suspicion of WCH is raised based on patient's clinical evaluation.

Given the limited resources for health care in most countries, the prevailing suggestion is that ABPM should be restricted to selected patients, such as those with a high probability of having WCE. These include patients with SBP values between 140 and 159 mm Hg and DBP between 90 and 99 mm Hg, with no evidence of target organ damage (e.g., normal left ventricular mass); women; nonsmokers; and those with a recent diagnosis of hypertension and with a limited number of office BP measurements available.[65] Another crucial issue for the diagnosis of WCH is the definition of "normal" out-of-office BP. CMS have proposed out-of-office BP values <140/90 mm Hg as a threshold to suspect WCH in patients with elevated office BP readings. However, most current recommendations indicate a level of 135/85 mm Hg as the threshold level to diagnose hypertension when considering either home BP or ambulatory daytime values,[22,24,66] thus suggesting that, in WCH, out-of-office BP should be lower than this value.

## ABPM AND ANTIHYPERTENSIVE TREATMENT

ABPM is commonly applied in the evaluation of antihypertensive drug efficacy. ABPM has several advantages in assessing the BP responses to treatment, for example, the absence of WCE and placebo effects and the possibility of assessing drug coverage over 24 hours, relevant both in clinical practice and in pharmacologic studies[44,67] (see Box 27-1). The usefulness of ABPM is further emphasized by the observation that assessments of the response to antihypertensive treatment obtained by office readings and ABPM often lead to discrepant conclusions.[68]

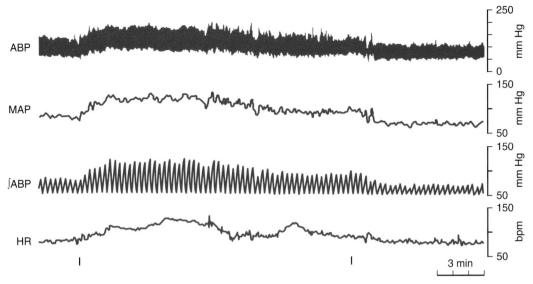

**Figure 27-12** Direct assessment of the white-coat effect. *Arrows* indicate the beginning and the end of a visit by the physician. (From Mancia G, Bertineri G, Grassi G, et al. Effects of blood pressure measured by the doctor on patient's blood pressure and heart rate. Lancet 2:695-698, 1983; by permission.)

An additional advantage of ABPM in assessing the BP effects of antihypertensive treatment is its capability to provide a detailed description of both the magnitude and the time distribution of the 24-hour BP reduction related to pharmacologic therapy. Given the contribution of enhanced BP variability to the cardiovascular consequences of hypertension, there is no doubt as to the theoretical advantages of ensuring a consistent and smooth treatment-induced reduction of BP over the entire 24-hour period.[69] Still, there is no agreement on the best method to assess whether and to what extent this goal has been achieved, either in drug studies or in individual patients. The most commonly used methods proposed include the trough/peak ratio, the morning/evening home BP ratio, and the smoothness index[70] (Figure 27-13). There is evidence that the smoothness index may be superior to the trough/peak ratio in predicting regression of cardiac and vascular damage.[70,71] The value of trough/peak ratio, morning/evening home BP ratio, and smoothness index in assessing the patterns of BP reduction by antihypertensive drug treatment were compared in a study by Stergiou et al.[72] The authors concluded that although the first two parameters can effectively demonstrate the duration of drug effect but not its magnitude, the smoothness index reflects both the degree and the homogeneity of the antihypertensive effect of a given therapeutic regimen, thus providing information that is complementary, rather than alternative to trough/peak ratio.[72]

**Box 27-2** Terminology of Alerting Reactions to Blood Pressure Measurement and Associated Phenomena

**Alerting reaction:** A complex, stereotypical reaction to an emotional, potentially threatening stimulus, characterized in the circulatory system by an increase in blood pressure (BP) and heart rate accompanied by vasoconstriction in the skin, splanchnic, and renal circulation, and by vasodilation in the skeletal muscle.

**White-coat effect (WCE), direct, "real"; also known as white-coat phenomenon:** Alerting reaction and pressor response of the patient to the measurement of BP in the clinic environment; can be quantified by continuous BP monitoring (invasive or noninvasive) before and during the physician's visit.

**White coat-effect (WCE), surrogate:** Difference between cuff BP measured in physician's office (clinic BP) and a measure of BP outside physician's office (daytime ambulatory BP, home BP); see text for its relation to direct WCE.

**Isolated office hypertension (IOH); also known as white-coat hypertension (WCH):** Condition characterized by persistently elevated clinic BP in a patient with normal daytime ambulatory or home BP values; 1999 WHO/ISH Guidelines suggest using the term "isolated office hypertension" instead of "white-coat hypertension" because of the evidence of a limited or absent correlation between the office-daytime average or the office-home BP difference and the real white-coat effect.

From Parati G, Bilo G, Mancia G. White coat effect and white coat hypertension: What do they mean? Cardiovasc Rev Rep 24:477-484, 2003. Copyright Cardiovascular Reviews and Reports, Inc.
WHO/ISH, World Health Organization/International Society of Hypertension.

## CLINICAL APPLICATIONS OF ABPM— CURRENT RECOMMENDATIONS AND FUTURE PERSPECTIVES

ABPM, as any other BP measurement technique available in clinical practice, has advantages and disadvantages, the latter including the possibility of artifacts and inaccurate readings, cost, and potential interference with daily life in a working day. In fact, current guidelines still recommend office measurements as the cornerstone for diagnosing high BP[22,24,66] and suggest that both ABPM and home BP measurement should be regarded as complementary rather than alternative approaches. Identification of situations where these methods might be suitably used in clinical practice is still matter of debate, although there is general agreement on the usefulness of either technique in a research setting.

Self–BP monitoring at home might provide accurate and prognostically relevant information on patients' BP levels by obtaining BP readings over a wide time window. Its main advantage is related to the possibility of offering an inexpensive solution to the need for repeated BP measurements, which are particularly useful in the follow-up of hypertensive patients over long time periods. On the other hand, as concluded by Hond et al., home BP measurements may not be sufficient for diagnosing hypertension and for an initial risk evaluation.[73]

Although ABPM is not (or at least not yet) recommended as a routine instrument in the clinical evaluation of the hypertensive patient, it is likely to be more and more frequently used, because of its demonstrated ability to more precisely evaluate BP-related cardiovascular risk and to quantify both the magnitude and distribution of treatment-related BP reduction over 24 hours. If the prognostic value of BP variability and of some of its specific components (e.g., morning rise, nocturnal fall) is confirmed, the ability of ABPM to quantify also these patterns will further emphasize its role in the management of hypertensive patients.

The clinical application of ABPM has been addressed in several sets of guidelines. The Seventh Report of the Joint National Committee on Prevention, Detection, Evaluation, and Treatment of High Blood Pressure (JNC 7) only briefly discusses the indications for ABPM in the evaluation of hypertensive patients, confirming the recommendations contained in the sixth report of the same committee (JNC VI).[66,74] White-coat hypertension, treatment resistance, hypotension, episodic hypertension, and autonomic failure are all situations in which ABPM should be used according to these guidelines. JNC 7 proposed ambulatory BP levels of 135/85 mm Hg for daytime and of 120/75 mm Hg for nighttime cutoffs for the diagnosis of hypertension. The European Society of Hypertension and European Society of Cardiology joint guidelines emphasize the superiority of ambulatory BP over office BP in terms of prognostic value.[24] Situations in which, according to the European guidelines, ABPM may be considered of additional clinical value are WCH, as suggested by excess variability of office BP; high office BP in patients otherwise at low global cardiovascular risk; and marked discrepancy between BP measured in the office and at home. Resistance to drug treatment and research applications are also considered other suitable conditions for ABPM use. Much more liberal are the suggestions for use of ABPM published by the European Society of Hypertension Working

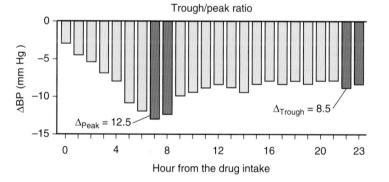

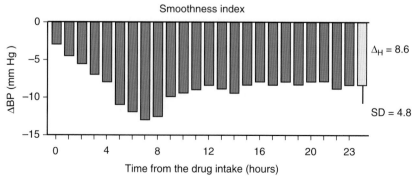

**Figure 27–13** Example to illustrate the calculation of the trough/peak ratio (T/P) and the smoothness index (SI) from hourly blood pressure (BP) values obtained before and during treatment by 24-hour ambulatory BP recordings. $\Delta_H$, average of treatment-induced pressure reductions for each hour over 24 hours; SD, standard deviation of the average of 24 hourly BP reductions. (From Parati G, Omboni S, Rizzoni D, Agabiti-Rosei E, Mancia G. The smoothness index: A new, reproducible and clinically relevant measure of the homogeneity of the blood pressure reduction with treatment for hypertension. J Hypertens 16:1685-1691, 1998; by permission.)

$$SI = \frac{\text{Average } \Delta_H}{\text{SD}} = 1.8$$

**Table 27–1** Recommendations for Ambulatory Blood Pressure Monitoring (ABPM) Use According to International Guidelines (JNC 7 Report, 2003 ESH-ESC Guidelines and Recommendations for BP Measurement from ESH Working Group on Blood Pressure Monitoring)

| Recommendation | JNC 7 | ESH-ESC | ESH WG |
|---|---|---|---|
| Patients with suspected white-coat hypertension | + | + | + |
| Suspected nocturnal hypertension, to establish a dipper status | – | – | + |
| Resistant hypertension | + | + | + |
| Elderly patients | – | – | + |
| Monitoring of antihypertensive drug treatment | – | – | + |
| Type 1 diabetes | – | – | + |
| Hypertension in pregnancy | – | – | + |
| Evaluation of hypotension | + | – | + |
| Episodic hypertension | + | – | + |
| Autonomic failure | + | – | – |
| Research | – | + | – |
| Normal levels (mm Hg): | | | |
| 24 hour | – | 125/80 | – |
| Awake | 135/85 | – | 135/85 |
| Asleep | 120/75 | – | 120/70 |

O'Brien E, Asmar R, Beilin L, et al. European Society of Hypertension recommendations for conventional, ambulatory and home blood pressure measurement. J Hypertens 21:821-848, 2003; 2003 European Society of Hypertension-European Society of Cardiology guidelines for the management of arterial hypertension. J Hypertens 21:1011-1053, 2003; Chobanian AV, Bakris GL, Black HR, et al. The Seventh Report of the Joint National Committee on Prevention, Detection, Evaluation, and Treatment of High Blood Pressure: The JNC 7 report. JAMA 289:2560-2572, 2003.
+, recommends; –, does not recommend.

Group on Blood Pressure Monitoring.[22] Table 27–1 compares these three sets of recommendations.

## SUMMARY

The expanding role of ABPM in clinical practice and in hypertension research is related to its advantages when compared with office readings. These consist in its ability to provide a large number of BP values devoid of any influence from the health care setting and to determine the dynamic changes of BP throughout 24 hours (see Box 27–1). Clearly, ABPM also carries some disadvantages (see Box 27–1), which need to be carefully considered for proper clinical use of this approach. In the light of these advantages and disadvantages, a cautious use of ABPM is recommended, while at the same time recognizing the need for more frequent and accurate office BP measurements. We cannot exclude, however, that an increasing amount of scientific evidence demonstrating the prognostic importance of ABPM might in the near future lead to a more extensive application of this diagnostic tool.

## References

1. Riva-Rocci S. Un nuovo sfigmomanometro. Gazzetta Medica di Torino 50:981-996, 1896.
2. O'Brien E. Replacing the mercury sphygmomanometer. BMJ 320:815-816, 2000
3. O'Brien E. Will mercury manometers soon be obsolete? J Hum Hypertens 9:933–934, 1995.
4. Mancia G, Parati G, Di Rienzo M, et al. Blood pressure variability. *In* Zanchetti A, Mancia, G (eds). Pathophysiology of Hypertension. [Vol. 17 of Handbook of Hypertension]. Amsterdam, Elsevier Science BV, 1997; pp. 117-169.
5. Bevan AT, Honour AJ, Stott FH. Direct arterial pressure recording in unrestricted man. Clin Sci 36:329-344, 1969.
6. Mancia G, Ferrari A, Gregorini L, et al. Blood pressure and heart rate variability in normotensive and hypertensive human beings. Circ Res 53:96-104, 1983.
7. Mancia G, Bertineri G, Grassi G, et al. Effects of blood pressure measured by the doctor on patient's blood pressure and heart rate. Lancet 2:695-698, 1983.
8. Mancia G, Parati G, Pomidossi G, et al. Alerting reaction and rise in blood pressure during measurement by physician and nurse. Hypertension 9:209-215, 1987.
9. Penaz J. Photoelectric measurement of blood pressure, volume, and flow in the finger. Digest 10th Int Conf Med Biol Eng Dresden 104 (abstract), 1973.
10. Parati G, Casadei R, Groppelli A, et al. Comparison of finger and intraarterial blood pressure monitoring at rest and during laboratory testing. Hypertension 13:647—655, 1989.
11. Imholz BPM, Langewouters GJ, van Montfrans GA, et al. Feasibility of ambulatory, continuous 24-hour finger arterial pressure recording. Hypertension 21:65-73, 1993.
12. Bos WJW, van Goudever J, van Montfrans GA, et al. Reconstruction of brachial artery pressure from non-invasive finger pressure measurements. Circulation 94:1870-1875, 1996.
13. Parati G, Ongaro G, Bilo G, et al. Non-invasive beat-to-beat blood pressure monitoring: New developments. Blood Press Monit 8:31-36, 2003.
14. Mancia G, Parati G, Castiglioni P, et al. Daily life blood pressure changes are steeper in hypertensive than in normotensive subjects. Hypertension. 42:277-282, 2003.
15. Parati G, Mancia G. Ambulatory blood pressure monitoring. *In* Mancia G, Chalmers J, Julius S, et al. (eds). Manual of Hypertension. London, Churchill Livingstone, 2002, pp 153-171.
16. Hinman AT, Engel BT, Bickford AF. Portable blood pressure recorder-Accuracy and preliminary use in evaluating intradaily variations in pressure. Am Heart J 63:663, 1962.
17. Sokolow M, Werdegar D, Kain HK, et al. Relationship between level of blood pressure measured casually and by portable

recorders and severity of complications in essential hypertension. Circulation 34:279-298, 1966.

18. Perloff D, Sokolow M, Cowan R. The prognostic value of ambulatory blood pressures. JAMA 249(20):2792-2798, 1983.

19. American National Standard. Electronic or automated sphygmomanometers. ANSI/AAMI SP 10-1992. Arlington, VA, Association for the Advancement of Medical Instrumentation, 1993; pp 40.

20. O'Brien E, Petrie J, Littler WA, et al. The British Hypertension Society Protocol for the evaluation of blood pressure measuring devices. J Hypertens 11(suppl 2):S43-S63, 1993.

21. O'Brien E, Pickering T, Asmar R, et al. [with the statistical assistance of Atkins N, Gerin W]; Working Group on Blood Pressure Monitoring of the European Society of Hypertension. International protocol for validation of blood pressure measuring devices in adults. Blood Press Monit 7:3-17, 2002.

22. O'Brien E, Asmar R, Beilin L, et al. European Society of Hypertension recommendations for conventional, ambulatory and home blood pressure measurement. J Hypertens 21: 821-848, 2003.

23. O'Brien E, Waeber B, Parati G, et al. Blood pressure measuring devices: Recommendations of the European Society of Hypertension. BMJ 322:531-536, 2001.

24. 2003 European Society of Hypertension-European Society of Cardiology guidelines for the management of arterial hypertension. J Hypertens 21:1011-1053, 2003.

25. Mancia G, Parati G. Ambulatory blood pressure monitoring and organ damage. Hypertension 36:894-900, 2000.

26. Devereux RB, Pickering TG. Relationship between variability of ambulatory blood pressure and target hypertension. J Hypertens. 8:S34-S38, 1991.

27. Parati G, Pomidossi G, Albini F, et al. Relationship of 24-hour blood pressure mean and variability to severity of target organ damage. J Hypertens 5:93-98, 1987.

28. Liu JE, Roman Mj, Pini R, et al. Cardiac and arterial target organ damage in adults with elevated ambulatory and normal office blood pressure. Ann Intern Med 131:564-572, 1999.

29. Pessina AC, Palatini P, Sperti G, et al. Evaluation of hypertension and related target organ damage by average day-time blood pressure. Clin Exp Hypertens [A] 7:267-78, 1985.

30. Rowlands DB, Ireland MA, Glover DR, et al. The relationship between ambulatory blood pressure and echocardiographically assessed left ventricular hypertrophy. Clin Sci (Lond) 61(Suppl 7):101S-103S, 1981.

31. Zanchetti A, Bomd MG, Hennig M, et al. Risk factors associated with alterations in carotid intima-media thickness in hypertension: Baseline data from the European Lacidipine Study on Atherosclerosis. J Hypertens 16:949-961, 1998.

32. Frattola A, Parati G, Cuspidi C, et al. Prognostic value of 24-hour blood pressure variability. J Hypertens 11:1133-1137, 1993.

33. Mancia G, Zanchetti A, Agabiti-Rosei E, et al. Ambulatory blood pressure is superior to clinic blood pressure in predicting treatment-induced regression of left ventricular hypertrophy. SAMPLE Study Group. Study on Ambulatory Monitoring of Blood Pressure and Lisinopril Evaluation. Circulation 95: 1464-1470, 1997.

34. Verdecchia P, Porcellati C, Schillaci G, et al. Ambulatory blood pressure: An independent predictor of prognosis in essential hypertension. Hypertension 24:793-801, 1994.

35. Redon J, Campos C, Narciso ML, et al. Prognostic value of ambulatory blood pressure monitoring in refractory hypertension: A prospective study. Hypertension 31:712-718, 1998.

36. Imai Y, Ohkubo T, Sakuma M, et al. Predictive power of screening blood pressure, ambulatory blood pressure and blood pressure measured at home for overall and cardiovascular mortality: A prospective observation in a cohort from Ohasama, Northern Japan. Blood Press Monit 1:251-254, 1996.

37. Staessen JA, Thijs L, Fagard R, et al. Predicting cardiovascular risk using conventional vs ambulatory blood pressure in older patients with hypertension. Systolic Hypertension in Europe Trial Investigators. JAMA 282:539-546, 1999.

38. Clement DL, De Buyzere ML, De Bacquer DA et al. Prognostic value of ambulatory blood-pressure recordings in patients with treated hypertension. N Engl J Med 348:2407-2415, 2003.

39. Palatini P, Mormino P, Santonastaso M, et al. Ambulatory blood pressure predicts end-organ damage only in subjects with reproducible recordings. HARVEST Study Investigators. Hypertension and Ambulatory Recording Venetia Study. J Hypertens 17:465-473, 1999.

40. Fagard RH, Staessen JA, Thijs L. Prediction of cardiac structure and function by repeated clinic and ambulatory blood pressure. Hypertension 29:22-29, 1997.

41. Fagard RH, Staessen JA, Thijs L. Relationships between changes in left ventricular mass and in clinic and ambulatory blood pressure in response to antihypertensive therapy. J Hypertens 15:1493-502, 1997.

42. Parati G, Mutti E, Ravogli A, et al. Advantages and disadvantages of non-invasive ambulatory blood pressure monitoring. J Hypertension 8(Suppl 6):S33-S38, 1990.

43. Mancia G, Di Rienzo M, Parati G. Ambulatory blood pressure monitoring: Use in hypertension research and clinical practice. Hypertension 21:500-524, 1993.

44. Parati G, de Leeuw P, Illyes M, et al. Blood pressure measurement in research. Blood Press Monit 7:83-87, 2002.

45. Parati G, Pomidossi G, Casadei V, et al. Lack of alerting reactions and pressor responses to intermittent cuff inflations during non-invasive blood pressure monitoring. Hypertension 7:597-601, 1985.

46. Mancia G, Omboni S, Parati G, et al. Lack of placebo effect on ambulatory blood pressure. Am J Hypertens 8:311-315, 1995.

47. Parati G, Bilo G, Vettorello M, et al. Assessment of overall blood pressure variability and its different components. Blood Press Monit 8:155-159, 2003.

48. Sander D, Kukla C, Klingelhofer J, et al. Relationship between circadian blood pressure patterns and progression of early carotid atherosclerosis: A 3-year follow-up study. Circulation 102:1536-1541, 2000.

49. Kikuya M, Hozawa A, Ohokubo T, et al. Prognostic significance of blood pressure and heart rate variabilities: The Ohasama Study. Hypertension 38:23-29, 2000.

50. Shimada K, Kawamoto A, Matsubayashi K, et al. Diurnal blood pressure variations and silent cerebrovascular damage in elderly patients with hypertension. J Hypertens 10:875-878, 1992.

51. Pringle E, Phillips C, Thijs L, et al. on behalf of the Syst-Eur Investigators. Systolic blood pressure variability as a risk factor for stroke and cardiovascular mortality in the elderly hypertensive population. J Hypertens. 21:2251-2257, 2003.

52. Liu JG, Xu LP, Chu ZX, et al. Contribution of blood pressure variability to the effect of nitrendipine on end-organ damage in spontaneously hypertensive rats. J Hypertens 21:1961-1967, 2003.

53. Verdecchia P. Prognostic value of ambulatory blood pressure: Current evidence and clinical implications. Hypertension 35:844-885, 2000.

54. Kario K, Matsuo T, Kobayashi H, et al. Nocturnal fall of blood pressure and silent cerebrovascular damage in elderly hypertensive patients. Advanced silent cerebrovascular damage in extreme dippers. Hypertension. 27:130-135, 1996.

55. Omboni S, Parati G, Palatini P, et al. Reproducibility and clinical value of nocturnal hypotension: Prospective evidence from the SAMPLE study. J Hypertens 16:733–738, 1998.

56. Rocco MB, Barry J, Campbell S, et al. Circadian variation of transient myocardial ischemia in patients with coronary artery disease. Circulation 75:395-400, 1987.

57. White W. Cardiovascular risk and therapeutic intervention for the early morning surge in blood pressure and heart rate. Blood Press Monit 6:63-72, 2001.

58. Kario K, Pickering TG, Umeda Y, et al. Morning surge in blood pressure as a predictor of silent and clinical cerebrovascular disease in elderly hypertensives: A prospective study. Circulation 107:1401-1406, 2003.

59. Sega R, Corrao G, Bombelli M, et al. Blood pressure variability and organ damage in a general population: Results from the PAMELA study (Pressioni Arteriose Monitorate E Loro Associazioni). Hypertension 39:710-714, 2002.

60. Verdecchia P, Borgioni C, Ciucci A, et al. Prognostic significance of blood pressure variability in essential hypertension. Blood Press Monit 1:3-11, 1996.

61. Di Rienzo M, Grassi G, Pedotti A, et al. Continuous vs intermittent blood pressure measurements in estimating 24-hour average blood pressure. Hypertension 5:264-269, 1983.

62. Pickering TG, James GD, Boddie C, et al. How common is white coat hypertension? JAMA 259:255-258, 1988.

63. Parati G, Bilo G, Mancia G. White coat effect and white coat hypertension: What do they mean? Cardiovasc Rev Rep 24:477-484, 2003.

64. CMS. Centers for Medicare & Medicaid Services. Medicare Coverage Policy. Decisions: ABPM monitoring (#CAG-00067N). *http://www.hcfa.gov/coverage/8b3-ff.htm*, 2001.

65. Verdecchia P, O'Brien E, Pickering T, et al.; European Society of Hypertension Working Group on Blood Pressure Monitoring. Statement from the working group on blood pressure monitoring of the European Society of Hypertension. Am J Hypertens 16:87-91, 2003.

66. Chobanian AV, Bakris GL, Black HR, et al. The Seventh Report of the Joint National Committee on Prevention, Detection, Evaluation, and Treatment of High Blood Pressure: The JNC 7 report. JAMA 289:2560-2572, 2003.

67. O'Brien E. Ambulatory blood pressure measurement is indispensable to good clinical practice. J Hypertens Suppl 21(Suppl 2):S11-S18, 2003.

68. Mancia G, Omboni S, Ravogli A, et al. Ambulatory blood pressure monitoring in the evaluation of antihypertensive treatment: Additional information from a large data base. Blood Press 4:148-156, 1995.

69. Mancia G. Clinical benefits of consistent reduction in the daily blood pressure of hypertensive patients. J Clin Hypertens (Greenwich) 4(Suppl 1):9-14, 2002.

70. Parati G, Omboni S, Rizzoni D, et al. The smoothness index: A new, reproducible and clinically relevant measure of the homogeneity of the blood pressure reduction with treatment for hypertension. J Hypertens 16:1685-1691, 1998.

71. Rizzoni D, Muiesan ML, Salvetti M, et al. The smoothness index, but not the trough-to-peak ratio predicts changes in carotid artery wall thickness during antihypertensive treatment. J Hypertens 19:703-711, 2001.

72. Stergiou GS, Efstathiou SP, Skeva II, et al. Comparison of the smoothness index, the trough: Peak ratio and the morning:evening ratio in assessing the features of the antihypertensive drug effect. J Hypertens 21:913-920, 2003.

73. Hond ED, Celis H, Fagard R, et al. Self-measured versus ambulatory blood pressure in the diagnosis of hypertension. J Hypertens 21:717-722, 2003.

74. The Sixth Report of the Joint National Committee on Prevention, Detection, Evaluation, and Treatment of High Blood Pressure (JNC VI). Arch Intern Med 157:2413-2446, 1997.

# White-Coat Hypertension

## George A. Mansoor, William B. White

The almost routine availability of ambulatory, office, and home blood pressure (BP) measurements has generated considerable debate into the relationships of these different measures and clinical outcomes.[1-8] Although these methods all attempt to obtain a measure of average BP, they do not provide results that are interchangeable. One commonly known disparity between office and ambulatory readings is the transient increase in BP observed in some individuals in the medical care environment. When the disparity persists in an untreated patient, this has been termed *isolated office* or *white-coat hypertension*.[1-3] In *treated* hypertensive patients, this increase in office over ambulatory BP has been termed the *white-coat effect* or *white-coat phenomenon*.[2] This latter group of patients is indeed hypertensive but the office BP readings overestimate their average daily BP.

Although it is accepted that the cause of the higher office than daytime pressure is not identical to the classically described white-coat effect[3] using intraarterial measurements, the terminology has taken root. The obvious question to clinical practitioners is whether it is ambulatory or office BP that should be used to diagnose hypertension and guide therapy in these patients. In the patient with untreated white-coat hypertension, should therapy be initiated based on high office readings when ambulatory readings are normal? In the treated patient, which measure of BP should guide changes in therapy?

Other important differences between the various types of BP measurements have also been observed. Office BP averages may be significantly *lower* than ambulatory BP.[4] This situation leads to possible underestimation of daily BP and can be considered a form of *hidden* or *masked hypertension*, perhaps leading to undertreatment of some patients (Figure 28–1).

These important discrepancies between office and average daily BP raise the question of the preferred indicator of overall BP burden and hence risk for that individual.[5] The clinical importance of white-coat hypertension has been recognized and most consensus groups recommend ambulatory monitoring for the patient with that diagnosis.[6] The Centers for Medicare and Medicaid Services, in recognition of the importance of ambulatory BP measurements, now reimburses for ambulatory BP monitoring, the indication of white-coat hypertension.[7]

There are many potential advantages in detecting white-coat hypertension: (1) Patients with white-coat hypertension may not require drug therapy and substantial cost savings may accrue, (2) a better diagnostic and prognostic risk assessment for individual patients may be possible, and (3) clinical drug studies can exclude white-coat hypertensives who may not respond to drug therapy in the same fashion as sustained hypertensive patients.[8] In patients with masked hypertension, the clinician may be alerted that office BP is an unreliable indicator of daily BP.

In this chapter, we examine the clinical features, prognosis, and treatment of white-coat or office-only hypertension and briefly discuss masked hypertension. The theme suggests that measurement of BP during daily activities more accurately predicts cardiovascular risk than measurement during office visits, and that incorporation of office, and out-of-office BP may optimize patient management.

## WHITE-COAT HYPERTENSION

### Background and Definition

A higher BP in the physician's presence compared with out-of-office BP was reported more than 60 years ago, but the observation lay dormant for many decades.[9] Today, clinicians are far more familiar with this concept but uncertainty remains about the optimal management of these patients. Many physicians feel uncomfortable not treating elevated office readings even when ambulatory readings are normal.

As a clinical issue, white-coat hypertension is important. The prevalence is reported to range widely from 10% to 60% of all newly diagnosed hypertensive patients.[10-17] However, the true prevalence is probably closer to 15%, because most studies that reported a higher prevalence used relatively high cut-off levels of ambulatory BP (>135/85 mm Hg) to define white-coat hypertension. The value of ambulatory BP in defining white-coat hypertension was highlighted by the demonstration of a several-fold variation in the prevalence of white-coat hypertension and left ventricular hypertrophy (LVH) with different criteria.[11] When conservative criteria are used (e.g., < 130/80 mm Hg), the prevalence of white-coat hypertension is 12% and the incidence of LVH is similar to that in normotensive subjects (3%).

To standardize research on white-coat hypertension, analyses should be consistent and follow generally accepted guidelines (Box 28–1). Although it is tempting to use home BP measurements alone to diagnose white-coat hypertension,[1] ambulatory BP remains the ideal method especially in employed subjects who often have higher average BPs at work than at home.[18]

The difference between office and daytime BP has been used by most researchers as an indicator of the white-coat effect, but this has been challenged.[3,19] Although the pathophysiologic cause behind the alerting reaction and the ambulatory-office BP difference may be different, the latter is more commonly available to the clinician. Undoubtedly, factors that lower or raise ambulatory BP will affect the daytime office BP difference, just as factors that elevate office BP will increase the difference.

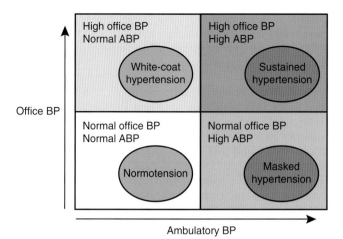

BP: blood pressure
ABP: ambulatory blood pressure

**Figure 28–1** Diagrammatic representation of how office and ambulatory BP values for defining hypertension lead to white-coat and masked hypertension.

## Pathophysiology of the White-Coat or Alerting Reaction

The pathophysiologic cause of the higher office than ambulatory BP is not certain.[20-29] It has been customary to use laboratory tests of reactivity[17,21,23,26] to infer causality of the white-coat effect, but this is likely to be an oversimplification. Suggestions about its etiology have included increased BP reactivity to the stress of clinical visits, as well as a conditioned response to the medical care environment.[1] Several groups could not find any substantial increase in BP variability in white-coat hypertensives compared with essential hypertensives. Furthermore, no consistent psychological or behavioral factors have been identified among white-coat hypertensives.[20-29] No differences have been found between white-coat

**Box 28–1** Considerations in Designing Cross-Sectional Studies of White-Coat Hypertension

- Definition should use both ambulatory SBP and DBP unless a population is studied in which one is obviously preferred (e.g., ISH).
- Define whether 24-hour averages or daytime averages are used.
- Define levels of nighttime BP hypertension.
- Define number of office visits to document high office BP (usually ≥2).
- Define normal ambulatory BP using a conservative criterion (e.g., 24-hour BP <130/80 mm Hg).
- If surrogate endpoint used, avoid effects of prior antihypertensive therapy and other factors that may influence measured outcome.
- Include both normotensive and sustained hypertensive comparison groups.
- Avoid using home BP alone to define white-coat hypertension.

SBP, systolic blood pressure; DBP, diastolic blood pressure; ISH, isolated systolic hypertension; BP, blood pressure.

hypertensives and normotensives in a battery of psychometric tests of anger and hostility and anxiety and depression.[20,24] Smith[29] used single and multiunit muscle sympathetic nerve activity to study the sympathetic nervous system in normotensives, white-coat hypertensives, and sustained hypertensives. They found that white-coat hypertensives had activity of the sympathetic system intermediate between that of normotensives and sustained hypertensives. Leary et al.[28] reported that increased BP reactivity to physical activity was associated with the white-coat effect. No clear psychological traits are consistently found in white-coat hypertension.

## Clinical and Demographic Predictors

Clinical identifiers are needed to be able to target persons with possible white-coat hypertension for ambulatory monitoring. Initial reports suggested that patients with white-coat hypertension were more likely to be young women with a short duration of hypertension.[14] However, subsequent studies have shown that a marked exaggeration of office BP may also occur in older patients irrespective of gender[30-32] and is common in older patients with isolated systolic hypertension (ISH).[33] Indeed, in a small group of generally older patients, reproducible, spectacular elevations of systolic blood pressure (SBP) were demonstrated in the office.[34] For untreated patients with newly diagnosed elevated office readings, ambulatory monitoring may be performed to detect white-coat hypertension in persons with office BP between 140/90 and 159/99 mm Hg, women, and nonsmokers.[32] In untreated patients, it is a reasonable strategy to consider the possibility of white-coat hypertension only after repeating the office readings on at least three occasions.

## Cross-Sectional Target Organ Studies in White-Coat Hypertension

Because left ventricular mass is reliably determined echocardiographically, this measurement has been used most often in evaluating target organ damage in white-coat hypertension. Other indicators of target organ damage that have been studied include microalbuminuria, arterial compliance, and cerebral white-matter lesions as indicators of silent cerebrovascular damage. Metabolic factors, homocysteine levels, and endothelial function have also been studied in white-coat hypertension.

### Left Ventricular Mass

Some studies[35-39] have found that left ventricular mass index in white-coat hypertensives is similar to that in a group of age- and sex-matched normotensive subjects but lower than that in a group of matched ambulatory hypertensives. One of the first studies in this area[35] compared three groups of matched and never-treated hypertensive patients; office hypertensives (n = 18, office BP >140/90 mm Hg, and awake BP <130/80 mm Hg); normotensives (n = 18, office BP <135/85 mm Hg, and awake BP <130/80 mm Hg); and sustained hypertensives (n = 18, office BP >140/90 mm Hg, and awake BP >140/90 mm Hg) with respect to left ventricular mass index and wall thicknesses. Office BP was similar for white-coat hypertensives and sustained hypertensives, and ambulatory BP was similar in normotensives and white-coat hypertensives. Left ventricular mass index was similar in the normotensive and white-coat group and significantly less than in the sustained hypertensive group. However, other researchers[40-46] have found that white-coat hypertensives have left ventricular mass higher than normotensives but consistently less than sustained hypertensives, perhaps placing them at intermediate risk. Many of the latter studies used an ambulatory diastolic blood pressure (DBP) of 90 mm Hg as the cut off for white-coat hypertension, a value likely to include many subjects with stage 1 hypertension.

Palatini[43] reported data from the Hypertension and Ambulatory Recording Venetia Study (HARVEST), in which 942 never-treated subjects with office BPs of 140 to 159/90 to 99 mm Hg were studied with echocardiography and ambulatory BP monitoring. The authors used three daytime BP criteria for isolated office hypertension: (1) <130/90 mm Hg, (2) <135/85 mm Hg, and (3) <130/80 mm Hg. Irrespective of the criterion used, both left ventricular mass index and wall thickness were higher in both the white-coat and sustained hypertensive group as compared with the normotensive group. There was a gradual increase in left ventricular mass from the normotensive group to the white-coat hypertensive group to the sustained hypertensive group, suggesting that white-coat group is at intermediate risk.

In support of this concept, Grandi[47] reported that white-coat hypertension based on an ambulatory value of <130/80 mm Hg was associated with higher left ventricular mass and reduced diastolic function indices compared with normotension. Compared with white-coat hypertensives the sustained hypertensives had higher left ventricular mass and lower diastolic function, suggesting an intermediate position of risk for the former group. Sega et al.[48] described similar findings.

In summary, available studies offer conflicting conclusions regarding cardiac mass in white-coat hypertension. These conflicting results reemphasize the need for prospective studies examining the merits of treating persons with white-coat hypertension.

### Renal Indices

Microalbuminuria is indicative of nephropathy in diabetic subjects and hypertensive patients. Hoegholm et al.[49] compared albumin excretion in 111 patients with white-coat hypertension (daytime DBP <90 mm Hg and office BP >90 mm Hg), 173 with established hypertension (office and daytime ambulatory DBP <90 mm Hg), and 127 normotensive controls (both office and ambulatory DBP <90 mm Hg). There was a graded increase in albumin excretion from normotensives to white-coat hypertensives to sustained hypertensives. These findings were not confirmed by Palatini[43] or by Pierdomenico,[50] who reported that white-coat hypertensives had urinary microalbumin levels similar to normotensives and lower than ambulatory hypertensives.

### Vascular Studies

A third target of inquiry has been the vascular system; the rationale being that if white-coat hypertension is indeed innocent, vascular involvement should be much less than in sustained hypertensive patients and similar to normotensive patients. Although the carotid system is amenable to examination by ultrasound, the extent to which properties of the carotid reflect hypertensive damage or the effects of other metabolic factors is not known. The findings from carotid arterial evaluations mirror other target organ studies, with some authors finding no increase in carotid wall thickness and others finding increases intermediate between those of normotensives and hypertensives.

Several studies[37,44,45,50] have found no evidence of increased carotid disease in white-coat hypertension. In contrast, Glen[36] concluded that both white-coat and sustained hypertensive subjects had abnormalities of elasticity, compliance, and stiffness that were different from normotensive subjects. Similarly, Muldoon[51] found increased carotid atherosclerosis in white-coat hypertension. Landray[52] cautioned that white-coat hypertension is associated with carotid atherosclerosis. In most of these studies, metabolic risk factors other than high BP were present in the white-coat hypertensive group and possibly contributed to the carotid pathology.

Other studies have focused on noninvasive evaluation of endothelial function. For example, Pierdomenico[53] compared brachial artery flow mediated dilation in 22 sustained hypertensives, 22 white-coat hypertensives, and 22 normotensive subjects matched for age, gender, and body mass index. They found that white-coat hypertensives had similar findings to normotensives, and that both had higher levels than sustained hypertensives. Similar results were reported when an older group of patients was studied.[54]

### Cerebrovascular Studies

Early effects of hypertension on cerebrovascular structures are difficult to measure, but magnetic resonance imaging (MRI) can detect small vessel occlusive disease. The two most commonly detected abnormalities are lacunae and periventricular white-matter lesions. Lacunae are in essence small infarcts, whereas hypertensive small vessel disease is thought to play a role in the genesis of periventricular white-matter lesions.

Shimada et al.[55] used these two patterns as indicators of silent cerebrovascular disease and compared their prevalence in elderly patients with sustained and white-coat hypertension with normotensives. The subjects had no history of overt stroke and underwent ambulatory BP monitoring and MRI studies of the brain, as well as office BP measurements. From the overall group of 73 patients, three age-matched groups were defined as follows: (1) sustained hypertensives (n = 26, office BP ≥140/90 mm Hg, 24-hour BP ≥135/80 mm Hg); (2) white-coat hypertensives (n = 14, office BP ≥140/90 mm Hg, 24-hour BP <135/80 mm Hg); and (3) normotensives (n = 28, office BP <140/90 mm Hg, 24-hour BP >135/80 mm Hg). MRI scans were graded by a neuroradiologist unaware of the BP data. The number of lacunae and the grade of periventricular white-matter hyperintensities were similar in the white-coat hypertensive and normotensive groups with both significantly less than the sustained hypertensive group. This was true even though the white-coat hypertensive group had higher ambulatory DBP than the normotensive group.

More recently, Eguchi[56] examined the effects of ambulatory BP and diabetes mellitus on silent cerebral infarcts. They studied 360 hypertensive patients with a mean age of 67 years with and without diabetes. All participants were studied using ambulatory BP and had brain MRI to quantitate silent cerebral infarcts. As expected, diabetic patients with elevated BP had more silent cerebral infarcts than the group with hypertension but without diabetes. The role of ambulatory BP was examined by stratification into four groups: (1) nondiabetic with white-coat hypertension, (2) nondiabetic with sustained hypertension, (3) diabetic with white-coat hypertension, and (4) diabetic with sustained hypertension. The most silent cerebral infarcts were seen in the group with combined diabetes and ambulatory hypertension, and the fewest in the white-coat hypertensive group who did not have diabetes mellitus.

### Cardiovascular Risk Factors

Additional cardiovascular risk factors are common in the patient with sustained hypertension. Therefore, several authors have measured metabolic parameters likely to confer or be associated with cardiovascular risk in white-coat hypertensives. Pierdominico[50] and Marchesi[57] found no metabolic derangements among white-coat hypertensives, but Weber et al.[40] found that white-coat hypertensives had slightly higher insulin, renin, aldosterone, and norepinephrine levels than did normotensives. Similar metabolic perturbations were also described in the white-coat hypertensive group of the Tecumseh study.[58] Circulating homocysteine levels have been shown to be similar in white-coat hypertensives and sustained hypertensives.[59] It is likely that many of the target organ measures used in research studies to assess the risk of white-coat hypertension are affected by these metabolic factors.

## Prognosis of White-Coat Hypertension

No randomized intervention study with morbidity and mortality as the endpoint has compared white-coat hypertensives, normotensives, and sustained hypertensives. However, an increasing number of studies in various types of populations have measured ambulatory and office BP at one point in time and then prospectively or retrospectively ascertained cardiovascular outcome several years later. These studies show that ambulatory monitoring of BP is superior to office-based measures of BP in predicting outcomes.[60-74] It should be noted that the majority of these studies either evaluated the effects of the circadian BP profile or the comparative effects of ambulatory versus office BP in predicting events. Only two studies using noninvasive ambulatory BP monitoring[61,67] and one using intraarterial monitoring[66] have specifically examined the outcome of white-coat hypertension.

Verdecchia[61] attempted to assess the prognosis of white-coat hypertension by initially studying 1187 patients with newly diagnosed essential hypertension compared with 205 healthy normotensive subjects. After a mean of 3.2 years cardiovascular endpoints were assessed retrospectively. They defined white-coat hypertension as daytime ambulatory BP <136/87 mm Hg for men and <131/86 mm Hg for women (the 90th percentiles of same gender normotensive groups). Patients were followed by their own physicians with the goal of reducing their office BP to <140/90 mm Hg. The ambulatory BP data were available to the doctors but probably played a small role in their management. Complete follow-up data were obtained on 99.1% of all participants. Combined cardiovascular morbidity and mortality per 100 patient-years were 0.47 in the normotensive group (4 events in 205 subjects), 0.49 in the white-coat hypertensive group (3 events in 228 subjects), 1.79 in the ambulatory hypertensive group with a dipping BP profile (37 events in 693 subjects), and 4.99 in the ambulatory hypertensive group with a nondipping BP profile (45 events in 266 subjects). Cardiovascular morbidity was

similar in the white-coat hypertension group and the normotensive group by multivariate analysis. A further analysis in which a daytime BP <130/80 mm Hg was used to define white-coat hypertension showed a difference in event-free survival between the two defined white-coat hypertension groups.[75]

The second outcome report of white-coat hypertension involved the data from the ambulatory BP substudy of the Systolic Hypertension in Europe (Syst-Eur) study.[67] Patients in the Syst-Eur study were 60 years or older and had office SBP between 160 and 219 mm Hg and DBP <95 mm Hg. After randomization, patients were treated either with active medication or placebo. In a subset of 808 patients, ambulatory monitoring was performed at baseline and again at 6 and 12 months. Data were available on 342 patients assigned to active treatment and 353 assigned to placebo. Three groups were defined according to daytime SBP: <140 mm Hg (nonsustained or white-coat hypertension), 140 to 159 mm Hg (mild sustained hypertension), and 160 mm Hg or more (moderate sustained hypertension). Nonsustained hypertensives taking placebo had three to four times lower stroke rates and cardiovascular complications compared with moderate sustained hypertensives. Patients in the mild sustained group were intermediate. Active treatment appeared to reduce outcomes only in the moderate sustained group. No comparison with a normotensive control group was possible. Khattar et al. used intraarterial BP monitoring[66] and had similar results.

To conduct a large outcome trial to evaluate the possible risks of white-coat hypertension is a complex matter. Event rates are low in this group of patients.[60] Thus any study would have to be exceedingly large and have long follow-up (>5 years) to show a difference compared with normotensives. Furthermore, pharmacologic therapy of white-coat hypertension may lead to reductions of office but not ambulatory BP,[76] further complicating the ability to conduct a trial and assess the results.

## Blood Pressure Evolution in White-Coat Hypertension

The natural history of persons labeled as white-coat hypertensives is not well studied. One approach has been to follow untreated patients over several years if ambulatory BP increases over time or to see if a surrogate marker of hypertension (e.g., left ventricular mass) changes. If white-coat hypertension is a prehypertensive state, then these persons should evolve into sustained hypertensives over time in excess of an age-matched normotensive group and may show increases of left ventricular mass. Polonia et al.[77] prospectively evaluated 36 untreated patients with white-coat hypertension (office BP >140/90 mm Hg and awake BP <132/84 mm Hg) and a control group of 52 normotensives (clinic BP <140/90 mm Hg and awake BP <132/84 mm Hg). Patients underwent repeat ambulatory and office BP measurements after a mean interval of 3.5 years. The two groups showed similar rates of evolution to sustained hypertension (22% and 15%, respectively). However, 17 of the original 88 patients studied at baseline had been started on drug therapy, making it difficult to be sure if they had evolved into sustained hypertensives.

White et al.[78] reported similar results, showing that when a restrictive definition of white-coat hypertension is used (awake ambulatory BP <135/85 mm Hg), the rate of evolution to sustained hypertension is similar to age-matched normotensives (12% vs 15%). Verdecchia[79] repeated clinic and ambulatory BP and echocardiographic evaluation of 83 untreated patients defined with white-coat hypertension after a mean period of 2.5 years, and they found that 37% became ambulatory hypertensives. In the group that evolved into sustained hypertension, there was a rise in left ventricular mass of 6.2%, whereas in the group that has persistent white-coat hypertension, there was a small decrease in left ventricular mass. This study had no control group, so that the proportion of age-matched normotensives who evolved into sustained hypertension could not be ascertained. In another study,[80] a high rate of progression to sustained hypertension was found, but this study used a liberal definition of white-coat hypertension and had no control group.

## MASKED HYPERTENSION

In some patients, office-based BP measurements may underestimate average daily BP. Although this phenomenon has not been well studied and many basic questions remain regarding the underlying mechanisms, some data suggest such persons are at high risk. This condition is seen in both young[81] and old patients[82] and is not rare. A few studies[48,81] show that masked hypertension is associated with a larger cardiac mass and more carotid atherosclerosis than true normotension. In a recent longitudinal follow-up study of men,[82] masked hypertension was associated with a twofold to threefold increase in cardiovascular morbidity.

## SUMMARY

There is continued uncertainty regarding the prognosis of patients with white-coat hypertension. The fully reported outcome studies suggest a relatively benign prognosis for white-coat hypertensives, and none has shown a worsened cardiovascular outcome compared with normotensives. Nevertheless, most investigators in the field would agree to a few general principles concerning the care of patients with white-coat hypertension. A strict definition using low ambulatory BP averages (e.g., daytime BP <130/80 mm Hg) is necessary to avoid misclassification of patients as white-coat hypertensives when they are actually sustained hypertensives. All coexistent cardiovascular risk factors should be treated. It is prudent to monitor such patients closely and reinforce lifestyle modifications while we await the results of a prospective randomized trial. In the case of masked hypertension, the possibility that out-of-office BP may be higher than office readings should be considered in smokers and in those with excessive target organ damage discordant to levels of office BP (e.g., unexplained LVH). Further study is needed to identify persons at high risk who may benefit from detection of masked hypertension.

### References

1. Pickering TG. Ambulatory Monitoring and Blood Pressure Variability. London, Science Press, 1991.
2. Pickering TG, Gerin W, Schwartz AR. What is the white-coat effect and how should it be measured? Blood Press Monit 7:293-300, 2002.
3. Parati G, Mancia G. White coat effect: Semantics, assessment and pathophysiological implications. J Hypertens 21:481-486, 2003.
4. Pickering TG, Davidson K, Gerin W, et al. Masked hypertension. Hypertension 40:795-796, 2002.
5. Mansoor GA, White WB. Ambulatory blood pressure and cardiovascular risk stratification. J Vas Med Biol 5:61-68, 1994.
6. Pickering TG. A review of national guidelines on the clinical use of ambulatory blood pressure monitoring. Blood Press Monit 1:151-156, 1996.
7. White WB. Clinical utility of ambulatory blood pressure: Perspectives for national insurance coverage. Blood Press Monit 7:27-31, 2002.
8. Mansoor GA, White WB. Contribution of ambulatory blood pressure monitoring to the design and analysis of antihypertensive therapy trials. J Cardiovasc Risk 1:136-142, 1994.
9. Ayman D, Goldshine AD. Blood pressure determination by patients with essential hypertension: The difference between clinical and home readings before treatment. Am J Med Sci 200:465-470, 1940.
10. Gosse P, Bougaleb M, Egloff P, et al. Clinical significance of white-coat hypertension. J Hypertens 12:S43-S47, 1994.
11. Verdecchia P, Schillaci F, Zampi I, et al. Variability between current definitions of normal ambulatory blood pressure. Hypertension 20:555-562, 1992.
12. Verdecchia P, Schillaci G, Borgioni C, et al. White coat hypertension and white coat effect. Am J Hypertens 8:790-798, 1995.
13. Palatini P, Mormino P, Santonastaso M, et al., on behalf of the HARVEST investigators. Target-organ damage in stage I hypertensive subjects with white-coat hypertension and sustained hypertension. Hypertension 31:57-63, 1998.
14. Pickering TG, James GD, Boddie C, et al. How common is white coat hypertension? JAMA 259:225-228, 1988.
15. Pierdomenico SD, Mezzetti A, Lapenna D, et al. White-coat hypertension in patients with newly diagnosed hypertension: Evaluation of prevalence by ambulatory monitoring and impact on cost of health care. Eur Heart J 16:692-697, 1995.
16. Waeber B, Jacot des Combes B, Porchet M, et al. Ambulatory blood pressure recording to identify truly hypertensive patients who truly need therapy. J Chron Dis 37:5-57, 1984.
17. Siegel WC, Blumenthal JA, Divine GW. Physiological, psychological, and behavioral factors and white coat hypertension. Hypertension 16:140-146, 1990.
18. Pieper C, Warren K, Pickering TG. A comparison of ambulatory blood pressure and heart rate at home and work on work and non-work days. J Hypertens 11:177-183, 1993.
19. Parati G, Omboni S, Staessen J, et al. Limitations of the difference between clinic and daytime blood pressure as a surrogate measure of the "white-coat" effect. Syst-Eur investigators. J Hypertens 16:23-29, 1998.
20. Lerman CE, Brody DS, Hui T, et al. The white-coat hypertension response: Prevalence and predictors. J Gen Intern Med 4:226-231, 1989.
21. Cardillo C, De Felice F, Campia U, et al. Psychophysiological reactivity and cardiac end-organ changes in white coat hypertension. Hypertension 21:836-844, 1993.
22. Ruddy MC, Bialy GB, Malka ES, et al. The relationship of plasma renin activity to clinic and ambulatory blood pressure in elderly people with isolated systolic hypertension. J Hypertens 6(S6):S412-S415, 1988.
23. Nakao M, Shimosawa T, Nomura S, et al. Mental arithmetic is a useful diagnostic evaluation in white-coat hypertension. Am J Hypertens 11:41-45, 1998.
24. Donner-Branzhoff N, Chan Y, Szalai JP, et al. Is the clinic-home blood pressure difference associated with psychological distress? A primary care-based study. J Hypertens 15:585-590, 1997.
25. Carels RA, Sherwood A, Blumenthal JA. High anxiety and white-coat hypertension. JAMA 279:197-198, 1998.

26. Lantelme P, Milon H, Gharib C, et al. White coat effect and reactivity to stress: Cardiovascular and autonomic nervous system responses. Hypertension 31:1021-1029, 1998.

27. Helmers KF, Baker B, O'Kelly B, et al. Anger expression, gender, and ambulatory blood pressure in mild un-medicated adults with hypertension. Ann Behav Med 22:60-64, 2000.

28. Leary AC, Donnan PT, MacDonald TM, et al. The white-coat effect is associated with increased blood pressure reactivity to physical activity. Blood Press Monit 7:209-213, 2002.

29. Smith PA, Graham LN, Mackintosh AF, et al. Sympathetic neural mechanisms in white-coat hypertension. J Am Coll Cardiol 40:126-132, 2003.

30. Myers MG, Reeves RA. White coat phenomenon in patients receiving antihypertensive therapy. Am J Hypertens 4:844-849, 1991.

31. Mansoor GA, McCabe EJ, White WB. Determinants of the white-coat effect in hypertensive subjects. J Hum Hypertens 10:87-92, 1996.

32. Verdecchia P, O'Brien E, Pickering T, et al. European Society of Hypertension Working Group on Blood Pressure Monitoring. When can the practicing physician suspect white coat hypertension? Statement from the Working Group on Blood Pressure Monitoring of the European Society of Hypertension. Am J Hypertens 16:87-91, 2003.

33. Thijs L, Amery A, Clement D, et al. Ambulatory blood pressure monitoring in elderly patients with isolated systolic hypertension. J Hypertens 10:693-699, 1992.

34. Mansoor GA, White WB. The patient with an exaggerated white-coat effect. Blood Press Monit 1:75-79, 1996.

35. White WB, Schulman P, McCabe EJ, et al. Average daily blood pressure, not office blood pressure determines cardiac function in patients with hypertension. JAMA 26:873-877, 1989.

36. Glen SK, Elliott HL, Curzio JL, et al. White-coat hypertension as a cause of cardiovascular dysfunction. Lancet 348:654-657, 1996.

37. Cavallini MC, Roman MJ, Pickering TG, et al. Is white coat hypertension associated with arterial disease or left ventricular hypertrophy? Hypertension 26:413-419, 1995.

38. Hoegholm A, Kristensen KS, Bang LE, et al. Left ventricular mass and geometry in patients with established hypertension and white-coat hypertension. Am J Hypertens 6:282-286, 1993.

39. Rizzo V, Cicconetti P, Bianchi A, et al. White-coat hypertension and cardiac organ damage in elderly subjects. J Hum Hypertens 10:293-298, 1996.

40. Weber MA, Neutel JM, Smith DHG, et al. Diagnosis of mild hypertension by ambulatory blood pressure monitoring. Circulation 90:2291-2298, 1994.

41. Kuwajima I, Suzuki Y, Fujisawa A, et al. Is white-coat hypertension innocent? Hypertension 22:826-831, 1993.

42. Soma J, Wideroe TE, Dahl K, et al. Left ventricular systolic and diastolic function assessed with two-dimensional and doppler echocardiography in "white-coat" hypertension. J Am Coll Cardiol 28:190-196, 1996.

43. Palatini P, Penzo M, Canali C, et al. Interactive action of the white-coat effect and the blood pressure levels on the cardiovascular complications in hypertension. Am J Med 103:208-216, 1997.

44. Cuspidi C, Marabini M, Lonati L, et al. Cardiac and carotid structure in patients with established hypertension and white-coat hypertension. J Hypertens 13:1707-1711, 1995.

45. Ferrara LA, Guida L, Pasanisi F, et al. Isolated office hypertension and end-organ damage. J Hypertens 15:979-985, 1997.

46. Pose-Reino A, Gonzalez-Juanatey JR, Pastor C, et al. Clinical implications of white-coat hypertension. Blood Press 5:264-273, 1996.

47. Grandi AM, Broggi R, Colombo S, et al. Left ventricular changes in isolated office hypertension: A blood pressure-matched comparison with normotension and sustained hypertension. Arch Intern Med 161:2677-2781, 2001.

48. Sega R, Trocino G, Lanzarotti A, et al. Alterations of cardiac structure in patients with isolated office, ambulatory, or home hypertension: Data from the general population (Pressione Arteriose Monitorate E Loro Associazioni [PAMELA] Study). Circulation 18(104):1385-1392, 2001.

49. Hoegholm A, Bang LE, Kristensen KS, et al. Microalbuminuria in 411 untreated individuals with established hypertension, white-coat hypertension, and normotension. Hypertension 24:101-105, 1994.

50. Pierdomenico SD, Lapenna D, Guglielmi MD, et al. Target organ status and serum lipids in patients with white-coat hypertension. Hypertension 26:801-807, 1995.

51. Muldoon MF, Nazzaro P, Sutton-Tyrrell K, et al. White-coat hypertension and carotid atherosclerosis. Arch Intern Med 160:1507-1512, 2000.

52. Landray MJ, Sagar G, Murray S, et al. White coat hypertension and carotid atherosclerosis. Blood Press 8:134-140, 1999.

53. Pierdomenico SD, Cipollone F, Lapenna D, et al. Endothelial function in sustained and white coat hypertension. Am J Hypertens 15:946-952, 2002.

54. Gomez-Cerezo J, Rios Blanco JJ, Suarez Garcia I, et al. Noninvasive study of endothelial function in white coat hypertension. Hypertension 40:304-309, 2002.

55. Shimada K, Kawamoto A, Matsubayashi K, et al. Silent cerebrovascular disease in the elderly: Correlation with ambulatory blood pressure. Hypertension 16:692-699, 1990.

56. Eguchi K, Kario K, Shimada K. Greater impact of coexistence of hypertension and diabetes on silent cerebral infarcts. Stroke 34:2471-2474, 2003.

57. Marchesi E, Perani G, Falaschi F, et al. Metabolic risk factors in white-coat hypertensives. J Hum Hypertens 8:475-479, 1994.

58. Julius S, Mejia A, Jones K, et al. "White-coat" verus sustained borderline hypertension in Tecumseh, Michigan. J Hypertens 16:617-623, 1990.

59. Pierdomenico SD, Bucci A, Lapenna D, et al. Circulating homocysteine levels in sustained and white coat hypertension. J Hum Hypertens 17:165-170, 2003.

60. Perloff D, Sokolow M, Cowan RM, et al. Prognostic value of ambulatory blood pressure measurements: Further analyses. J Hypertens 7:S3-S10, 1989.

61. Verdecchia P, Porcellati C, Schillaci G, et al. Ambulatory blood pressure; an independent predictor of prognosis in essential hypertension. Hypertension 24:793-801, 1994.

62. Ohkubo T, Imai Y, Tsuji I, et al. Relation between nocturnal decline in blood pressure and mortality. The Ohasama Study. Am J Hypertens 10:1201-1207, 1997.

63. Staessen JA, Thijs L, Fagard R, et al. Predicting cardiovascular risk using conventional vs ambulatory blood pressure in older patients with systolic hypertension. Systolic Hypertension in Europe Trial Investigators. JAMA 282:539-546, 1999.

64. Strandberg TE, Salomaa V. White coat effect, blood pressure and mortality in men: Prospective cohort study. Eur Heart J 21:1714-1718, 2000.

65. Clement DL, De Buyzere ML, De Bacquer DA, et al; Office versus Ambulatory Pressure Study Investigators. Prognostic value of ambulatory blood-pressure recordings in patients with treated hypertension. N Engl J Med 348:2407-2415, 2003.

66. Khattar RS, Senior R, Lahiri A. Cardiovascular outcome in white-coat versus sustained mild hypertension: A 10-year follow-up study. Circulation 98:1892-1897, 1998.

67. Fagard RH, Staessen JA, Thijs L, et al. Response to antihypertensive therapy in older patients with sustained and nonsustained systolic hypertension. Systolic Hypertension in Europe (Syst-Eur) Trial Investigators. Circulation 5(102):1139-1144, 2001.

68. Bjorklund K, Lind L, Zethelius B, et al. Isolated ambulatory hypertension predicts cardiovascular morbidity in elderly men. Circulation 107:1297-1302, 2000.

69. Kario K, Pickering TG, Matsuo T, et al. Stroke prognosis and abnormal nocturnal blood pressure falls in older hypertensives. Hypertension 38:852-857, 2001.

70. Redon J, Campos C, Narciso ML, et al. Prognostic value of ambulatory blood pressure monitoring in refractory hypertension: A prospective study. Hypertension 31:712-718, 1998.

71. Nakano S, Ogihara M, Tamura C, et al. Reversed circadian blood pressure rhythm independently predicts endstage renal failure in non-insulin-dependent diabetes mellitus subjects. J Diabetes Complications 13:224-231, 1999.

72. Zweiker R, Eber B, Schumacher M, et al. "Non-dipping" related to cardiovascular events in essential hypertensive patients. Acta Med Austriaca 21(3):86-89, 1994.

73. Celis H, Staessen JA, Thijs L, et al. Ambulatory Blood Pressure and Treatment of Hypertension Trial Investigators. Cardiovascular risk in white-coat and sustained hypertensive patients. Blood Press 11:352-356, 2002.

74. Yamamoto Y, Akiguchi I, Oiwa K, et al. Adverse effect of night-time blood pressure on the outcome of lacunar infarct patients. Stroke 29:570-576, 1998.

75. Verdecchia P, Angeli F, Gattobigio R, et al. Ambulatory blood pressure monitoring and prognosis in the management of essential hypertension. Expert Rev Cardiovasc Ther 1:79-89, 2003.

76. Hoegholm A, Wiinberg N, Kristensen KS. The effect of antihypertensive treatment with dihydropyridine calcium antagonists on white-coat hypertension. Blood Press Monit 1:375-382, 1996.

77. Polonia JJ, Santos AR, Gama GM, et al. Follow-up clinic and ambulatory blood pressure in untreated white-coat hypertensive patients. Blood Press Monit 2:289-295, 1997.

78. White WB, Daragjati C, Mansoor GA, et al. The management and follow up of patients with white-coat hypertension. Blood Press Monit 1(S2):S33-S36, 1996.

79. Verdecchia P, Schillaci G, Borgioni C, et al. Identification of subjects with white-coat hypertension and persistently normal ambulatory blood pressure. Blood Press Monit 1:217-222, 1996.

80. Bidlingemeyer I, Burnier M, Bidlingemeyer M, et al. Isolated office hypertension: A prehypertensive state? J Hypertens 14:327-332, 1996.

81. Liu JE, Roman MJ, Pini R, et al. Cardiac and arterial target organ damage in adults with elevated ambulatory and normal office blood pressure. Ann Intern Med 131:564-572, 1999.

82. Wing LM, Brown MA, Beilin LJ, et al. ANBP2 Management Committee and Investigators. Second Australian National Blood Pressure Study. "Reverse white-coat hypertension" in older hypertensives. J Hypertens 20:639-644, 2002.

# SECTION 5

# Treatment: General Considerations

## Chapter 29

# The Blood Pressure Lowering Treatment Trialists' Collaboration (BPLTTC)

### Fiona Turnbull, Jeffrey A. Cutler

## INTRODUCTION

### What is the Blood Pressure Lowering Treatment Trialists' Collaboration?

The Blood Pressure Lowering Treatment Trialists' Collaboration (BPLTTC) is an international collaboration of the principal investigators of large randomized trials of blood pressure–lowering regimens (see Appendix). The broad aim of the collaboration is to provide the most reliable evidence about the effects of commonly used blood pressure–lowering regimens on major cardiovascular events by using prospective meta-analyses (overviews) of individual trials.

The overviews are conducted and reported in accordance with a protocol[1] that prespecifies trial eligibility criteria, primary outcomes, and treatment comparisons. The size, scope, and conduct of these overviews generate precise estimates of the effects of different blood pressure–lowering agents that can then be used to inform clinical and health care policy decision making.

The day-to-day activities of the collaboration—including data management, statistical analysis, and report writing—are carried out by a secretariat (Appendix) based at the George Institute for International Health, a department of the University of Sydney, Australia. An executive committee (Appendix), comprising selected members of the collaboration and of the secretariat, oversees these activities. The secretariat takes primary responsibility for securing funding for the project and for coordinating collaborator meetings. These meetings allow investigators to have an active role in decisions about the direction of the collaboration.

### Background to the Formation of the BPLTTC

In the late 1970s and 1980s, newer and costlier agents, such as calcium antagonists and angiotensin-converting enzyme (ACE) inhibitors, were developed and approved for use as antihypertensive agents. However, even by the early 1990s, evi-

dence that might justify their use, particularly in preference to older classes of agents (diuretics and β-blockers), remained limited. The few studies that directly compared ACE inhibitors and calcium antagonists with conventional agents[2-5] failed to detect any clear differences, mainly because they were individually and collectively too small to detect any plausibly modest differences in the cause-specific effects of the regimens compared. Similar uncertainty also remained about the effects of different blood pressure–lowering regimens on other groups of patients not identified as being "hypertensive" but otherwise at high risk of cardiovascular events, such as those with diabetes or cerebrovascular or renal disease.

During the latter part of the 1990s, a number of new trials were started in an attempt to elucidate the role of newer agents in the prevention of major cardiovascular morbidity and mortality. However, reliable detection of differences of 15% or less would require an individual trial to record 1000 or more outcome events during follow-up, and few trials were likely to observe this number of events. Detection of such differences would require evidence from randomized trials involving many tens of thousands of patients and 1000 or more outcome events during the scheduled treatment period.

In July 1995, therefore, the principal investigators from many of the large-scale trials that were in progress or in advanced stages of planning met and agreed to collaborate in a program of prospectively planned overviews of randomized trials. The broad goal of the collaboration was to provide highly reliable evidence for the effects of commonly used blood pressure–lowering regimens on major cardiovascular events.

## METHODOLOGY

### Evidence-Based Medicine and the Value of Systematic Overviews/Meta-Analyses

Evidence-based medicine (EBM) is the "conscientious, explicit and judicious use of current best evidence in making decisions

**Appendix** Blood Pressure Lowering Treatment Trialists' Collaboration

L Agodoa (Bethesda, USA)
C Baigent (Oxford, UK)
H Black (Chicago, USA)
J-P Boissel (Lyon, France)
B Brenner (Boston, USA)
M Brown (Cambridge, UK)
C Bulpitt (London, UK)
R Byington (Winston-Salem, USA)
J Chalmers (Sydney, Australia)
R Collins (Oxford, UK)
J Cutler (Bethesda, USA)
B Dahlof (Göteborg, Sweden)
B Davis (Houston, USA)
J Dens (Leuven, Belgium)
R Estacio (Denver, USA)
R Fagard (Leuven, Belgium)
K Fox (London, UK)
R Holman (Oxford, UK)
L Hunsicker (Chicago, USA)
J Kostis (New Brunswick, USA)
K Kuramoto (Tokyo, Japan)
L Lindholm (Umea, Sweden)

J Lubsen (Lyon, France)
S MacMahon (Sydney, Australia)
E Malacco (Milan, Italy)
G Mancia (Monza, Italy)
B Neal (Sydney, Australia)
C Pepine (Gainsville, USA)
M Pfeffer (Boston, USA)
B Pitt (Ann Arbor, USA)
P Poole-Wilson (London, UK)
G Remuzzi (Bergamo, Italy)
A Rodgers (Auckland, New Zealand)
P Ruggenenti (Bergamo, Italy)
R Schrier (Denver, USA)
P Sever (London, UK)
P Sleight (Oxford, UK)
J Staessen (Leuven, Belgium)
K Teo (Edmonton, Canada)
P Whelton (New Orleans, USA)
L Wing (Adelaide, Australia)
Y Yui (Kyoto, Japan)
S Yusuf (Hamilton, Canada)
A Zanchetti (Milan, Italy)

*Executive Committee:* C Baigent, J Cutler, R Fagard, S MacMahon, B Neal, P Whelton, S Yusuf
*Secretariat:* C Algert, J Chalmers, S MacMahon, B Neal, F Turnbull, M Woodward
*Secretariat Office:* The George Institute for International Health
PO Box M201
Missenden Rd
Sydney NSW 2050
Australia
Tel: (61 2) 9993 4500
Fax: (61 2) 9993 4502
Website: www.thegeorgeinstitute.org/bplttc

about the care of individual patients."[6] An objective summary of the best available evidence can be provided by a systematic overview or meta-analysis, a statistical procedure that integrates the results of several independent studies that are "combinable."[7] Meta-analyses have become increasingly important tools in epidemiologic research because they are capable of assessing small risks[8] and, as a consequence of including many studies, the findings can be applied to a diverse range of patients.

In combining the results, individual trials are weighted according to size (numbers of clinical events) so that larger trials have more influence than smaller trials. The statistical techniques to combine the estimates of individual trials can be broadly classified into two models. The "fixed effects" model assumes that the variability between trials is entirely due to random variation. The "random effects" model takes into account an additional source of variation by assuming a different underlying effect for each study.[9] The differences between the models are reflected in the confidence intervals around the point estimate of effect (wider for the random effects model). Neither model is considered "correct," and substantial differences in the combined effect calculated by each method will be seen only if the findings of the individual, contributing studies are markedly different or "heterogeneous." Heterogeneity across studies can be formally examined by using statistical procedures. The more significant the test of homogeneity, the less likely it is that the observed differences in the size of the effect are due to chance alone.[10] A statistically significant test means that significant differences among the studies exist.

There are several different types of meta-analyses, but all share a requirement for a study protocol that clearly describes the research question and the design, including how studies are identified and selected, the statistical methods to be used, and how the results will be reported. Meta-analyses of published data can be performed without the cooperation or even agreement from study investigators. Although this is a relatively simple method for calculating a pooled estimate of effect, these meta-analyses are subject to a number of limitations, including publication bias and differences between contributing studies in their design and definitions of outcomes.[8] One variation of this type of meta-analysis is the "network meta-analysis," which combines trials conducting direct comparisons of different treatments with indirect comparisons derived from the use of similar comparator arms in different trials.[11,12] The Cochrane Collaboration also conducts meta-analyses if data from systematic reviews are of sufficient quality.[13] Searches for unpublished and non-English records reduce the risk of publication bias, but subsequent meta-analyses remain retrospective and are also subject to differences in the quality of the data from each study.

In meta-analyses using individual data, statistical reanalysis can be performed by using the same inclusion criteria for all studies and unified definitions for all variables. In prospectively designed overviews, the principal research hypotheses, criteria for inclusion of studies, and statistical analyses are all defined a priori in a formal protocol. By specifying these in advance of publication of trial results, retrospective outcome-dependent biases are avoided and the reliability of the estimates of the effects of the individual treatment regimens is increased. Examples of such prospective meta-analyses include the BPLTTC and the Cholesterol Treatment Trialists' (CTT) Collaboration.[14]

## The BPLTTC Study Protocol

In 1998, the Collaboration published a protocol[1] outlining plans for prospective overviews of major randomized trials of blood pressure–lowering treatments. The following section outlines the major components of this protocol, which guides ongoing work by the Collaboration.

### Eligible Trials and Their Identification

Trials are eligible for inclusion in the overviews if they satisfy one of the following criteria: (1) random allocation of patients to regimens based on different blood pressure–lowering agents, (2) random allocation of patients to a blood pressure–lowering agent or placebo, or (3) random allocation of patients to various blood pressure goals. In addition, eligible trials have to have a planned minimum follow-up of 1000 patient-years per treatment arm and could not have published or presented main trial results before July 1995. Although trials with factorial assignment to other interventions such as cholesterol-lowering treatment are eligible for inclusion, trials in which additional treatments are jointly assigned with blood pressure–lowering treatment are not eligible, because these other treatments act as potential confounders.

Eligible trials are identified by a number of methods, including computer-aided literature searches; scrutiny of the reference lists of trial reports and review articles; scrutiny of abstracts and meeting proceedings; and inquiry among colleagues, collaborators, and industry. Principal investigators of eligible studies are identified and invited to join the Collaboration on an ongoing basis.

### Data Collection

Both individual patient data and summary tabular data are sought from each trial. Although most trials provide tabular data in the first instance, individual patient data facilitate data checking and the conduct of more-comprehensive statistical analyses. The data requested include participant characteristics recorded at screening or randomization, selected measurements made during follow-up, and details of the occurrence of all prespecified BPLTTC outcomes during the scheduled follow-up period (Table 29–1). All data are reviewed for accuracy and completeness and, once tabulated, are sent to collaborating investigators for checking.

Table 29–1 Baseline, Follow-up, and Outcome Data Requested from Trials Participating in the BPLTTC

| Baseline (At or Before Randomization) | Follow-up (At Annual or Similar Intervals) | Outcomes (All Events in Each Category Recorded during Scheduled Follow-up period) |
|---|---|---|
| Patient identifier | Systolic blood pressure | Ischemic stroke |
| Date of randomization | Diastolic blood pressure | Cerebral hemorrhage |
| Treatment allocation | Weight | Subarachnoid hemorrhage |
| Date of birth/age | Serum cholesterol | Other stroke (including unknown) |
| Gender | Serum creatinine | Myocardial infarction |
| Ethnicity | Smoking status | Hospitalization for heart failure |
| Systolic blood pressure | Compliance | Hospitalization for renal disease |
| Diastolic blood pressure | | Hospitalization or transfusion for non-cerebral hemorrhage |
| Weight | | Arterial revascularization procedure |
| Height | | Major cancer (site-specific) |
| Smoking status | | Admission to hospital for any other cause |
| Serum total cholesterol | | Bone fracture |
| Serum creatinine | | Death (cause-specific) |
| Regular aspirin/antiplatelet drug | | Date for each event |
| Other blood pressure–lowering drug | | Date of last follow-up for fatal events |
| History of: | | Date of last follow-up for nonfatal events |
|   Hypertension | | |
|   Diabetes | | |
|   Left ventricular hypertrophy | | |
|   Heart failure | | |
|   Cerebrovascular disease | | |
| Planned end of scheduled treatment and follow-up | | |

## Prespecified Outcomes

The study outcomes chosen for these overviews represent the main cardiovascular outcomes likely to be affected by blood pressure–lowering treatment regimens and the main noncardiovascular disease (non-CVD) outcomes for which questions about the safety of some agents have arisen. The six prespecified primary outcomes are nonfatal stroke or death from cerebrovascular disease (codes 430-438 in the 9th revision of the International Classification of Diseases [ICD-9]); heart failure causing death or requiring hospitalization (ICD 428); total cardiovascular deaths (ICD 396-459); total major cardiovascular events (stroke, coronary heart disease [CHD] events, heart failure, other cardiovascular death); and total mortality. The secondary study outcomes include hemorrhagic stroke (ICD 431-432); ischemic stroke (ICD 433-434); death or hospitalization for renal disease (ICD 189, 403-404, 580-593); arterial revascularization procedure (ICD 36, 38.0, 38.1, and 38.4); any bone fracture (ICD 800-829); death, hospitalization, or transfusion for any noncerebral hemorrhage (ICD 459, 578.9, but not 430-432); or major site-specific cancer (lung [ICD 162], large bowel [ICD 153-154], breast [ICD 174-175], or prostate [ICD 185]); and admission to hospital for any cause.

## Prespecified Comparisons

The comparisons prespecified in the protocol can be broadly divided into two groups. The first group comprises comparisons of active blood pressure–lowering regimens with control regimens: ACE inhibitor–based regimens versus placebo, calcium antagonist–based regimens versus placebo, and regimens targeting different blood pressure goals (more- versus less-intensive blood pressure–lowering regimens). The second group comprises comparisons of different active regimens intended to produce similar blood pressure reductions: ACE inhibitor–based regimens versus diuretic- and/or β-blocker–based regimens; calcium antagonist–based versus diuretic-based or β-blocker–based regimens; and ACE inhibitor–based regimens versus calcium antagonist–based regimens. For each of these comparisons, the null hypothesis of no difference between regimens in their effects on primary outcomes is tested.

At the time of writing the protocol, there were insufficient trials of newer agents such as angiotensin receptor blockers to warrant separate analyses. However, provision was made to include comparisons of these agents as sufficient trials became available.

The protocol also prespecifies secondary analyses with tests of interaction performed to assess the association of any treatment differences with the following patient characteristics: age, sex, diabetes status, preexisting CVD, baseline serum creatinine level, baseline serum cholesterol level, baseline systolic and diastolic blood pressures, and nonstudy blood pressure–lowering treatment at study entry. These subgroup analyses are designed to answer whether there are important differences in the effects of different blood pressure–lowering regimens in younger and older patients, in patients with and without diabetes, and between the other prespecified comparator groups.

## Statistical Analyses

Analyses for each primary outcome are based on the first relevant outcome experienced by a participant. Each participant can contribute only one event to the calculation of one outcome analysis but more than one event to separate analyses of different outcomes. For each study, the relative risk and 95% confidence interval for each outcome are calculated according to the principle of intention to treat. Overall estimates of effect are calculated with a fixed effects model, where the log relative risk for each trial is weighted by the reciprocal of the variance of the log relative risk. The assumption of homogeneity between the treatment effects in different trials is tested with chi-square Q and more recently with the $I^2$ statistic.[15] If the assumption of homogeneity is rejected, then additional analyses are conducted with a random effects model. Mean levels of baseline characteristics and mean differences in follow-up blood pressure between randomized comparisons are calculated with estimates from individual trials weighted by the number of individuals in the study.

Since publication of the protocol, two cycles of overviews have been reported by the Collaboration. The first cycle, published in 2000, included results from 15 trials and nearly 75,000 individuals. More recently, the second cycle reported on the results from 29 trials and 160,000 individuals (Table 29–2).

## FIRST CYCLE FINDINGS: SETTING THE SCENE (FIGURES 29–1 THROUGH 29–6)

By 2000, sufficient data had become available to conduct the first cycle of BPLTTC overviews (Table 29–3).[16] These overviews showed conclusively that the benefits of blood pressure–lowering regimens were not limited to those based on diuretics and β-blockers but extended to newer agents (ACE inhibitors and calcium antagonists) and that these benefits were observed in a heterogeneous population of patients at high risk of CVD.

In the placebo-controlled trials of ACE inhibitors (12,000 individuals and 1800 major cardiovascular events), in which the weighted mean difference between randomized groups was 3/1 mm Hg, there was 20% to 30% reduction in the risk of stroke, CHD, major cardiovascular events, cardiovascular death, and total mortality with active treatment. There was no significant reduction in the risk of heart failure, although the 95% confidence intervals did not exclude a possible moderate advantage for patients receiving ACE inhibitor therapy.

Compared with placebo, calcium antagonist–based regimens producing blood pressure reductions of 9/5 mm Hg conferred clear 30% to 40% reductions in the risk of stroke and major cardiovascular events and nonsignificant trends toward benefits for the remaining outcomes. Although these analyses were limited by rather fewer data (5500 individuals and 380 major cardiovascular events), the estimates of treatment effect largely precluded adverse effects of calcium antagonists in hypertensive patients of the magnitude that had been suggested by earlier reviews in patients with acute myocardial infarction and unstable angina.[17,18]

Comparisons of regimens targeting different blood pressure goals (20,000 individuals and 1000 major cardiovascular events) showed that patients assigned the lowest diastolic blood pressure goals (75 to <85 mm Hg) experienced lower risks of stroke, CHD, and major cardiovascular events. These reductions in risk were on the order of 20%. However, the exact sizes of the differences remained uncertain because of the wide confidence intervals. There was also evidence of heterogeneity ($p = .02$) among the trials contributing to the more- versus less-intensive comparison, largely attributable to

**Table 29–2** Trials Included in Second Cycle of BPLTTC Overviews

| Trials | Main Treatments Compared | Entry Criteria* |
|---|---|---|
| **Trials comparing active treatment and control** | | |
| AASK | MAP ≤92 mm Hg vs 102-107 mm Hg | HBP + nephropathy, Afr |
| ABCD (H) | DBP ≤75 mm Hg vs ≤90 mm Hg | HBP + DM |
| ABCD (N) | DBP 10 mm Hg below baseline vs 80-89 mm Hg | DM |
| HOPE | Ramipril vs placebo | CHD, CVD, or DM + RF |
| HOT | DBP ≤80 mm Hg vs ≤85 or ≤90 mm Hg | HBP |
| IDNT | Amlodipine vs placebo | HBP + DM + nephropathy |
| NICOLE | Nisoldipine vs placebo | CHD |
| PART2 | Ramilpril vs placebo | CHD or CVD |
| PREVENT | Amlodipine vs placebo | CHD |
| PROGRESS | Perindopril (+/− indapamide) vs placebo(s) | Cerebrovascular disease |
| QUIET | Quinapril vs placebo | CHD |
| SCAT | Enalapril vs placebo | CHD |
| SYST-EUR | Nitrendipine vs placebo | HBP, ≥60 years |
| UKPDS-HDS | DBP <85 mm Hg vs <105 mm Hg | HBP + DM |
| **Trials comparing ARB-based regimens and "other" regimens** | | |
| IDNT | Irbesartan vs placebo | HBP + DM + nephropathy |
| LIFE | Losartan vs atenolol | HBP + CVD RF |
| RENAAL | Losartan vs placebo | DM + nephropathy |
| SCOPE | Candesartan vs placebo | HBP, 70-89 years |
| **Trials comparing regimens based on different drug classes** | | |
| AASK | Ramipril vs metoprolol vs amlodipine | HBP + nephropathy, Afr |
| ABCD (H) | Enalapril vs nisoldipine | HBP + DM |
| ABCD (N) | Enalapril vs nisoldipine | DM |
| ALLHAT | Lisinopril vs chlorthalidone vs amlodipine | HBP + RF |
| ANBP2 | Enalapril vs hydrochlorothiazide | HBP, 65-84 years |
| CAPPP | Captopril vs β-blocker or diuretic | HBP |
| CONVINCE | COER-verapamil vs hydrochlorothiazide or atenolol | HBP + RF |
| ELSA | Lacidipine vs atenolol | HBP |
| INSIGHT | Nifedipine GITS vs hydrochlorothiazide + amiloride | HBP + RF |
| JMIC-B | ACE inhibitor vs nifedipine | HBP + CHD |
| NICS-EH | Nicardipine vs trichlormethiazide | HBP, ≥60 years |
| NORDIL | Diltiazem vs β-blocker or diuretic | HBP |
| SHELL | Lacidipine vs chlorthalidone | HBP, ≥60 years |
| STOP-2 | Enalapril or lisinopril vs felodipine or isradipine vs atenolol or metoprolol or pindolol or hydrochlorothiazide + amiloride | HBP, 70-84 years |
| UKPDS-HDS | Captopril vs atenolol | HBP + DM |
| VHAS | Verapamil vs chlorthalidone | HBP |

ARB, angiotensin receptor blocker; MAP, mean arterial pressure; DBP, diastolic blood pressure; ACE, angiotensin-converting enzyme; HBP, high blood pressure; DM, diabetes mellitus; CHD, coronary heart disease; CVD, cardiovascular disease; RF, renal failure; Afr, African American.

trends in opposite directions of the treatment effects for Hypertension Optimal Treatment (HOT)[19] and United Kingdom Prospective Diabetes Study (UKPDS).[20]

The first cycle overviews of trials comparing regimens based on different active agents showed that where blood pressure differences between randomized groups were small (0-3 mm Hg), there was no evidence of a difference in the risk of composite events, major cardiovascular events, cardiovascular death, and total mortality. However, there was some evidence of moderate but potentially important differences between regimens for the cause-specific outcomes of stroke, CHD, and heart failure. In particular,

compared with regimens based on diuretics/β-blockers, calcium antagonist–based regimens appeared to afford greater protection against stroke but less against coronary heart disease. These findings were similar for trials of dihydropyridine and nondihydropyridine agents alike. In the comparisons of ACE inhibitor– and calcium antagonist–based regimens, there was a 20% reduction in the risk of both CHD and heart failure with ACE inhibitor–based regimens. However, for the outcome of CHD, there was significant ($p = .01$) heterogeneity among contributing trials, and for the outcome of heart failure, the risk reduction was of borderline significance.

**Table 29–3** Trials and Major Cardiovascular Events Contributing to the First and Second Cycle of BPLTTC Overviews

| Treatment Comparison | First Cycle Trials | Total Participants | Major Cardiovascular Events | Second Cycle Trials | Total Participants | Major Cardiovascular Events |
|---|---|---|---|---|---|---|
| **ACE-I vs PLACEBO** | | | | | | |
| | HOPE | 9297 | 1645 | | | |
| | PART2 | 617 | 81 | | | |
| | QUIET | 1750 | 104 | | | |
| | SCAT | 460 | 39 | PROGRESS | 6105 | 1062 |
| Cumulative totals | 4 trials | 12,124 | 1869 | 5 trials | 18,229 | 2931 |
| **CA vs PLACEBO** | | | | | | |
| | PREVENT | 825 | 54 | | | |
| | SYST-EUR | 4695 | 291 | IDNT | 1136 | 272 |
| | | | | NICOLE | 826 | NA |
| Cumulative totals | 2 trials | 5520 | 345 | 4 trials | 7482 | 617 |
| **MORE- vs LESS-INTENSIVE REGIMENS** | | | | | | |
| | ABCD (H) | 470 | 75 | | | |
| | HOT | 18,790 | 714 | | | |
| | UKPDS-HDS | 1148 | 246 | AASK | 1094 | 111 |
| | | | | ABCD (N) | 480 | 76 |
| Cumulative totals | 3 trials | 20,408 | 1035 | 5 trials | 21,982 | 1222 |
| **ARB vs 'OTHER' REGIMENS** | | | | | | |
| | — | — | | IDNT | 1148 | 282 |
| | — | — | | LIFE | 9193 | 1096 |
| | — | — | | RENAAL | 1513 | 515 |
| | — | — | | SCOPE | 4937 | 510 |
| Cumulative totals | — | — | | 4 trials | 16,791 | 2403 |
| **ACE-I vs DIURETIC/β-BLOCKER** | | | | | | |
| | CAPPP | 10,985 | 698 | | | |
| | STOP-2 | 4418 | 897 | | | |
| | UKPDS-HDS | 758 | 141 | AASK | 877 | 98 |
| | | | | ALLHAT | 24,309 | 3688 |
| | | | | ANBP2 | 6083 | 509 |
| Cumulative totals | 3 trials | 16,161 | 1736 | 6 trials | 47,430 | 6031 |
| **CA vs DIURETIC/β-BLOCKER** | | | | | | |
| | INSIGHT | 6321 | 407 | | | |
| | NICS-EH | 429 | 23 | | | |
| | NORDIL | 10,881 | 803 | | | |
| | STOP-2 | 4409 | 910 | | | |
| | VHAS | 1414 | 29 | AASK | 658 | NA |
| | | | | ALLHAT | 24,303 | 3704 |
| | | | | CONVINCE | 16,476 | 729 |
| | | | | ELSA | 2334 | 60 |
| | | | | SHELL | 1882 | 172 |
| Cumulative totals | 5 trials | 23,454 | 2172 | 10 trials | 69,107 | 6837 |

**Table 29-3** Trials and Major Cardiovascular Events Contributing to the First and Second Cycle of BPLTTC Overviews—cont'd

| Treatment Comparison | First Cycle Trials | Total Participants | Major Cardiovascular Events | Second Cycle Trials | Total Participants | Major Cardiovascular Events |
|---|---|---|---|---|---|---|
| **ACE-I vs CA** | | | | | | |
| | ABCD (H) | 470 | 75 | | | |
| | STOP-2 | 4401 | 887 | | | |
| | | | | AASK | 653 | NA |
| | | | | ABCD (N) | 480 | 76 |
| | | | | ALLHAT | 18,113 | 2838 |
| | | | | JMIC-B | 1650 | 88 |
| *Cumulative totals* | 2 trials | 4871 | 962 | 6 trials | 25,767 | 3964 |

ACE-I, angiotensin-converting enzyme inhibitor; CA, calcium antagonist; ARB, angiotensin receptor blocker.

## SECOND CYCLE FINDINGS: RESOLVING THE UNCERTAINTY

Although the first cycle of overviews provided many answers to questions they were designed to address, there remained some uncertainty about others—in particular the effects of active treatment with calcium antagonists (compared with none) on the risk of CHD and heart failure and about differences between active regimens in their cause-specific effects.

At the end of 2003, the Collaboration reported its second cycle of overviews.[21] This second cycle was able to resolve much of this persisting uncertainty. A doubling in the amount of data available for analyses substantially increased the evidence available and resulted in the generation of more-precise estimates of treatment effect, especially for comparisons of different active agents. The substantial increase in the amount of data also provided an opportunity to explore in more detail the association of blood pressure reduction and risk reduction. Furthermore, at the end of 2003, sufficient trials of angiotensin receptor blockers had been completed to warrant separate analyses of this important new class of blood pressure–lowering agent.

Because the second cycle of overviews provides the most recent and reliable evidence for the effects of different blood pressure–lowering agents, they are the major focus for the remainder of the chapter.

### Trials and Participants

Nine trials (25,000 individuals and 3500 major cardiovascular disease [CVD] events) provided data from placebo-controlled comparisons of ACE inhibitors and calcium antagonists, and five trials (22,000 individuals and 1200 major CVD events) provided data from trials targeting different blood pressure goals (Table 29–3). Sixteen trials (101,000 participants and 10,000 major CVD events) provided data on comparisons of different active regimens based on ACE inhibitors, calcium antagonists, and diuretics and/or β-blockers. For most trials, patients were selected on the basis of high blood pressure and an additional cardiovascular risk factor such as diabetes, renal disease, or increased age. The overall mean age of participants was 65 years, and just more than half (52%) were men. The mean duration of follow-up for contributing trials ranged from 2.0 to 8.4 years, resulting in more than 700,000 patient-years of follow-up.

### Stroke

In keeping with first cycle findings, there were significant reductions (30%-40%) in the risk of stroke with active regimens (ACE inhibitors, calcium antagonists, more intensive) as compared with control (placebo and less intensive) regimens (Figure 29–1, A). In the comparisons of different active regimens, where blood pressure differences between groups ranged from 0 to 2 mm Hg, there were some differences, but these were of borderline statistical significance. There was a trend toward a greater reduction in the risk of stroke associated with calcium antagonists when compared with regimens based on either ACE inhibitors or diuretic/β-blocker agents (Figure 29–1, B). Similarly, there was also a trend toward a greater protective effect associated with conventional therapy as compared with regimens based on ACE inhibitors. These findings, albeit of borderline significance, had not been apparent in the first cycle of overviews. Furthermore, in this second cycle of overviews based on more than 7500 stroke events, there was no evidence of significant heterogeneity between contributing trials in their estimates of treatment effect (all *p* homog >.1).

### Coronary Heart Disease

More than 10,000 CHD events contributed to the second cycle of overviews. These showed that ACE inhibitor–based regimens reduced the risk of CHD by 20% as compared with placebo (Figure 29–2, A). There was weaker evidence of a reduction with calcium antagonists, and for regimens targeting lower blood pressure goals, there was no clear evidence of benefit. Whereas the first cycle had suggested that there was some evidence of a greater protective effect from regimens based on both diuretics/β-blockers and ACE inhibitors as compared with calcium antagonists, in the second cycle, there was no evidence of any difference between any of the active regimens for the prevention of CHD. These findings were able to confirm conclusions from earlier reports[22,23] questioning the validity of claims of large increases in coronary risk in hypertensive patients treated with calcium antagonists. In the specific comparison of regimens based on ACE inhibitors and calcium antagonists for this outcome, there was evidence of heterogeneity among contributing trials, which had also been demonstrated in the first cycle of

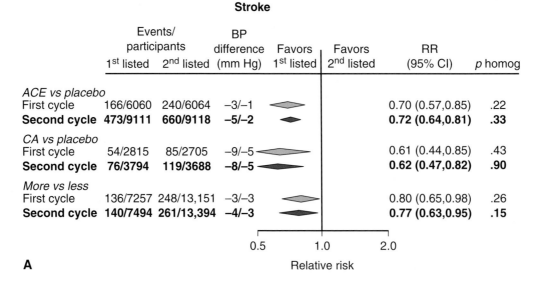

**Figure 29–1** Comparisons of active and control regimens **(A)** and comparisons of different active regimens **(B)** for the outcome of stroke. BP, blood pressure; RR, relative risk; CI, confidence interval; ACE, angiotensin-converting enzyme; CA, calcium antagonist; ACE-I, ACE inhibitor; D/BB, diuretic/β-blocker.

overviews. This heterogeneity was mainly due to one trial[24]; however, neither exclusion of this trial from the fixed-effects model nor the use of a random-effects model altered the conclusions for this outcome.

## Heart Failure

Heart failure events were defined as those resulting in death or admission to hospital. The second cycle of overviews demonstrated a greater protective effect against heart failure from regimens based on ACE inhibitors as compared with placebo but no evidence of a difference between regimens targeting different blood pressure goals. These results were broadly consistent with findings from the first cycle of overviews. Conversely, where first cycle findings indicated a trend toward a greater protective effect against heart failure from regimens

based on calcium antagonists compared with placebo, the second cycle demonstrated a trend in favor of placebo. However, the confidence intervals around the effect estimates for this comparison and for the comparison of more- and less-intensive regimens were wide, reflecting rather fewer data (318 events) available for these analyses.

Compared with regimens based on calcium antagonists, those based on diuretics and/or β-blockers and on ACE inhibitors produced greater reductions in risk of severe heart failure that were not easily accounted for by their comparative effects on blood pressure. Because heart failure events were restricted to those that resulted in death or hospitalization, minor side effects of calcium antagonists, such as peripheral edema, are unlikely to have been responsible for this finding.

The separation of trials that used dihydropyridine agents and those that used nondihydropyridine agents did not result

**Coronary heart disease**

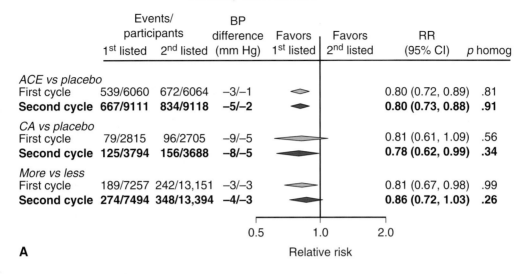

A

**Coronary heart disease**

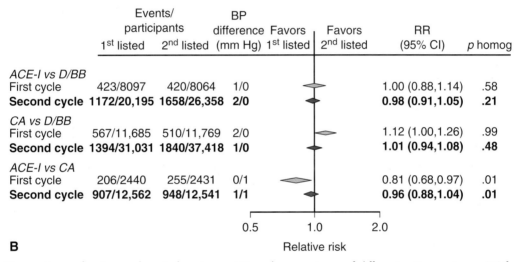

B

**Figure 29–2** Comparisons of active and control regimens **(A)** and comparisons of different active regimens **(B)** for the outcome of coronary heart disease. BP, blood pressure; RR, relative risk; CI, confidence interval; ACE, angiotensin-converting enzyme; CA, calcium antagonist; ACE-I, ACE inhibitor; D/BB, diuretic/β-blocker.

in any difference in the overall conclusions for this outcome (see Figure 29–3).

## Major Cardiovascular Events

A total of more than 17,000 major cardiovascular events (a composite outcome comprising stroke, CHD, and heart failure events plus death from any other cardiovascular cause) contributed to the second cycle of overviews, nearly double the number of events available at the time of the first cycle. In line with first cycle findings, there were significant reductions in the risk of this outcome with active treatment based on either ACE inhibitors (22%) or calcium antagonists (21%) as compared with placebo and for more-intensive as compared with less-intensive regimens (14%). There were no significant differences between regimens based on any of the active

agents (ACE inhibitors, calcium antagonists, or diuretics and/or β-blockers), and confidence intervals were narrow for the estimate for every comparison (see Figure 29–4).

## Cardiovascular Death

Compared with placebo, ACE inhibitors reduced the risk of cardiovascular death by 20%. There was a trend toward fewer deaths with calcium antagonist–based regimens but no clear evidence of a reduction in risk with regimens targeting lower blood pressure goals. These findings were comparable with those generated by the first cycle trials, as were the findings for the comparisons of different active agents, in which very precise estimates of effect indicated no difference between regimens based on ACE inhibitors, diuretics or β-blockers, or calcium antagonists (see Figure 29–5).

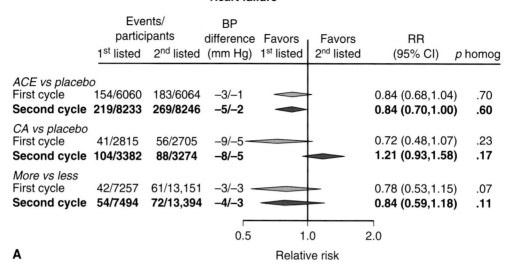

**Heart failure**

| | Events/participants | | BP difference | Favors | Favors | RR | |
|---|---|---|---|---|---|---|---|
| | 1st listed | 2nd listed | (mm Hg) | 1st listed | 2nd listed | (95% CI) | p homog |
| *ACE vs placebo* | | | | | | | |
| First cycle | 154/6060 | 183/6064 | –3/–1 | | | 0.84 (0.68,1.04) | .70 |
| **Second cycle** | **219/8233** | **269/8246** | **–5/–2** | | | **0.84 (0.70,1.00)** | **.60** |
| *CA vs placebo* | | | | | | | |
| First cycle | 41/2815 | 56/2705 | –9/–5 | | | 0.72 (0.48,1.07) | .23 |
| **Second cycle** | **104/3382** | **88/3274** | **–8/–5** | | | **1.21 (0.93,1.58)** | **.17** |
| *More vs less* | | | | | | | |
| First cycle | 42/7257 | 61/13,151 | –3/–3 | | | 0.78 (0.53,1.15) | .07 |
| **Second cycle** | **54/7494** | **72/13,394** | **–4/–3** | | | **0.84 (0.59,1.18)** | **.11** |

**A** Relative risk

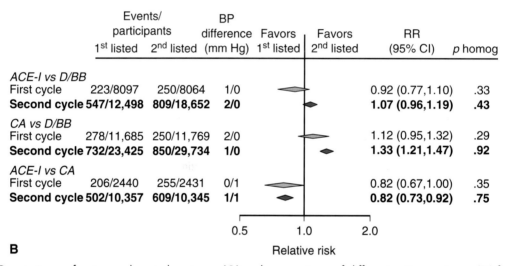

**Heart failure**

| | Events/participants | | BP difference | Favors | Favors | RR | |
|---|---|---|---|---|---|---|---|
| | 1st listed | 2nd listed | (mm Hg) | 1st listed | 2nd listed | (95% CI) | p homog |
| *ACE-I vs D/BB* | | | | | | | |
| First cycle | 223/8097 | 250/8064 | 1/0 | | | 0.92 (0.77,1.10) | .33 |
| **Second cycle** | **547/12,498** | **809/18,652** | **2/0** | | | **1.07 (0.96,1.19)** | **.43** |
| *CA vs D/BB* | | | | | | | |
| First cycle | 278/11,685 | 250/11,769 | 2/0 | | | 1.12 (0.95,1.32) | .29 |
| **Second cycle** | **732/23,425** | **850/29,734** | **1/0** | | | **1.33 (1.21,1.47)** | **.92** |
| *ACE-I vs CA* | | | | | | | |
| First cycle | 206/2440 | 255/2431 | 0/1 | | | 0.82 (0.67,1.00) | .35 |
| **Second cycle** | **502/10,357** | **609/10,345** | **1/1** | | | **0.82 (0.73,0.92)** | **.75** |

**B** Relative risk

**Figure 29–3** Comparisons of active and control regimens **(A)** and comparisons of different active regimens **(B)** for the outcome of heart failure. BP, blood pressure; RR, relative risk; CI, confidence interval; ACE, angiotensin-converting enzyme; CA, calcium antagonist; ACE-I, ACE inhibitor; D/BB, diuretic/β-blocker.

## Total Mortality

Compared with placebo, ACE inhibitor–based regimens reduced the risk of death by 12%. However, there were no significant differences in the risk of death for any of the five other treatment comparisons. There had been evidence of heterogeneity for this outcome in the comparison of more- and less-intensive regimens in the first cycle of analyses. This heterogeneity appeared to reflect a very large reduction in risk of death in favor of more-intensive regimens in the Appropriate Blood Pressure Control in Diabetes (ABCD) trial[24] and nonsignificant trends in the opposite direction from HOT[19] and UKPDS.[20] With the addition of two more trials[25,26] to this treatment comparison, the heterogeneity was less marked. Neither exclusion of the trial with the extreme result nor the use of the random effects model altered the conclusion for this outcome (see Figure 29–6).

## Angiotensin Receptor Blocker Trials

At the time of reporting the first cycle of overviews, there were insufficient data from trials of angiotensin receptor blockers (ARBs) to be included in the analyses. However, by 2003, data from four ARB trials were able to be included in the second cycle of overviews. These trials were Irbesartan Diabetic Nephropathy Trial (IDNT),[27] Reduction of Endpoints in NIDDM with the Angiotensin II Antagonist Losartan (RENAAL),[28] Study on Cognition and Prognosis in the Elderly (SCOPE),[29] and Losartan Intervention for Endpoint reduction in hypertension study (LIFE).[30] As the comparisons of these agents differed somewhat from other treatment comparisons, they were presented separately. Three trials[27-29] were placebo-controlled trials; however, in SCOPE, active treatment was initiated in a large proportion of the placebo group early in the study, and in IDNT and RENAAL, there was a

**Major cardiovascular events**

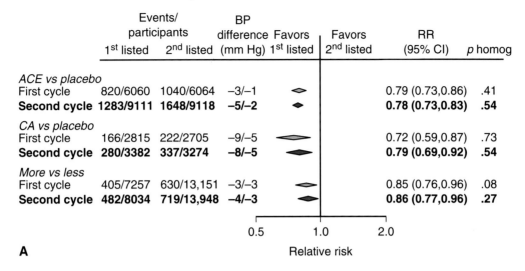

A

**Major cardiovascular events**

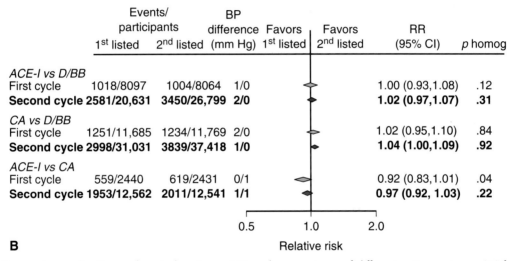

B

**Figure 29–4** Comparisons of active and control regimens **(A)** and comparisons of different active regimens **(B)** for the outcome of total major cardiovascular events. BP, blood pressure; RR, relative risk; CI, confidence interval; ACE, angiotensin-converting enzyme; CA, calcium antagonist; ACE-I, ACE inhibitor; D/BB, diuretic/β-blocker.

simultaneous attempt to achieve blood pressure reductions in both randomized groups. LIFE was the only trial designed as a head-to-head comparison (a comparison of an ARB and β-blocker). However, because all trials included control arms with active agents other than ARBs, they were analyzed as a single group.

There were significant reductions (10%-20%) in the risk of stroke, heart failure, and total major cardiovascular events with regimens based on ARBs as compared with control regimens (Figure 29–7). However, for the remaining outcomes, there was no significant difference, and it is possible that the differences in certain outcomes can be accounted for by differences in achieved blood pressure levels.

## KEY MESSAGES AND IMPLICATIONS FOR CLINICAL PRACTICE

i These overviews provide clinicians and their patients with uniquely reliable information about the relative benefits and risks of widely used classes of blood pressure–lowering drugs. The results are applicable to a broad population of hypertensive and nonhypertensive individuals at high risk of CVD.

ii Treatment with any commonly used regimen reduces the risk of total major cardiovascular events, and larger reductions in blood pressure produce larger reductions in risk. Direct evidence of this is provided by overviews of trials that compared more- with less-intensive blood pressure– lowering

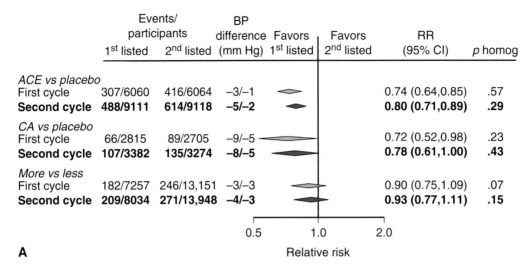

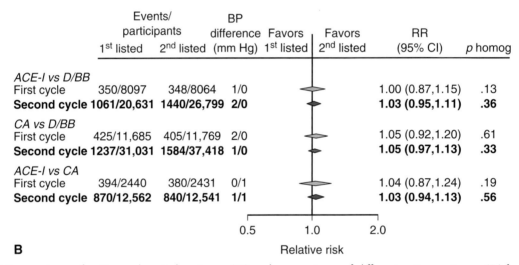

**Figure 29–5** Comparisons of active and control regimens (**A**) and comparisons of different active regimens (**B**) for the outcome of cardiovascular death. BP, blood pressure; RR, relative risk; CI, confidence interval; ACE, angiotensin-converting enzyme; CA, calcium antagonist; ACE-I, ACE inhibitor; D/BB, diuretic/β-blocker.

regimens. In these comparisons, the risk of stroke and of total major cardiovascular events was significantly reduced by regimens targeting lower blood pressure goals. Indirect evidence is provided by the association of weighted mean differences in blood pressure between randomized groups with differences in risk of an event (Figure 29–8). This direct association is true for all cardiovascular events except for heart failure.

iii There are some differences between regimens in their cause-specific effects that appear to be independent of blood pressure. Regimens based on ACE inhibitors and on diuretics and/or β-blockers are much more effective at preventing heart failure than regimens based on calcium antagonists—results that are broadly consistent with trials of both ACE inhibitors[31] and calcium antagonists[32] in heart failure patients. There remains less certainty about possible differences between regimens in their effects on stroke.

## THE COLLABORATION AND FUTURE CHALLENGES

Although the BPLTTC has been at the forefront of the field of collaborative overviews of trials and has achieved most of its objectives, it has also faced challenges regarding scope, methodology, logistics, and funding. With regard to scope, the protocol listed eight subgrouping variables, yet because of the complexity of describing results by subgroups, a paper based on one of these—diabetic status—has only recently been completed. To be most useful in informing practice and practice guidelines, it is desirable to report on as many subgroups as possible, because clinicians desire ensurance that the broad conclusions are applicable to a variety of patients. The ability to conduct such analyses is enhanced by the fact that early in its evolution the BPLTTC decided to include trials of blood pressure–lowering agents not restricted to hypertensive patients; thus the data set

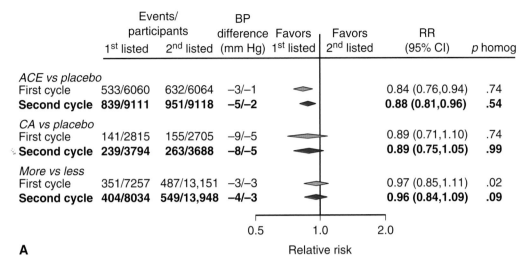

A

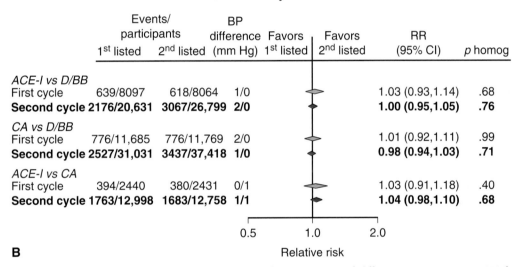

B

**Figure 29-6** Comparisons of active and control regimens **(A)** and comparisons of different active regimens **(B)** for the outcome of total mortality. BP, blood pressure; RR, relative risk; CI, confidence interval; ACE, angiotensin-converting enzyme; CA, calcium antagonist; ACE-I, ACE inhibitor; D/BB, diuretic/β-blocker.

is particularly enriched with patients having other vascular conditions. The decision not to be restricted to trials in hypertensive patients was based on the continuous, monotonic increase of cardiovascular risk with higher blood pressure levels starting below 115/75 mm Hg[33] and has not been challenged. However, it would be strengthened by analyses according to entry blood pressure levels. One non-prespecified subgrouping factor is race/ethnicity; completed trials have provided some basis for pursuing such analyses, albeit post hoc.[34]

Another issue of scope and methodology involves the treatment comparisons. The design decision to group diuretics and β-blockers as "traditional regimens" was based on results from a few completed large trials that compared diuretic-based with β-blocker–based treatments and found no differences in cardiovascular events or total mortality, along with the fact that several of the later large direct comparator trials adopted a "control" arm giving participating clinicians free choice between a diuretic, a β-blocker, or combined treat-

ment. A meta-analysis[35] published subsequent to the BPLTTC protocol suggested that these classes were not wholly equivalent in their effects and that larger reductions in CHD might be seen with diuretics. Although secondary analyses separating trials with these classes as traditional arms have been included in the second cycle papers, there are few trials contributing to these analyses.

With regard to endpoints, the protocol included definitions of the prespecified events according to ICD codes but did not specify clinical criteria, because such definitions would have been very difficult to apply to trials that had been independently designed and were largely ongoing already. Nevertheless, regional variations in diagnostic practices and medical management constitute a legitimate area for exploration regarding interpretations of overviews of this kind, although randomization largely protects against biased effect estimates. One post hoc decision needed to be made with regard to heart failure events in pursuit of greater uniformity—namely, to

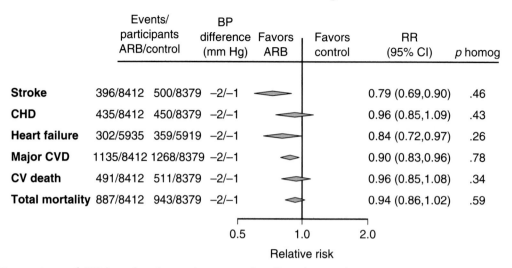

**Figure 29–7** Comparisons of ARB-based and control regimens for all cardiovascular outcomes. ARB, angiotensin receptor blocker; BP, blood pressure; RR, relative risk; CI, confidence interval; CHD, coronary heart disease; CVD, cardiovascular disease; CV, cardiovascular.

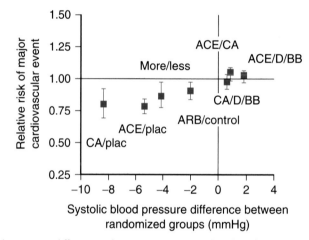

**Figure 29–8** Association of blood pressure differences between groups with risks of major cardiovascular events.

exclude cases diagnosed outside the hospital. Such a decision would influence absolute rates and therefore could affect the net effects on a composite such as major cardiovascular events if treatment regimens affect types of events in different ways (as appears to be the case). The same result could arise from medical care systems that lead to differential hospitalization rates for a variety of nonfatal events.

Finally, to be successful, the BPLTTC requires continuity of staff support and long-term funding. Clearly, an enterprise such as the Collaboration that seeks to inform practice policies broadly but is not likely to provide novel research findings nor serve any particular commercial interest inevitably faces continuing struggles for financial support. Nevertheless, it would appear to represent a valuable resource for informing national and international practice guidelines.[36-39]

## References

1. World Health Organisation-International Society of Hypertension Blood Pressure Lowering Treatment Trialists' Collaboration. Protocol for prospective collaborative overviews of major randomized trials of blood-pressure lowering treatments. J Hypertens 16:127-137, 1998.
2. Materson B. Department of Veteran Affairs single drug therapy of hypertension: Final results. JAMA 270:713-24, 1993.
3. Neaton J, Grimm RJ, Prineas R, et al. Treatment of Mild Hypertension Study. Final results. [Treatment of Mild Hypertension Study Research Group]. JAMA 270:713-24, 1993.
4. The GLANT Study Group. A 12-month comparison of ACE inhibitor and CA antagonist therapy in mild to moderate essential hypertension: The GLANT Study. Study Group on Long-term Antihypertensive Therapy. Hypertens Res 18:235-244, 1995.

5. Borhani N, Mercuri M, Borhani P, et al. Final outcome results of the Multicentre Isradipine Diuretic Atherosclerosis Study (MIDAS). A randomized controlled trial. JAMA 276:785-791, 1996.

6. Sackett D, Rosenberg W, Gray J, et al. Evidence based medicine: What it is and what it isn't. BMJ 312:71-2, 1996.

7. Egger M, Smith G, Phillips AN. Meta-analysis: Principles and procedures. BMJ 315:1533-1537, 1997.

8. Blettner M, Sauerbrei W, Schlehofer B, et al. Traditional reviews, meta-analyses and pooled analyses in epidemiology. Int J Epidemiol 28:1-9, 1999.

9. Der Simonian R, Laird N. Meta-analysis in clinical trials. Control Clin Trials 7:177-188, 1986.

10. Oxman A, Cook D, Guyatt G. Users' guides to the medical literature: VI. How to use an overview. JAMA 272:1367-1371, 1994.

11. Psaty B, Lumley T, Furberg C, et al. Health outcomes associated with various antihypertensive therapies used as first-line agents. JAMA 289:2534-2544, 2003.

12. Lumley T. Network meta-analysis for indirect treatment comparisons. Stat Med 21:2313-2324, 2002.

13. Chalmers I. The Cochrane collaboration: Preparing, maintaining, and disseminating systematic reviews of the effects of health care. Ann N Y Acad Sci 703:156-63, 1993.

14. Simes R. Prospective meta-analysis of cholesterol-lowering studies: The Prospective Pravastatin Pooling (PPP) Project and the Cholesterol Treatment Trialists (CTT) Collaboration. Am J Cardiol 76:122C-126C, 1995.

15. Higgins J, Thompson S. Quantifying heterogeneity in a meta-analysis. Stat Med 21:1539-58, 2002.

16. Blood Pressure Lowering Treatment Trialists' Collaboration. Effects of ACE inhibitors, calcium antagonists and other blood pressure lowering drugs: Results of prospectively designed overviews of randomised trials. Lancet 355:1955-1964, 2000.

17. Held P, Yusuf S, Furberg C. Calcium channel blockers in acute myocardial infarction and unstable angina: An overview. BMJ 229:1187-1192, 1989.

18. Yusuf S, Held P, Furberg C. Update of effects of calcium antagonists in myocardial infarction or angina in light of the Second Danish Verapamil Trial (DAVIT-II) and other recent studies. Am J Cardiol 67:1295-1297, 1991.

19. Hansson L, Zanchetti A, Carruthers S, et al. Effects of intensive blood-pressure lowering and low-dose aspirin in patients with hypertension: Principal results of the Hypertension Optimal Treatment (HOT) randomised trial. Lancet 351:1755-1762, 1998.

20. UK Prospective Diabetes Study Group. Tight blood pressure control and risk of macrovascular and microvascular complications in type 2 diabetes: UKPDS 38. BMJ 317:703-713, 1998.

21. Blood Pressure Lowering Treatment Trialists' Collaboration. Effects of different blood pressure lowering regimens on major cardiovascular events: Second cycle of prospectively designed overviews. Lancet 362:1527-1535, 2003.

22. Ad Hoc Subcommittee of the Liaison Committee of the World Health Organisation and the International Society of Hypertension. Effects of calcium antagonists on the risks of coronary heart disease, cancer and bleeding. J Hypertens 15:105-115, 1997.

23. MacMahon S, Collins R, Chalmers J. Reliable and unbiased assessment of the effects of calcium antagonists: Importance of minimizing both systematic and random errors. J Hypertens 15:1201-1204, 1997.

24. Estacio R, Jeffers B, Hiatt W, et al. The effect of nisoldipine as compared with enalapril on cardiovascular outcomes in patients with non-insulin dependent diabetes and hypertension. N Engl J Med 338:645-652, 1998.

25. Wright J, Bakris G, Green T, et al. Effect of blood pressure lowering and antihypertensive drug class on progression of hypertensive kidney disease: Results from the AASK trial. JAMA 288:2421-2431, 2002.

26. Schrier R, Estacio R, Esler A, et al. Effects of aggressive blood pressure control in normotensive type 2 diabetic patients on albuminuria, retinopathy and strokes. Kidney Int 61:1086-97, 2002.

27. Lewis E, Hunsicker L, Clarke W, et al. Renoprotective effect of the angiotensin-receptor antagonist irbesartan in patients with nephropathy due to type 2 diabetes. N Engl J Med 345:851-60, 2001.

28. Brenner B, Cooper M, De Zeeuw D, et al. Effects of losartan on renal and cardiovascular outcomes in patients with type 2 diabetes and nephropathy. N Engl J Med 345:861-9, 2001.

29. Lithell H, Hansson L, Skogg I, et al. The Study on Cognition and Prognosis in the Elderly (SCOPE). Principal results of a randomised double-blind intervention trial. J Hypertens 21:875-886, 2003.

30. Dahlof B, Devereux R, Kjeldsen S, et al. Cardiovascular morbidity and mortality in the Losartan Intervention For Endpoint reduction in hypertension study (LIFE): A randomised trial against atenolol. Lancet 359:995-1003, 2002.

31. Garg R, Yusuf S. Overview of randomized trials of angiotensin-converting enzyme inhibitors on mortality and morbidity in patients with heart failure. JAMA 273:1450-1456, 1995.

32. Cohn J, Ziesche S, Loss L, et al. Effect of felodipine on short-term exercise and neurohormone and long-term mortality in heart failure: Results of V-Heft III. Circulation 92:1-143, 1995.

33. Lewington S, Clarke R, Qizilbash N, et al. Age-specific relevance of usual blood pressure to vascular mortality: A meta-analysis of individual data for one million adults in 61 prospective studies. Lancet 360:1903-13, 2002.

34. ALLHAT Officers and Coordinators for the ALLHAT Collaborative Research Group. Major outcomes in high-risk hypertensive patients randomized to angiotensin-converting enzyme inhibitor or calcium channel blocker vs diuretic. JAMA 288:2981-97, 2002.

35. Psaty B, Smith N, Siscovick D, et al. Health outcomes associated with antihypertensive therapies used as first-line agents. A systematic review and meta-analysis. JAMA 277:739-745, 1997.

36. Chobanian A, Bakris G, Black H, et al. The seventh report of the Joint National Committee on prevention, detection, evaluation and treatment of high blood pressure. The JNC 7 report. JAMA 289:2560-2572, 2003.

37. World Health Organization. 2003 World Health Organization (WHO)/International Society of Hypertension (ISH) statement on management of hypertension. J Hypertens 21:1983-1992, 2003.

38. Williams B, Poulter N, Brown M, et al. British Hypertension Society Guidelines for management of hypertension: Report of the fourth working party of the British Hypertension Society, 2004-BHS IV. J Hum Hypertens 18:139-185, 2004.

39. Guidelines Committee. European Society of Hypertension: European Society of Cardiology Guidelines for the management of arterial hypertension. J Hypertens 21:1011-1053, 2003.

# Chapter 30

# The Antihypertensive and Lipid-Lowering Treatment to Prevent Heart Attack Trial (ALLHAT)

## Jackson T. Wright, Jr., Suzanne Oparil

## INTRODUCTION

The Antihypertensive and Lipid-Lowering treatment to prevent Heart Attack Trial (ALLHAT) is arguably the most important hypertension study since the demonstration that lowering blood pressure (BP) was associated with reduced adverse clinical outcomes. Its findings have also made it one of the most controversial trials.

Once the benefit of lowering BP in hypertensive patients was established, the next major issue was to determine the optimal treatment regimen to do so. Although thiazide diuretics and β-blockers (alone and in combination) and other sympatholytics and vasodilating drugs were the drugs originally used to demonstrate the benefit of BP lowering, they are also associated with adverse effects on markers associated with increased cardiovascular disease (CVD) risk (e.g., glucose, lipids, potassium, uric acid). Furthermore, evidence suggested that coronary heart disease (CHD) events in trials using these agents were reduced less effectively than predicted from epidemiologic studies.

Although previous trials were designed to examine the effect of treatment on either stroke or composite CVD, they did not have the statistical power to evaluate CHD. Thus the primary objective of ALLHAT was to determine whether antihypertensive drug therapy initiated with newer agents with more favorable metabolic profiles (i.e., angiotensin-converting enzyme inhibitors [ACEIs], α-blockers, or calcium channel blockers [CCBs]) was more effective in preventing CVD, especially CHD, than the older (and less costly) drugs represented by a thiazide-type diuretic. Another objective was to examine the effect of antihypertensive drug selection in populations known to suffer excessively from the hypertension and related target organ damage but who were underrepresented in previous studies. ALLHAT was the largest hypertension trial ever conducted, the first clinical outcome trial to evaluate newer agents in Blacks, and the largest clinical outcome trial in diabetics, and it had large numbers of women and participants older than age 65 years.

## METHODS

### Patient Selection

The rationale and design of ALLHAT have been presented elsewhere.[1] The goal was to recruit high-risk participants with relatively mild BP elevation and thus a high likelihood of successful control on monotherapy. Participants were men and women with either untreated systolic (≥140 mm Hg) and/or diastolic (≥90 mm Hg) hypertension (but ≤180/110 mm Hg at two visits) or treated hypertension (≤160/100 mm Hg on one to two antihypertensive drugs at visit 1 and ≤180/110 mm Hg at visit 2 when medication may have been withdrawn) and at least one additional risk factor for CHD events.[1,2] The risk factors included age ≥55 years, previous (>6 months) myocardial infarction (MI) or stroke, left ventricular hypertrophy (LVH) by electrocardiography or echocardiography, history of type 2 diabetes, current cigarette smoking, high-density lipoprotein cholesterol (HDLC) <35 mg/dl, or documentation of other atherosclerotic CVD. Individuals with a history of hospitalized or treated symptomatic heart failure (HF), serum creatinine >2.0 mg/dl, and/or known left ventricular ejection fraction <35% were excluded. Race was defined by self-report as Black, white, Asian, Native American, and other.

### Interventions

There was no washout period, and unless the drug regimen required tapering for safety reasons, individuals continued any prior antihypertensive medications until they received randomized study drug (after which previous antihypertensive medications were discontinued). Previous antihypertensive drug treatment was similar in participants across the randomized treatment groups. Participants were randomly assigned to chlorthalidone, amlodipine, doxazosin, or lisinopril in a ratio of 1.7:1:1:1, respectively.

Chlorthalidone was selected to represent the older therapy (thiazide-type diuretic) for several reasons. First, the largest experience in clinical outcome trials (especially in preventing CHD in older patients) was with this class of antihypertensive agents.[3-9] Previous data suggested similar endpoint reduction, regardless of the specific thiazide-type diuretic utilized. Although chlorthalidone was not the most common diuretic prescribed by providers, there was substantial experience with this agent in clinical trials.[7-9] Last, when ALLHAT was conceived, consistent with the contemporary emphasis on low-dose diuretic therapy, the dosages of 12.5 and 25 mg of chlorthalidone were thought to be more acceptable to potential clinical sites than 25 and 50 mg/day of hydrochlorothiazide.

Participants (n = 42,418) were recruited at 623 centers in the United States, Canada, Puerto Rico, and the U.S. Virgin Islands between February 1994 and January 1998. More than half of the clinical centers were private practice sites.[10] Closeout ended on March 31, 2002, for the amlodipine and lisinopril versus chlorthalidone comparison; closeout for the doxazosin arm ended approximately 2 years earlier on February 15, 2000.

BPs during the trial were measured by trained observers using standardized techniques.[11] Visit BP was the average of two seated measurements. Goal BP for all participants was both systolic BP (SBP) <140 mm Hg and diastolic BP (DBP) <90 mm Hg. This was achieved by titrating the assigned study drug (step 1), then adding open-label agents (step 2 or 3) when necessary. Non-pharmacologic approaches to treatment of hypertension were recommended according to contemporary national guidelines.[12]

The identity of the step 1 agents was double-masked at each dosage level. Dosages were 12.5, 12.5 (sham titration), and 25 mg/day for chlorthalidone; 2.5, 5, and 10 mg/day for amlodipine; and 10, 20, and 40 mg/day for lisinopril. In participants not controlled on monotherapy, open-label drugs were provided by the study. They included the following: step 2: atenolol, 25 to 100 mg/day; reserpine, 0.05 to 0.2 mg/day; or clonidine, 0.1 to 0.3 mg twice/day; step 3: hydralazine, 25 to 100 mg twice/day. Slow-release potassium chloride was also provided for serum potassium consistently <3.5 mEq/L. After randomization, if a clear indication arose, half doses of open-label step 1 drug classes were permitted along with blinded drugs.[1,11] After initial monthly titration visits, participants were seen every 3 months during the first year and every 4 months thereafter.

## Outcomes

The primary outcome was a composite of fatal CHD or nonfatal MI.[1] Previous primary prevention comparative outcome trials used a composite CVD outcome as the primary outcome. Designating fatal CHD and nonfatal MI as the primary outcome substantially increased the sample size required for the trial. Four major prespecified secondary outcomes were (1) all-cause mortality, (2) fatal and nonfatal stroke, (3) combined CHD (the primary outcome + coronary revascularization + hospitalized angina), and (4) combined CVD (combined CHD + stroke + nonhospitalized treated angina + HF [fatal, hospitalized, or treated nonhospitalized], and treated peripheral arterial disease). Individual components of the combined outcomes also were examined. Other pre-specified secondary outcomes included incident cancer, incident electrocardiogram (ECG) LVH, and end-stage renal disease (ESRD) (dialysis, renal transplant, or renal death). Change in estimated glomerular filtration rate (eGFR)[13] was examined posthoc.

Study endpoints were assessed at follow-up visits, reported to the Clinical Trials Center (CTC), and verified by several mechanisms.[1] Because of the large number of total events (>10,000), blinded review of all events was not feasible. A minimal goal was to ensure that no bias was introduced that favored any of the randomized treatment groups. Hospitalized outcomes were primarily based on clinic investigator reports, with copies of death certificates and hospital discharge summaries requested for central review. Among all combined CVD events that resulted in deaths and/or hospitalizations, the proportion with documentation (i.e., a death certificate or a hospital discharge summary) was 99% in the amlodipine and lisinopril versus chlorthalidone comparisons and 97% in the doxazosin versus chlorthalidone comparison. Searches for outcomes were also accomplished through the Centers for Medicare and Medicaid Services (CMS), the Department of Veterans Affairs (VA), the National Death Index, and the Social Security Administration databases. Medical reviewers at the CTC verified the clinician-assigned diagnoses of outcomes by using death certificates and hospital discharge summaries.

More-detailed information was collected on a random (10%) subset of CHD and stroke events to validate the procedure of using clinician diagnoses.[1] When a large excess of HF became evident in the doxazosin arm, a one-time sample of HF hospitalizations was reviewed by the ALLHAT Endpoints Subcommittee. Agreement rates between the subcommittee and clinic investigators were 90% (155/172) for the primary endpoint, 84% (129/153) for stroke, and 85% (33/39) for HF hospitalizations[14] and were similar in all treatment groups. Blinded review of 98% of the HF hospitalizations in 97% of the participants with HF has confirmed the validity of this outcome.[14,15]

## Statistical Analyses

Data were analyzed according to participants' randomized treatment assignments regardless of their subsequent medications (intent-to-treat analysis). ALLHAT had 83% power to detect a 16% reduction in nonfatal MI and fatal CHD at a two-sided $\alpha = 0.0178$.

## RESULTS

### Patient Characteristics

Table 30–1 presents baseline characteristics for the 42,418 participants in the trial. The mean age was 67 years; 47% were women, 35% were Black, 36% were diabetic. There were nearly identical distributions of baseline risk factors across the four treatment groups.[2]

### Visit and Medication Adherence

The mean duration of follow-up was 4.9 years in the chlorthalidone, amlodipine, and lisinopril arms and 3.2 years in the doxazosin arm.[16,17] Approximately 99% of expected person-years were observed for the chlorthalidone, amlodipine, and lisinopril arms, and in the doxazosin arm (which was stopped early), the figure was 95%. The maximum duration of follow-up was 8.0, 7.9, 8.1, and 5.9 years in the chlorthalidone, amlodipine, lisinopril, and doxazosin groups, respectively. Thus, ALLHAT had one of the longest periods of on-treatment follow-up of any clinical outcome trial. Despite the trial's size and length of follow-up, visit and medication adherence were excellent. At trial closeout, only 419 of 15,255 (2.7%) of the chlorthalidone group, 258 of 9048 (2.8%) of the amlodipine group, 276 of 9054 (3.0%) of the lisinopril group, and 449 of 9061 (4.9%) of the doxazosin group had unknown vital status. Visit adherence was 92% at 1 year and 84% to 87% at 5 years in the chlorthalidone, amlodipine, and lisinopril arms.[16] At 4 years, visit adherence was 80% for the doxazosin/chlorthalidone comparison.[17]

It is noteworthy that with the double-blind design, fewer participants randomized to ACEI or $\alpha$-blocker remained on their assigned drug than those randomized to the diuretic or CCB. Among participants in the chlorthalidone group who were contacted in the clinic or by telephone within 12 months of annual scheduled visits, 87.1% were taking chlorthalidone or another diuretic at 1 year, decreasing to 80.5% at 5 years. Among participants in the amlodipine group, 87.6% were taking amlodipine or another CCB at 1 year, decreasing to 80.4%

at 5 years. Among participants in the lisinopril group, 82.4% were taking lisinopril or another ACEI at 1 year, decreasing to 72.6% at 5 years. In the doxazosin group, 71% of participants were taking doxazosin or another α-blocker at 4 years. The most common reasons for not taking step 1 medication were unspecified refusals and symptomatic adverse effects in more than 50% of cases.

## Intermediate Outcomes

Mean seated BP at randomization was 146/84 mm Hg in all four groups, with 90% of participants reporting current antihypertensive drug treatment (Table 30–1). Among participants returning for follow-up visits, diastolic BP was reduced to a similar degree in all four treatment arms. However, mean systolic BP was ~1 mm Hg greater in the amlodipine arm than in the chlorthalidone arm and ~3 mm Hg greater in the lisinopril and doxazosin arms than in the chlorthalidone arm (Table 30–2). At the initial visit, the proportion of participants at or below the BP goal (<140/90 mm Hg) was ~27%; at 5 years, it was 68%, 66%, and 61% for the chlorthalidone, amlodipine, and lisinopril groups, respectively; and 58% for the doxazosin group at 4 years (Table 30–2).

The metabolic changes in the treatment groups were similar to what had been reported in multiple studies prior to ALLHAT. Mean total serum cholesterol levels at baseline were about 216 mg/dl in all four groups. At 4 years, the respective mean levels were 197.2 (chlorthalidone), 195.6 (amlodipine), 195.0 (lisinopril), and 187 mg/dl (Table 30–3). By 4 years, about 35% to 36% of participants in all three groups reported taking lipid-lowering drugs, largely hydroxymethylglutaryl coenzyme A reductase inhibitors, some as a result of participation in the ALLHAT lipid trial. Mean serum potassium levels at baseline were 4.3 to 4.4 mmol/L; at 4 years, the respective mean levels were 0.3 to 0.4 mmol/L lower for those in the chlorthalidone group than in the other groups.

Mean fasting serum glucose levels at baseline were similar (122-124 mg/dl) in the four groups; at 4 years, the respective mean levels were 126.3, 123.7, 121.5, and 117 mg/dl. Among individuals classified as nondiabetic at baseline, with baseline fasting serum glucose <126 mg/dl (7.0 mmol/L), the incidence of diabetes (fasting serum glucose ≥126 mg/dl) at 4 years was 11.6%, 9.8%, 8.1%, and 8.8%, respectively.

Mean eGFR at baseline was about 78 ml/min/1.73 m² in all groups. At 4 years, it was 70.0, 75.1, 70.7, and 72.8 ml/min/1.73 m² in the chlorthalidone, amlodipine, lisinopril, and doxazosin groups, respectively. The slopes of the reciprocal of serum creatinine over time were virtually identical in the chlorthalidone and lisinopril groups, whereas the decline in the amlodipine slope was less than that of the chlorthalidone slope.[16]

## Primary and Secondary Outcomes

The effects of the treatment regimens as compared with chlorthalidone are displayed in Table 30–4.

### Amlodipine Versus Chlorthalidone

No significant difference was observed between amlodipine and chlorthalidone for the primary outcome (relative risk [RR], 0.98; 95% confidence interval [CI] 0.90-1.07) or for the secondary outcomes of all-cause mortality, combined CHD, stroke, combined CVD, angina, coronary revascularization, peripheral arterial disease, cancer, or ESRD (Figure 30–1). The amlodipine group had a 38% higher risk of HF ($p <.001$) and a 35% higher risk of hospitalized/fatal HF ($p <.001$). The treatment effects for all outcomes were consistent across the predefined subgroups and by absence or presence of CHD at baseline.

### Lisinopril Versus Chlorthalidone

No significant difference was observed between lisinopril and chlorthalidone for the primary outcome (RR, 0.99; 95% CI 0.91-1.08) or for the secondary outcomes of all-cause mortality, combined CHD, peripheral arterial disease, cancer, or ESRD (Figure 30–2). The lisinopril group had a 15% higher risk for stroke ($p = .02$) and a 10% higher risk of combined CVD ($p <.001$). Included in this were a 19% higher risk of HF ($p <.001$), a 10% higher risk of hospitalized/fatal HF ($p = .11$), an 11% higher risk of hospitalized/treated angina ($p = .01$), and a 10% higher risk of coronary revascularization ($p = .05$). The treatment effects for all outcomes were consistent across subgroups by gender, diabetic status, and baseline CHD status. For stroke and combined CVD, there were significant differential effects by race ($p = .01$ and .04 for interaction, respectively). The relative risks (lisinopril versus chlorthalidone) for stroke were 1.40 ($p <.001$) in Blacks and 1.00 ($p = .96$) in non-Blacks; they were 1.19 ($p <.001$) and 1.06 ($p = .05$) for combined CVD in Blacks and non-Blacks, respectively.

The mean follow-up systolic BP for all participants was 2 mm Hg higher in the lisinopril group than in the chlorthalidone group, 4 mm Hg higher in Blacks, and 3 mm Hg higher in those age 65 years or older. Adjustment for follow-up BP as time-dependent covariates in a proportional hazards model slightly reduced the relative risks for stroke (RR 1.15 to 1.11) and HF (RR 1.20 to 1.17) overall and in the Black subgroup (stroke RR 1.40 to 1.36, and HF RR 1.32 to 1.28), but the results remained statistically significant.

### Doxazosin Versus Chlorthalidone

No significant difference was observed between doxazosin and chlorthalidone for the primary outcome (RR, 1.03; 95% CI 0.92-1.15) or for the secondary outcomes of all-cause mortality, combined CHD, peripheral arterial disease, cancer, or ESRD (Figure 30–3). The doxazosin group had a 26% higher risk for stroke ($p = .001$) and a 20% higher risk of combined CVD ($p <.001$). Included in this were an 80% higher risk of HF ($p <.001$), a 66% higher risk of hospitalized/fatal HF ($p <.001$), a 13% higher risk of hospitalized/treated angina ($p = .01$), and a 12% higher risk of coronary revascularization ($p = .05$). The treatment effects for all outcomes were consistent across subgroups by gender, diabetic status, baseline CHD status, and race.

### Primary Safety Outcomes

Six-year rates of hospitalization for gastrointestinal bleeding, available only for Medicare and VA participants, were similar in the chlorthalidone, amlodipine, and lisinopril treatment groups, with no significant differences. Angioedema occurred in 0.4% of persons in the lisinopril treatment group, a rate

**Table 30-1** Baseline Characteristics of the ALLHAT Antihypertensive Component Participants

|  | Chlorthalidone | Amlodipine | Lisinopril | Doxazosin |
|---|---|---|---|---|
| Number randomized | 15,255 | 9,048 | 9,054 | 9,061 |
| Age, mean (SD) years | 66.9 (7.7) | 66.9 (7.7) | 66.9 (7.7) | 66.8 |
| 55-64, n (%) | 6,471 (42.4) | 3,844 (42.5) | 3,869 (42.7) | 3,893 (43.1) |
| 65+, n (%) | 8,784 (57.6) | 5,204 (57.5) | 5,185 (57.3) | 5,148 (56.9) |
| White, non-Hispanic, n (%) | 7,202 (47.2) | 4,305 (47.6) | 4,262 (47.1) | 4,209 (46.5) |
| Black, non-Hispanic, n (%) | 4,871 (31.9) | 2,911 (32.2) | 2,920 (32.3) | 2,984 (32.9) |
| White Hispanic, n (%) | 1,912 (12.5) | 1,108 (12.2) | 1,136 (12.5) | 1,138 (12.6) |
| Black Hispanic, n (%) | 498 (3.3) | 302 (3.3) | 290 (3.2) | 308 (3.4) |
| Other, n (%) | 772 (5.1) | 422 (4.7) | 446 (4.9) | 421 (4.6) |
| Women, n (%) | 7,171 (47.0) | 4,280 (47.3) | 4,187 (46.2) | 4,203 (46.4) |
| Years of education, mean (SD) years | 11.0 (4.0) | 11.0 (3.9) | 11.0 (4.1) | 11.0 (4.0) |
| Antihypertensive treatment |  |  |  |  |
|   Treated, n (%) | 13,754 (90.2) | 8,171 (90.3) | 8,164 (90.2) | 8,175 (90.2) |
|   Untreated, n (%) | 1,500 (9.8) | 877 (9.7) | 890 (9.8) | 886 (9.8) |
| Blood pressure, mean(SD) mm Hg | 146(16)/84(10) | 146(16)/84(10) | 146(16)/84(10) | 146/84 |
|   Treated at baseline | 145(16)/83(10) | 145(16)/83(10) | 145(16)/84(10) | 145(16)/83(10) |
|   Untreated at baseline | 156(12)/89(9) | 157(12)/90(9) | 156(12)/89(9) | 157(12)/89(10) |
| Eligibility risk factors* |  |  |  |  |
|   Cigarette smoker, n (%) | 3,342 (21.9) | 1,980 (21.9) | 1,981 (21.9) | 1967 (21.7) |
|   Atherosclerotic cardiovascular disease,† n (%) | 7,900 (51.8) | 4,614 (51.0) | 4,684 (51.7) | 4,681 (51.7) |
|   History of MI or stroke, n (%) | 3,581 (23.5) | 2,098 (23.2) | 2,058 (22.7) | 2,079 (22.9) |
|   History of coronary revascularization, n (%) | 1,986 (13.0) | 1,106 (12.2) | 1,218 (13.5) | 1,159 (12.8) |
|   Other ASCVD, n (%) | 3,604 (23.6) | 2,145 (23.7) | 2,152 (23.8) | 2,241 (24.7) |
|   ST-T wave, n (%) | 1,572 (10.4) | 908 (10.1) | 940 (10.5) | 920 (10.2) |
|   Type 2 diabetes, n (%) | 5,528 (36.2) | 3,323 (36.7) | 3,212 (35.5) | 3,320 (35.5) |
|   HDLC <35 mg/dl, n (%) | 1,798 (11.8) | 1,018 (11.3) | 1,061 (11.7) | 1,048 (11.6) |
|   LVH by ECG, n (%) | 2,467 (16.2) | 1,533 (16.9) | 1,474 (16.3) | 1,478 (16.3) |
|   LVH by Echo, n (%) | 695 (4.6) | 411 (4.6) | 402 (4.5) | 405 (4.5) |
| History of CHD at baseline,‡ n (%) | 3,943 (26.0) | 2,202 (24.5) | 2,270 (25.3) | 249 (11.4) |
| Body mass index, mean (SD) kg/m² | 29.7 (6.2) | 29.8 (6.3) | 29.8 (6.2) | 29.7 (6.0) |
| Using aspirin, n (%) | 5,426 (35.6) | 3,268 (36.1) | 3,258 (36.0) | 3,271 (36.1) |
| Using estrogen supplementation (women only), n (%) | 1,273 (17.8) | 752 (17.6) | 727 (17.4) | 747 (18.0) |
| Lipid trial participants, n (%) | 3,755 (24.6) | 2,240 (24.8) | 2,167 (23.9) | 2,193 (24.2) |

*For trial eligibility, participants had to have at least one other risk factor in addition to hypertension. Thus the indicated risk factors are not mutually exclusive or exhaustive and may not represent prevalence.

†History of myocardial infarction (MI) or stroke; history of coronary revascularization; major ST segment depression or T wave inversion on any electrocardiogram (ECG) in the past two years; other ASCVD (history of angina pectoris; history of intermittent claudication, gangrene, or ischemic ulcers; history of transient ischemic attack; coronary, peripheral vascular, or carotid stenosis 50% or more documented by angiography or Doppler studies; ischemic heart disease documented by reversible or fixed ischemia on stress thallium or dipyridamole thallium, ST depression ≥1 mm for ≥1 minute on exercise testing or Holter monitoring; reversible wall motion abnormality on stress echocardiogram; ankle-arm index less than 0.9; abdominal aortic aneurysm detected by ultrasonography, CT scan, or X-ray; carotid or femoral bruits).

‡p = 0.03 for comparison of groups.

four times higher than in the other treatment groups. Significant differences were seen for the lisinopril versus chlorthalidone comparison overall (p <.001); in Blacks (2/5369 [<0.1%] for chlorthalidone, 23/3210 [0.7%] for lisinopril, p <.001) and in non-Blacks (6/9886 [0.1%] for chlorthalidone, 15/5844 for lisinopril [0.3%], p = .002). The only death from angioedema was in the lisinopril group.

## DISCUSSION

ALLHAT demonstrated that antihypertensive drug therapy initiated with ACEIs, α-blockers, and dihydropyridine-CCBs was not superior to that initiated with a thiazide-type diuretic in preventing CHD or any other CVD outcome.[16,17] Furthermore, the diuretic was superior to the CCB in pre-

**Table 30–2** Number of Participants, Mean (SD) BP, % at Goal, and BP Difference at Baseline and Annual Visits

| | Baseline | 1 Year | 2 Years | 3 Years | 4 Years | 5 Years |
|---|---|---|---|---|---|---|
| **N** | | | | | | |
| Chlorthalidone | 15,255 | 12,862 | 11,740 | 10,698 | 9,379 | 5,301 |
| Amlodipine | 9,048 | 7,609 | 6,883 | 6,381 | 5,637 | 3,195 |
| Lisinopril | 9,054 | 7,521 | 6,700 | 6,076 | 5,325 | 2,963 |
| Doxazosin | 9,061 | 7,513 | 6,725 | 4,570 | 2,424 | N/A |
| **Systolic blood pressure – mean (SD) mm Hg and comparisons, of amlodipine, doxazosin, and lisinopril with chlorthalidone** | | | | | | |
| Chlorthalidone | 146.2 (15.7) | 136.9 (15.8) | 135.9 (15.9) | 134.8 (15.4) | 133.9 (15.7) | 133.9 (15.2) |
| Amlodipine | 146.2 (15.7) | 138.5 (14.9) | 137.1 (15.0) | 135.6 (15.2) | 134.8 (15.0) | 134.7 (14.9) |
| | $p=.98$ | $p<.001$ | $p<.001$ | $p=.001$ | $p=.002$ | $p=.03$ |
| Lisinopril | 146.4 (15.7) | 140.0 (18.5) | 138.4 (17.9) | 136.7 (17.3) | 135.5 (17.2) | 135.9 (17.9) |
| | $p=.39$ | $p<.001$ | $p<.001$ | $p<.001$ | $p<.001$ | $p<.001$ |
| Doxazosin | 146.3 (15.7) | 140.1 (17.0) | 138.2 (16.7) | 137.6 (17.2) | 137.4 (17.5) | N/A |
| | $p=.73$ | $p<.001$ | $p<.001$ | $p<.001$ | $p<.001$ | N/A |
| **Diastolic blood pressure – mean (SD) mm Hg and comparisons, of amlodipine, doxazosin, and lisinopril with chlorthalidone** | | | | | | |
| Chlorthalidone | 84.0 (10.1) | 79.3 (9.9) | 78.3 (9.6) | 77.2 (9.5) | 76.5 (9.7) | 75.4 (9.8) |
| Amlodipine | 83.9 (10.2) | 78.7 (9.5) | 77.7 (9.6) | 76.4 (9.6) | 75.7 (9.6) | 74.6 (9.9) |
| | $p=.52$ | $p<.001$ | $p<.001$ | $p<.001$ | $p<.001$ | $p<.001$ |
| Lisinopril | 84.1 (10.0) | 79.9 (10.5) | 78.6 (10.3) | 77.3 (10.3) | 76.6 (10.4) | 75.4 (10.7) |
| | $p=.49$ | $p<.001$ | $p=.032$ | $p=.42$ | $p=.48$ | $p=.94$ |
| Doxazosin | 83.7 (10.1) | 79.5 (10.0) | 78.4 (9.9) | 76.9 (10.6) | 76.6 (10.8) | N/A |
| | $p=.47$ | $p=.60$ | $p=.80$ | $p=.10$ | $p=.90$ | N/A |
| **% <140/90 mm Hg (blood pressure goal)** | | | | | | |
| Chlorthalidone | 27.2% | 57.8% | 61.0% | 63.9% | 67.1% | 68.2% |
| Amlodipine | 27.6% $p=.56$ | 55.2% $p<.001$ | 57.4% $p<.001$ | 63.4% $p=.54$ | 65.8% $p=.15$ | 66.3% $p=.09$ |
| Lisinopril | 26.3% $p=.12$ | 50.6% $p<.001$ | 54.1% $p<.001$ | 59.2% $p<.001$ | 63.1% $p<.001$ | 61.2% $p<.001$ |
| Doxazosin | 27.3% $p=.95$ | 50.4% $p<.001$ | 54.8% $p<.001$ | 56.8% $p<.001$ | 57.6% $p<.001$ | N/A |
| **SBP/DBP Δ mm Hg (compared with the chlorthalidone group)** | | | | | | |
| Amlodipine | 0.0/−0.1 | 1.6/−0.6 | 1.2/−0.6 | 0.8/−0.8 | 0.9/−0.8 | 0.8/−0.8 |
| Lisinopril | 0.2/0.1 | 3.1/0.6 | 2.5/0.3 | 1.9/0.1 | 1.6/0.1 | 2.0/0.0 |
| Doxazosin | 0.1/−0.1 | 3.2/0.2 | 2.3/0.1 | 2.1/−0.4 | 2.1/0.1 | N/A |

**Table 30–3** Biochemical Changes by Treatment Group*

| | Baseline | p | 2 Years | p | 4 Years | p |
|---|---|---|---|---|---|---|
| **Cholesterol (mg/dl)** | | | | | | |
| Mean (SD, N) | | | | | | |
| Chlorthalidone | 216.1 (43.8, 14,483) | | 205.3 (42.1, 10,206) | | 197.2 (42.1, 8,495) | |
| Amlodipine | 216.5 (44.1, 8,586) | p = .47 | 202.5 (42.2, 6,025) | p <.001 | 195.6 (41.0, 5,025) | p = .009 |
| Lisinopril | 215.6 (42.4, 8,573) | p = .38 | 202.0 (42.8, 5,739) | p <.001 | 195.0 (40.6, 4,711) | p <.001 |
| Doxazosin | 215.0 (42.4, 8,567) | p = .10 | 195.8 (40.3, 4,697) | p <.001 | 187.4 (38.1, 1,435) | p <.001 |
| **% (n) ≥240 (mg/dl)** | | | | | | |
| Chlorthalidone | 26.5% (3,838) | | 18.6% (1,898) | | 14.4% (1,223) | |
| Amlodipine | 26.6% (2,284) | p = .89 | 16.9% (1,018) | p = .005 | 13.4% (673) | p = .13 |
| Lisinopril | 25.4% (2,178) | p = .06 | 17.0% (976) | p = .03 | 12.8% (603) | p = .005 |
| Doxazosin | 24.5% (2,137) | p = .008 | 13.2% (622) | p < .001 | 8.92% (128) | p <.001 |
| **Potassium (mmol/L)** | | | | | | |
| Mean (SD, N) | | | | | | |
| Chlorthalidone | 4.3 (0.7, 14,487) | | 4.0 (0.7, 9,877) | | 4.1 (0.7, 8,315) | |
| Amlodipine | 4.3 (0.7, 8,586) | p = .59 | 4.3 (0.7, 5,794) | p <.001 | 4.4 (0.7, 4,919) | p <.001 |
| Lisinopril | 4.4 (0.7, 8,573) | p = .001 | 4.5 (0.7, 5,516) | p <.001 | 4.5 (0.7, 4,616) | p <.001 |
| Doxazosin | 4.4 (0.7, 8,600) | p = .02 | 4.3 (0.6, 4,661) | p <.001 | 4.4 (0.8, 1,428) | p <.001 |
| **% (n) <3.5 mmol/L** | | | | | | |
| Chlorthalidone | 3.4% (493) | | 12.7% (1,254) | | 8.5% (707) | |
| Amlodipine | 3.4% (292) | p = .99 | 2.6% (151) | p <.001 | 1.9% (93) | p <.001 |
| Lisinopril | 2.6% (223) | p = .001 | 1.5% (83) | p <.001 | 0.8% (37) | p <.001 |
| Doxazosin | 2.8% (244) | p = .004 | 1.89% (88) | p <.001 | 1.75% (25) | p <.001 |
| **Fasting glucose (mg/dl)** | | | | | | |
| Mean (SD, N) | | | | | | |
| Chlorthalidone | 123.5 (58.3, 11,273) | | 127.6 (59.2, 5,980) | | 126.3 (55.6, 4,972) | |
| Amlodipine | 123.1 (57.0, 6,648) | p = .71 | 122.4 (54.2, 3,506) | p <.001 | 123.7 (52.0, 2,954) | p = .20 |
| Lisinopril | 122.9 (56.1, 6,752) | p = .54 | 120.8 (54.0, 3,333) | p <.001 | 121.5 (51.3, 2,731) | p = .002 |
| Doxazosin | 122.4 (56.2, 6,671) | p = .22 | 119.6 (51.9, 2,854) | p <.001 | 117.2 (48.4, 823) | p = .001 |
| **% (n) ≥126 mg/dl** | | | | | | |
| Chlorthalidone | 28.9% (3,258) | | 32.9% (1,967) | | 32.7% (1,626) | |
| Amlodipine | 29.2% (1,941) | p = .68 | 29.9% (1,048) | p <.001 | 30.5% (901) | p = .11 |
| Lisinopril | 29.4% (1,985) | p = .55 | 28.4% (947) | p <.001 | 28.7% (784) | p <.001 |
| Doxazosin | 29.0% (1,931) | p = .99 | 26.5% (757) | p <.001 | 26.1% (215) | p = .002 |

Continued

**Table 30–3** Biochemical Changes by Treatment Group*—cont'd

| | Baseline | | 2 Years | | 4 Years | |
|---|---|---|---|---|---|---|
| **Fasting glucose (mg/dl) among nondiabetics with a baseline fasting glucose <126 mg/dl** | | | | | | |
| *Mean (SD, N)* | | | | | | |
| Chlorthalidone | 93.1 (11.7, 6,766) | | 102.2 (27.1, 3,074) | | 104.4 (28.5, 2,606) | |
| Amlodipine | 93.0 (11.4, 3,954) | $p = .52$ | 99.0 (22.5, 1,787) | $p < .001$ | 103.1 (27.7, 1,567) | $p = .11$ |
| Lisinopril | 93.3 (11.8, 4,096) | $p = .45$ | 97.4 (20.0, 1,737) | $p < .001$ | 100.5 (19.5, 1,464) | $p < .001$ |
| Doxazosin | 93.0 (11.5, 4,029) | $p = .58$ | 97.1 (18.8, 1,505) | $p < .001$ | 99.7 (25.0, 469) | $p < .001$ |
| **% (n) ≥126 mg/dl** | | | | | | |
| Chlorthalidone | — | | 9.6% (295) | | 11.6% (302) | |
| Amlodipine | — | | 7.4% (132) | $p = .006$ | 9.8% (154) | $p = .04$ |
| Lisinopril | — | | 5.8% (101) | $p < .001$ | 8.1% (119) | $p < .001$ |
| Doxazosin | — | | 4.8% (72) | $p < .001$ | 8.7% (41) | $p = .30$ |

*SI unit conversions: serum cholesterol mg/dl × 0.0259 = mmol/L; serum potassium mEq/L × 1.0 = mmol/L; fasting glucose mg/dl × 0.0555 = mmol/L; serum creatinine mg/dl × 88.4 = μmol/L.

**Table 30-4** Clinical Outcomes in Blood Pressure Component of ALLHAT by Treatment Group

| | 6-Year Rates per 100 (SE) and Total Events | | | 4-Year Rates per 100 (SE) and Total Events | | Amlodipine/Chlorthalidone Relative Risk (A/C) (95% CI) z score p value | Lisinopril/Chlorthalidone Relative Risk (L/C) (95% CI) z score p value | Doxazosin/Chlorthalidone Relative Risk (D/C) (95% CI) z score p value |
|---|---|---|---|---|---|---|---|---|
| | Chlorthalidone | Amlodipine | Lisinopril | Chlorthalidone | Doxazosin | | | |
| **Primary Endpoint** | | | | | | | | |
| CHD (NF MI + F CHD)* | 11.5 (0.3) 1362 | 11.3 (0.4) 798 | 11.4 (0.4) 796 | 7.76 (0.30) 818 | 7.91 (0.39) 499 | 0.98 (0.90 – 1.07) z = −0.46 p = .65 | 0.99 (0.91 – 1.08) z = −0.24 p = .81 | 1.03 (0.92 – 1.15) z = .49 p = .62 |
| **Secondary Endpoints** | | | | | | | | |
| Total mortality | 17.3 (0.4) 2203 | 16.8 (0.5) 1256 | 17.2 (0.5) 1314 | 10.51 (0.32) 1258 | 11.04 (0.43) 769 | 0.96 (0.89 – 1.02) z = −1.27 p = .20 | 1.00 (0.94 – 1.08) z = 0.12 p = .90 | 1.03 (0.94 – 1.13) z = 0.68 p = .50 |
| Combined CHD† | 19.9 (0.4) 2451 | 19.9 (0.5) 1466 | 20.8 (0.5) 1505 | 14.87 (0.39) 1642 | 16.00 (0.53) 1040 | 1.00 (0.94 – 1.07) z = 0.04 p = .97 | 1.05 (0.98 – 1.11) z = 1.35 p = .18 | 1.07 (0.99 – 1.16) z = 1.82 p = .07 |
| Stroke | 5.6 (0.2) 675 | 5.4 (0.3) 377 | 6.3 (0.3) 457 | 0.79 (0.10) 92 | 1.25 (0.16) 76 | 0.93 (0.82 – 1.06) z = −1.09 p = .28 | 1.15 (1.02 – 1.30) z = 2.31 p = .02 | 1.26 (1.10 – 1.46) z = 3.20 p = .001 |
| Combined CVD‡ | 30.9 (0.5) 3941 | 32.0 (0.6) 2432 | 33.3 (0.6) 2514 | 25.1 (0.48) 2829 | 28.6 (0.64) 1947 | 1.04 (0.99 – 1.09) z = 1.55 p = .12 | 1.10 (1.05 – 1.16) z = 3.78 p <.001 | 1.20 (1.13 – 1.27) z = 6.13 p < .001 |
| ESRD | 1.8 (0.1) 193 | 2.1 (0.2) 129 | 2.0 (0.2) 126 | 1.10 (0.13) 104 | 1.08 (0.17) 64 | 1.12 (0.89 – 1.40) z = 0.98 p = .33 | 1.11 (0.88 – 1.38) z = 0.87 p = .38 | 1.04 (0.76 – 1.42) z = .26 p = .80 |
| Cancer | 9.7 (0.3) 1170 | 10.0 (0.4) 707 | 9.9 (0.4) 703 | 7.37 (0.30) 758 | 6.53 (0.36) 408 | 1.01 (0.92 – 1.11) z = 0.30 p = .77 | 1.02 (0.93 – 1.12) z = 0.42 p = .67 | 0.91 (0.80 – 1.02) z = −1.58 p = .11 |
| Hosp GI Bleed§ | 8.8 (0.3) 817 | 8.0 (0.4) 449 | 9.6 (0.4) 526 | 6.7 (0.30) 571 | 6.9 (0.4) 343 | 0.92 (0.82 – 1.03) z = −1.44 p = .15 | 1.11 (0.99 – 1.24) z = 1.82 p = .07 | 1.02 (0.90 – 1.17) z = .34 p = .74 |
| **Components of Secondary Endpoints** | | | | | | | | |
| HF (F/NF/Treated) | 7.7 (0.3) 870 | 10.2 (0.4) 706 | 8.7 (0.4) 612 | 5.35 (0.26) 546 | 8.89 (0.42) 584 | 1.38 (1.25 – 1.52) z = 6.29 p <.001 | 1.19 (1.07 – 1.31)‖ z = 3.33 p <.001 | 1.80 (1.61 – 2.02) z = 10.67 p = <.001 |
| Hosp Fatal HF | 6.5 (0.3) 724 | 8.4 (0.4) 578 | 6.9 (0.4) 471 | 4.41 (0.24) 440 | 6.63 (0.37) 434 | 1.35 (1.21 – 1.50) z = 5.37 p <.001 | 1.10 (0.98 – 1.23)‖ z = 1.59 p = .11 | 1.66 (1.46 – 1.89) z = 7.72 p <.001 |
| Angina (hosp or Tx) | 12.1 (0.3) 1567 | 12.6 (0.4) 950 | 13.6 (0.4) 1019 | 10.81 (0.33) 1227 | 11.82 (0.45) 811 | 1.02 (0.94 – 1.10) z = 0.42 p = .67 | 1.11 (1.03 – 1.20) z = 2.59 p = .01 | 1.13 (1.03 – 1.23) z = 2.65 p = .01 |

Continued

**Table 30–4** Clinical Outcomes in Blood Pressure Component of ALLHAT by Treatment Group—cont'd

| | 6-Year Rates per 100 (SE) and Total Events | | | 4-Year Rates per 100 (SE) and Total Events | | Amlodipine/ Chlorthalidone Relative Risk (A/C) (95% CI) z score p value | Lisinopril/ Chlorthalidone Relative Risk (L/C) (95% CI) z score p value | Doxazosin/ Chlorthalidone Relative Risk (D/C) (95% CI) z score p value |
|---|---|---|---|---|---|---|---|---|
| | Chlorthalidone | Amlodipine | Lisinopril | Chlorthalidone | Doxazosin | | | |
| **Components of Secondary Endpoints** | | | | | | | | |
| Angina (hosp) | 8.6 (0.3) 1078 | 8.4 (0.4) 630 | 9.6 (0.4) 693 | 6.8 (0.3) 796 | 7.2 (0.3) 513 | 0.98 (0.89 – 1.08) z = −0.41 p = .68 | 1.09 (0.99 – 1.20) z = 1.85 p = .06 | 1.09 (0.98 –1.22) z = 1.56 p = .12 |
| Coronary Revascularizations | 9.2 (0.3) 1113 | 10.0 (0.4) 725 | 10.2 (0.4) 718 | 7.08 (0.3) 770 | 8.0 (0.4) 508 | 1.09 (1.00 –1.20) z = 1.88 p = .06 | 1.10 (1.00 –1.21) z = 1.95 p = .05 | 1.12 (1.00 –1.25) z = 1.97 p = .05 |
| PVD (hosp or Tx) | 4.1 (0.2) 510 | 3.7 (0.2) 265 | 4.7 (0.4) 311 | 3.5 (0.2) 376 | 3.3 (0.3) 217 | 0.87 (0.75 –1.01) z = −1.86 p = .06 | 1.04 (0.90 –1.19) z = 0.48 p = .63 | 0.97 (0.82 –1.15) z = −0.31 p = .76 |

\* Nonfatal MI's comprise 64% to 66% of the primary endpoint.
† Combined CHD = CHD death, nonfatal MI, coronary revascularization procedures, and hospitalized angina.
‡ Combined CVD = CHD death, nonfatal MI, stroke, coronary revascularization procedures, hospitalized or treated angina, treated or hospitalized HF, and peripheral arterial disease (hospitalized or outpatient revascularization).
§ ICDA-9 codes for gastrointestinal bleeding are 459.0, 578.x, 531.0, 531.2, 531.4, 531.6, 532.0, 532.2, 532.4, 532.6, 533.0, 533.2, 533.4, 533.6, 534.0, 534.2, 534.4, 534.6, 535.01, 535.11, 535.21, 535.31, 535.41, 535.51, 535.61, 997.02, 998.1, 998.11, 998.12, 99.03, 99.04, 99.05.
|| Proportional hazards assumption violated; numbers given are relative risks from a 2 × 2 table.

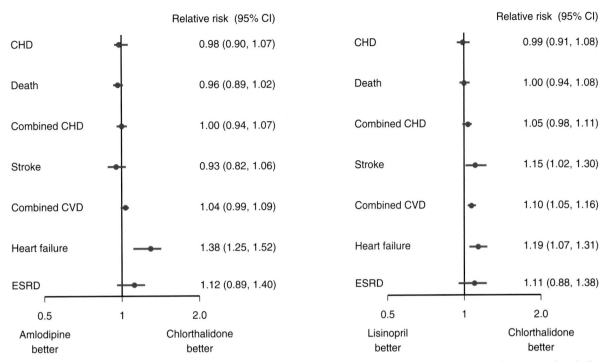

**Figure 30–1** The effects of amlodipine compared with those of chlorthalidone.

**Figure 30–2** The effects of lisinopril compared with those of chlorthalidone.

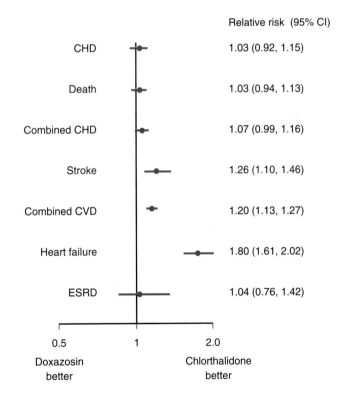

**Figure 30–3** The effects of doxazosin compared with those of chlorthalidone.

venting HF, superior to the ACEI in preventing HF and stroke (especially in Blacks), and superior to the α-blocker in preventing HF, stroke (in all subgroups), combined CHD, and combined CVD. Blood pressure adjustment by multiple procedures accounts for some of the differences in outcomes between the diuretic and the ACEI and α-blocker treatment groups. Finally, the diuretic was shown to be no less effective than the ACEI in preventing progression of kidney disease or development of ESRD. These findings were noted in all pre specified subgroups defined by age older than and younger than 65, gender, race, diabetic status, and the presence or absence of CHD or whether the participant was on previous antihypertensive therapy. Importantly, ALLHAT demonstrated these differences in outcomes despite the anticipated more-favorable metabolic effects that were seen with the newer agents.

ALLHAT also confirmed the increases in glucose and cholesterol and decrease in potassium seen in previous studies with diuretics as compared with other agents.[7,18] The increase in glucose in the diuretic arm resulted in a larger number of participants in this treatment arm reaching the threshold defining diabetes. These unfavorable metabolic characteristics of diuretic therapy were one of the major reasons for the hypothesized advantage of the newer agents in preventing CHD and a major motivation for the conduct of ALLHAT. However, despite having one of longest periods of follow-up of any antihypertensive trial (4-8 years), ALLHAT produced no evidence of this translating into more clinical (specifically CHD) events, as hypothesized by some authors.[18-23] Those who suggest that the risk of diabetes may overwhelm the early short-term benefit of diuretics must consider the increase in outcomes such as HF, stroke, and composite CVD that may occur while awaiting these hypothesized events.

It is worth noting that the selection of chlorthalidone to represent the thiazide-type diuretics represents an extreme test of diuretic therapy. Chlorthalidone is 1.5 to 2 times more potent than hydrochlorothiazide, has 2 to 3 times longer half-life, and is consequently more kaliuretic.[24] Thus the chlorthalidone dose (12.5-25 mg/day) administered in ALLHAT is higher than low-dose diuretic therapy. The hypokalemia seen with diuretics has been reported to result in worsened glucose tolerance, and potassium replacement ameliorates this effect.[25] Thus, more-aggressive potassium replacement may have lessened the effect of the diuretic on glycemic control in ALLHAT.

Although some of the findings of the trial surprised many, there is substantial support in the literature that could have foretold these results. ALLHAT confirmed the findings of trials such as (1) STOP-2 and CAPPP showing no difference in coronary events between ACEI, CCB, and diuretic therapy[26,27]; (2) SHEP as compared with Syst-Eur, CONVINCE, and INVEST showing a lower rate of HF with diuretic versus calcium channel blocker therapy[7,28-30]; (3) Syst-Eur and the Hypertension Optimal Treatment (HOT) trial showing excellent CVD protection in diabetic hypertensives with calcium channel blockers[28,31]; and (4) multiple studies documenting lesser BP lowering with ACEI monotherapy in Black hypertensive patients.[32]

The ALLHAT trial has clearly caused substantial controversy, and there have been misconceptions regarding the objectives of the trial. Despite having a randomized, double-blind design; clearly prespecified endpoints; and the largest and most-diverse study population of any antihypertensive trial, the design of ALLHAT has been criticized by some as flawed.[33-36] The primary objective of ALLHAT was to determine whether the newer agents are superior to diuretic-based therapy in preventing CHD when prescribed as initial therapy; the trial clearly demonstrated that they are not. Some have suggested that because there was no difference in the primary outcome, the trial was negative and no further conclusions can be drawn from it. In fact, the objectives of the trial were achieved, including the finding of no difference in the primary outcome. If they are few in number and prespecified, it is valid to consider secondary outcomes. Thus, the ALLHAT results demonstrate that the diuretic was either unsurpassed or superior in preventing mortality, stroke, combined CHD (consisting of the primary outcomes + coronary revascularization and hospitalized angina), and combined CVD (combined CHD + stroke + nonhospitalized treated angina + HF [fatal, hospitalized, or treated nonhospitalized], and treated peripheral arterial disease).

The difference in achieved BP between the diuretic and the ACEI and α-blocker arms has been the center of multiple commentaries. If the difference in achieved BP explained much of the favorable effect on outcomes of the diuretic, this would not suggest an advantage for initial therapy with agents that are less effective in lowering BP. If ACEIs and α-blockers require a diuretic to achieve adequate BP control but offer less benefit over diuretics in diuretic-free regimens, there is little reason to select them first. However, even in subgroups in which similar BP lowering was achieved (e.g., non-Blacks representing two thirds of the study population), the ACEI was not superior to the diuretic for any outcome.

Thus, ALLHAT definitively confmed that thiazide-type diuretics are unsurpassed in preventing the major complications of hypertension compared to three of the most promising newer classes of antihypertensive drugs. This finding, along with their unsurpassed BP lowering, tolerability, and cost, confirms the validity of the recommendations by most guideline panels that diuretics should remain the preferred first-step drug for treatment of hypertension.

# References

1. Davis BR, Cutler JA, Gordon DJ, et al. Rationale and design for the Antihypertensive and Lipid Lowering Treatment to Prevent Heart Attack Trial (ALLHAT). ALLHAT Research Group. Am J Hypertens 9(4 Pt 1):342-360, 1996.
2. Grimm RH Jr., Margolis KL, Papademetriou V, et al. Baseline characteristics of participants in the Antihypertensive and Lipid Lowering Treatment to Prevent Heart Attack Trial (ALLHAT). Hypertension 37(1):19-27, 2001.
3. Effects of treatment on morbidity in hypertension. Results in patients with diastolic blood pressures averaging 115 through 129 mm Hg. JAMA 202(11):1028-1034, 1967.
4. Effects of treatment on morbidity in hypertension. II. Results in patients with diastolic blood pressure averaging 90 through 114 mm Hg. JAMA 213(7):1143-1152, 1970.
5. Amery A, Birkenhager W, Brixko P, et al. Mortality and morbidity results from the European Working Party on High Blood Pressure in the Elderly trial. Lancet 1(8442):1349-1354, 1985.
6. Medical Research Council trial of treatment of hypertension in older adults: Principal results. MRC Working Party. BMJ 304(6824):405-412, 1992.
7. Prevention of stroke by antihypertensive drug treatment in older persons with isolated systolic hypertension. Final results of the Systolic Hypertension in the Elderly Program (SHEP). SHEP Cooperative Research Group. JAMA 265(24):3255-3264, 1991.
8. Five-year findings of the hypertension detection and follow-up program. I. Reduction in mortality of persons with high blood pressure, including mild hypertension. Hypertension Detection and Follow-up Program Cooperative Group. JAMA 242(23):2562-2571, 1979.
9. Mortality after 10 ½ years for hypertensive participants in the Multiple Risk Factor Intervention Trial. Circulation 82(5):1616-1628, 1990.
10. Wright JT Jr., Cushman WC, Davis BR, et al. The Antihypertensive and Lipid-Lowering Treatment to Prevent Heart Attack Trial (ALLHAT): Clinical center recruitment experience. Control Clin Trials 22(6):659-673, 2001.
11. Davis BR, Cutler JA, Furberg CD, et al. Relationship of antihypertensive treatment regimens and change in blood pressure

to risk for heart failure in hypertensive patients randomly assigned to doxazosin or chlorthalidone: Further analyses from the Antihypertensive and Lipid-Lowering treatment to prevent Heart Attack Trial. Ann Intern Med 137(5 Part 1): 313-320, 2002.

12. The fifth report of the Joint National Committee on Detection, Evaluation, and Treatment of High Blood Pressure (JNC V). Arch Intern Med 153(2):154-183, 1993.

13. Levey AS, Bosch JP, Lewis JB, et al. A more accurate method to estimate glomerular filtration rate from serum creatinine: A new prediction equation. Modification of Diet in Renal Disease Study Group. Ann Intern Med 130(6):461-470, 1999.

14. Piller LB, Davis BR, Cutler JA, et al. Validation of Heart Failure Events in the Antihypertensive and Lipid Lowering Treatment to Prevent Heart Attack Trial (ALLHAT) Participants Assigned to Doxazosin and Chlorthalidone. Curr Control Trials Cardiovasc Med 3(1):10, 2002.

15. Einhorn P, Davis BR, Pillar LB, et al. Review of heart failure events in the Antihypertensive and Lipid Lowering Treatment to Prevent Heart Attack Trial (ALLHAT): ALLHAT Validation Study. Circulation 108(Suppl IV): IV-399, 2003.

16. The ALLHAT Officers and Coordinators for the ALLHAT Collaborative Research Group. Major outcomes in high-risk hypertensive patients randomized to angiotensin-converting enzyme inhibitor or calcium channel blocker vs diuretic: The Antihypertensive and Lipid-Lowering Treatment to Prevent Heart Attack Trial. JAMA 288(23):2981-2997, 2002.

17. Diuretic versus alpha-blocker as first-step antihypertensive therapy: Final results from the Antihypertensive and Lipid-Lowering Treatment to Prevent Heart Attack Trial (ALLHAT). Hypertension 42(3):239-246, 2003.

18. Lithell HO. Effect of antihypertensive drugs on insulin, glucose, and lipid metabolism. Diabetes Care 14(3):203-209, 1991.

19. Messerli FH, Grossman E, Michalewicz L. Combination therapy and target organ protection in hypertension and diabetes mellitus. Am J Hypertens 10(9 Pt 2):198S-201S, 1997.

20. Ferrari P, Rosman J, Weidmann P. Antihypertensive agents, serum lipoproteins and glucose metabolism. Am J Cardiol 67(10):26B-35B, 1991.

21. Weber MA. Coronary heart disease and hypertension. Am J Hypertens 7(10 Pt 2):146S-153S, 1994.

22. Houston MC. New insights and new approaches for the treatment of essential hypertension: Selection of therapy based on coronary heart disease risk factor analysis, hemodynamic profiles, quality of life, and subsets of hypertension. Am Heart J 117(4):911-951, 1989.

23. Verdecchia P, Reboldi G, Angeli F, et al. Adverse prognostic significance of new diabetes in treated hypertensive subjects. Hypertension 43(5):963-969, 2004.

24. Carter BL, Ernst ME, Cohen JD. Hydrochlorothiazide versus chlorthalidone: Evidence supporting their interchangeability. Hypertension 43(1):4-9, 2004.

25. Davis BR, Furberg CD, Wright JT Jr., et al. ALLHAT: Setting the record straight. Ann Intern Med 141(1):39-46, 2004.

26. Hansson L, Lindholm LH, Ekbom T, et al. Randomised trial of old and new antihypertensive drugs in elderly patients: Cardiovascular mortality and morbidity the Swedish Trial in Old Patients with Hypertension-2 study. Lancet 354(9192):1751-1756, 1999.

27. Hansson L, Lindholm LH, Niskanen L, et al. Effect of angiotensin-converting-enzyme inhibition compared with conventional therapy on cardiovascular morbidity and mortality in hypertension: The Captopril Prevention Project (CAPPP) randomised trial. Lancet 353(9153):611-616, 1999.

28. Staessen JA, Thijs L, Celis H, et al. Dihydropyridine calcium-channel blockers for antihypertensive treatment in older patients: Evidence from the Systolic Hypertension in Europe Trial. S Afr Med J 91(12):1060-1068, 2001.

29. Black HR, Elliott WJ, Grandits G, et al. Principal results of the Controlled Onset Verapamil Investigation of Cardiovascular End Points (CONVINCE) trial. JAMA 289(16):2073-2082, 2003.

30. Pepine CJ, Handberg EM, Cooper-DeHoff RM, et al. A calcium antagonist vs a non-calcium antagonist hypertension treatment strategy for patients with coronary artery disease. The International Verapamil-Trandolapril Study (INVEST): A randomized controlled trial. JAMA 290(21):2805-2816, 2003.

31. Hansson L, Zanchetti A, Carruthers SG, et al. Effects of intensive blood-pressure lowering and low-dose aspirin in patients with hypertension: Principal results of the Hypertension Optimal Treatment (HOT) randomised trial. HOT Study Group. Lancet 351(9118):1755-1762, 1998.

32. Douglas JG, Bakris GL, Epstein M, et al. Management of high blood pressure in African Americans: Consensus statement of the Hypertension in African Americans Working Group of the International Society on Hypertension in Blacks. Arch Intern Med 163(5):525-541, 2003.

33. Messerli FH. ALLHAT, or the soft science of the secondary end point. Ann Intern Med 139(9):777-780, 2003.

34. Messerli FH, Weber MA. Long-term cardiovascular consequences of diuretics vs calcium channel blockers vs angiotensin-converting enzyme inhibitors. JAMA 289(16):2067-2068, 2003.

35. Flack JM, Nasser SA. The Antihypertensive and Lipid-Lowering Treatment to Prevent Heart Attack Trial (ALLHAT). Major outcomes in high-risk hypertensive patients randomized to angiotensin-converting enzyme inhibitor or calcium channel blocker vs diuretic. Curr Hypertens Rep 5(3):189-191, 2003.

36. Laragh JH, Sealey JE. Relevance of the plasma renin hormonal control system that regulates blood pressure and sodium balance for correctly treating hypertension and for evaluating ALLHAT. Am J Hypertens 16(5 Pt 1):407-415, 2003.

# Chapter 31

# The LIFE Study

Björn Dahlöf, Richard B. Devereux, Sverre E. Kjeldsen, Stevo Julius, D.G. Beevers, Ulf de Faire, Frej Fyhrquist, Hans Ibsen, Krister Kristianson, Ole Lederballe Pedersen, Lars H. Lindholm, Markku S. Nieminen, Per Omvik, Suzanne Oparil, Hans Wedel, Jonathan M. Edelman, Steve Snapinn, Katherine E. Harris, Gilbert W. Gleim

The Losartan Intervention For Endpoint Reduction (LIFE) in Hypertension Study represents a seminal clinical trial in patients with hypertension and evidence of target organ damage, manifest as electrocardiographic evidence of left ventricular hypertrophy (ECG LVH). LIFE had a double-blind, randomized design with an active control. LIFE achieved nearly identical goal blood pressure (BP) reductions in each treatment arm, permitting the assessment of features of losartan that are independent of its antihypertensive action.

LIFE was conceived in late 1993, and the first investigators' meeting was held in 1994. The first patient, from one of 945 clinical centers worldwide, entered the study in June of 1995 and the last patient was randomized in April, 1997. A total of 9222 patients, 29 of whom were excluded soon after randomization for irregularities, were randomized, leaving an analysis group of 9193. The study was terminated in September, 2001, when sufficient endpoints were predicted to have occurred, resulting in an average follow-up of 4.8 years. The primary composite endpoint was cardiovascular death, nonfatal myocardial infarction (MI), and stroke. The group assigned to treatment based on losartan, the first marketed angiotensin II receptor blocker (ARB), had fewer primary events (508, or 23.8/1000 patients × years) compared with the group assigned to the β-blocker, atenolol (588, or 27.9/1000 patients × years) ($p = .021$).[1] BP was kept nearly identical between the two treatment groups throughout the study, providing evidence that the benefit of losartan extends beyond its BP-lowering effects.

This chapter reviews many of the findings of the LIFE study, including the effects of treatment on the study population as a whole, in prespecified subgroups, and in post hoc analyses. Studies exploring the relationship of echocardiographic and electrocardiographic measurements of LVH to outcomes and differential responses to treatments have also been a major focus of the analyses of LIFE and are included here. Other issues relating to the pathology associated with hypertension among LIFE participants have been explored and are discussed in this chapter.

## LIFE STUDY BACKGROUND, DESIGN CONSIDERATIONS, AND METHODS

### Hypertension Treatment in the Early 1990s

Direct blockade of angiotensin II (Ang II) by ARBs was first accomplished with the octapeptide saralasin [Sar$^1$, Val$^5$, Ala$^8$] angiotensin-(1-8) by Pals et al. in 1971.[2] Saralasin had intrinsic pressor activity, and it was not until the development of losartan potassium ($C_{22}H_{22}ClKN_6O$), the first of a new class of orally active antihypertensive agents that block the Ang II type 1 (AT$_1$) receptor,[3] that an ARB became a viable agent for treating hypertension in humans. As a direct blocker of the AT$_1$ receptor, losartan did not delay catabolism of bradykinin, as had been seen with the angiotensin-converting enzyme (ACE) inhibitors. Perhaps as a consequence, losartan was associated with a lower incidence of cough and angioedema than the ACE inhibitors.

The Fifth Report of the Joint National Committee on Prevention, Detection, Evaluation, and Treatment of High Blood Pressure (JNC V), published in 1993, recommended diuretics or β-blockers for initial pharmacologic treatment of hypertension because these agents had been shown to reduce morbidity and mortality in randomized trials (Box 31–1).[3] Furthermore, as discussed by Frohlich[4] after JNC V was published, concurrent meta-analyses had demonstrated that there was a highly significant reduction in stroke[5] and MI[5,6] with β-blockers.

Other major points of interest to the designers of the LIFE study were the additional risk associated with LVH in patients with hypertension and the potential for an ARB to block the mitogenic and growth effects of Ang II.[7] Ample epidemiologic evidence from the Framingham Heart Study had documented the increased morbidity and mortality associated with LVH.[8-11] The Survival and Ventricular Enlargement (SAVE) trial had shown that blockade of the renin-angiotensin system (RAS) with an ACE inhibitor was associated with reduced mortality and less ventricular hypertrophy following MI.[12] These findings were also supported by the Studies of Left Ventricular Dysfunction (SOLVD) registry. Because it was known that Ang II could be formed locally in tissues as well as in the circulation,[13,14] blockade of the AT$_1$ receptor in the heart was an attractive target for preventing or regressing the LVH that accompanies chronic hypertension. Losartan had already been shown to prevent or ameliorate LVH in animal models of hypertension, perhaps because of blockade of the AT$_1$ receptor in the heart.[15,16]

A meta-analysis by Dahlof et al.[17] had shown that ACE inhibitors, β-blockers, calcium antagonists, and diuretics were all associated with reductions in left ventricular (LV) mass during treatment for hypertension. As discussed in the LIFE design paper, a β-blocker was chosen over a diuretic (both preferred agents in JNC V) as the active comparator because this class had a more favorable record in prevention (particularly secondary prevention) of coronary artery disease in control of arrhythmias.[7] The diuretic hydrochlorothiazide

**Box 31-1** Medical and Scientific Rationale at the Time of LIFE Design (1993-1994)

- JNC V published 1993: β-Blockers and diuretics *preferred* first-line agents in treatment of hypertension.
- Epidemiologic evidence for β-blockers and diuretics, not other classes.
- LVH associated with increased morbidity and mortality.
- Known trophic effects of renin-angiotensin system (RAS) on LV mass.
- Tissue sources of angiotensin II production, not only renal → pulmonary.
- Cardioprotective effects of β-blockers.
- Losartan, first marketed ARB, blocks $AT_1$ receptor.

**Box 31-2** Inclusion and Exclusion Criteria for the LIFE Study

**Inclusion**

Age 55 to 80 years.
Previously treated or untreated hypertension.
ECG LVH by Cornell product *or* Sokolow-Lyon criteria.
Sitting trough DBP 95-115 mm Hg or SBP of 160-200 mm Hg following 1 and 2 weeks of single blind placebo.

**Exclusion**

Known secondary hypertension.
DBP >115 mm Hg or SBP >200 mm Hg during 2-week placebo trial.
History of stroke or MI within 6 months.
Angina pectoris requiring treatment with β-blockers or calcium antagonists.
Severe renal impairment with serum creatinine ≥1.5 mg/dl or solitary kidney.
Severe liver impairment.
Significant known aortic stenosis (antegrade Doppler gradient ≥20 mm Hg).
Known hypersensitivity to losartan, atenolol, or hydrochlorothiazide (HCTZ).
Known condition requiring treatment with losartan, any β-blocker, ACE inhibitor, or HCTZ.
Serious concurrent disease expected to deteriorate patient's health in 4-6 years.
Current or recent history of alcohol or drug abuse.
Mental or legal incapacitation.
Participation in last 10 days in other investigational drug trial using nonapproved drug. (Participation in other drug trial providing it would not interfere was allowed.)
Low compliance at end of placebo—judged by the investigator.
Unwillingness to participate.

From Kannel WB, Gordon T, Castelli WP, et al. Electrocardiographic left ventricular hypertrophy and risk of coronary heart disease. The Framingham Study. Ann Intern Med 72:813-822, 1970.

(HCTZ) could be added to treatment with either a β-blocker or losartan. Atenolol was chosen as the β-blocker for the trial because it was the most widely used agent in its class and its efficacy and tolerability had been previously documented.[1]

## Design of the LIFE Study

LIFE was a prospective, multicenter, multinational, double-blind, double-dummy, randomized, active controlled study with two parallel groups. The primary objective was to study the effects of long-term treatment (≥4 years) with losartan compared with atenolol in patients with hypertension and ECG LVH. The primary composite outcome was cardiovascular morbidity and mortality defined as nonfatal, clinically evident MI or stroke and fatal MI, stroke, sudden death, progressive heart failure, or death due to other cardiovascular cause.[7] Several prespecified data analyses and protocols were approved prior to unblinding, including analysis of patients with diabetes mellitus (DM) at baseline, isolated systolic hypertension (ISH), cost-benefit analysis, new-onset DM, ECG substudy, echocardiographic substudy, microalbuminuria substudy, QT-dispersion substudy, insulin sensitivity and carotid ultrasound substudy (Insulin Carotids United States Scandinavia [ICARUS]), uric acid analysis, physical activity analysis, smoking analysis, and alcohol analysis.

Eligibility and exclusion criteria are shown in Box 31-2. Importantly, hypertension had to be documented following a 2-week single-blind placebo run-in period in order for a patient to qualify for the study. Patients were eligible with sitting trough diastolic blood pressure (DBP) of 95 to 115 mm Hg and/or systolic blood pressure (SBP) of 160 to 200 mm Hg, allowing for those with ISH. Entry criteria for ECG LVH changed during the study for women. Patients qualified initially by having a Cornell voltage (RaVL + $SV_3$) × QRS duration product >2440 mm × msec in men with an added gender adjustment of 8 mm for women. The adjustment was reduced to 6 mm for women on the basis of data published after the LIFE study had started.[18] Additionally, the Sokolow-Lyon voltage combination ($SV_1$ + $RV_5$ or $V_6$) >38 mm qualified men or women as having ECG LVH. Although these patients were at higher risk for cardiovascular events than those with hypertension without LVH, a noteworthy exclusion criterion was that enrollees could not have had a stroke or MI within 6 months of study entry.

Trough BPs (24 hours following the once-daily dosage of study medication, range 22-26 hours) were used to titrate study medication. Figure 31-1 schematizes the drug titration regimen. Following randomization and the 2-week placebo run-in period, patients received either 50 mg losartan or 50 mg atenolol daily. If goal BP (140/90 mm Hg) was not attained after 2 months, 12.5 mg HCTZ was added. After an additional 2 months, if goal BP was still not achieved, losartan or atenolol was doubled to 100 mg. Those still above target following an additional 2 months were to receive either an additional 12.5 mg HCTZ or other open-label antihypertensive agents, excluding ACE inhibitors, other ARBs, or β-blockers. Other open-label agents could be added after this time was necessary only if BP was ≥165/95 mm Hg.[7]

Analysis was done by intention-to-treat (ITT). LIFE was powered to detect a relative difference in the primary composite endpoint of 15% with 80% power and a two-sided significance level of 5%. Sample size was calculated so that with an absolute event rate of 15% over 5 years in the atenolol

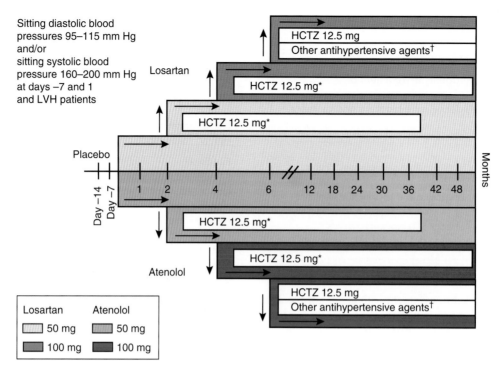

Figure 31–1 This schematic depicts the drug titration schedule employed in the LIFE study. With the exception of the placebo period, time is depicted in months.

group and 12.75% in the losartan group, 1040 primary endpoints over 4 years would be necessary. To demonstrate the effect of treatment time, the minimum follow-up was to be 4 years, regardless of the event rate. Background data to calculate a Framingham risk score[19] were obtained and these, as well as the degree of LVH, were prespecified to adjust hazard ratios associated with treatment.

All patients were followed even after they had a nonfatal endpoint. Therefore, full reporting of strokes and MIs allowed for true ITT analyses of those components of the endpoint. With stroke and MI, the intention was to analyze fatal and nonfatal occurrences together. If analyses were limited to nonfatal events, fatalities and nonevents would be grouped together, although the consequences of the two scenarios are vastly different (Figure 31–2). By analyzing fatal and nonfatal events together, as in the LIFE study, the potential inaccuracies of a separate accounting system for nonfatal events was avoided.

Endpoints were classified by two clinicians, masked to treatment, who reviewed clinical records of all cardiovascular events to determine whether they met endpoint criteria. Additionally, an independent safety and data board monitored interim trial results.

## Sample Demographics

The characteristics of all patients assigned to the losartan and atenolol groups are shown in Table 31–1, as are three subgroups of interest, ISH, DM, and no history of cardiovascular disease (CVD) (a posthoc analysis). Average DBP was roughly

8 mm Hg higher than the upper limit of normal (90 mm Hg), whereas SBP was nearly 25 mm Hg higher than the upper limit of normal (140 mm Hg), reflecting the high prevalence of systolic hypertension in older persons (average age 66.9 years). Many more patients satisfied the Cornell voltage-duration criterion for LVH than the Sokolow-Lyon definition,

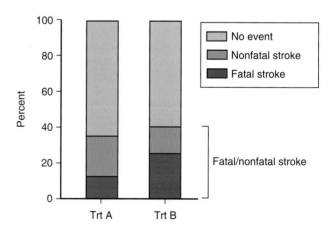

Figure 31–2 The bars indicate possible outcomes in a trial of two drugs: no event, fatal event, and nonfatal event. Studies counting only nonfatal events are in essence grouping fatalities and nonevents together, but these are very different outcomes. The LIFE study combined fatal and nonfatal events to avoid this problem.

Table 31–1 Patient Demographics and Characteristics in the Entire LIFE Sample and Selected Substudies

| Characteristics | LOS (Main LIFE) (n = 4605) | LOS, ISH (n = 660) | LOS, DM (n = 586) | LOS, No-CVD (n = 3402) | ATNL (Main LIFE) (n = 4588) | ATNL, ISH (n = 666) | ATNL, DM (n = 609) | ATNL, No-CVD (n = 3484) | Entire LIFE Sample (n = 9193) |
|---|---|---|---|---|---|---|---|---|---|
| Age (years) | 66.9 (7.0) | 70.2 (6.4) | 67.4 (6.8) | 66.3 (7.0) | 66.0 (7.0) | 70.4 (6.2) | 67.4 (7.0) | 66.3 (7.0) | 66.9 (7.0) |
| Women | 2487 (54%) | 388 (59%) | 302 (52%) | 1902 (56%) | 2476 (54%) | 409 (61%) | 332 (55%) | 1972 (57%) | 5963 (54%) |
| Ethnic origin | | | | | | | | | |
| White | 4258 (92%) | 606 (92%) | 506 (86%) | 3175 (93%) | 4245 (93%) | 616 (93%) | 519 (85%) | 3250 (93%) | 8503 (92%) |
| Black | 270 (6%) | 44 (7%) | 62 (11%) | 174 (5%) | 263 (6%) | 38 (5.7%) | 71 (12%) | 185 (5%) | 533 (6%) |
| Hispanic | 47 (1%) | 5 (0.8%) | 12 (2%) | 30 (0.9%) | 53 (1%) | 9 (1.4%) | 13 (2%) | 31 (0.9%) | 100 (1%) |
| Asian | 25 (0.5%) | 4 (0.6%) | 5 (0.9%) | 19 (0.6%) | 18 (0.4%) | 2 (0.3%) | 5 (0.8%) | 12 (0.6%) | 43 (0.5%) |
| Other | 5 (0.1%) | 1 (0.2%) | 1 (0.2%) | 4 (0.1%) | 9 (0.2%) | 1 (0.2%) | 2 (0.2%) | 6 (0.2%) | 14 (0.2%) |
| SBP (mm Hg) | 174 (14) | 174 (11) | 176 (14) | 174 (14) | 174 (14) | 174 (11) | 177 (14) | 174 (14) | 174 (14) |
| DBP (mm Hg) | 98 (9) | 83 (5) | 97 (9) | 98 (9) | 98 (9) | 82 (6) | 96 (10) | 98 (9) | 98 (9) |
| Heart rate (bpm) | 74 (11) | 72 (10) | 76 (12) | 74 (11) | 74 (11) | 72 (11) | 76 (11) | 74 (11) | 74 (11) |
| BMI (kg/m²) | 28.0 (4.8) | 27.2 (4.6) | 30.0 (5.3) | 28.1 (4.8) | 28.0 (4.8) | 27.7 (5.2) | 30.0 (5.6) | 28.1 (4.8) | 28.0 (4.8) |
| Cornell V (mm•ms) | 2834 (1065) | 2771 (1078) | 2885 (988) | 2789 (1006) | 2824 (1033) | 2821 (1158) | 2926 (995) | 2792 (1003) | 2829 (1049) |
| Sokolow-Lyon (mm) | 30.0 (10.6) | 30.8 (10.5) | 28.8 (10.3) | 29.7 (10.4) | 30.1 (10.4) | 31.4 (10.6) | 28.3 (10.2) | 29.8 (10.3) | 30.0 (10.5) |
| Framingham Risk Score | 0.223 (0.095) | 0.230 (0.103) | 0.304 (0.084) | 0.215 (0.092) | 0.225 (0.096) | 0.234 (0.098) | 0.312 (0.086) | 0.215 (0.092) | 0.224 (0.096) |
| Current smokers | 729 (16%) | 95 (14.4%) | 70 (12%) | 506 (15) | 770 (17%) | 101 (15%) | 92 (15%) | 551 (15) | 1499 (16%) |
| Any vascular disease | 1203 (26%) | 285 (43%) | 206 (35%) | NONE | 1104 (24%) | 281 (42%) | 214 (35%) | NONE | 2307 (25%) |
| Coronary heart Disease | 771 (17%) | 158 (23.9%) | 138 (24%) | NONE | 698 (15%) | 140 (21.0) | 145 (24%) | NONE | 1469 (16%) |
| Cerebrovascular Disease | 369 (8%) | 70 (10.6%) | 69 (12%) | NONE | 359 (8%) | 86 (12.9%) | 71 (12%) | NONE | 728 (8%) |
| Peripheral vascular Disease | 276 (6%) | 57 (8.6%) | 40 (7%) | NONE | 244 (5%) | 55 (8.3%) | 49 (8%) | NONE | 520 (6%) |
| Atrial fibrillation | 150 (3%) | 28 (4.2%) | 32 (5%) | 84 (2%) | 174 (4%) | 39 (5.9%) | 48 (8%) | 94 (3%) | 324 (4%) |
| ISH | 660 (14%) | ALL | 103 (18%) | 430 (13%) | 666 (15%) | ALL | 132 (22%) | 439 (13%) | 1326 (14%) |
| DM | 586 (13%) | 103 (16%) | ALL | 380 (11%) | 609 (13%) | 132 (20%) | ALL | 395 (11%) | 1195 (13%) |

Values in parentheses represent standard deviation or percent. *Abbreviations:* LOS, losartan; ATNL, atenolol; CVD, cardiovascular disease; Cornell V, Cornell voltage-duration product; ISH, isolated systolic hypertension; DM, diabetes mellitus. The **bolded cells** indicate the numbers for the primary study, as well as those factors that distinguished the subgroups of interest.

contributing to a mean voltage with the latter (30.0 ± 10.5 mm) that was lower than the entry criterion of 38 mm. Satisfaction of either criterion was necessary for inclusion and increased the sensitivity for detection of LVH. Characteristics of patients satisfying either criterion served as a topic for an interim publication[20] and is discussed later in the chapter. Patients were eligible based on their electrocardiogram at the screening visit, whereas the means in the interim publication were calculated based on the randomization visit.

Other important characteristics of the sample are the mean body mass index (BMI) of 28.0 kg/m², and that 92% of patients classified themselves ethnically as white, resulting in a sample with only 533 Blacks. Characteristics of the various subgroups presented in Table 31–1 are discussed later with the subgroup analyses. Inspection of the three subgroups in Table 31–1 indicates that they are not mutually exclusive. For example, some 20% of patients with DM also had ISH and would thus be counted in both studies.

## DIFFERENCES IN THERAPEUTIC OUTCOMES, LOSARTAN VERSUS ATENOLOL

### Blood Pressure Control and Medications Used

In keeping with the study design, BP was controlled similarly in the losartan and atenolol arms as shown in Figure 31–3. SBP at the end of follow-up or at the last visit before a primary event had fallen by 30.2 ± 18.5 mm Hg in the losartan group and by 29.1 ± 19.2 mm Hg in the atenolol group ($p = .017$). DBP had declined by 16.1 ± 10.1 mm Hg and 16.8 ± 10.1 mm Hg in the losartan and atenolol groups, respectively ($p = .37$). Mean arterial pressures (MAPs) at this point were nearly identical, 102.2 and 102.4 mm Hg, for the losartan and atenolol groups, respectively. In the three subgroup analyses (ISH, DM, and No-CVD), BP was controlled similarly in the two treatment groups (Table 31–2).

The average dosage of losartan during the study was 82 mg daily, and the average dosage for atenolol was 79 mg daily. As might be expected in treating patients with an initial mean SBP exceeding 170 mm Hg, the majority required the study medication plus HCTZ or another open-label medication (Table 31–3). In this regard, the LIFE study mimics the reality of treating patients with hypertension and can be viewed as a test of beginning therapy with losartan or atenolol in a stepped-care approach. The subgroup studies indicate a similar drug dosing profile to the entire LIFE cohort, but it must be remembered that current recommendations for BP control in patients with DM are SBP ≤130 mm Hg and DBP ≤80 mm Hg, likely necessitating a more consistent multidrug regimen than was used in this trial.

## Outcomes in the Main LIFE Study

LIFE is the first study in the treatment of hypertension, with equivalent BP control, to demonstrate therapeutic superiority of one treatment modality (losartan) over another established active treatment modality (atenolol) for preventing the combined primary outcome of cardiovascular death, nonfatal MI, and stroke. This finding to date has not been replicated by other studies, including Nordic Diltiazem (NORDIL),[21] Antihypertensive and Lipid-Lowering Treatment to Prevent Heart Attack Trial (ALLHAT),[22] Study on Cognition and Prognosis in the Elderly (SCOPE),[23] Controlled Onset Verapamil Investigation of Cardiovascular End Points (CONVINCE),[24] and International Verapamil/Trandolapril Study (INVEST),[25] using other antihypertensive agents. The main finding from LIFE was that 11% of participants treated with losartan compared with 13% treated with atenolol experienced a primary endpoint, with an adjusted (for LVH and Framingham Score) risk reduction of 13% ($p = .021$). The most significant contributor to the composite endpoint was fatal and nonfatal stroke, with the losartan group experiencing a rate of 10.8 of 1000 patients × years compared with a rate of 14.5 of 1000 patients × years for the atenolol group ($p = .001$ for adjusted hazard ratio). Figure 31–4 displays the Kaplan-Meier

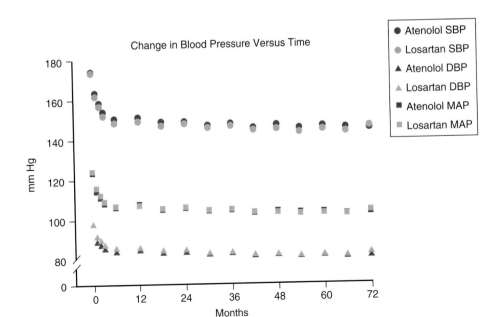

**Figure 31–3** The decline in systolic blood pressure (SBP), mean arterial pressure (MAP), and diastolic blood pressure (DBP) during the course of the LIFE study. Points on the graph that overlap are shown as only one point.

**Table 31–2** Change in Blood Pressure (mm Hg, Mean ± SD) Between Last Follow-up and Baseline, for the Entire LIFE Cohort and Subgroup Analyses

| Study | | Losartan | Atenolol | p-Value for Difference in Change from Baseline |
|---|---|---|---|---|
| LIFE | SBP | −30.2 ± 18.6 | −29.1 ± 19.2 | .015 |
| | DBP | −16.6 ± 10.2 | −16.8 ± 10.1 | .035 |
| | MAP | −21.1 ± 11.4 | −20.9 ± 11.4 | .435 |
| ISH | SBP | −28.4 ± 16.8 | −28.1 ± 19.7 | .761 |
| | DBP | −8.45 ± 9.3 | −8.9 ± 10.1 | .233 |
| | MAP | −15.1 ± 10.1 | −15.3 ± 11.2 | .591 |
| DM | SBP | −30.7 ± 18.6 | −28.4 ± 19.7 | .064 |
| | DBP | −17.4 ± 11.1 | −16.6 ± 11.0 | .291 |
| | MAP | −21.8 ± 11.8 | −20.5 ± 12.3 | .131 |
| No-CVD | SBP | −30.2 ± 18.1 | −29.3 ± 18.7 | .071 |
| | DBP | −16.7 ± 9.9 | −16.8 ± 9.8 | .549 |
| | MAP | −21.2 ± 11.0 | −21.0 ± 11.0 | .521 |

ISH, isolated systolic hypertension; DM, diabetes mellitus; No-CVD, no clinical history of cardiovascular disease.

plots for the primary composite endpoint and the three major individual endpoints: cardiovascular mortality, stroke, and MI. This figure depicts that when losartan was used to lower BP in patients with hypertension and LVH, it provided more protection from the composite endpoint, primarily because of its effect on stroke reduction (25%). The group randomized to atenolol, a drug associated with cardioprotective effects, did not differ from the losartan group in the endpoints of MI and cardiovascular mortality.

Table 31–4 depicts the other prespecified endpoints of interest in the main LIFE study, as well as in the substudies. New-onset DM was less common in the losartan-treated group (p = .001). To further examine this finding in a separate analysis, a risk model was developed to predict new-onset DM based on baseline serum glucose (nonfasting), BMI, serum high-density lipoprotein (HDL) cholesterol, SBP, and history of previous antihypertensive drugs. Independent of these factors, losartan was found to reduce the incidence of new-onset DM over the course of the LIFE trial.[26]

Other prespecified endpoints were in favor of the losartan group (cardiovascular mortality, total mortality, heart failure hospitalization, and revascularization), but did not attain statistical significance. Alternatively, those endpoints likely to be more influenced by the known cardioprotective actions of atenolol (MI, hospitalization for angina pectoris, and resuscitated cardiac arrest) were in favor of atenolol without attaining statistical significance in any case.

## ISH, DM, and No-CVD Substudies

Two higher-risk subgroups of the main LIFE cohort were topics of specific investigation from the LIFE study, namely those patients with ISH[27] and those patients with DM.[28] By contrast, a large posthoc subgroup analysis of patients without a history of clinically evident CVD (i.e., "No-CVD," defined as no previous diagnosis of coronary, cerebral, or peripheral vascular disease by either self-report or report of treating physicians) was also performed.[29] Importantly, the three subgroups are not mutually exclusive, as discussed previously. Figure 31–5 illustrates the event rates and hazard ratios for the primary composite endpoint and individual endpoints for the subgroups and for the main LIFE cohort.

By referring back to Table 31–1 and remembering that some overlap exists between the groups, certain baseline differences are apparent. Patients with ISH represented an older portion of the LIFE cohort, whereas those in the No-CVD group were

**Table 31–3** Drug Doses in the Main LIFE and LIFE Substudies (%) at Endpoint or Termination of Follow-up

| Drug Doses | LIFE | n = 9193 | ISH | n = 1326 | DM | n = 1195 | No CVD | n = 6886 |
|---|---|---|---|---|---|---|---|---|
| | Losartan | Atenolol | Losartan | Atenolol | Losartan | Atenolol | Losartan | Atenolol |
| 50 mg only | 9% | 10% | 10% | 9% | 8% | 5% | 10% | 10% |
| 50 mg + additional therapy* | 18% | 20% | 21% | 22% | 14% | 16% | 19% | 20% |
| 100 mg with or without HCTZ | 50% | 43% | 44% | 37% | 51% | 47% | 51% | 44% |
|   Alone | 2% | 2% | 2% | 1% | 1% | 1% | 2% | 2% |
|   With HCTZ only | 18% | 16% | 16% | 14% | 16% | 13% | 19% | 17% |
|   With other therapy only | 4% | 4% | 4% | 3% | 4% | 6% | 3% | 4% |
|   With HCTZ + other therapy | 26% | 22% | 22% | 19% | 30% | 27% | 27% | 22% |
| Discontinued therapy | 23% | 27% | 26% | 32% | 27% | 32% | 21% | 25% |

*Including hydrochlorothiazide (HCTZ).

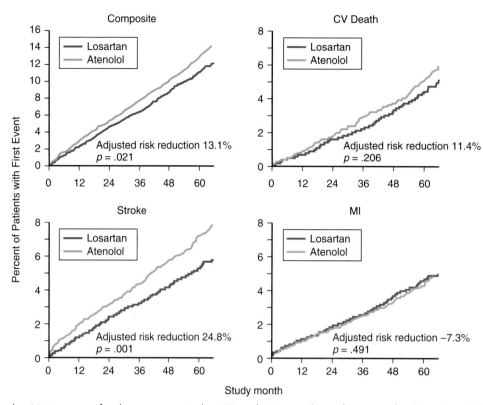

**Figure 31–4** Kaplan-Meier curves for the outcomes in the LIFE trial. Statistical significance is for the adjusted (for ECG LVH and Framingham Risk Score) risk reduction. Note that the ordinates for cardiovascular (CV) death, stroke, and myocardial infarction (MI) are half the magnitude as for the primary composite outcome.

**Table 31–4** Other Prespecified Endpoints in the Main LIFE and LIFE Substudies.*

| Study | Measure | Losartan Rate | Atenolol Rate | HR (95% CI) | p |
|---|---|---|---|---|---|
| LIFE-Main | Total mortality | 17.3 | 19.6 | 0.90 (0.78-1.03) | .128 |
| n = 9193 | Hospitalization for angina pectoris | 7.4 | 6.6 | 1.16 (0.92-1.45) | .212 |
| | Hospitalization for heart failure | 7.1 | 7.5 | 0.97 (0.78-1.21) | .765 |
| | Revascularization | 12.2 | 13.3 | 0.94 (0.79-1.11) | .441 |
| | New-onset DM | 13.0 | 17.4 | 0.75 (0.63-0.88) | .001 |
| LIFE-ISH | Total mortality | 21.2 | 30.2 | 0.72 (0.53-1.00) | .046 |
| n = 1326 | Hospitalization for angina pectoris | 11.3 | 7.6 | 1.48 (0.87-2.51) | .150 |
| | Hospitalization for heart failure | 8.5 | 13.3 | 0.66 (0.40-1.09) | .110 |
| | Revascularization | 16.4 | 14.4 | 1.17 (0.78-1.77) | .530 |
| | New-onset DM | 12.6 | 20.1 | 0.62 (0.40-0.97) | .040 |
| LIFE-DM | Total mortality | 22.5 | 37.2 | 0.61 (0.45-0.84) | .002 |
| n = 1195 | Hospitalization for angina pectoris | 11.1 | 11.1 | 1.06 (0.64-1.76) | .989 |
| | Hospitalization for heart failure | 11.8 | 20.7 | 0.59 (0.38-0.92) | .019 |
| | Revascularization | 23.5 | 26.6 | 0.90 (0.64-1.26) | .533 |
| | New-onset DM | NA | NA | NA | NA |
| LIFE-No-CVD | Total mortality | 13.5 | 15.9 | 0.85 (0.71-1.02) | .080 |
| n = 6886 | Hospitalization for angina pectoris | 4.7 | 4.4 | 1.09 (0.79-1.50) | .600 |
| | Hospitalization for heart failure | 4.7 | 4.4 | 1.06 (0.77-1.46) | .720 |
| | Revascularization | 7.6 | 9.0 | 0.85 (0.67-1.08) | .180 |
| | New-onset DM | 12.2 | 17.7 | 0.69 (0.67-0.84) | .001 |

ISH, isolated systolic hypertension; DM, diabetes mellitus; No-CVD, no clinical history of cardiovascular disease; HR, hazard ratio; CI, confidence interval; NA, not applicable.
*Rates are given per 1000 patients × years. Hazard ratios are adjusted for Framingham Risk Score and ECG LVH.

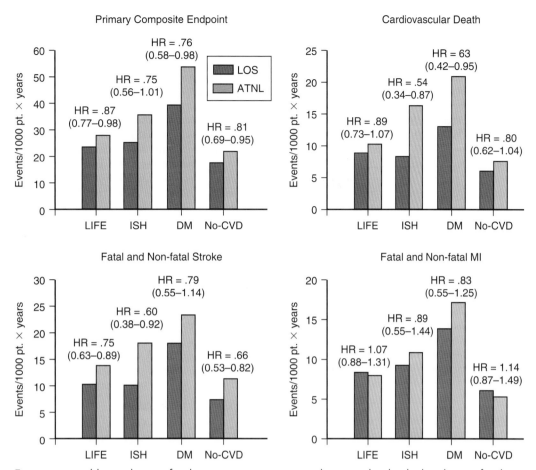

**Figure 31–5** Event rates and hazard ratios for the primary composite endpoint and individual endpoints for the main LIFE cohort and subgroups. Bar graphs depicting the rate of events in the main LIFE study and the isolated systolic hypertension (ISH), diabetic mellitus (DM), and no clinical history of cardiovascular disease (No-CVD) subgroup analyses. Hazard ratios (HR) are depicted followed by the 95% confidence interval and are adjusted for ECG LVH and Framingham Risk Score.

younger. Patients with DM had higher BMIs and higher Framingham Risk Scores. Although a very small portion of the LIFE cohort, Black patients comprised a greater percentage of those with DM. Sample sizes in the ISH and DM groups were smaller, decreasing the power to detect statistically significant results, than in the No-CVD group. Larger treatment effects are typically necessary for statistical significance as sample size decreases.

Figure 31–5 illustrates the event rates in the various subgroups and how they relate to the entire LIFE sample. Both the ISH and DM groups experienced a greater rate of outcomes than the entire LIFE sample and the No-CVD group, underscoring the more serious nature of systolic hypertension and the presence of DM as a concomitant risk factor. In addition, the LIFE study and its subgroup analyses corroborate the finding that stroke is a more common outcome than MI in patients with hypertension.[30]

For the primary composite endpoint, all subgroups responded more favorably to losartan than atenolol treatment, although statistical significance was not attained for the 25% reduction (95% confidence interval [CI]; –1% to 44%) in the ISH group. The subgroup analyses also demonstrated that losartan had the most consistent and dramatic impact on fatal and nonfatal stroke, most prominently the 40% reduc-

tion in the ISH group and least prominently (21%) in the DM group (heart rate = 0.79, 95% CI 0.55-1.14). As in the entire LIFE sample, there was no significant benefit of losartan over atenolol for fatal and nonfatal MI.

Not illustrated is the important exception that there was no evidence for a beneficial effect of losartan over atenolol in Black participants in the LIFE study.[31] Prespecified in the data analysis plan was a test for interaction by ethnic background. A statistical trend for interaction was noted and, when dichotomized to non-Blacks and Blacks, statistical significance was found. These findings revealed that Blacks in the LIFE study had more favorable outcomes with atenolol than losartan treatment.

In both the No-CVD and ISH patients, new-onset DM was significantly less in the losartan group (Table 31–4), paralleling the findings for the entire LIFE cohort. Whether this indicates a protective effect of losartan or a promoting effect of atenolol is not known from the results of the LIFE trial. However, evidence from the ICARUS substudy (n = 99) indicates that insulin sensitivity increased nonsignificantly in the group randomized to losartan, despite the aging that occurred during the study, but decreased significantly in the atenolol group.[32] Hospitalizations for angina were consistently nonsignificantly higher in all subgroups randomized to losartan, whereas in the DM group, fewer patients assigned to losartan were hospitalized for heart failure ($p = .019$).

The occurrence of sudden death was not significantly different between treatment groups in the overall LIFE cohort. In a posthoc analysis of patients with DM, there were 44 occurrences of sudden death that comprised 44% of all cardiovascular deaths. Fourteen of these deaths occurred in the losartan group compared with 30 in the atenolol group ($p = .027$). Less sudden death in patients with DM and atrial fibrillation was observed in the losartan group than in the atenolol group (6% vs. 13%).[33]

Prespecified adverse events (not necessarily drug related) and any other adverse events that attained statistical significance between treatments are shown in Table 31–5. Overall, losartan was associated with fewer adverse events in the main LIFE cohort and the subgroup analyses. Bradycardia is a known consequence of β-blockade, and the increased reporting of this as an adverse event is expected in the atenolol group. A consistent finding across all subgroups and the entire LIFE cohort was the observation of more reporting of albuminuria as an adverse event in the atenolol group compared with the losartan group. Dyspnea and lower extremity edema were consistently more common in the atenolol group, whereas the reporting of lower back pain was more common in the losartan group.

## Treatment-Related Differences in Markers of Hypertensive Disease

BP in the two treatment groups differed little throughout LIFE, making BP effect an unlikely cause of the difference in outcomes. Possible mechanisms for the outcome difference that were explored include differential effects on regression of LVH, on serum uric acid (SUA) levels, on protein excretion, and on vascular structure. Many of these findings have been published in either abstract or manuscript form and provide some insight into the mechanism of superiority of losartan over atenolol in the LIFE trial.

## ECG LVH Regression

A qualifying inclusion characteristic for the LIFE study was the presence of ECG LVH in addition to hypertension. It had previously been shown that regression of LVH in hypertension related to improved prognosis,[34] and attenuation of the actions of the RAS as a therapeutic intervention for preventing or regressing LVH had considerable historic precedent.[17] The LIFE study allowed for a direct test of the question, does it matter how BP is lowered when a goal of therapy is regression of LVH?

By 6 months of treatment, both the Cornell product and Sokolow-Lyon voltage had declined significantly, with statistically greater reductions in losartan group ($p < .001$).[35] The difference in the ECG LVH regression (after adjustment for baseline measures of either the Cornell product or Sokolow-Lyon voltage and in treatment SBP and DBP and for diuretics) was consistent and statistically significant at $p < .001$ over the 5 years of treatment. Because of different units for the Cornell product and Sokolow-Lyon voltage, Figure 31–6 demonstrates the difference between treatments as the percent change over the course of the study.

Although there was no difference in the prevalence of LVH at the outset of the study, beginning at 6 months of treatment and continuing throughout the study, significantly fewer patients in the losartan group had LVH by either criterion ($p < .001$, at all measurement intervals). Furthermore, regression lines plotting the change in SBP versus the change in either the Cornell product or Sokolow-Lyon voltage demonstrated that for any change in SBP, the decline of ECG LVH was consistently greater for the losartan group.[35]

The Framingham study demonstrated that the odds of having CVD were increased in those patients who had an increase in serial voltage change on the electrocardiogram as opposed to those who decreased.[36] Consequently, the greater decrease in ECG LVH evident in the losartan group may have contributed to the reduction of events in the composite outcome of the LIFE study. Furthermore, previous work has demonstrated that cerebrovascular events are more common in patients with ECG LVH.[37] The fact that losartan produced a greater regression of LVH, with similar BP control, provides a possible mechanism explaining the reduced occurrence of fatal and nonfatal stroke that was noted in the primary LIFE cohort and the subsequent subgroup analyses, as well. LVH can increase atrial size, possibly increasing the occurrence of atrial fibrillation, a major risk factor for cardioembolic stroke.

## Serum Uric Acid

Losartan is the only ARB with uricosuric properties, and SUA has been independently associated with cardiovascular morbidity and mortality. In the LIFE study, baseline SUA was significantly associated with increased cardiovascular risk (heart rate = 1.024, 95% CI; 1.017-1.032 per 10-μmol/L increase).[38] Losartan attenuated the age-related increase in SUA in comparison with atenolol ($17.0 \pm 69.8$ vs. $44.4 \pm 72.5$ μmol/L, $p < .0001$) over the duration of the study. Furthermore, 29% of the treatment effect of losartan on the primary composite endpoint could be explained by the SUA ($p = .004$).[38] A trend toward an interaction of gender with SUA was not significant; however, the association with time-varying SUA and risk was higher in women ($p < .0001$) than in men ($p = .0695$). In men, there was a strong relationship of the Framingham Risk Score (along with degree of LVH, a prespecified adjustment in the risk models) that complicates the interpretation of these results.

Lacking controlled intervention studies, only statistical adjustment has established SUA as an independent risk factor for CVD. The association between cardiovascular risk and SUA is well accepted, but the causality is not. In the LIFE trial, the effect of losartan on the relationship of cardiovascular risk to SUA was more profound in women than in men. The enigma presented by these findings adds further to the controversy surrounding cardiovascular risk and SUA. Nevertheless, the LIFE trial suggests that the unique uricosuric quality of losartan may be an added benefit of this particular ARB.

## Urinary Albumin Excretion

The association of microalbuminuria with "benign" essential hypertension was first documented in 1974[39] and only later was microalbuminuria associated with CVD and mortality.[40-42] Microalbuminuria was also found to be associated with LVH in the LIFE study.[43]

**Table 31–5** Prespecified Adverse Events and Any Other Adverse Events Attaining Statistical Significance Between Treatment Groups*

| | LIFE-LOS | LIFE-ATNL | ISH-LOS | ISH-ATNL | LOS | DM-ATNL | No-CVD-LOS | No-CVD-ATNL |
|---|---|---|---|---|---|---|---|---|
| | | | | Prespecified | | | | |
| Angioedema | 6 (1%) | 11 (0.2%) | 2 (0.3%) | 2 (0.3%) | 1 (0.2%) | 3 (0.5%) | 5 (0.1%) | 7 (0.2%) |
| Bradycardia | 66 (1%) | **391 (9%)** | 20 (3%) | **97 (15%)** | 6 (1%) | **50 (8%)** | 37 (1%) | **252 (7%)** |
| Cancer | 356 (8%) | 315 (7%) | 65 (10%) | 55 (8%) | 49 (8%) | 37 (6%) | 258 (8%) | 234 (7%) |
| Cold extremities | 178 (4%) | **269 (6%)** | 27 (4%) | **44 (7%)** | 25 (4%) | 24 (4%) | 153 (4%) | **242 (7%)** |
| Cough | 133 (3%) | 113 (2%) | 27 (4%) | 19 (3%) | 24 (4%) | 15 (3%) | 77 (2%) | 72 (2%) |
| Dizziness | 771 (17%) | 727 (16%) | 129 (20%) | 131 (20%) | 95 (16%) | 87 (14%) | 475 (14%) | 465 (14%) |
| Hypotension | **121 (3%)** | 75 (2%) | 29 (4%) | 18 (3%) | 12 (2%) | 7 (1%) | **71 (2%)** | 42 (1%) |
| Sexual dysfunction | 164 (4%) | **214 (5%)** | 16 (2%) | 21 (3%) | 22 (4%) | 23 (4%) | 110 (3%) | **161 (5%)** |
| Sleep disturbances | 30 (0.7%) | 38 (0.8%) | 6 (0.9%) | 5 (0.8%) | 4 (0.7%) | 8 (0.7%) | 24 (0.7%) | 30 (0.9%) |
| | | | | Additional | | | | |
| Albuminuria | 213 (5%) | **293 (6%)** | 23 (4%) | **53 (8%)** | 43 (7%) | **79 (13%)** | 160 (5%) | **213 (6%)** |
| Hyperglycemia | 239 (5%) | 300 (7%) | | | | | 184 (5%) | 233 (7%) |
| Asthenia/fatigue | 691 (15%) | **802 (17%)** | | | | | 483 (14%) | **589 (17%)** |
| Back pain | **568 (12%)** | 477 (10%) | | | | | | |
| Dyspnea | 457 (10%) | 648 (14%) | 75 (11%) | **126 (19%)** | | | **408 (12%)** | 348 (10%) |
| Lower extremity edema | 539 (12%) | **637 (14%)** | 82 (12%) | **124 (19%)** | | | 299 (9%) | **474 (14%)** |
| Pneumonia | 218 (5%) | **269 (6%)** | | | | | 391 (12%) | **474 (14%)** |
| Hypokalemia | | | | | 22 (4%) | **42 (7%)** | | |
| Chest Pain | | | | | **71 (12%)** | 51 (8%) | | |
| Vertigo | | | | | **68 (12%)** | 44 (7%) | | |

ISH, isolated systolic hypertension; LOS, losartan; ATNL, atenolol; DM, diabetes mellitus; No-CVD, no clinical history of cardiovascular disease.
*Bolded figures are significant at p <.05.

SERIAL PERCENT CHANGE IN ECG LVH

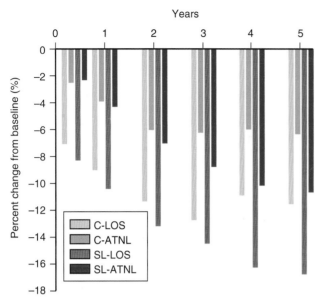

**Figure 31–6** Bar graphs depicting the percent change (decrease) in the ECG indicators of LVH over the course of the LIFE study. At all times, the differences between losartan (LOS) and atenolol (ATNL), for the mean adjusted values was significant at $p < .001$. The adjustments made were for baseline measurements of electrocardiographic evidence of left ventricular hypertrophy (ECG LVH) (Cornell product [C] or Sokolow-Lyon [SL] voltage); baseline in and in-treatment systolic blood pressure (SBP) and diastolic blood pressure (DBP); and diuretic use.

Losartan was associated with greater reductions in albuminuria than atenolol (33% greater after the first year, and 25% greater after the second year of study, both $p < .001$) in the 8206 LIFE patients who were studied. Baseline albuminuria did not clearly identify patients who benefited most from losartan, but ~20% of the differential benefits of losartan on the primary composite endpoint could be statistically accounted for by the greater effect of losartan on reducing albuminuria.[44] Thus the antiproteinuric effects of losartan exerted an apparent protection against cardiovascular outcomes in the LIFE cohort, adding to its known renal protective effect in patients with type 2 DM and nephropathy from the results of the Reduction of Endpoints in NIDDM with the Angiotensin II Antagonist Losartan (RENAAL) study.[45]

## Carotid Hypertrophy

As a part of the ICARUS substudy, measurements of carotid artery intima-media cross-sectional area were made at baseline and after 1, 2, and 3 years of treatment (n = 57).[46] Losartan decreased intima-media cross-sectional area indexed by height at every measurement interval compared with baseline (baseline = 11.2, year 1 = 10.6, year 2 = 10.2, and year 3 = 10.1 mm$^2$/m, all $p < .01$). Atenolol did not have a consistent effect (baseline = 11.9; year 1 = 11.6, not significant [NS], year 2 = 11.2; $p < .05$; and year 3 = 11.4, NS). Regression of carotid artery hypertrophy may have contributed to the observed reduced incidence of stroke in the losartan group.

## POOLED TREATMENT GROUP ANALYSES

The initial study design and baseline characteristics of the study population have been published previously.[7,47] The interrelationships of variables under study, most prominently echocardiographic characteristics, were examined by analyses of unblinded data. Following are important findings from LIFE that have contributed to our knowledge of patients with hypertension and LVH.

## Characteristics of LVH Determination by Electrocardiogram

Obesity can affect the magnitude of the voltage measured by surface electrocardiogram, and can lead to LVH, and many participants in the LIFE study were obese. Therefore, the LIFE investigators asked whether LVH determination by electrocardiogram was influenced by obesity. By analyzing the prevalence of LVH by both Cornell product and Sokolow-Lyon voltage against tertiles of BMI, the LIFE investigators demonstrated that obesity had a greater effect on LVH determination by the Sokolow-Lyon method than the Cornell product method.[20] A progressive increase in the Cornell product was noted, but a progressive decrease in the Sokolow-Lyon voltage was observed as BMI tertile increased.

Further examination of the characteristics of LVH determination by the Cornell product and Sokolow-Lyon voltage showed that the Cornell product criterion was satisfied by 65.9% of participants, whereas the Sokolow-Lyon voltage criterion was met by only 23.1% of the sample.[48] Multivariate analysis revealed that the best predictors of LVH by Cornell product criteria were higher BMI, increased age, and female gender. The Sokolow-Lyon criteria for LVH were predicted by lower BMI, male gender, and Black race.

The presence of albuminuria was also investigated in relation to the ECG LVH. In this examination, baseline albuminuria was associated independently with DM, higher BP, older age, serum creatinine, smoking, and ECG LVH.[43] Following 1 year of treatment, the decline in albuminuria was independently associated with ECG-measured regression of LVH,[49] leading the investigators to conclude that albuminuria represented generalized vascular damage.

## Echocardiography Substudies

A representative sample of 964 LIFE participants also enrolled in the echocardiographic substudy. Among 906 participants with measurable echocardiographic mass and baseline ECG measures, 75% had ECG LVH at screening and at baseline. Because of regression to the mean, 25% did not satisfy ECG criteria for LVH at baseline but did at screening. Those found to satisfy criteria at both time points had an increased prevalence of echocardiographic LVH (86% vs. 55%, $p < .001$).[50,51] The ECG criteria used to identify participants with LVH indicated a prevalence of >70% LVH by echocardiography.[49]

In 750 participants who had complete measures of LV dimensions and Doppler filling patterns, many correlates were observed.[52] Multiple regression analysis demonstrated that LV mass correlated with isovolumetric relaxation time, but LV mass and geometry were not related to peak early LV filling velocity (E), peak atrial filling velocity (A), or mitral valve

E peak deceleration time. The E/A ratio was independently correlated with isovolumetric relaxation time.

These LIFE patients were also compared with groups of 282 employed hypertensive and 366 apparently normal adults to study wall stress and myocardial oxygen demand (measured as a triple product of heart rate, mass, and wall stress).[53] The LIFE participants were heavier and older than the comparison groups and had substantially supranormal wall stresses and increased triple product compared with the other groups when compared by gender. These changes indicate an increased myocardial oxygen demand and predisposition for myocardial ischemia in the LIFE cohort. The main LIFE outcome study and substudies indicated no difference between the losartan and atenolol groups with respect to fatal and nonfatal MI, even though the β-blocking action of atenolol decreased heart rate, a component of the triple product and correlate of myocardial oxygen demand.

Systolic function was also a topic for the echocardiographic substudy analysis.[54] In this study, LV mass was the strongest correlate of impaired endocardial shortening and midwall shortening. In patients characterized with eccentric LVH, depressed endocardial shortening was most common, whereas patients with concentric remodeling or hypertrophy demonstrated impaired midwall shortening. As a follow-up to this study, it was later demonstrated in blinded treatment analyses that 3 years of antihypertensive therapy improved systolic LV performance, associated with decreases in LV mass, relative wall thickness, and BP and an increase in stroke volume.[55] In a separate analysis that addressed those participants with ISH versus those with combined hypertension, relative wall thickness was independently associated with ISH, supporting the concept that SBP is a stronger determinant of target organ damage than DBP.[56]

Because atrial fibrillation is strongly associated with stroke, correlates of left atrial size were also determined. It was found that 56% of women and 38% of men had enlarged left atria. Left atrial enlargement was found in multiple logistic regression to be related to LVH and eccentric geometry, increased BMI, SBP, age, mitral regurgitation, female gender, and atrial fibrillation.[57] Repolarization electrocardiogram correlates of ventricular arrhythmias, namely the QT interval and QT dispersion, were found to be significantly related to the LV mass index and LVH.[58]

## Insulin Carotids United States Scandinavia (ICARUS) Study

A small subset of LIFE participants (99, with 11 excluded from the analysis because of DM) underwent isoglycemic hyperinsulinemic clamp studies, forearm venous plethysmographic studies, and ultrasonic examination of the common carotid arteries during the placebo phase of the LIFE study.[59] The main finding from this examination was that high SBP was associated with common carotid vascular hypertrophy. Hyperinsulinemia and insulin resistance were related to carotid vascular distensibility, while minimal forearm vascular resistance was correlated with SBP and pulse pressure only in men.

Other smaller substudies have investigated issues surrounding insulin sensitivity, blood viscosity, and vascular changes, as well. In unmedicated LIFE-ICARUS participants, fasting insulin independently explained 12% of the variation in blood viscosity at high shear rate, whereas at low shear rates, baseline adrenaline independently explained 17% of the variance in blood viscosity.[60] Elevated DBP and serum low-density lipoprotein were found to be related to impaired acetylcholine-induced vasodilation independently from nitroprusside-induced vasodilation in small resistance arteries. These results suggested that, in 41 patients in the ICARUS study with previously treated hypertension, endothelial dysfunction was unrelated to structural changes in the vasculature.[61] In 43 patients, a low exercise capacity was documented and found to be related to increased LV mass (measured by magnetic resonance imaging), lower systemic vascular compliance, and higher minimal forearm vascular resistance.[62] Thus patients with longstanding hypertension had reduced exercise capacity perhaps due to cardiovascular hypertrophy and reduced systemic vascular compliance.

## SUMMARY

The LIFE study demonstrated that a treatment regimen based on losartan was superior to one based on atenolol in preventing cardiovascular endpoints in patients with hypertension and LVH, despite similar BP control during the 4.8 years of average follow-up. These effects were generally observed in the subsets of the LIFE cohort with higher risk, namely patients with ISH and DM, but also in those patients with no previous clinical history of CVD. The most profound treatment effect of losartan was on fatal and nonfatal stroke, whereas no significant differences between treatments were demonstrated for fatal and nonfatal MI.

Regression of ECG LVH was also greater in the group randomized to losartan, providing a possible mechanism for its protective action in comparison with atenolol. Reduction in endpoints in the losartan group could be related to blunting of the age-related increase in SUA. Furthermore, losartan reduced albuminuria to a greater extent than did atenolol.

In the future, we can expect to see a continuing flow of medical knowledge made possible by the persons who volunteered to participate in the LIFE study. The findings of this study have verified the importance of treatment with losartan in patients with hypertension and echocardiographic evidence of LVH.

## References

1. Dahlof B, Devereux RB, Kjeldsen SE, et al. Cardiovascular morbidity and mortality in the Losartan Intervention For Endpoint reduction in hypertension study (LIFE): A randomised trial against atenolol. Lancet 359:995-1003, 2002.
2. Blaschke TE, Melmon KL. Antihypertensive agents and the drug therapy of hypertension. *In* Gilman AG, Goodman LS, Gilman A (eds). The Pharmacological Basis of Therapeutics. New York, Macmillan Publishing Co., 1980; pp 793-818.
3. The Joint National Committee on the Detection, Evaluation, and Treatment of High Blood Pressure. The fifth report of the Joint national Committee on Detection, Evaluation, and Treatment of High Blood Pressure (JNC-V). Arch Intern Med 153: 154-183, 1993.
4. Frohlich ED. Continuing advances in hypertension: The Joint National Committee's fifth report. Am J Med Sci 310:S48-S52, 1995.
5. Collins R, Peto R, MacMahon S, et al. Blood pressure, stroke, and coronary heart disease. Part 2, short-term reductions in blood pressure: Overview of randomised drug trials in their epidemiological context. Lancet 335:827-838, 1990.

6. Thijs L, Fagard R, Lijnen P, et al. A meta-analysis of outcome trials in elderly hypertensives. J Hypertens 10:1103-1109, 1992.

7. Dahlof B, Devereux R, deFaire U, et al. The Losartan Intervention for Endpoint Reduction (LIFE) in Hypertension Study; rationale, design, and methods. Am J Hypertens 10: 705-713, 1997.

8. Kannel WB, Gordon T, Castelli WP, et al. Electrocardiographic left ventricular hypertrophy and risk of coronary heart disease. The Framingham Study. Ann Intern Med 72:813-822, 1970.

9. Levy D, Garrison RJ, Savage DD, et al. Prognostic implications of echocardiographically determined left ventricular mass in the Framingham Heart Study. N Engl J Med 322:1561-1566, 1990.

10. Kannel WB, Gordon T, Offutt D. Left ventricular hypertrophy by electrocardiogram. Prevalence, incidence, and mortality in the Framingham study. Ann Intern Med 71:89-105, 1969.

11. Koren MJ, Devereux RB, Casale PN, et al. Relation of left ventricular mass and geometry to morbidity and mortality in uncomplicated essential hypertension. Ann Intern Med 114:345-352, 1991.

12. Pfeffer MA. Mechanistic lessons from the SAVE study. Survival and ventricular enlargement. Am J Hypertens 7:106S-111S, 1994.

13. Campbell DJ. Circulating and tissue angiotensin systems. J Clin Invest 79:1-6, 1987.

14. Dzau VJ. Short- and long-term determinants of cardiovascular function and therapy: Contributions of circulating and tissue renin-angiotensin systems. J Cardiovasc Pharmacol 14(Suppl 4): S1-S5, 1989.

15. Dostal DE, Baker KM. Angiotensin II stimulation of left ventricular hypertrophy in adult rat heart. Mediation by the AT1 receptor. Am J Hypertens 5:276-280, 1992.

16. Qing G, Garcia R. Chronic captopril and losartan (DuP 753) administration in rats with high-output heart failure. Am J Physiol 263:H833-H840, 1992.

17. Dahlof B, Pennert K, Hansson L. Regression of left ventricular hypertrophy: A meta-analysis. Clin Exp Hypertens 14:173-180, 1992.

18. Norman JE, Levy D. Improved electrocardiographic detection of echocardiographic left ventricular hypertrophy: Results of a correlated data base approach. J Am Coll Cardiol 26:1021-1029, 1995.

19. Anderson KM, Wilson PW, Odell PM, et al. An updated coronary risk profile. A statement for health professionals. Circulation 83:356-362, 1991.

20. Okin PM, Jern S, Devereux RB, et al. Effect of obesity on electrocardiographic left ventricular hypertrophy in hypertensive patients: The Losartan Intervention For Endpoint (LIFE) Reduction in Hypertension Study. Hypertension 35:13-18, 2000.

21. Hansson L, Hedner T, Lund-Johansen P, et al. Randomised trial of effects of calcium antagonists compared with diuretics and [beta]-blockers on cardiovascular morbidity and mortality in hypertension: The Nordic Diltiazem (NORDIL) study. Lancet 356:359-365, 2000.

22. The ALLHAT Officers and Coordinators for the ALLHAT Collaborative Research Group; the Antihypertensive and Lipid-Lowering Treatment to Prevent Heart Attack Trial. Major outcomes in high-risk hypertensive patients randomized to angiotensin-converting enzyme inhibitor or calcium channel blocker vs diuretic. JAMA 288:2981-2997, 2002.

23. Lithell H, Hansson L, Skoog I, et al.: SCOPE Study Group. The Study on Cognition and Prognosis in the Elderly (SCOPE): Principal results of a randomized double-blind intervention trial. J Hypertens 21:875-886, 2003.

24. Black HR, Elliott WJ, Grandits G, et al. Principal results of the Controlled Onset Verapamil Investigation of Cardiovascular End Points (CONVINCE) trial. JAMA 289:2073-2082, 2003.

25. Pepine CJ, Handberg EM, Cooper-DeHoff RM, et al. A calcium antagonist vs a non-calcium antagonist hypertension treatment strategy for patients with coronary artery disease. The International Verapamil Trandolapril Study (INVEST): A randomized controlled trial. JAMA 290:2805-2816, 2003.

26. Lindholm LH, Ibsen H, Borch-Johnsen K, et al. Risk of new-onset diabetes in the Losartan Intervention For Endpoint reduction in hypertension study. J Hypertens 20:1879-1886, 2002.

27. Kjeldsen SE, Dahlof B, Devereux RB, et al. Effects of losartan on cardiovascular morbidity and mortality in patients with isolated systolic hypertension and left ventricular hypertrophy: A Losartan Intervention for Endpoint Reduction (LIFE) substudy. JAMA 288:1491-1498, 2002.

28. Lindholm LH, Ibsen H, Dahlof B, et al. Cardiovascular morbidity and mortality in patients with diabetes in the Losartan Intervention For Endpoint reduction in hypertension study (LIFE): A randomised trial against atenolol. Lancet 359:1004-1010, 2002.

29. Devereux RB, Dahlof B, Kjeldsen SE, et al. Effects of losartan or atenolol in hypertensive patients without clinically evident vascular disease: A substudy of the LIFE randomized trial. Ann Intern Med 139:169-177, 2003.

30. Kjeldsen, SE, Julius S, Hedner, T, et al. Stroke is more common than myocardial infarction in hypertension: Analysis based on 11 major randomized intervention trials. Blood Press 10: 190-192, 2001.

31. Julius S, Alderman MH, Beevers G, et al. Cardiovascular risk reduction in hypertensive black patients with left ventricular hypertrophy: The LIFE study. J Am Coll Cardiol 43(6): 1047-1055, 2004.

32. Olsen MH, Fossum E, Wachtell K, et al. Effect of losartan versus atenolol on insulin sensitivity and peripheral vascular hypertrophy in hypertension. ICARUS, a LIFE Substudy. Circulation 106:II-574, 2002.

33. Lindholm LH, Dahlof B, Edelman JM, et al. Less sudden cardiac death in diabetics treated with losartan—data from the LIFE trial. Lancet 362:619-620, 2003.

34. Verdecchia P, Schillaci G, Borgioni C, et al. Prognostic significance of serial changes in left ventricular mass in essential hypertension. Circulation 97:48-54, 1998.

35. Okin PM, Devereux RB, Sverker J, et al. Regression of Electrocardiographic left ventricular hypertrophy by losartan versus atenolol: The Losartan Intervention For Endpoint reduction in hypertension (LIFE) Study. Circulation 108:684-690, 2003.

36. Levy D, Salomon M, D'Agostino RB, et al. Prognostic implications of baseline electrocardiographic features and their serial changes in subjects with left ventricular hypertrophy. Circulation 90:1786-1793, 1994.

37. Verdecchia PM, Porcellati CM, Reboldi G, et al. Left ventricular hypertrophy as an independent predictor of acute cerebrovascular events in essential hypertension. Circulation 105: 2039-2044, 2001.

38. Hoieggen A, Alderman MH, Kjeldsen SE, et al., for the LIFE Study Group. The impact of serum uric acid on cardiovascular outcomes in the LIFE study. Kidney Int 65(3):1041-1049, 2004.

39. Parving HH, Mogensen CE, Jensen HA , et al. Increased urinary albumin-excretion rate in benign essential hypertension. Lancet 1:1190-1192, 1974.

40. Yudkin JS, Forrest RD, Jackson CA. Microalbuminuria as predictor of vascular disease in non-diabetic subjects. Islington Diabetes Survey. Lancet 2:530-533, 1988.

41. Damsgaard EM, Froland A, Jorgensen OD, et al. Microalbuminuria as predictor of increased mortality in elderly people. BMJ 300:297-300, 1990.

42. Kuusisto J, Mykkanen L, Pyorala K, et al. Hyperinsulinemic microalbuminuria. A new risk indicator for coronary heart disease. Circulation 91:831-837, 1995.

43. Wachtell K, Olsen MH, Dahlof B, et al. Microalbuminuria in hypertensive patients with electrocardiographic left ventricular hypertrophy: The LIFE Study. J Hypertens 20:405-412, 2002.

44. Ibsen H, Olsen MH, Wachtell K, et al. Does albuminuria predict cardiovascular outcome on treatment with losartan versus atenolol in patients with hypertension and left ventricular hypertrophy? The LIFE study. J Hypertens 21(suppl 4):S68, 2003.

45. Brenner BM, Cooper ME, de Zeeuw D, et al., for the RENAAL Study Investigators. Effects of losartan on renal and cardiovascular outcomes in patients with type 2 diabetes and nephropathy. N Engl J Med 345:861-869, 2001.

46. Olsen MH, Wachtell K, Neland K, et al. The effect of losartan versus atenolol on carotid artery hypertrophy in essential hypertension. A LIFE substudy. Circulation 106:II-574, 2002.

47. Dahlof B, Devereux RB, Julius S, et al. Characteristics of 9194 patients with left ventricular hypertrophy: The LIFE study. Hypertension 32:989-997, 1998.

48. Okin PM, Devereux RB, Jern S, et al., for the Investigators for the LIFE study. Baseline characteristics in relation to electrocardiographic left ventricular hypertrophy in hypertensive patients: The Losartan Intervention For Endpoint Reduction (LIFE) in Hypertension Study. Hypertension 2000; 36:766-773.

49. Olsen MH, Wachtell K, Borch-Johnsen K, et al. A blood pressure independent association between glomerular albumin leakage and electrocardiographic left ventricular hypertrophy. The LIFE Study. Losartan Intervention For Endpoint reduction. J Hum Hypertens 16:591-595, 2002.

50. Okin PM, Devereux RB, Jern S, et al. Relation of echocardiographic left ventricular mass and hypertrophy to persistent electrocardiographic left ventricular hypertrophy in hypertensive patients: The LIFE Study. Am J Hypertens 14:775-782, 2001.

51. Devereux RB, Bella J, Boman K, et al. Echocardiographic left ventricular geometry in hypertensive patients with electrocardiographic left ventricular hypertrophy: The LIFE Study. Blood Press 10:74-82, 2001.

52. Wachtell K, Smith G, Gerdts E, et al. Left ventricular filling patterns in patients with systemic hypertension and left ventricular hypertrophy (the LIFE study). Am J Cardiol 85:466-472, 2000.

53. Devereux RB, Roman MJ, Palmieri V, et al. Left ventricular wall stresses and wall stress-mass-heart rate products in hypertensive patients with electrocardiographic left ventricular hypertrophy: The LIFE study. J Hypertens 18:1129-1138, 2000.

54. Wachtell K, Rokkedal J, Bella JN, et al. Effect of electrocardiographic left ventricular hypertrophy on left ventricular systolic function in systemic hypertension (The LIFE Study). Am J Cardiol 87:54-60, 2001.

55. Wachtell K, Palmieri V, Olsen MH, et al. Change in systolic left ventricular performance after 3 years of antihypertensive treatment: The Losartan Intervention for Endpoint (LIFE) Study. Circulation 106:227-232, 2002.

56. Papademetriou V, Devereux RB, Narayan P, et al. Similar effects of isolated systolic and combined hypertension on left ventricular geometry and function: The LIFE Study. Am J Hypertens 14:768-774, 2001.

57. Gerdts E, Oikarinen L, Palmieri V, et al. Correlates of left atrial size in hypertensive patients with left ventricular hypertrophy: The Losartan Intervention For Endpoint Reduction in Hypertension (LIFE) Study. Hypertension 39:739-743, 2002.

58. Oikarinen L, Nieminen MS, Viitasalo M, et al. Relation of QT interval and QT dispersion to echocardiographic left ventricular hypertrophy and geometric pattern in hypertensive patients. The LIFE study. The Losartan Intervention For Endpoint Reduction. J Hypertens 19:1883-1891, 2001.

59. Olsen MH, Fossum E, Hjerkinn E, et al. Relative influence of insulin resistance versus blood pressure on vascular changes in longstanding hypertension. ICARUS, a LIFE substudy. Insulin Carotids US Scandinavia. J Hypertens 18:75-81, 2000.

60. Hoieggen A, Fossum E, Nesbitt SD, et al. Blood viscosity, plasma adrenaline and fasting insulin in hypertensive patients with left ventricular hypertrophy. ICARUS, a LIFE substudy. Insulin Carotids US Scandinavica. Blood Press 9:83-90, 2000.

61. Olsen MH, Wachtell K, Aalkjaer C, et al. Endothelial dysfunction in resistance arteries is related to high blood pressure and circulating low density lipoproteins in previously treated hypertension. Am J Hypertens 14:861-867, 2001.

62. Olsen MH, Wachtell K, Hermann KL, et al. Maximal exercise capacity is related to cardiovascular structure in patients with longstanding hypertension. A LIFE substudy. Am J Hypertens 14:1205-1210, 2001.

# The VALUE Trial

**Stevo Julius, Sverre E. Kjeldsen, Hans Brunner, Steffan Enkman, John H. Laragh, Pelle Stolt, Gordon T. McInnes, Beverly A. Smith, Francis Plat, M. Anthony Schork, Michael A. Weber, Alberto Zanchetti**

The benefits of antihypertensive treatment in terms of reduced morbidity and mortality are well established. However, the question whether there are differences between blood pressure (BP)–lowering agents beyond their direct antihypertensive effects remains undecided. Several large-scale hypertension trials have failed to show significant outcome differences when comparing different types of treatment (i.e., diuretics, β-blockers, calcium channel blockers, angiotensin-converting enzyme [ACE] inhibitors, or α-blockers), with respect to primary cardiovascular outcomes (Figure 32–1).[1-4] However, a growing number of trials have shown indications of benefits beyond BP lowering as a result of inhibiting the renin-angiotensin system (RAS). Two studies, CAPPP (the Captopril Prevention Project)[1] and HOPE (the Heart Outcomes Prevention Evaluation Study),[5] reported that treatment with ACE inhibitors conferred greater cardiovascular protection than other treatments, albeit the results relied on secondary analyses. In CAPPP, where patients were randomly assigned to captopril or to diuretic, β-blocker, or diuretic plus β-blocker, the incidence of diabetes was lower in the captopril group than in the conventional group (.86; p = .039). However, in many cases captopril (50-100 mg daily) was given once a day, which is contrary to the usual recommendation of two or three daily doses.[6] Another important point is that there were differences between the two treatment groups in prerandomization height, weight, BP, and the presence of diabetes. Furthermore, the higher (2 mm Hg) diastolic blood pressure (DBP) in the captopril group at baseline seemed to persist throughout the study and may have influenced outcomes.

In the HOPE study, 9297 men and women ≥ 55 years of age were eligible if they had a history of coronary disease, stroke, peripheral vascular disease, or diabetes mellitus, plus at least one other cardiovascular risk factor (smoking, hypertension, hyperlipidemia, or microalbuminuria). The eligible patients were randomized to either ramipril 10 mg daily or matching placebo.

The ramipril patients had lower rates of the primary composite endpoint of myocardial infarction (MI), stroke, or death from cardiovascular causes (relative risk, .78; p <.001). Risk reductions were also reported for death from cardiovascular causes (relative risk, .74; p <.001), MI (relative risk, .80; p <.001), stroke (relative risk, .68; p <.001), heart failure (relative risk, .77; p <.001), and complications related to diabetes (relative risk, .84; p = .03).

However, HOPE was not primarily directed at patients with hypertension and was not actively controlled. Ramipril was reported to have a small effect (–3/2 mm Hg) on BP, but this small difference between treatment groups has been questioned. The reported differences refer to office BP, whereas a substudy of HOPE showed a 15/6–mm Hg difference from placebo in 24-hour ambulatory BP.[7] If expressed as the reduction in cardiovascular events per mm Hg difference in BP, the benefits in HOPE were no greater than those seen in other high-risk populations treated with other forms of antihypertensive therapy.[8]

The Second Australian National Blood Pressure Study (ANBP2) reported reduced risk for cardiovascular events or death from any cause in elderly (65-84 years) hypertensive subjects treated with ACE inhibitors than with diuretics. A mean decrease of 26/12 mm Hg in the 6083 participants led to a risk ratio of .89 with borderline significance (p = .05).[9] However, this was an open-label study in family practices and thus not directly comparable with randomized double-blind controlled trials. The Antihypertensive and Lipid-Lowering treatment to prevent Heart Attack Trial (ALLHAT) failed to show outcome differences between the ACE inhibitor lisinopril and the thiazide-like diuretic chlorthalidone,[4] which may have been due to inadequate dose levels or to differences in systolic blood pressure (SBP) in disfavor of the ACE inhibitor throughout.

The strongest evidence for differences between antihypertensive therapies has come from trials with angiotensin receptor blockers (ARBs). The LIFE study (Losartan Intervention for Endpoint Reduction in Hypertension) compared the ARB losartan with the β-blocker atenolol in 9194 hypertensive patients with left ventricular hypertrophy (LVH).[10] The trial reported 13% reduction in the primary composite endpoint of death, MI, or stroke; 25% reduction in risk of stroke; and 25% reduction in new-onset diabetes in hypertensive patients treated with losartan compared with atenolol, for the same degree of BP reduction. The risk reduction was most prominent in patients with isolated systolic hypertension (ISH) (25% reduction in primary composite endpoint).[11] The equal BP reduction in both treatment groups in LIFE has not been challenged and the results were widely recognized as the first demonstration of BP independent differences between antihypertensive therapies. Mean BPs at the last visit were 144.1/81.3 mm Hg in the losartan group and 145.4/80.9 mm Hg in the atenolol group.[10]

Further support for the conclusions from LIFE came from SCOPE (Study on Cognition and Prognosis in the Elderly), which focused on elderly populations (70-89 years) with mild hypertension. In SCOPE, there was a statistically significant 28% reduction in stroke and a nonsignificant trend toward reduced rates of new-onset diabetes with the ARB candesartan compared with a non-ARB–based antihypertensive regimen.[12] However, the trial design was changed from the planned placebo-controlled to active-controlled for ethical reasons, and BP reductions at the end of study were not equal between

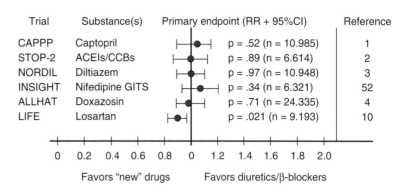

| Trial | Substance(s) | Primary endpoint (RR + 95%CI) | Reference |
|---|---|---|---|
| CAPPP | Captopril | p = .52 (n = 10.985) | 1 |
| STOP-2 | ACEIs/CCBs | p = .89 (n = 6.614) | 2 |
| NORDIL | Diltiazem | p = .97 (n = 10.948) | 3 |
| INSIGHT | Nifedipine GITS | p = .34 (n = 6.321) | 52 |
| ALLHAT | Doxazosin | p = .71 (n = 24.335) | 4 |
| LIFE | Losartan | p = .021 (n = 9.193) | 10 |

Favors "new" drugs     Favors diuretics/β-blockers

**Figure 32–1** Large hypertension trials with "new" versus "old" drugs. (Adapted from Kjeldsen SE, Westheim AS, Os I. INSIGHT and NORDIL. International Nifedipine GITS study: Intervention as a goal in hypertension treatment. Nordic Diltiazem Study. Lancet 356:1929-1930, 2000. © Elsevier Ltd; used with permission.)

the treatment groups (3.2/1.6 mm Hg greater reduction with candesartan). These two factors reduced the power and weakened the interpretation of SCOPE results.

Thus, to date, we have two trials indicating that ARBs confer cardiovascular protection, most dramatically against stroke, beyond that of lowering BP alone. This is a highly intriguing finding. Although traditionally hypertension has been associated with a higher incidence of coronary heart disease (CHD) than of stroke, an analysis of 11 major randomized antihypertensive intervention trials recently revealed stroke to be the more common event.[13] This strong association was seen not only for elderly patients, who tend to be more stroke-prone than younger people, but also in other age groups.[1,3,8] It is still possible that some of the differences in LIFE were due to negative effects of atenolol rather than to benefits from losartan, but this explanation is less plausible for the SCOPE results, in which the use of β-blockers was limited.[12] Atenolol and other β-blockers are reported to increase insulin resistance.[14] Other trials are needed to clarify this issue, as well as the mechanism of the possible beneficial effect of ARBs.

As to the stroke effects, there are data supporting the contention that the effects in LIFE and SCOPE are indeed due to positive actions of the ARBs. ARBs are known to have benefits on endothelial function. Losartan has been shown to improve maximal acetylcholine response as compared with atenolol.[15] A small crossover study with irbesartan and atenolol has shown that the media width:lumen ratio in resistance arteries decreased when hypertensive patients whose BP was controlled after 1 year of atenolol treatment were switched to the ARB irbesartan for 1 year.[16] Because these studies were comparisons with β-blocker treatment, a negative effect of the comparator drugs such as peripheral vasoconstriction cannot be excluded, but there are data showing that the ARB valsartan improves the vasodilator response to acetylcholine in hypertensive patients, whereas the effects of the calcium channel blocker amlodipine were neutral.[17] However, it needs to be established whether such data translate into clinical outcome benefits.

Furthermore, we still need data on the cardiac effects of angiotensin receptor blockade. The similar cardiac outcomes in both arms in LIFE are an interesting issue, because losartan reduced LVH to a significantly greater extent than atenolol, an effect that would have been expected to translate into cardiac protection. However, it is important to remember that the comparison in LIFE was against an active agent with proven cardiac benefits. A hypothesis is that the cardioprotective effects of the two treatments used

in LIFE were balanced; the reduced stroke work and antiarrhythmic effects conferred by atenolol may have compensated for the benefits from the LVH reduction in the losartan group.

Such unanswered questions and more raise high expectations of the Valsartan Antihypertensive Long-term Use Evaluation (VALUE) Trial of Cardiovascular Events in Hypertension,[18] one of the largest intervention studies in essential hypertension. VALUE is a multicenter, double-blind, randomized, prospective, active-controlled parallel group trial designed to compare the effects of valsartan with those of the calcium channel blocker amlodipine, in doses of 80 to 160 mg and 5 to 10 mg once daily, respectively, on coronary morbidity and mortality in patients with essential hypertension and at high risk for CHD. All primary endpoints in VALUE are cardiac endpoints, with the hypothesis that for the same level of BP control, valsartan will be significantly more effective than amlodipine in decreasing acute MI, congestive heart failure (CHF), and cardiac mortality.[18]

The choice of amlodipine as comparator in VALUE is highly appropriate, because calcium channel blockers are considered to have stroke-protective and possible cardioprotective effects. Recently, ALLHAT found similar stroke-protective effects from amlodipine as from a diuretic,[4] and thus there is a need for adequately designed trials addressing the issue. In contrast to the effects of valsartan or the ACE inhibitor enalapril, amlodipine has been shown to increase sympathetic activity.[19,20] Furthermore, amlodipine has a neutral effect on insulin resistance,[21] in contrast to atenolol. Such metabolic effects, possible confounders in LIFE, are unlikely in VALUE.

The stroke protection from calcium channel blockers has been attributed to direct effects on the structural integrity of the blood-brain barrier from reduced endothelial permeability[22] or to amelioration in the abnormal sensitivity of arterial smooth muscle cells to $Ca^{2+}$.[23] Other possible effects are inhibition of detrimental effects of oxygen radicals.[24] Among cardioprotective effects, amlodipine has been reported to improve myocardial function, to reduce the size of the myocardial infarct following ischemia-reperfusion,[25-27] and to protect against the postischemic impairment of coronary endothelium-dependent relaxation.[28] The mechanisms of some of these effects remain to be established.

The VALUE trial will provide important information on cardiac effects of valsartan and amlodipine, and is expected to resolve the issue of whether the lower rates of stroke with losartan in LIFE were due to negative effects of atenolol or positive effects of angiotensin receptor blockade.

## VALUE TRIAL DESIGN

VALUE is a prospective, multinational, multicenter, double-blind, randomized, active, controlled two-arm parallel group comparison trial with a response-dependent dose titration scheme. Eligible patients were men and women 50 years of age or older with essential hypertension previously untreated or treated. To be included, previously untreated patients had to have mean sitting SBP of 160 to 210 mm Hg (inclusive) and a mean DBP ≤115 mm Hg, or a mean sitting DBP of 95 to 115 mm Hg and SBP ≤210 mm Hg. For patients already taking antihypertensive treatment, there were no lower limits of BPs, but upper limits of ≤210/115 mm Hg. Exclusion criteria included cardiovascular conditions and obvious noncardiac diseases that may limit long-term survival or increase the likelihood of nonadherence to study medication. Patients already receiving antihypertensive treatment were directly rolled over to one of the two VALUE arms, discontinuing previous drugs and starting on the treatment drug, without a placebo run-in period.

Patients were randomized to either valsartan 80 mg once daily or amlodipine 5 mg once daily. The BP target is 140/90 mm Hg. After 4 weeks on the initial dose, patients were titrated to a dose of valsartan 160 mg or amlodipine 10 mg once daily (Figure 32–2). If the BP target was still not achieved, hydrochlorothiazide could be added at 12.5- or 25-mg doses. A fifth step of the protocol allowed for free add-on of antihypertensive drugs, with the exception of ACE inhibitors, calcium channel blockers, ARBs, or diuretics other than hydrochlorothiazide; however, in patients with impaired renal function or with CHF, thiazide diuretics could be replaced or supplemented by loop diuretics. The usual dose titration period of 4 weeks could be shortened if it was considered in the patient's best interest.

VALUE is endpoint driven and will run until 1450 patients have experienced a primary cardiac event. The primary endpoint is defined as composite sudden cardiac death, fatal MI, death during or following percutaneous transluminal coronary angioplasty (PTCA) or coronary artery graft bypass (CABG), death due to heart failure, MI on autopsy, new-onset heart failure or chronic heart failure requiring hospital management, nonfatal MI, emergency PTCA/CABG, or thrombolytic/fibrinolytic treatment to avoid MI. It was calculated that 14,400 enrolled patients were needed to give the study 90% power at a significance level of $p < .05$ to detect a 15% reduction in the primary endpoint rate from 12.5% in the amlodipine group to 10.6% in the valsartan group over an average of 5 years of treatment. As a comparison, LIFE had 80% power to detect differences in the primary endpoint rates. Altogether, 15,314 eligible patients in 31 countries were randomized by December 31, 1999.

Overall, BP reduction was similar with both treatments. However, the mean differences throughout the study were not consistent. The differences in BP between drug regimens were 4.0/2.1, 4.3/2.5, 3.0/2.0, 2.4/1.7, 2.1/1.6, and 2.0/1.5 mm Hg after months 1, 2, 3, 4, 6, and 12, respectively, and stabilized at 1.5/1.3 mm Hg thereafter. The target BP (<140/90 mm Hg) was achieved in 56% of the valsartan group and 62% of the amlodipine group. The cardiovascular event rate was 25.5 per 1000 patient-years in the valsartan group and 24.7 per 1000 patient-years in the amlodipine group. Cardiac mortality and morbidity were not significantly different in the two treatment groups (4.0% vs. 4.0% and 7.7% vs. 7.6%, respectively). Heart failure, stroke, and all-cause death were similar between valsartan- and amlodipine-randomized groups (4.6% vs. 5.3% $p = .12$; 4.2% vs. 3.7% $p = .08$; 11.0% vs. 10.8% $p = .45$, respectively). However, fatal and nonfatal MI were reduced with amlodipine compared with valsartan (4.8% vs. 4.1% $p = .02$, respectively), whereas new-onset diabetes was significantly reduced with valsartan compared with amlodipine (13.1% vs. 16.4% $p < .0001$). The VALUE study highlights the importance of BP lowering in a prompt manner. The early BP differences limit the ability to assess the BP-independent effects between these two drug treatments. Furthermore, achieving adequate BP control in high-risk patients often requires combination therapy early in the treatment period.

### Risk Stratification

A unique feature of VALUE is the use of a specially designed algorithm that takes into account risk factors and disease factors, to assess cardiovascular risk.[18] The risk factors include diabetes mellitus, cigarette smoking, hypercholesterolemia, LVH without strain diagnosed on ECG, proteinuria, and serum creatinine above 1.7 mg/dl. Disease factors include a documented history of MI, peripheral vascular disease, stroke or transient ischemic attack, or the presence of LVH with strain on ECG (Box 32–1). This combination of risk factors and disease factors, together with age and sex, makes it uniquely possible to assess the predictive power of an up-to-date cardiovascular risk scale in a large international population of treated hypertensive patients traditionally considered to be at high risk of a cardiovascular event.

The age/risk stratification criteria vary between patient groups according to age. For men aged 50 to 59 years, there is a requirement for at least three additional risk factors or one additional disease factor to be eligible for enrollment. Because of the lower risk profile of women of perimenopausal age, women between 50 and 59 years need to present with a minimum of two risk factors and one additional disease factor to qualify for enrollment. For patients ≥60 years of age, sex is not considered a factor influencing cardiovascular risk, and thus the requirements are identical for both sexes. Patients aged 60 to 69 years need at least two risk factors or one disease factor, whereas only one risk or one disease factor is required for patients ≥70 years. The requirements for this last group are based on the significantly increased predictive value of increasing age.

### Endpoints

As noted, all primary endpoints in VALUE are cardiac endpoints. The primary variable to be assessed is the time to the first cardiac morbidity or mortality event. Cardiac mortality was defined previously; cardiac morbidity is defined as new or chronic CHF requiring hospitalization, nonfatal acute MI, emergency thrombolysis, or any other interventional procedure performed to prevent a full-blown MI. Important secondary variables are all-cause mortality, cardiac mortality and cardiac morbidity (both defined as for the primary endpoint), stroke, cardiac morbidity plus stroke, worsening of chronic stable angina or unstable angina, routine cardiac interventional procedures, potentially lethal arrhythmias, syncope or near-syncope, silent MI, and end-stage renal disease.

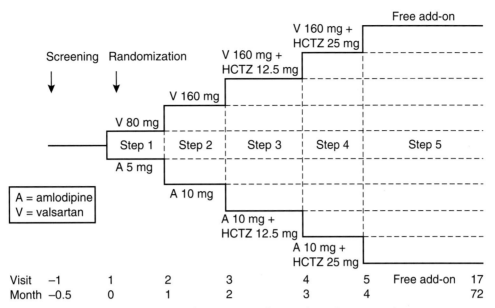

**Figure 32–2** VALUE trial design. (After Mann J, Julius S. The Valsartan Antihypertensive Long-Term Use Evaluation [VALUE] trial of cardiovascular events in hypertension. Rationale and design. Blood Press 7:176-183, 1998. © Taylor & Francis; used with permission.) HCTZ, hydrochlorothiazide.

---

**Box 32–1** Risk Factors and Disease Factors in the VALUE Trial

**Risk Factors**
- Diabetes mellitus (defined as overnight fasting plasma glucose concentration >7.8 mmol/L [140 mg/dl] on at least two separate occasions or as chronic intake of hypoglycemic agents with or without occasional intake of insulin)
- Current smoking (defined as smoking at least 10 cigarettes/day on a regular basis for at least 5 years before inclusion in the study; if the patient has quit smoking, he or she will be considered a smoker if he or she stopped less than 12 months before inclusion)
- High total cholesterol (>6.2 mmol/L or >240 mg/dl); left ventricular hypertrophy (LVH) as per ECG (Sokolow-Lyon criteria or Cornell criteria); proteinuria (1+ or more on dipstick in a morning urine specimen)
- Serum creatinine >150 µmol/L (>1.7 mg/dl)

**Disease Factors**
- History of MI verified by Q-wave ECG and/or hospital records, and/or cardiovascular revascularization; coronary heart disease (CHD) verified by angiography and/or hospital records
- History of peripheral arterial occlusive disease, verified by angiography or Doppler or hospital records or statement of angiologist
- History of stroke, transient ischemic attack (TIA), verified by angiography or Doppler or PET or CT scan or persistent hemiparesis (stroke) or hospital records
- LVH with strain pattern (ST-segment depression)

(After Mann J, Julius S. The Valsartan Antihypertensive Longterm Use Evaluation [VALUE] trial of cardiovascular events in hypertension. Rationale and design. Blood Press 3:176-183, 1998. © Taylor & Francis; used with permission.)
ECG, electrocardiogram; MI; myocardial infarction; PET, positron emission tomography; CT, computed tomography.

## VALUE BASELINE DATA

VALUE enrolled a total of 15,314 patients at 947 centers in 31 countries, with the largest numbers of patients randomized in the United States (n = 3676), Germany (n = 1557), Italy (n = 1095), United Kingdom (n = 887), and France (n = 841).[30] The average age at randomization was 67.2 years, and more than 80% of patients were older than the age of 60.

There are a large number of women (6496) in the trial population, although the majority of patients (57.6%) are men. Some significant differences in baseline characteristics exist between the sexes: Women were on average 3.7 years older than the men (p <.0001) and had higher levels of SBP (p <.0001) and DBP (p <.0001). Average SBP was 3.9 mm Hg higher in the female group. Women also had lower serum creatinine levels (Table 32–1). Rates of diabetes mellitus were higher in women (p <.0001), but the rates of CHD were higher in the male population (p <.0001; Table 32–2).

The population was slightly overweight at randomization, with an average body mass index of 28.6 kg/m². Most patients (>92%) were taking antihypertensive medication at the time of randomization and were started on the treatment drug without a placebo run-in period. Hence, BP at the time of randomization was only moderately elevated, averaging 154.7/87.5 mm Hg. The high rate of patients already on treatment is in contrast to the populations in large-scale trials such as the Hypertension Optimal Treatment (HOT) study[8] or the Nordic Diltiazem (NORDIL) study,[3] in which 48% and 56%, respectively, of participants were untreated at the time of enrollment. Elevated SBP tended to be more prevalent than elevated DBP: 37.5% of patients had SBP >160 mm Hg but only 10.4% had DBP >100 mm Hg.

As seen in Table 32–2, the prevalence of CHD (45.8%), high cholesterol (33.0%), type 2 diabetes mellitus (31.7%), smoking (24.0%), proteinuria (22.5%), cerebrovascular disease (19.8%), LVH including bundle branch block and strain (18.3%), and peripheral arterial disease (13.9%) were high in

**Table 32-1** Demographic and Biochemical Characteristics at Randomization of Patients in the VALUE Trial*

| Variable | Men (n = 8816) | Women (n = 6497) | Total (n = 15,314) |
|---|---|---|---|
| Age (years) | 65.7 ± 8.1 | 69.4 ± 7.6 | 67.2 ± 8.1 |
| Body mass index (kg/m²) | 28.5 ± 4.5 | 28.8 ± 5.6 | 28.6 ± 5.0 |
| Previously treated (%) | 92.2 | 92.6 | 92.3 |
| SBP (mm Hg) | 153.0 ±18.9 | 156.9 ± 18.9 | 154.7 ± 19.0 |
| DBP (mm Hg) | 87.8 ± 10.7 | 87.1 ± 10.9 | 87.5 ± 10.8 |
| Heart rate (beats/min) | 71.4 ± 10.9 | 73.7 ± 10.3 | 72.4 ± 10.7 |
| Race (%) | | | |
|   Caucasian | 89.3 | 88.9 | 89.1 |
|   Black | 3.7 | 5.2 | 4.3 |
|   Oriental | 4.0 | 2.8 | 3.5 |
|   Other | 3.0 | 3.1 | 3.1 |
| Serum potassium (mmol/L) | 4.4 ± 0.4 | 4.4 ± 0.5 | 4.4 ± 0.5 |
| Serum sodium (mmol/L) | 140.6 ± 2.6 | 140.7 ± 2.7 | 140.7 ± 2.7 |
| Serum creatinine (μmol/L)[†] | 108.1 ± 23.2 | 91.5 ± 21.2 | 101.1 ± 23.8 |
| Serum uric acid (μmol/L) | 393 ± 93 | 347 ± 92 | 373 ± 95 |
| Serum cholesterol (mmol/L)[‡] | 5.3 ± 1.0 | 5.9 ± 1.0 | 5.5 ± 1.0 |
| Serum glucose (mmol/L)[§] | 6.8 ± 2.7 | 6.9 ± 2.9 | 6.9 ± 2.8 |

After Kjeldsen S, Julius S, Brunner H, et al. [for the VALUE Trial Group]. Characteristics of 15,314 hypertensive patients at high coronary risk. The VALUE Trial. Blood Press 10:83-91, 2001. © Taylor & Francis; used with permission.
*Values are mean ± standard deviation or percentage of total.
[†]Conversion factor from μmol/L to mg/dl: 88.4.
[‡]Conversion factor from mmol/L to mg/dl: 38.664.
[§]Conversion factor from ml/L to mg/L: 181.8.

**Table 32-2** Additional Risk Factors and Disease History of Patients Randomized in the VALUE Trial*

| | Men (n = 8816) | Women (n = 6497) | Total (n = 15313) |
|---|---|---|---|
| **Qualifying Risk Factors** | | | |
| Serum cholesterol >6.2 mmol/L (>240 mg/dl) | 23.9 | 45.2 | 33.0 |
| Diabetes mellitus (mostly type 2) | 29.8 | 34.2 | 31.7 |
| Current smoking | 26.7 | 20.3 | 24.0 |
| Proteinuria | 22.1 | 23.2 | 22.5 |
| LVH[†] | 9.2 | 16.3 | 12.2 |
| Serum creatinine >150 μmol/L (>1.7 mg/dl) | 4.7 | 2.1 | 3.6 |
| **Qualifying Disease Factors** | | | |
| CHD | 53.5 | 35.4 | 45.8 |
| Stroke or TIA | 21.1 | 17.9 | 19.8 |
| Peripheral arterial disease | 15.5 | 11.6 | 13.9 |
| LVH with strain pattern | 6.2 | 6.0 | 6.1 |

After Kjeldsen S, Julius S, Brunner H, et al. [for the VALUE Trial Group]. Characteristics of 15,314 hypertensive patients at high coronary risk. The VALUE Trial. Blood Press 10:83-91, 2001. © Taylor & Francis; used with permission.
*Results are percentage of total.
[†]LVH including left bundle branch block.
LVH, left ventricular hypertrophy; CHD, coronary heart disease; TIA, transient ischemic attack.

the VALUE population. The high number of patients with diabetes is notable. This is a consequence of the use of diabetes as qualifying risk factor in VALUE, which was not the case for the LIFE trial (12% diabetic patients).[31] The number of patients with diabetes in VALUE (4854) is greater than the total number enrolled into the four trials that established ARBs as first-line treatment in diabetic hypertensive patients: Reduction of Endpoints in NIDDM with the Angiotensin II Antagonist Losartan (RENAAL; n = 1513),[32] Irbesartan Diabetic Nephropathy Trial (IDNT; n = 1715),[33] Irbesartan Microalbuminuria Type 2 (IRMA-2; n = 690),[34] and

Microalbuminuria Reduction with Valsartan (MARVAL; n = 332).[35] However, reduced renal function is of low frequency in VALUE (3.6%), indicating that patients are at earlier stages of the disease than the patients enrolled into the diabetes trials. This may well affect the benefits from treatment. In contrast to LIFE, in which there was a major reduction in mortality in the diabetic subgroup,[36] neither IRMA-2, IDNT, nor RENAAL showed mortality benefits from ARB treatment.[37] This has been attributed to the less advanced stages of renal disease in LIFE,[38] similar to the population in VALUE, as well as limited power of the diabetes trials related to small patient numbers.

The proportion of patients with LVH in VALUE is smaller than in LIFE, in which LVH was an inclusion criterion. There is a relatively high proportion of smokers (24%). Cross-sectional studies of the population indicate that the percentage of smokers is lower among patients with higher BP.[39] This can be interpreted as a greater success with smoking cessation attempts in patients with higher BP,[40] or alternatively, that smoking is particularly lethal in this population.[41]

An estimate of the total cardiovascular risk in the VALUE trial population puts patients at a similar risk level to the populations in the Swedish Trial in Old Patients with Hypertension (STOP),[42] or HOPE.[5] The main risk factors in the two STOP trials were age and hypertension, and there was a low proportion of CHD events. In contrast, the main risk in HOPE was due to history of CHD in about 80% of patients, almost half with treated hypertension, and one third with type 2 diabetes. Against these differences, it will be interesting to analyze the effects of the VALUE algorithm on the number of CHD events in VALUE.

An important issue in evaluating the trial results and their impact on future antihypertensive treatment patterns is to what extent the VALUE population is representative of patients at high cardiovascular risk in general.[43] Only the risk profile, but not the demographic characteristics, differed between the patients enrolled in VALUE and those who were

screened but who did not meet the criteria for high risk of CHD.[30] From the data available it seems reasonable to consider the randomized patients in the trial to reflect the risk profile of other hypertensive populations at high coronary risk.

## BLOOD PRESSURE CONTROL IN VALUE

VALUE is primarily an antihypertensive prevention trial, and thus it is important to achieve adequate BP reduction in both treatment arms and to ensure that there are no relevant differences between the degree of BP lowering between the patients receiving different treatments. Such differences between the treatment arms were responsible for the doubts about the possible BP-independent effects of ramipril in HOPE[7] and for the limited analysis that could be made from the SCOPE data.[12]

Because the VALUE trial is ongoing at the point of writing, there is no information on differences between the treatment arms. Data are currently available on BP control in 13,449 patients for whom there are complete BP records at baseline, who had in-study BP measurements at each point up to 24 months and for whom information about treatment status at 24 months is available. Similar data for BP control at 30 months are available for 12,570 patients,[44] but no analysis of the

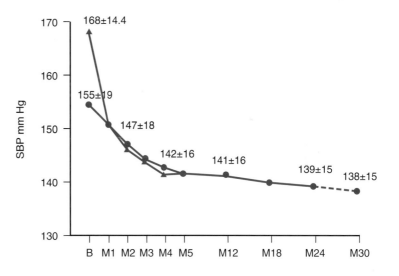

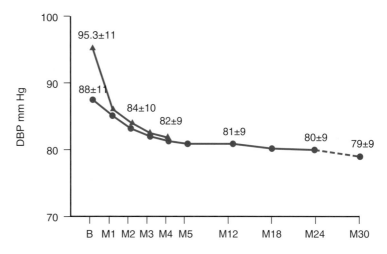

Figure 32-3 Blood pressure trends in the cohort of 13,449 patients who had baseline and 24-month data (dots) and in 12,750 patients who also had 30-month data (broken line). Triangles denote the pressures in 1051 patients who were not receiving antihypertensive treatment before the enrollment. (From Julius S, Kjeldsen SE, Brunner H, et al. VALUE trial: Long-term blood pressure trends in 13,449 patients with hypertension and high cardiovascular risk. Am J Hypertens 16:544-548, 2003. © Elsevier Ltd; used with permission.)

utilization of blinded drugs at 30 months has been published. Of the total of 15,314 patients, 1864 were not included in the 24-month report, mostly because of discontinuation for reasons other than death (n =1012) and because of death (n = 524).

A majority of patients with 24-month BP data (n = 12,398, 92.2%) received antihypertensive drugs prior to enrollment and were rolled over directly to study drugs. The baseline status of these patients gives an insight into how hypertension is treated in routine clinical practice. Among these patients, only 21.9% subjects had controlled (<140 mm Hg) SBP at baseline compared with a DBP control (<90 mm Hg) rate of 54.2%. These findings confirm other observations that practicing physicians are more attuned to controlling the diastolic than SBP.[6,45-49]

The baseline BP of the 1051 patients who were not receiving treatment prior to enrollment was 14.6/8.4 mm Hg higher than in the patients previously treated. However, both the treated and untreated groups achieved similar BP levels as early as at month 4, and by month 6 the BP readings of both groups were identical (Figure 32–3).

BP was rapidly reduced in the VALUE population during the initial medication up-titration phase over the first 6 months of the trial, but there was very little additional reduction between months 6 and 12, particularly in SBP. The response to this situation was a strong concerted effort at all organizational levels of the trial to improve control of BP, SBP in particular. Through an extensive information and monitoring effort, emphasizing the BP goals and the simple algorithm to achieve these goals, major reductions in SBP were achieved over the next 18 months. Between months 12 and 24, the reduction in SBP/DBP was 1.3/1.0 mm Hg ($p$ <.0001/.0001). A further reduction of 1.0/1.0 mm Hg was achieved between months 24 and 30 ($p$ <.0001/.0001; see Figure 32–3).

The percentage of patients with controlled SBP (<140 mm Hg) at baseline was 21.9%, rising to 59.5% at month 24 and to 62.2% at month 30. In addition to the 62.2% with controlled SBP, an additional 20.6% had "nearly controlled" (≥140 to <150 mm Hg) SBP and 9.3% had "inadequate" SBP control (≥150 to <160 mm Hg; Figure 32–4). Only 7.9% had "uncontrolled" systolic hypertension (≥160 mm Hg). The DBP control increased from 54.2% at baseline to 88.6% at month 24 and 90.2% at month 30. An additional 6.5% had "near control" values (≥90 to <95 mm Hg), and only 1.3% of patients had "inadequate" (≥95 to <100 mm Hg) or "uncontrolled" DBP (≥100 mm Hg; see Figure 32–4).

A comparison with other hypertension trials further illuminates the success of the SBP initiative. VALUE has achieved substantially greater reductions in BP than most published studies. The average achieved SBP level in VALUE is 16 mm Hg lower than in the STOP 2[2] and NORDIL[3] studies, 12 mm Hg lower than in Syst-Eur,[50] and 11 mm Hg lower than in CAPPP.[1] A comparison of the 30-month BP reduction rates in VALUE with final results of the Systolic Hypertension in the Elderly Program (SHEP)[51] and HOT[8] studies shows the rates in VALUE to be a couple of mm Hg lower than in the other two trials and similar to values reported at the end of the INSIGHT (Intervention as a Goal in Hypertension Treatment) study.[52] Finally, in perhaps the most relevant trial, LIFE, average SBPs at study end were 6 mm Hg higher in the losartan and 7.3 mm Hg higher in the atenolol group than the average SBP achieved at the 30-month point in VALUE.[10] The SBP control rate in the LIFE study was 48%, compared with a control rate of 62.2% in VALUE at 30 months. This is in spite of the use of a stricter definition of control in VALUE than in LIFE (<140 mm Hg vs ≤140 mm Hg).

At first glance, the BP reductions in the ALLHAT trial appear greater than in VALUE: In ALLHAT, SBP in the chlorthalidone, amlodipine, and lisinopril groups, were 135.9, 137.1, and 138.4 mm Hg, respectively, at study end.[4] However, if the higher baseline SBPs in VALUE are taken into account (155.2 vs. 146.2 mm Hg in ALLHAT), the BP reduction from baseline even in the most successful patient group in ALLHAT, the chlorthalidone group, was 10.3 mm Hg compared with a 16–mm Hg decrease at month 30 in the VALUE study. Thus, VALUE is on track to become one of the most successful trials ever conducted in terms of achieved reductions in BP.

The VALUE titration scheme aimed to achieve BP control by titrating to the maximum dose of monotherapy before adding hydrochlorothiazide and other medications. This is in contrast to LIFE, in which hydrochlorothiazide was added as a second step, before increasing doses of losartan or atenolol.[53] Such differences in trial design limit the comparisons of treatment status to BP control between trials. The number of patients still on monotherapy at month 24 in VALUE was

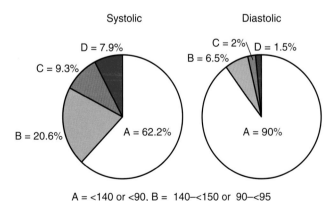

A = <140 or <90, B = 140–<150 or 90–<95
C = 150–<160 or 95–<100, D = 60 or 100

**Figure 32–4** Proportion of patients reaching different blood pressure targets in VALUE at 30 months. (After Julius S, Kjeldsen SE, Brunner H, et al. VALUE trial: Long-term blood pressure trends in 13,449 patients with hypertension and high cardiovascular risk. Am J Hypertens 16:544-548, 2003. © Elsevier Ltd; used with permission.)

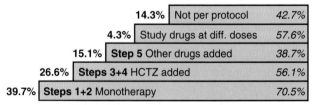

**Figure 32–5** Drug utilization and blood pressure control at 24 months in the VALUE study (n = 13,449). Numbers in **bold** are percentages of all patients at various drug steps. Numbers in *italics* are the percentages of patients whose blood pressure was controlled (<140/90 mm Hg) within each category. (After Julius S, Kjeldsen SE, Brunner H, et al. VALUE trial: Long-term blood pressure trends in 13,449 patients with hypertension and high cardiovascular risk. Am J Hypertens 16:544-548, 2003. © Elsevier Ltd; used with permission.)

5342 or 39.7% (Figure 32–5).[44] This is higher than in the differently designed LIFE trial, where only 9% to 10% of patients were on monotherapy at the end of the trial, but comparable with other large-scale trials. In the ALLHAT trial, 49.6% of patients were still receiving monotherapy at year 3,[54] and 37% of participants were still on single drug at the 5-year visit.[54] The corresponding figure at the end (median treatment period 4.1 years) of ANBP2 was 66%.[9] In national surveys, the proportion of treated hypertensive patients that receive monotherapy is typically 60% to 70%.[47]

A majority of the VALUE patients on monotherapy (70.5%) had their BP controlled, but almost one third of the patient group had inadequate BP control (≥140/90 mm Hg). Most of these inadequately controlled patients had acceptable DBP but elevated SBP, further illustrating the greater difficulties with controlling SBP than DBP.

The VALUE study protocol stipulated hydrochlorothiazide as the first added-on medication, and at month 24, 66.3% of patients were receiving either this combination or monotherapy. Further permitted add-on drugs were used in 15.1% of the population. In an additional 4.3% of patients, the physicians used drugs defined by the protocol but in different doses from those stipulated. A small number of patients (6.3%) received added drugs not foreseen by the protocol.

At the time of the analysis, there was clearly room for further improvement in the utilization of study medications. The control rates in the monotherapy group indicate that diuretics should be added to the regimens for a substantial percentage of patients. In the diuretics-added group, approximately 44% of patients had BP above the treatment goals, indicating that the fifth step of the protocol should be used (see Figure 32–5). Despite these options for further efficacy increases, in all probability some study subjects will have systolic hypertension refractory to treatment. An indication of this is that although the group receiving additional therapy in addition to full doses of treatment drugs and diuretics (step 5) comprised a rather low (15.1%) percentage of the VALUE population, this group had a relatively high percentage of patients (61.3%) with BP still above target. However, the true proportion and the clinical characteristics of patients whose SBP is resistant to treatment will be known only after all therapeutic options for controlling BP provided by the VALUE protocol have been exhausted.

## SUMMARY

VALUE is expected to be one of the most important hypertension trials. After the LIFE study showed differences between the ARB losartan and the β-blocker atenolol beyond that which could be attributed to lowering of BP, VALUE is expected to resolve several outstanding issues and to establish whether such benefits are due to vascular and cardiac effects of angiotensin receptor blockade or whether the reduction in outcomes in LIFE can be attributed to negative effects in the β-blocker group. In selecting the calcium channel blocker amlodipine as the comparator in VALUE, the design has ensured a substance with neutral effects on insulin resistance and with reported stroke-protective and cardioprotective actions, as well as beneficial effects on ISH. This sets the scene for a trial designed to decide the issues of whether ARBs are stroke-protective and cardioprotective beyond their effects on BP.

It should be reemphasized that VALUE is a BP trial and as such has already been very successful. The impressive rates of BP control achieved at months 24 and 30 demonstrate what is possible when practitioners work in a structured environment, with the help of explicit BP goals, a simple algorithm to achieve these goals, and education of both patients and practitioners on the importance of achieving stringent BP control.

## References

1. Hansson L, Lindholm LH, Niskanen L, et al. Effect of angiotensin-converting-enzyme inhibition compared with conventional therapy on cardiovascular morbidity and mortality in hypertension: The Captopril Prevention Project (CAPPP) randomised trial. Lancet 353:611-616, 1999.
2. Hansson L, Lindholm LH, Ekbom T, et al. Randomised trial of old and new antihypertensive drugs in elderly patients: Cardiovascular mortality and morbidity the Swedish Trial in Old Patients with Hypertension-2 study. Lancet 354:1751-1756, 1999.
3. Hansson L, Hedner T, Lund-Johansen P, et al. Results of the Nordic Diltiazem (NORDIL) Study. Effects of calcium antagonist-based treatment versus diuretics and beta-blockers on cardiovascular morbidity and mortality in hypertension. Lancet 356:359-365, 2000.
4. ALLHAT Officers and Coordinators for the ALLHAT Collaborative Research Group. The Antihypertensive and Lipid-Lowering Treatment to Prevent Heart Attack Trial. Major outcomes in high-risk hypertensive patients randomized to angiotensin-converting enzyme inhibitor or calcium channel blocker vs diuretic: The Antihypertensive and Lipid-Lowering Treatment to Prevent Heart Attack Trial (ALLHAT). JAMA 288: 2981-2997, 2002.
5. The Heart Outcomes Prevention Evaluation Study Investigators. Effects of an angiotensin-converting-enzyme inhibitor, ramipril, on cardiovascular events in high-risk patients. N Engl J Med 342:145-153, 2000.
6. The sixth report of the joint national committee on prevention, detection, evaluation, and treatment of high blood pressure. Arch Intern Med 157:2413-2446, 1997.
7. Svensson P, de Faire U, Sleight P, et al. Comparative effects of ramipril on ambulatory and office blood pressures: A HOPE Substudy. Hypertension 38:E28-E32, 2001.
8. Hansson L, Zanchetti A, Carruthers SG, et al. Effects of intensive blood-pressure lowering and low-dose aspirin in patients with hypertension: Principal results of the Hypertension Optimal Treatment (HOT) randomised trial. Lancet 351: 1755-1762, 1998.
9. Wing LM, Reid CM, Ryan P, et al. A comparison of outcomes with angiotensin-converting-enzyme inhibitors and diuretics for hypertension in the elderly. N Engl J Med 348:583-592, 2003.
10. Dahlöf B, Devereux RB, Kjeldsen SE, et al; tLIFE study group. Cardiovascular morbidity and mortality in the Losartan Intervention For Endpoint reduction in hypertension study (LIFE): A randomised trial against atenolol. Lancet 359: 995-1003, 2002.
11. Kjeldsen SE, Dahlöf B, Devereux RB, et al. Effects of losartan on cardiovascular morbidity and mortality in patients with isolated systolic hypertension and left ventricular hypertrophy: A Losartan Intervention for Endpoint Reduction (LIFE) substudy. JAMA 288:1491-1498, 2002.
12. Lithell H, Hansson L, Skoog I, et al. The Study on Cognition and Prognosis in the Elderly (SCOPE): Principal results of a randomised double-blind intervention trial. J Hypertens 21:875-886, 2003.

13. Kjeldsen SE, Julius S, Hedner T, et al. Stroke is more common than myocardial infarction in hypertension: Analysis based on 11 major randomised intervention trials. Blood Press 10: 190-192, 2001.

14. Poirier L, Cleroux J, Nadeau A, et al. Effects of nebivolol and atenolol on insulin sensitivity and haemodynamics in hypertensive patients. J Hypertens 19:1429-1435, 2001.

15. Schiffrin EL, Park JB, lntengan HD, et al. Correction of arterial structure and endothelial dysfunction in human essential hypertension by the angiotensin receptor antagonist losartan. Circulation 101:1653-1659, 2000.

16. Schiffrin EL, Park JB, Pu Q. Effect of crossing over hypertensive patients from a beta-blocker to an angiotensin receptor antagonist on resistance artery structure and on endothelial function. J Hypertens 1:71-78, 2002.

17. Tzemos N, Lim P, McDonald TM. Valsartan improves vascular endothelial dysfunction in essential hypertension. Am J Hypertens 14:66A, 2001.

18. Mann J, Julius S. The Valsartan Antihypertensive Long-term Use Evaluation (VALUE) trial of cardiovascular events in hypertension. Rationale and design. Blood Press 3:176-183, 1998.

19. Ligtenberg G, Blankestijn PJ, Oey PL, et al. Reduction of sympathetic hyperactivity by enalapril in patients with chronic renal failure. N Engl J Med 340:1321-1328, 1999.

20. Struck J, Muck P, Trubger D, et al. Effects of selective angiotensin II receptor blockade on sympathetic nerve activity in primary hypertensive subjects. J Hypertens 6:1143-1149, 2002.

21. Lithell HO. Insulin resistance and diabetes in the context of treatment of hypertension. Blood Press Suppl 3:28-31, 1998.

22. Nag S. Protective effect of flunarizine on blood-brain barrier permeability alterations in acutely hypertensive rats. Stroke 22: 1265-1269, 1991.

23. Jiang GC, Iwanov V, Moulds RF. Increased sensitivity to inhibition by nifedipine of responses of the mesenteric artery bed of the SHRSP to noradrenaline is not dependent on alpha1-adrenoceptor subtypes. J Cardiovasc Pharmacol 26:79-84, 1995.

24. Napoli C, Salomone S, Godfraind T, et al. 1,4-Dihydropyridine calcium channel blockers inhibit plasma and LDL oxidation and formation of oxidation-specific epitopes in the arterial wall and prolong survival in stroke-prone spontaneously hypertensive rats. Stroke 30:1907–1915, 1999.

25. Hoff PT, Tamura Y, Lucchesi BR. Cardioprotective effects of amlodipine in the ischemic-reperfused heart. Am J Cardiol 64:10H-16H, 1989.

26. Gross GJ, Farber NE, Pieper GM. Effects of amlodipine on myocardial ischemia-reperfusion injury in dogs. Am J Cardiol 64:941-1001, 1989.

27. Taylor SH. The efficacy of amlodipine in myocardial ischemia. Am Heart J 118:1123-1126, 1989.

28. Sobey CG, Dalipram RA, Woodman OL. Allopurinol and amlodipine improve coronary vasodilatation after myocardial ischaemia and reperfusion in anaesthetised dogs. Br J Pharmacol 108:342-347, 1993.

29. Julius S, Kjeldsen SE, Weber M, et al. Outcomes in hypertensive patients at high cardiovascular risk treated with regimens based on valsartan or amlodipine: The VALUE randomised trial. Lancet 363:2022-2031, 2004.

30. Kjeldsen SE, Julius S, Brunner H et al.;[for the VALUE Trial Group]. Characteristics of 15,314 hypertensive patients at high coronary risk. The VALUE Trial. Blood Press 10:83-91, 2001.

31. Dahlöf B, Devereux RB, Julius S, et al. Characteristics of 9194 patients with left ventricular hypertrophy: The LIFE study. Losartan Intervention For Endpoint Reduction in Hypertension. Hypertension 32:989-997, 1998.

32. Brenner BM, Cooper ME, de Zeeuw D, et al.; RENAAL Study Investigators. Effects of losartan on renal and cardiovascular outcomes in patients with type 2 diabetes and nephropathy. N Engl J Med 345:861-869, 2001.

33. Lewis EJ, Hunsicker LG, Clarke WR, et al.; Collaborative Study Group. Renoprotective effect of the angiotensin-receptor antagonist irbesartan in patients with nephropathy due to type 2 diabetes. N Engl J Med 345:851-860, 2001.

34. Parving HH, Lehnert H, Brochner-Mortensen J, et al.; Irbesartan in Patients with Type 2 Diabetes and Microalbuminuria Study Group. The effect of irbesartan on the development of diabetic nephropathy in patients with type 2 diabetes. N Engl J Med 345:870-878, 2001.

35. Viberti G, Wheeldon NM; MARVAL Study Investigators. Microalbuminuria reduction with valsartan in patients with type 2 diabetes mellitus. A blood pressure independent effect. Circulation 106:672-678, 2002.

36. Lindholm LH, Ibsen H, Dahlöf B, et al.; LIFE Study Group. Cardiovascular morbidity and mortality in patients with diabetes in the Losartan Intervention For Endpoint reduction in hypertension study (LIFE): A randomised trial against atenolol. Lancet 359:1004-1010, 2002.

37. Pourdjabbar A, Lapointe N, Rouleau JL. Angiotensin receptor blockers: Powerful evidence with cardiovascular outcomes? Can J Cardiol 18:7A-14A, 2002.

38. Ruilope L. Proven benefits of angiotensin receptor blockers in the progression of renal disease. Eur Heart J 5:C9-C12, 2003.

39. Mundal R, Kjeldsen SE, Sandvik L, et al. Predictors of 7-year changes in exercise blood pressure: Effect of smoking, physical fitness and pulmonary function. J Hypertens 15:245-249, 1997.

40. Kjeldsen SE, Dahlof B, Devereux RB, et al. Lowering of blood pressure and predictors of response in patients with left ventricular hypertrophy. The LIFE Study. Am J Hypertens 13:899-906, 2000.

41. Omvik P. How smoking affects blood pressure. Blood Press 5:71-77, 1996.

42. Dahlöf B, Lindholm LH, Hansson L, et al. Morbidity and mortality in the Swedish Trial in Old Patients with Hypertension (STOP-Hypertension). Lancet 338:1281-1285, 1991.

43. Ramsay LE, Williams B, Johnston GD, et al. Guidelines for management of hypertension: Report of the third working party of the British Hypertension Society. J Hum Hypertens 13:569-592, 1999.

44. Julius S, Kjeldsen SE, Brunner H, et al. "VALUE" trial: Long-term blood pressure trends in 13,449 patients with hypertension and high cardiovascular risk. Am J Hypertens 16:544-548, 2003.

45. Joffres MR, Ghadirian P, Fodor JG, et al. Awareness, treatment, and control of hypertension in Canada. Am J Hypertens 10:1097-1102, 1997.

46. De Henaw S, De Bacquer D, Fonteyne W, et al. Trends in the prevalence, detection, treatment and control of arterial hypertension in the Belgian adult population. J Hypertens 16: 277-284, 1998.

47. Colhoun HM, Dong W, Poulter NR. Blood pressure screening, management and control in England: Results from the health survey for England 1994. J Hypertens 16:747-752, 1998.

48. Kastarinen MJ, Salomaa VV, Variainen EA, et al. Trends in blood pressure levels and control of hypertension in Finland from 1982 to 1997. J Hypertens 16:1379-1387, 1998.

49. Coca Payeras A. Evolucion del control del la hipertension arterial en espana. Resultados del Estudio Controlpres 98. Hipertension 15:298-308, 1998.

50. Staessen JA, Fagard R, Thijs L, et al. Randomised double-blind comparison of placebo and active treatment for older patients with isolated systolic hypertension. Lancet 350:757-764, 1997.

51. SHEP Cooperative Research Group. Prevention of stroke by antihypertensive drug treatment in older persons with isolated systolic hypertension. Final results of the systolic hypertension in the elderly program (SHEP). JAMA 265:3255-3264, 1991.

52. Brown MJ, Palmer CR, Castaigne A, et al. Morbidity and mortality in patients randomised to double-blind treatment with a long-acting calcium-channel blocker or diuretic in the

International Nifedipine GITS study: Intervention as a Goal in Hypertension Treatment (INSIGHT). Lancet 356:366-372, 2000.

53. Dahlöf B, Devereux R, de Faire U, et al. The Losartan Intervention For Endpoint reduction (LIFE) in Hypertension study: Rationale, design, and methods. The LIFE Study Group. Am J Hypertens 7:705-713, 1997.

54. Cushman WC, Ford CE, Cutler JA, et al. ALLHAT Collaborative Research Group. Success and predictors of blood pressure control in diverse North American settings: The antihypertensive and lipid-lowering treatment to prevent heart attack trial (ALLHAT). J Clin Hypertens 4:393-404, 2002.

# Main Results from VALUE

Sverre E. Kjeldsen, Stevo Julius, Michael A. Weber, Pelle Stolt

The first results of the Valsartan Antihypertensive Long-term Use Evaluation (VALUE) were reported in mid-2004 and are summarized here.[1,2] The rationale of the trial and design were discussed in the previous chapter, together with details of baseline characteristics of the enrolled patients. Because the main results of VALUE were published so recently, no subgroup analyses or further details are available at the time of writing. The data are presented here in a brief format.

A total of 15,245 randomized patients were included in the analysis, and 68 patients in nine centers were excluded because of good clinical practice deficiencies. Only 90 patients (0.6%) were lost to follow-up. The mean duration of exposure to study medication was 3.6 years in both treatment groups. The median daily doses were 151.7 mg of valsartan and 8.5 mg of amlodipine. As indicated in the 30-month analysis, the majority of patients in both groups were on combination treatment by the end of the trial. Fewer patients in the valsartan-based group (27.0%) than in the amlodipine group (35.3%) remained on monotherapy during the course of the study.

Blood pressure control rates in VALUE were among the highest reported for an outcome trial: 56% of patients in the valsartan group and 62% of patients in the amlodipine group reached target blood pressure levels below 140/90 mm Hg. These numbers should be viewed in light of the fact that although 92% of patients were being treated for hypertension at baseline and most were receiving more than one drug, only 22% had their blood pressures controlled at that time.

## MAJOR OUTCOMES

However, particularly during the first 6 months' treatment-adjustment period, the effects of the amlodipine-based regimen in VALUE were more pronounced than those of the valsartan-based regimen (Figure 33–1). Differences in systolic blood pressure were 4.0/2.1 mm Hg after 1 month and were reduced to 1.5/1.3 mm Hg after 1 year ($p < .001$ between groups). Despite these differences, there was no difference in the primary outcome of composite cardiac endpoints between the valsartan and amlodipine groups (Figure 33–2).

The primary endpoint occurred in 10.6% of patients in the valsartan arm and in 10.4% of patients in the amlodipine arm: hazard ratio 1.04, 95% confidence interval (CI) .94-1.15, $p = .49$. Rates of all-cause death were not different between the groups: hazard ratio 1.04, 95% CI 0.94-1.14, $p = .45$. Of the secondary endpoints, fatal and nonfatal myocardial infarction occurred in more patients on valsartan-based therapy (hazard ratio 1.19, 95% CI 1.02-1.38, $p = .02$), although it should be noted that this was due to lower rates of nonfatal events with amlodipine (hazard ratio 1.22, 95% CI 1.04-1.44, $p = .02$) and that the rates of fatal events were not different between the treatment groups (hazard ratio 1.04, 95% CI 0.74-1.47, $p = .81$). There was a trend toward fewer heart failure hospitalizations in the valsartan group (hazard ratio 0.89, 95% CI 0.77-1.03, $p = .12$). Stroke rates were not significantly different between the groups (hazard ratio 1.15, 95% CI 0.98-1.35, $p = .08$).

Notably, new-onset diabetes developed in 690 patients on valsartan-based and in 845 patients on amlodipine-based regimens (odds ratio 0.77; 95% CI 0.69-0.86, $p < .0001$ (Figure 33–2). This is the first demonstration of benefits in the prevention of diabetes with an angiotensin receptor blocker as compared with a metabolically neutral antihypertensive agent.

The early differences in blood pressure appeared to have influenced the overall outcomes. During the treatment-adjustment period of the first 6 months, odds ratios tended to favor amlodipine-based treatment for all endpoints. This corresponded to the time of greatest differences in blood pressure between treatments. As blood pressure differences diminished during the following months, there was attenuation in odds ratios (Figure 33–3). For the endpoint of hospital admission for heart failure, there was a trend in favor of valsartan during the last 4 years.

## ADVERSE EVENTS

Tolerability was good in both groups, but the most common adverse event, edema, including peripheral edema, was twice as common in amlodipine-treated patients as in valsartan-treated patients. Hypokalemia was more common in the amlodipine group. Although they occurred with low frequency, dizziness, headache, and diarrhea were more frequently reported in patients on valsartan-based regimens. Discontinuation rates from adverse events were significantly lower with valsartan-based treatment (13.4% compared with 14.5%, $p = .045$). It should be noted that the rates of adverse events were somewhat higher than those reported previously for these drugs, almost certainly reflecting the influence of the agents that were added to the primary treatments.

## THE ROLE OF BLOOD PRESSURE

VALUE emphasizes the importance of prompt blood pressure control in hypertensive patients at high cardiovascular risk. This was reinforced by further analyses of the correlation between early blood pressure response and outcomes.[2] By 1 month of treatment, 32.6% of 7543 valsartan patients had systolic blood pressure higher than 160 mm Hg, a significantly greater proportion ($p < .0001$) than the 23.0% of 7504 taking amlodipine; at 6 months, the corresponding proportions (13.2% vs. 8.3%) were also different ($p < .0001$). Event rates in these uncontrolled patients in the valsartan and amlodipine groups, respectively, were as follows: at 1 month, 12.1% of 2456 and 12.3% of 1725 for the combined cardiac endpoints, 5.4% and 5.0% for stroke, and 12.7% and 13.7% for death; at

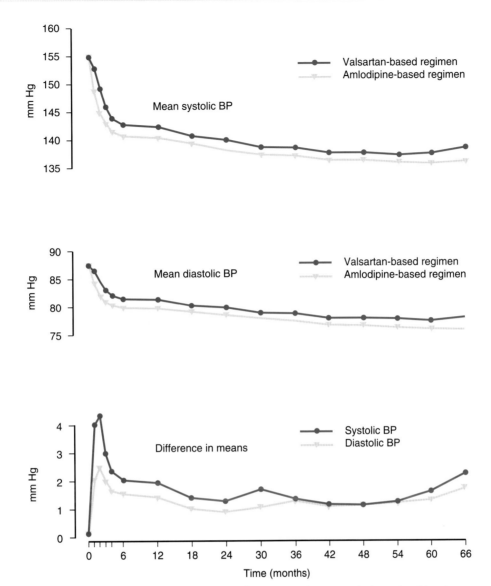

**Figure 33–1** Systolic and diastolic blood pressure (BP) and differences (valsartan-amlodipine) in blood pressure between the treatment groups during follow-up. (From Julius S, et al., Lancet 363:2022-2031, 2004.)

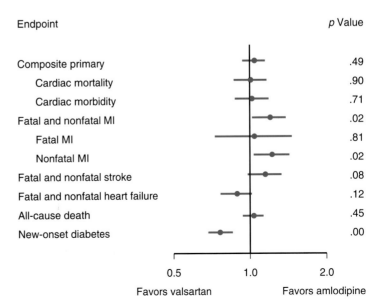

**Figure 33–2** Hazard ratios (odds ratio for new-onset diabetes) and 95% confidence intervals for the primary and secondary endpoints in VALUE, as well as for all-cause death and new-onset diabetes. MI, myocardial infarction.

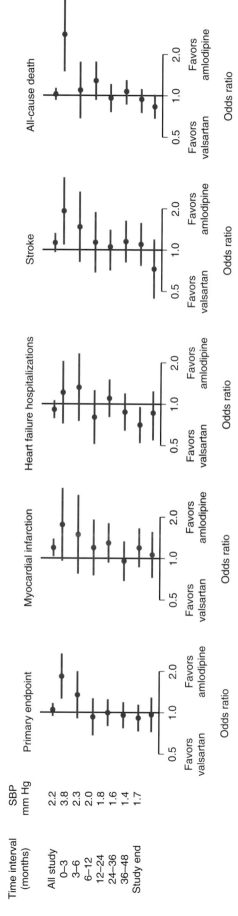

**Figure 33-3** Blood pressure differences between the treatment groups together with odds ratios and 95% confidence intervals in groups randomized to valsartan or amlodipine during consecutive time periods in the study. Data are presented for the primary endpoint, the secondary endpoints, and all-cause death. (From Julius S, et al., Lancet 363:2022-2031, 2004.)

6 months, 11.7% of 951 and 11.5% of 601 for the combined cardiac endpoints, 5.9% of 953 and 7.0% of 603 for stroke, and 12.4% of 964 and 15.5% of 606 for death. Event rates during the remainder of the study for patients in this hypertensive stratum were closely similar in the valsartan and amlodipine arms. These numbers indicate that achieved blood pressure rather than drug type was the main determinant of event rates in this high-risk population.

## ACHIEVING CONTROL

Because the aim of VALUE was to achieve control of blood pressure by 6 months, it was assessed whether reaching this goal affected outcomes for each of the drug groups. Hazard ratios for subsequent clinical events in patients with systolic blood pressure <140 mm Hg at 6 months were compared with those whose systolic blood pressure was not controlled, within each treatment group. Control of blood pressure was a powerful determinant for the primary and secondary endpoints (except myocardial infarction), as well as for all-cause death. The differences between the two groups were so minor that the data could be pooled to show the overall role of blood pressure control in optimizing outcomes independent of drug type (Table 33–1). These findings provide evidence to validate the target recommendations (140/90 mm Hg) in hypertension guidelines from both Europe and the United States for this high-risk population.

## TESTING THE HYPOTHESIS: SERIAL MEDIAN MATCHING

The early blood pressure differences between treatment groups in VALUE made the overall results difficult to interpret. In an attempt to test the hypothesis in a controlled population, the technique of serial median matching was applied to the dataset at 6 months. Although a posthoc analysis, this method should be considered in plans for new studies and perhaps even tested in previously reported studies with substantial blood pressure inequalities. The method selected the most

**Table 33–1** Controlled Compared with Noncontrolled Patients: Endpoint

| Endpoint | Hazard Ratio (95% CI) |
|---|---|
| Fatal and nonfatal cardiac events | 0.75 (0.67–0.83)* |
| Fatal and nonfatal stroke | 0.55 (0.46–0.64)* |
| All-cause death | 0.79 (0.71–0.88)* |
| Myocardial infarction | 0.86 (0.73–1.01) |
| Heart failure hospitalizations | 0.64 (0.55–0.74)* |

After Weber MA, et al., Lancet 363:2047-2049, 2004.
*Hazard ratios for events in controlled compared with noncontrolled patients. After Weber MA, et al., Lancet 363:2047-2049, 2004.

median patient (based on systolic blood pressure) within the valsartan group and paired this patient with one from the amlodipine group matched for systolic blood pressure (within 2 mm Hg); age; sex; and the presence or absence of previous coronary disease, stroke, and diabetes. The process was repeated until all eligible patients were included. In this way, 5006 comprehensively matched valsartan/amlodipine cohort pairs (a total of 10,012 patients) were created, with a mean systolic blood pressure of 139.9 mm Hg in each drug group. The analysis of this patient population, where essentially patients at the high and low extremes of achieved blood pressure were excluded, showed a nonsignificant trend in favor of valsartan for the combined cardiac endpoint. The rates of fatal and nonfatal myocardial infarction, stroke, and mortality were close to identical in both treatment groups. However, admission to hospital for heart failure was significantly ($p = 0.040$) lower with valsartan (Figure 33–4).

## SUMMARY

The results from VALUE underscore that in hypertensive patients at high risk for cardiac events, achieving blood pressure targets is a highly important determinant of outcomes. Most of these patients should be on combination therapies. If blood pressure is controlled, VALUE indicated that valsartan-

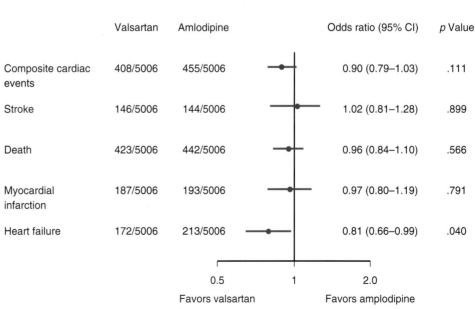

**Figure 33–4** Hazard ratios for major study endpoints in patients on valsartan- or amlodipine-based therapies for events occurring after a baseline translocated to the 6-month point of the trial and after treatment adjustment designed to achieve blood pressure control. Data are shown for 5006 treatment cohort pairs matched by systolic blood pressure; age; sex; and the presence or absence of prior coronary disease, stroke, and diabetes. (From Weber MA, et al., Lancet 363:2047-2049, 2004.)

| | Valsartan | Amlodipine | | Odds ratio (95% CI) | p Value |
|---|---|---|---|---|---|
| Composite cardiac events | 408/5006 | 455/5006 | | 0.90 (0.79–1.03) | .111 |
| Stroke | 146/5006 | 144/5006 | | 1.02 (0.81–1.28) | .899 |
| Death | 423/5006 | 442/5006 | | 0.96 (0.84–1.10) | .566 |
| Myocardial infarction | 187/5006 | 193/5006 | | 0.97 (0.80–1.19) | .791 |
| Heart failure | 172/5006 | 213/5006 | | 0.81 (0.66–0.99) | .040 |

0.5     1     2.0

Favors valsartan      Favors amplodipine

based therapy is associated with a reduced risk for heart failure hospitalizations and is otherwise closely similar to amlodipine for other cardiovascular endpoints. Furthermore, regardless of blood pressure, valsartan-based treatment was associated with a significantly reduced number of cases of new-onset diabetes. These data were obtained with a valsartan dose range of 80 to 160 mg, which is less than the 160 to 320 mg now recommended in the United States and is associated with the more complete blockade of the renin-angiotensin system. The findings of VALUE are likely to influence future guidelines for blood pressure control and drug selection in high-risk patients.

## References

1. Julius S, Kjeldsen SE, Weber MA, et al. Outcomes in hypertensive patients at high cardiovascular risk treated with regimens based on valsartan or amlodipine: The VALUE randomized trial. Lancet 363:2022-2031, 2004.
2. Weber MA, Julius S, Kjeldsen SE, et al. Blood pressure dependent and independent effects of antihypertensive treatment on clinical events in the VALUE Trial. Lancet 363:2047-2049, 2004.

# Chapter 34

# Clinical Outcome Trials of Hypertension with Angiotensin Receptor Blockers

## Shawna D. Nesbitt, Stevo Julius

Recent basic science research has revealed that the renin-angiotensin system (RAS) plays an integral role in the development and propagation of hypertension and related to target organ damage. Agents that block the deleterious effects of the RAS on the vasculature have the potential to ameliorate the cardiovascular consequences of hypertension. Angiotensin receptor blockers (ARBs) are the most recently developed class of antihypertensive agents. They are distinguished their high tolerability without compromising efficacy in blood pressure (BP) reduction. Another class of closely related agents, angiotensin-converting enzyme (ACE) inhibitors, has been shown to protect against renal, cardiac, and cerebrovascular morbidity and mortality associated with hypertension. Although ACE inhibitors are effective in blocking the RAS through limiting the conversion of angiotensin I to angiotensin II, ARBs may be even more selective in blocking the effects of angiotensin on the vasculature and target organs because they act directly on the angiotensin receptors. In this chapter we review the important completed and ongoing clinical outcome trials of ARBs in hypertension (Table 34–1).

## CARDIOVASCULAR OUTCOME TRIALS

The effect of lowering BP on cardiovascular mortality has been demonstrated with various antihypertensive agents. Meta-analysis of the early studies, including primarily β-blockers and diuretics, showed a 25% reduction in stroke and 14% reduction in coronary heart disease (CHD).[1] As newer therapies become available, it is necessary to study their effects on cardiovascular outcomes. Every agent in the ARB class has been shown to be efficacious in lowering BP but there is only one completed trial of cardiovascular outcomes with an ARB. Other important studies are in progress.

### LIFE Study

The Losartan Intervention for Endpoint Reduction in Hypertension Study (LIFE) is the only completed hypertension trial of an ARB to assess cardiovascular outcomes.[2] This landmark study was designed to establish whether the ARB losartan reduces cardiovascular morbidity and death to a greater extent than the β-blocker atenolol despite equal BP reduction. In this double-blinded, randomized, parallel group trial, 9193 participants aged 55 to 80 years with essential hypertension and left ventricular hypertrophy (LVH) by electrocardiographic criteria were assigned to losartan-based or atenolol-based antihypertensive treatment and followed for 4 years. BP was decreased by 30.2/16.6 (± standard deviation 18.5/10.1) mm Hg and 29.1/16.8 (± 19.2/10.1) mm Hg in the losartan and atenolol groups, respectively.

The cardiovascular event rate was 23.8 per 1000 patient-years in the losartan group and 27.9 per 1000 patient-years in the atenolol group, resulting in a 13% reduction in the losartan group. Assignment to losartan was associated with a 25% reduction in stroke and a 25% reduction in new-onset diabetes. These results were equally robust in the subset of participants who had no clinical evidence of vascular disease. Among the 1195 diabetics in the LIFE study, losartan reduced the primary endpoint by 24%, cardiovascular mortality by 37%, congestive heart failure (CHF) by 41%, and total mortality by 39% compared with atenolol.[3] In a subsequent analysis of the 533 African American participants in the LIFE study, although BP reduction was similar in both treatment groups, the greater reduction in cardiovascular endpoints was seen in the atenolol group, not the losartan group. This finding must be viewed with caution because the sample size was small.[4] Nevertheless, the LIFE study suggests that with equivalent BP control, treatment with losartan prevents more cardiovascular morbidity and death than atenolol, thus conferring benefits beyond BP reduction alone.

The largest ongoing outcome trials of ARBs are the Valsartan Antihypertensive Long-term Use Evaluation (VALUE) and the Ongoing Telmisartan Alone and in Combination with Ramipril Global Endpoint Trial (ONTARGET).[5-7] They have different foci, and their results will be instrumental in determining future standards of hypertension care.

### VALUE Study

The VALUE study is a multinational, multicenter, double-blind, randomized, prospective, active-controlled parallel group trial comparing the effects of two treatment modalities on BP and cardiovascular endpoints in hypertension.[5,6] The ARB valsartan at doses of 80 or 160 mg/day is compared with a calcium antagonist amlodipine at doses of 5 or 10 mg/day. Additional treatment may be given as open-label hydrochlorothiazide, 12.5 or 25 mg/day. If needed, additional antihypertensive agents may be added, with the exception of calcium antagonists, ACE inhibitors, or other ARBs, to reach a target BP of <140/90 mm Hg.

Patients are randomized to one of the treatment regimens and followed for 4 to 6 years or until 1450 primary events occur. The study is an endpoint-driven trial, and it has been calculated that 14,400 enrolled patients are needed to detect a 15% between-group difference in cardiovascular outcomes with a 90% power and a significance level of $p < .05$ during an average treatment period of 5 years.

VALUE includes men and women ≥50 years of age from 31 countries of any racial background with high-risk cardiovascular profile and systolic and/or diastolic hypertension. Those who were previously untreated must have seated systolic blood pressure (SBP) of 160 to 210 mm Hg and diastolic

Table 34–1 Clinical Trials of Angiotensin Receptor Blockers

| Trial | Expected Completed | Agents Used in Trial | Sample Size | Study Group | Length of Study (years) | Primary Endpoint | % Reduction ARB vs. Comparator Drug |
|---|---|---|---|---|---|---|---|
| LIFE | 2002 | Losartan vs. atenolol | 9193 | HTN + LVH | 4 | CVD mortality and morbidity | 13% |
| VALUE | 2004 | Valsartan vs. amlodipine | 15,314 | HTN | 5 | CVD morbidity and mortality | No difference in CV events |
| ONTARGET | 2007 | Telmisartan vs. ramipril vs. telmisartan + ramipril | 23,400 | High CV risk | 4 | CVD mortality and morbidity | In progress |
| TRANSCEND | 2007 | Telmisartan vs. placebo | 6000 | ACE intolerant, high CV risk | 4 | CVD mortality and morbidity | In progress |
| HOMED-BP | 2009 | ARB vs. ACE vs. CCB | 9000 | HTN | 7 | Fatal/nonfatal MI, fatal/nonfatal stroke, CVD death | In progress |
| TROPHY | 2005 | Candesartan vs. placebo | 809 | Prehypertension | 4 | Incidence of HTN | In progress |
| SCOPE | 2002 | Candesartan vs. placebo | 4964 | Elderly HTN | 2.5 | CV events, cognitive decline, dementia | No difference in CV events; stroke reduced by 23%; no difference in cognition |
| PRoFESS | 2007 | Telmisartan + ASA/dipyridamole vs. telmisartan + ASA + clopidogrel vs. placebo + dipyridamole/ASA vs. placebo + clopidogrel + ASA | 15,500 | Recent ischemic stroke, ≥55 years old | 4 | Recurrent stroke | In progress |
| IRMA | 2001 | Irbesartan 150 mg vs. irbesartan 300 mg vs. placebo | 590 | DM type 2, HTN | 2 | Diabetic nephropathy | 44% with irbesartan 150 mg; 68% with irbesartan 300 mg |
| RENAAL | 2001 | Losartan vs. placebo | 1513 | HTN, DM type 2 | 3.5 | Doubling serum creatinine, ESRD, and death | 16% by intent-to-treat analysis; 22% by per protocol analysis; 25% reduction in doubling serum creatinine; 28% reduction in ESRD |
| IDNT | 2001 | Irbesartan vs. amlodipine vs. placebo | 1713 | HTN, renal disease + proteinuria, DM type 2 | 2.6 | Doubling serum creatinine, ESRD, and death | 20% reduction with irbesartan compared with placebo; 23% reduction with irbesartan amlodipine |

ARB, angiotensin receptor blocker; HTN, hypertension; LVH, left ventricular hypertrophy; CVD, cardiovascular disease; CV, cardiovascular; ACE, angiotensin-converting enzyme; CCB, calcium channel blocker; MI, myocardial infarction; ASA, acetylsalicylic acid (aspirin); DM, diabetes mellitus; ESRD, end-stage renal disease.

blood pressure (DBP) <115 mm Hg; or SBP <210 mm Hg and DBP 95 to 115 mm Hg. For those patients already on antihypertensive treatment, the SBP should be <210 mm Hg and DBP <115 mm Hg; there is no lower BP limit for entry. These patients are then rolled over to one of the two treatment arms without a placebo run-in period, while discontinuing previous drugs.

The primary outcome in this study is time to first cardiac morbid or mortal event. Cardiac mortality is defined as sudden cardiac death, fatal acute myocardial infarction (MI), death during or post-percutaneous transluminal coronary angioplasty (PTCA) or post-coronary artery bypass graft (CABG), death due to CHF, and evidence of recent acute MI on autopsy. Cardiac morbidity is defined as new or chronic CHF requiring hospitalization, nonfatal acute MI, emergency thrombolysis, or any other interventional procedure performed to prevent a full-blown MI. Secondary outcomes include all-cause mortality, cardiac mortality or morbidity, cardiac morbidity with worsening of chronic stable angina or unstable angina, routine interventional procedures, potentially lethal arrhythmias, syncope or near-syncope, stroke, silent MI, and end-stage renal failure.

A total of 15,313 patients were randomized into the study at the close of recruitment in Novermber 1999. The key feature of the VALUE study is that it is the first to directly compare these two vastly different classes of antihypertensives on cardiac mortality and morbidity.

## ONTARGET Study

ONTARGET is designed to compare the effects of the ARB telmisartan, the ACE inhibitor ramipril, and the combination of ramipril and telmisartan on cardiovascular morbidity and mortality in high-risk patients similar to the Heart Outcomes Prevention Evaluation (HOPE) study participants.[7] This international, multicenter study of 23,400 participants is intended to include 35% diabetics and to have a significant recruitment from Asian countries. The study participants are aged ≥55 years and have a history of coronary artery disease, stroke or recent transient ischemic attack, peripheral vascular disease or diabetes mellitus with target organ damage, ankle brachial index of <0.8, or LVH. The study drugs are given in addition to other antihypertensive medications, thus the baseline BP <140/90 mm Hg. Recruitment was completed in June 2003 and the trial will be completed in 2007. ONTARGET is not a "classical" hypertension trial because the participants are not all hypertensive and stage 2 hypertensives (BP >160/100 mm Hg) will be excluded. Rather, this trial is more specifically designed to study the benefit of reducing the activity of the RAS on cardiovascular disease in high-risk patients, including stage 1 hypertensives. As in the HOPE study, BP will likely be lowered in these individuals regardless of hypertensive status. ONTARGET will attempt to discern the difference between the benefits of ACE inhibitors alone and those seen with ARBs alone and whether there is an advantage to combining of the two drug classes.

The related Telmisartan Randomized Assessment Study in ACE-I Intolerant Patients with cardiovascular disease (TRANSCEND) study will assess the effects of telmisartan compared with placebo on cardiovascular events in 6000 high-risk patients who are intolerant of ACE inhibitors.[7]

## HOMED-BP Study

The only completed trial that attempted to define an optimal BP goal for patients was the Hypertension Optimal Treatment (HOT) trial, which utilized a dihydropyridine calcium channel blocker–based therapy in all treatment groups.[8,9] The Hypertension Objective Treatment based on Measurement by Electrical Devices of Blood Pressure (HOMED-BP) study is a Japanese study of 9000 untreated essential hypertensives aged 40 to 78 years with home BPs of ≥135/85 mm Hg. HOMED-BP is designed to determine an optimal target BP level based on home self-measured BPs and the optimal initial antihypertensive agent to prevent cardiovascular events. It is a 2×3 factorial randomized controlled trial conducted with a prospective randomized open-blinded endpoint (PROBE) design. The participants will be randomized to an antihypertensive regimen based on a calcium antagonist, ACE, or ARB and to one of two levels of target home BP: 125 to 134/80 to 84 mm Hg or ≤125/80 mm Hg. Any drug within a randomized class of agents may be prescribed by the physician. Thus this trial is a study of class effect, rather than a specific drug. When the data are collected in the outpatient clinics, they will be transmitted to a host computer, which will determine the necessity for additional therapy or dose increments to reduce the bias in the study. The home BPs in this trial will be collected using an automated device. The primary outcome is a composite of nonfatal stroke, nonfatal MI, and cardiovascular death. The planned average follow-up is 7 years.

## TROPHY Study

The Trial of Preventing Hypertension (TROPHY) study is a randomized, placebo-controlled trial designed to assess the effects of treatment with the ARB candesartan cilexetil on the progression to hypertension in individuals with high-normal BP.[10] Between June 1999 and June 2001, 809 individuals were randomized to placebo or low-dose candesartan for 2 years followed by 2 years of placebo. They were qualified for the study by the average of three seated BP measurements taken on three separate clinic visits by an automated device (OMRON 706). Untreated individuals with SBPs between 130 and 139 mm Hg and DBPs between 85 and 89 mm Hg were included in the study. The primary outcome of the trial is the incidence of hypertension determined by clinic SBP >140 mm Hg and/or DBP >90 mm Hg on three visits during the study follow-up or SBP >160 mm Hg systolic and/or DBP >100 mm Hg on one occasion; secondary outcomes include the development of target organ damage requiring BP treatment.

## CEREBROVASCULAR OUTCOME TRIALS

In the LIFE study, the greatest benefit of losartan compared with atenolol in hypertensives with LVH was in stroke. Thus there is evidence that ARBs offer a benefit beyond BP reduction in cerebrovascular disease.

The Study on Cognition and Prognosis in the Elderly (SCOPE) is a prospective, double-blind, randomized, parallel group study designed to assess whether candesartan-based therapy in elderly hypertensives confers a reduction in cardiovascular events, cognitive decline, and dementia.[11] SCOPE included 4964 patients aged 70 to 89 years with SBP of 160 to

179 mm Hg and/or DBP 90 to 99 mm Hg with a Mini Mental State Examination (MMSE) score ≥24. Patients were assigned to candesartan or placebo in addition to other open label antihypertensive medications. The BP reduction in the study was 21.7/10.8 mm Hg in the candesartan group and 18.5/9.2 mm Hg in the control group, a net difference of 3.2/1.6 mm Hg. The MMSE score was equally well maintained in both the candesartan and placebo groups. The reduction in cardiovascular events was not statistically significant, but the reduction in nonfatal stroke was 27.8% ($p = .04$) and in overall stroke 23.6% ($p = .056$) with candesartan-based therapy compared with placebo.

The benefit of ACE inhibitors in the reduction of secondary stroke has been demonstrated in the Perindopril Protection against Recurrent Stroke Study (PROGRESS) utilizing perindopril in combination with indapamide.[12,13] However the individuals in this study were not all hypertensive. Another trial that may have further implications regarding the use of ARBs in the prevention of secondary stroke is the Prevention Regimen for Effectively Avoiding Second Strokes (PRoFESS) trial. In this trial telmisartan in combination with antiplatelet agents is compared with placebo with antiplatelet agents to assess the most effective regimen for preventing recurrent stroke. This is a randomized, parallel group, multinational, double-blind, double-dummy, active, and placebo-controlled study, which has a 2×2 factorial design with a target enrollment of 15,500 patients. The study arms include (1) dipyridamole extended-release/aspirin + telmisartan; (2) clopidogrel + aspirin + telmisartan; (3) dipyridamole extended-release/aspirin + placebo; and (4) clopidogrel + aspirin + placebo. The only entry criteria are that the individual must be male or female ≥55 years of age and have had an ischemic stroke within the previous 90 days. Thus the population will not be restricted to hypertensives, but it is likely that many of the participants will be hypertensive. The primary endpoint of PRoFESS is time to the first recurrent stroke. The secondary endpoints are composite endpoint of "vascular events" defined as time to first recurrent stroke (fatal or nonfatal), MI (fatal or nonfatal), or vascular death; major hemorrhagic events; and composite outcome of first occurrence of recurrent stroke or major hemorrhagic event. The study launched in 2003 and will be completed in 2007.

## RENAL OUTCOME TRIALS

The effectiveness of ARB treatment in renal disease has been demonstrated in several trials. Losartan, irbesartan, and valsartan have all been shown to reduce the progression of renal disease in type 2 diabetic hypertensives. In the Irbesartan for MicroAlbuminuria in type 2 Diabetes study (IRMA-2), 590 patients with 20 to 200 μg/min albuminuria, normal serum creatinine, hypertension (BP >135/85 mm Hg), and type 2 diabetes were randomized to placebo or irbesartan 150 or 300 mg daily for 2 years.[14] The participants were all Caucasian, 70% male, with mean age 58 years, mean baseline BP 153/90 mm Hg, baseline albuminuria 55 μg/min, glomerular filtration rate (GFR) 110 ml/min, and HgbA$_{1c}$ 7.2%. The 24-hour trough BP was 145/84, 143/84, and 142/84 mm Hg on placebo; 150 mg irbesartan; and 300 mg irbesartan, respectively. After adjustment for baseline microalbuminuria and the BP achieved during the study, the risk reduction for diabetic nephropathy was 44% in the 150-mg irbesartan group

and 68% in the 300-mg irbesartan group compared with placebo. In the placebo group, albuminuria decreased 2%, whereas it decreased 24% with the 150-mg irbesartan group and 38% with the 300-mg irbesartan group. Although the difference was not statistically significant, the rate of nonfatal cardiovascular disease was 8.7% in the placebo and 4.5% in the 300-mg irbesartan groups.

In the Reduction in Endpoints in NIDDM with the Angiotensin II Antagonist Losartan (RENAAL) trial of 1513 participants with type 2 diabetes and nephropathy, the study participants were randomized with losartan (50-100 mg) or placebo and treated with other antihypertensive agents to lower BP to <140/90 mm Hg.[15] This 4.5-year planned study was discontinued 1 year early because of the mounting evidence that blockade of the RAS conferred cardioprotective benefits in patients with renal disease. The study participants had a mean age of 60 years, 38% were female, and 48% were Caucasian. In the losartan group, 27% were taking 50 mg, whereas while 71% were taking 100 mg. BP was lowered from 152/82 versus 153/82 mm Hg at baseline to 140/74 versus 142/74 mm Hg at the study endpoint with losartan and placebo, respectively. The primary endpoint of doubling of serum creatinine, progression to end-stage renal disease (ESRD) or death was reduced in the losartan group by 16% in the intention-to-treat analysis and by 22% in the patients on treatment analysis. There was a 25% reduction in doubling of serum creatinine and 28% reduction in ESRD with losartan. Despite the −4/−2–mm Hg BP difference at the end of year 1 favoring losartan, the results remained statistically significant even after adjustment. Of note, 87% to 90% of the participants in the losartan group were also treated with a calcium channel blocker, which did not appear to adversely affect the benefits of the ARB treatment. Losartan prevented one case of ESRD for every 16 patients treated during the 3.5 years of the study.[16]

In RENAAL there were no significant differences between the groups in the composite endpoints of cardiovascular mortality and morbidity. However, first hospitalization for CHF was significantly reduced with losartan, and the number of MIs was less in the losartan group although not statistically significant.

The Irbesartan Diabetic Nephropathy Trial (IDNT) included 1713 participants age 30 to 70 years with type 2 diabetes; proteinuria (>900 mg/day); creatinine 1.0 to 3.0 mg/dl (women) and 1.2 to 3.0 mg/dl (men); hypertension (SBP >135 mm Hg or DBP >85 mm Hg or taking antihypertensives); and no recent active cardiovascular disease.[17,18] Participants were randomized to irbesartan 300 mg, amlodipine 10 mg, or placebo and followed for a mean of 2.6 years. Baseline mean age was 59 years; baseline BP was 160/87 mm Hg; creatinine was 1.7 mg/dl; proteinuria was 4 g/24 hours; and 30% had experienced at least one cardiovascular disease event >6 months before entering the study. The BP goal was 135/85 mm Hg. However, the mean achieved BP was 140/77 mm Hg in the placebo group. The relative risk of the primary endpoint, including doubling of serum creatinine, progression to ESRD or death, was reduced by 20% in the irbesartan group relative to the placebo group and by 23% relative to the amlodipine group. There was no significant difference between the amlodipine and placebo groups. The unadjusted relative risk of doubling serum creatinine in the irbesartan group was 33% lower than placebo and 37% lower than the amlodipine group. The unadjusted relative risk of ESRD was 23% lower in the irbesartan group than in the other groups. The effects of irbesartan remain significant after adjustment for BP differences between the groups. Based on this study, over 3 years, to prevent one patient from having a primary event, it is necessary to treat 15 patients with irbesartan 300 mg or 10 patients to prevent one patient from doubling serum creatinine.

There was no difference in all-cause mortality or composite cardiovascular disease endpoints among the study groups in IDNT. However, there were some differences in individual cardiovascular outcomes. Irbesartan reduced CHF 35% compared with amlodipine and 27% compared with placebo, whereas amlodipine compared with placebo showed no difference in CHF. Interestingly amlodipine significantly reduced nonfatal MI compared with placebo, yet irbesartan did not show the same effect. There were no differences in stroke between the treatment groups.[19] Small trials of other ARBs demonstrate similar effects on microalbuminuria, thus this may well be a class effect.[20]

An extensive series of clinical trials is being conducted to compare telmisartan with valsartan, losartan, amlodipine, and ramipril in patients at increased risk of target organ damage. Nine clinical studies will examine the effects of telmisartan in 5000 hypertensive patients with isolated systolic hypertension, type 2 diabetes, obesity, LVH, or renal disease. All of the studies will be conducted using state-of-the-art technology, including such techniques as ambulatory BP monitoring and magnetic resonance imaging.[21] This program will also investigate the effects of an ARB on key surrogate markers of target organ damage.

The earliest outcome trials of ARBs have shown an emerging role for this new class of antihypertensives in preventing cardiovascular, cerebrovascular, and renal outcomes in hypertension. The trials currently in progress may further expand the role of ARBs in hypertensive therapy.

## References

1. Collins R, Peto R, MacMahon S, et al. Blood pressure, stroke, and coronary heart disease. Part 2, Short-term reductions in blood pressure: Overview of randomized drug trials in their epidemiologic context. Lancet 335:1534-1535, 1990.
2. Dahlöf B, Devereux RB, Kjeldsen SE, et al. Cardiovascular morbidity and mortality in the Losartan Intervention For Endpoint reduction in hypertension study (LIFE): A randomised trial against atenolol. Lancet 359(9311):995-1003, 2002.
3. Lindholm LH, Ibsen H, Dahlöf B, et al. Cardiovascular morbidity and mortality in patients with diabetes in the Losartan Intervention for Endpoint reduction in hypertension study (LIFE): A randomised trial against atenolol. Lancet 359(9311):1004-1010, 2002.
4. Julius S, Alderman MH, Beevers G, et al. Cardiovascular risk reduction in hypertensive black patients with left ventricular hypertrophy: The LIFE Study. J Am Coll Cardiol 43(6):1047-1055, 2004.
5. Mann J, Julius S. The Valsartan Antihypertensive Long-term Use Evaluation (VALUE) trial of cardiovascular events in hypertension. Rationale and design. Blood Press 7(3):176-183, 1998.
6. Kjeldsen SE, Julius S, Brunner H, et al. Characteristics of 15,314 hypertensive patients at high coronary risk. The VALUE trial. The Valsartan Antihypertensive Long-term Use Evaluation. Blood Press 10(2):83-91, 2001.
7. Unger T. The ongoing Telmisartan alone and in combination with ramipril global endpoint trial program. Am J Cardiol 91(Suppl 10A):28G-34G, 2003.
8. Fujiwara T, Nishimura T, et al. Rationale and design of HOMED-BP Study: Hypertension objective treatment based on measurement by electrical devices of blood pressure study. Blood Press Monit 7(1):77-82, 2002.
9. Fujiwara T, Matsubara M, Ohkubo T, et al. Study design of HOMED-BP: Hypertension objective treatment based on measurement by electrical devices of blood pressure. Clin Exp Hypertens 25(3):143-144, 2003.
10. Nesbitt SD, Julius S. Prehypertension: A possible target for antihypertensive medication. Curr Hypertens Rep 2(4):356-361, 2000.
11. Lithell H, Hansson L, Skoog I, et al. The Study on Cognition and Prognosis in the Elderly (SCOPE): Principal results of a randomized double-blind intervention trial. J Hypertens 21(5):875-886, 2003.
12. PROGRESS Collaborative Group. Randomised trial of a perindopril-based blood-pressure-lowering regimen among 6105 individuals with previous stroke or transient ischaemic attack. Lancet 358(9287):1033-1041, 2001.
13. Staessen JA, Wang J. Blood-pressure lowering for the secondary prevention of stroke. Lancet 358(9287):1026-1027, 2001.
14. Parving HH, Lehnert H, Brochner-Mortensen J, et al. The effect of irbesartan on the development of diabetic nephropathy in patients with type 2 diabetes. N Engl J Med 345(12):870-878, 2001.
15. Brenner BM, Cooper ME, de Zeeuw D, et al. Effects of losartan on renal and cardiovascular outcomes in patients with type 2 diabetes and nephropathy. N Engl J Med 345(12):861-869, 2001.
16. Bloomgarden ZT. Angiotensin II receptor blockers and nephropathy trials. Diabetes Care 24(10):1834-1838, 2001.
17. Lewis EJ, Hunsicker LG, Clarke WR, et al. Renoprotective effect of the angiotensin-receptor antagonist irbesartan in patients with nephropathy due to type 2 diabetes. N Engl J Med 345(12):851-860, 2001.
18. Lewis EJ. The role of angiotensin II receptor blockers in preventing the progression of renal disease in patients with type 2 diabetes. Am J Hypertens 15(10 pt 2):123S-128S, 2002.
19. Berl T, Hunsicker LG, Lewis JB, et al. Cardiovascular outcomes in the Irbesartan Diabetic Nephropathy Trial of patients with type 2 diabetes and overt nephropathy. Ann Intern Med 138(7):542-549, 2003.
20. Viberti G, Wheeldon NM. Microalbuminuria reduction with valsartan in patients with type 2 diabetes mellitus: A blood pressure-independent effect. Circulation 106(6):672-678, 2002.
21. Weber M. The telmisartan programme of research to show telmisartan end-organ protection (PROTECTION) program. J Hypertens 21(Suppl 6):S37-S46, 2003.

# ACE Inhibitor Trials: Effects in Hypertension

**Irene Gavras, Haralambos Gavras**

The relationship between blood pressure (BP) levels and increased cardiovascular morbidity/mortality was recognized long ago. Oral antihypertensive drugs for chronic treatment of hypertension first became available in the 1950s with the appearance of reserpine, hydralazine, and methyldopa. A major advance was the introduction of thiazides in 1958, followed by the β-adrenergic blockers in the 1960s in the United Kingdom and the 1970s in the United States. As antihypertensive therapy became widespread, the benefits and adverse effects of various agents became a matter of debate: Although the treatment of malignant hypertension undoubtedly prolonged survival, the benefits of treating "benign" essential hypertension were less readily apparent, and there was a lingering notion that the age-related BP rise may be necessary to ensure adequate perfusion of vital organs. The Veterans Administration studies in 1967 and 1970[1,2] finally proved beyond doubt that successful BP lowering in essential hypertension could significantly decrease the rates of morbidity and mortality from heart failure, renal failure, stroke, and progression to malignant hypertension, although the rates of coronary events seemed to be less affected.

Several theories were proposed to explain this discrepancy between cardioprotection and protection of other target organs, including the fact that hypertension is one of several coronary risk factors and some antihypertensives tend to exacerbate other risk factors, offsetting the benefit of BP lowering. For example, thiazides and β-blockers tend to accentuate insulin resistance,[3,4] the defining feature of the metabolic syndrome, whose components are independent coronary risk factors.[5] Diuretics and direct vasodilators (including the dihydropyridine calcium channel blockers) also tend to trigger neurohormonal stimulation, and there is evidence that an activation of the renin-angiotensin system (RAS) increases cardiovascular risk.[6]

The angiotensin-converting enzyme (ACE) inhibitors that became available in the 1980s held the promise of overcoming this handicap. They were shown to be as effective as any other antihypertensive class in terms of BP-lowering capacity, with the added advantages of inhibiting the RAS and improving insulin sensitivity—the latter most likely attributable to their bradykinin-mediated actions.[7] Theoretically, the ACE inhibitors should be cardioprotective and nephroprotective, and both animal studies and clinical studies confirmed this.[8] It was noted that Black patients, who tend to have suppressed RAS and kinin systems, are less responsive to ACE inhibition in terms of both BP lowering and cardioprotection. Nevertheless, because of the mechanistic considerations indicated previously, it was postulated that most hypertensives would benefit from ACE inhibitors, at least to the same extent as, if not more than, from other antihypertensive drug classes.

Twenty years and several large controlled outcome trials later, this issue is still under debate. Many of these trials have shown better protection of target organs with an ACE inhibitor–based regimen than other antihypertensives, yet others, including the largest one, the Antihypertensive and Lipid-Lowering Treatment to Prevent Heart Attack Trial (ALLHAT), found either no difference or a better protection with a thiazide-based regimen.[9] The value of attaining BP control is well established and drugs from all antihypertensive classes are generally equally effective in lowering BP. It has been estimated that a 10– to15–mm Hg decrease in systolic BP should lead to a relative risk (RR) reduction of 15% for myocardial infarction (MI) and 40% for stroke.[10] Ideally, the magnitude of BP decrease and the level of BP attained should be identical in the ACE inhibitor–based arm and the comparator arm of each trial to permit a fair comparison of regimens, because a 3– to 4–mm Hg difference may translate into a 5% and 13% difference in RR of MI and stroke, respectively. In fact, small BP differences between treatment arms in outcome trials are common and may contribute to the results.

Following is a brief overview of some of the trials comparing ACE inhibitors with conventional therapies and an attempt to reconcile the discrepant results. Of note, several earlier trials in patients with congestive heart failure (CHF), cardiomyopathy, or post-MI, showed 20% to 25% reductions in RR of recurrent coronary events or hospitalizations for CHF. These trials, including the Survival and Ventricular Enlargement (SAVE) trial (testing captopril post-MI),[11] the Studies of Left Ventricular Dysfunction (SOLVD) trial (enalapril in CHF),[12] the Cooperative North Scandinavian Enalapril Survival Study (CONSENSUS) (enalapril in CHF),[13] the Acute Infarction Ramipril Efficacy (AIRE/AIREX) trial (ramipril in CHF),[14] and the Quinapril Ischemic Event Trial (QUIET) (quinapril in coronary disease)[15] enrolled patients selected for preexisting coronary disease or CHF. These trials are not included in this overview because the issue in question is whether ACE inhibitors have advantages over other drug classes in the treatment of hypertensive patients. Specifically, we evaluate studies testing whether antihypertensive treatment based on ACE inhibition compared with conventional therapies results in decreases in morbidity and mortality beyond those attributable to BP lowering per se (Box 35–1).

## THE HYPERTENSION TRIALS

The earliest prospective randomized outcome trials comparing ACE inhibitor–based antihypertensive therapy with therapy based on other drug classes were the Appropriate Blood Pressure Control in Diabetes (ABCD) trial[16] the Fosinopril versus Amlodipine Cardiovascular Events Trial (FACET),[17] and the UK Prospective Diabetes Study (UKPDS).[18] All three are small trials comprising a few hundred patients selected for the presence of type 2 diabetes and hypertension, a combination known to increase the risk of cardiovascular events and hence permit the detection of significant treatment-related differences with smaller numbers and in a shorter follow-up period.

**Box 35–1** Alphabetic List of Randomized Outcome Trials Comparing Morbidity/Mortality Reduction from BP Lowering with ACE Inhibitors Vs. Other Drug Classes (Year of Publication)

AASK (2002)—African American Study of Kidney Disease and Hypertension
ABCD (1998)—Appropriate Blood Pressure Control in Diabetics
ALLHAT (2002)—Antihypertensive and Lipid-Lowering Treatment to Prevent Heart Attack Trial
ANBP2 (2003)—Second Australian National Blood Pressure Trial
BPLT (2000)—Blood Pressure Lowering Treatment Trialists' Collaboration
CAPPP (1999)—Captopril Prevention Project
FACET (1998)—Fosinopril versus Amlodipine Cardiovascular Events Trial
HOPE (2000)—Heart Outcomes Prevention Evaluation
PROGRESS (2001)—Perindopril Protection Against Recurrent Stroke Study
STOP-2 (1999)—Swedish Trial in Old Patients with Hypertension, Part 2
UKPDS (1998)—United Kingdom Prospective Diabetes Study

The ABCD[16] compared enalapril with nisoldipine in 470 hypertensive diabetics. The nisoldipine arm was terminated early, when an interim evaluation revealed a risk ratio of 7.0 for MI in the nisoldipine arm compared with the enalapril arm. Although more detailed evaluation of additional cases in the next 2 years decreased this risk ratio to 4.2,[19] the conclusion remained the same (i.e., overall cardiovascular mortality was not statistically different), but the rate of MI was significantly lower with ACE inhibition. FACET[17] compared fosinopril with amlodipine in 380 hypertensive diabetics. Over the 3.5 years of follow-up, twice as many amlodipine patients experienced the combined cardiovascular endpoint of stroke, MI, or hospitalization for angina (27/191 vs. 14/189 on fosinopril, $p = .03$).

The UKPDS,[18] in contrast, showed no advantage of captopril compared with atenolol in preventing cardiovascular complications in diabetics. In a subset of 758 diabetic hypertensives allocated to "tight control" of BP with an average follow-up of 9 years, all cardiovascular endpoints, including total cardiovascular mortality (48/400 vs. 32/358, respectively), tended to be higher in the captopril than in the atenolol group, although none of the differences was statistically significant. What was highly significant was the overall 24% reduction in total endpoints in the group assigned to "tight control" (BP ≤150/≤85 mm Hg), which, by today's standards, seems inadequate. These results support the notion that the degree of BP control is the deciding factor for target organ protection, regardless of how it is achieved.

Subsequent trials, whose results are more directly applicable to the general population, comprised much larger numbers of hypertensive patients. The Scandinavian Captopril Prevention Project (CAPPP)[20] assigned 5492 patients to captopril and 5493 to a diuretic, β-blocker, or both. Overall, there

was no significant difference in the primary endpoints, including MI, although the rate of cardiovascular mortality tended to be lower with captopril (RR 23%, not significant) and the rate of stroke was higher (RR 25%, $p = .044$). In this, as in all subsequent large trials, the incidence of new-onset type 2 diabetes was significantly lower in the ACE inhibitor arm (RR 22%, $p = .04$). This trial has been criticized because the short-acting ACE inhibitor captopril was administered once daily, and the captopril arm had an average 2-mm higher systolic and diastolic BP throughout.

The Swedish Trial in Old Patients with Hypertension-2 (STOP-2)[21] comprised 6614 patients aged 70 to 84 years assigned to either an ACE inhibitor, a dihydropyridine calcium channel blocker, or a conventional (β-blocker and/or diuretic) arm. There was no difference in endpoints among the three arms, leading to the conclusion that the only important factor for the prevention of cardiovascular events was a decrease in BP.

In contrast, the Heart Outcomes Prevention Evaluation (HOPE) study,[22] which included 9297 persons older than age 55 with evidence of atherosclerotic cardiovascular disease (of whom 47% were nonhypertensives, but with other cardiovascular risk factors), found that treatment with ramipril decreased by 22% ($p < .001$) the combined RR of MI, stroke, or cardiovascular death, compared with placebo added to standard therapy. RR of stroke was decreased by 32%, of MI by 20%, of heart failure by 23%, of new-onset diabetes by 34%, of death from cardiovascular causes by 24%, and from any cause by 16% (all highly significant with $p < .001$).

Furthermore, a meta-analysis of 15 studies carried out by the Blood Pressure Lowering Treatment Trialists' Collaboration that collectively included 74,696 patients[23] compared treatment regimens based on different drug classes, including ACE inhibitors, as well as treatments of different intensity. Studies of ACE inhibitors and comparator regimens included more than 12,000 patients and revealed reductions in stroke by 30%, coronary heart disease (CHD) by 20%, and cardiovascular death by 26% with ACE inhibitors versus placebo. Both ACE inhibitors and placebo were added to standard therapy in these studies. In the same meta-analysis, treatment with calcium channel blockers was associated with a 19% higher risk of CHD and 18% higher risk of heart failure when compared with treatment with ACE inhibitors, both statistically significant. In this as in other meta-analyses,[24] calcium channel blockers seemed to have a small, nonstatistically significant advantage over other treatments in terms of protection from stroke.

The Perindopril Protection against Recurrent Stroke Study (PROGRESS)[25] was designed to evaluate the effect of the ACE inhibitor perindopril, alone or in combination with indapamide, on recurrence of stroke in 6105 patients who had suffered an ischemic or hemorrhagic stroke within the past 5 years. Of those, only half were hypertensive and all were receiving standard protective therapy, including antiplatelet agents, statins, and antihypertensives (other than ACE inhibitors) as needed. Patients were assigned to either perindopril alone, perindopril plus diuretic, or placebo; added to standard therapy; and followed for an average 3.9 years. Those on perindopril-based therapy had a 28% RR reduction in the primary outcome endpoint (i.e., total stroke), but this reduction was driven by the results in the perindopril plus diuretic group, who had a more pronounced

BP fall (12/5 mm Hg, compared with 5/3 mm Hg on the ACE inhibitor alone). It is also notable that among patients who did experience recurrent strokes, those taking perindopril were reported to have significantly lesser cognitive decline and dementia compared with those on standard therapy.[26]

Every RAS-inhibiting drug (whether ACE inhibitor or angiotensin II receptor blocker [ARB]), when first introduced, was compared for antihypertensive efficacy with a thiazide. The aforementioned large outcome trials were multinational collaborative studies conducted mostly in Europe and the Far East and comprising mainly Caucasian or Asian populations, who respond equally well or better to the RAS-inhibiting agent than to a diuretic. However, in Black patients the RAS-inhibiting drugs were found to be less effective for reasons that have remained largely elusive. An obvious explanation is that Blacks generally have a suppressed RAS. However, the same is true for elderly hypertensives, yet older patients respond readily to RAS-inhibiting treatment and, in fact, require on average lower doses of these drugs (as with most other drugs) than younger hypertensives.[27] Trials of the effects of RAS inhibition on the heart, such as SOLVD[12] and the Losartan Intervention For Endpoint Reduction in Hypertension (LIFE) trial,[28] have suggested that Black patients might not get the same degree of cardioprotection with these agents as Caucasian patients. However, the numbers of Black participants in these trials were not large enough to produce conclusive results, and the issue requires further study (see Chapter 56 for a discussion of hypertension in Blacks).

The National Institutes of Health (NIH)–sponsored African American Study of Kidney Disease and Hypertension (AASK)[29] was designed to evaluate the effects of BP lowering and of choice of antihypertensive drug on the rate of decline of renal function in African Americans (Blacks) with mild hypertensive (nondiabetic) renal disease. It evaluated 1094 patients randomized according to a 3×2 fractional design comparing higher (102-107 mm Hg) with lower (≤92 mm Hg) BP goals, as well as therapy based on ramipril, metoprolol, or amlodipine, with add-ons as needed to achieve goal BP. Surprisingly and contrary to previous experience, the level of BP attained did not affect rate of decline of renal function. However, the choice of antihypertensive class did: The ramipril group manifested reduced risk for the clinical composite outcome (reduction of GFR by ≥50% from baseline, end-stage renal disease, or death over 3 to 6 years of follow-up) by 22% versus metoprolol and by 38% versus amlodipine, both highly significant.

The ALLHAT trial,[9] also an NIH-sponsored outcome study, enrolled 42,416 hypertensives older than 55 years of age, of whom 35% were African Americans, making it the largest outcome study of antihypertensive treatment ever, and clearly the largest hypertension study involving African Americans. ALLHAT was designed to compare four drug classes—the diuretic chlorthalidone against the ACE inhibitor lisinopril, the calcium channel blocker amlodipine, and the peripheral $\alpha_1$–adrenoceptor blocker doxazosin. The α-blocker arm was interrupted prematurely, when an interim evaluation found that patients randomized to it had twice the rate of heart failure as the other three arms and because the probability of finding benefit beyond diuretic therapy was vanishingly small (a futility indication). After an average 4.9 years of follow-up, there was no difference between ACE inhibitor and calcium channel blocker versus diuretic treatments in the rate of primary outcome (CHD or MI) or of all-cause mortality.

Consistent with previous trials, there was a 30% lesser incidence of new-onset type 2 diabetes in the lisinopril group compared with the chlorthalidone group. However, the lisinopril group had a 20% higher RR of heart failure and 15% of stroke—the latter driven by a 40% higher RR in African Americans, who also had an average 4–mm Hg higher systolic BP throughout. Although subgroup analyses by age, race, and other clinical characteristics may help explain some of these results, the discrepancy between these findings and those of most previous trials will surely be debated for a long time.

The Second Australian National Blood Pressure Study (ANBP2)[30] enrolled an unselected hypertensive population of 6083 patients aged 65 to 84 years attending family practices throughout Australia. Comparison of ACE inhibitor–based or diuretic-based therapy over an average of 4.1 years, with add-on drugs as needed to normalize BP, revealed an advantage of the ACE inhibitor (any drug of this class) in overall reduction of the incidence of cardiovascular events or death by a modest, but statistically significant 11%, despite a slightly higher incidence of fatal strokes. For reasons difficult to explain, this result was driven by the 17% decrease in RR in men, whereas there was no discernible difference in women. The study population was mostly Caucasian.

## COMMENTARY AND SUMMARY

In spite of their disparate results, these trials have some things in common. One is that morbidity and mortality were affected first and foremost by the degree of BP reduction, and therefore insufficient BP lowering in one arm of a comparative trial would adversely affect the outcomes in that arm (e.g., the once-daily captopril dosing in CAPPP was probably inadequate for 24-hour BP control). A related issue is that of salt sensitivity and its impact on the reciprocal relationship between sodium retention and reactivity of the RAS.[31] The prevalence of salt-sensitive hypertension has been estimated at between 30% to 75%, depending on the population studied, with the higher percentages found in Black persons and in older individuals, because it is known to increase with age.[32] Hypertension in such patients is characterized by a suppressed RAS that is less reactive to salt depletion.

Clinical and experimental animal studies have established that a reciprocal relationship exists between the contributions of the RAS and sodium to the maintenance of a given BP level: When sodium intake is high, the RAS is suppressed and BP is maintained via salt-dependent mechanisms, whereas when sodium is removed, the RAS becomes activated and BP is maintained to a larger extent via angiotensin-induced vasoconstriction. Therefore, normotensive persons and normal- or high-renin hypertensive patients, when treated with diuretics and/or a low-salt diet, respond with activation of the RAS, which tends to limit the BP-lowering effect of salt depletion. Low-renin and salt-sensitive hypertensives are usually less responsive to treatment with RAS inhibition, but with vigorous diuresis to effectively remove a substantial proportion of their exchangeable sodium, these patients respond with a reactive hyperreninemia and exhibit a marked BP fall after blockade of the RAS.[27] This particularly efficacious combination of a diuretic with an RAS blocker has been used in many outcome trials that have demonstrated the target organ protection with ACE inhibitors or ARBs.

Existing knowledge of the pathophysiology of hypertension and its cardiovascular complications can thus reconcile some seemingly conflicting results: The STOP-2 trial in elderly Scandinavians used small doses of diuretics, which would fail to produce much reactive hyperreninemia—and the same would be true for amlodipine. Hence, these patients were not exposed to the detrimental influence of an activated RAS and were equally responsive to ACE inhibitors as to calcium channel blocker or diuretic/β-blocker treatment. On the other hand, Black patients in the ALLHAT trial had a poor BP response to lisinopril monotherapy. Combination with a diuretic, which would have enhanced the benefits of the ACE inhibitor, was not permissible on this protocol. A more detailed analysis and comparison of subgroups may explain some of these findings.

In general, trials in populations in whom the RAS is expected to contribute to high BP and target organ damage (younger, Caucasians, diabetics, or prediabetics) are more likely to show advantages of ACE inhibitors in protection against cardiovascular mortality, morbidity, and target organ damage. Populations with a suppressed and less reactive RAS seem to do as well or better on diuretic-based regimens. It is important to keep in mind that the best regimen is one that ensures optimal BP control with the least neurohormonal activation.

## References

1. Veterans Administration Cooperative Study Group on Antihypertensive Agents. Effects of treatment on morbidity in hypertension. Results in patients with diastolic blood pressures averaging 115 through 129 mm Hg. JAMA 202:1028-1034, 1967.
2. Veterans Administration Cooperative Study Group on Antihypertensive Agents. Effects of treatment on morbidity in hypertension. II. Results in patients with diastolic blood pressure averaging 90 through 114 mm Hg. JAMA 213:1143-1152, 1970.
3. Lewis PJ, Kohner EM, Petrie A, et al. Deterioration of glucose tolerance in hypertensive patients on prolonged diuretic treatment. Lancet 1:564-566, 1976.
4. Gress TW, Nieto FJ, Shahar E, et al. Hypertension and antihypertensive therapy as risk factors for type 2 diabetes mellitus. Atherosclerosis Risk in Communities Study. N Engl J Med 342:905-912, 2000.
5. Kaplan NM. The deadly quartet. Arch Int Med 149:1514-1520, 1989.
6. Gavras H, Brunner HR, Laragh JH. Renin and aldosterone and the pathogenesis of hypertensive vascular damage. Prog Cardiovas Dis 17:39-49, 1974.
7. Gavras I, Gavras H. Metabolic effects of angiotensin-converting enzyme inhibition: The role of bradykinin. Curr Opin Endocrinol Diab 9:323-328, 2002.
8. Gavras H. Angiotensin-converting enzyme inhibition and the heart. Hypertension 23:813-818, 1994.
9. The ALLHAT Officers and Coordinators for the ALLHAT Collaborative Research Group. Major outcomes in high-risk hypertensive patients randomized to angiotensin-converting enzyme inhibitor or calcium channel blocker vs diuretic. The antihypertensive and lipid-lowering treatment to prevent heart attack trial. JAMA 288:2981-2997, 2002.
10. Chalmers J, MacMahon S, Mancia G, et al. 1999 World Health Organization—International Society of Hypertension Guidelines for the management of hypertension. Guidelines subcommittee of the World Health Organization. Clin Exp Hypertens 21:1009-1060, 1999.
11. Pfeffer MA, Braunwald E, Moye LA, et al. Effect of captopril on mortality and morbidity in patients with left ventricular dysfunction after myocardial infarction. Results of the Survival and Ventricular Enlargement Trial. The SAVE Investigators. N Engl J Med 327:669-677, 1992.
12. The SOLVD Investigators. Effect of enalapril on mortality and the development of heart failure in asymptomatic patients with reduced left ventricular ejection fractions. N Engl J Med 327:685-691, 1992.
13. The CONSENSUS Trial Study Group. Effects of enalapril on mortality in severe congestive heart failure: Results of the Cooperative North Scandinavian Enalapril Survival Study (CONSENSUS). N Engl J Med 316:1429-1435, 1987.
14. Acute Infarction Ramipril Efficacy (AIRE) Study Investigators. Effect of ramipril on mortality and morbidity of survivors of acute myocardial infarction with clinical evidence of heart failure. Lancet 342:821-828, 1993.
15. Pitt B, O'Neill B, Feldman R, et al. QUIET Study Group. The Quinapril Ischemic Event Trial (QUIET): Evaluation of chronic ACE inhibitor therapy in patients with ischemic heart disease and preserved left ventricular function. Am J Cardiol 87: 1058-1063, 2001.
16. Estacio RO, Jeffers BW, Hiatt WR, et al. The effect of nisoldipine as compared with enalapril on cardiovascular outcomes in patients with non-insulin-dependent diabetes and hypertension. N Engl J Med 338:645-652, 1998.
17. Tatti P, Pahor M, Byington RP, et al. Outcome results of the Fosinopril Amlodipine Cardiovascular Events Randomized Trial (FACET) in patients with hypertension and NIDDM. Diabetes Care 21:597-603, 1998.
18. UK Prospective Diabetes Study Group. Efficacy of atenolol and captopril in reducing risk of macrovascular and microvascular complications in type 2 diabetes: UKPDS 39. BMJ 317:713-720, 1998.
19. Schrier RW, Estacio RO. Additional follow-up from the ABCD trial in patients with type 2 diabetes and hypertension. N Engl J Med 343:1969, 2000.
20. Hansson L, Lindholm LH, Niskanen L, et al. Effect of angiotensin-converting-enzyme inhibition compared with conventional therapy on cardiovascular morbidity and mortality in hypertension: The Captopril Prevention Project (CAPPP) randomised trial. Lancet 353:611-616, 1999.
21. Hansson L, Lindholm LH, Ekbom T, et al. Randomised trial of old and new antihypertensive drugs in elderly patients: Cardiovascular mortality and morbidity the Swedish Trial in Old Patients with Hypertension-2 study. Lancet 354:1751-1756, 1999.
22. Yusuf S, Sleight P, Pogue J, et al. Effects of an angiotensin-converting-enzyme inhibitor, ramipril, on cardiovascular events in high-risk patients. The Heart Outcomes Prevention Evaluation Study Investigators. N Engl J Med 342:145-153, 2000.
23. Blood Pressure Lowering Treatment Trialists' Collaboration. Effects of ACE inhibitors, calcium antagonists, and other blood pressure lowering drugs: Results of prospectively designed overviews of randomized trials. Lancet 356:1955-1964, 2000.
24. Blood Pressure Lowering Treatment Trialists' Collaboration. Effects of different blood pressure lowering regimens on major cardiovascular events: Second cycle of prospectively designed overviews. Lancet 362:1527-1535, 2003.
25. Progress Collaborative Group. Randomized trial of a perindopril-based blood-pressure-lowering regimen among 6105 individuals with previous stroke or transient ischaemic attack. Lancet 358:1033-1040, 2001.
26. Chalmers J, MacMahon S. On behalf of the PROGRESS Management Committee. PROGRESS—Perindopril Protection against Recurrent Stroke Study; main results. J Hypertens 19 (Suppl 2):260, 2001 (abstract).
27. Mulinari R, Gavras I, Gavras H. Efficacy and tolerability of enalapril monotherapy in mild-to-moderate hypertension in

older patients compared to younger patients. Clin Ther 9: 678-689, 1987.

28. Dahlof B, Devereux RB, Kjeldsen SE, et al. Cardiovascular morbidity and mortality in the Losartan Intervention For Endpoint reduction in hypertension study (LIFE): A randomised trial against atenolol. Lancet 359:995-1003, 2002.

29. Wright JT Jr, Bakris G, Greene T, et al. Effect of blood pressure lowering and antihypertensive drug class on progression of hypertensive kidney disease: Results from the AASK trial. JAMA 288:2421-2431, 2002.

30. Wing LMH, Reid CM, Ryan P, et al. Second Australian National Blood Pressure Study (ANBP2)—comparative outcome trial of ACE inhibitor- and diuretic-based treatment of hypertension in the elderly: Principal results. N Engl J Med 348:583-592, 2003.

31. Gavras H, Ribeiro A, Gavras I, et al. Reciprocal relation between renin dependency and sodium dependency in essential hypertension. N Engl J Med 295:1278-1283, 1976.

32. Weinberger MH, Miller JZ, Luft FC, et al. Definitions and characteristics of sodium sensitivity and blood pressure resistance. Hypertension 8 (Suppl II):127-134, 1986.

# Chapter 36

# Critical Assessment of Hypertension Guidelines

## Gordon T. McInnes

## INTRODUCTION

The delivery of care for individuals with hypertension is variable and often poor.[1] In the United States, control rates are much less than 50%, with a particular shortfall in the control of systolic blood pressure. Furthermore, 30% of those with high blood pressure are unaware that they have hypertension, and awareness has not changed in the last decade. As a consequence of the ageing population in most developed countries, the total number of stroke and coronary heart disease events is increasing or remains static. Also, a "second wave" epidemic of cardiovascular disease is flowing through developing countries and the former socialist republics. Thus, hypertension is an emerging public health problem on a global scale.

There is no shortage of well-meaning advice for clinicians treating hypertension. In 2003 alone, five major organizations published guidelines,[1-5] and revised British recommendations appeared early in 2004.[6] Authors of guidelines are quick to offer justification. More than 50% of countries lack formal guidelines for the management of hypertension,[7] and many lack the resources to make significant impact. Rather surprisingly, the recent World Health Organization–International Society of Hypertension (WHO-ISH) Guidelines[5] overlap substantially with those of the Joint National Committee (JNC)[1] and the European Society of Hypertension–European Society of Cardiology (ESH-ESC)[3] recommendations, which are aimed primarily at a North American or European audience, with little acknowledgment of problems in the developing countries that make up the vast bulk of the world population.

The guidelines essentially address three issues—when (or whom) to treat, what the target of treatment should be and how to treat. Discrepancies in detail are readily apparent, but the concordance of opinion is impressive. All guidelines emphasize the need for careful assessment before diagnosis and treatment, the early treatment of severe and accelerated hypertension, rigorous targets particularly in high-risk individuals, and the role of nonpharmacologic management. The choice of drugs for treatment of hypertension is perhaps the area where uniformity is least.

The need for advice on the management of hypertension is evident, but the dangers are seldom recognized. When an authoritative body makes specific recommendations, it is easy for deviation from the guidelines to be regarded as suboptimal or even negligent practice.

## WHEN (OR WHOM) TO TREAT

Traditionally, the threshold for treatment of hypertension has been based on blood pressure levels. "Hypertension should be defined in terms of a blood pressure level above which inves-tigation and treatment do more good than harm."[8] The threshold has to be set to select the individuals most likely to benefit. Reduction in risk is valuable only if it is appreciable in magnitude and in absolute terms.

Both systolic and diastolic blood pressure are recommended for guidance on treatment thresholds. Although the benefit of treating elevated systolic blood pressure is restricted to the elderly, the same systolic threshold is recommended at all ages. Some recent guidelines[1,5] recommend a treatment threshold for systolic blood pressure of 140 mm Hg and/or for diastolic blood pressure of 90 mm Hg, even in low-risk individuals. The evidence in support of this advice comes from observational data.[9,10]

Recommendations have been extended to those with high-normal blood pressure (130-139/85-89 mm Hg).[1-6] Because experimental support for blood pressure reduction in such individuals is so far limited to those with diabetes mellitus,[11-14] coronary heart disease,[12] and stroke,[15,16] antihypertensive drug treatment can be advised only for patients with high risk.[3]

JNC 7[1] has gone further by including a category termed pre-hypertension (120-139/80-89 mm Hg) because such individuals have twice the risk of developing hypertension as compared with those with lower blood pressures.[10] Prehypertension is intended to identify those in whom early adoption of healthy lifestyle could reduce blood pressure, decrease the rate of progression of blood pressure elevation to hypertension with age, or prevent hypertension entirely.[1] JNC 7 claims that prehypertension is not a disease category but that drug treatment is recommended when there is concomitant diabetes or renal disease if lifestyle intervention fails to reduce blood pressure to 130/80 mm Hg or less.[1]

Contemporary guidelines further extend the definition of threshold for intervention by advising ambulatory blood pressure monitoring (ABPM) or home blood pressure monitoring (HBPM) in some circumstances.[1-6] There is uncertainty about definitions and implications. Measurement of blood pressure outside the clinician's office (ABPM or HBPM) may have a role in some patients but should not be used indiscriminately in the routine evaluation of patients with hypertension. Although all guidelines provide considerable detail on how to use ABPM or HBPM to diagnose white coat (isolated office or clinic) hypertension, little practical advice is given on how such individuals should be managed. These approaches are not available in many developing countries.[4]

With successive guidelines, the blood pressure threshold has been reduced, often without trial evidence of benefit and without consideration for the practical issues of implementation. Small changes in thresholds can have a profound effect on the proportion of adults who will be given drug treatment. Even when using the cheapest antihypertensive drugs, current blood pressure thresholds have a massive economic impact on the healthcare system when additional labor costs are included in the equation.

Although there may be divergence about the appropriate blood pressure thresholds, there is unanimity that the presence of other cardiovascular risk factors (e.g., dyslipidemia, diabetes, smoking), target organ damage (e.g., left ventricular hypertrophy), and associated clinical conditions[1,3,5,6] should result in a lowering of the threshold for intervention (Table 36–1). It may be reasonable to delay drug treatment in individuals with mild hypertension unless there are other risk factors.[3,5] This recommendation is sensitive to circumstances where resources are limited.[4]

Guidelines for hypertension[1-6] and cardiovascular risk prevention[17] endorse the concept of risk stratification, but not all provide precise advice. Intuitive estimates of cardiovascular risk are crude and indiscriminate.[18] Risk stratification is more accurate when major risk factors are estimated and weighted by using risk functions derived from epidemiologic studies.[19] The categorical method recommended by WHO-ISH[5] and ESH-ESC[3] is less accurate than those using continuous variables such as British Hypertension Society (BHS),[6] based on the Framingham risk equation,[19] which has been shown to apply to U.S. and North European populations, although it is less predictive in other ethnic groups.

Although management based on a precise estimation of cardiovascular risk is logical, it requires consultation of relevant computer programs, charts, or tables before a decision is made about treatment. This approach determines short-term (10-year) risk and therefore favors treatment of the elderly (men) rather than the young (women). Restricting treatment to high- or very high-risk persons may be cost-saving for the practitioner but less than optimal for the patient. In some cases, strict adherence to these approaches would result in drug treatment being denied when blood pressure exceeds conventional thresholds. Although short-term risk of cardiovascular and renal morbidity and mortality may be low in younger patients with risk factors of only moderate severity, long-term risk can be unacceptably high. A decision not to treat should be reviewed regularly, because risk increases with age and may in time become sufficient to justify intervention.

When resources are limited, priority should be given to hypertensive patients with high and then moderate cardiovascular risk. In those with low cardiovascular risk, decisions should be based on estimated cardiovascular risk and patient choice.

The JNC 7 guidelines have largely abandoned the risk stratification approach and provide treatment recommendations primarily based on blood pressure levels.[1] The simplicity of this method may be useful for the busy clinician, but there are confusing inconsistencies. Treatment of all patients with mild hypertension is advised if either risk factors, target organ damage, or both are present. Furthermore, the Framingham risk score[19] is suggested as an aid to doctors and patients in demonstrating the benefits of treatment. The strategy advocated by JNC 7 is less logical than others but is also less expensive. It may provide a better service for countries where every penny counts.

## TARGET BLOOD PRESSURE

Until recently, detailed discussion about the threshold for treatment was not often matched by detailed consideration of the target for treatment—that is, the level of blood pressure that should be achieved. There is very good epidemiologic evidence that, within the usual range of systolic and diastolic blood pressure, the lower the pressure, the lower the risk of both stroke and coronary events.[20] However, there has been persistent concern that normalization of diastolic blood pres-

**Table 36–1** Factors Influencing Prognosis

| Risk Factors for Cardiovascular Disease | Target Organ Damage | Associated Cinical Conditions |
| --- | --- | --- |
| • Levels of systolic and diastolic blood pressure (grades 1–3) | • Left ventricular hypertrophy (electrocardiogram or echocardiogram) | • Diabetes |
| | | • Cerebrovascular disease |
| • M >55 years | • Microalbuminuria (20–300 mg/day) | Ischemic stroke |
| | | Cerebral hemorrhage |
| • F >65 years | • Radiologic or ultrasound evidence of extensive atherosclerotic plaque (aorta, carotid, coronary, iliac, and femoral arteries) | Transient ischemic attack |
| | | Heart disease |
| | | Myocardial infarction |
| | | Angina |
| | | Coronary revascularization |
| • Smoking | • Hypertensive retinopathy grade III or IV | Congestive heart failure |
| • Total cholesterol >6.1 mmol/L (240 mg/dl) or LDL cholesterol >4.0 mmol/L (160 mg/dl)* | | • Renal disease |
| • HDL cholesterol M <1.0, F <1.2 mmol/L (<40, <45 mg/dl) | | Plasma creatinine concentration: F >1.4, M >1.5 mg/dl (120, 133 μmol/l) |
| • History of cardiovascular disease in first-degree relatives before age 50 | | Albuminuria >300 mg/day |
| • Obesity, physical inactivity | | • Peripheral vascular disease |

From World Health Organization, International Society of Hypertension Writing Group World Health Organization [WHO]/International Society of Hypertension [ISH] Statement on management of hypertension. J Hypertens 21:1983-1992, 2003.
*Lower levels of total and low-density lipoprotein (LDL) cholesterol are known to delineate increased risk, but they were not used in the stratification table. HDL, high-density lipoprotein; M, male; F, female.

sure (80-85 mm Hg) may increase the risk of coronary death in patients with established coronary artery disease.[21]

The findings from the Hypertension Optimal Treatment (HOT) study[22] have been hugely influential in determining target blood pressure. Despite limitations, the HOT study provides reasonable support for contemporary recommendations that blood pressure should be reduced to less than 140/90 mm Hg in all treated individuals.[1-6] In the HOT study,[22] there was little additional benefit from reducing systolic blood pressure to below 150 mm Hg. Therefore, this systolic blood pressure target is an acceptable fall-back position[3,5,6] and is particularly appropriate when resources are limited.[5]

The evidence for more-rigorous blood pressure control is most robust for diastolic blood pressure in type 2 diabetes[22-25] but is extrapolated to include systolic blood pressure and patients with type 1 diabetes and other high-risk individuals including those with established cardiovascular disease where a target blood pressure of less than 130/80 mm Hg is recommended.[1,3,5,6] Even tighter blood pressure control is advised in diabetic patients with nephropathy and in nondiabetic renal disease. However, the quality of data in support of rigorous targets becomes weaker the lower the achieved blood pressure. Clinical trial evidence[26] questions the desirability of pressing below conventional levels even in patients at high risk of cardiovascular events and renal failure.

Despite best practice, blood pressure targets may be difficult to achieve. Particularly in the elderly, rigorous control of systolic blood pressure may prove impossible without severe detrimental influences on the individual's quality of life. Occasionally, there is no alternative to accepting poor blood pressure control. Under these circumstances, it is vitally important that the physician does not convey to the patient an impression of therapeutic failure or despair. Both the physician and the patient should recognize that partial blood pressure control reduces the risk posed by hypertension. Guidelines should pay more attention to this difficult but not infrequent clinical problem.

The primary goal of management is to obtain maximum reduction in total risk of cardiovascular and renal morbidity and mortality. Effective treatment requires management of all identified reversible risk factors and associated clinical conditions, as well as blood pressure. The burden of lifestyle modification and drug therapy can be overwhelming for the patient and the practitioner.

## HOW TO TREAT

There is universal agreement about the role of lifestyle modification in the management of hypertension, including those with high-normal blood pressure, particularly where there is a strong family history[1-6] (Box 36-1 and Table 36-2). Lifestyle modifications can be difficult to apply in the population at large and in the long-term, and the ability of nonpharmacologic interventions to reduce mortality and morbidity in hypertension has not been shown directly. Application of lifestyle intervention should not delay the introduction of drug therapy, especially in high-risk patients.

Practitioners who advocate rigorous lifestyle modifications can be considered by the recipient of advice as "warriors against pleasure." An individual's lifestyle is driven by personal performance and economic realities. Although the person

may accept that habits are harmful and should be improved, change is always difficult, and undue pressure may be resented. The consequence may be poor concordance with management plans. Overzealous lifestyle advice without immediate benefit can result in the individual declining further contact with the perceived persecutor.

Advocated lifestyle changes are chiefly of value in more-prosperous communities, although even then, success may be elusive. These lifestyle changes may not always be relevant to poorer countries where dietary approaches may be unaffordable. The most helpful approach for poorer areas[5] may be trying to influence the policies of government agencies and food manufacturers to reduce sodium consumption in these communities.

There is general agreement that lowering blood pressure is the main determinant of benefit and is more important than specific drug selection.[1-6] The major classes of antihypertensive agents—diuretics, β-blockers, calcium channel blockers, angiotensin-converting enzyme (ACE) inhibitors, and angiotensin receptor blockers—are suitable for initiation and maintenance of therapy. The emphasis on identifying the first class of drugs to be used has probably been superseded by the recognition that two or more drugs in combination are needed to achieve the goal blood pressure.

Despite these considerations, two influential recent guidelines[1,5] advocate therapy based on a specific drug class, thiazide, or thiazide-like diuretics, for all hypertensive patients unless there are compelling indications for another class. Findings from the Antihypertensive and Lipid-Lowering Treatment to Prevent Heart Attack Trial (ALLHAT)[27] are used to justify this policy, despite misgivings about the validity of its interpretation.[28] Diuretics are undoubtedly underused, enhance blood pressure lowering in multidrug regimens, and are often more affordable than other drugs.[29] It is probable that the last factor is decisive in determining the advice from JNC 7[1] and WHO-ISH.[5]

In settings where cost is the overriding consideration, this approach may not be unreasonable. This is particularly true in African countries,[4] because diuretics have strong blood pres-

**Box 36-1** Lifestyle Measures That Lower Blood Pressure and Cardiovascular Disease

**Lifestyle measures that lower blood pressure**
- Weight reduction
- Reduced salt intake
- Limitation of alcohol consumption
- Increased physical activity
- Increased fruit and vegetable consumption
- Reduced total fat and saturated fat intake

**Measures to reduce cardiovascular disease risk**
- Cessation of smoking
- Reduced total fat and saturated fat intake
- Replacement of saturated fats with mono-unsaturated fats
- Increased oily fish consumption

From Williams B, Poulter NR, Brown MJ, et al. Guidelines for management of hypertension: Report of the fourth working party of the British Hypertension Society, 2004-BHS IV. J Human Hypertens 18:139-185, 2004.

**Table 36–2** Lifestyle Modifications to Prevent and Manage Hypertension*

| Modification | Recommendation | Approximate SBP Reduction (Ranger)[†] |
|---|---|---|
| Weight reduction | Maintain normal body weight (body mass index 18.5-24.9 kg/m$^2$) | 5-20 mm Hg/10 kg |
| Adopt DASH eating plan | Consume a diet rich in fruits, vegetables, and low-fat dairy products with a reduced content of saturated and total fat | 8-14 mm Hg |
| Dietary sodium reduction | Reduce dietary sodium intake to no more than 100 mmol per day (2.4 g sodium or 6 g sodium chloride) | 2-8 mm Hg |
| Physical activity | Engage in regular aerobic physical activity such as brisk walking (at least 30 min/day, most days of the week) | 4-9 mm Hg |
| Moderation of alcohol consumption | Limit consumption to no more than 2 drinks (e.g., 24 oz beer, 10 oz wine, or 3 oz 80-proof whiskey) per day in most men and to no more than 1 drink per day in women and lighter-weight persons | 2-4 mm Hg |

From Chobanian AV, Bakris GL, Black HR, et al. Seventh Report of the Joint National Committee on Prevention, Detection, Evaluation, and Treatment of High Blood Pressure. Hypertension 42:1206-1252, 2003.
DASH, Dietary Approaches to Stop Hypertension.
*For overall cardiovascular risk reduction, stop smoking.
†The effects of implementing these modifications are dose- and time-dependent and could be greater for some individuals.

sure lowering effects in Blacks.[30] In low-risk patients, treatment may not be cost-effective unless the cheapest drugs are used, but in high-risk patients who gain large benefits from treatment, expensive drugs may be more cost-effective.[31] Because the focus of most recent guidelines is on identification and treatment of patients at high risk, a more-relaxed approach to treatment regimens may be more logical.

The average blood pressure fall induced by each of the different drug classes is similar, but there is considerable heterogeneity among patients. The appropriate choice for a patient may be determined by the individual's other characteristics, such as ethnicity and age. Diuretics and calcium channel blockers are particularly effective in Blacks and the elderly.[30,32] This is emphasized by the WHO-ISH guidelines,[5] but it is not pointed out that other drugs, such as ACE inhibitors and angiotensin receptor blockers, may be more efficacious in non-Blacks and younger individuals. Furthermore, certain high-risk conditions provide compelling indications for particular drugs (Table 36–3). In certain individuals there are contraindications and cautions for all classes of drugs (see Table 36–3).

If the first-choice therapy is well tolerated but blood pressure remains above target, all guidelines[1-6] give the option of switching to a different class of drugs (substitution) in mild and uncomplicated hypertension. Whether this should be continued if the second choice fails to control blood pressure is controversial. Rotational monotherapy is laborious and frustrating for doctors and patients and may reduce compliance. Moving to combination therapy achieves blood pressure control more efficiently.[1-6] Drugs can be added in a stepwise manner until blood pressure is controlled.

Simple algorithms can aid the prescriber in choosing the most appropriate sequence of drug combinations.[3,4,6] The most recent BHS guidelines[6] endorse the ABCD algorithm. This is based on the categorization of hypertensive patients into high- and low-renin groups. Younger patients (younger than 55 years) and Caucasians tend to have high-renin hypertension and respond well to A (ACE inhibitors or angiotensin receptor blockers) or B (β-blockers), which block the renin-angiotensin system,[33] whereas older patients and Blacks respond well to C (calcium channel blockers) or D (diuretics),[30,34-37] predicting responsiveness to first-line therapy. If control is not achieved, A (or B) can be combined with C or D with favorable effectiveness.[38,39] When there is no compelling indication for a particular drug class, the cheapest available drugs should be used. β-Blockers (B) in combination with diuretics (D) should be avoided in patients at high risk of diabetes[40,41]—that is, those with a strong family history of type 2 diabetes, obesity, impaired glucose tolerance, and/or the metabolic syndrome, and certain ethnic groups such as South Asians. The ABCD algorithm appears logical, but its utility needs to be tested in clinical practice.

Combination therapy is needed by most patients to achieve optimal blood pressure control. The most innovative recommendation of the recent guidelines[1-3] is to consider initiating therapy with combinations of two agents in those whose blood pressure is substantially elevated or where target organ damage or other risk factors demand an aggressive approach. In JNC 7,[1] combination therapy from the outset is an option if blood pressure is 160/100 mm Hg or greater. Thus, if baseline blood pressure is 20/10 mm Hg above target, prescribers might initiate therapy with two agents. This should help dispel the myth that most patients can be controlled with one agent.

The prompt initiation of combination therapy enhances efficacy, facilitates more-rapid achievement of goals, requires fewer visits to clinicians, and is particularly desirable in communities that lack adequate healthcare provisions. A disadvantage is the possible exposure to an unnecessary drug. There is also an increased risk of orthostatic hypotension, particularly in diabetics and older people. However, for the majority, combination therapy is an efficient approach to management.

**Table 36-3** Compelling and Possible Indications, Contraindications, and Cautions for the Major Classes of Antihypertensive Drugs

| Class of Drug | Compelling Indications | Possible Indications | Caution | Compelling Contraindications |
|---|---|---|---|---|
| α-Blockers | Benign prostatic hypertrophy | | Postural hypotension heart failure[a] | Urinary incontinence |
| ACE inhibitors | Heart failure, LV dysfunction, post-MI, type 1 diabetic nephropathy, 2° stroke prevention[e] | Chronic renal disease,[b] type 2 diabetic nephropathy, proteinuric renal disease | Renal impairment,[b] PVD[c] | Pregnancy, renovascular disease[d] |
| ARBs | ACE inhibitor intolerance, type 2 diabetic nephropathy, hypertension with LVH, heart failure in ACE-intolerant patients, post-MI | LV dysfunction post-MI, intolerance of other antihypertensive drugs, proteinuric renal disease, chronic renal disease[b] | Renal impairment,[b] PVD[c] | Pregnancy, renovascular disease[d] |
| β-Blockers | MI, angina | Heart failure[f] | Heart failure,[f] PVD, diabetes (except with CHD) | Asthma/COPD, heart block |
| CCBs (dihydropyridine) | Elderly, ISH | Elderly, angina | — | — |
| CCBs (rate limiting) | Angina | MI | Combination with β-blockade | Heart block, heart failure |
| Thiazide/thiazide-like diuretics | Elderly, ISH heart failure | | | Gout[g] |

From Williams B, Poulter NR, Brown MJ, et al. Guidelines for management of hypertension: Report of the fourth working party of the British Hypertension Society, 2004–BHS IV. J Human Hypertension 18:139-185, 2004.
[a]HF when used as monotherapy.
[b]ACE inhibitors or ARBs may be beneficial in chronic renal failure but should only be used with caution, close supervision, and specialist advice when there is established and significant renal impairment.
[c]Caution with ACE inhibitors and ARBs in peripheral vascular disease because of association with renovascular disease.
[d]ACE inhibitors and ARBs are sometimes used in patients with renovascular disease under specialist supervision.
[e]In combination with a thiazide/thiazide-like diuretic.
[f]β-Blockers are increasingly used to treat stable heart failure. However, β-blockers may worsen heart failure.
[g]Thiazide/thiazide-like diuretics may sometimes be necessary to control blood pressure in people with a history of gout, ideally used in combination with allopurinol.
COPD, chronic obstructive pulmonary disease; ISH, isolated systolic hypertension; PVD, peripheral vascular disease; LVH, left ventricular hypertrophy; ACE, angiotensin-converting enzyme; ARBs, angiotensin II receptor blockers; MI, myocardial infarction; CCBs, calcium channel blockers.

For reasons of convenience and increased patient compliance, preparations that contain two or more drugs in a single tablet or capsule may be appropriate if there are no cost disadvantages. The availability and cost of fixed-dose combinations vary greatly around the world. Optimal strategies should take into consideration local circumstances and needs.

When blood pressure is at goal and stable, follow-up every 3 months is reasonable.[1] If therapeutic goals are not achieved in 6 months, referral to a specialist is advised.[3] In many settings, this resource may not be available.

When appropriate, step-down of therapy is generally recommended.[1,3] This should be undertaken only after blood pressure has been controlled effectively for at least 1 year. Careful monitoring is required, and success is minimal if the initial diagnosis of hypertension was accurate.

Treatment of all other reversible risk factors for cardiovascular disease should be considered as an integral part of hypertension management. Recommended strategies include lifestyle modification, lipid lowering, glycemic control, and antiplatelet therapy.[1-6] Aspirin should be included only when blood pressure is controlled because of the increased risk of intracerebral bleeding in uncontrolled hypertension.

## SPECIAL CONSIDERATIONS

### Diabetes Mellitus

The main focus of treatment is generally considered to be systolic blood pressure, although it is not yet firmly established by clinical trial evidence. The systolic blood pressure target (<130 mm Hg) is particularly difficult to achieve.[42] Most trials have failed to reduce systolic blood pressure to 140 mm Hg or below.[43]

The choice of drugs is an area of great controversy, myths, and misconceptions.[44] ACE inhibitors are generally recommended as first-line treatment,[3] but the supporting evidence is weak. Findings from ALLHAT[24] and other trials[41,45,46] provide little indication that ACE inhibitor–based therapy offers advantages over other regimens. It is uncertain whether the renoprotective effect of ACE inhibitors in type 1 diabetes and of angiotensin receptor blockers in type 2 diabetes makes such agents first-line therapy in all patients with diabetes, as suggested by ESH.[3] JNC 7[1] and BHS[6] advise use of these agents only where there is established nephropathy or target organ damage, in line with existing evidence.[11,13,14,47-49]

Statins are recommended regardless of lipid levels. Aspirin should be used when reasonable blood pressure control has been achieved. Glycemic control should be optimized. Thus, hypertensive patients with diabetes can expect to be prescribed seven or more drugs, as well as strict lifestyle changes. It is little wonder that compliance is often poor.

## Chronic Kidney Disease

Strict blood pressure control is essential to retard progression of renal impairment, but the precise blood pressure goal for optimal renoprotection is uncertain.[26,50,51] The evidence for preferential use of drugs that block the renin-angiotensin system[3] in patients with chronic kidney disease is restricted to trials in African Americans.[51,52] In patients with overt proteinuria, the data in favor of blockade of the renin-angiotensin system is more compelling.[6,53-54] Because of high cardiovascular risk, statins and aspirin are usually indicated.[3,6]

## Cardiovascular Disease

In these high-risk individuals, antihypertensive therapy is indicated even if blood pressure is only marginally elevated. Tight blood pressure control is critical. The guidelines provide advice on appropriate agents.

## Cerebrovascular Disease

In the absence of evidence, it is reasonable to recommend a cautious approach after acute stroke until the patient and the blood pressure are stabilized.[1] Little additional advice is provided despite recent findings that strongly support rigorous control of blood pressure beyond the acute phase of stroke or transient ischemic attack.[16]

## Age

The guidelines give special consideration to hypertension in the elderly, because absolute risk is much greater than in younger people. Initiation of therapy beyond 80 years of age depends on the presence of comorbidities. If the individual is generally fit and especially if there are hypertensive complications or target organ damage, treatment should not be denied.[55] JNC 7 recommends treatment of systolic blood pressures of 140 to 159 mm Hg.[1] No consideration is given to the relative benefits and resource implications of treating all those older than 60 years of age with systolic blood pressure in this range. To avoid cognitive dysfunction, the optimal blood pressure appears to be particularly low (135-150/70-79 mm Hg).[56,57] Posthoc analysis of the Systolic Hypertension in the Elderly Program (SHEP)[58] suggests that it is advisable to avoid reducing diastolic blood pressure below 70 mm Hg or 60 mm Hg at the lowest.

In contrast, very little guidance is provided about management of hypertension in young individuals. Secondary hypertension is more common in the young but is still rare. In the absence of clinical clues or very high blood pressure, management should follow the usual protocol with further investigation if there is a poor response to therapy. Guidelines that advocate treatment based on short-term (usually 10-year) cardiovascular risk[3,5,6] lead to undertreatment of the young, who are left to develop increasing blood pressure and a lifetime risk of cardiovascular events far greater than that in the elderly.

## Minority Groups

Blacks respond particularly well to diuretics and calcium channel blockers that should form the basis of drug therapy. However, there is evidence of preferential renal protection with drugs that block the renin-angiotensin system in Black patients with renal impairment.[51] Individuals of South Asian origin are at high risk of the metabolic syndrome and require an aggressive multifactorial approach.[6] In ethnic subgroups, socioeconomic and lifestyle factors may be barriers to acceptance of treatment. People from African and South Asian communities are less willing to accept the disease label of hypertension, and the cost of management can be a disincentive.

## Resistant Hypertension

The guidelines do not deal adequately with the frequent clinical problem of the patient whose blood pressure falls short of the accepted target. More-complex treatment and specialist referral is suggested,[1,3,56] without indicating how the specialist should deal with the issue.

## SUMMARY

Current guidelines emphasize the importance of risk assessment in identifying individuals who merit antihypertensive treatment. Patients with established cardiovascular disease readily identify themselves to medical services, are at high risk, and gain considerable benefit from treatment. However, doctors are very poor at identifying high-risk individuals from clinical clues in the general "healthy" population, as can be seen from the continued failure to recognize and treat those at high risk.

A staged approach may be appropriate where resources are scarce. Priority is given to those with established vascular disease. Thereafter, intervention focuses on those with high cardiovascular risk, including patients with diabetes, target organ damage, and absolute cardiovascular risk above an agreed threshold.

Algorithms to initiate treatment on the basis of the level of risk rather than the level of blood pressure in individuals with the mildest hypertension represent an important new direction. This approach will require evaluation because it alters fundamentally the way in which doctors are encouraged to think about the treatment of hypertension. The future cannot be predicted with any real certainty for asymptomatic individuals. For 1000 persons with 20% cardiovascular risk, neither the 200 potential losers nor the 800 potential winners can be anticipated.

Short-term risk assessment favors treatment of older individuals, but older individuals without symptomatic disease can be classified among the winners, because they have tolerated risk factors for many years. Younger people with risk factors have relatively low short-term absolute risk yet stand to gain the most benefit in the long-term and are at increased risk of premature disease.

Costs of treatment are assuming greater importance as larger populations are being treated in healthcare systems that work within limited budgets. Even nonpharmacologic management may carry a heavy cost in advice and monitoring and may actually prove more expensive than drug therapy.[59] Thoughtful drug selection, even when the cost at first may seem painfully high, makes economic sense when compared with the expense of hospitalization or other major interventions for the serious consequences of inadequate management.

In developing countries, costs may make it difficult to afford diagnostic procedures and drug therapies. Some might be considered a luxury when healthcare systems are inadequate. For instance, countries in sub-Saharan Africa may spend only USD 10 per citizen annually on health. Despite those deficiencies, key recommendations of international guidelines[1,3,5] are accepted. However, concepts such as prehypertension are of questionable significance when healthcare is tightly constrained. The obstacles facing practitioners in developing countries should not be underestimated. These challenges appear beyond the capacity of authors of international guidelines.

The impact of guidelines in changing practice has been small.[60] There is little evidence that clinical practice has improved based on guidelines that are widely acknowledged but largely ignored. Most practitioners can hardly keep pace with advances in healthcare. They would have to read 20 articles every day to maintain present knowledge.[61] Although guidelines reduce the need to read original papers, it is still difficult to keep up.[62] Even if practitioners are aware and willing, change is difficult, particularly if the environment is nonconducive to improving standards of care.

To date, it may be argued that the major beneficiaries of guidelines are their authors, administrators/managers, and lawyers. The authors gain prestige, administrators and managers gain control over practitioners, and lawyers can sue those who do not follow the guidelines. Benefits do not necessarily extend to clinicians or, most importantly, to patients.

Management guidelines presume a simple algorithm in which clinical evidence is distilled into guidelines that will filter down into clinical practice. However, the flow is unlikely to be successful without efforts to improve implementation. Traditional approaches have focused on improving availability and presentation by producing "glossy" summary guidelines, reviews in clinical journals, and continuing medical education (conferences). Practitioners value management guidelines but consider those available to be too scientific, excessively demanding on resources and of impractical complexity, of limited local applicability, and also having a short shelf-life. Revised guidelines may be published before the generalist has come to terms with the earlier version. Guidelines appear to be updated every few years to follow contemporary fashion rather than to reflect important new evidence. Often,

the data supporting the revision appear marginal at most and may simply reflect expert opinion qualified by prejudice.

In addressing the problems of implementation, most guidelines are long on rhetoric but short on practical advice. Various strategies are needed to target obstacles to change.[63,64] Change in practice is only partially within the doctor's control.

Hypertension guidelines are unlikely to be successful unless concerted efforts are made to address public health issues.[7] The American Public Health Association has led the way in its resolution that food manufacturers and restaurants should reduce sodium in food by 50%. This important primary prevention initiative is endorsed by JNC 7[1] and echoed in other guidelines.[3,5,6]

# References

1. Chobanian AV, Bakris GL, Black HL, et al. Seventh report of the Joint National Committee on Prevention, Detection, Evaluation, and Treatment of High Blood Pressure. Hypertension 42: 1206-1252, 2003.
2. Consensus Statement at the Hypertension in African American Working Group of the International Society on Hypertension in Blacks. Management of High Blood Pressure in African Americans. Arch Intern Med 163:524-541, 2003.
3. Guidelines Committee 2003 European Society of Hypertension–European Society of Cardiology guidelines for the management of arterial hypertension. J Hypertens 21: 1011-1053, 2003.
4. Lemogoum D, Seedat YK, Mabadejc AFB, et al. on behalf of the International Forum for Hypertension control and prevention in Africa IFHA. Recommendations for prevention, diagnosis and management of hypertension and cardiovascular risk factors in sub-Saharan Africa. J Hypertens 21:1993-2000, 2003.
5. World Health Organization, International Society of Hypertension Working Group. 2003 World Health Organization (WHO)/International Society of Hypertension (ISH) statement on management of hypertension. J Hypertens 21:1983-1992, 2003.
6. Williams B, Poulter NR, Brown MJ, et al. Guidelines for management of hypertension: Report of the fourth working party of the British Hypertension Society, 2004–BHS IV. J Human Hypertens 18:139-185, 2004.
7. Weber MA. Yet more hypertension guidelines : What do they add? J Hypertens 21:1977-1981, 2000.
8. Evans JG, Rose G. Hypertension. Br Med Bull 27:37-42, 1971.
9. Van den Hoogen PCW, Feskens EJM, Nagekerke NJD, et al. for the Seven Countries Study Research Group. The relation between blood pressure and mortality due to coronary heart disease among men in different parts of the world. N Engl J Med 342:1-8, 2000.
10. Vasan RS, Larson MG, Leip EP, et al. Impact of high-normal pressure on the risk of cardiovascular disease. N Engl J Med 345:1291-1297, 2001.
11. Brenner BM, Cooper ME, De Zeeuw D, et al. for the RENAAL Study Investigators. Efforts of losartan on renal and cardiovascular outcomes in patients with type 2 diabetes and nephropathy. N Engl J Med 345:861-869, 2001.
12. The Heart Outcomes Prevention Evaluation Study Investigators: Effects of an angiotensin-converting-enzyme inhibitor, ramipril, on cardiovascular events in high-risk patients. N Engl J Med 342:145-153, 2000.
13. Lewis EJ, Hunsicker LG, Clarke WR, et al. for the Collaborative Study Group. Renoprotective effect of the angiotensin-receptor antagonist irbesartan in patients with nephropathy due to type 2 diabetes. N Engl J Med 345:851-860, 2001.

14. Parving H-H, Leinnert H, Bröchner-Mortensen J, et al. for the Irbesartan in Patients with Type 2 Diabetes and Micro-albuminuria Study Group. The effect of irbesartan on the development of diabetic nephropathy in patients with type 2 diabetes. N Engl J Med 345:870-878, 2001.

15. PATS Collaborative Group. Post-stroke antihypertensive treatment study: A preliminary result. Clin Med J 108:710-717, 1995.

16. PROGRESS Collaborative Group. Randomised trial of a perindopril-based blood-pressure-lowering regimen study among 6105 individuals with previous stroke or transient ischaemic attack. Lancet 3581:1033-1041, 2001.

17. Pearson TA, Blair SN, Daniels SP, et al. AHA guidelines for primary prevention of cardiovascular disease and stroke: 2002 update: Consensus panel guide to comprehensive risk reduction for adult patients with coronary and other atherosclerotic vascular diseases. American Heart Association Science Advisory and Coordinating Committee. Circulation 106:388-391, 2002.

18. Chatellier G, Blinowska A, Menard J, et al. Do physicians estimate reliably CVD risk in hypertensive patients? Medical Info 8:876-877, 1995.

19. Anderson KM, Wilson PWF, Odell PM, et al. An updated coronary risk profile: A statement for health professionals. Circulation 83:356-362, 1991.

20. Prospective Studies Collaboration. Age-specific relevance of usual blood pressure to vascular mortality: A meta-analysis of individual data for one million adults in 61 prospective studies. Lancet 360:1903-1913, 2002.

21. Cruickshank JM, Thorp JM, Zacharias FJ. Benefits and potential harm of lowering high blood pressure. Lancet i:581-584, 1987.

22. Hansson L, Zanchetti A, Carruthers SG, et al. for the HOT Study Group. Effects of intensive blood pressure lowering and low-dose aspirin in patients with hypertension: principal results of the Hypertension Optimal Treatment (HOT) randomised trial. Lancet 351:1755-1762, 1998.

23. Estacio RO, Jeffers BW, Hiatt WR, et al. The effect of nisoldipine as compared with enalapril on cardiovascular events in patients with non-insulin-dependent diabetes and hypertension. N Eng J Med 338:645-652, 1998.

24. Schrier RW, Estacio RO, Esler A, et al. Effects of aggressive blood pressure control in a normotensive type 2 diabetic patients on albuminuria. Kidney Int 61:1088-1097, 2002.

25. UK Prospective Diabetes Study Group. Tight blood pressure control and risk of macrovascular and microvascular complications in type 2 diabetes: UKPDS 38. BMJ 317:703-713, 1998.

26. Jafar TH, Stark PC, Schmid CH, et al. Progression of chronic kidney disease : The role of blood pressure control, proteinuria, and angiotensin-converting enzyme inhibition. A patient-level meta-analysis. Am Intern Med 139:244-252, 2003.

27. The ALLHAT Officers and Coordinators for the ALLHAT Collaborative Research Group. Major outcomes in high-risk hypertensive patients randomized to angiotensin-converting enzyme inhibitor or calcium channel blocker vs diuretic. The Antihypertensive and Lipid-Lowering Treatment to Prevent Heart Attack Trial (ALLHAT) JAMA 288:2981-2997, 2002.

28. McInnes GT. Size isn't everything—ALLHAT in perspective. J Hypertens 21:459-461, 2003.

29. Psaty BM, Manolio TA, Smith NL, et al. Time trends in high blood pressure control and the use of antihypertensive medications in older adults. Arch Intern Med 162:2325-2332, 2002.

30. Materson BJ, Reda DJ, Cushman WC, et al. Single-drug therapy for hypertension in men: A comparison of six antihypertensive agents with placebo. The Department of Veterans Affairs Comparative Study Group on Antihypertensive Agents. N Engl J Med 328:914-921, 1993.

31. Lindholm L, Hallgren CG, Boman K, et al. Cost-effectiveness analysis with defined budget: How to distribute resources for the prevention of cardiovascular disease? Health Policy 48: 155-170, 1999.

32. Cushman WC, Reda DJ, Perry HM, et al. Regional and racial difference in response to antihypertensive medication use in a randomised controlled trial of men with hypertension in the United States. Department of veterans Affairs Cooperative Study Group on Antihypertensive Agents. Arch Intern Med 160:825-831, 2000.

33. Dickerson JE, Hingorani AD, Ashby MJ, et al. Optimisation of antihypertensive treatment by crossover rotation of four major classes. Lancet 353:2008-2013, 1999.

34. Materson BJ, Reda DJ, Cushman WC. Department of Veterans Affairs single-drug therapy of hypertension study. Revised figures and new data. Department of Veterans Affairs Cooperative Study Group on Antihypertensive Agents. Am J Hypertens 8:189-192, 1995.

35. Gibbs CR, Beevers DG, Lip GY. The management of hypertensive disease in black patients. Q J Med 92:187-192, 1990.

36. He FJ, Markandu ND, Sagnella GA, et al. Importance of the renin system in determining blood pressure fall with salt restriction in black and white hypertensives. Hypertension 32:820-824, 1998.

37. Sagnella GA. Why is plasma renin activity lower in populations of African origin? J Human Hypertens 15:17-25, 2001.

38. Laragh JH. Renin system analysis defines the special value of combination antihypertensive therapy using an antirenin agent (CEI) with a long-acting calcium channel blocker (CCB). Am J Hypertens 11:170S-174S, 1998.

39. Tsutamoto T, et al. Effects of long-ac ting calcium channel antagonists on neurohumoral factors: Comparison of nifedipine coat-core with amlodipine. J Cardiovasc Pharmacol 41(Suppl 1):S77-S81, 2003.

40. Dahlöf B, Devereux RB, Kjeldson SE, et al. for the LIFE study group. Cardiovascular morbidity and mortality in the Losartan Intervention For Endpoint reduction in hypertension study (LIFE): A randomised trial against atenolol. Lancet 359: 995-1003, 2002.

41. Hansson L, Helmer T, Lund-Johannsen P, et al. for the NORDIL Study Group. Randomised trial of efforts of calcium antagonists compared with diuretics and a-blockers on cardiovascular morbidity and mortality in hypertension: The Nordic Diltiazem (NORDIL) Study. Lancet 356:359-365, 2000.

42. Brown MJ et al. Influence of diabetes and type of hypertension on response to antihypertensive therapy. Hypertension 35: 1038-1042, 2000.

43. Mancia G, Grassi G. Systolic and diastolic blood pressure control in antihypertensive drug trials. J Hypertens 29:1461-1464, 2002.

44. Zanchetti A, Ruilope L. Antihypertensive treatment in patients with type 2 diabetes mellitus: What guidance for recent controlled randomised trials. J Hypertens 20:2099-2110, 2002.

45. Brown MJ, Palmer CR, Castaigne A, et al. Morbidity and mortality in patients randomised to double-blind treatment with a long-acting calcium channel blocker or diuretic in the International Nifedipine GITS Study: Intervention as a Goal in Hypertension Treatment (INSIGHT). Lancet 356; 366-377, 2000.

46. Hansson L, Lindholm LH, Ekbom T, et al. Randomised trial of old and new antihypertensive drugs in elderly patients: Cardiovascular mortality and morbidity the Swedish Trial in Old Patients with Hypertension-2 Study. Lancet 354:1751-1756, 1999.

47. Lewis EJ, Hunsicker LG, Blain RP, et al. and the Collaborative Study Group. The effect of angiotensin-converting enzyme inhibition on diabetic nephropathy. N Engl J Med 329: 1456-1462, 1993.

48. Lindholm LH, Ibsen H, Dahlöf B, et al. for the LIFE study group. Cardiovascular morbidity and mortality in patients with diabetes in the Losartan Intervention For Endpoint reduction in hypertension study (LIFE): A randomised trial against atenolol. Lancet 359:1004-1010, 2002.

49. Lindholm LH, et al. Effects of losartan on sudden cardiac death in people with diabetes: Data from the LIFE study. Lancet 362:619-620, 2003.

50. Klahr S et al. for the Modification of Diet in Renal Disease Study Group. The effects of dietary protein restriction and blood pressure control on the progression of chronic renal disease. N Engl J Med 330:877-884, 1994.

51. Wright JT, Bakris J, Greene T, et al. for the American Study of Kidney Disease and Hypertension Study Group. Effect of blood pressure lowering and antihypertensive drug class on progression of hypertensive kidney disease: results from the AASK trial. JAMA 288:2421-2431, 2002.

52. Giatras I, Lau J, Levey AS for the Angiotensin-Converting-Enzyme Inhibition and Progressive Renal Disease Study Group. Effect of angiotensin-converting enzyme inhibitors on the progression of nondiabetic renal disease: A meta-analysis of randomized trial. Ann Intern Med 127:337-345, 1997.

53. Gruppo Italiano di Studi Epidemiologia in Nefrologia. Randomised placebo-controlled trial of effect of ramipril on decline in glomerular filtration rate and risk of terminal renal failure in proteinuric non-diabetic nephropathy. Lancet 349:1857-1863, 1997.

54. Jafar TH, Schmid CH, Landa M, et al. Angiotensin-converting enzyme inhibitors and progression of nondiabetic renal disease: A meta-analysis of patient-level data. Ann Intern Med 135: 73-87, 2001.

55. Gueyffier F, Bulpitt C, Brossel J-P, et al. Antihypertensive drugs in very old people: A subgroup meta-analysis of randomised controlled trials. Lancet 353:793-796, 1999.

56. Glynn RJ, Beckett LA, Hebert LE, et al. Current and remote blood pressure control and cognitive decline. JAMA 281: 438-445, 1999.

57. Sacktor N, Gray S, Kawas C, et al. Systolic blood pressure within an intermediate range may reduce memory loss in an elderly hypertensive cohort. J Geriatr Psychiatry Neurol 12: 1-16, 1999.

58. Somes GN, Pahor M, Schorr RJ, Cushman WC, Applegate WS. The role of diastolic blood pressure when treating systolic hypertension. Arch Intern Med 159:2004-2009, 1999.

59. Johannesson M, Fagerberg B. A health economic comparison of diet and drug treatment in obese men with mild hypertension. J Hypertens 10:1063-1070, 1992.

60. Oxman AD, Thomson MA, Davis DA, et al. No magic bullet: A systematic review of 102 trials or interventions to improve professional practice. Can Med Assoc J 153:1423-1430, 1995.

61. Shaneyfelt T. Building bridges to quality. JAMA 286:2600-2601, 2001.

62. Gyatt G, Meade M, Jaschke R, et al. Practitioners of evidence-based care. BMJ 320:954-955, 2000.

63. Grol R, Grimshaw J. From best evidence to best practice: Effective implementation of change in patients' care. Lancet 362:1225-1230, 2003.

64. Kottke TE, Stroebel RJ, Hoffman RS. JNC7: It's more than high blood pressure. JAMA 289:2573-2575.

# Current Prescribing Practices

## J. Jaime Caro, Krista A. Payne

That clinical decisions should be rational and based on the best evidence possible is the keystone of modern scientific medicine. Finding reality wanting, however, opinion leaders have increasingly called for a more determined effort to ensure that actual practice meets this standard. Criteria that have been proposed for the selection of studies that will provide this evidence emphasize the randomized clinical trial as a gold standard.[1,2] A physician faced with a common—and very well studied—condition such as hypertension is expected to turn to randomized trials (or corresponding meta-analyses), and the guidelines based on these, for information on which to base treatment choices.[3-9]

The sixth report of the Joint National Committee on Prevention, Detection, Evaluation, and Treatment of High Blood Pressure (JNC VI), published in 1997,[3] recommended that a diuretic or β-blocker be selected as first line pharmacologic therapy in the absence of special patient characteristics that indicate use of a specific drug. Moreover, it was suggested that a series of steps be followed, including adding or switching medications, if the response to the initial treatment was insufficient.[3] Published in December 2002, results of the landmark Antihypertensive and Lipid-Lowering Treatment to Prevent Heart Attack Trial (ALLHAT),[10] the first and only trial to compare, longitudinally, three classes of antihypertensive drug therapies with conventional thiazide therapy, validated the recommendation to initiate antihypertensive therapy with older versus newer medications. More specifically, in a clinical trial of 33,357 patients over a mean follow-up period of 4.9 years, it was observed that although each class of medication substantially reduced blood pressure (BP) and served equally well to decrease the risk of combined fatal coronary heart disease (CHD) or nonfatal myocardial infarction (MI; the primary trial endpoint), thiazide-type diuretics, the least expensive of the antihypertensives, were superior to either angiotensin-converting enzyme (ACE) inhibitors or α-blockers in the prevention of one or more major forms of cardiovascular disease (CVD). Although these results appear to have achieved mainstream acceptance, many have publicly refuted these findings, citing design-related biases that may be associated with better outcomes for the diuretic group, an apparent lack of concern on the part of the ALLHAT investigators for the higher rate of diuretic-related adverse events observed in the trial and the potential long-term clinical and economic sequelae of these events.[11-14] Given the flurry of editorials and publications related to both the merits and weaknesses of ALLHAT, it is anticipated that debate will continue for quite some time. One wonders if the ALLHAT trial raises more questions than it answers.[14]

Primarily as a result of the ALLHAT trial[10] and a published meta-analysis of clinical trials of antihypertensive treatments,[15] a seventh set of guidelines by the Joint National Committee on Prevention, Detection, Evaluation, and Treatment of High Blood Pressure (JNC 7) has been issued.[16]

Consequently, it is now recommended that pharmacologic treatment for uncomplicated hypertension *always* begin with a thiazide-type diuretic with the addition of a second drug from a different class if the BP goal is not achieved. Marking a major change from previous guidelines, β-blockers have now been relegated to second-line therapy. In contrast, the most recent set of European Society of Hypertension guidelines[17] do not recommend a specific class of antihypertensive drug as first-line therapy for uncomplicated hypertension. These guidelines, instead, encourage the practitioner to consider, at his or her own discretion, each patient and his/her optimal therapy on a case-by-case basis.

Although it will take some time before the full impact of studies like the ALLHAT trial and recent guidelines on physician prescribing practices can be observed, in this chapter we review recent hypertension treatment patterns from actual practice in several countries and examine how they have accorded with earlier guidelines. We also provide comment on the generalizability of clinical trial results, the gold standard upon which treatment guidelines are based, to the real world and reasons to start treatment for uncomplicated hypertension with drugs other than diuretics or β-blockers (in this chapter, referred to as *group 1* to connote "older" drugs). Only data from articles published since 1988 are included.

## INITIAL TREATMENT CHOICES

### United States

In the United States, antihypertensive treatment practice appears quite varied. For example, in a study of 377 newly diagnosed patients carried out in the Midwest over an 18-month period (1991-1992),[18] 55% received monotherapy, but only about a third started on a diuretic or β-blocker. The most common initial therapy was a calcium channel blocker given to 30%, followed by an ACE inhibitor in 22%. Sequential monotherapy was used in 18% of the patients, and stepped therapy (with more than one class of drug given at some point) in 22%; 5% were started on more than one drug. The picture was very different in patients beginning antihypertensive therapy who were part of a cohort of approximately 1700 patients examined annually between 1989 and 1993.[19] Consistently, about half started with regimens that incorporated a group 1 drug (55% of the 157 patients seen in 1989-1991; 49% of the 142 seen in 1990-1992; and 56% of the 120 seen in 1991-1993). Calcium channel blockers slightly led ACE inhibitors among the rest.

In contrast to these studies of actual practice, surveys of U.S. physicians find that they report much greater adherence to published treatment guidelines. For example, 69% of 128 family physicians and primary care internists in Iowa in 1988 reported choosing a group 1 drug as initial therapy for patients younger than 40 years of age.[20] Most of the rest (27%) would choose an ACE inhibitor. Similar results were obtained for older patients in a survey of more than 1000 New Jersey physicians in 1985: 78% reported choosing a group 1 drug as the initial treatment for patients older than 60 years with isolated systolic hypertension (ISH).[21] Even greater adherence to official guidelines was reported in a survey of 274 physicians in Minnesota in 1987,[22] where 91% stated that a group 1 drug was their first choice of medication.

Factors such as age and gender of the patient can influence the choice of antihypertensive treatment in the United States. Among 183 Minnesota physicians surveyed about initial therapy in 1992,[23] no drug class predominated as first choice, but group 1 drugs were more frequently selected for a 48-year-old man (30%) than for a 65-year-old (25%). Choice of a calcium channel blocker was much less common for the younger man (16% vs. 36%), whereas ACE inhibitors were more common (44% vs. 37%). For older women, however, the preferences were evenly distributed.

Studies have revealed changes in the level of adherence to the guidelines over time. A review of 8428 people aged 65 years and older, whose records were in the New Jersey Medicaid and Medicare databases from 1982 to 1988, found that the proportion starting treatment with a group 1 drug dropped from about 70% to 45%—most of the decline occurring in diuretic prescriptions.[24] Use of a calcium channel blocker increased from 7% to 28%, and of an ACE inhibitor from 0.3% to 16%, during the same 6-year period. Diuretic use was more common in patients older than 85 years, women, and African Americans.

Similar declines in preference for group 1 drugs were found among 241 primary care physicians in the Midwest surveyed in 1987 and again in 1989[25]—from 90% to 62%. In the latter survey, 30% chose an ACE inhibitor and the rest, a calcium channel blocker or other class. Physicians were also asked for their preferences for a group 2 medication. In 1987, 84% stayed within group 1, whereas only 60% did so by 1989, with ACE inhibitors chosen by about one quarter of physicians.

In a structured care setting, changes in preferences appear to parallel treatment guidelines more closely. This is evident in a study of 550 union members during the first year of a union-sponsored hypertension screening and follow-up program carried out between 1986 and 1992.[26] In the period before JNC IV guidelines, physicians treated 87% of their patients with group 1 drugs. After JNC IV (which recommended all four classes), 90% of patients were started with a calcium channel blocker or an ACE inhibitor, whereas publication of JNC V (which recommended group 1 drugs for initial treatment) saw practice even out to about 25% for each major class.

## Canada

Evidence from Canada also reveals much variation in antihypertensive prescribing practices and a tendency to disregard practice guidelines. In a review of the medical records of 711 newly diagnosed hypertensive patients seen in Edmonton, Alberta, between 1993 and 1995,[27] less than one third (31%) of those receiving medicines (531) were started on a group 1 drug. This remained less than 50% even when patients with a documented contraindication to one of these drugs were excluded. ACE inhibitors were the most common first choice (44%), whereas only 23% used a calcium channel blocker.

These prescribing patterns were reported to be very similar among physicians in many different types of practice. However, family physicians were found to choose the recommended classes of medication more often than did internists.

In a study of the records of more than 27,000 new patients in the neighboring province of Saskatchewan, carried out from 1990 through 1994,[28] nearly half (48%) were found to have started on a group 1 drug. Indeed, among the 24 different drugs prescribed initially to at least 100 patients each, the combination of triamterene and hydrochlorothiazide in a single tablet was more than three times more common than any given ACE inhibitor or calcium channel blocker. ACE inhibitors, however, were the second most frequent initial drug class, whereas only 13% of new patients began on a calcium channel blocker. The initial choice of drug among new patients varied according to the age and gender of the patient (Table 37-1). In females and older males, group 1 drugs remained the most common choice, with diuretics predominating. By contrast, in younger men, an ACE inhibitor was as common as a group 1 drug. Although choice of a β-blocker was infrequent in all groups, it was relatively more common in younger patients.

There was little variation over the 5 years of the study, however, with group 1 drugs consistently representing the initial choice in about 45% of new patients. ACE inhibitors also remained the second most common initial choice throughout the study period. Use of calcium channel blockers, other single drugs, combination drugs, and multiple drugs also remained stable during the study period.

These data on actual practice confirm the results of a Canadian survey of physicians' preferences in the province of Alberta in 1995.[29] In that study, physicians were asked for their choice of initial therapy for several hypothetical cases. In the case of a lower-risk patient, group 1 drugs were prescribed by 44% of physicians, ACE inhibitors by 46%, and calcium channel blockers by 5%. As risk factors increased, group 1 drugs dropped to 20%, ACE inhibitors increased to 67%, and calcium channel blockers increased to 10%. Only in the case of a patient with target organ damage, left ventricular hypertrophy (LVH), and previous MI did the preference shift to group 1 drugs (62%), primary β-blockers (56%).

The choice of medication can vary, as expected, with the clinical condition.[30] When ISH was the issue, the majority of 281 physicians surveyed in 1995 in Edmonton, Alberta, reported their choice of antihypertensive treatment to be a diuretic—74% among internists and 58% among family physicians; only 10% of internists and 26% of family physicians would choose an ACE inhibitor first in this situation.

## New Zealand

Physicians in New Zealand also reported less preference for group 1 drugs. In a 1992 survey of 100 physicians, only 48% would choose a group 1 drug for a 60-year-old man with essential hypertension and no contraindications.[31] Most of the remainder (39%) would choose an ACE inhibitor (9% chose a calcium channel blocker).

Actual practice data do not clearly address the issue of initial treatment choices, because they do not distinguish between new and established patients. For example, a 1988 survey of 37 general practitioners that included information on 2 months of prescriptions[32] found that nearly half of patients (44%) were receiving more than one drug. Thus,

**Table 37-1** Distribution of Initial Drug Regimens in Newly Diagnosed Hypertensives*

| Drug Class | Male (%) | | Female (%) | | Overall (%) |
| | Younger than 60 years (n = 5262) | 60+ years (n = 6653) | Younger than 60 years (n = 6046) | 60+ years (n=9403) | (n = 27,364) |
|---|---|---|---|---|---|
| Diuretics | 23 | 36 | 41 | 45 | 38 |
| β-Blockers | 15 | 8 | 13 | 8 | 10 |
| ACE inhibitors | 38 | 28 | 25 | 25 | 29 |
| Calcium channel blockers | 14 | 16 | 11 | 13 | 13 |
| Other single agent | 3 | 4 | 5 | 3 | 4 |
| Combinations | 3 | 3 | 3 | 2 | 3 |
| Multiples | 4 | 5 | 3 | 4 | 4 |

*Differences in distribution within gender and age group p <.001.

although diuretics were used in 47% and β-blockers in 48%, it is uncertain what their first prescription was. This problem applies as well to surveys in 1982 and 1987,[33] in which the use of diuretics was high initially but dropped between surveys (64%-47%), whereas β-blocker use remained constant (52%-55%), and use of calcium channel blockers (3%-13%) and ACE inhibitors increased (0%-13%).

## United Kingdom

In the United Kingdom, actual practice has conformed to guidelines—at least, according to surveys of physicians' opinions. In one survey of 360 general practitioners in Leicestershire, England, in 1991,[34] 62% reported they would start treatment with a thiazide diuretic in a 70-year-old hypertensive patient without target organ damage. Among the remainder, 17% reported they would use nonpharmacologic treatment. Another survey of 200 physicians in England (East Anglia) in 1993 found similar results: 85% of the respondents indicated that in the absence of contraindications, they would start therapy with a group 1 drug—nearly two thirds of these with a diuretic. Only 10% chose an ACE inhibitor and 5% a calcium channel blocker.[35] The tendency to favor a diuretic was even more pronounced among 92 physicians surveyed in Northamptonshire in 1993[36]: 83% reported that a thiazide diuretic would be their initial choice for a 70-year-old patient with no end-organ damage; another 5% reported choosing a β-blocker first.

Although there are some differences according to the type of physician, the preference for group 1 drugs persists. For example, a 1992 survey of 214 general practitioners and 127 hospital physicians in the northern region of England found that the former would choose a group 1 drug for an otherwise well, 75-year-old male nonsmoker 79% of the time, whereas the latter would do so only 62% of the time.[37] For the remainder, the split was similar, with a calcium channel blocker chosen almost three times as often as an ACE inhibitor.

These reported preferences for group 1 drugs are supported by actual practice data, although they are not specific to new patients. In a review of the database records of more than 37,000 hypertensive patients seen in 1992 to 1993, new courses of treatment were analyzed.[38] Among the 10,222

patients starting a new type of treatment, 86% received a group 1 drug, 32% a calcium channel blocker, and 27% an ACE inhibitor. The numbers add to more than 100%, because more than a third of patients received multiple new drugs.

## Australia

Survey data published in 1992 on 132 randomly selected general practitioners in South Australia indicate similarly high adherence to the guidelines: About three quarters would choose a group 1 drug for treating an uncomplicated moderately hypertensive patient.[39] Although this preference varied little with the age of the hypothetical patient, the balance between diuretics and β-blockers did. In a 75-year-old patient, the diuretics were heavily favored (68% vs. 9%) compared with a more even distribution for a 45-year-old patient (41% vs. 31%). Most of the physicians surveyed in Australia (80%) also indicated that if they failed to achieve control with the initial therapy, they would add another drug rather than switch therapies.

These reported preferences differ from the findings of an analysis over an 11-year period of the Commonwealth Department of Community Services and Health database, which covers 80% of community prescriptions (not including hospital dispensings or those paid by private insurance). According to these data, the use of diuretics decreased by nearly one third from 1982 to 1987, whereas the use of ACE inhibitors increased dramatically.[40] Unfortunately, as in the United Kingdom, the analysis did not distinguish new from established patients, and thus it is impossible to say whether this change in prescription patterns reflects a shift in the choice of initial medication or in the drugs used subsequently.

In an analysis of the Australian Pharmaceutical Benefits Scheme (PBS) and Repatriation Pharmaceutical Benefits Scheme (RPBS) data from 1994 to 1998, it was observed that in 1998, the most frequently prescribed antihypertensive medications were those acting on the renin-angiotensin system (RAS), followed by calcium channel blockers, and then group 1 drugs.[41] Results show a trend of decreasing rates of prescriptions to group 1 medications over this 5-year period, and the opposite for RAS agents and calcium channel blockers. Authors also note that this lack of adherence to guidelines has cost the Australian government $1.45 million annually due to the significantly higher cost of the newer medications.

## Germany

Physicians in Germany also reported remarkable adherence to published guidelines in the choice of initial therapy. In a 1988 survey of 315 general practitioners, 93% reported choosing a group 1 drug for a 45-year-old man; in contrast to the United Kingdom and Australia, nearly all (92%) would select a β-blocker.[42] Only 3% chose a calcium channel blocker and 1% an ACE inhibitor. For a 65-year-old man, a group 1 drug was chosen 71% of the time; most, however, chose a diuretic. A calcium channel blocker was chosen by 21%; an ACE inhibitor by 2%. The overall pattern of prescribing was very similar for internists and was not affected by the physician's age.

Again, these reported preferences are somewhat at odds with actual data—this time gathered in the Monitoring of Trends and Determinants of Cardiovascular Disease (MONICA) Augsburg project, which surveyed 3324 hypertensive men and women in 1984 to 1985 and again in 1987 to 1988.[43] There were 167 patients treated for hypertension in the second survey who were untreated in the first. Although these patients were considered "newly treated" by the authors, it is unlikely that the prescription information obtained consistently represented the first medication used. Thus, by the time they were surveyed, only 25% of these patients were on a β-blocker and just as many were on triple-agent therapy. Among men, calcium channel blockers, singly or in combination with another agent, accounted for one third of prescriptions, whereas among women, diuretics and diuretic combinations accounted for one third of prescriptions reported.

## Sweden

β-Blockers were reported to be the favorite in a survey of 126 general practitioners and specialists in the Uppsala-Orebro region in 1991.[44] The physicians were asked for their first choice of therapy for each of six hypothetical hypertensive patients. For a healthy, nonsmoking, 44-year-old man with a family history of diabetes and BP of 180/100 mm Hg, 40% indicated that they would choose a β-blocker, whereas less than 1% chose a diuretic. ACE inhibitors were the second most common choice (24%), but more so among specialists (34% vs. 18%). Calcium channel blockers were the choice of 18%, and 17% would not choose pharmacotherapy. In only two of the six hypothetical cases did diuretics account for more than 10% of the choices, and neither of these was a new patient.

This preference for β-blockers was reported to be even stronger in a 1991 survey of 236 physicians.[23] For an otherwise healthy 48-year-old man, 72% chose a β-blocker. The preference for a β-blocker was less pronounced for older patients and women: 57% of physicians chose a β-blocker for a 65-year-old man, but only 52% did for a 65-year-old woman. Preference for diuretics increased from less than 5% for a 48-year-old man to 20% for a 65-year-old man and 27% for older women. Physicians were surveyed about the hypothetical 48-year-old man again in 1993, and treatment preferences were found to have changed little.[45]

More data from Swedish actual practice[46] reveal that from 1981 to 1998 in patients who attended their annual follow-up visit to an outpatient hypertension clinic, rates of prescriptions of thiazides declined from 61% to 10%, whereas prescriptions of calcium channel blockers increased from 4% to 30% and ACE inhibitors from 0% to 23%. It was also reported that prescriptions of both calcium channel blockers and ACE inhibitors increased during 1990 to 1995, but that the former decreased significantly from 1996 to 1998 when concerns related to their safety emerged.

## Norway

Preferences for β-blockers did not hold in Norway. A 1989 survey of 235 Oslo physicians found that 51% would choose diuretics for an asymptomatic 75-year-old hypertensive man[47]; calcium channel blockers were a second choice at 25%. ACE inhibitors accounted for only 13%, and β-blockers and others accounted for the remaining 11%. Physicians older than 50 years of age were more apt to prescribe a diuretic, whereas a calcium channel blocker was more commonly chosen by physicians younger than age 40 years and by specialists. Female physicians were significantly less apt to choose an ACE inhibitor than were males.

## Italy

A physician preference for newer antihypertensive medications instead of group 1 drugs was observed in an Italian database analysis of data from 5061 elderly patients with hypertension from 1988 to 1997.[48] Group 1 drugs were prescribed to a minority of patients despite a significant increase in their use over time. ACE inhibitor prescriptions also increased over time and by 1997 became the most common class of antihypertensive prescribed (50%). With respect to diuretics, their use dipped between 1988 (3%) and 1991(3%) following publication of the JNC IV guidelines,[49] but over time reached rates of 4% in 1997, second only to ACE inhibitors. According to these authors, evidence-based medicine has had little impact on the hypertension management practices of Italian physicians.

## India

Two studies conducted in India[50,51] suggest that physician practice is more in accord with guideline recommendations than most other countries. In the first,[50] survey data of 1076 prescriptions written to patients attending an outpatient hypertension clinic (validated by medical records and patient interviews) revealed that β-blockers were the most frequently prescribed (51%), followed by calcium channel blockers (47%), and ACE inhibitors (46%). This study did not differentiate between patients with new versus chronic hypertension nor single and combination therapies.

The same pattern emerged in a second study[51] of 300 patients attending an internal medicine clinic: β-Blockers were the most frequently prescribed (46.7%), followed by calcium channel blockers (34.3%), and then ACE inhibitors (30%). Diuretics were prescribed only 13.2% of the time, which prompted a call by the authors for more frequent use of these agents given their low relative cost.

## Other Countries

Marked differences between countries were reported in a 1992 survey of general practitioners in Indonesia, Italy, United Kingdom, Croatia, Panama, France, and Belgium (each represented by at least 18 physicians).[52] Asked for their first choice for treating mild hypertension in the absence of contraindications, 63% of Italian physicians and 93% of Croatian physicians chose diuretics, compared with Indonesia and Belgium, where 40% and 94%, respectively, chose β-blockers.

## EFFECTS OF INITIAL TREATMENT CHOICES

The recommendations to choose group 1 drugs as initial therapy depend, at least in part, on two key assumptions: One is that at the start of therapy there is *no reason to expect that any one therapy will do better than others.* The second is that the initial treatment choice is not so important because, if it is not successful, changes can be made to optimize the regimen for a given patient and these *modifications will have no detrimental effects.* If these two assumptions hold, it makes sense to choose a drug from a class proven to reduce cardiovascular risk and with a lower acquisition cost. If they prove untenable, however, the appropriate first choice might turn out to be quite different. This might be the case if the likelihood of patients remaining compliant—and, thus, benefiting from treatment—differs according to the class of drug chosen initially. This could happen if the side effect profile of a class were less well tolerated by patients who, in the context of an otherwise asymptomatic condition, tend to stop treatment or if the therapeutic "turbulence" generated by changes in the regimen to deal with side effects or to achieve BP control bothers the patient in excess of the perceived benefits. The patient may ask, why put up with what appears to be troublesome trial and error to treat a condition with nebulous menace?

The assumptions underlying the choice of group 1 drugs as initial therapy for uncomplicated hypertension may seem reasonable to the physician, but they have been implemented virtually without testing in routine actual practice. The evidence for equivalent expectations has been based on controlled clinical trials and the evidence that treatment modifications, or therapeutic turbulence, will have no detrimental effects is actually quite scant. Even clinical trials as high profile as the ALLHAT study, which was designed to assess efficacy, are unable to address these assumptions because the very procedures implemented to ensure valid efficacy data so alter compliance that the trial no longer reflects true routine practice.

The essence of these two assumptions—that the drug classes are equivalent in the proportion of patients who can be expected to stay on therapy and thus achieve BP control—was tested in a study using the healthcare databases of Saskatchewan.[28,53] Saskatchewan Health funds the healthcare system of the province, including a prescription drug plan.[54] The records were examined of 27,364 Saskatchewan residents with a diagnosis of essential hypertension who received at least one antihypertensive agent listed in the Saskatchewan formulary between November 1, 1989, and December 31, 1994, but had no record of treatment in the preceding year. Men and women older than age 40 years without a diagnosis of malignant hypertension of hepatic, renal, or cardiovascular diseases other than hypertension were eligible.

The outpatient prescription drug plan database yielded all dispensings of an antihypertensive drug identified by its generic name, as well as the dispensing date, quantity, strength, and drug form. The database did not include information on the actual prescription nor on BP. A patient was considered persistent with therapy if it was estimated, based on a priori algorithm used to assess the dispensing records that he or she still had antihypertensive medication to take on the last day of follow-up. Whether the patient actually took the medication, or if it had been discontinued following physician's advice, could not be determined.

Persistence was analyzed for the 22,918 patients who were observed in the database for at least 6 months and who began treatment with one of the four major classes of medication. Almost one quarter of patients had discontinued all antihypertensive therapy within a year of starting it. The rate of persistence varied with class of drug: 74% of patients who started treatment with a diuretic were persistent at 1 year; the persistence rate among patients starting on a β-blocker was 78%, 81% for those starting on a calcium channel blocker, and 84% for those starting on an ACE inhibitor. At 2 years, persistence rates were even lower: 64% for a diuretic, 69% for a β-blocker, 71% for a calcium channel blocker, and 74% for an ACE inhibitor. Four years after starting antihypertensive therapy, only 46% of those starting on a diuretic were still on antihypertensive therapy; this figure was 54% for a β-blocker, 53% for a calcium channel blocker, and 58% for an ACE inhibitor. The increased persistence over time associated with ACE inhibitors compared with group 1 drugs remains significant, even when controlling for differences in age, gender, and use of healthcare resources in the prior year.

A higher frequency of changes in the therapeutic regimen was also significantly associated with decreasing persistence in each of the first 3 years of therapy ($p = .05$). For example, subjects who had two or more changes to their therapeutic regimen in any 6-month interval were 25% less likely to persist with medication in the next 6 months, and even a single change decreased persistence by 7%. These data indicate that the choice of first antihypertensive agent is an important determinant of the likelihood that the patient will continue with therapy.

These results from actual practice have been replicated. A comprehensive review that included the Saskatchewan analyses[53] and other similar database studies revealed that *all* studies of initial hypertension treatment in newly diagnosed patients reported very poor adherence in actual practice with observed rates of nonadherence ranging from 12% to 57% depending on the definition of nonadherence and time horizon employed.[55] It was also evident from this same review that initial treatment with newer classes of drugs in newly diagnosed hypertension patients was a significant factor favoring treatment adherence. More specifically, when the results by initial drug class for each of the 10 studies reviewed were rank ordered (i.e., lowest to highest rate of nonadherence), the following pattern emerged without exception: Adherence in the first year was greatest for patients initially prescribed ACE inhibitors, followed in descending order by those treated with calcium channel blockers, β-blockers, and diuretics. Results of more actual practice database studies, which include adherence profiles for the newest class of antihypertensives, the angiotensin II (Ang II) receptor antagonists, are consistent with earlier studies and reveal even higher rates of persistence for this class.[56-59]

The interpretation of these persistence data from actual practice has been hotly debated, with critics citing selection bias and effective marketing as factors to explain the observed results.[60,61] Although it is not possible to determine the validity of these arguments, in light of the international scope and replicability of these studies, at the very least this evidence from actual practice should not so easily be dismissed. The underlying premise of therapeutic guidelines, which suggests that drug classes are equivalent in terms of *effectiveness* outcomes and that changes in medication can be made without detriment, therefore, must be questioned. Evidence from actual practice also suggests that side effects associated with diuretics and other older drugs can lead to therapeutic inefficiency and nonpersistence, which dramatically diminish differences in treatment costs between older and newer agents.[62] The issue is not that observational data should replace data from clinical trials, but simply that results from studies in actual practice are also worth considering when weighing all of the evidence for the selection of a first-line therapy.[60] Curiously, neither JNC VI nor 7 make reference to this growing volume of data from actual practice.[3,17]

## SUMMARY

When physicians are surveyed about their hypertension treatment practices, adherence to guidelines is typically reported. Consistently, however, data from actual practice in numerous countries with diverse healthcare systems reveal that drugs other than diuretics or β-blockers are nevertheless being prescribed as first-line therapy in the majority of newly diagnosed cases of elevated BP. Whereas in some countries, such as Germany, India, and the United Kingdom, a diuretic or β-blocker is frequently used; an ACE inhibitor or calcium channel blocker is more common in others (United States, Canada, Sweden, and Italy). The choice of initial medication for treatment of hypertension in actual practice varies by country and by practitioner.

Although a general discussion of the full range of possible reasons why physicians do not adhere to guidelines is outside of the scope of this chapter,[63-65] some potential guideline-related barriers to such adherence have been hypothesized.[64] In a published critique of three current guidelines for hypertension treatment,[3,4,65] numerous shortcomings are highlighted that could account for the limited impact on physician practice that has been observed. The most significant of these reported were dissidence among guidelines, failure to address clinically relevant issues, format deficiencies, lack of implementation strategies, poor methodologic quality, and failure to incorporate patient-clinician values.

Generally, for patients without comorbidities, known drug sensitivity, or other factors that drive the decision, results from key clinical trials[10] and current guidelines suggest that treatment be started with a diuretic and that changes be made thereafter as needed. Data from actual practice studies, such as the Saskatchewan analysis,[28,53] indicate that there may be disadvantages to this process.[55] Although the interpretation of these data have been debated[60,61] and largely excluded from the pool of evidence drawn upon for the creation of treatment

guidelines, physicians, nevertheless, should weigh all the evidence. An increased probability of achieving BP control by ensuring that patients remain on medication could justify the initial choice of one of the newer agents, such as an ACE inhibitor Ang II receptor blocker.

## References

1. Evidence-Based Medicine Working Group. Evidence-based medicine: A new approach to teaching the practice of medicine. JAMA 268:2420-2425, 1992.
2. Editorial Staff. Purpose and procedure. Evidence-Based Med 1:98-99, 1996.
3. Joint National Committee on Prevention, Detection, Evaluation, and Treatment of High Blood Pressure. The sixth report. Arch Intern Med 157:2401-2402, 1997.
4. WHO/ISH Guidelines Sub-Committee: 1993 Guidelines for the management of mild hypertension: Memorandum from a WHO/ISH meeting. Bull World Health Organ 71:503-517, 1993.
5. Wright JM, Lee C-H, Chambers GK. Systematic review of antihypertensive therapies: Does the evidence assist in choosing a first-line drug? CMAJ 161:25-32, 1999.
6. Wright JM. Choosing a first-line drug in the management of elevated blood pressure: What is the evidence? 1: Thiazide diuretics. CMAJ 163:57-60, 2000.
7. Wright JM. Choosing a first line drug in the management of elevated blood pressure: What is the evidence? 2: Beta-blockers. CMAJ 163:188-192, 2000.
8. Wright JM. Choosing a first-line drug in the management of elevated blood pressure. What is the evidence? 3: Angiotensin-converting-enzyme inhibitors. CMAJ 163:293-296, 2000.
9. Jackson PR, Ramsay LE. First-line treatment for hypertension. Eur Heart J 232:179-182, 2002.
10. The ALLHAT officers and coordinators for the ALLHAT Collaborative Research Group. Major outcomes in high-risk hypertensive patients randomized to angiotensin-converting enzyme inhibitor or calcium channel blocker vs. diuretic: The Antihypertensive and Lipid-Lowering Treatment to Prevent Heart Attack Trial (ALLHAT). JAMA 288:2981-2997, 2002.
11. Messerli FH, Beevers DG, Franklin SS, et al. Beta-blockers in hypertension-the emperor has no clothes: An open letter to present and prospective drafters of new guidelines for the treatment of hypertension. Am J Hypertens 16:870-873, 2003.
12. Resnick LM. Why we can't translate clinical trials into clinical practice in hypertension. Am J Hypertens 16:421-425, 2003.
13. Julius S. The ALLHAT study: If you believe in evidence-based medicine, stick to it! J Hypertens 21:453-454, 2003.
14. McInnes GT. Size isn't everything—ALLHAT in perspective. J Hypertens 21:459-461, 2003.
15. Psaty BM, Lumley T, Furberg CD, et al. Health outcomes associated with various antihypertensive therapies used as first-line agents. A network meta-analysis. JAMA 289:2534-2544, 2003.
16. Chobanian AV, Bakris GL, Black H, et al. The seventh report of the Joint National Committee on Prevention, Detection, Evaluation, and Treatment of high blood pressure. The JNC7 report. JAMA 289:2560-2572, 2003.
17. Guidelines Committee. 2003 European Society of Hypertension—European Society of Cardiology guidelines for the management of arterial hypertension. J Hypertens 21:1011-1053, 2003.
18. Jerome M, Xakellis GC, Angstman G, et al. Initial medication selection for treatment of hypertension in an open-panel HMO. J Am Board Fam Pract 8:1-6, 1995.
19. Psaty BM, Koepsell TD, Yanez ND, et al. Temporal patterns of antihypertensive medication use among older adults, 1989 through 1992. JAMA 273:1436-1438, 1995.

20. Carter BI, Kriesel HT, Steinkraus L, et al. Antihypertensive drug-prescribing patterns of internists and family physicians, J Fam Prac 29:257-262, 1989.

21. Breckenridge MB, Kostis JB. Isolated systolic hypertension in the elderly: Results of a statewide survey of clinical practice in New Jersey. Am J Med 86:370-375, 1989.

22. Kofron PM, Rästam L, Pirie CB, et al. Physician practice for cardiovascular disease risk-factor reduction in six upper Midwestern communities. J Fam Pract 32:49-55, 1991.

23. Troein M, Arneson T, Rästam L, et al. Reported treatment of hypertension by family physicians in Sweden and Minnesota: A physician survey of practice habits. J Intern Med 238:215-221, 1995.

24. Monane M, Glynn RJ, Gurwitz, D, et al. Trends in medication choices for hypertension in the elderly. Hypertension 25:1045-1051, 1995.

25. Bostick RM, Luepker RV, Kofron PM, et al. Changes in physician practice for the prevention of cardiovascular disease. Arch Intern Med 151:478-484, 1991.

26. Alderman MH, Madhavan S, Cohen H. Antihypertensive drug therapy. The effect of JNC criteria on prescribing patterns on patient status through the first year. Am J Hypertens 9:413-418, 1996.

27. McAlister FA, Teo KK, Lewanczuk RZ, et al. Contemporary practice patterns in the management of newly diagnosed hypertension. CMAJ 157:23-30, 1997.

28. Caro JJ, Salas M, Speckman JL, et al. Persistence with treatment for hypertension in actual practice. CMAJ 160:31-37, 1999.

29. McAlister FA, Laupacis A, Teo KK, et al. A survey of clinician attitudes and management practices in hypertension. J Hum Hypertens 11:413-419, 1997.

30. McAlister FA, Teo KK, Laupacis A. A survey of management practices for isolated systolic hypertension. J Am Geriatr Soc 45:1219-1222, 1997.

31. Arroll B, Jenkins S, North D, et al. Management of hypertension and the core services guidelines: Results from interviews with 100 Auckland general practitioners. N Z Med J 108:55-57, 1995.

32. Kawachi I, Malcolm LA, Purdie G. Variability in antihypertensive drug therapy in general practice: Results from a national survey. N Z Med J 102:307-309, 1989.

33. Sinclair B, Jackson R, Beaglehole R. Patterns in the drug treatment of hypertension in Auckland, 1982-7. N Z Med J 102:491-493, 1989.

34. Fotherby MD, Harper GD, Potter JF. General practice: General practitioners' management of hypertension in elderly patients. BMJ 305:750-752, 1992.

35. Dickerson JEC, Garratt CJ, Brown MJ. Management of hypertension in general practice: Agreements with and variations from the British Hypertension Society guidelines. J Hum Hypertens 9:835-839, 1995.

36. Fahey T, Silagy C. General practitioners' knowledge of and attitudes to the management of hypertension in elderly patients. Br J Gen Pract 44:446-449, 1994.

37. Ford GA, Asghar MN. Management of hypertension in the elderly: Attitudes of general practitioners and hospital physicians. Br J Clin Pharmacol 1995;39:465-469.

38. Jones JK, Gorkin L, Lian JF, et al. Discontinuation of and changes in treatment after start of new courses of antihypertensive drugs: A study of a United Kingdom population. BMJ 311:293-295, 1995.

39. Steven ID, Wilson DH, Wakefield MA, et al. South Australian hypertension survey. General practitioner experiences with drug treatment. Med J Aust 156:641-644, 1992.

40. Hurley SF, Williams SL, McNeil JJ. Trends in prescribing of antihypertensive drugs in Australia, 1977-1987. Med J Aust 152:259-266, 1990.

41. Nelson MR, McNeil JJ, Peeters A, et al. PBS/RPBS cost implications of trends and guideline recommendations in the pharmacological management of hypertension in Australia, 1994-1998. Med J Aust 174:565-568, 2001.

42. Weiland SK, Keil U, Spelsberg A, et al. Diagnosis and management of hypertension by physicians in the Federal Republic of Germany. J Hypertens 9:131-134, 1991.

43. Hense HW, Tennis P. Changing patterns of antihypertensive drug use in a German population between 1984 and 1987. Eur J Clin Pharmacol 39:1-7, 1990.

44. Ribacke M. Treatment preferences, return visit planning and factors affecting hypertension practice amongst general practitioners and internal medicine specialists. J Intern Med 237:473-478, 1995.

45. Troein M, Gardell B, Selander S, et al. Guidelines and reported practice for the treatment of hypertension and hypercholesterolemia. J Intern Med 242:173-178, 1997.

46. Bog-Hansen E, Lindblad U, Ranstam J, et al. Antihypertensive drug treatment in a Swedish community: Skaraborg Hypertension and Diabetes Project. Pharmacoepidemiol Drug Saf 11:45-54, 2002.

47. Strømme HK, Botten G. Factors relating to the choice of antihypertensive and hypnotic drug treatment in old patients. Scand J Prim Health Care 10:301-305, 1992.

48. Onder G, Gambassi G, Landi F, et al. Trends in antihypertensive drugs in the elderly: The decline of thiazides. J Hum Hypertens 15:291-297, 2001.

49. Joint National Committee on Detection, Evaluation, and Treatment of High Blood Pressure. The 1988 report of the joint national committee on detection, evaluation and treatment of high blood pressure. Arch Intern Med 148:1023-1038, 1988.

50. Malhotra S, Karan RS, Pandhi P, et al. Pattern of use and pharmacoeconomic impact of antihypertensive drugs in a north Indian referral hospital. Eur J Clin Pharmacol 57:535-540, 2001.

51. Jhag R, Goel NK, Gautam CS, et al. Prescribing patterns and cost of antihypertension drugs in an internal medicine clinic. Indian Heart J 53(3):323-327, 2001.

52. Avanzini F, Tognini G, Alli C, et al., on behalf of the International Society of Drug Bulletins. How informed general practitioners manage mild hypertension: A survey of readers of drug bulletins in 7 countries. Eur J Clin Pharmacol 49:445-450, 1996.

53. Caro JJ, Speckman JL, Salas M, et al. The effect of initial drug choice on persistence with antihypertensive therapy: The importance of actual practice data. CMAJ 160:41-46, 1999.

54. Malcolm E, Downey W, Strand LM, et al. Saskatchewan Health's linkable data base and pharmacoepidemiology. Post Marketing Surveillance 6:175-264, 1993.

55. Payne KA, Esmonde-White S. Observational studies of antihypertensive medication use and compliance: Is drug choice a factor in treatment adherence? Curr Hypertens Rep 2:515-524, 2000.

56. Conlin PR, Gerth WC, Fax JF, et al. Four-year persistence patterns among patients initiating therapy with the angiotensin II receptor antagonist losartan versus other antihypertensive drug classes. Clin Ther 23:1999-2010, 2001.

57. Esposti LD, Esposti ED, Valpiani G, et al. A retrospective, population-based analysis of persistence with antihypertensive drug therapy in primary care practice in Italy. Clin Ther 24:1347-1357, 2002.

58. Esposti D, Sturani A, DeMartino M, et al. Long-term persistence with antihypertensive drugs in new patients. J Hum Hypertens 16:439-444, 2002.

59. Marentette MA, Gerth WC, Billings DK, et al. Antihypertensive persistence and drug class. Can J Cardiol 18:349-356, 2002.

60. Caro JJ, Payne K. The value of industry-sponsored studies of initial antihypertensive therapies [letter]; CMAJ 164:1832, 2001.

61. Wright JM. The value of industry-sponsored studies of initial antihypertensive therapies. CMAJ 164:1832-1833, 2001.

62. Payne KA, Caro JJ. Evaluating the true cost of hypertension management: Evidence from actual practice. Expert Rev Pharmacoeconomics Outcomes Res 4:179-187, 2004.

63. Cabana MD, Rand CS, Powe NR, et al. Why don't physicians follow clinical practice guidelines? A framework for improvement. JAMA 282:1458-1465, 1999.

64. Davis DA, Taylor-Vaisey A. Translating guidelines into practice. A systematic review of theoretic concepts, practical experience and research evidence in the adoption of clinical practice guidelines. CMAJ 157:408-416, 1997.

65. Logan J, Graham ID. Toward a comprehensive interdisciplinary model of health care research use. Sci Commun 20:227-246, 1998.

66. McAlister FA, Campbell NRC, Zarnke ML, et al. The management of hypertension in Canada: A review of current guidelines, their shortcomings and implications for the future. CMAJ 164:517-522, 2001.

67. Feldman RD, Campbell N, Larochelle P, et al. 1999 Canadian recommendations for the management of hypertension. CMAJ 161:S1-S17, 1999.

# Chapter 38

# Calcium Channel Blockers: Controversies, Lessons, and Outcomes

## Lionel H. Opie

Calcium channel blockers (CCBs) are powerful antihypertensive agents. Until relatively recently, however, there have been no trials showing long-term efficacy and safety of CCBs in reducing outcome measures such as stroke and heart disease. Efficacy of any group of drugs does not necessarily equal safety. The latter may be defined as the absence of significant adverse effects when the drug is used with due regard for its known contraindications.[1] In the case of CCBs, concerns have been expressed that these agents may have inherent safety problems, such as increases in myocardial infarction (MI), cancer, and gastrointestinal bleeding. The latter two fears have largely been discounted,[1] but the possible relationship of CCB use to acute myocardial infarction (AMI) has remained controversial[2] until recently. Results of three medium-sized (between 1000 and 10,000 participants) randomized controlled trials, STOP-2,[3] NORDIL,[4] and INSIGHT,[5] and three mega-trials, ALLHAT, CONVINCE, and INVEST (Table 38–1), have swollen the total number of subjects persons studied to more than 100,000 to allow an objective reappraisal of the role of CCBs in hypertension therapy based on solid trial data in more than 100,000 hypertensives. These extensive trial data weaken the conclusions of an earlier negative meta-analysis.[6] As summarized in Table 38–2, AMI is not increased with CCB treatment.[7] This chapter reevaluates the safety and efficacy of CCBs as antihypertensives with special emphasis on the randomized controlled trials and updates the information in the author's previous meta-analysis[8] and review.[9]

## HISTORICAL BACKGROUND TO CONTROVERSY

CCBs were initially hailed as very effective antianginal agents at a time when the coronary spasm theory of unstable angina held sway. The HINT (Holland Inter-university Nifedipine Trial) study was one of the first to test the safety and efficacy of a CCB in this condition.[10] Patients with unstable angina were allocated to one of several groups: placebo, CCB (short-acting nifedipine), β-blocker (metoprolol), or the combination (nifedipine plus metoprolol). The trial was stopped because nifedipine capsules doubled the rate of AMI within 48 hours of beginning therapy, the mechanism presumably being adrenergic activation because the addition of the CCB to preexisting β-blocker therapy gave benefit. By combining a number of trials using very high doses of short-acting nifedipine given to patients with largely unstable coronary disease, Furberg linked use of this agent to increased mortality in a widely cited meta-analysis.[11] Although his results have been

disputed by many, including myself and Messerli,[12] and although there were serious errors in the calculations, nonetheless Furberg correctly pointed out the need for large randomized controlled trials with the CCBs. In the case of hypertension, many adequate trials have now been undertaken, all with long-acting rather than short-acting CCBs, which is important because sustained blood levels of an antihypertensive agent are required for maximal antihypertensive effects over 24 hours. The results of these trials indicate that CCBs can be used in hypertension with reductions in cardiovascular mortality similar to those with conventional agents such as diuretics and β-blockers, and without evidence of increased cardiovascular risk (see Table 38–1). Going back to 1995,[13] observational studies have pointed to potential negative effects of CCBs, specifically the short-acting dihydopyridines (DHPs). The claimed adverse events included increased mortality, cardiovascular events, gastrointestinal bleeding, and cancer. These have often been reported in major U.S. newspapers, magazines, and even leading medical journals. Many other articles denied these claims. The result has been confusion that should now be dispelled by outcome and safety data on more than 100,000 patients. This chapter evaluates the controversies, the lessons that can be learned, and the outcomes.

## CONTROVERSY 1: DO CALCIUM CHANNEL BLOCKERS DECREASE MORTALITY IN HYPERTENSION?

To achieve a decrease in mortality with any antihypertensive requires either a very large trial, a very high-risk population, or a meta-analysis of several trials.[14] A number of nonrandomized cohort studies, available in the year 2000, tested the hypothesis that CCB therapy could increase mortality.[1] There was suggestive evidence for a mortality increase related to short-acting agents, chiefly nifedipine. However, in 13 placebo-controlled trials, there was a trend to reduced mortality rates. Currently there is much stronger evidence for the hypothesis that CCBs can reduce mortality in hypertension. Proof of this supposition comes from four trials—STOP-2,[3] NORDIL,[4] INSIGHT,[5] and ALLHAT[15] (see Table 38–1). In each case, the mortality in the CCB group equaled that of conventional therapy. When considering the elderly population, in the only trial that gave a clear-cut mortality reduction vs. placebo,[16] two thirds of the patients received combined β-blocker plus diuretic therapy after starting on one of these agents. The conventional therapy group in STOP-2 and NORDIL was similarly treated. In INSIGHT and ALLHAT, the CCB group gave similar mortality results to diuretic-based therapy. If conventional antihypertensive therapy reduces mortality,[16] then CCBs do likewise.

Lionel H. Opie, M.D., retains copyright to his original figures.

**Table 38–1** Key Features of Recent Large Outcome Trials, Each in More than 10,000 Personas, Comparing Calcium Channel Blockers (CCBs) with Other Agents in 82,355 Hypertensives

| | ALLHAT[15] | CONVINCE[49] | INVEST[40] | ASCOT[50] |
|---|---|---|---|---|
| Comparators | CCB (amlodipine); diuretic | CCB (verapamil); diuretic or β-B | CCB (verapamil ± ACEi); β-B ± diuretic | CCB (amlodipine ± ACEi); β-B ± diuretic |
| Numbers in trial, CCBs vs. non-CCBs | 9048; 15,255 respectively | 8179; 8297 respectively | 11,267; 11,309 respectively | >19,000 |
| Mean age at start | 67 years | 66 years | 66 years | To come |
| Trial design | Double-blind, randomized | Double-blind, randomized | PROBE, randomized open; blinded for endpoint | PROBE; randomized open; blinded for endpoint |
| Strong points of study | Patients at high risk for MI | Older than 55 years, high risk including obesity | 100% of patients had CAD | 1, 2, and 3 endpoints; event driven |
| Weak points of study | Low initial BP; practice-based endpoints | Stopped after 3 years instead of planned 5 | Not blinded for drugs | Not blinded for drugs |
| Mean initial BP | 146/84 mm Hg | 150/87 mm Hg; | 150/86 mm Hg; | Not known |
| Mean final BP | 135/75 mm Hg; 134/75 mm Hg; | 137/79; mm Hg; 137/78 mm Hg; | 131/76 mm Hg; | Not known |
| Duration (approximate) | 4 to 8 years | 5 years; forced early stop | Mean, 2.7 years | Up to 5 years |
| Primary endpoint(s) | Combined fatal CHD or nonfatal MI | Nonfatal MI, nonfatal stroke, CV-related death | All cause mortality, nonfatal MI, nonfatal stroke | Nonfatal MI, fatal CHF |
| Major results | Similar | Similar | Similar | Not known |

ALLHAT, Antihypertensive and Lipid-Lowering Treatment to Prevent Heart Attack Trial; CONVINCE, Controlled Onset Verapamil Investigation of Cardiovascular Endpoints; INVEST, International Verapamil SR/Trandolapril Study; ASCOT, Anglo-Saxon Cardiac Outcomes Trial; β-B, beta-blocker; MI, myocardial infarction; BP, blood pressure; CAD, coronary artery disease; CHD, coronary heart disease; CV, cardiovascular.

## CONTROVERSY 2: ARE CALCIUM CHANNEL BLOCKERS SAFE?

In a comprehensive review of 100 studies available in the year 2000, the safety and efficacy of CCBs were evaluated in evidence coming from a variety of types of studies, including case series, case control studies, cohort studies (both prospective and retrospective), randomized controlled trials, and meta-analyses.[1] Eighty-four of these studies gave enough detail to allow evaluation of adverse or beneficial effects. Of these, 25 studies claimed adverse effects, 37 studies showed a lack of adverse effects, and 22 showed beneficial effects. Two additional epidemiologic studies, one with 3511 participants followed for 6 years[17] and the other with 11,663 participants followed for 16 years,[18] showed no impact of CCBs on cancer. In the case of hypertensives treated with CCBs, data from randomized controlled trials show no increase in AMI, cancer, GI bleeding, or depression. Only increased heart failure remains a problem, as will be discussed.

Overall safety does not mean that CCBs can be used with impunity. Clear contraindications such as the use of dihydropyridines (DHPs) without β-blockers in acute coronary syndromes (unstable angina), cannot be ignored. In the case of the non-DHPs, sinus bradycardia and/or an excessively prolonged PR-interval are relative contraindications, and combined therapy with β-blockers is generally contraindicated.

## LESSONS FROM META-ANALYSES

### Blood Pressure Lowering Treatment Trialists' Collaboration (BPLTTC)

This meta-analysis compared results of treatment with different antihypertensives in 162,341 patients in 29 trials (see Table 38–2).[7] Trials comparing ACE inhibitors and CCBs with placebo, included much smaller numbers: 18,229 in five ACE inhibitor trials and only 6656 in four CCB trials. Nevertheless, this analysis provides strong evidence of benefits of each type of drug on stroke and major cardiovascular events, including coronary heart disease (CHD). When compared with placebo, CCBs reduced stroke by 38% (confidence intervals [CI], 0.47-0.82), and major cardiovascular events by 18% (CI, 0.71-0.93). Furthermore, CCBs, when compared with "conventional" (diuretic- or β-blocker–based) therapy, gave the same incidence of coronary mortality, cardiovascular death, and total mortality. However, as will be discussed, heart failure increased by 33% (CI, 1.21-1.47) with CCB treatment. The specific virtue of this meta-analysis is that it was prospectively started in 1995 by the principal investigators of the major trials then in progress. This procedure avoided one of the major problems of a retrospective meta-analysis, namely selection bias, resulting from the subjective judgment of which trials to include and which to exclude. This study also has the support of the World Health Organization–International Society of Hypertension. The major defect of the analysis is the grouping together of trials with totally different cardiovascular inclusion criteria, for example hypertension and coronary artery disease or diabetic nephropathy. This incongruity does not affect the comparison of CCBs with conventional agents in hypertension.

## Pahor-Furberg Meta-Analysis

The Pahor-Furberg meta-analysis of 27,743 individuals in nine trials compares longer acting CCBs with all other antihypertensive drugs, not only in the three major trials shown in Table 38–1, but also in several smaller trials.[6] Strength of this analysis include its comprehensive nature and the viewpoint of a group experienced in meta-analytic techniques. Several important points emerge. First, this meta-analysis agrees with that of the BPLTTC in that CCBs as a group do not alter total mortality when compared with other agents (see Table 38–2). This conclusion is in contrast to the influential meta-analysis of Furberg in 1995 that linked short-acting nifedipine to increased mortality in patients with CHD.[11] Second, when compared with all other agents, including ACE inhibitors, CCBs give a 26% (CI, 1.11-1.43) increase in AMI and very similar increase in heart failure.

There are also some problems with this meta-analysis. The first, as in any other retrospective study, is the difficulty of eliminating selection bias. Second, as Psaty and Furberg emphasize elsewhere,[19] the quality of a meta-analysis critically depends on the quality of the studies deemed to be eligible for that meta-analysis. "Trials with major design flaws carry little or no weight." If the major issue is the effect of different antihypertensives on outcome measures, then it is crucial that these should be clearly defined. In STOP-2,[3] NORDIL,[4] and INSIGHT[5] there were exact and detailed definitions of stroke, AMI, and heart failure. In INSIGHT, an independent critical events committee assessed all endpoints according to prespecified criteria. These therefore become the major studies, constituting a total of 21,611 patients versus 27,743 in the Pahor meta-analysis. The minor studies included by Pahor[6] cover

**Table 38–2** Major Differences Between Four Meta-Analyses Comparing Calcium Channel Blockers (CCBs) with Other Therapies in Hypertension

| | Pahor et al., 2000[6] | Opie and Schall, 2002[8] | BPLTTC, 2003[7] | Staessen, 2003[24] |
|---|---|---|---|---|
| Authors | Seven academics from three U.S. universities | Dual authorship | Committee of 48 under the aegis of the WHO-International Society of Hypertension | Three academics from one Belgian center |
| Type of study | Retrospective | Retrospective | Prospective | Retrospective |
| Entry point | All trials on hypertension meeting criteria | All high-quality trials on hypertension | All trials from initiation of study | All BP-lowering trials with no heart failure at start |
| Comparators | All non-CCB results taken together | CCBs with conventional; separate comparison with ACEi in diabetics | Separate comparisons of CCBs with placebo, conventional therapy, and ACEi | New (CCBs, ACEi or ARB) vs. old drugs (diuretics, β-blockers) |
| Number of trials | 9 | 6 | 18 | 7 |
| CCB numbers in study | 12,699 vs. non-CCBs | 12,116 CCBs vs. conventional; 1965 vs. ACEi in diabetics | 31,031 CCBs vs. conventional; 12,541 CCBs vs. ACEi | 32,864 CCBs vs. conventional |
| Major result | Mortality unchanged | Mortality unchanged | Mortality unchanged | Mortality unchanged |
| CV outcomes vs. conventional | ↑MI 26% (CI = 1.11-1.43); ↑CHF 25% (CI = 1.07-1.46); stroke unchanged | ↓stroke 12.7% (CI = 0.77-0.99); ↑MI 18% (CI = 1.04-1.35); NS↑ CHF15% (CI = 0.97-1.36) | CV mortality and MI unchanged; CHF↑ 33% (CI = 1.21-1.47) | ↓stroke 10%; CV mortality, MI unchanged; CHF ↑ 33% |

MI, myocardial infarction; CHF, congestive heart failure; CV, cardiovascular; NS, nonsignificant; CI, confidence intervals; ↑, increase; ↓, decrease; ACEi, ACE inhibitor; ARB, angiotensin type 1 receptor blocker.

6132 individuals. In MIDAS (Multicenter Isradipine Diuretic Atherosclerosis Study)[20] clinical endpoints were not predefined. In CASTEL (Cardiovascular Study in the Elderly)[21] the only predefined endpoints were total and cardiovascular mortality, with others not listed in the trial protocol. The outcome results of these other endpoints were not published. CASTEL has other defects. According to data given to the present author, nifedipine tablets were given once daily (correct dosage interval twice daily) and compared with two other agents given together, namely high-dose atenolol plus a diuretic. Thus it is inevitable that 24-hour blood pressure (BP) reduction would have been better in the double-dosed patients, thereby explaining the better outcome.

The Pahor meta-analysis[6] also relies on ABCD (Appropriate Blood Pressure Control in Diabetes), in which the outcome data have had to be revised[22] and on FACET (Fosinopril versus Amlodipine Cardiovascular Events Trial),[23] an open-label study without clearly predetermined outcome endpoints. This meta-analysis also includes clonidine in the non-CCB drugs, although clonidine was used only in the small CASTEL study (61 patients given clonidine of a total of 27,743 in the meta-analysis as a whole).[21]

## Opie-Schall Meta-Analysis

Based on the same data as the other meta-analyses, the Opie-Schall[8] approach differed in that the primary studies were subjected to quality control and divided into grade A (such as those in Table 38–1) and others. The statistical quality was increased by introducing the Bonferroni criteria for multiple comparisons. As the other meta-analyses had concluded that total and cardiovascular mortality was unchanged by CCBs compared with conventional treatment, we reasoned that the prime differences must lie in nonfatal events. We proposed that diabetics treated by ACE inhibitors were likely to be different from nondiabetics, because of the known hemodyamic effects of ACE inhibitors on the kidneys. The study concluded that CCBs balanced a relatively small increase in AMI by a very similar decrease in stroke.

## Staessen Meta-Analysis

Using virtually the same studies as the other meta-analyses, but updated to March 2003, Staessen et al.[24] set out to compare the "old" agents, diuretics and β-blockers, with the "new" therapy, namely ACE inhibitors and CCBs. They proposed that all the agents had roughly similar effects for the same BP reduction and outcomes, and that most of the benefit came with a fall of about 5 mm Hg in systolic blood pressure (SBP). The CCBs reduced stroke by 10%, whereas heart failure increased by 33%. The latter value is heavily dependent on the large numbers in ALLHAT, in which the criteria for heart failure were one symptom and one sign, hence open to criticism.[24]

## Pstay Meta-Analysis

In the Pstay meta-analysis[25] a network system was used to incorporate both direct comparisons and indirect evidence from trials that had one treatment in common. This meta-analysis showed that low-dose diuretics reduced heart failure by 26% versus CCBs. Although the indirect methodology is open to question, this effect on heart failure is in accord with direct comparisons as in ALLHAT[15] and INSIGHT.[5]

## LESSONS TO BE LEARNED FROM META-ANALYSES

Four major lessons may be learned from these meta-analyses. First, the much-publicized large percentage increase in AMI found in the CCB group by Pahor and Furberg could not be confirmed in the better and larger mega-trials with CHD as a primary endpoint (see Table 38–1). Due caution must be exercised in interpreting any meta-analysis, especially when it is at least in part based on imperfect trial data. Although the result of a meta-analysis may look very impressive, more and better trial data can and do change the picture. Second, all the meta-analyses showed that there are no differences in mortality between CCB and conventional therapy, by far the most important endpoint. This point of concordance, which is very seldom emphasized, means that it is BP reduction and little else that determines mortality,[24] apart from some special situations to be considered later. Third, it is very important to publicize both the relative and absolute changes thought to be due to any specific therapy. Percentage changes make small absolute changes seem much larger. Last, a meta-analysis is not infallible. There have been obvious statistical mistakes in at least two of meta-analyses.[8,11]

## BENEFITS AND DEFECTS OF CALCIUM CHANNEL BLOCKER THERAPY

### Benefits of Calcium Channel Blocker Therapy

CCB therapy has several benefits in addition to favorable effects on outcome. First, CCBs act within hours or days, which is useful to convince the patient that the BP can be controlled, thereby gaining the patient's confidence. Second, they often bring down the BP in otherwise refractory patients. Third, they may be used as initial therapy in salt-sensitive Black patients[26] who may not respond to initial therapy with a β-blocker or ACE inhibitor (for reservations emanating from the AASK study, see later). Fourth, CCBs may be especially useful in selected patients with stable effort angina, often giving a better quality of life than β-blockers.[27] Fifth, they are often required in combination therapy to reduce BP to the new goals now being suggested,[28] especially in diabetics.[29,30] Sixth, they have antihypertensive effects that are less influenced by indomethacin than in those of ACE inhibitors.[31] Seventh, they lessen the risk of new diabetes when compared with diuretic/β-blocker therapy.[15,32]

### Known Defects of Calcium Channel Blockers

What are the disadvantages of CCB therapy? These agents, especially the DHP group when given in high doses, often have nuisance side effects such as headache and ankle swelling that make it relatively common for patients to discontinue them. Nonetheless, in the Treatment of Mild Hypertension Study[33] amlodipine in a low dose of 5 mg was the best tolerated of the five types of agents used, including a β-blocker and a diuretic.[33] There are some important situations in which CCBs *should not be used* as initial antihypertensive therapy. In post-MI patients, there are no trials favoring the use of DHPs. Non-DHPs may be different, with good data for verapamil[34] and lesser data for diltiazem. In heart failure, there are no data favoring CCBs. In fact, in INSIGHT[5] and ALLHAT[15] the long-acting DHP used increased heart failure, as will be discussed. In renal disease and in diabetics with nephropathy, ACE inhibitors or angiotensin receptor blockers (ARBs) are generally preferred as initial therapy (see next section).

## OUTCOMES: CALCIUM CHANNEL BLOCKERS IN SPECIFIC SUBGROUPS OF PATIENTS

### Isolated Systolic Hypertension

There have been only a few trials with clearly defined isolated systolic hypertension (ISH) as the entry criterion. A long-acting CCB, nitrendipine, was used in the Syst-Eur study, a placebo-controlled double-blinded trial in the elderly that was stopped early because of the marked reduction in stroke.[35] Although very similar results were obtained in a diuretic-based trial, Systolic Hypertension in the Elderly Program (SHEP),[36] it is often forgotten that hypokalemia was relatively frequent in SHEP and, when it occurred, took away the cardiovascular benefit of treatment.[37] In the diabetic subgroups of these studies, the CCB was overall more effective (e.g., with a reduction in total mortality).[38] In the Syst-Eur study, the development of dementia was lessened by the CCB.[24] Furthermore, in the Systolic Hypertension in China (Syst-China) study,[39] nifedipine tablets gave a clear reduction in overall mortality, again in an elderly population.

### Coronary Heart Disease

Although earlier meta-analyses suggested increased CHD with CCB therapy,[6,8] two large trials with this primary endpoint showed no difference between CCB and diuretic or β-blocker therapy.[15,40] The updated meta-analysis of the BPLTTC[7] and Staessen[24] also showed no differences.

### Renal Disease

Regarding hypertensives with overt proteinuria, there is a caution in African Americans (and probably Black patients elsewhere) on the basis of results of the AASK Study (African-American Study of Kidney Disease and Hypertension).[41] The amlodipine arm of this study was stopped because of worsening renal function, but the ACE inhibitor and β-blocker arms continued in those with proteinuria >1 g per day. Here there is a pathophysiologic basis for preferring ACE inhibitors, which reduce both afferent and efferent arteriolar tone, whereas the DHPs tend to reduce only afferent arteriolar tone, with risk of increasing intraglomerular hypertension and worsening proteinuria. Nonetheless, there is no evidence for a blanket contraindication to DHPs in hypertensives with proteinuria. Of note, in INSIGHT, proteinuria of 0.5 g or more

per 24 hours was one the possible entry criteria to the trial.[5] It was the diuretic group rather than the CCB group that had the greater withdrawal rate because of impaired renal function (4.6% withdrawal in the diuretic group, 1.8% in the CCB group, *p* <.0001). CCBs are often combined with other antihypertensive agents such as ARBs or ACE inhibitors in the treatment of advanced renal disease, including diabetic nephropathy,[42] with the aim of achieving current standards for optimal BP reduction.

### Diabetic Hypertensives

In diabetic hypertensives with nephropathy, similar hemodynamic arguments indicate a preference for the use of ACE inhibitors or ARBs. A direct comparative study of the CCB amlodipine versus the ARB, irbesartan and a placebo has been carried out in patients with diabetic nephropathy.[43] The ARB gave better renoprotection than the CCB or placebo, without, however, altering overall mortality. In elderly diabetics without overt nephropathy, CCB and conventional therapy could not be distinguished in STOP-2.[44] Likewise, in the diabetic subgroups of the NORDIL and INSIGHT studies, no significant differences emerged between CCBs and conventional or diuretic-only therapy.[4,5] With new BP goals as low as 128/75 mm Hg[30] or even 120 mm Hg SBP emerging,[29] combination therapy including a CCB will almost always be required.

## FEWER NEW DIABETICS THAN WITH DIURETICS, BUT MORE HEART FAILURE

The INSIGHT study[5] compared long-acting nifedipine in an initial dose of 30 mg daily with a thiazide-potassium retaining combination diuretic in an initial dose of 25 mg hydrochlorothiazide plus 5 mg amiloride daily (equivalent to *half* a tablet of Moduretic [amiloride and hydrochlorothiazide]). Doses could be doubled if needed. The diuretic group showed increased blood sugar and uric acid, matched by increased development of diabetes and gout. In INSIGHT, the diuretic treatment group also had more hypokalemia, hyponatremia, hyperuricemia, hypoglycemia, and renal impairment than the CCB group. Hypokalemia occurred in 6.2% of the diuretic-treated group and 1.9% of the nifedipine group, even though a potassium-retaining agent was used. Even mild hypokalemia may be more serious than previously thought. In the INSIGHT study the thiazide dose was allowed to go up to 50 mg, "high" by current standards. In the meta-analysis that separately considered low-dose and high-dose diuretic versus β-blocker therapy, only low-dose diuretics clearly reduced mortality.[45] Thus, the metabolic advantages of the CCB versus the diuretic found in INSIGHT would probably be less obvious if the thiazide dose had been limited to 25 mg daily or lower.

In the ALLHAT study, the diuretic chlorthalidone, started in a low dose of 12.5 mg daily and titrated up to 25 mg had similar effects as amlodipine on total mortality and AMI, but with a small advantage to the diuretic in heart failure, a secondary endpoint. Concern remains about adverse metabolic effects of the diuretic, especially on potassium and blood sugar. In ALLHAT 12.7% and 8.5% of participants randomized to chlorthalidone developed low potassium values (K < 3.5 mmol/L) after 2 and 4 years, respectively. Furthermore, other metabolic changes in ALLHAT were in the same direction as in INSIGHT, with increased blood glucose and cholesterol levels in the chlorthalidone group. Particularly serious in ALLHAT was the increase in new diabetes from 9.8% at 4 years with the CCB to 11.6% with the diuretic. Because antihypertensive therapy is often lifelong, these metabolic changes cannot be ignored. On the contrary, and perhaps unexpectedly, the CCB nifedipine may improve insulin sensitivity.[46,47] Overall, four studies in 25,529 patients show that CCBs reduce new diabetes by 16% (CI, 0.78-0.91) versus conventional therapy.[32]

## Heart Failure

Compared with diuretics, DHPs increase heart failure. In the INSIGHT study heart failure was carefully defined and experienced observers individually confirmed each case.[5] The incidence was low (0.82% in the CCB group) and the absolute increase only 0.38%, although the relative increase was large (220%) compared with the diuretic. Diuretic therapy is known to benefit heart failure, whereas CCBs are contraindicated, in part because of their negative inotropic effects. Therefore, incipient heart failure is less likely to develop in a patient treated with a diuretic. In ALLHAT, the incidence of heart failure was inexplicably much higher in both the diuretic (5.7%) and the CCB (7.8%) groups. There are several other points of concern. First, ACE inhibitors, agents known to be effective in the treatment of all stages of heart failure, *increased* heart failure in ALLHAT by 19% (*p* <0.001) compared with the diuretic. Second, the diagnosis of heart failure was chiefly made by primary care physicians, and it is not sure how the ankle edema, known to be a side effect of DHP therapy, was dealt with diagnostically. Therefore, while noting the findings of ALLHAT, those of INSIGHT seem to be based on more reliable clinical observations and data. Nonetheless, both studies showed increased heart failure with a DHP. To prevent heart failure, combination of a CCB with an ACE inhibitor is likely to be successful.[40]

## INDIVIDUALIZED AND PATIENT-GUIDED CHOICE

Although the diuretic appeared to be the clear winner in ALLHAT, in reality there was overall equality of the primary outcome, fatal CHD and nonfatal AMI, between the CCB and the diuretic. Apart from the problematic heart failure issues, the CCB has advantages. In contrast to the diuretic, there are no metabolic side effects. Furthermore, an earlier Veterans Affairs study showed little or no BP response to diuretics in whites aged younger than 60 years.[48] In ALLHAT, the initial mean age (67 years) was well into the elderly category. The choice between CCBs and conventional treatment with a β-blocker or diuretic or other therapies such as ACE inhibitors should be carefully considered for each individual patient. In the elderly, a low-dose diuretic may be the first choice,[25] but a CCB has equally strong arguments.[24] A small reduction in stroke and a better metabolic profile with CCBs may be balanced by an increase in heart failure when compared with the diuretics. In many patients, combination therapy must be used to achieve current low BP goals, especially in diabetics and those with renal disease. In some cases CCBs are contraindicated, in oth-

ers they will be among the agents of first choice. The latter category includes those with effort angina or more severe hypertension, or the elderly with ISH.[35,38]

## SUMMARY

This chapter evaluates the current position of CCBs in antihypertensive treatment in the light of three mega-trials and five extensive meta-analyses. CCBs are equivalent to conventional (initial diuretic, diuretic/β-blocker, or β-blocker) therapy when total and cardiovascular mortality are the endpoints. With the mega-trial data, increased AMI can with confidence be eliminated as an unwanted effect of CCB therapy. Prior findings, largely from observational studies and mostly focused on short-acting capsular nifedipine, suggesting increases in cancer, gastrointestinal bleeding, and suicide can now be discounted by the results of randomized trials. When evaluating a CCB versus conventional treatment for first line therapy, β-blockers are preferred in postinfarct patients or in those with heart failure or unstable angina (a contraindication to DHPs in the absence of β-blockade). (See Chapter 54 for complete discussion of antihypertensives in the patient with ischemic heart disease.) CCBs are particularly useful when hypertension is accompanied by effort angina or when β-blockade is not likely to work well, as in African Americans or the elderly. Reductions in new-onset diabetes (by 16%) and stroke (by about 10%) with CCBs balance the increase in heart failure (versus thiazides). This increased risk of heart failure can probably be avoided by combining the CCB with an ACE inhibitor. Such choices should be individualized for each patient. Thus an open mind should be kept about the place of CCBs in current hypertension therapy. CCBs are neither better nor worse than conventional therapy, but act differently to achieve combined vasodilation and antianginal effects. CCBs remain a very valuable component of the antihypertensive armamentarium.

## Acknowledgment

This study was supported by (1) the Medical Research Council of South Africa by a grant to the Hatter Institute of the Cape Heart Center as part of the program of the Interuniversity Heart Research Group; (2) the Chris Barnard Fund of the Faculty of Health Sciences of the University of Cape Town; and (3) an educational grant from Servier Laboratories, Paris.

## References

1. Opie LH, Yusuf S, Kübler W. Current status of safety and efficacy of calcium channel blockers in cardiovascular diseases. A critical analysis based on 100 studies. Prog Cardiovasc Dis 43:171-196, 2000.
2. He J, Whelton PK. Selection of initial antihypertensive drug therapy (Commentary). Lancet 356:1942-1943, 2000.
3. Hansson L, Lindholm LH, Ekbom T, et al. Randomised trial of old and new antihypertensive drugs in elderly patients: Cardiovascular mortality and morbidity the Swedish Trial in Old Patients with Hypertension-2 Study. Lancet 354:1751-1756, 1999.
4. Hansson L, Hedner T, Lund-Johansen P, et al. For the Nordil Study Group. Randomised trial of effects of calcium antagonists compared with diuretics and beta-blockers on cardiovascular morbidity and mortality in hypertension: The Nordic Diltiazem (NORDIL) Study. Lancet 356:359-365, 2000.

5. Brown MJ, Palmer CR, Castaigne A, et al. Morbidity and mortality in patients randomised to double-blind treatment with a long-acting calcium-channel blocker or diuretic in the International Nifedipine GITS study: Intervention as a Goal in Hypertension Treatment. Lancet 356:366-372, 2000.

6. Pahor M, Psaty BM, Alderman MH, et al. Health outcomes associated with calcium antagonists compared with other first-line antihypertensive therapies: A meta-analysis of randomised controlled trials. Lancet 356:1949-1954, 2000.

7. Blood Pressure-Lowering Treatment Trialists' Collaboration. Effects of different blood-pressure-lowering regimens on major cardiovascular events: Results of prospectively designed overviews of randomised trials. Lancet 362: 1527-1535, 2003.

8. Opie LH, Schall R. Evidence-based evaluation of calcium channel blockers (CCBs) for hypertension. Equality of mortality and cardiovascular risk relative to conventional therapy. J Am Coll Cardiol 39:315-322, 2002. Erratum in: J Am Coll Cardiol 39:1409-1410, 2002.

9. Opie LH. Calcium channel blockers (CCBs) in hypertension. Reappraisal after new trials and major meta-analyses. Am J Hypertens 14:1074-1081, 2001.

10. HINT Study. Early treatment of unstable angina in the coronary care unit, a randomised, double-blind placebo controlled comparison of recurrent ischemia in patients treated with nifedipine or metoprolol or both. Holland Inter-university Nifedipine Trial. Br Heart J 56:400-413, 1986.

11. Furberg CD, Psaty BM, Meyer JV. Nifedipine dose-related increase in mortality in patients with coronary heart disease. Circulation 92:1326-1331, 1995.

12. Opie LH, Messerli FH. Nifedipine and mortality. Grave defects in the dossier. Circulation 92:1068-1073, 1995.

13. Pahor M, Guralnik JM, Corti M, et al. Long term survival and use of antihypertensive medications in older persons. J Am Geriat Soc 43:1191-1197, 1995.

14. Collins R, Peto R, MacMahon S, et al. Blood pressure, stroke and coronary heart disease. Part 2. Short term reductions in blood pressure: Overview of randomised drug trials in their epidemiological context. Lancet 335:827-838, 1990.

15. ALLHAT Collaborative Research Group. Major outcomes in high-risk hypertensive patients randomized to angiotensin-converting enzyme inhibitor or calcium channel blocker vs diuretic. The Antihypertensive and Lipid-Lowering Treatment to Prevent Heart Attack Trial (ALLHAT). JAMA 288:2981-2997, 2002.

16. Dahlöf B, Lindholm LH, Hansson L, et al. Morbidity and mortality in the Swedish Trial in Old Patients with Hypertension (STOP-Hypertension). Lancet 338:1281-1285, 1991.

17. Cohen H, Pieper CF, Hanlon JT, et al. Calcium channel blockers and cancer. Am J Med 15:210-215, 2000.

18. Stahl M, Bulpitt CJ, Palmer AJ, et al. Calcium channel blockers, ACE inhibitors, and the risk of cancer in hypertensive patients: A report from the Department of Hypertension Care Computing Project. J Human Hypertens 14:299-304, 2000.

19. Psaty BM, Furberg CD, Alderman M, et al. National guidelines, clinical trials and quality of evidence. Arch Intern Med 160:2577-2580, 2000.

20. Borhani N, Mercuri M, Borhani P, et al. Final outcome results of the Multicenter Isradipine Diuretic Atherosclerosis Study (MIDAS). A randomized controlled trial. JAMA 276:785-791, 1996.

21. Casiglia E, Spolaore P, Mazza A, et al. Effect of two different therapeutic approaches on total and cardiovascular mortality in a Cardiovascular Study of the Elderly (CASTEL). Jpn Heart J 35:589-600, 1994.

22. Schrier RW, Estacio RO. Additional follow-up from the ABCD trial in patients with type 2 diabetes and hypertension (letter). N Engl J Med 343:1969, 2000.

23. Tatti P, Pahor M, Byington RP, et al. Outcome results of the fosinopril versus amlodipine cardiovascular events randomized trial in patients with hypertension and NIDDM. Diabetes Care 21:597-603, 1998.

24. Staessen JA, Wang JG, Thijs L. Cardiovascular prevention and blood pressure reduction: A quantitative overview updated until 1 March 2003. J Hypertens 21:1055-1076, 2003.

25. Psaty BM, Lumley T, Furberg CD, et al. Health outcomes associated with various antihypertensive therapies used as first-line agents. JAMA 289:2534-2544, 2003.

26. Weir MR, Chrysant SG, McCarron DA, et al. Influence of race and dietary salt on the antihypertensive efficacy of an angiotensin-converting enzyme inhibitor or a calcium channel antagonist in salt-sensitive hypertensives. Hypertension 31:1088-1096, 1998.

27. Opie LH. First line drugs in chronic stable effort angina: The case for newer, longer-acting calcium channel blocking agents. J Am Coll Cardiol. 36:1967-1971, 2000.

28. Hansson L, Zanchetti A, Carruthers SG, et al. HOT Study Group. Effects of intensive blood-pressure lowering and low-dose aspirin in patients with hypertension: Principal results of the Hypertension Optimal Treatment (HOT) randomised trial. Lancet 351:1755-1762, 1998.

29. Adler AI, Stratton IM, Neil HAW, et al. On behalf of the UK Prospective Diabetes Study Group. Association of systolic blood pressure with macrovascular and microvascular complications of type 2 diabetes (UKPDS 36): Prospective observational study. BMJ 321:412-419, 2000.

30. Schrier RW, Estacio RO, Esler A, et al. Effects of aggressive blood pressure control in normotensive type 2 diabetic patients on albuminuria, retinopathy and strokes. Kidney Int 61: 1086-1097, 2002.

31. Morgan TO, Anderson A, Bertram D. Effect of indomethacin on blood pressure in elderly people with essential hypertension well controlled on amlodipine or enalapril. Am J Hypertens 13:1161-1167, 2000.

32. Opie LH, Schall R. Old antihypertensives and new diabetics. J Hypertens 22:1453-1458, 2004.

33. Neaton J, Grimm R, Prineas R, et al. Treatment of Mild Hypertension Study (TOMHS). Final results. JAMA 270: 713-724, 1993.

34. Pepine CJ, Faich GF, Makuch R. Verapamil use in patients with cardiovascular disease: An overview of randomized trials. Clin Cardiol 21:633-641, 1998.

35. Staessen JA, Fagard R, Celis LT, et al. Randomised double-blind comparison of placebo and active treatment for older patients with isolated systolic hypertension. Lancet 350:757-764, 1997.

36. SHEP Cooperative Research Group. Prevention of stroke by antihypertensive drug treatment in older persons with isolated systolic hypertension Final results of the Systolic Hypertension in the Elderly Program (SHEP). JAMA 265:3255-3264, 1991.

37. Franse LV, Pahor M, Di Bari M, et al. Hypokalemia associated with diuretic use and cardiovascular events in the Systolic Hypertension in the Elderly Program. Hypertension 35: 1025-1030, 2000.

38. Tuomilehto J, Rastenyte D, Birkenhager WH, et al. Effects of calcium-channel blockade in older patients with diabetes and systolic hypertension. N Engl J Med 340:677-684, 1999.

39. Liu L, Wang JG, Gong L, et al. For the Systolic Hypertension in China (Syst-China) Collaborative Group. Comparison of active treatment and placebo in older Chinese patients with isolated systolic hypertension. J Hypertens 16:1823-1829, 1998.

40. Pepine CJ, Handberg EM, Cooper-DeHoff RM, et al. A calcium antagonist vs a non-calcium antagonist hypertension treatment strategy for patients with coronary artery disease. The

International Verapamil-Trandolapril Study (INVEST): A randomized controlled trial. JAMA 290:2805-2816, 2003.

41. Agodoa LY, Appel L, Bakris GL, et al. For the African American Study of Kidney Disease and Hypertension (AASK) Group. Effect of ramipril vs amlodipine on renal outcomes in hypertensive nephrosclerosis. JAMA 285:2719-2728, 2001.

42. Brenner BM, Cooper ME, De Zeeuw D, et al. For the RENAAL Study Investigators. Effects of losartan on renal and cardiovascular outcomes in patients with type 2 diabetes and nephropathy. N Engl J Med 345:861-869, 2001.

43. Lewis EJ, Hunsicker LG, Clarke WR, et al. Renoprotective effect of the angiotensin-receptor antagonist irbesartan in patients with nephropathy due to type 2 diabetes. New Engl J Med 345:851-860, 2001.

44. Lindholm L, Hansson L, Ekbom T, et al. For the STOP Hypertension-2 Study Group. Comparison of antihypertensive treatments in preventing cardiovascular events in elderly diabetic patients: Results from the Swedish Trial in Old Patients with Hypertension-2. J Hypertens 18:1671-1675, 2000.

45. Psaty BM, Smith NL, Siscovick DS, et al. Health outcomes associated with antihypertensive therapies uses as first-line agents. A systemic review and meta-analysis. JAMA 277: 739-745, 1997.

46. Sheu W, Swislocki A, Hoffman B, et al. Comparison of the effects of atenolol and nifedipine on glucose, insulin, and lipid metabolism in patients with hypertension. Am J Hypertens 4:199-205, 1991.

47. Koyama Y, Kodama K, Suzuki M, et al. Improvement of insulin sensitivity by a long-acting nifedipine preparation (Nifedipine-CR) in patients with essential hypertension. Am Heart J 15: 927-931, 2002.

48. Materson BJ, Reda DJ, Cushman WC, et al. Single-drug therapy for hypertension in men. A comparison of six antihypertensive agents with placebo. The Department of Veterans Affairs Cooperative Study Group on Antihypertensive Agents. N Engl J Med 328:914-921, 1993.

49. Black HR, Elliott WJ, Grandits G, et al. For the CONVINCE Research Group. Principal results of the Controlled Onset Verapamil Investigation of Cardiovascular End Points (CONVINCE) Trial. JAMA 289:2073-2082, 2003.

50. ASCOT Investigators, Sever PS, Dahlhof B, et al. Rationale, design, methods and baseline demography of participants of the Anglo-Scandinavian Cardiac Outcomes Trial. J Hypertens 19:1139-1147, 2001.

| **Chapter 39**

# Nursing Clinics in the Management of Hypertension

## Nancy Houston Miller, Martha N. Hill

Nearly one in four Americans has hypertension. It is the single most common reason for a medical office visit.[1] While awareness and treatment of hypertension have improved over the past two decades, control rates have lagged far behind, leaving only one third of hypertensive patients achieving blood pressures (BPs) of less than 140/90 mm Hg.[2]

As we move into the twenty-first century, several important insights compel us to recognize the importance of hypertension as a major public health and medical problem. First, the lifetime risk of developing hypertension is very large. Investigators from the Framingham Heart Study[3] have reported the lifetime risk of hypertension to be 90% for men and women normotensive at 55 or 65 years, who survive to age 80 to 85. Moreover, there is a linear risk of ischemic heart disease and stroke mortality associated with increasing BP beginning at 115 systolic (SBP) and 75 mm Hg diastolic (DBP).[4] A doubling of mortality occurs for every 20–mm Hg and 10–mm Hg increase in systolic and diastolic pressures, respectively. Secondly, environmental factors associated with high BP in the United States and globally require us to acknowledge the impact of this public health problem. These include an obese population (50% are overweight or obese),[5] a high-sodium intake of 4100 mg/day for men and 2750 mg/day for women,[6] fewer than 20% of the population engaging in recommended physical activity of 30 min/day,[7] and less than a quarter of the population consuming five or more fruits and vegetables per day.[8] In addition to traditional clinical care of ambulatory patients with hypertension, population strategies may help to reduce BP in the population. These strategies include health education, professional education, and partnerships with national organizations, such as the food industry. Finally, important at-risk and high-risk populations, including those with multiple risk factors, diabetes, older age, and renal impairment, require meticulous BP control to lower risk of morbidity and mortality and the associated economic costs of hypertension care.

During the past three decades, nurses and other healthcare providers have played important roles in screening and managing patients with hypertension in inner-city areas, academic and community centers, multicenter research trials, and hypertension care management programs. Recognizing the enormity of the problems associated with hypertension today, their efforts to screen, identify cases, refer, follow-up, and educate patients is paramount. Moreover, their success in following protocols to achieve more timely and persistent BP control is significant. This chapter will focus on the success of nurses managing hypertension in a variety of healthcare settings.

## IMPLEMENTATION OF NURSE-RUN CLINICS

Management of an asymptomatic condition such as hypertension is challenging. Once individuals with hypertension are aware of their high BP, the first challenge is having them enter into and remain in treatment after initial screening and diagnosis. Many patients never make a first appointment after elevated BP is identified with screening or return for follow-up appointments after the initial diagnosis is made. Others do not undertake the lifestyle changes that could improve BP control or remain on medications. Moreover, it is well known that lifestyle changes cannot be adequately achieved without ongoing support during both the adoption and maintenance of these behaviors. The reasons for these patterns of medical care are many and discussed in other chapters.

Early efforts to involve nurses in hypertension management sought to offer more convenient options for supporting individuals with hypertension by bringing hypertension care to the home, local community, and work environment. In a landmark study by Runyan,[9] patients with hypertension, diabetes, or cardiac disease could choose to be followed by specially trained nurses in decentralized clinics close to their homes or in a hospital outpatient clinic for chronic disease staffed by internists. Patients in both groups were similar with regard to sociodemographic and clinical characteristics. At the end of 2 years, patients treated by nurses had lower BPs in all age groups except those aged 30 to 39 and older than 80 years of age. Moreover, by the end of the treatment period, patients treated in the nurse clinics had utilized approximately 50% fewer hospital admission days, while those treated in the outpatient clinics staffed by physicians showed an increase in hospital days for each of the disease categories. The authors attributed the success of the nurse-run clinics to the greater follow-up and greater time devoted by nurses to helping patients manage their condition.

In another study by Alderman et al.,[10] nurses played the central role in the screening and follow-up of patients in a worksite setting in New York City. In this successful program, nurses performed screening and enrollment in a New York department store. Hypertensive individuals who elected to participate in the program were followed by a nurse for 1 year. Nurses were responsible for taking the initial medical history, drawing preliminary laboratory data, and obtaining an electrocardiogram (ECG) upon entrance into the program. Approximately 1 week later, the medical director obtained a history, performed a physical exam, and reviewed laboratory data. Working closely with the medical director and using treatment algorithms, nurses initiated drug therapy and increased treatment in a step-wise fashion until the BP was <140/90 mm Hg. Diuretics were used as first-line therapy. The number and frequency of follow-up visits to the nurse were individualized based on patient's needs and control of BP. At these visits, which decreased in frequency to one every 3 months once BP was controlled, nurses monitored the BP, reviewed therapy and potential complications, checked medication and diet compliance, and helped to motivate patients to assume greater participation in and responsibility for their care. At the end of 1 year, the nurses' provision of care did not compromise program acceptability. In this worksite, 84% of the 1850 employees were screened, two thirds of those eligible for the hypertension treatment program sought care through the nurse program, and 97% of accepted patients remained in therapy, with 81% achieving acceptable BP reduction. Moreover, the direct annual per patient cost of $100 offset the costs associated with hypertension, including time lost from work, and allowed the health payer to offer this program as a union membership benefit.

In a study similar to that of Alderman, Logan et al.[11] found that hypertensive patients who were randomly allocated to receive care at work compared with those receiving standard care were significantly more likely to be put on antihypertensive medications (94.7% vs. 62.7%), to reach goal BP in the first 6 months of therapy (48.5% vs. 27.5%), and to take prescribed medications (67.6% vs. 49.1%). The authors claimed that the improvement in BP control was due to the fact that long-term care was more convenient, therapy was more vigorously applied, and compliance with therapy was more strongly encouraged by nurses.

Nurses have also made a major contribution to the management of hypertensive patients in national multisite clinical trials, many of which began in the late 1970s. The Hypertension Detection and Follow-up Program (HDFP)[12] and the Systolic Hypertension in the Elderly Program (SHEP)[13] are just two examples of large clinical trials conducted in the United States in which nurses provided screening, counseling, and medication management of hypertensive individuals. Most recently, nurses were part of the intervention team of the Antihypertensive and Lipid-Lowering Treatment to Prevent Heart Attack (ALLHAT) study.[14]

Evaluations of nurse-run clinics in which nurses saw patients alone or in collaboration with physicians show a level of BP control comparable with that achieved by physicians.[15] Similar results are seen where case-mix adjustment indicates nurses care for patients as complex as those seen by physicians.[16] Pheley et al.[17] reported on the screening, outcomes, and management of patients enrolled in a nurse-run hypertension management program in a large multispecialty practice in Minnesota. One year after entry into this program the proportion of patients who had their BP controlled to 140/90 mm Hg or less increased from 17% to 44%.

Nursing case management involving the use of telecommunication holds promise as an application for managing hypertensive individuals. In a study by Miller,[18] 78 patients were managed in a single face-to-face encounter and then systematically followed by telephone. During the initial encounter patients were educated about lifestyle changes and taught to measure BP using a home device. This session was followed by biweekly nurse-initiated telephone encounters of 10 minutes duration over a 6-month period, at which time SBPs and DBPs had declined by 10% and 8%, respectively, or 15 mm Hg and 7 mm Hg in absolute terms. The proportion of patients reach-

ing a goal BP increased from 22% to 48%. Importantly, the mean weight loss of patients enrolled in the study was 3.5 kg.

A similar pilot study conducted by Artenian et al.[19] highlights the value of a nurse-managed home telemonitoring system. Using a telephonic management system (Lifelink Monitoring, Inc.) to download BPs taken three times weekly at home by patients, nurses followed up with patients weekly through telephone calls to provide feedback on BP and counsel about lifestyle modification and adherence to medication regimens. This home-based nurse treatment intervention was compared with usual care and an intervention consisting of home BP measurement three times per week in a community center and feedback about lifestyle education by nurses. At the end of 3 months those in the home-based nurse treatment arm had the greatest improvement in BP.

More recently, Hill et al.[20,21] showed the benefit of incorporating a multidisciplinary team including a nurse-practitioner, community health worker, and physician in controlling BP in a high-risk population. Three hundred nine hypertensive African American males, mean age 41 ± 6 years, were randomly allocated to an intensive intervention consisting of nurse practitioner visits every 1 to 3 months for medications, and at least an annual visit by a community health worker versus a less intensive intervention. For those assigned to the intensive intervention, a community health worker provided referrals to social services, and offered job training and local housing resources. The physician offered consultation to the nurse practitioner about management and participated in case consultation. Those randomized to the less intensive intervention received education about the benefits of hypertension control, and referrals to hypertension care in the community. Men in both groups received an annual hypertension evaluation and a 6-month telephone call to assess health status and healthcare utilization. At 36 months, the mean change in SBP and DBP was −7.5/−10 mm Hg for the more intensive group, compared with +3.4/−3.7 mm Hg for the less intensive group ($p = .01$ and $.005$ for SBP and DBP, respectively). Moreover, the proportion of men reaching a controlled BP of <140/90 mm Hg was 44% in the intensive group compared with 31% in the less intensive group ($p = .45$), figures surpassing the national control rate. The authors suggest that, especially in high-risk populations, the traditional one-on-one physician-patient visit in an office practice setting needs to be supplanted by a more systematic patient-centered team approach.[21]

## NURSE MANAGEMENT—CLINICAL SETTINGS

### Roles and Responsibilities

The goals of managing hypertensive individuals are the same, whether the care is given in specialty clinics, private practice offices, worksite settings, primary care clinics, or neighborhood clinics. A team approach, bringing together physicians and nurses as well as community health workers, often produces better outcomes than a traditional medical approach. If nurse practitioners are caring for the patients, they practice quite independently, using protocols based upon guidelines and modified jointly with the physicians with whom they collaborate.[22] In settings in which the nurses do not have advanced practice credentials, physicians are responsible for making the diagnosis of hypertension and for determining secondary causes and comorbidities, which may influence decisions about appropriate treatment. Physicians help to formulate a treatment plan and provide consultation to nurses in managing complex cases. This shared collaborative practice arrangement allows physicians to use their time caring for sicker patients.

Nurses have shown that they can demonstrate critical clinical judgment in the management of patients within a hypertension clinic. In the worksite setting, they are often responsible for conducting screening programs to identify and refer hypertensive individuals. In programs to verify sustained elevated BP, nurses are responsible for determining the appropriateness of patients' ongoing management. For example, in the hypertension management program described by Pheley et al.,[17] more than three quarters of all patients referred for management of hypertension were deemed normotensive on the basis of a BP readings <140/90 mm Hg documented over three consecutive weekly screenings. Within this program nurses were responsible for seeing patients weekly to determine their level of BP and to provide the appropriate education for individuals with or at risk for hypertension. Screening and verification programs conducted by nurses enable them to identify individuals with sustained hypertension using standardized BP measurement techniques and to establish a database of individuals who can be followed for appropriate rescreening, as necessary. Such programs also help nurses identify patients who, based upon the multiple BP measurements, need lifestyle modification to lower high-normal pressures. By having nurses measure BP on multiple occasions, false positive diagnoses of hypertension and unnecessary treatment can be avoided.[23] This is important because previous studies have shown that physicians may base their treatment on a single measurement rather than making the diagnosis on at least two occasions with the appropriate attention to technique.[24] Moreover, having nurses use home BP measures taken by the patient or multiple measures more frequently in the clinic may obviate the "white coat" hypertension effect found by the physicians in office settings.[23]

In managing a cohort of patients within a hypertension clinic the nurse is responsible for taking a thorough medical history and for ordering appropriate blood chemistry tests such as sodium, potassium, creatinine, blood urea nitrogen, cholesterol, and a complete blood cell count; a urinalysis; and an electrocardiogram. This preliminary data collection allows physicians to devote their efforts either later in the visit or during a subsequent visit to performing the physical exam and formulating an appropriate treatment plan based upon the information and laboratory data provided by the nurse.

In the majority of hypertension clinics, nurses provide the education and counseling necessary to ensure that individuals are undertaking lifestyle changes that may favorably influence BP. Weight loss, the most successful nonpharmacologic technique to lower BP, requires behavior change for both eating and physical activity patterns. In addition, patients need help to limit calorie and sodium intake (to 100 Mmol/day) and alcohol consumption (to 1-2 drinks* per day).[22] In addition,

many hypertensive individuals present to the clinic with multiple risk factors for cardiovascular disease. The nurse can provide education and counseling for smoking cessation and dyslipidemia to help patients lower their overall risk of cardiovascular disease.

Why is the nurse's role so critical? Modifying lifestyle behaviors requires many clinical interventions: assessment of an individual's baseline behaviors, education about how to make the appropriate changes, counseling to develop strategies such as setting short-term goals and self-monitoring that will ensure the maintenance of the changes, constant rechecking with the individual to determine whether compliance is a problem and to resolve barriers, and reinforcement about progress toward the goal of change in behavior.[25] Success with any of these changes requires frequent interaction with the patient. Additional exchange of information to assess progress toward goals and provide feedback and reinforcement can be done by telephone, facsimile, e-mail, home visit, and face-to-face clinic visits. This is often best accomplished by a healthcare provider, such as the nurse, who has the requisite time for the education and counseling necessary to change behavior. Moreover, it has been shown that individuals who receive education and counseling on hypertension management exhibit increased adherence.[26] The important aspects of education and counseling that should be incorporated into the management of individuals with hypertension are noted in Box 39–1.

In many settings, nurses are also responsible for the pharmacologic aspects of hypertension management. Using well-defined protocols based upon national guidelines such as the seventh report of the Joint National Committee on Prevention, Detection, Evaluation, and Treatment of High Blood Pressure (JNC 7),[2] advanced practice nurses and specially trained nurse case managers can prescribe and titrate medications and help patients to manage the numerous steps in taking medications required for BP control. The ability to attain greater control of BP than is achieved with standard care has been demonstrated in numerous settings.[9,11,17,20] In many cases the improved outcomes have resulted from nurses placing a greater number of patients on medications, altering drug regimens more frequently in response to inadequate BP control, and prescribing more effectively. In some studies nurses have also been noted to place a higher proportion of patients on multiple drug regimens to achieve greater BP control.[16,27] Although changes may produce higher costs initially, as noted by Logan,[28] obtaining the best regimen for the patient must be paramount if patients are to remain in treatment and achieve greater adherence and BP control rates.

The effective development and implementation of protocols for medication management allow achievement of BP control, a significant factor in helping to offset some of the costs of providing a clinic. For example, more than 20 years ago more than 6000 treated patients within the Veterans Affairs Clinics,[27] were managed by nurses who used a successful combination of a thiazide diuretic and other agents, such as methyldopa and reserpine. At the end of five treatment visits, half of all patients had DBPs below 90 mm Hg, and two thirds of those who began treatment remained in treatment for at least 2.5 years. The total yearly cost for treating one patient was $221. Nurses have been shown to effectively manage other risk factors, such as dyslipidemia, using multiple drugs at lower cost than usual care.[29]

---

*A drink is defined as 1 oz of ethanol (e.g., 24 oz of beer, 10 oz of wine, or 2 oz of 100-proof whiskey).

**Box 39–1** Strategies for Patient Education

**Identify knowledge, attitudes, beliefs, and experience**
- Assess readiness to achieve blood pressure (BP) control
- Correct misinterpretations

**Educate about condition and treatment**
- Inform patient of his or her BP level
- Identify alternative treatment plans
- Provide simple oral and written information
- Teach self-monitoring skills

**Tailor the regimen to the patient**
- Include patient in decision making
- Agree on BP goal
- Incorporate treatment into patient's daily lifestyle
- Simplify the regimen
- Prioritize critical aspects of the regimen
- Implement the treatment plan in stages
- Encourage self-monitoring of BP in selected patients
- Encourage discussion of medication, side effects, and concerns
- Modify dosages or change medications to avoid side effects
- Minimize cost of therapy
- Schedule frequent visits for nonadherent patients

**Provide reinforcement**
- Hold exit interviews
- Arrange home visits
- Use appointment reminders
- Contact patients who miss appointments
- Consider clinician-patient contracts

**Promote social support**
- Include family and others in care
- Suggest group sessions

**Collaborate with other professionals**
- Recognize shared practice goals
- Draw upon the skills and knowledge of other providers

From Hill MH. Strategies for patient education. Clin Exp Hypertens A11(5&6):1187-1201, 1989. Courtesy of Marcel Dekker, Inc.

Another role of the nurse is to direct and coordinate the efforts of other team members who provide consultation or are practicing in the clinic. Whereas collaborative teams of physicians and nurses provide care in a typical outpatient setting, other healthcare providers such as nutritionists, pharmacists, and community healthcare workers also practice in some clinics. The role of community healthcare workers involved in underserved communities is discussed in Chapter 40. The nurse may also be responsible for training and supervising office personnel such as office assistants and the receptionists. The ability of office assistants to take BPs accurately can be helpful in screening and can also decrease costs. Receptionists also play a very helpful role by scheduling appointments, making reminder telephone calls, obtaining laboratory results, entering data to support evaluation of clinical outcomes, and ensuring that referring physicians receive timely correspondence about their patient's management.

## Clinic Needs and Setup

Most ambulatory settings, whether physician offices or clinics, in which nurses may provide hypertension management require no additional specialized equipment or space. An examination room and/or clinic office can be used to see patients and their families for education and counseling as well as patient care, thus avoiding additional space costs. Setting up neighborhood clinics, especially in underserved communities, minimizes the burdens of transportation, enabling many individuals to remain in care who might not otherwise do so. Although this may require additional resources for rental space in a neighborhood, improved hypertension care in high-risk individuals reduces hospitalizations and chronic illness management for heart failure, stroke, and renal failure.

Clinic staff must use equipment that is appropriately calibrated to ensure adequate measurement of BP. The clinic must be structured with a variety of cuff sizes and furniture that permits taking BPs appropriately. In addition, if a clinic provides patients with BP monitors for home use or access to a service for home monitoring, patients whose BP needs tighter control will benefit. Computers are necessary to track appointments and telephone contacts; collect medical, demographic, and billing information; and generate reports to physicians, payers, and patients. Moreover, documentation of clinical outcomes is increasingly important and necessary. Tracking the frequency of visits, medications, compliance, hospitalizations, and BPs through a computer program enables rapid evaluation of clinical outcomes and the costs incurred in providing antihypertensive treatment. A simple checklist for use in starting up a hypertension clinic is shown in Box 39–2.

## Caseload Size

Several factors influence the capability of nurses and others to manage a caseload of patients within a clinic setting. Caseload size is strongly influenced by the characteristics of the patient population. Patients with more severe hypertension often require more frequent and/or longer visits to regulate medications and manage target organ complications. Those with mild hypertension may require less frequent monitoring and reinforcement of education and counseling. Experience of a large clinic in Glasgow suggests that a single nurse practitioner working with a physician can manage up to 700 to 900 patients per year.[30] Within a worksite clinic, Alderman et al. observed that a nurse can see an average of 16 patients per day.[10] Nurses and other personnel may be able to shorten the length of clinic visits by increasing office efficiency. Efficiency also can be increased if staff order fewer unnecessary blood chemistry tests, lower the cost of medications, and provide education creatively within the clinic by offering education and counseling through videotapes, written materials, and other vehicles in the waiting rooms. Additional support can also be obtained by using volunteers to provide services that do not require the expertise of the nurse or physician.

## Reimbursement for Services

Reimbursement issues need to be understood by nurses and physicians wanting to establish a collaborative hypertension management program. Much of what has been learned in the

**Box 39–2** Outpatient Hypertension Clinic Start-up Checklist

1. Establish need and cost benefits
2. Assess and establish staff support and qualifications
3. Designate physician medical director and coordinator
4. Ensure efficient assessment and educational physical space
5. Develop written policies and procedures
   - Entry and referral criteria
   - Treatment algorithms
   - Exit criteria
   - Laboratory standards
   - Pricing
   - Fee-for-service schedule
   - Compute capitation rate or contribution to global rate for managed care contracts
   - Billing and corrections policy
   - Operational budget and proforma outcomes measures (JNC 7 goals)
6. Develop standard forms
   - Patient information (medical history, lifestyle)
   - Initial assessment and treatment plan
   - Return visit and progress report
   - Drug descriptions and patient administration instructions
   - Individual lifestyle counseling prescription (dietary, exercise, stress management)
   - Dietary and body fat assessment (BMI)

7. Determine sequence and pathway of patient visit flow
   - Schedule for new and return visit
   - Physician consultation schedule with new patients
8. Develop patient data storage and tracking system
   - Assess existing patient tracking software packages
   - Determine relevant patient data
   - Develop protocol for monitoring clinical events and associated costs
9. Acquire and maintain patient education materials
   - Pharmacologic information
   - Lifestyle information

Other resources
10. Marketing and promotion plan
    - Internal marketing and promotion: medical and ancillary staff
    - Patients
    - Referring physicians, PPOs, and HMOs
    - Business and industry
    - Alliances with hospitals, PPOs, and drug companies to form organized and efficient disease management programs
11. Develop continuing education schedule for clinic staff
    - New research funding
    - New reimbursement guidelines and legislation
12. Develop link and network with national hypertension organizations

Revised and adapted with permission from LaForge R, Thomas T. Outpatient management of lipid disorders. J Cardiovasc Nurs 11(1):39-53, 1996.
JNC 7, the seventh report of the Joint National Committee on the Prevention, Detection, Evaluation, and Treatment of High Blood Pressure; BMI, body mass index; PPOs, preferred provider organizations; HMOs, health maintenance organizations; BMI, body mass index.

establishment of lipid clinics, anticoagulation monitoring services, and diabetic education programs applies to obtaining coverage for services provided within a hypertension clinic.[31] Although a hypertension management clinic is not a covered service per se, many of the services provided within the clinic are covered under the Medicare and Medicaid guidelines set forth by the Centers for Medicare and Medicaid Services (CMS), formerly called the Health Care Finance Administration (HCFA), under Medicare. Hypertension clinic personnel should establish a fee structure using guidelines set forth by the CMS in Health Care Finance Administration Medicare Carriers Manual, Section 2050.[32] Because the "incident to" guidelines under Medicare are nationally recognized, many insurance carriers follow the rules developed by CMS. The guidelines indicate that nurses and other licensed personnel may provide follow-up services such as conducting physical examinations, taking medical histories, and providing medical decision making as long as the service is provided under the direct supervision of a physician or nurse practitioner. The physician or nurse practitioner must be in the same office setting, and must be immediately available to provide assistance. In these instances, the physician employs or contracts with the nurse and directly supervises the healthcare professional who provides the services. Some of the important issues that should be noted about

following the "incident to" ruling under Medicare are noted in Box 39–3. Clinic personnel should recognize that each CMS representative within a state may interpret the guidelines differently; therefore obtaining clarification through written guidelines is important to ensure that rules are followed and adequate coverage is obtained. When the registered nurse or other licensed personnel bills under the physician provider or nurse practitioner, the maximum billing code that may be used is a level I (99211).[32]

Several innovative mechanisms of payment may also provide a way to cover the costs incurred in running a hypertension clinic. Contracting to provide these services with a managed care organization may be a viable option. Developing relationships with pharmaceutical companies (e.g., to conduct small research projects) may offset some of the costs. Providing multiple services for cardiovascular disease management for patients with heart failure, lipid disorders, hypertension, and diabetes may also expand the scope and opportunities for success of specialized clinics. Additionally, if physicians or nurse practitioners spend more than half of their time in the visit educating or coordinating care, they may bill for a higher level of service even if a physical examination is not performed. This time must be actual time spent face-to-face with the patient and provider.[33]

**Box 39–3** Medicare "Incident To" Billings (What Is Important)

---

Service must be
- Integral part of physician's professional service
- Commonly included in physician's bill
- Furnished in physician's office or clinic under direct supervision
- Furnished by individual qualifying as an "employee" acting under scope of state licensure laws

Services are billed
- Under supervising physician's provider number using same CPT codes
- As one service per patient per day unless there is documentation of need

Documentation in the patient record to support level of service/coding is absolutely essential.

---

CPT, Current Procedural Terminology.

## MODIFICATION OF GLOBAL RISK AS PART OF NURSE MANAGEMENT OF HYPERTENSION

The magnitude and significance of multiple risk factors in the American population and globally is noteworthy. Treating hypertension is especially critical in the diabetic population, who are at high risk for coronary heart disease (CHD) and kidney failure. Importantly, a BP goal of <130/80 mm Hg for the diabetic population has been shown to be more difficult to achieve than a BP goal of <140/90 mm Hg.[33] Nurses can have a major impact on this population and positively influence their risk. In a study conducted in the United Kingdom where nurses have gained widespread acknowledgment for their efforts to reduce CVD risk, Denver et al.[34] followed 120 hypertensive men and women with type 2 diabetes and a BP >140/90 mm Hg, 71% of whom had increased urinary albumin excretion (UAE). Patients were randomized to conventional primary care whereby physicians received a letter stating the measured and target BP as well as recommendations for treatment according to guidelines or to a nurse-led hypertension clinic. Patients assigned to the nurse clinics saw nurses monthly for 3 months and then every 6 weeks for 3 months. At these visits BP was measured, compliance was reviewed, nonpharmacologic therapies were discussed, and medication changes were initiated based on physician orders through standing protocols. At 6 months of follow-up, the proportion of treatment changes was 88% in the nurse-led group compared with 15% in primary care; $p = .000$. While SBP and DBP fell in both groups, the fall in SBP was far greater (12.6 mm Hg, $p = .000$) in those assigned to the nurse clinics. No changes in CHD or stroke risk were noted in those assigned to primary care, while the reductions in 10-year CHD and stroke risk were significant in the nurse-led group ($p = .004$ and .000). These risk reductions were entirely due to the six times greater changes in medications in the nurse clinics compared with conventional care. Further studies are needed to support the approach of nurse-managed clinics and case management for populations at greatest risk of morbidity and mortality from CHD and stroke.

## SUMMARY

In two separate editorials in the mid-1970s,[35,36] Finnerty suggested that asymptomatic patients would not remain under care and on medication without proper motivation. He noted that once the initial diagnosis of hypertension was made, the care of the patient was an issue primarily of education. He further suggested that we should recognize the value of specially trained nurses in managing hypertension, just as we have relied on nurses' expertise in the coronary care unit. His suggestion was based on the reality that most physicians have been trained as diagnosticians responsible for managing complicated illness or treating the patient in an emergent situation. Today, recognizing that close to one third of hypertensive patients drop out of care and that only a third of all patients treated with hypertension achieve a goal BP of <140/90 mm Hg,[2] we should focus on the need for what Finnerty advocated and what we know improves patient care and outcomes. In a system that is highly focused on medical care of acute illness and on reducing costs, nurses practicing collaboratively with physicians in the outpatient setting can benefit large numbers of patients with hypertension and other chronic asymptomatic conditions, as well as the healthcare provider and the healthcare system.

## References

1. Cherry DK, Woodwill DA. National Ambulatory Medical Care Survey: 2000 Summary Advance Data. 328:1-32, 2002.
2. Chobanian AV, Bakris GL, Black HR, et al. The seventh report of the Joint National Committee on Prevention, Detection, Evaluation and Treatment of High Blood Pressure. JAMA 289:2560-2572, 2003.
3. Vasan RS, Beiser A, Seshadri S, et al. Residual lifetime risk for developing hypertension in middle-aged women and men: The Framingham Heart Study. JAMA 287:1003-1010, 2002.
4. Lewington S, Clarler R, Qizilbush N, et al. Age-specific relevance of usual blood pressure to vascular mortality: A meta-analysis of individual data for one million adults in 61 prospective studies. Prospective studies collaboration. Lancet 360:1903-1913, 2002.
5. Flegal KM, Carroll MD, Ogden CH, et al. Prevalence and trends in obesity among US adults. JAMA 288:1723-1727, 2002.
6. Cleveland LE, Goldman JD, Borrud LG. Data tables: Results from USDA's 1994 continuing survey of food intake by individuals and 1994 diet and health knowledge survey. Riverdale, MD, Agricultural Research Service, US Dept. of Agriculture, 1996.
7. US Department of Health and Human Services. Physical activity and health: A report of the surgeon general. Atlanta, GA, US Department of Health and Human Services. Centers for Disease Control and Prevention, National Center for Chronic Disease Prevention and Health Promotion, 1996.
8. Division of Adult and Community Health, National Center for Chronic Disease Prevention and Health Promotion Centers for Disease Prevention. 5 day surveillance behavioral risk factor surveillance system online prevalence data. 1995-2000.
9. Runyan KW Jr. The Memphis Chronic Disease Program. Comparisons in outcome and the nurse's extended role. JAMA 231(3):264-267, 1975.
10. Alderman MH, Schoenbaum EF. Detection and treatment of hypertension at the work site. N Engl J Med 293(2):65-68, 1973.
11. Logan AG, Milne BJ, Achber C, et al. Work-site treatment of hypertension by specially trained nurses. A controlled trial. Lancet 2(8153):1175-1178, 1979.

12. Hypertension Detection and Follow-up Program Cooperative Group. Five-year findings of the hypertension detection and follow-up program, I: Reduction in mortality of persons with high blood pressure, including mild hypertension. JAMA 242:2562-2571, 1979.

13. SHEP Cooperative Research Group. Prevention of stroke by antihypertensive drug treatment in older persons with isolated systolic hypertension. JAMA 261:3255-3264, 1991.

14. Furberg CD, Wright JT Jr, Davis BR, et al. Major outcomes in high-risk hypertensive patients randomized to angiotensin-converting enzyme inhibitor or calcium channel blocker vs. diuretic: The Antihypertensive and Lipid-Lowering Treatment to Prevent Heart Attack Trial (ALLHAT). JAMA 288:2981-2997, 2002.

15. Hill MN, Reichgott MJ. Achievement of standards for quality care of hypertension by physicians and nurses. Clin Exp Hypertens 1:665-684, 1979.

16. Reichgott MJ, Pearson S, Hill MN. The nurse practitioner's role in complex patient management: hypertension. J Natl Med Assoc 75(1):1197-1204, 1983.

17. Pheley AM, Terry P, Pietz L, et al. Evaluation of a nurse-based hypertension management program: Screening, management, and outcomes. J Cardiovasc Nurs 9(2):54-61, 1995.

18. Miller NH. Nurse case management–the MULTIFIT Program. Abstract. Am J Hypertension 9(4):194A, 1996.

19. Artenian NT, Washington OGM, Templin TN. Effects of home based telemonitoring and community-based monitoring on blood pressure control in urban African Americans: A pilot study. Heart Lung 30(3):191-199, 2001.

20. Hill MN, Hae-Ra H, Dennison CR, et al. Hypertension care and control in underserved urban African American men: Behavioral and physiologic outcomes at 36 months. Am J Hypertens 16:906-913, 2003.

21. Hall PS, Hill MN, Roary MC, et al. A look at hypertension in young African-American men. Nurse Pract 28(1):59-60, 2003.

22. Sox HC. Quality of patient care by nurse practitioners and physician's assistants: a ten-year perspective. Ann Intern Med 91:459-468, 1979.

23. La Batide AA, Chatellier G, Bobrie G, et al. Comparison of nurse- and physician-determined clinic blood pressure levels in patients referred to a hypertension clinic: implications for subsequent management. J Hypertens 18: 391-398, 2000.

24. Stason WB. Opportunities to improve the cost-effectiveness of treatment for hypertension. Hypertension 18(3 Suppl): I161-I166, 1991.

25. Miller NH, Taylor CB. Lifestyle Management for Patients with Coronary Heart Disease. Current Issues in Cardiac Rehabilitation, Monograph Number 2. Champaign, IL, Human Kinetics, 1995.

26. Levine DM, Green LW, Deeds SG, et al. Health education for hypertensive patients. JAMA 241:1700-1703, 1979.

27. Perry HM, Schnapner JW, Meyer G, et al. Clinical program for screening and treatment of hypertension in veterans. J Natl Med Assoc 74:433-444, 1982.

28. Logan AC, Milne BJ, Flanagan PT, et al. Clinical effectiveness and cost-effectiveness of monitoring blood pressure of hypertensive employees at work. Hypertension 5:828-836, 1983.

29. DeBusk RF, Miller NH, Superko HR, et al. A case management system for coronary risk factor modification following acute myocardial infarction. Ann Intern Med 120(9):721-729, 1994.

30. Curzio JL, Beevers M. The role of nurses in hypertension care and research. J Hum Hypertens 11:541-550, 1997.

31. Cahill NE, Thomas T. Reimbursement Planning for Lipid Clinic Services. Princeton NJ, Bristol-Myers Squibb Co, 1997.

32. Champagne MA, Berra K, Lamendola C, et al. A Guide to Developing a Successful Cardiovascular Risk Reduction Program. New York, NY, PCNA Phillips Healthcare Communications, 2002.

33. Pellegrini F, Belfiglio M, DeBerardis G, et al. Role of organizational factors in poor blood pressure control in patients with type 2 diabetes. Arch Intern Med 163:473-480, 2003.

34. Denver EA, Woolfson RG, Barnard M, et al. Management of uncontrolled hypertension in a nurse-led clinic compared with conventional care for patients with type 2 diabetes. Diabetes Care 26(8):2256-2260, 2003.

35. Finnerty FA Jr. Editorial: The nurse's role in treating hypertension. N Engl J Med 293:93-94, 1975.

36. Finnerty FA. The nurse and care of the hypertensive patient. Ann Intern Med 84:746, 1976.

# Community Outreach

**Martha N. Hill, Lee R. Bone, David M. Levine**

Community outreach is an essential component of comprehensive programs to promote health, as well as prevent and/or control disease and related risk factors. It complements other strategies and is especially effective in reaching individuals and populations who do not have access to healthcare and related human services and those who have discontinued care. Community outreach improves care and outcomes by providing state-of-the-art prevention and treatment interventions to the populations, as well as to individuals and families. Outreach has been utilized successfully to impact positively on a wide variety of health problems, including prenatal care, immunizations, hypertension, HIV/AIDS, tuberculosis, chronic obstructive pulmonary disease (COPD), asthma, diabetes, and mental health.

Effective hypertension control requires a comprehensive approach that integrates social, psychological, behavioral, and economic, as well as medical, strategies. Community outreach improves hypertension control by linking health professionals, healthcare organizations, and current or potential patients with resources in patients' communities. Clinical hypertension care and control programs, which include community outreach provide three important lessons:

1. Clinicians can use resources in the community to directly enhance their care of patients, thus improving long-term control of hypertension and reducing associated target organ damage.
2. Community programs provide reinforcement of the clinician's recommendations and teaching efforts.
3. Physicians, nurse practitioners, and other clinicians can provide community service and leadership by accepting referrals, promoting outreach programs, and acting as consultants.

## DEFINITION OF COMMUNITY OUTREACH

*Community outreach* is a health services, health education, and health promotion strategy directed to entire populations, as well as to specific high risk and underserved groups and individuals. It is an activity at the interface of medicine and public health, an area that is the focus of community nursing. It seeks to mobilize health and human resources at local, state, and national levels. Outreach can be defined differently depending on a program's purpose. Its goal, however, is to reach those who are not reached by usual methods for the purpose of increasing knowledge, information, and access to and utilization of health services. It inevitably has to address issues of health services availability, accessibility, acceptability, and affordability focusing on removing geographic, cultural, linguistic, administrative, and financial barriers to healthcare.[1] Outreach has been an integral part of public health for more than the past century. Traditionally, it has targeted meeting the needs of the underserved. In the past few decades, however, hospitals and academic health centers have begun to extend of medical and nursing care to patients' homes and communities, in part to respond to needs identified by surrounding communities. Outreach has thus become a way of providing community service to meet patient and population needs, health promotion and disease prevention objectives and marketing and public relations goals.

Key principles of community outreach are active community participation and/or partnership, careful diagnosis and planning program implementation, and evaluation. A needs assessment and definition of goals, aims, strategies, and resources are essential for success. The types of outreach programs vary widely and include screening, case finding, referral, education, and monitoring. Effective interventions combine persuasive communications, interpersonal relationships, skills training, and community organizing. Mass media can be used to deliver informative messages through local radio, television, and newspaper public service announcements; talk shows; celebrity guest features; and other methods. Additional outreach strategies include person-person contact, mailed postcards and letters, telephone calls, street contact, home visits, mobile units, and hot or warm lines. Outreach also can be provided at community events such as health fairs or in sites such as churches and recreation centers.[2]

Community participation and partnership are essential ingredients for productive sustained outreach programs. Organizing a group of respected community leaders as an advisory or coordinating committee can be constructive. Community organizers, politicians, physicians, clergy, and others with an interest can help design, implement, evaluate, and sustain an outreach program that will be acceptable and responsive to the community and directed at meeting their needs. Uncommon partners (e.g., dental school faculty) have joined outreach collaborations to help reduce health disparities.[3] Community involvement is invaluable in deciding who should participate, what they should do, and how they should be recognized for their contributions. While the good will and community service produced by many outreach activities is evident, it is important to evaluate the efficiency and cost effectiveness of such activities to compare various approaches prior to replication. Particularly in a time of scarce resources, outreach programs need to demonstrate achievement of objectives and impact on clinical outcomes.

# HISTORY OF OUTREACH PROGRAMS TO CONTROL HYPERTENSION

During the 1960s and the War on Poverty, outreach services became an integral part of many health and social service programs.[4] Grass roots organizing, community development and, more recently, economic development were seen as mechanisms to improve quality of life including social, emotional, and physical well-being. In an effort to reduce disparities in health status and outcomes, many hypertension outreach programs targeted African Americans whose high blood pressure (BP) was detected, treated, and controlled at rates that lagged behind rates of whites.[5-8]

The value of finding undetected cases of hypertension through community outreach was first demonstrated in the late 1960s. The purpose of these outreach programs was to motivate people to have their BP measured at a familiar and convenient site for little or no cost. Organized BP screenings found that an accessible location, community participation, referrals to care, and follow-up of referred people contributed to improved care and control of hypertension. Community-based screening programs became common place at sites where people congregate and space was available for staff or volunteers to measure BP and provide education and counseling. Firehouses, churches, barbershops, and work sites were frequently used.

In the early 1970s, household, community, and clinic surveys documented low rates of hypertension awareness, treatment, and control in Georgia, Virginia, Maryland, and Washington, DC.[9-13] In an effort to screen for undetected hypertension in inner city Washington, D.C., Finnerty et al. found house-to-house canvassing by trained interviewers to be ineffective, time consuming, and dangerous. Encouraged by civic leaders, trained allied personnel held screenings in churches and supermarkets, identified large numbers of hypertensive individuals, and referred them to care. In several care settings, low rates of appointment attendance and BP control and high rates of clinic dropouts were documented. Interviews with patients revealed three key findings affecting patients' attitudes about remaining in care: amount of time expended to receive care (transportation and waiting), understanding of all aspects of the disease, and "doctor/paramedical/patient" relationship. A new patient-centered hypertension care program was designed, including health aides trained to (1) serve as patient advocates; (2) deliver preappointment reminders by telephone, mail or in person (which led to a doubling of attendance); and (3) help resolve difficulties affecting compliance with visits and medication.[12,13]

The Hypertension Detection and Follow-up Program (HDFP) was designed to test the effectiveness of a comprehensive treatment program to control high BP and reduce its complications compared with usual care in the community.[14,15] Clinic-based care, community outreach, free transportation and medication, a multidisciplinary team approach to care, and a very committed staff, in addition to pharmacologic benefits of hypertension control, were demonstrated to be very effective in improving BP control, as well as morbidity and mortality rates. These methods, which were first published in the 1970s, have been generalized to the community and incorporated into all major multisite hypertension treatment and prevention clinical trials since the conclusion of, for example, MRFIT, TOHMS, and TOPH.[16-19] In a classic health education clinical trial designed to develop ways to improve physician care of hypertension, Green, Levine, and colleagues used a factorial design to test three supplementary interventions: physician visit exit interview with the nurse, home visits to a person identified by the patient as a source of social support with health matters, and group classes.[20,21] The home visits, which were found to be an effective outreach strategy, were conducted by nurse-supervised high school students from the community. Work-site programs—an additional type of outreach—were found to be very successful in improving rates of hypertension care and control. Schoenbaum et al., working with a labor union for department store employees, documented the high standard of care provided on site by nurse practitioners[22]; Foote and Erfurt documented the value of work-site interventions at Ford Motor Company.[23]

A broad definition of community outreach encompasses many of the efforts of the National Heart, Lung, and Blood Institute's (NHLBI) National High Blood Pressure Education Program founded in 1972. These outreach activities were directed to the public (through mass media campaigns), healthcare practitioners, professional societies, voluntary health organizations, industry, and individual patients. In the 1970s and early 1980s, seven state programs supported by NHLBI demonstrated the value of mobilizing and coordinating community-wide resources to increase the rates of hypertension awareness, treatment, and control.[24-27] In Maryland, a coordinating council served as the hub for the collaboration of professional groups, academic health centers, voluntary nonprofit organizations, and others who wanted to improve hypertension care and control. Committees were formed to carry out the project aims of the NHLBI funded program by providing outreach into many communities. The projects were numerous, varied, and included professional education; public information and communication; screening and monitoring at health departments, work sites, churches, and barbershops; and demonstration projects in inner city and rural areas of the state.[28,29,30] Professional education, which can disseminate consensus recommendations to improve practice and patient care, has been a national priority since the High Blood Pressure Education Program began. Over the following decades, the Joint National Committee reports have focused increasingly on diagnosis, evaluation, and initial medical treatment of hypertension and other risk factors with lessening emphasis on community programs, multidisciplinary approaches, and adherence strategies.[31] Outreach information is available in separate documents that have been disseminated primarily to the public health community.[32]

In the 1980s, the following comprehensive community-based cardiovascular risk reduction studies were conducted: The Stanford Five-Cities Project,[33] The Minnesota Heart Health Program,[34] and The Pawtucket Heart Health Program.[35] These major community-based programs to reduce cardiovascular and stroke risk utilized state-of-the-art communication and education strategies in combination with community organization, outreach, and social support.[36] This application of knowledge drew from the social and behavioral sciences complementing and supplementing knowledge from the biomedical sciences.[37] These programs demonstrated the complex challenges in improving outcomes through risk reduction at the community level.

Today, telecommunication technologies, including hand-held and personal computers, telephone, facsimile (FAX), and electronic mail (e-mail) are being used to collect, transmit, and store data. These technologies provide opportunities for creative models of outreach for diagnosis and treatment. These tools facilitate patient self-monitoring of BP and communication of information among patients in their homes, community laboratories, nurse case managers, primary care physicians, and specialist physicians, improving the diagnosis and management of hypertension.[38] In addition, home BP monitoring by the patient and review of the progress toward goal BP by the health provider with feedback by email, mail, or telephone, improves adherence by tailoring therapy promptly without office visits. Programs incorporating telecommunications, such as MULTIFIT, have earned high levels of patient and provider satisfaction and improved outcomes.[39-41]

## THE GAP BETWEEN RESEARCH AND PRACTICE

It is clear from these and other studies that a combination of lifestyle and pharmacologic interventions can control hypertension and reduce associated morbidity and mortality. These interventions are significantly more effective when based on an assessment of the education and skill building needed by patients, providers, and the public. The unmet challenge in hypertension control is to extend the health benefits of these interventions to the population at large and, in particular, to groups that are more diverse, less select, and at higher risk than those studied in the clinical trials that demonstrated the efficacy of the interventions. Despite our increased knowledge and subsequent improvements in the control of hypertension, national data indicate that the majority of Americans with hypertension do not have controlled BPs and that awareness, treatment, and control rates have not increased as much as had been assumed.[31,42] Community outreach that includes grassroots advocacy and education by voluntary health organizations, such as the American Heart Association, is necessary to eliminate the gap in the care and control of hypertension between majority and minority populations.[43] Evidence supports the value of community outreach activities designed with an understanding of the sociocultural context of patients' lives. Significant improvement in national hypertension control rates will require renewed commitment, a more comprehensive approach, and more clearly and strongly stated policy recommendations for effective culturally relevant community outreach.

## HOW COMMUNITY OUTREACH WILL MOVE US FORWARD TO ELIMINATE HEALTH DISPARITIES

### Community-Health System Partnership

Community outreach has contributed importantly to the detection and control of prevalent chronic diseases by incorporating the priorities and strategies of health professionals and those of the community.[44] This shared approach reflects a broader definition of health and its determinants, including the social, cultural, and economic context within which health is promoted. Community-health system partnerships allow for individual and collective empowerment. These partnerships also allow the community to participate in identifying health problems and strategies for addressing those problems at interpersonal, health care organization, community, and policy levels.[45] This partnership approach is recommended by the Task Force on Community Preventive Services and The Institute of Medicine's Committee on Capitalizing on Social and Behavioral Research to Improve the Public's Health.[46,47] Such partnership strategies are also important for addressing the Healthy People 2010 national objectives to enhance access and care management.[48]

Advocacy is one such important partnership effort. Recognizing needs, identifying solutions, securing resources, and influencing policy makers have been shown to improve national and local hypertension control activities. For example, securing the availability of malls and high school tracks for people to walk and providing more low fat, low calorie, and low sodium foods in grocery stores are examples of advocacy outcomes. "Lose Weight and Win," a church-based weight loss program for BP control among African American women, is an example of a successful community-based outreach program that operated independently from health care providers, systems, and settings with the goal of modifying lifestyle to complement, enhance, and reinforce medical recommendations.[49]

Academic health centers and their neighboring communities are increasingly investing in health by forming partnerships to address local environmental and social needs and maintain cohesive neighborhoods.[50] These partnerships also are one solution to the national health care issues concerning underserved minority populations.[51] Opportunities abound for integrating critical care, education and research and for translating best practices while providing patient care targeted to community health priorities.[47] Such initiatives further advance both institutional and community capacity to build meaningful partnerships and collaborative community health programs.[52]

### Ecological Multidisciplinary Approach

Hypertension care and control are complex challenges. Comprehensive multifactorial and multidisciplinary approaches are needed to eliminate the gap between what has been shown to be beneficial in clinical trials and what occurs in practice and in patients' daily lives.[43] The five-level Ecological Model (intrapersonal, interpersonal, organizational, community, and societal) is a useful way to organize responses to these challenges.[53] At the societal level, for example, more people are without health insurance or are underinsured than ever before. Those who do have health insurance are finding that their benefits are covering fewer services, including preventive services such as screening and risk factor management. Community outreach programs can provide information about available affordable services to uninsured and underinsured individuals. In addition, staff in outreach programs can advocate influencing policy makers to support the provision of effective hypertension care, if the disproportionate burden of hypertension among the lower socioeconomic groups is to be addressed.

At the level of the health care organization and the individual provider with responsibility for the care of hypertensive patients, the delivery of care needs to be culturally competent as well as evidence- and guideline-based. If desired patient outcomes are to be achieved long-term, administrators and clinicians need to invest their expertise wisely. By joining with others in a multidisciplinary team and including community health workers reaching out across geographic settings, physicians can maximize use of their medical expertise. We cannot afford to ignore the evidence supporting the important contributions of nurses, nurse practitioners, physician assistants, pharmacists, nutritionists, health educators, and outreach workers.[54] The compliance challenge is multileveled, and improving outcomes requires us to address behavior not only at patient level, but also at the provider and health care organization levels.[55] The fields of medicine, nursing, and public health have unique contributions to make and together can compliment one another to eliminate the gap between what we know controls hypertension and reduces its complications and what is happening daily in practice and patients' daily lives.[43]

## Use of Community Health Workers

A particularly important aspect of community-outreach and community-based team approaches is the inclusion of community health workers. Also called *health aides, lay advisors, natural helpers,* or *peer educators,* these members of the same cultural group as the patient population of interest, are receiving growing acceptance as valued members of the health care team.[56-58] Often working closely with nurses, community health workers provide basic primary care services in community settings, including the home.[59-64] Their role focuses on improving access to and continuity of care, educating patients and families, reinforcing adherence to treatment, and addressing needed human services, as well as promoting self-care skills and confidence. Additionally, they are advocates for the communities they serve. In research, as well as service delivery, community health workers strengthen community understanding and acceptability of medical care, and thereby the effectiveness of many outreach activities, including hypertension care programs.[65-68] The members of the healthcare team are trained to (1) provide health information to improve knowledge and skills with appointments and recommended treatment; (2) assist with referrals to community resources, including assistance with financial problems; (3) monitor BP and communicate with care providers in clinical settings; and

(4) facilitate the identification and involvement of a key support person to whom the patient turns to for help with health matters. Crucial qualifications include a desire to help others and to improve the health of the community and its residents. The worker, often a member of the neighborhood, understands the community's language, culture, and socioeconomic conditions and is able to help providers and patients better understand each other's expectations. This insight and linking function facilitates the development of an individualized plan for hypertension care that the patient can adhere to within the context of his/her daily life.

In inner city Baltimore, a program of research was developed to test the effectiveness of a nurse practitioner–community health worker–physician team approach to improving hypertension care and control in young African American men. Lack of health insurance, a primary care physician, and compliance with antihypertensive treatment, as well as dependence on emergency departments for episodic care, contributed to low rates of hypertension care and control in this underserved high-risk population.[65,69-71] Planning for the 5-year clinical trial was guided by an eclectic conceptual framework that represented an integration of models, particularly the PRECEDE-PROCEED model[72] This approach, which is presented in Figure 40–1, integrated health education, behavioral change and health maintenance principles, culturally sensitive strategies, social action, and social learning theory. It is essential that the conceptual approaches to hypertension control incorporate economic, psychosocial, and behavioral factors (individual lifestyles, self-management practices, and long-term adherence to treatment) in elegant ways. The PRECEDE-PROCEED model incorporates predisposing, reinforcing, and enabling factors for behavioral change. Predisposing factors are those antecedents to behavior that provide the rationale or motivation for the behavior, such as knowledge, beliefs, attitudes, or values. Enabling factors are those that allow a predisposition to be translated into behavior, such as accessing health care resources or acquiring appropriate skills. Reinforcing factors, such as family, peer, or health provider/community health worker support, and supportive services are subsequent to a behavior and provide the continuing reward or incentive for the behavior as well as contribute to its maintenance. The conceptual framework used in this trial emphasized adherence with treatment recommendations in the More Intensive Intervention Group in comparison with the Less Intensive Intervention Group with the intent of improving health outcomes (Figure 40–2). A team approach to

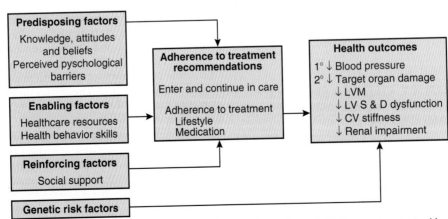

**Figure 40–1** Conceptual framework. (Modifield from Green LW, Kreuter MW. Health Promotion Planning: An Educational and Environmental Approach, 2nd ed. Mountain View, Mayfield, 1991.)

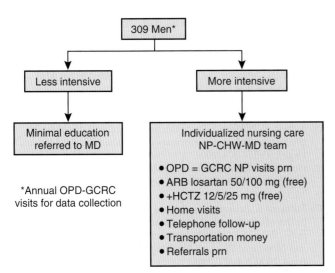

**Figure 40-2** Ongoing randomized clinical trial design.

care, in which a community health worker provided outreach services led to better BP care and control compared with traditional medical care over a 5-year period.[73,74]

An additional program in another area of inner city Baltimore focused on testing the effectiveness of nurse-supervised community health workers delivering home-based interventions.[71,74] Trained health workers were helpful members of the investigative teams in improving hypertension care and control in these programs. These individuals contributed their community perspective and experience, which helped balance the inevitable tension between standardizing an intervention to meet protocol needs and providing individualized culturally salient patient care and service. The training and employment of residents from the community strengthened the academic-community partnerships and provided excellent career opportunities for the community members.

## SUMMARY

We must redouble our efforts to improve U.S. rates of hypertension awareness, treatment and control. Community outreach offers proven strategies for complementing office- and clinic-based medical care of hypertension. Community outreach also offers strategies that increase entry into and remaining in continuous care, as well as adherence to treatment recommendations. For these reasons, one of the three major areas of focus in the NHLBI's plan to address health disparities is outreach and education. Of special importance, community-based participatory research is needed to further investigate the most cost-effective and efficient strategies in diverse populations with disproportionate burdens of hypertension and its complications.

## References

1. Veazie MA, Teufel-Shone NI, Silverman GS, et al. Building community capacity in public health: The role of action-oriented partnerships. J Public Health Manag Pract 7:21-32, 2001.

2. Lasater TM, Becker DM, Hill MN, et al. Synthesis of findings and issues from religious-based cardiovascular disease prevention trials. Ann Epidemiol 7:S46-S53, 1997.

3. Harper HJ. Buckle-up and smile for life: Uncommon partners find common ground to collaborate and eliminate disparities. Part 1. Dent Asst 72:8-12, 2003.

4. Colombo TJ, Freeborn DK, Mullooly JP, et al. The effect of outreach workers' educational efforts on disadvantaged preschool children's use of preventive services. Am J Public Health 69: 465-468, 1979.

5. Kong BW. Community-based hypertension control programs that work. J Poor & Underserved 8:409-415, 1997.

6. Bone LR, Hill MN, Stallings R, et al. Community health survey in an urban African American neighborhood: Distribution and correlates of evaluated blood pressure. Ethn Dis 10:87-95, 2000.

7. Levine DM, Bone LR, Hill MN, et al. The effectiveness of a community-Academic Health Center Partnership to Decrease the Level of Blood Pressure in an Urban African-American Population. Ethn Dis13(3):354-361, 2003.

8. Kong BW, Miller JM, Smoot RT. Churches as high blood pressure control centers. JNMA 74:920-923, 1982.

9. Wilber JA, Milward D, Baldwin A, et al. Atlanta community high blood pressure program methods of community hypertension screening. Circ Res 2;31:101-109, 1972.

10. Carey RM, Reid RA, Ayers CR, et al. The Charlottesville Blood-Pressure Survey. Value of repeated blood-pressure measurements. JAMA 236:847-851, 1976.

11. Entwistle G, Scott J, Apostoledes A, et al. A survey of blood pressure in the state of Maryland. Prev Med 12:695-708, 1983.

12. Finnerty FA Jr, Mattie EC, Finnerty FA III. Hypertension in the inner city, I: Analysis of clinic dropouts. Circulation 47:73-75, 1973.

13. Finnerty FA Jr, Shaw LW, Himmelsbach CK. Hypertension in the inner city, II: Detection and follow-up. Circulation. 47: 76-78, 1973.

14. Hypertension Detection and Follow-up Program Cooperative Group. Five-year findings of the Hypertension Detection and Follow-up Program. I. Reduction in mortality of persons with high blood pressure, including mild hypertension. JAMA 242:2562-2571, 1979.

15. Hypertension Detection and Follow-up Program Cooperative Group. Five year findings of the Hypertension Detection and Follow-up Program. II. Mortality by race-sex and age. JAMA 242:2572-2577, 1979.

16. Multiple Risk Factor Intervention Trial [MRFIT]. Risk factor changes and mortality results. Multiple Risk Factor Intervention Trial Research Group. JAMA 248:1465-1477, 1982.

17. Mortality rates after 10.5 years for participants in the Multiple Risk Factor Intervention Trial. Findings related to a prior hypotheses of the trial. The Multiple Risk Factor Intervention Trial Research Group. JAMA 263:1795-1801, 1990

18. The Trials of Hypertension Prevention Collaborative Research Group. The effects of nonpharmacological interventions on blood pressure of persons with high normal levels: Results of the Trials of Hypertension Prevention, phase I. JAMA 267: 1213-1220, 1992.

19. Treatment of Mild Hypertension Study Research Group. Treatment of mild hypertension study: Final results. JAMA 270:713-724, 1993.

20. Levine DM, Morisky DE, Bone LR, et al. Data-based planning for educational interventions through hypertension control programs for urban and rural populations in Maryland. Public Health Rep 97:107-112, 1982.

21. Morisky DE, Levine DM, Green LW, et al. Five-year blood pressure control and mortality following health education for hypertensive patients. Am J Public Health 73:153-162, 1983.

22. Schoenbaum EE, Alderman MH. Organization for long-term management of hypertension: The recruitment, training, and

responsibilities of the health team. Bull NY Academy Med 52:699-708, 1976.

23. Foote A, Erfurt JC. Development and dissemination of model systems for hypertension control in organizational settings. Institute of Labor and Industrial Relations, The University of Michigan–Wayne State University, Ann Arbor, Michigan, 1974.

24. Ware D, Leonard A, Southard J, et al. A coordination of statewide high blood pressure control activities: A study in four states. Prev Med 7:245, 1979.

25. Chiappini M, Henson M, Wilber J, et al. Statewide community high blood pressure control programs. J Med Assoc Ga 70:357-360, 1981.

26. Medical Care Development, Inc. Statewide household survey of prevalence and control of hypertension in Maine. Monograph; May, 1982.

27. Mills E. (ed). Coordination of High Blood Pressure Control in Michigan: Final Report, Vols. I and II. Lansing, MI, Michigan Dept. of Public Health, 1985.

28. Morisky D, Levine D, Green L, et al. The relative impact of health education for low and high-risk patients with hypertension. Prev Med 9:550-558, 1980.

29. Shanker B, Russell R, Southard J, et al. Patterns of care for hypertension among hospitalized patients. Public Health Rep 97:521-527, 1982.

30. Levine D, Bone L, Steinwachs D, et al. The physicians' role in improving patient outcome in high blood pressure control. MD St Med J 32:291-293, 1983.

31. Chobanian AV, Bakris GL, Black HR, et al. The seventh report of the Joint National Committee on Prevention, Detection, Evaluation, and Treatment of High Blood Pressure: The JNC 7 report. JAMA. 289:2560-2572, 2003.

32. Community Guide to High Blood Pressure Control. US Dept. of Health & Human Services. PHS, NIH, NHLBI, NHBPEP. NIH Publication #82-2333, May, 1982.

33. Fortmann SP, Winleby MA, Flora JA, et al. Effect of long-term community health education on blood pressure and hypertension control: The Stanford Five-City Project. Am J Epidemiol 132:629-646, 1990.

34. Luepker RV, Murray DM, Jacobs DR, et al. Community education for cardiovascular disease prevention: Risk factor changes in the Minnesota Heart Health Program. Am J Public Health 84:1383-1393, 1994.

35. Carleton RA, Lasater TM, Assaf AR, et al. The Pawtucket Heart Health Program: An experiment in population-based disease prevention. RI Med J 70:533-538, 1987.

36. Weiss SM. Community health promotion demonstration programs: Introduction. *In:* Matarrazo JD, Herd JA, Miller NE, Weiss SM (edis). Behavioral Health: A Handbook of Health Enhancement and Disease Prevention. New York, John Wiley, 1984;pp. 1137-1139.

37. Winkleby MA. The future of community-based cardiovascular disease intervention studies. Am J Public Health 84:1369-1372, 1994.

38. Rogers MA, Buchan DA, Small D, et al. Telemedicine improves diagnosis of essential hypertension compared with usual care. J Telemed Telecare 8:344-349, 2002.

39. DeBusk RF, Miller NH, Superko R, et al. A case-management system for coronary risk factor modification after acute myocardial infarction. Ann Intern Med 120:721-729, 1994.

40. Friedman RH, Kazis LE, Jette A, et al. A telecommunications system for monitoring and counseling patients with hypertension: Impact on medication adherence and blood pressure control. Ame J Hypertens 9:285-292,1996.

41. Artinian NT, Washington OG, Templin TN. Effects of home telemonitoring and community-based monitoring on blood pressure control in urban African Americans: A pilot study. Heart Lung 30:191-199, 2001.

42. Burt VL, Cutler JA, Higgins M, et al. Trends in the prevalence, awareness, treatment, and control of hypertension in the adult US population: Data from the Health Examination Survey, 1960-1991. Hypertension 26:60-69, 1995.

43. Hill MN. Behavior and biology: The basic sciences for AHA action. Circulation 97:807-810, 1998.

44. Robertson A, Minkler M. New health promotion movement: A critical examination. Health Educ Q 2:295-312, 1994.

45. Merzel, C, D'Affitti J. Reconsidering community-based health promotion: Promise, performance, and potential. Am J Public Health 93:557-574, 2003.

46. Gold MR, McCoy KI, Teutsch SM, et al. Assessing outcomes in population health: Moving the field forward. Am J Prev Med 13:3-5, 1997.

47. Emmans K. Behaviorial and social science contributions to the health of adults in the United States. *In:* Smedley B, Syme L (eds). Promoting Health: Intervention Strategies from Social and Behaviorial Research. Washington, DC, National Academy Press. 2000;254-321, 2000.

48. U.S. Department of Health and Human Services, Office of Disease Prevention and Health Promotion. Healthy People 2010, 2nd ed. Washington, DC, Government Printing Office, 2000.

49. Kumanyika SK, Charleston JB. Lose weight and win: A church-based weight loss program for blood pressure control among black women.. Patient Educ and Couns 19:19-32, 1992.

50. Thompson LS, Story M, Butler G. Use of a university-community collaboration model to frame issues and set an agenda for strengthening a community. Health Promot Pract 4:385-392, 2003.

51. Levine DM, Becker DM, Bone LR, et al. Community-academic health center partnerships for underserved minority populations-one solution to a national crisis. JAMA272:309-311, 1994.

52. Raczynski JM, Cornell CE, Stalker V, et al. Developing community capacity and improving health in African American communities. Am J Med Sci 322:269-275, 2001.

53. McLeroy KR, Bibeau D, Steckler A, et al. An ecological perspective on health promotion programs. Health Educ Q 15:351-377, 1988.

54. Hill MN, Miller NH. Compliance enhancement: A call for multidisciplinary team approaches. Circulation 93:4-6, 1996.

55. Miller NH, Hill MN, Kottke T, et al. The multilevel compliance challenge: Recommendations for a call to action. Circulation 95:1085-1090, 1997.

56. Pew Health Professions Commission. Community Health Workers: Integral Yet Often Overlooked Members of the Health Care Workforce. San Francisco, CA, USCF Center for the Health Professions, 1994.

57. Witmer W, Seifr SD, Finocchio L, et al. Community health workers: Integral members of the health care force. Am J Public Health 85:1055-1058, 1995.

58. Smedley BD, Stith AY, Nelson AR. Unequal treatment: Confronting racial and ethnic disparities in health care. Institute of Medicine of the National Academies. Washington, DC, National Academies Press, 2003.

59. Scherer JL. Neighbor to neighbor: Community health workers educate their own. Hosp Health Netw 52-56, 1994.

60. Hill MN, Becker DM. Roles of nurses and health workers in cardiovascular health promotion. Am J Med Sci 310:S123-S126, 1995.

61. Bray ML, Edwards LH. A primary care approach using Hispanic workers as nurse extenders. Public Health Nurs 11:7-11, 1994.

62. Fedder DO, Chang RJ, Curry S, et al. The effectiveness of a community health worker outreach program on healthcare utilization of west Baltimore City Medicaid patients with diabetes, with or without hypertension. Ethn Dis 13:22-27, 2003.

63. Crawford P, Maxey R, Dacosta K. Community0 outreach: A call for community action. J Natl Med Assoc 94(8 Suppl):63S-71S, 2002.

64. Hill MN, Bone LR, Butz AM. Maximizing the effectiveness of community health workers in research. IMAGE. J Nurs Scholarsh 25:221-226, 1996.

65. Bone LR, Mamon J, Levine DM, et al. Emergency department detection and follow-up of high blood pressure: Use and effectiveness of community health workers. Am J Emerg Med 7: 16-20, 1989.

66. Kreiger J, Collier C, Song L, et al. Linking community-based blood pressure measurements to clinical care: A randomized controlled trial of outreach and tracking by community health workers. Am J Pub Health 89:859-861, 1999.

67. Kotchen JM, Shakoor-Abdullah B, Walker W, et al. Planning for a community-based hypertension control program in the inner city. J Hum Hypertens Suppl 3:S9-S13, 1996.

68. Gary TL, Bone LR, Hill MN, et al. Randomized controlled trial of the effects of nurse case manager and community health worker interventions on risk factors for diabetes-related complications in urban African Americans. Prev Med 37:23-32, 2003.

69. Hill MN, Bone LR, Stewart MC, et al. A clinical trial to improve HBP care in young urban African American men. Am J Hypertension 9:1A-2A, 1996.

70. Hill MN, Han HR, Dennison CR, et al. Hypertension care and control in underserved urban African American men: Behavioral and physiologic outcomes at 36 months. Am J Hypertens 16:906-913, 2003.

71. Rose LE, Kim MT, Dennison CR, et al. The contexts of adherence for African Americans with high blood pressure. J Adv Nurs 32:587-594, 2000.

72. Green LW, Kreuter MW. Health Promotion Planning: An Educational and Environmental Approach, 2nd ed. Mountain View, Mayfield, 1991.

73. Dennison CR, Hill MN, Bone LR, et al. Comprehensive hypertension care in underserved urban black men: High follow-up rates and blood pressure improvement over 60 months. Circulation 108:IV-381, 2003.

74. Felix-Aaron KL, Bone LR, Levine DM, et al. Using participant information to develop a tool for the evaluation of community health worker outreach services. Ethn Dis 12:87-96, 2002.

# Chapter 41

# Medication Adherence for Antihypertensive Therapy

## Lars Osterberg, Peter Rudd

Hypertension remains a powerful contributor to cardiovascular diseases, which are the most common cause of death in the United States. Calculated to be the fourth largest risk factor for mortality, hypertension may predict 6% of all deaths worldwide.[1] Over the past four decades, the prevalence of hypertension has changed little (~24% of the U.S. population) despite improvements in its detection and treatment.[2] The importance of optimizing treatment adherence rises in proportion to the potential benefit from therapy. With successful treatment, the relative risks of fatal events fall by 40% for stroke and 26% for coronary heart disease (CHD).[3]

These promising results are not guaranteed. The benefits largely depend on achieving high rates of blood pressure (BP) control. National data, displayed in Figure 41–1, suggest the need for continued efforts and improvement, since less than 30% of American hypertensive patients are diagnosed, under treatment, and at goal BP. This leaves more than 30 million hypertensives in this country who remain suboptimally controlled.[4]

One of the critical factors that determines BP control is the patient's adherence to the prescribed regimen, also called *compliance*. In general, patient compliance refers to the willingness and ability of an individual patient to follow health-related advice, take medication as prescribed, attend scheduled clinic appointments, and complete recommended tests and consultations.[5] The sizable investment in diagnosing, evaluating, and prescribing treatment for individual hypertensive patients achieves value in proportion to how well they follow the prescription: taking medications, modifying diet and activity, and making other lifestyle changes.

## THERAPEUTIC PARADIGM

The path to improving BP control begins with steps taken by the clinician in evaluating, treating, and reassessing the patient's hypertension. Most clinicians titrate their patients' BP to a therapeutic goal level, which is most commonly ≤140/90 mm Hg and recently revised to ≤135/85 mm Hg[6] for uncomplicated hypertensives. The clinician has multiple tasks: deciding whom to treat, when to treat, how to treat, and how to adjust treatment to optimize the benefit/risk ratio. More than two decades ago, Sackett et al.[7-9] focused on the adjustment process. They formulated the clinician's dilemma as having to categorize the returning patient as falling into one of four mutually exclusive clusters, illustrated in Figure 41–2.

The clinician must decide whether to continue the current regimen, augment it, attenuate it, or withhold it altogether. For the busy clinician, the decision may appear deceptively simple. If the clinician considers only two possibilities (the regimen is satisfactory *or* the regimen needs to be augmented), he is following a simplified strategy. At least two other conditions may escape detection: (1) the patient has achieved goal BP despite not having fully complied with the prescription, and (2) the patient may have failed to achieve goal BP (in part) because of imperfect adherence. To be comprehensive, the clinician must consider all four possibilities.

Very limited data exist about the relative frequency distributions of the four groupings among ambulatory hypertensive patients. The McMaster group reported data from male steelworkers assessed by pill counts and home BP assessments.[8-10] Silas et al.[11] used quantitative urinary assays after calibration for the adherence measure. Their data appear together in Table 41–1.

Despite different methodologies, the two studies display remarkably similar patterns. Only a minority of studied patients achieved both goal BP and optimal adherence at the same time. Indeed, only about half of each group achieved satisfactory BP control. Perhaps most critically, more than half of those patients who failed to achieve goal BP exhibited suboptimal medication compliance. Finally, a small but definable minority achieved goal BP despite less than full adherence, perhaps because of overzealous diagnosis or prescription.

Box 41–1 enumerates some implications of these distributions. The first implication is that optimal compliance with prescribed antihypertensive medications should not be assumed, since it seems not to occur about half the time. Second, the clinician should resist automatic escalation of the drug regimen if the patient fails to achieve goal BP. About half the time, the reason for failure reflects suboptimal medication-taking behavior rather than the biology of the disease or the pharmacology of the regimen. Third, an important minority on chronic antihypertensive medication succeeds at combining full compliance without special interventions to attain goal BP levels. Finally, a small group achieves goal BP despite poor compliance but needs special assessments for detection.

There are consequences if the clinician misclassifies the patient, both in terms of risking toxic levels of drug exposure when full compliance occurs and in failing to achieve consistent BP reduction with imperfect cardiovascular risk reduction. The data indirectly support the conclusion that the impact of treatment, both positive and negative, is proportional to the amount of treatment actually received rather than to the amount prescribed.[12] Urquhart has phrased the matter succinctly: "The quality of execution of drug prescription is a patient attribute, not a drug attribute." (John Urquhart, MD, FRCP [Edin], Pharmaco-epidemiology Group, Maastricht University, Maastricht, NL, personal communication.)

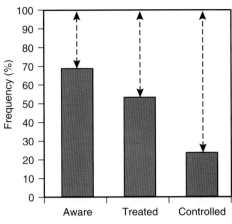

Figure 41-1 Status of antihypertensive management and opportunities for improvement: 1988-1991. Prevalence of hypertension by status of diagnosis, treatment, and BP control from the Third National Health and Nutrition Examination Survey (NHANES III; 1988-1991), based on a cross-sectional survey of the civilian, noninstitutionalized population of the United States after both an in-home interview and clinical examination for 9901 participants above age 18. The dashed arrows represent the opportunity still unrealized to optimize antihypertensive control. (From Burt VL, Whelton P, Roccella EJ, et al. Prevalence of hypertension in the US adult population. Results from the Third National Health and Nutrition Examination Survey, 1988-1991. Hypertension 25:305-313, 1995.)

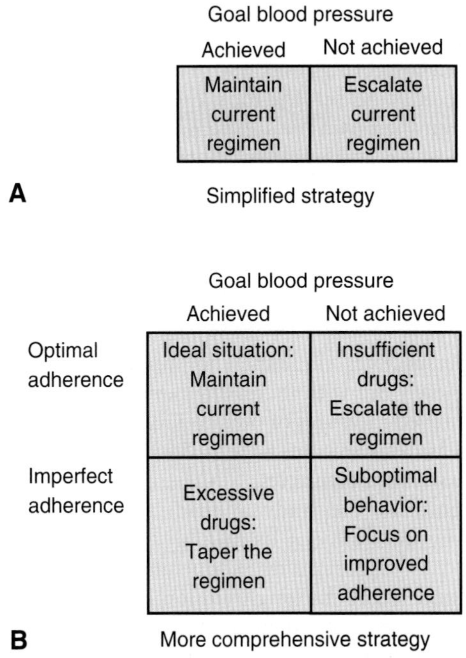

Goal blood pressure

| Achieved | Not achieved |
|---|---|
| Maintain current regimen | Escalate current regimen |

**A**    Simplified strategy

Goal blood pressure

|  | Achieved | Not achieved |
|---|---|---|
| Optimal adherence | Ideal situation: Maintain current regimen | Insufficient drugs: Escalate the regimen |
| Imperfect adherence | Excessive drugs: Taper the regimen | Suboptimal behavior: Focus on improved adherence |

**B**    More comprehensive strategy

Figure 41-2 Clinicians must decide when and how to respond to returning patients prescribed antihypertensive medication. A simplified strategy, **A,** uses regimen escalation when patients fail to achieve goal blood pressure (BP). **B** illustrates a more complex strategy, acknowledging the role that both patient and clinician play in achieving therapeutic goals. (Adapted from Sackett DL, Haynes RB, Tugwell P. Compliance. Clinical Epidemiology: A Basic Science for Clinical Medicine. Boston, Little, Brown, 1985; pp 199-222).

Table 41-1 Distributions of Adherence by Blood Pressure Achievement

| Adherence | BP Goal Achieved | BP Goal Not Achieved | Totals |
|---|---|---|---|
| Sackett et al.[9] | | | |
| **PILL COUNT ≥80%** | 43 (32%) | 32 (24%) | 75 (56%) |
| **PILL COUNT <80%** | 21 (16%) | 38 (28%) | 59 (44%) |
| Totals | 64 (48%) | 70 (52%) | 134 |
| (100%) | | | |
| Silas et al.[11] | | | |
| **[Debrisoquine]U ≥11 mg/dl** | 15 (41%) | 6 (16%) | 21 (57%) |
| **[Debrisoquine]U <11 mg/dl** | 6 (16%) | 10 (27%) | 16 (43%) |
| Totals | 21 (57%) | 16 (43%) | 37 (100%) |

Adapted from Rudd P. Clinicians and patients with hypertension: Unsettled issues about compliance. Am Heart J 130:572-579, 1995.

Box 41-1 Implications of the Adherence Distributions

1. Optimal adherence to the antihypertensive prescription should not be assumed.
   (a) Nonadherence occurs about half the time.
   (b) Overprescribing coupled with under-adhering may still produce satisfactory BP control.
2. Failure to achieve goal BP despite an adequate regimen and adequate time to respond may result from biologic, pharmacologic, behavioral factors or a combination of all three components.
   (a) About half the time when goal BP is not achieved, suboptimal medication-taking may be present.
   (b) Escalating the regimen in such a context will be incorrect half the time.
3. Only an important minority combines full compliance without special interventions to achieve goal BP in a consistent manner.

On the positive side, full compliance brings maximal reduction of BP and cardiovascular risk. On the negative side, full compliance also brings maximal drug-related side effects and other toxicities. All but the most naive patients quickly learn to carry out their own mini-experiments, seeking to optimize among positive and negative, short- and long-term, benefit and risk.[13] Not surprisingly, partial or complete nonadherence is a major contributor to "refractory" hypertension.[14]

## MEASURING COMPLIANCE

These perspectives on adherence and hypertension have evolved slowly but with increasing rapidity in the last decade with improved measures of medication-taking behavior. With better measures, clinicians have learned to broaden their focus and seize new opportunities.

For centuries, the study of medication-taking was constrained by the frailty of its measurements, as illustrated in Table 41–2.[15-20] Allusions by Hippocrates and Plato to nonadherence underscore the long tradition but provided few metrics except for global patient self-report or clinician opinion. Both of these techniques are easy and inexpensive but prone to subjectivity and easy distortion. They are examples of indirect measures, remote in time and space from the actual consumption of prescribed medication. Other measures similar in stature and similarly subject to error are short-recall patient self-report, self-monitoring by diary, and therapeutic outcome. The latter has the hidden complexity that other factors beside adherence may determine clinical outcomes with little foundation for teasing out the separate contribution of compliance on its own.

The arrival of pill counts has been a mixed blessing. On the one side, they appear to bring a degree of precision and quantitation to measuring adherence. But, on the other hand, the parking lots of many clinical study facilities may give evidence of pill-dumping as patients try to represent themselves as adherent and cooperative.[21] Some cynics have argued that pill counts have provided job security for a whole generation of research assistants without adding substantially to our knowledge of true compliance patterns.[22]

In contrast, several groups have confirmed the relative accuracy of prescription refill rates, especially when carried out over several months compared with a home inventory.[23,24] Important cautions, however, include discrepancies between the prescription and the medical record and using refill rates for periods less than 60 days.[25] Even more limiting is the need for a closed system of pharmacies for all refills and complete, computerized records. The method may also be distorted by the sharing of medications by the index patient and others taking the same drug.

Over nearly 30 years, several investigators have explored the use of medication monitors, capable of recording vial openings or discrete dispensings.[19,22,26-42] For the first time, one could track the day-to-day dynamics of medication-taking rather than relying on an imprecise average over days, weeks, or months and also minimize the likelihood of patients misrepresenting their own report card.[43] Lingering problems and disappointments include relatively high cost, need for vial returns or transmissions for downloading of data, and limited discreteness of tracking individual doses with some devices. Most clinicians and investigators quickly agreed that it was improbable that anyone would systematically dispense pills over several months as tracked by the monitor and then discard the doses without actually administering them. These indirect methods dramatically advanced our sophistication about the process of medication-taking.[44]

In contrast, the available direct measures like biologic assays[45,46] or tracer systems[47,48] do confirm drug administration but require collection of body fluids (e.g., blood, urine, saliva) and performing discrete quantitative assays while making assumptions about hepatic and/or renal function. Such measures still do not permit retrospective review beyond several pharmacokinetic half-lives. They further suffer from relatively high cost and difficulties of administration in exchange for superior sensitivity and specificity over the short periods reflected by point estimates of drug concentrations.[49]

## EPIDEMIOLOGY OF MEDICATION COMPLIANCE

### Patterns of Medication-Taking Behavior

Constrained by imperfect adherence measures, early studies concluded that chronic preventive treatments, such as those for hypertension, exhibit compliance rates approximating 50%.[50] More discrete measures, especially electronic medication monitors, revealed more granularity, clarity, and complexity from the data analysis. Most deviation from the prescription occurs as dose omissions rather than as dose insertions or misschedulings.[51,52] The dose omissions occur more frequently as the dosing frequency increases, as illustrated in Figure 41–3. Medication-taking patterns commonly improve significantly in the 5 days preceding and following schedule appointments, compared with 30 days after appointments, generating a "white-coat compliance" pattern.[35,53]

Although intuitive, the prescribing of very simple regimens (e.g., one pill once daily) does not ensure consistent adherence,[54] even among those with relatively frequent, reinforcing visits with the clinician.[36] There remains a core of 10% to 40% of subjects displaying imperfect dosing. The difference in compliance between once- and twice-daily dosing tends to be small in most studies, while adherence declines more dramatically as prescribed dosing frequency exceeds twice-daily.[36,54] Electronic monitoring has confirmed that the adherence varies inversely with dosing frequency. Those on a once-daily regimen display less dosing variability than with twice-daily dosing among 198 Canadian hypertensives randomized to diltiazem twice-daily vs. amlodipine once-daily.[55] Among diabetics on oral agents, the compliance rate fell from 79% on once-daily to 38% on three-times daily dosing.[51]

Similar patterns appear in adherence data from diverse medical conditions, whether compliance distributions come from patients with hypertension,[32,36,38,56] seizure disorders,[22,35] glaucoma,[33,40,57] or other clinical scenarios like hormone therapy and lipid-reducing agents.[58-60] Most of the available data come from settings of chronic therapy to prevent long-term negative consequences. Figure 41–4, although a hypothetical composite, reflects the similar J-shaped distributions reported by the respective investigator groups.

Closer inspection of Figure 41–4 reveals three principal subgroups. On the positive side, 50% to 60% of the patients are *full compliers* with trivial deviations from the prescription

**Table 41–2** Available Measures of Medication Adherence

| COMPLIANCE MEASURE | Marginal Cost | Difficulty of Use | | Approximate* Related to "Gold Standard" | | Comments |
|---|---|---|---|---|---|---|
| | | Patient | Investigator | Sensitivity<br>Noncompliance | Specificity<br>Compliance | |
| **INDIRECT** | | | | | | |
| 1. Self-report | + | + | + | 20%-55% | 80%-95% | Unspecified versus short (1-2 day) recall |
| 2. Self-monitoring | + | ++ | ++ | 40%-70% | 80%-95% | Prospective logging of drug-taking |
| 3. Clinician opinion | + | | + | 50%-65% | 40%-80% | Point estimates of dynamic process |
| 4. Pill/packet count | ++ | ++ | +++ | 60%-90% | 75%-90% | Pill vial return issues: nontrivial |
| 5. Prescription refill | ++ | | +++ | 60%-90% | 60%-90% | Central pharmacy or comprehensive records are critical |
| 6. Therapeutic outcome | + | | + | 20%-40% | 40%-80% | Implicit versus explicit criteria should be prede-fined |
| 7. Medication monitor | +++ | ++ | +++ | 85%-95% | 85%-95% | Often needs supple-mental pill count as well |
| **DIRECT** | | | | | | |
| 1. Direct supervision | ++ | + | +++ | 85%-95% | 85%-95% | Parenteral adminis tration versus oral drugs |
| 2. Bioassay of drug | +++ | ++ | +++ | 60%-90% | 80%-95% | Bioassays not always feasible or available |
| 3. Pharmacologic marker | +++ | ++ | +++ | 60%-90% | 80%-95% | Combination of marker and primary drug may need FDA approval |

Adapted from Hasford J. Compliance and the benefit/risk relationship of antihypertensive treatment. J Cardiovasc Pharmacol 20:S30-S34, 1992.
Arbitrary scale of degree: + = small; ++ = moderate; +++ = large

and remarkably consistent medication-taking behaviors from day to day. At the other extreme, the *noncompliers* exhibit extremely imperfect adherence, although sometimes misrepresenting their usual behavior by pill-dumping just before scheduled visits. In the middle are the *partial compliers*. Rather than a simple intermediate point, the partial compliers show a complicated mixture of nearly perfect pill-taking interspersed with periods of marked deviation from the prescription. Such a pattern suggests that they understand what they are supposed to do but have difficulty in performing the tasks in a consistent manner.[61] Although not a bell-shaped distribution, the average compliance for such groups approximates 60% to 75%, consistent with other reports.[62] Seeking more detail, Urquhart summarized the compliance distribution of a patient cohort as follows:

1. One sixth of the patients take their medications exactly as directed.
2. One sixth take nearly all the medications with some fluctuations in dose timing.
3. One sixth occasionally omit a single daily dose.
4. One sixth have a drug holiday (the sequential omission of 3 or more days' doses) 3 to 4 times per year, together with occasional omissions of 1 to 2 days' doses.
5. One sixth of the patients have a "drug holiday" monthly, together with frequent omissions of 1 to 2 days' doses.
6. One sixth take few or no doses while giving the impression of being completely compliant. (See Figure 41–5.)[63]

All but the full compliers display important gaps in medication-taking. The consequences of such nonadherence

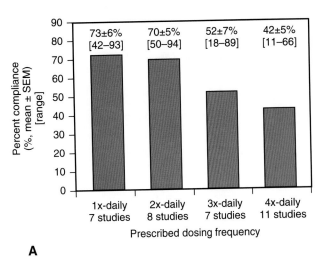

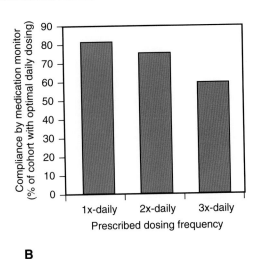

**A**

**B**

**Figure 41-3** Compliance rate by dosing schedule. Compliance rates tend to fall as the frequency of daily doses increases. **(A)** Greenberg performed a literature review in 1984, reflecting adherence assessments primarily by self-report and pill count. **(B)** Eisen and coworkers employed an electronic medication monitor among hypertensive patients. Both studies support an inverse relationship between adherence and dosing frequency with more modest differences between 1x- and 2x-daily dosing than with more frequent dosing schedules. (**A** from Greenberg RN. Overview of patient compliance with medication dosing: A literature review. Clin Ther 6:592-599, 1984; **B** from Eisen SA, Miller DK, Woodward RS, et al. The effect of prescribed daily dose frequency on patient medication compliance. Arch Intern Med 150:1881-1884, 1990.)

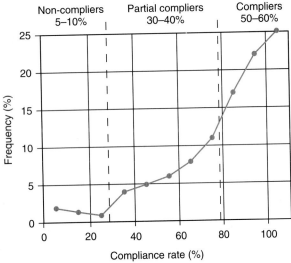

**Figure 41-4** Compliance distribution composite: hypertension, seizures, glaucoma, congestive heart failure (CHF). Several investigators have reported remarkably similar patterns of compliance among ambulatory patients monitored electronically for medication-taking behavior despite dissimilar diseases like hypertension, seizures, glaucoma, and CHF (see text for references). All the conditions exhibit three clusters: (1) *full compliers* (50%-60% of total) with negligible deviations from the prescription; (2) *partial compliers* (30%-40%) with periods of excellent adherence interspersed with poor adherence or "drug holidays"; and (3) *noncompliers* (5%-10%) with low levels of compliance. (Adapted from Rudd P, Hagar RW: Hypertension: Mechanisms, diagnosis, therapy. In Topol E (ed). Textbook of Cardiovascular Medicine, 1st ed. New York, Lippincott-Raven, 1997; pp 109-143.)

include subtherapeutic drug concentrations; imperfect BP control; submaximal cardiovascular risk reduction; unnecessary and potentially dangerous treatment escalation; avoidable tests, procedures, and hospitalizations; and threats of withdrawal, rebound, and first-dose phenomena.[64] None of these bad outcomes should be surprising if one acknowledges that drugs act episodically in patients who dose episodically, inadequately or not at all in patients who underdose, and hazardously when dosed in intermittent patterns.[65] At a more extreme level, drugs cannot work if (1) they are never prescribed, (2) the prescription is written but never filled, (3) the drug is never taken by the patient, or (4) the drug is taken but not absorbed. Overall, the pharmacologic impact, whether beneficial or toxic, is proportional to the drug exposure and the dose received.

## Predictors of Noncompliance

Given the high stakes, many groups have begun searches for predictors of noncompliance, so as to concentrate remedial resources on the groups most needy of change. Early efforts quickly concluded that no simple, nonadherent, personality profile existed. At the extremes of age, poverty, social isolation, and psychiatric dysfunction, increased noncompliance was observed. Symptom level, educational level, and objective seriousness of the medical condition provided little predictive value.[66] In contrast, Hill et al.,[67] focusing on disadvantaged, inner city populations, encountered high rates of no current antihypertensive care (49%), use of illicit drugs (45%), social isolation (47%), unemployment (40%), and lack of health insurance (51%). Low alcoholism risk and employment were identified as significant predictors of compliance with antihypertensive medication-taking behavior. Men currently using illicit drugs were 2.6 times less likely to have controlled BP compared with their counterparts who did not use illicit drugs.

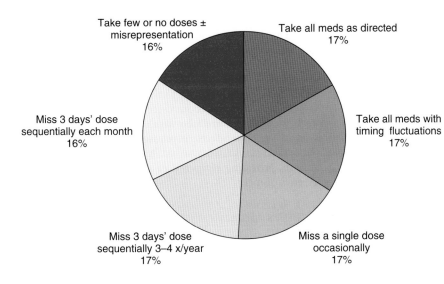

**Figure 41–5** Dose-taking distribution from unpublished series of diverse patients on chronic medications by electronic monitoring of dose dispensings. (Adapted from Urquhart J. The electronic medication event monitor. Lessons for pharmacotherapy. Clin Pharmacokinet 32:345-356, 1997.)

Despite limited success to date in finding predictors, the obvious broad areas for future focus include characteristics of the individual patient, the disease, the prescribed treatment, the patient-provider relationship, and the clinical setting.[68] Among patient characteristics, consistent patterns of superior adherence with electronic monitoring emerged from older rather than younger patients[69-72] except for the "old-old" up to age 87.[71] Among an ambulatory, hypertensive, Medicaid population, Bailey et al. reported that prescription refill compliance varied by drug class (α-blockers > ACE-inhibitors > calcium channel blockers > diuretics),[69] although others have recently reported no difference in the discontinuation rate of the various drug classes.[73] Independent predictors of nonadherence as measured by medication refill rates include younger age, multiple daily doses, fewer provider visits, and depressive symptoms.[69,74] In contrast, patient gender and regimen complexity hold little predictive value.[69]

Knowledge about the disease and familiarity with the regimen are necessary but not sufficient to ensure high levels of adherence.[7,75] Indeed, health professionals themselves are often cited to demonstrate that knowledge and education are no guarantee of compliance. Each individual, whether or not sophisticated about the medical condition and its management, must make hard choices to optimize among risks and benefits, hardships and conveniences, costs and rewards. Commonly cited barriers include simple forgetfulness, drug side effects, financial costs, confusion about the regimen, and interference with daily schedules.[76-78]

Some patients, especially the elderly, construct elaborate systems of locations and cues to facilitate remembering and adhering to the prescribed regimen.[76] Still others struggle with childproof vials, which functionally become person-proof.[79] Most of these coping mechanisms are highly personal and rarely emerge from routine clinical surveillance. Some advocates of patient self-management[80,81] have argued that three issues are key to improving adherence: (1) defining the key behaviors to be mastered and implemented, (2) providing consistent guidance and reinforcement, and (3) linking the behaviors to the desired clinical outcomes.

There appears to be something beneficial associated with compliant behaviors in general, even when they consist of taking placebos in clinical trials. Three of 12 studies comparing rates of hospitalization and mortality for chronic heart disease revealed better clinical outcomes with adherence versus nonadherence to placebo, suggesting that adherent behavior may be a marker for other behaviors with protective effects or otherwise confer an improved prognosis.[82]

On the other side, there are some definite negative consequences for nonadherence. Interruptions in antihypertensive prescription refills among California Medicaid patients greater than 40 years old were associated with higher costs, especially for hospitalization.[83] Among 602 women enrolled in the Beta Blocker Heart Attack Trial, nonadherence by appointment and medications conferred a 2.4-fold (95% CI 1.1-5.6) increase in postmyocardial infarction (post-MI) death rates Those who complied had a 2.4-fold reduction in mortality, whether or not they were randomized to receive propranolol as the active drug.[84]

## APPLICATION TO HYPERTENSION

Treatment of hypertension almost never occurs in isolation but arises as part of a more comprehensive strategy to reduce overall cardiovascular risk, such as from dyslipidemia, cigarette smoking, glucose intolerance, and obesity.[2] Unfortunately, the multiplicity of factors and resultant interventions may diminish rather than enhance some patients' motivation. The adherence burden rises when clinicians seek to have patients reduce salt, saturated fat, and alcohol intake at the same time as they have patients decrease stress and increase regular physical exercise. The sheer number of things to change may overwhelm all but the most focused, trusting, and dedicated patient.

Interactions among the treatments may create extra dilemmas and opportunities. As data emerge indicating circadian variation in cardiovascular risk, selection of specific antihypertensive agents and their optimal administration time becomes more complex.[85] The clinician must learn to choose drugs on the basis of their ability to reduce overall cardiovascular risk as well as to optimize antihypertensive efficacy, safety, quality of life, and adherence.[86,87] Partially abandoned, the old concept of "stepped care" has been largely replaced by evolving notions of more personalized, nearly customized treatment plans.[88]

Part of the rationale for more aggressive and presumably more effective treatment strategies is the growing appreciation of lost benefits and increased risks for poor antihypertensive management. Suboptimal compliance carries increased probabilities of extra hospitalizations,[89] sudden death,[90] and other cardiovascular morbidity, even when the elevated pressures are linked to white-coat phenomena.[91]

Several features about treating ambulatory hypertension pose special challenges to the treating clinician. Most day-to-day responsibilities for following the regimen rest squarely on the patient's shoulders, regardless of the amount of instruction, guidance, and support provided by physician, nurse, pharmacist, or family members (see Figure 41–6). Although many factors can contribute to a patient's nonadherence to medications, the patient is still the main player in attaining full compliance.

## FOCUS ON COMPLIANCE IN HYPERTENSION

### The Patient

There is a diverse array of problem areas for the hypertensive patient. Some investigators classify patients according to their readiness to accept the diagnosis and undertake active participation: deniers versus acceptors versus pragmatists.[92] Others focus on the perceived "net" barriers to full adherence, especially relevant and prevalent among younger patients and those most recently initiating treatment.[93] An unpublished telephone survey by the Angus Reid Group among 301 Canadian hypertensives reported that 62% of respondents admitted to not taking their prescribed antihypertensive medication as prescribed (cited in *Ontario Medicine,* June 1994, p. 19). Fully 47% of respondents acknowledged side effects from these drugs, and only 41% were aware that stroke was a major risk of hypertension. Perhaps most intriguing were the types of magical thinking among some respondents, who believed they could skip doses and remain protected, who rewarded themselves with drug holidays for good behavior, and who tended not to refill medications promptly because they were too busy.

Early studies on the effect of labeling patients as hypertensive demonstrated decreased perceived health, increased absenteeism from work, increased depressive symptoms, and a decreased quality of life, even when the "label" of hyperten-

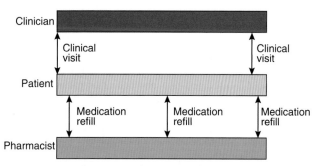

**Figure 41–6** Relative contribution to adherent behaviors. The clinician, patient, and pharmacist all contribute to the frequency, consistency, and degree of adherence to the clinical prescription for ambulatory hypertensive patients. The relative contribution of the patient is the greatest, both overall and on a daily basis, despite the frequency of clinical visits and medication refills.

sion was incorrect and when no antihypertensive therapy was given.[94] The principal factors associated with increased absenteeism reflected patients' becoming aware of their condition and low medication compliance.[94,95] Even in an academic family practice clinic, patients estimated that their recovery from an upper respiratory tract infection, urinary tract infection, or ankle sprain was about twice as long since the diagnosis of hypertension compared with those who had never had the diagnosis.[96] The adverse psychosocial impact may be tempered or even eliminated by avoiding forced screenings for the condition, providing reassurance, and offering a supportive work environment.[97,98]

### The Physician

Enlarging the focus of concern to include prescribing physicians has challenged several existing myths.[79] Many clinicians accept little if any responsibility for the complexity of the regimens they prescribe or for assisting their patients in minimizing drug-related side effects. They may overestimate their skill in detecting or preventing suboptimal adherence among their own patients and underestimate the several barriers which patients face in trying to comply.[99]

Surprising to some has been the correlation of patients' adherence to recommendations of lifestyle changes and the prescribing physician's own style. Predictors of patients' adherence include the physician's job satisfaction, the number of patients seen per week, the scheduling of follow-up appointments, and the tendency to answer patients' questions.[100]

#### Physicians Adherence to Clinical Guidelines

Physicians may themselves fail to adhere to evidence-based guidelines of diagnosis and treatment for hypertension. Such clinical guidelines arise from domain experts and opinion leaders and receive considerable emphasis and distribution.[72,101,102] Although existing clinical guidelines define explicit BP targets, physicians often display misinformation about the recommended BP goals for their patients.[103] Even more problematic is the clinical inertia or "knowledge-practice gap" when clinicians know guideline recommendations but fail to initiate or intensify treatment when indicated in their patients.[104,105] Such inertia may be particularly prevalent in treating conditions that are common and without limiting symptoms. As a consequence, prescribing clinicians may settle for BP levels above the recommendations rather than pushing themselves and their patients to attain the target range.[104,106]

One model of physician behavior outlines five necessary and sequential steps for successful adherence to practice guidelines: awareness, agreement, self-efficacy, outcome expectancy, and presence of a cueing mechanism.[107-109] Failures at any of these steps may lead to physician nonadherence to a guideline. By overcoming any of the barriers to achieving the five steps, physicians can attain improved guideline adherence.[110]

#### Effective Physician-Patient Communication

Still another physician-based opportunity arises in optimizing communication to and from patients.[78,111,112] The components may include identifying and problem solving about barriers to full adherence, using education about risks and benefits to increase motivation, and employing active listening to patients' concerns for teasing out remaining problems of adherence. Optimizing communication among the patient and provider team provides the essential foundation for patient compliance.[52,78,112-114]

## The Healthcare System

On a larger scale, the American healthcare system introduces other problems. At least 42 million Americans remain without medical insurance.[115] The absence of insurance alone or failure to link care with a principal provider does not in itself prevent good BP control. In fact, the multiplicity of influences obscures any simple correlation of poor access to health care to inadequate BP control.[116,117] Improved access to medications, in contrast, has been associated with improved adherence.[118] The growing dominance of managed care has brought pharmacy benefits management in an array of forms and formats that are sometimes helpful yet sometimes a barrier to patient compliance. The forced use of restrictive formularies, generic substitutions, and mail-away prescription-filling may exacerbate the hurdles to full adherence.[119,120]

## Opportunities for Collaboration

By defining adherence as the responsibility of several parties, new opportunities for collaboration and synergy emerge. The thoughtful clinician, concerned about optimizing a patient's BP, can bring skills, focus, and perseverance to the challenge of prescription adherence beyond proper diagnosis and evaluation. The health plan administrator, in turn, seeks to optimize outcomes for both the individual patient and the group of patients with similar characteristics and conditions. Pharmaceutical manufacturers wishes to differentiate their products from competitive medications for the optimal combination of therapeutic efficacy and quality of life, while minimizing symptomatic and biochemical toxicity.[121] Each constituency (patient, clinician, administrator, manufacturer) has its special priorities. Enhancing medication-taking for better outcomes will require a higher degree of sensitivity and collaboration among the principal parties than has existed in the past.[122]

## EVOLVING STRATEGIES FOR COMPLIANCE IMPROVEMENT

### Guiding Principles

The field of medication compliance has shown repetitively that a one-size solution does *not* fit all. Just as there is no single cause for suboptimal compliance, so there is no single fix. The reasons underlying noncompliance are multifaceted and therefore so must be the solutions.[123] As the field evolves, it has come to incorporate ethnocultural and psychosocial perspectives, as well as traditional sociodemographic, clinical, pharmacologic, and medical system issues. At the core of the broadened perspective is a realization that the patient with a chronic condition, even one with few symptoms such as hypertension, has special kinds of "work" to accomplish in living with the condition. The problem solving by physicians, nurses, pharmacists, and other health professionals must go beyond the simplistic sender-message-receiver communication model used as a default. As an alterna-

tive, the patient should actively participate in the selection of therapeutic ingredients and the pace of treatment.[124,125]

### New Skills and Collaboration

The effective prescriber-clinician should ask, simplify, tailor, and reinforce. Asking the patient for input early in the process immediately sets up a different and potentially far more useful dynamic than the traditional, autocratic stance. Minimizing the total number of daily doses usually arises as a priority. Selecting the most useful cues and location for the particular patient's life and lifestyle provides an added "fit."[126]

Optimization still requires a melding of patients' personal preferences with clinical and pharmacologic realities. Several recent reports emphasize the importance of effective 24-hour-a-day BP control, smooth antihypertensive effect with decreased variability in diurnal variation in BP, reduced early morning surge in BP, and minimal reflex activation of the sympathetic nervous system.[127] These characteristics assume even more prominence if medication-taking is imperfect and highly variable.

### Pharmacokinetics as a Guide for Adherence

A lively debate has arisen about the value and relevance of trough-to-peak variability in BP in comparing one antihypertensive agent with another. Some have argued that the optimal drug is one with a smooth concentration-time profile and long elimination half-life to maintain stable drug concentrations and stable antihypertensive effect despite imperfect medication-taking.[128] In this context, the trough-to-peak ratio reflects the duration of drug's action relative to its dosing interval, avoiding the use of inappropriately large drug doses simply to extend the apparent duration of action. At least two different clusters of drugs have been identified. In the first group, the concentration–effect relationship is essentially linear, and the trough-to-peak ratio is almost invariably dose-independent and therefore more stable. In the second grouping, the concentration–effect relationship is sigmoid-shaped, and the trough-to-peak ratio becomes dose-dependent and highly affected by compliance.[129] The data from Meredith and Elliott, shown in Figure 41–7, illustrate some interdrug differences among several antihypertensive agents.[130]

Drugs with linear relationships are more forgiving of imperfect adherence. They achieve therapeutic sufficiency with desirable and sustained reductions in BP in spite of variable pill-taking.[131] Using ambulatory BP monitoring, Leenen et al. confirmed that once-daily amlodipine provided more effective and consistent antihypertensive effect than twice-daily diltiazem in the face of interrupted therapy.[132] Some authors have used the same arguments in support of newly introduced combination products, when one of the components is especially long-lasting.[133,134]

### The New Paradigm: Challenges for the Decade

Ultimately, the clinician is the expert on the disorder and its treatment in general, but the patient remains the expert in his or her own disorder and his or her own experience with the treatment.[135] The principal challenges for the next decade will be to (1) forge strong foundations for collaboration among patient, clinician, and healthcare system; (2) reassess the

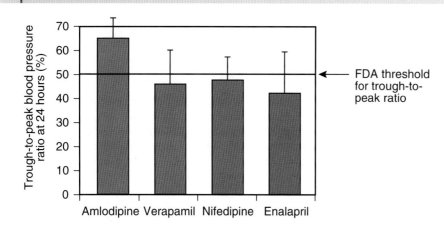

**Figure 41–7** Antihypertensive response reflects plasma drug concentrations. Trough-to-peak blood pressure (BP) ratios at 24 hours provide a useful index of sustained antihypertensive effect for once-daily medications. Meredith and Elliott report the ratios for four antihypertensive agents compared with the Food and Drug Administration (FDA) benchmark of 50% at 24 hours. (From Meredith PA, Elliott HL. Amlodipine: Clinical relevance of a unique pharmacokinetic profile. J Cardiovasc Pharmacol 22:S6-S8, 1993.)

traditional wisdoms about predictors of nonadherence and effective interventions; and (3) establish thresholds of therapeutic sufficiency for optimizing cardiovascular benefit to hypertensive patients despite sometimes imperfect adherence.

## Compliance-Enhancing Strategies for the Clinician

There are a cluster of discrete, effective, and feasible steps to detect, evaluate, and intervene among partial and noncompliant hypertensive patients, summarized in Box 41–2.[9] The remedial steps represent challenges because few clinicians have received training in how to be educators, motivators, and coaches. For their part, many practices and medical institutions have not readily accepted responsibility for these critical efforts.[136]

---

**Box 41–2** Compliance-Enhancing Strategies for Clinicians

1. Watch for nonattenders.
2. Watch for nonresponders.
3. Inquire without confrontation about compliance barriers.
4. Encourage the development and use of a medication-taking "system."
5. Provide simple, clear instruction.
6. Simplify the regimen as much as possible.
7. Provide substitutive and sequential steps.
8. Monitor progress to goal, both in blood pressure (BP) and in compliance.
9. Reinforce desirable behaviors and outcomes whenever possible.
10. Apply useful, relevant information and help from all possible sources.
11. Make explicit the potential value of the prescribed regimen and the impact of compliance.
12. Emphasize the importance of dose timing when appropriate.
13. Seek to customize the regimen to the patient's needs and preferences.

---

Partially adapted from Sackett DL, Haynes RB, Tugwell P. Compliance. Clinical Epidemiology: A Basic Science for Clinical Medicine. Boston, Little, Brown, 1985; p 218.

1. *Watch for nonattenders.*
   Those patients who fail initial or follow-up appointments are most at risk for dropping permanently out of care. This is especially likely to occur in the first year of treatment but may occur at any time.[137] Once detected, such patients should receive special handling to maximize the likelihood of their resuming regular visits and progress to goal.

2. *Watch for nonresponders.*
   Most patients will respond to antihypertensive medications with a relatively prompt and sustained reduction in BP, assuming selection of a rational and suitably aggressive regimen. Initial or secondary "resistance" to treatment carries its own differential diagnosis: secondary hypertension, interfering substances, biologic factors, suboptimal regimen, and medication nonadherence.[14] Retaining a low threshold for these possibilities helps promptly detect, address, and hopefully resolve any noncompliance.

3. *Inquire without confrontation about compliance barriers.*
   When exploring for nonadherence, the art may lie in establishing collaboration rather than confrontation. Few patients will openly admit to noncompliance if the clinician asks, "You're taking all your pills, aren't you?" More useful phrasings might include the following: "Many people have difficulty taking their medications as prescribed. What kinds of problems have you had in taking the pills?" In one study of a community pharmacy, 549 submitted prescriptions were never picked up over a 9-month interval. The stated reasons included transfer to another pharmacy, forgotten prescription, patient still had medication left over, or patient no longer needed the medication.[138] In another survey of general practice patients, prescribing physicians and assisting nurses, imperfect knowledge of the medications occurred in up to 60% of patients.[139] After a suitable open-ended inquiry, the clinician may use some follow-up questions:
   (a) "Some people experience awkward or embarrassing side effects, like leaking urine or having sexual problems. These problems may be hard to discuss.[140] Sometimes we can reduce or eliminate these problems if we know about them. Have you had any problems like these?"
   (b) "Other people have trouble remembering the pills or find that pill-taking interferes with their normal schedule. What kind of system do you use at home or work to stay on track with your pills?"

(c) "I once had a patient who came to see me regularly but never mentioned that he could not afford the medications I prescribed. As soon as I gave him sample drugs, his blood pressure was promptly controlled. Have you had any problems filling the prescription, opening the vials, or swallowing the pills?"

4. *Encourage the development and use of a medication-taking "system."*

Cramer has called for compliance enhancement by asking every patient at every visit about how the prescribed medications are taken.[126] The clinician may then encourage the selection of location, time, and/or activity cues, consistent with the patient's personal, daily routine. At each follow-up visit, the discussion may review how the selected method is working and lead to selective changes. In a survey of outpatients, Rudd and Marshall reported that the majority of patients had one or more systems of locations and cues for this purpose.[76]

5. *Provide simple, clear instructions.*

Learning theory indicates that patients will often recall the first and last things they are told but retain little of what comes in between. Uncomplicated, unambiguous directions are important, even when reinforced in writing or by review in the presence of the patient's significant other. Reliance on the pharmacist to provide more patient instruction, reinforcement, or reassurance may not always be realistic. On occasion, the addition of a pill dispenser aid facilitates following the instructions and highlights any missed doses.

6. *Simplify the regimen as much as possible.*

The number of dosings appears to be more of a stumbling block than the number of pills taken at any one time. In the elderly, such simplification may be particularly difficult but important when the reality is "polymedicine" for multiple, concurrent conditions rather than avoidable polypharmacy.[141,142] One useful strategy involves selecting, whenever possible, one drug to serve more than one function, such as using an $\alpha_1$-blocker for both prostatism and hypertension or an ACE-inhibitor for both congestive heart failure (CHF) and hypertension.

7. *Provide substitutive and sequential steps.*

Too often, the well-intentioned patient may be overwhelmed by requests to change several medications, modify diet, and increase exercise all at the same time. In most cases, urgency is unnecessary. If possible, the clinician should identify one behavior to substitute for another rather than add to the large and daunting number of requests. Well selected, the substitutive behavior takes no more work than the replaced behavior. The clinician can further assist by negotiating priorities for change in a manageable sequence rather than all at once.

8. *Monitor progress to goal, both in BP and in compliance.*

The clinician should specify the relation between prescribed medication and the attainment of goal BP, laying the foundation for further inquiry about adherence if the goal is not achieved or is not sustained. Introducing electronic monitoring of compliance alone can enhance antihypertensive control among patients with resistant hypertension, unmasking imperfect adherence.[143]

9. *Reinforce desirable behaviors and outcomes whenever possible.*

The key behaviors to reinforce include keeping appointments, taking medications as prescribed, avoiding running out of medication, and remaining willing to work out medication-taking and other clinical problems in a collaborative way. Secret efforts to titrate down one's medications to minimize side effects is a double loss: loss of maximal cardiovascular protection and loss of the opportunity to reduce the symptoms by adjusting the regimen. Another useful strategy is to reinforce desirable behaviors, so that they produce discomfort or dysphoria when missed, such as feeling ill at ease when going to bed without brushing one's teeth or riding in an automobile when a seatbelt is not available. Patients may learn both the dysphoria and how to avoid it by adhering to the prescription.

10. *Apply useful, relevant information and help from all possible sources.*

Family members and significant others may provide invaluable assistance and reinforcement for pill-taking, especially for patients with handicaps or cognitive impairment. For others, visiting nurse services and home health aides offer structure and support. Sometimes, important clues to nonadherence appear from failure to request prescription refills at indicated intervals. Other potential sources of key data include symptoms, signs, or laboratory test changes linkable to the specific, prescribed medications.[144] On a more ambitious scale, several successful programs have used nurse-mediated services with decision support by algorithm and frequent telephone contacts to yield improved compliance and better cardiovascular control.[145,146]

11. *Make explicit the potential value of the prescribed regimen and the impact of compliance.*

The clinician should emphasize the multiple benefits that can follow from optimal control of BP, including reduced risk of stroke, MI, heart failure, kidney failure, and peripheral vascular disease. There is a difference between an "average effect," based on the mean level of adherence, with that achievable with maximal compliance.[147] Figure 41–8 illustrates the difference of lipid-lowering efficacy for cholestyramine at average and maximal levels of compliance.

12. *Emphasize the importance of dose timing when appropriate.*

Unless told and reminded, many patients will not pay much attention to the precise timing of doses. For some medications and some dosing times, electronic monitoring has confirmed the superiority of morning versus evening dosing.[148,149]

13. *Seek to customize the regimen to the patient's needs and preferences.*

Most patients and most clinicians appear convinced that once-daily dosing will always be superior to more frequent dosing schedules. From a theoretical perspective, Levy has argued that more frequent dosings reduce the likelihood of having drug concentrations fall to subtherapeutic levels when lapses in pill-taking occur.[150] Figure 41–9 illustrates the relationship for a hypothetical drug prescribed once, twice, three, or four times daily. Empirically with electronic monitoring, Kruse et al. confirmed that once-daily dosing was more likely than twice-daily dosing to result in skipped days without any treatment, especially on weekends, and that evening doses were twice as likely as morning doses to be missed.[151] Although combination drug therapy might on one hand make a patient's medication regimen more complicated, it might be more appropriate to use

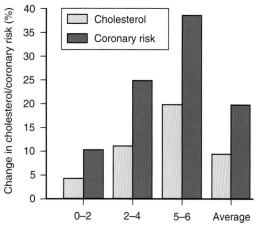

**Figure 41-8** Coronary heart disease (CHD) risk reduction by cholesterol change and medication compliance. The original report of the Lipid Research Clinics Coronary Primary Prevention Trial included the now famous relation of 10% reduction in cholesterol associated with 20% reduction in coronary risk. These data reflect the "average" level of adherence with cholestyramine packets. Maximum compliance (6 packets/day) leads to nearly a 20% reduction in cholesterol and almost a 40% reduction in coronary risk. Thus benefit may co-vary with compliance.

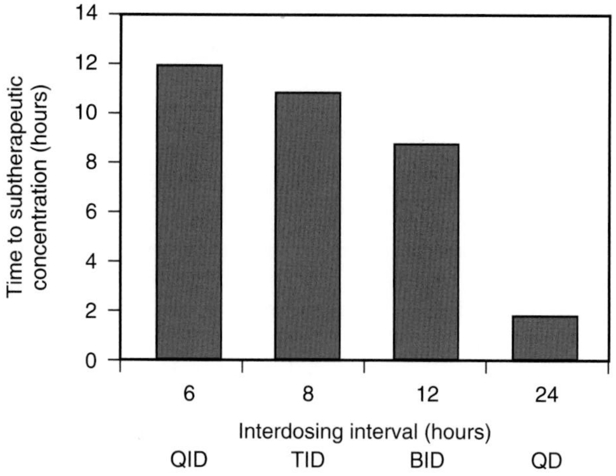

**Figure 41-9** Safety margin for dosing intervals using a hypothetical drug. Levy calculated the "safety margin" associated with different dosing intervals for a hypothetical drug with a half-life of 12 hours, volume of distribution of 1 L, dose of 10 mg/kg, 100% absorption, and minimum effective concentration of 3.0 mg/L. As dosing frequency decreases, the margin for error is reduced, even though drug concentrations remain therapeutic for once-daily dosing. (From Levy G. A pharmacokinetic perspective on medicament noncompliance. Clin Pharmacol Ther 54:242-244, 1994.)

lower doses of two drugs in some patients in order to limit the side effects that might be caused by using a higher dose of one drug.

## Compliance-Enhancing Strategies for Healthcare Systems

Health care systems themselves offer new opportunities for enhancing adherence. Two converging trends should assist the process: the emergence of vertically integrated health care systems and growing accountability for outcomes. The principal opportunities consist of reminder systems, technology applications, and aligning of incentives for patients, clinicians, and administrators. Among reminder systems, there are both paper and electronic methods to highlight and alert the prescribing clinician for missed events, whether appointments, prescription refills, scheduled monitorings, or aberrant test results. The use of an electronic medical record and a closed pharmacy system greatly facilitates the tracking and reporting functions. Such reminder systems have successfully improved rates of preventive service utilization.[152] Similarly, automated reminder cards for medication refills help identify poorly compliant patients and improve medication refill rates.[153,154] Telephone reminder systems can enhance patient medication compliance as measured by electronic medication monitors.[155,156]

Information technology may link traditional clinical practice with decision support and track progress to therapeutic goals. Decision-support software integrates disparate data sources, such as patient history, renal function, serum potassi-

um and most recent antihypertensive drug regimen, to guide drug and dose selections.[157-159] Even with such support, the clinician can often improve clinical outcomes for patients by specifying target outcomes with regular tracking of progress. Traditional progress notes and flowsheet tables are useful but gain impact for patient and clinician alike when data are graphed against the goals over time, as illustrated in Table 41-3 and Figure 41-10.

The final opportunity arises from aligning incentives among all the interested parties: patient, significant other(s), clinician, support staff, administrator, payers, and regulators. As with all complex issues, there are multiple levels of importance and relevance, especially in managed care and prepaid settings, as illustrated in Figure 41-11.

Presumably, all participants would agree on the common goals of achieving excellent BP control for as many patients as possible and thereby minimizing cardiovascular morbidity and mortality at acceptable cost. Beyond this simple agreement, consensus becomes more difficult. For example, does the clinician remain responsible for all patients eligible to come for care or only for those who actually present for care? Does the "acceptable cost" refer to that for the insurance carrier (premiums minus expenses), the employer (tax write-offs and employee benefits), the government (tax credits), or the patient (out-of-pocket expenses)?

Under the emerging expectation of professional accountability, payers and regulators will increasingly hold health professionals responsible for the medical outcomes they produce, including the rates of BP control, complications of the condition and its treatment, and the costs associated with these

**Table 41-3** Treatment to Goal

| Patient: John DOE | | | #123-45-67 | | Drug #1 | Drug #2 | Drug #3 | Serum |
| Date | SBP (mm Hg) | DBP (mm Hg) | Weight (lbs) | | HCTZ (mg/dl) | Lisinopril (mg/dl) | Atenolol (mg/dl) | Creatinine (mg/dl) |
|---|---|---|---|---|---|---|---|---|
| 2/15/00 | 159 | 104 | 212 | | | | | 1.0 |
| 3/2/00 | 164 | 102 | 210 | | 25 | | | |
| 4/12/00 | 154 | 99 | 209 | | 25 | 10 | | |
| 6/26/00 | 148 | 96 | 210 | | 25 | 20 | | 1.2 |
| 8/9/00 | 150 | 93 | 209 | | 25 | 40 | | |
| 10/4/00 | 144 | 90 | 207 | | 25 | 40 | 50 | 1.3 |

SBP, systolic blood pressure; DBP, diastolic blood pressure.

results. The most likely consequences of high expectations and constrained resources will include larger copayments and deductibles by patients for needed medical services, as well as cost- and risk-shifting from employers to insurance carriers and from insurance carriers to medical groups and provider institutions. All parties are searching for value rather than high quality of care regardless of cost. In this context, patients' low level of adherence to appointments, monitoring, and treatments become comparable to prescribing ineffective therapy.

To date, the validation of many proposed strategies and tactics to improve adherence for antihypertensive therapy remains imperfect. Haynes et al.'s review of compliance-enhancing interventions found 33 suitable randomized controlled trials in their computerized search of studies from 1967 through August, 2001. Half (19 of 39) of the interventions for long-term treatments were associated with improvements in adherence, and 17 interventions led to improvements in treatment outcomes. The most useful interventions for long-term care included complex combinations of more convenient care, information, counseling, reminders, self-monitoring, reinforcement, family therapy, and other forms of additional supervision or attention. Even the most effective interventions did not lead to substantial improvements in adherence.[160]

Even if a small core of effective interventions were identified, individual clinicians and their medical groups and support staff would need orientation, training, and reinforcement, so that all components of the health care team work together in a seamless and effective manner.[161]

Several new and promising approaches warrant close review and consideration. In a population of both psychotic and nonpsychotic patients, Cramer et al. used simple, focused steps to simplify drug regimens, scheduling dosings with tailoring to individual patients' daily patterns, helping patients select reminders or cues, and offering systematic monitoring, feedback, and reinforcement. Over 6 months, mean compliance by electronic monitoring remained relatively high among 32 intervention subjects (81%→76%), significantly higher than among 28 control subjects (68%→57%; $p = .008$).[162] Their intervention principles consisted of education, planning dosing regimens, clinic scheduling, and communication.[163]

In a similar manner, Burnier et al. achieved mean compliance rates of 94% in refractory hypertensive patients from among a highly noncompliant subset at baseline.[143] Urquhart et al. described a spreadsheet-based method to summarize patients' drug dosing patterns, based on electronic medication monitor data.[164] They went on to describe a "measurement-guided medication management" approach that uses electronic medication monitors to identify noncompliant individuals and then links them to instruction by clinician, pharmacist, or trained counselor on adherence-enhancing methods.[165]

The future path for optimizing patient, professional, and medical care system adherence for hypertension management remains largely uncharted. Its importance to ensure improved BP control becomes clearer as we examine the rate-limiting steps to bring full benefit to all hypertensive patients.

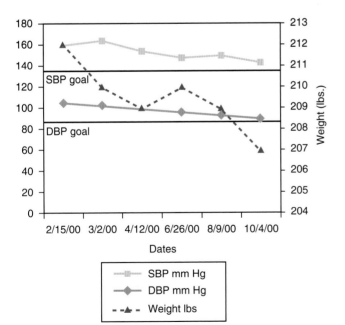

**Figure 41-10** Treatment to goal. The graphic representation of data may allow more prompt and intuitive capture of rates, goals, and opportunities for improvement than tabular summaries of the same information, illustrated here with data from a hypothetical hypertensive patient. In this example, the patient's serum creatinine data were not plotted.

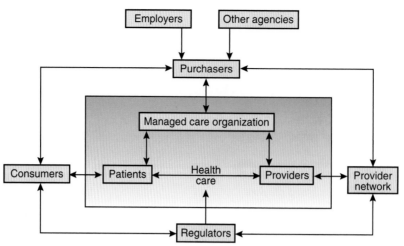

**Figure 41–11** Key participants in the managed care setting. Multiple individuals and groups participate in the managed care framework: *Purchasers,* who may represent employers or other agencies, contract with *managed care organizations* to provide health and medical care to patients who are *enrollees,* who come from the larger group of potential *consumers* of the services. The *managed care organization* contracts with some physician *providers* from a larger *provider network.* The key players are all subject to guidelines issued by *regulators,* who in turn impact both consumers and provider networks with both options and constraints. (Adapted from Hopkins J, Siu S, Cawley M, Rudd P. Drug therapy: The impact of managed care. Adv Pharmacol 44:2, 1998.)

## References

1. Julius S. Current trends in the treatment of hypertension: A mixed picture. Am J Hypertens 10:300S-305S, 1997.
2. Kannel WB. Blood pressure as a cardiovascular risk factor; Prevention and treatment. JAMA 275:1571-1576, 1996.
3. Mulrow C, Lau J, Cornell J, Brand M. Pharmacotherapy for hypertension in the elderly. Cochrane Database Syst Rev 2, 2000.
4. Burt VL, Whelton P, Roccella EJ, et al. Prevalence of hypertension in the US adult population. Results from the Third National Health and Nutrition Examination Survey, 1988-1991. Hypertension 25:305-313, 1995.
5. Murphy J, Coster G. Issues in patient compliance. Drugs 54: 797-800, 1997.
6. Hansson L, Zanchetti A, Carruthers SG, et al. Effects of intensive blood-pressure lowering and low-dose aspirin in patients with hypertension: Principal results of the Hypertension Optimal Treatment (HOT) randomised trial. HOT Study Group. Lancet 351:1755-1762, 1998.
7. Sackett DL, Haynes RB, Gibson ES, et al. Randomized clinical trial of strategies for improving medication compliance in primary hypertension. Lancet 1:1205-1208, 1975.
8. Sackett D. Hypertension in the real world: Public reaction, physician response, and patient compliance. *In:* Genest J, Koiw E, Kuchel O (eds). Hypertension: Physiopathology and Treatment. New York, McGraw-Hill, 1979; pp.1142-1149.
9. Sackett DL, Haynes RB, Tugwell P. Compliance. Clinical Epidemiology: A Basic Science for Clinical Medicine. Boston, Little, Brown, 1985; pp 199-222.
10. Taylor D, Sackett D, Haynes R, et al. Compliance with antihypertensive drug therapy. Ann NY Acad Sci 304:390-403, 1978.
11. Silas JH, Tucker GT, Smith AJ. Drug resistance, inappropriate dosing and non-compliance in hypertensive patients. Br J Clin Pharmacol 9:427-430, 1980.
12. Rudd P. Medication compliance: Correlation with clinical outcomes. P & T 19:10S-18S, 1994.
13. Wallenius SH, Vainio KK, Korhonen MJ, et al. Self-initiated modification of hypertension treatment in response to perceived problems. Ann Pharmacother 29:1213-1217, 1995.
14. Setaro JF, Black HR. Refractory hypertension. N Engl J Med 327:543-547, 1992.
15. Dunbar J. Adherence measures and their utility. Control Clin Trials 5:515-521, 1984.
16. Mattson ME, Friedman LM. Issues in medication adherence assessment in clinical trials of the National Heart, Lung, and Blood Institute. Control Clin Trials 5:488-496, 1984.
17. Roth HP. Historical review: Comparison with other methods. Control Clin Trials 5:476-480, 1984.
18. Dunbar J, Dunning EJ, Dwyer K. Compliance measurement with arthritis regimen. Arthritis Care Res 2:16-24, 1989.
19. Spilker B. Methods of assessing and improving patient compliance in clinical trials. *In* Cramer JA, Spilker B (eds). Patient Compliance in Medical Practice and Clinical Trials. New York, Raven Press, 1991; pp. 37-56.
20. Rudd P. The measurement of compliance: Medication-taking. *In* Krasnegor NA, Epstein L, Johnson SB, et al. (eds). Developmental Aspects of Health Compliance Behavior. Hillsdale, NJ, Lawrence Erlbaum Assoc, 1993; pp 185-213.
21. Rudd P, Byyny RL, Zachary V, et al. Pill count measures of compliance in a drug trial: Variability and suitability. Am J Hypertens 1:309-312, 1988.
22. Cramer JA, Mattson RH, Prevey ML, et al. How often is medication taken as prescribed? A novel assessment technique. JAMA 261:3273-3277, 1989.
23. Lau HS, de Boer A, Beuning KS, et al. Validation of pharmacy records in drug exposure assessment. J Clin Epidemiol 50: 619-625, 1997.
24. Steiner JF, Prochazka AV. The assessment of refill compliance using pharmacy records: Methods, validity, and applications. J Clin Epidemiol 50:105-116, 1997.
25. Christensen DB, Williams B, Goldberg HI, et al. Assessing compliance to antihypertensive medications using computer-based pharmacy records. Med Care 35:1164-1170, 1997.

26. Moulding TS. The potential uses of the medication monitor in the treatment of leprosy. Int J Lepr Other Mycobact Dis 47: 601-606, 1979.

27. Norell SE. Accuracy of patient interviews and estimates by clinical staff in determining medication compliance. Soc Sci Med 15E:57-61, 1981.

28. Kass MA, Meltzer DW, Gordon M. A miniature compliance monitor for eyedrop medication. Arch Ophthalmol 102: 1550-1554, 1984.

29. Norell SE. Methods in assessing drug compliance. Acta Med Scand Suppl 683:35-40, 1984.

30. Kass MA, Gordon M, Meltzer DW. Can ophthalmologists correctly identify patients defaulting from pilocarpine therapy? Am J Ophthalmol 101:524-530, 1986.

31. Spector SL, Kinsman R, Mawhinney H, et al. Compliance of patients with asthma with an experimental aerosolized medication: Implications for controlled clinical trials. J Allergy Clin Immunol 77:65-70, 1986.

32. Eisen SA, Hanpeter JA, Kreuger LW, et al. Monitoring medication compliance: Description of a new device. J Compliance Health Care 2:131-142, 1987.

33. Kass MA, Gordon M, Morley RJ, et al. Compliance with topical timolol treatment. Am J Ophthalmol 103:188-193, 1987.

34. Rudd P, Marshall G. Resolving problems of measuring compliance with medication monitors. J Compliance Health Care 2:23-35, 1987.

35. Cramer JA, Scheyer RD, Mattson RH. Compliance declines between clinic visits. Arch Intern Med 150:1509-1510, 1990.

36. Eisen SA, Miller DK, Woodward RS, et al. The effect of prescribed daily dose frequency on patient medication compliance. Arch Intern Med 150:1881-1884, 1990.

37. Kruse W, Schlierf G, Weber E. Monitoring compliance in clinical trials [letter; comment]. Lancet 335:803-804, 1990.

38. Rudd P, Ahmed S, Zachary V, et al. Improved compliance measures: Applications in an ambulatory hypertensive drug trial. Clin Pharmacol Ther 48:676-685, 1990.

39. Cramer JA, Mattson RH. Monitoring compliance with antiepileptic drug therapy. *In* Cramer JA, Spilker B (eds). Patient Compliance in Medical Practice and Clinical Trials. New York, Raven Press, 1991; pp 123-137.

40. Gordon ME, Kass MA. Validity of standard compliance measures in glaucoma compared with an electronic eyedrop monitor. *In* Cramer JA, Spilker B, (eds). Patient Compliance in Medical Practice and Clinical Trials. New York, Raven Press, 1991; pp 163-173.

41. Spector SL, Mawhinney H. Aerosol inhaler monitoring of asthmatic medication. *In:* Cramer JA, Spilker B (eds). Patient Compliance in Medical Practice and Clinical Trials. New York, Raven Press, 1991; pp 149-162.

42. Rudd P, Ramesh J, Bryant-Kosling C, et al. Gaps in cardiovascular medication taking: The tip of the iceberg. J Gen Intern Med 8:659-666, 1993.

43. Straka RJ, Fish JT, Benson SR, et al. Patient self-reporting of compliance does not correspond with electronic monitoring: An evaluation using isosorbide dinitrate as a model drug. Pharmacotherapy 17:126-132, 1997.

44. Urquhart J. Role of patient compliance in clinical pharmacokinetics. A review of recent research. Clin Pharmacokinet 27: 202-215, 1994.

45. Larkin JG, Herrick AL, McGuire GM, et al. Antiepileptic drug monitoring at the epilepsy clinic: A prospective evaluation. Epilepsia 32:89-95, 1991.

46. Wiseman IC, Miller R. Quantifying non-compliance in patients receiving digoxin—A pharmacokinetic approach. S Afr Med J 79:155-157, 1991.

47. Hardy E, Kumar S, Peaker S, et al. A comparison of a short half-life marker (low-dose isoniazid), a long half-life pharmacological indicator (low-dose phenobarbitone) and measurements of

48. Maenpaa H, Manninen V, Heinonen OP. Compliance with medication in the Helsinki Heart Study. Eur J Clin Pharmacol 42:15-19, 1992.

49. Pullar T, Kumar S, Tindall H, et al. Time to stop counting the tablets? Clin Pharmacol Ther 46:163-168, 1989.

50. Sackett DL, Snow JC. The magnitude of compliance and noncompliance. *In* Haynes RB, Taylor DW, Sackett DL (eds). Compliance in Health Care. Baltimore, Johns Hopkins, 1979; pp 11-22.

51. Paes AH, Bakker A, Soe-Agnie CJ. Impact of dosage frequency on patient compliance. Diabetes Care 20:1512-1517, 1997.

52. Burnier M. Long-term compliance with antihypertensive therapy: Another facet of chronotherapeutics in hypertension. Blood Press Monit 5:S31-S34, 2000.

53. Feinstein A. On white-coat effects and the electronic monitoring of compliance. Arch Intern Med 150:1377-1378, 1990.

54. Greenberg RN. Overview of patient compliance with medication dosing: A literature review. Clin Ther 6:592-599, 1984.

55. Leenen FH, Wilson TW, Bolli P, et al. Patterns of compliance with once versus twice daily antihypertensive drug therapy in primary care: A randomized clinical trial using electronic monitoring. Can J Cardiol 13:914-920, 1997.

56. Guerrero D, Rudd P, Bryant-Kosling C, et al. Antihypertensive medication-taking. Investigation of a simple regimen. Am J Hypertens 6:586-592, 1993. [Erratum appears in Am J Hypertens 6(11 Pt 1):982. 1993.]

57. Kass MA, Meltzer DW, Gordon M, et al. Compliance with topical pilocarpine treatment. Am J Ophthalmol 101:515-523, 1986.

58. Kruse W, Weber E. Dynamics of drug regimen compliance—Its assessment by microprocessor-based monitoring. Eur J Clin Pharmacol 38:561-565, 1990.

59. Kruse W, Effert-Kruse W, Rampmaier J, et al. Compliance with short-term high-dose ethinyl oestradiol in young patients with primary infertility. New insights from the use of electronic devices. Agents Actions Suppl:105-115, 1990.

60. Kruse WHH. Compliance with treatment of hyperlipoproteinemia in medical practice and clinical trials. *In* Cramer JA, Spilker B (eds). Patient Compliance in Medical Practice and Clinical Trials. New York, Raven Press, 1991; pp 175-186.

61. Rudd P. Clinicians and patients with hypertension: Unsettled issues about compliance. Am Heart J 130:572-579, 1995.

62. Urquhart J. Patient compliance with crucial drug regimens: Implications for prostate cancer. Eur Urol 2:124-131, 1996.

63. Urquhart J. The electronic medication event monitor. Lessons for pharmacotherapy. Clin Pharmacokinet 32:345-356, 1997.

64. Rand CS, Wise RA. Measuring adherence to asthma medication regimens. Am J Respir Crit Care Med 149:S69-S78, 1994.

65. Urquhart J. Patient non-compliance with drug regimens: Measurement, clinical correlates, economic impact. Eur Heart J 17:8-15, 1996.

66. Haynes RB. Determinants of compliance: The disease and the mechanisms of treatment. *In* Haynes RB, Taylor DW, Sackett DL (eds). Compliance in Health Care. Baltimore, Johns Hopkins, 1979; pp 49-62.

67. Hill MN, Bone LR, Kim MT, et al. Barriers to hypertension care and control in young urban black men. Am J Hypertens 12: 951-958, 1999.

68. Ickovics JR, Meisler AW. Adherence in AIDS clinical trials: A framework for clinical research and clinical care. J Clin Epidemiol 50:385-391, 1997.

69. Bailey JE, Lee MD, Somes GW, et al. Risk factors for antihypertensive medication refill failure by patients under Medicaid managed care. Clin Ther 18:1252-1262, 1996.

70. Curtin RB, Svarstad BL, Andress D, et al. Differences in older versus younger hemodialysis patients' noncompliance with oral medications. Geriatr Nephrol Urol 7:35-44, 1997.

a controlled release 'therapeutic drug' (metoprolol, Metoros) in reflecting incomplete compliance by volunteers. Br J Clin Pharmacol 30:437-441, 1990.

71. Morrell RW, Park DC, Kidder DP, et al. Adherence to antihypertensive medications across the life span. Gerontologist 37:609-619, 1997.

72. Joint National Committee on Prevention Detection, Evaluation, and Treatment of High Blood Pressure. The sixth report of the Joint National Committee on prevention, detection, evaluation, and treatment of high blood pressure. Arch Intern Med 157:2413-2446, 1997.

73. Benson S, Vance-Bryan K, Raddatz J. Time to patient discontinuation of antihypertensive drugs in different classes. Am J Health Syst Pharm 57:51-54, 2000.

74. Wang PS, Bohn RL, Knight E, et al. Noncompliance with antihypertensive medications. J Gen Intern Med 17:504-511, 2002.

75. Haynes RB, Sackett DL, Gibson ES, et al. Improvement of medication compliance in uncontrolled hypertension. Lancet 1:1265-1268, 1976.

76. Rudd P, Marshall G. Antihypertensive medication-taking behavior: Outpatient patterns and implications. In Rosenfeld J (ed). Hypertension Control in the Community. London, John Libbey, 1985; pp 232-236.

77. Col N, Fanale JE, Kronholm P. The role of medication noncompliance and adverse drug reactions in hospitalizations of the elderly. Arch Intern Med 150:841-845, 1990.

78. DiMatteo MR. Patient adherence to pharmacotherapy: The importance of effective communication. Formulary 30:596-598;601-602;605, 1995.

79. Rudd P. Maximizing compliance with antihypertensive therapy. Drug Ther 22:25-32, 1992.

80. Bandura A. Self-efficacy mechanism in human agency. Am Psychol 37:122-130, 1982.

81. Lorig KR, Mazonson PD, Holman HR. Evidence suggesting that health education for self-management in patients with chronic arthritis has sustained health benefits while reducing health care costs. Arthritis Rheum 36:439-446, 1993.

82. McDermott MM, Schmitt B, Wallner E. Impact of medication nonadherence on coronary heart disease outcomes. A critical review. Arch Intern Med 157:1921-1999, 1997.

83. McCombs JS, Nichol MB, Newman CM, et al. The costs of interrupting antihypertensive drug therapy in a Medicaid population. Med Care 32:214-226, 1994.

84. Gallagher EJ, Viscoli CM, Horwitz RI. The relationship of treatment adherence to the risk of death after myocardial infarction in women. JAMA 270:742-744, 1993.

85. Flack JM, Yunis C. Therapeutic implications of the epidemiology and timing of myocardial infarction and other cardiovascular diseases. J Hum Hypertens 11:23-28, 1997.

86. Schueler K. Cost-effectiveness issues in hypertension control. Can J Public Health 85:S54-S56, 1994.

87. Gandhi SK, Kong SX. Quality-of-life measures in the evaluation of antihypertensive drug therapy: Reliability, validity, and quality-of-life domains. Clin Ther 18:1276-1295, 1996.

88. Rudd P, Dzau VJ. Hypertension: Evaluation and management. In Loscalzo J, Creager MA, Dzau VJ (eds). Vascular Medicine. Boston, Little, Brown, 1996; pp 609-638.

89. Maronde RF, Chan LS, Larsen FJ, et al. Underutilization of antihypertensive drugs and associated hospitalization. Med Care 27:1159-1166, 1989.

90. Psaty BM, Koepsell TD, Wagner ED, et al. The relative risk of incident coronary heart disease associated with recently stopping the use of beta-blockers. JAMA 263:1653-1657, 1990.

91. Mezzetti A, Pierdomenico SD, Costantini F, et al. White-coat resistant hypertension. Am J Hypertens 10:1302-1307, 1997.

92. Adams S, Pill R, Jones A. Medication, chronic illness and identity: The perspective of people with asthma. Soc Sci Med 45:189-201, 1997.

93. Richardson MA, Simons-Morton B, Annegers JF. Effect of perceived barriers on compliance with antihypertensive medication. Health Educ Q 20:489-503, 1993.

94. Bloom JR, Monterossa S. Hypertension labeling and sense of well-being. Am J Publ Health 71:1228-1232, 1981.

95. Haynes RB, Sackett DL, Taylor DW, et al. Increased absenteeism from work after detection and labeling of hypertensive patients. N Engl J Med 299:741-744, 1978.

96. Mold JW, Hamm RM, Jafri B. The effect of labeling on perceived ability to recover from acute illnesses and injuries. J Fam Pract 49:437-440, 2000.

97. Harlan LC, Polk BF, Cooper S, et al. Effects of labeling and treatment of hypertension on perceived health. Am J Prev Med 2:256-261, 1986.

98. Rudd P, Price MG, Graham LE, et al. Consequences of work-site hypertension screening. Differential changes in psychosocial function. Am J Med 80:853-860, 1986.

99. Rudd P. Compliance with antihypertensive therapy: Raising the bar of expectations. Am J Man Care 4:600-609, 1998.

100. DiMatteo MR, Sherbourne CD, Hays RD, et al. Physicians' characteristics influence patients' adherence to medical treatment: Results from the Medical Outcomes Study. Health Psychol 12:93-102, 1993.

101. Leape LL. Practice guidelines and standards: An overview. QRB Qual Rev Bull 16:42-49, 1990.

102. Kennerly DMM, Moore V. Development and dissemination of minimum standards of care for asthma. J Healthc Qual 22:22-28, 2000.

103. Hagemeister J, Schneider CA, Barabas S, et al. Hypertension guidelines and their limitations—the impact of physicians' compliance as evaluated by guideline awareness. J Hypertens 19:2079-2086, 2001.

104. Phillips LS, Branch WT, Cook CB, et al. Clinical inertia. Ann Intern Med 135:825-834, 2001.

105. Amsterdam EA, Laslett L, Diercks D, et al. Reducing the knowledge-practice gap in the management of patients with cardiovascular disease. Prev Cardiol 5:12-15, 2002.

106. Oliveria SA, Lapuerta P, McCarthy BD, et al. Physician-related barriers to the effective management of uncontrolled hypertension. Arch Intern Med 162:413-420, 2002.

107. Pathman DE, Konrad TR, Freed GL, et al. The awareness-to-adherence model of the steps to clinical guideline compliance. The case of pediatric vaccine recommendations. Med Care 34:873-889, 1996.

108. Cabana M. Barriers to guideline adherence. Based on a presentation by Michael Cabana, MD. Am J Manag Care 4:S741-S744; discussion S745-S748, 1998.

109. Cabana MD, Rand CS, Powe NR, et al. Why don't physicians follow clinical practice guidelines? A framework for improvement. JAMA 282:1458-1465, 1999.

110. Rossi RA, Every NR. A computerized intervention to decrease the use of calcium channel blockers in hypertension. J Gen Intern Med 12:672-678, 1997.

111. Kjellgren KI, Ahlner J, Saljo R. Taking antihypertensive medication—controlling or co-operating with patients? Int J Cardiol 47:257-268, 1995.

112. Svensson S, Kjellgren KI, Ahlner J, et al. Reasons for adherence with antihypertensive medication. Int J Cardiol 76:157-163, 2000.

113. Ambrosioni E, Leonetti G, Pessina AC, et al. Patterns of hypertension management in Italy: Results of a pharmacoepidemiological survey on antihypertensive therapy. Scientific Committee of the Italian Pharmacoepidemiological Survey on Antihypertensive Therapy. J Hypertens 18:1691-1699, 2000.

114. Betancourt JR, Carrillo JE, Green AR. Hypertension in multicultural and minority populations: Linking communication to compliance. Curr Hypertens Rep 1:482-488, 1999.

115. Shaw DV. Solving the problem of the uninsured. J Med Pract Manage 16:179-183, 2001.

116. Hyman DJ, Pavlik VN. Characteristics of patients with uncontrolled hypertension in the United States. N Engl J Med 345:479-486, 2001.

117. Shea S, Misra D, Ehrlich MH, et al. Predisposing factors for severe, uncontrolled hypertension in an inner-city minority population. N Engl J Med 327:776-81, 1992.

118. Johnson MJ, Williams M, Marshall ES. Adherent and nonadherent medication-taking in elderly hypertensive patients. Clin Nurs Res 8:318-335, 1999.

119. Strandberg LR. Pharmacy benefits management and ambulatory pharmacy services. Pharm Pract Manag Q 15:19-26, 1996.

120. Sanchez LA. Pharmacoeconomics and formulary decision making. Pharmacoeconomics 1:16-25, 1996.

121. Urquhart J. Correlates of variable patient compliance in drug trials: Relevance in the new health care environment. Adv Drug Res 26:237-257, 1995.

122. Cramer JA. Relationship between medication compliance and medical outcomes. Am J Health Syst Pharm 52:S27-S29, 1995.

123. Crespo-Fierro M. Compliance/adherence and care management in HIV disease. J Assoc Nurses Aids Care 8:43-54, 1997.

124. Lewis RK, Lasack NL, Lambert BL, et al. Patient counseling—A focus on maintenance therapy. Am J Health Syst Pharm 54:2084-2098; quiz 2125-2126, 1997.

125. Montgomery AA, Harding J, Fahey T. Shared decision making in hypertension: The impact of patient preferences on treatment choice. Fam Pract 18:309-313, 2001.

126. Cramer JA. Optimizing long-term patient compliance. Neurology 45:S25-S28, 1995.

127. Meredith PA, Perloff D, Mancia G, et al. Blood pressure variability and its implications for antihypertensive therapy. Blood Press 4:5-11, 1995.

128. Meredith PA, Elliott HL. Therapeutic coverage: Reducing the risks of partial compliance. Br J Clin Pract Symp Suppl 73:13-17, 1994.

129. Meredith PA, Elliott HL. Concentration-effect relationships and implications for trough-to-peak ratio. Am J Hypertens 9:66S-70S; discussion 87S-90S, 1996.

130. Meredith PA, Elliott HL. Amlodipine; clinical relevance of a unique pharmacokinetic profile. J Cardiovasc Pharmacol 22:S6-S8, 1993.

131. Rudd P, Ahmed S, Zachary V, et al. Issues in patient compliance: The search for therapeutic sufficiency. Cardiology 1:2-10, 1992.

132. Leenen FH, Fourney A, Notman G, et al. Persistence of antihypertensive effect after 'missed doses' of calcium antagonist with long (amlodipine) vs short (diltiazem) elimination half-life. Br J Clin Pharmacol 41:83-88, 1996.

133. Waeber B, Brunner HR. Combination antihypertensive therapy: Does it have a role in rational therapy? Am J Hypertens 10:131S-137S, 1997.

134. Prisant LM, Doll NC. Hypertension: The rediscovery of combination therapy. Geriatrics 52:28-30, 33-38, 1997.

135. Frank E, Kupfer DJ, Siegel LR. Alliance not compliance: A philosophy of outpatient care. J Clin Psychiatry 1:11-16; discussion 16-17, 1995.

136. Miller NH, Hill M, Kottke T, et al. The multilevel compliance challenge: Recommendations for a call to action. A statement for healthcare professionals. Circulation 95:1085-1090, 1997.

137. Rudd P, Tul V, Brown K, et al. Hypertension continuation adherence: Natural history and role as an indicator condition. Arch Intern Med 139:545-549, 1979.

138. Hamilton WR, Hopkins UK. Survey on unclaimed prescriptions in a community pharmacy. J Am Pharm Assoc 3:341-345, 1997.

139. McCormack PM, Lawlor R, Donegan C, et al. Knowledge and attitudes to prescribed drugs in young and elderly patients. Ir Med J 90:29-30, 1997.

140. Lip GY, Beevers DG. Doctors, nurses, pharmacists and patients—The Rational Evaluation and Choice in Hypertension (REACH) survey of hypertension care delivery. Blood Press Suppl 1:6-10, 1997.

141. Colley CA, Lucas LM. Polypharmacy: The cure becomes the disease. J Gen Intern Med 8:278-283, 1993.

142. Monane M, Monane S, Semla T. Optimal medication use in elders. Key to successful aging [see comments]. West J Med 167:233-237, 1997.

143. Burnier M, Schneider MP, Chiolero A, et al. Electronic compliance monitoring in resistant hypertension: The basis for rational therapeutic decisions. J Hypertens 19:335-341, 2001.

144. Haynes RB, Taylor DW, Sackett DL, et al. Can simple clinical measurements detect patient noncompliance? Hypertension 2:757-764, 1980.

145. DeBusk RF. MULTIFIT: A new approach to risk factor modification. Cardiol Clin 14:143-157, 1996.

146. West JA, Miller NH, Parker KM, et al. A comprehensive management system for heart failure improves clinical outcomes and reduces medical resource utilization. Am J Cardiol 79:58-63, 1997.

147. Urquhart J. Patient compliance as an explanatory variable in four selected cardiovascular studies. In Cramer JA, Spilker B (eds). Patient Compliance in Medical Practice and Clinical Trials. New York, Raven Press, 1991; pp 301-322.

148. Mengden T, Binswanger B, Spuhler T, et al. The use of self-measured blood pressure determinations in assessing dynamics of drug compliance in a study with amlodipine once a day, morning versus evening. J Hypertens 11:1403-1411, 1993.

149. Vrijens B, Goetghebeur E. Comparing compliance patterns between randomized treatments. Control Clin Trials 18:187-203, 1997.

150. Levy G. A pharmacokinetic perspective on medicament noncompliance. Clin Pharmacol Ther 54:242-244, 1994.

151. Kruse W, Rampmaier J, Ullrich G, et al. Patterns of drug compliance with medications to be taken once and twice daily assessed by continuous electronic monitoring in primary care. Int J Clin Pharmacol Ther 32:452-457, 1994.

152. Murphy DJ, Gross R, Buchanan J. Computerized reminders for five preventive screening tests: Generation of patient-specific letters incorporating physician preferences. Proc AMIA Symp 600-604, 2000.

153. Brown DJ, Ellsworth A, Taylor JW. Identification of potentially noncompliant patients with a mailed medication refill reminder system. Contemp Pharm Pract 3:244-248, 1980.

154. Ascione FJ, Brown GH, Kirking DM. Evaluation of a medication refill reminder system for a community pharmacy. Patient Educ Couns 7:157-165, 1985.

155. Fulmer TT, Feldman PH, Kim TS, et al. An intervention study to enhance medication compliance in community-dwelling elderly individuals. J Gerontol Nurs 25:6-14, 1999.

156. Friedman RH, Kazis LE, Jette A, et al. A telecommunications system for monitoring and counseling patients with hypertension. Impact on medication adherence and blood pressure control. Am J Hypertens 9:285-292, 1996.

157. Degoulet P, Chatellier G, Devries C, et al. Computer-assisted techniques for evaluation and treatment of hypertensive patients. Am J Hypertens 3:156-163, 1990.

158. Caironi PV, Portoni L, Combi C, et al. HyperCare: A prototype of an active database for compliance with essential hypertension therapy guidelines. Proc AMIA Annu Fall Symp 288-292, 1997.

159. Peleska J, Svejda D, Zvarova J. Computer supported decision making in therapy of arterial hypertension. Int J Med Inf 45:25-29, 1997.

160. McDonald HP, Garg AX, Haynes RB. Interventions to enhance patient adherence to medication prescriptions: Scientific review. JAMA. 288:2868-2879, 2002.

161. Thormodsen M, Fonnelop H, Rytter E, et al. ["To be used as directed by your physician"—reasons why patients do not use

prescribed medicines]. Tidsskr Nor Laegeforen 117:3521-3525, 1997.

162. Cramer JA, Rosenheck R. Enhancing medication compliance for people with serious mental illness. J Nerv Ment Dis 187: 53-55, 1999.

163. Cramer JA. Practical issues in medication compliance. Transplant Proc 31:7S-9S, 1999.

164. de Klerk E, van der Linden S, van der Heijde D, et al. Facilitated analysis of data on drug regimen compliance. Stat Med 16:1653-1664, 1997.

165. Urquhart J. The odds of the three nons when an aptly prescribed medicine isn't working: Non-compliance, non-absorption, non-response. J Clin Pharmacol 54:1-9, 2002.

# SECTION 6

# Diet and Nutrition

## Chapter 42

## Diet: Micronutrients

### David A. McCarron, Molly E. Reusser

## SO MANY DATA, SO LITTLE CONSENSUS

Decades of research have focused on the role of specific dietary nutrients in blood pressure regulation. Sodium, potassium, calcium, and magnesium have each been examined extensively in epidemiologic surveys, in clinical trials, and in laboratory investigations.[1] Yet the debates continue.[2] Despite years of investigative effort and volumes of publications, the effects on blood pressure of these individual dietary factors remain subjects of scientific controversy and public confusion.

The most obvious example is sodium chloride, which, for reasons both rational and otherwise,[2] has long been considered the foremost dietary cause of high blood pressure. This presumption first received "factual" support from Dahl's classic epidemiologic study published in 1960, which included a graph with very few data points indicating an almost perfect, linear relationship between the prevalence of hypertension and salt intake among five separate populations around the world.[3] Although that often-cited study has been discounted on the basis of severe design and methodologic flaws,[4] and although the vast body of medical literature regarding the contribution of dietary salt to the worldwide prevalence of hypertension is plagued with conflicting results, the controversy surrounding the sodium–blood pressure relationship continues to engage and enrage nutrition and cardiovascular scientists.[2,5-9]

Although not at the same magnitude and intensity as for sodium, studies of other micronutrients in association with blood pressure control are similarly equivocal. Inadequate intakes of potassium, calcium, and magnesium have all been individually implicated in increased hypertension risk in population studies and in some but not all clinical trials. Studied in isolation, each of these micronutrients has been reported to decrease blood pressure, to increase blood pressure, and to have no effect on blood pressure.[10,11] The one similarity these studies share is that of heterogeneity; that is, modifications in nutrient intake consistently induce inconsistent responses in blood pressure.

The lack of consensus regarding the blood pressure effects of these nutrients, the discrepancies in the results of the studies, and the heterogeneity of response commonly observed in clinical trials assessing electrolytes have a number of possible, related explanations. It is likely that the antihypertensive effects of single nutrients are small and require large-scale trials for their detection. In contrast, the results of epidemiologic surveys and of clinical trials that include modifications of more than one nutrient may reflect larger, more easily detected additive effects, as evidenced by the results of recent studies assessing overall diet patterns.[12-14] Interactions among coexisting nutrients may also play a major role in the inconsistency of results in all studies in which intake levels of one or more nutrients are manipulated. Additional confounding factors in dietary studies include the degree to which baseline intake of the nutrient under study may influence individual blood pressure responses and the likely possibility that the supplemental form of nutrients used in many studies does not have an effect on blood pressure that is comparable to that seen with nutrients naturally occurring in foods.

## NUTRIENT INTERACTIONS

Each of these explanations likely contributes in some part to the unresolved questions regarding the role of specific nutrients in blood pressure regulation. However, we now have available both indirect and direct evidence of the paramount role of nutrient interactions in the prevention and treatment of high blood pressure. Preliminary evidence comes from animal and human studies of sodium effects on blood pressure. Kotchen et al.[15] first reported that the hypertensive effect of sodium chloride in Dahl salt-sensitive rats is preceded by the emergence of disturbances in calcium homeostasis. Kurtz et al.[16] postulated that the induction of a calciuresis may indicate the mechanism(s) by which sodium chloride raises blood pressure in humans. In laboratory models of hypertensive cardiovascular disease known to be salt-sensitive, Tobian et al.[17,18] demonstrated the protective effect of dietary potassium on blood pressure increases. Their data are supported by the clinical observation of Krishna et al.[19] that short-term, severe potassium restriction induces salt sensitivity in normotensive humans and the epidemiologic data of Khaw and Barrett-Connor[20] indicating that adequate potassium intake protected against the potential adverse effects of sodium chloride on blood pressure regulation.

In the index report that characterized the calciuresis of essential hypertension, it was noted that this metabolic defect was more evident at greater levels of urinary sodium excretion.[21] This report was strikingly similar to observations reported in both the Dahl salt-sensitive rat[15] and the rat model of deoxycorticosterone acetate-salt hypertension[22] and has also been demonstrated in humans.[23,24] Subsequent studies have shown that reducing sodium chloride intake does not eliminate the renal defect. In the spontaneously hypertensive rat, an animal with well-characterized disturbances of calcium metabolism including a renal calcium leak,[25] the antihypertensive effect of increasing dietary calcium has been shown to require a normal or high-normal concurrent intake of sodium chloride.[26,27] In humans, Hamet et al.[28] have reported that individuals consuming higher levels of sodium chloride could fall into the highest or lowest blood pressure group depending on whether they were consuming inadequate amounts of calcium or amounts that met recommended dietary allowances.

Similar to the relationship between sodium and other nutrients, interactions among calcium, potassium, and magnesium have also been reported. However, as emphasized by Reed et al.[29] in their analyses of the Honolulu Heart Study, identifying these interactions is complicated by multicollinearity that makes it inherently difficult to clearly isolate the effects of one nutrient from the effects of those consumed concurrently. From the Nurses Health Study, Witteman et al.[30] observed that dietary calcium and magnesium both had strong and independent inverse associations with hypertension and that adjusting for calcium and magnesium intake eliminated the observed crude inverse association of dietary potassium and fiber with hypertension risk. It was reported in the Health Professionals Follow-up Study that nutrient effects on blood pressure observed when assessed individually were obliterated when the nutrients were considered together.[31] In the case of calcium specifically, meta-analysis of randomized controlled trials noted that the effects of food sources appear to be more effective than calcium supplements,[32] likely caused in part by the presence of the other nutrients in food that track with calcium.

Thus numerous studies in recent years have examined relationships between nutrients and have identified some of the interdependencies that exist among the major electrolytes. We now recognize that nutrients function interactively both in the body and in their impact on blood pressure regulation. Considering that nutrients are not ingested in isolation but as combined constituents of a total diet, it is not surprising that manipulations of a single nutrient would produce inconsistent and often contradictory results. If one accepts the hypothesis that micronutrients express their physiologic actions through integrated pathways, it is paradoxical to expect a uniform benefit in terms of blood pressure control by altering the intake of any one of them.

## DIETARY NUTRIENT PATTERNS

Whenever the consumption of a single nutrient is significantly altered, an entirely new dietary pattern is created. Nutrients occur in clusters in the typical human diet and may therefore act synergistically to alter physiologic variables such as blood pressure. In a study assessing blood pressure effects of calcium carbonate as compared with increased calcium in the diet, up to 1500 mg calcium per day, Karanja et al.[33] observed signifi-

cant simultaneous increases in consumption of magnesium, potassium, phosphorus, riboflavin, and vitamin D. In a review of the effect of sodium restriction on overall nutrient intake, Morris[34] found that most of the published studies did not address concomitant nutrient changes, but those that did reported significant decreases in a number of essential dietary components. Although improvements were frequently observed in energy and fat intake, these were offset by reductions in calcium, potassium, fiber, and protein intake. Interestingly, each of the first three of these dietary components has a purported role in blood pressure regulation, and all three are known to be typically consumed at less-than-adequate levels in the general population.

## COMPREHENSIVE DIETARY CLINICAL TRIALS

### Vanguard Studies

As a result of our increasing awareness of the impact and complexity of dietary interactions, nutrition research has expanded in recent years to include assessment of overall dietary patterns as they contribute to lower cardiovascular disease risk through the treatment or the prevention of hypertension. The Cardiovascular Risk Reduction Dietary Intervention Trial was a 4-year series of multicenter, randomized clinical studies to evaluate multiple health effects of a complete nutrition program on persons at high risk of cardiovascular disease. Free-living adults with established hypertension, dyslipidemia, and/or type 2 diabetes mellitus were provided with a prepared meal plan formulated to include levels of vitamins and minerals that meet the recommended dietary allowances (RDA) of the Food and Nutrition Board[35] and the levels of micronutrients and macronutrients recommended by major health organizations.[36-39] The clinical effects of the total nutrition plan were compared with those of a self-selected diet based on the exchange list system.[39]

The results of the first 14-week study in the series demonstrated significant improvements from both diet plans in blood pressure, lipid levels, glycemic control, homocysteine levels, weight, overall nutrient intake, and quality of life, with greater improvements in most of these measures observed with the prepared meal plan as compared with a self-selected diet.[40] The second Vanguard study assessed the same endpoints by using similar dietary interventions for 10 weeks but reduced the amount of contact with participants to the level more likely to occur in clinical practice when dietary therapy is recommended.[41] A third trial used a 52-week intervention and reported similar results.[42] These studies demonstrated that consumption of a nutritionally complete and balanced dietary pattern, which provides appropriate levels of multiple nutrients, can improve blood pressure as well as multiple other risk factors for cardiovascular disease, even in persons with high-normal risk profiles. Subsequent analysis of the Vanguard data identified highly predictive correlations between various electrolytes and the hormones controlling them and the observed changes in blood pressure (Figure 42–1).[43]

### DASH Trial

To specifically address the relationship between total dietary patterns and blood pressure, the National Heart, Lung, and

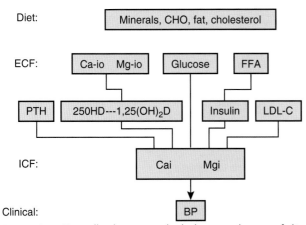

Diet:
Minerals, CHO, fat, cholesterol

ECF:
Ca-io  Mg-io  Glucose  FFA

PTH  250HD---1,25(OH)₂D  Insulin  LDL-C

ICF:
Cai  Mgi

Clinical:
BP

**Figure 42–1** Overall scheme in which the contribution of diet to blood pressure is determined by the net effect of individual dietary components on steady-state levels of cytosolic free mineral ions such as calcium and magnesium. These effects are due both to direct ionic effects of circulating nutrient levels, such as glucose or calcium, and to ionic effects of hormones responsible for regulating the metabolism of these dietary components such as insulin, PTH, and 1,25D. ECF, extracellular fluid; ICF, intracellular fluid; CHO, carbohydrates; Ca-io, ionized calcium; Mg-io, ionized magnesium; FFA, free fatty acids; Cai, intracellular calcium; Mgi, intracellular magnesium. (From Resnick LM, Oparil S, Chait A, et al. Factors affecting blood pressure responses to diet: the Vanguard Study. Am J Hypertens 13:956-965, 2000.)

Blood Institute (NHLBI) initiated the multicenter, randomized, controlled Dietary Approaches to Stop Hypertension (DASH) clinical trial.[12] This carefully designed and executed study provides dramatic evidence of the effect and importance of the dietary pattern of nutrients, as they occur together in food, on blood pressure regulation. Three diets were assessed in the trial: (1) a typical American diet (control), with four daily servings of fruits and vegetables and half a serving of dairy products; (2) the fruits-and-vegetables diet, with 8.5 servings/day of these foods; and (3) the combination, or DASH, diet, which included 10 fruit and vegetable servings and 2.7 daily servings of low-fat dairy products.

Highly significant blood pressure reductions among all participants were achieved with the DASH diet; systolic pressure was reduced by 5 mm Hg more and diastolic pressure by 3.0 mm Hg more than with the control diet. Blood pressure reductions with the fruits-and-vegetables diet as compared with the control were also highly significant, but only about half (2.8 mm Hg systolic and 1.1 mm Hg diastolic) of those achieved with the combination diet. The reductions with both intervention diets were observed within the first 2 weeks of study and were sustained for the remaining 6 weeks of the intervention.

Of notable clinical significance, blood pressure reductions in hypertensive participants on the DASH combination diet were 11.4 mm Hg systolic and 5.5 mm Hg diastolic as compared with the control diet and 4.1 mm Hg systolic and 2.26 mm Hg diastolic as compared with the fruits-and-vegetables diet.[12] In a subsequent publication, the investigators reported that the DASH diet was particularly effective in older persons

with systolic hypertension,[44] such that in almost 80% of these participants, blood pressure would have been controlled by the DASH diet alone. The observed blood pressure reductions with the DASH diet in hypertensive participants were similar in magnitude to those reported in pharmacologic trials of treatment of mild hypertension.[45]

The diet-related factors most commonly associated with blood pressure management—sodium, alcohol, and weight—were held constant throughout the DASH study and were similar across the three diets. Thus they were not accountable for the blood pressure changes observed in this trial and suggest a protective blood pressure effect of comprehensive nutrient intake patterns on known dietary blood pressure determinants. As we reported in *Science*,[1] the results of the DASH Trial are remarkably consistent with the epidemiologic evidence we published 20 years ago[46] that identified a close association of dietary calcium and potassium in the American diet with blood pressure control (Figure 42–2). Our 1984 article was the first to report that a diet rich in dairy foods, fruits, and vegetables was the dietary pattern associated with lower levels of blood pressure in the United States.

## DASH-Sodium Trial

The publication of the DASH Trial[12] and the Trials of Hypertension Prevention, Phase II (TOHPS II; 47) within a few months of one another raised the question of whether the DASH diet alone was more effective than sodium restriction alone. NHLBI thus initiated a second DASH study, the DASH-Sodium Trial, in which the blood pressure effects of the DASH diet alone and in combination with sodium restriction were assessed in a study population at higher risk for salt sensitivity, that is, with overrepresentation of overweight, hypertensive adults of African American descent.[13]

The DASH-Sodium investigators concluded that the DASH diet in conjunction with sodium restriction was more effective than either of the approaches alone in reducing blood pressure in both hypertensive and normotensive persons. They stated further that their findings "provide a scientific basis for a lower goal for dietary sodium than the level currently recommended."[13] These interpretations of the DASH-Sodium data have been met with controversy and challenge.[48-50] The actual effect of the DASH diet alone in this high-risk population was virtually identical to that observed in the first DASH Trial, supporting the reproducible, generalizable, and beneficial effect across the entire population of a diet rich in low-fat dairy foods, fruits, and vegetables.

In a subsequent publication of the subgroup analysis of the DASH-Sodium Trial, the investigators acknowledged that the effect of sodium restriction on blood pressure was significant only among hypertensive African Americans ≥45 years of age.[51] Based on those findings and the initial concerns expressed regarding the interpretation of the DASH-Sodium Trial,[49] it is apparent that a diet that emphasizes low-fat dairy products, fruits, and vegetables has a significant effect on all adults regardless of their blood pressure status and that sodium restriction has a minimal effect isolated to older, overweight African American patients with high blood pressure.

Although there has not yet been full publication of all the data that should be made available from the DASH-Sodium Trial,[48] the data that have been shown provide critical evidence of where our priorities should be placed with regard to

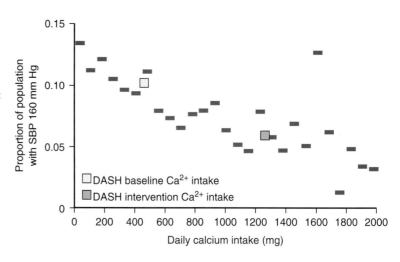

**Figure 42–2** National Health and Nutrition Examination Survey I data portraying the relationship between dietary calcium and systolic blood pressure[46] in relation to values (boxes) at baseline and end of the DASH combination diet intervention for dietary calcium intake and systolic blood pressure.[12] (From McCarron DA, Morris CD, Henry HJ, Stanton JL. Blood pressure and nutrient intake in the United States. Science 224:1392-1398, 1984.)

nutritional guidelines to prevent and to manage hypertension. The DASH-Sodium Trial confirmed that (1) the beneficial blood pressure effect of the DASH diet is generalizable to the entire population and not limited to people with hypertension, (2) the effects of the DASH diet are substantial and significantly greater than any that have been reported for sodium restriction, (3) sodium sensitivity is ablated by the DASH diet in most people who would otherwise be categorized as salt sensitive, and (4) recommendation of the DASH diet should be the first step for high blood pressure management for all individuals with hypertension.

## TOWARD A NEW PARADIGM

Our efforts to understand the blood pressure effects of micronutrients, as individual components as well as interactive constituents of the human diet, have revealed several important and easily adopted answers to long-standing questions in this area. While experts in the fields of nutrition and blood pressure may continue to argue the merits of altering the intake of one nutrient or another, we have available to us today the body of appropriate and definitive data to resolve the conflicting results and to lay to rest the scientific controversies surrounding the role of dietary nutrients in preventing and managing high blood pressure. For even the most vitriolic debate, that of the sodium–blood pressure relationship,[2] the data now exist that could finally produce consensus on this issue.

Using established analytical standards to assess the "pool effect" of randomized controlled trials of sodium restriction, the Cochrane Collaboration[52] recently provided a conclusive statistical evaluation of the clinical trial data addressing the role of dietary sodium in hypertension. Hooper and colleagues concluded that there was not sufficient evidence that sodium restriction was an effective therapeutic modality in the hypertensive population and that it was not appropriate as a preventive measure in the general population. They left open the possibility that future studies might demonstrate a benefit in a subset of individuals with hypertension, but no convincing data exist to support such a recommendation at this time. Furthermore, these investigators acknowledged that the available data suggest that broad application of low-sodium diets to either the general population or hypertensive individuals may actually contribute to cardiovascular events and mortali-

ty, an issue first raised a decade ago[53] that still needs to be resolved conclusively with properly controlled long-term clinical trials.

The importance of first ensuring that hypertensive patients improve the overall quality of their diets was recently addressed by the Seventh Report of the Joint National Committee on Prevention, Detection, Evaluation, and Treatment of High Blood Pressure (JNC 7).[54] In their recommendations, the National High Blood Pressure Education Program ranked the DASH diet as a primary nutritional intervention in the management of this common medical disorder. However, that transition in nutritional guidance for the patient with high blood pressure leaves several important issues to be resolved, including whether it is possible for adults at risk of hypertension and its cardiovascular consequences to incorporate the DASH diet into the multiple lifestyle adjustments these patients often have to make and whether adherence to the DASH diet will reduce cardiovascular events and lower mortality rate.

As recently reported,[55] the cumulative body of evidence from randomized controlled trials and prospective observational studies strongly suggests that, at least with regard to the dairy component of the DASH diet, the prevalence of several common cardiovascular risk factors can be reduced by regular dairy consumption with 3 to 4 servings per day, a range consistent with the DASH diet and current national dietary recommendations. The risk factors that have been shown to be improved with adequate dairy consumption include body weight, insulin-resistant syndrome, blood pressure, and serum lipids. Incorporating regular dairy food intake into the diets of at-risk young adults has been demonstrated to also lead to increased fruit and vegetable consumption[56]—that is, a nutritional pattern consistent with the DASH diet.

While implementation of dietary and lifestyle changes can be a challenge for individual patients, the evidence we have today clearly indicates that improved diet quality can be the single means of managing blood pressure for many patients and that, for others, improved diets can reduce their antihypertensive medication requirements. Furthermore, it is now well recognized that positive diet and lifestyle alterations can prevent the development of hypertension. As stated in JNC 7, lifestyle modifications—including improved nutrient intake, weight loss, and increased physical activity—"are critical for the prevention of high blood pressure...decrease blood pressure, enhance antihypertensive drug efficacy, and decrease cardiovascular risk."[54] Although some patients may require more aggressive management, for those with mild to moderate hypertension, as well as for the population at large, improving the overall quality of the diet should be the primary focus of nutritional guidance for optimal blood pressure management.

# References

1. McCarron DA. Diet and blood pressure: The paradigm shift. Science 281:933-934, 1998.
2. Taubes G. The (political) science of salt. Science 281:898-907, 1998.
3. Dahl LK. Possible role of salt intake in the development of essential hypertension. In Bock KD, Cottier PT (eds). Essential Hypertension. Berlin, Springer Verlag, 1960;53-65.
4. National Kidney Foundation Nonpharmacologic Management of Hypertension Organizing Committee. NKF Nonpharmacologic Management of Hypertension Program Syllabus. New York: NKF, 1996.
5. Freedman DA, Petitti DB. Salt and blood pressure: Conventional wisdom reconsidered. Evaluation Rev 25:267-287, 2001.
6. McCarron DA. The dietary guideline for sodium: Should we shake it up? Yes! Am J Clin Nutr 71:1013-1019, 2000.
7. Kaplan NM. The dietary guideline for sodium: Should we shake it up? No. Am J Clin Nutr 71:1020-1026, 2000.
8. Chrysant GS, Bakir S, Oparil S. Dietary salt reduction in hypertension: What is the evidence and why is it still controversial? Prog Cardiovasc Dis 42:23-38, 1999.
9. Alderman MH, Anderson S, Bennett WM, et al. Scientists' statement regarding data on the sodium-hypertension relationship and sodium health claims on food labeling. Nutr Rev 55:172-175, 1997.
10. Luft FC. Heterogeneity of hypertension: The diverse role of electrolyte intake. Annu Rev Med 42:347-355, 1991.
11. Luft FC, Weinberger MH. Heterogeneous responses to changes in dietary salt intake: The salt-sensitivity paradigm. Am J Clin Nutr 65:S612-S617, 1997.
12. Appel LJ, Moore TJ, Obarzanek E, et al. A clinical trial of the effects of dietary patterns on blood pressure. N Engl J Med 336:1117-1124, 1997.
13. Sacks FM, Svetkey LP, Vollmer WM, et al. Effects on blood pressure of reduced dietary sodium and the Dietary Approaches to Stop Hypertension (DASH) diet. N Engl J Med 344:3-10, 2001.
14. Appel LJ, Champagne CM, Harsha DW, et al. Effects of comprehensive lifestyle modification on blood pressure control: main results of the PREMIER clinical trial. JAMA 289:2083-2093, 2003.
15. Kotchen TA, Ott CE, Whitescarver SA, et al. Calcium and calcium regulating hormones in the "prehypertensive" Dahl salt sensitive rat (calcium and salt sensitive hypertension). Am J Hypertens 2:747-753, 1989.
16. Kurtz TW, Morris RC. Dietary chloride as a determinant of "sodium-dependent" hypertension in men. N Engl J Med 317:1043-1048, 1987.
17. Tobian L. High potassium diets markedly protect against stroke deaths and kidney disease in hypertensive rats: A possible legacy from prehistoric times. Can J Physiol Pharmacol 64:840-848, 1986.
18. Tobian L, Lange J, Ulm K, et al. Potassium reduces cerebral hemorrhage and death rate in hypertensive rats, even when blood pressure is not lowered. Hypertension 7(suppl I):I-110-I-114, 1985.
19. Krishna GG, Miller E, Kapoor S. Increased blood pressure during potassium depletion in normotensive men. N Engl J Med 320:1177-1182, 1989.
20. Khaw K-T, Barrett-Connor E. Dietary potassium and stroke-associated mortality. A 12-year prospective population study. N Engl J Med 316:235-240, 1987.
21. McCarron DA, Pingree PA, Rubin RJ, et al. Enhanced parathyroid function in essential hypertension: A homeostatic response to a urinary calcium leak. Hypertension 2:162-168, 1980.
22. Kurtz TW, Morris RC Jr. Dietary chloride as a determinant of disordered calcium metabolism in salt-dependent hypertension. Life Sci 36:921-929, 1985.
23. Luft FC, Zemel MB, Sowers JR, et al. Sodium carbonate and sodium chloride: Effects on blood pressure and electrolyte homeostasis in normal and hypertensive men. J Hypertens 8:663-670, 1990.
24. Strazzullo P, Nunziata V, Cirillo M, et al. Abnormalities of calcium metabolism in essential hypertension. Clin Sci 65:137-141, 1983.
25. Young EW, Bukoski RD, McCarron DA. Calcium metabolism in essential hypertension. Proc Soc Exp Biol Med 187:123-141, 1988.
26. McCarron DA, Lucas PA, Shneidman RJ, et al. Blood pressure development of the spontaneously hypertensive rat after concurrent manipulations of dietary $Ca^{2+}$ and $Na^+$: Relation to intestinal $Ca^{2+}$ fluxes. J Clin Invest 76:1147-1154, 1985.
27. Hamet P, Skuherska R, Cherkaouil L, et al. Calcium levels and platelet responsiveness in spontaneously hypertensive rats on high calcium diet [abstract]. J Hypertens 4(Suppl 6):S716, 1986.
28. Hamet P, Mongeau E, Lambert J, et al. Interactions among calcium, sodium, and alcohol intake as determinants of blood pressure. Hypertension 17(suppl I):I-150-I-154, 1991.
29. Reed D, McGee D, Yano K, et al. Diet, blood pressure, and multicollinearity. Hypertension 7:405-410, 1985.
30. Witteman JCM, Willett WC, Stampfer MJ, et al. A prospective study of nutritional factors and hypertension among US women. Circulation 80:1320-1327, 1989.
31. Ascherio A, Rimm EB, Giovannucci EL, et al. A prospective study of nutritional factors and hypertension among US men. Circulation 86:1475-1484, 1992.
32. Bucher HC, Cook RJ, Guyatt GH, et al. Effects of dietary calcium supplementation on blood pressure: A meta-analysis of randomized controlled trials. JAMA 275:1016-1022, 1996.
33. Karanja N, Morris CD, Rufolo P, et al. The impact of increasing dietary calcium intake on nutrient consumption, plasma lipids and lipoproteins in humans. Am J Hypertens 59:900-907, 1994.
34. Morris CD. Effect of dietary sodium restriction on overall nutrient intake. Am J Clin Nutr 65(Suppl):687S-691S, 1997.
35. National Research Council (U.S.) Subcommittee on the Tenth Edition of the RDAs. Recommended Dietary Allowances. Washington DC, National Academy Press, 1989.
36. Krauss RM, Deckelbaum RJ, Ernst N, et al. Dietary guidelines for healthy American adults: A statement for health professionals from the Nutrition Committee, American Heart Association. Circulation 94:1795-1800, 1996.
37. National Cholesterol Education Program. Report of the Expert Panel on Population Strategies for Blood Cholesterol Reduction: executive summary. Arch Intern Med 151:1071-1084, 1991.
38. Franz MJ, Horton ES, Bantle JP, et al. Nutrition principles for the management of diabetes and related complications [technical review]. Diabetes Care 17:490-518, 1994.
39. American Dietetic Association and American Diabetes Association. Exchange Lists for Weight Management. Chicago IL, American Dietetic Association, 1989.
40. McCarron DA, Oparil S, Chait A, et al. Nutritional management of cardiovascular risk factors: A randomized clinical trial. Arch Intern Med 175:169-177, 1997.
41. Haynes RB, Kris-Etherton P, McCarron DA, et al. Nutritionally complete prepared meal plan to reduce cardiovascular risk factors: A randomized clinical trial. J Am Diet Assoc 99:1077-1083, 1999.
42. Metz JA, Stern JS, Kris-Etherton P, et al. Randomized trial of improved weight loss with a prepared meal plan in overweight and obese patients: Impact on cardiovascular risk-reduction. Arch Intern Med 160:2150-2158, 2000.

43. Resnick LM, Oparil S, Chait A, et al. Factors affecting blood pressure responses to diet: The Vanguard Study. Am J Hypertens 13:956-965, 2000.

44. Conlin PR, Chow D, Miller ER, et al. The effect of dietary patterns on blood pressure control in hypertensive patients: Results from the Dietary Approaches to Stop Hypertension (DASH) trial. Am J Hypertens 13:949-955, 2000.

45. The Treatment of Mild Hypertension Research Group. The Treatment of Mild Hypertension Study: A randomized, placebo-controlled trial of a nutritional-hygienic regimen along with various drug monotherapies. Arch Intern Med 151:1413-1423, 1991.

46. McCarron DA, Morris CD, Henry HJ, et al. Blood pressure and nutrient intake in the United States. Science 224:1392-1398, 1984.

47. Trials of Hypertension Prevention Collaborative Research Group. Effects of weight loss and sodium reduction intervention on blood pressure and hypertension incidence in overweight people with high-normal blood pressure. Arch Intern Med 157:657-667, 1997.

48. McCarron DA. DASH-Sodium Trial: Where are the data? Am J Hypertens 16:92-94, 2003.

49. Alderman M, McCarron DA, Petitti DB, et al. Dietary sodium and blood pressure [letter]. N Engl J Med 344:1716-1717, 2001.

50. Jürgens G, Graudal N. Subgroup results in the DASH-Sodium Trial [letter]. Ann Intern Med 137:772, 2002.

51. Vollmer WM, Sacks FM, Ard J, et al. Effects of diet and sodium intake on blood pressure: Subgroup analysis of the DASH-Sodium Trial. Ann Intern Med 135:1019-1028, 2001.

52. Hooper L, Bartlet C, Davey Smith G, et al. Systematic review of long term effects of advice to reduce dietary salt in adults. Br Med J 325:628-637, 2002.

53. Alderman MH, Madhavan S, Cohen H, et al. Low urinary sodium is associated with greater risk of myocardial infarction among treated hypertensive men. Hypertension 25:1144-1152, 1995.

54. Chobanian AV, Barkis GL, Black HR, et al. The seventh report of the Joint National Committee on Prevention, Detection, Evaluation, and Treatment of High Blood Pressure: The JNC 7 Report. JAMA 289:2560-2572, 2003.

55. McCarron DA, Heaney RP. Estimated healthcare savings associated with adequate dairy food intake. Am J Hypertens 17:88-97, 2004.

56. Pereira MA, Jacobs DR, Van Horn L, et al. Dairy consumption, obesity, and the insulin resistance syndrome in young adults. JAMA 287:2081-2089, 2002.

# Dietary Approaches to Hypertension Management: The DASH Studies

## Heather L. McGuire, William L. Fan, Laura P. Svetkey

Nonpharmacologic measures have been widely recommended for the prevention and treatment of high blood pressure (BP). Weight loss, increased physical activity, moderation of alcohol consumption, and dietary sodium reduction are discussed in Chapters 42 and 45 to 47. Several other nonpharmacologic, nutritional factors are associated with reductions in BP levels. Epidemiologic data suggest that low BP is associated with high dietary intake of potassium, magnesium, calcium, fiber, and protein and with low intake of fat. However, trials of alterations in the intake of individual nutrients or the use of nutrient supplements have led to small, inconsistent, and/or inconclusive BP effects. Combinations of nutrients or the dietary pattern itself may be more important than individual nutrients. Indeed, the Dietary Approaches to Stop Hypertension (DASH) study demonstrated that adoption of a specific dietary pattern (the "DASH dietary pattern") lowers BP as much as single drug antihypertensive therapy.[1,2] The DASH dietary pattern also enhances the BP-lowering effect of antihypertensive therapy.[3] In individuals with prehypertension, the BP-lowering effect of the DASH dietary pattern is of a magnitude sufficient to prevent the development of hypertension. In addition, the DASH dietary pattern has beneficial effects on other cardiovascular risk factors, such as lipid profiles[4] and homocysteine.[5]

These effects of the DASH dietary pattern were established in feeding studies and a clinical trial addressing the ability of free-living individuals to adopt the DASH dietary pattern.[6] Similar to other nonpharmacologic interventions, there are no data directly demonstrating the ability of the DASH dietary pattern to reduce morbidity and mortality, but favorable effects of interventions on outcomes in hypertensive patients are presumed to be due to BP lowering and modulation of other cardiovascular disease (CVD) risk factors. Consequently, since 1997, national guidelines for the prevention and treatment of high BP have included the DASH dietary pattern.[7] In this chapter we review the rationale, design, and findings of the DASH studies, consider possible mechanisms of action, and discuss strategies for implementation. Widespread implementation of the DASH dietary pattern has the potential to reduce the CVD burden attributable to BP and to reduce the rising health care costs associated with the large burden of prehypertension and hypertension in the United States and around the world.

## BACKGROUND

### Vegetarian Diet, Nutrients, and Blood Pressure

Observational studies have demonstrated that vegetarians have lower BP levels than comparable nonvegetarian populations.[8,9] In addition, vegetarian diets seem to blunt the rise in BP observed with aging.[8,10] In a randomized controlled trial, when nonhypertensive, nonvegetarian volunteers ate a vegetarian diet, systolic BP (SBP) decreased by an average of 5 to 6 mm Hg and diastolic BP (DBP) by 2 to 3 mm Hg.[9] Similar effects were seen when a vegetarian diet was eaten by a mildly hypertensive population.[11] A slight increase in SBP was found when strict vegetarians were fed isocaloric amounts of beef, but there was no change in DBP.[12] Animal products are apparently not the main culprit, however, since a BP-lowering effect is not seen when they are replaced by starch and sugar.[13,14] Specific dietary components of a vegetarian diet (e.g., plant foods and dairy products) may be responsible for its BP-lowering effect. These dietary components include several micronutrients (namely potassium, magnesium, and calcium) that have been linked to BP regulation and that are discussed in Chapter 43. Meta-analyses suggest a relatively consistent BP-lowering effect of potassium,[15] but smaller and less consistent effects of calcium and magnesium.[16-19] Micronutrients have generally been tested individually and often in the form of supplement pills, leaving open the possibility that BP may be influenced by the micronutrient content of foods. In addition to these micronutrients, a vegetarian diet frequently has a macronutrient profile that is epidemiologically associated with lower BP, namely high fiber and low fat.

Small epidemiologic studies have found a weak inverse relationship between fiber intake and BP.[20] However, this relationship may be confounded by the correlation between fiber intake and intake of other nutrients. When other dietary components are held stable, fiber supplementation has no significant effect on BP.[21] Similarly, epidemiologic data suggest that low intake of total fat and saturated fat, and a high ratio of polyunsaturated fat to saturated fatty acids, is associated with lower BP, but clinical trial evidence, generally from underpowered and/or confounded studies, does not demonstrate consistent or clinically significant BP-lowering effects of decreased fat intake by itself (i.e., without weight loss).[20] High protein has also been associated with lower stroke risk in certain populations.[22,23] However, vegetarian diets tend to be low in protein,[8] and protein supplements have no effect on BP[13] even when the protein is from vegetable sources.[14]

There are several possible reasons that alterations in single micronutrients or macronutrients have not been associated with significant BP effects. First, single nutrients may individually have small effects on BP that would require a very large study to be detectable. The small effects of individual nutrients may be additive and therefore will only be detected if several nutrient changes are tested simultaneously. Second, interactions among nutrients may exist that amplify their effects when eaten in combination. Third, nutrient supplements may not affect BP in the same manner as the naturally occurring nutrients found in food, possibly because of increased bioavailability in naturally occurring foods. Finally, the BP effects of a vegetarian diet may be due to unknown or untested nutrients that are generally found in this dietary pattern.[24]

In summary, epidemiologic and interventional evidence suggests that elements in a vegetarian diet lead to lower BP levels, but studies that alter individual micronutrients or macronutrients have not produced consistent, significant BP effects. This apparent paradox suggests that there is a complex interaction between multiple dietary components and BP level.

## Development of the DASH Dietary Pattern

The DASH dietary pattern was developed to contain the micronutrient and macronutrient profile that had been posited to be beneficial for BP—high potassium, magnesium, calcium, fiber, and polyunsaturated:saturated fatty acid ratio; and low total and saturated fat. Other goals of the diet were to contain enough animal products to make it palatable to nonvegetarians and to contain commonly available foods that were not supplemented with nutrients beyond what would normally be added as part of common food manufacturing practice.[25] Consequently, it emphasizes fruits, vegetables, and low-fat dairy products. It includes whole grains, poultry, fish, and nuts and is reduced in fats, red meat, sweets, and sugar-containing beverages. Its sodium content is slightly below average U.S. consumption. For a 2100 kcal diet, 18% of the energy intake comes from protein, 58% from carbohydrate, 27% from total fat, 7% from saturated fatty acids, and 10% from monounsaturated fatty acids. The DASH dietary pattern includes 31g/day of fiber, 150 mg/day of cholesterol, 4700 mg/day of potassium, 500 mg/day of magnesium, and 1240 mg/day of calcium.

## THE DASH STUDIES

The first DASH study tested the BP effects of the DASH dietary pattern compared with other dietary patterns.[24] By controlling for energy expenditure and keeping weight and sodium intake stable, the DASH study was able to observe the effect of dietary patterns on BP without confounding from other lifestyle modifications known to influence BP. The second DASH study tested the combined effects of the DASH dietary pattern and reduced sodium intake on BP.[26]

## The Dietary Approaches to Stop Hypertension Trial

### Design

The initial DASH trial was a multicenter, randomized feeding study that tested the effects of three dietary patterns on BP: a Control diet, a diet rich in fruits and vegetables (F/V), and the DASH dietary pattern (Table 43–1). In the Control diet, micronutrient content approximated the twenty-fifth percentile of population intake, and macronutrient content was set at average American intake.[27] The F/V diet was rich in fruits and vegetables, but similar in macro- and micronutrient content to the Control diet. The DASH dietary pattern, as noted above, mimicked the micronutrient and macronutrient contents found to lower BP in epidemiologic studies, approximating the seventy-fifth percentile of population intake of

**Table 43-1** Nutrient Composition of the Experimental Diets in the DASH Study

| Nutrient | Treatment Group | | |
|---|---|---|---|
| | Control | Fruits and Vegetables | DASH |
| Fat | 37 | 37 | 27 |
| Saturated | 16 | 16 | 6 |
| Monounsaturated | 13 | 13 | 13 |
| Polyunsaturated | 8 | 8 | 8 |
| P/S ratio | 0.5 | 0.5 | 1.33 |
| Carbohydrates (g) | 48 | 48 | 55 |
| Protein (g) | 15 | 15 | 18 |
| Potassium (mg) | 1700 | 4700 | 4700 |
| Magnesium (mg) | 165 | 500 | 500 |
| Calcium (mg) | 450 | 450 | 1240 |
| Fiber (g) | 9 | 31 | 31 |
| Cholesterol (mg) | 300 | 300 | 150 |
| Sodium (mg) | 3000 | 3000 | 3000 |

From Appel LJ, Moore TJ, Obarzanek E, et al. A clinical trial of the effects of dietary patterns on blood pressure. DASH Collaborative Research Group. N Engl J Med 336(16): 1117-1124, 1997.

potassium, magnesium and calcium. To achieve this nutrient profile, the DASH dietary pattern contained 9 to 12 servings/day of fruits and vegetables; 2 to 3 servings/day of low-fat dairy products; whole grains; less than 2 servings/day of meat, fish and poultry; and minimal sweets and sugary beverages (Figure 43–1). In all three dietary patterns, sodium intake was the same and not restricted (about 3000 mg/day). Energy intake was adjusted to maintain the baseline body weight of each participant.

All meals consumed by DASH trial participants were prepared in metabolic kitchens using standardized procedures. The nutrient content of the meals was confirmed by chemical analysis.[28] Participants ate one meal each weekday, preferably lunch or dinner, at the clinical center, and carried out all other weekday meals, snacks, and all weekend meals. Thus all foods consumed during the study were provided. Each weekday, body weight was measured, and calorie intake was adjusted if weight increased or decreased by more than 2%.

The study population consisted of adults with high-normal BP or stage 1 hypertension who were not taking antihypertensive medication. Specifically, eligibility criteria were DBP 80 to 95 mm Hg and SBP less than 160 mm Hg, based on the average of readings obtained over three screening visits. Exclusion criteria were use of vitamin or food supplements; alcoholic beverage intake >14 drinks per week; poorly controlled diabetes mellitus; severe dyslipidemia; renal insufficiency; recent CVD event; chronic illness; and body mass index (BMI) >35 kg/m². Because of the disproportionate burden of hypertension in African Americans, the study was designed to include two-thirds minority participants, predominantly African Americans.

The DASH study consisted of two phases: run-in and intervention. After eligibility was established, participants entered a run-in phase of 3 weeks during which they were fed the Control dietary pattern. Participants were then randomly assigned to one of the three dietary interventions: Control, F/V, or DASH. The intervention phase began the day after the run-

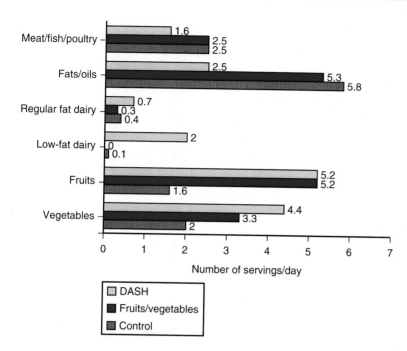

**Figure 43-1** Intake of food groups in the DASH study. (From Vogt TM, Appel LJ, Obarzanek E, et al. Dietary Approaches to Stop Hypertension: Rationale, design, and methods. DASH Collaborative Research Group. J Am Diet Assoc 99[8 Suppl]:S12-S18, 1999, with permission from the American Dietetic Association.)

in feeding period ended and lasted for 8 weeks (Figure 43–2). Adherence to the study diet was assessed by observation at the on-site meal, by self-report of study participants, and by biochemical measurement. As an objective estimate of adherence, sodium, potassium, calcium, urea nitrogen, and magnesium were measured in 24-hour urine collections.

The primary outcome was the change in DBP from the end of run-in to the end of the intervention phase. Secondary end points included the change in SBP and in 24-hour ambulatory BP. Other outcomes assessed included changes in levels of serum lipids, calcium, vitamin D, and effects of baseline characteristics on BP response to intervention. All analyses were performed using the intention-to-treat principle. The study was powered to detect a difference in DBP between treatment groups of 2.0 mm Hg ($\beta = 0.15$).

## Results

A total of 459 participants were randomized in the DASH trial. The mean age was 44 years; approximately 60% of participants

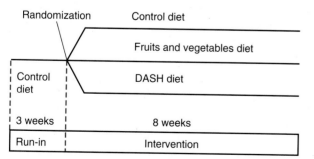

**Figure 43-2** DASH study design. (From Vogt TM, Appel LJ, Obarzanek E, et al. Dietary Approaches to Stop Hypertension: Rationale, design, and methods. DASH Collaborative Research Group. J Am Diet Assoc 99[8 Suppl]:S12-S18, 1999, with permission from the American Dietetic Association.)

were African American, 50% were women, and 29% were classified as hypertensive. Baseline characteristics were similar in the three diet groups.[1] The percentages of participants who completed the intervention phase in the Control, F/V, and DASH groups were 95.5%, 97.4%, and 98.7%, respectively. Dietary adherence was excellent: more than 95% attended the required meals and ate all the meals. Urinary potassium increased in proportion to the intended increase in dietary intake of fruits and vegetables, with significant increases in both the F/V diet and the DASH diet. Urinary magnesium, phosphorus, and urea nitrogen also increased significantly in the DASH diet, reflecting the increased intake of low-fat dairy products and protein. As intended, urinary sodium excretion and body weight were unchanged from baseline.

Both intervention diets significantly lowered BP compared with the Control diet, with greater effects in the DASH diet group than in the F/V group. (Figure 43–3). The full BP effects were seen after 2 weeks and were sustained for the subsequent 6 weeks of the intervention. Compared with Control, the DASH diet reduced SBP by 5.5 mm Hg and DBP by 3.0 mm Hg ($p <.001$ for both). The F/V diet reduced SBP by 2.8 mm Hg and DBP by 1.1 mm Hg more than the Control diet ($p <.001, .07$ respectively). The DASH diet significantly reduced the SBP (2.7 mm Hg, $p = .001$) and DBP (1.9 mm Hg, $p = .002$) more than the F/V diet. Based on 24-hour ambulatory BP measurements, the BP effects of the DASH diet were also noted throughout the day and night, with retention of the diurnal pattern.[29]

Subgroup analysis demonstrated similar improvements in BP in all groups. The DASH diet reduced BP more than the Control or F/V diet in subgroups defined by gender, race, age, hypertension status, education level, BMI, annual family income, physical activity, family history of hypertension, and alcohol intake.[30] The DASH dietary pattern was equally effective in men and women. It lowered BP more in participants with hypertension than in those with high-normal BP (11.6/5.3 vs. 3.5/2.2 mm Hg) (Figure 43–4). Regardless of hypertension status, African Americans had a larger BP

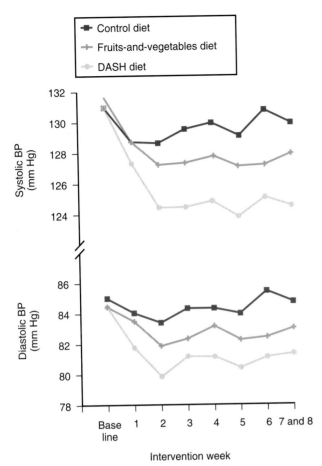

**Figure 43-3** Change in blood pressure (BP) by treatment group in the DASH study. (Reprinted with permission from Appel LJ, Moore TJ, Obarzanek E, et al. A clinical trial of the effects of dietary patterns on blood pressure. DASH Collaborative Research Group. N Engl J Med 336(16):1117-1124, 1997. Copyright © 1997 Massachusetts Medical Society.)

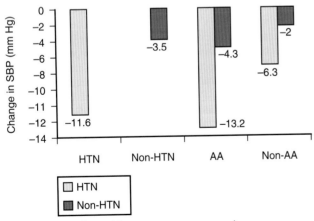

**Figure 43-4** Effect of hypertension status and race on systolic blood pressure (SBP) response to the DASH dietary pattern. HTN hypertensive; AA, African American. (Adapted from Svetkey LP, Simons-Morton D, Vollmer WM, et al. Effects of dietary patterns on blood pressure: Subgroup analysis of the Dietary Approaches to Stop Hypertension [DASH] randomized clinical trial. Arch Intern Med 159(3):285-293, 1999. Copyright © 1999 American Medical Association. All rights reserved.)

response to the DASH dietary pattern than did non–African Americans. The effect in hypertensive African Americans was a 13.2/6.1 mm Hg decrease in BP.

Among the 459 participants in the DASH trial, there were 72 with stage 1 isolated systolic hypertension (ISH). The DASH diet proved to be effective as first-line therapy for stage 1 ISH. Compared with the Control diet, use of the DASH diet lowered SBP by 11.2 mm Hg in these study participants ($p$ <.001, 95% confidence interval (CI) −6.1 to −16.2 mm Hg). The systolic response was highly consistent, occurring in virtually every individual with ISH assigned to the DASH dietary pattern. Seventy-eight percent of these individuals achieved SBP goal (<140 mm Hg).[31]

### Conclusions

The DASH dietary pattern lowers both SBP and DBP in a broad range of individuals with high-normal BP and stage 1 hypertension. DASH is particularly effective in hypertensives and African Americans. The magnitude of effect is sufficient to potentially prevent hypertension in those with prehypertension and to serve as first-line therapy in those with stage 1 hypertension.

Given the design of the DASH trial, the effects of this complex dietary pattern on BP could be evaluated, but the specific dietary components responsible for changes in BP could not be identified. However, because of the partial efficacy of the F/V diet, it is clear that the effect of DASH was not simply attributable to the increase in either dietary potassium or calcium. It is possible that the total macronutrient and micronutrient composition of the DASH dietary pattern is necessary to achieve its full BP-lowering effect.

## The Dietary Approaches to Stop Hypertension-Sodium Trial

### Rationale and Design

After the publication of the DASH study results, national guidelines for lifestyle interventions for preventing and treating hypertension included the DASH dietary pattern.[7] However, the effect of the DASH dietary pattern in combination with other recommendations was unknown. Of particular interest was the combined effect of DASH with reduced sodium intake. Additive effects of these two BP-lowering dietary strategies would be advantageous. On the other hand, previous research demonstrated that the effect of potassium on BP is greatest when sodium intake is high,[32,33] suggesting that, to the extent that the DASH effect was due to increased potassium intake, its effects might be mitigated by simultaneously reducing sodium intake. The DASH-Sodium trial was conducted to determine the BP effect of three levels of sodium intake in combination with either the DASH or the Control dietary pattern. The three sodium levels were defined as higher (150 mM/day), intermediate (100 mM/day), and lower (50 mM/day). The higher level reflects the typical American diet, the intermediate level represents the upper limit of national recommendations, and the lower sodium level was chosen as a potentially optimal level that might produce further BP-lowering effects.

Similar to the DASH trial, the DASH-Sodium study was a multicenter, randomized feeding trial. Entry criteria and minority enrollment were also similar. The trial consisted of a run-in period during which all individuals consumed the higher-sodium Control diet. Participants were then randomly assigned to follow either the DASH diet or the Control diet for 90 days. Within this parallel design, a crossover design provided participants each of the three sodium levels for 30 consecutive days in random order (Figure 43–5).

The primary outcome was SBP at the end of each 30-day period of dietary intervention, with DBP the secondary outcome. The study assessed sodium effects within each diet and the effects of diet at each sodium level, using an intention-to-treat analysis. The study was powered to detect a 2.1 mm Hg difference in SBP between sodium levels within each diet and 3.0 mm Hg between diets at a given sodium level ($\beta = 0.1$). Adherence was assessed by the methods described in the DASH trial above.

### Results

Four hundred twelve participants were randomized. Baseline characteristics were similar in those assigned to the Control diet and those assigned to the DASH dietary pattern. The mean age was 48 years, approximately 56% were African American, and just over half were women. Forty-one percent had hypertension at baseline. A total of 95% (198 of 208) of the individuals in the DASH diet group and 94% (192 of 204) of those assigned to the Control diet group completed the study and provided BP measurements during each intervention period. Analysis of 24-hour urine collections showed that those assigned to the various levels of sodium intake nearly achieved their goals. Mean urine sodium averaged 142 mM/day during the higher-sodium period, 107 mM/day during the intermediate-sodium period, and 65 mM/day during the lower-sodium period. As expected, urinary potassium, magnesium, phosphorus, and urea nitrogen were higher in the DASH group and were stable across all three sodium levels. By design, weight remained stable throughout the intervention phase.

Both the DASH diet and reduced sodium intake led to BP lowering. BP was lower on the DASH than the Control diet at each level of sodium intake, and decreasing sodium intake reduced SBP and DBP in the context of both the DASH and the Control diets (Figure 43–6). On the Control diet, BP was reduced by 2.1/1.1 mm Hg going from the higher sodium

intake to the intermediate sodium intake and by 4.6/2.4 mm Hg when the sodium intake was further reduced to the lower level. On the DASH diet, reducing sodium intake from the higher to the intermediate level resulted in a BP-lowering effect of 1.30/0.6 mm Hg. When these participants were fed the lower-sodium diet, BP was further reduced by 1.7/1.0 mm Hg. The effect of reducing sodium was not linear: the approximately 40-mM decrease in sodium from the intermediate to the lower-sodium diet resulted in a larger decrease in BP than the similar decrease in sodium from the higher to the intermediate level.

The largest BP effect was observed with the combination of DASH diet and lower sodium intake, although the effects were not fully additive. Participants eating the lower-sodium DASH diet had a BP reduction of 8.9/4.5 mm Hg compared with participants consuming the higher-sodium Control diet.

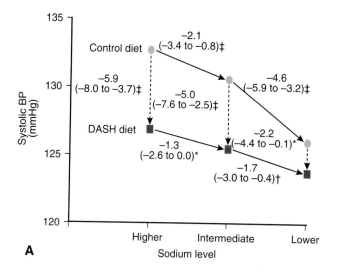

**A**

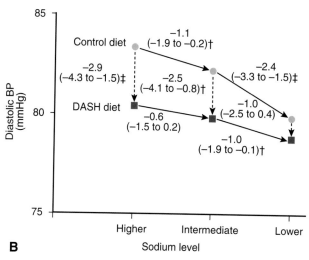

**B**

**Figure 43–6** Blood pressure (BP) effects of the DASH diet and sodium intake. *$p <.05$; †$p <.01$; ‡$p <.001$ (Significant difference between groups or dietary sodium categories.) (Reprinted with permission from Sacks FM, Svetkey LP, Vollmer WM, et al. Effects on blood pressure of reduced dietary sodium and the Dietary Approaches to Stop Hypertension [DASH] diet. DASH-Sodium Collaborative Research Group. N Engl J Med 344(1):3-10, 2001. Copyright © 2001 Massachusetts Medical Society.)

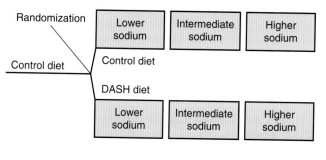

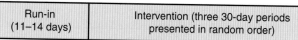

**Figure 43–5** DASH-Sodium study design. (From Svetkey, LP, Sacks FM, Obarzanek E, et al. The DASH Diet, Sodium Intake and Blood Pressure Trial [DASH-sodium]: Rationale and design. DASH-Sodium Collaborative Research Group. J Am Diet Assoc 99(8 Suppl):S96-S104, 1999, with permission from the American Dietetic Association.)

The DASH-Sodium results were consistent across subgroups defined by race, sex, age, and baseline hypertension status.[2] The effects of sodium were greater in participants with hypertension, in African Americans on the Control diet compared with non–African Americans on that diet, and in women on the DASH diet compared with men on that diet. In individuals with hypertension, the combination of the DASH diet and the lower sodium intake reduced SBP by 11.5 mm Hg. This effect was larger in African Americans (12.6 mm Hg vs. 9.5 mm Hg for others). The combination of the two dietary interventions had similar, but smaller, effects in individuals without hypertension (7.1 mm Hg), men (6.8 mm Hg), and women (10.5 mm Hg).[2] Older patients appeared to be more salt sensitive, with lower (vs. higher) sodium intake reducing BP more in older (>45 years), nonhypertensive participants fed the Control diet, compared with younger participants. However, this effect was not seen in hypertensive individuals.[34]

### Conclusions

The DASH-Sodium trial demonstrated that the DASH dietary pattern reduced BP at all levels of sodium intake compared with the Control diet, confirming and extending the findings of the DASH trial. This benefit was seen across subgroups defined by age, race, and hypertension status. In addition, sodium reduction alone decreased BP in persons eating a diet similar to the average American diet. The greatest BP-lowering effect was seen with the combination of the DASH diet and reduced sodium intake, leading to BP reductions similar to single-drug antihypertensive therapy. These findings support the use of the DASH dietary pattern and reduced sodium intake for the prevention and treatment of high BP.

## OTHER EFFECTS OF DASH

### Effects in Patients with More Severe Hypertension and/or Those on Antihypertensive Medication

The DASH trials reviewed previously were limited to a study population with high-normal BP (prehypertension in the Seventh Report of the Joint National Committee on Prevention, Detection, Evaluation, and Treatment of High Blood Pressure [JNC 7]) or unmedicated stage 1 hypertension. Within that range, participants with higher BP had a greater BP reduction from the DASH diet[30] (Figure 43–7). The effects of DASH in persons with higher than stage 1 hypertension and/or those on BP medications is largely unknown. Conlin et al. randomly assigned participants with stage 1 or 2 hypertension to an 8-week trial of the Control or DASH diet.[3] These individuals were also assigned to the angiotensin receptor blocker (ARB) losartan or placebo in an embedded double-blind crossover design. Mean baseline BP in the DASH group was 151/95 mm Hg. (compared with mean BP of 131.9/83.6 mm Hg in the DASH trial[1]). During the placebo phase, the DASH dietary pattern reduced ambulatory SBP by 5.3 mm Hg ($p$ <.05) compared with participants eating the Control diet, with no significant effect on DBP. Thus, the DASH diet is effective at lowering SBP in individuals with stage 1 or 2 hypertension. This study also demonstrated that the BP-lowering effect of losartan was greater in the setting of the DASH dietary pattern than when the Control diet was

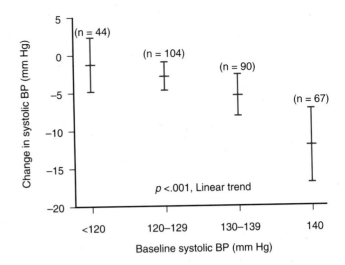

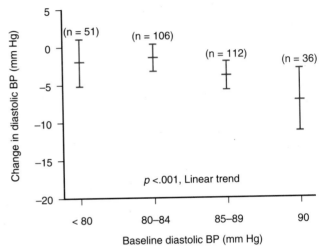

**Figure 43–7** Change in blood pressure (BP) with the DASH diet as a function of baseline BP. (*Bars* indicate 95% confidence intervals.) (Reprinted with permission from Svetkey P, Simons-Morton D, Vollmer WM, et al. Effects of dietary patterns on blood pressure: Subgroup analysis of the Dietary Approaches to Stop Hypertension [DASH] randomized clinical trial. Arch Intern Med 159(3):285-293, 1999. Copyright © 1999 American Medical Association. All rights reserved.)

consumed (Figure 43–8). This trial suggests that the DASH diet enhances the BP response to antihypertensive medication that blocks the renin-angiotensin system (RAS) and raises the possibility that it also will enhance the effects of other classes of antihypertensive medication.

### Effects on Other Cardiovascular Disease Risk Factors

In the DASH studies, the DASH dietary pattern, in which saturated fats are replaced by carbohydrates, monounsaturated fats, and polyunsaturated fats, reduced total and LDL-cholesterol by 13.7 mg/dl and 10.7 mg/dl, respectively[4] (Figure 43–9). Triglycerides increased slightly. HDL-Cholesterol decreased by 3.7 mg/dl, but the total:HDL and LDL:HDL ratios were improved. These effects were observed in subgroups defined by race, sex, age, and baseline lipids. The implication of decreased HDL levels needs to be further studied, but the finding was not unexpected given the known

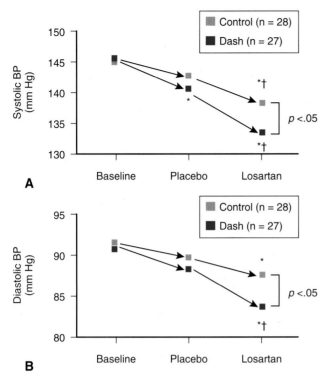

**A**

**B**

**Figure 43–8** Twenty-four hour ambulatory **(A)** systolic and **(B)** diastolic blood pressures (BPs) at baseline and during placebo and losartan treatment. *p <.05 vs. baseline; †p <.05 vs. placebo. (From Conlin PR, Erlinger TP, Bohannon A, et al. The DASH diet enhances the blood pressure response to losartan in hypertensive patients. Am J Hypertens 16(5 Pt 1):337-342, 2003, with permission from The American Journal of Hypertension, Ltd.)

decrease in HDL levels associated with low-fat diets.[35] There was no effect of sodium level on lipids.[36]

The DASH diet also lowers homocysteine levels. A substantial body of observational data suggests that homocysteine is an independent risk factor for atherosclerotic cardiovascular disease (CVD). The DASH diet is rich in nutrients known to

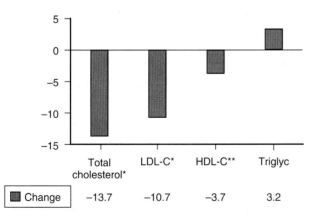

**Figure 43–9** Effect of DASH dietary pattern on lipids, *p <compared with control diet effects, **no significant change in LDL/HDL or total cholesterol/HDL ratios. (Reprinted with permission from Obarzanek E, Sacks FM, Vollmer WM, et al. Effects on blood lipids of a blood pressure-lowering diet: The Dietary Approaches to Stop Hypertension [DASH] Trial. Am J Clin Nutr 74(1):80-89, 2001.)

influence homocysteine metabolism, including folate, vitamin B6, and vitamin B12. In 118 patients in the DASH trial, preintervention and postintervention serum folate, pyridoxal 5′ phosphate (the coenzyme form of vitamin B6), and homocysteine were measured.[5] Compared with the Control diet, there was a 0.8-μM/L reduction in homocysteine level in the DASH diet group (p = .03) (Figure 43–10).

## Effects on Bone Health

Calcium intake is associated with bone health. In addition, cross-sectional studies demonstrate that a diet rich in fruits and vegetables is associated with higher bone mineral density, possibly related to promotion of a positive calcium balance from increased intake of potassium and magnesium.[37] In contrast, high sodium intake is associated with increases in urinary calcium excretion,[38,39] which, in combination with inadequate calcium intake, may result in disturbances in calcium metabolism and bone loss mediated by a rise in parathyroid hormone (PTH).[40] Therefore, the DASH diet alone would be expected to improve bone health. Lin et al. studied the effect of the DASH diet and sodium intake on markers of bone turnover and calcium metabolism.[41] Bone turnover was assessed using the serum marker of bone formation, osteocalcin, which is released by the osteoblast into circulation during the mineralization of newly synthesized collagen. Bone resorption was measured using the serum marker of bone resorption, C-terminal N-telopeptide (CTX), which is released from bone collagen into circulation following its degradation by osteoclasts. At all three sodium levels in the DASH-Sodium trial, the DASH diet reduced bone turnover, as indicated by decreased serum osteocalcin (8%-11%) and CTX (16%-18%). Reduction in bone turnover was significant in all subgroups regardless of hypertension status, race, gender, and age. Although there was a higher calcium intake in the DASH group, urinary calcium was similar to Control, suggesting greater calcium retention. The suppression of bone turnover observed in this study appears to be similar to or greater than that observed with calcium supplementation

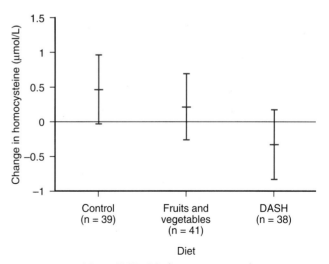

**Figure 43–10** Mean (95% CI) change in serum homocysteine (μm/L) from end of run-in to end of intervention in the DASH study. (Reprinted with permission from Appel LJ, Miller ER 3rd, Jee SH, et al. Effect of dietary patterns on serum homocysteine: Results of a randomized, controlled feeding study. Circulation 102(8):852-857, 2000.)

alone. Thus, the DASH dietary pattern, with or without reduced sodium intake, significantly, reduces bone turnover, which if sustained, may improve bone mineral status and reduce the risk of osteoporosis.

## MECHANISM OF ACTION

The BP-lowering mechanism of the DASH diet remains unknown, but there is some evidence for genetic modulation as well as effects on the RAS and sodium homeostasis.

Genetic modulation of the BP response to dietary intervention has been previously demonstrated. Both reduced sodium intake and weight loss[42] are more effective in lowering BP in individuals with the AA genotype of the G-6A angiotensinogen (ANG) polymorphism compared with other ANG genotypes. This polymorphism is also associated with the greatest BP response to the DASH dietary pattern, with an average decrease of 6.93/3.68 mm Hg (compared with 2.80/0.20 mm Hg in those with the GG genotype).[43] Most of this genetic association is explained by data in whites, since African Americans have a very low prevalence of the GG genotype. The effect of the DASH diet in relationship to other BP-modulating genes is under investigation.

In the losartan study by Conlin noted above, the larger BP response to losartan experienced by non–African Americans compared with African Americans was substantially neutralized when the African American participants were eating the DASH diet.[3] The fact that BP reduction is comparable in African Americans and whites on losartan when it is taken in the context of the DASH dietary pattern is reminiscent of the racial parity in BP effects of angiotensin-converting enzyme (ACE) inhibitor or ARBs when combined with diuretics.[44,45] Indeed, there is evidence that the DASH diet may have diuretic effects. Akita et al.[46] demonstrated that the DASH diet increases the slope of the pressure natriuresis curve, a measure of the relationship between arterial pressure and urinary sodium excretion, without shifting the curve along the BP axis. These findings are consistent with a natriuretic action.

The DASH diet is high in potassium and calcium. Previous studies suggest that these micronutrients play a role in the function of the renin-angiotensin-aldosterone system (RAAS). Hollenberg et al.[47] showed that a low potassium intake (40 mmol/day) reduced renal blood flow and blunted the vascular response to angiotensin II, consistent with an increase in RAAS function. Potassium supplementation lowers BP and increases plasma renin activity (PRA).[15] A relationship between calcium supplementation, calcium regulating hormones, and the RAAS also exists.[48] Administration of oral calcium significantly increases PRA and suppresses calcium-regulating hormones. These findings suggest that there is an interaction between the DASH diet and the RAAS in BP control. The other micronutrients and macronutrients involved in BP control could not be identified because of the study design. Further studies are required in order to understand the precise mechanisms and the specific dietary components that contribute to the BP-lowering effect of the DASH diet.

## IMPLEMENTATION

The DASH and DASH-Sodium trials were relatively short-term feeding studies. They were not designed to assess either adherence to the diet among people selecting their own food or the long-term effects of the DASH dietary pattern. The PREMIER trial attempted to address the feasibility of implementing the DASH diet along with other established recommendations for lowering BP in free-living persons.[6] PREMIER was a multicenter randomized trial that included 810 adults with above-optimal BP or stage 1 hypertension who were not taking antihypertensive medications. The participants were randomly assigned to one of three intervention groups: (1) the "Established" intervention, a behavioral intervention that implemented long-standing recommendations (weight loss, sodium reduction, increased physical activity, and limited alcohol intake); (2) the "Established Plus DASH" intervention, which also implemented the DASH diet; and (3) an "Advice Only" comparison group. The main outcome was BP measurement and hypertension status at 6 months, with continued intervention and follow-up for a total of 18 months postrandomization. Results demonstrated gradients in BP and hypertension status across the groups. The mean net reduction in SBP was 3.7 mm Hg ($p$ <.001 compared with Advice Only) in the Established group and 4.3 mm Hg ($p$ <.001 compared with Advice Only) in the Established Plus DASH group. The prevalence of hypertension was decreased from the baseline of 37% to 26% in the Advice Only group, 17% in the Established group, and 12% in the Established Plus DASH group (Figure 43–11). In addition, the percent of individuals with optimal BP, defined as

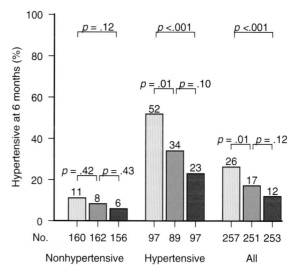

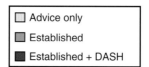

**Figure 43–11** Percentage of participants in the PREMIER study with hypertension at 6 months by randomized group, by hypertension status at baseline. (Reprinted with permission from Appel LJ, Champagne CM, Harsha DW, et al. Effects of comprehensive lifestyle modification on blood pressure control: Main results of the PREMIER clinical trial. JAMA 289(16):2083-2093, 2003. Copyright © 2003 American Medical Association. All rights reserved.)

less than 120/80 mm Hg,[7] went from 0% to 19% in Advice Only, 30% in Established, and 35% in Established Plus DASH (Figure 43–12). The trial demonstrated that free-living adults can adopt multiple lifestyle changes with improvement in BP control. Lifestyle modifications were effective in preventing the development of hypertension and increasing the number of individuals with optimal BPs.

A potential limitation of the PREMIER study was the unexpected reduction in BP in the Advice Only group, making it difficult to estimate the true effects of the active interventions (Established and Established Plus DASH). Participants randomized to the Advice Only "control" group made lifestyle changes similar to (but to a lesser extent than) the active intervention groups, suggesting that the advice that was provided conferred a less intense but still active behavioral intervention. A smaller, randomized controlled feeding trial, the Diet, Exercise, and Weight Loss Intervention Trial (DEW-IT), found that multiple lifestyle modifications including the DASH dietary pattern are effective in reducing BP compared with control (no intervention).[49] After a 9-week intervention of a hypocaloric DASH diet, moderate-intensity exercise program, and 100 mM/day sodium intake, participants assigned to the intervention arm had a reduction in mean ambulatory BP of 9.5/5.3 mm Hg ($p < .001$, $p < .002$ respectively) compared with the controls. This feeding trial confirmed the efficacy of multiple lifestyle interventions but did not address effectiveness. DEW-IT does provide evidence that the DASH dietary pattern in combination with other lifestyle modification reduces BP compared with a true control. Taken together, the PREMIER and DEW-IT trials show that the currently recommended lifestyle modifications, including the DASH dietary pattern, are feasible and improve BP control.

Implementation outside of the research context requires that the study results be broadly applicable and that the interventions be feasible. The DASH dietary pattern was tested in a population that was demographically heterogeneous, consisting of approximately 50% women, and 37% with household incomes less than $30,000. African Americans were overrepresented in order to ensure that the interventions were effective in this population at increased risk of BP-related morbidity and mortality. With the exception of minority composition, the participants were similar to the U.S. adult population.[30] The range of baseline BP in the study populations represents at least 40% of U.S. adults.[50] The feeding trials used commonly available foods. However, the DASH dietary pattern, for daily energy consumption of 2000 kcal, includes 8 to 10 servings of fruits and vegetables a day, twice the current average amount consumed by U.S. adults[51] and higher than the U.S. Department of Agriculture's *Dietary Guidelines for Americans'*[52] recommended 5 to 7 servings. DASH includes 2 to 3 servings of low-fat diary products, consistent with current recommendations, but again approximately twice the current intake.[53] Further, to be feasible, the recommended dietary pattern must be reasonably priced. Based on U.S. Department of Agriculture estimates of food bills for a typical American family of four in January 1997, the estimated cost of a week of food for the DASH dietary pattern falls between "low cost" and "moderate."[30] Adoption of the DASH dietary pattern may be facilitated by descriptions based on a recommended number of food group servings per day rather than on goals for consumption of targeted nutrients. Meal plans and DASH recipes are readily available on the Internet (http://www.nhlbi.nih.gov/health/public/heart/hbp/dash/) and in a book written for the general public.[54]

## IMPLICATIONS

The DASH dietary pattern is an effective nonpharmacologic treatment for high BP. In the participants with hypertension, the reduction in BP with the DASH diet is similar in magnitude to that observed in trials of drug monotherapy for stage 1 hypertension.[55] Further, the DASH dietary pattern improves the BP response to the antihypertensive medication losartan, especially in the African American population. It seems reasonable to predict that the DASH dietary pattern would have similar interactions with other medications that affect the RAAS. Adoption of the DASH dietary pattern by patients with hypertension could decrease medication costs by reducing the amount of medication required to control BP and limiting the side effects of hypertension treatment due to numerous drugs.

Individuals with prehypertension[56] and high-normal BP[7] also achieve reductions in BP with the DASH dietary pattern. Despite nonhypertensive BP, these individuals have excess BP-related cardiovascular risk.[57] In addition, because BP increases with age, it is the population with prehypertension now that is most likely to develop hypertension in the future.[58] Despite the expected benefits of lowering BP in the population with prehypertension or high-normal BP, pharmacologic interventions in this very large segment of the population have not been tested and may not be cost-effective. Widespread adoption of the DASH dietary pattern could prevent the development of hypertension in this group and subsequently lower CVD risk.

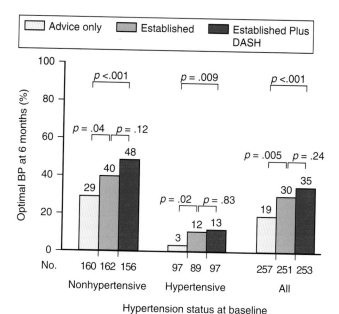

**Figure 43–12** Percentage of participants in the PREMIER study with optimal blood pressure (BP) at 6 months, by treatment group and baseline hypertension status. (Reprinted with permission from Appel LJ, Champagne CM, Harsha DW, et al. Effects of comprehensive lifestyle modification on blood pressure control: Main results of the PREMIER clinical trial. JAMA 289(16):2083-2093, 2003. Copyright © 2003 American Medical Association. All rights reserved.)

The DASH studies and PREMIER demonstrated a significant BP-lowering effect of the DASH dietary pattern. However, these relatively short studies did not directly assess the expected consequences of the observed BP changes (i.e., reduced cardiovascular outcomes). If applied population-wide, the DASH dietary pattern could lead to a small decrease in the population distribution of BP that would result in a large decrease in the number of cardiovascular events. It is estimated that a population-wide reduction in SBP or DBP of the magnitude observed with the DASH diet would reduce incident coronary heart disease (CHD) by approximately 15% and stroke by approximately 27%.[59]

Erlinger et al. used the Framingham risk equation and data from the Third National Health and Nutrition Survey (NHANES III) to estimate the number of CHD events that would be prevented in the United States by a population-wide adoption of the DASH diet.[60] Applying an overall uniform SBP reduction of 5.5 mm Hg (the mean reduction in DASH), there was a predicted reduction of 668,426 CHD events over 10 years. After accounting for differential BP effects by race and baseline SBP, there was a predicted reduction of 416, 514 CHD events (94,828 in African Americans and 321,080 in whites). This represents a decrease in CHD events of 9% in African Americans and 3% in whites. The greatest risk reduction occurred in African Americans with hypertension. These data imply that adoption of a healthy dietary pattern could have a substantial impact on the incidence of CHD in the United States, especially among African Americans.

The DASH dietary pattern may also have health benefits beyond its role in BP reduction. Several observational studies suggest that a prudent diet similar to DASH may reduce CHD events and total mortality. The Nurses' Health Study identified two dietary patterns: "prudent" and "Western."[61] The prudent diet was similar to the DASH diet, while the Western diet was similar to the Control diet. After 8 years of follow-up, the prudent diet was associated with a relative risk of 0.64 for cardiovascular events (95% CI 0.44-0.92) comparing those at the extremes of either diet. A similar study in men without known CVD at baseline found a similar decrease in the risk of CVD events in those eating the DASH-like diet.[62] Further, observational data suggest that a healthy dietary pattern similar to DASH is associated with a 20% to 30% reduction in total mortality.[63] Based on these observational studies, there may be additional benefits of the DASH dietary pattern beyond its favorable effects on BP, cholesterol, and homocysteine levels.

## References

1. Appel LJ, Moore TJ, Obarzanek E, et al. A clinical trial of the effects of dietary patterns on blood pressure. DASH Collaborative Research Group. N Engl J Med 336(16):1117-1124, 1997.
2. Sacks FM, Svetkey LP, Vollmer WM, et al. Effects on blood pressure of reduced dietary sodium and the Dietary Approaches to Stop Hypertension (DASH) diet. DASH-Sodium Collaborative Research Group. N Engl J Med 344(1):3-10, 2001.
3. Conlin PR, Erlinger TP, Bohannon A, et al. The DASH diet enhances the blood pressure response to losartan in hypertensive patients. Am J Hypertens 16(5 Pt 1):337-342, 2003.
4. Obarzanek E, Sacks FM, Vollmer WM, et al. Effects on blood lipids of a blood pressure-lowering diet: The Dietary Approaches to Stop Hypertension (DASH) Trial. Am J Clin Nutr 74(1): 80-89 2001.
5. Appel LJ, Miller ER 3rd, Jee SH, et al. Effect of dietary patterns on serum homocysteine: Results of a randomized, controlled feeding study. Circulation 102(8):852-857, 2000.
6. Appel LJ, Champagne CM, Harsha DW, et al. Effects of comprehensive lifestyle modification on blood pressure control: Main results of the PREMIER clinical trial. JAMA 289(16): 2083-2093, 2003.
7. The sixth report of the Joint National Committee on prevention, detection, evaluation, and treatment of high blood pressure. Arch Intern Med 157(21):2413-2446, 1997.
8. Sacks FM, Rosner B, Kass EH. Blood pressure in vegetarians. Am J Epidemiol 100(5):390-398, 1974.
9. Rouse, IL, Beilin LJ, Armstrong BK, et al. Blood-pressure-lowering effect of a vegetarian diet: Controlled trial in normotensive subjects. Lancet 1(8314-5):5-10, 1983.
10. Ophir O, Peer G, Gilad J, et al. Low blood pressure in vegetarians: The possible role of potassium. Am J Clin Nutr 37(5): 755-762, 1983.
11. Margetts BM, Beilin LJ, Armstrong BK, et al. Vegetarian diet in the treatment of mild hypertension: A randomized controlled trial. J Hypertens 3:S429-S431, 1985.
12. Sacks FM, Donner A, Castelli WP, et al. Effect of ingestion of meat on plasma cholesterol of vegetarians. JAMA 246(6): 640-644, 1981.
13. Sacks FM, Kass EH. Low blood pressure in vegetarians: Effects of specific foods and nutrients. Am J Clin Nutr 48(3 Suppl):795-800, 1988.
14. Sacks FM, Beilin LJ, Armstrong BK, et al. Lack of an effect of dietary saturated fat and cholesterol on blood pressure in normotensives. Hypertension 6(2 Pt 1):193-198, 1984.
15. Whelton PK, He J, Cutler JA, et al. Effects of oral potassium on blood pressure. Meta-analysis of randomized controlled clinical trials. JAMA 277(20):1624-1632, 1997.
16. Jorde R, Bonaa KH. Calcium from dairy products, vitamin D intake, and blood pressure: The Tromso Study. Am J Clin Nutr 71(6):1530-1535, 2000.
17. Bostick RM, Fosdick L, Grandits GA, et al. Effect of calcium supplementation on serum cholesterol and blood pressure. A randomized, double-blind, placebo-controlled, clinical trial. Arch Fam Med 9(1):31-38, 2000.
18. Kawano Y, Matsuoka H, Takishita S, et al. Effects of magnesium supplementation in hypertensive patients: Assessment by office, home, and ambulatory blood pressures. Hypertension 32(2):260-265, 1998.
19. The effects of nonpharmacologic interventions on blood pressure of persons with high normal levels. Results of the Trials of Hypertension Prevention, Phase I. JAMA 267(9): 1213-1220, 1992.
20. Beilin LJ. Vegetarian and other complex diets, fats, fiber, and hypertension. Am J Clin Nutr 59(5 Suppl):1130S-1135S, 1994.
21. Margetts BM, Beilin LJ, Vandongen R, et al. A randomized controlled trial of the effect of dietary fibre on blood pressure. Clin Sci (Lond) 72(3):343-350, 1987.
22. Kagan A, Popper JS, Rhoads GG, et al. Dietary and other risk factors for stroke in Hawaiian Japanese men. Stroke 16(3): 390-396, 1985.
23. Kimura N. Atherosclerosis in Japan. Epidemiology, Atheroscler Rev 2:209-221, 1977.
24. Sacks FM. Obarzanek E, Windhauser MM, et al. Rationale and design of the Dietary Approaches to Stop Hypertension trial (DASH). A multicenter controlled-feeding study of dietary patterns to lower blood pressure. Ann Epidemiol 5(2): 108-118, 1995.
25. Karanja NM, Obarzanek E, Lin PH, et al. Descriptive characteristics of the dietary patterns used in the Dietary Approaches to Stop Hypertension Trial. DASH Collaborative Research Group. J Am Diet Assoc 99(8 Suppl):S19-S27, 1999.

26. Svetkey LP, Sacks FM, Obarzanek E, et al. The DASH Diet, Sodium Intake and Blood Pressure Trial (DASH-sodium): Rationale and design. DASH-Sodium Collaborative Research Group. J Am Diet Assoc 99(8 Suppl): S96-S104, 1999.

27. Carroll MD, Abraham S, Dresser, CM. Dietary intake source data: United States, 1976-80. Vital Health Stat 11 11(231):1-483, 1983.

28. Vogt TM, Appel LJ, Obarzanek E, et al. Dietary Approaches to Stop Hypertension: Rationale, design, and methods. DASH Collaborative Research Group. J Am Diet Assoc 99(8 Suppl):S12-S18, 1999.

29. Moore TJ, Vollmer WM, Appel LJ, et al. Effect of dietary patterns on ambulatory blood pressure: Results from the Dietary Approaches to Stop Hypertension (DASH) Trial. DASH Collaborative Research Group. Hypertension 34(3):472-477, 1999.

30. Svetkey LP, Simons-Morton D, Vollmer WM, et al. Effects of dietary patterns on blood pressure: Subgroup analysis of the Dietary Approaches to Stop Hypertension (DASH) randomized clinical trial. Arch Intern Med 159(3):285-293, 1999.

31. Moore TJ, Conlin PR, Ard J, et al. DASH (Dietary Approaches to Stop Hypertension) diet is effective treatment for stage 1 isolated systolic hypertension. Hypertension 38(2):155-158, 2001.

32. Addison W. The use of sodium chloride, potassium chloride, sodium bromide and potassium bromide in cases of arterial hypertension which are amenable to potassium chloride. Can Med Assoc J 18:281-185, 1928.

33. McQuarrie I, Anderson JA. Effects of excessive ingestion of sodium and potassium salts on carbohydrate metabolism and blood pressure in diabetic children. J Nutr 11:77-101, 1936.

34. Vollmer WM, Sacks FM, Ard J, et al. Effects of diet and sodium intake on blood pressure: Subgroup analysis of the DASH-sodium trial. Ann Intern Med 135(12):1019-1028, 2001.

35. Knopp RH, Walden CE, Retzlaff BM, et al. Long-term cholesterol-lowering effects of 4 fat-restricted diets in hypercholesterolemic and combined hyperlipidemic men. The Dietary Alternatives Study. JAMA 278(18):1509-1515, 1997.

36. Harsha DW, Sacks FM, Obarzanek E, et al. Effect of dietary sodium intake on blood lipids: Results from the DASH–Sodium trial. Hypertension 43:393-398, 2004.

37. New SA, Robins SP, Campbell MK, et al. Dietary influences on bone mass and bone metabolism: Further evidence of a positive link between fruit and vegetable consumption and bone health? Am J Clin Nutr 71(1):142-151, 2000.

38. Shortt C. Sodium-calcium inter-relationships with specific reference to osteoporosis. Nutr Res Rev 3:101-115, 1990.

39. Massey L. Dietary salt, urinary calcium, and bone loss. J Bone Miner Metab 11:731-736, 1996.

40. McCarron DA, Morris, CD. Epidemiological evidence associating dietary calcium and calcium metabolism with blood pressure. Am J Nephrol 6(Suppl 1):3-9, 1986.

41. Lin PH, Ginty F, Appel LJ, et al. The DASH diet and sodium reduction improve markers of bone turnover and calcium metabolism in adults. J Nutr 133(10):3130-3136, 2003.

42. Hunt, SC, Cook NR, Oberman A, et al. Angiotensinogen genotype, sodium reduction, weight loss, and prevention of hypertension: Trials of hypertension prevention, phase II. Hypertension 32(3):393-401, 1998.

43. Svetkey LP, Moore TJ, Simons-Morton DG, et al. Angiotensinogen genotype and blood pressure response in the Dietary Approaches to Stop Hypertension (DASH) study. J Hypertens 19(11):1949-1956, 2001.

44. Weir MR, Smith DH, Neutel JM, et al. Valsartan alone or with a diuretic or ACE inhibitor as treatment for African American hypertensives: Relation to salt intake. Am J Hypertens 14(7 Pt 1):665-671, 2001.

45. Racial differences in response to low-dose captopril are abolished by the addition of hydrochlorothiazide. Br J Clin Pharmacol 14:1947-1953, 1982.

46. Akita S, Sacks FM, Svetkey LP, et al. Effects of the Dietary Approaches to Stop Hypertension (DASH) diet on the pressure-natriuresis relationship. Hypertension 42(1):8-13, 2003.

47. Hollenberg NK, Williams G, Burger B, et al. The influence of potassium on the renal vasculature and the adrenal gland, and their responsiveness to angiotensin II in normal man. Clin Sci Mol Med 49(6):527-534, 1975.

48. Petrov V, Lijnen P. Modification of intracellular calcium and plasma renin by dietary calcium in men. Am J Hypertens 12(12 Pt 1-2):1217-1224, 1999.

49. Miller ER 3rd, Erlinger TP, Young DR, et al. Results of the Diet, Exercise, and Weight Loss Intervention Trial (DEW-IT). Hypertension 40(5):612-618, 2002.

50. Burt VL, Whelton P, Roccella EJ, et al. Prevalence of hypertension in the US adult population. Results from the Third National Health and Nutrition Examination Survey, 1988-1991. Hypertension 25(3):305-313, 1995.

51. Krebs-Smith SM, Cook A, Subar AF, et al. US adults' fruit and vegetable intakes, 1989 to 1991: A revised baseline for the Healthy People 2000 objective. Am J Public Health 85(12): 1623-1629, 1995.

52. Department of Agriculture, Nutrition and Your Health: Dietary Guidelines for Americans, 4th ed. Washington, DC, Government Printing Office, 1995.

53. Cleveland LE, G[MC5]J, Borrud LG. Data tables: Results from USDA's 1994 Continuing Survey of Food Intakes by Individuals and the 1994 Diet and Health Knowledge Survey. F.S.R. Group, 1996.

54. Moore T, Svetkey LP, Lin P-H, et al. The DASH Diet: Lower Your Blood Pressure in 14 Days without Drugs. New York, Simon & Schuster, 2001.

55. The treatment of mild hypertension study. A randomized, placebo-controlled trial of a nutritional-hygienic regimen along with various drug monotherapies. The Treatment of Mild Hypertension Research Group. Arch Intern Med 151(7): 1413-1423, 1991.

56. Chobanian, AV, Bakris GL, Black HR, et al. The Seventh Report of the Joint National Committee on Prevention, Detection, Evaluation, and Treatment of High Blood Pressure: The JNC 7 report. JAMA 289(19):2560-2572, 2003.

57. Vasan RS, Larson MG, Leip EP, et al. Impact of high-normal blood pressure on the risk of cardiovascular disease. N Engl J Med 345(18):1291-1297, 2001.

58. Vasan RS, Larson MG, Leip EP, et al. Assessment of frequency of progression to hypertension in non-hypertensive participants in the Framingham Heart Study: A cohort study. Lancet 358(9294):1682-1686, 2001.

59. Cutler JA, Psaty BM, MacMahon S, et al. Public health issues in hypertension control: What has been learned from clinical trials. In Laragh JH, Brenner BM (eds). Hypertension: Pathophysiology, Diagnosis, and Management, ed 2. New York, Raven Press, 1995; pp 253-270.

60. Erlinger TP, Vollmer WM, Svetkey LP, et al. The potential impact of nonpharmacologic population-wide blood pressure reduction on coronary heart disease events: Pronounced benefits in African-Americans and hypertensives. Prev Med 37(4):327-333, 2003.

61. Hajjar IM, Grim CE, George V, et al. Impact of diet on blood pressure and age-related changes in blood pressure in the US population: Analysis of NHANES III. Arch Intern Med 161(4):589-593, 2001.

62. Hu FB, Rimm EB, Stampfer MJ, et al. Prospective study of major dietary patterns and risk of coronary heart disease in men. Am J Clin Nutr 72(4):912-921, 2000.

63. Kant AK, Schatzkin A, Graubard BI, et al. A prospective study of diet quality and mortality in women. JAMA 283(16):2109-2115, 2000.

# Obesity and Hypertension: Impact on Cardiovascular and Renal Systems

**John E. Hall, Daniel W. Jones, Jay J. Kuo, Alexandre A. da Silva, Jiankang Liu, Lakshmi Tallam**

Obesity and physical inactivity are estimated to cause more than 300,000 premature deaths each year in the United States, especially from cardiovascular disease.[1] Excess weight gain increases the risk for cardiovascular disease through multiple mechanisms, including hypertension, diabetes, dyslipidemia, atherosclerosis, and chronic renal dysfunction, many of which are interdependent.[2-4] This cluster of disorders is often referred to as the "metabolic syndrome," although excess weight gain is the primary cause in most patients.

Although kidney disease has not, in the past, been widely recognized as a major consequence of the metabolic syndrome or obesity per se, there is little doubt that excess weight gain is a major cause of hypertension and type 2 diabetes, which together account for approximately 70% of end-stage renal disease (ESRD). Accumulating evidence also suggests that even in nondiabetic obese patients, there is some degree of renal dysfunction that can lead to more serious renal injury as metabolic and hemodynamic disturbances worsen with prolonged obesity.[5]

The overall impact of obesity on hypertension and kidney disease is likely to become even more important in the future, as the prevalence of obesity continues to increase, especially in children and adolescents. Currently, more than 64% of adults in the United States are overweight, with a body mass index (BMI) greater than 25, and almost one third of the population is obese, with a BMI greater than 30.[6] Similar trends have been reported in most industrialized countries and there appears to be no abatement of this worldwide "epidemic." In children and adolescents the prevalence of obesity is rising even more rapidly, suggesting that obesity-associated medical problems are likely to worsen in the future unless these trends can be slowed or reversed.[7,8]

## OVERWEIGHT AND OBESITY—PRIMARY CAUSES OF ESSENTIAL HYPERTENSION

Population studies have shown that excess weight gain (as estimated by BMI, waist:hip ratio, abdominal diameter, and other indices of adiposity) is one of the best predictors for development of hypertension.[9-11] The relationships between BMI and systolic blood pressure (SBP) and diastolic blood pressure (DBP) are almost linear and have been observed in diverse populations throughout the world.[9-12] Moreover, the association between BMI and arterial pressure occurs not only for obese hypertensive subjects, but also for nonobese normotensive subjects.[9-10] In general, the relationship between BMI and arterial pressure appears to be continuous, extending from the range of very lean to very obese.[10] The strength of the association between BMI and blood pressure (BP), however,

may vary in different ethnic groups, possibly because of differences in body fat distribution or other factors that influence the susceptibility of BP to increased adiposity.

The full impact of obesity on hypertension has been difficult to estimate from cross-sectional population studies because its effects on BP are likely to worsen as obesity is sustained for many years and as injury to various target organs develops. Also, nonlinear, synergistic relationships may exist among the multiple effects of obesity (e.g., hyperlipidemia, glucose intolerance, and hypertension) in increasing the risk for cardiovascular and renal disease. Although these complex, time-dependent effects of obesity are difficult to assess in population studies, risk estimates from the Framingham Heart Study suggest that approximately 78% of hypertension in men and 65% in women can be attributed to obesity.[11]

Clinical studies also suggest that obesity is an important cause of increased BP in many patients with essential hypertension, and the therapeutic value of weight loss in reducing BP has been demonstrated in normotensive as well as hypertensive obese subjects.[9,13-15] (For a comprehensive discussion of the management of obesity, see Chapter 46.) Even modest weight loss of 5% to 10% of baseline weight may lower BP and reduce the need for antihypertensive medication.[14] Clinical trials have also demonstrated the effectiveness of weight loss in primary prevention of hypertension.[15] Weight loss does not always completely normalize BP in obese hypertensive patients, however. This is perhaps not surprising in view of the many pathologic changes that occur as excess adiposity is maintained for long periods of time. For example, prolonged obesity may lead to glomerular injury, loss of functional nephrons, and resetting of renal-pressure natriuresis to higher BPs.[4,5]

Although some overweight or obese persons may not have BPs greater than 140/90 mm Hg and are therefore not considered to be "hypertensive" by the usual standards, weight loss usually lowers their BP. Excess weight gain shifts the frequency distribution of BP toward higher levels, increasing the probability of a person's BP falling into the hypertensive range. This suggests that in these "normotensive" obese persons, BP is higher than it would be at a lower body weight, and that many are likely to be "prehypertensive," a term introduced by the Seventh Report of the Joint National Committee on Prevention, Detection, Evaluation, and Treatment of High Blood Pressure (JNC 7).[16] It is increasingly recognized that, in prehypertensive persons, reducing BP may provide protection against future development of cardiovascular disease,[16] especially when additional risk factors are present, as is the case for most obese subjects.

Studies in experimental animals have provided mechanistic insights into the cardiovascular and renal changes associated with excess weight gain. In dogs and rabbits a reproducible rise in BP is observed with weight gain induced by a high-fat diet.[17-19] Moreover, the metabolic, endocrine, cardiovascular, and renal changes caused by diet-induced obesity in experimental animals closely mimic the changes observed in obese humans[3,20] (Table 44–1). Some of these changes are time dependent, occurring rapidly after weight gain and later becoming obscured by pathologic changes associated with prolonged obesity. For example, the glomerular hyperfiltration, characteristic of the early phases of obesity, may eventually subside as renal injury and nephron loss occur in association with obesity-induced hypertension.

## HEMODYNAMIC, CARDIAC, AND VASCULAR CHANGES IN OBESITY

### Increased Heart Rate and Cardiac Output

In experimental animals and humans, obesity induces a rise in resting heart rate due primarily to withdrawal of parasympathetic tone rather than increased sympathetic activity or increased intrinsic heart rate.[21,22] Obesity also causes extracellular volume expansion and higher blood flows to many tissues.[3,17,18] These elevated tissue blood flows summate to raise venous return and cardiac output.

Part of the increased cardiac output observed with weight gain is due to additional blood flow required for the excess adipose tissue. However, obesity also increases blood flow in nonadipose tissue, including the heart, kidneys, gastrointestinal tract, and skeletal muscles.[17,18,23] The mechanisms responsible for increased regional blood flows have not been fully elucidated but are probably due, in part, to higher oxygen consumption and metabolic rate, accumulation of local vasodilator metabolites, and growth of the organs and tissues in response to increased metabolic demands associated with obesity.

### Cardiac Hypertrophy and Impaired Systolic and Diastolic Function

Obesity is associated with eccentric and concentric cardiac hypertrophy.[24,25] Moreover, cardiac hypertrophy is more severe in obese than in lean subjects with comparable hypertension.[26] Because blood volume and venous return are increased, there is increased preload, cardiac dilation, and development of eccentric left ventricular hypertrophy (LVH) in obese subjects.

The rise in BP also increases cardiac afterload, leading to increased left ventricular wall thickness. Thus, when obesity is combined with increased BP, cardiac workload is greatly amplified, leading to marked LVH. High sodium chloride intake, which often occurs concurrently with high caloric intake, exacerbates obesity-induced cardiac hypertrophy, even when the high-salt diet does not raise arterial pressure.[27]

Functional changes in the heart also occur rapidly after excess weight gain. In animals fed a high-fat diet for 12 weeks, cardiac filling pressures were increased, and diastolic dysfunction, associated with decreased left ventricular compliance, was evident even at this early stage of obesity.[28] With more prolonged obesity, impaired systolic function may also occur. The mechanisms responsible for cardiac diastolic and systolic dysfunction in obesity are not well understood, but they probably involve structural changes in the heart, such as fibrosis, as well as functional changes, such as impaired β-adrenergic receptor signaling.[29] There may also be increases in intramyocellular lipids that lead to increased formation of reactive oxygen species, apoptosis, and deposition of collagen.[30] All of these structural and functional changes in the heart combine to greatly increase the risk for congestive heart failure (CHF) in obese persons.[31]

## ENDOTHELIAL DYSFUNCTION AND ARTERIAL STIFFNESS IN OBESE SUBJECTS

Obesity is associated with impaired endothelial-mediated vasodilation,[32] and weight reduction improves flow-mediated vasodilation in obese individuals.[33] Accelerated arterial stiffening also occurs in elderly, middle-aged, and even young adults (20-40 years of age) who have excess adiposity, as estimated by increased BMI, abdominal visceral fat, larger waist circumference, and increased waist:hip ratio.[34] Moreover, higher aortic pulse-wave velocity, a measure of aortic stiffness, strongly correlates with increases in BMI, waist circumference, and waist:hip ratio independent of SBP, race, and sex.[34] Important effects of excess weight gain that impair vascular function may be apparent even in children.[35]

The mechanisms responsible for the deleterious effects of obesity on the vasculature are likely to be due to interactions of multiple disorders, including increased BP, inflammation, "lipotoxicity" caused by excessive non–β-oxidative

Table 44–1 Hemodynamic, Neurohumoral, and Renal Changes in Experimental Obesity Caused by a High-Fat Diet and in Human Obesity

| Model | Arterial Pressure | Heart Rate | Cardiac Output | Renal Sympathetic Activity | Renal Renin Activity | Na+ Balance | Renal Tubular Reabsorption | GFR* |
|---|---|---|---|---|---|---|---|---|
| Obese rabbits (high-fat diet) | ↑ | ↑ | ↑ | ↑ | ↑ | ↑ | ↑ | ↑ |
| Obese dogs (high-fat diet) | ↑ | ↑ | ↑ | ↑ | ↑ | ↑ | ↑ | ↑ |
| Obese humans | ↑ | ↑ | ↑ | ↑ | ↑ | ↑ | ↑ | ↑ |

*The GFR changes refer to the early phases of obesity before major loss of nephron function has occurred. GFR, glomerular filtration rate.

metabolism of fatty acids, oxidative stress, and activation of multiple neurohumoral systems. There is increasing evidence that adipose tissue itself is an important source of cytokines and other factors that create a vascular milieu of inflammation and oxidative stress and may contribute to endothelial dysfunction, vascular stiffening, and eventually atherosclerosis.[36]

## MECHANISMS OF OBESITY HYPERTENSION—IMPAIRED RENAL-PRESSURE NATRIURESIS

Excess renal sodium reabsorption appears to play a major role in initiating the rise in BP associated with weight gain, and obese subjects require higher-than-normal arterial pressure to maintain sodium balance, indicating impaired renal-pressure natriuresis.[4,37] With chronic obesity, increases in arterial pressure, glomerular hyperfiltration, neurohumoral activation, and metabolic changes may cause renal injury, further impairment of pressure natriuresis, and greater increases in BP.

Three mechanisms appear to be especially important in mediating increased sodium reabsorption, impaired renal-pressure natriuresis, and hypertension associated with weight gain (Figure 44–1): (1) increased sympathetic nervous system (SNS) activity, (2) activation of the renin-angiotensin-aldosterone system (RAAS), and (3) compression of the kidneys by fat accumulation within the kidneys and around the renal capsule and by increased abdominal pressure. As obesity is sustained and as metabolic disturbances (e.g., hyperlipi-

demia, glucose intolerance) worsen, renal injury may occur, resulting in progressive impairment of renal-pressure natriuresis and further increases in arterial pressure.

## Sodium Retention Caused by Obesity-Induced Sympathetic Nervous System Activation

Several observations suggest that increased SNS activity contributes to obesity hypertension[3,4,38,39]: (1) Obese persons have elevated SNS activity, as assessed by microneurography, tissue catecholamine spillover, or other methods; (2) pharmacologic blockade of adrenergic activity reduces BP to a greater extent in obese than in lean subjects; and (3) renal denervation markedly attenuates sodium retention and the development of obesity hypertension associated with a high-fat diet in experimental animals.

### Obesity-Induced Sympathetic Nervous System Activation May Be Differentiated

Cardiac sympathetic activity does not appear to be substantially elevated in obese humans,[40,41] and the high heart rate observed in obese persons appears to be related mainly to decreased parasympathetic activity.[21,22] In contrast, SNS activity is usually increased in skeletal muscle and kidneys of obese rather than lean subjects.[40-42]

SNS responses to weight gain may vary depending on ethnicity and factors such as fat distribution. In Pima Indians, who have a high prevalence of obesity but a relatively low prevalence of hypertension, muscle SNS activity is lower than in whites and does not track well with adiposity.[43] In African American men, however, the prevalence of increased SNS activity and hypertension is higher than in white men despite comparable levels of obesity.[44] In young, overweight African American women, adiposity is associated with high SNS activity.[44]

The mechanisms for ethnic differences in SNS responses to obesity are unclear but may be related to factors such as differences in fat mass distribution. For reasons that are still unclear, abdominal obesity may elicit greater SNS activation than lower body obesity.[45] Almost all human studies have measured muscle SNS activity rather than renal SNS activity, the primary pathway by which the SNS causes chronic hypertension.[4] Because there is considerable heterogeneity in the control of autonomic outflow to different organs, measurements of muscle SNS activity may not necessarily reflect renal SNS activity. No comprehensive analysis of the multiple factors that influence the relationships among obesity, SNS activity, and hypertension in diverse populations has been conducted.

### Adrenergic Blockade or Renal Denervation Attenuates Obesity Hypertension

Studies in experimental animals fed a high-fat diet indicate that combined α- and β-adrenergic blockade markedly attenuates the rise in BP during the development of obesity.[46] Clonidine, a drug that stimulates central $\alpha_2$ receptors and reduces sympathetic activity, also prevents most of the rise in BP in dogs fed a high-fat diet.[47] In obese hypertensive patients, combined α- and β-adrenergic blockade for 1 month reduced ambulatory BP significantly more than in lean essential hypertensive patients.[48]

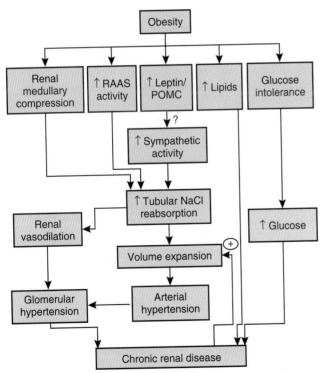

**Figure 44–1** Summary of mechanisms by which obesity causes hypertension and renal injury by activating the sympathetic nervous system, the renin-angiotensin-aldosterone system (RAAS), by physical compression of the kidneys, and by metabolic abnormalities. POMC, proopiomelanocortin pathway; NaCl, sodium chloride.

These findings suggest that increased adrenergic activity contributes to the development and maintenance of obesity hypertension in experimental animals and in humans.

The renal sympathetic efferent nerves mediate much of chronic effects of SNS activation on BP in obesity. In obese dogs fed a high-fat diet, bilateral renal denervation greatly attenuated sodium retention and hypertension.[49] Thus, obesity increases renal tubular sodium reabsorption, impairs pressure natriuresis, and causes hypertension, in part, by increasing renal SNS activity.

## Mechanisms of Sympathetic Nervous System Activation in Obesity

Although the mechanisms that increase renal SNS activity in obesity have not been fully elucidated, several potential mediators have been suggested, including (1) hyperinsulinemia, (2) fatty acids, (3) angiotensin II (Ang II), (4) hyperleptinemia, (5) impaired baroreceptor reflexes, and (6) activation of chemoreceptor-mediated reflexes associated with sleep apnea. Some of these mechanisms have been reviewed previously.[50-53]

Evidence supporting direct cause-and-effect relationships for most of these mechanisms in obesity-induced SNS activation is scanty. For example, multiple studies in experimental animals and humans have shown that hyperinsulinemia, although closely correlated with hypertension, cannot account for increased arterial pressure in obese subjects.[51] In fact, chronic hyperinsulinemia caused by insulin infusion or insulinoma in dogs and humans is often associated with reduced, rather than increased, BP.[51] Likewise, studies from our laboratory do not support a major role for increased levels of fatty acids in causing chronic SNS activation associated with obesity.[54] Studies in experimental animals and in humans suggest that obesity is associated with impaired ability of baroreceptor reflexes to suppress SNS activity during acute increases in BP induced by pharmacologic agents.[50] However, whether these acute measures of baroreflex sensitivity reflect the long-term influence of arterial baroreceptors on SNS activity in obesity hypertension is unclear.

## *Possible Role of Leptin and Hypothalamic Melanocortins in Sympathetic Nervous System Activation*

Leptin may be an important link between obesity and SNS activation[55] (Figure 44-2). Leptin is secreted by adipocytes in proportion to the degree of adiposity and crosses the blood-brain barrier via a saturable receptor-mediated transport system. Leptin binds to its receptor in various regions of the hypothalamus and activates signaling pathways, especially in the arcuate nucleus, that regulate body weight by decreasing appetite and increasing energy expenditure.[56] Evidence that leptin acts as a powerful controller of body weight comes from genetic studies of mice and humans demonstrating that missense mutations of the leptin gene cause extreme, early-onset obesity.[56] Mutations of the leptin gene, however, are very rare in humans, and the importance of abnormalities of leptin production or sensitivity of leptin receptors in contributing to obesity is still unclear.

There is substantial evidence in rodents that high levels of leptin can activate SNS activity and increase arterial pressure.[3,55,57,58] The rise in BP with hyperleptinemia is slow in

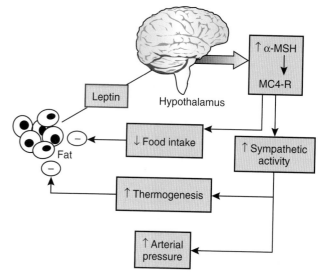

**Figure 44-2** Possible links between leptin and its effects on the hypothalamus, sympathetic activation, and hypertension. Leptin may mediate much of its effects on appetite and sympathetic activity by stimulating other neurochemical pathways, including α-melanocyte stimulating hormone (α-MSH), which activates melanocortin 4-receptors (MC4-R).

onset and occurs over a period of several days despite decreased food intake, which would otherwise tend to lower BP.[58] Moreover, the hypertensive effects of leptin are enhanced when nitric oxide synthesis is inhibited,[59] as often occurs in obese subjects with endothelial dysfunction. The chronic effects of leptin to raise arterial pressure are completely abolished by α- and β-adrenergic blockade, indicating that they are mediated by adrenergic activation.[60]

An observation that points toward leptin as a potential link between obesity and hypertension is the finding that mice with leptin deficiency and rats with mutations of the leptin receptor usually have little or no increase in arterial pressure despite severe obesity when compared with their lean controls.[3,61] There have been few studies in which BP has been measured in obese children with leptin gene mutations. In one study by Ozata et al.,[62] four young patients with homozygous missense mutations of the leptin gene were found to have early-onset, morbid obesity but no indication of hypertension. Each of these children also had impaired sympathetic activity, postural hypotension, and attenuated RAAS responses to upright posture.[62] Moreover, hypertension was absent in spite of severe insulin resistance and hyperinsulinemia. These observations are consistent with those in leptin-deficient mice and suggest that hyperleptinemia may be an important factor in linking obesity with SNS activation and hypertension in humans as well as in rodents. However, these studies do not rule out the possibility that prolonged obesity may also activate other mechanisms that raise BP, such as renal injury.[4]

The stimulatory effect of leptin on SNS activity may be mediated, in part, by interaction with other hypothalamic factors, especially the proopiomelanocortin (POMC) pathway. Antagonism of the melanocortin 3/4 receptor (MC3/4-R) completely abolished the acute effects of leptin on renal SNS activity.[63] In addition, chronic blockade of the MC3/4-R in rats caused rapid weight gain but little or no increase in arterial pressure and a decrease in heart rate.[64] As weight gain usually raises BP and heart rate, these findings are consistent with the possibility that a functional MC3/4-R is important in linking excess weight gain with increased SNS activity and hypertension. However, the importance of the POMC pathway and MC3/4-R in controlling SNS activity and raising BP in obese humans has not, to our knowledge, been investigated.

## Renin-Angiotensin-Aldosterone System Activation in Obesity

Even though excess weight gain is associated with sodium retention and expansion of extracellular fluid volume, obese subjects often have small increases in plasma renin activity (PRA), angiotensinogen, angiotensin-converting enzyme (ACE) activity, Ang II, and aldosterone levels.[3,65] Possible mechanisms for increased renin secretion and activation of the RAAS include (1) increased loop of Henle sodium chloride reabsorption and reduced sodium chloride delivery to the macula densa and (2) activation of the renal sympathetic nerves. Increased angiotensinogen formation by adipose tissue has also been suggested to contribute to elevated Ang II levels in obesity.[65] Although the quantitative importance of these different pathways for forming Ang II in obesity is uncertain, activation of the RAAS appears to contribute to elevated BP and target organ damage in obese persons.

### Role of Ang II in Obesity Hypertension and Renal Injury

A significant role for Ang II in stimulating sodium reabsorption, impairing renal-pressure natriuresis, and causing hypertension in obesity is supported by the finding that treatment of obese dogs with an Ang II antagonist or an ACE inhibitor blunted sodium retention, volume expansion, and increased arterial pressure.[66,67] Also, ACE inhibitors are effective in reducing BP in obese humans, particularly in young patients.[68] Whether the effects of Ang II to raise BP in obesity are due primarily to direct actions on the kidneys or to SNS activation is unclear. The direct renal sodium-retaining effects of Ang II are well known, as are the direct effects of Ang II on SNS activity.[69]

Activation of the RAAS may also contribute to the glomerular injury and nephron loss associated with obesity. Increased Ang II formation, by constricting efferent arterioles, exacerbates the rise in glomerular hydrostatic pressure caused by systemic arterial hypertension.[69] Studies in type 2 diabetic patients, who are usually obese, clearly indicate that ACE inhibitors or Ang II antagonists slow the progression of renal disease.[70-73] However, further studies are needed in nondiabetic, obese subjects to determine the efficacy of RAAS blockers compared with other antihypertensive agents in reducing the risk of renal injury.

### Role of Aldosterone in Obesity Hypertension and Renal Injury

Studies in experimental animals and in humans have provided evidence that antagonism of aldosterone may provide an important therapeutic tool not only for lowering BP, but also for attenuating target organ injury in hypertension.[74] However, few studies have examined the role of aldosterone in contributing to sodium retention, hypertension, or renal

injury in obesity. We have shown in obese dogs fed a high-fat diet that antagonism of aldosterone markedly attenuated sodium retention, hypertension, and glomerular hyperfiltration (Figure 44–3).[75] Moreover, this protection against

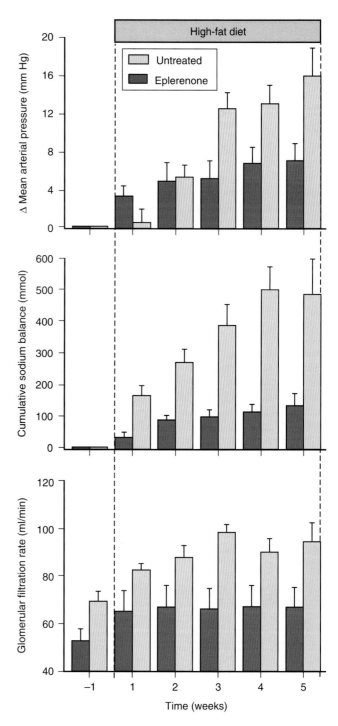

**Figure 44–3** Changes (Δ) in mean arterial pressure (mm Hg), cumulative sodium balance (mmol), and glomerular filtration rate (ml/min) in control, untreated, and eplerenone-treated (10 mg/kg, twice daily) dogs that were fed a high-fat diet for 5 weeks to develop obesity. (Redrawn from data in de Paula RB, da Silva AA, Hall JE. Aldosterone antagonism attenuates obesity-induced hypertension and glomerular hyperfiltration. Hypertension 43:41-47, 2004.)

sodium retention and hypertension occurred despite marked increases in PRA, suggesting that combined blockade of aldosterone and Ang II might be even more effective in preventing obesity-induced sodium retention and hypertension.

The fact that aldosterone antagonism markedly attenuated glomerular hyperfiltration associated with obesity may have important implications for renal protection. Although there are no studies, to our knowledge, that have tested this concept directly in obese subjects, previous studies in various experimental models of hypertension have provided evidence that aldosterone antagonism attenuates renal injury.[74]

## Renal Compression Caused by Visceral Obesity

Visceral obesity initiates several changes that lead to compression of the kidneys and increased intrarenal pressures.[3,5] For example, intraabdominal pressure rises in proportion to sagittal abdominal diameter, reaching levels as high as 35 to 40 mm Hg in some subjects.[76] In addition, retroperitoneal adipose tissue often encapsulates the kidneys and penetrates the renal hilum into the renal medullary sinuses, causing additional compression and increased intrarenal pressures.[3,5] Obesity also causes increased formation of a renal medullary extracellular matrix that could exacerbate intrarenal compression and sodium retention.[3,5] Although these physical changes in the kidneys cannot account for the initial increase in arterial pressure that occurs with rapid weight gain, they may help to explain why abdominal obesity is much more closely associated with hypertension than lower body obesity.

## OBESITY AND CHRONIC RENAL DISEASE

Although obesity is not widely recognized as a major cause of renal disease, its impact becomes obvious if we consider that the two most important causes of ESRD are diabetes and hypertension, both of which are closely associated with excess weight gain. Moreover, the rapid rise in the prevalence of ESRD in the past two decades has been paralleled by increasing obesity and diabetes.[77] In fact, most of the increasing prevalence of ESRD has been attributed to increasing type 2 diabetes.

## Obesity Exacerbates Development of Nondiabetic Renal Diseases

In addition to causing renal injury through diabetes and hypertension, obesity also exacerbates the effects of other primary renal insults, even those that are often considered to be relatively benign, such as unilateral nephrectomy.[78] In patients who underwent unilateral nephrectomy an average of 13.6 ± 8.6 years before, 92% of those with a BMI >30 developed proteinuria or renal insufficiency, whereas only 12% with a BMI <30 developed these disorders[78] (Figure 44–4).

In patients with immunoglobulin A (IgA) nephropathy, those with a BMI >25 at the time of renal biopsy had more severe renal lesions and increased proteinuria, as well as a much faster decline of renal function and progression to chronic renal failure compared with patients with a BMI <25.[79] Moreover, moderate weight loss in overweight patients with chronic nondiabetic proteinuric nephropathies markedly reduced proteinuria, whereas in overweight subjects who

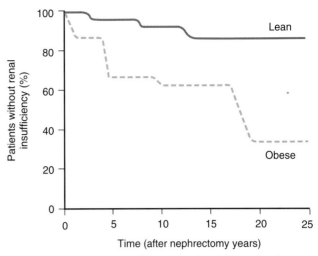

**Figure 44–4** Percentage of patients who did not develop renal insufficiency after unilateral nephrectomy and who were lean (BMI <25, solid line) or obese (BMI >30, dashed line) at the time of unilateral nephrectomy. (Redrawn from data in Praga M, Hernandez E, Herrero JC, et al. Influence of obesity on the appearance of proteinuria and renal insufficiency after unilateral nephrectomy. Kidney Int 58:2111-2118, 2000.)

did not lose weight, renal function worsened with time.[80] These observations indicate that obesity greatly exacerbates loss of renal function in patients with preexisting glomerulopathies, and that weight loss may lessen the impact of renal injury from other causes.

## Early Structural and Functional Renal Changes in Obese Subjects

Even in the absence of preexisting renal disease, excess weight gain causes early structural and functional changes in the kidneys that may eventually lead to more serious renal disorders. Significant structural changes in the kidneys were observed in dogs placed on a high-fat diet for only 7 to 9 weeks.[81] These changes included enlargement of Bowman's space, increased glomerular cell proliferation, increased mesangial matrix, thicker basement membranes, and increased expression glomerular transforming growth factor β.[81] Moreover, these early changes occurred with only modest hypertension, no evidence of diabetes, and only mild metabolic abnormalities.

Obese humans often develop proteinuria, frequently in the nephrotic range, that may be followed by progressive loss of kidney function even in the absence of diabetes or severe hypertension.[80] The most common types of lesions observed in renal biopsies of obese subjects are focal and segmental glomerulosclerosis and glomerulomegaly.[82] A review of 6818 biopsies indicated that the incidence of obesity-related glomerulopathy, defined as combined focal glomerulosclerosis and glomerulomegaly, rose tenfold from 1990 to 2000, coincident with the rapid increase in the prevalence of obesity during this period.[82]

The mechanisms of obesity-induced renal injury likely involve a combination of hemodynamic and metabolic abnormalities. Obesity causes marked glomerular hyperfiltration and preglomerular vasodilation that permits greater transmission of the increased arterial pressure to the glomerular capillaries.[83] These renal hemodynamic changes, along with the metabolic abnormalities, such as hyperglycemia and hyperlipidemia, likely exacerbate the effects of increases in arterial pressure to cause renal injury.

A synergistic relationship may exist between the metabolic abnormalities and increased glomerular pressure in causing chronic renal vascular disease and nephron loss. Results of the Prospective Cardiovascular Munster (PROCAM) study suggest that this is the case for coronary artery disease.[84] For example, the risk for myocardial infarction (MI) was increased about twofold by hypertension and twofold by diabetes. However, when hypertension and diabetes occurred together the risk was increased more than eightfold. When hypertension, diabetes, and hyperlipidemia were all present, as occurs in most obese patients, the risk for MI increased almost 20-fold. Similar synergistic relationships between glomerular pressure and metabolic abnormalities may also exist for renal vascular disease, although there are no large-scale studies that have addressed this issue.

## Do Caloric Restriction and Weight Loss Prevent or Attenuate Renal Disease?

There is compelling evidence in experimental animals that excess caloric intake causes progressive nephron loss and that caloric restriction protects against glomerular injury. Modest food restriction (8%-18% below the usual ad lib amounts) in the obese Zucker rat, for instance, reduces renal injury and increases life span by approximately 30%.[85] Similar beneficial effects of food restriction have been observed in other models of obese and nonobese rodents, indicating that food restriction can largely prevent chronic renal disease in rats.

In nondiabetic obese humans, short-term weight loss also produces marked reductions in proteinuria. An antiproteinuric effect of weight loss is also evident in overweight persons with nephropathies caused by factors other than obesity.[80] The renal benefits of weight loss appear to occur whether they are induced by diet and exercise or by surgical methods (e.g., gastroplasty), although there have been no large studies directly comparing the effectiveness of different methods of weight loss on progression of renal dysfunction. Also, most studies have lasted only a few weeks or months. Studies lasting for at least a year, however, have shown remarkable reductions in proteinuria (>80%) with a weight loss of about 12%.[86] Although the long-term consequences of weight loss in protecting against renal disease have not been rigorously tested in humans, there is little doubt that weight loss reduces hypertension and prevents or reverses the development of type 2 diabetes, the two main risk factors for development of ESRD.

## TREATMENT OF OBESITY HYPERTENSION AND RENAL DISEASE

### Weight Loss and Lifestyle Modification

The numbers of people affected and the severity of the consequences are rapidly making obesity the most important and most prevalent health care problem of the modern world. Few effective treatments are available to prevent or treat obesity (see Chapter 46). For morbidly obese patients (BMI >40) or

for patients with a BMI >35 and comorbid conditions, various surgical procedures, especially gastric bypass surgery, are becoming increasingly popular and usually produce significant weight loss. However, the long-term consequences of these procedures in reversing cardiovascular and renal disease and on overall mortality are still uncertain.

Only two drugs, sibutramine (a sympathomimetic that induces satiety and increases thermogenesis) and orlistat (a gastrointestinal lipase inhibitor), are currently approved by the U.S. Food and Drug Administration (FDA) to promote weight loss. Both of these drugs have significant side effects that limit their use in many patients, and their long-term effects on morbidity and mortality are unknown.

Until more effective and safer pharmacologic treatments are available, voluntary weight loss associated with lifestyle modifications, including increased physical activity, is still the best option for most overweight patients.[87] Several studies have demonstrated that weight loss lowers BPs in normotensive or hypertensive obese subjects[88,89] and may prevent the development of hypertension in persons with "high normal" BPs.[88] Even modest weight reductions of 5% to 10% can improve control of BP and reduce the amount of medication necessary to achieve goal BPs.[14,90,91] Weight loss also is effective in reducing other risk factors for cardiovascular and renal disease (e.g., blood glucose and lipids) in many hypertensive patients.

Current guidelines for achieving weight loss usually recommend as a first step the development of an individualized plan to reduce caloric intake and increase energy expenditure by behavioral modification.[87] A major obstacle, however, in successful prevention and treatment of obesity has apparently been the lack of adequate involvement of health care professionals. Fewer than half of obese adults report that their physicians advised them to lose weight.[92] Patients whose physicians advised them to lose weight, however, were three times more likely to attempt weight loss as those who were not so advised.[93] The successful management of obesity will require the same attention and planning for effective treatment as other important medical conditions, such as hypertension.

## Drug Therapy of Hypertension in Obese Patients

Until effective strategies for preventing and treating obesity are developed, physicians will be left with the responsibility of managing the cardiovascular, metabolic, and renal consequences of obesity. Selection of specific drugs for antihypertensive therapy in obese subjects is often empiric or based on clinical experience and knowledge of the physiology of obesity hypertension.[83,94] No large clinical trials have tested the effectiveness of different drugs in reducing BP and preventing cardiovascular and renal disease in obese compared with lean subjects. The Antihypertensive Therapy and Lipid-Lowering Heart Attack Trial (ALLHAT), however, included many overweight subjects and may provide some useful information about the relative effectiveness of the four main classes of antihypertensive drugs tested: diuretics, α-adrenergic blockers, ACE inhibitors, and calcium antagonists.[95] Also, some inferences may be drawn from other randomized, controlled clinical trials of drug therapy in essential hypertension, because most of these trials have included many participants who were overweight or obese.

The potential advantages and disadvantages of different antihypertensive drugs in obese patients have been previously discussed.[94,96] However, it is important to point out that adequate BP control in obese patients may not be the usual <140/90 mm Hg. For many, lower levels of BP should be the goal because of the coexistence of other risk factors, such as hyperlipidemia, glucose intolerance or diabetes, and atherosclerosis. Another important consideration for obese persons is that hypertension may often be difficult to control with one drug. Therefore, combination therapy is often required for the effective management of obese hypertensive patients.

## Diuretics

Because of their ability to reduce renal sodium and water reabsorption and decrease extracellular fluid volume, diuretics may be useful in lowering BP in many obese hypertensive patients.[97] Some clinicians prefer diuretics in obese patients because of the strong evidence from randomized controlled clinical trials indicating that reducing BP with diuretics lowers cardiovascular morbidity and mortality.[16] Because obese patients often have glucose intolerance and dyslipidemia, some clinicians avoid diuretics to prevent worsening these metabolic abnormalities.[98] Although studies using high doses of diuretics have demonstrated significant adverse metabolic effects, such as increases in insulin resistance and plasma lipids, low-dose diuretics are less frequently associated with these effects, and, when used in combination with other agents, can be very useful in treating obesity hypertension.[16]

## β-Adrenergic Blockers

There is strong outcome evidence for treatment of essential hypertension with β-blockers.[16] In obese patients, β-blockers may be useful in countering some effects of obesity-induced sympathetic activation, such as stimulation of renin secretion. β-blockers are also especially beneficial in patients after MI, and studies have demonstrated that these drugs decrease morbidity and mortality in diabetic patients, most of whom are overweight or obese.[99] However, β-blockers may make it more difficult for the obese patient to lose weight and, in some studies, are associated with worsening glucose control, higher lipid levels, and increased body weight.[94] Thus, although β-blockers may be indicated in obese hypertensive patients with ischemic heart disease and/or arrhythmias, other drugs may be preferable for initial therapy in obese patients who have no evidence of heart disease.

## Angiotensin-Converting Enzyme Inhibitors

ACE inhibitors offer some theoretical advantages in treating obesity-related hypertension. As discussed previously, the RAAS is activated in obesity, suggesting that blockers of this system should be effective in lowering BP. The ability of ACE inhibitors to attenuate glomerular hyperfiltration and urinary protein excretion provide an advantage in managing BP in obese patients who are particularly prone to renal disease. The improved insulin sensitivity associated with ACE inhibitors is also a positive feature. One of the few randomized, controlled trials in obese hypertensive patients included an ACE inhibitor. The Treatment of Obese Patients with Hypertension (TROPHY) study compared the BP responses to the ACE inhibitor lisinopril and the diuretic hydrochlorothiazide in obese hypertensives.[68] Both agents effectively lowered SBP and DBP after 12 weeks of therapy. African Americans and older participants were more likely to respond favorably to the diuretic, while the white and younger participants were more likely to respond to the ACE inhibitor.

Studies in patients with hypertension and/or CHF have demonstrated that the response to ACE inhibitors depends on sodium intake and volume status. These drugs can be used in combination with diuretics in the obese hypertensive patient for optimal BP responses, even in patients who do not have elevated PRA.[16]

## Angiotensin II Receptor Antagonists

Ang II receptor antagonists have not been studied extensively in obese hypertensive patients. Studies in patients with essential hypertension suggest that they have BP-lowering effects similar to ACE inhibitors.[16] Some differences between these two classes (e.g., the effect of ACE inhibitors to increase kinin levels) may be responsible for subtle differences in the incidence of complications such as angioedema and cough. It is likely that obese patients have similar BP responses to ACE inhibitors and Ang II antagonists. Extensive trials have been completed in hypertensive patients, including those with diabetes, to examine the effects of Ang II antagonists on cardiovascular morbidity and mortality and on progression of renal disease. Two different Ang II antagonists were shown to prevent or decrease proteinuria in hypertensive patients with type 2 diabetes mellitus.[71-73]

## α₁-Adrenergic Blocking Agents

Results of ALLHAT suggest that $\alpha_1$-adrenergic blockers are not as effective as diuretics in preventing heart failure and cardiovascular disease.[100] Therefore, these drugs will likely be used less as monotherapy for patients with essential hypertension, including those who are obese. Because they lower plasma lipids, they may continue to play a role in combination therapy for managing obese hypertensive patients with dyslipidemia.[101] They may also be useful as part of a combination of medications in many patients with resistant hypertension, which is common among obese persons.[102]

## Calcium Channel Blockers

These drugs are frequently used to treat obese hypertensive patients. Their effectiveness does not seem to be very dependent on the status of blood volume, the RAAS, or SNS activity. Because calcium channel blockers are effective in a broad range of hypertensive patients, including obese patients, they have gained popularity.[16] However, some studies suggest that calcium channel blockers are less effective in obese than in lean hypertensive patients.[94,103] The dihydropyridine calcium antagonists have the potential disadvantage of further increasing heart rate in obese patients. The nondihydropyridine calcium antagonists, in contrast, lower heart rate.[16]

It is clear that a randomized controlled outcome trial is needed to guide drug selection for obese hypertensive patients. In the meantime, clinicians should continue to use their best judgment, based on their understanding of the pathophysiology of obesity hypertension and the characteristics of the individual patient, in selecting a regimen of pharmacologic therapy appropriate to control BP, attenuate the development of cardiovascular and renal disease, and avoid worsening of other metabolic disorders associated with obesity.

## SUMMARY

There has been an alarming increase in the prevalence of overweight and obesity in most industrialized countries, resulting in increasing diabetes mellitus, hypertension, and renal disease. Excess weight gain is the key risk factor for increased BP in most patients with essential hypertension and also appears to be a major cause of chronic kidney disease. Obesity initially raises BP by increasing renal tubular reabsorption, impairing pressure natriuresis, and causing volume expansion. These changes are due to activation of the SNS and RAAS and to physical compression of the kidneys when visceral obesity is present. Blockade of the SNS and RAAS is therefore effective in reducing BP in obese subjects. With prolonged obesity, there may be progressive renal dysfunction that worsens the hypertension. In some obese individuals, renal injury may progress to ESRD, especially if other preexisting glomerulopathies are present. Weight reduction is an essential first step in the management of obesity-associated hypertension and renal disease. There are, however, few drugs available to produce significant long-term weight loss and few guidelines for treating obesity-associated hypertension, other than the recommendation of reducing weight. Special considerations for the obese patient, in addition to controlling the BP, include correcting the metabolic abnormalities and protecting the kidneys from further injury. More emphasis should be placed on prevention of obesity and on lifestyle modifications that help patients to maintain a healthier weight.

## References

1. US Department of Health and Human Services, Centers for Disease Control and Prevention, Office of Communications. Obesity epidemic increases dramatically in the United States: CDC director calls for national prevention effort. 26 October 1999. Available at: *http://www.cdc.gov/od/oc/media/pressrel/r991026.htm* Accessed January 5, 2004.

2. Eckel RH, Krauss RM. American Heart Association call to action: Obesity as a major risk factor for coronary heart disease. Circulation 97:2099-2100, 1998.

3. Hall JE, Jones DW, Kuo JJ, et al. Impact of obesity on hypertension and renal disease. Curr Hypertens Rep 5:386-392, 2003.

4. Hall JE. The kidney, hypertension, and obesity. Hypertension 41:625-633, 2003.

5. Hall JE, Henegar JR, Dwyer TM, et al. Is obesity a major cause of chronic renal disease? Adv Ren Replace Ther 11:41-54, 2004.

6. Flegal KM, Carroll MD, Ogden CL, et al. Prevalence and trends in obesity among US adults 1999-2000. JAMA 288:1723-1727, 2002.

7. Ogden CL, Flegal KM, Carroll MD, et al. Prevalence and trends in overweight among US children and adolescents. JAMA 288:1728-1732, 2002.

8. Sorof J, Daniels S. Obesity hypertension in children: A problem of epidemic proportions. Hypertension 40:441-447, 2002.

9. Alexander J, Dustan HP, Sims EAH, et al. Report of the Hypertension Task Force, US Department of Health, Education, and Welfare Publication 70-1631 (NIH). Washington, DC, US Government Printing Office, 1979; pp 61-77.

10. Jones DW, Kim JS, Andrew ME, et al. Body mass index and blood pressures in Korean men and women: The Korean National Blood Pressure Survey. J Hypertens 12:1433-1437, 1994.

11. Garrison RJ, Kannel WB, Stokes J, et al. Incidence and precursors of hypertension in young adults: The Framingham Offspring Study. Prev Med 16:234-251, 1987.

12. Cooper, RS, Potimi CN, Ward R. The puzzle of hypertension in African-Americans. Sci Am 280:56-63, 1999.

13. Reisen E, Abel R, Modan M, et al. Effect of weight loss without salt restriction on the reduction of blood pressure in overweight hypertensive patients. N Engl J Med 198:1-6, 1978.

14. Jones DW, Miller ME, Wofford MR, et al. The effect of weight loss interventions on antihypertensive medication requirements in the Hypertension Optimal Treatment (HOT) Study. Am J Hypertens 12:1175-1180, 1999.

15. Stevens VJ, Obarzanek E, Cook NR, et al. Long-term weight loss and changes in blood pressure: Results of the Trials of Hypertension Prevention, phase II. Ann Intern Med 134:1-11, 2001.

16. Chobanian AV, Bakris GL, Black HR, et al; Joint National Committee on Prevention, Detection, Evaluation, and Treatment of High Blood Pressure. National High Blood Pressure Education Program Coordinating Committee. Seventh Report of the Joint National Committee on prevention, detection, evaluation, and treatment of high blood pressure. Hypertension 42:1206-1252, 2003.

17. Hall JE, Brands MW, Dixon WN, et al. Obesity-induced hypertension: Renal function and systemic hemodynamics. Hypertension 22:292-299, 1993.

18. Carroll JF, Huang M, Hester RL, et al. Hemodynamic alterations in obese rabbits. Hypertension 26:465-470, 1995.

19. Rocchini AP, Mao HZ, Babu K, et al. Clonidine prevents insulin resistance and hypertension in obese dogs. Hypertension 33:548-553, 1999.

20. Messerli FH, Christie B, DeCarvalho JG, et al. Obesity and essential hypertension. Hemodynamics, intravascular volume, sodium excretion and plasma renin activity. Arch Intern Med 141:81-85, 1981.

21. Van Vliet BN, Hall JE, Mizelle HL, et al. Reduced parasympathetic control of heart rate in obese dogs. Am J Physiol 269:H629-H637, 1995.

22. Arrone LJ, MacKintosh R, Rosenbaum M, et al. Autonomic nervous system activity in weight gain and weight loss. Am J Physiol 269:222-225, 1995.

23. Rocchini AP. The influence of obesity in hypertension. News Physiol Sci 5:245-249, 1990.

24. Carroll JF, Braden DS, Cockrell K, et al. Obese rabbits develop concentric and eccentric hypertrophy and diastolic filling abnormalities. Am J Hypertens 10:230-233, 1997.

25. Alpert MA. Obesity cardiomyopathy and the evolution of the clinical syndrome. American J Med Sci 321:225-236, 2001.

26. Gottdiener JS, Reda DJ, Materson BJ, et al. Importance of obesity, race and age to the cardiac structural and functional effects of hypertension. J Am Coll Cardiol 24:1492-1498, 1994.

27. Carroll JF, Braden DS, Henegar JR, et al. Dietary sodium chloride (NaCl) worsens obesity-related cardiac hypertrophy. FASEB J 12:A708(Abstract), 1998.

28. Carroll JF, Summers RL, Dzielak DJ, et al. Diastolic compliance is reduced in obese rabbits. Hypertension 33:811-815, 1999.

29. Carroll JF. Post-beta receptor defect in isolated hearts of obese-hypertensive rabbits. Int J Obes Relat Metab Disord 23:863-866, 1999.

30. Unger RH. Weapons of lean body mass destruction: The role of ectopic lipids in the metabolic syndrome. Endocrinology 144:5159-5165, 2003.

31. Kenchaiah S, Evans JC, Levy D, et al. Obesity and the risk of heart failure. N Engl J Med 347:305-313, 2002.

32. Steinberg HO, Chaker H, Leaming R, et al. Obesity/insulin resistance is associated with endothelial dysfunction. Implications for the syndrome of insulin resistance. J Clin Invest 97:2601-2610, 1996.

33. Raitakari M, Ilvonen T, Ahotupa M, et al. Weight reduction with very low-caloric diet and endothelial function in overweight adults: Role of plasma glucose. Arterioscler Thromb Vasc Biol 24:124-128, 2004.

34. Wildman RP, Mackey RH, Bostom A, et al. Measures of obesity are associated with vascular stiffness in young and older adults. Hypertension 42:468-473, 2003.

35. Tounian P, Aggoun Y, Dubern B, et al. Presence of increased stiffness of the common carotid artery and endothelial dysfunction in severely obese children: A prospective study. Lancet 358:1400-1404, 2001.

36. Lyon CJ, Law RE, Hsueh WA. Adiposity, inflammation, and atherogenesis. Endocrinology 144:2195-2200, 2003.

37. Hall JE. Mechanisms of abnormal renal sodium handling in obesity hypertension. Am J Hypertens 10:S49-S55, 1997.

38. Eslami P, Tuck M. The role of the sympathetic nervous system in linking obesity with hypertension in white versus black Americans. Curr Hypertens Rep 5:269-272, 2003.

39. Landsberg L, Krieger DR. Obesity, metabolism, and the sympathetic nervous system. Am J Hypertens 2:1255-1325, 1989.

40. Rumantir MS, Vaz M, Jennings GL, Collier G, et al. Neural mechanisms in human obesity-related hypertension. J Hypertens 17:1125-1133, 1999.

41. Esler M. The sympathetic system and hypertension. Am J Hypertens 13:99S-105S, 2000.

42. Grassi G, Servalle G, Cattaneo BM, et al. Sympathetic activity in obese normotensive subjects. Hypertension 25:560-563, 1995.

43. Weyer C, Pratley RE, Snitker S, et al. Ethnic differences in insulinemia and sympathetic tone as links between obesity and blood pressure. Hypertension 36(4):531-537, 2000.

44. Abate NI, Mansour YH, Arbique D, et al. Overweight and sympathetic activity in black Americans. Hypertension 38:379-383, 2001.

45. Alvarez GE, Beske SD, Ballard TP, et al. Sympathetic neural activation in visceral obesity. Circulation 106:2533-2536, 2002.

46. Antic V, Kiener-Belforti F, Tempini A, et al. Role of the sympathetic nervous system during the development of obesity hypertension in rabbits. Am J Hypertens 13:556-559, 2000.

47. Rocchini AP, Mao HZ, Babu K, et al. Clonidine prevents insulin resistance and hypertension in obese dogs. Hypertension 33:548-553, 1999.

48. Wofford MR, Anderson DC, Brown CA, et al. Antihypertensive effect of alpha and beta adrenergic blockade in obese and lean hypertensive subjects. Am J Hypertens 14:694-698., 2001.

49. Kassab S, Kato T, Wilkins C, et al. Renal denervation attenuates the sodium retention and hypertension associated with obesity. Hypertension 25:893-897, 1995.

50. Grassi G, Seravalle G, Dell'Oro R, et al. Adrenergic and reflex abnormalities in obesity-related hypertension. Hypertension 36:538-542, 2000.

51. Hall JE. Hyperinsulinemia: A link between obesity and hypertension? Kidney International 43:1402-1417, 1993.

52. Narkiewicz K, Kato M, Pesek CA, et al. Human obesity is characterized by selective potentiation of central chemoreflex sensitivity. Hypertension 33:1153-1158, 1999.

53. Wolk R, Shamsuzzaman ASM, Somers VK. Obesity, sleep apnea, and hypertension. Hypertension 42:1067-1074, 2003.

54. Hildebrandt DA, Kirk D, Hall JE. Renal and cardiovascular responses to chronic increases in cerebrovascular free fatty acids. FASEB J 13:A780 (Abstract), 1999.

55. Hall JE, Hildebrandt DA, Kuo JJ. Obesity hypertension: Role of leptin and sympathetic nervous system. Am J Hypertens 14:103S-115S, 2001.

56. Jequier E. Leptin signaling, adiposity, and energy balance. Ann N Y Acad Sci 967:379-388, 2002.

57. Correia MLG, Morgan DA, Sivitz WI, et al. Leptin acts in the central nervous system to produce dose-dependent changes in arterial pressure. Hypertension 27:936-942, 2001.

58. Shek EW, Brands MW, Hall JE. Chronic leptin infusion increases arterial pressure. Hypertension 31:409-414, 1998.

59. Kuo J, Jones OB, Hall JE. Inhibition of NO synthesis enhances chronic cardiovascular and renal actions of leptin. Hypertension 37:670-676, 2001.

60. Carlyle M, Jones OB, Kuo JJ, Hall JE. Chronic cardiovascular and renal actions of leptin-role of adrenergic activity. Hypertension 39:496-501, 2002.

61. Mark AL, Shaffer RA, Correia ML, et al. Contrasting blood pressure effects of obesity in leptin-deficient ob/ob mice and agouti yellow mice. J Hypertens 17:1949-1953, 1999.

62. Ozata M, Ozdemir IC, Licinio J. Human leptin deficiency caused by a missense mutation: Multiple endocrine defects, decreased sympathetic tone, and immune system dysfunction indicate new targets for leptin action, greater central than peripheral resistance to the effects of leptin, and spontaneous correction of leptin-mediated defects. J Clin Endocrinol Metab 10:3686-3695, 1999.

63. Haynes WG, Morgan DA, Djalali A, et al. Interactions between the melanocortin system and leptin in control of sympathetic nerve traffic. Hypertension 33:542-547, 1999.

64. Kuo JJ, Silva AA, Hall JE. Hypothalamic melanocortin receptors and chronic regulation of arterial pressure and renal function. Hypertension 41:768-774, 2003.

65. Engeli S, Sharma AM. The renin angiotensin system and natriuretic peptides in obesity associated hypertension. Journal of Molecular Medicine 79:21-29, 2001.

66. Hall JE, Henegar JR, Shek EW, et al. Role of renin-angiotensin system in obesity hypertension. Circulation 96:I-33 (Abstract), 1997.

67. Robles RG, Villa E, Santirso R, et al. Effects of captopril on sympathetic activity, lipid and carbohydrate metabolism in a model of obesity-induced hypertension in dogs. Am J Hypertens 6:1009-1019, 1993.

68. Reisen E, Weir M, Falkner B, et al. Lisinopril versus hydrochlorothiazide in obese hypertensive patients: A multicenter placebo-controlled trial. Hypertension 30:140-145, 1997.

69. Hall JE, Brands MW, Henegar JR. Angiotensin II and long-term arterial pressure regulation: The overriding dominance of the kidney. J Am Soc Nephrol 10:S258-S265, 1999.

70. Ravid M, Lang R, Rachmani R, et al. Long-term renoprotective effect of angiotensin-converting enzyme inhibition in non-insulin-dependent diabetes mellitus. A 7-year follow-up study. Arch Intern Med 156:286, 1996.

71. Lewis EJ, Hunsicker LG, Clark WR, et al. Renoprotective effect of the angiotensive receptor antagonist irbesartan in patients with nephropathy due to type 2 diabetes. N Engl J Med 345:851-860, 2001.

72. Brenner BM, Cooper ME, deZeeuw D, et al. Effects of losartan on renal and cardiovascular outcomes in patients with type 2 diabetes and nephropathy. N Engl J Med 345:861-869, 2001.

73. Parving HH, Lehnert H, Brochner-Mortensen J, et al. The effect of irbesartan on the development of diabetic nephropathy inpatients with type 2 diabetes. N Engl J Med 345:870-878, 2001.

74. Rocha R, Stier CT Jr. Pathophysiological effects of aldosterone in cardiovascular tissues. Trends Endocrinol Metab 12:308-314, 2001.

75. de Paula RB, da Silva AA,. Hall JE. Aldosterone antagonism attenuates obesity-induced hypertension and glomerular hyperfiltration. Hypertension 43:41-47, 2004.

76. Sugarman HJ, Windsor ACJ, Bessos MK, et al. Intra-abdominal pressure, sagittal abdominal diameter and obesity co-morbidity. J Intern Med 241:71-79, 1997.

77. Hall JE, Crook ED, Jones DW, et al. Mechanisms of obesity-associated cardiovascular and renal disease. Am J Med Sci 324:127-137, 2002.

78. Praga M, Hernandez E, Herrero JC, et al. Influence of obesity on the appearance of proteinuria and renal insufficiency after unilateral nephrectomy. Kidney Int 58:2111-2118, 2000.

79. Bonnet F, Deprele C, Sassolas A, et al. Excessive body weight as a new independent risk factor for clinical and pathological progression in primary IgA nephritis. Am J Kidney Dis 37: 720-727, 2001.

80. Morales E, Valero MA, Leon M, et al. Beneficial effects of weight loss in overweight patients with chronic proteinuric nephropathies. Am J Kidney Dis 41:319-327, 2003.

81. Henegar JR, Bigler SA, Henegar LK, et al. Functional and structural changes in the kidney in the early stages of obesity. J Am Soc Nephrol 12:1211-1217, 2001.

82. Kambham N, Markowitz GS, Valeri AM, et al. Obesity related glomerulopathy: An emerging epidemic. Kidney Int 59:1498-1509, 2001.

83. Hall JE, Jones DW, Henegar J, et al. Obesity hypertension and renal disease. *In:* Eckel RH (ed). Obesity: Mechanisms and Clinical Management. Philadelphia, Lippincott, Williams & Wilkins, 2003; pp 273-300.

84. Assmann G, Schulte H. The Prospective Cardiovascular Munster study (PROCAM): Prevalence of hyperlipidemia in persons with hypertension and/or diabetes mellitus and the relationship to coronary artery disease. Am Heart J 1116: 1713-1724, 1988.

85. Stern JS, Gades MD, Wheeldon CM, et al. Calorie restriction in obesity: Prevention of kidney disease in rodents. J Nutr 131:913S-917S, 2001.

86. Praga M. Obesity-a neglected culprit in renal disease. Nephrol Dial Transplant 17:1157-1159, 2002.

87. National Institutes of Health Clinical guidelines on the identification, evaluation, and treatment of overweight and obesity in adults: The evidence report. National Heart, Lung, and Blood Institute and National Institute of Diabetes and Digestive and Kidney Diseases. Bethesda, MD, 1998. Available at: *http://www.nhlbi.nih.gov/guidelines/index.htm*

88. The Trials of Hypertension Prevention Collaborative Research Group. The effects of nonpharmacologic interventions on blood pressure of persons with high normal levels. Results of the Trials of Hypertension Prevention, Phase I. JAMA 267:1213-1220, 1992.

89. Whelton PK, Appel LJ, Espeland MA, et al. For the TONE Collaborative Research Group. Sodium reduction and weight loss in the treatment of hypertension in older persons: A ran domized controlled trial of nonpharmacologic interventions in the elderly (TONE). JAMA 279:839-846, 1998.

90. Davis BR, Blaufox MD, Oberman A, et al. Reduction in long-term antihypertensive medication requirements. Effects of weight reduction by dietary intervention in overweight persons with mild hypertension. Archi Intern Med 153: 1773-1782, 1993.

91. Imai Y, Sato K, Abe K, et al. Effects of weight loss on blood pressure and drug consumption in normal weight patients. Hypertension 8:223-228, 1986.

92. Galuska DA, Will JC, Serdula MK, et al. Are health care professionals advising obese patients to lose weight? JAMA 282:1576-1578, 1999.

93. Serdula MK, Mokdad AH, Williamson DF, et al. Prevalence of attempting weight loss and strategies for controlling weight. JAMA 282:1353-1358, 1999.

94. Sharma AM, Pischon T, Engeli S, et al. Choice of drug treatment for obesity-related hypertension: Where is the evidence? J Hypertens 19:667-674, 2001.

95. Oparil S. Antihypertensive and lipid-lowering treatment to prevent heart attack trial (ALLHAT): Practical implications. Hypertension 41:1006-1009, 2003.

96. Zanella MT, Kohlmann Jr O, Ribeiro AB. Treatment of obesity hypertension and diabetes syndrome. Hypertension 38: 705-708, 2001.

97. Reisin E, Weed SG. The treatment of obese hypertensive black women: A comparative study of chlorthalidone versus clonidine. J Hypertens 10:489-493, 1992.

98. Bakris GL, Weir MR, Sowers JR. Therapeutic challenges in the obese diabetic patient with hypertension. Am J Med 101(suppl 3A):33S-46S, 1996.

99. UK Prospective Diabetes Study Group. Efficacy of atenolol and captopril in reducing risk of both macrovascular and microvascular complications in type 2 diabetes (UKPDS 39). BMJ 317:713-720, 1998.

100. The ALLHAT Officers and Coordinators for the ALLHAT Collaborative Research Group. Major cardiovascular events in hypertensive patients randomized to doxazosin vs. chlorthalidone: The Antihypertensive and Lipid-Lowering treatment to prevent Heart Attack Trial (ALLHAT). JAMA 283: 1967-1975, 2000.

101. Black HR. The addition of doxazosin to the therapeutic regimen of hypertensive patients inadequately controlled with other antihypertensive medications. Am J Hypertens 13: 468-474, 2000.

102. Kaplan NM. Obesity in hypertension: Effects on prognosis and treatment. J Hypertens 16:S35-S37, 1998.

103. Stoa-Birketvedt G, Thom E, Aarbakke J, et al. Body fat as a prediction of the antihypertensive effect of nifedipine. J Intern Med 237:169-173, 1995.

# Alcohol and Hypertension

## Ian B. Puddey, Lawrence J. Beilin

The relationship between regular alcohol consumption and hypertension that was first described by Lian[1] in 1915 in young French ex-servicemen was largely ignored until the latter half of the twentieth century, when interest in the phenomenon reemerged with case series of higher blood pressures (BPs) in problem drinkers.[2,3] In one such study, heavy drinkers who abstained were noted to have a higher prevalence of persisting hypertension following alcohol withdrawal than those who resumed drinking.[4] Subsequent reports from hypertension clinics in Scotland[5,6] and Sweden[7] noted an increase in the prevalence of abnormal liver function tests among hypertensives, which the authors attributed to heavy alcohol consumption. In the Swedish study, patients with hypertension who were resistant to antihypertensive drug therapy were noted to include a high proportion of heavy drinkers in whom compliance with treatment was thought to be a major issue.[7] In 1976 Matthews[8] noted a positive association between death rates from stroke and cirrhosis and an inverse relation with coronary heart deaths in England and Wales and speculated that alcohol consumption might be the key to these relationships. However, it was not until Klatsky et al.[9] published the Kaiser Permanente Insurance data relating current alcohol consumption to the prevalence of hypertension in over 80,000 contributors to a health insurance plan that the issue really claimed the attention of the medical scientific community.

## CROSS-SECTIONAL STUDIES

The Kaiser Permanente data showed a J-shaped relationship between alcohol and BP in both men and women in the three ethnic groups studied, whites, African Americans, and those of Asian origin (Figure 45–1). The effect was also seen in both smokers and nonsmokers and in obese and nonobese participants and with all types of alcoholic beverage commonly drunk in the United States. Those drinking on average 3 or more standard drinks a day had twice the prevalence of hypertension (>160/90 mm Hg) compared with current non-drinkers. Ex-drinkers seemed to have similar BP to abstainers. Approximately 100 cross-sectional population studies from around the world have now confirmed a relationship between alcohol and increased BP.

Many of the population studies have not had alcohol as a primary focus, and there have been concerns about underreporting of consumption, particularly in heavier or problem drinkers and in women, because of the perceived social stigma. Arkwright et al.[10] evaluated the relative importance of the effects of alcohol on BP in relation to other lifestyle factors in a younger population of working men. In 491 men aged 20 to 44 years, alcohol consumption, assessed by 7-day retrospective diaries, was found to be linearly related to BP and the prevalence of mild hypertension (Figure 45–2). The effect was

independent of all other lifestyle factors studied, including smoking, physical activity, and tea and coffee consumption. The effects were additive to those of body mass index (BMI) and were seen equally in smokers and nonsmokers. Ex–heavy drinkers had similar BPs to lifelong abstainers, suggesting that the effects of alcohol on BP were reversible. Fifty percent of the men who averaged 3 or more standard drinks (1 standard drink estimated at 10 g ethanol equivalent) a day, principally as beer, had three to four times the prevalence of systolic hypertension (140 mm Hg or more) compared with current nondrinkers. In multivariate analysis, alcohol consumption equated with BMI in the magnitude of its contribution to population variation in BP levels, presumably reflecting the relatively high levels of alcohol drinking in this young male Australian population.

The relation between alcohol and BP is by no means restricted to heavier-drinking populations and has been demonstrated in studies from nations in all five continents. Although most of these reports come from acculturated societies, alcohol use has also been an important factor in relation to elevated BP in unacculturated populations with low mean BP. For example, in a community sample of urban and rural Chinese, it was estimated that 33% of hypertension could be attributed to alcohol in the Yi farmers compared with 9.5% in the urban-living Han.[11]

A number of issues have arisen out of the earlier population studies. These include the linearity of the dose-response relationship between alcohol and BP; possible gender differences in the responses; interactions between the effects of alcohol, smoking, and age on BP; whether the association in cross-sectional studies really represents cause and effect; mechanisms of any alcohol-related pressor effect; and possible effects of different patterns of drinking and of types of alcoholic beverage on both BP and clinical manifestations of cardiovascular disease.

The pressor effects of alcohol appeared to increase with age at least up to the 1960s[12] but have been demonstrated in adolescent men and women as young as 18 years who reported drinking patterns outside Australian National guidelines for safe drinking.[13] Despite the fact that clinic BPs tend to be lower in smokers, some studies suggest a greater pressor effect of regular alcohol with smoking.[14,15]

The shape of the dose–response relationship between alcohol and BP has been questioned, as some of the population studies have shown a J-shaped relationship (e.g., the original Kaiser Permanente study),[9] with a threshold of around 2 drinks a day in men, while others, such as that by Arkwright et al.[10] and others,[16-18] have shown a linear relationship.

Ambulatory BP measurements have provided further insights into the effects of alcohol on BP. The Harvest study[19] in 1100 Italians is the largest population study that has used ambulatory BP to examine factors influencing the daily variation of BP. Participants aged 18 to 45 years with clinical

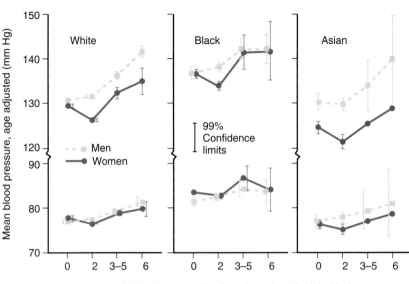

**Figure 45-1** Mean systolic blood pressures (upper bar graph) and mean diastolic blood pressures (lower bar graph) of white, African American, and Asian men and women with known drinking habits. Small circles represent data based on fewer than 30 persons. (Reproduced with permission from Klatsky A, Friedman G, Siegelaub A, et al. Alcohol consumption and blood pressure: Kaiser-Permanente Multiphasic Health Examination Data. N Engl J Med 296:1194-2000, 1977; copyright © 1977 Massachusetts Medical Society.)

diastolic blood pressures (DBP) of 90 to 99 mm Hg or isolated systolic hypertension (ISH) were enrolled. Alcohol intake was linearly related to daytime BP and heavier drinkers showed greater BP variability. Alcohol intake, as well as family history of hypertension, obesity, smoking, coffee consumption, physical activity, oral contraceptive use, and environmental temperature, influenced ambulatory BPs to a greater extent than office pressures.

## TYPES OF ALCOHOLIC BEVERAGE

The Kaiser Permanente study reported similar effects on BP in North Americans drinking beer, wine, or spirits,[9] and studies from countries drinking predominantly sake,[20] wine[21,22] or beer[10,23,24] have shown similar relationships. However, wine drinking has been associated with smaller effects on BP. For example, in the Lipid Clinics Prevalence Study[25] in the United States, regression data from participants who reported drinking only one type of alcoholic beverage showed significant positive regression coefficients for wine and spirits and BP but no significant relationships for wine drinkers. The PRIME study also found a weaker association for wine and BP compared with beer.[26] Such studies should be regarded with a high degree of circumspection given the potentially confounding effects of differences in diet and other behaviors between groups drinking predominantly wine, beer, or spirits.[27] Although both of the aforementioned studies adjusted for obvious confounders such as age and BMI, neither adjusted for diet, and this and other lifestyle differences may have accounted for the findings. Moreover, in a recent 4 × 4-week crossover trial in Perth comparing effects of wine, dealcoholized red wine, beer, and water on 24-hour ambulatory BP in 26 men, similar increases in BP were observed with the two alcohol-containing beverages (Zilkens et al., personal communication). The effect of red wine and beer was predominantly on awake systolic blood pressure (SBP) with significant increases of 2.9 mm Hg for red wine and 1.9 mm Hg for beer compared with water.

## PROSPECTIVE POPULATION STUDIES

Prospective studies such as Framingham and others from North America have shown a strong association between levels of alcohol consumption and the subsequent risk of developing hypertension in men or women with initially normal BP. In 1999 a meta-analysis of three prospective studies reported a 40% increase in the relative risk of developing hypertension in those drinking more than 25 g alcohol per day and a more than fourfold increase in risk in those drinking more than 100 g/day.[28] Subsequently, large-scale prospective studies from Japan[29-31] and the United States, have reported up to a twofold risk of hypertension with intakes of 30 to 50 g/day or more. In the ARIC study it was estimated that in participants drinking 30 g/day or more, one in five cases of hypertension could be attributed to alcohol consumption.[32] In young middle-aged Swedish males, alcohol intake emerged as an important determinant of the development of hypertension over a period of 6 years.[33] Increases in BP have also been reported in those who initiate drinking[34,35] and decreases in those who decrease intake or stop consuming alcohol.[31,36]

## GENDER EFFECTS

The nature of the alcohol–BP relationship is less certain in women. As in men, heavier drinking has been associated with an increased prevalence of hypertension, and some Australian[37] and South American studies[38] indicate that this relationship is linear. The pressor effect of alcohol also seemed additive to that of oral contraceptives in the Lipid Research Clinic Prevalence Study[39] conducted in the United States when higher dose estrogens were in vogue. However, other reports describe a depressor effect of lower levels of alcohol consumption in women, with a greater curvilinearity of the alcohol–BP relationship compared with men.[9,40] Moreover, a meta-analysis of 11 population studies up to 1993[41] suggested that BPs and the risk of hypertension were decreased in women drinking low levels of alcohol compared with non-

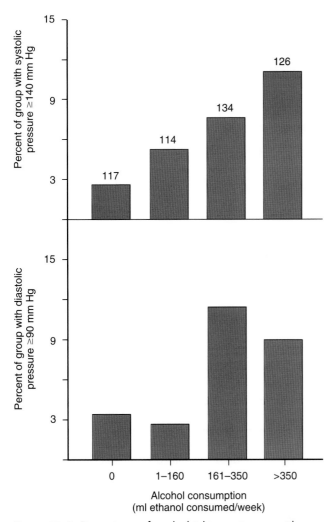

**Figure 45-2** Percentage of each drinking category with systolic or diastolic hypertension. Numbers in columns refer to total in the population subgroup. The $\chi_0^2$ trend for systolic hypertension and alcohol consumption = 8.09, $p$ <.005; for diastolic hypertension, $\chi_0^2$ trend = 5.84, $p$ <.025. (Reproduced with permission from Arkwright PD, Beilin LJ, Rouse I, et al. Effects of alcohol use and other aspects of lifestyle on blood pressure (BP) levels and prevalence of hypertension in a working population. Circulation 66: 60-66, 1982.)

drinkers. However, women have generally been underrepresented in population studies of the effects of alcohol, especially in heavier drinking categories. A cross-sectional survey of 19,000 persons in the United States found that women reporting a prior diagnosis of hypertension also reported drinking less alcohol than those not reporting hypertension,[42] whereas the opposite was true of hypertensive men. In a United Kingdom–based study of 14,000 female employees of the firm Marks and Spencer,[43] the prevalence of hypertension was decreased with consumption of up to 14 drinks a week. These findings could largely be explained by confounding effects of age, BMI, physical activity, and family history of premature coronary artery disease. The NHANES III study,[44] which included more than 9000 women, found that associations between alcohol intake and BP and pulse pressure were

weaker in women than men, whereas a smaller Brazilian study[38] showed the opposite. Greater sensitivity about admitting heavy drinking in different cultures may account for this variability, but the issue remains to be resolved.

Prospective population studies also leave uncertainty as to gender differences in the alcohol–BP relationship. A Canadian report[45] that compared the effects of drinking 8 or more drinks in one sitting with a nonbinge drinking pattern found that only the binge-drinking men showed an increased risk of hypertension after 8 years of follow-up. However, in the ARIC study[32] the relative risks for those drinking more than 210 g alcohol per week were increased similarly for men and women. The largest prospective study, the Nurses Health Study,[46] reported a biphasic effect of alcohol in female nurses aged 25 to 42 at baseline. There was a 14% decrease in the risk of developing hypertension in those consuming 2 to 3.5 drinks per week compared with nondrinkers and a 20% increased risk in those drinking more than 14 drinks a week.

Randomized controlled trials demonstrating the effects on BP of changing alcohol consumption in regular drinkers have so far either been confined to men or included too few women for assessment of a gender effect of alcohol on the direction or magnitude of BP change.

## RANDOMIZED CONTROLLED TRIALS

Randomized controlled trials in drinkers have shown unequivocally that regular alcohol consumption can raise BP in men. The first of these trials, conducted by Puddey et al.[47] in Western Australia, used a crossover design in normotensive drinkers who reduced their alcohol intake for a period of 6 weeks by consuming low-alcohol (0.9% ethanol) beer as a control for the normal-alcohol (5% ethanol) beer from which it was distilled. This enabled the volunteers to reduce their alcohol consumption by at least 80% while retaining their usual intake of fluid, electrolytes, and other nutrients and micronutrients. The study demonstrated a pressor effect of alcohol, which was at least partially reversible, with the major fall in BP evident within 1 to 2 weeks of reducing alcohol intake and continuing over 4 to 6 weeks. The time course of the changes indicated that any BP-raising effect of alcohol could not be solely attributed to acute alcohol withdrawal. A pressor effect of regular drinking of similar magnitude was subsequently shown to occur in both untreated[48] and treated[49] hypertensives in further crossover intervention trials. Based on clinic BP measurements, the trials suggest that the magnitude of this pressor effect equates to around 0.6 to 1.0 mm Hg systolic for each standard drink per day in those with normal BP or mild hypertension.

This pressor effect was confirmed in a recent meta-analysis of 15 randomized controlled trials of effects of changing alcohol consumption on BP[50] (Figure 45–3). Seven of the trials came from the Perth group, including the first to assess effects of patterns of alcohol consumption on ambulatory BP.[51] Men were the sole participants in 12 of these studies and predominated in the remaining three. Seven of the trials studied hypertensives; six studied only normotensives; two studied both normotensive and hypertensive; and six trials studied hypertensives who were taking antihypertensive medication. The duration of most of these studies ranged from 4 to 18 weeks with a median duration of 8 weeks and a

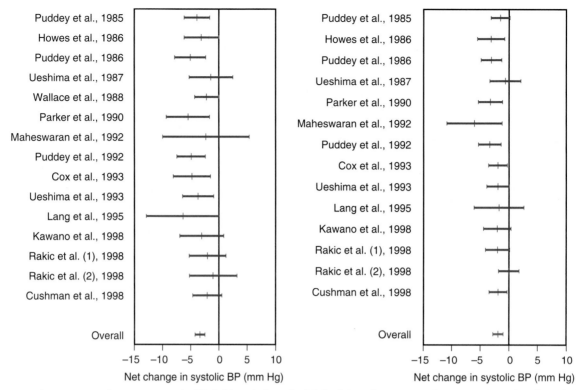

**Figure 45-3** Average net change in systolic BP (left) and diastolic BP (right) and corresponding 95% CIs related to alcohol reduction intervention in 15 randomized controlled trials. Net change was calculated as the difference of the baseline minus follow-up levels of BP for the intervention and control groups (parallel trials) or the difference in BP levels at the end of the intervention and control treatment periods (crossover trials). The overall effect represents a pooled estimate obtained by summing the average net change for each trial, weighted by the inverse of its variance. (Reprinted with permission from Xin X, He J, Frontini MG, et al. Effects of alcohol reduction on blood pressure: a meta-analysis of randomized controlled trials. Hypertension 38:1112-1117, 2001.)

median 76% reduction in alcohol intake from a baseline of 3 to 6 standard drinks a day. The meta-analysis indicated that this reduction resulted in a mean fall in BP of 3.3/2.0 mm Hg, with similar reductions seen in normotensive and hypertensive (treated and untreated) participants. There was a significant positive relationship between the mean percentage reduction in alcohol intake and the corresponding net reductions in SBP and DBP, consistent with a dose-response effect. The mean fall in BP corresponded well with estimates predicted from large cross-sectional population studies such as Intersalt,[52] where BPs in nondrinkers were 2.7/1.6 mm Hg lower than in those drinking 2.8 to 4.8 drinks a day.

In contrast, the largest long-term randomized controlled intervention study, the Prevention and Treatment of Hypertension Study,[53] carried out in 641 moderate- to heavy-drinking men with baseline DBPs 80 to 99 mm Hg, showed small and nonsignificant (0.9/0.6 mm Hg) reduction in SBP and DBP in the intervention compared with the control group. This negative result was attributed to the fact that both groups reduced alcohol consumption so that the intervention group averaged only 1.3 drinks a day less than controls. However, in a work-site program in France in which 129 hypertensives considered to be excessive drinkers were randomized to intervention or control groups for counseling, there was a 7 mm Hg greater fall in SBP in the active group at the end of the 8-week intervention and 6 mm Hg systolic difference at 2 years of follow-up.[54] This was despite

a difference of only 1.2 units/day in the reduction in alcohol consumption between the two groups. Advice on moderation of alcohol intake has also been shown to be effective in a hypertension clinic setting in Britain, resulting in a halving of reported alcohol consumption over 18 months in association with significantly greater reductions in DBP and liver enzymes in the treatment group than in controls.[55]

A number of potential interactions between the effects of alcohol reduction and other lifestyle changes have been studied in randomized controlled trials in Perth. A factorial study of alcohol moderation and 5 kg weight reduction by calorie restriction in overweight drinkers who averaged 5 to 6 standard drinks a day at baseline found independent and additive effects on BP reduction.[56] At the end of 5 months, BPs had fallen by 5 mm Hg systolic with alcohol or weight loss alone and by 9 to 14 mm Hg systolic in the group that reduced both weight and alcohol (Figure 45-4). The latter group also showed the greatest improvement in blood lipids and in left ventricular diastolic function as assessed by echocardiography. The study demonstrated the potential power of lifestyle changes to produce sustained reductions in BP in overweight persons who consume large amounts of alcohol, many of whom have high normal BP or mild hypertension. In contrast, a factorial study of the effects of sodium restriction and alcohol moderation only showed an effect of reducing alcohol consumption in treated hypertensives, suggesting that dietary salt played no part in the BP elevation of these moderately

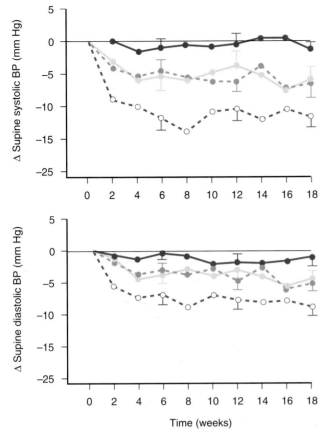

**Figure 45–4** Line graphs show change in mean ± SEM systolic (top) and diastolic (bottom) blood pressure (BP) in four study groups. ●–● (dark color), normal alcohol intake/normal caloric intake (n = 20); ●––●, normal alcohol intake/low caloric intake (n = 22); ●–● (light color), low alcohol intake/normal caloric intake (n = 21); ○––○, low alcohol intake/low caloric intake (n = 23). (Reproduced with permission from Puddey IB, Parker M, Beilin LJ, et al. Effects of alcohol and caloric restrictions on blood pressure and serum lipids in overweight men. Hypertension 20:533-541, 1992.)

heavy drinkers.[57] Similarly, a factorial study of exercise training and alcohol moderation showed only an effect of alcohol reduction on BP.[58] However, in a large cross-sectional population study, the pressor effect of alcohol was partly ameliorated by increased physical fitness.[59]

Several studies from Japan demonstrated a biphasic effect of drinking on BP in hypertensives, with acute BP falls lasting for up to 8 hours following evening drinking, followed by a sustained pressor effect.[60] Kawano et al.[61] used home BP recording in 52 essential hypertensives in a randomized crossover trial to show that when alcohol was reduced from a mean daily intake of 66.5 to 10.2 ml, morning BPs rose by 4.4/2.9 mm Hg while evening pressures fell by 7.4/5.7 mm Hg.

## MECHANISTIC STUDIES IN ANIMALS

The cause of alcohol-related hypertension remains elusive, and animal (predominantly rat) models have been utilized to gain further insights. Findings of animal studies have proved controversial because of inconsistencies in BP outcomes

between studies. One of the first such studies demonstrated no significant effects on BP of chronic ethanol feeding in either normotensive Wistar-Kyoto (WKY) rats or spontaneously hypertensive rats (SHR).[62] Chan et al.,[63-65] on the other hand, have consistently identified a pressor response in Wistar rats following 12 weeks of alcohol feeding. They have described a slight increase in calcium pump activity together with decreased membrane cholesterol content in association with the increase in BP.[64] Such changes were interpreted as compensatory to the known acute fluidizing effects of alcohol on cell membranes, with altered lipid composition ultimately resulting in increased $Ca^{2+},Mg^{2+}$-ATPase activity. Similarly, our group has reported changes in red cell membrane lipid composition with alterations in the polyunsaturated to saturated fatty acid ratio in red cells, which were directly related to alcohol-induced increases in BP.[66] These findings suggest altered membrane function or diminished availability of arachidonic acid precursors as potential mechanisms for alcohol-induced hypertension.

Increases in vascular smooth muscle calcium uptake and BP have been seen in WKY rats chronically fed even lower doses of alcohol.[67] Renal arteriolar vascular smooth muscle hyperplasia occurred in the alcohol-fed rats and could be reversed by coadministration of the calcium entry blocker verapamil.[68] The increases in BP and intracellular calcium and the renal vascular changes in this model could be reversed by coadministration of n-acetyl cysteine,[69] suggesting an important role for the metabolism of alcohol to acetaldehyde in alcohol-induced hypertension. In another report, a pressor response to alcohol in WKY rats was identified with as little as 1% alcohol v/v in the drinking water ad libitum over a period of 14 weeks.[70] Coadministration of dietary vitamin B6 (which augments methionine metabolism to cysteine) decreased tissue acetaldehyde conjugates, prevented an increase in intracellular calcium levels, and counteracted both the increase in BP and renal arteriolar changes. Hsieh et al.[71] have reported that magnesium supplementation can also prevent the development of hypertension in Wistar rats chronically fed alcohol. They postulated that the magnesium counteracted an alcohol-induced increase in intracellular calcium and suppressed sodium pump activity. In the same rat model, more severe hypertension has been induced by the combination of chronic alcohol feeding with chronic heat stress, suggesting that this synergistic increase in BP is mediated by chronic activation of the sympathetic nervous system.[72]

Chronic alcohol administration to male Sprague Dawley rats had no effect on basal BP but impaired arterial baroreceptor responses,[73] likely providing a pathophysiologic basis for subsequent BP elevation. After 12 weeks of alcohol administration, this mechanism was clearly identified in Wistar rats but less evident in Sprague Dawley rats,[74] although in both strains chronic alcohol feeding led to modest increases in BP.

In contrast to findings in the Wistar rat and those of Vasdev et al.[67-70] in WKY rats with low doses of alcohol, high-dose alcohol has usually produced hypotensive effects in SHR, stroke-prone SHR, and WKY rats.[75-77] Sanderson et al.[75] found reductions in BP after feeding SHR 20% alcohol solutions for 16 weeks, while Howe et al.[76,77] reported a retardation of the rise in BP normally seen with aging in both SHR and stroke-prone SHR. Reductions in BP after alcohol feeding occur in these strains despite heightened heart rate responses to stress[78] and enhanced vascular contractility,[79] possibly due to a myocardial depressant effect of alcohol, a phenomenon known to be augmented in the setting of hypertension in these strains.[80,81] The alcohol-induced BP reductions may also have resulted from the lower weight gain characteristically observed when rats are fed alcohol ad libitum.[78] In this regard, the previously discussed increases in BP after chronic alcohol feeding in Wistar rats have not been confirmed when animals were pair fed with control animals to maintain identical calorie and fluid intakes.[79]

Some of the differences between rat models may relate to the dose of alcohol and its means of administration as well as the timing of BP measurement in relation to the last intake of alcohol. Howe et al.[76] reported an increase in BP lasting several days after sudden withdrawal of alcohol in SHR; in Sprague Dawley rats, a hypertensive response has also been reported 24 hours after cessation of alcohol feeding.[82] An acute increase in BP is also characteristic of the alcohol withdrawal syndrome in humans.

Gender may have been a further confounding factor in animal studies. Despite achieving identical blood alcohol concentrations, the acute administration of ethanol intragastrically resulted in hypotensive responses in female but not male Sprague Dawley rats, together with evidence of myocardial depression.[83] These differences are clearly estrogen dependent,[84] but their mechanisms have yet to be fully elucidated.

## MECHANISTIC STUDIES IN HUMANS

The phenomenon of alcohol-related hypertension is something of a paradox in view of the acute vasodilator and BP-lowering responses that occur within minutes of ingesting alcohol and last several hours. Acute alcohol withdrawal in heavy drinkers is often associated with a rise in BP along with increases in circulating catecholamines, renin, and vasopressin. This observation has led to suggestions that the effects observed in population studies might be due to transient effects of acute alcohol withdrawal under survey circumstances where participants abstain after previous consumption.[85,86] There is some support for this interpretation in heavy drinkers from the British Heart Survey,[87] in whom hypertension was more likely to be diagnosed on a Monday than at the end of the week (the assumption being that on Monday the drinkers were exhibiting withdrawal pressor effects following heavy weekend drinking). Different alcohol drinking and weekday BP relationships were observed between men in France and Northern Ireland.[88] In the Irishmen, many of whom binge drank on weekends, BPs were highest on Monday, whereas no such weekday effect was seen in the French, whose alcohol consumption was assumed to be more homogeneous through the week. However, as reviewed elsewhere,[89] other authors have reported that the overall consumption of alcohol averaged over a week or more is more important than the pattern of intake with regard to BP elevation.[90,91]

To help resolve this controversy, we conducted a randomized controlled crossover trial in 55 men, 14 of whom drank more than 60% of their alcohol on weekends and the remainder of whom were daily drinkers.[51] Baseline 24 hour BPs were higher on Mondays than Thursdays in weekend but not daily drinkers, an effect that was lost after switching to low-alcohol beer (Figure 45–5). Both groups showed a fall in 24 hour ambulatory BP when changing from normal to low alcohol

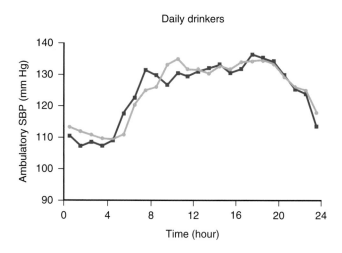

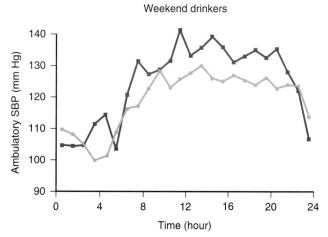

**Figure 45–5** The 24-hour ambulatory systolic blood pressure (SBP) profile by day of assessment for daily drinkers compared with weekend drinkers. -■-, Monday SBP; -●-, Thursday SBP. (Reproduced with permission from Rakic V, Puddey IB, Burke V, et al. Influence of pattern of alcohol intake on blood pressure in regular drinkers: A controlled trial. J Hypertens 16:165-174, 1998.)

beer, an effect that was evident after 1 week in the weekend drinkers but not until the fourth week in daily drinkers. This study indicated there are elements of both acute withdrawal hypertension and more sustained BP elevation in weekend drinkers, whereas those who drink throughout the week show a more sustained pressor response.

Studies indicate that sustained alcohol ingestion likely induces hypertension in humans through effects on the autonomic nervous system. In case control studies, measurements of circulating catecholamines, renin activity, angiotensin II, and cortisol have shown no differences between regular drinkers and age-matched controls,[92] but direct sympathetic nerve recordings in muscle show increased activity during drinking compared with nondrinking periods.[93] In controlled trials, reductions in alcohol consumption are associated with reductions in heart rate.[47,49] Drinkers also show increased BP variability,[19,94] and studies in humans suggest that acute ethanol ingestion leads to impaired baroreceptor function, which may contribute to hypertension.[95]

Pseudo-Cushing's syndrome has been reported in heavy drinkers,[96] raising a question as to whether increased ACTH and cortisol could contribute to alcohol-induced hypertension. However, studies comparing regular drinkers and abstainers[97] suggest that normally there is no increase in cortisol production in age- and obesity-matched participants. Cases of pseudo-Cushing's syndrome in heavy drinkers appear to be the exception rather than the rule.

Alcohol causes acute vasodilation, but more prolonged use may result in direct vasoconstrictor effects. However, most studies of effects of alcohol on vascular function in humans have involved acute alcohol administration.[98,99] A study of the effects of 4 days of alcohol ingestion on forearm vascular function demonstrated decreased responsiveness to noradrenaline, which the authors interpreted as being mediated through $\alpha$-adrenoreceptors.[100] More recently attention has focused on possible effects of alcohol on endothelial vasodilator function.[101] A case control study in chronic alcohol abusers showed decreased flow-mediated dilation (FMD) in the brachial artery after 3 months of abstinence compared with nondrinking controls.[102] In contrast, a study in 108 Japanese men with coronary artery disease, 54 of whom consumed alcohol on at least 1 day per week, revealed better endothelial function of the brachial artery in the drinkers despite a worse coronary risk factor profile.[103] Further, a randomized controlled crossover trial of reducing alcohol consumption from beer from 72.4 to 7.9 g/day in 16 healthy Perth-based male drinkers showed no changes in either FMD of the brachial artery or biomarkers of endothelial function.[104] These noninvasive studies do not exclude vasoconstrictor or endothelial effects of alcohol on selective vascular beds, as has been suggested from some animal studies.[105]

Effects of drinking on large artery stiffness have been implied from changes in augmentation index assessed by radial artery applanation tonometry. Acute and chronic alcohol consumption had differential effects on arterial stiffness, the augmentation index being higher in 67 men drinking more than 21 units of alcohol a week than in 156 lesser drinkers or abstainers.[106] In contrast, in a small substudy of 8 participants drinking red wine (alcohol 0.8 g/kg), augmentation index fell acutely along with BP and pulse wave velocity.[106] There was no effect of dealcoholized wine.[106]

In summary, although the mechanism of BP elevation with regular alcohol consumption is unclear, a central nervous system effect leading to impaired baroreceptor function, increased sympathetic outflow, and greater BP and heart rate responses to environmental stress seems most compatible with the data. A balance between these effects and the peripheral vasodilator actions of alcohol may account for some of the individual variability in BP responses, while in heavy drinkers myocardial depressant effects may further influence the final levels of BP attained.

## γ-GLUTAMYLTRANSPEPTIDASE

γ-Glutamyltranspeptidase (γGT) has long been utilized as a biomarker for alcohol intake. Its serum level has been consistently associated with level of BP in cross-sectional[107] and longitudinal population studies,[108] as well as poor BP control in treated hypertensive drinkers.[7] However, the association of γGT with BP in several studies persisted even after adjustment for alcohol intake, leading to the hypothesis that an increase in

γGT may reflect individual susceptibility to the pressor effect of regular alcohol consumption. One cross-sectional study in Japanese male workers in a metal products factory[109] and a second large prospective study in Korean steel workers[110] support this concept. In both studies, when drinking and nondrinking participants were categorized on the basis of high or low levels of γGT, only drinkers with a high γGT demonstrated increasing levels of BP and increased risk of hypertension with increasing alcohol intake. Moreover, in both normotensive and hypertensive Japanese drinkers, following a 4-week period of moderation of alcohol intake, BP levels decreased more markedly in those who initially had the highest γGT levels.[111]

Why γGT should be an independent predictor for alcohol-related hypertension, hypertriglyceridemia and other elements of the metabolic syndrome,[112,113] type 2 diabetes mellitus,[114] coronary artery disease,[115] and stroke[116,117] is unknown. It is clearly more than just a reflection of underlying hepatic damage or induction of the enzyme by alcohol (the commonly accepted explanations). γGT is a membrane-bound ectopeptidase that cleaves the glutamyl group from glutathione, the first step in the uptake of extracellular glutathione. Nitric oxide also increases intracellular glutathione levels in aortic endothelial cells through a pathway that is γGT dependent, and both nitric oxide and the glutathione cycle appear to be coordinately regulated.[118] Maintenance of intracellular glutathione levels is integral to redox homeostasis and an increase in γGT with chronic alcohol ingestion may be a marker for those participants who develop increased oxidative stress and/or nitric oxide depletion with alcohol. Such oxidative stress may be an important pathogenic mechanism for the subsequent development of hypertension[119] and atherosclerosis.[120,121] γGT has also been shown, at least in T lymphocytes,[122] to control the rate of nitric oxide production from the naturally occurring nitrosothiol, S-nitrosoglutathione, a mechanism that may markedly affect the physiologic response to this compound. This suggests an additional mechanism of the pathogenesis of alcohol-related hypertension.

## GENE-ENVIRONMENT INTERACTIONS

Particularly in Japanese subjects, a point mutation with a G to A substitution at −357 of the promoter region of the gene coding for the aldehyde dehydrogenase isozyme, ALDH2, leads to a deficiency in metabolism of the major metabolite of ethanol, acetaldehyde. This ALDH*2/2 genotype results in high levels of acetaldehyde after drinking, leading to acute increases in the pulse rate, facial flushing, and decreases in BP.[123] A role for this polymorphism in the pathogenesis of alcohol-induced hypertension has been investigated in several Japanese studies.[124-127] The first examined a large cohort of 4000 male participants, and found that those with the ALDH*2/2 genotype consumed less alcohol and as a result were significantly less likely to have hypertension.[124] A similar conclusion was drawn in 2 smaller studies in middle-aged men where influences of the mutant gene on drinking behavior also confounded the results.[125,126] A recent study that included only participants who consumed >300 g per week[127] has suggested a significantly higher odds ratio for higher SBP in those with the ALDH*2/2 genotype, even after adjustment for alcohol consumption, as well as for other potential demographic and lifestyle confounders.

In high alcohol consumers, metabolism of ethanol via the mitochondrial cytochrome P450 oxidase is an important metabolic pathway. Investigation of a polymorphism of CYP2E1, the c2 allele, has suggested that this mutation predisposes to higher BP, possibly as a consequence of higher acetaldehyde levels.[126] Polymorphisms of another important alcohol-metabolizing enzyme, alcohol dehydrogenase, have not yet been widely evaluated in relation to the alcohol–BP relationship. An alcohol dehydrogenase type 2 polymorphism did not predict risk of alcohol-related hypertension in a Japanese study.[126] Among men in the Physicians' Health Study,[128] slow metabolism of alcohol due to presence of an alcohol dehydrogenase type 3 polymorphism was associated with decreased risk of myocardial infarction (MI), probably because of higher HDL-cholesterol levels, but the implications of this polymorphism for alcohol-related hypertension were not reported. Apolipoprotein E polymorphisms have also been investigated as determinants of alcohol-related hypertension.[129] The E2/E3 and E3/E3 genotypes were identified with stronger alcohol—BP relationships than E4/E3 genotypes in Finnish participants. However, in an intervention study, we found no relationship between the apolipoprotein E genotype and the magnitude of the reductions in BP with alcohol restriction.[130]

## ALCOHOL AND HYPERTENSIVE TARGET-ORGAN DISEASE

In contrast to its tendency to increase BP, regular consumption of alcohol is associated with a decreased risk for coronary artery disease, as shown in a recent meta-analysis.[131] A J-shaped curve was observed with its nadir at 20 g ethanol per day, where the mean decrease in relative risk was approximately 20%. This protective effect was lost at the level of 72 g/day, and at intakes greater than 89 g/day there was a mean 5% increase in relative coronary risk. A putative antiatherosclerotic effect of alcohol has been supported by the observation that light regular alcohol consumption decreases the incidence of atherosclerotic peripheral vascular[132,133] and renal vascular disease.[134] These protective effects may be related to alcohol-induced increases in high-density lipoprotein cholesterol (HDL-C) and its major apolipoproteins A-I and A-II,[135] decreases in fibrinogen levels,[136] and reductions in platelet adhesiveness.[137] Loss of these protective effects and the increase in cardiovascular risk with heavy alcohol consumption may reflect the influence of alcohol-related hypertension, as well as increases in triglyceride and plasma homocysteine levels and increased risk of cardiac arrhythmias and sudden cardiovascular death. When data from the Honolulu Heart Program[138] were subjected to statistical modeling, estimates indicated that while 50% of the decrease in coronary risk with alcohol could be attributed to the increase in HDL-C, there was a corresponding 17% increase in risk due to higher SBP.

A comprehensive systematic review of the association between alcohol and stroke included 41 studies where careful categorization of the type of stroke and amount of alcohol consumed had been performed.[139] For ischemic stroke, the authors observed a J-shaped relationship similar to that reported for coronary heart disease events. The evidence linking light to moderate alcohol consumption with a reduction in risk was thought to be inconsistent, while that linking increased consumption, especially recent consumption and binge drinking,[140] to increased risk of both ischemic and hemorrhagic

stroke was considered strong. Alcohol-induced hypertension may be in the causal pathway for this increase in stroke risk, although in some reports the increase in risk has persisted after adjustment for BP.[141] In a Japanese study,[142] heavy drinking acted synergistically with hypertension to increase the risk of cerebral hemorrhage and infarction twofold and threefold, respectively. In contrast, in the Department of Health Hypertension Care Computing Project, including over 10,000 British patients attending a hypertension clinic,[143] there was a 40% decrease in relative risk of stroke in drinkers, with the lowest risk of stroke mortality at intakes of 1 to 10 units (8 to 80 g alcohol) per week. This population included few heavy drinkers and the beneficial effects of alcohol were offset at intakes >21 units/wk by an increasing incidence of noncirculatory causes of death.

Alcohol consumption has been associated with increased echocardiographically determined left ventricular mass[144,145] and electrocardiographic evidence of left ventricular hypertrophy.[146] These associations have persisted after controlling for BP, suggesting that direct trophic effects of ethanol on the myocardium may be a more important determinant than alcohol-related hypertension. Such hypertrophic changes are a feature of the alcoholic cardiomyopathy characteristic of prolonged heavy alcohol abuse. In contrast, recent large population-based studies have emphasized the protective effects of light to moderate consumption of alcohol against heart failure. In the Framingham Heart Study[147] there was an approximate halving of the hazard ratio for congestive heart failure among men who consumed 8 to 14 drinks/wk and women who consumed 3 to 7 drinks/wk compared with those who consumed less than 1 drink/wk. A prospective cohort study of elderly participants showed a similar halving of the relative risk for heart failure among moderate drinkers,[148] while in the Studies of Left Ventricular Dysfunction (SOLVD), among patients with established ischemic left ventricular dysfunction, light-to-moderate alcohol consumption was independently associated with a reduced risk of all-cause mortality, particularly for death from MI.

Effects of alcohol on the kidney have not been well characterized. Several reports suggest that heavy alcohol use can increase the risk of microalbuminuria,[145,149] an effect that in at least one of these studies appeared to be mediated by alcohol-related hypertension.[145] In a case control study in Maryland,[150] the finding of an increased risk of end-stage renal disease with increasing alcohol intake was independent of any effects of alcohol on hypertension. Results from postmortem studies in the Honolulu Heart Program[134] indicate that alcohol intake is negatively associated with the degree of renal arteriolar hyalinization, suggesting that effects of alcohol to reduce the risk of intrarenal atherosclerotic vascular disease may counteract any potential for hypertensive nephrosclerosis due to alcohol-related hypertension.

## PUBLIC HEALTH IMPLICATIONS AND RECOMMENDATIONS

The importance of the relation between alcohol consumption and hypertension has been recognized in national and international guidelines on the prevention and management of hypertension.[151-153] However, from the point of view of cardiovascular disease, alcohol is a two-edged sword. Despite predisposing to

BP elevation, regular mild-to-moderate drinking appears to protect against coronary events, and possibly ischemic stroke, while higher-level consumption increases the risk of hemorrhagic and ischemic stroke, cardiac arrhythmias, and sudden cardiovascular death.[154] The "benefits" in this equation are less in populations with a low risk of atherosclerosis. Heavier drinking is also a significant factor in resistance to antihypertensive drug therapy and alcohol-related cardiomyopathy. From the point of view of cardiovascular risk, an intake averaging 1 to 2 standard drinks a day in men and up to 1 a day in women seems optimal for those who can control drinking habits. Binge drinking appears to carry a particular risk for several cardiovascular outcomes. Outstanding issues include possible mechanisms for alcohol-related hypertension, gender differences, effects on endothelial function, and the relation between moderate alcohol consumption, diabetes, and congestive cardiac failure. Because alcohol may contribute to hypertension in up to 30% of heavier drinkers and because heavy and binge drinking increase the risk of stroke in particular, the potential for prevention by moderation of consumption should be a major medical and public health priority.

# References

1. Lian C. L'alcoolisme, cause d'hypertension arterielle. Bull Acad Med 74:525-528, 1915.
2. Gruntzig A, Blohmke M, Depner R, et al. Alcohol consumption and social, physiological and medical data. Quart J Stud Alc 33:283, 1972.
3. Ashley MJ, Rankin JG. Alcohol consumption and hypertension: the evidence from hazardous drinking and alcoholic populations. Aust NZ J Med 9:201-206, 1979.
4. Saunders J, Beevers D, Paton A. Alcohol-induced hypertension. Lancet ii:653-656, 1981.
5. Beevers DG. Alcohol and hypertension. Lancet ii:114-115, 1977.
6. Ramsay L. Alcohol and hypertension. Lancet ii:300, 1977.
7. Henningsen NC, Ohlsson O, Mattiasson I, et al. Hypertension, levels of serum gamma glutamyl transpeptidase and degree of blood pressure control in middle-aged males. Acta Med Scand 207:245-251, 1980.
8. Matthews JD. Alcohol use as a possible explanation for socioeconomic and occupational differentials in mortality from hypertension and coronary heart disease in England and Wales. Aust NZ J Med 6:393-397. 1976.
9. Klatsky A, Friedman G, Siegelaub A, et al. Alcohol consumption and blood pressure: Kaiser-Permanente Multiphasic Health Examination Data. N Engl J Med 296:1194-1200, 1977.
10. Arkwright PD, Beilin LJ, Rouse I, et al. Effects of alcohol use and other aspects of lifestyle on blood pressure levels and prevalence of hypertension in a working population. Circulation 66:60-66, 1982.
11. Klag MJ, He J, Whelton PK, et al. Alcohol use and blood pressure in an unacculturated society. Hypertension 22:365-70, 1993.
12. Krogh V, Trevisan M, Jossa F, et al. Alcohol and blood pressure. The effect of age, findings from the Italian Nine Communities Study. Ann Epidemiol 3:245-249, 1993.
13. Burke V, Milligan RA, Beilin LJ, Dunbar D, Spencer M, Balde E, Gracey MP. Clustering of health-related behaviors among 18-year-old Australians. Prev Med 26:724-733, 1997.
14. Cairns V, Keil U, Kleinbaum D, et al. Alcohol consumption as a risk factor for high blood pressure. Munich Blood Pressure Study. Hypertension 6:124-131, 1984.
15. Keil U, Chambless L, Filipiak B, et al. Alcohol and blood pressure and its interaction with smoking and other behavioural variables: results from the MONICA Augsburg Survey 1984-1985. J Hypertens 9:491-498, 1991.
16. Cooke K, Frost G, Stokes G. Blood pressure and its relationship to low levels of alcohol consumption. Clin Exp Pharmacol Physiol 10:229-233, 1983.
17. Milon H, Froment A, Gaspard P, et al. Alcohol consumption and blood pressure in a French epidemiological study. Eur Heart J 3(Suppl C):59-64, 1982.
18. Dyer A, Cutter G, Liu K, et al. Alcohol intake and blood pressure in young adults: The Cardia Study. J Clin Epidemiol 43: 1-13, 1990.
19. Palatini P. Factors affecting the daily variation of blood pressure. The HARVEST study. Cardiovasc Risk Factors 7:206-213, 1997.
20. Ueshima H, Shimamoto T, Iida M, et al. Alcohol intake and hypertension among urban and rural Japanese populations. J Chron Dis 37:585-592, 1984.
21. Lang T, Degoulet P, Aime F, et al. Relationship between alcohol consumption and hypertension prevalence and control in a French population. J Chron Dis 40:713-720, 1987.
22. Trevisan M, Krogh V, Farinaro E, et al. Alcohol consumption, drinking pattern and blood pressure: analysis of data from the Italian National Research Council Study. Int J Epidemiol 16:520-527, 1987.
23. Keil U, Chambless L, Remmers A. Alcohol and blood pressure: results from the Luebeck blood pressure study. Prev Med 18: 1-10, 1989.
24. Cairns V, Keil U, Kleinbaum D, et al. Alcohol consumption as a risk factor for high blood pressure - Munich Blood Pressure Study. Hypertension 6:124-131, 1984.
25. Criqui MH, Wallace RB, Mishkel M, et al. Alcohol consumption and blood pressure. The Lipid Research Clinics Prevalence Study. Hypertension 3:557-565, 1981.
26. Marques-Vidal P, Montaye M, Haas B, et al. Relationships between alcoholic beverages and cardiovascular risk factor levels in middle-aged men, the PRIME study. Atherosclerosis 157:431-440, 2001.
27. Tjonneland A, Gronbaek M, Stripp C, et al. Wine intake and diet in a random sample of 48763 Danish men and women. Am J Clin Nutr 69:49-54, 1999.
28. Corrao G, Bagnardi V, Zambon A, et al. Exploring the dose-response relationship between alcohol consumption and the risk of several alcohol-related conditions: a meta-analysis. Addiction 94:1551-1573, 1999.
29. Nakanishi N, Yoshida H, Nakamura K, et al. Alcohol consumption and risk for hypertension in middle-aged Japanese men. J Hypertens 19:851-855, 2001.
30. Tsuruta M, Adachi H, Hirai Y, et al. Association between alcohol intake and development of hypertension in Japanese normotensive men: 12-year follow-up study. Am J Hypertens 13: 482-487, 2000.
31. Okubo Y, Suwazono Y, Kobayashi E, et al. Alcohol consumption and blood pressure change: 5-year follow-up study of the association in normotensive workers. J Hum Hypertens 15: 367-372, 2001.
32. Fuchs FD, Chambless LE, Whelton PK, et al. Alcohol consumption and the incidence of hypertension: The Atherosclerosis Risk in Communities Study. Hypertension 37:1242-1250, 2001.
33. Henriksson KM, Lindblad U, Gullberg B, et al. Development of hypertension over 6 years in a birth cohort of young middle-aged men: the Cardiovascular Risk Factor Study in southern Sweden (CRISS). J Intern Med 252:21-26, 2002.
34. Gordon T, Kannel W. Drinking and its relation to smoking, BP, blood lipids, and uric acid - The Framingham Study. Arch Int Med 143:1366-1374, 1983.
35. Gordon T, Doyle JT. Alcohol consumption and its relationship to smoking, weight, blood pressure, and blood lipids. The Albany Study. Arch Int Med 146:262-265, 1986.
36. Curtis AB, James SA, Strogatz DS, et al. Alcohol consumption and changes in blood pressure among African Americans : The Pitt County Study. Am J Epidemiol 146:727-733, 1997.

37. Cooke KM, Frost GW, Stokes GS. Blood pressure and its relationship to low levels of alcohol consumption. Clin Exp Pharmacol Physiol 10:229-233, 1983.

38. Moreira LB, Fuchs FD, Moraes RS, et al. Alcohol intake and blood pressure: the importance of time elapsed since last drink. J Hypertens 16:175-180, 1998.

39. Wallace R, Barrett-Connor E, Criqui M, et al. Alteration in blood pressures associated with combined alcohol and oral contraceptive use - The Lipid Research Clinics Prevalence Study. J Chron Dis 35:251-257, 1982.

40. Harburg E, Ozgoren F, Hawthorne V, et al. Community norms of alcohol usage and blood pressure: Tecumseh, Michigan. Am J Pub Health 70:813-820, 1980.

41. Holman CDJ, English DR, Milne E, et al. Meta-analysis of alcohol and all-cause mortality: A validation of NHMRC recommendations. Med J Aust 164:141-145, 1996.

42. Laforge R, Williams GD, Dufour MC. Alcohol consumption, gender and self-reported hypertension. Drug Alcohol Depend 26:235-249, 1990.

43. Nanchahal K, Ashton WD, Wood DAE. Alcohol consumption, metabolic cardiovascular risk factors and hypertension in women. Int J Epidemiol 29:57-64, 2000.

44. Hajjar IM, Grim CE, George V, et al. Impact of diet on blood pressure and age-related changes in blood pressure in the US population: analysis of NHANES III. Arch Int Med 161:589-593, 2001.

45. Murray RP, Connett JE, Tyas SL, et al. Alcohol volume, drinking pattern, and cardiovascular disease morbidity and mortality: Is there a U-shaped function? Am J Epidemiol 155:242-248, 2002.

46. Thadhani R, Camargo CA Jr, Stampfer MJ, et al. Prospective study of moderate alcohol consumption and risk of hypertension in young women. Arch Int Med 162:569-574, 2002.

47. Puddey IB, Beilin LJ, Vandongen R, et al. Evidence for a direct effect of alcohol consumption on blood pressure in normotensive men. A randomized controlled trial. Hypertension 7:707-713, 1985.

48. Ueshima H, Mikawa K, Baba S, et al. Effect of reduced alcohol consumption on blood pressure in untreated hypertensive men. Hypertension 21:248-252, 1993.

49. Puddey IB, Beilin LJ, Vandongen R. Regular alcohol use raises blood pressure in treated hypertensive subjects. A randomised controlled trial. Lancet 1:647-651, 1987.

50. Xin X, He J, Frontini MG, et al. Effects of alcohol reduction on blood pressure: a meta-analysis of randomized controlled trials. Hypertension 38:1112-1117, 2001.

51. Rakic V, Puddey IB, Burke V, et al. Influence of pattern of alcohol intake on blood pressure in regular drinkers: A controlled trial. J Hypertens 16:165-174, 1998.

52. Marmot MG, Shipley MJ, Elliott P, et al. Alcohol and blood pressure: The INTERSALT study. Br Med J 308:1263-1267, 1994.

53. Cushman WC, Cutler JA, Hanna E, et al. Prevention and Treatment of Hypertension Study (PATHS): Effects of an alcohol treatment program on blood pressure. Arch Int Med 158:1197-207, 1998.

54. Lang T, Nicaud V, Darne B, et al. Improving hypertension control among excessive alcohol drinkers: a randomised controlled trial in France. J Epidemiol Comm Health 49:610-616, 1995.

55. Maheswaran R, Beevers M, Beevers DG. Effectiveness of advice to reduce alcohol consumption in hypertensive patients. Hypertension 19:79-84, 1992.

56. Puddey IB, Parker M, Beilin LJ, et al. Effects of alcohol and caloric restrictions on blood pressure and serum lipids in overweight men. Hypertension 20:533-541, 1992.

57. Parker M, Puddey IB, Beilin LJ, et al. Two-way factorial study of alcohol and salt restriction in treated hypertensive men. Hypertension 16:398-406, 1990.

58. Cox KL, Puddey IB, Morton AR, et al. The combined effects of aerobic exercise and alcohol restriction on blood pressure and serum lipids: A two-way factorial study in sedentary men. J Hypertens 11:191-201, 1993.

59. Hartung GH, Kohl HW, Blair SN, et al. Exercise tolerance and alcohol intake. Blood pressure relation. Hypertension 16:501-507, 1990.

60. Abe H, Kawano Y, Kojima S, et al. Biphasic effects of repeated alcohol intake on 24-hour blood pressure in hypertensive patients. Circulation 89:2626-2628, 1994.

61. Kawano Y, Pontes CS, Abe H, et al. Effects of alcohol consumption and restriction on home blood pressure in hypertensive patients: Serial changes in the morning and evening records. Clin Exp Hypertens 24:33-39, 2002.

62. Khetarpal V, Volicer L. Effects of ethanol on blood pressure of normal and hypertensive rats. J Stud Alcohol 40(7):732-736, 1979.

63. Chan TC, Sutter MC. The effects of chronic ethanol consumption on cardiac function. Can J Physiol Pharmacol 60:777-782, 1982.

64. Chan TC, Sutter MC. Ethanol consumption and blood pressure. Life Sci 33:1965-1973, 1983.

65. Chan TC, Godin DV, Sutter MC. Erythrocyte membrane properties of the chronic alcoholic rat. Drug Alcohol Depend 12:249-257, 1983.

66. Puddey IB, Burke V, Croft K, et al. Increased blood pressure and changes in membrane lipids associated with chronic ethanol treatment of rats. Clin Exp Pharmacol Physiol 22:655-657, 1995.

67. Vasdev S, Sampson CA, Prabhakaran VM. Platelet-free calcium and vascular calcium uptake in ehtanol-induced hypertensive rats. Hypertension 18:116-122, 1991.

68. Vasdev S, Gupta IP, Sampson CA, et al. Ethanol induced hypertension in rats: reversibility and role of intracellular cytosolic calcium. Artery 20:19-43, 1993.

69. Vasdev S, Mian T, Longerich L, et al. N-acetyl cysteine attenuates ethanol induced hypertension in rats. Artery 21:312-336, 1995.

70. Vasdev S, Wadhawan S, Ford CA, et al. Dietary vitamin B6 supplementation prevents ethanol-induced hypertension in rats. Nutr Metab Cardiovasc Dis 9:55-63, 1999.

71. Hsieh ST, Sano H, Saito K, et al. Magnesium supplementation prevents the development of alcohol-induced hypertension. Hypertension 19:175-182, 1992.

72. Chan TC, Wall RA, Sutter MC. Chronic ethanol consumption, stress, and hypertension. Hypertension 7:519-524, 1985.

73. Abdel-Rahman A-RA, Dar MS, Wooles WR. Effect of chronic ethanol administration on arterial baroreceptor function and pressor and depressor responsiveness in rats. J Pharmacol Exp Ther 232:194-201, 1984.

74. Abdel-Rahman AA, Wooles WR. Ethanol-induced hypertension involves impairment of baroreceptors. Hypertension 10:67-73, 1987.

75. Sanderson JE, Jones JV, Graham DI. Effect of chronic alcohol ingestion on the heart and blood pressure of spontaneously hypertensive rats. Clin Exp Hypertens 5:673-689, 1983.

76. Howe PRC, Rogers PF, Smith RM. Effects of chronic alcohol consumption and alcohol withdrawal on blood pressure in stroke-prone spontaneously hypertensive rats. J Hypertens 7:387-393, 1989.

77. Howe PR, Rogers PF, Smith RM. Antihypertensive effect of alcohol in spontaneously hypertensive rats. Hypertension 13:607-611, 1989.

78. Beilin LJ, Hoffmann P, Nilsson H, et al. Effect of chronic ethanol consumption upon cardiovascular reactivity, heart rate and blood pressure in spontaneously hypertensive and Wistar-Kyoto rats. J Hypertens 10:645-650, 1992.

79. Hatton DC, Bukoski RD, Edgar S, et al. Chronic alcohol consumption lowers blood pressure but enhances vascular contractility in Wistar rats. J Hypertens 10:529-537, 1992.

80. Jones JV, Raine AEG, Sanderson JE, et al. Adverse effect of chronic alcohol ingestion on cardiac performance in spontaneously hypertensive rats. J Hypertens 6:419-422, 1988.

81. Ren J, Brown RA. Hypertension augments ethanol-induced depression of cell shortening and intracellular Ca(2+) transients in adult rat ventricular myocytes. Biochem Biophys Res Commun 261:202-208, 1999.

82. Crandall DL, Ferraro GD, Lozito RJ, et al. Cardiovascular effects of intermittent drinking: assessment of a novel animal model of human alcoholism. J Hypertens 7:683-687, 1989.

83. el-Mas MM, Abdel-Rahman A-RA. Sexually dimorphic hemodynamic effects of intragastric ethanol in conscious rats. Clin Exp Hypertens 21:1429-1445, 1999.

84. El Mas MM, Abdel-Rahman AA. Estrogen-dependent hypotensive effects of ethanol in conscious female rats. Alcohol Clin Exp Res 23:624-632, 1999.

85. Potter JF, Beevers DG. Two possible mechanisms for alcohol associated hypertension. Scand J Lab Clin Med 45:92-99, 1985.

86. Maheswaran R, Gill JS, Beevers DG. The effect of alcohol on blood pressure is due to recent alcohol intake. Clin Sci 72:70P, 1987.

87. Wannamethee G, Shaper AG. Alcohol intake and variations in blood pressure by day of examination. J Human Hypertens 5:59-67, 1991.

88. Marques-Vidal P, Arveiler D, Evans A, et al. Different alcohol drinking and blood pressure relationships in France and Northern Ireland: The PRIME Study. Hypertension 38:1361-1366, 2001.

89. Puddey IB, Rakic V, Dimmitt SB, et al. Influence of pattern of drinking on cardiovascular disease and cardiovascular risk factors: A review. Addiction 94:649-63, 1999.

90. Puddey IB, Jenner DA, Beilin LJ, et al. An appraisal of the effects of usual vs recent alcohol intake on blood pressure. Clin Exp Pharmacol Physiol 15:261-264, 1988.

91. Seppa K, Laippala P, Sillanaukee P. Drinking pattern and blood pressure. Am J Hypertens 7:249-254, 1994.

92. Arkwright PD, Beilin LJ, Vandongen R, et al. The pressor effect of moderate alcohol consumption in man: a search for mechanisms. Circulation 66:515-519, 1982.

93. Grassi GM, Somers VK, Renk WS, et al. Effects of alcohol intake on blood pressure and sympathetic nerve activity in normotensive humans: a preliminary report. J Hypertens 7:S20-S21, 1989.

94. Puddey IB, Jenner DA, Beilin LJ, et al. Alcohol consumption, age and personality characteristics as important determinants of within-subject variability in blood pressure. J Hypertens 6:S617-S619, 1988.

95. Abdel-Rahman A-RA, Merrill RH, Wooles WR. Effect of acute ethanol administration on the baroreceptor reflex control of heart rate in normotensive human volunteers. Clin Sci 72:113-122, 1987.

96. Smals AG, Njo KT, Knoben JM, et al. Alcohol-induced Cushingoid syndrome. J Roy Coll Phys Lond 12:36-41, 1977.

97. Mori TA, Puddey IB, Wilkinson SP, et al. Urinary steroid profiles and alcohol-related blood pressure elevation. Clin Exp Pharmacol Physiol 18:287-290, 1991.

98. Howes LG, Reid JL. Changes in blood pressure and vascular reactivity in normotensives following regular alcohol consumption. J Hypertens 3(Suppl 3):S443-S445, 1985.

99. Puddey IB, Vandongen R, Beilin LJ, et al. Alcohol stimulation of renin release in man: its relation to the hemodynamic, electrolyte, and sympatho-adrenal responses to drinking. J Clin Endocrinol Metab 61:37-42, 1985.

100. Howes LG, Reid JL. The effects of alcohol on local, neural and humoral cardiovascular regulation. Clin Sci 71:9-15, 1986.

101. Puddey IB, Zilkens RR, Croft KD, et al. Alcohol and endothelial function: a brief review. Clin Exp Pharmacol Physiol 28:1020-1024, 2001.

102. Maiorano G, Bartolomucci F, Contursi V, et al. Noninvasive detection of vascular dysfunction in alcoholic patients. Am J Hypertens 12:137-144, 1999.

103. Teragawa H, Fukuda Y, Matsuda K, et al. Effect of alcohol consumption on endothelial function in men with coronary artery disease. Atherosclerosis 165:145, 2002.

104. Zilkens RR, Burke V, Beilin LJ, et al. The effect of alcohol intake on endothelial function: A randomized controlled trial in men. J Hypertens 21:97-103, 2003.

105. Knych ET. Endothelium-dependent tolerance to ethanol-induced contraction of rat aorta: Effect of inhibition of EDRF action and nitric oxide synthesis. Alcohol Clin Exp Res 16:58-63, 1992.

106. Mahmud A, Feely J. Divergent effect of acute and chronic alcohol on arterial stiffness. Am J Hypertens 15:240-243, 2002.

107. Henningsen NC, Janzon L, Trell E. Influence of carboxyhemoglobin, gamma-glutamyl-transferase, body weight, and heart rate on blood pressure in middle-aged men. Hypertension 5:560-563, 1983.

108. Nilssen O, Forde OH. Seven-year longitudinal population study of change in gamma-glutamyltransferase: The Tromso Study. Am J Epidemiol 139:787-192, 1994.

109. Yamada Y, Ishizaki M, Kido T, et al. Alcohol, high blood pressure and serum gamma-glutamyl transpeptidase level. Hypertension 18:819-826, 1991.

110. Lee DH, Ha MH, Kim JR, Gross M, Jacobs DR, Jr. Gamma-glutamyltransferase, alcohol, and blood pressure. A four year follow-up study. Ann Epidemiol 12:90-96, 2002.

111. Yamada Y, Tsuritani I, Ishizaki M, et al. Serum gamma-glutamyl transferase levels and blood pressure falls after alcohol moderation. Clin Exp Hypertens 19:249-268, 1997.

112. Cucuianu M. Serum gamma-glutamyltransferase and/or serum cholinesterase as markers of the metabolic syndrome. Diab Care 22:1381-1382, 1999.

113. Hashimoto Y, Futamura A, Nakarai H, Nakahara K. Relationship between response of gamma-glutamyl transpeptidase to alcohol drinking and risk factors for coronary heart disease. Atherosclerosis 158:465-470, 2001.

114. Perry IJ, Wannamethee SG, Shaper AG. Prospective study of serum gamma-glutamyltransferase and risk of NIDDM. Diab Care 21:732-737, 1998.

115. Jousilahti P, Vartiainen E, Alho H, et al. Opposite associations of carbohydrate-deficient transferrin and gamma-glutamyl-transferase with prevalent coronary heart disease. Arch Int Med 162:817-821, 2002.

116. Jousilahti P, Rastenyte D, Tuomilehto J. Serum gamma-glutamyl transferase, self-reported alcohol drinking, and the risk of stroke. Stroke 31:1851-1855, 2000.

117. Emdin M, Passino C, Donato L, et al. Serum gamma-glutamyl-transferase as a risk factor of ischemic stroke might be independent of alcohol consumption. Stroke 33:1163-1164, 2002.

118. Moellering D, Mc AJ, Patel RP, et al. The induction of GSH synthesis by nanomolar concentrations of NO in endothelial cells: a role for gamma-glutamylcysteine synthetase and gamma-glutamyl transpeptidase. FEBS Lett 448:292-296, 1999.

119. Romero JC, Reckelhoff JF. State-of-the-Art lecture. Role of angiotensin and oxidative stress in essential hypertension. Hypertension 34:943-949, 1999.

120. Puddey IB, Croft K. Alcoholic beverages and lipid peroxidation: Relevance to cardiovascular disease. Addict Biol 2:269-276, 1997.

121. Croft KD, Puddey IB, Rakic V, et al. Oxidative susceptibility of low-density lipoproteins: Influence of regular alcohol use. Alcohol Clin Exp Res 20:980-984, 1996.

122. Henson SE, Nichols TC, Holers VM, et al. The ectoenzyme gamma-glutamyl transpeptidase regulates antiproliferative effects of S-nitrosoglutathione on human T and B lymphocytes. J Immunol 163:1845-1852, 1999.

123. Minami J, Todoroki M, Yamamoto H, et al. Effects of alcohol intake on ambulatory blood pressure, heart rate and heart rate variability in Japanese men with different ALDH2 genotypes. J Human Hypertens 16:345-351, 2002.

124. Takagi S, Baba S, Iwai N, et al. The aldehyde dehydrogenase 2 gene is a risk factor for hypertension in Japanese but does not alter the sensitivity to pressor effects of alcohol: The Suita study. Hypertens Res 24:365-370, 2001.

125. Tsuritani I, Ikai E, Date T, et al. Polymorphism in ALDH2-genotype in Japanese men and the alcohol-blood pressure relationship. Am J Hypertens 8:1053-1059, 1995.

126. Yamada Y, Sun F, Tsuritani I, et al. Genetic differences in ethanol metabolizing enzymes and blood pressure in Japanese alcohol consumers. J Human Hypertens 16:479-486, 2002.

127. Hashimoto Y, Nakayama T, Futamura A, et al. Relationship between genetic polymorphisms of alcohol-metabolizing enzymes and changes in risk factors for coronary heart disease associated with alcohol consumption. Clin Chem 48:1043-1048, 2002.

128. Hines LM, Stampfer MJ, Ma J, et al. Genetic variation in alcohol dehydrogenase and the beneficial effect of moderate alcohol consumption on myocardial infarction. N Engl J Med 344:549-555, 2001.

129. Kauma H, Savolainen MJ, Rantala AO, et al. Apolipoprotein E phenotype determines the effect of alcohol on blood pressure in middle-aged men. Am J Hypertens 11:1334-1343, 1998.

130. Puddey IB, Rakic V, Dimmitt SB, et al. Apolipoprotein E genotype and the blood pressure raising effect of alcohol. Am J Hypertens 12:946-947, 1999.

131. Corrao G, Rubbiati L, Bagnardi V, et al. Alcohol and coronary heart disease: a meta-analysis. Addiction 95:1505-1523, 2000.

132. Djousse L, Levy D, Murabito JM, et al. Alcohol consumption and risk of intermittent claudication in the Framingham Heart Study. Circulation 102:3092-3097, 2000.

133. Mingardi R, Avogaro A, Noventa F, et al. Alcohol intake is associated with a lower prevalence of peripheral vascular disease in non-insulin dependent diabetic women. Diabetologia 38:A268, 1995.

134. Burchfiel CM, Tracy RE, Chyou PH, et al. Cardiovascular risk factors and hyalinization of renal arterioles at autopsy: The Honolulu Heart Program. Arterioscler Thromb Vasc Biol 17:760-768, 1997.

135. Masarei JR, Puddey IB, Rouse IL, et al. Effects of alcohol consumption on serum lipoprotein-lipid and apolipoprotein concentrations. Results from an intervention study in healthy subjects. Atherosclerosis 60:79-87, 1986.

136. Dimmitt SB, Rakic V, Puddey IB, et al. The effects of alcohol on coagulation and fibrinolytic factors: A controlled trial. Blood Coagul Fibrinolysis 9:39-45, 1998.

137. Renaud SC, Beswick AD, Fehily AM, et al. Alcohol and platelet aggregation: the Caerphilly Prospective Heart Disease Study. Am J Clin Nutr 55:1012-1017, 1992.

138. Langer RD, Criqui MH, Reed DM. Lipoproteins and blood pressure as biological pathways for effect of moderate alcohol consumption on coronary heart disease. Circulation 85:910-915, 1992.

139. Mazzaglia G, Britton AR, Altmann DR, et al. Exploring the relationship between alcohol consumption and non-fatal or fatal stroke: a systematic review. Addiction 96:1743-1756, 2001.

140. Hansagi H, Romelsjo A, Gerhardsson de Verdier M, et al. Alcohol consumption and stroke mortality. 20-year follow-up of 15,077 men and women. Stroke 26:1768-1773, 1995.

141. Gill JS, Shipley MJ, Tsementzis SA, et al. Alcohol consumption: A risk factor for hemorrhagic and non-hemorrhagic stroke. Am J Med 90:489-497, 1991.

142. Kiyohara Y, Kato I, Iwamoto H, et al. The impact of alcohol and hypertension on stroke incidence in a general Japanese population. The Hisayama Study. Stroke 26:368-372, 1995.

143. Palmer AJ, Fletcher AE, Bulpitt CJ, et al. Alcohol intake and cardiovascular mortality in hypertensive patients: report from the Department of Health Hypertension Care Computing Project. J Hypertens 13:957-964, 1995.

144. Manolio TA, Levy D, Garrison RJ, et al. Relation of alcohol intake to left ventricular mass: The Framingham Study. J Am Coll Cardiol 17:717-721, 1991.

145. Vriz O, Piccolo D, Cozzutti E, et al. The effects of alcohol consumption on ambulatory blood pressure and target organs in subjects with borderline to mild hypertension. Am J Hypertens 11:230-234, 1998.

146. Ishimitsu T, Yoshida K, Nakamura M, et al. Effects of alcohol intake on organ injuries in normotensive and hypertensive human subjects. Clin Sci 93:541-547, 1997.

147. Walsh CR, Larson MG, Evans JC, et al. Alcohol consumption and risk for congestive heart failure in the Framingham Heart Study. Ann Int Med ALC2009:181-191, 2002.

148. Abramson JL, Williams SA, Krumholz HM, et al. Moderate alcohol consumption and risk of heart failure among older persons. JAMA 285:1971-1977, 2001.

149. Klein R, Klein BE, Moss SE. Prevalence of microalbuminuria in older-onset diabetes. Diab Care 16:1325-1330, 1993.

150. Perneger TV, Whelton PK, Puddey IB, et al. Risk of end-stage renal disease associated with alcohol consumption. Am J Epidemiol 150:1275-1281, 1999.

151. Campbell NR, Burgess E, Choi BC, et al. Lifestyle modifications to prevent and control hypertension. 1. Methods and an overview of the Canadian recommendations. Canadian Hypertension Society, Canadian Coalition for High Blood Pressure Prevention and Control, Laboratory Centre for Disease Control at Health Canada, Heart and Stroke Foundation of Canada. CMAJ 160:S1-S6, 1999.

152. WHO-ISH Liaison Committee. 1999 World Health Organization : International Society of Hypertension Guidelines for the Management of Hypertension. J Hypertens 17:151-183, 1999.

153. Pearson TA, Blair SN, Daniels SR, et al. AHA Guidelines for primary prevention of cardiovascular disease and stroke: 2002 Update: consensus panel guide to comprehensive risk reduction for adult patients without coronary or other atherosclerotic vascular diseases. American Heart Association Science Advisory and Coordinating Committee. Circulation 106:388-391, 2002.

154. Beilin LJ, Puddey IB, Burke V. Alcohol and hypertension: Kill or cure. J Human Hypertens 10:S1-S5, 1996.

# Obesity in Hypertension: Role of Diet and Drugs

## Panagiotis Kokkoris, Xavier Pi-Sunyer

Obesity is very common in the United States. The prevalence of obesity and overweight has increased during the last decade. It is estimated that more than 100 million Americans are obese or overweight.[1] The Third National Health and Nutrition Examination Survey (NHANES III) reported that 59.4% of men and 50.7% of women are obese or overweight.[2]

It is known that obesity may lead to many serious disorders, including myocardial infarction, dyslipidemia, diabetes mellitus, gallbladder disease, osteoarthritis, sleep apnea, heart failure, stroke, end stage renal disease, and hypertension.[3-5] Hypertension is especially common among obese people. In addition, hypertensive patients have a higher incidence of obesity compared with normotensive people.[6] The Framingham Heart Study showed that obese individuals have a twofold increase in the prevalence of hypertension compared with normal weight individuals and that for every 10% increase in relative body weight there is an increase in systolic blood pressure (SBP) of 6.5 mm Hg.[7]

The pathogenesis of obesity-related hypertension is not completely understood. Hyperinsulinemia and insulin resistance, very common findings in obese patients, may be reasons for the rise in the blood pressure (BP). Hyperinsulinemia may cause hypertension through different mechanisms, such as increased sympathetic nervous system activity, increased renal sodium reabsorption, proliferation of the vascular smooth cells, and alterations in the renin-angiotensin-aldosterone (RAAS) system.[8-11]

Measurement of BP can be difficult in obese persons, so special care should be taken in this group of patients. A common error is use of a cuff that is too small, which gives a falsely high BP. The cuff must be wide enough to cover 80% of the circumference and 75% of the length of the upper arm. The patient should rest for about 5 minutes before the measurement and the final BP measurement should be the average of two or more readings in both the lateral and the contralateral arm.

It is important to know the total fat burden and the fat distribution of a patient for the management of BP elevation. A simple and relatively accurate way to estimate total fat burden is to calculate the body mass index (BMI), which is (weight in kg)/(height in m²) (Box 46–1). The BMI correlates fairly well with the degree of obesity except in very muscular individuals.[12] According to the World Health Organization, BMI of 18.5 to 24.9 kg/m² is defined as normal, 25 to 29.9 kg/m² as overweight, and more than 30 kg/m² as obese, with 30-34.5 kg/m² class I obesity, 35-39.9 kg/m² class II obesity, and more than 40 kg/m² class III or extreme obesity[13] (Table 46–1). Central fat distribution is also correlated with high BP. Central obesity can be evaluated by measuring the waist circumference or the waist:hip ratio (WHR). Waist circumference should be measured at the uppermost lateral border of the iliac crest. A waist circumference greater than 102 cm (40 inches) in men and 88 cm (35 inches) in women is considered abnormal and indicates increased risk for type 2 diabetes, hypertension, and cardiovascular disease (CVD). Waist circumference is especially useful in estimating the CVD risk in patients with a BMI between 25 and 34.9 kg/m², since patients with a BMI greater than 35 kg/m² are already at an increased risk.[1] A WHR greater than 1.0 in men and greater than 0.85 in women is considered abnormally high.

Weight loss has been associated with a decrease in BP in many studies. It is estimated that for every kg of weight loss there is a reduction of 0.45 mm Hg in both SBP and diastolic blood pressure (DBP).[14] Weight loss can be achieved with lifestyle interventions such as diet and exercise, with pharmacotherapy, and with surgery. The initial target of weight loss therapy should be the reduction of body weight by 10% to 15%. This weight loss goal, which can reasonably be achieved with a combination of lifestyle modification and drug therapy, is associated with significant improvement in BP. With weight loss, hypertensive patients may be able to discontinue antihypertensive medications.[15-17]

## OVERVIEW OF WEIGHT LOSS THERAPY

Before starting a weight loss program, a careful preliminary assessment has to be made. This should include the patient's usual diet, food preferences, and eating habits. Also, a history of previous weight loss attempts and the reason why they failed has to be taken. Losing weight is a difficult and time-consuming process, so the patient has to be appropriately motivated. Behavior modification is focused mainly on changing eating habits, increasing physical activity, altering attitude, and developing support systems.

Patient motivation is a prerequisite for achieving the target of weight loss. Motivation can be increased by describing to the patient the health risks of obesity. Some things that have to be considered before starting the weight loss procedure include the following:

1. How serious and determined to lose weight is the patient?
2. How well does the patient understand the dangers of being obese?
3. Can the patient's family and friends help him or her in the attempt to lose weight?
4. Is the patient prepared to start exercise along with diet therapy?
5. Does the patient have adequate time to spend in the attempt to lose weight?

It is very important for the patient to trust the physician or other health care provider involved in the weight loss process and for the physician to show respect and concern for the

**Box 46-1** Calculation of Body Mass Index (BMI)

**You Can Calculate BMI as Follows:**

$$BMI = \frac{weight\ (kg)}{height\ squared\ (m^2)}$$

If pounds and inches are used:

$$BMI = \frac{weight\ (pounds) \times 703}{height\ squared\ (inches^2)}$$

**Calculation Directions and Sample**
Here is a shortcut method for calculating BMI.
(Example: A person who is 5 feet 5 inches tall weighing 180 lbs.)
1. Multiply weight (in pounds) by 703
   $$180 \times 703 = 126{,}540$$
2. Multiply height (in inches) by height (in inches)
   $$65 \times 65 = 4225$$
3. Divide the answer in step 1 by the answer in step 2 to get the BMI
   $$126{,}540/4225 = 29.9$$
   $$BMI = 29.9$$

patient. This patient–physician partnership is basic for the success of the weight loss program.

First, the physician and the patient must set an achievable goal. Some patients set unrealistic goals (for example, to lose half of their weight). They must be counseled to set goals that are easier to achieve (to lose 10% of their initial weight in a certain period of time). If they achieve this goal and maintain it for a year, they can then set another goal to lose more weight.

The behavior of an obese patient has to be changed gradually, following reasonable steps. This program has to be individualized for each case. The first step is to determine what exactly has to be modified. Usually this requires the patient to self-monitor to allow him or her to understand his or her eating and activity patterns. For example, keeping records of food choices, food quantity, and times of meals helps both the patient and the physician to identify and correct what can be changed. The mood of the patient and its relation to the type and the amount of food can also be recorded in the same diary. Everyday physical activity and weight change should also be included in the diary.

The second step is to control stimuli that affect eating behavior. The patient learns how to identify situations that are

**Table 46-1** Classification of Obesity and Overweight by Body Mass Index (BMI)

| Classifications | BMI |
| --- | --- |
| Underweight | <18.5 kg/m$^2$ |
| Normal weight | 18.5-24.9 kg/m$^2$ |
| Overweight | 25-29.9 kg/m$^2$ |
| Obesity (Class I) | 30-34.9 kg/m$^2$ |
| Obesity (Class II) | 35-39.9 kg/m$^2$ |
| Extreme obesity (Class III) | ≥40 kg/m$^2$ |

associated with unnecessary eating, for example, periods of increased stress and anxiety. The specific stimulus has to be identified and the patient has to learn to stay away from it. For example, when a patient finds that he or she eats a lot of unnecessary food while watching television, he or she has to make an effort to stop eating in front of the television.[18]

The third step is to find ways to control eating. This might include the places where the patient eats, the speed of eating, or the frequency of meals. All these things can be identified and modified. In finding ways to control eating, it is sometimes helpful to reward a patient. For example, if the patient achieves a specific goal, then he or she receives a small reward (for example, a small amount of money). These rewards help the patient to gradually achieve small goals and increase or maintain motivation.

Another step is stress management. Stress management with different techniques (for example, meditation or relaxation) can help keep the patient from overeating. Finally, social support from family members, friends, and/or colleagues can be very helpful to the obese individual in losing weight.

Once some weight has been lost, the most difficult thing for an individual is to maintain the weight loss. Most patients regain a part or all of the weight they have lost.[19] Furthermore, after a 6-month weight loss period, the rate of weight loss usually declines. It is important to prevent weight regain particularly at this point. A weight maintenance program is considered successful when weight regain is not more than 3 kg in 2 years.[1] This can be done with the same tools the patients used to lose weight, that is, diet, physical activity, and behavior therapy. Successful weight loss and weight maintenance both require long-term effort by the patient. Especially in the weight maintenance period, the importance of physical activity has to be stressed.

## DIET

The most important aspect of a weight reduction program is the diet. A hypocaloric diet combined with increased physical activity can result in significant weight loss and a decrease in BP in obese hypertensive individuals. The typical American diet consists of approximately 15% protein, 35% fat, and 50% carbohydrates.[20] Fat should be reduced and portion sizes should also be decreased. Heavy intake of sugar should be discouraged, while fiber consumption should be increased. Alcohol consumption should also be eliminated or drastically reduced, because alcohol not only provides excess calories but also elevates BP. The target is a 500 to 1000 kcal deficit for the weight loss phase. In specific individuals it may be helpful to use a low-calorie liquid formula diet for a limited time (usually 12 to 16 weeks).

The basic target of a weight loss program is the reduction of fat mass, rather than lean tissue. However, during a weight loss period there is always a reduction in lean body mass. In order to minimize lean body mass reduction, the protein that is consumed must be of high biologic value (e.g., egg whites, fish, poultry, lean meat, low-fat dairy products). The remaining calories should come from carbohydrates and fat. It is very important that an individual on a weight-loss diet take adequate amounts of vitamins and micronutrients. Fat is a high-energy food, containing 9 calories per gram, while carbohydrate and protein have only 4 calories per gram. Thus, reducing high-fat foods in the diet provides a significant caloric decrease.

Total fat should not exceed 30% of total daily caloric intake, with saturated fatty acids not more than 8% to 10% of total calories. Monounsaturated and polyunsaturated fatty acids should be up to 15% and 10% of total calories, respectively. Protein should be approximately 15% of total calories. Either plant protein or lean animal protein should be used. Carbohydrates should be approximately 55% of total calories. The daily carbohydrate intake should include 20 to 30 grams of fiber from fruits, vegetables, whole grains, and legumes. Fiber helps in weight loss by increasing satiety at lower levels of calorie intake.[21]

A low-calorie diet (LCD) includes 800 to 1500 calories per day and is the cornerstone of a dietary treatment program. A caloric deficit of 500 to 1000 calories per day can result in a weight loss of 70 to 140 grams per day, or 0.5 to 1 kg per week (about 1-2 pounds per week).[21] A diet of 1200 to 1500 calories per day for men and 1000 to 1200 calories per day for women seems reasonable, but this should be individualized according to the differing needs of each person. It is important for a diet to contain the necessary amounts of vitamins and micronutrients. LCDs usually contain the daily vitamin and mineral requirements. LCDs can achieve the target of a 10% reduction in body weight over a 6-month period. Studies have shown that this weight loss is approximately 75% fat and 25% lean tissue.[22]

A very low-calorie diet (VLCD) is a diet with fewer than 800 calories per day (300 to 800 calories per day). VLCDs are usually given in the form of liquid formulas with a known caloric content. VLCDs should never be used without medical supervision. Their duration is usually 12 to 16 weeks. During that time the obese individuals have 4 to 5 portions per day. After that time, regular food can be added and substituted in the daily schedule. VLCDs may produce a rapid weight loss. However, this weight loss is generally not permanent and the obese individuals tend to regain a part of the weight they have lost. Studies have shown that VLCDs are not more effective than LCDs in long-term weight loss.[23] Also, VLCDs usually do not contain all the necessary vitamins and micronutrients, so supplementation with these components is necessary. Side effects of the VLCD are gallstones, gout, and cardiac arrhythmias.

## EFFECT OF DIET ON BLOOD PRESSURE

The Dietary Approaches to Stop Hypertension (DASH) trial was a multicenter, randomized, controlled-feeding trial that was designed to test the effect of specific dietary patterns on BP. In this trial, 459 adults with untreated SBP less than 160 mm Hg and DBP between 80 and 95 mm Hg were randomized into three different diet groups, after an initial 3-week period when they all had the same "control" diet low in fruits, vegetables, and dairy products, with a fat content typical of the average American diet. After this introductory period the first group continued the same diet; the second group received a diet rich in fruits and vegetables, and the third group received a combination diet including fruits, vegetables, low-fat dairy products, whole grains, poultry, fish, and nuts. Sodium intake and body weight were maintained at the same

levels. After 8 weeks of following these diets, there was no weight loss, but the combination diet reduced SBP and DBP by 5.5 and 3.0 mm Hg respectively compared with the control group, while the "fruits and vegetables" diet reduced SBP by 2.8 mm Hg and DBP by 1.1 mm Hg compared with the control diet (Figure 46–1).[24-28] Thus, dietary modifications can reduce BP, even without weight loss or dietary sodium reduction.

Another study looked at the effects of reducing dietary sodium in conjunction with the DASH diet.[29] A total of 412 individuals were randomized into two groups following either a control diet or the DASH diet. In each group there were three subgroups with high, intermediate, and low sodium consumption. The weight of the participants was maintained during the 30-day study. At the end of the study the group on the DASH–low sodium diet had 7.1 mm Hg lower SBP and 3.7 mm Hg lower DBP for normotensive participants and 11.5 mm Hg lower SBP and 5.7 mm Hg lower DBP for hypertensive participants, compared with the control diet group.

The Diet, Exercise, and Weight Loss Intervention Trial (DEW-IT) examined the effects of combined dietary and physical activity interventions on BP in 44 overweight, hypertensive adults on a single antihypertensive medication.[30] Lifestyle changes consisted of a moderately intense exercise program three times per week and a hypocaloric DASH diet with restriction of sodium intake. At the end of the 9-week study, there was a reduction in body weight of 4.9 kg in the

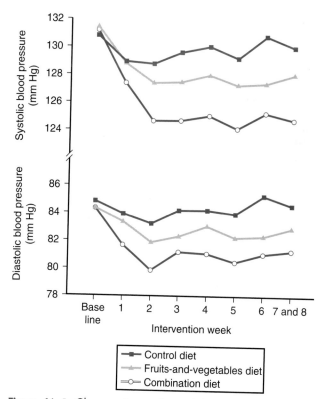

**Figure 46–1** Changes in systolic and diastolic blood pressures during the intervention period in the DASH Study. (From Appel LJ, Moore TJ, Obarzanek E, et al. A clinical trial of the effects of the dietary patterns on blood pressure. DASH Collaborative Research Group. N Engl J Med 336: 1117-1124, 1997; copyright © 1977 Massachusetts Medical Society.)

lifestyle group compared with the control group and a reduction in SBP and DBP of 12.1 mm Hg and 6.6 mm Hg, respectively compared with the control group.

Similar results were found in another study that examined the impact of nonpharmacologic interventions on the treatment of hypertension in older individuals.[31] The 975 hypertensive persons aged 60 to 80 years old who participated received a single antihypertensive medication and had a BP of less than 145 mm Hg (systolic) and less than 85 mm Hg (diastolic). Of these, 585 were obese, and they were randomized into four groups. The first had a diet low in sodium; the second was assigned to a weight loss; program with diet and physical exercise; the third had both salt restriction and diet for weight loss; and the fourth was the control group (Figure 46–2). The 390 nonobese participants were assigned either to the reduced sodium group or to the usual care group. After a period of time, a medication withdrawal was attempted. Before the medication withdrawal, the mean SBPs and DBPs were significantly lower in all intervention groups compared with the usual care group. There was a mean decrease of 3.4 mm Hg in SBP and 1.9 in DBP compared with the baseline in the sodium reduction group, and a decrease of 4.0 mm Hg in SBP and 1.1 in DBP in the weight loss group, and a decrease of 5.3 mm Hg in SBP and 3.4 in DBP in the combined intervention group, but only a slight decrease of 0.8 mm Hg in both SBP and DBP in the usual care group. The average weight loss at 9 months of the study was 3.8 kg for the patients assigned to weight loss versus an average of 0.9 kg for the patients not assigned to weight loss groups.

The Trial of Hypertension Prevention (TOHP-Phase I and II) investigated the effect of weight loss in the prevention of hypertension. The aim of TOHP-Phase I was to determine the efficacy of nonpharmacologic interventions in reducing or preventing an increase in the DBP. Participants in this study were overweight or obese individuals (body weight was 15% to 65% above the desirable for their height), with DBP 80 to 89 mm Hg. They were randomly assigned to either an 18-month weight loss intervention program (with caloric reduction and increase in physical activity) or a control condition. The average weight loss for the intervention group at 6, 12, and 18 months was 6.5, 5.6, and 4.7 kg for men and 3.7, 2.7, and 1.6 kg for women, respectively. The mean change in the DBP and SBP for the intervention group was −2.8 mm Hg and −3.1 mm Hg for the men and −1.1 mm Hg and −2.0 mm Hg for the women, respectively, compared with the control group. BP reduction was greater among those individuals who lost more weight.[32]

TOHP Phase II investigated the long-term effects of weight loss on BP. In this phase, 595 individuals were assigned to a weight loss group, and another 596 individuals were assigned to the control group. The participants' baseline BMI was 31 kg/m² for both men and women in the weight loss group and 31 kg/m² for the men and 30.8 kg/m² for the women in the control group. The average SBP and DBP were 127.6 mm Hg and 86.0 mm Hg, respectively, for the intervention group, and 127.3 mm Hg and 85.8 mm Hg for the control group. The mean weight loss from baseline in the intervention group was 4.4 kg, 2.0 kg, and 0.2 kg at 6, 18, and 36 months respectively,

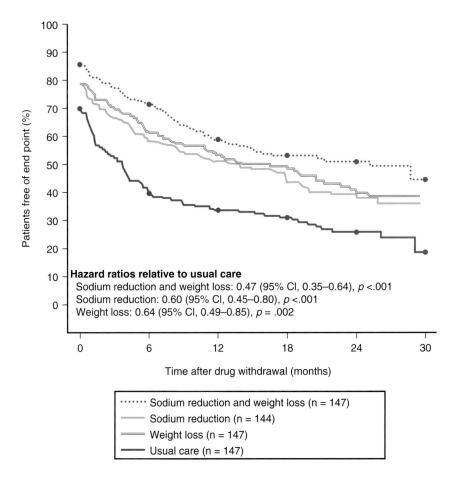

**Figure 46–2** Percentages of obese participants in the TONE study who remained free of cardiovascular events and hypertension and did not have an antihypertensive drug prescribed during follow-up. (From Whelton PK, Appel LJ, Espeland MA, et al. Sodium reduction and weight loss in the treatment of hypertension in older persons: A randomized controlled trial of nonpharmacologic interventions in the elderly (TONE). TONE Collaborative Research Group. JAMA 279:839-846, 1998.)

**Hazard ratios relative to usual care**
Sodium reduction and weight loss: 0.47 (95% CI, 0.35–0.64), $p < .001$
Sodium reduction: 0.60 (95% CI, 0.45–0.80), $p < .001$
Weight loss: 0.64 (95% CI, 0.49–0.85), $p = .002$

Time after drug withdrawal (months)

.......... Sodium reduction and weight loss (n = 147)
——— Sodium reduction (n = 144)
——— Weight loss (n = 147)
——— Usual care (n = 147)

while in the control group at the same time points there was an increase in body weight of 0.1, 0.7, and 1.8 kg. BP was significantly lower in the intervention group compared with the control group at all time points (Figure 46–3). Participants who lost at least 4.5 kg at 6 months and maintained this weight for the next 30 months had the best results in their BP. The final result of this trial is that even modest weight reduction may lead to a significant decrease in BP.[33]

The Trial of Antihypertensive Interventions and Management (TAIM) and the Treatment of Mild Hypertension Study (TOMHS) investigated the effects of combining lifestyle intervention and pharmacologic treatment on BP control in hyper-

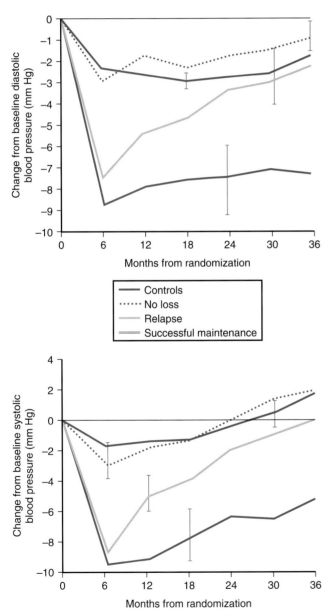

**Figure 46–3** Mean change in diastolic and systolic blood pressures during the intervention period in the TOHP II study. (From Stevens VJ, Obarzanek E, Cook NR, et al. Long-term weight loss and changes in blood pressure: Results of the Trials of Hypertension Prevention, phase II. Ann Intern Med 134:1-11, 2001.)

tensive individuals, either obese or nonobese. In the TAIM study, 692 obese or overweight individuals with DBP between 90 mm Hg and 100 mm Hg were randomized into nine different groups according to diet (usual, low sodium, weight loss) and antihypertensive medication (placebo, chlorthalidone, atenolol). Six months later there was a significant decrease in both SBP and DBP in the diet intervention groups, especially in the weight loss group.[34]

TOMHS compared the effectiveness of five different antihypertensive medications in combination with lifestyle changes in lowering BP. All 902 participants were advised to lose weight and decrease sodium and alcohol consumption and increase physical activity. Then they were randomized into one of the six groups according to antihypertensive medication (placebo, chlorthalidone, acebutolol, doxazocin, amlodipine, and enalapril). At the end of the study there was a reduction in BP in all six groups, although less in the placebo group, indicating that weight loss and other lifestyle interventions play an important role in BP control.[35]

The Hypertension Control Program was a 4-year study that investigated whether patients with modestly elevated BPs could discontinue antihypertensive drug therapy with the help of dietary modification. One hundred eighty-four patients were randomized to three groups. Patients in the first group discontinued antihypertensive drugs and modified their diet, reducing salt and alcohol and losing weight, while patients in the second group discontinued drug treatment without dietary modification. Patients in the third group continued their usual antihypertensive therapy. At the end of the study, 39% of the patients in the first group remained off hypertensive medication, while only 5% of the second group remained normotensive without medication.[36]

Similar results were found in the Dietary Intervention Study in Hypertension (DISH). In this study 496 patients who were normotensive while receiving antihypertensive drugs were randomized into seven groups. The overweight patients were randomized into four groups (antihypertensive drugs, no drugs or diet, no drugs but sodium restriction, and no drugs but weight reduction) and the normal weight patients were randomized into three groups (drugs, no drugs or diet, and no drugs but sodium restriction). At 56 weeks, the weight reduction group had the highest percentage (59.5%) of patients off medication. The average weight loss in this group was −4 ± 5 kg.[37]

In a trial of 421 participants with hypertension on the Optifast program, a commercial weight loss program using a hypocaloric formula diet, 54% had a decrease in their BP. More than half of those who achieved a weight loss of more than 20% of the initial body weight achieved normal BP at the end of the study, but resolution of the hypertension required weight loss of more than 10% of initial body weight.[38]

A summary of some of the studies that examined the effect of weight loss on BP is shown in Table 46–2.

## PHYSICAL ACTIVITY

Physical activity is very important for the maintenance of weight loss over time. In the absence of a contraindication such as a cardiac, orthopedic, or metabolic reason, exercise should be encouraged. The role of physical activity in BP control is discussed in Chapter 47.

**Table 46-2** Summary of the Studies of the Effects of Weight Loss on Blood Pressure

| Study Name | Participants' Characteristics | Study Duration | Treatment Groups | Weight Change (kg) | Systolic/Diastolic BP Change |
|---|---|---|---|---|---|
| DASH[24] | 459 adults with untreated hypertension | 8 weeks after a 3-week introductory period | Usual diet<br>Fruits/vegetables<br>Fruits/vegetables and low fat | -0.1<br>-0.3<br>-0.4 | -2.8/-1.1 mm Hg*<br>-5.5/-3.0 mm Hg* |
| DEWIT[30] | 44 obese hypertensive adults | 9 weeks | Control<br>DASH diet-low salt-exercise | -0.6<br><br>-5.5 | -12.1/-6.6 mm Hg* |
| TONE[31] | 975 adults 60-80 years old on a single antihypertensive medication | 15-36 months (median 29 months) | 1. Usual care<br>2. Low sodium<br>3. Weight loss diet<br>4. Low sodium and weight loss | -0.9 for groups 1 and 2<br><br>-3.8 for groups 3 and 4 | -0.8/-0.8 mm Hg†<br>-3.4/-1.9 mm Hg†<br>-4.0/-1.1 mm Hg†<br>-5.3/-3.4 mm Hg† |
| TOHP-I[32] | 564 obese adults with high-normal BP | 18 months | Control group<br>Diet and exercise | -4.7 for men and -1.6 for women | -3.1/-2.8 mm Hg (men)<br>-2.0/-1.1 mm Hg (women) |
| TOHP-II[33] | 1191 obese adults | 36 months | Control group<br>Intervention group | +1.8<br>-0.2 | -1.3/-0.9 mm Hg* |
| HCP[36] | 184 patients on antihypertensive drugs | 4 years | Discontinue drugs and diet<br>Discontinue drugs<br>Continue drugs | -1.8<br>+2.0<br>+2.0 | +10.8/+5.2 mm Hg†<br>+11.4/+6.7 mm Hg<br>+2.5/+1.0 mm Hg |
| DISH[37] | 496 patients on antihypertensive drugs | 56 weeks | 1. Overweight, on antihypertensive drugs<br>2. Overweight, no drugs or diet<br>3. Overweight, salt restriction, no drugs<br>4. Overweight, weight loss, no drugs<br>5. Normal weight, on drugs<br>6. Normal weight, no drugs<br>7. Normal weight, less salt | -0.46<br><br>-0.46<br><br>0<br><br>-4.0<br>+0.46<br>0<br>+0.46 | *% not taking drugs at the end of the study*<br>0<br><br>35.3%<br><br>44.9%<br><br>59.5%<br>0<br>45.0%<br>53.4% |

*Compared with control.
†From baseline.
BP, blood pressure.

# DRUG TREATMENT FOR WEIGHT LOSS

Currently, the only medications available in the United States for the treatment of obesity are orlistat and sibutramine.

## Orlistat

Orlistat is an inhibitor of pancreatic intestinal lipase.[39] The result of this inhibition is that about 30% percent of the daily ingested fat intake is not absorbed. This would lead to a 200-calorie deficit per day in an individual who consumed a diet of 2000 calories per day with 30% of calories as fat. The most common side effects of orlistat are gastrointestinal, such as fatty or oily stools, more frequent defecation, and fecal incontinence. Another side effect is a slight reduction in fat-soluble vitamins, generally not outside of the normal range.

Several studies have confirmed the efficacy of orlistat in losing weight. The European Multicenter Orlistat Group carried out a double-blind study in which 688 obese individuals (average BMI 36 kg/m$^2$) were assigned to orlistat or placebo for 1 year, in combination with a hypocaloric diet (minimum energy intake 1000-1200 kcal/day). At the end of the first year they were reassigned randomly to either orlistat or placebo for another year. At the end of the first year of the study the mean weight loss was 10.2% for the orlistat group and 6.1% for the placebo group. During the second year of the study, the participants who were switched to placebo gained twice as much weight as those who continued on orlistat. Participants who were switched from placebo to orlistat lost 0.9 kg more than in the first year of the trial.[40]

Similar results were found in another U.S. study.[41] In this trial, 892 obese individuals (BMI 30-43 kg/m$^2$) who were previously on a 4-week controlled-energy diet plus placebo were randomized into either continuing placebo or starting orlistat 120 mg three times in a day (tid). After 52 weeks, the participants started a weight maintenance diet, and those in the orlistat group were rerandomized to continuing orlistat (60 mg or 120 mg tid) or placebo for another 52 weeks. Participants who were already on placebo continued taking placebo. At the end of the first year the participants on orlistat had lost more weight than those on placebo (8.76 ± 0.37 kg vs. 5.81 ± 0.67 kg). At the end of the second year participants on orlistat 120 mg tid regained less weight than those on orlistat 60 mg tid or placebo (3.2 ± 0.45 kg, 4.26 ± 0.57 kg, and 5.63 ± 0.42, respectively).

These studies showed that there is a significant weight loss with the use of orlistat in combination with diet during the first year, and that the tendency for weight regain that occurs during the second year is less with the use of orlistat.

Weight loss with orlistat also helps in the treatment of comorbidities, including high BP. A U.S. trial investigated the effect of orlistat on BP.[42] The participants were randomized to either orlistat plus diet or placebo plus diet. After 1 year of treatment, participants in the orlistat group had greater reductions in BMI and DBP than the placebo group (−1.9 kg/m$^2$ vs. 0.9kg/m$^2$, and −11.4 mm Hg vs. −8.4 mm Hg, respectively).

Another multicenter trial investigated the effect of orlistat on obese hypertensive patients.[43] Participants in this study (n = 628) were randomly assigned to orlistat plus diet or placebo plus diet. At the end of the study the decreases in SBP and DBP were 9.4/7.7 mm Hg for the orlistat group and 4.6/5.6 mm Hg for the placebo group.

## Sibutramine

The other drug that can be used for the treatment of obesity is sibutramine. Sibutramine is a serotonin and norepinephrine reuptake inhibitor that decreases body weight by reducing food intake (by decreasing appetite).

The effect of sibutramine on weight loss was investigated in a multicenter dose-ranging study.[44] Participants (n = 1047) were randomly assigned to either sibutramine (1-30 mg) or placebo. After 6 months a dose-dependent weight loss was observed (1.2% weight loss with placebo compared with 2.7% with sibutramine 1 mg, 3.9% with 5 mg, 6.1% with 10 mg, 7.4% with 15 mg, 8.8% with 20 mg, and 9.4% with 30 mg).

Another study investigated the effect of sibutramine on weight loss, using VLCD and sibutramine, compared with the same diet and placebo.[45] In the sibutramine group, 86% of the participants lost at least 5% of their initial body weight compared with 55% of the placebo group 6 months after the study entry. At month 12, 75% of the sibutramine group maintained at least 100% of their weight loss, compared with 42% of the placebo group.

The Sibutramine Trial in Obesity Reduction and Maintenance (STORM) investigated the effect of sibutramine in maintaining weight that was lost on a hypocaloric formula diet.[46] In this trial, 605 obese patients, after losing weight, received 10 mg sibutramine daily for 6 months. After this period, participants who achieved at least 5% reduction in their body weight were randomly assigned either to continue with sibutramine for 18 more months or to receive placebo. Of the participants who completed the study, 43% of the sibutramine group maintained more than 80% of their original weight loss, while in the placebo group only 16% maintained this level of weight loss.

Sibutramine's side effects include dry mouth, headache, insomnia, and constipation, but, most important, it can increase heart rate by 4 to 6 beats per minute and elevate DBP by 2 to 3 mm Hg. Sibutramine should not be used in patients with a history of coronary heart disease, arrhythmias, or heart failure. Although some studies support sibutramine use in obese hypertensive patients,[47-48] it must be used with great caution or not at all in patients with uncontrolled hypertension. Patients taking sibutramine should regularly be monitored for their heart rate and BP.

## Antihypertensive Drugs

Although weight loss may reduce BP, there are many obese hypertensive patients who either cannot lose weight or having lost weight still have elevated BP. These individuals need treatment with antihypertensive drugs.

Thiazides have been used for many years for the treatment of hypertension. BP lowering with the use of these medications has been shown in obese hypertensive patients, but usually higher doses (up to 50 mg/day hydrochlorothiazide) are required to achieve this effect. One of the side effects of the thiazides is causing or worsening of insulin resistance. Since many obese patients are insulin resistant, thiazide diuretics should be used with caution in these patients, or in combination with other antihypertensive drugs, such as ACE inhibitors. β-Blockers may be effective in decreasing BP in obese hypertensive patients. However, β-blockers may decrease insulin sensitivity and increase glucose intolerance, so they are not the first-choice treatment for these patients. β-blockers may decrease the early insulin response and increase insulin sensitivity, so they might be a good choice for obese hypertensive patients. However, they do not protect against heart failure, which occurs commonly in obese hypertensive individuals, so they have limited use as monotherapy or initial therapy for controlling hypertension in these patients. Used in combination with other antihypertensive drugs, α-blockers are helpful in the management of hypertension in obese patients.

Calcium antagonists lower BP by reducing peripheral vascular resistance. Unlike diuretics and β-blockers, they have no effect on insulin sensitivity, glucose uptake, or lipid profile. However, they frequently cause lower extremity edema, which may be especially troublesome to obese people.

ACE inhibitors reduce peripheral resistance, increase insulin sensitivity, decrease left ventricular mass, and protect the kidney, so they have theoretical advantages over other classes of antihypertensive agents for treating obese people with high BP. Angiotensin II receptor blockers (ARBs) have similar advantages with respect to intermediate endpoints. However, no particular advantage or disadvantage of any class of antihypertensive drug for treatment of obese patients has been demonstrated in outcome trials.

## SUMMARY

Obese patients who are hypertensive should undergo a program of behavior modification to decrease caloric intake and increase physical activity. Numerous studies have documented that this will lower BP. The weight loss drugs orlistat and sibutramine may be used to enhance and maintain the weight loss process, but sibutramine must be used with extreme caution in hypertensive patients. If hypertension is not controlled with weight loss, antihypertensive therapy should be initiated. An algorithm for the treatment of obese hypertensive patients is shown in Figure 46–4.

## References

1. Clinical guidelines on the identification, evaluation and treatment of overweight and obesity in adults. The evidence report. NIH Publication, September 1998.
2. Kuczmarski RJ, Carrol MD, Flegal KM, et al. Varying body mass index cut-off points to describe overweight prevalence among U.S. adults: NHANES III Obes. Res 5:542-548, 1997.
3. Pi-Sunyer FX. Health implications of obesity. Am J Clin Nutr 53:1595S-1603S, 1991.
4. Pi-Sunyer FX. Medical hazards of obesity. Ann Intern Med 119:655-660, 1993.
5. Pi-Sunyer FX . A review of long-term studies evaluating the efficacy of weight loss in ameliorating disorders associated with obesity. Clin Ther 18:1006-1035, 1996.
6. Thompson D, Edelsberg J, Colditz GA. Lifetime health and economic consequences of obesity. Arch Intern Med 159: 2177-2183, 1999.
7. Hubert HB, Feinleib M, McNamara PM, et al. Obesity as an independent risk factor for cardiovascular disease: A 26-year follow-up of participants in the Framingham Heart Study. Circulation 67:968-977, 1983.
8. Hall JE. Renal and cardiovascular mechanisms of obesity. Hypertension 23:381-394, 1994.
9. Modan M, Halkin H, Almog S, et al. Hyperinsulinemia: A link between hypertension, obesity and glucose intolerance. J Clin Invest 75:809-817, 1985.
10. De Fronzo RA, Ferrannini E. Insulin Resistance. A multifaceted syndrome responsible for NIDDM, obesity, hypertension, dyslipidemia, and atherosclerotic cardiovascular disease. Diabetes Care 14:173-194, 1991.
11. Rocchini AR. Obesity and blood pressure regulation. *In:* Bray GA, Bouchard C, James WPT (eds). Handbook of Obesity. New York, Marcel Dekker, 1998; pp 677-695.
12. Gallagher D, Visser M, Sepulveda D, et al. How useful is body mass index for comparison of body fatness across age, sex, and ethnic groups? Am J Epidemiol 143:228-239, 1996.
13. World Health Organization. Obesity: Preventing and managing the global epidemic. Report of a WHO consultation of obesity. Geneva, June 1997.
14. Reisin E, Frohlich ED, Messerli FH, et al. Cardiovascular changes after weight reduction in obesity hypertension. Ann Intern Med 98:315-319, 1983.

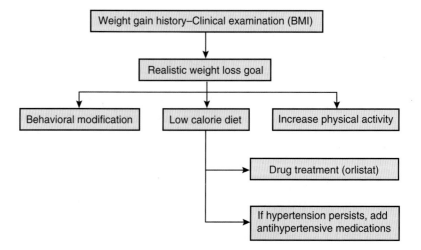

**Figure 46–4** Algorithm for the treatment of obese hypertensive patients.

15. Joint National Committee. The 1998 report of the Joint National Committee on Detection, Evaluation and Treatment of High Blood Pressure. Arch Intern Med 148:1023-1038, 1988.

16. Corrigan SA, Raczynski JM, Swencionis C, et al. Weight reduction in the prevention and treatment of hypertension: A review of representative clinical trials. Am J Health Promot. 5:208-214, 1991.

17. Eliahou HE, Iaina A, Gaon T, et al. Body weight reduction necessary to attain normotension in the overweight hypertensive patient. Int J Obes 5 (Suppl 1):157-163, 1981.

18. Wadden T, Foster D. Behavioral assessment and treatment of markedly obese patients. In: Wadden T, Van Itallie T (eds). Treatment of the Seriously Obese Patient. New York, Guilford Press, 1992; pp 290-330.

19. Methods for voluntary weight loss and control. NIH Technology Assessment Conference Panel. Ann Intern Med 116:942-949, 1992.

20. Dietary Intake of Macronutrients, Micronutrients, and Other Dietary Constituents, USA 1988-94. Centers of Disease Control and Prevention. Vital and Health Statistics: Series 11, Number 245, July 2002.

21. Identification, Evaluation and Treatment of Overweight and Obesity in Adults. The Practical Guide. NIH Publication January 2002; pp 26-27.

22. Yang M, Van Itallie TB. Effect of energy restriction on body composition and nitrogen balance in obese individuals. In: Wadden T, Van Itallie T (eds). Treatment of the Seriously Obese Patient. New York, Guilford Press, 1992; pp 83-106.

23. Wadden TA, Foster GD, Letizia KA. One-year behavioral treatment of obesity: Comparison of moderate and severe caloric restriction and the effects of weight maintenance therapy. J Consult Clin Psychol 49:824-831, 1994.

24. Appel LJ, Moore TJ, Obarzanek E, et al. A clinical trial of the effects of the dietary patterns on blood pressure. DASH Collaborative Research Group. N Engl J Med. 336: 1117-1124, 1997.

25. Conlin PR. The dietary approaches to stop hypertension (DASH) clinical trial: Implications for lifestyle modifications in the treatment of hypertensive patients. Cardiol Rev 7:284-288, 1999.

26. Moore TJ, Vollmer WM, Appel LJ, et al. Effect of dietary patterns on ambulatory blood pressure: Results from the Dietary Approaches to Stop Hypertension (DASH) Trial. DASH Collaborative Research Group. Hypertension 34:472-477, 1999.

27. Conlin PR, Chow D, Miller ER 3rd, et al. The effect of dietary patterns on blood pressure control in hypertensive patients: Results from the Dietary Approaches to Stop Hypertension (DASH) trial. Am J Hypertens 13:949-955, 2000.

28. Moore TJ, Conlin PR, Ard J, et al. DASH diet is effective treatment for stage 1 isolated systolic hypertension. Hypertension 38:155-158, 2001.

29. Sacks FM, Svetkey LP, Vollmer WM, et al.; DASH-Sodium Collaborative Research group. Effects on blood pressure of reduced dietary sodium and the Dietary Approaches to Stop Hypertension (DASH) diet. N Engl J Med. 344:3-10., 2001.

30. Miller ER 3rd, Erlinger TP, Young DR, et al. Results of the Diet, Exercise, and Weight loss Intervention Trial (DEW-IT). Hypertension 40:612-618, 2002.

31. Whelton PK, Appel LJ, Espeland MA, et al. Sodium reduction and weight loss in the treatment of hypertension in older persons: A randomized controlled trial of nonpharmacologic interventions in the elderly (TONE). TONE Collaborative Research Group. JAMA 279:839-846, 1998.

32. Stevens VJ, Corrigan SA, Obarzanek E, et al. Weight loss intervention in phase I of the Trials of Hypertension Prevention. The TOHP Collaborative Research Group. Arch Intern Med 153:849-858, 1993.

33. Stevens VJ, Obarzanek E, Cook NR, et al. Trials for the Hypertension Prevention Research Group. Long-term weight loss and changes in blood pressure: Results of the Trials of Hypertension Prevention, phase II. Ann Intern Med 134: 1-11, 2001.

34. Wassertheil-Smoller S, Blaufox MD, Oberman AS, et al. The Trial of Antihypertensive Interventions and Management (TAIM) Study. Arch Intern Med. 152:131-136, 1992.

35. Neaton JD, Grimm RH Jr, Prineas RJ, et al. Treatment of Mild Hypertension Study. Final Results. JAMA 270:713-724, 1993.

36. Stamler R, Stamler J, Grimm R, et al. Nutritional therapy for high blood pressure. Final report of a four-year randomized controlled trial-the Hypertension Control Program. JAMA 257:1484-1491, 1987.

37. Langford HG, Blaufox MD, Oberman A, et al. Dietary therapy slows the return of hypertension after stopping prolonged medication. JAMA 253:657-664, 1985.

38. Kanders BS, Blackburn GL, Lavin P, et al. Weight loss outcome and health benefits associated with the Optifast program in the treatment of obesity. Int J Obes 13 (Suppl 2):131-134, 1989.

39. Heck AM, Yanovski JA, Calis KA. Orlistat, a new lipase inhibitor for the management of obesity. Pharmacotherapy 20: 270-279, 2000.

40. Sjostrom L, Rissanen A, Andersen T, et al. Randomised placebo-controlled trial of orlistat for weight loss and prevention of weight regain in obese patients. European Multicenter Orlistat Study Group. Lancet 352:167-172, 1998.

41. Davidson MH, Hauptman J, Di Girolamo M, et al. Weight control and risk factor reduction with orlistat: A randomized control trial. JAMA 281:235-242, 1999.

42. Bakris G, Calhoun D, Egan B, et al. Orlistat improves blood pressure control in obese subjects with treated but inadequately controlled hypertension. J Hypertens 20:2257-2267, 2002.

43. Sharma AM, Golay A. Effect of orlistat-induced weight loss on blood pressure and heart rate in obese patients with hypertension. J Hypertens 20:1873-1878, 2002.

44. Bray GA, Blackburn GL, Ferguson JM, et al. Sibutramine produces dose-related weight loss. Obes Res 7:189-198, 1999.

45. Apfelbaum M, Vague P, Ziegler O, et al. Long-term maintenance of body weight loss after a very-low-calorie diet: A randomized blinded trial of the efficacy and tolerability of sibutramine. Am J Med 106:179-184, 1999.

46. Hansen D, Astrup A, Toubro S, et al. Predictors of weight loss and maintenance during 2 years of treatment by sibutramine in obesity. Results from the European multicenter STORM trial (Sibutramine Trial of Obesity Reduction and Maintenance). Int J Obes Relat Metab Disord 25:496-501, 2001.

47. McMahon FG, Weinstein SP, Rowe E, et al. Sibutramine is safe and effective for weight loss in obese patients whose hypertension is well controlled with angiotensin-converting enzyme inhibitors. J Hum Hypertens 16:5-11, 2002.

48. Sramek JJ, Leibowitz MT, Weinstein SP, et al. Efficacy and safety of sibutramine for weight loss in obese patients with hypertension well controlled by beta-adrenergic blocking agents: A placebo-controlled, double-blind, randomised trial. J Hum Hypertens 16:13-19, 2002.

# Exercise and Hypertension

## Garry L. R. Jennings

Regular exercise is an increasingly rare component of modern living. With the advent of electronic communication and transportation, large amounts of physical movement no longer underpin everyday life. Recreational activities and many forms of work can now be undertaken from the comfort of the home or office. This societal trend toward sedentary lifestyles is affecting many spheres of health, including osteoporosis and its complications, metabolic syndromes such as diabetes, coronary heart disease (CHD), and other consequences of atherosclerosis. It is also significantly influencing the prevalence and management of hypertension.

As seen in a wide range of communities throughout the world, individuals with hypertension are more likely to have sedentary lifestyles than their normotensive counterparts. While hypertension is much more than an exercise deficiency condition, the link between the two is evident. Researchers have found that hypertensive children undertake less physical activity when playing games than normotensive children. In animal models, this link also exists. Genetically hypertensive strains of rats voluntarily undertake less physical activity than normotensive strains when a treadmill is introduced into their cage. Resting blood pressure (BP) is inversely related to objective indices of physical fitness. It is likely that these benefits to BP are contributing to the observed lower cardiovascular mortality in the more active members of the general population.

Nevertheless, it was not very long ago that doctors recommended that hypertensive patients avoid strenuous physical activity. The basis of this was probably the observation every clinician has made that BP falls as soon as patients are admitted to hospital and rest in bed. This view may have also reflected the fact that BP increases acutely during isometric exercise and to a lesser extent during isotonic exercise. There are also frequently publicized, although rare, instances of sudden cardiac death among athletes. These events are more likely to occur during competition than between. The purpose of this chapter is to review some of the bases for the complete aboutface that has occurred in professional attitudes toward regular physical activity among hypertensives.

Strong recommendations have ensued among hypertension guidelines such as the Seventh Report of the Joint National Committee on Prevention, Detection, Evaluation, and Treatment of High Blood Pressure (JNC 7)[1] and the World Health Organization/International Society of Hypertension (WHO/ISH)[2] Committee and authoritative national reports, including the U.S. Surgeon General's Report on Physical Activity,[3] to encourage regular physical activity for the entire community, including those with hypertension.

In considering this issue several paradoxes are apparent. The change in BP with acute exercise is largely dependent on the type of activity undertaken. In some forms, such as power lifting, the increase in systolic blood pressure (SBP) is profound. With others it is minimal depending on where and how the BP is measured (see discussion in sections that follow).

After acute exercise, BP generally falls for some hours. With repeated bouts of exercise there is increased physical fitness and also lower BP than before training, even when BP is measured at a considerable time after the last bout of exercise.

It is important to emphasize that even if regular aerobic exercise had no effect on BP whatsoever, there would be strong grounds for recommending it in the hypertensive population. Regular exercise is broadly efficacious in providing cardioprotection, acting not just through BP regulation but also through metabolic systems affecting cardiovascular risk, including insulin resistance and lipids, a powerful sympatholytic activity and effects on other neurohormonal systems.

Hypertensives are a high-risk population susceptible to multiple adverse cardiovascular risk factors. They are therefore most likely to benefit from regular exercise. On a population basis the association between exercise and BP may be particularly important to public health. The greatest threat associated with the slight decrease in prevalence of hypertension in developed communities is the rapidly increasing prevalence of obesity and its associated metabolic and other consequences. There is a strong argument that diminishing physical activity in the community is a major contributor to obesity and that increasing body weight is not just a consequence of excessive energy intake, but also of diminished energy expenditure through occupational and leisure time physical activity.

## ISOTONIC AND ISOMETRIC EXERCISE

Many forms of exercise in normal daily life are a mixture of isotonic and isometric forms. Isotonic exercise involves shortening and lengthening of various muscle groups. Typical forms include running, cycling, and swimming. When performed for more than a few minutes these involve an increase in maximum oxygen uptake by the body. The body matches the increase in oxygen consumption mainly by exercising skeletal muscle. Isometric exercise, by definition, is skeletal muscle contraction without shortening. Resistance exercises such as power lifting involve a high degree of isometric and a limited isotonic component. The effects of acute isotonic and acute isometric exercise on BP are reviewed in the next sections.

## ACUTE ISOTONIC EXERCISE

### Blood Pressure during Exercise

To the clinician performing exercise stress testing, the BP response to acute isotonic exercise may seem straightforward. SBP measured indirectly at the brachial artery with a sphygmomanometer increases linearly in relation to workload. This is seen universally in healthy participants and in most patients with cardiovascular disease. However, in a few patients with poor left ventricular function and/or major coronary artery disease, SBP does not increase, and in some cases it may even fall. The latter carries grave prognostic implications unless successful therapeutic intervention occurs. There is some variation in the extent to which BP increases with workload in the healthy population, leading to suggestions that an exaggerated rise in SBP with exercise may be a portent of hypertension later in life.

Factors affecting brachial systolic pressure determined sphygmomanometrically include cardiac output, which increases linearly with workload, and the properties of large arteries. A stiffer proximal vasculature will be associated with higher SBP. Pulse wave reflection from the periphery also contributes to SBP, having different effects at different levels of the arterial system. It is responsible for considerable amplification of the arterial pulse wave from the aortic valve to the brachial artery and beyond. In fact, much of the increase in brachial systolic pressure during exercise is due to increased effects of pulse wave velocity on the brachial systolic pressure as exercise progresses. When central BP is measured directly and invasively at the aortic root, there is very little change in aortic systolic pressure across the range of 25% to 100% of maximal oxygen uptake, even though brachial or radial artery systolic pressure increases considerably. Mean arterial pressure changes very little during progressive aerobic exercise[4,5] (Figure 47–1).

Diastolic blood pressure (DBP) is not measurable by any of the conventional noninvasive means during exercise. Even invasively measured DBPs may be unreliable unless great care and attention is given to the frequency response and other characteristics of the apparatus used. DBP tends to slightly fall during progressive aerobic exercise (see Figure 47–1). As a consequence of this, high SBPs seen by clinicians using a sphygmomanometer in patients with hypertension during acute exercise do not translate into the expected increases in afterload. The heart experiences a vastly increased preload due to increased blood flow to and from the heart related to profound vasodilation in working skeletal muscle. Increased load

on the heart is also brought about by the tachycardia of exercise, which results from a combination of vagal withdrawal and cardiac sympathetic stimulation. The latter also increases cardiac contractility.

Although increased brachial systolic pressure during exercise is in a sense artifactual (it does not reflect increased central arterial pressures), there have been many proponents for the notion that exercise BP is a useful predictor of both hypertension and cardiovascular morbidity and mortality. The evidence for this is reviewed in the next sections.

### Systemic Hemodynamic Changes during Exercise

BP is regulated closely during exercise, as can be understood by looking at the overall systemic hemodynamic changes. As stated previously, a primary hemodynamic driver during aerobic exercise is vasodilation in working skeletal muscle. This serves to meet the increased oxygen and nutrient demands at the local level. Increased oxygen is also extracted by exercising muscles. It is likely that the maximum vasodilatory capacity of skeletal muscle is never reached in normal healthy participants during aerobic exercise, because flows of 240 mm Hg per minute to the exercising quadriceps muscle alone have been measured during leg exercise.[4,6]

If vasodilation in working skeletal muscle were the only hemodynamic change during exercise, BP would fall considerably. The fact is that active vasoconstrictor tone is maintained in both exercising and resting skeletal muscle, as well as in splanchnic and other beds during exercise. The net result is the redistribution of blood flow to exercising skeletal muscle away from other organs, some more than others. With persisting exercise, other factors become important, including demand for blood flow to the respiratory muscles, which may account for as much as 10% of total oxygen uptake at near maximal exercise. In the cutaneous circulation, there is dilation, which assists in the dissipation of heat generated by exercise.

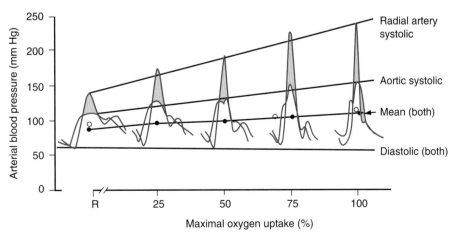

**Figure 47–1** Simultaneously measured radial arterial and aortic pressures during rest (R) and upright exercise. Note the similarities in mean aortic pressures at a given percentage of VO₂ max from two studies on participants whose absolute values of VO₂ max varied widely. Peripheral wave amplification caused large increases in radial arterial pulse pressure. Pressure waveforms were traced from direct simultaneous recordings from a representative subject. (Redrawn from Rowell LB. Human Cardiovascular Control. New York, Oxford University Press, 1993; p 183. Used by permission of Oxford University Press, Inc.)

The heart responds to the increase in venous return with an increase in diastolic volume that tends to increase stroke volume by the Frank Starling mechanism.[7] Cardiac output increases linearly with exercise workload, but the mechanism is different at lower and higher exercise levels. At lower levels, stroke volume increases. At higher levels, exercise tachycardia is more important, and both end-diastolic and end-systolic volume decrease despite increases in filling pressure.[8-10]

There has been a considerable amount of experimental work on the role of the arterial baroreflex in BP responses to acute aerobic exercise. Early workers considered that the reflex must be inhibited during such exercise. An apparent simultaneous increase in heart rate and arterial BP seemed to indicate that the arterial baroreflex was ineffective under these conditions. However, more recent data suggest that the arterial baroreflex remains active, albeit working at different operating points, so that vascular conductance and cardiac output are matched over the entire range from rest to maximum exercise.[4,11]

## Blood Pressure after Exercise

BP generally falls after an acute bout of exercise. This occurs within a few minutes and may last several hours. The mechanism probably involves reduction in peripheral resistance below preexercise levels, in part related to sympathetic inhibition.

In the longer term, engaging in a regular exercise program will reduce both resting BP and exercise-related BP increases (Figure 47–2). These effects can be seen after 2 weeks, with a further reduction in resting BP noted after 4 weeks of training.

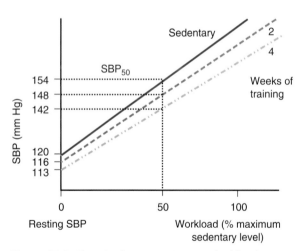

**Figure 47–2** Exercise lowers resting systolic blood pressure (SBP) and SBP during acute exercise, both at any given absolute workload or at workloads expressed as percent of maximum work (e.g., SBP$_{50}$ = SBP at 50% of maximum workload achieved during a graded exercise test). Lower blood pressure at any given level of exercise reflects both carryover of the effects at rest and a reduction in the slope of the relationship between workload and SBP. (Data [fitted to linear regression equations] from Jennings G, Nelson L, Nestel P, et al. The effects of changes in physical activity on major cardiovascular risk factors, hemodynamics, sympathetic function, and glucose utilisation in man: A controlled study of four levels of activity. Circulation 73:30-40, 1986.)

## Other Changes with Acute Exercise
### Metabolic

In addition to its effects on BP, exercise is associated with a number of other changes, chiefly metabolic, that contribute to reduced cardiovascular risk. These changes occur with different intensities and durations of exercise. A reduction in BP can be seen with a relatively low threshold of around 50% of maximum oxygen expenditure. At these levels, insulin resistance measurements show a biphasic response, with a very transient impairment followed by many hours of improved insulin sensitivity. Lipid measurements also change acutely with exercise. A fall in triglycerides and increase in high-density lipoprotein (HDL) cholesterol is consistently observed. These changes appear to be dependent on the intensity and duration of exercise. Transient efflux of HDL cholesterol can be measured from exercising skeletal muscle, probably reflecting a reduction in intracellular triglyceride levels due to metabolism. Prolonged exercise seems to be necessary for an acute effect of exercise on low-density lipoprotein (LDL) cholesterol levels.

There is, of course, a nexus between the acute and chronic effects of exercise. For example, some of the long-term effects of chronic exercise may be due to repeated acute effects. Moreover, exercise training increases exercise capacity, permitting more intense and prolonged exercise sessions, which may compound the acute effects.[12]

### Implications of Hypertension on the Blood Pressure Responses to Acute Exercise

Hypertension is associated with left ventricular hypertrophy (LVH), which involves both cardiomyocyctes and the cardiac interstitium. With early LVH in young participants, the effects of the cardiomyocyte hypertrophy may be the main determinant of the hemodynamic performance. There is evidence that at given levels of preload and afterload, cardiac contractility is higher with LVH than without. Thus, younger patients with mild LVH may have increased cardiac output during exercise and consequently higher SBP both centrally and in the periphery. More profound LVH in older participants is associated with stiffening of the ventricle, left ventricular diastolic dysfunction, and, if progressive, diminished left ventricular function and even cardiac dilation and failure. These changes would tend to lessen the BP responses to aerobic exercise.

Hypertension is also associated with impairment of the buffering effects of the arterial baroreflex. As mentioned previously, recent data indicate that the baroreceptor–heart rate reflex remains intact and operative, contributing to BP regulation during acute bouts of exercise, albeit operating at different set points as exercise progresses. However, reflex buffering of BP is impaired in the setting of ageing and hypertension, likely altering BP responses during and after exercise in this population.

## ACUTE ISOMETRIC EXERCISE

The cardiovascular response, particularly the change in BP during isometric exercise, is quite different from that seen during isotonic aerobic exercise. In the contracting skeletal muscle bed there is a large increase in vascular resistance, mainly due to extravascular constriction of the vessels. This elicits a powerful reflex, resulting in an increase in BP that is largely sympathetically mediated. Systolic, diastolic, and mean BP, as well as cardiac output, increase.

Observers suggested that this major increase in BP during acute isometric exercise might account for a small but significant increase in the likelihood of stroke due to intracerebral hemorrhage in susceptible individuals. This is the main reason why many authorities in the past have suggested that patients with hypertension and other cardiovascular disease should avoid heavy straining. However, there are also likely health benefits that arise from regular and repeated episodes of resistance exercise.

## EXERCISE, BLOOD PRESSURE, AND CARDIOVASCULAR DISEASE MORTALITY

There has been considerable interest over many years in the extent to which differences in BP during acute exercise reflect prognosis. As outlined previously, the primary physiologic mediators of exercise BP include cardiac performance, which may be influenced by the prevailing levels of sympathetic activity, by cardiac hypertrophy, and by the presence of underlying cardiac disease. The second important mediator of exercise BP is the characteristics of the major arteries, including arterial compliance and the influences of wave reflection. Peripheral mechanisms that play a role include total peripheral resistance, which affects mean BP and DBP specifically, and cardiac preload, which is affected by the properties of the venous circulation. Other determinants of exercise BP are listed in Box 47–1.

A large number of studies have looked at the long-term outcome in relation to various indices of exercise BP at an initial exercise test. The results of some of these studies[13-16] are shown in Figure 47–3.

Overall, the studies show an inconsistent relationship between exercise BP and subsequent mortality, although some of the better designed and controlled studies show a significantly positive relationship with a hazard ratio of around 2 for patients with high exercise BP compared with those without. Whether this is a useful finding applicable to clinical practice and whether any relationship between exercise BP and cardiovascular disease or mortality is causal or an indirect measure of other more important predictors is uncertain.

One consideration is the very strong interdependence of BP variables. In any population of hypertensive or normotensive participants, there are generally strong relationships between various BP variables, including SBP, DBP and/or mean BP,

resting BP, and submaximal or maximal exercise BPs. The linearity of the SBP response measured at the brachial artery at different workloads determines that the relationship can be described by an intercept (resting BP) and slope of the BP workload relationship. At any given slope of this relationship, a higher intercept (resting BP) will result in higher absolute BPs at each level of absolute work, including maximum work capacity. Thus, one explanation of the relationship between exercise BP and cardiovascular disease or mortality is that it indirectly reflects the known relationship between resting BP and outcome.

However, mortality has been shown to be independent of resting BP in several recent studies. At present the utility of the putative prognostic information arising from measurement of exercise BP is limited, not only because of the lack of a clear conceptual framework but also due to the lack of agreed measurement techniques and established normal values in local populations.

### Long-Term Effects of Regular Aerobic Exercise on Blood Pressure

To some extent the question of whether exercise per se has a long-term antihypertensive benefit becomes less important in the light of strong epidemiologic, experimental, and clinical evidence that, irrespective of the effects on BP, regular exercise reduces mortality from CHD. It is not our purpose to review in detail the studies relating to regular exercise and CHD outcome, as these have been reviewed elsewhere.[17-20] However, studies using a range of measures of physical activity or fitness have consistently shown benefits, particularly those conducted since the late 1980s, in which greater attention has been paid to methodologic rigor. Classic studies contributing to this knowledge base have included those of Harvard alumni,[21-22] Framingham,[23] UK civil servants,[24] and major trial patients,[25] as well as health screening programs in Texas.[26]

The relationship between physical activity and morbidity or mortality in hypertensive or normotensive subgroups has been compared in a number of epidemiologic studies. In Harvard alumni,[21] sedentary hypertensives had about twice the risk of death compared with those who were normotensive over the follow-up period of 12 to 16 years. The age-adjusted death rate per 10,000 man-years of observation was 173 in hypertensives and as low as 79 in normotensives. The relative risk of hypertension in sedentary participants throughout the follow-up period was 2.18, considerably higher than the figure of 1.58 observed in the most active alumni participants. Designation to the most active groups in this study required an estimated additional 2000 kcal/wk in work or leisure time exercise. This is a fairly substantial increment over sedentary levels, and more recent studies have examined milder increases in weekly exercise. These data suggest that hypertensives may benefit more from increased physical activity than those in the community who have normal BP.

By analogy with drug therapy, any benefit of regular exercise on BP should be reflected in reduced stroke rates. Wannamethee and Shaper[27] followed 7735 men for 9.5 years and observed an inverse relationship between physical activity and stroke risk. This persisted after statistically controlling for age, coronary risk factors, alcohol intake, and known vascular disease. The relative risk of stroke (assessed by questionnaire) was 0.6 for moderate activity compared with inactivity

**Box 47–1** Determinants of Exercise Blood Pressure

Age
Exercise habits
Obesity and diet
Cardiac and vascular disease
Resting blood pressure
Reflexes
Testing methods

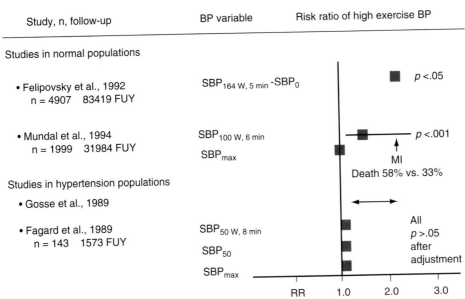

**Figure 47–3** Exercise blood pressure (BP) and cardiovascular mortality. FUY, years of patient follow-up; n, number of subjects; W, workload in watts; $SBP_n$, systolic BP at n% of maximum workload; $SBP_{nw}$, systolic BP at an absolute workload of n watts.

and 0.3 for vigorous activity. However, the vigorous exercise group had a somewhat higher risk of myocardial infarction (MI). The lowest combined risk of stroke and MI was seen in the group with a moderate level of physical activity.

Epidemiologic data also support the benefit of regular exercise in primary prevention of hypertension. Blair et al.[26] determined physical activity indirectly by measuring physical fitness by treadmill testing. They followed more than 7000 men and women for a median of 4 years (range 1-12 years). Those with low levels of physical fitness at the outset of the study had a risk of 1.52 of developing hypertension relative to physically fit individuals even after adjustment for sex, age, duration of follow-up, baseline BP, and body mass index (BMI).

Epidemiologic approaches have also been used to determine whether a dose-response relationship exists between physical activity and cardiovascular mortality. However, interpretation of cross-sectional studies can be difficult, because there is a need to account for possible confounding effects of differences in body weight, diet, and other lifestyle habits in those who voluntarily and habitually adopt a lifestyle involving regular exercise. Although a general consensus is emerging from the epidemiologic data that moderate levels of physical activity are most protective, individual studies can be found in the literature to support the views that a very low,[28-32] a medium, or a high level[21] of exercise is optimal. This question is better assessed in longitudinal studies using either crossover or parallel group designs where BP can be measured in exercising participants compared with appropriate controls.

## Clinical Studies

If regular aerobic exercise were an antihypertensive drug, widespread recommendation of its use would require knowl-

edge of a full therapeutic profile, including indications, contraindications, side effects, precautions, interactions, adverse reactions, optimal dosage, and form of administration. Many clinical trials have been performed using exercise training as an intervention and many conclusions can be drawn. However, there are so many ways in which the level of physical activity can be altered in the course of normal daily life that it is not possible to provide a complete picture from clinical studies. Nor have major clinical outcome trials of the kind performed with antihypertensive drugs been feasible for studying the effects of regular exercise on BP and cardiovascular outcomes. The design and measurement challenges of such a study are formidable. Under these circumstances it is likely that the most complete picture will be obtained from carefully designed and conducted clinical studies using intermediate endpoints, particularly BP itself, and other measures of cardiovascular risk supported by coherent data from epidemiologic, experimental, and observational studies.

## Major Design and Measurement Considerations

Many studies have investigated the effect of regular exercise on BP. Variability in the results of efficacy studies can largely be attributed to study design. Major design factors include the following:

1. *Controls*
   The effect of regular exercise as an intervention cannot be measured in a double-blind, placebo-controlled trial. Nevertheless, to have no control intervention[33] is unacceptable. The general perception of exercise as a healthy activity ensures that there is likely to be a significant placebo contribution to any result where exercise has been involved. Some studies have used normal sedentary activity

as the control intervention[34-36]; others have used specific sedentary activities such as reading[37] or light exercises that were thought to be below the threshold for any possible active benefit of exercise.[38-40] In an early meta-analysis, an average fall of BP in control groups in exercise studies was calculated at 2/2 mm Hg.[41]

2. *Selection and randomization*

   Many members of the community regularly engage in physical activity during their work or recreation. There is a known tendency for health-conscious groups to volunteer for clinical trials. In order to diminish the contrast between active and inactive groups or trial phases, it is important that only sedentary participants be enrolled in controlled trials. Nevertheless, many previous studies have used athletes, who have been a convenient sample, but this has reduced the contrast between baseline, or control, and active groups or phases of the study.

3. *Blood pressure measurement*

   It is clearly good clinical trial practice to measure BP using a method that is free of observer bias. There are several ways in which this can occur. Ambulatory BP measurements are now being used fairly routinely in clinical trials of antihypertensives. In the case of exercise studies, ambulatory BP recording avoids common biases from clinic measurements and has a limited placebo effect. However, it is important to recognize and account for the effect of physical activity performed during the day, as this is the major determinant of variance in ambulatory BP in a given individual. Even if BP recordings are not disrupted during the day of measurement by the acute BP effects during an exercise bout, variations in daily physical activity are important determinants of the variation in ambulatory BP. It has been observed that the level of physical activity that free-living individuals perform in the community depends to some extent on their physical fitness, so the group that has been engaged in the exercise intervention may be more active on rest days than the group that has not.

   The timing of BP measurements is clearly important in relation to the most recent bout of acute exercise. Some studies have avoided the postacute exercise phase of up to 24 to 48 hours after the last bout of exercise.

4. *Method of training*

   It is mandatory for good trial design that training be both quantitated and supervised. In many studies the level of exercise prescribed during the training phase has been expressed as a percentage of maximum work capacity or maximum oxygen uptake. However, as participants progress through the exercise program and their fitness improves, this translates to a higher absolute workload if work is adjusted according to the change in maximum capacity, or a diminishing fraction of maximum capacity if it is not. Therefore, whatever is done, the exercise-training stimulus will be different at the end of a period of regular exercise training from at the beginning.

   It is particularly difficult to quantitate the amount of exercise performed in mixed programs involving different forms of exercise. However, these have been commonly used in longitudinal studies assessing the benefits of exercise on BP with the justification that they are more realistic and acceptable to the participants than laboratory-based studies.

5. *Confounding factors*

   Regular exercise is always part of a general lifestyle package. The trial analysis and design must be able to account for major confounding influences such as changes in body weight, alcohol consumption, and sodium intake that might occur as the imposition of the exercise program impacts other aspects of daily life.

## Summary and Meta-Analyses of Longitudinal Studies of Exercise Training on Blood Pressure

In the absence of a major outcome study, the best clinical trial evidence comes from meta-analyses that selectively include the studies with the design characteristics outlined previously. The earliest exercise studies were conducted from the early to middle 1970s, particularly in Japan,[42] but most were flawed by inadequate or absent controls, nonrandom allocation of participants, or inadequate blinding of BP measurements. There have now been a number of systematic reviews of these data dating back to 1990.[41,43-49]

Reports from more highly controlled studies now exist, including both males and females over a wide age range from teenagers to those older than 70 years. The exercise periods have varied from 1 to 8 or more months, and typical training frequency has been three times a week with a session time of 30 to 120 minutes. More frequent and less frequent exercise bouts have also been studied. Studies now exist on the effects of isotonic training, including bicycling, walking, jogging, running, calisthenics, and various combinations. The training intensity has usually been 40% to 80% of maximum oxygen consumption, and most have been in the 50% to 60% range.

Normotensive, borderline, and established hypertensive patient populations have all been studied. The presence of hypertension may be an important factor in determining the magnitude of BP change, although this remains somewhat controversial. Fagard[41] reported that in early studies in normotensive participants, the average reduction in BP with exercise training was 4/4 mm Hg. In those with higher BPs (>140 mm Hg systolic), the average reduction was 11/6 mm Hg when corrected for reductions in the control groups. Several studies have shown that the BP reduction with exercise training is independent of changes in body weight or sodium consumption.[50,51]

Most studies have been of longitudinal design. Crossover studies are more challenging, particularly if a larger number of participants are to have exercise intervention. However, they do avoid influences due to genetic and other confounding environmental factors acting on BP. In crossover studies, a standard exercise intervention of three 40-minute periods of cycling on a bicycle ergometer at 60% to 70% of maximum work capacity for 4 weeks reduced the BP in participants with mild hypertension by 11/9 mm Hg. The same protocol reduced the BP of normotensives by slightly less (10/7 mm Hg).[50,51] These changes are at the upper limit of what has been observed in most well-controlled studies investigating the effects of exercise training on BP. This may have reflected population characteristics such as an extremely sedentary prestudy lifestyle and/or the improved contrast allowed by a crossover and a balanced Latin square design.

Whelton et al.[47] published a meta-analysis using English-language articles published before September 2001 as the data source. Using predetermined selection criteria, the authors identified 104 original reports, including 121 trials. Of these, 54 trials from 38 reports met the requirements for the systematic analysis. These requirements included provision of adequate controls, limited ability for confounding factors to influence results, enrollment of participants older than 18 years old, and follow-up for more than 2 weeks. The median number of participants in each trial was 28 and the largest study included 247 people. In total, 2419 participants contributed data; 12 trials included predominantly men and 17 included predominantly women. Although most of the participants were white, six trials were conducted in Asian populations and four in African American. About half of the studies were performed in normotensive participants. The median duration of the trials was 12 weeks, ranging from 3 weeks to 2 years. The trial designs varied, and five had some kind of active intervention in the control group.

Baseline SBP varied from 101 to 168 mm Hg, with a median of 126.5 mm Hg. Corresponding diastolic values were 61 to 104 mm Hg, with a median of 77 mm Hg.

Overall the pooled effect of aerobic exercise on SBP was −3.84 mm Hg. The 95% confidence limits were between −4.97 and −2.72, $p < .001$. The pooled effect on DBP was a reduction of 2.58 mm Hg (95% confidence intervals −3.35 to −1.81; $p < .001$). It is interesting that when only studies where the exercise intervention was supervised were included, the net change in BP increased, on average, to −4.13 mm Hg over −2.68 mm Hg. The mean change also increased when studies in which antihypertensive medications were allowed were excluded.

It is difficult to draw conclusions from subgroup analyses with such a relatively small number of trials and study participants. However, there appeared to be a greater reduction in BP in studies of shorter duration (<10 weeks).[47] In trials of longer duration, participants were allowed to exercise without supervision. It is likely that failure to adhere to the prescribed exercise intervention therapy contributed to this result.

## MECHANISMS OF BLOOD PRESSURE REDUCTION BY REGULAR EXERCISE

The mechanisms contributing to the antihypertensive effects of exercise have proven difficult to elucidate. There has been some debate over whether the fall in BP is due to a reduction in cardiac output[52-55] or total peripheral resistance.[37,50,51] Methodologic and population differences may be responsible, and these have been reviewed previously.[46] Possible mechanisms include changes in neural regulation of the circulation, various hormonal systems, including the renin-angiotensin-aldosterone system (RAAS), and altered regulation by ion channels, growth, or endothelial factors. It has been proposed that exercise-elevated prostaglandin E levels[56] or increased intrinsic depressor systems, including atrial natriuretic peptide (ANP),[57] play a role. However, other studies have failed to show any change in cardiac secretion or renal extraction of ANP with 4 weeks of moderate training.[58] Other work has shown increased serum taurine in conjunction with training,[58] with consequent natriuretic[59] and sympatholytic[60] changes.

The most consistent response to regular exercise is reduction in resting heart rate. This is brought about by both reduced sympathetic activity[61,62] and enhanced parasympathetic activity.[63,64] It is highly likely that sympathetic modulation plays a role in other longer-term hemodynamic effects of regular exercise. As mentioned previously, there is a reduction in sympathetic nerve activity after a single acute bout of exercise.[65] Many studies have shown that venous plasma norepinephrine concentration is reduced after training.[34,37,50,51] More detailed catecholamine kinetic studies at the Baker Heart Research Institute have confirmed that there is substantial reduction in sympathetic efferent activity with regular exercise. Regional norepinephrine spillover studies[66] have shown that norepinephrine spillover into the circulation is substantially reduced after training compared with control periods. The majority of this effect is seen in the renal bed, which contributes two thirds to the fall in norepinephrine spillover.

Although these and many other changes associated with exercise training may contribute to the antihypertensive effect, it is difficult to determine which are causal and which are consequential. Meredith et al.[37] determined the time course of changes in BP in norepinephrine spillover and cardiac structure in healthy participants in a crossover study of training and sedentary periods. Interestingly, the reduction in BP was a relatively early phenomenon, being evident and statistically significant after only a little more than a week from commencement of a 4-week period of moderate exercise, three times per week. On the other hand, reduction in norepinephrine spillover took longer, being evident after approximately 3 weeks of training, at the same time as increased cardiac dimensions were noted using echocardiography. This suggests that other factors are responsible for the initiation of BP reduction after exercise training, although sympathetic inhibition may contribute over the longer term, perhaps as a consequence of altered cardiac afferent activity when the heart dilates. Inhibition of renin secretion with regular exercise may follow the sympathetic responses as reduction in renal norepinephrine spillover accounts for the major proportion of the total change in spillover.[56]

Of several mechanisms proposed for the early reduction of BP by regular exercise, change in vascular function is supported. Systemic arterial compliance falls after a single bout of exercise and is seen to be below pretraining levels in the first week of a training program (three times per week). This has reflex effects on the circulation, particularly the baroreceptor heart rate reflex, probably by altering afferent input from the carotid baroreceptors. Exercise training has been consistently shown to reduce the maximum tachycardia response to BP reduction.[67-69] This may be a factor in the orthostatic intolerance reported occasionally by athletes.[70] The reflex effects of training are slightly different when autonomic function is impaired, as in hypertension. In hypertension reduction there is a deficit in the parasympathetic component of the baroreceptor heart rate reflex.[71-73] In the context of hypertension and heart failure, baroreflex failure has been reported to be a marker of high risk of sudden cardiac death.[74] Regular exercise tends to improve reflex function. Interestingly, regular exercise, particularly when combined with a weight loss program, has been demonstrated to reduce BP under both resting and stress (laboratory mental stress) conditions.[75]

There has been considerable interest in the possibility that the vascular effects of regular exercise involve alterations in nitric oxide (NO) action on large and small arteries. Short-term diet and exercise intervention in healthy participants was associated with reductions in BP, measures of oxidative stress, and NO availability, as well as alterations in the metabolic profile, including fasting insulin and improvement in the HDL cholesterol ratio.[76] Kingwell et al. reviewed the influence of regular exercise on endothelially mediated vasodilation[77] and found consistent evidence that exercise training enhances endothelial NO release. However, there is a difference between short- and longer-term exercise in the balance of effects on basal NO release and that stimulated by agonists such as acetylcholine.[77]

A likely sequence of events, at least with a moderate exercise training program three times a week at an intensity of about 60% of maximum work capacity, is an early fall in BP due to reduced compliance of large arteries and NO-mediated vasodilation of peripheral resistance vessels. As a result, increased vascular perfusion, particularly in skeletal muscle during acute exercise, increases venous return with a consequent increase in central blood volume. Over a period of about 3 weeks this is associated with left and right ventricular dilation and increased cardiac output. Altered cardiopulmonary afferent input to the brain as a result of this cardiac remodeling reduces brain stem sympathetic efferent activity, particularly to the renal circulation, causing a reduction in renin production and natriuresis (Figure 47–4).

After 4 weeks, a three-times-weekly exercise program on a bicycle ergometer in normal and hypercholesterolemic participants[78] is associated with higher basal NO release than in sedentary controls, but stimulated release is similar. Constrictor responses to the endothelium-dependent agonist acetylcholine are seen in cross-sectional studies in athletes compared with sedentary participants. It is possible that there is progressive adaptation in the NO system during long-term training. In the study referred to previously,[52] a single bout of

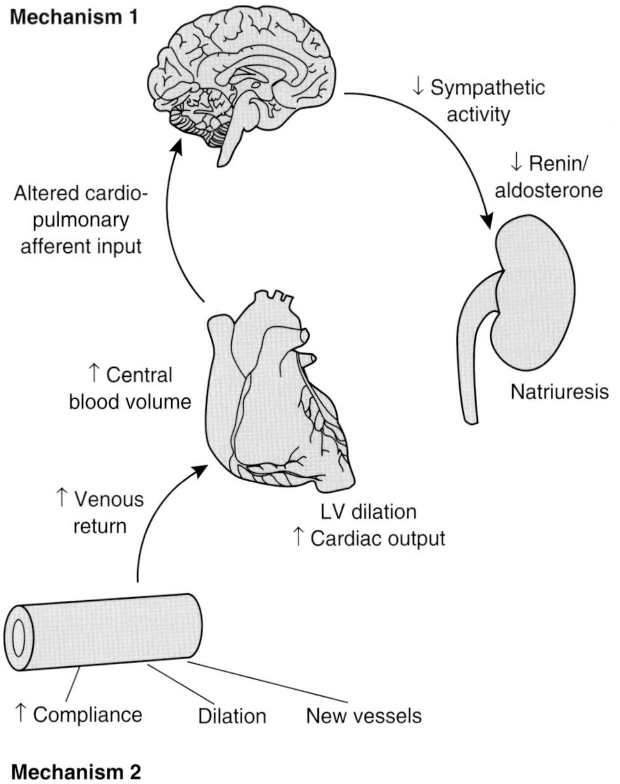

leg exercise increased forearm sheer stress, a pertinent factor in the up-regulation of endothelial NO synthase. This may be responsible for the early demonstration of increased NO production and vasodilation between exercise bouts over the first few weeks. Over months, adaptations to meet increased metabolic demands during exercise may develop, involving changes in metabolic enzymes and perhaps vascular structural modification along the lines of that referred to previously for the heart. Another factor in free-living individuals is that over the long term, there are likely to be changes in the lipid profile, which will have beneficial effects on endothelial function. Endothelial function may be an important initiating factor and prognostic marker in vascular disease, and changes induced by regular exercise could be an important component of its protective effect.

Over the longer term a program of regular aerobic exercise can reduce LVH in hypertensive participants.[79,80] It is not clear whether this reflects long-term BP lowering and is afterload dependent or whether there are specific effects of regular exercise on myocardial hypertrophy and/or the cardiac interstitium.

## Effects of Resistance Exercise on Blood Pressure

Historically there has been concern over persons with hypertension performing more than moderate levels of resistance exercise because of the acute rise in BP, which exceeds that occurring with isotonic aerobic exercise. On the other hand, there are a number of likely benefits of resistance exercise that should apply to hypertensive patients as well as to the general population. These include maintenance of muscle bulk in later years, particularly in the upper limbs, which may be important in maintaining quality of life. There are also metabolic benefits in relation to, for example, glucose utilization that may differ from those seen with regular isotonic exercise.

Few data address whether progressive resistance exercise has effects on BP in the long term. Kelley and Kelley have reviewed studies that were indexed between January 1966 and December 1998 and required resistance exercise as the only intervention for at least 4 weeks.[81] Only 12 studies met the criteria, and one of these was excluded from the final analysis because of missing BP data. Six of these studies were published in journals and five as part of doctoral theses. The 11 studies analyzed had a total of 320 participants, 182 of whom received the exercise intervention. The average number of participants in each group ranged from 6 to 31 in the exercises. Both males and females were included, and some studies had patients on antihypertensive medications. Training programs were variable. The overall pooled effects using fixed effects modeling in this study showed a decrease of approximately 2% and 4% for SBP and DBP, respectively. Both of these reductions were statistically significant. The authors concluded that progressive resistance exercise is efficacious for reducing resting SBP and DBP "in adults" but noted the need for additional data in hypertensive persons.

**Mechanism 1**

↓ Sympathetic activity
↓ Renin/aldosterone
Altered cardiopulmonary afferent input
↑ Central blood volume
Natriuresis
↑ Venous return
LV dilation
↑ Cardiac output
↑ Compliance    Dilation    New vessels

**Mechanism 2**
→ ?    ↓ Central blood volume → ↓ Cardiac output → ↓ BP

**Figure 47–4** Potential mechanisms for the mediation of exercise training–induced blood pressure reduction. LV, left ventricular.

## THE SAFETY OF EXERCISE

Hypertensives are a high-risk group for underlying CHD and other manifestations of atherosclerosis, particularly in later life. In patients with CHD, whether it is overt or latent, sudden cardiac death may occur at any time. That it sometimes occurs during physical exercise is not surprising. The risks are lower with moderate exercise programs, beginning slowly and gradually progressing the workload level.

Supervised maximal exercise testing may be warranted before patients at high risk (i.e., severe hypertension [BP >180/110 mm Hg] or mild to moderate hypertension with additional risk factors) engage in an exercise program of moderate intensity (40%-60% of maximum work capacity). For patients who have CHD, heart failure, or stroke, exercise is best initiated under direct medical supervision.

By far the most common complications of an exercise program are associated with the musculoskeletal system, involving sprains, muscle tears, and soft tissue injury. Again these can be minimized by relatively simple measures, particularly by gradual and progressive increase in the intensity of exercise, and by not doing too much too soon.

## SUMMARY OF CURRENT RECOMMENDATIONS

It is no longer considered beneficial for hypertensives to avoid physical activity. The available evidence[3] supports the widespread adoption of regular aerobic exercise in the general population, including those with hypertension. Regular exercise lowers resting BP and has a positive impact on cardiovascular health. The existing trend toward sedentary lifestyles may be reversed through a concerted effort to increase the uptake of regular exercise in the community. Likely consequences include a reduction in the prevalence of hypertension, as well as lower mortality from CHD. An optimal exercise program in hypertensives may be on the order of 30 to 45 minutes of aerobic exercise about three times a week at a level of 50% to 70% of maximum work capacity. It is not clear whether all forms of regular exercise are similarly effective. These recommendations certainly apply to walking, running, cycling, and mixed programs. There are conflicting data on swimming, as some studies show BP lowering and others do not. Nevertheless, swimming has considerable overall health benefits and specific advantages, since the lack of weight bearing may be the only form of exercise available to some participants with musculoskeletal disorders.

It should be emphasized that the studies reviewed in this chapter involved participants who were generally adherent to the programs. This will clearly not apply in the general community. Strategies for improving adherence to nonpharmacologic measures for cardiovascular risk reduction have been reviewed.[82] The issue is complex, and there are relatively few solutions. One important issue that emerges from the literature is the key role of clinicians in providing their imprimatur on the adoption of nonpharmacologic measures, including exercise, by their patients. Data suggest that if the doctor does not mention the benefits of exercise, weight loss, stopping smoking, or other hygienic measures during a consultation, many patients assume that it is not necessary for them to change. In the light of the present data, clinicians should consider and articulate their exercise and lifestyle prescriptions as clearly and carefully as they do a drug prescription for their patients.

## References

1. The Seventh Report of the Joint National Committee on Prevention, Detection, Evaluation and Treatment of High Blood Pressure. The JNC 7 Report. JAMA 289:2560-2572, 2003.
2. Guidelines Subcommittee of the World Health Organization-International Society of Hypertension (WHO-ISH). 1999 World Health Organization-International Society of Hypertension Guidelines for the Management of Hypertension. J Hypertens 17:151-183, 1999.
3. US Department of Health and Human Services. Physical Activity and Health. A Report of the Surgeon General. Atlanta, GA, US Department of Health and Human Services, Centers for Disease Control and Prevention, National Centre for Chronic Disease Prevention and Health Promotion, 1996.
4. Rowell LB. Human Circulation: Regulation during Physical Stress. New York, Oxford University Press, pp 213-256, 1986.
5. Rowell LB. Human Cardiovascular Control. New York:, Oxford University Press, 1993.
6. Anderson P, Saltin B. Maximal perfusion of skeletal muscle in man. J Physiol (Lond) 366:233-249, 1985.
7. Sonnenblick EH, Braunwald E, Williams JF. Effects of exercise on myocardial force-velocity relations in intact unanaesthetised man: Relative roles of changes in heart rate, sympathetic activity and ventricular dimensions. J Clin Invest 44:2051-2061, 1965.
8. Higginbotham MB, Morris KG, Williams RS, et al. Regulation of stroke volume during submaximal and maximal upright exercise in normal man. Circ Res 58:281-291, 1986.
9. Plotnick GD, Becker LC, Fisher ML, et al. Use of the Frank-Starling mechanism during submaximal versus maximal upright exercise. Am J Physiol 251(Heart Circ Physiol 20):H1101-H1105, 1986.
10. Poliner LR, Dehmer GJ, Lewis SE, et al. Left ventricular performance in normal subjects: A comparison of the responses to exercise in the upright and supine positions. Circulation 2:528-534, 1980.
11. Ludbrook J. Reflex control of blood pressure during exercise. Ann Rev Physiol 45:155-168, 1983.
12. Thompson PD, Crouse SF, Goodpaster B, et al. The acute versus the chronic response to exercise. Med Sci Sports Exerc 33(Suppl 6):S438-S545, 2001.
13. Filipovsky J, Ducimetiere P, Safar ME. Prognostic significance of exercise blood pressure and heart rate in mid aged men. Hypertension 20(3):333, 1992.
14. Mundal R, Kjeldsen SE, Sandvik L, et al. Exercise blood pressure predicts cardiovascular mortality in middle-aged men. Hypertension 24(1):56-62, 1994.
15. Gosse P, Desrumeau GC, Roudaut R, et al. Left ventricular mass in normotensive subjects. Importance of blood pressure response to activity. Am J Hypertens 2(2 Pt 1):78-80, 1989.
16. Fagard R, Van den Broeke C, Amery A. Left ventricular dynamics during exercise in elite marathon runners. J Am Coll Cardiol 14(1):112-118, 1989.
17. Eichner E. Exercise and heart disease; epidemiology of the "exercise hypothesis." Am J Med 75:1008-1023, 1983.
18. Kannel WB, Wilson P, Blair S. Epidemiological assessment of the role of physical activity and fitness in development of cardiovascular disease. Am Heart J 109:876-885, 1985.
19. Powell KE, Thompson PD, Casperson CJ, et al. Physical activity and the incidence of coronary heart disease. Ann Rev Public Health 8:253-287, 1987.
20. Paffenbarger RS Jr, Jung DL, Leung RW, et al. Physical activity and hypertension: An epidemiological view. Ann Med 23(3):319-327, 1991.
21. Paffenbarger RS, Hyde PH, Wing AL, et al. Physical activity, all-cause mortality, and longevity of college alumni. N Engl J Med 314:605-613, 1986.

22. Paffenbarger RS, Hyde PH, Wing AL, et al. The association of changes in physical-activity level and other lifestyle characteristics with mortality among men. N Engl J Med 328: 538-545, 1993.

23. Kannel WB, Belanger A, D'Agostino RD, et al. Physical activity and physical demand on the job and risk of cardiovascular disease and death: The Framingham Study. Am Heart J 112: 820-836, 1986.

24. Morris JN, Adam C, Chave SPW, et al. Vigorous exercise in leisure-time and the incidence of coronary heart disease. Lancet i:333-339, 1973.

25. Ekelund LG, Haskell WL, Johnson JL, et al. Physical fitness as a predictor of the cardiovascular mortality in asymptomatic North American men. N Engl J Med 319(21):1379-1384, 1988.

26. Blair SN, Goodyear NN, Gibbons LW, et al. Physical fitness and incidence of hypertension in healthy normotensive men and women JAMA 252:487-490, 1984.

27. Wannamethee G, Shaper AG. Physical activity and stroke in British middle aged men. Brit Med J 304:597-601, 1992.

28. Leon AS, Blackburn H. Physical activity and heart disease. Ann NY Acad Sci 301:561-578, 1977.

29. Leon AS. Comparative cardiovascular adaptations to exercise in animals and man and its relevance to coronary heart disease. In: Comparative Pathophysiology of Circulatory Disturbance. C M Bloom (ed). New York, Plenum, 1973; pp 143-174.

30. Zukal WJ, Lewis RH, Enterline RC, et al. A short time community study of the epidemiology of coronary heart disease Am J Public Health 49:1630-1639, 1959.

31. Leon AS, Connett J, Jacobs DR, et al. Leisure-time physical activity levels and risk of coronary heart disease and death: The Multiple Risk Factor Intervention Trial. JAMA 258: 2388-2395, 1987.

32. Slattery ML, Jacobs DR Nichaman MZ. Leisure time physical activity and coronary heart disease death: The US Railroad Study. Circulation 79:304-311, 1989.

33. Choquette G, Ferguson RJ. Blood pressure reduction in 'borderline' hypertensives following physical training. Canad Med Ass J 108:699-703, 1973.

34. Urata H, Tanabe Y, Kiyonaga A, et al. Antihypertensive and volume-depleting effects of mild exercise on essential hypertension. Hypertension 9:245-252, 1987.

35. Kinoshita A, Urata H, Tanabe Y, et al. What types of hypertensives respond better to mild exercise therapy? J Hypertens 6(Suppl 4):S631-S633, 1988.

36. Hagberg JM, Montain SJ, Martin WH, et al. Effect of exercise training in 60- to 69-year-old persons with essential hypertension. Am J Cardiol 64:348-353, 1989.

37. Meredith IT, Jennings GL, Esler MD, et al. Time-course of the antihypertensive and autonomic effects of regular endurance exercise in human subjects. J Hypertens 8:859-866, 1990.

38. Martin JE, Dubbert PM, Cushman WC. Controlled trial of aerobic exercise in hypertension. Circulation 81:1560-1567, 1990.

39. Allen DH, Puddey IB, Morton AR, et al. A controlled study of the effects of aerobic exercise on antihypertensive drug requirements of essential hypertensive patients in general practice. Clin Exp Pharmacol Physiol 18(5):279-282, 1991.

40. Cox KL, Puddey IB, Morton AR, et al. The effects of calorie restriction and exercise on blood pressure in overweight, sedentary males. J Hypertens 10(Suppl 4):S5, 1992.

41. Fagard R, Bielen P, Hespel P, et al. Physical exercise in hypertension. In: Hypertension: Pathophysiology, Diagnosis and Management. Laragh JH, Barry M, Brenner BM (eds). New York, Raven Press, 1990; pp 1985-2010.

42. Shindo M, Tanaka H, Ohara S, et al. Training of 50% VO$_2$ max on healthy middle aged men by bicycle ergometer. Rep Res Cen Phys Ed 2:139-152, 1974.

43. Tipton CM. Exercise, training and hypertension: An update. Exerc Sport Sci Rev 19:447-505, 1991.

44. Seals DR, Hagberg JM. The effect of exercise training on human hypertension: A review. Med Sci Sports Exerc 16(3): 207-215, 1984.

45. Arroll B, Beaglehole R. Does physical activity lower blood pressure: A critical review of the clinical trials. J Clin Epidemiol 45(5):439-447, 1992.

46. Jennings G, Kingwell B. Exercise. In: Textbook of Hypertension. Swales J (ed). Oxford, Blackwell Scientific Publications, 1994; pp 593-604.

47. Whelton SP, Chin A, Xin X, et al. Effect of aerobic exercise on blood pressure: A meta-analysis of randomised controlled trails. Ann Intern Med 136:493-503, 2002.

48. Fagard RH. Physical fitness and blood pressure. J Hypertens 11(Suppl 5):S47-S52, 1993.

49. Kelley GA. Aerobic exercise and resting blood pressure among women: A meta-analysis. Prev Med 28:264-75, 1999.

50. Jennings G, Nelson L, Nestel P, et al. The effects of changes in physical activity on major cardiovascular risk factors, hemodynamics, sympathetic function, and glucose utilisation in man: A controlled study of four levels of activity. Circulation 73:(1) 30-40, 1986.

51. Nelson L, Jennings GL, Esler MD, et al. Effect of changing levels of physical activity on blood pressure and hemodynamics in essential hypertension. Lancet 2:473-476.

52. Hanson JS, Nedde WH. Preliminary observations on physical training for hypertensive males. Circ Res 26(Suppl. 1): 149-153, 1970.

53. Johnson WP, Grover JA. Hemodynamic and metabolic effects of physical training in four patients with essential hypertension. Can Med Assoc J 96:842-846, 1967.

54. Sannerstedt R, Wasir H, Henning R, et al. Systemic hemodynamics in mild arterial hypertension before and after physical training. Clin Sci Molec Med 45:S145-S149, 1973.

55. De Plaen JE, Detry JM. Hemodynamic effects of physical training in established hypertension. Acta Cardiol 35:179-188, 1980.

56. Kiyonaga A, Arakawa K, Tanaka H, et al. Blood pressure and hormonal responses to aerobic exercise. Hypertension 7: 125-131, 1985.

57. Kinoshita A, Koga M, Matsusaki M, et al. Changes of dopamine and atrial natriuretic factor by mild exercise for hypertensives. Clin Exp Hypertens A. A13:1275-1290, 1991.

58. Sudhir K, Meredith IT, Jennings GL, et al. Effect of endurance exercise on cardiac secretion and renal clearance of atrial natriuretic peptide in normal humans. Clin Exp Hypertens Theory Pract A12:1223-1235, 1990.

59. Okabayashi T, Kohashi N, Yagi T, et al. The differences in natriuretic effect of taurine between healthy volunteers and patients with essential hypertension. Med J Kinki Univ 9:73-84, 1984.

60. Fujita T, Sato Y, Ando K. Role of the sympathetic nervous system in the antihypertensive effect of taurine in DOCA-salt hypertensive rats. Jpn Circ J 48:792, 1984.

61. Lin Y-C, Horvath SM. Autonomic nervous control of cardiac frequency in the exercise trained rat. J Appl Physiol 33: 796-799, 1972.

62. Ekblom B, Kilbom A, Soltysiak. Physical training, bradycardia, and autonomic nervous system. Scand J Clin Lab Invest 32: 251-256, 1973.

63. Tipton CM, Taylor B. Influence of atropine on heart rates of rats. Am J Physiol 208(3):480-484, 1965.

64. Frick MH, Elovainio RO, Somer T. The mechanism of bradycardia evoked by physical training. Cardiologia 51:46-54, 1967.

65. Floras JS, Sinkey CA, Aylward PE, et al. Postexercise hypotension and sympathoinhibition in borderline hypertensive men. Hypertension 14:28-35, 1989.

66. Meredith IT, Frieberg P, Jennings GL, et al. Exercise training lowers resting renal but not cardiac sympathetic activity. Hypertension 18:575-582, 1991.

67. Kingwell BA, Dart AM, Jennings GL, et al. Exercise training reduces the sympathetic component of the blood pressure-heart rate baroreflex in man. Clin Sci (Lond)82:357-362, 1992.

68. Stegemann J, Busert A, Brock D. Influence of fitness on the blood pressure control system in man. Aerospace Med 45: 45-48, 1974.

69. Smith ML, Graitzer HM, Hudson DL, et al. Baroreflex function in endurance- and static exercise-trained men. J Appl Physiol 64(2):585-591, 1988.

70. Kingwell BA, Gillies KJ, Cameron JC, et al. Elevated arterial compliance in athletes may mediate autonomic reflex changes. Proc Aust Physiol Pharmacol Soc p38P, 1993.

71. Korner PI, West MJ, Shaw J, et al. 'Steady-state' properties of the baroreceptor heart rate reflex in essential hypertension in man. Clin Exp Pharmacol Physiol 1:65-76, 1974.

72. Pagani M, Somers V, Furlan R, et al. Changes in autonomic regulation induced by physical training in mild hypertension. Hypertension 12:600-610, 1988.

73. Somers VK, Conway J, Sleight P. Physical training and ambulatory and sleep blood pressures in borderline hypertensive patients. *In* Abstract book of the 12th Scientific Meeting of the International Society of Hypertension. 1988; p 420.

74. Schwartz PJ, La Rovere MT, Vanoli E. Autonomic nervous system and sudden cardiac death: Experimental basis and clinical observations for post-myocardial infarction risk stratification. Circulation 85(Suppl I):I77-I91, 1992.

75. Georgiades A, Sherwood A, Gullette ECD, et al. Effects of exercise and weight loss on mental stress-induced cardiovascular responses in individuals with high blood pressure. Hypertension 36:171-176, 2000.

76. Roberts CK, Vaziri ND, Barnard RJ. Effect of diet and exercise intervention on blood pressure, insulin, oxidative stress, and nitric oxide availability. Circulation 106:2530-2532, 2002.

77. Kingwell B A, Sherrard B, Jennings GL, et al. Four weeks of cycle training increases basal production of nitric oxide from the forearm. Am J Physiol 272:H1070-H1077, 1997.

78. Lewis TV, Dart AM, Chin-Dusting JP, et al. Exercise training increases basal nitric oxide production from the forearm in hypercholesterolaemic patients. Arterioscler Thromb Vasc Biol 19(11):2782-2787, 1999.

79. Jennings G, Dart A, Meredith I, et al. Effects of exercise and other non-pharmacological measures on blood pressure and cardiac hypertrophy. J Cardiovasc Pharmacol 17(Suppl 2): S70-S74, 1991.

80. Hinderliter A, Sherwood A, Gullette ECD, et al. Reduction of left ventricular hypertrophy after exercise and weight loss in overweight patients with mild hypertension. Arch Intern Med 162:1333-1339, 2002.

81. Kelley GA, Kelley KS. Progressive resistance exercise and resting blood pressure: A Meta-analysis of randomised controlled trials. Hypertension 35:838-843, 2000.

82. Jennings G. The patient with multiple risk factors. *In* Manual of Hypertension. Mancia G, Chalmers J, Julius S, et al. (eds). London; New York, Churchill Livingstone, 2002; pp 555-564.

# SECTION 7

# Pharmacologic Treatment

## Chapter 48

# Initial Choices in the Treatment of Hypertension

## Myron H. Weinberger

A plethora of important studies conducted during the 1990s have provided an incredible database of new information concerning the benefits of antihypertensive therapy, the comparative effects of various classes of antihypertensive agents, and even information concerning optimal blood pressure (BP) levels in both uncomplicated and complex hypertensive patient groups. This information is slowly being analyzed, evaluated, published, reevaluated, compared, and considered by the medical community ranging from researchers and specialists, to primary care physicians, and even by the lay public. In many cases the results have formed the basis of recommendations for optimal levels of BP and for specific forms of therapy for some individuals, promulgated by a variety of national and international medical organizations, ranging from specialty groups to national and international health and policy-making bodies. As a result of the ever-increasing size, complexity, and costs of these studies, media publicity aimed at the consumer has often followed and, in some cases, even preceded the presentation of the results to the scientific community. This barrage of information has led to much confusion on the part of the practitioners as well as the general public. This chapter attempts to survey the most important and largest of these endeavors to assist physicians in making a rational and beneficial choice for initial antihypertensive therapy. Other chapters are devoted to specific classes of antihypertensive agents and particular subgroups of patients and provide much more detailed and comprehensive information.

## WHEN AND WHOM TO TREAT

Evidence regarding the impact of BP on morbidity and mortality has undergone drastic reevaluation on the basis of several important studies that have provided new insight into the importance of this major risk factor for cardiovascular disease. For example, observational data from more than 1 million individuals participating in a variety of studies has indicated that the risk of cardiovascular morbidity and mortality begins to increase at BP levels of 115/75 mm Hg and doubles at each increment of 20/10 mm Hg above that level.[1]

When considering the traditional criteria of 140/90 mm Hg for the definition of hypertension, it is important to recognize that the Framingham Heart Study has demonstrated that individuals with a BP between 130 and 139 mm Hg systolic and 80 to 89 mm Hg diastolic are at twice the risk for the development of future hypertension as those with "normal" BP.[2] Thus we have two compelling prospective observations documenting the increased risk of cardiovascular events in persons with BPs below 140/90 mm Hg. Moreover, individuals with normal BP at the age of 55 years have a 90% chance of developing hypertension in their lifetime.[3] Thus those fortunate enough to reach the age of 55 without becoming hypertensive have an overwhelming likelihood of doing so as they age. These convincing and compelling findings led the seventh report of the Joint National Committee on Prevention, Detection, Evaluation, and Treatment of High Blood Pressure (JNC 7) to draw attention to lower BP levels than had previously been of concern, by defining BP levels between 120/80 mm Hg and 139/89 mm Hg as "prehypertensive" and by recommending nonpharmacologic therapy as a means of reducing those levels.[4] These nondrug approaches will be discussed subsequently.

The guidelines of 120-139/80-89 mm Hg for nonpharmacologic intervention and drug treatment for those above 140/90 mm Hg, the traditional point for initiation of drug treatment for those not adequately controlled with nondrug approaches, apply to uncomplicated individuals. However, there are several subgroups with evidence of, or at high risk for, vascular disease or other conditions such as diabetes mellitus or renal disease, for whom BP levels even lower than the traditional 140/90 mm Hg are desirable. These persons should require antihypertensive drug therapy to achieve more aggressive BP goals. The most recent guidelines suggest that the goal for diabetics should be a BP consistently below 130/80 mm Hg and for those with renal disease of any form, below 125/75 mm Hg. Individuals with congestive heart failure (CHF) comprise another group for whom BP levels lower than the traditional 140/90 mm Hg have been advocated, but specific levels have not been precisely defined.

## NONPHARMACOLOGIC THERAPY FOR THOSE WITH "PREHYPERTENSION"

The nonpharmacologic approaches that have been shown to lower BP, and which have been advocated as initial therapy for the stage 1 hypertensive, do not have universal efficacy in all individuals. For example, weight loss for the obese person is usually associated with a reduction in BP. Curiously, BP tends to fall early in the weight loss program, if it falls at all. Thus massive weight loss, even for the grossly obese individual, is not always required for a beneficial reduction in BP. As with all interventions, maintaining the weight loss is more difficult than initially achieving it.[5] The benefit of aerobic exercise on BP is less consistent. Some of the earlier studies of exercise failed to control for the effect of weight loss on BP, and thus the effects of uncontrolled weight loss accompanying the exercise regimens may have confounded the results. Nonetheless, a regular exercise program aids in maintaining weight loss and improves cardiovascular fitness and is thus to be recommended as a nondrug approach whenever possible. In general, weight loss has been associated with greater decreases in BP than those reported with exercise alone.[6] Another lifestyle alteration that has been shown to reduce BP is a decrease in alcohol consumption for those who drink more than 2 ounces of alcohol daily.[7] Monitoring adherence to this recommendation is often difficult in view of the central nervous system effects of alcohol and the need to precisely limit the quantity consumed.

The greatest reductions in BP among the nondrug approaches have been seen in salt-sensitive individuals who reduce their sodium intake to levels at or below 100 mM/dl (2.3 g/day). Salt sensitivity is essentially a research definition but its prevalence has been observed to be greater among older individuals (older than 60 years of age), African Americans, diabetics, and those with a family history of hypertension in a first-degree relative.[8] In many individuals who are salt sensitive, a deficient intake of potassium has been noted, and thus potassium supplementation has been shown to lower BP. In fact, a recent study that incorporated both sodium restriction and potassium supplementation by dietary means (the Dietary Approaches to Stop Hypertension [DASH] diet) was effective in reducing BP in those with "high-normal" and stage 1 BP elevation.[9] This study demonstrated that the BP lowering effect of the original DASH diet was enhanced by reduction of sodium intake from 100 mM/dl to 65 mM/dl (1.5 g/day).

The decision of when and how to treat BP is sometimes influenced by factors other than the office or clinic BP measurements. Patients have been identified who manifest higher BP readings in the office or clinic than outside the medical environment, the so-called white-coat hypertension syndrome. This phenomenon may not be as innocuous as many believe, since it may be associated with early evidence of target organ disease and with the progression to established hypertension with the passage of time. Given the new prehypertension category, such individuals certainly will require closer scrutiny and earlier treatment. The decision of whether to embark on nonpharmacologic or drug therapy may require 24-hour ambulatory BP monitoring, which should include careful attention to the presence or absence of the typical nocturnal decline in BP. Individuals in whom this nocturnal "dip" is not present are exposed to a greater pressure load over the 24-hour period and thus are more apt to demonstrate early

target organ changes.[10] The diagnosis of hypertension is made when the average awake ambulatory BP exceeds 135/85 mm Hg and the nocturnal average is more than 120/75 mm Hg.

Another consideration that may influence the decision to begin antihypertensive drug therapy is the presence of other risk factors for cardiovascular disease. Diabetes mellitus and renal disease have already been mentioned as conditions in which lower BP levels have been clearly shown to be beneficial. Elevated BP or even prehypertension represents only one of many risk factors requiring attention in many other patient types. As examples, the patient with a history of cigarette smoking who can not be induced to quit, the dyslipidemic patient, the individual with the metabolic syndrome ("X"), and the obese patient all represent individuals for whom even a mild increase in BP above the "normal" level of 120/80 mm Hg represents increased risk for cardiovascular events and for whom drug therapy may be considered appropriate. Moreover, the impact antihypertensive drugs on these other risk factors requires particular consideration as will be outlined in the next section. A drug that lowers BP but has an adverse effect on glucose tolerance or lipids will be less beneficial in reducing the risk of cardiovascular events than a drug that reduces BP to the same degree without an undesirable effect on the other risk factors.[11-13]

## FACTORS TO CONSIDER IN CHOOSING INITIAL DRUG THERAPY

When the decision has been made to begin antihypertensive therapy, several considerations are appropriate in selecting the agent. The BP level provides an initial clue regarding whether a single agent is likely to produce adequate BP lowering to achieve the desired goal. Individuals with BPs above 160 mm Hg systolic and/or 100 diastolic mm Hg will generally require more than a single drug to reach goal levels. A detailed discussion of such combination therapies will follow consideration of monotherapy, which is generally more appropriate for those with elevations of BP less than 160/100 mm Hg. Because factors such as age, ethnicity, cigarette smoking, and concomitant risk factors and disorders influence the response to, and benefit of, specific drug therapy, such factors need to be identified and considered.

In persons younger than age 50 and in those with evidence of increased sympathetic drive as manifest by a hyperdynamic chest wall and/or a resting tachycardia, β-adrenergic blocking drugs are a good initial choice. Such agents are also effective in patients with a history of angina or migraine, and those with familial tremor. The more lipid-soluble agents such as propranolol and nadolol seem to be the most effective in the latter two situations, while virtually all β-blockers have been reported to be effective in reducing angina. A history of asthma represents a contraindication to the administration of β-blockers. In patients with symptomatic peripheral vascular disease, agents that act by inducing peripheral vasodilation are preferable to β-adrenergic blocking drugs, which may worsen the symptoms of peripheral vascular insufficiency.

In salt-sensitive subjects,[8] BP is most responsive to agents that have a diuretic and/or natriuretic effect. Diuretics fall into this category but for reasons suggested in the previous section and discussed in more detail subsequently, they may not always be an ideal initial choice for antihypertensive monotherapy. An alternative consideration for the salt-sensitive hypertensive is the administration of a calcium channel blocker, because such agents have been shown to have a diuretic and natriuretic effect[14-16] in addition to their vasodilator action, reducing peripheral resistance. Comparative studies have demonstrated equivalent efficacy for diuretics such as hydrochlorothiazide and chlorthalidone and calcium channel blockers such as amlodipine in reducing BP in older hypertensives and those with the characteristics of salt sensitivity.[17] The Antihypertensive and Lipid-Lowering Treatment to Prevent Heart Attack Trial (ALLHAT) was composed of a highly salt-sensitive hypertensive cohort that included mild hypertensives, 36% Black, and 36% diabetic and with an average age of 67 years. The ALLHAT trial demonstrated equivalent BP reduction in the groups randomized to chlorthalidone and amlodipine, which is significantly greater than the reduction achieved by the group assigned to initial therapy with lisinopril. At the end of this 5-year study, however, only one third of the participants were receiving monotherapy, while the remaining majority required multiple drugs to reach the BP goal of 140/90 mm Hg or less.

In contrast to the findings of the ALLHAT trial, observations from a study in almost exclusively white hypertensives in Australia showed greater benefit from initial treatment with an angiotensin-converting enzyme (ACE) inhibitor than a diuretic.[18] This would seem to confirm earlier observations suggesting that diuretics and calcium channel blockers are preferred *initial* therapeutic choices for the older hypertensive, the Black hypertensive, and the diabetic hypertensive, about whom more detail will be provided shortly. In contrast, β-adrenergic blockers, ACE inhibitors, and angiotensin II receptor blockers (ARBs) are more effective in younger persons, particularly in white hypertensives as *initial* therapy. For example, the Veterans Administration Cooperative Study Group showed that in an older, male population with the typical characteristics of individuals obtaining their care at such facilities, diuretics and calcium channel blockers were more effective than β-adrenergic blocking drugs and ARBs.[19] Not surprisingly, these observations are consistent with the findings of the ALLHAT trial, because many of the ALLHAT sites were Veterans Administration Hospital clinics.

Most studies examining the effect of gender have failed to reveal a significant difference in the responses of men and women to specific antihypertensive monotherapy when other factors such as age, ethnicity, and diabetes are considered. These important studies then permit a broad, general summary of the likely BP efficacy of the major antihypertensive drug classes. However, the treatment of hypertension involves much more than lowering BP. Thus the major antihypertensive drug trials emphasize cardiovascular and other outcomes.

What have we learned from the large, long, and expensive antihypertensive drug trials conducted since the original Veterans Administrative Cooperative Study,[20] which first documented the beneficial effects of lowering BP in severe hypertensives compared with placebo more than 40 years ago? First and foremost, we have learned that lowering BP reduces cardiovascular events, including stroke, heart attacks, and CHF, as well as renal impairment and failure. All of these events have not consistently been shown to be reduced in the earlier trials, some of which may not have been conducted for a sufficiently long period of time to document benefit in reducing events other than stroke, for which BP reduction has consistently been shown to be beneficial. The ALLHAT trial con-

firmed the benefit of BP reduction in preventing stroke by demonstrating that stroke was significantly (40%; $p < .001$) more common among Black hypertensives assigned to lisinopril as initial therapy compared with those whose first drug was chlorthalidone.[17] An important contributor to this dramatic finding is higher BP (4 mm Hg systolic and 2 mm Hg diastolic) in the Black subgroup randomized to lisinopril compared with the groups assigned to chlorthalidone. Although it is difficult to believe that such small differences in BP could account for such a large relative increase in stroke, the very large size and tremendous statistical power of the ALLHAT trial provide confidence in the relevance of the finding. Thus it would appear that no antihypertensive regimen will provide cardioprotective benefit unless it lowers BP to a degree comparable with other agents.

Beyond BP reduction, there are other benefits of antihypertensive therapy. Although stroke incidence decreases almost immediately after effective BP reduction in hypertensive subjects, a reduction in coronary artery disease events has not always been observed. There is considerable debate about the reasons for this. Some have suggested that BP is less important in the prevention of coronary disease than in stroke. Others have proposed that while the benefit of antihypertensive drug treatment in decreasing stroke incidence is primarily due to pressure reduction per se, coronary disease results from a much more complex array of factors and is more insidious in its development. Thus the relatively short duration of most antihypertensive trials may not have been sufficient to disclose beneficial effects on this endpoint. Exclusion of persons at high risk for vascular events from many studies may have also influenced the impact on heart disease events.

It has also been suggested that the potential adverse metabolic effects of some antihypertensive drugs on insulin sensitivity and lipids, both well-recognized risk factors for coronary artery disease, may have counterbalanced the benefit of BP reduction on coronary events. Thus it has been more difficult to demonstrate a reduction in heart disease than stroke by BP lowering. Evidence from several large trials that were conducted for sufficient time to examine these issues in detail has revealed some support for the latter hypothesis. For example, in the ALLHAT trial, which had an average 5-year follow-up period, the chlorthalidone-assigned group had a 40% greater incidence of new-onset diabetes ($p < .001$) at the end of the study compared with the group assigned to lisinopril, which had an incidence not significantly different from the amlodipine group.[17] Although this increase in diabetes was not reflected in more coronary events during the course of the trial, the longer-term implications of the development of de novo diabetes must be a consideration in choosing initial antihypertensive therapy. Two other trials that compared a β-adrenergic blocking regimen with either an ARB (the Losartan Intervention for Endpoint Reduction in Hypertension Study [LIFE])[21] or a calcium channel blocker (the International Verapamil-Trandolapril Study [INVEST])[22] regimen also demonstrated a significantly ($p < .01$) greater incidence of new onset diabetes in the group randomized to β-adrenergic blocking drug.

Dyslipidemia is another important risk factor for cardiovascular disease, particularly coronary artery disease. Antihypertensive drugs have been shown to have variable effects on the lipid profile, which may impact on these risks.[11-13] Some have argued that the effects of diuretics on the lipid profile are only transient. However, the observation of significantly ($p$ <.01) higher total cholesterol levels at the end of 5 years of follow-up for those participants in the ALLHAT trial assigned to a chlorthalidone compared with the lisinopril and amlodipine groups indicates that these changes, although small, are certainly persistent and clinically relevant. Similarly, β-adrenergic blocking agents can also reduce high-density lipoproteins, increase triglycerides, and thus raise the risk for cardiovascular events.[11,13]

Another surprising finding from the ALLHAT trial relates to the effects of the assigned drug regimens on renal function in this cohort without renal dysfunction at baseline (serum creatinine in the normal range was one of the entry criteria for the study). At the end of the 5 years of the study, the chlorthalidone and lisinopril groups evidenced a significantly ($p$ <.05) greater decrease in glomerular filtration rate (GFR) than the amlodipine group.[17] This was surprising in view of the evidence of a beneficial effect of ACE inhibitors and more consistently, ARBs, in the stabilization of renal function in those with chronic kidney disease.[23-26]

## IS THERE A BEST SINGLE DRUG?

It should be clear from the experience of these large trials, supported by a tremendous older literature, than no single drug class will provide an optimal choice for all patients. The overriding message from these studies is that the majority of even mild and uncomplicated hypertensive patients will require multiple drug therapy to reach the new recommendations for BP goals as stated by JNC 7.[4] In fact, JNC 7 recommends beginning with two drugs when the BP is above 160 mm Hg systolic and/or 100 mm Hg diastolic. Even among the 10% of ALLHAT participants who were untreated at entry to the study and who had an average baseline BP of 157/90 mm Hg, more than 60% required three drugs to reach treatment goals.[17] Thus arguments concerning which agent is best for the initiation of therapy are often moot because multiple drug therapy will usually be required. Moreover, because reducing the dose of diuretics decreases both their dose-dependent adverse effects and their BP-lowering efficacy, it seems appropriate to consider combination therapy as a means of achieving BP goals and minimizing adverse effects.

What then are the two-drug combinations that have proven to be effective? Are there any particular benefits to specific combinations? The literature on these issues is too extensive for a detailed discussion in this chapter and thus their implications will simply be summarized. One of the major limitations of the large and important ALLHAT trial resided in the treatment algorithm. Because the primary aim of the study was to determine whether any of the three newer classes of antihypertensive drugs assignments was better than a thiazide-type diuretic in reducing fatal and nonfatal heart attack, the design attempted to minimize "crossover" of the test drugs (amlodipine, chlorthalidone, doxazosin, and lisinopril).[17] For this reason, participants who did not reach the goal BP of <140/90 mm Hg (almost two thirds of the study population) could be given an open-label or third-step agent at the discretion of the investigator. For the second-step, drugs working by interfering with the sympathetic nervous system (reserpine, clonidine, or atenolol) were recommended. Such agents are not generally effective in reducing BP in salt-sensitive hypertensives, who

comprised the majority of the ALLHAT cohort. Therefore participants assigned to lisinopril who did not achieve the BP goal on monotherapy would not be expected to achieve that goal with one of the second step agents. Thus the third-step drug, hydralazine, a short-acting direct vasodilator would be recommended. However, this agent causes salt and water retention and volume expansion and would also not likely be effective in salt-sensitive subjects. In other words, the treatment algorithm employed in this study was flawed from the standpoint of physiologic factors and pharmacologic efficacy. In general, low-dose diuretic therapy increases the efficacy of drugs from the sympatholytic and vasodilator classes. Although the combination of diuretic and β-adrenergic blocking agent has greater BP-lowering efficacy than either monotherapy, the adverse effects of both agents on insulin sensitivity, glucose, and lipids make this a less-than-ideal choice for most uncomplicated hypertensives.

Combining ACE inhibitors or ARBs with low-dose diuretic therapy is a very effective antihypertensive approach that has an added benefit of blocking many of the adverse metabolic effects of diuretic therapy, which are largely mediated by activations of the renin-angiotensin-aldosterone system.[27] The combination of calcium channel blockers with diuretics has questionable additive efficacy on the basis of relatively few studies with small numbers of subjects.[28] This is not surprising when it is recognized that both agents have diuretic and natriuretic effects, while calcium channel blockers have an additional vasodilator effect, accounting for greater efficacy. In contrast, the combination of calcium channel blockers with ACE inhibitors or ARBs has a powerful additive efficacy. Moreover, such combinations are devoid of adverse metabolic actions and each of the components has been shown to have beneficial effects on cardiovascular disease outcomes.

α-Adrenergic blocking drugs have fallen into disfavor because of a lack of benefit on cardiovascular disease outcomes reported in the ALLHAT trial.[29] However, that may be a short-sighted conclusion in view of the fact that most patients require the addition of a low-dose diuretic for antihypertensive efficacy with this class of drugs. α-Adrenergic blockers are very useful in the treatment of the symptoms of benign prostatic hyperplasia, a disorder frequently found in older hypertensive men.[30] In addition to the combination of α-adrenergic blocker and diuretic, the combination of α- and β-adrenergic blocker has been shown to be effective for many individuals. Aldosterone antagonists, represented by the older agent, spironolactone, and the new generation drug, eplerenone, which has side effects, have recently been shown to be effective antihypertensive agents.[31]

## COMPELLING INDICATIONS FOR SPECIFIC DRUG THERAPY

There are several subgroups of hypertensive patients for whom specific antihypertensive drugs should be prescribed. Examples include diuretics, β-adrenergic blocking agents, ACE inhibitors, ARBs, and aldosterone antagonists for the patient with heart failure; β-adrenergic blocking agents, ACE inhibitors, and aldosterone antagonists for postmyocardial infarction; diuretics, ACE inhibitors, ARBs, and calcium channel blockers for diabetics; ACE inhibitors and ARBs for chronic kidney disease; diuretics, calcium channel blockers, and ACE inhibitors for stroke prevention (primary or recurrent); and diuretics, β-adrenergic blocking agents, ACE inhibitors, and calcium channel blockers for those at high risk for coronary artery disease.[4] It should be recognized that not *all* of these recommended agents need to be given in combination to every patient with the problems indicated, but rather that treatment with these agents requires special and individualized consideration. Moreover, many of these drugs will not be efficacious in lowering BP unless combined with other agents, such as those suggested previously.

# References

1. Lewington S, Clarke R, Qizilbash N, et al. Age-specific relevance of usual blood pressure to vascular mortality: a meta-analysis of individual data for one million adults in 61 prospective studies. Lancet 360:1903-1913, 2002.
2. Vasan RS, Larson MG, Leip EP, et al. Assessment of frequency of progression to hypertension in nonhypertensive participants in the Framingham heart Study: A cohort study. Lancet 358: 1682-1686, 2001.
3. Vasan RS, Beiser A, Seshadri S, et al. Residual lifetime risk for developing hypertension in middle-aged women and men: The Framingham Heart Study. JAMA 287:1003-1010, 2002.
4. Chobanian AV, Bakris GL, Black HR, et al. and the National High Blood Pressure Education Program Coordinating Committee. The seventh report of the Joint National Committee on Prevention, Detection, Evaluation and Treatment of High Blood Pressure. The JNC 7 report. JAMA 289:3560-3572, 2003.
5. He J, Whelton PK, Appel LJ, et al. Long-term effect of weight loss and dietary sodium reduction on incidence of hypertension. Hypertension 35:544-549, 2000.
6. Blumenthal JA, Sherwood A, Gullette ECD, et al. Exercise and weight loss reduce blood pressure in men and women with mild hypertension. Arch Intern Med 160:1947-1958, 2000.
7. Xin X, He J, Frontini MG, et al. Effects of alcohol reduction on blood pressure: a meta-analysis of randomized controlled trials. Hypertension 38:1112-1117, 2001.
8. Weinberger MH, Miller JZ, Luft FC, et al. Definitions and characteristics of sodium sensitivity and blood pressure resistance. Hypertension 8(Suppl II):127-134, 1986.
9. Sacks FM, Svetkey LP, Vollmer WM, et al. Effects on blood pressure of reduced dietary sodium and the Dietary Approaches to Stop Hypertension (DASH) diet. DASH-sodium Collaborative Research Group. N Engl J Med 344:3-10, 2001.
10. Pickering T. Recommendations for the use of home (self) and ambulatory blood pressure monitoring. American Society of Hypertension Ad Hoc Panel. Am J Hypertens 9:1-11, 1996.
11. Weinberger MH. Antihypertensive drugs and lipids: Evidence, mechanisms and implications. Arch Intern Med 145:1102-1105, 1985.
12. Weinberger MH. Diuretics and their side effects: Dilemma in the treatment of hypertension. Hypertens 11(Suppl II): 16-20, 1988.
13. Weinberger MH. The treatment of hypertension in the 1990s: Optimizing the benefit of blood pressure reduction by minimizing risk factors for cardiovascular disease. Am J Med 82(1A):44-49, 1987.
14. Luft FC, Aronoff GR, Fienberg NS, et al. Calcium channel blockade with nitrendipine. Hypertension 7:438-442, 1985.
15. Luft FC, Aronoff GR, Fineberg NS, et al. Facilitation of natriuresis with nifedipine in normal humans. J Cardiovasc Pharmacol 12(Suppl 6):120-122, 1988.
16. Luft FC, Fienberg NS, Weinberger MH. Long-term effect of nifedipine and hydrochlorothiazide on blood pressure and sodium homeostasis at varying levels of salt intake in mildly hypertensive patients. Am J Hypertens 4:752-760, 1991.
17. The ALLHAT Officers and Co-ordinators for the ALLHAT Collaborative Group. Major outcomes in high-risk hypertensive patients randomized to angiotensin converting enzyme inhibitor or calcium channel blocker vs. diuretic. The Antihypertensive and Lipid-Lowering Treatment to Prevent Heart Attack Trial (ALLHAT). JAMA 288:1981-1997, 2002.
18. Wing LMH, Reid CM, Ryan P, et al. for the Second Australian National Blood Pressure Study Group. A comparison of outcome with angiotensin-converting enzyme inhibitors and diuretics for hypertension in the elderly. N Engl J Med 348: 583-592, 2003.
19. Materson BJ, Reda DJ, Cushman WC, et al. Single-drug therapy for hypertension in men: a comparison of six antihypertensive agents with placebo: The Department of Veterans Affairs Cooperative Study Group on Antihypertensive Agents. N Engl J Med 328:914-921, 1993.
20. Veterans Administration Cooperative Study Group on Antihypertensive Agents. Effects of treatment on morbidity in hypertension. I. Results in patients with diastolic pressures averaging 115 through 129 mm Hg. JAMA 202:1028-1035, 1967.
21. Dahlof B, Devereux RB, Kjeldsen SE, et al. Cardiovascular morbidity and mortality in the Losartan Intervention For Endpoint reduction in hypertension study (LIFE): A randomized trial against atenolol. Lancet 359:995-1003, 2002.
22. Pepine CJ, Handberg EM, Cooper-DeHoff RM et al.; INVEST Investigators. A calcium antagonist vs a non-calcium antagonist hypertension treatment strategy for patients with coronary artery disease. The International Verapamil-Trandolapril Study (INVEST): A randomized controlled trial. JAMA 290(21): 2805-2816, 2003.
23. The ACE Inhibitors in Diabetic Nephropathy Trialist Group. Should all patients with type 1 diabetes mellitus and microalbuminuria receive angiotensin-converting enzyme inhibitors? A meta-analysis of individual patient data. Ann Intern Med 134:370-379, 2001.
24. Wright JT Jr, Bakris G, Greene T, et al., for the African American Study of Kidney Disease and Hypertension Study Group. Effect of blood pressure lowering and antihypertensive drug class on the progression of hypertensive kidney disease: Results from the AASK trial. JAMA 288:2421-2431, 2002.
25. Brenner BM, Cooper ME, de Zeeuw D, et al. Effects of losartan on renal and cardiovascular outcomes in patients with type 2 diabetes and nephropathy. N Engl J Med 345:861-869, 2001.
26. Lewis EJ, Hunsicker LG, Clarke WR, et al. Renoprotective effect of the angiotensin-receptor antagonist irbesartan in patients with nephropathy due to type 2 diabetes. N Engl J Med 345:851-860, 2001.
27. Weinberger MH. The influence of an angiotensin converting enzyme inhibitor captopril on diuretic-induced metabolic effects in hypertension. Hypertension 5:III132-III138, 1983.
28. Weinberger MH. Additive effects of diuretics or sodium restriction with calcium channel blockers in the treatment of hypertension. J Cardiovasc Pharmacol 12:S72-S75, 1988.
29. The ALLHAT Officers and Coordinators for the ALLHAT Collaborative Research Group. Major cardiovascular events in hypertensive patients randomized to doxazosin vs chlorthalidone: The Antihypertensive and Lipid-Lowering Treatment to Prevent Heart Attack Trial (ALLHAT). JAMA 283(15): 1967-1975, 2000.
30. Weinberger MH, Fawzy A. Doxazosin in elderly patients with hypertension. Int J Clin Prac 54:181-189, 2000.
31. Weinberger MH, Roniker B, Krouse SL, et al. Eplerenone, a selective aldosterone blocker (SAB) in mild to moderate hypertension. Am J Hypertension 15:709-716, 2002.

# Pharmacokinetics of Antihypertensive Drugs
## Alexander M. M. Shepherd

## INTRODUCTION

The previous edition of this book did not contain a chapter dedicated to the disposition of the drugs used in the treatment of hypertension. I considered whether clinicians need to know much about the kinetics of this group of drugs. After all, we can readily measure the response to them and alter the administered dose to achieve the desired antihypertensive response.

On reflection, however, I created a fairly long list of reasons why knowledge of drug disposition and mode of action was essential to a clinician using drug therapy to treat hypertension. This list includes the following:

1. Knowledge of the route and manner of elimination from the body would permit dose alteration in disease states; for example, accumulation of a drug in hepatic failure or of its active metabolites in renal failure could increase toxicity or efficacy.
2. This knowledge would also be of use in predicting drug interactions; for example, knowing that verapamil is broken down in the liver by the Phase 1 microsomal isoenzyme cytochrome P450 3A4 would predict the possibility of an interaction with some of the "statins" used to treat the hypercholesterolemia that commonly accompanies the hypertension. This interaction could increase the blood level of the statin and make toxicity more likely.
3. Knowledge of the plasma half-life of a drug can aid in determining the dosing schedule, for example, furosemide should be used twice daily because its duration of action is relatively short and blood pressure control may be lost if the drug is given once a day. Caution must be exercised in predicting duration of effect from plasma half-life. We tend to dose many drugs once every half-life because we can easily tolerate swings in blood levels of around 50%. With antihypertensive drugs, the effect tends to last longer than would be predicted—sometimes much longer. Examples include the hydralazine plasma half-life of around 90 minutes, which does not easily translate into the twice-daily regimen effective in many patients. Also, propranolol has a plasma half-life of less than 5 hours but can be given twice daily.
4. Knowledge of whether a drug is lipid or water soluble may help in determining whether it will cause central nervous system side effects, whether it will be well absorbed when given by mouth, and whether it will be rapidly metabolized in the liver. An example of this is the β-adrenergic blocker group, of which some (e.g., propranolol and metoprolol) are lipid soluble and therefore more likely to be rapidly eliminated from the body, requiring twice-daily dosing, and also may be more likely to cause insomnia and nightmares.
5. Knowledge of whether the drug has first- or zero-order elimination may aid in deciding on dose escalations. Doubling the dose of a drug with first-order (a fixed proportion of the drug is eliminated per unit time) elimination will approximately double the antihypertensive effect, whereas the same escalation in a drug with zero-order (a fixed amount of the drug is eliminated per unit time) elimination could produce much greater effect and side effects than expected.
6. Knowledge of the mode of action of the drug is also important, because this permits the appropriate drug to be given to match the pathophysiology of the hypertension in a particular patient. For example, use of a β-blocker may benefit a young patient with systolic hypertension but may actually elevate the blood pressure in an old patient with systolic hypertension. The first patient is more likely to have elevated cardiac output (reduced by the drug) and the second to have reduced compliance in the large arteries (worsened by the drug). Also, beneficial drug combinations can be predicted from knowledge of the mode of action. For example, addition of a diuretic to therapy with an angiotensin-converting enzyme inhibitor (ACEI) is predicted to—and does—enhance efficacy by plasma volume reduction, thus increasing the reliance of the blood pressure on the renin angiotensin system. Finally, nothing damages the confidence of a patient in his physician more than to have the physician prescribe a first drug that does not cause blood pressure reduction but that does cause symptomatic side effects. This can often be prevented by knowing both the mode of action and the pathophysiology of the disease. After all, about half of the patients can be controlled with one drug and about half of the remainder with the addition of a second drug. The physician must start with the correct drug.

This chapter addresses the clinically important aspects of the pharmacokinetics of the different drug classes used for the treatment of hypertension.

These classes are as follows:

1. Diuretics (thiazides, loop diuretics, and potassium-sparing diuretics)
2. β-Adrenergic blockers
3. $\alpha_1$-Adrenergic blockers
4. Central $\alpha_2$ agonists
5. ACEIs
6. Angiotensin receptor blockers
7. Direct-acting vasodilators
8. Calcium channel blockers (CCBs)
9. Selective aldosterone receptor antagonists
10. Drug classes under development

## DIURETICS

### Thiazides

There are many drugs in this class. Some are described in Table 49–1.

**Table 49-1** Thiazides

| Drug | Plasma $t_{1/2}$ (hours) | Dose Frequency (time/day) | Usual Dose (mg/day) | Maximum Dose (mg/day) |
|------|------|------|------|------|
| Chlorothiazide | 1-2 | 2 | 125-500 | 1000 |
| Chlorthalidone | 40-60 | 1 | 12.5-25 | 50 |
| Hydrochlorothiazide | 10-12 | 1 | 6.25-25 | 50 |
| Indapamide | 14-15 | 1 | 1.25-2.5 | 5 |
| Methyclothiazide | ? | 1 | 2.5-5.0 | 10 |
| Metolazone | 8-14 | 1 | 0.5-1.0 | 1 |
| Polythiazide | 25 | 1 | 1-2 | 4 |
| Trichlormethiazide | 2-3 | 1 | 1-2 | 4 |

$t_{1/2}$, half-life.

It can readily be seen from the table that there is little correlation between plasma half-life and effect half-life. All can be given once daily, except chlorothiazide, which should usually be given twice daily. The side effect profiles are similar between the drugs, and most clinicians will choose based on price rather than on drug disposition, side effects, or effectiveness.[1]

The drugs as a group have good (60%-80%) absorption after oral administration, independent of dose, apart from chlorothiazide, which has poor, saturable absorption that therefore decreases further with dose increases. Giving two 250-mg tablets produces about the same blood levels as one 250-mg tablet.

These drugs have distribution volumes of 3 to 25 L/kg of body weight, indicating that most of the drug is present in the tissues rather than in the circulating compartment. This makes it unlikely that hemodialysis will remove much of the drug.

This class is defined as the "low ceiling" class of diuretics because most of the blood pressure lowering effect occurs at lower doses. Increasing the dose above this level will produce little or no additional lowering of blood pressure. On the other hand, adverse effects continue to increase in a dose-related manner. For example, hypokalemia will become more pronounced as the dose increases above 25 mg/day of hydrochlorothiazide, whereas most of the hypotensive effect occurs at 25 mg/day or less. It makes sense, therefore, to use these drugs at lower doses and to add a second drug if adequate effect is not obtained.

Blood potassium levels will stabilize about 2 weeks after a dose change, so continued measurement of blood potassium levels is usually not necessary after that time. Prevention of significant fall in blood potassium level will prevent a portion of the increased insulin resistance that is sometimes seen with the thiazide diuretics. This can most easily be done by measuring blood potassium before and 1 month after starting or changing the dose of the drug.

In the past it was thought that thiazides induced an increase in total and low-density lipoprotein (LDL) cholesterol and in triglycerides in the blood. This is true in the short term, but after 1 year of therapy, the thiazides have the same effect on lipid levels as ACEIs and CCBs.

Several troublesome but relatively rare adverse effects must also be mentioned. All the thiazides contain -SH groups and cause reactions in patients who are sensitive. The alternative is ethacrynic acid, which does not have such a group.

Many of the thiazides can cause photoallergies, resulting in itchy skin rashes in the sun-exposed areas of the body. Stopping the drug does not always result in regression of the rash.

## Loop Diuretics

Loop diuretics are shown in Table 49-2.

This group of drugs is used in the treatment of hypertension, but thiazides are preferable in all but a few clinical situations (e.g., concomitant heart failure or renal failure, or when minoxidil is also being used), as the thiazides have longer duration of action, more gradual blood pressure reduction, and fewer adverse effects.

Absorption of furosemide is incomplete and erratic, with large intersubject variation. Absorption is lower in heart failure and in renal failure, making parenteral administration (usually intravenous) a more certain way to achieve a clinical response in the short term. Absorption of the other drugs in the group does not appear to be significantly affected by these conditions.[2]

These drugs have high protein binding and small distribution volumes. They reach their site of action in the ascending limb of the loop of Henle by first being filtered in the glomerulus and passing from the luminal side of the tubule into the cells. This means that when renal function is reduced, there will be resistance to its diuretic effects because the drug cannot get to the site of action. Increased doses are used in this clinical situation to achieve the desired effect. Because the drug is now distributed systemically in the body but not in the urine, there is increased risk of adverse effects, particularly hearing loss with furosemide. This must be monitored when the drug is used for long periods of time at high doses.

## Potassium-Sparing Diuretics

Potassium-sparing diuretics are described in Table 49-3.

Amiloride is chemically unrelated to other diuretics but has structural similarities to triamterene. The mechanism of action of amiloride, and of triamterene, is interference with the potassium-sodium exchange mechanism in the distal convoluted tubule.[3] Spironolactone has a different mode of action. It is a synthetic steroid aldosterone antagonist and

**Table 49–2** Loop Diuretics

| Drug | F (%) | Vd (L/kg) | Protein Binding (%) | Plasma $t_{1/2}$ (hours) | Dose Frequency (times/day) | Usual Dose (mg/day) | Maximum Dose (mg/day) |
|------|-------|-----------|---------------------|--------------------------|----------------------------|---------------------|------------------------|
| Bumetanide | 90 | 0.2 | 95 | 1.5 | 1 | 0.5-1.0 | 2 |
| Ethacrynic acid | 100* | ? | 90 | 1-4 | 2 | 50-100 | 600 |
| Furosemide | 65 | 0.2 | 95 | 0.5-2 | 2 | 40 | 160† |
| Torsemide | 85 | 0.2 | 99 | 3 | 1 | 5 | 10 |

F, systemic availability after oral administration; Vd, distribution volume; $T_{1/2}$, terminal phase plasma half-life.
*A small study has measured absolute oral bioavailability and found it to be much lower (21%) when it is compared with the levels seen after intravenous administration.
†Doses up to 640 mg/day have been used, but a better approach would be to add alternative drugs to the antihypertensive regimen.

**Table 49–3** Potassium-Sparing Diuretics

| Drug | F (%) | Vd (L/kg) | Protein Binding (%) | Plasma $t_{1/2}$ (hours) | Dose Frequency (times/day) | Usual Dose (mg/day) | Maximum Dose (mg/day) |
|------|-------|-----------|---------------------|--------------------------|----------------------------|---------------------|------------------------|
| Amiloride | 60 | 5 | Low | 7 | 1 | 10 | 20 |
| Spironolactone | 75 | ? | 90 | 1.3 | 1-2 | 25 | 50 |
| Triamterene | 50 | 1.5 | 60 | 2 | 2 | 100 | 300 |

inhibits aldosterone effect by competing drwith aldosterone for mineralocorticoid receptors.

All of these drugs are well absorbed after oral administration and can be given on a once- or twice-a-day basis despite short plasma half-lives. Because of their actions, they will tend to increase plasma potassium levels and to conserve potassium. In hypertension, they are usually given with a loop or a thiazide diuretic to prevent or remedy a fall in plasma potassium levels. This is especially important in patients with concomitant heart failure, in whom circulating aldosterone levels will be high. Given alone, they are not very effective in causing reduction in blood pressure.

## β-ADRENERGIC BLOCKERS

The β-blockers that are used in the emergent, or maintenance, treatment of hypertension are shown in Table 49–4.

Their antihypertensive action is probably related to their $β_1$-adrenergic blocking action on the heart and on the juxtaglomerular apparatus in the kidney. The effect on the heart will reduce cardiac output and the renal effect will reduce renin secretion.

All except esmolol (given parenterally) have reasonable oral bioavailability, ranging from 30% of the administered dose of carvedilol up to about 100% for penbutolol. Complete absorption would be more desirable, as there would be less inter- and intra-subject variability in plasma levels. Some, such as propranolol, have high first-pass uptake in the liver as they pass from the gut to the systemic circulation, particularly after the first dose. This results in very high inter-subject variability in plasma levels.[4]

The degree of lipid solubility varies from low to high in this group of drugs. A low degree of lipid solubility is preferable, because there may be less likelihood of the central nervous system adverse effects of insomnia and nightmares. Nadolol and atenolol, both of which have low lipid solubility, are renally excreted and have fairly long half-lives. All of the others require hepatic metabolism for all or a major portion of their excretion. Despite a wide range of plasma half-lives, all except pindolol can be dosed on a once- or twice-a-day basis.

Many have active metabolites formed in the liver that will tend to prolong the activity of the drug, especially when given on a chronic basis. *Cardioselectivity* is a term used to describe the presence of more $β_1$- than $β_2$-adrenergic blocking activity. About half of this group is classified as cardioselective, but this selectivity tends to disappear as dose is increased. A cardioselective drug should have fewer adverse effects because there will be less blockade of $β_2$ receptors in the lungs, resulting in less bronchoconstriction, and in the peripheral blood vessels, resulting in vasoconstriction, both potentially undesirable effects.

Only two, carvedilol and labetalol, have significant α-adrenergic blocking activity to go along with the β-blocking effect. This is potentially useful because it means that there will be less likelihood of a reflex vasoconstriction to oppose the acute reduction of cardiac ouput. This permits these two drugs to be used in the acute reduction of blood pressure. However, it must be remembered that the β-to-α-blocking effect is at least three to one for labetalol and more than that for carvedilol, so that the afterload reducing effect is much less than the negative chronotropic and inotropic effect on the heart in patients with congestive heart failure.

Several β-blockers, including carvedilol and propranolol, stabilize membranes. This provides a theoretical advantage in

Table 49–4 β-Blockers Used in the Emergent, or Maintenance, Treatment of Hypertension

| Drug | F (%) | Lipid Solubility | Protein Binding (%) | Vd (L/kg) | t$_{1/2}$ (hours) | Dosing (times/day) | Main Route of Elimination | Active Meta-Bolites? | Cardio-Selective? | α-Adrenergic Block? | MSA? | ISA? |
|---|---|---|---|---|---|---|---|---|---|---|---|---|
| Acebutolol | 40 | Low | 18 | 3 | 6 | 1-2 | H/R | Y | Y | N | Low | Low |
| Atenolol | 53 | Low | <5 | 0.9 | 6.5 | 1 | R | N | Y | N | N | N |
| Betaxolol | 45 | Low | 55 | 9 | 17 | 1 | H | N | Y | N | Low | N |
| Bisoprolol | 88 | Moderate | 33 | 3 | 11 | 1 | H/R | N | Y | N | N | N |
| Carteolol | 84 | Low | 27 | 4 | 6.5 | 1 | H/R | Y | N | N | N | Moderate |
| Carvedilol | 30 | High | 96 | 1.8 | 8 | 1-2 | H | Y | N | Y | Moderate | N |
| Esmolol | NA | Low | 55 | 3.4 | 0.15 | NA | O | N | Y | N | N | N |
| Labetalol | 32 | Moderate | 50 | 7.3 | 6.5 | 2 | H | N | N | Y | N | Weak |
| Metoprolol | 50 | Moderate | 12 | 5.6 | 5 | 2 | H | N | Y | N | Weak | N |
| Nadolol | 30 | Low | 29 | 2 | 22 | 1 | R | N | N | N | N | N |
| Penbutolol | 100 | High | 89 | 0.5 | 21 | 1 | H/R | Y | N | N | N | Low |
| Pindolol | 88 | Moderate | 50 | 1.6 | 3.5 | 1-3 | H/R | N | N | N | N | High |
| Propranolol | 50 | High | 93 | 6 | 3.5 | 2 | H | Y | N | N | Moderate | N |
| Timolol | 61 | Low | 10 | 1.5 | 3 | 1-2 | H/R | ? | N | N | N | N |

MSA, membrane stabilizing ability; ISA, intrinsic sympathomimetic activity; NA, drug always given parenterally, usually as a one-time dose.
Main route of elimination: H, hepatic; R, renal; O, metabolized by esterases in the cytosol of red blood cells.

potentially reducing the likelihood of cardiac arrhythmias. These benefits have not been seen in clinical practice, however.

Another difference within this group is whether they are partial agonists at the $\beta_1$ receptor. The term *partial agonist* means that when the drug attaches to the receptor, it stimulates the receptor to a lesser degree than if a full agonist were to attach to it. Pindolol is the most potent partial agonist, and when the patient is resting, it results in less reduction in heart rate than other $\beta$-blockers. When the patient is undergoing even moderate exercise, this difference disappears. A second potential advantage of partial agonist activity is that it may cause less increase in triglycerides and less decrease in HDL levels. Whether this is of clinical significance is not clear. It may be of use in hypertensive patients who need a $\beta$-blocker but experience an excessive bradycardic response to other $\beta$-blockers.

Esmolol differs from the other $\beta$-blockers in having a very short plasma half-life. It is broken down in the cytoplasm of the circulating red blood cells even before it gets to the liver. This means that it has to be given by the intravenous route, which limits its use in hypertension to the emergent and operative situations. It is useful in limiting the hypertensive response to laryngoscopy and to endotracheal intubation.

## $\alpha_1$-ADRENERGIC ANTAGONISTS

$\alpha_1$-Adrenergic antagonists used in the treatment of hypertension are described in Table 49–5.

Each has good and reliable absorption after oral administration. Protein binding to albumin in the blood is high, resulting in much of the drug being localized in the central compartment. Plasma half-life of the prototype drug prazosin is short, resulting in the need for administration three times a day. For an asymptomatic disorder such as hypertension, few patients can reliably take a drug long term on such a frequent schedule. Subsequent drugs doxazosin and terazosin, with the same mechanism of action, have longer residence in the blood, permitting a much easier dosing schedule to be followed. All are extensively metabolized in the liver with subsequent excretion in the urine and feces as a combination of parent drug and metabolites.[5]

The mechanism of action is competitive antagonism at postsynaptic $\alpha_1$-adrenergic receptors on the vasculature. This can result in orthostasis by preventing reflex vasoconstriction, especially in the elderly and in diabetic patients who have peripheral autonomic dysfunction. The selective blockade of postsynaptic $\alpha_1$-adrenergic receptors permits continued activation of the $\alpha_2$ receptors. This results in less catecholamine release and less cardiac stimulation, which tends to reduce the compensatory increase in cardiac output.

This group of drugs has potentially beneficial biochemical effects: improvement in the lipid profile and reduction in insulin resistance. Whether these effects translate into improved morbidity and mortality has not been shown. The only outcome trial to test this hypothesis, the Antihypertensive and Lipid-Lowering Treatment to Prevent Heart Disease (ALLHAT) trial, showed no benefit in heart attack prevention and harm in terms of increased heart failure and stroke with doxazosin as compared with the diuretic chlorthalidone (see Chapter 30). An infrequent but distressing adverse effect is the occurrence of priapism, which must be treated rapidly by surgical intervention if erectile function is to be preserved.

These drugs must be started in low doses and titrated in small steps to prevent the occurrence of the "first dose phenomenon," which results in a much greater fall in blood pressure after the first dose than is seen with subsequent doses of the same size. The effect is seen in the first hour or two after dosing and can last for up to 8 hours. Optimally, the first dose is given at bedtime to prevent exacerbation of this effect by standing upright.

## CENTRAL $\alpha_2$-ADRENERGIC AGONISTS

Central $\alpha_2$-adrenergic agonists used in hypertension are described in Table 49–6.

This group of drugs has good oral bioavailability and a wide range of distribution volumes, plasma protein binding, and plasma half-lives, as shown in Table 49-6. The two older drugs can each be given on a twice- or three-times-a-day basis[6]; the newer drugs, guanfacine and guanabenz, can be given on a once- or twice-a-day basis. Potency ranges from low for methyldopa to high for clonidine, and the daily dose requirements reflect this range. All have sedation and dry mouth as common side effects, and this seems to be inseparable from the therapeutic $\alpha_2$-agonist effect in the central nervous system. This high incidence of adverse effects limits the use of this class of agents.

Clonidine may be given as a transdermal patch that minimizes the peak plasma drug concentrations and reduces the incidence of the adverse effects. It may also be given by the intravenous route, but this can cause transient hypertensive effects as the drug acts peripherally before it penetrates into the central nervous system.

$\alpha$-Methyldopa forms the false neurotransmitter $\alpha$-methyl norepinephrine in the central nervous system, and this substance stimulates inhibitory central $\alpha_2$-adrenergic receptors and reduces central sympathetic outflow. In addition, it may have a peripheral ganglionic blocking effect, which would explain its tendency to cause orthostatic falls in blood pressure. A Coombs' positive hemolytic anemia is seen uncommonly, and rebound hypertension may be seen when higher doses of both $\alpha$-methyldopa and clonidine (more than 0.8 mg daily) are withdrawn suddenly. The same rebound may be seen when more than 32 mg/day of guanabenz is withdrawn suddenly, although the likelihood may be less than that for clonidine.

## ANGIOTENSIN RECEPTOR ANTAGONISTS

Angiotensin receptor antagonists are shown in Table 49–7.

Losartan is the first of this class of nonpeptide angiotensin receptor blockers. It was introduced to overcome the disadvantages of the earlier peptide (and therefore, not orally active) drugs that antagonized both angiotensin II type 1 ($AT_1$) and angiotensin II type 2 ($AT_2$) receptors.[7] This class of drugs has poor to moderate oral bioavailability and high plasma protein binding that, for those without avid tissue binding, means that the volume of distribution is small. The dosing frequency is once a day, even for those with a short plasma

**Table 49-5** $\alpha_1$-Adrenergic Antagonists Used in the Treatment of Hypertension

| Drug | F (%) | Vd (L/kg) | Protein Binding (%) | Plasma $t_{1/2}$ (hours) | Dose Frequency (times/day) | Usual Dose (mg/day) | Maximum Dose (mg/day) |
|------|-------|-----------|---------------------|--------------------------|----------------------------|---------------------|-----------------------|
| Doxazosin | 65 | 3 | 99 | 15 | 1 | 8 | 16 |
| Prazosin | 63 | 1.3 | 95 | 3 | 3 | 8 | 20 |
| Terazosin | 90 | 0.4 | 92 | 12 | 1 | 5 | 20 |

**Table 49-6** Central $\alpha_2$-Adrenergic Agonists Used in Hypertension

| Drug | F (%) | Vd (L/kg) | Protein Binding (%) | Plasma $t_{1/2}$ (hours) | Dose Frequency (times/day) | Usual Dose (mg/day) | Maximum Dose (mg/day) |
|------|-------|-----------|---------------------|--------------------------|----------------------------|---------------------|-----------------------|
| Clonidine | 85 | 2 | 30 | 14 | 3 | 0.6 | 1.8 |
| $\alpha$-Methyldopa | 45 | 0.6 | 0 | 1.7 | 2 | 500 | 2000 |
| Guanabenz | 75 | 10 | 90 | 6 | 2 | 32 | 64 |
| Guanfacine | 90 | 6 | 72 | 17 | 1 | 2 | 6 |

**Table 49-7** Angiotensin Receptor Antagonists

| Drug | F (%) | Vd (L/kg) | Protein Binding (%) | Plasma $t_{1/2}$ (hours) | Dose Frequency (times/day) | Usual Dose (mg/day) | Maximum Dose (mg/day) |
|------|-------|-----------|---------------------|--------------------------|----------------------------|---------------------|-----------------------|
| Candesartan | 15 | 0.13 | 99 | * | 1 | 16 | 32 |
| Eprosartan | 70 | 1 | 90 | 6 | 1-2 | 400 | 600 |
| Irbesartan | 26 | 0.24 | 99 | 13† | 1 | 150 | 300 |
| Losartan | 30 | 0.5 | 99 | 2‡ | 1-2 | 50 | 100 |
| Olmesartan | 20 | 0.25 | 95 | 15 | 1 | 20 | 40 |
| Telmisartan | 42 | 7 | 99 | 24 | 1 | 40 | 80 |
| Valsartan | 13 | 4.4 | 98 | 6 | 1-2 | 160 | 320 |

*Dose-dependent half-life, 7-16 hours; active metabolite half-life, 7.5 hours.
†Active metabolite half-life, 10 hours.
‡Active metabolite half-life, 7 hours.

half-life, partly because candesartan, irbesartan, and losartan, which have short half-lives, have active metabolites that prolong their action. Also, because they are competitive antagonists, the duration of effect will depend more on residence time on the receptors than on the time in the plasma.

The mode of action is to competitively inhibit the binding of angiotensin II to its $AT_1$ receptors, which are found throughout the cardiovascular and renal systems.

Displacement of angiotensin II from $AT_1$ receptors opposes its biologic effects including smooth muscle contraction, aldosterone and catecholamine release, arginine vasopressin release, stimulation of thirst, and hypertrophy of smooth muscle in the vascular tree. The effects of the drugs depend on the activity of the renin-angiotensin system in maintaining cardiovascular homeostasis. Antihypertensive efficacy will therefore be expected to be more pronounced in younger rather than older patients.

Because this class of drugs (unlike the ACEIs) does not prevent bradykinin breakdown, there is lower likelihood of them causing cough and angioedema. At present, many clinicians regard their place in therapy as being in patients who need an ACEI but do not tolerate them. Because they act through the renin angiotensin system, they cause greater reductions in blood pressure in patients who are volume depleted and whose blood pressure depends more on the renin angiotensin system. This has the disadvantage of introducing uncertainty about the magnitude of antihypertensive response on initial dosing but the advantage of permitting greater efficacy when they are combined with a diuretic.

## ANGIOTENSIN-CONVERTING ENZYME INHIBITORS

ACEIs are shown in Table 49–8. Most of the ACEIs are given by mouth as the prodrug to ensure adequate absorption into the systemic circulation. Captopril and lisinopril are the exceptions. Enalaprilat, the active metabolite of enalapril, is

**Table 49–8** Angiotensin-Converting Enzyme Inhibitors

| Drug | F (%) | Vd (L/kg) | Protein Binding (%) | Plasma $t_{1/2}$ (hours) | Dose Frequency (times/day) | Usual Dose (mg/day) | Maximum Dose (mg/day) |
|---|---|---|---|---|---|---|---|
| Benazepril* | 37 | 0.12 | 97 | 0.6 | 1-2 | 20 | 40 |
| Captopril | 70 | 0.7 | 25 | 2 | 3 | 150 | 450 |
| Enalapril* | 60 | ? | 55 | 1.3 | 1-2 | 20 | 40 |
| Enalaprilat | † | ? | 55 | 11§ | 4 | 0.625 | 1.25 |
| Fosinopril* | 33 | 0.14‡ | 95 | 4‡ | 1 | 40 | 80 |
| Trandolapril* | 10‡ | 0.25‡ | 80 | 20‡ | 1 | 2 | 4 |
| Lisinopril | 25 | 1.8 | Low | 12 | 1 | 40 | 80 |
| Moexipril* | 18 | 2.6 | 60‡ | 6‡ | 1 | 20 | 60 |
| Perindopril* | 75 | 0.16‡ | 60‡ | 25‡ | 1 | 8 | 16 |
| Quinapril* | 50 | 0.7 | 97 | 25‡ | 1 | 40 | 80 |
| Ramipril* | 60 | ? | 73 | 15‡ | 1 | 10 | 20 |

*Prodrug.
†Drug given intravenously for severe hypertension.
‡Data for active metabolite.
§After administration of enalapril.

given by the intravenous route as emergent treatment of severe hypertension or when oral drugs cannot be given. Limitations of enalaprilat in this clinical situation include variability in response (depending on whether the patient is volume depleted or not), a rather modest magnitude of antihypertensive effect, and a relatively slow attainment of peak antihypertensive effect.

As is usual with any class of drugs, the first one (captopril) has the same efficacy as the latter members of the class but has less-convenient pharmacokinetics. Captopril has the shortest efficacy half-life and requires three-times-a-day administration in hypertension. This has the disadvantage of reducing compliance with therapy but the advantage of a shorter duration of action. The latter effect is of use when starting therapy, because the response may be unpredictable and the short duration of effect will limit the duration of hypotension if it occurs, particularly in patients with heart failure or reduced intravascular volume. Most ACEIs have relatively small distribution volumes, indicating that much of the drug and the metabolite are concentrated in the central compartment. Captopril is the only ACEI that contains a sulphydryl group. This has been blamed for the higher likelihood of neutropenia and proteinuria seen with large doses of captopril. Adverse affects common to the class include a dry, irritating, principally nocturnal cough in about 10% of patients. If it occurs, trial with another member of the class may not produce the same adverse effect. Angioedema of the upper respiratory tract may also be seen in about 0.1% of patients, and very rarely angioedema of the pancreatic duct may occur, causing pancreatic pseudocysts if the drug is not rapidly discontinued.

## DIRECT-ACTING VASODILATORS

Direct-acting vasodilators are described in Table 49–9.

Both of these drugs are very effective when given by the oral route. They dilate the arteries but not the veins. Because they cause the anticipated homeostatic effects of reflex tachycardia and fluid retention, they are now given in combination with a diuretic and a sympathetic antagonist. Because of the particularly severe fluid retention with minoxidil, most patients will require a loop diuretic when started on this drug.[8]

Despite its short plasma half-life, hydralazine may be given on a twice-daily basis, or sometimes three times a day when higher doses are given. This is probably because the drug binds covalently to its site of action on vascular smooth muscle.[9]

The anticipated adverse effects of both drugs are headache, palpitations, and edema that may be prevented by using these drugs in combination with a diuretic and β-blocker, as indicated above. In addition, hydralazine is metabolized partly by N-acetylation, and that portion of the drug that is not acetylated will interact with cell constituents, eventually resulting in a lupus-like syndrome. This syndrome is more likely in patients with the slow acetylator phenotype and less likely in patients of African descent. It is less likely than systemic lupus erythematosis to involve the kidneys. Patients taking hydralazine should have an antinuclear antibody test performed annually.

Minoxidil is likely to cause hirsutism. This is a major problem for younger women, particularly those with dark hair and pale skin. Silently accumulating pericardial effusions have been seen in patients with end-stage renal disease who are treated with minoxidil.

**Table 49-9** Direct-Acting Vasodilators

| Drug | F (%) | Vd (L/kg) | Protein Binding (%) | Plasma t$_{1/2}$ (hours) | Dose Frequency (times/day) | Usual Dose (mg/day) | Maximum Dose (mg/day) |
|------|-------|-----------|---------------------|--------------------------|----------------------------|---------------------|----------------------|
| Hydralazine | 20-50* | 0.5 | 90 | 1.5 | 2 | 50 | 300 |
| Minoxidil | 95 | 2.5 | Low | 42 | 1 | 10 | 80 |

*Bioavailability is lower in fast acetylators and higher in slow acetylators because of differences in first-pass uptake in the liver.

## CALCIUM CHANNEL BLOCKERS

CCBs are described in Table 49-10.

From a functional point of view, there are two groups of CCBs: those that block the action of the sinoatrial and the atrioventricular nodes in the heart—diltiazem and verapamil—and those that do not—the dihydropyridine group. The CCBs block voltage-dependent calcium entry of the vascular smooth muscle cells and to a lesser extent, cardiac myocytes and smooth muscle cells in the gastrointestinal tract. The latter effects are responsible for some adverse effects, namely negative inotropic effects on the heart and constipation. All CCBs will cause negative inotropic effects, which are only significant in patients with impaired ventricular function. Amlodipine and felodipine are less likely to do this than are other CCBs, possibly because of less distribution into cardiac tissue. Blood pressure lowering occurs because of reduced calcium entry into vascular smooth muscle, which relaxes the arterioles, reducing peripheral resistance.[10]

All CCBs are fairly well absorbed from the gut, but because of extensive first-pass uptake by the liver, systemic availability tends to be low. Amlodipine is the best absorbed CCB and has the lowest first-pass uptake. There is a significant drug interaction between grapefruit juice taken within several hours of ingesting several CCBs. Flavonoids in grapefruit juice inhibit the metabolism of the three dihydropyridine CCBs—nisoldipine, felodipine, and nifedipine. This inhibition occurs in the cytochrome P450 enzymes in the gut wall, so that there is greater systemic availability of the drugs. Verapamil inhibits cytochrome P450 3A4 and will therefore cause higher blood levels of other drugs metabolized by this route, such as many of the hydroxymethylglutaryl coenzyme A inhibitors (statins?).

All CCBs in clinical use have high plasma protein binding, but displacement from protein by other drugs is not a significant source of interactions. The CCBs also cause ankle edema in a significant number of patients. This edema is not associated with weight gain and is not effectively treated by diuretics. CCB-induced edema has been attributed to precapillary dilation, thus raising the intravascular pressure in the capillaries and inducing extravasation of fluid.

The first three CCBs in clinical use—verapamil, nifedipine and diltiazem—had short plasma and therapeutic half-lives and had to be taken three times a day. This reduced patient compliance with therapy. For this reason, and because of questions about the safety of short-acting dehydropyridine CCBs, these drugs are used as controlled release preparations and may all be given once a day. Because absorption occurs only when the drug is in the small intestine, changes in gastrointestinal motility could significantly alter systemic availability of these controlled-release drugs. In contrast, felodipine and amlodipine have sufficiently long plasma half-lives to permit once-a-day dosing.

**Table 49-10** Calcium Channel Blockers

| Drug | F (%) | Vd (L/kg) | Protein Binding (%) | Plasma t$_{1/2}$ (hours) | Dose Frequency (times/day) | Usual Dose (mg/day) | Maximum Dose (mg/day) |
|------|-------|-----------|---------------------|--------------------------|----------------------------|---------------------|----------------------|
| Amlodipine | 65 | 21 | 95 | 45 | 1 | 5 | 10 |
| Diltiazem | 42 | 5.3 | 85 | 3.9 | 1* | 240 | 540 |
| Felodipine | 15 | 10 | 99 | 13 | 1 | 10 | 10 |
| Isradipine | 19 | 1.6 | 97 | 8 | 2 | 10 | 20 |
| Nicardipine | 35† | 0.6 | 96 | 8.6 | 2* | 90 | 120 |
| Nifedipine | 50 | 1 | 95 | 2.5‡ | 1* | 60 | 120 |
| Nisoldipine | 6 | 4.5 | 99 | 9.5 | 1* | 30 | 60 |
| Verapamil | 30 | 3.8 | 91 | 8 | 1* | 240 | 480 |

*Controlled release preparation.
†Also used as intravenous preparation.
‡Apparent plasma half-life is up to 28 hours from controlled release preparation because of continued absorption from the gut.

## SELECTIVE ALDOSTERONE RECEPTOR ANTAGONISTS

Spironolactone, a nonselective aldosterone receptor antagonist, has been used for almost 20 years in treating high blood pressure. However, it is a nonselective antagonist and binds to other steroid receptors. This results in significant side effects such as gynecomastia. Eplerenone is the first of a new class of selective competitive antagonists of the aldosterone receptor. It is administered by mouth, and its oral bioavailability is approximately 98%. The distribution volume is 1 L/kg and is approximately 60% bound to plasma proteins. It is broken down in the liver to inactive metabolites, primarily cytochrome P450 3A4. This results in the potential for significant interactions with other drugs broken down by the same pathway. The plasma half-life is 5 hours. The usual daily dose is 50 to 100 mg, administered twice daily. Adverse effects are similar to those with placebo, but there is, as would be expected, a tendency for hyperkalemia.

## DRUG GROUPS UNDER DEVELOPMENT

Classes under development include potassium channel openers, dopamine agonists, serotonin-related agents, renin inhibitors, imidazolines, endothelin antagonists, and neutral endopeptidase inhibitors. Perhaps the most interesting are the neutral endopeptidase inhibitors. These drugs, which include omapatrilat and sampatrilat, are dual inhibitors of both angiotensin-converting enzyme and neutral endopeptidase. These drugs have good efficacy in lowering blood pressure and cause very few adverse effects. They have desirable pharmacokinetic profiles. However, there may be a predisposition to cause angioedema, and this has resulted in delay in obtaining FDA approval.

## DRUGS USED IN THE EMERGENT TREATMENT OF HYPERTENSION

Oral drugs, such as clonidine and labetalol, are described previously. Other drugs, apart from phenoxybenzamine, are given parenterally and are described in Table 49–11. (For a complete discussion of the management of hypertensive emergencies and urgencies, see Chapter 78.)

As may be seen from the table, much of the pharmacokinetic information is missing. These are old drugs that are not used extensively now and have not been subjected to the detailed investigation that is now routine with newer drugs.

Fenoldopam mesilate is a benzazepine derivative with selective postsynaptic dopamine-1 (DA-1) receptor agonist properties and minimal adrenergic effects. Blood pressure is lowered by peripheral vasodilation and with renal artery dilation. Because of the renal artery dilation, this drug is of use in patients with severe hypertension and impaired renal function. The short plasma and therapeutic half-life require that the drug be given as an intravenous infusion, at a dose of 40 µg/ml in dextrose or saline solution. Fenoldopam is metabolized extensively in the liver, principally to inactive metabolites, by conjugation rather than by cytochrome P450 mechanisms.

Diazoxide is a direct-acting vasodilator that was formerly given orally for the treatment of severe hypertension. It caused sufficient hyperglycemia that physicians would start an oral hypoglycemic agent contemporaneously with the diazoxide. It is now used only in the emergent treatment of hypertension as an intravenous preparation. Its half-life is long and its time to peak hypotensive effect is short, so it is given as a series of small bolus injections, with measures of blood pressure prior to each bolus. As with other direct-acting arterial vasodilators, a common adverse effect is hirsutism, with vellus hair growth affecting all normally hairy areas of the body except the pubic and axillary regions.

Sodium nitroprusside is a direct acting vasodilator that acts on the arterial and venous sides of the circulation by releasing NO into the vascular smooth muscle cells. It is light sensitive, and both the infusion bag and the tubing must be shielded from light. It should be diluted in dextrose solution and, because of its very short half-life, administered with an infusion pump with the blood pressure measured by an intraarterial probe. Metabolism in the vessel walls releases cyanide, which is rapidly detoxified by endogenous thiosulphate to thiocyanate. The body can detoxify the cyanide at a rate equivalent to infusion at a rate of about 2 µg/kg/min. Faster infusion rates of nitroprusside can be safely used if exogenous thiosulphate is administered. Thiocyanate has its own toxicity, because it blocks iodine uptake by the thyroid gland and causes hypothyroidism if long-term infusions of nitroprusside are used. Blood levels of thiocyanate should be measured if nitroprusside is given for more than 48 hours and, because of the renal excretion of thiocyanate, if there is renal dysfunction.

**Table 49–11** Drugs Used in the Emergent Treatment of Hypertension

| Drug | Vd (L/kg) | Protein Binding (%) | Plasma $t_{1/2}$ | Initial Dose | Maximum Dose |
|---|---|---|---|---|---|
| Fenoldopam | 0.6 | ? | 5 minutes | 0.1 µg/kg/min | 1.6 µg/kg/min |
| Diazoxide | 0.2 | 90 | 28 hours | 100 mg | Repeat every 10 minutes until DBP less than 100 mm Hg |
| Nitroprusside | ? | ? | 4 minutes | 0.3 µg/kg/min | 10 µg/kg/min |
| Phentolamine | ? | 70 | 19 minutes | 5 mg | 5 mg every 2 hours to total of 20 mg |
| Phenoxy-benzamine | ? | ? | 24 hours* | 10 mg po bid | 40 mg po tid |

*After intravenous administration; not known after oral administration.
po, orally; bid, two times per day; tid, three times per day.

Toxicity is associated with circulating thiocyanate levels of more than 10 mg/dl.

Phentolamine is a nonselective reversible α-adrenergic antagonist that is used to treat patients with pheochromocytoma, particularly during surgery to remove the tumor. It may also be of use in clonidine withdrawal rebound hypertension. It has a short duration of action and is extensively metabolized in the liver. Because the α-adrenergic block is nonselective, presynaptic α-adrenergic receptor blockade will remove the negative feedback inhibition of catecholamine release, and cardiac output will rise to oppose the fall in blood pressure. This limits the utility of phenotolamine in essential hypertension. The mode of action of both phentolamine and phenoxybenzamine means that most of the antihypertensive effect is orthostatic, and the patient may remain hypotensive when in the supine position but be hypertensive when standing or sitting. Both drugs cause severe nasal stuffiness in some patients.

Phenoxybenzamine has similar actions to phentolamine but binds covalently and therefore irreversibly to the α-receptors. Its onset of action is slow and its effect lasts for more than 24 hours. The duration of action is a function of the rate of synthesis of new α-adrenergic receptors rather than of the concentration and persistence of the drug in the plasma. Oral bioavailability is 25%, and it may be used by either the oral or the intravenous route. It is used to treat pheochromocytoma on a chronic basis.

## SUMMARY

There are now many effective and safe antihypertensive agents. For most, the duration of antihypertensive effect is much longer than would be predicted from the plasma half-life of the drug.

## References

1. Costanzo LS. Mechanism of action of thiazide diuretics. Semin Nephrol 8(3):234-241, 1988.
2. Brater DC. Clinical pharmacology of loop diuretics. Drugs 41(Suppl 3):14-22, 1991.
3. Vidt DG. Mechanism of action, pharmacokinetics, adverse effects, and therapeutic uses of amiloride hydrochloride, a new potassium-sparing diuretic. Pharmacotherapy 1:179-187, 1981.
4. Frishman WH, Alwarshetty M. Beta-adrenergic blockers in systemic hypertension: Pharmacokinetic considerations related to the current guidelines. Clin Pharmacokinet 41(7):505-516, 2002.
5. Harada K. Fujimura A. Clinical pharmacology of alpha1A selective and nonselective alpha1 blockers. BJU International 86(Suppl 2):31-35, 2000.
6. Khan ZP, Ferguson CN, Jones RM. Alpha-2 and imidazoline receptor agonists: Their pharmacology and therapeutic role. Anaesthesia 54(2):146-165, 1999.
7. Schachter M. ACE inhibitors, angiotensin receptor antagonists and bradykinin. J Renin Angiotensin Aldosterone Sys 1(1): 27-29, 2000.
8. Adams MH, Poynor WJ, Garnett WR, et al. Pharmacokinetics of minoxidil in patients with cirrhosis and healthy volunteers. Biopharmaceutics and Drug Disposition 19(8):501-515, 1998.
9. Shepherd AM, Irvine NA, Ludden TM, et al. Effect of oral dose size on hydralazine kinetics and vasodepressor response. Clin Pharmacol Ther 36(5):595-600, 1984.
10. van Zwieten PA, Pfaffendorf M. Pharmacology of the dihydropyridine calcium antagonists: Relationship between lipophilicity and pharmacodynamic responses. J Hypertens 11(Suppl 6):S3-S8, 1993.

# Fixed Combination Antihypertensive Therapy

Joel M. Neutel

The aggressive use of fixed-dose combination therapy early in the management of hypertension may be the most important change clinicians can make in their attempt to achieve adequate blood pressure control in hypertensive patients. Hypertension has been identified as the most powerful modifiable risk factor for the development of cardiovascular disease,[1] and its control has been shown to significantly decrease cardiovascular morbidity and mortality.[2-4] Despite this knowledge, only one third of the hypertensive patients in the United States achieve the conservative goals of 140/90 mm Hg.[5] Because inadequate blood pressure control remains an important risk factor for coronary artery disease, it is not surprising that the reductions in coronary artery disease among hypertensive patients have been disappointing. Achieving optimal blood pressure control is the most important issue in the management of hypertension, and in the majority of hypertensive patients, it is difficult or impossible to control blood pressure with one drug.[6-9] The use of combination therapy as first-line treatment, or early in the management of hypertension, will substantially enhance blood pressure control rates[5] and ultimately have a significant impact on coronary artery disease among hypertensive patients.

## THE IDEAL ANTIHYPERTENSIVE AGENT

The ideal antihypertensive agent would have the following qualities:

1. Highly efficacious—providing the ability to achieve adequate blood pressure control with a single agent in the majority of hypertensives
2. Provide 24-hour efficacy with once-a-day dosing
3. A high response rate—works in all groups of hypertensive patients: young, elderly, African Americans, and diabetics
4. Minimal symptomatic adverse effects
5. Minimal metabolic adverse effects
6. Affordable
7. Supported by outcomes data

No such drug exists for the management of hypertension. If it did, physicians would be using only one or two agents to manage this condition. There are in excess of 81 approved drugs for the management of hypertension,[5] testament to the fact that the ideal antihypertensive agent does not exist. Although several new drugs and drug classes are being developed for hypertension—including renin inhibitors, aldosterone antagonists, endothelin antagonists, and vasopepidase inhibitors—early clinical data suggest that none of these newer agents will be more effective (as monotherapy) than the drugs already available (see Chapters 11, and 69-72). Thus we must face the fact that, in terms of efficacy, we currently have what we are going to have for the next 10 years for treating hypertension.

With this in mind, the concept of combination therapy is, Can we create, from the drugs we have, the ideal antihypertensive agent? Is it possible to combine complementary agents to provide maximal efficacy and at the same time minimize side effects?

## RATIONALE FOR THE USE OF COMBINATION THERAPY

The two qualities most important to physicians in their selection of antihypertensive agents are efficacy and safety. Use of combination therapy potentially optimizes these qualities.

### Efficacy

The most important reason for use of combination therapy in clinical practice is that combining two complementary antihypertensive agents produces significantly greater efficacy than either of the components as monotherapy.[10-12] This is not surprising because the cause of hypertension is multifactorial, and many pathophysiologic factors contribute to high blood pressure. In most patients, blocking one system will activate counter-regulatory mechanisms and result in persistence of elevated blood pressure. However, when two physiologic systems are interrupted, counter-regulatory mechanisms are frequently neutralized, enabling greater reductions in blood pressure.

For example, diuretics, which stimulate the renin-angiotensin system, are ideally combined with angiotensin-converting-enzyme (ACE) inhibitors or angiotensin receptor blockers (ARBs). Alternatively, diuretics may be combined with β-blockers, which inhibit the release of renin. Dihydropyridine calcium channel blockers (CCBs) increase circulating catecholamines, which also tend to activate the renin-angiotensin system. Thus, dihydropyridine CCBs may be logically combined with ACE inhibitors. On the other hand, nondihydropyridine CCBs decrease circulating catecholamines, so combination with β-blockers is not logical. Similarly, ACE inhibitors and β-blockers both seem to interrupt the renin-angiotensin system and so are not a logical combination.

The combination of two complementary antihypertensive agents often results in blood pressure reductions that are additive, and in some cases, such as low-dose bisoprolol added to low-dose hydrochlorothiazide, may be synergistic.[13] All of the currently available fixed-dose combination products are significantly more effective than each of their components. Indeed, this is a major requirement of the U.S. Food and Drug Administration (FDA) for approval of a combination agent.

### Safety

Safety and efficacy tend to move in opposite directions as we increase the dose of antihypertensive agents (Figure 50-1).

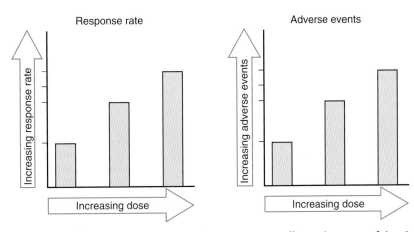

**Figure 50–1** Increasing doses of antihypertensive agents result in increasing efficacy because of the dose response curve of antihypertensive agents, but it also results in increasing dose-dependant adverse events.

This frequently results in physicians accepting less-effective blood pressure control to minimize adverse effects. Most of the adverse effects of antihypertensive drugs are dose dependent, with the exception of ACE inhibitor–induced cough and angioedema. Thus, combinations that use smaller drug doses in hypertensive patients will cause fewer adverse effects. Combination therapy provides adequate blood pressure control with smaller doses of each of the components, thereby reducing dose-dependent adverse effects. For example, use of a low-dose combination of a β-blocker and a diuretic results in less fatigue, impotence, and bradycardia than higher doses of each of the components.[13]

In the management of hypertension it is better to reduce blood pressure in a physiologic manner, thus reducing adverse events. For example, dihydropyridine CCBs are powerful arterial vasodilators. Although useful in the management of hypertension, these drugs reduce blood pressure by affecting only the arterial side of the circulation, leading to frequent adverse events—for example, peripheral edema and increased proteinuria in diabetic patients with renal disease. Adding an ACE inhibitor to a dihydropyridine CCB now provides venous dilation, and the combination produces a more physiologic reduction in blood pressure involving the entire vascular tree. This combination reduces not only CCB-induced edema[12] but also proteinuria in diabetic patients with renal disease, often to a greater extent than an ACE inhibitor given as monotherapy.[14] In some instances combination therapy results in fewer adverse effects than the same dose of the components given as monotherapy despite significantly greater reductions in blood pressure.[12,15]

## ADVERSE METABOLIC SIDE EFFECTS

Adverse metabolic effects of antihypertensive agents are generally dose dependent. For example, the effects of diuretics on potassium are dose dependent, as are their effects on lipids and insulin.[16] Use of combination therapy facilitates blood pressure control with lower doses of diuretics, thus minimizing their metabolic effects. For example, while high doses of thiazides frequently require potassium supplementation to prevent hypokalemia, combining a thiazide diuretic with an ACE inhibitor provides adequate blood pressure control with lower doses of hydrochlorothiazide (12.5 mg in many of the available combinations),[17,18] thus preventing decreases in potassium. In addition, ACE inhibitors are potassium sparing, further reducing the risk of potassium loss and the need for potassium supplementation.

## TWENTY-FOUR-HOUR EFFICACY WITH COMBINATION THERAPY

Use of once-a-day medication in the management of hypertension is critical to obtain patient compliance. Once-a-day agents must provide true 24-hour blood pressure control, including the last 4 to 6 hours of the dosing interval. The same principle applies to combination therapy. Most of the commercially available fixed-dose combinations have been carefully selected to include drugs that have 24-hour efficacy as monotherapy. The duration of action of the combination must be at least similar to that of the components. In some instances[19] the combination of two agents results in a lengthening of the duration of action as compared with the individual components. For example, captopril as monotherapy is a short-acting ACE inhibitor, which should be dosed two or three times per day, but combining it with hydrochlorothiazide significantly lengthens its duration of action. Ambulatory blood pressure monitoring data should be used to determine the duration of action of combination antihypertensive agents.

## RESPONSE RATES

Use of combination therapy results in greater efficacy across all subgroups of hypertensive patients and may have additional cardiovascular benefits. For example, ACE inhibitors and ARBs are generally less effective in African American patients, who tend to have lower plasma renin activity than Caucasian patients. Addition of a diuretic or CCB to an ACE inhibitor or ARB will stimulate the renin-angiotensin system and enhance the efficacy of the renin-angiotensin system blocker in African Americans. The blood pressure reductions seen with the combination are then similar in African American and Caucasian patients.[20]

ACE inhibitor/ARB-diuretic combinations in African American patients also have cardiovascular benefits independent of blood pressure reduction. African Americans have often been denied renin-angiotensin system blockers because of a perceived lack of antihypertensive efficacy. This is an important misconception, particularly in light of the African American Study of Kidney Disease and Hypertension.[21] African Americans should be treated with an ACE inhibitor or ARB to achieve the vascular protective benefits of these agents, which are independent of blood pressure. Adding a diuretic can achieve both antihypertensive efficacy and cardiovascular protection. (See Chapter 56 for a more complete discussion of the management of hypertension in African Americans.)

## CONVENIENCE

There is a clear inverse relationship between the complexity of the dosing regimen and patient compliance. Clinicians recognize that polypharmacy is not well tolerated by patients and try hard to avoid it in the management of hypertension, frequently at the expense of adequate blood pressure control.

Thus, in the selection of antihypertensive drugs, two properties need to be considered to enhance convenience and compliance:

1. *Once-daily dosing.* Adherence to antihypertensive agents that are dosed once daily is greater than drugs that are dosed twice daily.[22] There is little reason to prescribe antihypertensive drugs that must be taken three times a day. Many antihypertensive drugs can be safely and effectively given once daily. It is important for clinicians to select drugs that provide adequate blood pressure control over the entire 24-hour dosing interval. Some agents marketed as once-a-day preparations tend to lose efficacy during the final few hours of the dosing interval.[23] Because most antihypertensive drugs are dosed in the morning, loss of blood pressure control tends to coincide with the rapid increase in blood pressure during arousal from sleep, at the time at which the peak incidence of stroke and myocardial infarction occurs.[24,25] It is believed, although not proven, that optimal blood pressure control during this early morning period is needed to prevent ischemic events.

   Duration of action can be assessed clinically by instructing patients to omit dosing on the morning of their clinic visit. If blood pressure remains controlled 24 to 26 hours after dosing, this is good evidence of once-a-day efficacy. As discussed, most of the available fixed-dose combination drugs include agents that provide 24-hour blood pressure control as monotherapy, and the added blood pressure reduction of the combination product is sustained for 24 hours. In some cases, combining agents may even prolong the hemodynamic effect of the components.[19]

2. *Polypharmacy.* There is an inverse relationship between the number of drugs that patients have to take and their adherence to a regimen. This decrease in compliance is related to the following:

   a. Convenience—It is easier to forget to take multiple drugs.
   b. Confusion—Patients often become confused by multiple drugs with difficult dosing regimens and frequently dose incorrectly.

   c. Cost—There is higher cost with multiple drugs.

For these reasons, many physicians believe that monotherapy is more convenient and will improve compliance in the management of hypertension. However, the availability of increasing numbers of fixed-dose combination agents provides dosing that is no less convenient than monotherapy. In fact, it is more convenient to use combination therapy than monotherapy in that it is possible to decrease polypharmacy, which simplifies the dosing regimen and in many instances may reduce medication costs.[26]

Many clinicians believe that as long as the dosing of antihypertensive medication is once daily, the number of drugs given does not influence compliance. This has been shown to be incorrect in a recent study performed in more than 6000 patients.[27] When patients were given amlodipine and benazepril as a single tablet, the compliance rate was significantly greater than if they were given the same drugs as two separate pills dosed once daily. Not surprisingly, the control rate was greater in the patients taking the combination product.[39]

## COST

In most instances combination therapy is no more expensive than monotherapy. Use of combination agents requires only one copayment and one dispensing fee, which may be less costly than multiple drug therapy. In addition, low-dose combination agents are usually marketed as a "package deal" in that they are more expensive than each of the components individually but less expensive than both components administered separately. High-dose monotherapy may be more expensive than combination agents. Furthermore, many patients are limited to a certain number of drugs by their medical plans (e.g., Medicaid). If they exceed this number, they are responsible for paying for their drugs. A combination agent represents only one drug and its use allows another drug to be covered by the plan, resulting in decreased cost for the patient.

Higher blood pressure is associated with higher management costs. To the extent that blood pressure can be controlled more quickly with combination therapy, the cost of treating hypertension is reduced.

## OUTCOMES DATA

More outcomes data are available for combination therapy than for monotherapy. Virtually all recent outcomes studies in hypertension have utilized combination therapy, although the second, third, and fourth drugs in the regimens were usually "add ons" to an initial agent to which patients were randomized.[3,4,6-9] One of the requirements of outcomes studies is to provide their participants adequate blood pressure control. To achieve accepted blood pressure goals, the majority of patients enrolled in outcome studies require two or more drugs.[5-9] Importantly, studies such as the United Kingdom Prospective Diabetes Study and Hypertension Optimal Treatment[29] have shown a significant reduction in cardiovascular disease outcomes in patients with tight control compared with those with less tight control.

The Fosinopril versus Amlodipine Cardiovascular Events Randomized Trial (FACET) was one of the few outcomes studies that compared combination therapy to mono-therapy.[30] Patients with type 2 diabetes and hypertension were randomized to fosinopril or amlodipine. If their blood pressure was not adequately controlled, the alternative drug could be added. Patients were followed for 36 months to assess the development of cardiovascular disease. At the end of the study, patients treated with the ACE inhibitor had less cardiovascular disease than those treated with the CCB, but patients treated with the combination of the two drugs had the greatest reduction of cardiovascular disease incidence, probably related to the greater blood pressure reduction achieved with two agents.

In the ALERT study (A Lotrel Evaluation of Hypertensive Patients with Arterial Stiffness and Left Ventricular Hypertrophy),[31] patients were treated with a low-dose combination of amlodipine plus benazepril (5/20 mg) or with high-dose amlodipine (10 mg) or high-dose benazepril (40 mg) as monotherapy. Blood pressure reductions were similar in patients treated with the combination agents or the high-dose amlodipine but slightly less in those treated with high-dose benazepril. However, patients treated with the combination therapy had greater improvement in arterial compliance and greater regression of left ventricular hypertrophy (LVH) than those treated with either high-dose monotherapy. This study demonstrates that the combination of two complementary drugs results in greater cardiovascular benefits than high-dose monotherapy. Importantly, although blood pressure reduction in patients treated with the combination therapy was not different from that in patients treated with high-dose amlodipine, the ACE inhibitor in the combination treatment resulted in greater improvement in arterial compliance and greater regression of LVH. This clearly demonstrates the benefit of an ACE inhibitor, beyond blood pressure control, on cardiovascular protection. Furthermore, the combination of amlodipine and benazepril resulted in greater improvement in arterial compliance and greater regression of LVH than high-dose benazepril, demonstrating that the higher dose of the ACE inhibitor could not offset the benefit afforded by the greater reduction in blood pressure achieved with the combination in terms of vascular protection.

These findings suggest that an ACE inhibitor, even at smaller doses, in a combination product that provides larger blood pressure reductions has a greater cardiovascular protective effect than a high-dose ACE inhibitor with smaller reductions in blood pressure. Thus, greater cardiovascular protection is achieved by adding a second drug to a patient inadequately controlled on an ACE inhibitor than by uptitrating the ACE inhibitor. Additional benefit may also be associated with more complete blockade of the renin-angiotensin system, achieved by including high doses of an ACE inhibitor in combination treatment. Findings of the ALERT study illustrate the principle that both blood pressure control and vascular protective effects of an antihypertensive regimen are critical in the attempt to achieve target organ protection.

## ACHIEVING RAPID BLOOD PRESSURE CONTROL

The common teaching is that there is no great urgency to achieve blood pressure control and that this process can take 3 to 6 months. It is believed that there may be fewer side effects with a slower, smooth reduction in blood pressure over several months. However, there is now convincing evidence that "the longer you take to achieve blood pressure control, the less likely you are to get to goal blood pressure"[32] and, more importantly, the more likely your patient is to suffer a cardiovascular event related to uncontrolled blood pressure.[9] Many obstacles to the management of hypertension entice physicians to accept inadequate blood pressure control (Figure 50-2). It has been clearly shown that there is a negative association between the number of changes that a physician makes in antihypertensive treatment and patient compliance at 1 year.

Achieving rapid control has several benefits:

1. Patients tend to have more confidence in their physicians.
2. Patients believe that their drugs are working effectively if they get to the goal blood pressure outlined by their physicians more rapidly, and so they tend to be more compliant. On the other hand, if a patient is started on a low dose of a drug, which has minimal effects on his or her blood pressure, but has a potential for adverse events (as outlined in a package insert), the patient is likely to be disheartened and discontinue the drug in favor of nonpharmacologic treatment, which is perceived to be just as effective.
3. Reluctance of doctors to titrate. Many physicians prefer the flexibility of being able to titrate monotherapies and feel that this is limited by the use of fixed combination therapy. However, in actual practice, most physicians do not uptitrate doses of antihypertensive and lipid-lowering drugs for patients whose blood pressures and/or lipid levels are uncontrolled. Physicians often avoid titration over concerns of cost, adverse events, polypharmacy, metabolic side effects, patient perception (higher doses mean they are sicker), or because they may have improved (but not controlled) blood pressure and so refocus on another disease entity.[33] Undertreatment results in inadequate blood pressure control and its associated cardiovascular risks. Early use of combination therapy often avoids these problems.
4. Cardiovascular protection. Earlier blood pressure control affords cardiovascular protection by reducing the stress of elevated blood pressure on the vasculature, thus lowering the risk of an acute event. Data from the Antihypertensive and Lipid-Lowering Treatment to Prevent Heart Attack Trial (ALLHAT) and Valsartan Antihypertensive Long-term Use Evaluation (VALUE) provide convincing evidence that protection from cardiovascular disease outcomes is greatest in patients who achieve blood pressure control most rapidly.[7,9] This is particularly true in patients who are at high risk because of coexistent cardiovascular disease or multiple risk factors.

The concern over achieving rapid blood pressure control is whether it is associated with a greater number of adverse events caused by precipitous reductions in blood pressure. Several factorial studies have compared low-dose combination agents with each of their components given first line in achieving blood pressure control. These multifactorial studies are required by the FDA to gain approval for a combination product. As is shown in Tables 50-1 and 50-2, despite significantly greater reductions in blood pressure achieved with the combination agent, there were no significant differences in adverse effects. Thus, blood pressure reduction over days to weeks (as occurs with combination therapy) is well tolerated and has benefits as compared with blood pressure reduction that requires months. This should be distinguished from

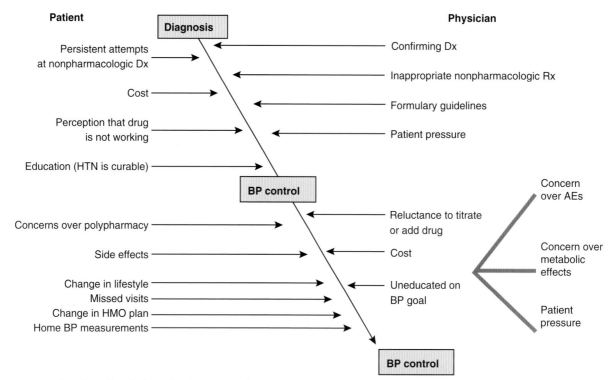

**Figure 50-2** The clinical path from the diagnosis of hypertension to BP control is fraught with many potential obstacles, which may result in the acceptance of inadequate BP control. To the extent that BP is controlled earlier *(hatched box)*, several of the obstacles are potentially eliminated, increasing the chance of achieving adequate BP control.

**Table 50-1** BP Reductions and AEs with First-Line Use of Amlodipine, Benazepril, or the Combination

| Placebo (77) | Amlodipine 5 mg (77) | Benazepril 20 mg (77) | Benazepril 5/20 mg (77) |
|---|---|---|---|
| **Changes in BP (mm Hg)** | | | |
| Systolic — | −16.2 | −12.4 | −24.7 |
| Diastolic — | −8.8 | −6.7 | −13.2 |
| **AEs (%)** | | | |
| Dizziness 0 | 1.3 | 3.9 | 5.2 |
| Edema 5.2 | 16.9 | 1.3 | 7.8 |
| Cough 0 | 0 | 0 | 5.2 |
| Headache 7.8 | 2.6 | 3.9 | 2.6 |

From Kuschnir E, Acuna E, Sevilla D, et al. Treatment of patients with essential hypertension: Amlodipine 5 mg/benazepril 20 mg compared with amlodipine 5 mg, benazepril 20 mg, and placebo. Clin Ther 18:1213-1224, 1996.
BP, blood pressure; AEs, adverse effects.

**Table 50-2** BP Reductions and AEs with First-Line Use of Verapamil SR, Trandolapril, or the Combination

| Placebo (n = 152) | Verapamil SR 240 mg (155) | Trandolapril 4 mg (155) | Verapamil SR/ Trandolapril 240/4 mg (77) |
|---|---|---|---|
| **Changes in BP (mm Hg)** | | | |
| Systolic — | −8.0 | −9.0 | −12.9 |
| Diastolic — | −4.5 | −4.3 | −8.1 |
| **AEs (%)** | | | |
| Dizziness 2.6 | 3.8 | 2.5 | 4.3 |
| Edema 3.3 | 1.3 | 1.3 | 0.6 |
| Cough 2.6 | 0.6 | 0.6 | 5.5 |
| Headache 10.5 | 12.1 | 10.7 | 6.7 |

From Messerli F, Frishman WH, Elliott WJ. Effects of verapamil and trandolapril in the treatment of hypertension. Trandolapril Study Group. Am J Hypertens 11[3 Pt 1]:322-327, 1998.
BP, blood pressure; AEs, adverse effects; SR, sustained release.

blood pressure reduction that occurs in minutes to hours, as with sublingual nifedipine. Extremely rapid blood pressure reduction with this agent has been shown to cause adverse effects and serious cardiovascular outcomes, including acute myocardial infarction.

Caution should be exercised with first-line use of combination therapy in the elderly. Despite frequently requiring multiple drugs to control their blood pressures, these patients are prone to postural hypotension and may take longer to reset their baroreceptors. A slower, more cautious approach to blood pressure reduction may be prudent in these patients. It is important to mention that although the recommended goal in the elderly is a systolic blood pressure of <140 mm Hg, in many cases older people cannot tolerate this blood pressure. This is the one instance in which we should back off to a point where patients have no adverse effects and accept inadequate blood pressure control, with the knowledge that for every 20–mm Hg reduction in systolic blood pressure, the rate of cardiovascular disease is halved.[4]

## IMPROVING WORLD-WIDE BLOOD PRESSURE CONTROL

One of the most important issues facing us in clinical medicine is the fact that fewer than one third of hypertensive patients have adequately controlled blood pressure when using a blood pressure of 140/90 mm Hg as goal, which many would argue is too high. This is troubling, considering that hypertension is the most important modifiable cardiovascular risk factor and that coronary artery disease is the most common cause of death in the industrialized world. Inadequately controlled blood pressure seen in patients on antihypertensive medication remains an important risk factor for coronary artery disease.

Complementary antihypertensive agents—for example, an ARB plus hydrochlorothiazide, an ACE inhibitor plus a dihydropyridine CCB, or a β-blocker plus hydrochlorothiazide—achieve rates greater than 70%. Thus, use of complementary combination agents has the potential to sharply increase control rates by 30% to 40%. This would have a dramatic impact on the incidence of cardiovascular disease worldwide. Earlier and more aggressive use of combination therapy for hypertension may be one of the most important changes that we can make in our approach to antihypertensive management.

Outcomes studies have shown that diastolic blood pressure goals can be achieved in >90% of patients and systolic goals in >60% of patients.[7-9,35] This clearly demonstrates that we have the tools to control hypertension in most patients. These studies have also shown that in more than 75% of patients, two or more drugs are required to achieve blood pressure goals.

## AVAILABLE COMBINATION AGENTS

Multiple fixed-dose combination agents are available for use in the management of hypertension (Table 50–3). All combination agents contain drugs that are complementary in action and provide an additive or even synergistic reduction in blood pressure, as well as side effect profiles that are better than or not different from their components. Over the next few years, many more antihypertensive combination agents will be added to the market, including three-drug combinations, and even combinations of agents for different disease processes—for example, hypertension and dyslipidemia. To provide physicians maximum flexibility in dosing, new combination agents are being developed by using all the recommended doses of each of the components.

The realization that cardiovascular risk factors seldom occur in isolation and that the presence of two or more cardiovascular risk factors are synergistic in their ability to cause cardiovascular disease has resulted in development of combination agents, which include drugs for the treatment of different disease processes. This represents a whole new era in combination therapy. For example, it is estimated that there are 27 million hypertensive patients in the United States[36] who also have dyslipidemia and require treatment of both conditions. However, frequently only the hypertension is treated pharmacologically and the dyslipidemia is treated nonpharmacologically in an effort to reduce polypharmacy. A novel new single-pill combination of atorvastatin plus amlodipine has become available in the United States.[37] This will enable clinicians to treat both conditions with a convenient single-drug preparation and will almost certainly decrease cardiovascular risk in these patients and improve patient compliance for these two important cardiovascular risk factors. Other similar combination agents are currently being developed, and it is likely that combination agents that include drugs for the treatment of other cardiovascular risk factors will be developed in the future. These advances in available therapeutic agents will facilitate achieving goals in patients with the metabolic syndrome.

## SUMMARY

Combination therapy provides a modality of treatment that is much closer to the "ideal antihypertensive" agent than anything we have currently or will have in the foreseeable future for the treatment of hypertension. The success rate in achieving blood pressure goals and decreasing cardiovascular events in hypertensive patients is greater with combination therapy than with monotherapy.

Hypertension is a multifactorial disorder that is difficult to control with monotherapy in many patients. Blocking two or more blood pressure regulatory systems provides a more effective and more physiologic reduction in blood pressure that is more likely to get patients to goal. This is critical in the prevention of cardiovascular disease. Use of combination therapy as first-line treatment, or early in the management of hypertension, is perhaps the most important change that can be made in attacking the major public health problem of poorly treated hypertension.

**Table 50–3** Antihypertensives Available as a Fixed-Dose Combination Product

| Class | Combination | Trade Name |
|---|---|---|
| β-Adrenergic Blockers and Diuretics | Atenolol 50-100 mg/clorthalidone 25 mg | Tenoretic |
| | Bisoprolol 2.5-10 mg/HCTZ 6.25 mg | Ziac* |
| | Metoprolol 50-100 mg/HCTZ 25-50 mg | Lopressor HCT |
| | Nadolol 40-80 mg/bendroflumethiazide 5 mg | Corzide |
| | Propranolol 40-80 mg/HCTZ 25 mg | Inderide |
| | Propranolol ER 80-160 mg/HCTZ 50 mg | Inderide LA |
| | Timolol 10 mg/HCTZ 25 mg | Timolide |
| ACE Inhibitors and Diuretics | Benazepril 5-20 mg/HCTZ 6.25-25 mg | Lotensin HCT |
| | Captopril 25-50 mg/HCTZ 15-25 mg | Capozide* |
| | Enalapril 5-10 mg/HCTZ 12.5-25 mg | Vaseretic |
| | Lisinopril 10-20 mg/HCTZ 12.5-25 mg | Zestoretic; Prinzide |
| Angiotensin II Receptor Blockers and Diuretics | Losartan 50 mg/HCTZ 12.5-25 mg | Hyzaar |
| | Valsartan 80-160 mg/HCTZ 12.5-25 mg | Diovan HCT |
| | Irbesartan 150-300 mg/HCTZ 12.5 mg | Irbesartan HCT |
| | Telmisartan 40-80 mg/HCTZ 12.5 mg | Telmisartan HCT |
| | Olmesartan 20-40 mg/HCTZ 12.5-25 mg | Olmesartan HCT |
| | Candesartan 16-32 mg/HCTZ 12.5 mg | Candesartan HCT |
| Calcium Antagonists and ACE Inhibitors | Amlodipine 2.5-10 mg/benazepril 10-20 mg | Lotrel |
| | Diltiazem 180 mg/enalapril 5 mg | Teczem |
| | Felodipine 5 mg/enalapril 5 mg | Lexxel |
| | Verapamil 180-240 mg/trandolapril 1-4 mg | Tarka |
| Other Combinations | Clonidine HCl 0.1-0.3 mg/chlorthalidone 15 mg | Combipres |
| | Deserpidine 0.25-0.5 mg/methyclothiazide 5 mg | Enduronyl (Forte) |
| | Guanethidine 10 mg/HCTZ 25 mg | Esimil |
| | Hydralazide 25-100 mg/HCTZ 25-50 mg | Apresazide |
| | Hydralazide 25 mg/reserpine 0.1 mg/HCTZ 15 mg | Ser-Ap-Es; Unipres; Tri-Hydroserpine |
| | Methyldopa 250 mg/chlorothiazide 150-250 mg | Aldoclor |
| | Methyldopa 250-500 mg/HCTZ 30-50 mg | Aldoril |
| | Prazosin 1-5 mg/polythiazide 0.5 mg | Minizide |
| | Rauwolfia 50 mg/bendroflumethiazide 4 mg | Rauzide |
| | Reserpine 0.125 mg/Chlorthalidone 25 mg | Demi-Regroton |
| | Reserpine 0.125 mg/chlorothiazide 250-500 mg | Diupres |
| | Reserpine 0.125 mg/HCTZ 25-50 mg | Hydropres; Hydroserpin |
| | Reserpine 0.125 mg/hydroflumethiazide 50 mg | Salutensin (-Demi) |
| | Reserpine 0.25 mg/polythiazide 2 mg | Renese-R |
| | Reserpine 0.1 mg/trichlormethiazide 2-4 mg | Metatensin |

ACE, angiotensin-converting enzyme; HCTZ, hydrochlorothiazide.

# References

1. World Health Report 2002: Reducing risks, promoting healthy life. Geneva, Switzerland: World Health Organization, 2002. *http://www.who.int/whr/2002.*
2. Collins R, Peto R, MacMahon S, et al. Blood pressure, stroke, and coronary heart disease. Part 2, short-term reductions in blood pressure: Overview of randomized drug trials in their epidemiological context. Lancet 335:827-839, 1990.
3. Effects of ACE inhibitors, calcium antagonists, and other blood-pressure lowering drugs: Results of prospectively designed overviews of randomized trials. Lancet 355:1955-1964, 2000.
4. Blood Pressure Lowering Treatment Trialists' Collaboration, Effect of different blood-pressure lowering regimens on major cardiovascular events: results of prospectively-designed overviews of randomized trials. Lancet 362:1527-1535, 2003.
5. The Seventh Report of the Joint National Committee on Prevention, Detection, Evaluation, and Treatment of High Blood Pressure. JAMA 289:2560-2572, 2003.
6. Dahlöf B, Devereux RB, Kjeldsen SE, et al. Cardiovascular morbidity and mortality in the Losartan Intervention For Endpoint reduction in hypertension study (LIFE): A randomized trial against atenolol. Lancet 359:995-1003, 2002.
7. Furberg CD, Wright JT, Davis BR, et al. Major outcomes in high-risk hypertensive patients randomised to angiotensin-converting enzyme inhibitor or calcium channel blocker vs

diuretic: The Antihypertensive and Lipid-Lowering Treatment to Prevent Heart Attack Trial (ALLHAT). JAMA 288:2981-2997, 2002.

8. Black H, Elliot W, Grandits G, et al. Principal results of the Controlled Onset Verapamil Investigation of Cardiovascular Endpoints (CONVINCE) trial. JAMA 289:2073-2082, 2003.

9. Julius S, Kjeldsen SE, Weber M, et al. Outcomes in hypertensive patients at high cardiovascular risk treated with regimens based on valsartan or amlodipine: The VALUE randomized trial. Lancet 363:2022-2031, 2004.

10. Frishman WH, Bryzinski DS, Coulson LR, et al. A multifactorial trial design to assess combination therapy in hypertension. Treatment with bisoprolol and hydrochlorothiazide. Arch Intern Med 154:1461-1468, 1994.

11. Prisant LM, Weir MR, Papademetriou V, et al. Low-dose drug combination therapy: An alternative first-line approach to hypertension treatment. Am Heart J 130:359-366, 1995.

12. Kuschair E, Acura E, Sevilla D. Treatment of patients with essential hypertension: Amlodipine 5mg/benazepril 20mg compared with benazepril 20mg and placebo. Clin Therapeutics 18:6-12, 1996.

13. Neutel JM, Rolf CM, Valentine SN, et al. Low-dose combination therapy as first line treatment of mild to moderate hypertension: The efficacy and safety of bisoprolol/HCTZ versus amlodipine, enalapril, and placebo. Cardiovasc Rev Rep 17:1-9,171-175, 1996.

14. Fogari R, Zoppi A, Mugellini A, et al. Effect of benazepril plus amlodipine vs. benazepril alone on urinary albumin excretion in hypertensive patients with type II diabetes and microalbuminuria. Clinical Drug Invest 13(suppl 1):50-55, 1997.

15. Messerli F, Frishman WH, Elliott WJ. Effects of verapamil and trandolapril in the treatment of hypertension. Trandolapril Study Group. Am J Hypertens 11(Part I):322-327, 1998.

16. Neutel JM, Back HR, Weber MA. Combination therapy with diuretics: An evolution of understanding. Am J Med. 101(suppl 3A):61S-70S, 1996.

17. Neutel JM. Metabolic manifestations of low-dose diuretics. Am J Med 101(3A):71S-82S, 1996.

18. Chrysant SG. Antihypertensive effectiveness of low-dose lisinopril-hydrochlorothiazide combination. A large multicenter study. Lisinopril-Hydrochlorothiazide Group. Arch Intern Med 154:737-743, 1994.

19. Cheung D, Gasster JL, Weber MA. Hypertension in the aged: A pathophysiologic basis for treatment. Am J Cardiol 65:25H-32H, 1989.

20. McGill JB, Reilly PA. Combination treatment with telmisartan and hydrochlorothiazide in black patients with mild to moderate hypertension. Clin Cardiol 24:66-72, 2001.

21. Agodoa LY, Appel L, Bakris GL, et al. Effect of ramipril vs amlodipine on renal outcomes in hypertensive nephrosclerosis: A randomized controlled trial. JAMA 285:2719-2728, 2001.

22. Sica DA. Fixed dose combination antihypertensive drugs. Do they have a role in rational therapy? Drugs 48:16-24, 1994.

23. Neutel JM, Schnaper HW, Cheung DG, et al. Evaluation of the 24-hour blood pressure effects of beta blockers given once daily. Am J Hypertens 3:114A, 1990.

24. Cohen MC, Rohtla KM, Lavery CE, et al. Meta-analysis of the morning excess of acute myocardial infarction and sudden cardiac death. Am J Cardiol 79:1512-1516, 1997.

25. Elliot WJ. Circadian variation in the timing of stroke onset a meta-analysis. Stroke 29:992-996, 1998.

26. Neutel JM, Smith DHG, Weber MA. Low-dose combination therapy: An important first-line treatment in the management of hypertension. Am J Hypertens 14:286-292, 2001.

27. Shoheiber O. Oral presentation 37th Annual American Society of Health System Pharmacists. Mid Year Clinical Meeting. December 8-12th, 2002; Atlanta, GA.

28. Tight blood pressure control and risk of macrovascular and microvascular complications in type 2 diabetes: UKPDS 38. UK Prospective Diabetes Study Group. BMJ 317:703-713, 1998.

29. Hasson L, Zanchetti A. Carruthers SG, et al. Effects of intensive blood-pressure lowering and low-dose aspirin in patients with hypertension: Principal results of the Hypertension Optimal Treatment (HOT) randomised trial. Lancet 351:1755-1762, 1998.

30. Tatti P, Pahor M, Byington RP, et al. Outcome results of the Fosinopril Versus Amlodipine Cardiovascular Events Randomized Trial (FACET) in patients with hypertension and NIDDM. Diabetes Care 21:597-603, 1998.

31. Neutel JM, Smith DHG, Weber MA. Effect of antihypertensive monotherapy and combination therapy on arterial dispensability and left ventricular mass. Am J Hypertens 17:37-42, 2004.

32. Caro JJ, Soeckman JL, Salas M, et al. Effects of initial drug choice on persistence with antihypertensive therapy: The importance of actual practice data. CMAJ 160:41-46, 1999.

33. Neutel JM, Smith DHG. Improving patient compliance: A major goal in the management of hypertension. J Clin Hypertens 5:127-132, 2003.

34. Lewington S, Clarke R, Qizilbash N, et al. Age-specific relevance of usual blood pressure to vascular mortality: A meta-analysis of individual data for one million adults in 61 prospective studies. Prospective Studies Collaboration. Lancet 360:1903-1913, 2002.

35. Cushman WC, Ford CE, Cutler JA, et al. Success and predictors of blood pressure control in diverse North American settings: The Antihypertensive and Lipid-Lowering Treatment to Prevent Heart Attack Trial (ALLHAT). J Clin Hypertens 4:393-404, 2002.

36. National Health and Nutrition Examination Survey III (NHANES III), 1988-1994, CDC/NCHS.

37. Blank R, LaSalle J, Reeves R, et al. Amlopidine/atorvastatin single pill dual therapy improves goal attainment in the treatment of concomitant hypertension and dyslipidemia: The Gemini Study. J Am Coll Cardiol 43 (Suppl A):447A(Abstr# 1008-190), 2004.

# Chapter 51

# Chronotherapeutics in the Treatment of Hypertension

## Michael H. Smolensky, Ramon C. Hermida, Francesco Portaluppi, Erhard Haus, Alain Reinberg

Chronotherapeutics is the purposeful timing of medications, with or without the utilization of special drug-release technology, to proportion serum and tissue concentrations in synchrony with known circadian rhythms in disease processes and symptoms as a means of enhancing beneficial outcomes and/or attenuating or averting adverse effects.[1] The concept of chronotherapeutics, although relatively new to hypertension and cardiovascular medicine, was first introduced and proven worthy in clinical medicine in the 1960s; the morning alternate-day corticosteroid tablet dosing schedule was introduced as a convenient means of minimizing the adverse effects of such antiinflammatory medications as prednisone and methylprednisolone.[2,3] The chronotherapy of hypertension takes into account the clinically relevant features of the 24-hour pattern of blood pressure (BP) (i.e., the accelerated morning rise at the commencement of diurnal activity and the extent of decline during nighttime sleep) plus potential administration-time (circadian rhythm) determinants of the pharmacokinetics and dynamics of individual antihypertensive medications. Herein, we focus on the chronotherapy of hypertension; however, as necessary background we first present the major concepts and mechanisms of biologic timekeeping.

## BIOLOGIC RHYTHMS AND BIOLOGIC TIME STRUCTURE

Biologic processes and functions are organized in time as rhythms of discrete periods. Ultradian rhythms, exemplified by neural and neuroendocrine activities, exhibit periods in the range of seconds, minutes, or hours. Infradian rhythms, characteristic of many biologic processes and functions, exhibit periods much longer than 24 hours, in the range of days (~week), weeks (~month, e.g., menstrual cycle), and months (~year). Circadian (*circa* = about; *dies* = day) rhythms, characteristic of nearly every life process, exhibit 24-hour or near-24-hour variation and are important to clinical medicine. They play a role in the pathophysiology of many chronic disease states, and they may influence the response to diagnostic tests, as well as the therapeutic efficiency and side-effect profile of prescribed treatments.[1,4]

The body's circadian rhythms are controlled by an endogenous master clock network composed of the paired suprachiasmatic nuclei (SCN), located within the hypothalamus, and the pineal gland through its 24-hour cycle of melatonin synthesis and secretion.[5,6] The activities of specific genes (e.g., per[1], per[2], per[3], bmal, clock, and CRY) and their gene products along with the cyclic (nocturnal) circulation of melatonin constitute the mechanism of circadian timekeeping.[6,7] This master clock network orchestrates the period and staging of the multitude of subservient peripheral circadian clocks located in cells, tissues, and organ systems. The end effect is an ordered temporal organization of the biology during each 24-hour period in support of peak functioning during diurnal activity and of rest and repair during nocturnal sleep.

Circadian rhythms are generated and coordinated by the genetically inherited brain clock network. Interestingly, the inherited period of circadian clocks, for as yet unknown reasons, is not precisely 24 hours.[8] The inherited period of the master clock of most persons is slightly greater than 24 hours (e.g., 24.2 hours), while in some it is slightly less than 24 hours. The master and subservient peripheral circadian clocks are synchronized to an exact 24-hour ambient and social cycle by specific external time cues, the most important being the environmental light-dark cycle.[9,10] The features of the natural light and dark cycle vary predictably both over the 24 hours and year. The central clock network relies on the 24-hour environmental light-dark cycle to titrate its period to exactly 24 hours. It also relies on information derived from sensing the duration of the daily environmental photoperiod to adjust the biology seasonally as circannual (~1-year) rhythms. Ambient light-dark time cues sensed by specialized noncone, nonrod photoreceptor cells of the retina are conveyed to the SCN and pineal gland via the retinohypothalamic neural tract.[10] Serum melatonin concentration displays a prominent circadian rhythm, with its synthesis and secretion occurring almost exclusively during nighttime sleep. Exposure to light at an atypical time—during the middle of the night, which is the case when working nights or when rapidly traveling across time zones—induces compensatory adjustment of the SCN-pineal gland clock network during the several days thereafter and in turn the staging of the circadian time structure.[11,12] Daytime light exposure exerts no effect on the SCN-melatonin clock network, while light exposure very late at night or during the initial hours of sleep delays the body clock and melatonin rhythm and ultimately the staging of all the other circadian rhythms. In contrast, light exposure in the early morning hours, close to the end of the sleep span, advances the melatonin and other circadian rhythms.

The integrity of the circadian time structure is central to efficient biological and cognitive functioning. This is amply illustrated by the acute feelings and complaints—the symptoms of jet lag—that result from the abrupt alteration of the habitual sleep-wake cycle and ensuing transient disruption of the circadian time structure following the rapid transmeridian displacement of travelers by jet aircraft.[13] Recurrent and chronic disturbance of the circadian time structure, common in career shift and night workers, is associated with elevated risk of sleep disorders, peptic ulcer, coronary heart disease

(CHD), cancer, and other medical problems.[14-16] Some of these health problems may result, at least in part, from the inhibition of melatonin production due to light exposure during night work.[15,16] Substantiation of the health risks of career shift workers implies that therapeutic interventions should preserve the circadian timekeeping network and the body's temporal organization. Indeed, the integrity and strength of the circadian time structure of cancer patients has been shown to be a sensitive predictor of the response to and outcome of chemotherapy.[17]

## CIRCADIAN BLOOD PRESSURE RHYTHM IN HYPERTENSION

Twenty-four hour intraarterial and ambulatory BP monitoring (ABPM) studies clearly reveal the circadian pattern and features of systolic blood pressure (SBP) and diastolic blood pressure (DBP) (Figure 51–1, A). In diurnally active normotensive persons the pattern is characterized by a decline during nighttime sleep of 10% to 20% from the daytime mean, sharp morning rise coincident with the commencement of daily activity, elevated level during the daytime and descending level in the evening. This day-night BP cycle results both from endogenous factors (circadian rhythms in autonomic nervous system and endocrine function) and exogenous factors (predictable-in-time differences in posture, stress, and activity).[18,19] The 24-hour BP pattern is much the same in the majority of uncomplicated essential (primary) hypertension patients except that either the temporal oscillation occurs around an abnormally elevated 24-hour mean or the amplitude of change is exaggerated resulting in an abnormally high level of pressure during a significant portion of the day. The BP pattern in secondary hypertension is often different. The extent of the nocturnal decline, relative to the daytime mean, may be blunted (less than 10%) or even reversed, with the sleep-time BP being higher than the daytime BP.[20]

Hypertension is a well-known risk factor for cerebrovascular and cardiovascular accidents. During the past two decades specific features of the 24-hour BP pattern have been assessed as potential sources of injury to target tissues and as triggers of cardiac and cerebrovascular events in hypertensive patients. Indeed, the prominent 24-hour variation in the occurrence of a variety of acute cardiovascular events, such as myocardial infarction (MI), angina, cardiac arrest, sudden cardiac death, and pulmonary embolism, has been shown to be closely related to the circadian BP pattern of hypertensive persons.[21] For example, the rate of rise of BP coincident with the commencement of diurnal activity has been identified as an independent predictor of one's risk of morning stroke and acute coronary syndrome, and is also hypothesized to be a trigger for MI at this time of day.[22-27] Interestingly, recent studies reveal that the 24-hour pattern and the characteristic morning peak in the occurrence of both ischemic[28] and hemorrhagic[29] stroke is the same in normotensive and hypertensive persons. Moreover, other cardiovascular events, such as acute aortic dissection, display prominent 24-hour variation, with a significant morning peak both in hypertensive and normotensive persons.[30] Taken together, all of these observations strengthen the suggestion that the morning surge in BP (whether in the presence or absence of hypertension) is a crucial determinant of the rupture of a vulnerable and critically weakened arterial wall.[31]

A growing number of studies also indicates that the extent of the nocturnal BP decline is deterministic of cardiovascular injury and risk. Absence of the normal 10% to 20% sleep-time BP decline is associated with elevated risk of target organ injury, particularly to the heart (left ventricular hypertrophy [LVH] and MI), brain (stroke), and kidney (albuminuria, progression to end-stage renal disease [ESRD]).[20,32-35] On the other hand, too great a decline in the sleep-time BP by more than 20% of the daytime mean (i.e., superdipping) may result in nocturnal hypotension, with heightened risk of nighttime stroke, ischemic ocular disorder, and perhaps falls with resultant fractures due to syncope with sudden change in posture (e.g., on bathroom use).[36-39] The chronotherapy of hypertension takes into account the epidemiology of the various features of the day-night BP pattern. The specific goals of chronotherapy are discussed in the next section

## CHRONOTHERAPY OF BLOOD PRESSURE–LOWERING MEDICATIONS

The pharmacotherapy of hypertension has been strongly influenced by the concept and assumptions of homeostasis. Until the last 10 years or so, the vast majority of the medical community believed SBP and DBP to be relatively constant throughout the 24 hours.[40] Consequently, it was deduced that a major goal of antihypertensive pharmacotherapy ought to be constancy of medication level throughout the 24-hour dosing interval. The application of intraarterial and ABPM methods during the past 10 to 15 years has clearly documented the prominence of the 24-hour variation in both SBP and DBP. In essential hypertension, as schematically represented in Figure 51–1, B, the relatively constant medication level achieved by conventional (homeostatically styled) antihypertensive therapies may be lower than required in the morning when SBP and DBP surge to peak or near-peak levels, whereas it may be higher than required during nighttime sleep when SBP and DBP decline to their lowest level.

The goals of the chronotherapy of essential hypertension are significant moderation of the morning accelerated rise in BP and reduction of abnormally elevated daytime, nighttime, and 24-hour BP means, without overcorrection (induction of superdipping) of sleep-time SBP and DBP. One way to achieve these goals is to utilize special drug-delivery technologies. The chronotherapeutic perspective of 24-hour BP control entails the purposeful tailoring of medication level over the 24 hours in close synchrony with the known (and expected) day-night pattern in SBP and DBP to optimize effect. A key premise of the chronotherapy of essential hypertension is that some 15% to 20% of each dose of once-a-day conventional medications is wasted by maintaining greater than required drug concentration during nocturnal sleep when BP is lowest, and not uncommonly normal in mild hypertension (Figure 51–1, B). Chronotherapeutic formulations rely on unique technology to redistribute this proportion of the daily dose to the time of day when BP rises to peak or near-peak levels and when the greatest concentration of antihypertensive is required for BP control. Unique drug-delivery technology, or in some instances bedtime dosing times of certain conventional medications, is thus utilized to ensure that peak and trough concentrations of antihypertensive medications are circulated in synchrony with predicted greatest and lowest SBP and DBP,

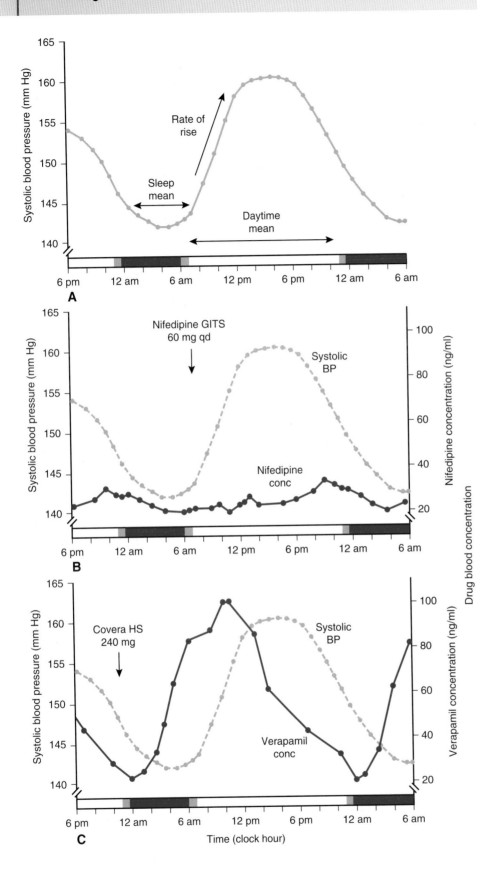

**Figure 51-1 A,** Clinically important features of the circadian rhythm of blood pressure (BP) in essential hypertension (EH): rate of rise and level of BP in the morning, sleep-time, diurnal, and 24-hour BP means and dipping status (mean daytime BP – mean sleep-time BP/mean daytime BP × 100%). **B,** BP circadian rhythm in EH relative to the steady-state nearly constant nifedipine concentration produce by morning ingestion of 60 mg of the (homeostatically styled) conventional nifedipine GITS formulation. The nearly constant blood drug concentration is likely to be too low in the morning to adequately control peak or near-peak values of SBP and DBP in EH that occur at this time of day, and it is likely to be greater than needed to control SBP and DBP during nighttime sleep when they decline to lowest levels of the 24 hours. **C,** The circadian BP rhythm in EH is depicted in relation to the 24-hour temporally modulated verapamil concentration following ingestion of 240 mg of COER-verapamil chronotherapy at bedtime. Note that the 24-hour pattern in verapamil concentration varies purposefully during the 24 hours in close synchrony with the expected circadian BP variation in EH to enhance control of the elevated morning and afternoon SBP and DBP and to avoid their excessive reduction during sleep when they are lowest during the 24 hours. Dark and light regions of the horizontal time axis indicate, respectively, the spans of nighttime sleep and daytime activity.

respectively, during the day and night. In the following section, we review those specific formulations that are now marketed—at least in the United States—as chronotherapies of hypertension.

## MARKETED CHRONOTHERAPIES OF HYPERTENSION

### Calcium Channel Blockers

The calcium channel blocker (CCB), controlled-onset, extended-release (COER)–verapamil was the first special drug-delivery tablet used for chronotherapy of hypertension (and stable angina pectoris[41,42]). COER–verapamil (United States: Covera HS; other markets: Chronovera) was approved in the United States by the Food and Drug Administration (FDA) in 1996 for marketing by the Searle Pharmaceutical Company. The drug-delivery technology of this tablet medication delays the release of verapamil for approximately 4 to 5 hours following bedtime ingestion as recommended. Medication is released thereafter so the highest blood concentration is achieved in the morning around the time of awakening, generally between 6 and 10 A.M., with an elevated level sustained throughout diurnal activity (Figure 51–2, A). The half-life kinetics of verapamil results in a progressive decline of drug level in the evening and over night, so the reduced (trough) concentration occurs during nighttime sleep when BP in essential hypertension is lowest.[43]

Multicenter clinical trials[44] of this verapamil chronotherapy utilizing 24-hour ABPM methods document the enhanced control of the morning BP rate of rise and level (Figure 51–3, A). Moreover, a statistically significant dose (placebo and 120, 180, 360, 540 mg)-dependent reduction of SBP and DBP was verified, both at the peak (between 6 and 10 A.M.) and trough (between 6 and 10 P.M.) drug concentration times. COER–verapamil has been shown to be therapeutic for both dipper and nondipper hypertensive patients; in nondippers, it effectively reduces abnormally elevated morning as well as nocturnal BP, particularly SBP, in a dose-dependent manner.[45] Furthermore, it is as effective in African Americans as in Caucasians.[46] COER–verapamil compared with the CCB nifedipine GITS formulation, which utilizes a special drug-delivery system to achieve near-constancy in drug concentration throughout the 24 hours, achieves significantly better BP control during the morning when BP typically rises to highest or near-highest levels.[47] Clinical trials show that COER–verapamil is safe. No significant differences were detected in reported side effects between COER–verapamil and placebo, apart from dose-related constipation and second-/third-degree atrioventricular block with the highest (540 mg) dose.[44]

Chronotherapeutic oral drug absorption system (CODAS)–verapamil is a second special drug-delivery–based CCB chronotherapy of hypertension. CODAS–verapamil (Verelan PM, Schwarz Pharma) was approved by the FDA in 1999. Release of verapamil from the polymer-coated beads of this capsule medication following recommended bedtime ingestion is delayed for approximately 4 hours (Figure 51–2, B). Medication is then dispersed in increasing amount so that peak blood concentration is achieved in the morning, between 6 and 10 A.M., when SBP and DBP are expected to rise to peak or near-peak levels.[48]

Two placebo-controlled, parallel-design, double-blind 24-hour ABPM trials involving stages 1 and 2 essential hypertensive patients document the exaggerated reduction of BP during the initial hours of diurnal activity (see Figure 51–3, B). Furthermore, they substantiate the dose (placebo and 100, 200, 300, 400 mg)-dependent reduction of SBP and DBP both at the peak, between 6 and 10 A.M. when BP is typically greatest, and at the trough, between 6 and 10 P.M. when BP declines to near low levels, drug concentration times.[49,50] The results of a large community-based trial (CHRONO[51]) involving almost 2400 previously treated and nontreated essential hypertensive patients further confirm the efficacy and safety of the CODAS–verapamil chronotherapy. Study participants received a starting dose of 200-mg; if the target clinic BP of <140/90 mm Hg was not achieved after 4 weeks of treatment, the dose was up-titrated to 300-mg for another 4 weeks. Patients who failed to attain goal BP with this dose were again up-titrated to 400-mg for an additional 4 weeks. In total, 62.6% of the participants achieved the target BP goal with this monotherapy; 36.7% achieved it with the 200-mg dose; 18.9% with the 300-mg dose, and 6.9% with the 400-mg dose. CODAS–verapamil chronotherapy was effective in both previously untreated and treated patients no matter their age, gender, or race, and it was well tolerated; the most frequent adverse events being gastrointestinal (8.2% of patients), primarily constipation.

Graded-release long-acting diltiazem (Cardizem LA, Biovail Pharmaceuticals) was approved by the FDA in 2003 for once-daily dosing either in the morning or evening. Multiple-dose studies[52] show that ingestion of the 360-mg dose of this special diltiazem medication at 10 P.M. results in the desired kinetic profile for the chronotherapy of essential hypertension. Trough blood diltiazem concentration occurs during nighttime sleep (~2 A.M.) and peak concentration during the morning (between ~10 A.M. and noon), with maintenance of an elevated drug level during the afternoon and early evening (Figure 51–2, C). In contrast, multiple-dose studies show the ingestion of 360 mg of this medication in the morning at 8 A.M., as opposed to at bedtime, results in trough drug level in the morning between 8 and 10 A.M. (when SBP and DBP in essential hypertension reach highest or near highest levels) and peak drug level in the evening between 6 and 8 P.M. (when SBP and DBP are declining) (Figure 51–2, C). The discordance between the timing of the peak and trough diltiazem blood concentrations relative to the circadian pattern of BP in essential hypertension, as exemplified by the ingestion of diltiazem at the improper time of the day, emphasizes the critical importance of patient and physician compliance to the recommended bedtime dosing of this and other BP chronotherapies. (See Glasser et al. 2003[53] for details of the extent and nature of the dosing-time differences in BP control by diltiazem.)

A multicenter 24-hour ABPM study of 429 essential hypertensive patients documents the statistically significant reduction of both peak and trough-time SBP and DBP for the 120-, 240-, 360- and 540-mg doses of diltiazem when ingested at bedtime.[53] Substantially enhanced BP reduction was achieved between 6 A.M. and noon across all the dose strengths. A substudy involving the 360-mg dose, a dose that is claimed to control BP in 85% of hypertensive patients,[54] illustrates the statistically significantly greater SBP- and DBP-lowering effect of diltiazem between 6 A.M. and noon when ingested at

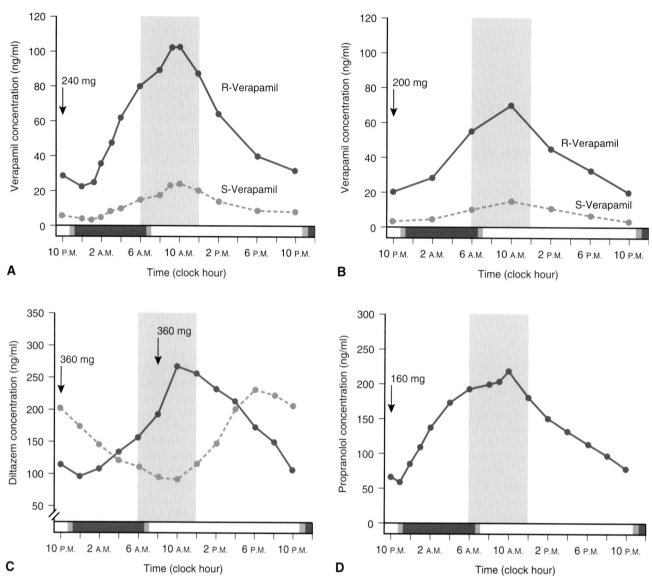

**Figure 51–2** Steady-state pharmacokinetics of the hypertension chronotherapies of **A,** 240 mg COER–verapamil; **B,** 200 mg CODAS–verapamil; **C,** 360 mg diltiazem; and **D,** 160 mg propranolol. Bedtime ingestion of the chronotherapies as recommended results in peak drug concentrations in the morning during the initial hours of daytime activity, generally between 6 and 10 A.M. when SBP and DBP in EH attain peak or near-peak values, and in trough drug concentration during the first 4 to 5 hours of nighttime sleep when SBP and DBP decline to lowest or near-lowest values during the 24 hours. Note that dosing diltiazem chronotherapy at the wrong time of the day (i.e., in the morning at 8 A.M.) results in mismatch of diltiazem concentration relative to biologic need as defined by the circadian BP rhythm in EH. Studies show dosing this, and presumably any other, chronotherapy of hypertension at an inappropriate time of the day (e.g., morning) significantly compromises BP control in the morning and afternoon.* Dark and light regions of the horizontal time axis indicate, respectively, the spans of nighttime sleep and daytime activity. (**A** adapted from Gupta SK, Yih BM, Atkinson L, et al. The effect of food, time of dosing and body composition on the pharmacokinetics and pharmacodynamics of verapamil and norverapamil. J Clin Pharmacol 35:1083-1093, 1995; **B** adapted from Prisant LM, Devane JG, Butler J. A steady state evaluation of the bioavailability of chronotherapeutic oral drug absorption system verapamil PM after nighttime dosing vs. immediate-acting verapamil dosed every eight hours. Am J Ther 7:345-251, 2000; **C** adapted from Sista S, Chi-Keung Lai, J, Eradiri O, et al. Pharmacokinetics of a novel diltiazem HCL extended-release tablet formulation for evening administration. J Clin Pharmacol 43:1149-1157, 2003; **D** adapted from Sica D, Frishman WH, Manowitz N. Pharmacokinetics of propranolol after single and multiple dosing with sustained-released propranolol or propranolol CR [Innopran XL], a new chronotherapeutic formulation. Heart Disease 5:176-181, 2003; *Glasser S, Neutel JM, Gana TJ, et al. Efficacy and safety of a once daily graded-release diltiazem formulation in essential hypertension. Am J Hypertens 16:51-58, 2003.)

**Figure 51-3** Steady-state BP-lowering activity assessed by 24-hour ambulatory blood pressure monitoring (ABPM) at baseline and again after 2 or more months of treatment with one of the following calcium channel blocker (CCB) chronotherapies ingested at bedtime: **A,** 360 mg COER–verapamil; **B,** 300 mg CODAS–verapamil; and **C,** titrated doses in steps from 240 mg to 360 mg to 540 mg diltiazem. Note the common features among the four chronotherapies of enhanced reduction of SBP and DBP in the morning between 6 A.M. and noon (when BP of essential hypertensive patients rapidly rise to near-peak or peak values) and the continuing significant attenuation of BP throughout the remainder of the 24-hour dosing interval, during the afternoon, evening, and nighttime. Dark and light regions of the horizontal time axis indicate, respectively, the spans of nighttime sleep and daytime activity. (**A** adapted from White WB, Anders RJ, MacInyre JM, et al. Nocturnal dosing of a novel delivery system of verapamil for systemic hypertension. Am J Cardiol 76:375-380, 1995; **B** adapted from Smith DHG, Neutel JM, Weber MA. A new chronotherapeutic oral drug absorption system for verapamil optimizes blood pressure control in the morning. Am J Hypertens 14:14-19, 2001; **C** from White WB, LaCourciere Y, Gana T, et al. The effects of graded-release diltiazem vs. ramipril dosed at bedtime on the early morning blood pressure, heart rate and the rate-pressure product. Am Heart J 148:628-634, 2004.)

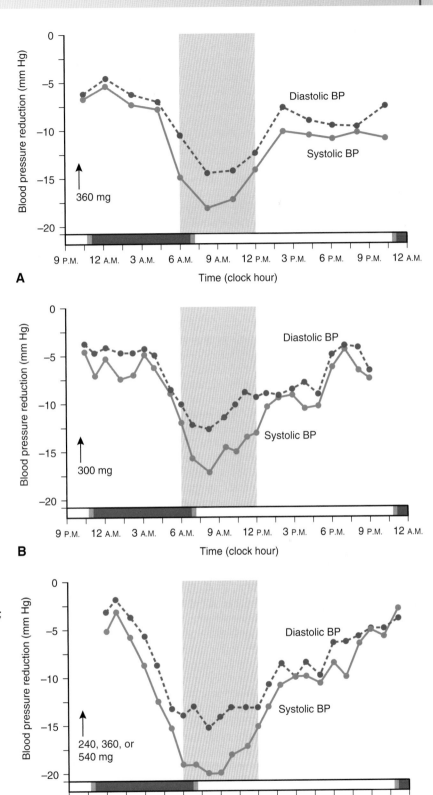

bedtime as opposed to in the morning on awakening.[53] Bedtime dosing of diltiazem has been found to be safe; the incidence of adverse events in the 120-, 240-, 360-, and 540-mg treatment groups was dose-independent and comparable with that of the placebo-treated groups. The most frequent side effects, independent of dose, were headache (11.7%), upper respiratory infection (5.6%), and lower limb edema (5.4%). No episodes of bradycardia and no episodes of first-degree atrioventricular heart block requiring dismissal from the clinical trials occurred in any of the diltiazem treatment groups.[55] Finally, another multicenter trial found bedtime diltiazem in doses of up to 540 mg/day to be significantly more effective in controlling morning SBP, DBP, heart rate (HR), and rate-pressure product (SBP × HR = surrogate measure of left ventricular work and myocardial oxygen demand) than the angiotensin-converting enzyme inhibitor (ACEI) ramipril ingested at bedtime in doses of up to 20 mg/day.[56]

### β-Antagonist

The β-antagonist propranolol (Innopran XL, Reliant Pharmaceuticals) was approved by the FDA in 2003 for use in chronotherapy. Multiple-dose study[57] of this capsule medication shows that its ingestion at bedtime as recommended results in trough drug concentration toward the latter hours of nighttime sleep (~4 A.M.) due to the intentional delay of propranolol release for 4 to 5 hours, peak drug concentration between 4 and 10 A.M., and an elevated plateau of drug concentration in the afternoon and early evening (Figure 51–2, D). Unpublished findings (Dr. Joel Neutel, Integrium, Tustin, CA, personal communication) from 24-hour ABPM trials of this β-antagonist chronotherapy document its potent SBP and DBP reduction in the morning with persistence of significant BP-lowering activity for the entire 24-hour dosing interval.

## CHRONOPHARMACOLOGY IN THE BLOOD PRESSURE–LOWERING EFFECTS OF CONVENTIONAL ONCE-A-DAY ANTIHYPERTENSIVE MEDICATIONS

Appreciable administration-time differences in the kinetics (i.e., chronokinetics) of BP-lowering and cardiac medications are well known.[58-62] They result from circadian rhythms in gastric pH and emptying; gastrointestinal motility; biliary function and circulation; blood flow to the duodenum, liver, and kidney; and liver enzyme activity, among other factors.[63,64] In some instances it is the chemistry and/or physics of the drug-delivery system of the tablet and capsule medications that is vulnerable to circadian influences, while in others it is the chemistry of the medication that is vulnerable. Clinically relevant administration-time differences in the beneficial and adverse effects (termed *chronodynamics*) of BP-lowering medications are also known. These result from the chronokinetics of the medications as well as circadian rhythms in the drug-free fraction, rate-limiting steps of key metabolic pathways, receptor number and conformation and/or second messenger dynamics, culminating in temporal disparities in the concentration-effect relationship.[65] Examples of administration-time differences in the BP-lowering effects of various types of antihypertensive medications—CCBs, ACEIs, angiotensin receptor blockers (ARBs), $\alpha_1$-adrenoceptor antagonists, and even aspirin—are presented

in Table 51–1. The dosing time–dependent difference in the BP-lowering effect of some of these medications is so great that it merits detailed discussion in the following sections.

### Morning vs. Evening Isradipine Therapy of Nondipper Pattern Hypertension

Nocturnal hypertension, characterized by the loss or even reversal of the expected 10% to 20% sleep-time BP decline, increases the risk of cardiovascular and cerebrovascular events, nephrosclerosis, and progression to ESRD in renal patients. Nondipper BP patterns are more frequent in hypertension secondary to specific medical conditions, such as chronic renal failure, diabetes, and autonomic nervous system dysfunction, than in uncomplicated primary hypertension. Normalization of the circadian BP rhythm is considered to be an important clinical goal of pharmacotherapy because it may slow the advance of renal injury and avert ESRD.[66-68]

One of us[69] explored the relative advantage of evening vs. morning once-a-day treatment with a conventional sustained-release isradipine formulation on the nondipping 24-hour pattern of SBP and DBP in 16 chronic renal failure patients. Participants were randomized into two groups according to the order, morning at 8 A.M. vs. evening at 8 P.M., of the 4-week-long, 5-mg/day isradipine treatment regimen. The 24-hour pattern of BP was determined by ABPM before and after each treatment-time schedule. Both isradipine treatment schedules were equally effective in reducing the mean 24-hour BP. However, it was the 8 P.M. dosing schedule that best reduced and normalized nocturnal SBP and DBP.

The findings of this study demonstrate that in nondipping chronic renal failure patients, an evening, as compared with a morning, 5-mg/day sustained-release isradipine treatment schedule is more likely to effectively reduce the 24-hour mean SBP and DBP and restore the normal nocturnal dipping and circadian BP patterning.

### Low-Dose Aspirin Chronoprevention of Preeclampsia/Gestational Hypertension in High-Risk Pregnancy Patients

Several small investigations established that low-dose aspirin (acetylsalicylic acid [ASA]) is safe to use in pregnancy and suggested that it might reduce the risk of preeclampsia in high-risk pregnancies. However, several subsequent large randomized clinical trials, while documenting the safety of low-dose ASA use in pregnancy, were unable to corroborate its protective action against preeclampsia.[70] Review of the published studies revealed several potential methodologic flaws. Trials did not always involve high-risk obstetric patients; low-dose ASA intervention often was not initiated until late in pregnancy, not until 28 to 32 weeks' gestation; and nowhere in the published articles was the ingestion time of the daily ASA dose specified.

Hermida et al.[70] wondered if the time of drug ingestion might have significantly affected the outcome of the previous clinical trials. He and his colleagues conducted a prospective double-blind, randomized, controlled-trial of the administration-time–dependent differences in the protective effect of low-dose ASA initiated early in pregnancy. A total of 341 pregnant (181 primipara) normotensive women, at high risk of developing gestational hypertension and preeclampsia, were recruited. These medication-free women were

**Table 51–1** Administration Time Differences in BP-Lowering Effects of Various Antihypertensive Medications

| Medication (authors) | Dose (mg) | Dosing Times (conditions) | Subjects (no. and type) | Differential Rx Time Effect on 24 BP Pattern |
|---|---|---|---|---|
| Benazepril (Palatini et al., 1993)[86] | 10 | 9 A.M. vs. 9 P.M. (single dose) | 10 EH | 9 A.M. dose exerted greater BP-lowering effect. Duration of therapeutic effect shortened by 5 hours with 9 P.M. dosing. |
| Ramipril (Myburgh et al., 1995)[87] | 2.5 | 8 A.M. vs. 8 P.M. (4 weeks) | 33 EH | 8 P.M. dosing improved nocturnal BP-lowering effect. |
| Enalapril (Witte et al., 1993)[88] | 10 | 7 A.M. vs. 7 P.M. (single dose) | 8 EH | 7 A.M. dose significantly reduced daytime but not nighttime BP; 7 P.M. dose exerted stronger BP-lowering overnight and morning but had no effect on afternoon BP. |
| Quinapril (Palatini et al., 1992)[89] | 20 | 8 A.M. vs. 10 P.M. (4 weeks) | 18 EH | No dosing-time difference on daytime BP; 10 P.M. dosing reduced nocturnal BP more than 8 A.M. dosing. |
| Perindopril (Morgan et al, 1997)[90] | 4 | 9 A.M. vs. 9 P.M. (4 weeks) | 18 EH | 9 P.M. dosing markedly lowered BP (particularly SBP) during nocturnal sleep but was associated with ~33% shortening of SBP and DBP-lowering effect during the 24-hour dosing interval. |
| Captopril + HTZ (Middeke et al., 1991)[91] | 25/12.5 | 7–8 A.M. vs. 6–8 P.M. (3 weeks) | 13 EH | Evening dosing resulted in attenuation of daytime BP-lowering. Evening dose reduced BP during daytime (6 A.M.–6 P.M.) equal to that achieved by a q12h dosing schedule (equal to twice the dose/24 hours) of the combination medication. |
| Diltiazem Retard (Kohno et al., 1997)[92] | 100–200 | 8 A.M. vs. 7 P.M. (3 weeks) | 7 EH | 8 A.M. dosing better reduced BP during nighttime sleep; 8 P.M. dosing exerted greater daytime BP-lowering effect and inhibition of morning BP rise. |
| Isradipine (Portaluppi et al., 1995)[69] | 5 | 8 A.M. vs. 8 P.M. (4 weeks) | 16 RP | 8 P.M. dosing best lowered both day and nighttime BP and normalized the non-dipping circadian BP pattern of renal patients. |
| Cilnidipine (Kitahara et al., 2004)[93] | ~10 | Morning vs. bedtime | 13 EH | Bedtime, but not morning, dosing significantly reduced nocturnal SBP and DBP. Daytime BP lowering was not dosing-time dependent. |
| Valsartan (Hermida et al., 2003c)[94] | 160 | Morning vs. bedtime (3 months) | 90 EH | No dosing-time difference in reduction of 24-hour mean BP. Bedtime dosing best normalized nondipper BP patterns. |
| Doxazosin (Hermida et al., 2004)[95] | 4 | Morning vs. bedtime (3 months) | 91 EH | Morning dosing exerted little nocturnal BP-lowering and had only minor effect on 24-hour mean BP. Bedtime dosing exerted full 24-hour BP control and, compared with morning dosing, several-fold greater reduction in 24-hour mean BP. |
| Aspirin (Hermida et al., 2003a)[70] | 100 | Morning vs. afternoon vs. bedtime (~6 months) | 174 pregnant women at risk for preeclampsia and gestational hypertension | Bedtime, but not morning, dosing commencing ~12–16 weeks' gestation reduced the occurrence of preeclampsia, gestational hypertension, intrauterine-growth retardation, and preterm delivery. |

*Continued*

**Table 51–1** Administration Time Differences in BP-Lowering Effects of Various Antihypertensive Medications—cont'd

| Medication (authors) | Dose (mg) | Dosing Times (conditions) | Subjects (no. and type) | Differential Rx Time Effect on 24 BP Pattern |
|---|---|---|---|---|
| Aspirin (Hermida et al., 2003b)[71] | 100 | Awakening vs. bedtime (3 months) | 50 stage 1 EH | Morning dosing had little effect on BP, while bedtime dosing significantly reduced 24-hour mean SBP and DBP by 6 and 4 mm Hg, respectively. |

EH, essential hypertensive patients; RP, renal (nondialysis) hypertensive patients; BP, blood pressure; SBP, systolic blood pressure; DBP, diastolic blood pressure.

randomized to one of six different groups, each composed of 55 to 59 pregnant women, specific to the types of treatment: placebo or 100 mg ASA and the times of treatment: on awakening in the morning, 8 hours after awakening (lunch), or before going to bed. BP was assessed every 20 minutes between 7 A.M. and 11 P.M. and every 30 minutes overnight for 48 hours by ABPM first at the time of recruitment, between 12 to 16 weeks' gestation, and thereafter at 4-week intervals until delivery.

The BP-lowering effect of the low-dose ASA was nil and comparable with the placebo when ingested on awakening. In contrast, the daily ingestion of ASA in the early afternoon (8 hours after morning awakening) resulted in significantly lower average 24-hour mean SBP and DBP compared to placebo after the first month of dosing, with the difference between the two treatments at the time of the delivery amounting to decreases of 4.4 mm Hg for SBP and 3.5 mm Hg for DBP. The BP-lowering effect of ASA compared with placebo was strongest when it was dosed at bedtime; the effect of ASA on the 24-hour mean SBP and DBP was again apparent after the first month of treatment, with the difference between the two treatments at the time of delivery now amounting to decreases of 9.7 mm Hg for SBP and −6.5 mm Hg for DBP.

The protective effect of the low-dose ASA against preeclampsia, gestational hypertension, intrauterine growth retardation, and preterm birth varied dramatically according to its time of ingestion. The incidence of preeclampsia was roughly 12% on average in the placebo-treated groups. Morning low-dose ASA was not at all protective (15% incidence), whereas afternoon and bedtime dosing was very protective (1% incidence). Gestational hypertension occurred in nearly 30% of the placebo-treated women. Morning ASA dosing again exerted little protection (25% incidence), whereas afternoon (9% incidence) and bedtime (7% incidence) dosing did protect against gestational hypertension. Intrauterine growth retardation occurred in roughly 18% of the placebo-treated women. As before, morning ASA dosing exerted little protection (16% incidence), whereas afternoon (7% incidence) and, especially, bedtime (3% incidence) dosing did protect. Finally, the incidence of preterm birth was approximately 14% in the placebo-treated women. Morning low-dose ASA again was not protective (12% incidence), whereas afternoon (3% incidence) and, in particular, bedtime (0% incidence) dosing was protective.

## Morning vs. Evening Low-Dose Aspirin in Stage 1 Hypertension

Hermida et al.,[71] motivated by the findings of the ASA study of high-risk pregnancies, assessed the potential BP-lowering effect of conventional low-dose (100 mg/day) ASA tablet therapy in mild hypertension as a function of its ingestion time. A total of 170 (66 men and 104 women) stage 1 hypertensives were randomly divided into three groups. One group served as a control and was prescribed an exercise and diet regimen (EDR), a second group was prescribed the identical EDR plus 100 mg/day ASA on awakening, and a third group was prescribed the identical EDR plus 100 mg/day ASA at bedtime. BP was assessed by ABPM for 48 hours, both before and after 3 months of treatment. The 3-month EDR intervention in the control group had no BP-lowering effect. Moreover, EDR plus morning low-dose ASA treatment exerted but little BP-lowering effect; the average decrease in the 24-hour mean SBP and DSP amounted to only 2.2 and 1.1 mm Hg, respectively. In contrast, EDR plus bedtime low-dose ASA reduced BP significantly; the average decline in the 24-hour mean SBP and DBP amounted to 7.1 and 4.4 mm Hg, respectively.

The studies by Hermida and colleagues involving low-dose ASA clearly demonstrate just how important the ingestion time of medications can be in determining their therapeutic effects. In the case of low-dose ASA, the dosing time determined whether it was protective against gestational hypertension and preeclampsia in high-risk pregnancies and whether it exerted a meaningful BP-lowering effect in stage 1 hypertension.

## DISCUSSION

The concepts of chronopharmacology and chronotherapeutics are not new to clinical medicine. The chronotherapy of conventional tablet corticosteroid medications, daily or alternate-day morning prednisone and methylprednisolone dosing, was introduced in the United States in the 1960s[2] and is still extensively used today. In the 1980s, special drug-delivery technology made possible the chronotherapy of theophylline (Uniphyl, Purdue Pharma in the United States; Uniphyllin, Knapp in England/Munipharma in Germany; Euphylong, Byk Gulden in Germany) to achieve highest drug concentration during nighttime sleep to avert nocturnal asthma.[60] Knowledge of the circadian rhythms in symptom intensity of chronic diseases,[4] along with the chronopharmacology of medications, has been used to optimize conventional once-a-day $H_2$-receptor antagonists for peptic ulcer disease,[72] $H_1$-receptor antagonists for allergic rhinitis,[73] nonsteroid antiinflammatory drugs for rheumatoid arthritis and osteoarthritis,[74] cholesterol-lowering agents such as simvastatin,[75] and even cancer medications to lessen their toxicity and enhance therapeutic outcome.[76]

The chronotherapy of hypertension commenced in 1996 with the introduction of COER–verapamil. Three other chronotherapies of hypertension (a diltiazem calcium antagonist, a propranolol β-antagonist, and another verapamil calcium antagonist) have since been introduced in the United States. The common features of these four chronotherapies are bedtime dosing, reliance on unique drug-delivery technology to retard the dispersal of medication for approximately 4 to 5 hours following ingestion, graded or slow release of medication thereafter during a portion of the 24-hour dosing interval, and drug half-life that makes possible the progressive stepwise reduction of morning peak blood level in close synchrony with the expected circadian pattern of BP in essential hypertension. Improved BP control at the beginning of daily activity may also benefit from a more favorable concentration-response relationship in the morning as compared with other times of the day as exemplified by the β-antagonist medication propranolol.[77] Clinical trials show that the chronotherapies of hypertension are much more effective than most conventional medications in attenuating both the morning rate of rise and level of BP and are as effective as most conventional BP formulations in maintaining BP control throughout the remainder of the 24-hour dosing interval. Enhancement of morning BP-lowering is accomplished by incorporating a roughly 4- to 5-hour delay in drug-release following bedtime ingestion of the chronotherapy. The equivalent 15% to 20% of the 24-hour dose that would ordinarily circulate from continuous release once-a-day conventional formulations during this time span, when BP is typically lowest in essential hypertension, is redistributed by design to the morning when more aggressive antihypertensive therapy is required to manage expected peak or near-peak SBP and DBP. Clinical trials show that the four chronotherapies are well tolerated, perhaps better than the respective conventional formulations of the same dose when routinely ingested in the morning as recommended. The major side effect of the verapamil chronotherapies is dose-dependent constipation. Bradycardia and heart block with the verapamil and diltiazem chronotherapies are uncommon, even with the very highest dose of 540 mg/day. The low incidence of this side effect with these CCB dosage forms may be related to the purposeful reduction in drug concentration during the sleep span when heart rate and impulse conduction through the cardiac tissue are slowest.

The awareness by clinicians of the temporal variation in BP and potential role of its accelerated rise in the morning as a trigger of cardiovascular events has increased significantly in recent years.[40] Indeed, an unpublished 2002 Gallup poll of 200 American family practitioners (Biovail Pharmaceuticals, personal communication) found that 99% of them knew that BP varied during the 24 hours, and 97% believed the temporal variation resulted, at least to some degree, from circadian rhythms. The 2002 survey further revealed that the majority of doctors today believe that highest BP is achieved in the morning (55%) or afternoon (19%). The survey also found that 88% of the surveyed clinicians recommended that patients take their antihypertensive medications at a certain time of day. Most of those who gave such advice recommended their patients take antihypertensive medicines either immediately on awakening (22%) or sometime in the morning (46%). However, studies show that the dosing of many popular conventional once-a-day antihypertensive medications immediately on awakening or later during the morning is too late to optimally attenuate the peak or near-peak BP at this time of the day; this is especially true for medications with short half-lives that do not maintain therapeutic effects for the full 24 hours.[47]

Even though a majority of doctors recommend that their hypertensive patients take BP-lowering medications on awakening or later in the morning, the idea of dosing antihypertensive medicines at bedtime is gaining popularity with American clinicians. At the time of the 2002 Gallup poll, about 15% of the surveyed American family practitioners stated they recommended dosing antihypertensive agents at night, presumably even conventional slow-release once-a-day drugs. A separate yet unpublished pharmaceutical company-sponsored Gallup poll of 600 American hypertensive patients (Biovail Pharmaceuticals, personal communication) found that, although most people take their BP-lowering medications on awakening (19%) or sometime in the morning (64%), an appreciable proportion do so either at night (7%) or at bedtime (7%). The 18% of patients surveyed who took antihypertensive medications twice a day stated that they ingested their second dose of medication either in the afternoon (9%), in the evening (50%), or at bedtime (27%). Many doctors and patients are unaware that the effects of certain antihypertensive medications may differ significantly according to the (circadian) time they are ingested, as exemplified by the entries of Table 51–1 for ACEIs, CCBs, and angiotensin receptor antagonists. Even low-dose ASA shows dramatic administration-time–dependent differences in its effect on the 24-hour BP mean of stage 1 essential hypertensive patients, and the administration-time–dependent differences in the effect of low-dose of aspirin in the prevention of preeclampsia and gestational hypertension of at-risk pregnancies are even more dramatic.

Our knowledge of the therapeutic potency and safety of antihypertensive medications is derived from the conduct of clinical trials designed and sponsored by pharmaceutical companies. The goal of these trials is to demonstrate to governmental agencies that the therapy in question is effective and safe for the indication trialed and that it is suitable for marketing to consumers. The labeling instructions regarding the dose and timing of medications are based on the conditions and findings of such trials. Generally, once-a-day medications that are proven to be efficacious and safe are approved and labeled for the dosing time selected for the clinical trials. Unless a pharmaceutical company seeks and substantiates its claim for bedtime labeling, information about the efficacy and safety of the medication when taken at this time will be unknown. Adherence to the recommended time of day of dosing on the drug label is seldom appreciated by clinicians and patients as a crucial attribute of compliance.[59]

Only a very few conventional medications have been studied for their therapeutic impact and safety when dosed at different times of the day.[56,78,79] Knowledge of the extent to which the safety and therapeutic effect of the majority of conventional once-a-day antihypertensive medications are affected by ingestion (circadian) time is far too sparse to support any broadscale practice of bedtime dosing of the large number of BP-lowering formulations. In fact, nocturnal hypotension, perhaps aggravated by the dosing of certain antihypertensive medications at bedtime, increases the risk of ischemic ocular disorders in glaucoma patients[36] and perhaps nocturnal stroke.[37] Moreover, evening ingestion of certain β-adrenoceptor blocker medications, such as atenolol and propranolol, has been shown to attenuate or even abolish the nocturnal secretion of melatonin,[80-82] a key component of the circadian clock network. The consequence of a chronically attenuated or altered circadian rhythm of melatonin awaits clinical assessment.

Sander and Klingelhofer[83] using conventional medications showed that drug-induced normalization of the pathologic circadian BP profile of patients with hemodynamic brain infarction resulted in progressive recovery of the blood-brain barrier. In addition, several endpoint studies document that normalization of the nondipping circadian BP rhythm of hypertensive patients may slow the advance of renal injury and avert ESRD.[66-68] Numerous clinical trials of the marketed chronotherapies of hypertension clearly document their improved control of morning SBP and DBP without compromise of BP control throughout the remainder of the 24-hour dosing interval. Moreover, COER–verapamil and long-acting diltiazem, which are approved for the management of chronic stable angina pectoris, evidence enhanced control of coronary ischemia in the morning—when it is most common—without loss of effect during the remainder of the 24 hours.[41,42,55] Yet at present there are no data to substantiate the hypothesis that these special chronotherapeutic formulations are more effective than conventional ones in the prevention of cardiovascular events in at risk patients.

The first proposed large-scale assessment of verapamil chronotherapy was the 5-year international multicenter (Controlled Onset Verapamil INvestigation of Cardiovascular Endpoints: CONVINCE) trial involving 15,000 hypertensive patients with identified cardiovascular risk. This trial was designed to compare the degree of BP control and protection against cardiovascular events afforded by a regimen of conventional β-blocker and diuretic medications vs. the COER–verapamil chronotherapy.[84] This community-based outcomes study was terminated prematurely not because of inadequate performance of the chronotherapy, but because of financial and corporate considerations of the pharmaceutical company that acquired the rights to the medication. Because the trial was terminated early, there were far too few cardiovascular events to carry out a valid scientific assessment of the advantage, if any, of verapamil chronotherapy in hypertension.[85] Thus, the relative merit of chronotherapy vs. conventional therapy in preventing cardiovascular events remains unresolved. The great majority of doctors, pharmacists, and public health officials have misinterpreted the premature termination of the CONVINCE trial and lack of significant differences in cardiovascular events between the trialed medications as evidence against the utility of chronotherapeutics in hypertension. Obviously, well-designed future trials are required to gauge the merit of the chronotherapy of hypertension in reducing the risk of morning cardiovascular accidents and improving patient quality of life.

## References

1. Smolensky MH, Haus E. Circadian rhythms in clinical medicine with applications to hypertension. Am J Hypertens 9(part 2): 280S-290S, 2001.
2. Harter JG, Reddy WJ, Thorn GW. Studies on an intermittent corticosteroid dosage regimen. N Engl J Med 296:591-595, 1963.
3. Reinberg AE. The chronopharmacology of corticosteroids and ACTH. *In* Lemmer B (ed). Chronopharmacology. Cellular and Biochemical Interactions. Dekker, New York, 1989; pp 137-167.
4. Smolensky MH, Lamberg L. Body Clock Guide to Better Health. New York, Henry Holt, 2000.
5. Reppert SM, Weaver DR. Molecular analysis of mammalian circadian rhythms. Ann Rev Physiol 63:647-676, 2001.
6. Paul KN, Fukuhara C, Tosini G, et al. Transduction of light in the suprachiasmatic nucleus: Evidence for two different neurochemical cascades regulating the levels of per1 mRNA and pineal melatonin. Neuroscience 119:137-144, 2003.
7. Hastings MH, Reddy AB, Garabette M, et al. Expression of clock gene products in the suprachiasmatic nucleus in relation to circadian behavior. Novartis Found Symp 253:203-217, 2003.
8. Wever RA. The Circadian System of Man. Results of Experiments under Temporal Isolation. Heidelberg, Springer-Verlag, 1979.
9. Duffy JF, Kronauer RE, Czeisler CA. Phase-shifting human circadian rhythms: influence of sleep timing, social contact and light exposure. J Physiol 495(Pt1):289-297, 1996.
10. Golombek DA, Ferreyra GA, Agostino PV, et al. From light to genes: Moving the hands of the circadian clock. Front Biosc 8:S285-S289, 2003.
11. Khalsa SB, Jewett ME, Cajochen C, et al. A phase response curve to single light pulses in human subjects. J Physiol 549(Pt3): 945-952, 2003.
12. Parry B. Jet lag: Minimizing its effect with critically timed bright light and melatonin administration. J Mol Microbiol Biotechnol 4:463-466, 2002.
13. Klein KE, Wegmann HM. The effect of transmeridian and transequatorial air travel on psychological well being. *In* Scheving LE, Halberg F (eds). Chronobiology: Principles and Applications to Shifts in Schedules. Sijthoff and Noorddhoff, The Netherlands, NATO Advanced Study Institutes Series. Series D: Behavioral and Social Sciences, 1980; pp 339-352.
14. Knutsson A. Health disorders of shift workers. Occup Med 53:103-108, 2003.
15. Scherhammer ES, Laden F, Speizer FE, et al. Rotating night shifts and risk of breast cancer in women participating in the nurses' health study. J Natl Cancer Inst 93:1563-1568, 2002.
16. Schernhammer ES, Laden F, Speizer FE, et al. Night-shift work and risk of colorectal cancer in the nurses' health study. J Natl Cancer Inst 95:825-828, 2003.
17. Mormont MC, Waterhouse JM, Bleuzen P, et al. Marked 24-h rest/activity rhythms are associated with better quality of life, better response and longer survival in patients with metastatic colorectal cancer and good performance status. Clin Cancer Res 6:3038-3045, 2000.
18. Portaluppi F, Waterhouse J, Minors D. The rhythms of blood pressure in humans. Exogenous and endogenous components and implications for diagnosis and treatment. Ann NY Acad Sci 783:1-9, 1996.
19. Portaluppi F, Smolensky, MH. Circadian rhythm and environmental determinants of blood pressure regulation in normal and hypertensive conditions. *In* White WB (ed). Blood Pressure Monitoring in Cardiovascular Medicine and Therapeutics. Totowa, NJ, Humana Press, 2001; pp 79-138.
20. Verdecchia P, Porcellati C Schillaci G, et al. Ambulatory blood pressure: An independent predictor of prognosis in essential hypertension. Hypertension 24:793-801, 1994.
21. Portaluppi F, Manfredini R, Fersini C. From a static to a dynamic concept of risk: The circadian epidemiology of cardiovascular events. Chronobiol Int 16:33-49, 1999.
22. Deedwania PC, Nelson J. Pathophysiology of silent ischemia during daily life. Circulation 82:1296-1304, 1990.
23. Deedwania PC (ed). Circadian Rhythms of Cardiovascular Disorders. Armonk, NY, Futura Publishing, 1997.

24. Chasen C, Muller JE. Cardiovascular triggers and morning events. Blood Press Monit 3:35-42, 1998.

25. Cohen MC, Rohtla KM, Lavery CE, et al. Meta analysis of the morning excess of acute myocardial infarction and sudden cardiac death. Am J Cardiol 79:1512-1516, 1997.

26. Elliot W J. Circadian variation in the timing of stroke onset. A meta-analysis. Stroke 29:992-996, 1998.

27. Kario K, Pickering TG, Umeda Y, et al. Morning surge in blood pressure as a predictor of silent and clinical cerebrovascular disease in elderly hypertensives: a prospective study. Circulation 107:1401-1406, 2003.

28. Manfredini R, Gallerani M, Portaluppi F, et al. Chronobiological patterns of onset of acute cerebrovascular diseases. Thromb Res 88:451-463, 1997.

29. Casetta I, Granieri E Portaluppi F, et al. Circadian variability in hemorrhagic stroke. JAMA 287:1266-1267, 2002.

30. Mehta HR, Manfredini R, Hassan F, et al. Chronobiological patterns of acute aortic dissection. Circulation 106:1110-1115, 2002.

31. Manfredini R, Boari B, Portaluppi F. Morning surge in blood pressure as a predictor of silent and clinical cerebrovascular disease in elderly hypertensives (Letter). Circulation 108: E72-E73, 2003.

32. Verdecchia P, Schillaci G. Prognostic value of ambulatory blood pressure monitoring. *In* White WB (ed). Blood Pressure Monitoring in Cardiovascular Medicine and Therapeutics. Humana Press, Totowa, NJ, 2001; pp 191-218.

33. O'Brien E, Sheridan J, O'Malley K. Dippers and non-dippers (Letter). Lancet 2:397, 1988.

34. Staessen JA, Thijs L, Fagard R, O'Brien ET, et al., for Systolic Hypertension in Europe (Syst-Eur) trial investigators. Predicting cardiovascular risk using conventional vs. ambulatory blood pressure in older patients with systolic hypertension. JAMA 282:539-546, 1999.

35. Ohkubo T, Hozawa A, Yamaguchi J, et al. Prognostic significance of the nocturnal decline in blood pressure in individuals with and without high 24-h blood pressure: The Ohasama study. J Hypertens 20:2183-2189, 2002.

36. Hayeh SS, Zimmerman B, Podhajsky P, et al. Nocturnal arterial hypotension and its role in optic head nerve and ocular ischemic disorders. Am J Ophthalmol 117:603-624, 1994.

37. Kario K, Matsuo T, Kobayashi H, et al. Nocturnal fall of blood pressure and silent cerebrovascular damage in elderly patients: advanced silent cerebrovascular damage in extreme dippers. Hypertension 27:130-135, 1996.

38. Tinetti ME. Preventing falls in elderly persons. N Engl J Med 348:42-49, 2003.

39. Oliver D, Daly F, Martin FC, et al. Risk factors and risk assessment tools for falls in hospital in-patients: a systematic review. Age Ageing 33:122-130, 2004.

40. Smolensky MH. Knowledge and attitudes of American physicians and public about medical chronobiology and chronotherapeutics. Findings of two 1996 Gallup surveys. Chronobiol Int 15:377-394, 1998.

41. Cutler NR, Anders RJ, Jhee SS, et al. Placebo-controlled evaluation of three doses of a controlled-onset, extended-release formulation of verapamil in the treatment of stable angina pectoris. Am J Cardiol 75:1102-1106, 1995.

42. Frishman WH, Glasser S, Stone P, et al. Comparison of controlled-onset, extended-release verapamil with amlodipine and amlodipine plus atenolol on exercise performance and ambulatory ischemia with chronic stable angina pectoris. Am J Cardiol 83:507-514, 1999.

43. Gupta SK, Yih BM, Atkinson L, et al. The effect of food, time of dosing and body composition on the pharmacokinetics and pharmacodynamics of verapamil and norverapamil. J Clin Pharmacol 35:1083-1093, 1995.

44. White WB, Anders RJ, MacInyre JM, et al. Nocturnal dosing of a novel delivery system of verapamil for systemic hypertension. Am J Cardiol 76:375-380, 1995.

45. White W, Mehrotra D, Black HR, et al. Effects of controlled-onset extended-release verapamil on nocturnal blood pressure (dippers versus nondippers). Am J Cardiol 80:469-474, 1997.

46. White WB, Johnson MF, Black HR, et al. Effects of the chronotherapeutic delivery of verapamil on circadian blood pressure in African-American patients with hypertension. Ethn Dis 9:341-349, 1999.

47. White WB, Black HR, Weber M, et al. Comparison of effects of controlled onset extended release verapamil at bedtime and nifedipine gastrointestinal therapeutic system on arising on early morning blood pressure, heart rate, and heart rate-blood pressure product. Am J Cardiol 81:424-431, 1998.

48. Prisant LM, Devane JG, Butler J. A steady state evaluation of the bioavailability of chronotherapeutic oral drug absorption system verapamil PM after nighttime dosing versus immediate-acting verapamil dosed every eight hours. Am J Ther 7: 345-351, 2000.

49. Smith DHG, Neutel JM, Weber MA. A new chronotherapeutic oral drug absorption system for verapamil optimizes blood pressure control in the morning. Am J Hypertens 14: 14-19, 2001.

50. Prisant LM, Weber, M, Black HR. The role of circadian rhythm in cardiovascular function-Efficacy of a chronotherapeutic approach to controlling hypertension with Verelan PM (verapamil HCl). Today's Therapeutic Trends 21:201-213, 2003.

51. Prisant LM, Black HR, Messerli F, et al. CHRONO: A community-based hypertension trial of a chronotherapeutic formulation of verapamil. Am J Ther 9:476-483, 2002.

52. Sista S, Chi-Keung Lai, J, et al. Pharmacokinetics of a novel diltiazem HCL extended-release tablet formulation for evening administration. J Clin Pharmacol 43:1149-1157, 2003.

53. Glasser SP, Neutel JM, Gana TJ, et al. Efficacy and safety of a once daily graded-release diltiazem formulation in essential hypertension. Am J Hypertens 16:51-58, 2003.

54. Pool PE. Anomalies in the dosing of diltiazem. Clin Card 23: 18-23, 2000.

55. Glasser SP, Gana TJ, Pascual LG, et al. Efficacy and safety of a chronotherapeutic graded-release diltiazem hydrochloride formulation dosed at bedtime compared to placebo and to morning dosing in chronic stable pectoris (Abstract). Am J Hypertens 16:133A, 2003.

56. White WB, LaCourciere Y, Gana T, et al. The effects of graded-release diltiazem versus ramipril dosed at bedtime on the early morning blood pressure, heart rate and the rate-pressure product. Am Heart J 148:628-634, 2004.

57. Sica D, Frishman WH, Manowitz N. Pharmacokinetics of propranolol after single and multiple dosing with sustained released propranolol or propranolol CR (Innopran XL™), a new chronotherapeutic formulation. Heart Disease 5:176-181, 2003.

58. Smolensky MH. Chronobiology and chronotherapeutics: Applications to cardiovascular medicine. *In* Deedwania PC (ed). Circadian Rhythms of Cardiovascular Disorders. Armonk, NY, Futura Publishing, 1997; pp 173-206.

59. Smolensky MH. Compliance to prescription medications entails respect for treatment timing (Letter). Chronobiol Int 19: 502-505, 2002.

60. Smolensky MH, D'Alonzo GE. Progress in the chronotherapy of nocturnal asthma. *In* Redfern PH, Lemmer B (eds.) Physiology and Pharmacology of Biological Rhythms. Handbook of Experimental Pharmacology series, vol 125. Berlin-New York, Springer-Verlag, 1997; pp 205-249.

61. Lemmer B, Portaluppi F. Chronopharmacology of cardiovascular diseases. *In* Redfern P, Lemmer B (eds).

Physiology and Pharmacology of Biological Rhythms. Berlin-New York, Springer Verlag, 1997; pp 251-297.

62. Lemmer, B. Cardiovascular chronobiology and chronopharmacology. Importance of timing of dosing. *In* White WB (ed). Blood Pressure Monitoring in Cardiovascular Medicine and Therapeutics. Totowa, NJ, Humana Press, 2001; pp 255-271.

63. Bélanger PM, Bruguerolle B, Labrecque G. Rhythms in pharmacokinetics: Absorption, distribution, metabolism. *In* Redfern PH, Lemmer B (eds.) Physiology and Pharmacology of Biological Rhythms. Handbook of Experimental Pharmacology series, vol 125. Berlin-New York, Springer-Verlag, 1997; pp 177-204.

64. Labrecque G, Beauchamp D. Rhythms and pharmacokinetics. *In* Redfern P (ed). Chronotherapeutics. London, Pharmaceutical Press, 2003; pp 75-110.

65. Witte K, Lemmer B. Rhythms and pharmacodynamics. *In,* Redfern P (ed). Chronotherapeutics. London, Pharmaceutical Press, 2003; pp 111-126.

66. Timio M, Lolli S, Verdura C, et al. Circadian blood pressure changes in patients with chronic renal insufficiency: A prospective study. Ren Fail 15:231-237, 1993.

67. Bianchi S, Bigazzi R, Baldari G, et al. Diurnal variations of blood pressure and microalbuminuria in essential hypertension. Am J Hypertens 7:23-29, 1994.

68. Del Rosso G, Amoroso L, Santoferrara A, et al. Impaired blood pressure nocturnal decline and target organ damage in chronic renal failure (Abstract). J Hypertens 12(Suppl 3):S15, 1994.

69. Portaluppi F, Vergnani L, Manfredini R, et al. Time-dependent effect of isradipine on the nocturnal hypertension in chronic renal failure. Am J Hypertens 8:719-726, 1995.

70. Hermida RC, Ayala DE, Iglesias M. Administration time-dependent influence of aspirin on blood pressure in pregnant women. Hypertension 41(part 2):651-656, 2003.

71. Hermida RC, Ayala DE, Calvo C, et al. Administration time-dependent effects of aspirin on blood pressure in untreated hypertensive patients. Hypertension 41:1259-1267, 2003.

72. Moore JG, Merki H. Gastrointestinal tract. *In* Redfern PH, Lemmer B (eds). Physiology and Pharmacology of Biological Rhythms. Handbook of Experimental Pharmacology Series, vol 125. Berlin-New York, Springer-Verlag, 1997; pp 351-373.

73. Reinberg A. Chronopharmacology of $H_1$-receptor antagonists: Experimental and clinical aspects (allergic disease). *In* Redfern PH, Lemmer B (eds). Physiology and Pharmacology of Biological Rhythms. Handbook of Experimental Pharmacology Series, vol 125. Berlin-New York, Springer-Verlag, 1997; pp 589-606.

74. Labrecque G, Reinberg AE. Chronopharmacology of nonsteroid anti-inflammatory drugs. *In* Lemmer B (ed). Chronopharmacology: Cellular and Biochemical Interactions. New York, Dekker, 1989; pp 545-579.

75. Stalenhoef AF, Mol MJ, Stuyt PM. Efficacy and tolerability of simvastatin (MK-733). Am J Med 87(Suppl 4A):39S-43S, 1989.

76. Lévi F. From circadian rhythms to cancer chronotherapeutics. Chronobiol Int 19:1-19, 2002.

77. Langner B, Lemmer B. Circadian changes in the pharmacokinetics and cardiovascular effects of oral propranolol in healthy subjects. Eur J Clin Pharmacol 33:619-624, 1988.

78. Svensson P, de Faire U, Sleight P, et al. Comparative effects of ramipril on ambulatory and office blood pressure: A HOPE substudy. Hypertension 38:E28-E32, 2001.

79. Kario K, Schwartz JE, Pickering TG. Changes of nocturnal blood pressure dipping status in hypertensives by nighttime

80. dosing of α-adrenergic blocker, doxazosin. Hypertension 35:787-794, 2000.

80. Cowen PJ, Bevan JS, Gosden B, et al. Treatment with beta-adrenoceptor blockers reduces plasma melatonin concentration. Br J Clin Pharmacol 19:258-60, 1985.

81. Nathan PJ, Maguire KP, Burrows GD, et al. The effect of atenolol, a beta1-adrenergic antagonist, on nocturnal plasma plasma melatonin secretion: Evidence for a dose-response relationship in humans. J Pineal Res 23:131-135, 1997.

82. Stoschitzky K, Sakotnik K, Lercher P, et al. Influence of beta-blockers on melatonin release. Eur J Clin Pharmacol 55: 111-115, 1999.

83. Sander D, Klingelhofer J. Circadian blood pressure patterns in four cases with hemodynamic brain infarction and prolonged blood-brain barrier disturbance. Clin Neurol Neurosurg 95:221-229, 1993.

84. Black HR, Elliot WJ, Neaton JD, et al. Rationale and design for the Controlled ONset Verapamil INvestigation of Cardiovascular Endpoints (CONVINCE) trial. Control Clin Trials 117:603-624, 1998.

85. Black HR, Elliott WJ, Grandits G, et al., for Convince Research Group. Principle results of the Controlled Onset Verapamil Investigation of Cardiovascular Endpoints (CONVINCE) Trial. JAMA 289:2073-2087, 2003.

86. Palatini P, Mos L, Motolese M, et al. Effect of evening versus morning benazepril on 24-hour blood pressure: A comparative study with continuous intraarterial monitoring. Int J Clin Pharmacol Ther Toxicol 31:295-300, 1993.

87. Myburgh DP, Verho M, Botes JH, et al. 24-hr pressure control with ramipril: Comparison of once daily morning and evening administration. Curr Ther Res 56:1298-1306, 1995.

88. Witte K, Weissser K, Neubeck M, et al. Cardiovascular effects, pharmacokinetics, and converting enzyme inhibition of enalapril after morning versus evening administration. Clin Pharmacol Ther 54:177-186, 1993.

89. Palatini P, Racioppa A, Raule G, et al. Effect of timing of administration on the plasma ACE inhibitory activity and the antihypertensive effect of quinapril. Clin Pharmacol Ther 52:378-383, 1992.

90. Morgan T, Anderson A, Jones E. The effect on 24 h blood pressure of an angiotensin converting enzyme inhibitor (perindopril) administered in the morning or at night. J Hypertens 15:205-211, 1997.

91. Middeke M, Klüglich M, Holzgreve H. Chronopharmacology of captopril plus hydrochlorothiazide in hypertension: Morning versus evening dosing. Chronobiol Int 8:506-510, 1991.

92. Kohno I, Iwasaki H, Okutani M, et al. Administration-time-dependent effects of diltiazem on the 24-hour blood pressure profiles of essential hypertension patients. Chronobiol Int 14:71-84, 1997.

93. Kitahara Y, Saito F, Akao M, et al. Effect of morning and bedtime dosing with cilnidipine on blood pressure, heart rate, and sympathetic nervous activity in essential hypertensive patients. Cardiovasc Pharmacol 43:68-73, 2004.

94. Hermida RC, Calvo C, Ayala DE, et al. Administration time-dependent effects of valsartan on ambulatory blood pressure in hypertensive subjects. Hypertension 42:283-290, 2003.

95. Hermida RC, Calvo C, Ayala DE, et al. Administration-time-dependent effects of doxazosin GITS on ambulatory blood pressure in hypertension subjects. Chronobiol Int 21:277-296, 2004.

# SECTION 8

# Comorbid Conditions and Special Populations in Hypertension

## Chapter 52

## Diabetes Mellitus and the Cardiovascular Metabolic Syndrome: Reducing Cardiovascular and Renal Events

### Jay Lakkis, Matthew R. Weir

This chapter provides perspective about identifying and treating patients with diabetes mellitus and the cardiovascular metabolic syndrome. Most patients are diagnosed late in the course of disease, which creates substantial difficulties in managing their cardiovascular disease (CVD) burden. This often requires multiple medications and complex medical care requirements. We need better screening tests to recognize higher-risk patients sooner so that prevention strategies can be optimized. It is likely that this will be the most cost-effective approach.

Our chapter is laid out in three parts. First, we define the problem and address the epidemiologic factors that are involved. Next, we focus on risk stratification and look at the individual factors that contribute to total risk. We conclude with a section focused on strategies to curb cardiovascular and renal disease risks in these patients.

## DEFINITIONS

### Diabetes Mellitus

In January 2004, the Expert Committee on the Diagnosis and Classification of Diabetes Mellitus of the American Diabetes Association (ADA) published a set of practice recommendations, including criteria for the diagnosis of diabetes mellitus modified from those previously recommended by the World Health Organization (WHO) (Box 52–1). These revised criteria are symptoms of diabetes plus random plasma glucose (PG) concentration ≥200 mg/dl (classic symptoms of diabetes include polyuria, polydipsia, and unexplained weight loss); fasting plasma glucose (FPG) ≥110 mg/dl, with fasting defined

as no caloric intake for at least 8 hours; or 2-hour PG ≥200 mg/dl during an oral glucose tolerance test (OGTT) performed using a glucose load containing the equivalent of 75-g anhydrous glucose dissolved in water. The Committee did not recommend the OGTT for routine clinical use, however. In the absence of unequivocal hyperglycemia with acute metabolic decompensation, these criteria should be confirmed by repeat testing on a different day.

The Expert Committee also identified an intermediate group of persons whose glucose levels, although not meeting criteria for diabetes, are nevertheless too high to be considered altogether normal. This group is defined as having impaired fasting glucose with FPG levels ≥110 mg/dl but <126 mg/dl or impaired glucose tolerance with 2-hour values on OGTT of ≥140 mg/dl but <200 mg/dl.[1]

Type 1 diabetes comprises approximately 10% of all cases of diabetes and its hallmark is total dependence on exogenous insulin for survival. Type 2 diabetes comprises 90% of all people with diabetes and is characterized by insulinopenia and/or insulin resistance.

### The Metabolic Syndrome

The metabolic syndrome, originally described by Reaven in 1988 (see Chapter 13), refers to a clustering of several component disorders, at the center of which lay central obesity and insulin resistance. Two definitions have been proposed: one by the National Cholesterol Education Program's Third Report of the Expert Panel on the Detection, Evaluation and Treatment of High Blood Cholesterol in Adults (NCEP-ATP III) and another by the WHO (Table 52–1). The clinical spectrum of this syndrome has been defined by the NCEP-ATP III

**Box 52–1** Criteria for the Diagnosis of Diabetes Mellitus*

1. Symptoms of diabetes plus casual plasma glucose concentration ≥200 mg/dl (11.1 mmol/L). Casual is defined as any time of day without regard to time since last meal. The classic symptoms of diabetes include polyuria, polydipsia, and unexplained weight loss.

   *or*

2. FPG ≥126 mg/dl (7.0 mmol/L). Fasting is defined as no caloric intake for at least 8 hours.

   *or*

3. 2-hour postload glucose ≥200 mg/dl (11.1 mmol/L) during an OGTT. The test should be performed as described by WHO, using a glucose load containing the equivalent of 75-g anhydrous glucose dissolved in water.

Adapted with permission from Expert Committee on the Diagnosis and Classification of Diabetes Mellitus. American Diabetes Association: Clinical practice recommendations 2004. Diabetes Care 27:S5-S10, 2004.
*In the absence of unequivocal hyperglycemia, these criteria should be confirmed by repeat testing on a different day. The third measure (OGTT) is not recommended for routine clinical use.

to include abdominal obesity defined by a waist circumference >102 cm or 40 inches in men and >88 cm or 35 inches in women, androgenic dyslipidemia reflected by an elevated triglyceride level >150 mg/dl, small low-density lipoprotein (LDL) particles or low high-density lipoprotein (HDL) cholesterol level (<40 mg/dl in men and <50 mg/dl in women), raised blood pressure (BP) >130/85 mm Hg, insulin resistance with or without glucose intolerance or fasting blood sugar >110 mg/dl, and prothrombotic and proinflammatory states.[2] The WHO defines the metabolic syndrome as either

impaired glucose tolerance or diabetes or an FPG >110 mg/dl, hyperinsulinemia or insulin resistance plus at least two other components: hypertension defined by an arterial BP >140/90 mm Hg or the administration of antihypertensive drugs; dyslipidemia defined as a serum triglyceride >150 mg/dl or an HDL cholesterol <35 mg/dl in men or <39 mg/dl in women; abdominal central obesity defined by a waist:hip ratio >0.90 in men or >0.85 in women or a waist circumference >94 cm or 37 inches or a body mass index (BMI) >30 kg/m², or microalbuminuria >20 μg/min or an albumin:creatinine ratio >30 mg/g.[3]

This constellation of metabolic disorders makes the affected individual highly prone to develop CVD, including coronary heart disease (CHD), cerebrovascular disease, and peripheral vascular disease, and hence the nomenclature has been appropriately expanded to "the *cardiovascular* metabolic syndrome." In the NHANES III (Third National Health and Nutrition Examination Survey 1988-1994) data set, the cardiovascular metabolic syndrome has also been linked to an increased risk for both microalbuminuria and chronic kidney disease (CKD; estimated GFR <60 ml/min/1.73 m²).[4]

## EPIDEMIOLOGY

### Diabetes Mellitus

The prevalence of diabetes has been rising over the past few decades.[5,6] NHANES III (1988-1994) data from a subsample of 6587 adults, 20 years of age or older, for whom FPG values were obtained, and a subsample of 2844 adults between 40 and 74 years of age who received an OGTT, demonstrated that the prevalence of diagnosed diabetes was estimated to be 5.1% (10.2 million people). Using ADA criteria, the prevalence of undiagnosed diabetes (FPG ≥126 mg/dl) was 2.7% (5.4 million), and the prevalence of impaired fasting glucose (110-125

**Table 52–1** Clinical Identification of the Cardiovascular Metabolic Syndrome

| Risk Factor | Defining Level |
|---|---|
| Abdominal obesity* (waist circumference)† | |
| Men | >102 cm (>40 in) |
| Women | >88 cm (>35 in) |
| Triglycerides | ≥150 mg/dl |
| High-density lipoprotein cholesterol | |
| Men | <40 mg/dl |
| Women | <50 mg/dl |
| Blood pressure | ≥130/≥85 mm Hg |
| Fasting glucose | ≥110 mg/dl |

Adapted with permission from Expert Panel on Detection, Evaluation, and Treatment of High Blood Cholesterol in Adults. Executive Summary of the Third Report of The National Cholesterol Education Program (NCEP) Expert Panel on Detection, Evaluation, and Treatment of High Blood Cholesterol In Adults (Adult Treatment Panel III). JAMA 285(19):2486-2497, 2001.
*Overweight and obesity are associated with insulin resistance and the cardiovascular metabolic syndrome. However, the presence of abdominal obesity is more highly correlated with the metabolic risk factors than is an elevated body mass index (BMI). Therefore, the simple measure of waist circumference is recommended to identify the body weight component of the syndrome.
†Some male patients can develop multiple metabolic risk factors when the waist circumference is only marginally increased (e.g., 94-102 cm [37-40 inches]. Such patients may have strong genetic contribution to insulin resistance and they should benefit from changes in life habits, similarly to men with categorical increases in waist circumference.

mg/dl) was 6.9% (13.4 million). Based on ADA criteria, the prevalence of diabetes (diagnosed plus undiagnosed) in the total population 40 to 74 years of age increased from 8.9% in the period 1976-1980 to 12.3% by 1988-1994. A similar increase from 11.4% and 14.3% was found when WHO criteria were applied.[6]

The National Diabetes Clearing House estimates that 16.9 million or 8.6% of adults, 20 years of age or older, have diabetes, and the prevalence increases among adults, age 65 years or older, to 7 million or 20.1%.[7]

## Cardiovascular Metabolic Syndrome

Several analyses of data from the NHANES III data set provide insight into the magnitude of the problem presented by the cardiovascular metabolic syndrome. With the adoption of the NCEP-ATP III definition, analysis of data from 8814 men and women aged 20 years or older estimated the unadjusted and age-adjusted prevalences of the syndrome to be 21.8% and 23.7%, respectively. The syndrome was more prevalent among Mexican Americans (31.9%) and the prevalence seemed to increase proportionally with age. Prevalence of the cardiovascular metabolic syndrome increased from 6.7% among participants aged 20 through 29 years to 43.5% and 42.0% for participants aged 60 through 69 years and aged at least 70 years, respectively. Using 2000 census data, about 47 million U.S. residents have the cardiovascular metabolic syndrome.[8] Another analysis adopting the NCEP-ATP III definition evaluated 3305 Black, 3477 Mexican American, and 5581 white men and women aged 20 years and older and revealed a prevalence of 22.8% and 22.6% of U.S. men and women, respectively. Similarly, the age-specific prevalence was highest in Mexican Americans and lowest in Blacks of both sexes.[9] In a third analyses of data from 8608 participants aged 20 years or older, the age-adjusted prevalence overall was 23.9% using the NCEP-ATP III definition and 25.1% using the WHO definition. Estimates differed substantially for some subgroups; for example, in African American men, the WHO estimate was 24.9%, compared with the ATP III estimate of 16.5%.[10]

## Comorbid Conditions: Obesity and Overweight

The epidemic of obesity and overweight is one of the most alarming health disorders in the United States and the Western hemisphere today. Obesity and overweight may be assessed by BMI, waist circumference, or waist:hip ratio. The Clinical Guidelines on the Identification, Evaluation, and Treatment of Overweight and Obesity in Adults recommend that waist circumference be measured and compared with sex-specific cutoffs (>102 cm or 40 inches in men and >88 cm or 35 inches in women) in adults with a BMI between 25 and 34.9 kg/m².[11]

The prevalence of obesity and overweight was evaluated in the NHANES among 4115 adult men and women recruited in 1999 and 2000. The age-adjusted prevalence of obesity was 30.5% in NHANES compared with 22.9% in NHANES III (1988-1994); the prevalence of overweight also increased during this period from 55.9% to 64.5%, and extreme obesity (BMI ≥40) also increased from 2.9% to 4.7%. Such an increase occurred in both sexes, all age

groups, and all racial and ethnic groups. Among women, the prevalences of obesity and overweight were highest among non-Hispanic Black women, with more than half of those aged 40 years or older being obese and more than 80% overweight.[12]

## Comorbid Conditions: Hypertension

It has been estimated that 24% of the U.S. adult population, representing 43.186 million persons, had hypertension, based on NHANES III data (1988-1994) from 9901 participants 18 years of age and older.[13] The prevalence of hypertension is rising, as subsequent data showed an increase in age-adjusted hypertension prevalence among NHANES participants (1999-2000) to 28.7%.[14]

High BP is more prevalent in the diabetic population. In fact, 100% of diabetic patients that progress to end-stage renal disease (ESRD) are hypertensive; 55% of diabetics are not controlled to a goal of <140/90 mm Hg; and only 12% patients are controlled to <130/85.[15] Even fewer diabetics reach the ADA recommended goal of 130/80 mm Hg.[16]

## Comorbid Conditions: Dyslipidemia

Similarly, dyslipidemia tends to be more prevalent in the diabetic population and in patients with the cardiovascular metabolic syndrome.

## RISK STRATIFICATION

It should be emphasized that the presence of one of these components of the syndrome almost always puts the patient at a higher risk for clustering of the other components, the end result being that these disorders individually or interactively affect cardiovascular and renal outcomes. In fact, the risk of these disorders is additive if not synergistic. Based on this and on the evidence to be presented, it is essential that all affected patients, be it with diabetes mellitus or the cardiovascular metabolic syndrome, must be stratified in the highest risk category for cardiovascular and renal disease.

### Diabetes Mellitus, Impaired Glucose Tolerance, Hyperinsulinemia, and Insulin Resistance

Diabetes mellitus is an established independent risk factor for microvascular disease and macrovascular disease, namely CVD. The presence of diabetes mellitus or the cardiovascular metabolic syndrome in a patient enhances the risk of thrombotic events and atherosclerosis, especially in the coronary arteries, and is associated with endothelial dysfunction, both of which may contribute to myocardial ischemia. CVD is the leading cause of mortality in diabetic persons. A diabetic person has at least a twofold to fourfold higher risk for a cardiovascular event than an age-matched nondiabetic subject, and if he or she does have an event, will fare worse. CVD is ominous in this population for being premature, more extensive, and diffuse at time of diagnosis and carries a higher mortality and morbidity after a myocardial infarction (MI) than age-matched controls.[17] Consequently, diabetes is considered a CVD-equivalent.

However, a definite causal relationship between diabetes mellitus and macrovascular disease or CVD has not been fully elucidated in major clinical trials, that is, the Diabetes Control and Complications Trial (DCCT) and the United Kingdom Prospective Diabetes Study (UKPDS).

The ADA and the American College of Cardiology published a Consensus Development Conference Report, including indications for cardiac testing in diabetic subjects and choosing the most appropriate test to detect CVD in each individual patient (Figures 52–1 and 52–2). They added that the presence of autonomic cardiac dysfunction in a patient, aged more than 35 years, with diabetes for more than 25 years warrants cardiac testing.[17]

Hyperinsulinemia, often viewed as a surrogate of insulin resistance, is also an independent risk factor for CHD in patients with diabetes mellitus,[18-27] as well as an independent risk factor and predictor of the development of type 2 diabetes mellitus and hypertension.[18,21]

Similarly, diabetes mellitus (both type 1 and 2) is an established risk factor for microvascular complications, including renal disease.[28,29] In fact, diabetes mellitus is the major cause of ESRD in the United States.[30] The incidence of ESRD would increase at an even greater rate were not the competing hazards of CVD and stroke causing mortality in these patients. Furthermore, as mentioned earlier, the majority of patients with diabetes have hypertension as an important contributing factor to the progression of their kidney and heart disease.

## Obese or Overweight Patient

Insulin resistance, hyperinsulinemia, diabetes mellitus, hypertension, and dyslipidemia are all much more prevalent in persons with central obesity than in nonobese subjects. Obesity causes cardiac and vascular disease through hypertension, type 2 diabetes, and dyslipidemia; furthermore, obesity is an independent predictor of cardiovascular risk factors, morbidity, and mortality.[31-34] Other contributing factors to this increased risk may include mediators of chronic inflammation and hypercoagulation.

Obesity is a cause as well as a consequence of abnormal kidney function (see Chapter 44). In the obese patient, there is an increase in renal tubular sodium reabsorption, resulting in volume expansion, elevated arterial pressure, and a hypertensive shift of pressure natriuresis associated with activation of the renin-angiotensin and sympathetic nervous systems, as well as physical compression of the kidneys due to accumulation of intrarenal fat and extracellular matrix.[35] With time, glomerular hyperfiltration and increased arterial pressure increase glomerular capillary wall stress, which along with activation of neurohumoral systems and obesity-associated dyslipidemia and glucose intolerance, cause glomerular cell proliferation and matrix accumulation, with the end result of glomerulosclerosis and loss of nephron function in the early phases of obesity. This creates a slowly developing vicious cycle that requires additional increases in arterial pressure to maintain sodium balance and therefore makes effective antihypertensive therapy more difficult.[35] Elevated circulating leptin levels may play a role in the sympathetic activation. Elevation in leptin was also associated with impaired vascular function in healthy adolescents, independent of the metabolic and inflammatory disturbances associated with obesity.[36] In addition, obesity increases the risk of renal cancer and is a known cause of proteinuria, focal segmental glomerulosclerosis and occult diabetic nephropathy.[37]

## Hypertension

The Seventh Report of the Joint National Committee on Prevention, Detection, Evaluation, and Treatment of High Blood Pressure (JNC 7) recommends a goal BP in patients with diabetes mellitus or CKD of less than 130/80 mm Hg.[38] In the diabetic population, hypertension increases the risk and accelerates the progression of CHD, left ventricular hypertrophy (LVH), congestive heart failure (CHF), cerebrovascular disease, peripheral vascular disease, and kidney disease. Studies in animal models reveal that hyperinsulinemia and hyperleptinemia occur concurrently in obese subjects, and

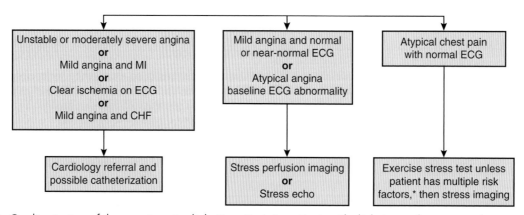

**Figure 52–1** Cardiac testing of the symptomatic diabetic patient. In patients with diabetes and symptoms that are either clearly related to ischemia or atypical in nature but suspected to be of cardiac origin, testing can be undertaken using this algorithm. *A multiple risk factor patient is defined as an individual with two or more risk factors. MI, myocardial infarction; ECG, electrocardiogram; CHF, congestive heart failure. (Adapted from Consensus Development Conference on the Diagnosis of Coronary Heart Disease in People with Diabetes: 10-11 February 1998, Miami, Florida. American Diabetes Association. Diabetes Care 21:1551-1559, 1998.)

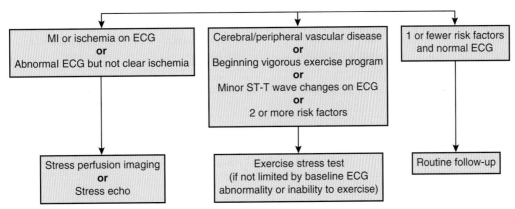

**Figure 52–2** Cardiac testing of the asymptomatic diabetic patient. Asymptomatic patients with diabetes and one or fewer risk factors and a normal ECG do not require cardiac testing. Patients with two or more risk factors or those beginning a vigorous exercise program should have an exercise stress test. In patients with clear or suggestive evidence of ischemia or myocardial infarction (MI) on ECG, stress perfusion imaging or stress echo should be used. If expertise with both modalities is available, perfusion imaging would be preferred. MI, myocardial infarction; ECG, electrocardiogram. (Adapted from Consensus Development Conference on the Diagnosis of Coronary Heart Disease in People with Diabetes: 10-11 February 1998, Miami, Florida. American Diabetes Association. Diabetes Care 21:1551-1559, 1998.)

both have been suggested to mediate increased BP associated with excess weight gain.[39]

There is a clear relationship between higher levels of BP and increased cardiovascular morbidity and mortality in the general population.[40-42] Epidemiologic studies demonstrate clearly that increasing systolic BP (SBP) and diastolic BP (DBP) correlate with increasing cardiovascular morbidity and mortality for the first 50 years of life with no evidence of any "threshold" below which lower levels were not associated with lower risks of stroke and of CHD. These results suggest that for the large majority of individuals, a lower BP should eventually confer a lower risk of vascular disease.[43] However, after 50 years of age, SBP is a more valid measure of cardiovascular risk; wider pulse pressure associated with higher SBP correlates well with cardiovascular morbidity and mortality[40-42] (see Chapters 3 and 22). Similarly, data from the Framingham Risk Study indicate that there is a graded relationship between BP and cardiovascular events, which extends below the traditional hypertensive threshold. Persons with SBP <120 mm Hg had fewer cardiovascular events than their counterparts with SBP of 120 to 129 or 130 to 139 mm Hg.[44] Although these are observational and not interventional studies, they do suggest that lower BP goals may be advantageous. This is likely the case in patients with more cardiovascular risk factors, such as diabetics.

Hypertension is both a cause and a consequence of renal disease. BP elevation is a strong independent risk factor for ESRD as has been shown by several trials.[45,46] Hypertension is the second most common cause of ESRD in the United States and the most common in the African American population.[30] In fact, results from the Multiple Risk Factor Intervention Trial (MRFIT) showed that the increase in risk for ESRD associated with higher BP was graded and continuous throughout the distribution of BP readings above the optimal level.[45] This raises some question about what are optimal BP goals in the diabetic. Schrier et al.[47] reported a 5-year prospective, randomized controlled trial of 480 "normotensive" type 2 diabetic patients. Compared with a group with mean BP controlled to 137/81 mm Hg, patients with intensive BP control of 128/75 mm Hg had not only slowed progression from normoalbuminuria to microalbuminuria, and microalbuminuria to overt albuminuria, but also decreased their risk for stroke and progression of retinopathy. In a study by Viberti et al.,[48] a modest 4/2–mm Hg reduction of BP with angiotensin-converting enzyme (ACE) inhibitor therapy in type 1 and type 2 diabetics with a baseline BP of 124/77 mm Hg resulted in a 50% reduction in progression from microalbuminuria to clinical proteinuria.[48,49]

## Microalbuminuria or Macroalbuminuria

Microalbuminuria is defined >30 mg but <300 mg albumin excreted per 24 hours (Table 52–2). The presence of microalbuminuria is the most important factor in predicting progression to macroalbuminuria or overt nephropathy in both type 1 and type 2 diabetics.[50-52] Microalbuminuria is also predictive of cardiovascular mortality in both diabetic and nondiabetic populations.[50,53-55]

To screen for microalbuminuria, a spot urine albumin:creatinine ratio is preferred due to its simplicity and reduced probability of collection error compared with timed urine specimens.[56-58] However, it should be noted that as a screening test, it is a poor predictor of quantitative albuminuria, and has a higher false-positive rate in older populations. Repetitive measurements (at least three) of first morning void urines provide a more accurate assessment. The ratio of albumin to creatinine in a spot or timed-urine collection can be helpful for quantifying 24-hour urine albumin excretion, because the creatinine output in the urine on a daily basis remains relatively constant.

Microalbuminuria may ultimately prove to be one of the most important risk factors for predicting cardiovascular events in both diabetic and nondiabetic patients. This has certainly been demonstrated to be the case in the Heart Outcomes Prevention Evaluation (HOPE) study (Figure 52–3).[59]

**Table 52–2** Definitions of Abnormalities in Albumin Excretion

| Category | Spot Specimen (mg/g creatinine) | 24-Hour Specimen (mg/24 hour) | Timed Collection (mg/min) |
|---|---|---|---|
| Normal | <30 | <30 | <20 |
| Microalbuminuria | 30-300 | 30-300 | 20-200 |
| Clinical albuminuria | >300 | >300 | >200 |

*Because of variability in urinary albumin excretion, two of three specimens collected over a 3- to 6-month period should be abnormal before considering a patient to have crossed these diagnostic thresholds. Exercise within 24 hours, infection, fever, congestive heart failure, marked hyperglycemia, marked hypertension, pyuria, and hematuria may elevate urinary albumin excretion over baseline values.

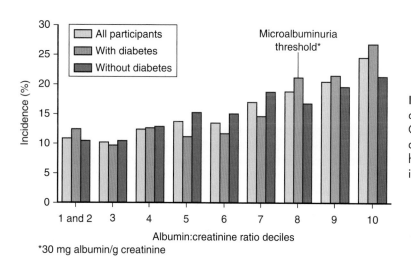

**Figure 52–3** Cardiovascular events by the degree of albuminuria in the HOPE study. (From Gerstein HC, Mann JF, Yi Q, et al. Albuminuria and risk of cardiovascular events, death, and heart failure in diabetic and nondiabetic individuals. JAMA 286:421-426, 2001.)

## Dyslipidemia

NCEP-ATP III recommends that diabetes mellitus should be considered a CHD risk equivalent, for risk factor management. The Expert Panel recommended the treatment of LDL cholesterol in patients with diabetes mellitus to levels <100 mg/dl.[2]

In type 2 diabetes, the most characteristic pattern of dyslipidemia is elevated triglycerides and decreased HDL cholesterol levels, although all lipoproteins have compositional abnormalities. Surprisingly few good prospective studies of lipoprotein levels in relation to CHD have been performed in diabetic subjects. Available observational studies suggest that low HDL cholesterol may be the most important risk factor for CHD. In studies in which total cholesterol and triglycerides were measured, both were risk factors for CHD, with triglycerides often a stronger predictor. The strength of triglycerides as a risk factor for CHD may depend partially on their association with other variables (e.g., hypertension and plasminogen activator inhibitor 1 [PAI-1]).[60]

Experimental evidence suggests that lipid abnormalities may contribute to the progression of kidney disease. In humans, there is limited clinical trial evidence for this hypothesis.[61]

## STRATEGIES TO REDUCE CARDIOVASCULAR RISK

Having established that all patients with diabetes mellitus or the cardiovascular metabolic syndrome are at highest risk for cardiovascular and renal events, it is imperative to devise preventive and therapeutic strategies to reduce such events and disease progression in this patient population.

### Nonpharmacologic Interventions: Dietary Modification

Dietary modification in the diabetic population should include reductions in carbohydrates, in salt for those with associated hypertension, and in fat for those with dyslipidemia.

### Nonpharmacologic Interventions: Physical Activity and Weight Loss

Over the past few decades, there have been trends in the general population towards more sedentary lifestyles. This has contributed to the epidemic of obesity and the cardiovascular metabolic syndrome. Initiation of a graded exercise program is highly recommended.[62,63] However, in diabetic patients, aged 35 years or older, who have been previously sedentary, it is recommended that cardiac testing be performed prior to initiation of a vigorous exercise program.[17]

## Nonpharmacologic Interventions: Tobacco Cessation

Tobacco use is an established independent risk factor for cardiovascular morbidity and mortality in all patients. Furthermore, there is evidence from several clinical trials of an enhanced risk for microvascular and macrovascular disease, as well as premature mortality from the combination of smoking and diabetes. Patients with diabetes should be continuously counseled about smoking cessation, the combined risks of smoking and diabetes for morbidity and mortality; and the proven efficacy and cost-effectiveness of cessation strategies.[64]

## Pharmacologic Interventions: Aspirin Therapy

Atherosclerosis and vascular thrombosis are major contributors to cardiovascular morbidity and mortality in patients with diabetes and the cardiovascular metabolic syndrome. Aspirin blocks the synthesis of thromboxane, a potent vasoconstrictor and platelet aggregant, by acetylating platelet cyclooxygenase. The Early Treatment Diabetic Retinopathy Study (ETDRS) proved the safety of aspirin use in the diabetic population.[65] The ADA published a Position Statement on Aspirin Use in Diabetes recommending enteric-coated aspirin in doses of 81 to 325 mg/day as a secondary prevention strategy in diabetics with evidence of large vessel disease, such as a history of MI, vascular bypass procedure, stroke or transient ischemic attack, peripheral vascular disease, claudication, or angina. Aspirin therapy should also be utilized for primary prevention in high-risk diabetic patients with a family history of CHD, cigarette smoking, hypertension, obesity defined by >120% desirable weight or a BMI >27.3 kg/m² in women or >27.8 kg/m² in men, microalbuminuria or macroalbuminuria, total cholesterol >200 mg/dl, LDL cholesterol ≥100 mg/dl, HDL cholesterol <45 mg/dl in men and <55 mg/dl in women, triglycerides >200 mg/dl, and age >30 years.[66,67]

## Pharmacologic Interventions: Glycemic Control

Atherosclerosis occurs earlier in people with diabetes than it does in those without elevated blood glucose levels. In the Diabetes Control and Complications Trial (DCCT), 1441 patients with type 1 diabetes were randomized to either standard or intensive care. Mean follow-up was 6.5 years. The intensive treatment group achieved a mean hemoglobin $A_{1c}$ ($HbA_{1c}$) of approximately 7%, whereas the standard care group maintained an approximate $HbA_{1c}$ of 9%. Improved glycemic control was associated with reduced cardiovascular events, but the difference was not statistically significant. However, this may be because the population studied consisted of young adults and therefore the event rate was very low.[28]

The UKPDS, which recruited 5102 patients with newly diagnosed type 2 diabetes between 1977 and 1991 and followed them for an average of 10 years, showed no increase in cardiovascular events or death with either insulin or sulfonylurea

drugs, despite the fact that both agents led to greater weight gain and higher plasma insulin levels than conventional treatment. The UKPDS showed strong associations between better blood glucose control and lower risk of CVD morbidity and mortality, but no statistically significant effect of lowering blood glucose on cardiovascular complications. There was a 16% reduction (not statistically significant, $p = .052$) in the risk of combined fatal or nonfatal MI and sudden death in the intensively treated group and a continuous association between the risk of cardiovascular complications and glycemia, such that for every percentage point decrease in $HbA_{1c}$, there was a 25% reduction in diabetes-related deaths, a 7% reduction in all-cause mortality, and an 18% reduction in combined fatal and nonfatal MI.[29]

In obese patients with diabetes mellitus type 2, the UKPDS has shown that initial single-agent intensive therapy with metformin results in a risk reduction of combined diabetes-related endpoints, diabetes-related deaths, all-cause deaths, and MI by about one third when compared with the conventionally treated patients. This risk reduction rate was statistically significant. Metformin was notably associated with an absence of weight gain.[68]

In the Diabetes Mellitus Insulin-Glucose Infusion Acute Myocardial Infarction (DIGAMI) study, 620 diabetic patients with acute MI were randomized to receive insulin-glucose infusion followed by multidose subcutaneous insulin for at least 3 months, and 314 to conventional therapy. After 1 year, the group that received insulin-glucose infusion followed by a multidose insulin regimen had a 29% reduction in mortality.[69]

In conclusion, both the DCCT and the UKPDS showed trends in reducing the risk of cardiovascular events with better glycemic control, but these trends were not statistically significant. Neither study proved definitively that intensive therapy, which lowered blood glucose levels, reduced the risk of cardiovascular complications compared with conventional therapy. Thus, the role of hyperglycemia in cardiovascular complications of diabetes is still unclear.

## Pharmacologic Interventions: Blood Pressure Control

The UKPDS showed that in the "tight blood pressure control group," lowering BP to a mean of 144/82 mm Hg significantly reduced stroke, diabetes-related death, and heart failure, and there was a continuous relationship between the risk of such outcomes and SBP (i.e., there was no evidence of a threshold for these complications above an SBP of 130 mm Hg). However, the risk reduction rate seen in MI (21%) was not statistically significant.[70]

The UKPDS also compared antihypertensive treatment with an ACE inhibitor to that with a β-blocker. Both drugs were equally effective in lowering BP, although patients on β-blockers had slightly better BP control (a 1–mm Hg systolic and 2–mm Hg diastolic improvement). Neither drug was superior to the other in any outcome measured, including diabetes-related death, MI, and all microvascular endpoints. Also, there were no significant differences in microalbuminuria or proteinuria ($p = .09$ for microalbuminuria to microalbuminuria for captopril vs. β-blocker). However, because of the low prevalence of nephropathy in the population studied, it is unclear whether there were sufficient events to observe a protective effect of either drug on the progression of nephropathy. We conclude that both drugs used to reduce BP are equally effective and safe, and that either can be used with great benefit to treat uncomplicated hypertension in patients with type 2 diabetes. Both conventionally and intensively treated blood glucose study patients had equal benefit from BP lowering. Likewise, the tightly and less tightly controlled BP study patients had equal benefit from blood glucose lowering.[71]

In the Captopril Prevention Project (CAPPP) subanalysis, captopril was found to be superior to a diuretic/β-blocker antihypertensive treatment regimen in preventing cardiovascular events in hypertensive diabetic patients.[72] Similar results have been observed in the Reduction of Endpoints in NIDDM with the Angiotensin II Antagonist Losartan (RENAAL) study, which included 1513 type 2 diabetic patients with early renal insufficiency and macroalbuminuria. Compared with placebo, the angiotensin receptor blocker (ARB) losartan was shown to reduce new onset CHF, with a statistically insignificant trend for reducing MI.[73] A meta-analysis of the data from the IRMA-2 (IRbesartan MicroAlbuminuria Type II Diabetes in Hypertensive Patients), IDNT (Irbesartan Diabetic Nephropathy Trial), and RENAAL trials demonstrated that ARB-based therapy provided a 15% risk reduction ($p = .03$) for cardiovascular events in type 2 diabetics compared with conventional antihypertensive therapy despite equal BP reduction.[74] Overall, these studies suggest that using a renin-angiotensin-aldosterone system (RAAS) blocking drug as part of an effective antihypertensive regimen in type 2 diabetics provides more cardiovascular risk reduction than a non-RAAS blocker–based medical regimen.

Using an ACE inhibitor or an ARB as part of the antihypertensive regimen clearly provides a distinct advantage for preventing progression of cardiovascular or renal disease, particularly in diabetics. However, it is important to remember that most patients will require multiple drugs for BP control, and that strong data support the use of thiazide diuretics to reduce cardiovascular events in diabetics in both the Systolic Hypertension in the Elderly Program (SHEP) and the Antihypertensive and Lipid-Lowering Treatment to Prevent Heart Attack Trial (ALLHAT).[75,76] The reality is, most diabetic hypertensive patients will likely require anywhere from two to five drugs to achieve a SBP goal of 130 mm Hg. Based on the clinical trial evidence, thiazide diuretics and a RAAS-blocking drug are indicated. Many patients will gain additional benefits from both β-blocker and calcium channel blocker (CCB) therapy to achieve lower BP goals. For example, when combined with an ACE inhibitor, the CCB amlodipine was shown to reduce BP, as well as morbidity and mortality, in diabetic hypertensives.[77] Moreover, the results of ALLHAT validated amlodipine as a useful drug to reduce CVD mortality and a safe antihypertensive drug. In addition, an analysis from the RENAAL study demonstrated that CCB therapy did not attenuate the risk reduction for renal disease progression associated with losartan.[78] In RENAAL, most patients taking CCBs were on a dihydropyridine.

## Pharmacologic Interventions: Microalbuminuria or Macroalbuminuria

Microalbuminuria is predictive of cardiovascular mortality in both diabetic and nondiabetic populations.[50,53-55] The presence of microalbuminuria indicates a widespread disturbance of endothelial function, resulting in an enhanced risk for the development of atherosclerosis.[79-82] It may thus serve as a useful biomarker for systemic vascular disease.

Once a patient is diagnosed with microalbuminuria, a lower BP goal should be considered because of the greater risk for cardiovascular events. Subgroup analyses of diabetics enrolled in major outcome trials indicate that more intensive control of BP, particularly SBP to <130 mm Hg with blockade of the RAAS as part of the regimen, provides the optimal strategy for both cardiovascular risk reduction[72,77] and preventing progression from microalbuminuria to macroalbuminuria, and from macroalbuminuria to overt nephropathy.[83]

Microalbuminuria is a very useful and important screening technique for CVD. It also indicates a need for more intensive BP control, <130/80 mm Hg, preferably including agents that block the RAAS. The presence of microalbuminuria indicates a need for more intensive cardiovascular risk reducing strategies, including attention to lipids, glucose, and platelet function. The ADA recommends yearly microalbuminuria screening for all diabetics. It may also be appropriate to recommend expansion of screening to include all patients in whom we suspect the cardiovascular metabolic syndrome.

## Pharmacologic Interventions: Correction of Dyslipidemia

In clinical trials that included diabetics, LDL reduction with statins has led to significant improvements in CHD incidence and cardiovascular and overall mortality. The Helsinki Heart Study recruited 4081 asymptomatic middle-aged men (40 to 55 years of age) with primary dyslipidemia and randomized them to gemfibrozil versus placebo. Gemfibrozil led to a 34% reduction in the incidence of CHD in all patients. Similar results were observed in the 135 diabetic participants in posthoc subgroup analysis, were not statistically significant perhaps, because of small sample size.[84,85] The Scandinavian Simvastatin Survival Study (4S) recruited 4444 patients with angina pectoris or previous MI, 202 of whom were diabetics, and randomized them to simvastatin or placebo. The statin was associated with a 42% reduction in cardiovascular mortality and a 30% reduction in overall mortality among all subjects.[86] Posthoc subgroup analyses showed a 55% reduction in major coronary events in diabetic subjects.[87] These results were reproduced in the Cholesterol and Recurrent Events Trial (CARE), which recruited 4159 patients with MI, 586 of whom were diabetic. Pravastatin resulted in a 24% reduction in CHD events in all patients, and posthoc subgroup analyses showed similar reduction rates in diabetics (25%) and nondiabetics (23%).[88,89]

The very positive results of statin trials point to LDL cholesterol as being a major predictor of CHD risk in diabetic patients. Therefore, the primary target of therapy in diabetic patients is lowering LDL cholesterol (and possibly, non-HDL cholesterol). Based on the aforementioned results, statins are the preferred pharmacologic agent in this situation. Reduction of LDL levels should take priority over reduction of triglycerides in combined hyperlipidemia because of the proven safety of the statin class of drugs, as well as greater reduction in CHD incidence. Once LDL cholesterol levels have been lowered, attention can be given to treatment of residual hypertriglyceridemia and low HDL.[60] However, it is still not known whether an LDL goal below the currently recommended 100 mg/dl, such as 70, 80, or 90 mg/dl will provide more cardiovascular risk reduction in the diabetic.

# STRATEGIES TO REDUCE KIDNEY DISEASE RISK

## Nonpharmacologic Interventions to Preserve Kidney Function in Diabetics

Lifestyle intervention should focus on dietary modification, including low-saturated fat and low-salt diets, weight reduction and increased physical activity, cessation of tobacco use, and moderation in alcohol consumption. Because the majority of patients with diabetes have hypertension, nonpharmacologic interventions to assist in the reduction of BP will help preserve kidney function.

Increasing salt intake attenuates the antihypertensive and antiproteinuric effects of ACE inhibitors and ARBs.[90] In hypertensive humans, high-salt intake increases glomerular filtration fraction.[91,92] In a diabetic rat model of renal insufficiency, salt restriction reduces hyperfiltration, renal enlargement, and albuminuria.[93] Thus, salt restriction should be encouraged in the hypertensive diabetic patient. Clinical trials need to assess the relationship of salt intake and risk for renal disease progression in diabetics to provide specific guidelines for optimal dietary approaches.

Moderate protein restriction has been shown to reduce albuminuria, progression of renal disease, and improve outcome in type 1 and type 2 diabetes. This benefit is described in addition to the beneficial effect of antihypertensive treatment.[94,95] A 4-year follow-up of 82 type 1 diabetic patients with macroalbuminuria suggested that patients on a low-protein diet (0.6 g/kg/day) had significantly slower ($p = .01$) progression to death, dialysis, or transplant compared with a usual protein diet group (1.02 g/kg/day).[96] Increasing protein in the diet causes glomerular capillary hypertension, which provides the rationale as to why lower protein intake is beneficial in reducing progression of renal disease in diabetics. However, the implementation of protein restriction in patients with kidney disease is controversial in part, because many patients with advanced kidney disease have poor nutrition. While theoretical reasons and some clinical data support the benefits of this intervention, this recommendation has not been uniformly accepted in the United States.

## Pharmacologic Interventions: Glycemic Control

Several major trials have shown that glycemic control preserves kidney function and delays the development of renal damage in diabetics. This, along with the fact that hypertension is far more prevalent in the diabetic population, highlight two major strategic interventions to preserve kidney function in these patients: strict glycemic control and optimal BP control.

In patients with type 2 diabetes, the UKPDS confirmed that improved blood glucose control reduces the risk of developing microvascular complications, including nephropathy. The overall microvascular complication rate decreased by 25% in patients receiving intensive therapy (median $HbA_{1c}$ 7.0%) versus conventional therapy (median $HbA_{1c}$ 7.9%). There was

a continuous relationship between the risk of microvascular complications and glycemia, such that for every percentage point decrease in $HbA_{1c}$, there was a 35% reduction in the risk of microvascular complications. There was no evidence of any glycemic threshold above a normal $HbA_{1c}$ level of 6.2%; therefore the results of the UKPDS mandate that treatment of type 2 diabetes include aggressive efforts to lower blood glucose levels as close to normal as possible.

## Pharmacologic Interventions: Blood Pressure Control

As mentioned earlier, JNC 7 recommends a goal BP in patients with diabetes mellitus of <130/80 mm Hg.[38] JNC 7 estimates that most patients with hypertension will require two or more antihypertensive medications to achieve this goal BP; if the BP is more than 20/10 mm Hg above goal, it is best to consider initiating therapy with two agents.[38] In fact, the average number of antihypertensive agents needed to achieve optimal BP control in patients with CKD is estimated at 2.6 to 4.3 agents.[97] Several clinical trials have supported the conclusion that the vast majority of hypertensive patients, even in the absence of diabetes, will need more than one antihypertensive medication to control their BP. In diabetic patients, there is evidence that the achievement of optimal BP is a major strategy to preserve renal function and delay the progression of renal disease.

The UKPDS showed that lowering BP by 10/5 mm Hg to a mean of 144/82 mm Hg significantly reduced microvascular complications that there was a reduction in the risk of microvascular outcomes compared with less aggressive treatment. They also noted that there was a continuous relationship between the risk of microvascular outcomes and SBP; that is, there was no evidence of a threshold for these complications above a SBP of 130 mm Hg.[70]

The choice of the appropriate antihypertensive agent for the individual patient should be based on an educated decision after evaluating evidence from controlled clinical trials. In the treatment of the diabetic patient, the antihypertensive regimen should include an ACE inhibitor or an ARB. Aldosterone receptor antagonists also might have a role but need to be studied in more detail.[98,99]

There are excellent clinical data demonstrating the advantage of lower BP goals in preventing renal disease progression in diabetics. A series of studies in microalbuminuric patients clearly provide evidence of the advantage of lower BP goals combined with RAAS blockade. Viberti et al.[48] studied 92 normotensive type 1 and type 2 diabetic patients whose mean BP before therapy was 124/77 mm Hg. After 2 years of follow-up, captopril-treated patients (BP reduction of 4/2 mm Hg) had significantly decreased progression to clinical proteinuria compared with a placebo group.[48] In another study, 94 patients with a mean pretreatment BP of 130/80 mm Hg were followed for 7 years. Patients on enalapril 10 mg had a 42% risk reduction for nephropathy compared with those taking a placebo.[100] Similar data have shown that ARB (irbesartan 300 mg) therapy provided a 70% risk reduction versus placebo for progression of microalbuminuria to clinical proteinuria in hypertensive type 2 diabetics.[101] Another trial in type 2 diabetics compared valsartan and amlodipine and demonstrated a BP-independent antimicroalbuminuric effect of the ARB.[102] In patients with clinical proteinuria the Collaborative Study

Group conducted the definitive trial demonstrating the advantage of the ACE inhibitor captopril in preventing ESRD in the type 1 diabetic.[103]

Studies with ARBs confirm the renoprotective effects of these drugs in patients with nephropathy associated with type 2 diabetes. The RENAAL study included 1513 type 2 diabetic patients with early renal insufficiency and macroalbuminuria. Compared with placebo, the ARB (losartan) was demonstrated to reduce proteinuria and ESRD.[73] RENAAL was the first trial to show that any therapy could significantly reduce the incidence of ESRD in type 2 diabetes (Figure 52–4). The IDNT trial also demonstrated the significant benefit of a multidrug regimen including irbesartan 300 mg compared with traditional multidrug therapy or an amlodipine-based regimen to reduce the composite endpoint of doubling of serum creatinine, ESRD, or death in 1715 patients with type 2 diabetes, clinical proteinuria, and early renal insufficiency (Figure 52–5).[103,104]

Because diabetic hypertensive patients often require multidrug regimens for adequate BP control, one needs to consider other therapies that are safe, well tolerated, and work well with the ACE inhibitor or ARB in reducing blood BP. Thiazides, or loop diuretics if there is renal insufficiency, facilitate the antihypertensive properties of the ACE inhibitor or ARB. Likewise, CCBs have demonstrated important and robust antihypertensive effects,[77] which make them useful adjuvant therapy in most diabetic hypertensives. β-Blockers are also useful adjuvants in the diabetic because of their important effects in reducing cardiovascular events, particularly in patients with angina, post-MI, and with systolic dysfunction.

Microalbuminuria is one of the most important factors in predicting progression to macroalbuminuria or overt nephropathy in both type 1 and type 2 diabetics.[50-52] Microalbuminuria indicates early renal damage, and the consequent need for more stringent BP control, preferably with drugs that block the RAAS, as these drugs provide both antihypertensive and antiproteinuric effects. Microalbuminuria is also an indicator of systemic vascular disease, as well as a risk factor for cardiovascular events. Consequently, once a patient is diagnosed with microalbuminuria, a lower BP goal should be applied, in addition to intensive control of glucose

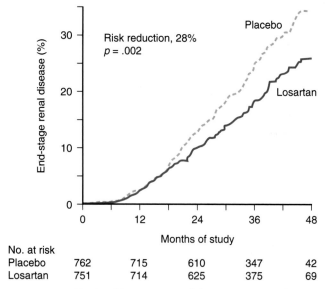

**Figure 52–4** Kaplan-Meier curves of the percentage of patients with end-stage renal disease (ESRD). (Adapted from Brenner BM, Cooper ME, de Zeeuw D, et al. Effects of losartan on renal and cardiovascular outcomes in patients with type 2 diabetes and nephropathy [RENAAL]. N Engl J Med 345:861-869, 2001.)

and lipids, with the ultimate goal being to prevent cardiovascular events. Normalization of urine microalbumin may serve as a clinical clue that optimal BP control is being achieved. This theoretical construct is based on evidence from clinical trials that reduction of microalbuminuria is associated with less likelihood for progression to macroalbuminuria and diminished risk for progression of kidney disease.

## Pharmacologic Interventions: Correction of Dyslipidemia

Bianchi et al.[61] conducted a prospective, controlled open-label study to evaluate the effects of 1-year treatment with atorvastatin versus no treatment on proteinuria and progression of

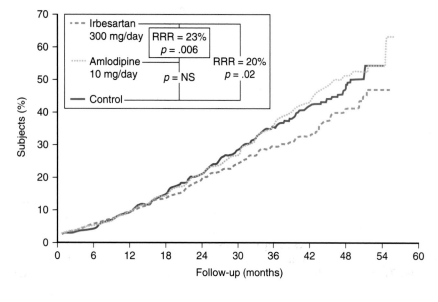

**Figure 52–5** IDNT primary endpoint: time to doubling of serum creatinine, end-stage renal disease (ESRD), or death. (From Lewis EJ, Hunsicker LG, Clarke WR, et al., for Collaborative Study Group. Renoprotective effect of the angiotensin-receptor antagonist irbesartan in patients with nephropathy due to type 2 diabetes. N Engl J Med 345:851-860, 2001.)

kidney disease in 56 patients with CKD. Before randomization, all patients had already been treated for 1 year with ACE inhibitors or ARBs and other antihypertensive drugs. By the end of 1 year of treatment, urine protein excretion decreased from 2.2 ± 0.1 g to 1.2 ± 1.0 g every 24 hours ($p$ <.01) in patients treated with atorvastatin in addition to ACE inhibitors or ARBs. By contrast, urinary protein excretion did not decrease significantly (from 2.0 ± 0.1 g to 1.8 ± 0.1 g every 24 hours, $p$ = not significant) in patients who did not receive atorvastatin in addition to an ACE inhibitor or ARB. During this time, creatinine clearance decreased only slightly and not significantly (from 51 ± 1.8 ml/min to 49.8 ± 1.7 ml/min) in patients treated with atorvastatin. By contrast, during the same period of observation, creatinine clearance decreased from 50 ± 1.9 to 44.2 ± 1.6 ml/min (p <.01) in patients who did not receive atorvastatin. The authors concluded that treatment with atorvastatin in addition to a regimen including ACE inhibitors or ARBs may reduce proteinuria and the rate of progression of kidney disease in patients with CKD, proteinuria, and hypercholesterolemia.[61] Although these patients were not all diabetic, it is likely that the benefit would be extrapolatable to diabetic populations. The same could be said for improving glycemic control, as a recent study comparing intensive versus less intensive strategies to control BP, lipids, and glucose by the Steno group demonstrated the benefit of intensive therapy on the development of nephropathy, autonomic neuropathy and cardiovascular death (Figure 52–6).[105]

## SUMMARY

The approach to the patient with diabetes mellitus or cardiovascular metabolic syndrome should combine early detection of comorbid risk factors and target organ damage, design of prevention strategies and lifestyle modification, and multitargeted pharmacologic interventions. This requires that all such patients should have their BMI, and waist circumference, and waist:hip ratio checked periodically. They should also be screened periodically for tobacco use, presence of high BP, dyslipidemia, and microalbuminuria or macroalbuminuria.

Prevention strategies should aim at a well-designed exercise program and weight loss to achieve a BMI <30 kg/m$^2$, a waist:hip ratio <0.90 in men and <0.85 in women, or a waist circumference <102 cm or 40 inches in men and <88 cm or 35 inches in women. Cardiac evaluation may be needed in diabetic patients 35 years or older who have been previously

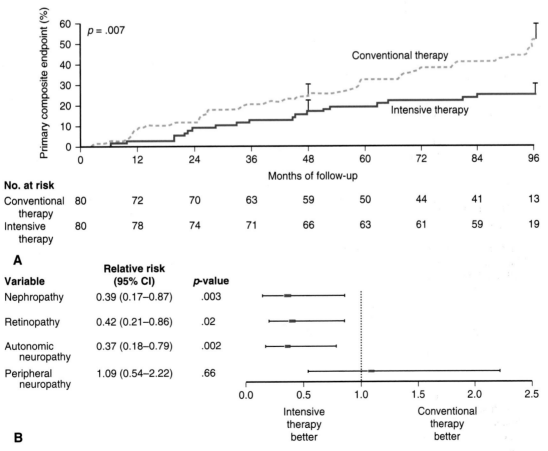

**Figure 52–6 (A),** Kaplan-Meier estimates of the composite endpoint of death from cardiovascular causes. **(B),** Relative risk for each variable based on type of therapy. (From Gaede P, Vedel P, Larsen N, et al. Multifactorial intervention and cardiovascular disease in patients with type 2 diabetes. N Engl J Med 348:383-393, 2003.)

sedentary. Dietary modification should aim at salt reduction in the hypertensive patient, low-carbohydrate diet in the diabetic patient, and low-fat diet in the dyslipidemic patient. Moderate protein reduction is also recommended. Alcohol consumption should be reduced to moderate levels or abstinence. Patients should be counseled at every clinic visit about tobacco cessation and all possible help should be offered to achieve it.

Pharmacologic interventions should include aspirin in doses of 81 to 325 mg/day. Glycemic control should target a goal $HbA_{1c}$ <7%. Metformin may be of added benefit in the obese patient when compared with other agents. BP control to a goal <130/80 mm Hg and normalization of microalbuminuria or macroalbuminuria with a multidrug regimen to include an ACE inhibitor in type 1 diabetics and an ARB in type 2 diabetics should be aggressively pursued. Dyslipidemia should be corrected; hydroxymethylglutaryl-coenzyme A reductase inhibitors (statins) may be used to achieve an LDL cholesterol level <100 mg/dl. Once LDL cholesterol levels is lowered to optimal levels, lowering non-LDL cholesterol to <130 mg/dl and lowering triglycerides to normal, and increasing HDL cholesterol level to >40 mg/dl in males and >45 mg/dl in women should be pursued. Fibrates may be a useful adjunct for the latter purposes, with special attention to the increased risk of myositis with these agents.

Diabetic patients will derive greater cardiovascular and renal risk reduction benefits from these approaches if they are initiated early. This will require multiple medications, good compliance, and a multidisciplinary effort.

## References

1. American Diabetes Association. clinical practice recommendations 2004. Diabetes Care 27:S1-143, 2004.
2. Executive Summary of The Third Report of The National Cholesterol Education Program (NCEP) Expert Panel on Detection, Evaluation, And Treatment of High Blood Cholesterol In Adults (Adult Treatment Panel III). JAMA 285:2486-2497, 2001.
3. World Health Organization. Definition, diagnosis, and classification of diabetes mellitus and its complications: Report of a WHO consultation: Part 1. Diagnosis and classification of diabetes mellitus. Geneva, World Health Organization, 1999. WHO, 2003.
4. Chen J, Muntner P, Hamm LL, et al. The metabolic syndrome and chronic kidney disease in US adults. Ann Intern Med 140:167-174, 2004.
5. Mokdad AH, Ford ES, Bowman BA, et al. The continuing increase of diabetes in the US. Diabetes Care 24:412, 2001.
6. Harris MI, Flegal KM, Cowie CC, et al. Prevalence of diabetes, impaired fasting glucose, and impaired glucose tolerance in US adults. The Third National Health and Nutrition Examination Survey, 1988-1994. Diabetes Care 21:518-524, 1998.
7. National Institute of Diabetes and Digestive and Kidney Diseases. National Kidney and Urologic Diseases Information Clearinghouse. Bethesda, MD, US Department of Health and Human Services, National Institutes of Health, NIH Publication No. 03-4572, July 2003.
8. Ford ES, Giles WH, Dietz WH. Prevalence of the metabolic syndrome among US adults: Findings from the third National Health and Nutrition Examination Survey. JAMA 287:356-359, 2002.
9. Park YW, Zhu S, Palaniappan L, et al. The metabolic syndrome: Prevalence and associated risk factor findings in the US population from the Third National Health and Nutrition Examination Survey, 1988-1994. Arch Intern Med 163:427-436, 2003.
10. Ford ES, Giles WH. A comparison of the prevalence of the metabolic syndrome using two proposed definitions. Diabetes Care 26:575-581, 2003.
11. Executive summary of the clinical guidelines on the identification, evaluation, and treatment of overweight and obesity in adults. Arch Intern Med 158:1855-1867, 1998.
12. Brown CD, Higgins M, Donato KA, et al. Body mass index and the prevalence of hypertension and dyslipidemia. Obes Res 8:605-619, 2000.
13. Burt VL, Whelton P, Roccella EJ, et al. Prevalence of hypertension in the US adult population: Results from the third National Health and Nutrition Examination Survey, 1988-1991. Hypertension 25:305-313, 1995.
14. Hajjar I, Kotchen TA. Trends in Prevalence, Awareness, Treatment, and Control of Hypertension in the United States, 1988-2000. JAMA 290:199-206, 2003.
15. Geiss LS, Rolka DB, Engelgau MM. Elevated blood pressure among US adults with diabetes, 1988-1994. Am J Prev Med 22:42-48, 2002.
16. Harris M. Health care and health status and outcomes for patients with type 2 diabetes. Diabetes Care 23:754-758, 2000.
17. Consensus Development Conference on the Diagnosis of Coronary Heart Disease in People with Diabetes: 10-11 February 1998, Miami, Florida. American Diabetes Association. Diabetes Care 21:1551-1559, 1998.
18. Zavaroni I, Bonini L, Gasparini P, et al. Hyperinsulinemia in a normal population as a predictor of non-insulin-dependent diabetes mellitus, hypertension, and coronary heart disease: The Barilla factory revisited. Metabolism 48:989-994, 1999.
19. Pyorala M, Miettinen H, Laakso M, et al. Hyperinsulinemia predicts coronary heart disease risk in healthy middle-aged men: The 22-year follow-up results of the Helsinki Policemen Study. Circulation 98:398-404, 1998.
20. Despres JP, Lamarche B, Mauriege P, et al. Hyperinsulinemia as an independent risk factor for ischemic heart disease. N Engl J Med 334:952-957, 1996.
21. Zavaroni I, Bonora E, Pagliara M, et al. Risk factors for coronary artery disease in healthy persons with hyperinsulinemia and normal glucose tolerance. N Engl J Med 320:702-706, 1989.
22. Strutton DR, Stang PE, Erbey JR, et al. Estimated coronary heart disease attributable to insulin resistance in populations with and without type 2 diabetes mellitus. Am J Manag Care 7:765-773, 2001.
23. Haffner SM, D'Agostino R Jr, Mykkanen L, et al. Insulin sensitivity in subjects with type 2 diabetes. Relationship to cardiovascular risk factors: The Insulin Resistance Atherosclerosis Study. Diabetes Care 22:562-568, 1999.
24. Abbasi F, Brown BW Jr, Lamendola C, et al. Relationship between obesity, insulin resistance, and coronary heart disease risk. J Am Coll Cardiol 40:937-943, 2002.
25. Golden SH, Folsom AR, Coresh J, et al. Risk factor groupings related to insulin resistance and their synergistic effects on subclinical atherosclerosis: The Atherosclerosis Risk in Communities Study. Diabetes 51:3069-3076, 2002.
26. Hanley AJ, Karter AJ, Festa A, et al. Factor analysis of metabolic syndrome using directly measured insulin sensitivity: The Insulin Resistance Atherosclerosis Study. Diabetes 51:2642-2647, 2002.
27. Howard G, O'Leary DH, Zaccaro D, et al. Insulin sensitivity and atherosclerosis. The Insulin Resistance Atherosclerosis Study (IRAS) Investigators. Circulation 93:1809-1817, 1996.
28. The effect of intensive treatment of diabetes on the development and progression of long-term complications in insulin-dependent diabetes mellitus. The Diabetes Control and Complications Trial Research Group. N Engl J Med 329:977-986, 1993.

29. Intensive blood-glucose control with sulphonylureas or insulin compared with conventional treatment and risk of complications in patients with type 2 diabetes (UKPDS 33). UK Prospective Diabetes Study (UKPDS) Group. Lancet 352: 837-853, 1998. Erratum in Lancet 354(9178):602, 1999.

30. US Renal Data System. USRDS 2002 Annual Data Report. Bethesda, MD, The National Institutes of Health, National Institute of Diabetes and Digestive and Kidney Diseases, 2002.

31. Katzmarzyk PT, Craig CL, Bouchard C. Underweight, overweight and obesity: Relationships with mortality in the 13-year follow-up of the Canada Fitness Survey. J Clin Epidemiol 54:916-920, 2001.

32. Seidell JC, Visscher TL, Hoogeveen RT. Overweight and obesity in the mortality rate data: Current evidence and research issues. Med Sci Sports Exerc 31:S597-S601, 1999.

33. Calle EE, Thun MJ, Petrelli JM, et al. Body-mass index and mortality in a prospective cohort of US adults. N Engl J Med 341:1097-1105, 1999.

34. Stevens J, Cai J, Pamuk ER, et al. The effect of age on the association between body-mass index and mortality. N Engl J Med 338:1-7, 1998.

35. Hall JE, Brands MW, Henegar JR. Mechanisms of hypertension and kidney disease in obesity. Ann NY Acad Sci 892:91-107, 1999.

36. Singhal A, Farooqi IS, Cole TJ, et al. Influence of leptin on arterial distensibility: A novel link between obesity and cardiovascular disease? Circulation 106:1919-1924, 2002.

37. Kasiske BL, Crosson JT. Renal disease in patients with massive obesity. Arch Intern Med 146:1105-1109, 1986.

38. Chobanian AV, Bakris GL, Black HR, et al. The Seventh Report of the Joint National Committee on Prevention, Detection, Evaluation, and Treatment of High Blood Pressure: The JNC 7 report. JAMA 289:2560-2572, 2003.

39. Kuo JJ, Jones OB, Hall JE. Chronic cardiovascular and renal actions of leptin during hyperinsulinemia. Am J Physiol Regul Integr Comp Physiol 284:R1037-R1042, 2003.

40. Franklin S, Gustin W, Wong N, et al. Hemodynamic patterns of age-related changes in blood pressure: The Framingham Heart Study. Circulation 96:308-315, 1997.

41. Franklin S, Shehzad A, Khan B, et al. Is pulse pressure useful in predicting risk for coronary heart disease? The Framingham Heart Study. Circulation 100:354-360, 1999.

42. National High Blood Pressure Education Program Working Group. National High Blood Pressure Education Program Working Group Report on Hypertension in the Elderly. Hypertension 23:275-285, 1994.

43. Lewington S, Clarke R, Qizilbash N, et al. Age-specific relevance of usual blood pressure to vascular mortality: A meta-analysis of individual data for one million adults in 61 prospective studies. Lancet 360:1903-1913, 2002.

44. Vasan R, Larson M, Leip E, et al. Impact of high-normal blood pressure on the risk for cardiovascular disease. N Engl J Med 345:1291-1297, 2001.

45. Klag MJ, Whelton PK, Randall BL, et al. Blood pressure and end-stage renal disease in men. N Engl J Med 334:13-18, 1996.

46. Hunsicker LG, Adler S, Caggiula A, et al. Predictors of the progression of renal disease in the Modification of Diet in Renal Disease Study. Kidney Int 51:1908-1919, 1997.

47. Schrier R, Estacio R, Esler A, et al. Effect of aggressive blood pressure control in normotensive type 2 diabetic patients on albuminuria, retinopathy and strokes. Kidney Int 61: 1086-1097, 2002.

48. Viberti G, Mogensen C, Groop L, et al.; European Microalbuminuria Captopril Study Group. Effect of captopril on progression to clinical proteinuria in patients with insulin-dependent diabetes mellitus and microalbuminuria. JAMA 271:275-279, 1994.

49. O'Hare P, Bilbous R, Mitchell T, et al., for the ACE-Inhibitor Trial to Lower Albuminuria in Normotensive Insulin-Dependent Subjects Study group. Low-dose ramipril reduces microalbuminuria in type 1 diabetic patients without hypertension: Results of a randomized controlled trial. Diabetes Care 23: 1823-1829, 2000.

50. Mogensen C. Microalbuminuria predicts clinical proteinuria and early mortality in maturity-onset diabetes. N Engl J Med 310:356-360, 1984.

51. Mogensen C, Keane W, Bennett P, et al. Prevention of diabetic renal disease with special reference to microalbuminuria. Lancet 346:1080-1084, 1995.

52. Mogensen C. Diabetic nephropathy: Natural history and management. In Meguid El Nahas A, Harris KPG, Anderson S (eds). Mechanisms and Clinical Management of Chronic Renal Failure, 2nd ed. New York, Oxford University Press, 2000; pp 211-240.

53. Ruggenenti P, Remuzzi G. Nephropathy of type 2 diabetes mellitus. J Am Soc Nephrol 9:2157-2169, 1998.

54. Agrawal B, Berger A, Wolf K, et al. Microalbuminuria screening by reagent predicts cardiovascular risk in hypertension. J Hypertens 14:223-228, 1996.

55. Mann J, Gerstein H, Pogue J, et al. Renal insufficiency as predictor of cardiovascular outcomes and impact of ramipril: The HOPE randomization trial. Ann Intern Med 134:629-636, 2001.

56. Connel S, Hollis S, Tieszen K, et al. Gender and the clinical usefulness of the albumin creatinine ratio. Diabet Med 11:32-36, 1994.

57. Houlihan C, Tsalamandris C, Akdeniz A, et al. Albumin to creatinine ratio: A screening test with limitations. Am J Kidney Dis 39:1183-1189, 2002.

58. Keane W, Eknoyan G. Proteinuria, albuminuria, risk, assessment, detection, elimination (PARADE): A position paper of the National Kidney Foundation. Am J Kidney Dis 33:1004-1010, 1999.

59. Gerstein HC, Mann JF, Yi Q, et al. Albuminuria and risk of cardiovascular events, death, and heart failure in diabetic and non-diabetic individuals. JAMA 286:421-426, 2001.

60. Haffner SM. Management of dyslipidemia in adults with diabetes. Diabetes Care 21:160-178, 1998.

61. Bianchi S, Bigazzi R, Caiazza A, et al. A controlled, prospective study of the effects of atorvastatin on proteinuria and progression of kidney disease. Am J Kidney Dis 41:565-570, 2003.

62. Wasserman DH, Zinman B. Exercise in individuals with IDDM. Diabetes Care 17:924-937, 1994.

63. Exercise and NIDDM. Diabetes Care 13:785-789, 1990.

64. Haire-Joshu D, Glasgow RE, Tibbs TL. Smoking and diabetes. Diabetes Care 22:1887-1898, 1999.

65. Aspirin effects on mortality and morbidity in patients with diabetes mellitus. Early Treatment Diabetic Retinopathy Study report 14. ETDRS Investigators. JAMA 268:1292-1300, 1992.

66. Colwell JA. Aspirin therapy in diabetes. Diabetes Care 26S87-S88, 2003.

67. Colwell JA. Aspirin therapy in diabetes. Diabetes Care 20: 1767-1771, 1997.

68. Effect of intensive blood-glucose control with metformin on complications in overweight patients with type 2 diabetes (UKPDS 34). UK Prospective Diabetes Study (UKPDS) Group. Lancet 352:854-865, 1998.

69. Malmberg K, Ryden L, Efendic S, et al. Randomized trial of insulin-glucose infusion followed by subcutaneous insulin treatment in diabetic patients with acute myocardial infarction (DIGAMI study): Effects on mortality at 1 year. J Am Coll Cardiol 26:57-65, 1995.

70. Tight blood pressure control and risk of macrovascular and microvascular complications in type 2 diabetes: UKPDS 38. UK Prospective Diabetes Study Group. BMJ 317:703-713, 1998.

71. Efficacy of atenolol and captopril in reducing risk of macrovascular and microvascular complications in type 2 diabetes: UKPDS 39. UK Prospective Diabetes Study Group. BMJ 317:713-720, 1998.

72. Niskanen L, Hedner T, Hansson L, et al. Reduced cardiovascular morbidity and mortality in hypertensive diabetic patients on first-line therapy with an ACE inhibitor compared with a diuretic/beta-blocker-based treatment regimen: A subanalysis of the Captopril Prevention Project. Diabetes Care 24: 2091-2096, 2001.

73. Brenner BM, Cooper ME, de Zeeuw D, et al. Effects of losartan on renal and cardiovascular outcomes in patients with type 2 diabetes and nephropathy (RENAAL). N Engl J Med 345:861-869, 2001.

74. Pourdjabbar A, Lapointe N, Rouleau J. Angiotensin receptor blockers: Powerful evidence with cardiovascular outcomes? Can J Cardiol 18:7A-14A, 2002.

75. Tuomilehto J, Rastenyte D, Birkenhager WH, et al., for Systolic Hypertension in Europe Trial Investigators. Effects of calcium-channel blockade in older patients with diabetes and systolic hypertension. N Engl J Med 340:766-684, 1999.

76. ALLHAT Collaborative Research Group. Major outcomes in high-risk hypertensive patients randomized to angiotensin-converting enzyme inhibitor or calcium channel blocker vs diuretic: The Antihypertensive and Lipid-Lowering Treatment to Prevent Heart Attack Trial (ALLHAT). JAMA 288:2981-2997, 2002.

77. Tatti P, Pahor M, Byington R, et al. Outcome results of the Fosinopril versus Amlodipine cardiovascular events trial (FACET) in patients with hypertension and NIDDM. Diabetes Care 21:597-603, 1998.

78. Bakris GL, Weir MR, Shanifar S, et al. Effects of blood pressure level on progression of diabetic nephropathy: Results from the RENAAL study. Arch Intern Med 163:1555-1565, 2003.

79. Schiffrin E. Beyond blood pressure: The endothelium and atherosclerosis progression. Am J Hypertens 15:S115, 2002.

80. Deckert T. Nephropathy and coronary death—the fatal twins in diabetes mellitus. Nephrol Dial Transplant 9:1069-1071, 1994.

81. Parving H, Nielsen F, Bang L, et al. Endothelial dysfunction in NIDDM patients with and without nephropathy (Abstract). J Am Soc Nephrol 5:380, 1994.

82. Ruilope L, Rodicio J. Microalbuminuria in clinical practice: A current survey of world literature. Kidney Int 4:211-216, 1995.

83. Effects of ramipril on cardiovascular and microvascular outcomes in people with diabetes mellitus: Results of the HOPE study and MICRO-HOPE substudy. Heart Outcomes Prevention Evaluation Study Investigators. Lancet 355:253-259, 2000. Erratum in Lancet 356(9232):860, 2000.

84. Frick MH, Elo O, Haapa K, et al. Helsinki Heart Study: Primary-prevention trial with gemfibrozil in middle-aged men with dyslipidemia. Safety of treatment, changes in risk factors, and incidence of coronary heart disease. N Engl J Med 317:1237-1245, 1987.

85. Koskinen P, Manttari M, Manninen V, et al. Coronary heart disease incidence in NIDDM patients in the Helsinki Heart Study. Diabetes Care 15:820-825, 1992.

86. Randomised trial of cholesterol lowering in 4444 patients with coronary heart disease: The Scandinavian Simvastatin Survival Study (4S). Lancet 344:1383-1389, 1994.

87. Pyorala K, Pedersen TR, Kjekshus J, et al. Cholesterol lowering with simvastatin improves prognosis of diabetic patients with coronary heart disease. A subgroup analysis of the Scandinavian Simvastatin Survival Study (4S). Diabetes Care 20:614-620, 1997.

88. Goldberg RB, Mellies MJ, Sacks FM, et al. Cardiovascular events and their reduction with pravastatin in diabetic and glucose-intolerant myocardial infarction survivors with average cholesterol levels: Subgroup analyses in the cholesterol and recurrent events (CARE) trial. The Care Investigators. Circulation 98:2513-2519, 1998.

89. Sacks FM, Pfeffer MA, Moye LA, et al. The effect of pravastatin on coronary events after myocardial infarction in patients with average cholesterol levels. Cholesterol and Recurrent Events Trial investigators. N Engl J Med 335: 1001-1009, 1996.

90. Heeg J, de Jong P, van der Hem G, et al. Efficacy and variability of the antiproteinuric effect of ACE inhibition by lisinopril. Kidney Int 36:272-279, 1989.

91. Mallamaci F, Leonardis D, Bellizzi V, et al. Does high salt intake cause hyperfiltration in patients with essential hypertension? J Hum Hypertens 10:157-161, 1996.

92. Weir MR, Dengel DR, Behrens MT, et al. Salt-induced increases in systolic blood pressure affect renal hemodynamics and proteinuria. Hypertension 25:1339-1344, 1995.

93. Allen T, Waldron M, Casley D, et al. Salt restriction reduces hyperfiltration, renal enlargement, and albuminuria in experimental diabetes. Diabetes 46:19-24, 1997.

94. Walker J, Bending J, Dodds R, et al. Restriction of dietary protein and progression of renal failure in diabetic nephropathy. Lancet 16:1411-1415, 1989.

95. Pedrini M, Levey A, Lau J, et al. The effect of dietary protein restriction on the progression of diabetic and nondiabetic renal diseases: A meta-analysis. Ann Intern Med 124:627-632, 1996.

96. Hansen H, Tauber-Lassen E, Jensen B, et al. Effect of dietary protein restriction on prognosis in patients with diabetic nephropathy. Kidney Int 62:220-228, 2002.

97. Bakris GL. Maximizing cardiorenal benefit in the management of hypertension: Achieve blood pressure goals. J Clin Hypertens (Greenwich) 1:141-147, 1999.

98. Sato A, Hayashi K, Naruse M, et al. Effectiveness of aldosterone blockade in patients with diabetic nephropathy. Hypertension 41:64-68, 2003.

99. Epstein M, Buckalew V, Martinez F, et al. Antiproteinuric efficacy of eplerenone, enalapril, and eplerenone/enalapril combination in diabetic hypertensives with microalbuminuria (Abstract). Am J Hypertens 15:24A, 2002.

100. Ravid M, Savin H, Jutrin I, et al. Long-term stabilizing effect of angiotensin-converting enzyme inhibition on plasma creatinine and on proteinuria in normotensive type II diabetic patients. Ann Intern Med 118:577-581, 1993.

101. Parving HH, Lehnert H, Brochner-Mortensen J, et al. The effect of irbesartan on the development of diabetic nephropathy in patients with type 2 diabetes. Irbesartan Microalbuminuria Type II Diabetes in Hypertensive Patients (IRMA 2). N Engl J Med 345:870-878, 2001.

102. Viberti G, Wheeldon N; MicroAlbuminuria Reduction with VALsartan (MARVAL) Study Investigators. Microalbuminuria reduction with valsartan in patients with type 2 diabetes mellitus: A blood pressure-independent effect. Circulation 106: 672-678, 2002.

103. Lewis EJ, Hunsicker LG, Clarke WR, et al.; Collaborative Study Group. Renoprotective effect of the angiotensin-receptor antagonist irbesartan in patients with nephropathy due to type 2 diabetes. N Engl J Med 345: 851-860, 2001.

104. Lewis EJ, Hunsicker LG, Bain RP, et al. The effect of angiotensin-converting-enzyme inhibition on diabetic nephropathy. The Collaborative Study Group. N Engl J Med 329:1456-1462, 1993.

105. Gaede P, Vedel P, Larsen N, et al. Multifactorial intervention and cardiovascular disease in patients with type 2 diabetes. N Engl J Med 348:383-393, 2003.

# Hypertension in Patients on Renal Replacement Therapy

## Todd W. B. Gehr, Domenic A. Sica

## PREVALENCE OF HYPERTENSION IN DIALYSIS PATIENTS

The prevalence of hypertension in patients with end-stage renal disease (ESRD) ranges between 70% and 90%.[1,2] Hypertension prevalence in ESRD (in other comorbid conditions such as diabetes) is definitionally dependent. In a survey of 2535 clinically stable adult hemodialysis patients, hypertension—as defined by either a systolic blood pressure (SBP) of >150 mm Hg or a diastolic blood pressure (DBP) >85 mm Hg or use of antihypertensive medications—was documented in 86% of the cohort.[1] These prevalence rates are in striking contrast to those of the general U.S. population for whom National Health and Nutrition Examination Survey (NHANES) data report a hypertension prevalence rate of 28.7%.[3]

The prevalence of hypertension in ESRD also appears to vary in keeping with population demographics. In the ESRD population, not unlike the general population, males and African Americans have a higher prevalence of hypertension. Also, during the first year of dialysis the prevalence of hypertension often declines only to return as dialysis goes on. The timing of specific blood pressure (BP) measurements (as determinants of the presence of hypertension) in ESRD can complicate the designation of a patient as being hypertensive. The point in time of BP measurement becomes less of an issue when ambulatory BP monitoring (ABPM) is employed as the diagnostic medium.[4] ABPM can be both a diagnostic tool and a means for determining adequacy of BP control in ESRD. For example, in a cohort of 53 hypertensive ESRD patients, only 15% maintained BP readings consistently <150/90 mm Hg over a 48-hour interdialytic period despite being actively treated for their hypertension.[5]

## HYPERTENSION AND DIALYSIS MODALITY

The prevalence of hypertension in renal replacement therapy (RRT) patients may also be dependent on the dialysis modality. For example, the prevalence of hypertension in peritoneal dialysis (PD) is viewed as being less than in hemodialysis (HD) patients with early reports showing that continuous ambulatory peritoneal dialysis (CAPD) provided more effective control of volume overload and hypertension.[6,7] PD also appeared to offer some distinct advantages over intermittent HD in that the hemodynamic perturbations with PD were less disruptive and antihypertensive medication pharmacokinetics more predictable.[8] Accordingly, in the short term, BP control on CAPD proved superior (particularly as relates to SBP)[9] to that of HD as long as the CAPD patient maintained some residual renal function[10] and peritoneal ultrafiltration capacity was intact.[11]

However, peritoneal transport characteristics may be important in determining the BP pattern of the CAPD patient. For example, when 24-hour ABPM was performed in a group of 25 CAPD patients and related to peritoneal transport characteristics, patients who were "high transporters" (reflecting high glucose absorption and poor ultrafiltration) had higher SBP and DBP values both during the day and at night. Left ventricular mass index was also higher in this group when compared with "low transporters."[12] Thus, it is not surprising that more long-term studies have shown a less-favorable hemodynamic profile for CAPD patients, particularly since the common scenario of insidious volume expansion would be expected to lead to BP increase and thereby left ventricular hypertrophy (LVH) more than with intermittent HD.[13,14] However, this deterioration in hemodynamic profile (compared with HD patients) can be prevented if volume status is strictly controlled in the long-term CAPD patient.[15]

A number of factors favorably influence both the prevalence and severity of hypertension in the HD patient. Two such modifications of the dialysis prescription include quotidian (daily) forms of dialysis: (1) short daily or (2) long nocturnal dialysis, 6 times per week.[16,17] Because the interdialytic period is shorter with quotidian dialysis, fluid shifts are minimized, as are the negative effects on cardiac function and hemodynamics. Patients on daily hemodialysis have been shown to obtain better BP control and a greater reduction in LVH.[18] The London Daily/Nocturnal Hemodialysis Study has also shown that patients treated with quotidian dialysis experienced significant reductions in BP even as they took fewer antihypertensive medications.[16] Observational studies with nocturnal hemodialysis bear out these findings.[19,20]

## CARDIOVASCULAR DISEASE IN END-STAGE RENAL DISEASE

Cardiovascular disease (CVD) and cerebrovascular disease account for more than 50% of all ESRD deaths, a figure that is remarkably similar around the world[21,22] (Figure 53–1). In fact, Clyde Shields, the first patient on long-term dialysis, died from a myocardial infarction (MI) in 1970, aged 50 years, 11 years after starting hemodialysis.[23] LVH is the most frequent cardiac abnormality in patients with ESRD[24] and, if left untreated, all too often progresses through phases of diastolic dysfunction, ventricular dilation, and systolic dysfunction, to death.[25] In addition to hypertension, episodic sodium and water retention, chronic volume and flow overload, associated with anemia and/or arteriovenous shunting, as well as nonhemodynamic factors, such as hyperparathyroidism and increases in angiotensin II (Ang II) and endothelin, also contribute to the development of LVH.[26]

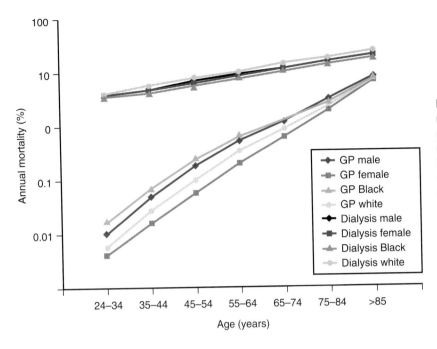

**Figure 53–1** Annual cardiovascular mortality by age group in the general population (GP) and in patients on dialysis. (From Foley RN, Parfrey PS, Sarnat MJ. Clinical epidemiology of cardiovascular disease in chronic renal disease. Am J Kidney Dis 32:S112-S119, 1998.)

## HYPERTENSION AND CARDIOVASCULAR DISEASE IN END-STAGE RENAL DISEASE

Whereas the general population has experienced a significant reduction in age-adjusted risk of death from CVD and cerebrovascular disease, this has not been the case for ESRD patients.[27,28] Any direct relationship between hypertension and cardiovascular mortality remains poorly defined, in part, because there are no prospective interventional trials in dialysis patients examining this issue.[29,30] Because of the increased number of cardiovascular risk factors in patients on dialysis, it would seem reasonable that lowering the BP in these persons would reduce cardiovascular risk. In one study of a select group of ESRD patients, normal BP values without antihypertensive therapy (in the setting of a higher than usual dose of dialysis) were associated with a reduction in cardiovascular mortality.[31] However, few observational studies have associated hypertension with a shorter survival and good/excellent BP control with increased survival.[32]

Surprisingly, several studies have even suggested the contrary (i.e., they have failed to identify hypertension as having a major influence on cardiovascular risk in large cohorts of ESRD patients[33-34] and have often found "U-shaped" correlation for more frequent cardiovascular deaths at very high and very low BP values.[35] This relationship was explored for predialysis and postdialysis SBP/DBP in an observational study of 4499 U.S. hemodialysis patients as part of the Case Mix Adequacy Study of the U.S. Renal Data System (USRDS). Patients with a predialysis SBP <110 mm Hg had an elevated adjusted mortality rate; however, predialysis systolic hypertension was not associated with excess mortality risk, although there was an increase in cerebrovascular deaths in this group. Low and high (>180 mm Hg) postdialysis SBP values (as compared with midrange SBP) were associated with increased mortality.[30]

The relationship between BP and cardiovascular risk is further confounded by the lack of agreement on which BP values—predialysis, postdialysis, off-dialysis day, and/or pulse pressure—provide the greatest predictive accuracy for cardiovascular risk/protection.[36,37] A large representative sample of patients undergoing maintenance hemodialysis have been found to have an increased risk of death in association with a widened pulse pressure (Figure 53–2).[38] Further confusing this issue is the observation that routine dialysis unit BP determinations (oftentimes obtained by poorly trained staff) can systematically exceed standardized readings. In one study, 55% of surveyed patients were noted to have postdialysis SBP measurements greater by at least 10 mm Hg than standardized readings obtained by trained evaluators.[39]

## PATHOGENESIS

A number of pathogenic factors contribute to the development of and/or persistence of hypertension in patients on RRT. Because mean arterial pressure is a product of both cardiac output and peripheral vascular resistance, both factors play an important role in the pathogenesis of ESRD-related hypertension. Another important determinant of BP (in particular, SBP and pulse pressure) in ESRD is vessel compliance and pressure wave reflectance.[40]

In most dialysis patients, multiple factors typically contribute to the pathogenesis of their hypertension. Despite this, a sensible approach to sorting out the pathogenesis of hypertension in a dialysis patient can be arrived at by classifying it into volume-dependent and volume-independent categories based on the response to ultrafiltration. Volume-dependent hypertension is by far the more common of the two and is usually characterized by normal to low plasma renin activity with a reduction in BP with either dietary sodium restriction or gradual net volume removal during consecutive dialysis sessions. Volume-independent forms of hypertension in ESRD are accompanied by a relative, if not, an absolute increase in the activity of the renin-angiotensin system (RAS), as well as limited BP reduction in response to volume removal and/or

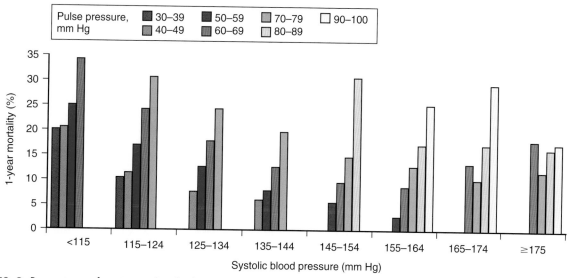

**Figure 53–2** Percentage of patients who died at 1 year within categories of postdialysis systolic blood pressure (SBP) and pulse pressure. Categories with fewer than 10 patients are not shown. Within each category of SBP, the grouped columns indicate death percentage as pulse pressure increases. Within each pulse pressure category, the death percentage can be followed across categories of increasing SBP. (From Klassen PS, Lowrie EG, Reddan DN, et al. Association between pulse pressure and mortality in patients undergoing maintenance hemodialysis. JAMA 287:1548-1555, 2002; with permission.)

dietary sodium restriction. In its most extreme form, bilateral nephrectomy has been required to control BP in ESRD.[41]

Although it is clinically useful to divide ESRD hypertension into these broad categories, additional factors play a role in its pathogenesis. Such factors should always be considered in the context of a patient's prevailing volume status/hemodynamic profile. Moreover, ESRD-related hypertension can reflect a carryover of pathogenic factors from the pre-ESRD period. As mentioned, volume and sodium excess are prime factors in the pathogenesis of hypertension in chronic kidney disease (CKD) and persist in ESRD.

Early phases of hypertension in CKD are generally marked by an increase in cardiac output and low to normal peripheral vascular resistance. Progressive renal disease is regularly accompanied by the onset of anemia and/or creation of an arteriovenous fistula, circumstances that reinforce the high cardiac output state. Changes in cardiac output can be attenuated with correction of anemia,[42] in which case the continued presence of hypertension becomes a function of increased peripheral vascular resistance, which positively correlates with the increase in exchangeable sodium that underscores the progression to ESRD.[43] Finally, the BP response to changes in sodium/volume status may be influenced by disturbances in the activity of and response to various neurohumoral pathways.[44]

Activation of the renin-angiotensin-aldosterone axis is a frequently cited factor in the pathogenesis of ESRD-related hypertension, but it is the predominant factor in only a handful of patients. The significance of this activation lies more in failure of appropriate renin suppression in the volume-expanded environment, typical of most ESRD patients.[45] Tissue-based Ang II production may also be implicated in the hypertension and CVD of the ESRD patient; however, this has not been directly studied.[46] Aldosterone (as both an autocrine and paracrine substance) is also increasingly viewed as a con-

tributor to the pathobiology of CVD. However, its exact pathogenic role in the ESRD patient has yet to be determined.[47]

Increased activity of the sympathetic nervous system (SNS) may be either directly or indirectly involved in ESRD-related hypertension.[48,49] Simple techniques for measurement of sympathetic activity are not available; and much has been wrongly inferred from relatively nonspecific indicators of sympathetic activity, such as the physical findings BP and pulse rate and/or the biomarker plasma norepinephrine concentration. The latter is particularly difficult to interpret in CKD, because plasma catecholamine concentrations are approximately doubled in the advanced stage of this disease.[50] Sympathetic nerve recordings are more accurate measures of sympathetic activation. Converse et al.[51] found that peroneal nerve sympathetic discharge was 2.5 times higher in hemodialysis patients than in normal persons and could be normalized by bilateral nephrectomy, suggesting that reduced sympathetic nerve discharge may be one mechanism by which bilateral nephrectomy reduces BP. Moreover, neuropeptide Y, a 36-amino acid vasoactive peptide, is released during sympathetic stimulation, as in volume overload[52] and is independently associated with LVH and systolic dysfunction in ESRD.[53] An increase in neuropeptide Y is one of several pathways by which SNS activation indirectly influences cardiovascular structure and function.

A host of other factors have been suggested as contributors to the pathogenesis of hypertension in ESRD. A full discussion of all such factors would exceed the scope of this chapter, and the reader is directed to several authoritative reviews on this theme.[2,44] The roles of nitric oxide (NO), circulating inhibitors of $Na^+,K^+$-ATPase and the calcium-phosphate axis in the pathogenesis of hypertension in ESRD are discussed briefly here.

NO deficiency occurs in ESRD and has been proposed as one of several factors contributing to hypertension in this population.[54] NO production by the vascular endothelium is inhibited by asymmetric dimethylarginine (ADMA). Levels of ADMA are 6- to 10-fold higher in hemodialysis patients than in healthy persons. Although ADMA levels are reduced by up to 65% during a standard 5-hour hemodialysis session, any reduction in plasma levels is transient.[55] In persons whose plasma ADMA levels fall with dialysis, a decrease in mean 24-hour ambulatory BP has been observed.[56] Of note, higher levels of exhaled NO are found in hemodialysis patients prone to low BP.[57]

Circulating natriuretic substances (including digoxin-like immunoreactive substances) appear to accumulate in CKD and in so doing could bring about a generalized inhibition of $Na^+,K^+$-ATPase. The ensuing rise in intracellular $Na^+$ concentration in vascular smooth muscle cells could then diminish $Na^+/Ca^{2+}$ exchange and thereby increase intracellular calcium concentration, resulting in a persistent state of vasoconstriction.[58] Consistent with these data, both false-positive digoxin levels (relating to digoxin-like immunoreactive substances)[59] and circulating $Na^+,K^+$-ATPase inhibitors have been identified in hemodialysis patients and are correlated with interdialytic weight gain.[60]

Defects in calcium metabolism are ubiquitous in dialysis patients and are typically manifest by secondary hyperparathyroidism, which may increase BP via entry of calcium into vascular smooth muscle cells.[61] Allosteric activators of the calcium-sensing receptor, which reduce parathyroid hormone levels in the setting of secondary hyperparathyroidism, are associated with a reduction in BP.[62]

## TREATMENT AND BLOOD PRESSURE GOALS IN HYPERTENSIVE END-STAGE RENAL DISEASE PATIENTS

BP goals in ESRD patients remain controversial, since no randomized, prospective outcome trials have expressly examined the issue of what represents an optimal BP in ESRD patients. This information void makes an evidence-based medicine approach to BP control unfeasible in ESRD patients. Recommendations advising BP goals below those currently advocated for the general population are occasionally forthcoming. These suggestions should not be widely applied based on the unique and highly individualized nature of the hypertension in this population.

The target BP in hypertensive ESRD patients with classic systolic/diastolic hypertension (without intradialytic hypotension) should not differ from that recommended for the general population, <140/90 mm Hg.[63] Certain high-risk patient groups such as diabetics should be treated to the currently suggested goal BP of <130/80 mm Hg. However, this recommendation often requires a deft touch in clinical practice since orthostatic hypotension is not uncommon in the hypertensive ESRD patient with diabetes.[64]

Hypertension in ESRD patients is mainly systolic, reflecting a loss of aortic distensibility and premature vascular aging.[65] The recommended BP goal for ESRD patients with predominantly systolic hypertension (with a widened pulse pressure) is a matter of personal opinion. These patients can be treated empirically to a goal SBP according to current guidelines, with the final SBP goal being influenced by several factors, including: drug tolerance, coexisting coronary and/or cerebrovascu-lar disease, and/or how much the SBP is reduced. The clinician should be mindful of the U-shaped correlation for cardiovascular mortality in this population.

## Nonpharmacologic Treatment

Irrespective of the individual patient's "mechanism" of hypertension, the first step in the nonpharmacologic management of hypertension is to set and achieve a true target or "dry weight." The term *dry weight* does not have a consensus definition, however.[58] Various definitions have been employed: (1) the weight at which there is an absence of overt physical findings of volume overload, such as peripheral edema, rales, or neck vein distension; (2) the weight at which the patient cannot tolerate the associated BP and symptom profile[66]; and (3) the postdialysis weight at which the patient is persistently normotensive without antihypertensive medications and despite interdialytic weight gain.[67,68] Noninvasive methods, such as ultrasound measurement of inferior vena cava diameter and multifrequency bioimpedance hold some promise for evaluating volume status, but access to these techniques, proficiency of use by staff, and cost are limiting factors in their application.[69,70]

The most stringent criterion for having reached a patient's "dry weight" is that of BP being controlled throughout the interdialytic period without the need for antihypertensive medications, but even this has several caveats attached to its broad-based application, including (1) There is a limited correlation between interdialytic weight gain and BP.[71] (2) Excessive weight reduction can activate the RAS and SNS and alter cardiac hemodynamics in such a way that certain patients experience a paradoxical increase in BP despite falling below their dry weight.[72,73] (3) The nutritional status of the ESRD patient is ever-changing and it is not uncommon that lean body weight occasionally decreases; however, unlike normal renal function patients where such lean body weight loss can be recognized by a fall in body weight, the ESRD patient sees no such fall in body weight since interdialytic volume gains "substitute" for muscle mass lost. Consequently, maintenance of a constant body weight in such an ESRD patient reflects an ongoing gradual expansion of extracellular volume replacing lost muscle weight.[58,66] (4) Reduction in extracellular volume via ultrafiltration does not immediately translate into BP reduction because there is a nonlinear relationship between extracellular volume status and BP. This "lag phase" is such that BP is not immediately controlled after ultrafiltration to a dry weight, especially in patients who are chronically volume overloaded.[5,58,74]

As previously mentioned, the initial phase of hypertension therapy in the ESRD patient entails the clinical assessment of volume status and an attempt to reach a patient's dry weight with a combination of dietary sodium restriction and dialysis-related ultrafiltration. During the initiation stage of hemodialysis, a patient's true dry weight is probed as weight begins to fall in tandem with efforts at ultrafiltration. It is of the essence that antihypertensive medications be tapered and withheld as this optimal weight is being sought. Failure to withhold medications can lead to a confusing picture characterized by assorted clinical scenarios of hypotension and hypertension. There can be a lag phase of several weeks before the full effect of volume removal on the BP is evident (Figure 53–3).

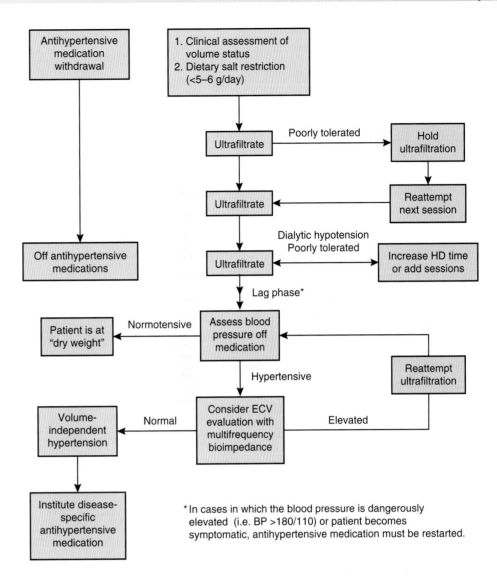

**Figure 53–3** Schematic for the control of blood pressure (BP) in the end-state renal disease (ESRD) patient on hemodialysis. (From Khosla UM, Johnson RJ. Hypertension in hemodialysis patients and the "lag phenomenon": Insights into pathophysiology and clinical management. Am J Kidney Dis 43:739-751, 2004.)

* In cases in which the blood pressure is dangerously elevated (i.e. BP >180/110) or patient becomes symptomatic, antihypertensive medication must be restarted.

Several alternatives to traditional dialysis may facilitate BP control. For example, thrice-weekly hemodialysis is the most commonly used form of RRT; however, there is an emerging body of evidence that frequent intensive hemodialysis—such as short daily or nocturnal dialysis, six times a week—offers superior uremic toxin clearance, BP control, and improvement in cardiovascular outcomes.[16-20] Such departures from the routine dialysis prescription have been integrated into the treatment plan for hypertension in only a handful of ESRD patients.

BP control may seem simplified in patients receiving CAPD because of the continuous nature of fluid removal; however, this impression proves to be an oversimplification of the real situation in these patients. Suboptimal fluid removal remains a clinical problem in many CAPD patients translating into higher BP values and the need for additional antihypertensive medications. For example, in a retrospective study of 66 CAPD patients selected for symptomatic fluid retention, peripheral edema, pulmonary congestion, pleural effusions, and systolic/diastolic hypertension occurred in the large majority of patients, resulting in a significant increase in hospitalization rate.[75] In addition, numerous studies have documented poor BP control in CAPD patients despite extensive use of antihypertensive medications.[76,77]

Traditional nonpharmacologic measures that assist in BP management are often overlooked in the dialysis population. These include a reduction in body weight in obese patients, regular exercise and the careful use (if not avoidance) of drugs causing hypertension such as nasal decongestants, migraine headache medications, and weight loss compounds.[78,79] In one study by Miller et al.,[79] patients performed stationary cycling during each hemodialysis treatment. Predialysis BPs, postdialysis BPs, and antihypertensive medication use were recorded during a 6-month period. Costs of the medication were analyzed at the end of the study. The average relative benefit of exercise was a 36% reduction in antihypertensive medications with an average annual cost savings of $885 per patient per year in the exercise group compared with a nonexercise control group (Figure 53–4).[79]

## Pharmacologic Management of Hypertension

When volume control through aggressive ultrafiltration and/or sodium and fluid restriction fails to control BP, pharmacologic therapy becomes necessary. These patients represent volume-independent hypertensives and are in the minority of all

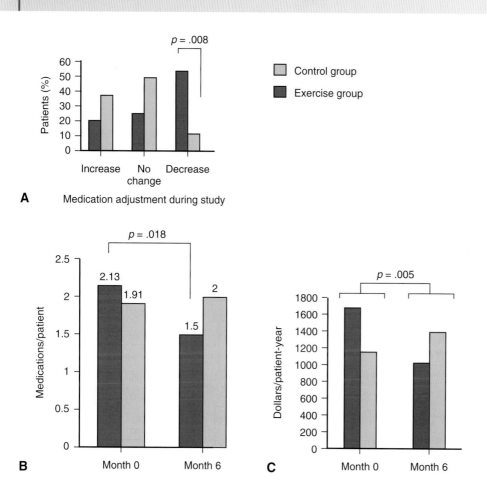

**Figure 53–4 (A)** Status of patients' antihypertensive medication at 6 months compared with baseline. p = .008 by chi-square test among exercise and control group at 6 months. **(B)** Number of antihypertensive medications taken per patient at month 0 and month 6 for exercise and control groups. **(C)** Annualized cost of antihypertensive medications per patient based on use at month 0 and month 6. Exercise patients (n = 24); control patients (n = 32). (From Miller BW, Cress CL, Johnson ME, et al. Exercise during hemodialysis decreases the use of antihypertensive medications. Am J Kidney Dis 39:828-833, 2002.)

hypertensive ESRD patients. Antihypertensive therapy should be directed toward the presumed underlying mechanism of the hypertension, but is often easier said than done, because an explicit mechanism is often hard to identify. That being said, considerable treatment experience exists with many of the more commonly used antihypertensive drug classes, and some comment will be provided for the more commonly used drug classes. However, the final medication regimen settled on should be individualized and directed towards decreasing patient morbidity and mortality while assisting in the management of comorbid conditions (Table 53–1).

### Diuretics

As long as some level of residual renal function exists in an ESRD patient, diuretics may be employed to aid in the short-term regulation of fluid balance and thereby facilitate BP control.[80] Diuretics have not been shown to reduce BP in ESRD patients independent of their ability to promote diuresis.[81] Typically, high doses of a loop diuretic, alone or together with a thiazide diuretic, are needed to establish and sustain a diuretic response. Diuretic therapy can provide an interdialytic bridge for fluid removal, reducing the need for an overly restrictive fluid prescription. However, the initial and sometimes rewarding diuretic effect in the ESRD patient will gradually taper off as the underlying renal disease advances. The progression of renal disease in an ESRD patient should be expected, and generally is marked by a decrease in interdialytic urine volume, signaling the need to discontinue diuretic therapy.[80]

### β-Blockers

β-Blockers are used regularly in the patient with ESRD for the treatment of hypertension[1,82-85] and/or for their cardioprotective effects.[85-88] The BP-lowering effect of β-blockers in the ESRD population can be attenuated by interdialytic weight gain.[83] The selection of a β-blocker in an ESRD patient should take place with some knowledge of the elimination characteristics (renal, hepatic, hepatic/renal) of the selected drug, as well as whether the compound is dialyzable and/or has active metabolites.[89,90] Accumulation of a β-blocker in an ESRD patient does not generally improve BP control, but β-blocker accumulation can be associated with more frequent side effects. If such side effects occur, two options exist: first, to continue the offending β-blocker with empiric dose reduction, or second, to convert to a hepatically cleared β-blocker such as metoprolol. Data from the USRDS Waves 3 and 4 Study show β-blocker use to be associated with lower mortality with and without adjustment for comorbidities.[85] Several pharmacologic features of β-blockers can be offered as possible explanations for these protective effects, including: decreasing sympathetic hyperactivity, reducing stroke volume, remodeling the myocardium, having antiarrhythmic effects, and/or (for nonselective β-blockers) increasing fasting serum potassium concentration.[49,86,87,91]

### Calcium Channel Blockers

Calcium channel blockers (CCBs) have demonstrated efficacy in patients with diverse cardiovascular conditions, including

**Table 53–1** Pharmacokinetic Properties of Antihypertensive Agents in Patients with End-Stage Renal Disease

| | | Half-Life (hr) | Dose Change | Removal with Dialysis | |
|---|---|---|---|---|---|
| | **Normal** | **ESRD** | **With ESRD** | **Hemodialysis** | **Peritoneal** |
| **α-Adrenergic Antagonists** | | | | | |
| Doxazosin | 22 | | None | None | Unlikely |
| Prazosin | 2-4 | | None | None | Unlikely |
| Terazosin | 12 | | None | None | Unlikely |
| **β-Adrenergic Antagonists** | | | | | |
| Acebutolol | 7-9 | Prolonged | 30-50% | Yes | ? |
| Atenolol | 6-7 | Prolonged | 25% | Yes | None |
| Bisoprolol | 12-13 | Prolonged | 50% | Yes | None |
| Betaxolol | 15-20 | Prolonged | 50% | Yes | ? |
| Carteolol | 7 | Prolonged | 25% | ? | ? |
| Carvedilol | 5-8 | | None | None | ? |
| Esmolol | 7-15 min | No Data | None | None | Unlikely |
| Labetolol | 3-9 | | None | ? | ? |
| Propranolol-LA | 10 | | None | None | Unlikely |
| Propranolol | 2-6 | | None | None | Unlikely |
| Metoprolol tartrate | 3-7 | | None | Yes | ? |
| Metoprolol succinate | 3-7 | | None | Yes | ? |
| Nadolol | 20-24 | Prolonged | 25% | Yes | None |
| Pindolol | 3-4 | | None | Unlikely | Unlikely |
| Timolol | 3-4 | | None | None | None |
| Penbutolol | 5 | | None | Unlikely | Unlikely |
| **Angiotensin Receptor Blockers** | | | | | |
| Candesartan | 9-12 | | No | Minimal | ? |
| Eprosartan | 5-9 | | No | None | ? |
| Irbesartan | 11-15 | | No | None | ? |
| Losartan | 4-6 | | No | None | ? |
| Olmesartan | 13 | | No | Unknown | ? |
| Telmisartan | 24 | | No | None | ? |
| Valsartan | 6 | | No | None | ? |
| **Vasodilators** | | | | | |
| Hydralazine | 2-5 | Prolonged | None | None | None |
| Minoxidil | 3-4 | | None | None | ? |
| **ACE Inhibitors** | | | | | |
| Benazepril | 10-11 | Prolonged | 25-50% | Unlikely | Unlikely |
| Captopril | 2-3 | Prolonged | 50% | Yes | None |
| Enalapril | 11-24 | Prolonged | 50% | Yes | None |
| Fosinopril | 12 | | None | No | None |
| Moexipril | 2-9 | Prolonged | 25-50% | ? | ? |
| Lisinopril | 12 | Prolonged | 25-50% | Yes | ? |
| Quinapril | 1-2 | Prolonged | 75% | ? No | ? |
| Perindopril | 5 | Prolonged | 50% | Yes | ? |
| Ramipril | 5-8 | Prolonged | 25-50% | Yes | None |
| Trandolapril | 16-24 | Prolonged | 50% | ? | ? |
| **Central α-Adrenergic Agonists** | | | | | |
| Clonidine | 6-23 | | None | None | Unlikely |
| **Calcium Channel Blockers** | | | | | |
| Amlodipine | 30-50 | | None | None | Unlikely |
| Diltiazem | 2-8 | | None | None | Unlikely |
| Felodipine | 10-14 | | None | None | Unlikely |
| Isradipine | 2-5 | | None | None | Unlikely |
| Nicardipine | 5 | | None | None | Unlikely |
| Nifedipine | 4-5.5 | | None | None | Unlikely |
| Nimodipine | 1-3 | | None | None | Unlikely |
| Nisoldipine | 7-8 | | None | None | Unlikely |
| Verapamil | 3-7 | | None | None | Unlikely |

ESRD, end-stage renal disease; LA, long-acting; ACE, angiotensin-converting enzyme.

hypertension, angina pectoris, supraventricular arrhythmias, and diastolic dysfunction. These cardiovascular conditions are widely prevalent in the ESRD patient, which explains the liberal use of CCBs in this population.[1,84,92,93] In general, the pharmacokinetics of CCBs are comparable in CKD/ESRD patients and persons with normal renal function. Therefore, dose adjustment based on pharmacokinetic considerations and/or dialysis clearance is not necessary with CCBs.[92]

In an analysis of the USRDS Wave 2 cohort, nondihydropyridine CCBs were associated with a reduced risk of cardiovascular death (hazard ratio, 0.78; 95% confidence interval, 0.62-0.97), and among ESRD patients with preexisting cardiovascular disease, both dihydropyridine and nondihydropyridine CCBs were associated with reduced risk of all-cause and cardiovascular mortality.[84] These data are important because they lessen the reliance in this patient population on medical evidence extrapolated from non-ESRD populations.

CCB-related side effects may be particularly bothersome in these patients. ESRD patients tend to be constipated, and this can be aggravated by verapamil.[92] Also, CCBs can produce peripheral edema on a vasodilatory basis. This form of peripheral edema is not distinguished by weight gain. When a true volume-expanded form of peripheral edema exists—as is often the case in ESRD—and a CCB is administered, any edema that develops cannot be viewed as an accurate reflection of the patient's volume status unless it is accompanied by weight gain.[94]

### ACE Inhibitors and Angiotensin Receptor Blockers

ACE inhibitors and more recently angiotensin receptor blockers (ARBs) have become popular therapies for the ESRD patient.[95,96] The ability of either of these drug classes to reduce BP in the ESRD patient is well accepted; however, there is considerably less information available to guide the clinician in the safe and effective use of these drugs in the ESRD patient with congestive heart failure (CHF) and/or coronary artery disease.

Head-to-head comparisons of BP effects and/or target organ protection in the ESRD patient are lacking for both drug classes. ACE inhibitor therapy has been suggested to decrease access failure rate and to improve survival in the ESRD population (see references cited here for a more comprehensive discussion).[95,96] However, drug classes other than ACE inhibitors appear to offer survival benefits, and it is not yet proven that ACE inhibitors are superior to other drug classes—such as CCBs—in survival benefits for patients with ESRD.

Several pharmacokinetic factors, including dialyzability and the propensity for systemic accumulation, can influence drug selection. ACE inhibitors and ARBs have nonpressor effects that are beneficial for patients with ESRD. These include their ability to decrease thirst drive and erythropoiesis.[95] The ACE inhibitors have a unique adverse effect profile, which includes cough and, less frequently, angioneurotic edema. In the ESRD population, so-called anaphylactoid dialyzer reactions can occur in conjunction with ACE inhibitor use.[95] ARBs carry less risk than ACE inhibitors and have a preferred pharmacokinetic profile—limited dialyzability and minimal systemic accumulation. These attributes favor the increased use of ARBs in this population.[96]

## SUMMARY

Hypertension in the RRT patient is a common phenomenon. Its pathophysiologic basis relates to a unique set of hemodynamic and volume changes, which are characteristic of ESRD. The treatment of ESRD-related hypertension is at the start heavily dependent on the adequacy of ultrafiltration and the stepwise attainment of a patient's target weight. Thereafter, as pharmacotherapy may become necessary, any of the full range of medication choices provides suitable options. Heavy emphasis is generally placed on the use of CCBs, ACE inhibitors, and/or ARBs, although outcomes data supporting the preferential use of one or the other of these drug classes are currently lacking. Choosing specific antihypertensive agents for a hypertensive ESRD patient is as much an art as a science—issues such as a patient's dialysis shift, dialyzer drug clearance, and altered drug pharmacokinetics are some of the factors that make consistent 24-hour BP control difficult. The goal BP for the hypertensive ESRD patient is a matter of debate, because specific outcomes studies have yet to be performed in this patient population. Moreover, there is evidence of a U-shaped relationship for BP reduction and mortality in the ESRD patient.

## References

1. Agarwal R, Nissenson AR, Battle D, et al. Prevalence, treatment, and control of hypertension in chronic hemodialysis patients in the United States. Am J Med 115:291-297, 2003.
2. Horl MP, Horl WH. Hemodialysis-associated hypertension: Pathophysiology and therapy. Am J Kid Dis 39:227-244, 2002.
3. Hajjar I, Kotchen TA. Trends in prevalence, awareness, treatment, and control of hypertension in the United States, 1988-2000. JAMA 290:199-206, 2003.
4. Peixoto AJ, Sica DA. Ambulatory blood pressure monitoring in end-stage renal disease. Blood Press Monit 2:275-282, 1997.
5. Cheigh JS, Milite C, Sullivan JF, et al. Hypertension is not adequately controlled in hemodialysis patients. Am J Kidney Dis 19:453-459, 1992.
6. Saldanha LF, Elmar WJ, Weiler WJ, et al. Effect of continuous ambulatory peritoneal dialysis on blood pressure. Am J Kidney Dis 21:184-188, 1993.
7. Cannata JB, Isles CG, Briggs JD, et al. Comparison of blood pressure control during hemodialysis and CAPD. Dial Transplant 15:675-679, 1986.
8. Taylor CA 3rd, Abdel-Rahman E, Zimmerman SW, et al. Clinical pharmacokinetics during continuous ambulatory peritoneal dialysis. Clin Pharmacokinet 31:293-308, 1996.
9. Menon MK, Naimark DM, Bargman JM, et al. Long-term blood pressure control in a cohort of peritoneal dialysis patients and its association with residual renal function. Nephrol Dial Transplant 16:2207-2213, 2001.
10. Khandelwal M, Kothari J, Krishnan M, et al. Volume expansion and sodium balance in peritoneal dialysis patients. Part II: Newer insights in management. Adv Perit Dial 19:44-52, 2003.
11. Bos WJ, Struijk DG, van Olden RW, et al. Elevated 24-hour blood pressure in peritoneal dialysis patients with ultrafiltration failure. Adv Perit Dial 14:108-110, 1998.
12. Tonbul Z, Altintepe L, Sozlu C, et al. The association of peritoneal transport properties with 24-hour blood pressure levels in CAPD patients. Perit Dial Int 23:46-52, 2003.
13. Enia G, Mallamaci F, Benedetto FA, et al. Long-term CAPD patients are volume expanded and display more severe left ventricular hypertrophy than haemodialysis patients. Nephrol Dial Transplant 16:1459-1465, 2001.

14. Takeda K, Nakamoto M, Hirakata H, et al. Disadvantage of long-term CAPD for preserving cardiac performance: An echocardiographic study. Am J Kidney Dis 32:482-487, 1998.
15. Gunal AI, Ilkay E, Kirciman E, et al. Blood pressure control and left ventricular hypertrophy in long-term CAPD and hemodialysis patients: A cross-sectional study. Peritoneal Dial Int 23:563-567, 2003.
16. Nesrallah G, Suri R, Moist L, et al. Volume control and blood pressure management in patients undergoing quotidian hemodialysis. Am J Kidney Dis 42(1 Suppl):13-17, 2003.
17. Lindsay RM; Daily/Nocturnal Dialysis Study Group. The London, Ontario, Daily/Nocturnal Hemodialysis Study. Semin Dial 17:85-91, 2004.
18. Buoncristiani U, Fagugli RM, Pinciaroli MR, et al. Reversal of left ventricular hypertrophy in uremic patients by treatment with daily hemodialysis. Cont Nephrol 1119:152-156, 1996.
19. Pierratos A, Ouwendyk M. Nocturnal hemodialysis: Five years later. Semin Dial 12:419-423, 1999.
20. Lockridge RS, Anderson HK, Coffey LT, et al. Nightly home hemodialysis in Lynchburg, Virginia: Economic and logistic considerations. Semin Dial 12:440-447, 1999.
21. USRDS: The United States Renal Data System. Am J Kidney Dis 42 (Suppl 5):1-230, 2003.
22. Rostand SG. Coronary heart disease in chronic renal insufficiency: Some management considerations. J Am Soc Nephrol 11:1948-1956, 2000.
23. Drukker W. Haemodialysis: A historical review. In Maher JF (ed). Replacement of Renal Function by Dialysis, 3rd ed. Boston, Kluwer Academic, 1989; p 20.
24. London GM. Left ventricular hypertrophy: Why does it happen? Nephrol Dial Transplant 18(Suppl 8):2-6, 2003.
25. London GM, Pannier B, Guerin AP, et al. Alterations of left ventricular hypertrophy in and survival of patients receiving hemodialysis: Follow-up of an interventional study. J Am Soc Nephrol 12:2759-2767, 2001.
26. London GM. Left ventricular alterations and end-stage renal disease. Nephrol Dial Transplant 17(Suppl 1):29-36, 2002.
27. 2004 Heart Disease and Stroke Statistics, American Heart Association.
28. USRDS. The United States Renal Data System. Am J Kidney Dis 42(Suppl 5):1-230.
29. Covic A, Gusbeth-Tatomir P, Goldsmith DJ. The challenge of cardiovascular risk factors in end-stage renal disease. J Nephrol 16:476-486, 2003.
30. Port FK, Hulbert-Shearon TE, Wolfe RA. Predialysis blood pressure and mortality risk in a national sample of maintenance hemodialysis patients. Am J Kid Dis 33:507-517, 1999.
31. Charra B, Calemard E, Ruffet M, et al. Survival as an index of adequacy of dialysis. Kidney Int 41:1286-1291, 1992.
32. Fernandez JM, Carbonell ME, Mazzuchi N, et al. Simultaneous analysis of morbidity and mortality factors in chronic hemodialysis patients. Kidney Int 41:1029-1034, 1992.
33. Iseki K, Miyasato F, Tokuyama K. Low diastolic blood pressure, hypoalbuminemia, and risk of death in a cohort of chronic hemodialysis patients. Kidney Int 51:1212-1217, 1997.
34. Duranti E, Imperiali P, Sasdelli M. Is hypertension a mortality risk factor in dialysis? Kidney Int 55:S173-S174, 1996.
35. Zager PG, Nikolic J, Brown RH. "U" curve association of blood pressure and mortality in hemodialysis patients. Kidney Int 54:561-569, 1998.
36. Mittal SK, Kowalski E, Trenkle J, et al. Prevalence of hypertension in a hemodialysis population. Clin Nephrol 51:77-82, 1999.
37. Kooman JP, Gladziwa U, Bocker G, et al. Blood pressure during the interdialytic period in haemodialysis patients: Estimation of representative blood pressure values. Nephrol Dial Transplant 7:917-923, 1992.
38. Klassen PS, Lowrie EG, Reddan DN, et al. Association between pulse pressure and mortality in patients undergoing maintenance hemodialysis. JAMA 287:1548-1555, 2002.
39. Rahman M, Griffin V, Kumar A, et al. A comparison of standardized versus "usual" blood pressure measurements in hemodialysis patients. Am J Kidney Dis 39:1226-1230, 2002.
40. London GM, Marchais SJ, Safar ME, et al. Aortic and large artery compliance in end-stage renal failure. Kidney Int 37:137-142, 1990.
41. Nuutinen M, Lautala P, Remes M, et al. Nephrectomy in severe hypertension. Clin Nephrol 54:342-346, 2000.
42. Neff MS, Kim KE, Persoff M, et al. Hemodynamics of uremic anemia. Circulation 43:876-883, 1971.
43. Safar ME, London GM, Weiss YA, et al. Overhydration and renin in hypertensive patients with terminal renal failure: A hemodynamic study. Clin Nephrol 5:183-188, 1975.
44. Kooman JP, Van Der Sande FM, Leunissen KM. Role of sodium and volume in the pathogenesis of hypertension in dialysis patients. Reflections on pathophysiological mechanisms. Blood Purif 22:55-59, 2004.
45. Mailloux LU. Hypertension in chronic renal failure and ESRD: Prevalence, pathophysiology, and outcomes. Semin Nephrol 21:146-156, 2001.
46. Agarwal R. Proinflammatory effects of oxidative stress in chronic kidney disease: Role of additional angiotensin II blockade. Am J Physiol Renal Physiol 284:F863-F869, 2003.
47. McLaughlin N, Gehr TWB, Sica DA. Aldosterone receptor antagonism and end-stage renal disease. Curr Hypertens Rep 6:327-330, 2004.
48. Campese VM, Romoff MS, Levitan D, et al. Mechanisms of autonomic nervous system dysfunction in uremia. Kidney Int 20:246-253, 1981.
49. Neumann J, Ligtenberg G, Klein II, et al. Sympathetic hyperactivity in chronic kidney disease: Pathogenesis, clinical relevance, and treatment. Kidney Int 65:1568-1576, 2004.
50. Laederach K, Weidmann P. Plasma and urinary catecholamines in relation to renal function in man. Kidney Int 31:107-111, 1987.
51. Converse RL Jr, Jacobsen TN, Toto RD, et al. Sympathetic overactivity in patients with chronic renal failure. N Engl J Med 327:1912-1918, 2002.
52. Odar-Cederlof I, Ericcson F, Theodorsson E, et al. Is neuropeptide Y a contributor to volume-induced hypertension? Am J Kidney Dis 31:803-808, 1998.
53. Zoccali C, Mallamaci F, Tripepi G, et al. Neuropeptide Y, left ventricular mass and function in patients with end stage renal disease. J Hypertens 21:1355-1362, 2003.
54. Schmidt RJ, Yokota S, Tracy T, et al. Nitric oxide production is low in end-stage renal disease patients on peritoneal dialysis. Am J Physiol 276:F794-F797, 1999.
55. Kielstein JT, Boger RH, Bode-Boger SM, et al. Asymmetric dimethylarginine plasma concentrations differ in patients with end-stage renal disease: Relationship to treatment method and atherosclerotic disease. J Am Soc Nephrol 10:594-600, 1999.
56. Scroider M, Riedel E, Beck W, et al. Increased reduction of dimethylarginines and lowered interdialytic blood pressure by the use of biocompatible membranes. Kidney Int 78: S19-S24, 2001.
57. Nishimura M, Takahashi H, Maruyama K, et al. Enhanced production of nitric oxide may be involved in acute hypotension during maintenance hemodialysis. Am J Kidney Dis 31:809-817, 1998.
58. Khosla UM, Johnson RJ. Hypertension in hemodialysis patients and the "lag phenomenon": Insights into pathophysiology and clinical management. Am J Kidney Dis 43:739-751, 2004.
59. Avendano C, Alvarez JS, Sacristan JA, et al. Interference of digoxin-like immunoreactive substances with TDx digoxin II assay in different patients. Ther Drug Monit 13:523-527, 1991.

60. Bisordi JE, Holt S. Digitalis-like immunoreactive substances and extracellular fluid volume status in chronic hemodialysis patients. Am J Kidney Dis 13:396-403, 1989.

61. Rostand SG, Drueke TB. Parathyroid hormone, vitamin D, and cardiovascular disease in chronic renal failure. Kidney Int 56:383–392, 1999.

62. Ogata H, Ritz E, Odoni G, et al. Beneficial effects of calcimimetics on progression of renal failure and cardiovascular risk factors. J Am Soc Nephrol 14:959-967, 2003.

63. Chobanian AV, Bakris GL, Black HR, et al. Seventh Report of the Joint National Committee on Prevention, Detection, Evaluation, and Treatment of High Blood Pressure. Hypertension 42:1206-1252, 2003.

64. Savica V, Musolino R, Di Leo R, et al. Autonomic dysfunction in uremia. Am J Kidney Dis 38(Suppl 1):S118-121, 2001.

65. Agarwal R. Systolic hypertension in hemodialysis patients. Semin Dial 16:208-213, 2003.

66. Jaeger JQ, Mehta RL. Assessment of dry weight in hemodialysis: An overview. J Am Soc Nephrol 10:392-403, 1999

67. Charra B, Chazot C. Volume control, blood pressure and cardiovascular function. Lessons from hemodialysis treatment. Nephron Physiol 93:94-101, 2003.

68. Laurent G. How to keep the dialysis patients normotensive? What is the secret of Tassin? Nephrol Dial Transplant 12:1104, 1997.

69. Tetsuka T, Ando Y, Ono S, et al. Change in inferior vena caval diameter detected by ultrasonography during and after hemodialysis. ASAIO J 41:105-110, 1995.

70. Chamney PW, Kramer M, Rode C, et al. A new technique for establishing dry weight in hemodialysis patients via whole body bioimpedance. Kidney Int 61:2250-2258, 2002.

71. Sherman RA, Daniel A, Cody RP. The effect of interdialytic weight gain on predialysis blood pressure. Artif Organs 17:770-774, 1993.

72. Gunal AI, Karaca I, Celiker H, et al. Paradoxical rise in blood pressure during ultrafiltration is caused by increased cardiac output. J Nephrol 15:42-47, 2002.

73. Kursat S, Ozgur B, Alici T. Effect of ultrafiltration on blood pressure variability in hemodialysis patients. Clin Nephrol 59:289-292, 2003.

74. Charra B, Bergstrom J, Scribner BH. Blood pressure control in dialysis patients: Importance of the lag phenomenon. Am J Kidney Dis 32:720-724, 1998.

75. Tzamaloukas AH, Saddler MC, Murata GH, et al: Symptomatic fluid retention in patients on continuous peritoneal dialysis. J Am Soc Nephrol 6:198-206, 1995.

76. Frankenfield DL, Prowant BF, Flanigan MJ, et al: Trends in clinical indicators of care for adult peritoneal dialysis patients in the United States from 1995 to 1997. ESRD Core Indicators Workgroup. Kidney Int 55:1998-2010, 1999.

77. Cocchi R, Esposti ED, Fabbri A, et al: Prevalence of hypertension in patients on peritoneal dialysis: Results of an Italian multicentre study. Nephrol Dial Transplant 14:1536-40, 1999.

78. O'Hare AM, Tawney K, Bacchetti P, et al. Decreased survival among sedentary patients undergoing dialysis: Results from the dialysis morbidity and mortality study wave 2. Am J Kidney Dis 41:447-454, 2003.

79. Miller BW, Cress CL, Johnson ME, et al. Exercise during hemodialysis decreases the use of antihypertensive medications. Am J Kidney Dis 39:828-833, 2002.

80. Sica DA, Gehr TW. Diuretic use in stage 5 chronic kidney disease and end-stage renal disease. Curr Opin Nephrol Hypertens 12:483-490, 2003.

81. Bennett WM, McGonald WJ, Kuehnel E, et al. Do diuretics have antihypertensive properties independent of natriuresis? Clin Pharmacol Ther 22:499-504, 1977.

82. Vlassopoulos DA, Mentzikof DG, Hadjiyannakos DK, et al. Long-term control of hypertension in dialysis patients by low dose atenolol. Int J Artif Organs 25:269-275, 2002.

83. Agarwal R. Supervised atenolol therapy in the management of hemodialysis hypertension. Kidney Int 55:1528-1535, 1999.

84. Griffith TF, Chua BSY, Allen AS, et al. Characteristics of treated hypertension in incident hemodialysis and peritoneal dialysis patients. Am J Kid Dis 42:1260-1269, 2003.

85. Foley RN, Herzog CA, Collins AJ. Blood pressure and long-term mortality in United States hemodialysis patients: USRDS Waves 3 and 4 Study. Kidney Int 62:1784-1790, 2002.

86. Hara Y, Hamada M, Shigematsu Y, et al. Beneficial effect of beta-adrenergic blockade on left ventricular function in haemodialysis patients. Clin Sci (London) 101:219-225, 2001.

87. McCullough PA, Sandberg KR, Borzak S, et al. Benefits of aspirin and beta-blockade after myocardial infarction in patients with chronic kidney disease. Am Heart J 144:226-232, 2002.

88. Ishani A, Herzog CA, Collins AJ, et al. Cardiac medications and their association with cardiovascular events in incident dialysis patients: Cause or effect? Kidney Int 65:1017-1025, 2004.

89. Frishman WH, Alwarshetty M. Beta-adrenergic blockers in systemic hypertension: Pharmacokinetic considerations related to the current guidelines. Clin Pharmacokinet 41:505-516, 2002.

90. Sica DA. Drug dosing in renal disease. In Bakris G (ed). The Kidney and Hypertension. London, Martin Dunitz, 2003; pp 127-138.

91. Nowicki M, Miszczak-Kuban J. Nonselective beta-adrenergic blockade augments fasting hyperkalemia in hemodialysis patients. Nephron 91:222-227, 2002.

92. Sica DA, Gehr TWB. Calcium channel blockers and end-stage renal disease: Pharmacokinetic and pharmacodynamic considerations. Curr Opin Nephrol Hypertens 12:123-131, 2003.

93. Sarnak MJ, Levey AS, Schoolwerth AC, et al. Kidney disease as a risk factor for development of cardiovascular disease: A statement from the American Heart Association Councils on Kidney in Cardiovascular Disease, High Blood Pressure Research, Clinical Cardiology, and Epidemiology and Prevention. Hypertension 42:1050-1065, 2003.

94. Sica DA. Calcium-channel blocker peripheral edema–Can it be resolved? J Clin Hypertens 5:291-294, 2003.

95. Sica DA, Gehr TWB, Fernandez A. Risk-benefit ratio of angiotensin receptor blockers versus angiotensin converting enzyme inhibitors in end-stage renal disease. Drug Saf 22:350-359, 2000.

96. Sica DA, Gehr TWB. The pharmacokinetics and pharmacodynamics of angiotensin receptor blockers in end-stage renal disease. J Renin Angio Aldo Sys 3:247-254, 2002.

# Chapter 54

# Ischemic Heart Disease

## George S. Chrysant, Suzanne Oparil

Cardiovascular disease (CVD) continues to be the leading cause of death in the United States, accounting for 946,000 deaths in the year 2000, which represents 39% of all deaths for that year. Many of the 62 million Americans with CVD have both coronary heart disease (CHD) (13 million) and hypertension (50 million). CHD was responsible for 515,000 deaths in the United States in 2000 representing approximately 75% of all CVD deaths that year.[1] Although the burden of CHD, including all forms of angina and myocardial infarction (MI), remains great, there has been a steady decline in CHD death rates since 1950. Between 1970 and 2000, the CHD death rate declined by 51.2%. Acute myocardial infarction accounted for 193,000 deaths in the year 2000. The indirect and direct costs of CHD to the United States are a staggering $111.8 and $58.2 billion, respectively.[1] For hypertension, the indirect and direct costs are $47.2 and $34.4 billion, respectively.[2] Hypertension is a major risk factor for CHD, as well as other forms of target organ damage. It both accelerates the progression of atherosclerotic disease and leads to left ventricular hypertrophy (LVH), which results in a diminished coronary reserve that exacerbates the ischemic effects of obstructive CHD. Through its associated target organ damage, hypertension can contribute to CHD and overall CVD mortality (between 200,000 and 205,000 deaths in 2000).[1]

## EVALUATION OF CORONARY HEART DISEASE AND HYPERTENSION

The first step in evaluating persons with hypertension and CHD is to perform a thorough history and physical examination. This should include evaluation of risk factors and family history. The frequency, intensity, and duration of anginal episodes should be determined with the knowledge that 2% to 4% of the general population will have silent ischemia. Routine laboratory tests, including hemoglobin/hematocrit, potassium, creatinine, calcium, fasting lipid profile, and a urinalysis should be obtained, as recommended by the Seventh Report of the Joint National Committee on Prevention, Detection, Evaluation, and Treatment of High Blood Pressure (JNC 7).[3] An electrocardiogram (ECG) should be performed because of its potential to predict in-hospital complications as well as long-term prognosis in patients with CHD. The most powerful predictor of poor prognosis on the initial ECG is sinus tachycardia. In the setting of an acute coronary syndrome (ACS), the sum of ST deviation (− and +), Q waves, and prolonged QRS duration has been correlated with an increase in mortality.[4,5]

Exercise ECG testing is the initial diagnostic test in patients at intermediate risk for having CHD. However, the ECG may be uninterpretable in individuals with preexcitation, left bundle branch block, pacing rhythm, LVH with >1 mm ST depression, or taking digoxin, and these patients should undergo stress testing with an imaging component. The Duke Treadmill Score gives prognostic information in terms of 4-year survival.[6] The 379 individuals studied with a score of ≥5, had a 4-year survival rate of 99% (low risk). The survival rate was 95% for the 211 persons scoring between −10 and +4 (intermediate risk). The individuals scoring <−10 had a 79% 4-year survival rate (high risk). Thus, a reasonable strategy would be to send high-risk patients for coronary angiography and revascularization if indicated, and to treat low-risk patients with medical therapy. For intermediate-risk patients, clinical judgment with the possibility of a stress imaging test could be used to guide decision making in regard to coronary angiography referral.

Echocardiography is the gold standard for detecting LVH, as well as the mechanical complications of MI, such as free wall rupture, pseudoaneurysm, papillary muscle rupture, and/or ventricular septal defect. Stress echocardiography combined with either exercise or dobutamine is widely used for the noninvasive detection of myocardial ischemia. The sensitivity of stress echocardiography (exercise ~85%, dobutamine ~88%) is lower than comparable nuclear cardiac stress tests; however, the specificity is higher, particularly for dobutamine stress echocardiography (Table 54–1). Dobutamine stress echocardiography is a valuable tool for predicting functional improvement in patients who undergo revascularization procedures.[7,8] Nuclear cardiac imaging with exercise, adenosine/dipyridamole, or dobutamine for stress combined with thallium and/or technetium sestamibi ($^{99m}$Tc) is another widely used noninvasive modality for detecting myocardial ischemia. These tests are usually more sensitive and less specific than stress echocardiography.

Newer modalities such as cardiac magnetic resonance imaging (MRI) and computed tomography (CT) have emerged as future contenders with the current "gold standard" of coronary imaging, conventional coronary angiography with fluoroscopic guidance. Although most of the literature on electron beam CT (EBCT) focuses on its role in coronary artery calcification scoring, some data support its potential use in coronary imaging. EBCT has been shown to identify lesions >50% with reasonable sensitivity (74%-92%) and specificity (79%-100%) compared with invasive coronary angiography.[9,10] Multirow detector CT (MDCT) or spiral CT has also been used with some success to image coronary arteries (Figure 54–1). Approximately 73% of the proximal segments of the coronary arteries can be visualized without significant motion artifacts. Sensitivity and specificity for 4-detector-row MDCT range from 37% to 85% and 76% to 99%, respectively, for the detection of >50% stenoses compared with invasive coronary angiography.[11,12] This is likely to improve with 16-, 32-, and 64-detector-row MDCT. MDCT is currently being evaluated for possible use in the detection of in-stent restenosis.[13] Major problems with EBCT include motion artifacts, breathing artifacts, and limited views of vessels due to heavy calcification. Distal arteries are difficult to visualize with EBCT and MDCT.

**Table 54–1** Sensitivity and Specificity of Noninvasive Tests for the Detection of Coronary Artery Disease

| Diagnostic Test | Sensitivity % (range) | Specificity % (range) | Number of Studies Analyzed | Number of Patients |
|---|---|---|---|---|
| Thallium scintigraphy | 89 | 80 | 2 | 28,751 |
| Exercise echocardiography | 85 | 79 | 58 | 5000 |
| Persantine thallium | 85 | 91 | 11 | <1000 |
| Dobutamine echocardiography | 88 | 84 | 5 | <1009 |

From Poon M, Fuster V, Fayad Z. Cardiac magnetic resonance imaging: A "one-stop-shop" evaluation of myocardial dysfunction. Curr Opin Cardiol 17:663-670, 2002.

MDCT has several drawbacks, including breathing and motion artifacts and a requirement for a high dose of radiation (6-10 mSv per study). Successful studies with MDCT usually require administration of a β-blocker to slow the heart rate to below 70 beats/min. Another problem is that both CT modalities require nephrotoxic contrast agents in the dose range of 125 to 150 ml.

Coronary MRI has been evaluated more extensively than CT angiography (Figure 54–2). Nine studies comparing MRI with invasive coronary angiography in 387 patients have revealed a sensitivity of 77% and a specificity of 71% for stenoses >50%.[9,14,15] The requirement for multiple long breath holds, claustrophobia, breathing and motion artifacts, and the presence of any metal such as a pacemaker, automatic implantable cardioverter defibrillator, aneurysm clips, or metal prostheses limit the ability to perform the test and the success of the test. Intracoronary stents do not appear to be affected in any way by MRI, contrary to the package inserts that accompany the stents. No heating, migration, or subacute thrombosis of the stents during MRI has been reported.[16,17] Both CT and MRI are used in many centers around the world to diagnose CHD; however, they are currently not an alternative to invasive coronary angiography (Table 54–2).

Cardiac MRI is emerging as a viable method for the evaluation and diagnosis of ischemic heart disease. Cardiac chamber structure (left ventricular mass), function (contractile function), flow (shunts), and both myocardial perfusion and myocardial viability can all be examined with cardiac MRI techniques. This makes cardiac MRI a potential "one-stop shop" as Fayad and Fuster have postulated.[8] Detection of infracted tissue by delayed hyperenhancement of contrast agent (gadolinium) has been demonstrated in several teaching centers and appears to be very sensitive. Stress imaging with dobutamine and adenosine has also been demonstrated effectively; however, this discussion is beyond the scope of this chapter.

Coronary angiography is the "gold standard" for coronary imaging. In the 20 years from 1979 to 2000, the number of cardiac catheterizations increased by 341%. More than 2 million of these procedures were performed in 2000 at a cost of $23 billion.[18,19] The overall risk of the procedure is <2%, with only the inability to consent freely being an absolute contraindication if needed urgently or emergently.[20] The guide-

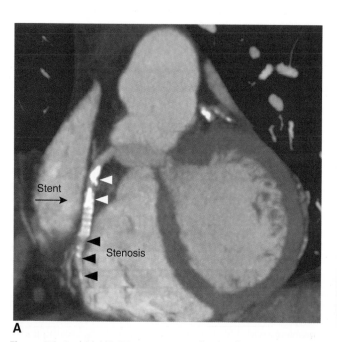

**A**

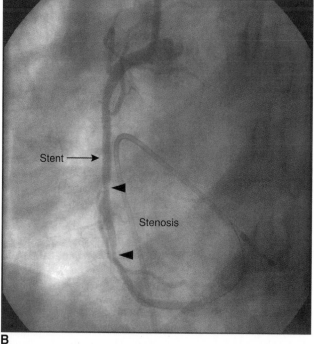

**B**

**Figure 54–1** **(A)** MDCT angiogram of RCA showing the presence of an intracoronary stent and a 50% stenosis. **(B)** X-ray angiogram of RCA of the same patient as in part **A.**

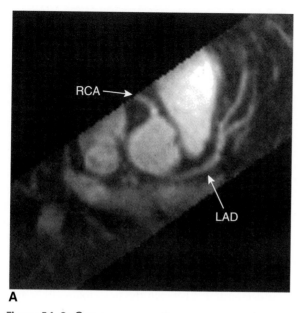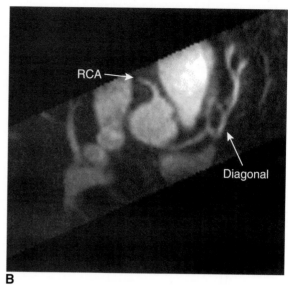

A                            B

**Figure 54–2** Coronary magnetic resonance angiograms of the proximal RCA, LAD, and diagonal arteries

lines for coronary angiography published by the American College of Cardiology are explicit in outlining the indications for performance of the procedure.[21] Coronary angiography requires the injection of nephrotoxic iodinated contrast, which has become increasingly safer over the last several years. There is also exposure to radiation for both the patient and the operator and staff. In spite of these drawbacks, coronary angiography continues to be widely used and is currently the definitive way to image the coronary arterial tree.

## TREATMENT OF CORONARY HEART DISEASE AND HYPERTENSION

### Medical Therapy

#### Chronic Stable Angina and Silent Ischemia

Angina pectoris is characterized as chest discomfort of short duration (minutes) that is usually retrosternal in location and relieved by rest, removal of stress, and/or the administration of nitroglycerin.[22] Approximately 24% of the male and 26% of the female population of the United States have angina pectoris.[1] As many as 40% of those persons with CHD experience

**Table 54– 2** Comparison of Coronary Magnetic Resonance Angiography and Computed Tomography Angiography with Angiography for the Detection of Coronary Artery Disease

| Modality | Subjects | Sensitivity (mean) | Specificity (mean) |
|----------|----------|--------------------|--------------------|
| MRA | 387 | 38-94 (77) | 42-95 (71) |
| EBCT | 583 | 74-92 (87) | 82-100 (91) |
| MDCT | 513 | 37-85 (59) | 76-99 (89) |

MRA, magnetic resonance angiography; EBCT, electron beam computed tomography; MDCT, multi-row detector computed tomography.

silent ischemic episodes (>1-mm ST-segment depression for at least 1 minute on 48-hour Holter monitoring).[23] Silent ischemic episodes have been demonstrated in clinical studies using 24- to 48-hour ambulatory monitoring in persons with known stable angina on antianginal drug regimens.[24] The choice of treatment depends on the underlying pathophysiologic process, concomitant risk factors, and comorbid conditions that could exacerbate anginal symptoms and potentially lead to adverse cardiac events. Treatment of hypertension, correction of lipoprotein abnormalities, and smoking cessation are important aspects of risk factor modification and therapy.[25] All persons with CHD should be taking aspirin in a dose between 81 mg and 325 mg unless contraindicated or an allergy is present. Aspirin is well studied and has a proven mortality benefit, as well as benefit in the prevention of CHD-related events.

Due to the enhanced myocardial oxygen demand created by increases in blood pressure (BP)—systolic BP (SBP) in particular—and heart rate, hypertensive patients with chronic stable angina are at particular risk. A study of 25 patients with known CHD who underwent simultaneous electrocardiographic and ambulatory BP monitoring (ABPM) showed that a majority of silent ischemic episodes were preceded by an average increase in SBP of 10 mm Hg, as well as a significant increase in heart rate.[26] Therefore, persons with both stable angina (with or without silent ischemic episodes) and hypertension derive particular benefit from treatment with β-blockers and calcium channel blockers (CCBs).

The goals of treating patients with CHD and hypertension are to lower BP, relieve angina, reduce ischemia, and prevent future cardiovascular (CV) events (Figure 54–3). First-line therapy should be with a β-blocker without intrinsic sympathomimetic activity unless contraindicated, because these agents are indicated as first-line treatment for both hypertension and CHD. β-Blockers reduce myocardial oxygen consumption and heart rate and help enhance coronary flow. Thus, they are particularly helpful in reducing angina in the hypertensive patient.

If angina continues on β-blocker therapy, then long-acting CCBs can be added to the regimen. CCBs decrease total

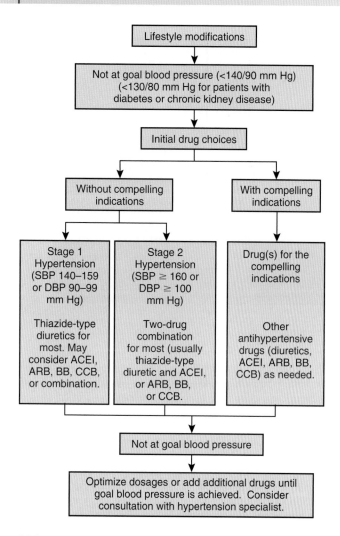

DBP, diastolic blood pressure; SBP, systolic blood pressure.

Drug abbreviations: ACEI, angiotensin-converting enzyme inhibitor; ARB, angiotensin receptor blocker; BB, β-blocker; CCB, calcium channel blocker.

**Figure 54–3** JNC 7 algorithm for the treatment of hypertension.

peripheral resistance, which leads to decreases in BP and in wall tension, thus reducing myocardial $O_2$ consumption. CCBs also decrease coronary resistance (helpful in relieving spasm, which may be associated with Prinzmetal's angina) and enhance poststenotic coronary perfusion, which increases myocardial $O_2$ supply. Nondihydropyridine CCBs have the additional benefit of decreasing heart rate. Short-acting dihydropyridine CCBs should be avoided due to increased mortality, particularly in the setting of acute MI.[27] Although nondihydropyridine CCBs can be used as antianginals in combination with a β-blocker, there is associated risk due to the potential for severe bradycardia and/or heart block. Long-acting dihydropyridine CCBs are effective antianginal agents and do not share the disadvantage of bradycardia/heart block. Therefore, if a CCB is needed in addition to a β-blocker to control angina in a hypertensive patient, it should be a long-acting dihydropyridine CCB. If angina is still not controlled on this two-drug regimen, nitrates can be added.[28]

The use of angiotensin-converting enzyme (ACE) inhibitors as antiischemic therapy continues to be controversial. More than 20 studies have examined whether these agents are or are not useful in preventing ischemia, but only two of these included large groups of patients. In the Perindopril Therapeutic Safety Collaborative Research Group study, 490 hypertensive patients with CVD and/or risk factors for CVD were randomized to treatment with an ACE inhibitor (perindopril) or placebo. Persons in the perindopril group had significantly less ST depression during maximal treadmill exercise testing and fewer anginal episodes ($p < .05$ for both anginal episodes and maximal ST depression).[29] The quinapril antiischemia and symptoms of angina reduction (QUASAR) trial was a study of 336 patients with stable CHD who were randomized to an ACE inhibitor (quinapril) or placebo. Approximately half of the study population had medically treated hypertension, and all were examined for ischemic events with treadmill testing, ambulatory ECG monitoring, and the Seattle Angina Questionnaire. No significant difference was demonstrated between the two groups either at 8 or 16 weeks.[30] Based on currently available evidence, the use of ACE inhibitors as antiischemic/antianginal agents is not indicated.

### Acute Coronary Syndromes: Unstable Angina, Non-ST-Elevation Myocardial Infarction, and ST-Elevation Myocardial Infarction

In the setting of an acute coronary syndrome (ACS), the goal of therapy is to pacify the unstable coronary plaque, relieve anginal pain, control BP and heart rate, and assist in the restoration of flow in the coronary arterial system. All patients with an ACS should immediately receive a crushed aspirin, oxygen, and an intravenous β-blocker (unless contraindicated). If the ACS is an ST-elevation acute MI in a setting where primary percutaneous coronary intervention cannot occur within 1 to 2 hours, reperfusion therapy with thrombolytics is indicated; otherwise, primary percutaneous coronary intervention should be performed (Figure 54–4).[31] Intravenous heparin should also be administered. If BP is appropriate and right ventricular infarction has been ruled out, intravenous nitroglycerin and narcotic agents can be given safely. If the ACS is unstable angina/non-ST-elevation MI, and certain features such as dynamic ECG changes, positive cardiac biomarkers, and/or uncontrolled pain are present, the use of a GP IIb/IIIa agent (either enoxaparin or tirofiban, not abciximab) is indicated[32,33] (Figure 54–5). The Thrombolysis in Myocardial Infarction (TIMI) risk score has been used to guide therapy and to predict future events and outcomes.[34] CV events increase dramatically with each increment in the TIMI Risk Score.

β-Blockers (nonintrinsic sympathomimetic activity) are first-line agents for both acute MI and hypertension (Figure 54–6). They help limit infarct size, decrease the risk of recurrent MI, improve survival, and decrease the incidence of sudden cardiac death secondary to fatal arrythmias.[35-39] Patients should receive early intravenous β-blocker therapy (metoprolol 5 mg every 5 minutes for three doses) within 12 hours of onset of the event, followed by an oral β-blocker (within the first 2 days) unless contraindicated (e.g., by bradycardia, bronchospasm, or hypotension). Both intravenous and oral β-blockers during and after acute MI have been studied extensively and have been proven to reduce mortality and the incidence of reinfarction.[31] The choice of agent, and the short-

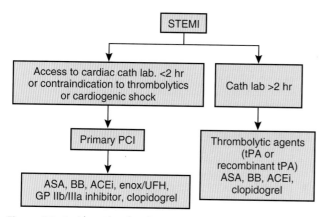

**Figure 54–4** Algorithm for the management of patients with ST-segment elevation myocardial infarction.

and long-term dosing goal, have varied substantially in clinical trials. In general, the dose of β-blocker should be that which achieves adequate reduction in heart rate and BP while still being tolerated by the patient.

The Carvedilol Post-Infarct Survival Control in Left Ventricular (LV) Dysfunction (CAPRICORN) trial, carried out in 1959 post-MI patients with LV dysfunction, is the first study to demonstrate the beneficial effects of β-blockers post-MI in the postreperfusion era, and in patients with LV dysfunction (a population excluded from prior β-blocker trials in acute MI).[40] All participants had a proven MI and LV ejection fraction (LVEF) ≤40%, and >50% had hypertension. After a mean follow-up of 1.3 years, all-cause mortality ($p$ = .031), CVD mortality ($p$ = .024), nonfatal MI ($p$ = .014), and all-cause mortality or nonfatal MI ($p$ = .002) were lower in the carvedilol group than in the placebo (usual therapy) group. The 23% observed reduction in mortality was in addition to ACE inhibitor (prescribed in 98% of participants) and reperfusion (prescribed in 46%) therapies.

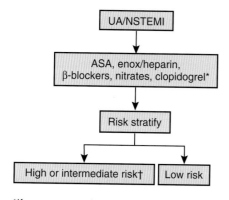

*If coronary arteriography >24 hours.

†Recurrent ischemia; ↑ Trop; ↓ ST; LV failure/dysf.;
hemodynamic instability; VT; prior CABG.

**Figure 54–5** Algorithm for the management of patients with unstable angina or non-ST-segment myocardial infarction. (From Braunwald E. Application of current guidelines to the management of unstable angina and non-ST-elevation myocardial infarction. Circulation 108:III28-III37, 2003.)

CCBs can be used for acute MI in situations in which β-blocker therapy is inadequately controlling angina, BP, and/or heart rate (e.g., supraventricular tachycardia), or if β-blockers are poorly tolerated or contraindicated. In the setting of unstable angina and concomitant β-blocker use, long-acting dihydropyridine CCBs are preferred over nondihydropyridine CCBs due to the possibility of excessive bradycardia or heart block associated with the latter agents. Short-acting dihydropyridine CCBs should be avoided in patients with acute MI, pulmonary edema, or LV dysfunction.[40a-43] Several trials have demonstrated that these agents increase mortality and the rate of reinfarction. Specifically, compared with patients treated with other antihypertensive agents (diuretics and β-blockers), hypertensive patients treated with short-acting CCBs have been shown to have a 60% higher risk of MI.[27]

Randomized trials of nondihydropyridine CCBs (verapamil and diltiazem) in patients with acute MI have shown benefit in preventing CVD events, but no significant influence on overall mortality. In the Danish Verapamil Infarction Trial II, verapamil use was associated with a 20% ($p$ = .03) reduction in first major CVD event (death and reinfarction).[44] In a meta-analysis of 28 randomized trials in approximately 19,000 post-MI patients, verapamil use resulted in a significant 19% decrease in reinfarction (relative risk, 0.81; 95% confidence interval, 0.67-0.98).[45] However, in these and other trials, no significant decrease in mortality has been shown. A large trial of diltiazem therapy (the Multicenter Diltiazem Postinfarction Trial [MDPIT]) demonstrated no reduction in mortality or reinfarction.[46] In patients with depressed LV function and/or pulmonary edema, diltiazem use was associated with a 41% increase in CVD events (death from a cardiac cause and nonfatal MI). Therefore, CCBs are not recommended in the setting of acute MI except in situations in which β-blockers are poorly tolerated or inadequate to control concomitant conditions (e.g., BP, angina, or supraventricular tachycardia).[32]

ACE inhibitors are indicated in all patients with acute MI who can tolerate them. In a hemodynamically stable (SBP ≥90-100 mm Hg) patient post-MI, an oral ACE inhibitor should be initiated, generally within 24 hours of onset of the event, particularly if the infarct is anterior and associated with depressed LV function (LVEF <40% ) and/or heart failure.[47-50] Creatinine and electrolytes should be checked prior to initiation of ACE inhibitor therapy and periodically until the highest tolerated dose of the agent has been given and the patient has shown stable renal function. Use of ACE inhibitors after acute MI has led to significant reductions in mortality.[51-53] The large clinical trials have shown that the greatest benefit occurs in patients who are at highest risk (Killip class 2 or 3, heart rate ≥100 beats/min). The hemodynamic effects and overall benefit of ACE inhibition are seen early. Approximately 40% of the 30-day increase in survival is observed in days 0 to 1, 45% in days 2 to 7, and approximately 15% after day 7.[47,50] These findings help support the current recommendation that ACE inhibitors should be initiated routinely after acute MI and continued for an indefinite period.[32]

Angiotensin receptor blockers (ARBs) have been proven to be effective as antihypertensive agents for both hypertension and heart failure and are now used in persons who are ACE inhibitor intolerant or allergic. Emerging data appear to support the use of ARBs in MI. The ARB valsartan was compared with the ACE inhibitor captopril in the (VALIANT) trial, a double-blind trial in which patients were randomized to

| Compelling indication* | Recommended drugs† | | | | | | Clinical trial basis‡ |
|---|---|---|---|---|---|---|---|
| | Diuretic | BB | ACEI | ARB | CCB | AldoANT | |
| Heart failure | ● | ● | ● | ● | | ● | ACC/AHA Heart Failure Guideline,[40] MERIT-HF,[41] COPERNICUS,[42] CIBIS,[43] SOLVD,[44] AIRE,[45] TRACE,[46] ValHEFT,[47] RALES[48] |
| Postmyocardial infarction | | ● | ● | | | ● | ACC/AHA Post-MI Guideline,[49] BHAT,[50] SAVE,[51] Capricorn,[52] EPHESUS[53] |
| High coronary disease risk | ● | ● | ● | | ● | | ALLHAT,[33] HOPE,[34] ANBP2,[36] LIFE,[32] CONVINCE[31] |
| Diabetes | ● | ● | ● | ● | ● | | NKF-ADA Guideline,[21,22] UKPDS,[54] ALLHAT[33] |
| Chronic kidney disease | | | ● | ● | | | NKF Guideline,[22] Captopril Trial,[55] RENAAL,[56] IDNT,[57] REIN,[58] AASK[59] |
| Recurrent stroke prevention | ● | | ● | | | | PROGRESS[35] |

\* Compelling indications for antihypertensive drugs are based on benefits from outcome studies or existing clinical guidelines; the compelling indication is managed in parallel with the BP.

† Drug abbreviations: ACEI, angiotensin-converting enzyme inhibitor; ARB, angiotensin receptor blocker; AldoANT, aldosterone antagonist; BB, β-blocker; CCB, calcium channel blocker.

‡ Conditions for which clinical trials demonstrate benefit of specific classes of antihypertensive drugs.

**Figure 54–6** JNC 7 recommendations for the initial drug choice for hypertensive persons with compelling indications.

valsartan (4909 patients), valsartan plus captopril (4885 patients), or captopril (4909 patients).[54] During the 2-year follow-up, 979 patients in the valsartan group died compared with 941 in the combination group and 958 in the captopril group. There was no statistically significant difference in the primary endpoint of death from any cause, and valsartan was shown to have noninferiority compared with captopril in regard to mortality ($p = .004$). The combination group had the most drug-related adverse events and did not show improved survival.

Aldosterone receptor antagonists have been proven to reduce mortality and morbidity in patients with severe heart failure who are already on ACE inhibitor therapy. Aldosterone blockade is believed to prevent ventricular remodeling and collagen formation in the ventricles of persons with severe LV dysfunction.[55] A large randomized, double-blind, controlled trial comparing eplerenone (a newer and more selective aldosterone antagonist) with placebo (conventional therapy) in 6632 patients who were less than 2 weeks from an MI complicated by LV dysfunction demonstrated a mortality and morbidity reduction in favor of eplerenone.[56] Total deaths, deaths from a CV cause, and the combined endpoint of CV death or hospitalization for CV illness were all significantly lower in the eplerenone group ($p = .008$, $p = .005$, $p = .002$, respectively). Hypertensive patients ($p = .05$) and those with a widened pulse pressure ($p = .01$) experienced a significant benefit. This important study has led to the U.S. Food and Drug Administration's approval of this novel agent for use as

an alternative to conventional therapy in the setting of acute MI with LV dysfunction.

### Other General Considerations

#### Antiplatelet Therapy

Antiplatelet therapy is a mainstay of medical therapy for CHD and ACS regardless of whether or not an invasive strategy is planned. Multiple studies have proven the benefit of aspirin, a cyclooxygenase-1 inhibitor. The most striking data supporting the use of aspirin come from the Second International Study of Infarct Survival (ISIS-2) trial in which aspirin and streptokinase, a thrombolytic agent, were found to independently equally reduce mortality (9.2% for streptokinase, 9.4% for aspirin).[57] Thienopyridine therapy has also become a mainstay of therapy, particularly in those patients who go on to percutaneous coronary intervention (PCI) with coronary stenting. Ticlopidine and clopidogrel are equally effective, but clopidogrel is better tolerated and exhibits a more favorable side effect profile.[58] The Clopidogrel in Unstable Angina to Prevent Recurrent Events (CURE) and Clopidogrel for the Reduction of Events During Observation (CREDO) trials have provided convincing evidence of benefit from clopidogrel treatment in preventing CVD events in the setting of ACS, coronary artery bypass grafting (CABG), or PCI (Figure 54–7).[59-61] The length of clopidogrel treatment and the decision of when to start the drug remain controversial. If the coronary anatomy is unknown, there is a risk that

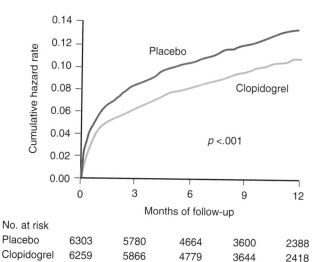

**Figure 54–7** Cumulative hazard rates for the first primary outcome of cardiovascular death, nonfatal myocardial infarction, or stroke during the 12 months of the CURE trial. (From Yusuf S, Zhao F, Mehta SR, et al. Effects of clopidogrel in addition to aspirin in patients with acute coronary syndromes without ST-segment elevation. N Engl J Med 345:494-502, 2001.)

urgent CABG may be needed and will have to be delayed due to clopidogrel use. Therefore, it is recommended that clopidogrel be administered to patients with ACS in combination with aspirin unless the patient has undefined coronary anatomy and/or is at risk of excess bleeding.[32,33]

### Low-Molecular-Weight Heparin and Glycoprotein IIb/IIIa Receptor Antagonists

Low-molecular-weight heparin (LMWH) has been shown to be more effective than unfractionated heparin (UFH) in ACS because it has a higher anti-Xa:IIa ratio than UFH and is very predictable and easy to use.[62-64] The Efficacy and Safety of Subcutaneous Enoxaparin in Unstable Angina and Non-Q-Wave MI (ESSENCE) trial compared the LMWH enoxaparin with UFH in 3000 patients with ACS.[62] Outcome (death, MI, repeat revascularization) rates were significantly lower for enoxaparin at 14 and 30 days.

A higher risk group of 3910 patients (ST-segment depression, positive cardiac enzymes) with ACS was randomized to enoxaparin or UFH in the TIMI 11B trial.[63] The primary endpoint of death, MI, recurrent ischemia, and need for revascularization was significantly reduced by enoxaparin treatment. A subsequent meta-analysis of ESSENCE and TIMI 11B showed an advantage for enoxaparin over several time points up to 43 days.[64] A meta-analysis of clinical trials involving 13,320 patients with non-ST-elevation ACS comparing LMWH and UFH demonstrated no significant differences in either efficacy or safety.[65]

A presumed advantage of LMWH is a reduction in the "rebound" phenomenon that was associated with abrupt cessation of UFH. An increase in CV events presumed to be due to increased platelet adhesion has been shown in the first 24 to 48 hours after UFH has been stopped. However, it appears that cardiac ischemic events occur within 24 hours of LMWH cessation, as well. This was demonstrated in an analysis of the TIMI 11B and ESSENCE trials.[66] Groups receiving UFH and

short-term enoxaparin (≤8 days) were compared with a group that received long-term enoxaparin (43 days). The long-term LMWH group had significantly fewer ischemic events following cessation compared with the UFH group (*p* <.0001) and the short-term enoxaparin group (*p* <.0003). LMWH is recommended by the ACC/AHA guidelines for use in unstable angina, non-ST-elevation MI, and acute MI. UFH may also be used. In the setting of PCI, LMWH and UFH can be used safely and effectively.

The use of platelet glycoprotein IIb/IIIa inhibitors in unstable angina/non-ST-elevation MI is controversial. Persons who are going to be treated with an early invasive strategy and who have positive cardiac enzymes and/or ECG changes benefit the most from the use of these agents. In a meta-analysis of more than 30,000 patients with unstable angina or non-ST-elevation MI, the 5847 patients who underwent early invasive management with revascularization had a 21% reduction in death or MI when treated with these agents. The 25,000+ patients who did not undergo an early invasive procedure had only a 3% reduction in death or MI with glycoprotein IIb/IIIa inhibitor treatment.[67] The ACC/AHA guidelines support the use of glycoprotein IIb/IIIa inhibitors in high-risk patients (particularly troponin positive) who are likely to have early angiography.

### HMG-CoA Reductase Inhibitors

All patients with an ACS should be discharged on an hydroxymethyl glutaryl-coenzyme A (HMG-CoA) reductase inhibitor (i.e., statin) because this class of medications has been shown to decrease CHD events and mortality.[68-70] Current National Cholesterol Education Program (NCEP) guidelines specify a goal LDL level in patients with known CHD of <100 mg/dl. A great number of patients will require pharmacologic intervention to achieve this goal.[71] Above and beyond LDL lowering, studies are now demonstrating positive effects of statins on endothelial function, oxidative stress, and biomarkers of inflammation.[72-74] Statin therapy has been shown in trials to significantly lower levels of C-reactive protein, in association with a significant reduction in CVD event rates.[75,76]

### Invasive Therapy

In patients presenting with ACS, there is now ample evidence to support an early invasive strategy whereby individuals are taken to the cardiac catheterization laboratory for coronary angiography within the first 24 to 48 hours, followed by revascularization as dictated by the anatomy. Prior to the "stent era," prospective randomized trials showed no benefit from an early invasive strategy compared with early conservative therapy.[77,78] Both TIMI IIIB and the Veterans Affairs non–Q-wave infarction strategies in hospital (VANQWISH) trial showed no significant difference between the two strategies.

"Stent-era" trials including the Fragmin and Fast Revascularization During Instability in Coronary Artery Disease (FRISC) II trial, the Randomized Intervention Trial of Unstable Angina (RITA) III trial, and the Treat Angina with Aggrastat and Determine Cost of Therapy with an Invasive or Conservative Strategy—Thrombolysis in Myocardial Infarction (TACTICS-TIMI) 18 trial, showed benefit (reduction in death or MI) at 4 to 12 months of follow-up in patients randomized to an early invasive strategy.[79-81] These studies support an early invasive strategy for all patients with ACS who do not have a contraindication to cardiac catheterization (Figure 54–8). Adjunctive therapy to PCI after diagnostic angiography includes several proven

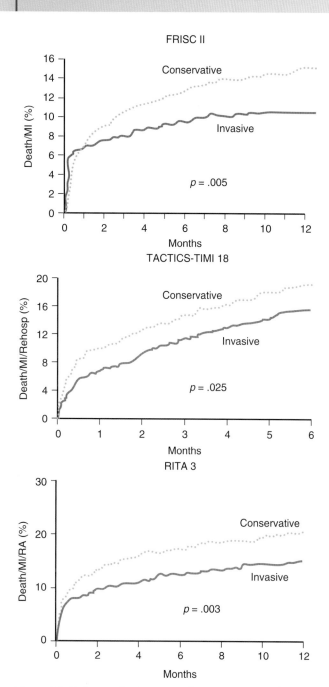

**Figure 54–8** Rates of adverse cardiac events according to assignment to either a conservative strategy or an early invasive strategy over time (6-12 months) in the FRISC II study, the TACTICS-TIMI 18 trial, or the RITA 3 trial. (From Wallentin L, Lagerqvist B, Husted S, et al. Outcome at 1 year after an invasive compared with a noninvasive strategy in unstable coronary artery disease: The FRISC II invasive randomized trial. Lancet 356:9-16, 2000; Cannon CP, Weintraub WS, Demopoulos LA, et al. Comparison of early invasive and conservative strategies in patients with unstable coronary syndromes treated with the glycoprotein IIb/IIIa inhibitor tirofiban. N Engl J Med 344:1879-1887, 2001; and Fox KAA, Poole-Wilson PA, Henderson RA, et al. Interventional versus conservative treatment for patients with unstable angina or non-ST-elevation myocardial infarction: The British Heart Foundation RITA 3 randomized trial. Lancet 360:743-71, 2002.)

pharmacologic agents. However, a formal discussion of the pros and cons of using GP IIb/IIIa inhibitors, LMWH, or bivalirudin in their setting is very controversial and beyond the scope of this chapter.

### Percutaneous Coronary Intervention versus Coronary Artery Bypass Grafting

Limited clinical trial data support the use of multivessel stenting as an alternative to CABG in patients with multivessel CHD[82-84] (Table 54-3). With the emergence of drug-eluting stent technology, the higher rates of revascularization in the PCI groups will decrease, making multivessel stenting an even more attractive alternative to CABG. In the setting of acute MI, only the "culprit" vessel should undergo PCI. According to ACC/AHA guidelines, intervening on a "nonculprit" vessel in the setting of acute MI is a class III indication.[85]

### Drug-Eluting Stents

Drug-eluting stents such as the sirolimus-eluting Cypher stent and the paclitaxel-eluting Taxus stent have revolutionized PCI by keeping in-stent restenosis in the single digits; thus, helping to eliminate PCI's Achilles heel, the need for repeat intervention and target vessel revascularization (Figure 54–9). Studies involving the sirolimus-eluting stent have demonstrated mortality rates <2%, target vessel revascularization rates of <9%, and in-stent restenosis rates <3% at 6 months.[86,87] At 2 years, the in-stent lumen assessed with intravascular ultrasound has remained essentially unchanged in a group of 30 patients with sirolimus-eluting stents.[88] Similarly, rates of restenosis (0% at 6 months), target vessel revascularization (3% at 6 months), and major adverse cardiac events such as death and MI (0% at 12 months) for the paclitaxel-eluting stent have been very low.[89] In the setting of acute MI, the sirolimus-eluting stent was shown to be safe in 96 patients enrolled over 6 months.[90] At 300 days post-MI, sirolimus-eluting stents have had lower overall adverse event rates compared with bare stents without an increase in subacute stent thrombosis.[91] Now that the "stent era" has developed into "the drug-eluting stent era," it is likely that PCI will become an option for even more patients previously thought to require CABG (Figure 54–10).

## HYPERTENSION AND PERIPHERAL VASCULAR DISEASE

Persons with symptomatic peripheral vascular disease (PVD) have a 15-fold increased rate of mortality from CVD and a high rate of concomitant coronary artery disease and/or cerebrovascular disease.[92] Hypertension, diabetes, and smoking are major risk factors for PVD. CHD and renovascular disease often occur together, with as many as 28% of hypertensive patients undergoing cardiac catheterization having renal artery disease. Therefore, the threshold for noninvasive screening for both disease processes in these persons should be low[93] (Table 54-4).

Relatively little attention has been devoted to PVD as an endpoint in controlled trials of antihypertensive therapy, and the sparse data that are available are disappointing. For example, in the United Kingdom Prospective Diabetes Study Group (UKPDS) trial, tight BP control (mean achieved BP = 144/82 mm Hg vs. 154/87 mm Hg in the less tight control group) in patients with hypertension and diabetes led to

**Table 54–3** Comparison of Coronary Artery Bypass Grafting with Multivessel Stenting

| Trial | CABG | MVS Mortality | CABG TVR Mortality | MVS TVR |
|-------|------|---------------|--------------------|---------|
| ERACI I/II | 4.7-7.5% | 3.1-4.7% | 4.8-6.3%* | 16.8-37% |
| ARTS | 10.8% | 10.2% | 4.8%† | 19.7% |
| SoS | 9% | 10% | 6%‡ | 21% |

*p <.002; †p <.001; ‡p <.0001.
CABG, coronary artery bypass grafting; MVS, multivessel stenting; TVR, target vessel revascularization.

significant reductions in risk of death ($p = .019$) and in complications related to diabetes ($p = .005$), stroke ($p = .013$), and microvascular disease ($p = .009$), but no significant decrease in PVD risk ($p = .17$).[94]

Antihypertensive drug treatment is also ineffective in relieving symptoms of PVD. Vasodilator agents such as ACE inhibitors, CCBs, α-adrenergic blockers, and direct vasodilators have not been shown to improve walking distance or symptoms of claudication in patients with PVD.[95-97] Whether this is due to the inability of diseased vessels to dilate further because they are maximally dilated during exercise, to a "steal" phenomenon, and/or to the possibility that systemic BP reduction decreases forward blood flow due to a loss of "driving" pressure is unknown. β-Blockers are generally thought to precipitate peripheral vasoconstriction and increase the frequency of intermittent claudication, and thus to be relatively contraindicated in patients with PVD. However, studies have shown that β-blockers do not reduce walking distance or calf blood flow in patients with intermittent claudication due to PVD.[98] Thus, if needed for CHD, β-blockers can be used in these patients.

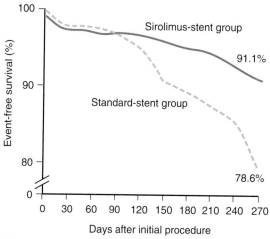

**Figure 54–10** Actuarial rate of survival free from target vessel failure among patients receiving either a sirolimus-eluting stent or a bare metal stent. (From Moses JW, Leon MB, Popma JJ, et al., for SIRIUS Investigators. Sirolimus-eluting stents versus standard stents in patients with stenosis in a native coronary artery. N Engl J Med 349:1315-1323, 2003.)

Because no class of antihypertensive medications offers particular benefits to the patient with PVD, treatment choices should be made based on concomitant conditions (CHD, diabetes, heart failure). In patients with PVD and no concomitant condition, a thiazide diuretic is the agent of first choice, followed by a β-blockers. If CHD is present, a β-blocker should be the first choice, followed by a thiazide diuretic. In patients with CHD, diabetes and/or heart failure, ACE inhibitor therapy is indicated. Renovascular disease should be excluded in this high-risk population before initiation of ACE inhibitor treatment. If the aforementioned agents fail to control BP and/or are poorly tolerated, or if the patient has Raynaud's phenomenon, CCBs (preferably nondihydropyridine CCBs) can be used.[99]

**Table 54–4** Percentage of Patients with Coronary Artery Disease or Peripheral Vascular Disease Who Have Atherosclerotic Renal Artery Disease

| Patients | ARAD |
|----------|------|
| PVD | 45-59% |
| Aortoiliac | 28-38% |
| CAD | 15-28% |

From Schreiber MJ, Pohl MA, Novick AC. The natural history of atherosclerotic and fibrous renal artery disease. Urol Clin North Am 11:383-392, 1984; and Aqel RA, Zoghbi GJ, Baldwin SA, et al. Prevalence of renal artery stenosis in high-risk veterans referred to cardiac catheterization. J Hypertens 21:1157-1162, 2003.
ARAD, atherosclerotic renal artery stenosis; PVD, peripheral vascular disease; CAD, coronary artery disease.

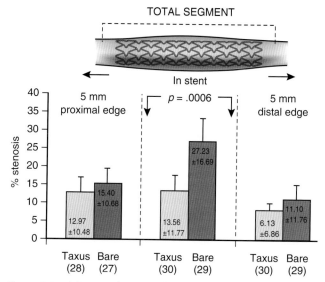

**Figure 54–9** Six-month stent edge analysis: % diameter stenosis. (From Grube Silber S, Hauptmann KE, et al. TAXUS-1: Six- and twelve-month results from a randomized double-blind trial on a slow-release paclitaxel-eluting stent for de novo coronary lesions. Circulation 107:38-42, 2003.).

# References

1. National Institutes of Health, National Heart, Lung, and Blood Institute. Morbidity and Mortality: 2002 Chart Book on Cardiovascular, Lung, and Blood Diseases. Bethesda. MD, National Institutes of Health, National Heart, Lung, and Blood Institute, May 2002.

2. National Institutes of Health, National Heart, Lung, and Blood Institute. Morbidity and Mortality: 2002 Fact Book Fiscal Year 2002. Bethesda, MD, National Institutes of Health, National Heart, Lung, and Blood Institute, February 2003.

3. Chobanian AV, Bakris GL, Black HR, et al. The Seventh Report of the Joint National Committee on Prevention, Detection, Evaluation, and Treatment of High Blood Pressure: The JNC 7 report. JAMA 289:2560-2572, 2003.

4. Hathaway WR, Peterson ED, Wagner GS, et al. Prognostic significance of the initial electrocardiogram in patients with acute myocardial infarction. JAMA 279:387, 1998.

5. Schroder R, Dissmann R, Bruggeman, et al. Extent of early ST segment resolution: A simple but strong predictor of outcome in patients with acute myocardial infarction. J Am Coll Cardiol 24:384, 1994.

6. Mark DB, Shaw L, Harrell FE, et al. Prognostic value of a treadmill exercise score in outpatients with suspected coronary artery disease. N Engl J Med 325:849-853, 1991.

7. Bax JJ, Wijns W, Cornel JH, et al. Accuracy of currently available techniques for prediction of functional recovery after revascularization in patients with left ventricular dysfunction due to chronic coronary artery disease: Comparison of pooled data. J Am Coll Cardiol 30:1451-1460, 1997.

8. Poon M, Fuster V, Fayad Z. Cardiac magnetic resonance imaging: A "one-stop-shop" evaluation of myocardial dysfunction. Curr Opin Cardiol 17:663-670, 2002.

9. Budoff MJ, Achenbach S, Duerinckx A. Clinical utility of computed tomography and magnetic resonance techniques for noninvasive coronary angiography. J Am Coll Cardiol 42:1867-1878, 2003.

10. Moshage WE, Achenbach S, Seese B, et al. Coronary artery stenosis: Three-dimensional imaging with electrocardiographically triggered contrast agent enhanced, electron beam CT. Radiology 196:707-714, 1995.

11. Ropers D, Baum U, Pohle K, et al. Detection of coronary artery stenoses with thin-slice multi-detector row spiral computed tomography and multiplanar reconstruction. Circulation 107:664-666, 2003.

12. Nieman K, Cademartiri F, Lemos PA, et al. Reliable noninvasive coronary angiography with fast submillimeter multislice spiral computed tomography. Circulation 106:2051-2054, 2002.

13. Hong C, Chrysant GS, Woodard PK, et al. Coronary artery stent patency assessed with in-stent contrast enhancement measurement in multi-detector row CT angiography. Radiology 233(1):286-291, 2004.

14. Hutter A, Kedan I, Srokowski TP, et al. Coronary magnetic resonance angiography. Semin Roentgenol 38:330-341, 2003.

15. Fayad ZA, Fuster V, Nikolaou K, et al. Computed tomography and magnetic resonance imaging for noninvasive coronary angiography and plaque imaging. Circulation 106:2026-2034, 2002.

16. Gerber TC, Fasseas P, Lennon RJ, et al. Clinical safety of magnetic resonance imaging early after coronary artery stent placement. J Am Coll Cardiol 42:1295-1298, 2003.

17. Nagel E, Thouet T, Klein C, et al. Noninvasive determination of coronary blood flow velocity with cardiovascular magnetic resonance in patients after stent deployment. Circulation 107:1738-1743, 2003.

18. American Heart Association. Heart and Stroke Facts: 2003 Statistics Supplement. Dallas, American Heart Association, 2003; pp 1-46.

19. Agency for Healthcare Research and Quality, Department of Health and Human Services. Available at www.AHRQ.gov/data. Accessed December 12, 2003.

20. Baim DS, Grossman W. Complications of cardiac catheterization. In Baim DS, Grossman W (eds). Grossman's Cardiac Catheterization, Angiography & Intervention, 6th ed. Philadelphia, Lippincott, Williams & Wilkins, 2000; pp 35-68.

21. Bashore TM, Bates ER, Berger PB, et al. American College of Cardiology/Society for Cardiac Angiography and Interventions Clinical Expert Consensus Document on Cardiac Catheterization Laboratory standards. J Am Coll Cardiol 37:2170-2214, 2001.

22. Gersh BJ, Braunwald E, Bonow RO. Chronic coronary artery disease. In Braunwald E (ed). Heart Disease: A Textbook of Cardiovascular Medicine, 6th ed. Philadelphia, WB Saunders Company, 2001; pp 1272-1352.

23. Deedwania PC, Carbajal EV. Role of beta blockade in the treatment of myocardial ischemia. Am J Cardiol 80:23J-28J, 1997.

24. Deedwania PC, Carbajal EV. Prevalence and patterns of silent myocardial ischemia during daily life in stable angina patients receiving conventional anti-anginal drug therapy. Am J Cardiol 65:1090-1096, 1990.

25. Gibbons RJ, Chatterjee K, Daley J, et al. ACC/AHA/ACP-ASIM guidelines for the management of patients with chronic stable angina: Executive summary and recommendations. Circulation 99:2829-2848, 1999.

26. Deedwania PC, Nelson JR. Pathophysiology of silent myocardial ischemia during daily life. Hemodynamic evaluation by simultaneous electrocardiographic and blood pressure monitoring. Circulation 82:1296-1304, 1990.

27. Psaty BM, Heckbert SR, Koepsell TD, et al. The risk of myocardial infarction associated with antihypertensive drug therapies. JAMA 274:620-625, 1995.

28. Chrysant GS, Oparil S. Treatment of hypertension in the patient with cardiovascular disease. In Antman EM (ed). Cardiovascular Therapeutics: A Companion to Braunwald's Heart Disease. Philadelphia, WB Saunders, 2002; pp 768-796.

29. Overlack A, Adamczak M, Bachmann W, et al. ACE-inhibition with perindopril in essential hypertensive patients with concomitant diseases. Am J Med 97:126-134, 1994.

30. Pepine CJ, Rouleau JL, Annis K, et al. Effects of angiotensin-converting enzyme inhibition on transient ischemia. J Am Coll Cardiol 42:2049-2059, 2003.

31. Ryan TJ, Antman EM, Brooks NH, et al. 1999: Update: ACC/AHA guidelines for the management of patients with acute myocardial infarction. J Am Coll Cardiol 34:890-911, 1999.

32. Braunwald E, Antman EM, Beasley JW, et al. ACC/AHA guidelines for the management of patients with unstable angina/non-ST segment elevation myocardial infarction. A report of the American College of Cardiology/American Heart Association Task Force on Practice Guidelines (Committee on the Management of Patients with Unstable Angina). J Am Coll Cardiol 36:970-1062, 2000.

33. Braunwald E. Application of current guidelines to the management of unstable angina and non-ST elevation myocardial infarction. Circulation 108:III28-III37, 2003.

34. Antman EM, Cohen M, Bernink PJLM, et al. The TIMI risk score for unstable angina/non-ST elevation myocardial infarction: A method for prognostication and therapeutic decision making. JAMA 284:835-842, 2000.

35. Goldstein S. β-Blockers in hypertensive and coronary heart disease. Arch Intern Med 156:1267-1276, 1996.

36. Frishman WH, Cheng A. Secondary prevention of myocardial infarction: Role of β-adrenergic blockers and angiotensin-converting enzyme inhibitors. Am Heart J 137:S25-S34, 1999.

37. Viskin S, Kitzis I, Lev E, et al. Treatment with beta-adrenergic blocking agents after myocardial infarction: From randomized trial to clinical practice. J Am Coll Cardiol 25:1327-1332, 1995.

38. Yusuf S, Peto R, Lewis J, et al. Beta blockade during and after myocardial infarction: An overview of the randomized trials. Prog Cardiovasc Dis 27:337-371, 1985.

39. Randomised trial of intravenous atenolol among 16,027 cases of suspected acute myocardial infarction: ISIS-1. First international study of Infarct Survival Collaborative Group. Lancet 2:57-66, 1986.

40. Dargie HJ. Effect of carvedilol on outcome after myocardial infarction in patients with left ventricular dysfunction: The CAPRICORN randomised trial. Lancet 357:1385-1390, 2001.

40a. Furberg C, Psaty BM, Meyer JV. Ni fedipine. Dose-related increase in mortality in patients with coronary heart disease. Circulation 92(5):1326-1331, 1995.

41. Hennekens CH, Albert CM, Godfried SL, et al. Adjunctive drug therapy of acute myocardial infarction: Evidence from clinical trials. N Engl J Med 335:1660-1667, 1996.

42. Hager WD, Davis BR, Riba A, et al. Absence of a deleterious effect of calcium channel blockers in patients with left ventricular dysfunction after myocardial infarction: The SAVE study experience. Am Heart J 135:406-413, 1998.

43. Alderman MH, Cohen H, Roque R, et al. Effect of long-acting and short-acting calcium antagonists on cardiovascular outcomes in hypertensive patients. Lancet 349:594-598, 1997.

44. The Danish Study Group on Verapamil in Myocardial Infarction. Effect of verapamil on mortality and major events after acute myocardial infarction (the Danish Verapamil Infarction Trial II (DAVIT II). Am J Cardiol 66:779-785, 1990.

45. Yusuf S. Verapamil following uncomplicated myocardial infarction: Promising, but not proven. Am J Cardiol 77:421-422, 1996.

46. The Multicenter Diltiazem Postinfarction Trial Research Group. The result of diltiazem on mortality and reinfarction after myocardial infarction. N Engl J Med 319:385-392, 1988.

47. Indications for ACE inhibitors in the early treatment of acute myocardial infarction: Systematic overview of individual data from 100,000 patients in randomized trials. Circulation 97:2202-2212, 1998.

48. Gruppo Italiano per lo Studio della Sopravvivenza nell'Infarto Miocardico III (GISSI-3). Effects of lisinopril and transdermal glyceryl trinitrate singly and together on 6-week mortality and ventricular function after acute myocardial infarction. Lancet 343:669-685, 1994.

49. International Study of Infarct Survival (ISIS-4). A randomized factorial trial assessing early oral captopril, oral mononitrate, and intravenous magnesium sulphate in 58050 patients with suspected acute myocardial infarction. Lancet 345:669-685, 1995.

50. Lonn EM, Yusuf S, Jha P, et al. Emerging role of angiotensin-converting enzyme inhibitors in cardiac and vascular protection. Circulation 90:2056-2069, 1994.

51. Flather MD, Yusuf S, Kober L, et al. Long-term ACE-inhibitor therapy in patients with heart failure or left-ventricular dysfunction: A systematic overview of data from individual patients. Lancet 355:1575-1581, 2000.

52. Pfeffer MA, Braunwald E, Moye LA, et al. Effect of captopril on mortality and morbidity in patients with left ventricular dysfunction after myocardial infarction. N Engl J Med 327:669-677, 1992.

53. Effect of ramipril on form mortality and morbidity of survivors of acute myocardial infarction with clinical evidence of heart failure. The Acute Infarction Ramipril Efficacy (AIRE) Study investigators. Lancet 342:821-828, 1993.

54. Pfeffer MA, McMurray JJV, Velazquez EJ, et al. Valsartan, captopril, or both in myocardial infarction complicated by heart failure, left ventricular dysfunction, or both. N Engl J Med 349:1893-1906, 2003.

55. Pitt B, Zannad F, Remme WJ, et al. The effect of spironolactone on morbidity and mortality in patients with severe heart failure. N Engl J Med 341:709-717, 1999.

56. Pitt B, Remme W, Zannad F, et al. Eplerenone, a selective aldosterone blocker, in patients with left ventricular dysfunction after myocardial infarction. N Engl J Med 348:1309-1321, 2003.

57. ISIS-2 (Second International Study of Infarct Survival) Collaborative Group. Randomized trial of intravenous streptokinase, oral aspirin, both or neither among 17,187 cases of suspected acute myocardial infarction. Lancet 2:349-396, 1998.

58. Taniuchi M, Kurz HI, Lasala JM. Randomized comparison of ticlopidine and clopidogrel after intracoronary stent implantation in a broad patient population. Circulation 104(5):539-543, 2001.

59. Yusuf S, Zhao F, Mehta SR, et al. Effects of clopidogrel in addition to aspirin in patients with acute coronary syndromes without ST-segment elevation. N Engl J Med 345:494-502, 2001.

60. Hongo RH, Ley J, Dick SE, et al. The effect of clopidogrel in combination with aspirin when given before coronary artery bypass grafting. J Am Coll Cardiol 40:231-237, 2002.

61. Steinhubl SR, Berger PD, Mann JT III, et al., for CREDO Investigators. Early and sustained dual oral antiplatelet therapy following percutaneous intervention: A randomized controlled trial. JAMA 288:2411-2420, 2002.

62. Cohen M, Demers C, Gurfinkel EP, et al., for Efficacy and Safety of Subcutaneous Enoxaparin in Non-Q-Wave Coronary Events Study Group. A comparison of low-molecular-weight heparin with unfractionated heparin for unstable coronary artery disease. N Engl J Med 337:447-452, 1997.

63. Antman EM, McCabe CH, Gurfinkel EP, et al., for TIMI 11B Investigators. Enoxaparin prevents death and cardiac ischemic events in unstable angina/non-Q-wave myocardial infarction: Results of the Thrombolysis in Myocardial Infarction (TIMI) 11B Trial. Circulation 100:1593-1601, 1999.

64. Antman EM, Cohen M, Radley D, et al. Assessment of the treatment effect of enoxaparin for unstable angina/non-Q-wave myocardial infarction: TIMI 11B ESSENCE meta-analysis. Circulation 100:1602-1608, 1999.

65. Le Nguyen MT, Spencer FA. Low molecular weight heparin and unfractionated heparin in the early pharmacologic management of acute coronary syndromes: A meta-analysis of randomized clinical trials. J Thromb Thrombolysis 12(3):289-295, 2001.

66. Bijsterveld NR, Peters RJG, Murphy SA, et al. Recurrent cardiac ischemic events early after discontinuation of short-term heparin treatment in acute coronary syndromes. J Am Coll Cardiol 42:2083-2089, 2003.

67. Boersma E, Harrington RA, Moliterno DJ, et al. Platelet glycoprotein IIb/IIIa inhibitors in acute coronary syndromes: A meta-analysis of all major randomized clinical trials. Lancet 359:189-198, 2002.

68. Scandinavian Simvastatin Survival Study Group. Randomised trial of cholesterol lowering in 4444 patients with coronary heart disease: The Scandinavian Simvastatin Survival Study (4S). Lancet 344:1383-1389, 1994.

69. Shepherd J, Cobbe SM, Ford I, et al. Prevention of coronary heart disease with pravastatin in men with hypercholesterolemia. N Engl J Med 333:1301-1307, 1995.

70. Sacks FM, Pfeffer MA, Moye LA, et al. The effect of pravastatin on coronary events after myocardial infarction in patients with average cholesterol levels. N Engl J Med 335:1001-1009, 1996.

71. Expert Panel on Detection, Evaluation, and Treatment of High Blood Cholesterol in Adults. Executive Summary of the Third Report of the National Cholesterol Education Program (NCEP) Expert Panel on Detection, Evaluation, and Treatment of High Blood Cholesterol in Adults (Adult Treatment Panel III). JAMA 285:2486-2497, 2001.

72. Wassmann S, Faul A, Hennen B, et al. Rapid effect of 3-hydroxy-3-methylglutaryl coenzyme A reductase inhibition on coronary endothelial function. Circ Res 93(9):E98-E103, 2003.

73. Berkels R, Nouri SK, Taubert D, et al. The HMG-CoA reductase inhibitor cerivastatin enhances the nitric oxide bioavailability of the endothelium. J Cardiovasc Pharmacol 42:356-363, 2003.

74. Kinlay S, Schwartz GG, Olsson AG, et al. High-dose atorvastatin enhances decline in inflammatory markers in patients with acute coronary syndromes in the MIRACL study. Circulation 108:1560-1566, 2003.

75. Libby P. Current concepts of the pathogenesis of the acute coronary syndromes. Circulation 104:365-372, 2001.

76. Fenster B, Tsao PS, Rockson SG. Endothelial dysfunction: Clinical strategies for treating oxidant stress. Am Heart J 146(2):218-226, 2003.

77. TIMI III Study Group. Effects of tissue plasminogen activator and a comparison of early invasive and conservative strategies in unstable angina and non-Q-wave MI: Results of the TIMI IIIb trial. Circulation 89:1545-1556, 1994.

78. Boden WE, O'Rourke RA, Crawford MH, et al. Outcomes in patients with acute non-Q-wave myocardial infarction randomly assigned to an invasive as compared to with a conservative management strategy. Veterans Affairs Non-Q-Wave Infarction Strategies in Hospital (VANQWISH) Trial Investigators. N Engl J Med 338:1785-1792, 1998.

79. Wallentin L, Lagerqvist B, Husted S, et al. Outcome at 1 year after an invasive compared with a noninvasive strategy in unstable coronary artery disease: The FRISC II invasive randomized trial. Lancet 356:9-16, 2000.

80. Cannon CP, Weintraub WS, Demopoulos LA, et al. Comparison of early invasive and conservative strategies in patients with unstable coronary syndromes treated with the glycoprotein IIb/IIIa inhibitor tirofiban. N Engl J Med 344:1879-1887, 2001.

81. Fox KAA, Poole-Wilson PA, Henderson RA, et al. Interventional versus conservative treatment for patients with unstable angina or non-ST elevation myocardial infarction: The British Heart Foundation RITA 3 randomized trial. Lancet 360:743-751, 2002.

82. Rodriguez A, Bernardi V, Navia J, et al. Argentine randomized study: Coronary angioplasty with stenting versus coronary bypass surgery in patients with multiple vessel disease (ERACI II): 30 day and one year follow-up results. J Am Coll Cardiol 37:51-58, 2001.

83. Serruys PW, Unger F, Sousa JE, et al. Comparison of coronary bypass surgery and stenting for the treatment of multivessel disease. N Engl J Med 344:117-124, 2001.

84. The SOS Investigators. Coronary artery bypass surgery versus percutaneous coronary intervention with stent implantation in patients with multivessel coronary artery disease (the stent or surgery trial): A randomized controlled trial. Lancet 360:965-970, 2002.

85. Smith SC, Dove JT, Jacobs AK, et al. ACC/AHA Guidelines for Percutaneous Coronary Intervention (Revision of 1993 PTCA Guidelines)–Executive Summary. Circulation 103:3019-3041, 2001.

86. Morice MC, Serruys PW, Sousa JE, et al. A randomized comparison of a sirolimus-eluting stent with a standard stent for coronary revascularization. N Engl J Med 346:1773-1780, 2002.

87. Regar E, Serruys PW, Bode C, et al. Angiographic findings of the multicenter randomized study with the sirolimus-eluting Bx Velocity balloon expandable stent (RAVEL). Circulation 106:1949-1956, 2002.

88. Sousa JE, Costa MA, Sousa AGMR, et al. Two year angiographic and intravascular ultrasound follow-up after implantation of sirolimus-eluting stents in human coronary arteries. Circulation 107:381-383, 2003.

89. Grube E, Silber S, Hauptmann KE, et al. TAXUS-1: Six- and twelve-month results from a randomized double-blind trial on a slow-release paclitaxel-eluting stent for de novo coronary lesions. Circulation 107:38-42, 2003.

90. Saia F, Lemos PA, Lee CH, et al. Sirolimus-eluting stent implantation in ST-elevation acute myocardial infarction. Circulation 108:1927-1929, 2003.

91. Lemos PA, Saia F, Hofma SH, et al. Short- and long-term clinical benefit of sirolimus-eluting stents compared to bare stents for patients with acute myocardial infarction. J Am Coll Cardiol 43(4):704-708, 2004.

92. Criqui MH, Langer RD, Fronek A, et al. Mortality over a period of 10 years in patients with peripheral vascular disease. N Engl J Med 326:381-386, 1992.

93. Aqel RA, Zoghbi GJ, Baldwin SA, et al. Prevalence of renal artery stenosis in high-risk veterans referred to cardiac catheterization. J Hypertens 21:1157-1162, 2003.

94. UK Prospective Diabetes Study Group. Tight blood pressure control and risk of macrovascular and microvascular complications in type 2 diabetes: UKPDS 38. BMJ 317:703-713, 1998.

95. UK Prospective Diabetes Study Group. Efficacy of atenolol and captopril in reducing risk of macrovascular and microvascular complications in type 2 diabetes: UKPDS 39. BMJ 317:713-720, 1998.

96. Coffman JD. Drug therapy: Vasodilator drugs in peripheral vascular disease. N Engl J Med 300:713-717, 1979.

97. Roberts DH, McLoughlin GA, Tsao Y, et al. Placebo-controlled comparison of captopril, atenolol, labetalol, and pindolol in hypertension complicated by intermittent claudication. Lancet 1:650-653, 1987.

98. Solomon SA, Ramsey LE, Yeo WW, et al. Beta-blockade and intermittent claudication: Placebo-controlled trial of atenolol and nifedipine and their combination. BMJ 303:1100-1104, 1991.

99. Radack K, Deck C. Beta-adrenergic blocker therapy does not worsen intermittent claudication in subjects with peripheral vascular disease. A meta-analysis of randomized controlled trials. Arch Intern Med 151:1769-1776, 1991.

# Hypertension in the Elderly
## Jan N. Basile, Renee P. Meyer

The elderly, defined as individuals 65 years of age and older, represent the most rapidly growing segment of the U.S. population. In 1990, they accounted for 13% of the population and are expected to account for 20% of the population by the year 2040.[1] While approximately 40 million Americans will be 65 years or older by the year 2010, the number of "old elderly" (i.e., those older than age 85) is projected to reach 16 million by the middle of the twenty-first century.[2]

Hypertension, defined as a systolic blood pressure (SBP) at or above 140 mm Hg and a diastolic blood pressure (DBP) at or above 90 mm Hg, remains the most common primary office diagnosis in the United States, with more than 35 million visits per year.[3] Hypertension is a powerful, independent, and modifiable risk factor whose presence increases the risk of atherosclerotic cardiovascular disease (CVD), including stroke, coronary heart disease (CHD), congestive heart failure (CHF), peripheral vascular disease (PVD), renal failure, dementia, and death.[3] Affecting approximately 58 million Americans, elevations in blood pressure (BP) exert a strong, continuous, and graded relationship with no threshold of risk for developing CVD.[3] High BP in the elderly confers a threefold to fourfold increase in risk for CVD compared with younger individuals.[3] In 1999-2000, prevalence data from the National Health and Nutrition Examination Survey (NHANES) found that about 30% of Americans 40 to 59 years of age and 65% of Americans older than 60 years of age were hypertensive, with 80% of older Blacks and 70% of older Mexican Americans and whites affected.[4] In addition, the prevalence of hypertension has increased significantly in older Americans between 1988 and 2000.[4] More than 90% of people will develop hypertension within their lifetime, usually after 55 years of age.[5] For persons 40 to 70 years of age, the risk of CVD begins at 115/75 mm Hg and doubles with each increase of 20/10 mm Hg up to 185/115 mm Hg.[6] While both SBP and DBP are independently predictive of cardiovascular risk up to age 50, for those older than 50 years of age, SBP is a better predictor of CVD risk than DBP.[7]

More people today are aware of and are on therapy for their hypertension than in previous years. Since the late 1970s, the minimum goal for BP reduction for patients with hypertension has been less than 140/90 mm Hg. In its seventh report on the Prevention, Detection, Evaluation, and Treatment of High Blood Pressure (JNC 7), the Joint National Committee recommended an even lower goal, to less than 130/80 mm Hg, for higher-risk patients, including diabetics and those with renal impairment.[3] While BP control rates are improving, BP is controlled in only one in every three persons in the United States, with control rates even worse in the elderly, of whom only 27% are controlled.[4]

## ISOLATED SYSTOLIC HYPERTENSION

As we age, elevation of SBP predicts the risk of CVD better than increases in DBP.[7] Although this was observed more than three decades ago, no attempt was made to translate this evidence into practice until 1993, when the Fifth Joint National Committee Report (JNC V) recognized isolated systolic hypertension (ISH) as an important target for BP control.[8,9] ISH, defined as a SBP of ≥140 mm Hg and a DBP of <90 mm Hg, represents the most common form of hypertension in the elderly and its prevalence increases with age; two thirds of individuals 60 years of age and older, and three fourths of those older than 75 years of age, have ISH.[10] In NHANES III, among persons 70 years of age and older, more than 90% of those who were inadequately treated had ISH, whereas in those less than 40 years of age who were inadequately treated, only 22% had ISH.[11] More than 25% of adults 60 years of age or older have stage 1 ISH (SBP of 140-159 mm Hg with DBP <90 mm Hg). It is the predominant form of hypertension in the elderly and often goes untreated.[11]

SBP is easier to measure than DBP in the elderly, and knowing the SBP allows more appropriate risk stratification. In an analysis of the Framingham Heart Study, knowing only the SBP correctly classified the stage of BP in 99% of adults older than the age of 60, while knowing only the DBP allowed 66% to be correctly classified.[12]

Age-related pathophysiologic changes explain the frequent development of ISH. While DBP elevation is caused by constriction of the smaller arterioles, ISH is caused by the loss of distensibility of the larger arteries, especially the aorta.[13] In younger persons, the aorta is highly distensible, expanding during systole to minimize the rise in BP. The majority of elderly individuals, however, develop progressive stiffening of their arterial tree with age. This reduces the compliance of the aorta during systole and leads to a progressive elevation in SBP. Because the smaller arterioles are not involved in this process, the DBP remains normal or tends to decrease, contributing to a higher pulse pressure (SBP-DBP) with age.[13] Accordingly, the elevated SBP increases both left ventricular work and the risk for left ventricular hypertrophy (LVH), while the decreased DBP may compromise coronary blood flow.[14] This increase in pulse pressure is a stronger predictor of cardiovascular risk than either SBP or DBP elevation in the elderly. As there is no trial-based evidence that a reduction in pulse pressure reduces cardiovascular risk, and because SBP reduction improves CVD outcomes and remains the major risk component of pulse pressure, treatment of SBP should continue to be targeted to reduce cardiovascular risk in the elderly patient.[15]

# APPROPRIATE GOALS OF THERAPY IN THE ELDERLY

## Treatment Benefits

The optimal BP level in the elderly individual with hypertension has not yet been conclusively determined.[3] In general, BP goals depend on the type of elevation (isolated systolic versus systolic/diastolic) and the presence of diabetes or renal disease. Clinical trials over the past 35 years have proven the benefits of antihypertensive therapy in reducing the rates of stroke, heart failure, and heart attack. Several large, prospective clinical trials conducted over the past several decades in older patients with combined systolic-diastolic hypertension have demonstrated the benefits of treating hypertension in the elderly (Table 55–1). Based on diastolic entry criteria, they showed significant decreases in the rates of stroke, heart failure, and heart attack, as well as mortality when treating to a DBP goal of less than 90 mm Hg. These treatment benefits are notably greater in older compared with younger individuals, due to the greater absolute risk for CVD outcomes in older individuals.[16] Small reductions in BP are associated with large reductions in cardiovascular events and stroke.[17] While cardiovascular events have been decreased by treatment of hypertension in the elderly, the demonstrated benefit has been even larger for the prevention of stroke and stroke-related mortality. Several meta-analyses found a 38% reduction in stroke, 16% reduction in heart attack, 52% reduction in heart failure, 21% reduction in cardiovascular death, and a 35% reduction in LVH in drug-treated compared with placebo or control participants.[18-21] The Blood Pressure Treatment Trialists' Collaboration evaluated 29 trials (162,341 participants with a mean age of 65 years) and found that reduction in BP with any of the commonly used regimens reduced the risk of cardiovascular events, and the larger the reduction in SBP, the larger the reduction in risk.[22]

In the most recent controlled clinical trials, including the Hypertension Optimal Treatment (HOT),[23] Antihypertensive, and Lipid-Lowering Treatment to Prevent Heart Attack Trial (ALLHAT),[24] and the Controlled Onset Verapamil Investigation of Cardiovascular Endpoints (CONVINCE)[25] trials, 90% of participants had their DBP reduced to <90 mm Hg, but only about 60% had SBPs reduced to <140 mm Hg. Accordingly, it is usually the inability to reduce SBP effectively that prevents BP targets from being reached.

Randomized placebo-controlled trials have demonstrated significant benefit from drug treatment in elderly patients with ISH. In those with a SBP ≥160 mm Hg and a DBP <90 to 95 mm Hg at baseline, a 35% to 40 % reduction in stroke, up to a 50% reduction in heart failure, a 30% reduction in coronary events, and a 10% to 15% reduction in mortality were achieved with antihypertensive treatment (Table 55–2). In order to achieve this benefit, SBP was reduced by at least 20 mm Hg from baseline, to a level below 150 or 160 mm Hg. In none of the trials was an average SBP <140 mm Hg achieved (Table 55–3).

Is there clinical trial evidence to recommend a goal SBP of <140 mm Hg in patients with ISH? Only a few clinical trials have specifically attempted to randomize patients to different target levels of BP as a primary intervention. Many recommendations to achieve a specific target BP come from epidemiologic observation or posthoc analyses of clinical trial data. One such posthoc analysis was published almost 10 years after the original results of the SHEP trial.[26] In this analysis, performed on the original 4736 participants 60 years of age or older with SBP of ≥160 mm Hg and DBP <90 mm Hg, the risk of stroke was calculated according to on-treatment BP during follow-up. With a targeted SBP <160 mm Hg and at least a 20–mm Hg reduction from baseline, those on-treatment had a 33% reduction in stroke. The patients who achieved a SBP <150 mm Hg did even better, with a 38% reduction in stroke risk. The group who achieved a SBP <140 mm Hg had a 22% reduction in stroke risk, which did not reach statistical significance because of the smaller numbers of participants involved. These data should not be interpreted to mean that achieving SBP <140 mm Hg is less beneficial than achieving a higher SBP level. They do suggest, however, that if SBP is reduced by at least 20 mm Hg from baseline, even if not to the presently recommended goal of <140 mm Hg, clinical outcome is improved.

**Table 55–1** Percent Event Reduction in Clinical Hypertension Trials in Older Patients

|  | **Stroke** | **CAD** | **CHF** | **All CVD** |
|---|---|---|---|---|
| Australian | 33 | 18 | — | 31 |
| EWPHE | 36 | 20 | 22 | 29* |
| STOP | 47* | 13† | 51* | 40* |
| MRC | 25* | 19 | — | 17* |
| HDFP | 44* | 15* | — | 16* |

*Statistically significant.
†Myocardial infarction only.
CAD, coronary artery disease; CHF, congestive heart failure; CVD, cardiovascular disease.

**Table 55–2** Major Clinical Trials Showing Benefit of Treating Isolated Systolic Hypertension

|  | **SHEP (n = 4736)** | **Syst-Eur (n = 4695)** | **Syst-China (n = 2394)** |
|---|---|---|---|
| Baseline SBP/DBP (mm Hg) | 160-219/<90 | 160-219/<95 | 160-219/<95 |
| BP reduction: SBP/DBP (mm Hg) | 27/9 | 23/7 | 20/5 |
| Drug therapy | Chlorthalidone Atenolol | Nitrendipine Enalapril HCTZ | Nitrendipine Captopril HCTZ |
| **Outcomes (%) ↓** | | | |
| Stroke | 33 | 42 | 38 |
| CAD | 27 | 30 | 27 |
| CHF | 55 | 29 | — |
| All CVR disease | 32 | 31 | 25 |

Reproduced from the Journal of Clinical Hypertension Vol II, No. 5, page 336, September/October.
HCTZ, hydrochlorothiazide; CAD, coronary artery disease; CHF, congestive heart disease; CVR, cardiovascular.

**Table 55-3** Blood Pressure in SHEP and Syst-Eur (mm Hg)

|  | SHEP | Syst-Eur |
|---|---|---|
| Entry | 160-219/<90 | 160-219/<95 |
| Goal (SBP) | <160 + ≥21 ↓ | <150 + ≥20 ↓ |
| Baseline | 170/77 | 174/86 |
| Achieved: Rx | 143/68 | 151/79 |
| Achieved: Placebo | 155/72 | 161/84 |
| Difference; Rx-Placebo | 12/4 | 10/5 |

Reproduced with permission for the Journal of Clinical Hypertension, Vol II, No. 5, page 336. March/April 2000.

The cardiovascular risk associated with stage 1 ISH (140-159 mm Hg) is well established, but no outcome-based trial has tested whether treatment reduces event rates. Nevertheless, JNC 7[3] and a consensus statement from the National High Blood Pressure Education Program recommend achieving a SBP <140 mm Hg based on epidemiologic rather than trial-based data.[10]

It should be noted that clinical trials in elderly patients with hypertension tend to underestimate the actual benefit of treatment for several reasons. First, patients with severe hypertension, who stand to benefit the most from treatment because of their greater absolute risk, are often excluded. In addition, many study protocols follow an "intention-to-treat" design, where patients in the placebo group are treated once their BP reaches a designated threshold, thus minimizing the treatment benefits in the active therapy group. In the Systolic Hypertension in the Elderly Program (SHEP), for example, by the end of the study, 44% of patients in the placebo group were receiving active treatment. Finally, a relatively short (3-5 year) trial duration may not allow treatment-related reductions in CHD events to be realized, because cerebrovascular endpoint benefits may occur sooner and cause the trial to be stopped early.[27] Accordingly, benefits of antihypertensive treatment seen in practice may be greater than those achieved in clinical trials.

Is there any age at which one would not treat the elderly patient with hypertension? A subgroup meta-analysis of effects of antihypertensive treatment on very old participants enrolled in randomized controlled trials supports the benefit of antihypertensive therapy even in patients 80 years of age and older, at least with respect to prevention of stroke, major cardiovascular events, and heart failure.[28] There was no treatment benefit for cardiovascular death, and a nonsignificant excess of all-cause mortality in the active treatment group, suggesting a need for a large-scale trial of antihypertensive treatment in the very elderly. In the interim, there is no justification for withholding antihypertensive treatment based on advanced age (Box 55-1).

## Clinical Evaluation

A thorough history and physical examination should be performed, as in the younger patient with hypertension. Patients should be specifically questioned about the use of any prior antihypertensive medication and how well their BP was controlled. In addition, they should be asked about the use of nonsteroidal antiinflammatory agents and over-the-counter medications, including nasal sprays and cold remedies, both of which may

**Box 55-1** General Guidelines Related to Antihypertensive Treatment in the Elderly

- Therapy in older individuals with hypertension should begin with lifestyle modification.
- Weight loss and sodium restriction may decrease the need for antihypertensive medication in this population.
- The starting dose of medication should be one half of that used in younger patients.
- In the elderly patient with hypertension and no compelling indications, a thiazide-type diuretic is recommended as initial therapy.
- α-Blocker therapy should not be used as initial therapy but it can be used as additive therapy to further help reduce blood pressure (BP).
- Although BP reduction should occur more gradually in the older patient with hypertension, the goal for effective BP control is similar to those younger in age.
- The minimum goal for BP control is <140/90 mm Hg; while in those with diabetes and renal disease the goal is <130/80 mm Hg.
- Patients with ISH should reduce their SBP to <140 mm Hg.
- Caution should be exercised when lowering DBP to <55 mm Hg when treating the older patient with ISH
- The effects of hormone replacement therapy (HRT) on BP are unclear. BP should be monitored closely if the patient is on HRT.
- HRT should not be used for cardiovascular disease (CVD) prevention. HRT should only be considered for the short-term treatment of menopausal symptoms.

raise BP. Questioning should also occur concerning alternative therapies, including ephedrine-containing neutraceuticals such as Ma Huang, which has been associated with stroke.

As in the younger patient, the diagnosis of hypertension should be based on the average of two standardized measurements taken over separate office visits. This is even more important in the elderly because BP is often more variable in this group than in younger persons. In addition, measurement of BP can pose special problems in the elderly. Pseudohypertension should be suspected in those with persistently high BP without any evidence of target organ damage or when antihypertensive medication causes hypotensive symptoms in elderly patients with continually elevated cuff-determined BP. In these individuals, the brachial arteries may be thickened and stiff and the BP measurement may be an overestimation of actual intraarterial pressure.

BP should be measured in the supine, sitting, and standing positions as the elderly are more prone to postural hypotension, especially after a meal. The occurrence of postural hypotension often limits the ability to control systolic hypertension and affects the ability to use sitting pressures to determine BP control. The standing BP, therefore, should often be used in the elderly to determine the dose of antihypertensive medication required and if BP is controlled.

Most elderly patients with hypertension are asymptomatic. Target organ damage is more likely to occur in the elderly, but very few elderly patients have a reversible, secondary form of hypertension. When an elderly patient presents with new-onset of severe hypertension or the sudden loss of what was previously well-controlled hypertension, a secondary cause should be considered. It is neither cost-effective nor rewarding to perform an extensive workup on every elderly patient with hypertension in hopes of finding a secondary cause. Although renovascular hypertension is more common and often unrecognized in the elderly, it is rarely cured by surgical or percutaneous (angioplasty with stent) intervention. Accordingly, if BP is controlled and renal function remains normal, there is little benefit from knowing that renal artery stenosis is present.

Two often unrecognized conditions in the elderly that lead to poor BP control are sleep apnea and obstructive uropathy. To make a presumptive diagnosis of sleep apnea, ask the patient and his or her sleeping partner whether the patient snores or gasps for air while sleeping, and whether the patient has daytime hypersomnolence. A positive answer indicates that the patient may need further evaluation such as a formal sleep study (see Chapter 73 ). A second cause of poor BP control is obstructive uropathy. A full bladder can cause discharge of sympathetic neurons and make BP control difficult. Catheterization is often curative.

The initial dose of antihypertensive drug(s) in the elderly should often be one half that used in the younger subject. This allows for the reduced renal or hepatic drug metabolism that often occurs in the elderly. The dose should be slowly increased until the maximum BP reduction occurs at the dose with the fewest side effects. Additional agents should be added until the BP goal is attained.

## Options for Therapy: Lifestyle (Nonpharmacologic) Changes

Lifestyle changes—in particular, weight loss and reduced sodium intake— are beneficial in controlling BP in the elderly hypertensive and are associated with a reduced need for pharmacologic therapy. Weight reduction is the most effective lifestyle intervention for lowering BP, especially in the elderly hypertensive who is overweight. Older hypertensive patients are often more salt sensitive than younger ones, and successful salt reduction can be achieved, in part by limiting a variety of high-salt–containing processed foods. The Trial of Nonpharmacologic Interventions in the Elderly (TONE) during 30-months of follow-up found that restricting salt to 80 mmol (2 g) per day reduced SBP by 4.3 mm Hg and DBP by 2 mm Hg. The combination of weight loss and salt restriction reduced BP more than either strategy by itself, and, when used together, enabled almost half the elderly participants to stop antihypertensive drug therapy. These individuals were unsuccessful in long-term weight reduction, with a high recidivism rate at 6 to 12 months.[29]

Additional lifestyle changes include adopting the Dietary Approaches to Stop Hypertension (DASH) diet. This diet, which is low in fat but rich in fruits, vegetables, and low-fat dairy products, has been successful in reducing BP in older hypertensive patients even when consuming an average salt intake.[30] Reducing alcohol intake and increasing physical activity should also be integral parts of BP control in the elderly.

## Options for Therapy: Pharmacologic Treatment of ISH

Several placebo-controlled randomized outcome trials have tested whether pharmacologic treatment of ISH can reduce cardiovascular events and stroke. In the SHEP trial, performed in 4736 patients at least 60 years of age with a SBP 160 mm Hg or above and a DBP below 90 mm Hg, initial therapy with a thiazide-type diuretic with or without a β-blocking agent reduced first stroke by 36%, and cardiovascular events by 27%.[31] Heart failure was reduced by 49% overall, with an 81% reduction in those with either a history or evidence of a prior myocardial infarction (MI) on the electrocardiogram.[32] In the 583 SHEP patients with type 2 diabetes, major cardiovascular events were reduced by 34%.[33] The benefit of diuretic therapy was lost if the serum potassium level was not kept above 3.5 mg/dl.[34]

The European Trial on Isolated Systolic Hypertension (Syst-Eur) in the elderly randomized 4695 patients 60 years of age or older with SBP 160 to 219 mm Hg and DBP <95 mm Hg (European definition of ISH) to the moderately long-acting dihydropyridine calcium channel blocker (CCB) nitrendipine, with the addition of the angiotensin-converting enzyme (ACE) inhibitor enalapril, and a thiazide-type diuretic as necessary, or to matching placebos. Over a median of 2 years of follow-up, active treatment reduced stroke by 42% and all cardiovascular events by 31%.[27]

A meta-analysis of eight placebo-controlled trials in the elderly with ISH, which included 15,693 patients 60 years of age and older followed for an average of 3.8 years, found that active treatment reduced coronary events by 23%, stroke by 30%, cardiovascular death by 18%, and total death by 13%.[35] In those patients older than 70 years of age, the absolute benefit was particularly high. Treating 19 patients for 5 years prevented one major fatal or nonfatal cardiovascular event.

In a prespecified subgroup analysis of the Losartan Intervention For Endpoint Reduction (LIFE) trial, losartan-based therapy was superior to β-blocker (atenolol) based therapy in the 14% of patients with ISH. All participants enrolled in LIFE had electrocardiographic evidence of LVH (ECG LVH). Over 4.7 years of follow-up, a 25% reduction in the combined endpoint of cardiovascular death, acute MI, and stroke occurred in the group randomized to losartan. Of note, hydrochlorothiazide was added in almost all patients in both treatment groups.[36]

In summary, in those with ISH, initial therapy with a thiazide-type diuretic or dihydropyridine-type calcium-antagonist therapy has been found to be superior to placebo-based therapy. In addition, in those with ECG-LVH, an angiotensin receptor blocker (ARB)–based strategy was more effective than a β-blocker–based regimen. Only 60% of elderly patients treated for ISH were controlled on a single agent in reported clinical trials. Accordingly, the majority of elderly patients with hypertension, including those with ISH, will require at least 2 to 3 drugs to achieve the SBP goal of <140 mm Hg.

## Pharmacologic Treatment of Systolic/Diastolic Hypertension

Although all classes of antihypertensive agents effectively lower combined SBP/DBP elevation in the elderly, the majority of outcome-based trials showing a reduction in cardiovascular morbidity and mortality have used diuretics and, when necessary, additional β-blocker therapy. A meta-analysis of outcome trials of antihypertensive treatment has suggested that the initial agent chosen likely does not have a unique status for event rate reduction, and that the SBP reduction achieved appears more important.[22]

The open-label Second Swedish Trial in Old Patients with Hypertension (STOP-2) compared the use of an ACE inhibitor, a CCB, or a diuretic with or without β-blocker therapy in 6628 participants 70 to 84 years of age with combined SBP/DBP elevation.[37] Similar BP reduction was achieved in all three treatment groups. There was no difference in cardiovascular mortality (the primary outcome) among the three randomized groups.

The open-label Nordic Diltiazem (NORDIL) trial, with an average participant age of 60 years, found a similar rate for the primary outcome of combined fatal and nonfatal stroke, MI, and cardiovascular death in participants randomized to the CCB diltiazem compared with those assigned to diuretic and/or β-blocker therapy.[38] Although fewer strokes occurred in the diltiazem arm, there was a trend toward more MIs and heart failure with diltiazem.

The double-blinded International Study of Intervention as a Goal In Hypertension Treatment (INSIGHT) trial enrolled men and women 55 to 80 years of age, 75% of who were older than the age of 60. It found that nifedipine GITS (GastroIntestinal Therapeutic System) and diuretic therapy had similar overall CVD outcomes.[39]

The Antihypertensive and Lipid-Lowering Treatment to Prevent Heart Attack Trial (ALLHAT), the largest outcome trial of antihypertensive therapy ever performed, was designed to determine whether the occurrence of fatal CHD or nonfatal MI (primary outcome) in high-risk patients with hypertension is lower when treated with a representative dihydropyridine CCB (amlodipine), or a representative ACE inhibitor (lisinopril), each compared with a representative long-acting thiazide-type diuretic (chlorthalidone).[24] The third active comparator arm involving an α-blocker (doxazosin) was stopped early because of a 25% greater cardiovascular event rate, principally a twofold greater risk of heart failure when compared with chlorthalidone, as well as a vanishingly small chance of finding a difference in the primary endpoint between the two treatment groups. Those results were interpreted as showing that an α-blocker should not be used as first-line therapy for hypertension in a relatively high risk, ALLHAT-like population.[40]

ALLHAT, with a mean follow-up of 4.9 years, enrolled 33,357 men and women aged 55 years or older (mean age 67) with at least one additional coronary risk factor. On entry, participants had stage 1 or stage 2 hypertension (BPs 140-180/90-110 mm Hg). More than 90% of patients were on one or two BP-lowering agents that were stopped prior to entry into the study. In the final analysis, 15,255 patients were randomized to chlorthalidone (12.5-25 mg once a day); 9048 to amlodipine (2.5-10 mg once a day); and 9054 to lisinopril (10-40 mg once a day). If the participant did not achieve the goal BP of <140/90 mm Hg after up-titration to the highest dose of the step 1 drug open-label step 2 drugs were added. Step 2 drugs included atenolol (25-100 mg/day), clonidine (0.1-0.3 mg twice a day), or reserpine (0.05-0.2 mg/day);

the only step 3 agent was hydralazine (25-100 mg twice a day). Amlodipine and lisinopril were both compared with chlorthalidone. No comparison was valid between amlodipine and lisinopril.[24]

Baseline risk factors were nearly identical in the three treatment groups. Of the participants, 47% were women, 35% were Black, 19% were Hispanic, 22% were smokers, 36% were diabetic, 25% had preexisting CHD, and 47% had preexisting CVD.[41] Mean seated BP on entry (usually on some antihypertensive medications) was 146/84 mm Hg in all three groups and was 134/75 mm Hg, 135/74 mm Hg, and 136/75 mm Hg in the chlorthalidone, amlodipine, and lisinopril groups respectively, at 5 years of follow-up. At the initial visit, 27% were at or below the BP goal of <140/90 mm Hg. After 5 years of follow-up, 68%, 66%, and 61% were below SBP goal in the chlorthalidone, amlodipine, and lisinopril groups, respectively.[24] In contrast, more than 90% had reached the DBP goal, reinforcing the relative unimportance of DBP in older hypertensive patients.

Adherence to therapy fell from 87% to 80% for chlorthalidone, 88% to 80% for amlodipine, and 82% to 73% for lisinopril from the first through the fifth year of follow-up. Adherence to initial therapy was different only between those on lisinopril and chlorthalidone.

A total of 2956 patients experienced a primary outcome event and there was no difference among the groups. Neither amlodipine nor lisinopril was superior to chlorthalidone in preventing major coronary events or improving overall survival. For both the primary and secondary outcomes, there was no difference between the amlodipine and chlorthalidone groups except that those randomized to chlorthalidone had a significant 38% reduction in the risk of heart failure that was seen within all the prespecified subgroups (old and young, men and women, Black and non-Black, diabetic and nondiabetic). Compared with chlorthalidone, amlodipine was not associated with excess gastrointestinal bleeding or cancer death—concerns that had been raised from past observations.

In comparing chlorthalidone and lisinopril, those on chlorthalidone had a 15% reduction in the risk of stroke with a mean 2–mm Hg lower SBP overall. In Blacks, who had a 4–mm Hg greater reduction in SBP on chlorthalidone compared with lisinopril, a 40% reduction in stroke risk occurred in those randomized to chlorthalidone compared with the lisinopril group. The risk of heart failure was reduced by 19% in those on chlorthalidone compared with lisinopril.

Thiazide-type diuretics were unsurpassed in reducing clinical events and lowering BP and were as well tolerated as CCB and ACE inhibitor therapy in ALLHAT. Accordingly, they are recommended as initial therapy in the elderly patient with hypertension. If a compelling comorbid condition exists, other initial therapy may be justified.[3] If not used initially, a thiazide-type diuretic should be included in most regimens to enhance the efficacy of other BP-lowering agents.

BP control rates can be improved, but more than one drug will usually be required to do so. Although two of every three ALLHAT participants were controlled to <140/90 mm Hg, only 30% were controlled on single-agent therapy.[42] The degree of BP (particularly SBP) reduction and not the individual antihypertensive drug used appears more important for improving outcome in the older individual.[22]

## J-CURVE HYPOTHESIS

The J-curve hypothesis describes the concern that lowering DBP below a certain critical value increases the risk of cardiovascular death and morbid events in the elderly hypertensive. Prospective data validating this hypothesis are lacking. The bulk of the evidence available comes from retrospective trials, which are associated with inherent observational bias.[43] As an increased occurrence of ischemic events has been prospectively observed in both placebo and actively treated patients with very low DBP, a low DBP is thought to serve more as a marker than a cause of cardiovascular events in those with underlying coronary disease.[44,45]

The Hypertension Optimal Treatment (HOT) study was designed to test whether intensive BP lowering was helpful or harmful in preventing cardiovascular events and death.[46] This Prospective, Randomized, Open with Blinded Endpoint evaluation (PROBE) trial randomly assigned 18,790 hypertensive patients (mean age 61.5 years) from 26 countries to a target DBP <80 mm Hg, <85 mm Hg, or <90 mm Hg and followed them for an average of 3.8 years. It found no increased cardiovascular risk for the DBP goal <80 versus <90 mm Hg.

A retrospective analysis of the SHEP trial, however, suggested that in the few patients whose DBP was lowered to <55 mm Hg with drug treatment, there was no benefit in outcome when compared with the placebo group.[47] This suggests that we exercise caution in lowering DBP to <55 mm Hg when treating older individuals with ISH.

## Hormone Replacement Therapy and Hypertension

After years of observational studies supporting use of hormone replacement therapy (HRT) in postmenopausal women for prevention of CVD, controlled clinical trials have provided no evidence for cardiovascular benefit and have noted the occurrence of serious adverse effects for those on HRT. The Hormone Estrogen Replacement Study (HERS) followed 2763 postmenopausal women with known CHD who were randomized to estrogen and progestin or placebo. It found an increased incidence of CHD for those on active therapy in the first year of follow-up and a reduction of CHD in years 3 through 5. No overall benefit in preventing cardiovascular events could be identified.[48] To determine whether the later risk reduction for CHD seen during years 3 though 5 in the HERS trial persisted, HERS II followed women from the original study for a total duration of 6.8 years. No significant decrease in cardiovascular events was seen during HERS II. The authors of the study stated that their findings support not recommending HRT to reduce CHD risk in postmenopausal women.[49]

Subsequent analysis of HERS data identified 11 risk factors for CVD among the participants, and assessed preventative measures.[50] Six factors that increased risk were identified by history: nonwhite ethnicity, lack of exercise, treated diabetes, angina, CHF, and more than one previous MI. The remaining five were obtained by measurement: uncontrolled hypertension, elevated low-density lipoprotein cholesterol, low high-density lipoprotein cholesterol, elevated Lp(a) lipoprotein level, and low creatinine clearance. Controlled hypertension was not a risk factor. In this cohort with known CHD, and therefore already at risk for another cardiovascular event, these 11 risk factors increased subsequent risk sixfold. Only three of the risk factors were potentially reversible: lipid lowering, exercise, and BP control. BP

and lipid-lowering agents were used in a minority of qualified enrollees at the onset of the HERS study and continued during the 4-year follow-up. The underuse of proven therapies in the HERS middle-aged to elderly female population is an important but not isolated finding. Inadequate secondary prevention measures have been observed in other studies of the elderly.[51-53]

The Women's Health Initiative (WHI) included in its complex design a randomized, double-blind clinical trial that compared a combination of 0.625 mg equine estrogen and 2.5 mg medroxyprogesterone acetate with placebo in more than 16,000 apparently healthy women 50 to 79 years of age.[54] The trial was stopped early after an average follow-up of 5.2 years because of an increased incidence of breast cancer in the estrogen plus progestin group. The number of cases of CHD (CHD deaths plus nonfatal MIs), stroke, pulmonary embolism, and venous thromboembolic disease were all increased in those on combined hormone replacement. HRT was associated with a 44% increased risk of ischemic stroke in women with and without hypertension.[55] A slight increase in SBP was noted in the HRT treatment group: 1 mm Hg higher after 1 year, increasing to 1.5 mm Hg at 2 years. Analysis of BP data at the time of enrollment in the trial revealed that current HRT use was associated with a 25% greater likelihood of developing hypertension than nonuse when adjusted for age, smoking, alcohol intake, cholesterol, physical activity, body mass index, family history, and other comorbidities.[53] The same report, focusing on the adequacy of BP control among WHI participants with hypertension, found that despite the fact that those 70 to 79 years of age were as likely to be on antihypertensive treatment as the younger 50 to 69 year old participants, a significantly lower percentage of the older age group had adequate BP control, with almost two thirds of the oldest women having BPs >140/90 mm Hg despite the fact that they had often seen a healthcare provider in the past year (Figure 55–1).

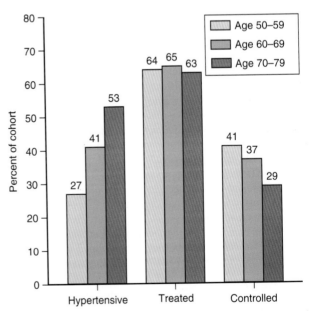

**Figure 55–1** The Women's Health Initiative—prevalence and treatment status by age. From Wassertheil-Smoller S, Anderson G, Psaty B, et al. Hypertension and its treatment in postmenopausal women. Baseline data from the Women's Health Initiative Hypertension 36:780-789, 2000.

In contrast to the aforementioned studies, which found an increase in BP on HRT, the Postmenopausal Estrogen/Progestin Interventions (PEPI) trial, which studied younger post-menopausal women who were normotensive on entry, found no difference in BP among any of four HRT treatment groups and placebo after 3 years of follow-up.[56] Furthermore, in the Baltimore Longitudinal Study on Aging, which followed 226 healthy postmenopausal women over an average 5.7 years, SBP increased 3 mm Hg more in the two thirds of participants on placebo compared with those that received HRT, with no change in DBP noted.[57]

There is no clear consensus about the direct effects of HRT on BP. HRT-related changes in BP are likely to be modest and should not preclude hormone use in normotensive or hypertensive women. Because of the adverse cardiovascular outcomes noted previously, HRT should not be given to prevent any adverse cardiovascular outcome in postmenopausal women[58] regardless of the presence of hypertension. If used, HRT should only be used for the short-term treatment of menopausal symptoms. In those with hypertension, BP should be monitored closely, both on initiation of HRT therapy and at 6-month intervals thereafter.[3]

# References

1. U.S. Census Bureau. Persons 65 Years Old and Over—Characteristics by Sex: 1980 to 2000. Statistical Abstracts of the United States: 2002. Washington, DC, U.S. Census Bureau, 2001; p 43.
2. Heart and Stroke Statistical Update. Dallas, TX, American Heart Association, 2003.
3. The Seventh Report of the Joint National Committee on Prevention, Detection, Evaluation, and Treatment of High Blood Pressure The JNC 7 Report. JAMA 289:2560-2572, 2003.
4. Hajjar I, Kotchen T. Trends in prevalence, awareness, treatment, and control of hypertension in the United States, 1988-2000. JAMA 290:199-206, 2003.
5. Vasan R, Beiser A, Seshadri S, et al. Residual lifetime risk for developing hypertension in middle-aged women and men: The Framingham Heart Study. JAMA 287:1003-1010, 2002.
6. Lewington S, Clarke R, Qizilbash N, et al. Age-specific relevance of usual blood pressure to vascular mortality. Lancet 360:1903-1913, 2002.
7. Kannel WB. Elevated systolic blood pressure as a cardiovascular risk factor. Am J Cardiol 15:251-255, 2000.
8. Kannel WB, Schwartz MJ, McNamara PM. Blood pressure and risk of coronary heart disease. The Framingham Study. Dis Chest 56:43-62, 1969.
9. Fifth Report of the Joint National Committee on Detection, Evaluation, and Treatment of High Blood Pressure. (JNC V). Arch Intern Med 153:154-183, 1993 .
10. Izzo J, Levy D, Black HR. Importance of systolic blood pressure in older Americans. Hypertension 35:1021-1024, 2000.
11. Franklin S, Jacobs M, Wong N, et al. Predominance of isolated systolic hypertension among middle-aged and elderly USA hypertensives: Analysis based on National Health and Nutrition Examination Survey (NHANES III). Hypertension 37:869-874, 2001.
12. Lloyd-Jones DM, Evans JC, Larson MG, et al. Differential impact of systolic and diastolic blood pressure level on JNC-VI staging. Hypertension 34:381-385, 1999.
13. Tonkin A, Wing L. Management of isolated systolic hypertension. Drugs 51:738-749, 1996.
14. Madhaven S, Ooi H, Cohen H, et al. Relation of pulse pressure and blood pressure reduction to the incidence of myocardial infarction. Hypertension 23:395-401, 1994.
15. Franklin S, Khan S, Wong D, et al. Is pulse pressure useful in predicting risk for coronary heart disease? The Framingham Heart Study. Circulation 100:354-360, 1999.
16. Black HR. New concepts in hypertension: Focus on the elderly. Am Heart J 135:S2-S7, 1998.
17. Staessen J, Wang J, Thijs L. Cardiovascular prevention and blood pressure reduction: A quantitative overview updated until 1 March 2003. J Hypertens 21:1055-1076, 2003.
18. Moser M, Hebert PR. Prevention of disease progression, left ventricular hypertrophy and congestive heart failure in hypertension treatment trials. J Am Coll Cardiol 27:1214-1218, 1996.
19. Psaty BM, Smith NL, Siscovick DS, et al. Health outcomes associated with antihypertensive therapies used as first-line agents: A systematic review and meta-analysis. JAMA 277:739-745, 1997.
20. Blood Pressure Lowering Treatment Trialists' Collaborative. Effects of ACE-inhibitors, calcium antagonists, and other blood-pressure-lowering drugs: Results of prospectively designed overviews of randomised trials. Lancet 356:1955-1964, 2000.
21. Hebert PR, Moser M, Mayer J, et al. Recent evidence on drug therapy of mild to moderate hypertension and decreased risk of coronary heart disease. Arch Intern Med 153:578-581, 1993.
22. Blood Pressure Lowering Treatment Trialists' Collaboration. Effects of different blood-pressure-lowering regimens on major cardiovascular events: Results of prospectively-designed overviews of randomized trials. Lancet 362:1527-1535, 2003.
23. Hansson L, Zanchetti A, Carruthers SG, et al. Effects of intensive blood-pressure lowering and low-dose aspirin in patients with hypertension: Principal results of the Hypertension Optimal Treatment (HOT) randomized trial. HOT Study Group. Lancet 351:1755-1762, 1998.
24. Major outcomes in high-risk hypertensive patients randomized to angiotensin-converting enzyme inhibitor or calcium channel blocker vs diuretic. The Antihypertensive and Lipid-Lowering Treatment to Prevent Heart Attack Trial (ALLHAT). JAMA 288:2981-2997, 2002.
25. Black HR, Elliot WJ, Grandits G, et al., for CONVINCE Research Group. Principal results of the Controlled Onset Verapamil Investigation of Cardiovascular Endpoints (CONVINCE) trial. JAMA 289:2073-2082, 2003.
26. Perry HM Jr, Davis BR, Price TR, et al. Effect of treating isolated systolic hypertension on the risk of developing various types and subtypes of stroke. The Systolic Hypertension in the Elderly Program (SHEP). JAMA 284:465-471, 2000.
27. Staessen JA, Fagard R, Thijs L, et al. Randomised double-blind comparison of placebo and active treatment for older patients with isolated systolic hypertension. The Systolic Hypertension in Europe (Syst-Eur) Trial Investigators. Lancet 350:757-764, 1997.
28. Gueyffier F, Bulpitt C, Boissel JP, et al. Antihypertensive drugs in very old people: A subgroup meta-analysis of randomized controlled trials. INDANA Group. Lancet 353:793-796, 1999.
29. Whelton PK, Appel LJ, Espeland MA, et al. Sodium restriction and weight loss in the treatment of hypertension on older persons: A randomized controlled trial of non pharmacologic interventions in the elderly (TONE). TONE collaborative Research Group. JAMA 279:839-846, 1998.
30. Appel L, Moore T, Obarzanek E, et al. The effect of dietary patterns on blood pressure: Results from the Dietary Approaches to Stop Hypertension (DASH) randomized clinical trial. N Engl J Med 336:1117-1124, 1997.
31. SHEP Cooperative Research Group. Prevention of stroke by antihypertensive drug treatment in older persons with isolated systolic hypertension. JAMA 265:3255-3264, 1996.
32. Kostis JB, Davis BR, Cutler JA, et al., for SHEP Cooperative Research Group. Prevention of heart failure by antihypertensive drug treatment in older persons with isolated systolic hypertension. JAMA 278:212-216, 1997.

33. Curb JD, Pressel SL, Cutler JA, et al. Effect of diuretic-based antihypertensive treatment on cardiovascular disease risk in older diabetic patients with isolated systolic hypertension. JAMA 276:1886-1892, 1996.

34. Franse LV, Pahor M, Di Bari M, et al. Hypokalemia associated with diuretic use and cardiovascular events in the systolic hypertension in the elderly program. Hypertension 35:1025-1030, 2000.

35. Staessen JA, Gasowski J, Wang JG, et al. Risk of untreated and treated isolated systolic hypertension in the elderly: Meta-analysis of outcome trials. Lancet 355:865-872, 2000.

36. Kjeldsen S, Dahlof B, Devereux R, et al. Effects of losartan on cardiovascular morbidity and mortality in patients with isolated systolic hypertension and left ventricular hypertrophy: A Losartan Intervention For Endpoint Reduction (LIFE) substudy. JAMA 288:1491-1498, 2002.

37. Hansson L, Lindholm LH, Ekbom T, et al., for STOP-Hypertension-2 Study Group. Randomized trial of old and new antihypertensive drugs in elderly patients: Cardiovascular mortality and morbidity in the Swedish Trial in Old Patients with Hypertension-2 (STOP-2) study. Lancet 354:1751-1756, 1999.

38. Hansson L, Hedner T, Lund-Johansen P, et al., for the NORDIL Study Group. Randomised trial of effects of calcium antagonists compared with diuretics and β-blockers on cardiovascular morbidity and mortality in hypertension: The Nordic Diltiazem (NORDIL) study. Lancet 356:359-365, 2000.

39. Brown MJ, Palmer CR, Castaigne A, et al. Morbidity and mortality in patients randomised to double-blind treatment with a long-acting calcium-channel blocker or diuretic in the International Nifedipine GITS study: Intervention as a Goal in Hypertension Treatment (INSIGHT). Lancet 356:366-372, 2000.

40. The ALLHAT Officers and Coordinators for the ALLHAT Collaborative Research Group. Major cardiovascular events in hypertensive patients randomized to doxazosin vs chlorthalidone: The Antihypertensive and Lipid-Lowering Treatment to Prevent Heart Attack Trial (ALLHAT). JAMA 283:1967-1975, 2000.

41. Grimm RH, Margolis KL, Papademetriou VV, et al., for ALLHAT Collaborative Research Group. Baseline characteristics of participants in the Antihypertensive and Lipid Lowering Treatment to Prevent Heart Attack Trial (ALLHAT). Hypertension 37:19-27, 2001.

42. Cushman WC, Ford CE, Cutler JA, et al. Success and predictors of blood pressure control in diverse North American settings: The Antihypertensive and Lipid-Lowering Treatment to Prevent Heart Attack Trial (ALLHAT). J Clin Hypertens 4:393-404, 2002.

43. Farnett L, Mulrow CD, Linn WD, et al. The J-curve phenomenon and the treatment of hypertension: Is there a point beyond which blood pressure reduction is dangerous? JAMA 265:489-495, 1991.

44. Coope J, Warrender TS. Randomized trial of treatment of hypertension in elderly patients in primary care. Br Med J (Clin Res Ed) 293:1145-1151, 1986.

45. Staessen J, Bulpitt C, Clement D, et al. Relation between mortality and treated blood pressure in elderly patients with hypertension: Report of the European Working Party on High Blood Pressure in the Elderly. BMJ 298:1552-1556, 1989.

46. Hansson L, Zanchetti A, Carruthers SG, et al. Effects of intensive blood-pressure lowering and low-dose aspirin in patients with hypertension: Principal results of the Hypertension Optimal Treatment (HOT) randomized trial. Lancet 351:1755-1762, 1998.

47. Somes G, Pahor M, Shorr RI, et al. The role of diastolic blood pressure when treating isolated systolic hypertension. Arch Intern Med 159:2004-2009, 1999.

48. Hulley S, Grady D, Bush T, et al. Randomized trial of estrogen plus progestin for secondary prevention of coronary heart disease in postmenopausal women. Heart and Estrogen/progestin Replacement Study (HERS) Research Group. JAMA 280:605-613, 1998.

49. Grady D, Herrington D, Bittner V, et al. Cardiovascular disease outcomes during 6.8 years of hormone therapy. JAMA 288:49-57, 2002.

50. Vittinghof E, Shilpak MG, Varosy PD, et al. Risk factors and secondary prevention in women with heart disease: The Heart and Estrogen/Progestin Replacement Study. Ann Intern Med 138:81-89, 2003.

51. Giugliano R, Camargo, CA, Lloyd-Jones DM, et al. Elderly patients receive less aggressive medical and invasive management of unstable angina. Arch Intern Med 158:1113-1120, 1998.

52. Hyman DJ, Pavlik VN. Characteristics of patients with uncontrolled hypertension in the United States. N Engl J Med 345:479-486, 2001.

53. Wassertheil-Smoller S, Anderson G, Psaty B, et al. Hypertension and its treatment in postmenopausal women: Baseline data from the Women's Health Initiative. Hypertension 36:780-789, 2000.

54. Manson JE, Hsia J, Johnson KC, et al., for Women's Health Initiative Investigators. Estrogen plus progestin and the risk of coronary heart disease. N Engl J Med 349:523-534, 2003.

55. Wassertheil-Smoller S, Hendrix SL, Limacher M, et al. Effect of estrogen plus progestin on stroke in post-menopausal women. The Women's Health Initiative: A randomized trial. JAMA 289:2673-2684, 2003.

56. Writing Group for the PEPI trial. Effects of estrogen or estrogen/progestin Regimens on heart disease risk factors in postmenopausal women. JAMA 273:199-208, 1995.

57. Scuteri A, Bos A, Brant LJ, et al. Hormone replacement therapy and longitudinal changes in blood pressure in postmenopausal women. Ann Intern Med 135:229-238, 2001.

58. Mosca L, Appel LJ, Benjamin EJ, et al., for American Heart Association. Evidence-based guidelines for cardiovascular disease prevention in women. Expert Panel Writing Group. J Am Coll Cardiol 43:900-921, 2004.

# Management of Hypertension in Black Populations

## Ernest F. Johnson III, Jackson T. Wright, Jr.

Hypertension is the major risk factor for cardiovascular morbidity and mortality in African Americans.[1] An estimated 50 million Americans are affected with roughly 2 million new diagnoses annually. With almost 6 million hypertensives, African Americans have the highest rate of hypertension, among the lowest rates of control to goal blood pressure (BP), and the highest risk of complications from hypertension of any ethnic group in the United States. Multiple theories have been proposed to explain this disparity. Potential patient-related barriers include lack of awareness, socioeconomic status, and genetic predisposition. Physician-related barriers have included an overall lower expectation of treatment as well as the limitation of available clinical trial data to guide management. This chapter reviews the epidemiology, potential mechanisms, and management of hypertension in the African American population.

## EPIDEMIOLOGY

African Americans, compared with U.S. whites, develop hypertension at an earlier age, have more severe hypertension, and manifest more clinical sequelae of target organ damage. In the most recent National Health and Nutrition Examination Survey (NHANES), a total of 5448 participants were surveyed, including 1049 non-Hispanic Blacks (Table 56–1).[2] Non-Hispanic Blacks had a higher age-adjusted prevalence of hypertension than the general population in 2000 (33.5% vs. 28.7%). Consistent with previous NHANES data, both non-Hispanic Black men (30.9%) and women (35.8%) had a higher prevalence of hypertension compared with non-Hispanic white men (27.7%) and women (30.2%). Despite concerted efforts, hypertension awareness in the African American community has remained virtually unchanged since 1988, with rates of 73.3% and 73.9% in phases I and III of NHANES III. Although overall treatment rates in the United States have improved from 55.8% to 63.0%, a smaller percentage (28.1% vs. 33.4%) of African American hypertensives was controlled to BP <140/90 mm Hg. Among African American hypertensives, women (29.4%) had higher control rates than men (26.5%). As in other populations, both systolic BP (SBP) and diastolic BP (DBP) increase with age through the fifth decade of life (Figure 56–1). Subsequently, DBP stabilizes or trends downward while SBP (and thus pulse pressure) continues to increase.

The Atherosclerosis Risk in Communities (ARIC) study evaluated cardiovascular risk factors in 14,062 participants including 3694 African Americans, aged 45 to 64 between 1987 and 1997.[3] ARIC reported a hypertension prevalence of 56% in African American women and 53% in African American men, compared with 25% in whites. The

African American component of ARIC continues to be followed as part of the Jackson Heart Study.[4] The Meharry Cohort Study (MCS) was begun in 1958 as a longitudinal study of the incidence of hypertension in 433 African American medical students at Meharry Medical College.[5] A parallel study was conducted at Johns Hopkins University with white students. The prevalence of hypertension rose to 44% in the Meharry cohort compared with 7% in the Johns Hopkins cohort over 26 years of follow-up.

Differences in prevalence of hypertension and stroke have also been noted by race and region of the country, suggesting that southern residence is associated with increases in both hypertension and stroke. Obisesan analyzed regional and urbanized data from NHANES III in 6278 non-Hispanic whites and Blacks age 40 to 79 to determine whether differences in hypertension prevalence might explain the disproportionate number of strokes in the southeastern part of the United States known as the "Stroke Belt."[6] A significant regional difference in hypertension prevalence was noted between southern and nonsouthern non-Hispanic Black males age 40 to 59 (44.1% vs. 36.7%), as well as a trend toward higher rates in southern versus nonsouthern African American females in the same age group (45.6% vs. 39.4%). Regional differences were also reported in 5115 men and women age 18 to 30 (~39% African American) in the Coronary Artery Disease Risk Development In Young Adults (CARDIA) study, extending the regional disparity to younger African American adult males.[7] Although there was no baseline regional difference in hypertension, both African American and white men in Birmingham, Alabama had significantly higher incidences of elevated BP (>130/85 mm Hg) by the seventh year compared with men in the Midwest and far West. This was especially true for African American men in Birmingham, who had the highest incidence (20%) of hypertension of any racial/gender/regional group.

Because most surveys of secondary hypertension prevalence have used clinic-based rather than population-based data, the epidemiology of secondary hypertension in African Americans is uncertain. Thus, the true incidence of renovascular disease in African Americans remains a matter of controversy.[8-10] Svetkey et al.[10] prospectively evaluated 167 hypertensives with clinical features of renovascular hypertension. Renal artery stenosis was found in 27% of whites and 19% of African Americans, and renovascular hypertension (defined by BP response to intervention) was diagnosed in 18% of whites and only 9% of African Americans. However, the criteria used to select patients for evaluation for secondary hypertension (i.e., resistant hypertension and early onset of hypertension) more commonly occur with essential hypertension in African Americans. Therefore, surveys using these selection criteria tend to oversample essential hypertension in African Americans.

**Table 56-1** Trends in Hypertension Prevalence, Awareness, Treatment, and Control in the United States (NHANES)

| Ethnic Group | Prevalence % | Awareness % | Treated % | Controlled % |
|---|---|---|---|---|
| **Non-Hispanic White** | | | | |
| 1988-1991 | 25.9 | 70.6 | 53.9 | 25.6 |
| 1991-1994 | 25.6 | 67.5 | 51.9 | 22.7 |
| 1999-2000 | 28.9 | 69.5 | 60.1 | 33.4 |
| **Mexican American** | | | | |
| 1988-1991 | 17.2 | 54.4 | 34.1 | 13.7 |
| 1991-1994 | 17.8 | 62.0 | 43.5 | 16.3 |
| 1999-2000 | 20.7 | 57.8 | 40.3 | 17.7 |
| **Non-Hispanic Black** | | | | |
| 1988-1991 | 28.9 | 73.3 | 55.8 | 24.4 |
| 1991-1994 | 32.5 | 72.6 | 56.4 | 23.3 |
| 1999-2000 | 33.5 | 73.9 | 63.0 | 28.1 |

From Hajjar I, Kotchen TA. Trends in prevalence, awareness, treatment, and control of hypertension in the United States, 1988-2000. JAMA 290:199-206, 2003.

## MECHANISMS OF HYPERTENSION

Multiple theories have been proposed to account for the higher incidence and severity of hypertension in African American persons. These include differences in socioeconomic status (SES) and other environmental factors, increased sympathetic nervous system activity, deficiency of renal vasodilators, higher rates of low birth weight (LBW), increased salt sensitivity, and genetic susceptibility (Box 56-1). No single mechanism is fully explanatory. On the contrary, it is likely that the true explanation will involve a combination of factors.

SES has received a considerable amount of attention over the years.[11-13] The MCS attempted to eliminate the potential role of SES by including only physicians, thus individuals with roughly equivalent income and living environment. The racial difference in hypertension incidence was unaffected.[5] Other studies have reported that controlling for differences in SES dramatically reduces the racial differences in the epidemiology of hypertension and its consequences.[14] The effect of SES on health outcomes is complex and gross estimates provided by current markers (e.g., income, education, employment, insurance status, place of residence) probably oversimplify its significance.

Increased release of endothelin-1 (ET-1), a 21-residue peptide, has been associated with hypertension in African Americans.[15-17] Ergul et al.[16] measured resting plasma concentrations of ET-1 in African American and white hypertensives. In 50 hypertensive and 50 normotensive individuals, divided into categories by race and ethnicity, blood ET-1 levels in African American hypertensives were nearly eightfold higher compared with their normotensive counterparts and nearly fourfold higher compared with white hypertensives. Treiber et al.,[18] in 23 white and 18 African American adolescent males with family histories of hypertension, reported greater cardiovascular reactivity and higher levels of ET-1 in African Americans in response to acute physical or mental stress.

Lower activity of endogenous renal vasodilators such as kallikrein, atrial natriuretic peptide (ANP), prostaglandin, and

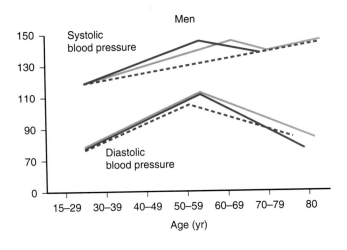

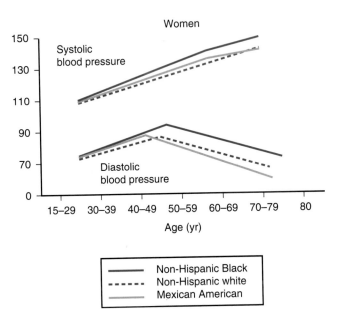

**Figure 56-1** Changes in systolic (SBP) and diastolic blood pressure (DBP) with age, SBP and DBP by age and race or ethnicity for men and women over 18 years of age in the U.S. population. (Data from Burt VL, Whelton P, Roccella EJ, et al. Prevalence of hypertension in the US adult population. Results from the Third National Health and Nutrition Examination Survey, 1988-1991. Hypertension 25:305-313, 1995.)

nitric oxide has also been reported in African Americans. African Americans, regardless of BP, were found to excrete less urinary kallikrein than whites.[19-22] This association may be familially aggregated, as Zinner et al.[23] found that kallikrein excretion tends to be lower in children of families with the highest BPs. In another study, Ferrari et al.[24] observed markedly reduced levels of ANP during salt loading in children of hypertensive compared with normotensive parents. In addition, salt-sensitive African Americans have been found to exhibit a paradoxical decrease in ANP in response to increased dietary-salt intake.[25] Further exploration of the potential role of these systems in the development of essential hypertension may prove important.

**Box 56-1** Proposed Mechanisms of African American Hypertension

SES
Increased endothelin-1
Low birth weight
Salt sensitivity
Obesity
Physical inactivity
Low dietary potassium
Genetic susceptibility
Decreased activity of renal vasodilators
Obstructive sleep apnea

Multiple studies have reported lower activity of the renin-angiotensin system (RAS) in African Americans compared with whites in response to changes in vascular volume or BP.[26-29] Thus, hypertension in African Americans is more often classified as low renin; this is associated with a lesser response to antihypertensives directed at inhibiting the RAS.

Several epidemiologic studies have raised the possibility that LBW may influence disease later in life.[30-32] The increased incidence of hypertension in African Americans has been proposed to be related to a higher incidence of LBW and an associated nephron deficit acquired in utero that is not recovered after birth.[32] The nephron deficit is postulated to lead to the development of glomerular sclerosis, salt sensitivity, and subsequent hypertension. This hypothesis was supported by a study in almost 5000 persons that reported a statistically significant inverse relationship between SBP at all ages beyond birth and LBW.[31] Babies weighing ≤3180 g at birth had a 4- to 12-mm Hg higher SBP than those weighing >3860 g, and by ages 64 to 71 there was a 5.2-mm Hg increase in SBP for every 1-kg decrease in birth weight.[31,32]

Racial differences in salt handling have been described and are proposed as a potential explanation for the increased incidence of African American hypertension. An abnormal renal pressure–natriuresis relationship resulting in altered sodium handling has been suggested by multiple studies reporting that African Americans have a higher incidence of salt sensitivity and low plasma renin activity compared with white Americans.[33-36] Luft et al.[35] studied 68 age-matched persons before and after a 2-L saline infusion and reported that African Americans not only excreted sodium less effectively following the salt load, but also had lower renin levels 20 hours after salt load despite identical levels immediately postsaline.

Weinberger et al.,[34] using a similar protocol, evaluated 198 essential hypertensives and reported a salt sensitivity prevalence of 73% in African Americans compared with 56% in whites. However, many previous studies reporting racial differences in salt sensitivity either did not report or control for differences in age, hypertension severity, renal function, and levels of obesity. Differences in these characteristics may result in differences in salt sensitivity. A study in which gender, age, renal function, hypertension status, and weight were closely matched found no racial difference in prevalence of salt sensitivity.[37] However, the magnitude of BP increase was greater in African American than white hypertensives; this racial difference was not seen in normotensive persons.

A defect in sodium transport is one proposed mechanism for the altered sodium metabolism.[38] African American adults have 10% to 20% higher intracellular sodium than whites.[39,40] African Americans also have up to a 30% depression in $Na^+$, $K^+$-ATPase pump activity.[41] Elevated intracellular sodium may trigger a cascade of compensatory events that lead to elevated intracellular calcium, increased vascular reactivity, and eventual hypertension.[42] The clinical implication of all of these findings is that multiple factors other than race per se may contribute to the racial difference in salt sensitivity and the lower renin levels seen in African Americans.

The question of whether or not there is a genetic contribution to African American hypertension remains to be answered. As a major component of the RAS, angiotensinogen (AGT) has a major influence on both salt and water homeostasis and vascular tone. The AGT gene has been linked to essential hypertension in families of European descent.[43] Moreover, a molecular variant of AGT known as T235 has been associated with higher AGT levels, as well as essential hypertension.[44] Although the frequency of T235 is twice as high in African Americans as in whites,[45] an association with hypertension has been found only in peoples of African origin living in the Caribbean.[46] T235 may not be a surrogate marker in African Americans due to its high prevalence.[47] Bloem et al.[47] investigated potential haplotypes more likely to serve as potential markers based on their ability to increase AGT levels. Of the three haplotypes examined, only T-1074 showed a significant association with serum AGT level. African Americans heterozygous for T-1074 had higher AGT levels than those with no copy. In addition, African Americans had a higher frequency (0.2 vs. 0.12) of T-1074 compared with whites. Therefore, AGT remains a candidate gene contributing to hypertension in both racial groups.

## CLINICAL SEQUELAE OF HYPERTENSION

African Americans have the highest morbidity and mortality from hypertension of any population group in the United States.[48] Mortality related to hypertension is four to five times higher in the African American community, and the risk of end-stage renal disease (ESRD), left ventricular hypertrophy (LVH), coronary heart disease (CHD), congestive heart failure (CHF), and stroke is increased two to four times in African Americans compared with U.S. whites. Better understanding of the potential mechanisms of hypertension in conjunction with earlier initiation of effective treatment is needed to reduce or prevent hypertension-related complications.

Ethnic minorities, especially African Americans and Native Americans have a threefold to fourfold higher prevalence of ESRD than whites. Of the 335,915 total and 60,923 new ESRD patients in the United States in 2002, African Americans comprised 28.9% of the entire ESRD population and 16,568 of all new diagnoses. In 2001, this rate was 4.4 times higher for African Americans compared with whites. Hypertension has been a long established risk factor for the development of chronic kidney disease (CKD) and ultimately ESRD.[48-52] Until the turn of the century, when overtaken by diabetes, hypertension was the most common cause of ESRD in African Americans. Therefore, suboptimal BP control in African Americans may have a dual negative effect on renal function via the development of hypertensive nephrosclerosis, as well as exacerbating other underlying disease.

In the year 2000, cardiovascular disease (CVD) resulted in 33.5% and 40.6% of African American male and female total deaths, respectively. LVH is a major independent risk factor for CVD. Several studies, including Evans County and the Hypertension Detection and Follow-up Program (HDFP), have reported a higher prevalence of LVH in African American than in white hypertensives using electrocardiogram (ECG) criteria.[48] Other studies using echocardiogram have shown a similar prevalence in both races.[53-56] As a result, the validity of ECG to determine LVH in hypertensive African Americans is now in question. Using echocardiogram as the reference standard, Lee et al.[54,56] assessed this racial difference in ECG accuracy in 122 African American and 148 white hypertensives. Although the prevalence of ECG LVH was 2.4 to 6 times higher in African Americans, specificity was consistently lower and ranged from 73% to 94% compared with 95% to 100% in whites. The reason for this overestimation is unknown, but the data suggest that using ECG algorithms for defining LVH in African American patients will require restandardization.

CHD, CHF, and stroke are also more prevalent in African Americans than in whites due in part to hypertension. Among non-Hispanic Blacks older than age 20, 7.1% of men and 9.0% of women have CHD as opposed to 6.9% and 5.4% of white men and women (American Heart Association [AHA], Stat Fact Sheet 2000). Whereas the overall death rate for CHD was 186.9 in 100,000 in 2000, death rates for African Americans were 262.4 in 100,000 for men and 187.5 in 100,000 for women. Furthermore, CHD tends to develop nearly 5 years earlier in African Americans.[1] The prevalence rate for CHF is 1.3% for African Americans aged 35 to 44 versus 0.4% and 0.3% for similar-aged white men and women.

Hypertension is a major risk factor for stroke, the third leading cause of death in the United States. (AHA, Stat Fact Sheet 2000) The overall death rate for stroke in 2000 was 60.8 of 100,000. The relative risk of a first event in African Americans is almost twofold greater than in whites. Despite declining total stroke mortality in the United States, African Americans have maintained a higher stroke mortality rate than whites, with African American males experiencing the highest rate (87.1 of 100,000 vs. 78.1 of 100,000 for women). This increased risk is most notable among African Americans aged 35 to 54 (4.0 times higher) and diminishes in the elderly (1.2 times higher for ages 75-84).

## TREATMENT OPTIONS

### Lifestyle Modification

Clinical trial data have shown that lifestyle modification (especially salt and caloric restriction, the Dietary Approaches to Stop Hypertension [DASH] eating plan, regular physical activity, and moderation of alcohol) is effective in lowering BP in African Americans.[37,58-60] Weight loss is a particularly important lifestyle modification in the African American population because of the greater prevalence of obesity, especially among women. More than 60% of non-Hispanic Black men and 77% of non-Hispanic Black women are overweight (body mass index ≥25).[61] African Americans also exercise less often than whites. Approximately half of African American adults (44.1% of men, 55.2%

of women) report no participation in any leisure-time physical activity.[62] Furthermore, African Americans, like whites, consume excess salt.[63] Lifestyle modification is essential in treating African Americans with hypertension.

The DASH study included 459 participants (60% African American), who were randomized to one of the following diets: a control diet typical of the average American; a diet rich in fruits and vegetables; or a combination diet low in fat and rich in fruits, vegetables, and low-fat diary products—the DASH eating plan (see Chapter 43).[64] The combination diet yielded the greatest BP-lowering effect. This effect was most notable in African American hypertensives, who exhibited a decrease of BP of 13.2/6.1 mm Hg (Figure 56–2). A subsequent study combining the DASH eating plan with sodium restriction found an additional BP-lowering effect.[58] This benefit again was more pronounced in African Americans.

### Pharmacologic Intervention

The majority of patients with hypertension, especially African Americans, will require two or more antihypertensive drugs to achieve their BP goal.[59,65-67] However, studies clearly document that a majority of hypertensives, including African American hypertensives, can achieve even the most aggressive BP goal.[59,65,66] Although multiple studies have shown that all of the available antihypertensive agents are effective in African Americans, monotherapy with drugs that inhibit the RAS (i.e., angiotensin-converting enzyme [ACE] inhibitors, angiotensin receptor blockers [ARBs], and β-blockers) consistently produces attenuated BP lowering in this population.[59,68-71] Saunders et al.[68] compared the efficacy of atenolol, captopril, and verapamil sustained-release (SR) in a cohort of 394 African American patients with mild to moderate hypertension over a period of 11 to 13 weeks. Goal BP (<140/90 mm Hg or <10 mm Hg decrease) was achieved in 65.2% of those randomized to verapamil SR compared with 55.1% and 43.8% of those randomized to atenolol and captopril, respectively. Likewise, the Veterans Affairs (VA) Cooperative Studies Group followed 1092 men (533 African Americans) included in the VA Cooperative Trial to compare the efficacy of hydrochlorothiazide, atenolol, diltiazem SR, captopril, prazosin, and clonidine in BP reduction by region of the country.[69,70] African Americans were less likely to achieve target BP with atenolol or captopril. This racial difference is eliminated when RAS blockers and β-blockers are used in combination with diuretics or calcium channel blockers (CCBs).[48,72-74]

The VA Cooperative trial, with 42% African American participants employing a regimen of hydrochlorothiazide, reserpine, and hydralazine and conducted more than 35 years ago, and the HDFP trial, with 44% African Americans completed 25 years ago using chlorthalidone, reserpine, methyldopa, and hydralazine, both documented the benefit on clinical outcomes of lowering elevated BP in African American hypertensives with a thiazide-type diuretic-based regimen.[75,76] The Systolic Hypertension in the Elderly Program (SHEP) trial (14% African American) using chlorthalidone and atenolol also produced similar results in both African Americans and whites with isolated systolic hypertension.[77] Results of hypertension outcome trials involving nondiuretic-based treatment with significant minority representation have become available more recently. Because of data indicating reduced BP-lowering efficacy in African Americans, evaluation of the effects of RAS

**Figure 56-2** Joint effect of race and hypertension status on blood pressure (BP) response to the Dietary Approaches to Stop Hypertension (DASH) combination diet. HF, heart failure; CKD, chronic kidney disease; MI, myocardial infarction; CCB, calcium channel blocker; ACEI, angiotensin-converting enzyme inhibitor; ARB, angiotensin receptor blocker; BB, β-blocker. (From Svetkey LP, Simons-Morton D, Vollmer WM, et al. Effects of dietary patterns on blood pressure: Subgroup analysis of the Dietary Approaches to Stop Hypertension [DASH] randomized clinical trial. Arch Intern Med 159:285-293, 1999.)

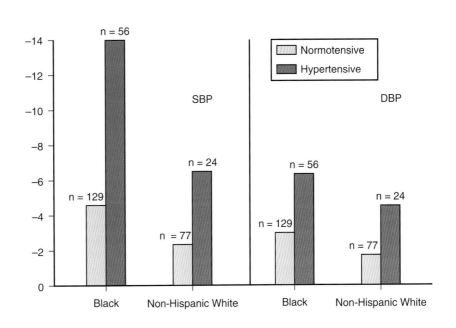

inhibitors on clinical outcomes in African Americans are especially important.

The African American Study of Kidney Disease (AASK) was the first to evaluate the effect of a CCB and an ACE inhibitor on a clinical outcome in African Americans.[78] The objectives of AASK were to determine whether lowering of BP below the goal recommended to prevent cardiovascular events or choice of antihypertensive regimen mattered in slowing the progression of hypertensive kidney disease. A total of 1094 African Americans with hypertensive renal disease (glomerular filtration rate 20-65 ml/min) were randomized to receive either ramipril or amlodipine, comparing both with metoprolol. Participants were also randomized to a usual mean arterial pressure goal of 102 to 107 mm Hg or a lower goal of 92 mm Hg or less. No significant difference in renal outcomes was detected between the two BP groups. However, the ACE inhibitor ramipril was significantly more effective in slowing the progression of kidney disease compared with amlodipine or metoprolol. Thus, the benefit of ACE inhibitors in preventing renal outcomes in African American hypertensives was demonstrated.

The effects of ACE inhibitors and other nondiuretic-based regimens in preventing cardiovascular events in African Americans were not addressed by AASK. The Antihypertensive and Lipid-Lowering Treatment to Prevent Heart Attack Trial (ALLHAT) was the first study to evaluate the relative benefit of newer agents on cardiovascular outcomes in African American hypertensives.[79,80] A total of 42,418 participants (35% African American) aged 55 or older were randomized to receive chlorthalidone, amlodipine, lisinopril, or doxazosin. Compared with amlodipine, SBP averaged 1 mm Hg lower in the chlorthalidone arm in both African Americans and whites. The chlorthalidone-lisinopril difference was 2 mm Hg in white and 4 mm Hg in Black ALLHAT participants. Although there was no difference between treatments in occurrence of the primary outcome (myocardial infarction or fatal CHD) or on all-cause mortality, chlorthalidone proved superior in reducing CHF versus doxazosin, amlodipine, and lisinopril. Chlorthalidone also reduced combined CVD and stroke compared with doxazosin and lisinopril. These differences in outcome were even greater in the African American cohort. Additionally, the higher risk of angioedema in African Americans treated with ACE inhibitors was also confirmed in this trial. Thus, ALLHAT did not support the use of α-blockers or ACE inhibitors in African American hypertensives over diuretics or CCBs (in hypertensives unable to take a diuretic) as initial treatment in the absence of CKD or CHF.

The Losartan Intervention for Endpoint (LIFE) Reduction in Hypertension study was the first to compare ARB-based treatment with an active comparator (β-blocker–based treatment) in reducing cardiovascular morbidity and mortality in a high-risk population that included more than 9000 patients (11% African American) with essential hypertension and LVH by ECG.[81] Participants were randomized to 50 to 100 mg/dl of either atenolol or losartan to achieve a target BP of <140/90. Additional antihypertensive drugs were added as necessary, and approximately 90% of participants were also receiving a thiazide-type diuretic by the end of the trial. BP reduction was similar between groups, with 49% of the losartan group and 46% of the atenolol group reaching the target. Contrary to the overall results of the study, losartan was less effective than atenolol in reducing cardiovascular risk (17% vs. 11%) in African Americans.[82] This difference in outcome of African Americans versus whites was independent of BP and had no other biologically plausible explanation. This finding must be viewed with caution, since the size of the African American sample and the number of events occurring in African Americans were small. The mechanism of this apparent racial difference in outcome is unclear and merits further investigation in trials that include larger numbers of African Americans.

## RECOMMENDATIONS

The recommendations outlined in JNC 7 are especially pertinent to the African American hypertensive (Figure 56–3). The definition of prehypertension and emphasis on lifestyle modification as integral to the treatment and prevention of hypertension in African Americans are shared by JNC 7 and the guidelines of the International Society of Hypertension in Blacks (ISHIB).[59,60] African Americans have a higher prevalence of obesity and physical inactivity, and the effects of sodium restriction and the DASH diet were greatest in the African American population. The consideration of multi-drug therapy as initial treatment for those more than 20/10 mm Hg above target BP is also consistent with both guidelines.

ACE inhibitors and ARBs should be used as first-line therapy in hypertensives, including African American hypertensives, with CKD or CHF. Along with the α-blockers and all other agents in the antihypertensive armamentarium, ACE inhibitors and ARBs should be used as needed as add-on agents to achieve the BP goal in African Americans. The JNC 7 recommends that thiazide-type diuretics should be considered first and form the cornerstone of pharmacologic therapy in most hypertensives. This recommendation especially applies to the African American hypertensive.[59,71,79] In African American hypertensives, a thiazide-type diuretic was unsurpassed in lowering BP and in preventing clinical events.[79] A CCB produced similar lowering of BP and was equally effective in preventing most clinical outcomes, but was associated with a substantially greater risk of CHF. CCBs are a reasonable alternative first-line choice in African American hypertensives unable to take a diuretic. Although recommended as equivalent or preferable to diuretics in African American diabetics in the ISHIB guidelines,[60] in the absence of renal disease or CHF, it is difficult to justify the selection of an ACE inhibitor or ARB over a diuretic (or CCB) as initial therapy in this patient population.

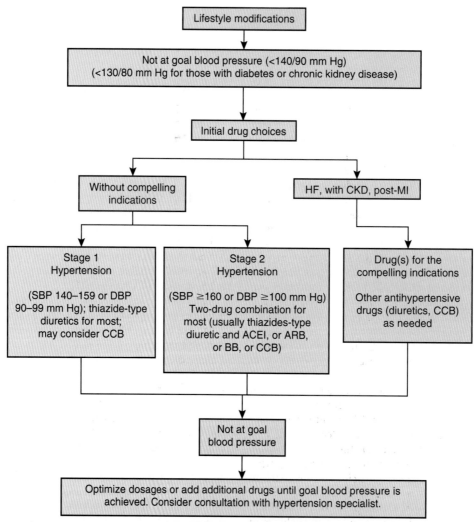

**Figure 56–3** Algorithm for treatment of hypertension. HF, heart failure; CKD chronic kidney disease; MI, myocardial infarction. (Modified from JNC 7, JAMA 2003.)

## SUMMARY

African Americans develop hypertension at an earlier age and with a higher overall prevalence than whites. Despite similar rates of awareness, African American hypertensives not only are more likely to have more severe hypertension, but are also less well controlled once treatment is initiated. The etiology of hypertension in African Americans remains unknown. The approach to treatment should be multidisciplinary and should include both lifestyle modification and pharmacologic intervention. For the majority of hypertensives, especially African Americans, multiple agents will be required to achieve target BP. Although all classes of antihypertensive are effective, thiazide-based regimens should be considered as first line treatment in the absence of compelling indications for alternative regimens. CCBs are recommended as initial therapy in African American hypertensives who cannot take a diuretic. Monotherapy with ACE inhibitors, ARBs, or β-blockers is less effective in African Americans compared with other population groups. This racial difference disappears with the addition of a diuretic or CCB. ACE inhibitors or ARBs should be included in antihypertensive regimens prescribed for African American hypertensives with renal disease or CHF. In the absence of these conditions, ACE inhibitors or ARBs should be added to a regimen containing a thiazide-type diuretic and/or CCB in order to achieve the desired BP goal. Aggressive treatment of BP to recommended goals can have a significant impact on preventing CVD, stroke, and ESRD in African Americans.

## References

1. Flack JM, Ferdinand KC, Nasser SA. Epidemiology of hypertension and cardiovascular disease in African Americans. J Clin Hypertens (Greenwich) 5(1 Suppl 1):5-11, 2003.
2. Hajjar I, Kotchen TA. Trends in prevalence, awareness, treatment, and control of hypertension in the United States, 1988-2000. JAMA 290:199-206, 2003.
3. Krop JS, Coresh J, Chambless LE, et al. A community-based study of explanatory factors for the excess risk for early renal function decline in blacks vs whites with diabetes: The Atherosclerosis Risk in Communities study. Arch Intern Med 159:1777-1783, 1999.
4. Sempos CT, Bild DE, Manolio TA. Overview of the Jackson Heart Study: A study of cardiovascular diseases in African American men and women. Am J Med Sci 317:142-146, 1999.
5. Thomas J, Semenya KA, Neser WB, et al. Risk factors and the incidence of hypertension in black physicians: The Meharry Cohort Study. Am Heart J 110:637-645, 1985.
6. Obisesan TO, Vargas CM, Gillum RF. Geographic variation in stroke risk in the United States. Region, urbanization, and hypertension in the Third National Health and Nutrition Examination Survey. Stroke 31:19-25, 2000.
7. Kiefe CI, Williams OD, Bild DE, et al. Regional disparities in the incidence of elevated blood pressure among young adults: The CARDIA study. Circulation 96:1082-1088, 1997.
8. Emovon OE, Klotman PE, Dunnick NR, et al. Renovascular hypertension in blacks. Am J Hypertens 9:18-23, 1996.
9. Sica DA, Hansen KJ, Deitch JS, et al. Renovascular disease in blacks: Prevalence and result of operative management. Consortium of Southeastern Hypertension Control. Am J Med Sci 315:337-342, 1998.
10. Svetkey LP, Kadir S, Dunnick NR, et al. Similar prevalence of renovascular hypertension in selected blacks and whites. Hypertension 17:678-683, 1991.
11. Rooks RN, Simonsick EM, Miles T, et al. The association of race and socioeconomic status with cardiovascular disease indicators among older adults in the health, aging, and body composition study. J Gerontol B Psychol Sci Soc Sci 57:S247-S256, 2002.
12. Howard G, Anderson RT, Russell G, et al. Race, socioeconomic status, and cause-specific mortality. Ann Epidemiol 10:214-223, 2000.
13. James SA. Primordial prevention of cardiovascular disease among African-Americans: A social epidemiological perspective. Prev Med 29(6 Pt 2):S84-S89, 1999.
14. Matthews KA, Kiefe CI, Lewis CE, et al. Socioeconomic trajectories and incident hypertension in a biracial cohort of young adults. Hypertension 39:772-776, 2002.
15. Grubbs AL, Anstadt MP, Ergul A. Saphenous vein endothelin system expression and activity in African American patients. Arterioscler Thromb Vasc Biol 22:1122-1127, 2002.
16. Ergul S, Parish DC, Puett D, et al. Racial differences in plasma endothelin-1 concentrations in individuals with essential hypertension. Hypertension 28:652-655, 1996.
17. Grubbs AL, Ergul A. A review of endothelin and hypertension in African-American individuals. Ethn Dis 11:741-748, 2001.
18. Treiber FA, Musante L, Braden D, et al. Racial differences in hemodynamic responses to the cold face stimulus in children and adults. Psychosom Med 52:286-296, 1990.
19. Margolius HS. Urinary kallikreins and prostaglandins in blacks. J Clin Hypertens 3(3 Suppl):51S-56S, 1987.
20. Levy SB, Lilley JJ, Frigon RP, et al. Urinary kallikrein and plasma renin activity as determinants of renal blood flow. The influence of race and dietary sodium intake. J Clin Invest 60:129-138, 1977.
21. Gainer JV, Brown NJ, Bachvarova M, et al. Altered frequency of a promoter polymorphism of the kinin B2 receptor gene in hypertensive African-Americans. Am J Hypertens 13:1268-1273, 2000.
22. Wong CM, O'Connor DT, Martinez JA, et al. Diminished renal kallikrein responses to mineralocorticoid stimulation in African Americans: Determinants of an intermediate phenotype for hypertension. Am J Hypertens 16:281-289, 2003.
23. Zinner SH, Margolius HS, Rosner B, et al. Familial aggregation of urinary kallikrein concentration in childhood: Relation to blood pressure, race and urinary electrolytes. Am J Epidemiol 104:124-132, 1976.
24. Ferrari P, Weidmann P, Ferrier C, et al. Dysregulation of atrial natriuretic factor in hypertension-prone man. J Clin Endocrinol Metab 71:944-951, 1990.
25. Campese VM, Tawadrous M, Bigazzi R, et al. Salt intake and plasma atrial natriuretic peptide and nitric oxide in hypertension. Hypertension 28:335-340, 1996.
26. Channick BJ, Adlin EV, Marks AD. Suppressed plasma renin activity in hypertension. Arch Intern Med 123:131-140, 1969.
27. Chrysant SG, Danisa K, Kem DC, et al. Racial differences in pressure, volume, and renin interrelationship in essential hypertension. Hypertension 1:136-141, 1979.
28. Holland OB, Gomez-Sanchez C, Fairchild C, et al. Role of renin classification for diuretic treatment of black hypertensive patients. Arch Intern Med 139:1365-1370, 1979.
29. Fray JC, Russo SM. Mechanism for low renin in blacks: Studies in hypophysectomised rat model. J Hum Hypertens 4:160-162, 1990.
30. Barker DJ, Martyn CN. The fetal origins of hypertension. Adv Nephrol Necker Hosp 26:65-72, 1997.
31. Law CM, de Swiet M, Osmond C, et al. Initiation of hypertension in utero and its amplification throughout life. BMJ 306(6869):24-27, 1993.
32. Lopes AA, Port FK. The low birth weight hypothesis as a plausible explanation for the black/white differences in hypertension, non-insulin-dependent diabetes, and end-stage renal disease. Am J Kidney Dis 25:350-356, 1995.
33. Channick BJ, Adlin EV, Marks AD. Suppressed plasma renin activity in hypertension. Arch Intern Med 123:131-140, 1969.

34. Weinberger MH. Salt sensitivity of blood pressure in humans. Hypertens 27:481-490, 1996.

35. Luft FC, Grim CE, Higgins JT Jr, et al. Differences in response to sodium administration in normotensive white and black subjects. J Lab Clin Med 90:555-562, 1977.

36. Falkner B. Sodium sensitivity: A determinant of essential hypertension. J Am Coll Nutr 7:35-41, 1988.

37. Wright JT Jr, Rahman M, Scarpa A, et al. Determinants of salt sensitivity in black and white normotensive and hypertensive women. Hypertension 42:1087-1092, 2003.

38. Laurenzi M, Trevisan M. Sodium-lithium countertransport and blood pressure: The Gubbio Population Study. Hypertension 13:408-415, 1989.

39. Cooper RS, Borke JL. Intracellular ions and hypertension in blacks. *In* Fray JCS, Douglas JG (eds). Pathophysiology of Hypertension in Blacks. New York, Oxford, 1993; pp 181-213.

40. Cooper R, Aina O, Chaco L, et al. Cell cations and blood pressure in U.S. whites, U.S. blacks and West African blacks. J Hum Hypertens 4:477-484, 1990.

41. Rygielski D, Reddi A, Kuriyama S, et al. Erythrocyte ghost Na$^+$,K$^+$-ATPase and blood pressure. Hypertension 10:259-266, 1987.

42. Douglas JG, Thibonnier M, Wright JT. Essential hypertension: Racial/ethnic differences in pathophysiology. J Assoc Acad Minor Phys 7:16-21, 1996.

43. Caulfield M, Lavender P, Farrall M, et al. Linkage of the angiotensinogen gene to essential hypertension. N Engl J Med 330:1629-1633, 1994.

44. Jeunemaitre X, Soubrier F, Kotelevtsev YV, et al. Molecular basis of human hypertension: Role of angiotensinogen. Cell 71: 169-180, 1992.

45. Bloem LJ, Manatunga AK, Tewksbury DA, et al. The serum angiotensinogen concentration and variants of the angiotensinogen gene in white and black children. J Clin Invest 95:948-953, 1995.

46. Caulfield M, Lavender P, Newell-Price J, et al. Linkage of the angiotensinogen gene locus to human essential hypertension in African Caribbeans. J Clin Invest 96:687-692, 1995.

47. Bloem LJ, Foroud TM, Ambrosius WT, et al. Association of the angiotensinogen gene to serum angiotensinogen in blacks and whites. Hypertension 29:1078-1082, 1997.

48. Rahman M, Douglas JG, Wright JT. Pathophysiology and treatment implications of hypertension in the African-American population. Endocrinol Metab Clin North Am 26:125-144, 1997.

49. Gassman JJ, Greene T, Wright JT Jr et al. Design and statistical aspects of the African American Study of Kidney Disease and Hypertension (AASK). J Am Soc Nephrol 14(7 Suppl 2):S154-S165, 2003.

50. Appel LJ, Middleton J, Miller ER III, et al. The rationale and design of the AASK cohort study. J Am Soc Nephrol 14(7 Suppl 2):S166-S172, 2003.

51. Feldman HI, Appel LJ, Chertow GM, et al. The Chronic Renal Insufficiency Cohort (CRIC) Study: Design and methods. J Am Soc Nephrol 14(7 Suppl 2):S148-S153, 2003.

52. Klag MJ, Whelton PK, Randall BL, et al. End-stage renal disease in African-American and white men: 16-year MR-FIT findings. JAMA 277:1293-1298, 1997.

53. Rautaharju PM, Park LP, Gottdiener JS, et al. Race- and sex-specific ECG models for left ventricular mass in older populations. Factors influencing overestimation of left ventricular hypertrophy prevalence by ECG criteria in African-Americans. J Electrocardiol 33:205-218, 2000.

54. Lee DK, Marantz PR, Devereux RB, et al. Left ventricular hypertrophy in black and white hypertensives. Standard electrocardiographic criteria overestimate racial differences in prevalence [published erratum appears in JAMA 268:3201, 1992] JAMA 267:3294-3299, 1992.

55. Gottdiener JS, Reda DJ, Materson BJ, et al. Importance of obesity, race and age to the cardiac structural and functional effects of hypertension. The Department of Veterans Affairs Cooperative Study Group on Antihypertensive Agents. J Am Coll Cardiol 24:1492-1498, 1994.

56. Okin PM, Wright JT, Nieminen MS, et al. Ethnic differences in electrocardiographic criteria for left ventricular hypertrophy: The LIFE study. Am J Hypertens 15:663-671, 2002.

57. Liebson PR, Grandits GA, Dianzumba S, et al. Comparison of five antihypertensive monotherapies and placebo for change in left ventricular mass in patients receiving nutritional-hygienic therapy in the Treatment of Mild Hypertension Study (TOMHS). Circulation 91:698, 1995.

58. Sacks FM, Svetkey LP, Vollmer WM, et al. Effects on blood pressure of reduced dietary sodium and the Dietary Approaches to Stop Hypertension (DASH) diet. DASH-Sodium Collaborative Research Group. N Engl J Med 344:3-10, 2001.

59. Chobanian AV, Bakris GL, Black HR, et al. Seventh report of the Joint National Committee on Prevention, Detection, Evaluation, and Treatment of High Blood Pressure. Hypertension 42:1206-1252, 2003.

60. Douglas JG, Bakris GL, Epstein M, et al. Management of high blood pressure in African Americans: Consensus statement of the Hypertension in African Americans Working Group of the International Society on Hypertension in Blacks. Arch Intern Med 163:525-541, 2003.

61. Flegal KM, Carroll MD, Ogden CL, et al. Prevalence and trends in obesity among US adults, 1999-2000. JAMA 288:1723-1727, 2002.

62. American Heart Association. Heart Disease and Stroke Statistics—2004 Update. Dallas, TX, American Heart Association, 2004. *www.americanheart.org/downloadable/heart/1079736729696HDSStats2004UpdateREV3-19-04.pdf.*

63. Svetkey LP, Simons-Morton D, Vollmer WM, et al. Effects of dietary patterns on blood pressure: Subgroup analysis of the Dietary Approaches to Stop Hypertension (DASH) randomized clinical trial. Arch Intern Med 159:285-293, 1999.

64. Appel LJ, Moore TJ, Obarzanek E, et al. A clinical trial of the effects of dietary patterns on blood pressure. DASH Collaborative Research Group. N Engl J Med 336:1117-1124, 1997.

65. Wright JT Jr, Agodoa L, Contreras G, et al. Successful blood pressure control in the African American Study of Kidney Disease and Hypertension. Arch Intern Med 162:1636-1643, 2002.

66. Cushman WC, Ford CE, Cutler JA, et al. Success and predictors of blood pressure control in diverse North American settings: The Antihypertensive and Lipid-Lowering Treatment to Prevent Heart Attack Trial (ALLHAT). J Clin Hypertens (Greenwich) 4:393-405, 2002.

67. Black HR, Elliott WJ, Grandits G, et al. Principal results of the Controlled Onset Verapamil Investigation of Cardiovascular End Points (CONVINCE) trial. JAMA 289:2073-2082, 2003.

68. Saunders E, Weir MR, Kong BW, et al. A comparison of the efficacy and safety of a beta-blocker, a calcium channel blocker, and a converting enzyme inhibitor in hypertensive blacks. Arch Intern Med 150:1707-1713, 1990.

69. Materson BJ, Reda DJ, Cushman WC, et al. Single-drug therapy for hypertension in men. A comparison of six antihypertensive agents with placebo. The Department of Veterans Affairs Cooperative Study Group on Antihypertensive Agents. N Engl J Med 328:914-921, 1993.

70. Cushman WC, Reda DJ, Perry HM, et al. Regional and racial differences in response to antihypertensive medication use in a randomized controlled trial of men with hypertension in the United States. Department of Veterans Affairs Cooperative Study Group on Antihypertensive Agents. Arch Intern Med 160:825-831, 2000.

71. Wright JT Jr, Douglas J. Optimal treatment of hypertension and cardiovascular risk reduction in African Americans: Treatment approaches for outpatients. J Clin Hypertens (Greenwich) 5(1 Suppl 1):18-25, 2003.

72. Veterans Administration Cooperative Study Group on Antihypertensive Agents. Efficacy of nadolol alone and combined with bendroflumethiazide and hydralazine for systemic hypertension. Am J Cardiol 52:1230-1237, 1983.

73. Frishman WH, Bryzinski BS, Coulson LR, et al. A multifactorial trial design to assess combination therapy in hypertension. Treatment with bisoprolol and hydrochlorothiazide. Arch Intern Med 154:1461-1468, 1994.

74. Soffer BA, Wright JT Jr, Pratt JH, et al. Effects of losartan on a background of hydrochlorothiazide in patients with hypertension. Hypertension 26:112-117, 1995.

75. Veterans Administration Cooperative Study Group on Antihypertensive Agents. II. Results in patients with diastolic blood pressure averaging 90 through 114 mm Hg. JAMA 213:1143-1152, 1970.

76. Five-year findings of the Hypertension Detection and Follow-up Program. II. Mortality by race-sex and age. Hypertension Detection and Follow-Up Program Cooperative Group. JAMA 242:2572-2577, 1979.

77. SHEP Cooperative Research Group. Prevention of stroke by antihypertensive drug treatment in older persons with isolated systolic hypertension: Final results of the Systolic Hypertension in the Elderly Program (SHEP). JAMA 265:3255-3264, 1991.

78. Wright JT Jr, Bakris G, Greene T, et al. Effect of blood pressure lowering and antihypertensive drug class on progression of hypertensive kidney disease: Results from the AASK trial. JAMA 288:2421-2431, 2002.

79. The ALLHAT Officers and Coordinators for the ALLHAT Collaborative Research Group. Major outcomes in high-risk hypertensive patients randomized to angiotensin-converting enzyme inhibitor or calcium channel blocker vs diuretic: The Antihypertensive and Lipid-Lowering Treatment to Prevent Heart Attack Trial (ALLHAT). JAMA 288:2981-2997, 2002.

80. The ALLHAT Officers and Coordinators for the ALLHAT Collaborative Research Group. Major cardiovascular events in hypertensive patients randomized to doxazosin vs chlorthalidone: The antihypertensive and lipid-lowering treatment to prevent heart attack trial (ALLHAT). ALLHAT Collaborative Research Group [see comments]. JAMA 283:1967-1975, 2000.

81. Dahlof B, Devereux RB, Kjeldsen SE, et al. Cardiovascular morbidity and mortality in the Losartan Intervention For Endpoint reduction in hypertension study (LIFE): A randomized trial against atenolol. Lancet 2002;359(9311):955-1003.

82. Julius S, Alderman MH, Beevers G, et al. Cardiovascular risk reduction in hypertensive Black patients with left ventricular hypertrophy: The LIFE Study. J Am Coll Cardiol 43:1047-1055, 2004.

# Chapter 57

# Hypertension in Pregnancy

## Sandra J. Taler

## INTRODUCTION

The key to managing hypertension in pregnancy rests on early detection and accurate disease classification to distinguish preeclampsia, a pregnancy-specific syndrome of reduced organ perfusion, from preexisting chronic hypertension. Although the cause of preeclampsia remains unknown, the pathophysiologic mechanisms and associated risks and therefore management differ from chronic hypertension. Classification is based on the work of the American College of Obstetricians and Gynecologists Committee on Terminology, with minor revisions by the U.S. National High Blood Pressure Education Program in 2000. Hypertension in pregnancy is classified into one of five categories (Table 57–1): chronic hypertension, preeclampsia-eclampsia, preeclampsia superimposed on chronic hypertension, gestational hypertension, and transient hypertension.[1]

Hypertensive disorders are estimated to occur in 6% to 8% of pregnancies in the United States Preeclampsia is more common in nulliparous women, occurring in up to 10% of first-time pregnancies. Chronic hypertension occurs in up to 5% of pregnant women, although rates may vary by the population studied. With recent societal trends to delay childbearing to older maternal ages and the increasing use of fertility drugs resulting in multiple gestation pregnancies, the incidence of preeclampsia increased 40% between 1990 and 1999 and will likely continue to rise.[2] Risk factors for preeclampsia are listed in Box 57–1. Older maternal age may contribute to preeclampsia risk because of an increased frequency of chronic hypertension. The prevalence of preeclampsia increases to 25% in women with chronic hypertension and is even higher in the setting of renal or other systemic diseases.

Following their initial presentation, hypertensive disorders have a high rate of recurrence (20%-50%) in subsequent pregnancies.[3] Risk factors for recurrence are shown in Box 57–2. Although gestational hypertension has long been known to predict subsequent essential hypertension, studies suggest that women with preeclampsia also have a greater tendency than women with normotensive pregnancies to develop hypertension later in life.[3,4]

## CHRONIC HYPERTENSION IN PREGNANCY

Chronic hypertension complicates pregnancy by increasing the risk of adverse outcomes, including premature birth, intrauterine growth retardation, fetal death, placental abruption, and cesarean delivery. The incidence of these conditions is related to the severity and duration of the hypertension prior to conception, the presence of target organ damage or coexistent renal disease, and the higher risk for superimposed preeclampsia. Pregnancy may present additional risks to the woman with chronic hypertension by the added stress of volume expansion on compromised cardiac function or by increases in proteinuria that accelerate renal decline. Women with chronic hypertension may be at higher risk for adverse neonatal outcomes independent of the development of preeclampsia.[5,6] The risks of fetal loss and acceleration of maternal renal disease increase at serum creatinine levels above 1.4 mg/dl at conception, although it may be difficult to delineate the effects of pregnancy from progression of the underlying renal disease.[7,8]

## PREPREGNANCY EVALUATION

Ideally, women with chronic hypertension should seek evaluation prior to pregnancy to define the severity of their hypertension, adjust medications, and plan for potential lifestyle changes (Table 57–2). If the systolic blood pressure is ≥180 mm Hg or diastolic pressure is ≥110 mm Hg or if treatment requires multiple antihypertensive agents, it is particularly important to search for a potentially reversible cause. Some practitioners would change to antihypertensive medications known to be safe during pregnancy even before conception. Angiotensin-converting enzyme (ACE) inhibitors and angiotensin receptor blockers (ARBs) may cause oligohydramnios, fetal renal failure, and neonatal death and should be discontinued before conception or as soon as pregnancy is confirmed.

Women with a history of hypertension over several years should be evaluated for target organ damage, including retinopathy, left ventricular hypertrophy, and renal disease. If present, they should be advised that pregnancy may worsen these conditions. Risk factors for superimposed preeclampsia include renal insufficiency, a history of hypertension for more than 4 years, or hypertension in a previous pregnancy.

Planning for pregnancy may require lifestyle changes. Hypertensive women are advised to restrict aerobic exercise during pregnancy based on theoretical concerns that reduced placental blood flow may increase the risk of preeclampsia.[9] Weight reduction is not recommended during pregnancy, even in obese women. Sodium restriction may be continued for women who have been successfully treated by this approach prior to pregnancy. As in all pregnancies, alcohol and tobacco use is strongly discouraged.

## TREATMENT OF CHRONIC HYPERTENSION IN PREGNANCY

Most women with chronic hypertension in pregnancy have stage 1 hypertension (systolic blood pressure of 140-159, diastolic pressure of 90-99 mm Hg, or both). In the short time frame of pregnancy, the risk of cardiovascular complications

**Table 57-1** Classification of Hypertension in Pregnancy

| | |
|---|---|
| Chronic hypertension | • BP ≥140 mm Hg systolic or 90 mm Hg diastolic before pregnancy or before 20 weeks' gestation<br>• Persists >12 weeks postpartum |
| Preeclampsia | • BP ≥140 mm Hg systolic or 90 mm Hg diastolic with proteinuria (>300 mg/24 hr) after 20 weeks' gestation<br>• Can progress to eclampsia (seizures)<br>• More common in nulliparous women, multiple gestation, women with hypertension for ≥4 years, family history of preeclampsia, hypertension in previous pregnancy, renal disease |
| Chronic hypertension with superimposed preeclampsia | • New-onset proteinuria after 20 weeks in a woman with hypertension<br>• In a woman with hypertension and proteinuria before 20 weeks' gestation:<br>    Sudden twofold to threefold increase in proteinuria<br>    Sudden increase in BP<br>    Thrombocytopenia<br>    Elevated AST or ALT |
| Gestational hypertension | • Hypertension without proteinuria occurring after 20 weeks' gestation<br>• Temporary diagnosis (only during pregnancy)<br>• May represent pre-proteinuric phase of preeclampsia or recurrence of chronic hypertension abated in midpregnancy<br>• May evolve to preeclampsia<br>• If severe, may result in higher rates of premature delivery and growth retardation than mild preeclampsia |
| Transient hypertension | • Retrospective diagnosis (only after pregnancy)<br>• BP normal by 12 weeks' postpartum<br>• May recur in subsequent pregnancies<br>• Predictive of future essential hypertension |

AST, aspartate aminotransferase; ALT, alanine aminotransferase.

is low. Because there is no evidence that pharmacologic treatment leads to improved neonatal outcomes and blood pressure usually falls during the first half of pregnancy, these women can be monitored with no or reduced drug therapy.[10] Some centers manage chronic hypertensives by stopping antihypertensive medications under close observation. Women with evidence for target organ damage or taking multiple agents may be able to taper medications based on blood pressure readings. Medications should be continued if needed to maintain blood pressure control. There is evidence that antihypertensive treatment will prevent progression of chronic hypertension to severe levels during pregnancy. Treatment should be reinstituted if blood pressure reaches levels of 150 to 160 mm Hg systolic or 100 to 110 mm Hg diastolic.

Complete secondary hypertension evaluation is usually postponed during pregnancy. All hypertensive women should still be screened for pheochromocytoma at the time of hypertension diagnosis because of the high morbidity and mortality associated with this condition if not diagnosed before delivery. When the hypertension is severe, further evaluation for secondary causes may be indicated and treatment may save the life of the fetus. Ultrasound and magnetic resonance scanning techniques offer safe modalities for renal artery or adrenal imaging. Laparoscopic adrenalectomy has been successfully performed during the second trimester in settings of primary aldosteronism, resulting in excellent fetal survival.[11,12]

## ANTIHYPERTENSIVE DRUG SELECTION

The goal of treating chronic hypertension is to reduce maternal risk by using agents that are safe for the fetus. Methyldopa

**Box 57-1** Maternal Risk Factors for Preeclampsia

Primigravida
Positive family history (maternal or paternal)
Multiple gestations
Diabetes mellitus
Insulin resistance/obesity
Chronic hypertension
Preexisting renal disease
Extremes of reproductive age
Hydatidiform disease
History of severe early preeclampsia in a prior pregnancy
Collagen vascular disease
Black race
Increased circulating testosterone
Thrombophilias

**Box 57-2** Risk Factors for Recurrent Hypertension in Pregnancy

Early onset of hypertension in a prior pregnancy
Chronic hypertension
Persistent hypertension beyond 5 weeks postpartum
High baseline blood pressure early in pregnancy

**Table 57-2** Management of Chronic Hypertension in Pregnancy

| | |
|---|---|
| **Before conception** | |
| Evaluation for secondary hypertension | Pheochromocytoma |
| | Other causes if severe |
| Evaluation for target organ damage | Cardiac function, LVH (echocardiography) |
| | Renal disease (serum creatinine, proteinuria) |
| Change to medications safe for pregnancy | Taper early |
| | Titrate later |
| Lifestyle planning | Restrict aerobic exercise |
| | Avoid weight reduction |
| | Moderate sodium intake |
| | Avoid all alcohol and tobacco |
| Baseline laboratory testing | Hematocrit, hemoglobin, platelet count, serum creatinine, uric acid, urinalysis |
| **During pregnancy** | |
| Selection of medications safe for pregnancy | Table 57-3 |
| Thresholds for treatment | 150-160 mm Hg systolic |
| | 100-110 mm Hg diastolic |
| Laboratory monitoring | Hematocrit, hemoglobin, platelet count, serum creatinine, uric acid, AST, ALT, quantification of urine protein, serum albumin, LDH, peripheral blood smear, coagulation studies |
| **Delivery** | |
| Maternal indications | Gestational age ≥38 weeks |
| | Platelet count <100,000 cells/mm$^3$ |
| | Deterioration in hepatic or renal function |
| | Suspected placental abruption |
| | Severe headache or visual changes |
| | Severe epigastric pain, nausea, or vomiting |
| Fetal indications | Severe fetal growth restriction |
| | Concerning fetal testing results |
| | Oligohydramnios |
| Acute/parenteral therapy | Table 57-5 |
| **Postpartum** | |
| Lactation | Withhold antihypertensive medication |
| | Taper medication dosage |
| | Selection of safe medications |
| | Close monitoring for adverse effects |
| **Late issues after hypertensive pregnancy** | |
| Persistent hypertension | Evaluation for secondary causes |
| | Change medication |
| Long-term risk | Monitor blood pressure for future hypertension |
| | Treat cardiovascular risk factors |

LVH, left ventricular hypertrophy; AST, aspartate aminotransferase; ALT, alanine aminotransferase; LDH, lactate dehydrogenase.

is preferred by many as first-line therapy, based on reports of stable uteroplacental blood flow and child development studies out to 7.5 years showing no long-term adverse effects.[13] Other treatment options are listed in Table 57-3. For all medication choices, there are concerns regarding safety in pregnancy. In a meta-analysis of 45 randomized controlled trials of treatment of mild to moderate hypertension in pregnancy when using methyldopa, β-blockers, thiazide diuretics, hydralazine, calcium antagonists, and clonidine, there was a direct linear relationship between treatment-induced fall in mean arterial pressure and the proportion of small-for-gestational-age infants.[14] Neither type of hypertension, type of agent, nor duration of therapy explained this relationship.

There are no placebo-controlled trials evaluating the treatment of severe hypertension in pregnancy, and none are like-

ly to be performed because of ethical concerns. Historical experience with severe chronic hypertension in the first trimester describes fetal loss rates of 50% and significant maternal mortality, primarily occurring in pregnancies complicated by superimposed preeclampsia.[15]

## PREGNANCY IN WOMEN WITH RENAL DISEASE

Women with renal diseases likely to progress should be encouraged to complete their childbearing while their renal function is well preserved. For women with mild renal disease (serum creatinine below 1.4 mg/dl), fetal survival is moderately reduced and the underlying disease does not generally

**Table 57–3** Oral Treatment of Hypertension in Pregnancy

| Agent | Comments |
|-------|----------|
| Methyldopa | Preferred based on stable utero-placental blood flow and long-term child development studies[13] |
| β-Blockers | Reports of intrauterine growth retardation (atenolol)[42,43]<br>Generally safe |
| Labetalol | Increasingly preferred to methyldopa due to reduced side effects |
| Clonidine | Limited data |
| Calcium antagonists | Limited data<br>Most experience with nifedipine and isradipine<br>No increase in major teratogenicity with exposure[44] |
| Diuretics | Not first-line agents<br>Probably safe<br>Most experience with thiazide diuretics |
| Angiotensin-converting enzyme inhibitors, angiotensin II receptor antagonists | Contraindicated[45,46]<br>Reports of fetal toxicity and death |

worsen. In moderate or severe renal insufficiency, pregnancy may accelerate the hypertension and the renal disease.[7,16,17] A decrease in birthweight correlates directly with rising maternal serum creatinine concentration.[17] As renal failure progresses, hypertension may worsen because of volume overload, requiring treatment with diuretics or dialysis. Conception should be discouraged in chronic dialysis patients, as pregnancy is associated with significant maternal morbidity. Renal transplant recipients are advised to wait 1.5 to 2 years after successful transplantation and undertake pregnancy only if renal function is stable, with creatinine of 2.0 mg/dl or less. All pregnancies in transplant recipients are considered high risk, with high rates of prematurity. No increase in structural malformations has been reported in these infants, and in the majority of cases, maternal graft function does not deteriorate.[18]

## PREECLAMPSIA

Preeclampsia is a pregnancy-specific syndrome of reduced organ perfusion caused by vasospasm and activation of the coagulation cascade. Although the pathologic changes are primarily ischemic, the cause of preeclampsia remains unknown. Current hypotheses focus on impaired placentation of the trophoblast and incomplete vascular remodeling as underlying pathogenic processes. Failure to develop the normal low-resistance, high-flow vascular connections between endovascular trophoblasts and the maternal spiral arteries results in reduced placental perfusion and a generalized disturbance in endothelial function. Postulated causes include inadequate immune tolerance, activation of inflammatory cytokines, and genetic mechanisms. Research efforts have been restricted by the lack of a de novo animal model and the difficulties inherent in predicting which women will develop preeclampsia before it presents.

Clinically preeclampsia is manifest by hypertension and proteinuria. Generalized vasoconstriction and reduced plasma volume lead to systemic hypoperfusion and reduced blood flow to multiple organs. The degree of blood pressure elevation may be mild, not reflective of the severity of the disease in the various vascular beds. Proteinuria is defined as the urinary excretion of 300 mg protein or greater in a 24-hour urine collection (usually equivalent to a dipstick measure of 30 mg/dl, "1+ dipstick" or more). A random urine protein:creatinine ratio has been shown to correlate closely with 24-hour urine protein measurements in pregnancy.[19] Preeclampsia should be suspected in the absence of proteinuria when other symptoms or signs are present (Table 57–4).

## PREVENTION

Prevention of preeclampsia has been frustrated by lack of knowledge of its underlying cause. Current strategies focus on identifying women at higher risk as targets for early disease recognition, close monitoring, and delivery when indicated. Although early small trials suggested benefit, several large multi-center trials of low-dose aspirin failed to demonstrate a protective effect over placebo.[20-22] Based on subgroup analysis, selective treatment for certain women at higher risk (specifically women with the antiphospholipid syndrome) may be reasonable. Calcium supplementation has effectively reduced the incidence of preeclampsia in third world women with low calcium intake but offers no benefit for low-risk women in the United States.[23,24] Recent attention has focused on a potential role for antioxidant vitamins to defend against oxidative stress as a mediator of preeclampsia.

## TREATMENT

Treatment for preeclampsia is palliative, because it does not alter the underlying pathophysiology of the disease. Delivery is always appropriate therapy for the mother but may not be so for the fetus, particularly when the fetus is very premature (< 32 weeks' gestation). For a preterm fetus without evidence of fetal compromise in a woman with mild disease, valuable time may be gained by postponing delivery under close monitoring. Regardless of gestational age, delivery should be strongly considered when there are signs of fetal distress or intrauterine growth retardation or signs of maternal risk, including severe hypertension, hemolysis, elevated liver enzymes, and low platelet count (termed the *HELLP syndrome*), deteriorating renal function, visual disturbance, headache, or epigastric pain (see Table 57–4). Vaginal delivery is preferable to cesarean delivery to avoid the added stress of surgery. Antihypertensive therapy is prescribed only for maternal protection. It does not improve perinatal outcomes and may reduce uteroplacental blood flow. The choice of agent and route of administration depend on anticipated timing of delivery. If it is likely to be more than 48 hours until delivery, an oral agent is selected (see Table 57–3). Methyldopa is preferred based on its safety record, with labetalol increasingly used as an effective alternative with few side effects. If delivery is imminent, parenteral agents are used. Appropriate agents and initial dosages are listed in Table 57–5.

**Table 57–4** Clinical Characteristics and Laboratory Tests Used to Discriminate Preeclampsia from Chronic Hypertension

|  | Preeclampsia | Chronic Hypertension |
|---|---|---|
| Age | Extremes of age | Older (≥30 yrs) |
| Parity | Nulliparous | Often multiparous |
| Time of diagnosis of hypertension | After 20 weeks | Before 20 weeks |
| Maternal risk factors for preeclampsia | Yes | No |
| Hypertension/ preeclampsia in prior pregnancies | Yes | Yes |
| Proteinuria (>300 mg/24 hours) | Yes | No |
| Serum uric acid | Elevated (≥5.5 mg/dl) | Normal to low |
| Elevated liver enzymes | Yes | No |
| Thrombocytopenia | Yes | No |
| Headache, blurred vision, epigastric abdominal pain | Yes | No |
| Persistent hypertension >12 weeks postpartum | No | Yes |

Treatment is initiated for persistent diastolic levels of 105 to 110 mm Hg or higher before induction, aiming for diastolic pressures of 95 to 105 mm Hg. Although hydralazine has been considered first-line parenteral therapy, a recent meta-analysis of randomized trials of short-acting antihypertensive treatment suggested greater maternal and fetal complication rates with hydralazine as compared with labetalol or nifedipine.[25]

## TREATING HYPERTENSION DURING LACTATION

Although all studied antihypertensive agents are excreted into human breast milk, differences in lipid solubility and extent of ionization of the drug at physiologic pH affect the milk:plasma ratio.[26] Breast-feeding can usually be done safely with attention to antihypertensive drug choices. For mildly hypertensive mothers who wish to breast-feed for a few months, medication may be withheld with close monitoring of blood pressure. Following discontinuation of nursing, therapy can be restarted. For patients with more severe blood pressure elevation, the clinician may consider reducing drug dosages while monitoring mother and infant. No short-term adverse effects have been reported from exposure to methyldopa or hydralazine. If a β-blocker is

**Table 57–5** Acute/Parenteral Treatment of Hypertension in Preeclampsia

| Hydralazine | 5-mg IV bolus, then 10 mg every 20 to 30 minutes to a maximum of 25 mg, repeat in several hours as necessary |
|---|---|
| Labetalol (second-line) | 20-mg IV bolus, then 40 mg 10 minutes later, 80 mg every 10 minutes for two additional doses to a maximum of 220 mg |
| Nifedipine (controversial) | 10 mg PO, repeat every 20 minutes to a maximum of 30 mg Caution when using nifedipine with magnesium sulfate, can see precipitous blood pressure drop Short-acting nifedipine is not approved by FDA for managing hypertension |
| Sodium nitroprusside (rarely when others fail) | 0.25 μg/kg/min to a maximum of 5 μg/kg/min Fetal cyanide poisoning may occur if used for more than 4 hours |

indicated, propanolol and labetalol are preferred. Diuretics may reduce milk volume and thereby suppress lactation. ACE inhibitors and ARBs should be avoided based on reports of adverse fetal and neonatal renal effects. Given the scarcity of data, it is important to monitor all breast-fed infants of mothers taking antihypertensive agents for potential adverse effects.

## RISK FOR HYPERTENSION AND ATHEROSCLEROSIS AFTER A HYPERTENSIVE PREGNANCY

Past epidemiologic studies failed to relate preeclampsia or eclampsia with first pregnancy to a greater future risk of hypertension or cardiovascular disease.[27-29] Rates of subsequent hypertension among women who had eclampsia as multiparas were higher, but the prevalence among nulliparous eclamptic women was reported to be no greater than in the general population. Hypertension or preeclampsia/eclampsia in any subsequent pregnancy predicted a threefold to fourfold higher rate of cardiovascular death.[28] In contrast, it is well established that transient hypertension recurs in a high proportion of subsequent pregnancies and predicts later development of chronic hypertension at recurrence rates of 80% to 90%.[30-32]

A growing body of evidence indicates higher risk for future development of hypertension after a hypertensive pregnancy for women with a family history of hypertension, more severe hypertension during pregnancy, and multiparity.[33-35] Of 238 women followed 7 to 12 years after a hypertensive pregnancy, 26% had hypertension and another 10% borderline hypertension as compared with 2% and 6.5%, respectively, in a group of matched controls.[36] Systolic blood pressure in early pregnancy was the single most important factor predicting systolic blood pressure at follow-up. In contrast, in a series of 26 pairs of primiparous women matched for age, race, weight, and year of delivery, no difference in frequency of hypertension was reported at a mean of 10 years later.[37] Microalbuminuria, a marker of increased risk for cardiovascular disease, has been reported at higher frequency after preeclampsia than after normotensive pregnancy with or without hypertension in women with no evidence for diabetes mellitus.[38,39] Preeclampsia has been linked to other markers of persistent endothelial dysfunction including increased plasma levels of von Willebrand factor, fibrinogen, cholesterol, triglycerides, and very-low-density lipoprotein.[40]

Few data address the late cardiovascular consequences of hypertensive pregnancy. A review of maternity records on 7543 Icelandic women reported higher death rates from ischemic heart disease (IHD) among women with any hypertension in pregnancy (RR 1.47, 95% CI 1.05-2.02), based on death certificates, autopsy, and hospital records over the next 43 to 60 years.[41] In contrast to earlier reports, the relative risk of IHD death was higher among eclamptic women and those with preeclampsia than those with hypertension alone. These data suggest that the endothelial dysfunction seen in the uterine spiral arteries during a hypertensive pregnancy may manifest as ischemic heart disease later in life. It is evident from a number of follow-up studies that women whose pregnancies are normotensive are a select group, less likely to develop chronic hypertension than the general population. Thus, pregnancy may be considered a screening test for chronic hypertension. Based on these findings, a recent consensus document concluded that women who have had preeclampsia are more prone to hypertensive complications in subsequent pregnancies; the risk is higher for recurrence with earlier presentation during the index pregnancy; recurrence rates are higher for those experiencing preeclampsia as multiparas as compared with nulliparous women; and preeclampsia reappearance rates may be population specific.[1]

# References

1. Gifford RW, August PA, Cunningham G, et al. Report of the National High Blood Pressure Education Program Working Group on High Blood Pressure in Pregnancy. Am J Obstet Gynecol 183:S1-S22, 2000.
2. Ventura SJMJ, Curtin SC, Menaker F, et al. Births: Final data for 1999. National Vital Statistics Reports 2001:49.
3. Zhang J, Troendle JF, Levine RJ. Risks of hypertensive disorders in the second pregnancy. Paediatric and Perinatal Epidemiology 15:226-231, 2001.
4. Hannaford P, Ferry S, Hirsch S. Cardiovascular sequelae of toxemia of pregnancy. Heart 77:154-158, 1997.
5. Rey E, Couturier A. The prognosis of pregnancy in women with chronic hypertension. Am J Obstet Gynecol 171: 410-416, 1994.
6. Buchbinder A, Sibai BM, Caritis S, et al. Adverse perinatal outcomes are significantly higher in severe gestational hypertension than in mild preeclampsia. Am J Obstet Gynecol 186: 66-71, 2002.
7. Jones DC, Hayslett JP. Outcome of pregnancy in women with moderate or severe renal insufficiency. N Engl J Med 335: 226-232, 1996.
8. Jungers P, Chauveau D, Choukroun G, et al. Pregnancy in women with impaired renal function. Clin Nephrol 47:281-288, 1997.
9. Clapp III JF, Simonian S, Lopez B, et al. The one-year morphometric and neurodevelopmental outcome of the offspring of women who continued to exercise regularly throughout pregnancy. Am J Obstet Gynecol 178:594-599, 1998.
10. Sibai BM, Mabie WC, Shamsa F, et al. A comparison of no medication versus methyldopa or labetalol in chronic hypertension during pregnancy. Am J Obstet Gynecol 162:960-967, 1998.
11. Solomon CG, Thiet M, Moore F Jr, et al. Primary hyperaldosteronism in pregnancy. A case report. J Reprod Med 41:255-258, 1996.
12. Aboud E, de Swiet M, Gordon H. Primary aldosteronism in pregnancy: Should it be treated surgically? Irish J Med Sci 164:279-280, 1995.
13. Cockburn J, Moar VA, Ounsted M, et al. Final report of study on hypertension during pregnancy: The effects of specific treatment on the growth and development of the children. Lancet 1:647-649, 1982.
14. von Dadelszen P, Ornstein MP, Bull SB, et al. Fall in mean arterial pressure and fetal growth restriction in pregnancy hypertension: A meta-analysis. Lancet 355:87-92, 2000.
15. Sibai BM, Anderson GD. Pregnancy outcome of intensive therapy in severe hypertension in first trimester. Obstet Gynecol 67:517-522, 1986.
16. Hou SH, Grossman SD, Madias NE. Pregnancy in women with renal disease and moderate renal insufficiency. Am J Med 78:185-194, 1985.
17. Cunningham FG, Cox SM, Harstad TW, et al. Chronic renal disease and pregnancy outcome. Am J Obstet Gynecol 163: 453-459, 1990.
18. Armenti VT, Radomski JS, Moritz MJ, et al. Report from the National Transplantation Pregnancy Registry (NTPR): Outcomes of pregnancy after transplantation. Clinical Transplants 121-130, 2002.
19. Robert M, Sepandj F, Liston RM, et al. Random protein-creatinine ratio for the quantification of proteinuria in pregnancy. Obstet Gynecol 90:893-895, 1997.
20. Caritis S, Sibai B, Hauth J, et al. Low-dose aspirin to prevent preeclampsia in women at high risk. National Institute of Child Health and Human Development Network of Maternal-Fetal Medicine Units (Comments). N Engl J Med 338:701-705, 1998.
21. ECPPA (Estudo Colaborativo para Prevencao da Pre-eclampsia com Aspirina) Collaborative Group. ECPPA: Randomised trial of low dose aspirin for the prevention of maternal and fetal complications in high risk pregnant women. Br J Obstet Gynaecol 103:39-47, 1996.
22. CLASP (Collaborative Low-dose Aspirin Study in Pregnancy) Collaborative Group. CLASP: A randomised trial of low-dose aspirin for the prevention and treatment of pre-eclampsia among 9364 pregnant women. Lancet 343:619-629, 1994.
23. Carroli G, Duley L, Belizan JM, et al. Calcium supplementation during pregnancy: A systematic review of randomised controlled trials. Br J Obstet Gynaecol 101:753-758, 1994.
24. Levine RJ, Hauth JC, Curet LB, et al. Trial of calcium to prevent preeclampsia (Comments). N Engl J Med 337:69-76, 1997.
25. Magee LA, Cham C, Waterman EJ, et al. Hydralazine for treatment of severe hypertension in pregnancy: Meta-analysis. Br Med J 327:955-964, 2003.
26. White WB. Management of hypertension during lactation. Hypertension 6:297-300, 1984.
27. Bryans CI Jr. The remote prognosis in toxemia of pregnancy. Clin Obstet Gynecol 9:973-990, 1966.
28. Chesley LC, Annitto JE. Pregnancy in the patient with hypertensive disease. Am J Obstet Gynecol 53:372, 1947.
29. Fisher KA, Luger A, Spargo BH, et al. Hypertension in pregnancy: Clinical-pathological correlations and late prognosis. Medicine 60:267-287, 1981.
30. Herrick WW, Tillman AJB. The mild toxemias of late pregnancy: Their relation to cardiovascular and renal disease. Am J Obstet Gynecol 31:832-844, 1936.
31. Adams EM, MacGillivray I. Long-term effect of pre-eclampsia on blood pressure. Lancet 2:1373-1375, 1961.
32. Chesley LC, Annitto JE, Cosgrove RA. The remote prognosis of eclamptic women: Sixth periodic report. Am J Obstet Gynecol 124:446-459, 1976.
33. Selvaggi L, Loverro G, Schena FP, et al. Long term follow-up of women with hypertension in pregnancy. Int J Gynaecol Obstet 27:45-49, 1988.

34. Lindeberg S, Axelsson O, Jorner U, et al. A prospective controlled five-year follow-up study of primiparas with gestational hypertension. Acta Obstet Gynecol Scand 67:605-609, 1988.

35. Nisell H, Lintu H, Lunell NO, et al. Blood pressure and renal function seven years after pregnancy complicated by hypertension. Br J Obstet Gynaecol 102:876-881, 1995.

36. Svensson A, Andersch B, Hansson L. Prediction of later hypertension following a hypertensive pregnancy. J Hypertens 1:94-96, 1983.

37. Carleton H, Forsythe A, Flores R. Remote prognosis of preeclampsia in women 25 years old and younger. Am J Obstet Gynecol 159:156-160, 1988.

38. Bar J, Kaplan B, Wittenberg C, et al. Microalbuminuria after pregnancy complicated by pre-eclampsia. Nephrol Dial Transplant 14:1129-1132, 1999.

39. North RA, Simmons D, Barnfather D, et al. What happens to women with preeclampsia? Microalbuminuria and hypertension following preeclampsia. Aust NZ J Obstet Gynaecol 36:233-238, 1996.

40. He S, Silveira A, Hamsten A, et al. Haemostatic, endothelial and lipoprotein parameters and blood pressure levels in women with a history of preeclampsia. Thromb Haemost 81:538-542, 1999.

41. Jonsdottir LS, Arngrimsson R, Geirsson RT, et al. Death rates from ischemic heart disease in women with a history of hypertension in pregnancy. Acta Obstet Gynecol Scand 74:772-776, 1995.

42. Rubin PC, Clark DM, Sumner DJ, et al. Placebo-controlled trial of atenolol in treatment of pregnancy-associated hypertension. Lancet 1:431-434, 1983.

43. Butters L, Kennedy S, Rubin PC. Atenolol in essential hypertension during pregnancy. Br Med J 301:587-589, 1990.

44. Magee LA, Schick B, Donnenfeld AE, et al. The safety of calcium channel blockers in human pregnancy: A prospective, multicenter cohort study. Am J Obstet Gynecol 174:823-828, 1996.

45. Hulton SA, Thomson PD, Cooper PA, et al. Angiotensin-converting enzyme inhibitors in pregnancy may result in neonatal renal failure. S Afr Med J 78:673-676, 1990.

46. Schubiger G, Flury G, Nussberger J. Enalapril for pregnancy-induced hypertension: Acute renal failure in a neonate. Ann Intern Med 108:215-216, 1988.

# Hypertension in Children
## Bonita Falkner

Hypertension may occur at any phase of childhood, from the newborn period through adolescence. The literature on hypertension generally regards hypertension in children and adolescents as a "special population" problem that should be approached as a unique issue. Compared with hypertension in adults, childhood hypertension is defined differently and occurs less frequently. Secondary causes of hypertension are detected more frequently in children than in adults, which often requires a different approach in evaluation of the hypertension. Childhood hypertension also has some striking similarities to hypertension in adults. Severe untreated hypertension in children has as poor an outcome as it does in adults.[1] Children with essential hypertension can express the same risk factors for cardiovascular disease (CVD) as adults; and children with hypertension can benefit from interventions to control the blood pressure (BP). An important aspect of BP surveillance in the young is to distinguish between elevated BP signaling an underlying disease (i.e., secondary hypertension), and when elevated BP in childhood is an early expression of primary (essential) hypertension.

## DEFINITION OF HYPERTENSION IN CHILDHOOD

The definition of hypertension in adults is based on the level of BP that is linked with an increase in risk for cardiovascular events. Although the risk for cardiovascular events increases as systolic blood pressure (SBP) rises above 115 mm Hg,[2] hypertension continues to be defined as BP that exceeds 140/90 mm Hg regardless of adult age or gender. However, in children, with the exception of extreme hypertension noted previously, there are not yet data that link a level of BP with subsequent cardiovascular events. In the absence of such data, hypertension is defined statistically. The results of several large epidemiologic studies that measured BP in healthy children[3-7] provide data from which the normal distribution of BP in healthy children and adolescents in the United States has been established.[5] An analysis of BP data on healthy children in Europe describes a very similar BP distribution pattern in childhood.[8,9]

There is a progressive rise in the BP level with increasing age concurrent with the normal age-related increase in height and weight throughout childhood. Thus there is a consistent relationship of BP with body size in childhood, and there is a normal upward shift in BP with growth. A gender difference in BP distribution emerges in adolescence that is concurrent with a gender difference in height.

Hypertension is defined as BP at or above the 95th percentile on the BP distribution for age and sex.[3] This definition delineates the top segment of the normal BP distribution at each phase of childhood. With the expansion of the epidemiologic data, and with further analysis of the growth-related determinants of BP in childhood, the 95th percentile is further adjusted for height.[5] The present definition of hyperten-sion in children and adolescents is SBP and/or diastolic blood pressure (DBP) that is equal to or greater than the 95th percentile for age, sex, and height. High normal BP or "prehyper-tension" is SBP or DBP that is between the 90th and 95th percentile for age, sex, and height. Normal BP is SBP and DBP that is less than the 90th percentile for age, sex, and height. Table 58–1 provides the level of BP for the 95th and 90th per-centile for age, sex, and height for boys, and Table 58–2 provides the same percentile levels for girls.[5]

Hypertension can also occur in newborn infants. There are limited data on normal levels of BP in newborns and very young infants.[6,7,10] When daily BP measurement in healthy newborns is examined, there is a rapid and consistent increase in BP from day of birth through the first 5 days of life.[11] This upward shift in BP over a few days reflects the normal hemo-dynamic transition from intrauterine to extrauterine life. Similar observations were made in a larger study on newborn infants that included a broad range of birth weight and gesta-tional age.[12] There is a direct relationship of BP with both birth weight and gestational age at birth. Regardless of birth weight or gestational age at birth, there is a transition, reflect-ed by a progressive increase in BP that occurs during the first 5 days of postnatal life. Subsequently, BP is directly related to body weight and age, in terms of gestation or postconception-al age. This relationship is depicted in Figure 58–1. As can be seen in the figure, the upper 95% confidence limit (CL) for a term infant (40 weeks' postconceptional age) is 90 mm Hg for SBP. BP levels that exceed 90 mm Hg are considered to be hypertensive in a term infant, and by 4 to 6 weeks of age (44 to 46 weeks postconceptional age), a SBP that exceeds 100 mm Hg is hypertension.

## MEASUREMENT OF BLOOD PRESSURE IN THE YOUNG

Measurement of BP in children and adolescents should be performed in a standardized manner that is similar to the methods used in the development of the BP tables. In the ambulatory clinic setting, the preferred method for BP meas-urement in children is by auscultation with a standard sphyg-momanometer.

Correct BP measurement in children requires the use of a cuff that is appropriate for the size of the child's upper arm.[13] A technique that can be used to select a BP cuff size of appro-priate size is to select a cuff that has a bladder width that is approximately 40% of the arm circumference midway between the olecranon and the acromion. This will usually be a cuff bladder that will cover 80% to 100% of the circumfer-ence of the arm. Most manufacturers of BP cuffs provide lines on the cuff that are useful in choosing the correct cuff size for a given child. The equipment necessary to measure BP in chil-dren 3 years of age through adolescence includes three pedi-atric cuffs of different size, as well as a standard adult cuff, an

**Table 58–1** Blood Pressure Levels for Boys by Age and Height Percentile

| Age, Yr | Blood Pressure Percentile | Systolic Blood Pressure by Percentile of Height, mm Hg† | | | | | | | Diastolic Blood Pressure by Percentile of Height, mm Hg† | | | | | | |
|---|---|---|---|---|---|---|---|---|---|---|---|---|---|---|---|
| | | 5th | 10th | 25th | 50th | 75th | 90th | 95th | 5th | 10th | 25th | 50th | 75th | 90th | 95th |
| 1 | 50th | 80 | 81 | 83 | 85 | 87 | 88 | 89 | 34 | 35 | 36 | 37 | 38 | 39 | 39 |
| | 90th | 94 | 95 | 97 | 99 | 100 | 102 | 103 | 49 | 50 | 51 | 52 | 53 | 53 | 54 |
| | 95th | 98 | 99 | 101 | 103 | 104 | 106 | 106 | 54 | 54 | 55 | 56 | 57 | 58 | 58 |
| | 99th | 105 | 106 | 108 | 110 | 112 | 113 | 114 | 61 | 62 | 63 | 64 | 65 | 66 | 66 |
| 2 | 50th | 84 | 85 | 87 | 88 | 90 | 92 | 92 | 39 | 40 | 41 | 42 | 43 | 44 | 44 |
| | 90th | 97 | 99 | 100 | 102 | 104 | 105 | 106 | 54 | 55 | 56 | 57 | 58 | 58 | 59 |
| | 95th | 101 | 102 | 104 | 106 | 108 | 109 | 110 | 59 | 59 | 60 | 61 | 62 | 63 | 63 |
| | 99th | 109 | 110 | 111 | 113 | 115 | 117 | 117 | 66 | 67 | 68 | 69 | 70 | 71 | 71 |
| 3 | 50th | 86 | 87 | 89 | 91 | 93 | 94 | 95 | 44 | 44 | 45 | 46 | 47 | 48 | 48 |
| | 90th | 100 | 101 | 103 | 105 | 107 | 108 | 109 | 59 | 59 | 60 | 61 | 62 | 63 | 63 |
| | 95th | 104 | 105 | 107 | 109 | 110 | 112 | 113 | 63 | 63 | 64 | 65 | 66 | 67 | 67 |
| | 99th | 111 | 112 | 114 | 116 | 118 | 119 | 120 | 71 | 71 | 72 | 73 | 74 | 75 | 75 |
| 4 | 50th | 88 | 89 | 91 | 93 | 95 | 96 | 97 | 47 | 48 | 49 | 50 | 51 | 51 | 52 |
| | 90th | 102 | 103 | 105 | 107 | 109 | 110 | 111 | 62 | 63 | 64 | 65 | 66 | 66 | 67 |
| | 95th | 106 | 107 | 109 | 111 | 112 | 114 | 115 | 66 | 67 | 68 | 69 | 70 | 71 | 71 |
| | 99th | 113 | 114 | 116 | 118 | 120 | 121 | 122 | 74 | 75 | 76 | 77 | 78 | 78 | 79 |
| 5 | 50th | 90 | 91 | 93 | 95 | 96 | 98 | 98 | 50 | 51 | 52 | 53 | 54 | 55 | 55 |
| | 90th | 104 | 105 | 106 | 108 | 110 | 111 | 112 | 65 | 66 | 67 | 68 | 69 | 69 | 70 |
| | 95th | 108 | 109 | 110 | 112 | 114 | 115 | 116 | 69 | 70 | 71 | 72 | 73 | 74 | 74 |
| | 99th | 115 | 116 | 118 | 120 | 121 | 123 | 123 | 77 | 78 | 79 | 80 | 81 | 81 | 82 |
| 6 | 50th | 91 | 92 | 94 | 96 | 98 | 99 | 100 | 53 | 53 | 54 | 55 | 56 | 57 | 57 |
| | 90th | 105 | 106 | 108 | 110 | 111 | 113 | 113 | 68 | 68 | 69 | 70 | 71 | 72 | 72 |
| | 95th | 109 | 110 | 112 | 114 | 115 | 117 | 117 | 72 | 72 | 73 | 74 | 75 | 76 | 76 |
| | 99th | 116 | 117 | 119 | 121 | 123 | 124 | 125 | 80 | 80 | 81 | 82 | 83 | 84 | 84 |
| 7 | 50th | 92 | 94 | 95 | 97 | 99 | 100 | 101 | 55 | 55 | 56 | 57 | 58 | 59 | 59 |
| | 90th | 106 | 107 | 109 | 111 | 113 | 114 | 115 | 70 | 70 | 71 | 72 | 73 | 74 | 74 |
| | 95th | 110 | 111 | 113 | 115 | 117 | 118 | 119 | 74 | 74 | 75 | 76 | 77 | 78 | 78 |
| | 99th | 117 | 118 | 120 | 122 | 124 | 125 | 126 | 82 | 82 | 83 | 84 | 85 | 86 | 86 |
| 8 | 50th | 94 | 95 | 97 | 99 | 100 | 102 | 102 | 56 | 57 | 58 | 59 | 60 | 60 | 61 |
| | 90th | 107 | 109 | 110 | 112 | 114 | 115 | 116 | 71 | 72 | 72 | 73 | 74 | 75 | 76 |
| | 95th | 111 | 112 | 114 | 116 | 118 | 119 | 120 | 75 | 76 | 77 | 78 | 79 | 79 | 80 |
| | 99th | 119 | 120 | 122 | 123 | 125 | 127 | 127 | 83 | 84 | 85 | 86 | 87 | 87 | 88 |
| 9 | 50th | 95 | 96 | 98 | 100 | 102 | 103 | 104 | 57 | 58 | 59 | 60 | 61 | 61 | 62 |
| | 90th | 109 | 110 | 112 | 114 | 115 | 117 | 118 | 72 | 73 | 74 | 75 | 76 | 76 | 77 |
| | 95th | 113 | 114 | 116 | 118 | 119 | 121 | 121 | 76 | 77 | 78 | 79 | 80 | 81 | 81 |
| | 99th | 120 | 121 | 123 | 125 | 127 | 128 | 129 | 84 | 85 | 86 | 87 | 88 | 88 | 89 |
| 10 | 50th | 97 | 98 | 100 | 102 | 103 | 105 | 106 | 58 | 59 | 60 | 61 | 61 | 62 | 63 |
| | 90th | 111 | 112 | 114 | 115 | 117 | 119 | 119 | 73 | 73 | 74 | 75 | 76 | 77 | 78 |
| | 95th | 115 | 116 | 117 | 119 | 121 | 122 | 123 | 77 | 78 | 79 | 80 | 81 | 81 | 82 |
| | 99th | 122 | 123 | 125 | 127 | 128 | 130 | 130 | 85 | 86 | 86 | 88 | 88 | 89 | 90 |
| 11 | 50th | 99 | 100 | 102 | 104 | 105 | 107 | 107 | 59 | 59 | 60 | 61 | 62 | 63 | 63 |
| | 90th | 113 | 114 | 115 | 117 | 119 | 120 | 121 | 74 | 74 | 75 | 76 | 77 | 78 | 78 |
| | 95th | 117 | 118 | 119 | 121 | 123 | 124 | 125 | 78 | 78 | 79 | 80 | 81 | 82 | 82 |
| | 99th | 124 | 125 | 127 | 129 | 130 | 132 | 132 | 86 | 86 | 87 | 88 | 89 | 90 | 90 |
| 12 | 50th | 101 | 102 | 104 | 106 | 108 | 109 | 110 | 59 | 60 | 61 | 62 | 63 | 63 | 64 |
| | 90th | 115 | 116 | 118 | 120 | 121 | 123 | 123 | 74 | 75 | 75 | 76 | 77 | 78 | 79 |
| | 95th | 119 | 120 | 122 | 123 | 125 | 127 | 127 | 78 | 79 | 80 | 81 | 82 | 82 | 83 |
| | 99th | 126 | 127 | 129 | 131 | 133 | 134 | 135 | 86 | 87 | 88 | 89 | 90 | 90 | 91 |

*Blood pressure percentile was determined by a single reading.
† Height percentile was determined by standard growth curves.

**Table 58-1** Blood Pressure Levels for Boys by Age and Height Percentile—cont'd

| Age, Yr | Blood Pressure Percentile | Systolic Blood Pressure by Percentile of Height, mm Hg[†] | | | | | | | Diastolic Blood Pressure by Percentile of Height, mm Hg[†] | | | | | | |
|---|---|---|---|---|---|---|---|---|---|---|---|---|---|---|---|
| | | 5th | 10th | 25th | 50th | 75th | 90th | 95th | 5th | 10th | 25th | 50th | 75th | 90th | 95th |
| 13 | 50th | 104 | 105 | 106 | 108 | 110 | 111 | 112 | 60 | 60 | 61 | 62 | 63 | 64 | 64 |
| | 90th | 117 | 118 | 120 | 122 | 124 | 125 | 126 | 75 | 75 | 76 | 77 | 78 | 79 | 79 |
| | 95th | 121 | 122 | 124 | 126 | 128 | 129 | 130 | 79 | 79 | 80 | 81 | 82 | 83 | 83 |
| | 99th | 128 | 130 | 131 | 133 | 135 | 136 | 137 | 87 | 87 | 88 | 89 | 90 | 91 | 91 |
| 14 | 50th | 106 | 107 | 109 | 111 | 113 | 114 | 115 | 60 | 61 | 62 | 63 | 64 | 65 | 65 |
| | 90th | 120 | 121 | 123 | 125 | 126 | 128 | 128 | 75 | 76 | 77 | 78 | 79 | 79 | 80 |
| | 95th | 124 | 125 | 127 | 128 | 130 | 132 | 132 | 80 | 80 | 81 | 82 | 83 | 84 | 84 |
| | 99th | 131 | 132 | 134 | 136 | 138 | 139 | 140 | 87 | 88 | 89 | 90 | 91 | 92 | 92 |
| 15 | 50th | 109 | 110 | 112 | 113 | 115 | 117 | 117 | 61 | 62 | 63 | 64 | 65 | 66 | 66 |
| | 90th | 122 | 124 | 125 | 127 | 129 | 130 | 131 | 76 | 77 | 78 | 79 | 80 | 80 | 81 |
| | 95th | 126 | 127 | 129 | 131 | 133 | 134 | 135 | 81 | 81 | 82 | 83 | 84 | 85 | 85 |
| | 99th | 134 | 135 | 136 | 138 | 140 | 142 | 142 | 88 | 89 | 90 | 91 | 92 | 93 | 93 |
| 16 | 50th | 111 | 112 | 114 | 116 | 118 | 119 | 120 | 63 | 63 | 64 | 65 | 66 | 67 | 67 |
| | 90th | 125 | 126 | 128 | 130 | 131 | 133 | 134 | 78 | 78 | 79 | 80 | 81 | 82 | 82 |
| | 95th | 129 | 130 | 132 | 134 | 135 | 137 | 137 | 82 | 83 | 83 | 84 | 85 | 86 | 87 |
| | 99th | 136 | 137 | 139 | 141 | 143 | 144 | 145 | 90 | 90 | 91 | 92 | 93 | 94 | 94 |
| 17 | 50th | 114 | 115 | 116 | 118 | 120 | 121 | 122 | 65 | 66 | 66 | 67 | 68 | 69 | 70 |
| | 90th | 127 | 128 | 130 | 132 | 134 | 135 | 136 | 80 | 80 | 81 | 82 | 83 | 84 | 84 |
| | 95th | 131 | 132 | 134 | 136 | 138 | 139 | 140 | 84 | 85 | 86 | 87 | 87 | 88 | 89 |
| | 99th | 139 | 140 | 141 | 143 | 145 | 146 | 147 | 92 | 93 | 93 | 94 | 95 | 96 | 97 |

The 90th percentile is 1.28 SD, the 95th percentile is 1.645 SD, and the 99th percentile is 2.326 SD over the mean.
Reproduced from National High Blood Pressure Education Program Working Group on High Blood Pressure in Children and Adolescents. The fourth report on the diagnosis, evaluation, and treatment of high blood pressure in children and adolescents. Pediatrics 114:555-576, 2004.

oversized cuff, and a thigh cuff for leg BP measurement. The latter two cuffs may be needed for use in obese adolescents.

BP measurement in children should be conducted in a quiet and comfortable environment after 3 to 5 minutes of rest. With the exception of acute illness, the BP should be measured with the child in the seated position with the cubital fossa supported at heart level. It is preferable that the child has her or his feet on the floor while the BP is measured, rather than her or his feet dangling from an examination table. Overinflation of the cuff should be avoided due to discomfort, particularly in younger children. The BP should be measured and recorded at least twice on each measurement occasion.

SBP is determined by the onset of the auscultated pulsation or first Korotkoff sound. The disappearance of Korotkoff sounds or fifth Korotkoff sound (K5) is the definition of DBP in adults. In children, particularly preadolescents, a difference of several millimeters of mercury is often present between the fourth Korotkoff sound, the muffling of Korotkoff sounds, and K5.[14] The substantial body of normative BP data in children indicates that K5 can be used as the measure of DBP in children, as well as adults.

The measured BP level in a child is interpreted by comparing the child's BP to the BP tables. Precise interpretation requires plotting the BP according to the child's height percentile, as well as age and sex. The child's height is measured and plotted on the standard child growth curves. The height percentile is used in the tables, wherein the BP level for the 90th and 95th percentile at the child's age, sex, and height percentile are compared with the child's measured BP.

Elevated BP measurements in a child or adolescent must be confirmed on repeated visits before characterizing a child as having hypertension. A more accurate characterization of an individual's BP level is an average of multiple BP measurements taken for weeks or months. A notable exception to this general guideline for asymptomatic generally well children would be situations in which the child is symptomatic or has profoundly elevated BP. Children with elevated BP on repeated measurement should also have the BP measured in the leg as a screen for coarctation of the aorta. To measure the BP in the leg, a thigh cuff or an oversized cuff should be placed on the thigh and the BP measured by auscultation over the popliteal fossa. Coarctation is suspected if the SBP measured in the thigh is 10 mm Hg or more lower than the SBP measured in the arm.

There continues to be an increase in the use of automated devices to measure BP in children. Situations in which use of automated devices is acceptable include BP measurement in newborn and young infants in whom auscultation is difficult, as well as in an intensive care setting, where frequent BP measurement is necessary. The reliability of these instruments in an ambulatory clinical setting is less clear because of the need for frequent calibration of the instruments and the current lack of established reference standards.

**Table 58–2** Blood Pressure Levels for Girls by Age and Height Percentile

| Age, Yr | Blood Pressure Percentile | Systolic Blood Pressure by Percentile of Height, mm Hg[†] | | | | | | | Diastolic Blood Pressure by Percentile of Height, mm Hg[†] | | | | | | |
|---|---|---|---|---|---|---|---|---|---|---|---|---|---|---|---|
| | | 5th | 10th | 25th | 50th | 75th | 90th | 95th | 5th | 10th | 25th | 50th | 75th | 90th | 95th |
| 1 | 50th | 83 | 84 | 85 | 86 | 88 | 89 | 90 | 38 | 39 | 39 | 40 | 41 | 41 | 42 |
| | 90th | 97 | 97 | 98 | 100 | 101 | 102 | 103 | 52 | 53 | 53 | 54 | 55 | 55 | 56 |
| | 95th | 100 | 101 | 102 | 104 | 105 | 106 | 107 | 56 | 57 | 57 | 58 | 59 | 59 | 60 |
| | 99th | 108 | 108 | 109 | 111 | 112 | 113 | 114 | 64 | 64 | 65 | 65 | 66 | 67 | 67 |
| 2 | 50th | 85 | 85 | 87 | 88 | 89 | 91 | 91 | 43 | 44 | 44 | 45 | 46 | 46 | 47 |
| | 90th | 98 | 99 | 100 | 101 | 103 | 104 | 105 | 57 | 58 | 58 | 59 | 60 | 61 | 61 |
| | 95th | 102 | 103 | 104 | 105 | 107 | 108 | 109 | 61 | 62 | 62 | 63 | 64 | 65 | 65 |
| | 99th | 109 | 110 | 111 | 112 | 114 | 115 | 116 | 69 | 69 | 70 | 70 | 71 | 72 | 72 |
| 3 | 50th | 86 | 87 | 88 | 89 | 91 | 92 | 93 | 47 | 48 | 48 | 49 | 50 | 50 | 51 |
| | 90th | 100 | 100 | 102 | 103 | 104 | 106 | 106 | 61 | 62 | 62 | 63 | 64 | 64 | 65 |
| | 95th | 104 | 104 | 105 | 107 | 108 | 109 | 110 | 65 | 66 | 66 | 67 | 68 | 68 | 69 |
| | 99th | 111 | 111 | 113 | 114 | 115 | 116 | 117 | 73 | 73 | 74 | 74 | 75 | 76 | 76 |
| 4 | 50th | 88 | 88 | 90 | 91 | 92 | 94 | 94 | 50 | 50 | 51 | 52 | 52 | 53 | 54 |
| | 90th | 101 | 102 | 103 | 104 | 106 | 107 | 108 | 64 | 64 | 65 | 66 | 67 | 67 | 68 |
| | 95th | 105 | 106 | 107 | 108 | 110 | 111 | 112 | 68 | 68 | 69 | 70 | 71 | 71 | 72 |
| | 99th | 112 | 113 | 114 | 115 | 117 | 118 | 119 | 76 | 76 | 76 | 77 | 78 | 79 | 79 |
| 5 | 50th | 89 | 90 | 91 | 93 | 94 | 95 | 96 | 52 | 53 | 53 | 54 | 55 | 55 | 56 |
| | 90th | 103 | 103 | 105 | 106 | 107 | 109 | 109 | 66 | 67 | 67 | 68 | 69 | 69 | 70 |
| | 95th | 107 | 107 | 108 | 110 | 111 | 112 | 113 | 70 | 71 | 71 | 72 | 73 | 73 | 74 |
| | 99th | 114 | 114 | 116 | 117 | 118 | 120 | 120 | 78 | 78 | 79 | 79 | 80 | 81 | 81 |
| 6 | 50th | 91 | 92 | 93 | 94 | 96 | 97 | 98 | 54 | 54 | 55 | 56 | 56 | 57 | 58 |
| | 90th | 104 | 105 | 106 | 108 | 109 | 110 | 111 | 68 | 68 | 69 | 70 | 70 | 71 | 72 |
| | 95th | 108 | 109 | 110 | 111 | 113 | 114 | 115 | 72 | 72 | 73 | 74 | 74 | 75 | 76 |
| | 99th | 115 | 116 | 117 | 119 | 120 | 121 | 122 | 80 | 80 | 80 | 81 | 82 | 83 | 83 |
| 7 | 50th | 93 | 93 | 95 | 96 | 97 | 99 | 99 | 55 | 56 | 56 | 57 | 58 | 58 | 59 |
| | 90th | 106 | 107 | 108 | 109 | 111 | 112 | 113 | 69 | 70 | 70 | 71 | 72 | 72 | 73 |
| | 95th | 110 | 111 | 112 | 113 | 115 | 116 | 116 | 73 | 74 | 74 | 75 | 76 | 76 | 77 |
| | 99th | 117 | 118 | 119 | 120 | 122 | 123 | 124 | 81 | 81 | 82 | 82 | 83 | 84 | 84 |
| 8 | 50th | 95 | 95 | 96 | 98 | 99 | 100 | 101 | 57 | 57 | 57 | 58 | 59 | 60 | 60 |
| | 90th | 108 | 109 | 110 | 111 | 113 | 114 | 114 | 71 | 71 | 71 | 72 | 73 | 74 | 74 |
| | 95th | 112 | 112 | 114 | 115 | 116 | 118 | 118 | 75 | 75 | 75 | 76 | 77 | 78 | 78 |
| | 99th | 119 | 120 | 121 | 122 | 123 | 125 | 125 | 82 | 82 | 83 | 83 | 84 | 85 | 86 |
| 9 | 50th | 96 | 97 | 98 | 100 | 101 | 102 | 103 | 58 | 58 | 58 | 59 | 60 | 61 | 61 |
| | 90th | 110 | 110 | 112 | 113 | 114 | 116 | 116 | 72 | 72 | 72 | 73 | 74 | 75 | 75 |
| | 95th | 114 | 114 | 115 | 117 | 118 | 119 | 120 | 76 | 76 | 76 | 77 | 78 | 79 | 79 |
| | 99th | 121 | 121 | 123 | 124 | 125 | 127 | 127 | 83 | 83 | 84 | 84 | 85 | 86 | 87 |
| 10 | 50th | 98 | 99 | 100 | 102 | 103 | 104 | 105 | 59 | 59 | 59 | 60 | 61 | 62 | 62 |
| | 90th | 112 | 112 | 114 | 115 | 116 | 118 | 118 | 73 | 73 | 73 | 74 | 75 | 76 | 76 |
| | 95th | 116 | 116 | 117 | 119 | 120 | 121 | 122 | 77 | 77 | 77 | 78 | 79 | 80 | 80 |
| | 99th | 123 | 123 | 125 | 126 | 127 | 129 | 129 | 84 | 84 | 85 | 86 | 86 | 87 | 88 |
| 11 | 50th | 100 | 101 | 102 | 103 | 105 | 106 | 107 | 60 | 60 | 60 | 61 | 62 | 63 | 63 |
| | 90th | 114 | 114 | 116 | 117 | 118 | 119 | 120 | 74 | 74 | 74 | 75 | 76 | 77 | 77 |
| | 95th | 118 | 118 | 119 | 121 | 122 | 123 | 124 | 78 | 78 | 78 | 79 | 80 | 81 | 81 |
| | 99th | 125 | 125 | 126 | 128 | 129 | 130 | 131 | 85 | 85 | 86 | 87 | 87 | 88 | 89 |
| 12 | 50th | 102 | 103 | 104 | 105 | 107 | 108 | 109 | 61 | 61 | 61 | 62 | 63 | 64 | 64 |
| | 90th | 116 | 116 | 117 | 119 | 120 | 121 | 122 | 75 | 75 | 75 | 76 | 77 | 78 | 78 |
| | 95th | 119 | 120 | 121 | 123 | 124 | 125 | 126 | 79 | 79 | 79 | 80 | 81 | 82 | 82 |
| | 99th | 127 | 127 | 128 | 130 | 131 | 132 | 133 | 86 | 86 | 87 | 88 | 88 | 89 | 90 |

*Blood pressure percentile was determined by a single reading.
[†] Height percentile was determined by standard growth curves.

**Table 58-2** BP Levels for Girls by Age and Height Percentile—cont'd

| Age, Yr | Blood Pressure Percentile | Systolic Blood Pressure by Percentile of Height, mm Hg† | | | | | | | Diastolic Blood Pressure by Percentile of Height, mm Hg† | | | | | | |
|---|---|---|---|---|---|---|---|---|---|---|---|---|---|---|---|
| | | 5th | 10th | 25th | 50th | 75th | 90th | 95th | 5th | 10th | 25th | 50th | 75th | 90th | 95th |
| 13 | 50th | 104 | 105 | 106 | 107 | 109 | 110 | 110 | 62 | 62 | 62 | 63 | 64 | 65 | 65 |
| | 90th | 117 | 118 | 119 | 121 | 122 | 123 | 124 | 76 | 76 | 76 | 77 | 78 | 79 | 79 |
| | 95th | 121 | 122 | 123 | 124 | 126 | 127 | 128 | 80 | 80 | 80 | 81 | 82 | 83 | 83 |
| | 99th | 128 | 129 | 130 | 132 | 133 | 134 | 135 | 87 | 87 | 88 | 89 | 89 | 90 | 91 |
| 14 | 50th | 106 | 106 | 107 | 109 | 110 | 111 | 112 | 63 | 63 | 63 | 64 | 65 | 66 | 66 |
| | 90th | 119 | 120 | 121 | 122 | 124 | 125 | 125 | 77 | 77 | 77 | 78 | 79 | 80 | 80 |
| | 95th | 123 | 123 | 125 | 126 | 127 | 129 | 129 | 81 | 81 | 81 | 82 | 83 | 84 | 84 |
| | 99th | 130 | 131 | 132 | 133 | 135 | 136 | 136 | 88 | 88 | 89 | 90 | 90 | 91 | 92 |
| 15 | 50th | 107 | 108 | 109 | 110 | 111 | 113 | 113 | 64 | 64 | 64 | 65 | 66 | 67 | 67 |
| | 90th | 120 | 121 | 122 | 123 | 125 | 126 | 127 | 78 | 78 | 78 | 79 | 80 | 81 | 81 |
| | 95th | 124 | 125 | 126 | 127 | 129 | 130 | 131 | 82 | 82 | 82 | 83 | 84 | 85 | 85 |
| | 99th | 131 | 132 | 133 | 134 | 136 | 137 | 138 | 89 | 89 | 90 | 91 | 91 | 92 | 93 |
| 16 | 50th | 108 | 108 | 110 | 111 | 112 | 114 | 114 | 64 | 64 | 65 | 66 | 66 | 67 | 68 |
| | 90th | 121 | 122 | 123 | 124 | 126 | 127 | 128 | 78 | 78 | 79 | 80 | 81 | 81 | 82 |
| | 95th | 125 | 126 | 127 | 128 | 130 | 131 | 132 | 82 | 82 | 83 | 84 | 85 | 85 | 86 |
| | 99th | 132 | 133 | 134 | 135 | 137 | 138 | 139 | 90 | 90 | 90 | 91 | 92 | 93 | 93 |
| 17 | 50th | 108 | 109 | 110 | 111 | 113 | 114 | 115 | 64 | 65 | 65 | 66 | 67 | 67 | 68 |
| | 90th | 122 | 122 | 123 | 125 | 126 | 127 | 128 | 78 | 79 | 79 | 80 | 81 | 81 | 82 |
| | 95th | 125 | 126 | 127 | 129 | 130 | 131 | 132 | 82 | 83 | 83 | 84 | 85 | 85 | 86 |
| | 99th | 133 | 133 | 134 | 136 | 137 | 138 | 139 | 90 | 90 | 91 | 91 | 92 | 93 | 93 |

The 90th percentile is 1.28 SD, the 95th percentile is 1.645 SD, and the 99th percentile is 2.326 SD over the mean. Reproduced from National High Blood Pressure Education Program Working Group on High Blood Pressure in Children and Adolescents. The fourth report on the diagnosis, evaluation, and treatment of high blood pressure in children and adolescents. Pediatrics 114:555-576, 2004.

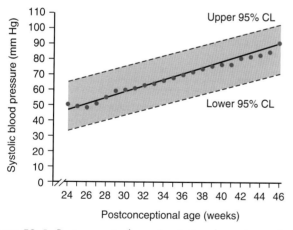

**Figure 58-1** Postconceptual age (gestational age in weeks + weeks after delivery) is computed daily for each infant (8566 daily records) and regressed against mean SBP and DBP. Regression lines and equations are presented in terms of postconceptional weeks, which is more useful clinically. Regression equations are SBP = (0.255 × postconceptional age in weeks × 7) + 6.34, r = 0.61, p <.0001 and DBP = (0.151 × postconceptional age in weeks × 7) + 3.32, r = 0.46, p <.0001. Observed means of SBP and DBP for each postconceptional week are also plotted. CL, confidence limits. (From Zubrow AB, Hulman S, Kushner H, et al. Determinants of blood pressure in infants admitted to neonatal intensive care units: A prospective multicenter study. J Perinatol 15:470-479, 1995.)

## CAUSES OF HYPERTENSION IN THE YOUNG

### Secondary Hypertension

Underlying causes of hypertension, or secondary hypertension due to an underlying renal or endocrine disorder, occur more frequently during childhood than in adults. Prior to the development of normative data on BP levels in children, BP was measured infrequently. When elevated BP was detected in children, the hypertension was, by current standards, quite severe. Because secondary hypertension is generally characterized by marked BP elevation, this led to the belief that hypertension in children was *always* secondary. This concept has now changed, largely due to better understanding of normal levels of BP in the young and the practice of regularly measuring the BP in children as part of health assessment and health maintenance. The prevalence of secondary hypertension in the young varies according to the age and severity of hypertension. Hana et al.[15] identified a secondary cause of hypertensive in 90% of children that were younger than 10 years of age and only 10% of these young children were considered to have essential hypertension. A report on a series that included both children and adolescents with hypertension describes secondary hypertension in 65% of the adolescents, with 35% of the adolescents having essential hypertension.[16]

Young children, younger than 12 years of age, with sustained hypertension are more likely to have a secondary cause for the hypertension. The degree of hypertension is also an important clue, as severe BP elevation in a young child is most likely to be due to an underlying abnormality. In general, a child that has either SBP or DBP that is consistently 8 to 10 mm Hg above the 95th percentile has significant hypertension, and a child that has either SBP or DBP that is consistently 15 mm Hg or more above the 95th percentile has severe hypertension. Children and adolescents with this degree of hypertension should have a careful evaluation for a possible cause of the hypertension and also for evidence of target organ damage from the hypertension. Although the list of conditions that can cause hypertension in the young is quite long, the majority of the identifiable causes of hypertension in the young are related to renal disorders. Box 58–1 provides a list of underlying causes for chronic hypertension in the young, as well as the conditions associated with acute hypertension in the young.

Hypertension is uncommon in healthy newborn infants. However, certain infants have conditions that increase the risk for hypertension. Some newborn infants require treatment in intensive care units where umbilical artery catheterization may be required for vascular access. The umbilical artery catheters are a risk for thromboembolic events.[17,18] Low-birth-weight infants, with respiratory distress syndrome, can progress to bronchopulmonary dysplasia and develop sodium retention from chronic steroid therapy.[19] The most commonly identified causes of hypertension in the newborn infant are renal artery thrombosis, renal artery stenosis, congenital renal malformations, coarctation of the aorta, and bronchopulmonary dysplasia.[4] In some critically ill newborn infants with hypertension, an underlying cause may not be identified. Regardless of whether a cause for the hypertension is determined, BP control and monitoring in these infants is important.

For children up to 10 years of age, the leading causes of hypertension are renal parenchymal diseases, coarctation of the aorta, and renal artery stenosis. Coarctation of the aorta, a congenital cardiac anomaly that can be missed in infants and toddlers, should be considered in a hypertensive child.[20-22] In later childhood, essential hypertension also occurs. The disorders that cause acute hypertension include postinfectious glomerulonephritis and hemolytic uremic syndrome. Some conditions such as hemolytic uremic syndrome may cause permanent renal scarring that results in chronic hypertension.

During the adolescent years the most common cause of hypertension is essential hypertension. The secondary causes of hypertension that are detected most frequently in adolescents are renal parenchymal diseases, such as chronic pyelonephritis, focal segmental glomerulosclerosis (FSBS), and other types of chronic glomerulonephritis. Adolescent behaviors that may contribute to high BP are illicit substance

---

**Box 58–1** Secondary Causes of Hypertension

**Chronic Hypertension**

*Renal*
- Chronic glomerulonephritis
- Interstitial nephritis
- Collagen vascular diseases
- Reflux nephropathy
- Polycystic kidney disease
- Medullary cystic disease
- Hydronephrosis
- Hypoplastic/dysplastic kidney

*Cardiac and Vascular*
- Coarctation of aorta
- Renal artery stenosis
- Takayasu arteritis

*Endocrine*
- Hyperthyroidism
- Pheochromocytoma
- Primary aldosteronism

*Drugs*
- Corticosteroids
- Alcohol
- Appetite suppressants
- Anabolic steroids
- Oral contraceptive
- Nicotine

*Syndromes*
- Alport's syndrome
- Williams syndrome (renovascular lesions)
- Turner's syndrome (coarctation or renovascular)
- Neurofibromatosis (renovascular)
- Adrenogenital syndromes
- Little syndrome

**Acute Hypertension**

*Renal*
- Postinfectious glomerulonephritis
- Schönlein-Henoch purpura
- Hemolytic uremic syndrome
- Acute tubular necrosis

*Vascular*
- Renal or renal vascular trauma

*Neurogenic*
- Increased intracranial pressure
- Guillain-Barré syndrome

*Drugs*
- Cocaine
- Phencyclidine
- Amphetamines
- Jimson weed

*Miscellaneous*
- Burns
- Orthopedic surgery
- Urologic surgery

use, especially cocaine and amphetamine-related compounds.[23,24] Other substances that have been associated with high BP in adolescents include appetite suppressants (both prescription and over-the-counter remedies), oral contraceptives, excessive alcohol intake, and use of anabolic steroids for body building.[25]

## Essential Hypertension

Essential hypertension has been considered to be a disorder of adulthood. The concept that essential hypertension has its roots in childhood can be inferred from BP tracking data that demonstrate that children with elevated BP will continue to have elevated BP as adults.[5] Classic risk factors for hypertension such as overweight and a positive family history of hypertension or CVD may be present in childhood. The combination of higher BP and typical risk factors has been considered indicative of risk for future hypertension. Recent reports indicate, however, that this condition is more than a risk for future problems. Effects of high BP on left ventricular mass in children and adolescents have been investigated. Using echocardiography and appropriate childhood reference values for cardiac structure, left ventricular hypertrophy (LVH) has been reported in 30% to 40% of children and adolescents with hypertension.[26,27] Longitudinal data are now becoming available that demonstrate a direct link between risk factors in childhood, including BP level, with evidence of target organ injury, including greater intima-media thickness of carotid arteries.[26,28,29] Essential hypertension in childhood should be considered an early phase of a chronic disease.

Children and adolescents with essential hypertension generally demonstrate several clinical characteristics or associated risk factors. The degree of BP elevation is generally mild, approximating the 95th percentile and there is often considerable variability in BP over time. Laboratory and observational studies have demonstrated a marked cardiovascular response to stress, characterized by increased heart rate and BP responses to stimuli.[30-33] A consistent clinical observation in children exhibiting mild essential hypertension is a positive history of hypertension in parents and/or grandparents.[30,34,35]

In both children and adults, greater body weight and increases in body weight correlate with higher BP.[36,37] Essential hypertension in children is frequently associated with obesity, which appears to be a contributory factor because even a modest reduction in excess adiposity is associated with a reduction in BP.[38,39] The cluster of mild BP elevation, a positive family history of hypertension, and obesity is a typical pattern in children and adolescents with essential hypertension.[40]

Currently the prevalence of childhood obesity is increasing[41] and has more than doubled in the past 20 years.[42] Obesity has an adverse effect on risk for CVD and warrants attention for disease prevention and health promotion. In a study by Daniels et al.[27] cardiac structure was examined by echocardiography in young adolescents with essential hypertension. These investigators found a significant incidence of LVH. The adolescents who had echo criteria of cardiac hypertrophy, despite mild BP elevation, were all obese. Rocchini et al.[38,39] have demonstrated augmented BP sensitivity to sodium intake in obese adolescents, and a significant dampening in the BP response to sodium following weight reduction.

Over the past two decades, the literature on hypertension and CVD in adults has focused on the overlap of hypertension, non–insulin-dependent diabetes mellitus, atherosclerosis, and obesity. This constellation within individuals and within populations has been described as the insulin-resistance syndrome.[43-45] Children, as well as adults, may exhibit characteristics of the insulin-resistance syndrome.[39,46,47] Some investigators have detected the insulin-resistance syndrome in nonobese offspring of hypertensive parents,[48,49] indicating a hereditary component to the syndrome. The characteristics of the insulin-resistance syndrome are also congruent with the overweight child having a strong family history of hypertension or early heart disease. These children often have high BP.[50] Although these children are not at risk for immediate adverse effects of the higher than normal BP, they should be considered at risk for future CVD.[51] These children can benefit from health behavior changes that improve insulin action, including an increase in physical activity, diet modifications, and control of excess adiposity.

The cause of essential hypertension is believed to be multifactorial and the outcome of an interplay of genetic and environmental factors. Barker et al.[52] have proposed an alternative cause of hypertension based on observations of an association of hypertension and ischemic heart disease in adults with a low recorded birth weight. These investigators propose that lower birth weight reflects alteration in the intrauterine nutritional environment. Impaired fetal growth effects an alteration in organ structure and impairment in organ function in later life.[52,53] Higher BP is the link between compromised intrauterine growth and the long term risk for CVD.[52] Despite the reports, based on retrospective data that support the low-birth-weight–high BP hypothesis,[52-55] this concept is in conflict with the body of data in childhood, as well as adulthood, which consistently demonstrates a direct relationship between body weight and BP,[56-59] and BP tracking in childhood.[34,60-65] Reports from studies on small cohorts have not detected a significant correlation.[58,59] When the body of reports on the association of birth weight with future BP is examined, the effect of birth weight on future BP is in the range of 2– to 3–mm Hg BP reduction for each 1-kg increase in birth weight. When the current child or adult weight is taken into consideration the birth weight effect is minimal.[66] Although the birth weight hypothesis has some appeal, clinical investigations have not yet firmly demonstrated that birth weight has a substantial effect on future BP.

## EVALUATION OF HYPERTENSION IN CHILDREN AND ADOLESCENTS

When sustained hypertension is established in a child by repeated BP measurements that are at or above the 95th percentile, additional evaluation is needed. The extent of the diagnostic evaluation is determined by the type of hypertension that is suspected. When a secondary cause is considered, a more extensive evaluation may be necessary. On the other hand, when the patient's elevated BP is more likely to be an early expression of essential hypertension, a few screening studies may be sufficient. The medical history and physical examination is key in determining whether the characteristics of a patient's presentation indicate essential hypertension or reflect a secondary, and potentially correctable, cause.

Children or adolescents with severe hypertension, in particular very young children, generally have an identifiable underlying cause. As noted previously, the higher the BP and the younger the child, the more likely a secondary cause is present.

A particular symptom complex revealed in the history or findings on physical examination may also prompt a thorough investigation. In these patients, the direction of the evaluation is dictated by the particular symptom or physical examination findings. Any pediatric patient who is hypertensive and is not growing normally should also undergo an evaluation for secondary causes. A sudden onset of elevated BP in a previously normotensive child should always prompt a search for secondary causes. Absence of a positive family history of hypertension should increase the level of suspicion for an underlying disorder.

Another set of findings characterizes children and adolescents with essential hypertension. These characteristics include slight to mild elevations in BP, a strong family history of essential hypertension, elevated resting heart rate, variable BP readings on repeated measurement, and obesity. If no other abnormalities are found on history or physical examination, these children require less extensive evaluations than those in whom secondary causes are suspected.

## Medical History

The medical history and physical examination are used to detect clues to determine whether the BP elevation is secondary or essential. It is also helpful to determine whether the hypertension is longstanding or of acute onset. The family history is particularly important. In both first- and second-degree relatives, the family history of essential hypertension, myocardial infarction (MI), stroke, renal disease, diabetes, and obesity should be obtained. It can be relevant to the diagnosis in a hypertensive child if relatives had an onset at an early age of any of the aforementioned conditions. Parents should also be asked about conditions in family members that are inheritable and have hypertension as a component (e.g., polycystic kidney disease, neurofibromatosis, pheochromocytoma). Another familial type of hypertension is glucocorticoid-remediable aldosteronism, an autosomal-dominant condition that should be considered when multiple family members have early-onset hypertension associated with hypokalemia or stroke.[67,68]

Details about previous health problems such as history of urinary tract infections are important as there may be associated reflux nephropathy, renal scarring, and resultant hypertension. A history of medications and over-the-counter products used can be helpful.[69,70] Information should be obtained about health-related behaviors such as usual diet, amount of physical activity, or athletic participation. Other adverse adolescent lifestyles to consider are use of "street" drugs, smokeless tobacco, oral contraceptive pills, cigarette smoking, diet aids, ethanol, and anabolic steroids.

## Physical Examination

The physical examination of a hypertensive child should be comprehensive. An assessment of the child's general growth rate and growth pattern should be made. Weight, height, and body mass index (BMI) should be plotted according to age and sex on the child growth charts. Abnormalities in growth that are associated with hypertension can be seen with chronic renal disease, hyperthyroidism (causing primarily systolic

hypertension), pheochromocytoma, adrenal disorders, or certain genetic abnormalities such as Turner's syndrome.

To rule out coarctation of the aorta, the evaluation of every child for hypertension should include upper- and lower-extremity BP measurements taken with appropriately sized cuffs. Normally the leg BP levels are slightly higher than the arm BP levels. A child with coarctation will have systolic hypertension in an upper extremity, sometimes absent or decreased femoral pulses, and a BP differential greater than 10 mm Hg between the upper and lower extremities.[20,22]

There are other physical clues that could suggest a secondary etiology for child hypertension.[71] Abnormal facies or dysmorphic features may suggest a syndrome, some of which are associated with specific lesions causing hypertension. For example, both Turner's and Williams syndromes are associated with renovascular or cardiac lesions that cause hypertension. Renal vascular lesions may sometimes cause an audible abdominal bruit detectable by auscultation of the abdomen. Skin lesions are sometimes the first manifestations of disorders such as tuberous sclerosis and systemic lupus erythematosus.

## Diagnostic Testing

When the history and physical examination provide clues for a specific underlying cause for the hypertension, such as an endocrine or cardiac disorder, the testing should be directed to the area of clinical suspicion. Other important historical information such as a history of urinary tract infections might dictate studies to evaluate vesicoureteral reflux and renal scarring. In the absence of clues, however, renal parenchymal disease should be considered a likely cause, because this diagnosis is the most frequent cause of secondary hypertension in the pediatric population. The initial studies to screen for renal abnormalities include a full urinalysis, electrolytes, creatinine, complete blood count, urine culture, and renal ultrasound.

The other component of the evaluation includes an assessment of target organ injury. The presence of target organ injury provides a measure of chronicity and severity (characteristics sometimes difficult to ascertain from the history) and will aid in deciding whether pharmacologic therapy should be instituted. Echocardiography is a sensitive means to detect interventricular septal and posterior ventricular wall thickening.[72-75] Chest radiograph and electrocardiography (ECG) are much less sensitive measures of LVH in children. An ophthalmologic examination can also be helpful. In a study of 97 children and adolescents with essential hypertension, Daniels et al.[76] found that 51% displayed retinal abnormalities. The usefulness of microalbuminuria, sometimes used as a marker for renal injury in adults,[77] has not been determined for children. The remainder of the evaluation should be directed by specific findings on history and physical examination, as well as results of initial screening studies.

The use of 24-hour ambulatory BP monitoring (ABPM) has become increasingly common in the evaluation of adults with hypertension.[78] Some population standards for ambulatory BP values in children and adolescents are now available,[79] and there are some situations in which this information can be quite helpful.[80] ABPM is useful in determining how consistently BP readings are elevated over a 24-hour period and can aid in assessing the need for implementing pharmacologic therapy.

# TREATMENT OF HYPERTENSION IN CHILDREN AND ADOLESCENTS

Health-related behavior changes in diet, physical activity, and weight control improve BP control in adults. Children may also benefit in these lifestyle changes. Children and adolescents with a mild elevation of BP and without target organ damage, should begin treatment with nonpharmacologic interventions that include weight reduction or control, exercise, and diet modification.

Obesity is often associated with mild hypertension in childhood and weight reduction has benefit in obese children. Using a program of both behavior modification and parental involvement, Brownell et al.[81] showed that weight loss in obese adolescents was associated with a significant decrease in BP. There is also evidence that exercise training lowers BP in both school-aged children and adolescents.[82-84] Rocchini et al.[38] showed that a program that included both caloric restriction and exercise produced a decrease in BP and a reversal of structural changes in forearm resistance vessels. Weight reduction can be extremely difficult and generally requires multiple strategies that include the input of a nutritionist, dietary education, emotional support, information about exercise, and family involvement. Power weight-lifting should be discouraged in hypertensive adolescents due to its potential to induce marked BP elevation. Participation in other sports should be encouraged as long as BP is under reasonable control, regular monitoring of BP occurs, and a thorough examination has been conducted to exclude cardiac conditions.[25]

The guidelines for dietary modifications in the pediatric population are less clear than in adults. Information on the effects of salt on BP in children are not as definitive as in adults. There does seem to be a subset of adolescents, particularly those who are obese, who demonstrate BP sensitivity to salt as well as other risk factors for hypertension.[38] Because the usual dietary intake of sodium for most children and adolescents in the United States far exceeds nutrient requirements, it is reasonable to restrict sodium intake to less than 4 g/day by decreasing fast-food consumption and refraining from adding salt to cooked foods.[85]

Current information on the effects of potassium and calcium intake on BP in children is even less definitive. Some reports suggest that a diet high in potassium and calcium may help lower BP,[86] yet no study has definitively shown this effect in children or adolescents. The dietary intervention clinical trial, Dietary Approach to Stop Hypertension (DASH) reported results that could be relevant to diet benefits in children. This study, which was conducted in adults with normal BP or stage 1 hypertension, demonstrated a significant reduction in both SBP and DBP when a diet high in fruits, vegetables, and low-fat dairy products was consumed compared with the BP in the same subjects when consuming the usual diet. These results indicate that a benefit in BP occurs from diets that are high in potassium, calcium, magnesium, and other vitamins.[87] A similar approach may be of benefit for children and investigations to examine this issue would be appropriate.

Pharmacologic therapy is indicated if nonpharmacologic approaches are unsuccessful, or when a child is symptomatic, has severe hypertension, or target organ damage. Children with diabetes mellitus or chronic renal disease may receive renoprotective benefits from BP reduction. For children with these disorders it is reasonable to use pharmacologic therapy to lower BP to a level that is below the 90th percentile for age, sex, and height.

Most of the medications used for adults can be used for children. However, efficacy data, as well as long-term safety data, are limited for the pediatric population. The choice of antihypertensive medication must be individualized and depends on the child's age, the cause of the hypertension, the degree of BP elevation, adverse effects, and concomitant medical conditions. In most patients therapy is begun with a single agent. The dose is titrated upward until control of the BP is attained. BP control, in most instances, is defined as maintaining SBP and DBP below the 90th percentile. If control cannot be achieved using the maximum dose of a single agent, a second medication can be added or, alternatively, another agent from a different class selected. The more commonly used medications for chronic antihypertensive therapy in children are listed in Table 58-3 and those for use in acute, hypertensive emergencies in Table 58-4. Presently, the dosing recommendations for children have been largely based on practitioner experience, not on large, multicenter trials. Some clinical trial work is now being conducted on the medications that are already approved and prescribed for hypertension in adults. This information, as it becomes available will provide more information on efficacy, safety, and dosing in children.

β-Adrenergic blockers, such as propranolol, metoprolol, and atenolol, are good choices in some nonasthmatic children, but may not be well tolerated by athletes in whom exercise capacity could be decreased. More frequently, first-line medications are either angiotensin-converting enzyme (ACE) inhibitors or calcium channel blockers (CCBs). ACE inhibitors rarely cause side effects (e.g., cough, rash, neutropenia) in children, are usually well tolerated, and many formulations have the advantage of once-a-day dosing. Not only are they effective at controlling BP, but may have beneficial effects on renal function, peripheral vasculature, and cardiac function.[88] Importantly, children with diabetes and those with chronic renal disease may be at special risk for progressive renal deterioration and may benefit from ACE inhibitors.[89,90] Because of their vasodilator effects on the efferent arteriole, ACE inhibitors can severely reduce glomerular filtration and should therefore be used with caution in patients with renal artery stenosis, a solitary kidney, or a transplanted kidney.[91] ACE inhibitors are contraindicated during pregnancy because of teratogenic effects on the lungs, kidneys, and brain of the fetus.[92] Therefore, these agents should be used with special caution in adolescent females. Angiotensin receptor blockers (ARBs) also interact with the renin-angiotensin system (RAS) and have benefits similar to the ACE inhibitors. Some experience is now being developed with these agents in treatment of children with hypertension.

Several of the CCBs are being used in children. In children, the CCBs can be used as initial therapy or as the second or third medication when more than one drug is needed to control BP. As with most of the oral antihypertensive preparations, the appropriate dose for small children is often lower than the strength of available tablets, which makes initial dose determinations challenging. Both short-acting and longer-acting forms are available. Use of short-acting CCBs should be limited to children with acute hypertension, such as occurs with acute glomerulonephritis. When CCBs are

**Table 58–3** Treatment of Chronic Hypertension in Children

| Drug | Dose | Frequency | Available Preparations |
|------|------|-----------|------------------------|
| **Diuretics** | | | |
| Chlorothiazide | 20-30 mg/kg/day Max: 500 mg/day | q12-24h | Tablets: 250, 500 mg<br>Solution: 250 mg/5 ml |
| Hydrochlorothiazide | 1-4 mg/kg/day Max: 50 mg/day | q12-24h | Tablets: 25, 50, 100 mg |
| Metolazone | 0.1-0.5 mg/kg/day Max: 20 mg/day (Zaroxolyn) | q24h | Tablets: 2.5, 5, 10 mg (Zaroxolyn) |
| | 0.5-1 mg/day (Mykrox) | q24h | Tablets: 0.5, 1.0 mg (Mykrox) |
| Furosemide | 0.5-4 mg/kg/day Max: 80 mg/dose | q6-24h | Tablets: 20, 40, 80 mg<br>Solution: 10 mg/ml, 40 mg/5 ml, 80 mg/10 ml |
| Spironolactone | 1-3.0 mg/kg/day Max: 100 mg/day for hypertension | q8-24h | Tablets: 25, 50, 100 mg |
| **β-Adrenergic Antagonists** | | | |
| Nonselective:<br>  Propranolol | 0.5-5 mg/kg/day Max: 640 mg/day | q6-12h | Tablets: 10, 20, 40, 60, 80 mg<br>Long-acting capsules: 60, 80, 120, 160 mg<br>Solution: 20, 40 mg/5 ml |
| Nadolol* | 40-240 mg/day | q24h | Tablets: 20, 40, 80, 120, 160 mg |
| Selective:<br>  Atenolol | 0.5-2 mg/kg/day Max: 100 mg/day | q24h | Tablets: 25, 50, 100 mg |
| Metoprolol | 1-6 mg/kg/day Max: 200 mg/day | q12-24h | Tablets: 50, 100 mg |
| Bisoprolol/HCTZ | 2.5/6.25 mg/day Max: 10/6.25 mg/day | q24h | Tablets: 2.5/6.25, 5/6.25, 10/6.25 mg |
| **α-Adrenergic Antagonists** | | | |
| Prazosin | 0.02-0.5 mg/kg/day Max: 20 mg/day | q6-12h | Tablets: 1, 2, 5 mg |
| **Complex Adrenergic Antagonists** | | | |
| Labetalol | 2-3 mg/kg/day initially Max: 20 mg/kg/day | q8-12h | Tablets: 100, 200, 300 mg |
| **Central α-Adrenergic Agonists** | | | |
| Clonidine | 0.05-0.1 mg/dose Max: 2.4 mg/day | q6-12h | Tablets: 0.1, 0.2, 0.3 mg<br>Patches: 0.1, 0.2, 0.3 mg/week |
| Methyldopa | 10-65 mg/kg/day Max: 3 g/day | q6-12h | Tablets: 125, 250, 500 mg<br>Solution: 250 mg/5 ml |
| **Angiotensin-Converting Enzyme Inhibitors** | | | |
| Captopril | 0.05-6 mg/kg/day Max: 200 mg/day | q8-12h | Tablets: 12.5, 25, 50, 100 mg |
| Enalapril | 0.1-0.6 mg/kg/day Max: 40 mg/day | q12-24h | Tablets: 2.5, 5.0, 10, 20 mg |
| Lisinopril* | 0.07-0.6 mg/kg/day Max: 40 mg/day | q24h | Tablets: 5, 10, 20 mg |
| Quinapril* | 5-80 mg/day | q24h | Tablets: 5, 10, 20 mg |
| Ramipril* | 1.25-20 mg/day | q12-24h | Capsules: 1.25, 2.5, 5, 10 mg |
| Fosinopril | 0.1-0.6 mg/kg/day Max: 40 mg/day | q24h | Tablets: 10, 20, 40 mg |
| Benazepril | 0.2-0.6 mg/kg/day Max: 40 mg/day | q24h | Tablets: 5, 10, 20, 40 mg |
| **Vasodilators** | | | |
| Hydralazine | 1-8 mg/kg/day Max: 200 mg/day | q12-24h | Tablets: 10, 25, 50, 100 mg |
| **Calcium Antagonists** | | | |
| Nifedipine | 0.25-3 mg/kg/day Max: 180 mg/day | q6-24h | Capsules: 10, 20 mg<br>Extended release: 30, 60, 90 mg |
| Isradipine | 0.15-0.8 mg/kg/day | q8-12h | Capsules: 2.5, 5, 10 mg |
| Amlodipine* | 0.06-0.34 mg/kg/day Max: 10 mg/day | q24h | Tablets: 2.5, 5, 10 mg |
| Felodipine ER | 2.5-20 mg/day | q24h | Tablets: 2.5, 5, 10 mg |
| **Angiotensin II Receptor Blockers** | | | |
| Losartan | 0.75-1.44 mg/kg/day Max: 100 mg/day | q24h | Tablets: 25, 50, 100 mg |
| Irbesartan* | 75-300 mg/day | q24h | Tablets: 75, 150, 300 mg |
| Telmisartan* | 20-80 mg/day | q24h | Tablets: 40, 80 mg |
| Candesartan* | 2-32 mg/day | q24h | Tablets: 4, 8, 16, 32 mg |
| Valsartan* | 80-160 mg/day | q24h | Tablets: 80, 160 mg |

*The pediatric dose is under investigation.

**Table 58–4** Treatment of Hypertensive Emergencies in Children

| Drug | Dose | Route | Comments |
|------|------|-------|----------|
| Furosemide | 1-4 mg/kg/dose<br>Max: 160 mg/dose | IV, IM, or PO | Nephrotoxic, ototoxic<br>When administered IV, infuse slowly to avoid ototoxicity<br>Onset: 5-20 min |
| Hydralazine | 0.1-0.5 mg/kg/dose<br>Max: 50 mg/dose | IV, IM | Tachycardia, flushing, salt retention<br>Onset: 10-20 min |
| Diazoxide | 1-5 mg/kg/dose q5-15min<br>Max: 150 mg/dose | IV | Pain at injected vein, sodium retention<br>Onset: 2 min |
| Sodium nitroprusside | 0.3-10 μg/kg/min by continuous infusion | IV | Cyanide poisoning in patients with renal failure<br>Onset: seconds |
| Nifedipine | 0.2-0.5 mg/kg/dose<br>Max: 10 mg/dose | PO, sublingual, bite, and swallow | Headaches, edema<br>Onset: 2-3 min |
| Nicardipine | 1-3 μg/kg/min | IV | Dizziness, flushing |
| Labetalol | 0.2-1 mg/kg/dose by bolus over 2-min period<br>or | IV q10min | Contraindicated in congestive heart failure, diabetes mellitus, and asthma |
| | 0.25-3.0 mg/kg/hr<br>Max: 80 mg/dose or 300 mg/total dose | Continuous IV infusion | Onset: 5-10 min |
| Enalapril | 0.05-0.1 mg/kg/dose<br>Max: 1.25 mg/dose | IV bolus | Cough, angioedema, renal failure, hyperkalemia<br>Onset: 15 min |

IV, intravenously; IM, intramuscularly; PO, orally.

needed for BP control in chronic hypertension, long-acting preparations are preferred, provided that the correct dosage preparation can be used.

Diuretics are generally recommended as initial drug therapy for uncomplicated hypertension in adults. This recommendation is based on a vast amount of clinical trial data in adults. No such information is available to guide recommendations for pharmacologic management of hypertension in children and adolescents. Unless there is clinical evidence of fluid retention in a hypertensive child, such as may occur when the elevated BP is related to chronic steroid use, diuretics are usually not the preferred first step in drug treatment. Although some hypertensive children may achieve adequate BP control with a thiazide diuretic alone, most will not. Children receiving thiazide diuretics will often develop hypokalemia and require potassium supplements; and for children, taking the potassium supplements is extremely unpleasant. The need to take potassium supplements in turn can lead to compliance problems. Although not favored as an initial drug to treat hypertension in children, low-dose diuretics can be very useful as a second or third drug in those children who require multiple drugs to achieve BP control.

## SUMMARY

Essential, or primary, hypertension can occur in childhood. Due to the rising rates of childhood obesity, the expression of essential hypertension in childhood will increase. Despite this trend, the possibility of secondary hypertension should be considered in a child with documented hypertension. Children with suspected secondary hypertension may require a more extensive evaluation compared with children and adolescents expressing characteristics of essential hypertension. Whether the hypertension is determined to be secondary or essential, these children require careful monitoring, interventions to control the BP, and long-term follow-up. Considering the long-term morbidity and mortality associated with essential hypertension, interventions, including preventive interventions that focus on BP control beginning in the young are needed. Essential hypertension may be found to encompass several distinct pathophysiologic entities, each with its own genetic basis and management approach. As new information develops, improved management strategies can be created for hypertension in the young as well as in adults.

## References

1. Still JL, Cottom D. Severe hypertension in childhood. Arch Diseases Child 42:34-39, 1967.
2. Chobanian AV, Bakris GL, Black HR, et al., for National Heart, Lung, and Blood Institute Joint National Committee on Prevention, Detection, Evaluation, and Treatment of High Blood Pressure; National High Blood Pressure Education Program Coordinating Committee. The Seventh Report of the Joint National Committee on Prevention, Detection, Evaluation, and Treatment of High Blood Pressure: The JNC 7 report. JAMA 289:2560-2572, 2003.
3. Blumenthal S, Epps RP, Heavenrich R, et al. Report of the Task Force on Blood Pressure Control in Children. Pediatrics 59:797-820, 1977.

4. Task Force on Blood Pressure Control in Children: Report of the Second Task Force on Blood Pressure Control in Children—1987. Pediatrics 79:1-25, 1987.

5. National High Blood Pressure Education Program Working Group on High Blood Pressure in Children and Adolescents. The fourth report on the diagnosis, evaluation, and treatment of high blood pressure in children and adolescents. Pediatrics 114:555-576, 2004.

6. de Swiet M, Fayers P, Shinebourne EA. Blood pressure survey in a population of newborn infants. Br Med J 2:9-11, 1976.

7. Schachter J, Kuller LH, Perfetti C. Blood pressure during the first five years of life: Relation to ethnic group (black or white) and to parental hypertension. Am J Epidemiol 119:541-553, 1984.

8. Menghetti E, Virdis R, Strambi M, et al., for the Study Group on Hypertension of the Italian Society of Pediatrics'. Blood pressure in childhood and adolescence: The Italian normal standards. J Hypertens 17:1363-1372, 1999.

9. Pall D, Katona E, Fulesdi B, et al. Blood pressure distribution in a Hungarian adolescent population: Comparison with normal values in the USA. J Hypertens 21:41-47, 2003.

10. Zinner SH, Rosner B, Oh WO. Significance of blood pressure in infancy. Hypertension 7:411-416, 1985.

11. Hulman S, Edwards R Chen Y, et al. Blood pressure patterns in the first three days of life. J Perinatol 11:231-234, 1991.

12. Zubrow AB, Hulman S, Kushner H, et al. Determinants of blood pressure in infants admitted to neonatal intensive care units: A prospective multicenter study. J Perinatol 15:470-479, 1995.

13. Prineas RJ, Elkwiry ZM. Epidemiology and measurement of high blood pressure in children and adolescents. *In* Loggie JMH (ed). Pediatric and Adolescent Hypertension. Boston, MA, Blackwell Scientific Publications, 1992; pp 91-103.

14. Sinaiko AR, Gomez-Martin O, Prineas RJ. Diastolic fourth and fifth phase blood pressure in 10–15 year old children: The Children and Adolescent Blood Pressure Program. Am J Epidemiol 132:647-655, 1990.

15. Hanna JD, Chan JCM, Gill JR, Jr. Hypertension and the kidney. J Pediatr 118:327-340, 1991.

16. Arar MY, Hogg RI, Arant BS Jr, et al. Etiology of sustained hypertension in children in the southwestern United States. Pediatr Nephrol 8:186, 1994.

17. Plumer LB, Kaplan GW, Mendoza SA. Hypertension in infants - a complication of umbilical arterial catheterization. J Pediatr 89:802-805, 1976.

18. Vailas GN, Brouillette RT, Scott JP, et al. Neonatal aortic thrombosis: Recent experience. J Pediatr 109:101-108, 1986.

19. Abman SH, Warady BA, Lum GM, et al. Systemic hypertension in infants with bronchopulmonary dysplasia. J Pediatr 104:928-931, 1984.

20. Ing FF, Starc TJ, Griffiths SP, et al. Early diagnosis of coarctation of the aorta in children: A continuing dilemma. Pediatrics 98:378-382, 1996.

21. Stafford MA, Griffiths SP, Gersony WM. Coarctation of the aorta: A study in delayed detection. Pediatrics 69:159-163, 1982.

22. Thoele DG, Muster AJ, Paul MH. Recognition of coarctation of the aorta. Am J Dis Child 141:1201-1204, 1987.

23. Adelman RD. Smokeless tobacco and hypertension in an adolescent. Pediatrics 79:837-838, 1987.

24. Blachley JD, Knochel JP. Tobacco chewer's hypokalemia: Licorice revisited. N Eng J Med 302:784-785, 1980.

25. Committee on Sports Medicine and Fitness. Athletic participation by children and adolescents who have systemic hypertension. Pediatrics 99:637-638, 1997.

26. Sorof JM, Alexandrov AV, Dardwell G, et al. Carotid artery intimal-medial thickness and left ventricular hypertrophy in children with elevated blood pressure. Pediatrics 111:61-66, 2003.

27. Daniels SR, Loggie JM, Khoury P, et al. Left ventricular geometry and severe left ventricular hypertrophy in children and adolescents with essential hypertension. Circulation 97:1907-1911, 1998.

28. Li S, Chen W, Srinivasan SR, et al. Childhood cardiovascular risk factors and carotid vascular changes in adulthood. The Bogalusa Heart Study. JAMA 290:2271-2276, 2003.

29. Raitakari OT, Juonala M, Kahonen M, et al. Cardiovascular risk factors in childhood and carotid artery intima-media thickness in adulthood. The Cardiovascular Risk in Young Finns Study. JAMA 290:2277-2283, 2003.

30. Falkner B, Onesti G, Angelakos ET, et al. Cardiovascular response to mental stress in normal adolescents with hypertensive parents. Hypertension 1:23-30, 1979.

31. Warren P, Fischbein C. Identification of labile hypertension in children and hypertensive parents. Conn Med 44:77-79, 1980.

32. Matthews KA, Manuck SB, Saab PG. Cardiovascular responses of adolescents during a naturally occurring stressor and their behavioral and psychophysiological predictors. Psychophysiology 23:198, 1984.

33. Falkner B, Kushner H. Racial differences in stress induced reactivity in young adults. Health Psychol 8:613-617, 1989.

34. Shear CL, Burke GL, Freedman DS, et al. Value of childhood blood pressure measurements and family history in predicting future blood pressure status: Results from 8 years of follow-up in the Bogalusa Heart Study. Pediatrics 1986; 77:862-869.

35. Munger R, Prineas R, Gornez-Marin O. Persistent elevation of blood pressure among children with a family history of hypertension: The Minneapolis children's blood pressure study. J Hypertension 6:647-653, 1988.

36. Himes JH, Dietz WH. Guidelines for overweight in adolescent preventive services: Recommendations from an expert committee. Am J Clin Nutr 1994; 59:307-316.

37. Havlik R, Hubert H, Fabsity R, et al. Weight and hypertension. Ann Intern Med 98 855-859, 1983.

38. Rocchini AP, Katch V, Anderson J, et al. Blood pressure in obese adolescents: Effect of weight loss. Pediatrics 82:16-23, 1988.

39. Rocchini AP, Key J, Bondie D, et al. The effect of weight loss on the sensitivity of blood pressure to sodium in obese adolescents. N Eng J Med 321:580-585, 1989.

40. Sinaiko AR. Hypertension in children. N Engl J Med 35:1968-1973, 1996.

41. Troiano RP, Flegal KM, Kuczmarski RJ, et al. Overweight prevalence and trends for children and adolescents. Arch Pediatr Adolesc Med 149:1085-1091, 1995.

42. Ogden CL, Flegal KM, Carroll MD, et al. Prevalence and trends in overweight among US children and adolescents, 1999-2000. JAMA 288:1728-1732, 2002.

43. DeFronzo R, Tobin JD, Andres R. Glucose clamp technique: A method for quantifying insulin secretion and resistance. Am J Physiol 237:E214-E223, 1979.

44. Ferrannini E, Buzzigoli G, Bonadonna R, et al. Insulin resistance in essential hypertension. N Engl J Med 317:350-357, 1987.

45. Reaven GM. Role of insulin resistance in human disease. Diabetes 37:1595-1607, 1988.

46. Berenson GS, Wattigney WA, Bao W, et al. Epidemiology of early primary hypertension and implication for prevention: The Bogalusa Heart Study. J Human Hypertension 8:303 311, 1994.

47. Falkner B, Hulman S, Tannenbaum J, et al. Insulin resistance and blood pressure in young Black men. Hypertension 16:706-711, 1990.

48. Ferrari P, Weidmann P, Shaw S, et al. Altered insulin sensitivity, hyperinsulinemia, and dyslipidemia in individuals with a hypertensive parent. Am J Med 91:589 596, 1991.

49. Grunfeld B, Balzareti M, Romo M, et al. Hyperinsulinemia in normotensive offspring of hypertensive parents. Hypertension 23(Suppl.1):12-15, 1994.

50. Sorof J, Daniels S. Obesity hypertension in children. Hypertension 40:441-455, 2002.

51. Bao W, Srinivasan SR, Wattigney WA, et al. Persistence of multiple cardiovascular risk clustering related to syndrome X from childhood to young adulthood. Arch Intern Med 154:1842-1847, 1994.

52. Barker DJP, Osmond C, Golding J, et al. Growth in utero, blood pressure in childhood and adult life, and mortality from cardiovascular disease. Br Med J 298:564-567, 1989.

53. Law CM, Shiell AW. Is blood pressure inversely related to birth weight? The strength of evidence from a systematic review of the literature. J Hypertension 14:935-941, 1996.

54. Barker DJP, Gluckman PD, Godfrey KM, et al. Fetal nutrition and cardiovascular disease in adult life. Lancet 341:938-941, 1993.

55. Osmond C, Barker DJP, Winter PD, et al. Early growth and death from cardiovascular disease in women. BMJ 307:1519-1524, 1993.

56. Harlan WR, Cornoni Huntley J, et al. Blood pressure in childhood. National Health Examination Survey. Hypertension 1:566-571, 1979.

57. Katz SH, Hediger MC, Schall HI, et al. Blood pressure, growth and maturation from childhood to adolescence. Hypertension 2(Suppl):1-55-69, 1980.

58. Falkner B, Hulman S, Kushner H. Birth weight vs childhood growth as determinants of adult blood pressure. Hypertension 31(1):145-150, 1998.

59. Hulman S, Kushner H, Katz S, et al. Can cardiovascular risk be predicted by newborn, childhood, and adolescent body size? An examination of longitudinal data in urban African Americans. J Pediatr 132:90-97, 1998.

60. Lauer RM, Clarke WR, Beaglehole R. Level, trend, and variability of blood pressure during childhood. The Muscatine Study. Circulation 69:242-249, 1984.

61. Michels V, Bergstralh E, Hoverman V, et al. Tracking and prediction of blood pressure in children. Mayo Clin Proc 62:875-881, 1987.

62. Julius S, Jamerson K, Mejia A, et al. The association of borderline hypertension with target organ changes and higher coronary risk. Tecumseh Blood Pressure Study. JAMA 264:354-358, 1990.

63. Mahoney LT, Clarke WR; Burns TL, et al. Childhood predictors of high blood pressure. Am J Hypertens 4:6085, 1991.

64. Nelson M, Ragland D, Syme S. Longitudinal prediction of adult blood pressure from juvenile blood pressure levels. Am J Epidemiol 136:633-645, 1992.

65. Lauer RM, Clarke WR, Maloney LT, et al. Childhood predictors for high adult blood pressure: The Muscatine Study. Pediatr Clin North Am 40:23-40, 1993.

66. Huxley R, Neil A, Collins R. Unraveling the fetal origins hypothesis: Is there really an inverse association between birthweight and subsequent blood pressure? Lancet 31:360:659-665, 2002.

67. Rich GM, Ulick S, Cook S, et al. Glucocorticoid-remediable aldosteronism in a large kindred: Clinical spectrum and diagnosis using a characteristic biochemical phenotype. Ann Intern Med 116:813-820, 1992.

68. Lifton RP, Dluhy RG, Powers M, et al. Hereditary hypertension caused by chimeric gene duplications and ectopic expression of aldosterone synthase. Nature Genet 2:66-74, 1992.

69. Kroenke K, Omori DM, Simmons JO, et al. The safety of phenylpropanolamine in patients with stable hypertension. Ann Intern Med 111:1043-1044, 1989.

70. Lake CR, Gallant S, Masson E, et al. Adverse drug effects attributed to phenylpropanolamine: A review of 142 case reports. Am J Med 89:195-208, 1990.

71. Hurley JK. A pediatrician's approach to the evaluation of hypertension. Pediatr Ann 18:542, 544-546, 548-549, 1989.

72. Laird WP, Fixler DE. Left ventricular hypertrophy in adolescents with elevated blood pressure: Assessment by chest roentgenography, electrocardiography and echocardiography. Pediatrics 67:255-259, 1981.

73. Shieken RM, Clark WR, Lauer RM. Left ventricular hypertrophy in children with blood pressures in the upper quintile of the distribution: The Muscatine Study. Hypertension 3:669-675, 1981.

74. Zahka KG, Neill CA, Kidd L, et al. Cardiac involvement in adolescent hypertension. Hypertension 3:664-668, 1981.

75. Culpepper WS, Sodt PC, Messerli FH, et al. Cardiac status in juvenile borderline hypertension. Ann Intern Med 98:1-7, 1983.

76. Daniels SR, Lipman MJ, Burke MJ, et al. The prevalence of retinal vascular abnormalities in children and adolescents with essential hypertension. Am J Ophthalmol 111:205-208, 1991.

77. Yudkin JS, Forrest RD, Jackson CA. Microalbuminuria as predictor of vascular disease in non-diabetic subjects. Lancet ii:530-533, 1988.

78. Townsend RR, Ford V. Ambulatory blood pressure monitoring: Coming of age in nephrology. J Am Soc Nephrol 7 2279-2287, 1996.

79. Soergel M, Kirschstein M, Busch C, et al. Oscillometric 24-hour ambulatory blood pressure values in healthy children and adolescents: A multicenter trial including 1141 subjects. J Pediatr 130:178-184, 1997.

80. Harshfield GA, Alpert BS, Pulliam DA, et al. Ambulatory blood pressure recordings in children and adolescents. Pediatrics 94:180-184, 1994.

81. Brownell KD, Kelman JH, Stunkard AJ. Treatment of obese children with and without their mothers: Changes in weight and blood pressure. Pediatrics 71:515-523, 1983.

82. Hagberg JM, Goldring D, Ehsani AA, et al. Effect of exercise training on the blood pressure and hemodynamic features of hypertensive adolescents. Am J Cardiol 52:763-768, 1983.

83. Hansen HS, Froberg K, Hyldebrandt N, et al. A controlled study of eight months of physical training and reduction of blood pressure in children: The Odense Schoolchild Study. Br Med J 303:682-685, 1991.

84. Shea S, Basch CE, Gutin B, et al. The rate of increase in blood pressure in children 5 years of age is related to changes in aerobic fitness and body mass index. Pediatrics 94:465-470, 1994.

85. Falkner B, Michel S. Blood pressure response to sodium in children and adolescents. Am J Clin Nutr 65(Suppl):618S~621S, 1997.

86. Sinaiko AR, Gomez-Marin O, Prineas RJ. Effect of low sodium diet or potassium supplementation on adolescent blood pressure. Hypertension 21:989-994, 1993.

87. Appel LJ, Moore TJ, Obarzanek B, et al., for the DASH Collaborative Research Group. A clinical trial of the effects of dietary patterns on blood pressure. N Engl J Med 336(16):1117-1124, 1997.

88. Doyle AK. Angiotensin-converting enzyme (ACE) inhibition: Benefits beyond blood pressure control. Am J Med 92(4B):1S-107S, 1992.

89. Krolewski AS, Canessa M, Warram JH, et al. Predisposition to hypertension and susceptibility to renal disease in insulin-dependent diabetes mellitus. N Engl J Med 318:140-145, 1988.

90. National High Blood Pressure Education Program. Working group report on hypertension and diabetes. Hypertension 23:145-158, 1994.

91. Hricik DE, Dunn MJ. Angiotensin-converting enzyme inhibitor-induced renal failure: Causes, consequences, and diagnostic uses. J Am Soc Nephrol 1:845-858, 1990.

92. Pryde PG, Sedman AB, Nugent CE, et al. Angiotensin-converting enzyme inhibitor fetopathy. J Am Soc Nephrol 3:1575-1582, 1993.

# Resistant Hypertension
## David A. Calhoun

## DEFINITION

Resistant hypertension has traditionally been defined as failure of concomitant use of three or more different antihypertensive agents to achieve goal blood pressure (BP). This definition has generally required that one of the agents be a diuretic and/or that all of the prescribed agents be at maximal or near-maximal doses.[1] It is more practical; however, to define resistant hypertension as concomitant need of three or more antihypertensive agents prescribed at pharmacologically effective doses. The latter definition has several advantages. First, it does not exclude patients who, because of real or perceived adverse effects, are intolerant of diuretics. Second, it is more realistic in not requiring use of maximal doses of all prescribed agents, as adverse effects often preclude titration to the highest recommended dose of a medication. Last, such a definition allows for use of recent clinical trials to estimate the prevalence of resistant hypertension. Such trials provide our best estimates of the true frequency of resistant hypertension, as continued drug titration is mandated by protocol, medications are generally provided at no charge, and adherence is closely monitored with pill counts. Also, as in real-world treatment of hypertension, these outcome studies have not generally required use of a diuretic in all participants.

## PREVALENCE

Using the aforementioned definition of concomitant prescription of three or more antihypertensive medications, recent clinical trials indicate that resistant hypertension is common, affecting 20% to 30% of the different study populations. Given the size and diversity of the study population, the Antihypertensive and Lipid-Lowering Treatment to Prevent Heart Attack Trial (ALLHAT) may provide the best estimation of the prevalence of resistant hypertension.[2] In ALLHAT, more than 33,000 persons 55 years of age or older with a history of hypertension and one other cardiovascular risk factor were randomized to chlorthalidone, amlodipine, or lisinopril. The dose of the randomized medication as titrated first and then nonstudy antihypertensive medications were added as long as the BP was above 140/90 mm Hg. After 5 years of follow-up, 34% of subjects had not achieved goal BP and overall, 27% of participants were receiving three or more medications.[3]

Other recent outcome studies have documented that resistant hypertension is not rare. In the Controlled Onset Verapamil Investigation of Cardiovascular End Points Trial (CONVINCE), more than 16,600 participants were randomized to COER–verapamil or conventional antihypertensive therapy (atenolol or hydrochlorothiazide [HCTZ]), with other medications added as necessary to reduce BP below 140/90 mm Hg.[4] After a mean follow-up of 3 years, 33% of participants had not achieved goal BP and 17% to 18% were receiving three or more antihypertensive medications. In the International Verapamil-Trandolapril Study (INVEST), over 22,500 persons with hypertension and known coronary artery disease were enrolled.[5] At 2 years follow-up, 29% of participants remained uncontrolled at >140/90 mm Hg and approximately 50% required three or more antihypertensive agents. In studies of even more complicated hypertensive patients, controls rates are even worse. In the LIFE Study, which enrolled hypertensive patients with left ventricular hypertrophy (LVH), only 46% to 49% of participants had a BP of <140/90 mm Hg after almost 5 years of intensive antihypertensive treatment.[6]

The above studies, on one hand, likely overestimate the prevalence of resistant hypertension, as they were limited to older, higher-risk patients. However, on the other hand, they likely underestimate the frequency of resistant hypertension, as persons with severe or known drug resistance were excluded from enrolling; a percentage of enrollees were not titrated in spite of lack of BP control; and control rates were not based on recommended lower BP goals for diabetics and/or persons with chronic kidney disease.

Overall, these recent outcome studies suggest that resistant hypertension is not rare with approximately 30% of subjects never achieving goal BP because of drug resistance and/or nonadherence and 20% to 30% enrollees requiring three or more antihypertensive medications.

## PATIENT CHARACTERISTICS

In the large majority of patients, resistant hypertension is a consequence of the systolic blood pressure (SBP) remaining uncontrolled. This is indicated by both epidemiologic data and clinical trial results. Cross-sectional data from the Framingham Heart Study demonstrated that among patients being treated for hypertension, 90% had a diastolic blood pressure (DBP) of <90 mm Hg, whereas only 49% had a SBP <140 mm Hg.[7] Similar discrepancies between systolic and diastolic control rates are seen in clinical trials. In ALLHAT, 92% of participants achieved goal DBP but only 67% achieved goal SBP.[2] In LIFE, 89% of enrollees a SBP <90 mm Hg, while 45% to 48% had a systolic <140 mm Hg.[6] These studies clearly demonstrate that the poor BP control is overwhelmingly due to lack of SBP control in treated patients.

Uncontrolled hypertension, which includes untreated and under-treated persons as well as treatment-resistant patients, increases with age. Analyzing data from the third National Health and Nutrition Examination Survey III (NHANES III), Hyman and Pavlik reported that among persons being treated, hypertension was controlled in 65% of those between 25 to 44 years of age, 52% 45 to 64 years of age, and 34% 65 years or older.[8] In this analysis, the largest relative risk of uncontrolled hypertension was associated with being 65 years of age or older. In the Framingham Heart Study, cross-sectional analysis indicated that increasing age was significantly associated with lack of SBP control, whereas prospectively, participants ≥55 years of age were two thirds as likely to have controlled BP as participants <55 years age.[8,9] In ALLHAT, older age predicted a lower likelihood of achieving BP control.[3] In participants 55 to 59 years of age, the control rate of SBP was 62%. In those older than 80 years of age, the systolic control rate fell to 49%.

Although there is wide individual variation, in general, the more severe the hypertension, the more medications it will require to effectively reduce BP to goal. In the Framingham Heart Study, higher levels of SBP predicted lower BP control rates. Participants with SBP 140 to 159 mm Hg were 50% as likely to be achieve BP control as participants with SBP <140 mm Hg, whereas participants with SBP ≥160 mm Hg were only 25% as likely to be controlled.[9] In ALLHAT, similar effects were seen, with higher baseline SBP being strongly associated with a lower likelihood of achieving BP control.[3]

Other characteristics associated with resistant hypertension include obesity, diabetes, Black race, renal insufficiency, and presence of LVH (Box 59–1). Obesity predicts need for an increasing number of antihypertensive medications and increased likelihood of never achieving adequate BP control.[3,8] In ALLHAT, Black participants had overall worse BP control than non-Blacks.[3] The best control rate was in non-Black men (70%) and the lowest in Black women (59%). Clinical trials indicate that diabetics are more resistant to antihypertensive treatment than nondiabetics, requiring more medications to achieve the same level of BP control.[3,10,11] Renal insufficiency increases BP, presumably through increased sodium retention and corresponding volume expansion and through increased release of vasoconstrictors such as angiotensin II and norepinephrine. In general, as renal function deteriorates, BP control becomes more difficult to treat.[3] Last, LVH is associated with an increased resistance to BP reduction.[3,7] Whether LVH contributes to drug resistance or reflects underlying severity of hypertension is unknown.

## DIAGNOSIS AND EVALUATION

The evaluation of patients with resistant hypertension is generally the same as for all patients with primary hypertension, except that there should be a higher level of suspicion for secondary causes of hypertension. In this regard, acquisition of a 24-hour urine during ingestion of the patient's normal salt diet is recommended. This will allow for simultaneous assessment of sodium and aldosterone excretion, as well as calculation of creatinine clearance. Special attention should be paid to use of good BP measurement technique, including obtaining the BP after 5 minutes of rest and use of appropriately sized cuffs as falsely high readings may result. Degree of target organ damage should be documented.

## ADHERENCE

Poor adherence undoubtedly contributes substantially to poor BP control. In one study based on patient self-report, BP was controlled in 81% of patients who reported taking more than 75% of their medications, but in only 37% of patients who took less than 75% of their pills.[12] In other studies, lack of BP control has been attributed to poor adherence to the prescribed regimen in approximately 50% of cases.[13] Need for multiple medications and frequent medication changes, as often typifies treatment of resistant hypertension, worsens adherence. In specialty clinics, poor adherence may be less of a problem than among generalized hypertension patients. In an evaluation of patients referred to a university-based hypertension clinic, it was estimated that poor adherence was a contributing factor to treatment resistance in only 10% of patients.[14]

Ultimately, poor adherence in the clinical setting can only be confirmed by the patient's self-report. Accordingly, establishing and maintaining good rapport is essential to maintaining effective clinician-patient dialog. Adherence should be queried in a nonthreatening manner, including questions of out-of-pocket costs, dosing convenience, and possible adverse experiences. Input from family members (in the patient's presence) can be solicited. Poor adherence might be suspected in a patient chronically unfamiliar with prescribed medications or dosing regimens or in whom anticipated adverse experiences are absent or denied.

## PSEUDOHYPERTENSION

Pseudohypertension refers to the phenomenon whereby vascular stiffening results in falsely high auscultatory BP measurements. Such an occurrence could result in the misdiagnosis of resistant hypertension when intraarterial pressures are actually normal or below normal. Small studies suggest that pseudohypertension may be common among the elderly, but definitive evaluation is lacking.[15,16] Use of Osler's maneuver (ability to palpate the brachial or radial artery despite ipsilateral occlusion of the artery by a BP cuff inflated to suprasystolic values) has been recommended as a method to screen for pseudohypertension,[17] but other investigators have found the maneuver to have questionable predictive value.[18] Use of infrasonic or oscillometric measurement devices may more accurately reflect intraarterial pressure, but whether this translates into an effective clinical screen for pseudohypertension has not been determined.[16,19] Pseudohypertension might be suspected if auscultatory BP values remain high in the absence of demonstrable target organ deterioration (i.e., LVH, retinopathy, renal insufficiency) or if patients with seemingly resistant hypertension manifest symptoms of hypotension. Confirmation of pseudohypertension requires direct intraarterial measurement of BP.

**Box 59–1** Patient Characteristics Associated with Development of Resistant Hypertension

High baseline blood pressure
Obesity
Older age
Black race
Chronic kidney disease
Diabetes
Left ventricular hypertrophy

## WHITE-COAT PHENOMENA

A small number of studies suggest that white-coat or isolated clinic hypertension is as least as common in patients with resistant hypertension as the general hypertensive population, with a prevalence ranging from 28% to 52%.[20-22] As in the general hypertensive population, persons with resistant clinic hypertension but normal ambulatory BP are at lower cardiovascular risk than those with sustained ambulatory hypertension. For example, in a study of 86 patients with resistant hypertension, defined as a clinic SBP >100 mm Hg during concomitant treatment with at least three antihypertensive agents that included a diuretic, one third were found to have an ambulatory SBP <88 mm Hg.[23] This group had a generally benign prognosis in terms of cardiovascular events during a mean follow-up of 49 months.

White-coat hypertension should be suspected if the patient reports consistently lower home BP levels than is recorded in clinic, if BP elevations persist in the absence of target organ damage, or if symptoms of hypotension develop in spite of persistently high clinic BP measurements. In these situations, ambulatory BP assessment is appropriate to look for a significant white-coat effect. If present, use of home and work BP values should be relied upon to guide therapy.

## DIETARY SODIUM

Population-based studies suggest a weak positive relationship between dietary-salt ingestion and BP.[24-26] However, there are subsets of patients more likely to manifest increased salt-sensitivity, including Blacks, the elderly, and in particular, patients with underlying renal insufficiency. In any patient, excessive sodium ingestion can blunt the antihypertensive benefit of most classes of agents, especially angiotensin-converting enzyme (ACE) inhibitors, angiotensin receptor blockers (ARBs), and diuretics. Accordingly, dietary-salt reduction should be recommended to all patients with resistant hypertension. In patients with renal insufficiency, an assessment of 24-hour urinary sodium excretion may be helpful in guiding adherence to reduced salt intake. Urinary sodium excretion should be maintained at <100 mEq/24 hours in persons with resistant hypertension.

## EXOGENOUS SUBSTANCES

Exogenous substances most often compromising hypertension control include nonsteroidal antiinflammatory drugs (NSAIDs), alcohol, oral contraceptives, decongestants, and less commonly, certain psychotropic drugs (Box 59–2). There is wide individual variation in BP response to the different agents, with most persons being able to tolerate them without significant hypertensive effects. However, a minority of patients may be particularly sensitive to certain agents and withdrawal from the potentially interfering medication should be attempted if possible.

NSAIDs, presumably through inhibition of vasodilating prostaglandins in the kidney, impair natriuresis and induce fluid retention and volume expansion. They can also acutely worsen renal function, particularly in patients with underlying renal insufficiency, including elderly and diabetics, in

**Box 59–2** Exogenous Substances That Can Contribute to Development of Resistant Hypertension

Nonsteroidal antiinflammatory drugs including selective COX-2 inhibitors
Alcohol
Oral contraceptives
Sympathomimetic agents (decongestants, diet pills)
Caffeine
Anabolic steroids
Licorice
Chemotherapeutic agents
Corticosteroids
Cyclosporine
Erythropoietin
Tricyclic antidepressants

whom renal dysfunction may be subtle or unrecognized. In addition to directly raising BP, NSAIDs may blunt the antihypertensive effects of certain agents, particularly diuretics, β-blockers, and ACE inhibitors. Although selective cyclooxygenase-2 (COX-2) inhibitors seem to have renal effects similar to nonselective NSAIDs,[27,28] adverse effects on BP may be less likely, particularly with celecoxib.[29-31]

In general, the pressor effects of NSAIDs are dose dependent and modest, with an anticipated increase in mean BP of 4 to 6 mm Hg.[32,33] However, on an individual basis the compounds can induce acute renal insufficiency, pronounced fluid retention, and severe BP elevations. These effects are more likely to occur in patients with preexisting renal insufficiency. BP and renal function should be monitored closely when initiating NSAIDs use in patients with hypertension. In patients presenting with resistant hypertension, NSAIDs should be withdrawn if possible. Acetaminophen can be substituted for analgesic effect, although it does not provide antiinflammatory benefit.

Sympathomimetic compounds such as decongestants or certain diet pills can elevate pressure and should be avoided in patients with resistant hypertension. Oral contraceptives tend overall to induce a modest increase in BP, but the effect can be more severe in some individuals. Corticosteroids induce fluid retention and consequently may worsen BP control. Tricyclic antidepressants can blunt the efficacy of sympatholytic compounds such as clonidine. Erythropoietin and cyclosporine have well-documented pressor effects, but the option to withdraw such therapies is often limited.

## ALCOHOL

Epidemiologic studies indicate that alcohol ingestion is associated with increases in BP with heavy drinking, increasing the risk of hypertension remaining uncontrolled.[34,35] In a group of patients referred to a Finnish hypertension clinic, 38.5% had elevated γ-glutamyltransferase (GGT) levels, a marker of heavy alcohol ingestion, and among those patients, 22.5% failed to achieve BP control over the subsequent 2 years.[36] In contrast, in patients with normal GGT levels, only 7.1% failed to achieve BP control. Among patients with self-admitted heavy alcohol ingestion (>80 g/day), BP remained uncontrolled in 46.1%. In a prospective study, cessation of heavy daily alcohol ingestion reduced 24-hour systolic and SBP by 7.2 and 6.6 mm Hg, respectively.[37]

Whether through physiologic effects and/or improvements in adherence, cessation of heavy drinking does improve BP control. Accordingly, in all patients with resistant hypertension, alcohol consumption should to limited to ≤1 ounce ethanol/day (i.e., 24 ounces of beer, 10 ounces of wine, or 2 ounces of 100 proof liquor).

## OBESITY

BP and weight are directly related, with each 10% increase in weight associated with a 6.5–mm Hg increase in SBP.[38] This relationship is continuous throughout the entire range of body weight. The mechanism by which weight gain increases BP is not fully known. Likely contributing factors include increases in cardiac output, peripheral resistance, and sympathetic activation, and increases in circulating insulin, which may induce salt sensitivity.

In observational studies, obesity correlates with lack of BP control. The Framingham investigators have reported that body mass indexes (BMIs) greater than 25 and 30 kg/m$^2$ are associated with lack of control of DBP and SBP, respectively.[7] Cross-sectional studies indicate that increasing BMI independently correlates with increasing number of prescribed antihypertensive medications.[39] Last, in ALLHAT, obese subjects, despite receiving more medications, were less likely to achieve goal BP.[3] While weight reduction is difficult to accomplish and maintain, it should be recommended to overweight patients with resistant hypertension, because it will likely reduce the need for antihypertensive treatment.

## SLEEP APNEA

Epidemiologic studies clearly demonstrate a significant association between obstructive sleep apnea and hypertension. Two large cross-sectional studies have shown that the prevalence of hypertension increases with increases in sleep-disordered breathing.[40,41] In a prospective evaluation, patients with a high number of nocturnal respiratory events characteristic of sleep apnea were more than three times as likely to develop hypertension as those with no respiratory events.[42] Furthermore, Logan et al. reported that sleep apnea was very common in patients with drug-resistant hypertension.[43] In their study of 41 patients with resistant hypertension, 96% of the men and 65% of women were diagnosed to have previously unrecognized sleep apnea. In a separate study, sleep apnea was found to be an independent predictor of uncontrolled hypertension in patients <50 years of age.[44] Furthermore, the more severe the sleep apnea, the more likely the accompanying high BP will be resistant to pharmacologic therapy.[45]

Treatment of sleep apnea has generally shown associated reductions in BP, with the benefit being most demonstrable on reductions in nighttime BP.[46] In one prospective evaluation, nasal continuous positive airway pressure (CPAP) reduced both daytime and nighttime mean BP, but only the nighttime reduction was significantly different from placebo treatment.[47] While CPAP seems to improve BP control in general, the benefit may be modest, particularly in patients with severe and/or resistant hypertension. There are other cardiovascular and neurocognitive benefits of CPAP, so it should be prescribed when appropriate, even though large reductions in BP may not occur. For a more complete discussion of sleep apnea, see Chapter 73.

## SECONDARY HYPERTENSION

The most common secondary causes of resistant hypertension are hyperaldosteronism, renal parenchymal disease, renal artery stenosis, and sleep apnea (Box 59–3). Retrospective reports have suggested that the prevalence of secondary causes of hypertension among patients referred to a hypertension specialty clinic is approximately 20%.[48] The prevalence of secondary hypertension increases with age, largely due to the increased prevalence of renovascular disease and renal insufficiency in older persons.[49] Recent prospective studies indicate that hyperaldosteronism is the most common cause of secondary hypertension.

### Hyperaldosteronism

A growing body of evidence indicates that primary aldosteronism (PA) is much more common than thought historically. In an extensive evaluation that included more than 600 hypertensive persons, Mosso et al. found that the prevalence of PA increases according to the severity of the hypertension (Figure 59–1).[50] Applying JNC VI (Sixth Report of the Joint National Committee on Prevention, Detection, Evaluation, and Treatment of High Blood Pressure) staging criteria to untreated patients, PA was diagnosed in 2% of those with stage 1 hypertension (140-159/90-99 mm Hg), 8% of those with stage 2 hypertension (160-179/100-109 mm Hg), and 13% among patients with stage 3 hypertension (>180/110 mm Hg). Earlier, Lim et al. had reported a PA rate, based on an elevated plasma aldosterone:plasma renin activity ratio (ARR), of 14% among hypertensive patients randomly selected from a family physician database.[51] Loh et al.[52] reported a prevalence of 18% among 350 unselected hypertensive patients attending primary care clinics in Singapore.

These studies are just a few of many that report PA to be a common cause of hypertension. PA is particularly common in

**Box 59–3** Secondary Causes of Resistant Hypertension

**Common Causes**
Primary aldosteronism
Renal artery stenosis (fibromuscular dysplasia, atherosclerotic)
Renal parenchymal disease
Sleep apnea

**Rare Causes**
Cushing's disease
Pheochromocytoma
Coarctation of the aorta
Hypercalcemia
Carcinoid syndrome
Central nervous system tumors
Acromegaly

patients with resistant hypertension. In a prospective evaluation of Black and white patients with resistant hypertension, defined as uncontrolled hypertension in spite of use of three or more antihypertensive agents, Calhoun et al.[53] found an overall prevalence of PA of approximately 20% (see Figure 59–1). These results are consistent with a study from separate investigators reporting a prevalence of PA of 17% among patients referred to hypertension specialists for uncontrolled hypertension.[54]

The reason for the increased prevalence of PA is unknown. Early studies of aldosteronism may have underestimated the prevalence of PA by evaluating small numbers of selected patients, such as those presenting with hypokalemia. The high prevalence of PA is also likely related to expanded screening of hypertensive patients. Recently described associations between obesity, sleep apnea, and aldosteronism suggest a possible mechanistic relationship between body weight and aldosterone excess, but such a relation remains speculative.[55,56]

As indicated by the aforementioned reports, PA has become the most common secondary cause of hypertension. Accordingly, PA should be excluded in all patients with resistant hypertension. PA responds well to treatment, particularly in the absence of long-standing hypertension, with either resection of the hypersecreting adenoma or with use of aldosterone antagonists such as spironolactone or eplerenone. (See Chapter 75 for a more complete discussion.)

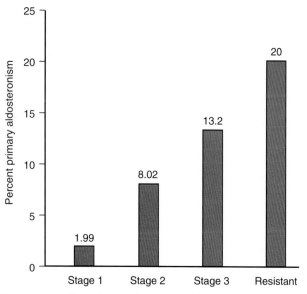

**Figure 59–1** Prevalence of primary aldosteronism (PA) according to severity of hypertension (JNC VI stage 1, 140-159/90-99 mm Hg; stage 2, 160-179/100-109 mm Hg; stage 3, >180/>110 mm Hg; resistant, >140/90 mm Hg on three or more antihypertensive medications). (Modified from Mosso L, Carvajal C, Gonzalez A, et al. Primary aldosteronism and hypertensive disease. Hypertension 42:161-165, 2003; and Calhoun DA, Nishizaka MK, Zaman MA, et al. High prevalence of primary aldosteronism among black and white subjects with resistant hypertension. Hypertension 40:892-896, 2002.)

## Renovascular Disease

Fibromuscular dysplasia accounts for less than 10% of cases of renal artery stenosis. It typically affects young women between the ages of 15 and 50. Angioplasty is successful in up to 100% of patients, the majority of whom will have significant improvement in BP.[57] Restenosis occurs in approximately 10% of cases postangioplasty. Captopril renography is very sensitive in screening for fibromuscular dysplasia.[57]

Atherosclerosis accounts for 90% of the cases of renal artery stenosis. It generally occurs in patients >50 years of age and is more common in smokers and in patients with other atherosclerotic disease, particularly peripheral vascular disease. Patients will often present with exacerbation of previously controlled hypertension. Angioplasty of atherosclerotic renal artery lesions is less successful than with fibromuscular dysplastic lesions, however, with use of stents, short-term success rates approach 100% with restenosis occurring to 11% to 23% of patients at 1 year follow-up.[58,59] Captopril renography has diminished sensitivity in patients with renal insufficiency, such as elderly patients or those with long standing hypertension. Duplex ultrasonography, gadolinium-enhanced magnetic resonance angiography, or computed tomographic angiography can provide effective screening of atherosclerotic renal disease, depending on institutional experience.

Although revascularization helps preserve renal function, the BP response to angioplasty of atherosclerotic lesions is often limited. Studies suggest that less than one third of those will be cured of their hypertension.[57] This response rate may be improved with stenting, but prospective studies evaluating outcomes following angioplasty and stenting are needed. (See Chapter 74 for a more complete discussion of renovascular hypertension.)

## Renal Parenchymal Disease

Renal insufficiency secondary to renal parenchymal disease commonly contributes to resistant hypertension. The most common causes of renal insufficiency are diabetes and poorly controlled hypertension. Such patients are often volume expanded and have increased sensitivity to salt. Renal insufficiency is generally indicated by an elevated serum creatinine. In patients with reduced muscle mass, such as some elderly patients, significant renal disease may be unrecognized unless creatinine clearance is estimated. An estimate of creatinine clearance in the absence of 24-hour urine collection can be obtained based on prediction equations corrected for age, gender, and body size.[1,60]

## Pheochromocytoma

Pheochromocytoma is a rare cause of resistant hypertension. In the report by Anderson et al.,[49] pheochromocytoma was diagnosed in 0.3% of 4429 patients referred to their hypertension clinic. Pheochromocytoma is easily screened for by assessment of 24-hour urinary excretion of catecholamines or plasma metanephrines.[61] It should be suspected in patients with sustained or episodic hypertension complicated by headache, palpitations, or diaphoresis. (See Chapter 76 for a comprehensive discussion of pheochromocytoma.)

# TREATMENT FOR RESISTANT HYPERTENSION

The best treatment for resistant hypertension is based on identification and reversal of contributing factors. Accordingly, there should be a thorough screening for poor adherence, use of interfering substances, renal insufficiency, and secondary causes of hypertension, in particular aldosteronism. Obesity and sleep apnea, if present, should be treated.

In an evaluation of patients referred to a hypertension specialty clinic, failure of treatment after excluding secondary causes of hypertension, was attributed to ineffective regimens, most commonly inadequate dosing of prescribed agents and lack of appropriate use of long-acting diuretics.[14] Antihypertensive agents should be prescribed in the maximum tolerated dose. Use of combination products improves adherence by reducing pill burden, simplifying the dosing regimen, and reducing out-of-pocket costs to the patient. Unless poorly tolerated, use of long-acting diuretics will significantly enhance BP control, particularly in patients already receiving vasodilators. Unless there is significant renal insufficiency (creatinine clearance <60 ml/min), thiazide diuretics are appropriate. Loop diuretics may be needed in patients with renal insufficiency or who are receiving potent vasodilators. Long-acting agents are preferred; if a short-acting agent such as furosemide is prescribed, it should be taken twice a day.

Use of aldosterone antagonists may provide additional BP reduction, even in patients already receiving a diuretic. It has been observed that low-dose spironolactone, 12.5 to 50 mg daily, when added to a regimen that included a diuretic, ACE inhibitor or ARB, and a calcium channel blocker (CCB) provided significant additional BP reduction (Figure 59–2).[62] It is interesting to note that BP reduction was achieved even in patients without true PA, suggesting additional diuretic effects of the aldosterone antagonist when added to multidrug regimens, and/or a role for aldosterone in causing resistant hypertension even in the absence of excess hormone levels (Figure 59–3).

In patients in whom BP remains uncontrolled in spite of use of three or more medications, referral to a hypertension specialist is appropriate. A focused evaluation of contributing factors and especially exclusion of secondary causes of hypertension, along with expert tailoring of the prescribed medications should serve to maximize treatment.[48,63]

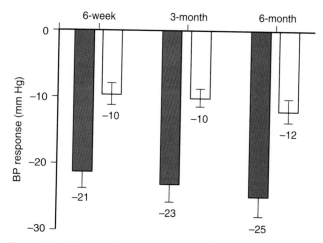

**Figure 59-2** Spironolactone-induced reduction in systolic blood pressure (SBP) *(filled bars)* and diastolic blood pressure (DBP) *(open bars)* at 6-week, 3-month, and 6-month follow-up in patients with resistant hypertension. BP reduction was significant at all time points compared with the baseline. (Nishizaka MK, Zaman MA, Calhoun DA. Efficacy of low-dose spironolactone in subjects with resistant hypertension. Am J Hypertens 16:925-930, 2003.)

## SUMMARY

Resistant hypertension is most often a consequence of poorly controlled systolic hypertension. Common reversible contributing factors include nonadherence, obesity, heavy alcohol consumption, and NSAID use. Prevalent secondary causes of resistant hypertension include hyperaldosteronism, renal insufficiency, renal artery stenosis, and sleep apnea. Of these, hyperaldosteronism may be the most common. Pharmacologic treatment of resistant hypertension requires use of maximum tolerated doses of multiple agents including, if possible, a long-acting diuretic. Addition of aldosterone antagonists to multidrug regimens may provide greater BP reduction.

**Figure 59-3** Spironolactone-induced reduction in systolic blood pressure (SBP) and diastolic blood pressure (DBP) at 6-week, 3-month, and 6-month follow-up in patients with primary aldosteronism (PA) *(filled bars)* and without PA *(open bars)*. Blood pressure (BP) reduction was not significantly different between patients with and without hyperaldosteronism.

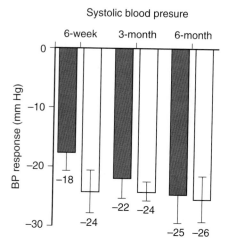
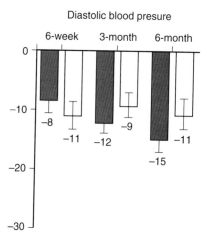

# References

1. Chobanian AV, Bakris GL, Black HR, et al. National High Blood Pressure Education Program Coordinating Committee. Seventh Report of the Joint National Committee on Prevention, Detection, Evaluation, and Treatment of High Blood Pressure. Hypertension 42:1206-1252, 2003.

2. The ALLHAT Officers and Coordinators for the ALLHAT Collaborative Research Group. Major outcomes in high-risk hypertensive patients randomized to angiotensin-converting enzyme inhibitor or calcium channel blocker vs. diuretic. The Antihypertensive and Lipid-Lowering Treatment to Prevent Heart Attack Trial (ALLHAT). JAMA 288:2981-2997, 2002.

3. Cushman WC, Ford CE, Cutler JA, et al. ALLHAT Collaborative Research Group. Success and predictors of blood pressure control in diverse North American settings: The Antihypertensive and Lipid-Lowering Treatment to Prevent Attack Trial (ALLHAT). J Clin Hypertens 4:393-404, 2002.

4. Black HR, Elliott WJ, Grandits G, et al. CONVINCE Research Group. Principal results of the Controlled onset Verapamil Investigation of Cardiovascular End Points (CONVINCE) Trial. JAMA 289:2073-2082, 2003.

5. Pepine CJ, Handberg EM, Cooper-DeHoff RM, et al. INVEST Investigators. A calcium antagonist vs a non-calcium antagonist hypertension treatment strategy for patients with coronary artery disease. The International Verapamil-Trandolapril Study (INVEST): A randomized controlled trial. JAMA 290:2805-2816, 2003.

6. Dahlöf B, Devereux RB, Kjeldsen SE, et al. LIFE study group. Cardiovascular morbidity and mortality in the Losartan Intervention For Endpoint reduction in hypertension study (LIFE): A randomized trial against atenolol. Lancet 359:995-1003, 2002.

7. Lloyd-Jones DM, Evans JC, Larson, et al. Differential control of systolic and diastolic blood pressure: Factors associated with lack of blood pressure control in the community. Hypertension 36:594-599, 2000.

8. Hyman DJ, Pavlik VN. Characteristics of patients with uncontrolled hypertension in the United States. N Engl J Med 345:479-486, 2001.

9. Lloyd-Jones DM, Evans JC, Larson MG, et al. Treatment and control of hypertension in the community. A prospective analysis. Hypertension 40:640-646, 2002.

10. Mancia G, Brown M, Castaigne A, et al. Outcomes with nifedipine GITS or Co-Amilozide in hypertensive diabetics and nondiabetics in Intervention as a Goal in Hypertension (INSIGHT). Hypertension 41:431-436, 2003.

11. Kjeldsen SE, Dahlöf B. Devereux RB, et al. LIFE Study Group. Lowering of blood pressure and predictors of response in patients with left ventricular hypertrophy: The LIFE Study. Am J Hypertens 13:899-906, 2000.

12. Inui TS, Carter WB, Pecoraro RE. Screening for noncompliance among patients with hypertension: Is self-report the best available measure? Med Care 19:1061-1064, 1981.

13. Sackett DL, Haynes RB, Gibson ES, et al. Randomized clinical trial of strategies for improving medication compliance in primary hypertension. Lancet 1:1205-1207, 1975.

14. Yakovlevitch M, Black HR. Resistant hypertension in tertiary care clinic. Arch Intern Med 151:1786-1792, 1991.

15. Zuschke CA, Pettyjohn FS. Pseudohypertension. S Med J 88:1185-1190, 1995.

16. Anazal M, Palmer AJ, Starr J, et al. The prevalence of pseudohypertension in the elderly. J Hum Hypertens 10:409-411, 1996.

17. Messerli FH, Ventura HO, Amodeo C. Osler's maneuver and pseudohypertension. N Engl J Med 312:1548-1551, 1985.

18. Hla K, Samsa G, Stoneking H, et al. Observer variability of Osler's maneuver in detection of pseudohypertension. J Clin Epidemiol 44:513-518, 1991.

19. Hla KM, Feussner JR. Screening for pseudohypertension: A quantitative, noninvasive approach. Arch Intern Med 148:673-676, 1988.

20. Brown MA, Buddle ML, Martin A. Is resistant hypertension really resistant? Am J Hypertens 14:1263-1269, 2001.

21. Mezzetti A, Pierdomenico SD, Costantini F, et al. White-coat resistant hypertension. Am J Hypertens 10:1302-1307, 1997.

22. Hernandez del-Ray R, Armario P, Martin-Baranera M, et al. Target-organ damage and cardiovascular risk profile in resistant hypertension. Influence of the white-coat effect. Blood Pressure Monitoring 3:331-337, 1998.

23. Redon J, Campos C, Narciso ML, et al. Prognostic value of ambulatory blood pressure monitoring in refractory hypertension: A prospective study. Hypertension 31:712-718, 1998.

24. Elliott P, Stamler J, Nichols R, et al. Intersalt Cooperative Research Group. Intersalt revisited: Further analyses of 24-hour sodium excretion and blood pressure within and across populations. BMJ 312:1249-1253, 1996.

25. Elliott P. Observational studies of salt and blood pressure. Hypertension 17(suppl I):I3-I8, 1991.

26. Weinberger MH. Salt-sensitivity of blood pressure in humans. Hypertension 27(part 2):481-490, 1996.

27. Brater DC, Harris C, Redfern JS, et al. Renal effects of COX-2-selective inhibitors. Am J Nephrol 21:1-15, 2001.

28. Swan SK, Rudy DW, Lasseter KC, et al. Effect of cyclooxygenase-2 inhibition on renal function in elderly persons receiving a low-salt diet. A randomized, controlled trial. Ann Intern Med 133:1-9, 2000.

29. Whelton A, White WB, Bello A, et al. SUCCESS-VII Investigators. Effects of celecoxib and refecoxib on blood pressure and edema in patients ≥65 years of age with systemic hypertension and osteoarthritis. Am J Cardiol 90:959-963, 2002.

30. Palmer R, Weiss R, Zusman RM, et al. Effects of nabumetone, celecoxib, and ibuprofen on blood pressure control in hypertensive patients on angiotensin converting enzyme inhibitors. Am J Hypertens 16:135-139, 2003.

31. White WB, Kent J, Taylor A, et al. Effects of celecoxib on ambulatory blood pressure in hypertensive patients on ACE inhibitors. Hypertension 39:929-934, 2002.

32. Johnson AG, Nguyen TV, Day RO. Do nonsteroidal anti-inflammatory drugs affect blood pressure? A meta-analysis. Ann Intern Med 121:289-300, 1994.

33. Radack KL, Deck CC, Bloomfield SS. Ibuprofen interferes with the efficacy of antihypertensive drugs. Ann Intern Med 107:628-635, 1987.

34. MacMahon S. Alcohol consumption and hypertension. Hypertension 9:111-121, 1987.

35. de Gaudemaris R, Lang T, Chatellier G, et al. Socioeconomic inequalities in hypertension prevalence and care. The IHPAF Study. Hypertension 39:1119-1125, 2002.

36. Henningsen NC, Ohlsson O, Mattiasson I, et al. Hypertension, levels of serum gamma glutamyl transpeptidase and degree of blood pressure control in middle-aged males. Acta Med Scand 207:245-251, 1980.

37. Aquilera MT, de la Sierra A, Coca A, et al. Effect of alcohol abstinence on blood pressure: Assessment by 24-hr ambulatory blood pressure monitoring. Hypertension 33:653-657, 1999.

38. Ashley FW Jr, Kannel WB. Relation of weight change to changes in atherogenic traits: The Framingham Study. J Chronic Dis 27:103-114, 1974.

39. Modan M, Almog S, Fuchs Z, et al. Obesity, glucose intolerance, hyperinsulinemia, and response to antihypertensive drugs. Hypertension 17:656-673, 1991.

40. Grote L, Ploch T, Heitmann J, et al. Sleep-related breathing disorder is an independent risk factor for systemic hypertension. Am J Respir Crit Care Med 160:1875-1882, 1999.

41. Nieto FJ, Young TB, Lind BK, et al., for the Sleep Heart Health Study. Association of sleep disordered breathing, sleep apnea,

and hypertension in a large community-based study. JAMA 283:1829-1836, 2000.

42. Peppard PE, Young T, Palta M, et al. Prospective study of the association between sleep-disordered breathing and hypertension. N Engl J Med 342:1378-1384, 2000.

43. Logan AG, Perlikowski SM, Mente A, et al. High prevalence of unrecognized sleep apnea in drug-resistant hypertension. J Hypertens 20:1-7, 2002.

44. Grote L, Hedner J, Peter JH. Sleep-related breathing disorder is an independent factor for uncontrolled hypertension. J Hypertens 18:679-685, 2000.

45. Lavie P, Hoffstein V. Sleep apnea syndrome: A possible contributing factor to resistant hypertension. Sleep 24:721-725, 2001.

46. Silverberg DS, Oksenberg A. Are sleep-related breathing disorders important contributing factors to the production of essential hypertension? Curr Hypertens Rep 3:209-215, 2001.

47. Dimsdale JE, Loredo JS, Profant J. Effect of continuous positive airway pressure on blood pressure: A placebo trial. Hypertension 35:144-147, 2000.

48. Bansal N, Tendler BE, White WB, et al. Blood pressure control in the hypertension clinic. Am J Hypertens 16:878-880, 2003.

49. Anderson GH Jr, Blakeman N, Streeten DHP. The effect of age on prevalence of secondary forms of hypertension in 4429 consecutively referred patients. J Hypertens 12:609-615, 1994.

50. Mosso L, Carvajal C, Gonzalez A, et al. Primary aldosteronism and hypertensive disease. Hypertension 42:161-16, 2003.

51. Lim PO, Dow E, Brennan G, et al. High prevalence of primary aldosteronism in the Tayside hypertension clinic population. J Human Hypertens 14:311-315, 2000.

52. Loh K-C, Koay ES, Khaw M-C, et al. Prevalence of primary aldosteronism among Asian hypertensive patients in Singapore. J Clin Endocrinol Metab 85:2854-2859, 2000.

53. Calhoun DA, Nishizaka MK, Zaman MA, et al. High prevalence of primary aldosteronism among black and white subjects with resistant hypertension. Hypertension 40:892-896, 2002.

54. Galley BJ, Ahmad S, Xu L, et al. Screening for primary aldosteronism without discontinuing hypertensive medications: The plasma aldosterone-renin ratio. Am J Kidney Dis 37:699-705, 2001.

55. Goodfriend TL, Calhoun DA. Resistant hypertension, obesity, sleep apnea, and aldosterone: Theory and therapy. Hypertension 43:518-24, 2004. [Epub 2004 Jan 19.]

56. Calhoun DA, Nishizaka MK, Zaman MA, et al. Aldosterone excretion among subjects with resistant hypertension and symptoms of sleep apnea. Chest 125:112-117, 2004.

57. Safian RD, Textor S. Renal-artery stenosis. N Engl J Med 344:431-442, 2001.

58. Bonelli FS, McKusick MA, Textor SC, et al. Renal artery angioplasty: Technical results and clinical outcome in 320 patients. Mayo Clin Proc 70:1041-1052, 1995.

59. Canzanello VJ, Millan VG, Spiegel JE, et al. Percutaneous transluminal renal angioplasty in management of atherosclerotic renovascular hypertension: Results in 100 patients. Hypertension 13:163-172, 1989.

60. Levey AS, Bosch JP, Lewis JB, et al. A more accurate method to estimate glomerular filtration rate from serum creatinine: A new prediction equation. Modification of Diet in Renal Disease Study Group. Ann Intern Med 130:461-470, 1999.

61. Lenders JWM, Pacak K, Walther MM, et al. Biochemical diagnosis of pheochromocytoma: Which test is best? JAMA 287:1427-1434, 2002.

62. Nishizaka MK, Zaman MA, Calhoun DA. Efficacy of low-dose spironolactone in subjects with resistant hypertension. Am J Hypertens 16:925-930, 2003.

63. Singer GM, Izhar M, Black HR. Goal-oriented hypertension management: Translating clinical trials to practice. Hypertension 40:464-469, 2002.

# Chapter 60

# Orthostatic Hypotension and Autonomic Dysfunction Syndromes

## Satish R. Raj, David Robertson

Patients with dysfunction of autonomic cardiovascular regulation often present with extremes of blood pressure (BP) or heart rate (HR), especially when they assume an upright posture. Some have disorders with a well-understood pathophysiologic substrate, whereas others are less well understood and their mechanisms are under intensive investigation. In this chapter we focus on three major dysautonomic categories: (1) severe dysautonomias (pure autonomic failure [PAF] and multiple system atrophy [MSA]), rare conditions in which orthostatic hypotension is present; (2) mild dysautonomias (orthostatic intolerance/postural tachycardia syndrome [POTS] and neurally mediated syncope [NMS]), more common disorders, but with poorly characterized pathophysiologies, in which orthostatic hypotension is intermittent or absent, and in which tachycardia may be present; and (3) baroreflex failure, in which exaggerated BP and HR swings are exacerbated by emotional or physical stress (as opposed to gravity). Clinical features of some autonomic disorders are shown in Table 60–1.

## SEVERE DYSAUTONOMIAS

### Pure Autonomic Failure (Idiopathic Orthostatic Hypotension)

In 1925, Bradbury and Eggleston[1] described the clinical presentation of severe autonomic failure: orthostatic hypotension with an unchanging HR, supine hypertension, reduced sweating, reduced basal metabolic rate, impotence, nocturia, constipation, and anemia. They demonstrated pharmacologically the failure of both sympathetic and parasympathetic nervous systems, together with denervation hypersensitivity to respective agonists. In these cases, garments that prevented pooling of blood in the lower part of the body helped the patients, and successful symptomatic pharmacotherapy with sympathomimetic amines was soon reported.[2]

PAF is a disease process primarily involving the ganglion and the postganglionic neurons; central nervous system (CNS) involvement is rare. Lewy bodies have been found in autonomic neurons. The disease tends to progress slowly and has a good prognosis. Compared with normal individuals, patients with PAF have a significantly lower supine level of plasma norepinephrine.

### Multiple System Atrophy (Shy-Drager Syndrome)

MSA is a sporadic, progressive, neurodegenerative disease of uncertain cause characterized by predominant autonomic dysfunction and various combinations of extrapyramidal, pyramidal, and cerebellar dysfunction.[3] MSA is characterized by a progressive loss of neuronal and oligodendroglial cells in multiple sites in the CNS. The cause of MSA is unknown. This rare disorder (prevalence 2-15 per 100,000; men affected more commonly than women) has an age of onset of 55 years with median survival of only 9 years from the first symptom.[4] Autonomic symptoms often develop first—orthostatic hypotension, urinary incontinence, or erectile dysfunction. Patients who develop Parkinsonian symptoms often demonstrate a poor or temporary response to levodopa therapy. PAF and MSA are compared in Table 60–2.

## Orthostatic Hypotension

The orthostatic hypotension in PAF is often extraordinarily severe [5] (Figure 60–1), being greatest early in the day and after a large meal. In mildly affected individuals, orthostatic hypotension may be present only after a meal. It may be present in the morning but not later in the day or only after climbing stairs or walking up a hill. Even small body temperature elevation (e.g., due to infection) greatly reduces BP. Patients learn to avoid hot environments because they lower BP.[6]

The upright BP may fall by 60/30 mm Hg or more in the most severely affected patients and cannot be accurately measured sphygmomanometrically. For this reason, it is useful to monitor disease severity with the standing time (the length of time a patient can stand motionless before the onset of symptoms of orthostatic hypotension). As soon as the herald symptom of orthostatic hypotension appears, the patient is allowed to sit down and the time is recorded. If the patient is able to stand for 3 minutes without symptoms, a reliable BP determination can then usually be obtained.[7] Many patients who have small increases in standing time (e.g., from 30-120 seconds) may have a substantial increase in functional capacity. It is important to remember to treat the patient and not the standing BP. Patients can sometimes tolerate a standing systolic blood pressure (SBP) as low as 70 mm Hg without dizziness or syncope, probably because their cerebral blood flow is maintained at an adequate level because of the capacity of their cerebral circulation to undergo autoregulation.[8]

### Supine Hypertension in Pure Autonomic Failure/Multiple System Atrophy

Many patients with PAF or MSA also have supine hypertension, even when they are not taking pressor medications. Supine hypertension can be undetected if BP is measured only in the seated position. In a study of 117 autonomic failure patients at our institution, 56% had supine diastolic blood pressure ≥90 mm Hg, and in 43% it was ≥95 mm Hg.[9] Supine BPs as high as 228/140 mm Hg were observed. The results of

**Table 60-1** Clinical Features of Autonomic Disorders

| Feature | PAF | POTS | BF |
|---|---|---|---|
| Orthostatic hypotension | +++ | +/− | +/− |
| Postprandial hypotension | +++ | − | − |
| Episodic hypotension | + | ++ | +++ |
| Supine hypertension | ++ | +/− | + |
| Chronic hypertension | − | − | ++ |
| Labile hypertension | − | +/− | +++ |
| Orthostatic tachycardia | +/− | +++ | + |
| Episodic tachycardia | − | ++ | +++ |
| Syncope | +++ | +/− | + |
| Diaphoresis | − | + | +++ |
| Flushing | − | ++ | +++ |
| Emotional volatility | − | ++ | +++ |

(Adapted from Robertson D. Disorders of autonomic cardiovascular regulation: Baroreflex failure, autonomic failure, and orthostatic intolerance syndromes. *In* Laragh JH, Brenner BM [eds]. Hypertension: Pathology, Diagnosis and Management. New York, Raven Press, 1995; pp 941-959.)
PAF, pure autonomic failure; POTS, postural tachycardia syndrome; BF, baroreceptor failure.

**Table 60-2** Characteristics of Pure Autonomic Failure and Multiple System Atrophy

| Feature | Pure Autonomic Failure | Multiple System Atrophy |
|---|---|---|
| CNS involvement | No | Multiple |
| Lesion location | Ganglionic/ postganglionic | Central/ preganglionic |
| Progression | Slow | Fast |
| Prognosis | Good | Poor |
| Cerebellar signs | No | Common |
| Extrapyramidal signs | No | Common |
| Supine plasma NE | Low | Normal |
| Standing plasma NE | Low | Low |
| Lewy bodies | Noradrenergic cells | None |
| BP response to water | ↑↑ | ↑↑↑ |

CNS, central nervous system; NE, norepinephrine; BP, blood pressure.

this study show that supine hypertension is common in autonomic failure and frequently can be severe. The mechanisms responsible for supine hypertension in these patients are not known. It has been reported that patients with autonomic failure have a normal plasma volume,[10] so an increase in intravascular volume is not likely to be responsible for supine hypertension. We previously found that autonomic failure patients with supine hypertension had a normal cardiac output, so their hypertension was due to increased peripheral vascular resistance.[11] Because plasma norepinephrine and renin are low in these patients, it is unlikely that they play a substantial role in this increased vascular resistance. Other mediators that increase smooth muscle tone (vasopressin, endothelin,

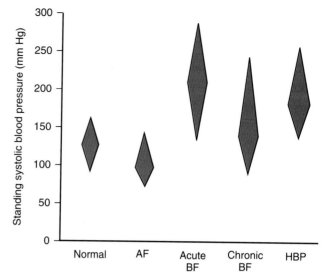

**Figure 60-1** Blood pressures (BP) in patients with various dysautonomic syndromes. Standing systolic blood pressures (SBPs) in normal persons and in patients with autonomic failure (AF), acute baroreceptor failure (Acute BF), chronic baroreceptor failure (Chronic BF), and severe essential hypertension (HBP). The widest part of each diamond depicts the most common standing SBP seen in typical patients, while the height depicts the range of pressures seen throughout the day. Patients with AF have the lowest standing BP. Extremely high BPs are seen in acute BF, and these can exceed the BPs seen in severe hypertension. After several months (Chronic BF), the standing SBP is usually near normal, but great variability is still seen. (Reprinted from Robertson RM. Baroreflex failure. *In* Robertson D, Low PA, Polinsky RJ [eds]. Primer on the Autonomic Nervous System. San Diego, CA, Academic Press, 1996; with permission).

decreased nitric oxide production) need to be addressed in future studies.

## Treatment in Pure Autonomic Failure/Multiple System Atrophy

Patients with asymptomatic orthostatic hypotension require no treatment. They should, however, be closely observed for the development of symptoms. Symptomatic patients can be treated nonpharmacologically by applying external support (by bandages firmly wrapped around the legs or by custom-fitted counter-pressure support stockings) and by using physical counter-maneuvers (leg-crossing, squatting, abdominal compression, bending forward or placing one foot on a chair) to reduce venous pooling in upright position.[12] Patients with PAF and MSA demonstrate a very significant pressor response to drinking 16 fluid ounces (480 ml) of room temperature water. This simple therapy can be used throughout the day as needed.[13] If orthostatic symptoms continue, pharmacologic treatment consisting of the mineralocorticoid fludrocortisone,[14] pressor drugs,[15] or pyridostigmine[16] can be added. As patients with severe autonomic failure have a high incidence of anemia, which may contribute to their symptoms, erythropoietin has been used. This treatment has reversed anemia and improved upright BP.[17] An approach to

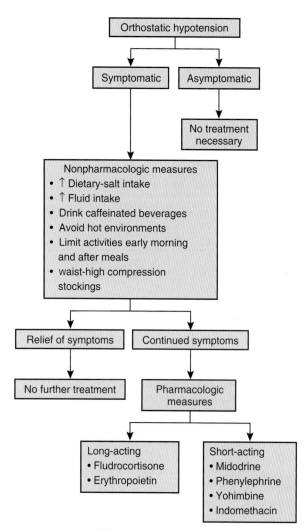

**Figure 60–2** A useful strategy for the treatment of orthostatic hypotension. (Adapted from Jordan J, Shannon JR, Biaggioni I, et al. Contrasting actions of pressor agents in severe autonomic failure. Am J Med 105:116-124, 1998; with permission.)

**Table 60–3** Contrasting Features Between Pure Autonomic Failure and Postural Tachycardia Syndrome

| Feature | Pure Autonomic Failure | Postural Tachycardia Syndrome |
|---|---|---|
| Hemodynamic perturbation | Hypotension | Tachycardia |
| Syncope on standing | Early | Late |
| Age at onset | >50 years | <35 years |
| Gender | Male = Female | Female >> Male |
| Upright norepinephrine | Low | High |

treatment of orthostatic hypotension is schematically shown in Figure 60–2.[18]

However, these agents also aggravate supine hypertension. One approach for treating orthostatic hypotension in patients with supine hypertension is to use only short-acting pressor agents early in the day.[19] Transdermal nitrates, oral clonidine, and oral hydralazine at bedtime are sometimes effective for the treatment of overnight supine hypertension. Patients are also encouraged to sleep with the head of the bed elevated 6 to 10 inches to avoid supine hypertension.[9]

## MILD DYSAUTONOMIAS

### Orthostatic Intolerance/Postural Tachycardia Syndrome

Orthostatic intolerance/POTS is the most common disorder of the regulation of BP after essential hypertension. It is present in approximately 500,000 Americans. It tends to occur in younger individuals (most are younger than age 35) and women are affected most often. Homeostatic adjustments to the upright posture[20] for some reason fail, and disabling symptoms may occur.[21] The symptoms are described as dizziness, visual changes, head or neck discomfort, throbbing of the head, poor concentration, tiredness or weakness. Palpitations, tremulousness, fatigue, and anxiety are also seen. Generally, there is little or no fall in BP[5] (see Figure 60–1). These symptoms are attributed to inadequate perfusion of the CNS.

POTS is very poorly characterized in terms of pathophysiology. In the 1920s it was shown that orthostatic symptoms occur in patients now considered to have PAF.[1] Over the subsequent 80 years, our understanding of the heterogeneity of orthostatic disorders and autonomic failure has improved.[7] The contrasting features of PAF and orthostatic intolerance/POTS are presented in Table 60–3.

Postural tachycardia, the most constant feature of POTS, has caused investigators to consider several possibilities to explain the syncope. If there were a circulating vasodilator,[22] or a reduced "effective" blood volume,[23-25] the orthostatic tachycardia might be an appropriate autonomic compensatory response mediated through the baroreflex to maintain adequate BP and cardiac output.[26] It is possible that this hemodynamic response may not be sufficient to adequately perfuse the CNS, but a more likely explanation may be dysregulation in local vascular beds. A number of possible vasodilators have been investigated: bradykinin,[22] atrial natriuretic factor,[27] histamine, and prostaglandin D$_2$.[28] However, it does not appear that vasodilators are a common cause for this disorder.

These largely negative studies have caused investigators to look elsewhere to explain POTS. Some proposed that an abnormally sensitive cardiac β$_1$-adrenoreceptor could result in orthostatic tachycardia in situations in which the sympathetic nervous system (SNS) is activated.[29] Orthostatic intolerance occurs in many patients with the mitral valve prolapse syndrome.[30] Some investigators reported an apparent "supercoupling" of β$_2$-adrenoreceptors: Although receptor number and affinity were not abnormal, activation of lymphocyte β$_2$-adrenoreceptors from patients resulted in greater cyclic adenosine monophosphate accumulation than in normal persons,[31] suggesting an abnormal coupling of the receptors to the guanine nucleotide regulatory complex. All of these observations strongly suggest that the major abnormality underlying POTS remains undiscovered.

The elevated normal and raised plasma norepinephrine levels[32] and elevated urinary norepinephrine excretion[33] found in some patients with POTS supports the view that increased SNS activation is responsible for the disorder. On the other hand, the observation of delayed recovery from the bradycardia of phase IV of the Valsalva maneuver and increased HR variability[30] suggests that there might be an imbalance in central autonomic regulation, a view that has been strengthened by evidence that there is raised muscle sympathetic nerve traffic even at rest in some patients with POTS.[34]

It has also been suggested that POTS may be explained, perhaps paradoxically, by impairment in sympathetic function. Loss of the galvanic skin response (a sympathetic marker) on the soles of the feet has been noted.[35] The cause of orthostatic intolerance might thus be partial (or selective) denervation of the lower extremities that allows pooling of blood with upright posture. This hypothesis is based on an analogy to certain sensory and motor neurologic disorders, in which selective impairment of neurons may occur distally, with or without more proximal progression. Viral and/or immunologic causes could be operative.[36] In addition, patchy impairment of autonomic neuronal function could occur so that some areas remain intact. The heart might, for example, remain normally innervated while the distal extremities could have innervation impaired.[37] Observations of reduced clearance of norepinephrine from the circulation in some patients with POTS support this view.[38]

No pharmacotherapy of POTS is generally effective, although individual agents may be somewhat helpful in selected patients.[39] The most widely employed agents are the β-adrenoreceptor antagonists, given to attenuate the symptomatic tachycardia on standing. Patients often respond to very low doses of nonselective β-blockers (e.g., propranolol 1-20 mg two to three times per day). Another approach is to use the $\alpha_2$-adrenoreceptor agonists (e.g., clonidine) to minimize sympathetic activation.[40] Finally, fludrocortisone has been employed in an attempt to increase blood volume.[41] It is noteworthy that all of these drugs have a well-established capacity to lower plasma renin activity in normal persons. If low plasma renin activity contributes to the pathophysiology of orthostatic intolerance,[42] it is possible that the currently used agents are marginally effective precisely because, along with the primary actions that constitute the rationale for their use, they also have a counterproductive action at the level of the juxtaglomerular apparatus. If this were true, it would mean that therapeutic alternatives that did not suppress renin ought to be sought. One potential alternative that is known to raise renin levels is exercise.[43]

In summary, orthostatic intolerance/POTS is a final common clinical expression of multiple pathophysiologic processes that alter the normal response to upright posture. Two pathophysiologies seem to represent a substantial proportion of patients with POTS: (1) a partial dysautonomia due to impairment of the peripheral autonomic system and (2) a hyperadrenergic orthostatic intolerance in which the abnormality is in the CNS. With improved dissection of these and other pathophysiologies and improved matching of therapy to pathophysiology, improved therapeutic strategies for management of these patients will emerge.

## Neurally Mediated Syncope

Syncope is a sudden, transient loss of consciousness with spontaneous recovery that is associated with a loss of postural tone. It is very common, with conservative estimates that

3% of the general population has experienced at least 1 syncopal spell and is responsible for more than 1% of hospital admissions.[44] Neurally mediated syncope (NMS), or reflex fainting, is the most common cause of syncope, especially in those patients without evidence of structural heart disease. NMS most commonly occurs following prolonged sitting or standing, although it can also occur with exercise (initiation or peak exercise) or with emotional/psychologic triggers (e.g., phlebotomy). In contrast to POTS, NMS is associated with intermittent postural hypotension, with normal orthostatic BPs more than 99% of the time.

The pathophysiology of NMS is not completely understood, but a frequently used pathophysiologic model is shown in Figure 60–3.[45] The most common hypothesis argues that the initiating event is a pooling of blood in the legs (from prolonged sitting or standing) with a resultant reduction in venous return (preload) to the heart. The fall in BP leads to a baroreceptor-mediated increase in sympathetic tone, with a subsequent increase in chronotropic and inotropic effect. The vigorous cardiac contraction, in the setting of an underfilled ventricle, is thought to stimulate ventricular afferents in the left ventricle that trigger a reflex loss of sympathetic tone and an associated increase in vagal tone. The adrenal gland also releases epinephrine in response to this stress. The result is clinical hypotension and/or bradycardia.

The history and physical examination are at the heart of the diagnosis. A clinical diagnosis can be made with these alone in most cases. The history should focus on the circumstances surrounding the syncope, the associated symptoms before and after the event, and any collateral history from witnesses. The past medical history may contain evidence of structural heart disease and coexisting medical conditions, which both point away from NMS. Medications may provoke syncope, and a family history of sudden death may point to an arrhythmic cause. Historical features of NMS have been found to include a female gender, younger age, associated diaphoresis, nausea, or palpitation, and postsyncopal fatigue.[44] A long duration of spells (from the first lifetime spell) also suggests NMS. The physical examination should focus on ruling out structural heart disease and focal neurologic lesions.

Tilt table testing involves subjecting patients to head-up tilt at angles of 60 to 80 degrees, in an attempt to induce either syncope or intense presyncope, with a reproduction of presenting symptoms.[46] Passive tilt tests simply use upright tilt for up to 45 minutes to induce vasovagal syncope.[44] Provocative tilt tests use a simultaneous combination of orthostatic stress and drugs such as isoproterenol, nitroglycerin, or adenosine to provoke syncope with a slightly higher sensitivity, but reduced specificity. There is little agreement about the best protocol. Recent studies with implantable loop recorders have called the value of tilt testing into question.[47] Tilt tests are contraindicated in patients with severe aortic or mitral stenosis, or critical coronary or cerebral artery stenosis.

## Treatment of Neurally Mediated Syncope

Most patients should simply be reassured about the usual benign course of NMS and instructed to avoid those situations that precipitate fainting. They should be taught to recognize an impending faint and urged to lie down (or sit down if that is not possible) quickly. This will not be enough for some patients, and other treatment options may be necessary.

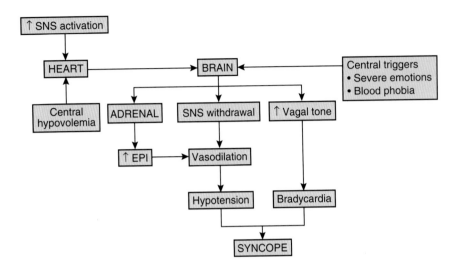

**Figure 60–3** Pathophysiologic model of neurally mediated syncope. Multiple potential triggers lead to a loss of sympathetic tone, an increase in vagal parasympathetic tone, and the adrenomedullary release of epinephrine with resultant hypotension and bradycardia leading to syncope. SNS, sympathetic nervous system. (Adapted from Raj SR, Robertson RM. Neurally mediated syncope. *In* Robertson D, Biaggioni I, Burnstock G, et al. [eds]. Primer on the Autonomic Nervous System. San Diego, CA, Academic Press; 2003; pp 249-251; with permission.)

Pharmacologic therapy has only inconsistent results.[44] Although salt replenishment and fludrocortisone have not been rigorously studied, they are both commonly used because of low side effect profile and probable efficacy. β-Adrenergic antagonists are commonly used for this disorder, but with only poor evidence of effectiveness.[48] The α₁-agonist midodrine has been found to decrease the rate of recurrent syncope among frequent fainters,[49] but other agents in this class have not had the same results.[50] In one well-designed study, the selective serotonin reuptake inhibitor paroxetine was found to be effective.[51] Orthostatic training has been described as an effective nonpharmacologic therapy for patients with recurrent NMS,[52] but this therapy has not been properly studied. Permanent dual-chamber pacemakers were initially a very promising therapy,[53] but recent evidence suggests only a modest benefit.[54] Pacemaker implantation is not currently a front-line therapy for NMS.

## BAROREFLEX FAILURE

Arterial baroreflexes maintain arterial pressure within a narrow range. The baroreflex arc can be damaged at any site: at the baroreceptors (stretch-receptors) in the vasculature (mainly in the carotid sinus), in the course of the glossopharyngeal or vagal nerves, or at the nuclei in the brain stem. In humans, baroreflex failure is a rare disorder, which is usually related to neck surgery, neck irradiation therapy for malignant tumors, brain stem lesions, or bilateral carotid body tumors.[55] Failure of the baroreflex at any point produces a characteristic clinical syndrome. It is presumably caused by an inability to buffer supramedullary input to cardiovascular control centers in the brain stem.[55] It has been shown in numerous animal studies and in humans that nearly complete denervation of the carotid and aortic baroreceptors is necessary to cause flagrant baroreflex failure, (i.e., all baroreceptors, both glossopharyngeal and vagus nerves or the brain stem nuclei have to be damaged).[55,56]

At Vanderbilt University's Autonomic Dysfunction Center we identified 36 patients with arterial baroreflex failure (out of approximately 2700 referred with severe disorders of autonomic function). Reasons for referral were evaluation of essential hypertension, suspicion of pheochromocytoma,

uncontrolled severe hypertension, and assumption that glossopharyngeal or vagal nerves had been damaged. The causes for baroreflex failure included surgery and irradiation of throat carcinoma in three patients, surgical section of the glossopharyngeal nerve for glossopharyngeal neuralgia in a patient with previously sustained injury to the contralateral glossopharyngeal and vagus nerves, the familial paraganglioma syndrome in four patients, and a marked bilateral cell loss in the nuclei of the solitary tract (found at subsequent autopsy) in the setting of a degenerative neurologic disease of medullary and higher structures in one patient. The familial paraganglioma syndrome is a genetic disorder in which affected individuals develop multiple benign noncatecholamine-producing tumors. These tumors physically damage the glossopharyngeal and vagus nerves, leading to baroreflex failure. In two patients no cause could be documented.

Patients usually present with arterial hypertension, usually episodic but occasionally sustained. Labile, episodic hypertension is often seen in patients who develop baroreflex failure gradually (e.g., years after neck irradiation) or with a chronic disorder. In contrast, sustained hypertension is especially severe in patients with acute interruption of the baroreflex arc (see Figure 60–1). Arterial pressures of 310/150 mm Hg have been seen, with resultant hypertensive crises. The clinical picture is often similar to that of pheochromocytoma, where arterial hypertension and tachycardia also occur together. Patients have the same subjective sensations of warmth or flushing, palpitations, headache, and diaphoresis. The diagnosis of pheochromocytoma[57] can be ruled out by computed tomography scanning, metaiodobenzylguanidine (MIBG) scanning, adrenal arteriography, or venous norepinephrine sampling (see Chapter 76). In contrast to patients with a pheochromocytoma, patients with baroreflex failure show stability or improvement in their hypertension over time.

There is sometimes emotional lability or nervousness in patients with baroreflex failure, more prominent at the time of BP elevation.[55] The loss of the baroreflex buffering capacity causes much more pronounced effects of cortical influences on the vasomotor centers in patients with baroreflex failure. Pain, emotion, visual attention, or mental arithmetic may have a much greater effect in patients than in normal subjects. Cold pressor test (placing the patient's hand in ice water for 1 minute) in normal persons caused an increase in systolic arterial pressure of 24 ± 7 mm Hg with the BP normalizing within a few minutes of hand rewarming; in patients with baroreflex failure, responses of 56 ± 14 mm Hg were noted,[58] and these sometimes persisted for 30 minutes despite hand rewarming (Figure 60–4).

The hallmark diagnostic feature of baroreflex failure is a parallel increase in BP and HR with stress and a substantial parallel decrease with sedation or rest. There is no reflex decrease in HR after pressor agents and no reflex increase in HR after vasodilators. In normal persons an increase in BP of 20 mm Hg with phenylephrine will decrease the HR by 7 to 21 beats per minute (bpm), and a decrease in BP of 20 mm Hg with sodium nitroprusside will increase the HR by 9 to 28 bpm. Patients with baroreceptor failure, however, do not alter their HR by more than 4 bpm with either drug.[58]

Plasma norepinephrine levels parallel the BP changes. During surges of sympathetic activity associated with hypertensive-tachycardic episodes, plasma norepinephrine levels as high as 2260 pg/ml (13.36 nM) have been seen. During quiescent periods, norepinephrine levels may be normal (111-360 pg/ml [0.66-2.13 nM]). There can be diagnostic confusion with POTS, because POTS is sometimes also associated with elevated catecholamines and volatile BP.

Acute administration of clonidine decreases BP, HR, and plasma catecholamine levels in patients with baroreflex failure and is therefore useful as a diagnostic test to distinguish baroreflex failure from pheochromocytoma.[59] Clonidine is the most effective drug in terms of decreasing the number and the severity of hypertensive crises. Diazepam is used to control stress.

In contrast to the majority of patients with nonselective baroreflex failure (with loss of parasympathetic efferent discharge), occasional patients with this syndrome have intact parasympathetic control of the HR. They have a lesion involving only the afferent arc of the baroreflex (selective baroreceptor failure). In addition to undamped sympathetic tone, they can also have excessive vagotonic reactions. Such patients have phases of severe hypertension and tachycardia alternating with prolonged episodes of severe bradycardia and asystole.[60] They require unique therapeutic strategies, including medications that attenuate sympathetic nerve traffic, medications that increase BP, and, in some cases, implantation of a cardiac pacemaker.

## ACKNOWLEDGMENTS

This work was supported in part by National Institutes of Health grants 2P01 HL56693, R01 HL071784, and M01 RR00095 (General Clinical Research Center) from the National Institutes of Health. Dr. Raj is a Vanderbilt Clinical Research Scholar, supported by a K12 grant from the National Institutes of Health.

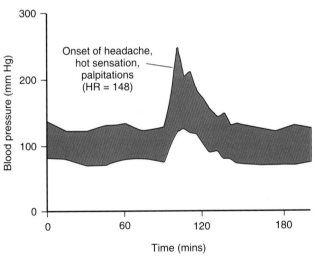

**Figure 60–4** Blood pressure (BP) in acute baroreflex failure. BP monitoring over a 200-minute period in a 43-year-old man approximately 2 weeks following surgical removal of a second carotid body tumor, 5 years after removal of the initial (contralateral) carotid body tumor. While BP was being monitored at normal baseline levels, a cold pressor test (immersion of the hand in ice water for 60 seconds) was performed. The BP immediately rose and continued to rise for several minutes following of the cold stimulus. The symptoms appeared during his time and resolved as BP and heart rate (HR) returned to normal over the succeeding half-hour. On some occasions, paroxysms of similar magnitude occurred without obvious exogenous causative stimuli. (Reprinted from Robertson D, Hollister AS, Biaggioni I, et al. The diagnosis and treatment of baroreflex failure. N Engl J Med 329:1449-1455, 1993. Copyright © 1993 Massachusetts Medical Society. All rights reserved.)

## References

1. Bradbury S, Eggleston C. Postural hypotension with syncope: A report of three cases. Am Heart J 1:75-86, 1925.
2. Ghrist DG, Brown GE. Postural hypotension with syncope: Its successful treatment with ephedrine. Am J Med Sci 175: 336-349, 1928.
3. Gilman S, Low P, Quinn N, et al. Consensus statement on the diagnosis of multiple system atrophy. American Autonomic Society and American Academy of Neurology. Clin Auton Res 8:359-362, 1998.
4. Diedrich A, Robertson D. Multiple system atrophy. eMedicine Journal 2, 2001.
5. Robertson D. Hypotension. In Carruthers SG, Hoffman BB, Melmon KL, et al. (eds). Melmon and Morrelli's Clinical Pharmacology. New York, McGraw-Hill, 2000; pp 95-113.
6. Bannister R, Mathias CJ. Clinical features and evaluation of the primary chronic autonomic failure syndromes. In Mathias CJ, Bannister R (eds). Autonomic Failure: A Textbook of Clinical Disorders of the Autonomic Nervous System. Oxford, Oxford University Press, 1999; pp 307-316.
7. Robertson D. Disorders of autonomic cardiovascular regulation: Baroreflex failure, autonomic failure, and orthostatic intolerance syndromes. In Laragh JH, Brenner BM (eds). Hypertension: Pathology, Diagnosis and Management. New York, Raven Press, 1995; pp 941-959.
8. Bannister R, Mathias CJ. Management of postural hypotension. In Mathias CJ, Bannister R (eds). Autonomic Failure: A Textbook of Clinical Disorders of the Autonomic Nervous System. Oxford, Oxford University Press, 1999; pp 307-316.
9. Shannon J, Jordan J, Costa F, et al. The hypertension of autonomic failure and its treatment. Hypertension 30:1062-1067, 1997.
10. Wilcox CS, Puritz R, Lightman SL, et al. Plasma volume regulation in patients with progressive autonomic failure during changes in salt intake or posture. J Lab Clin Med 104:331-339, 1984.

11. Kronenberg MW, Forman MB, Onrot J, et al. Enhanced left ventricular contractility in autonomic failure: Assessment using pressure-volume relations. J Am Coll Cardiol 15:1334-1342, 1990.

12. Weiling W. Nonpharmacological management of autonomic disorders. In Robertson D, Biaggioni I, Burnstock G, et al. (eds). Primer of the Autonomic Nervous System. New York, Academic Press, 2004.

13. Jordan J, Shannon JR, Black BK, et al. The pressor response to water drinking in humans: A sympathetic reflex? Circulation 101:504-509, 2000.

14. Robertson D. Fludrocortisone. In Robertson D, Biaggioni I, Burnstock G, et al. (eds). Primer of the Autonomic Nervous System. New York, Academic Press, 2004.

15. Freeman R. Midodrine and other pressor drugs. In Robertson D, Biaggioni I, Burnstock G, et al. (eds). Primer of the Autonomic Nervous System. New York, Academic Press, 2004.

16. Singer W, Opfer-Gehrking TL, McPhee BR, et al. Acetylcholinesterase inhibition: A novel approach in the treatment of neurogenic orthostatic hypotension. J Neurol Neurosurg Psychiatry 2003;74:1294-1298.

17. Biaggioni I, Robertson D, Krantz S, et al. The anemia of primary autonomic failure and its reversal with recombinant erythropoietin. Ann Intern Med 121:181-186, 1994.

18. Jordan J, Shannon JR, Biaggioni I, et al. Contrasting actions of pressor agents in severe autonomic failure. Am J Med 105:116-124, 1998.

19. Biaggioni I, Onrot J, Stewart CK, et al. The potent pressor effect of phenylpropanolamine in patients with autonomic impairment. JAMA 258:236-239, 1987.

20. Jacob G, Ertl AC, Shannon JR, et al. Effect of standing on neurohumoral responses and plasma volume in healthy subjects. J Appl Physiol 84:914-921, 1998.

21. Robertson D. Genetics and molecular biology of hypotension. Curr Opin Nephrol Hypertens 3:13-24, 1994.

22. Streeten DH, Kerr CB, Kerr LP, et al. Hyperbradykininism: A new orthostatic syndrome. Lancet 2:1048-1053, 1972.

23. Fouad FM, Tadena-Thome L, Bravo EL, et al. Idiopathic hypovolemia. Ann Intern Med 104:298-303, 1986.

24. el Sayed H, Hainsworth R. Relationship between plasma volume, carotid baroreceptor sensitivity and orthostatic tolerance. Clin Sci (Lond) 88:463-470, 1995.

25. Jacob G, Biaggioni I, Mosqueda-Garcia R, et al. Relation of blood volume and blood pressure in orthostatic intolerance. Am J Med Sci 315:95-100, 1998.

26. Cryer PE, Silverberg AB, Santiago JV, et al. Plasma catecholamines in diabetes. The syndromes of hypoadrenergic and hyperadrenergic postural hypotension. Am J Med 64:407-416, 1978.

27. Hollister AS, Tanaka I, Imada T, et al. Sodium loading and posture modulate human atrial natriuretic factor plasma levels. Hypertension 8:II106-III111, 1986.

28. Roberts LJ, Oates JA. Mastocytosis. In Wilson JD, Foster DW (eds). Williams Textbook of Endocrinology. Philadelphia, Saunders, 1985; pp 1363-1379.

29. Feldman RD, Limbird LE, Nadeau J, et al. Dynamic regulation of leukocyte beta adrenergic receptor-agonist interactions by physiological changes in circulating catecholamines. J Clin Invest 72:164-170, 1983.

30. Coghlan HC, Phares P, Cowley M, et al. Dysautonomia in mitral valve prolapse. Am J Med 67:236-244, 1979.

31. Davies AO, Mares A, Pool JL, et al. Mitral valve prolapse with symptoms of beta-adrenergic hypersensitivity. Beta 2-adrenergic receptor supercoupling with desensitization on isoproterenol exposure. Am J Med 82:193-201, 1987.

32. Low PA, Opfer-Gehrking TL, Textor SC, et al. Postural tachycardia syndrome (POTS). Neurology 45:S19-S25, 1995.

33. Boudoulas H, Reynolds JC, Mazzaferri E, et al. Metabolic studies in mitral valve prolapse syndrome. A neuroendocrine—cardiovascular process. Circulation 61:1200-1205, 1980.

34. Furlan R, Jacob G, Snell M, et al. Chronic orthostatic intolerance: A disorder with discordant cardiac and vascular sympathetic control. Circulation 98:2154-2159, 1998.

35. Hoeldtke RD, Davis KM. The orthostatic tachycardia syndrome: Evaluation of autonomic function and treatment with octreotide and ergot alkaloids. J Clin Endocrinol Metab 73:132-139, 1991.

36. Fujii N, Tabira T, Shibasaki H, et al. Acute autonomic and sensory neuropathy associated with elevated Epstein-Barr virus antibody titre. J Neurol Neurosurg Psychiatry 45:656-657, 1982.

37. Streeten DH. Pathogenesis of hyperadrenergic orthostatic hypotension. Evidence of disordered venous innervation exclusively in the lower limbs. J Clin Invest 86:1582-1588, 1990.

38. Jacob G, Shannon JR, Costa F, et al. Abnormal norepinephrine clearance and adrenergic receptor sensitivity in idiopathic orthostatic intolerance. Circulation 99:1706-1712, 1999.

39. Jacob G, Shannon JR, Black B, et al. Effects of volume loading and pressor agents in idiopathic orthostatic tachycardia. Circulation 96:575-580, 1997.

40. Gaffney FA, Lane LB, Pettinger W, et al. Effects of long-term clonidine administration on the hemodynamic and neuroendocrine postural responses of patients with dysautonomia. Chest 83:436-438, 1983.

41. Freitas J, Santos R, Azevedo E, et al. Clinical improvement in patients with orthostatic intolerance after treatment with bisoprolol and fludrocortisone. Clin Auton Res 10:293-299, 2000.

42. Jacob G, Robertson D, Mosqueda-Garcia R et al. Hypovolemia in syncope and orthostatic intolerance role of the renin-angiotensin system. Am J Med 103:128-133, 1997.

43. Convertino VA. Blood volume: Its adaptation to endurance training. Med Sci Sports Exerc 23:1338-1348, 1991.

44. Raj SR, Sheldon AR. Syncope: Investigation and treatment. Curr Cardiol Rep 4:363-370, 2002.

45. Raj SR, Robertson RM. Neurally mediated syncope. In Robertson D, Biaggioni I, Burnstock G, Low PA (eds). Primer of the Autonomic Nervous System. New York, Academic Press, 2004; pp 249-251.

46. Benditt DG, Ferguson DW, Grubb BP, et al. Tilt table testing for assessing syncope. American College of Cardiology. J Am Coll Cardiol 28:263-275, 1996.

47. Moya A, Brignole M, Menozzi C, et al. Mechanism of syncope in patients with isolated syncope and in patients with tilt-positive syncope. Circulation 104:1261-1267, 2001.

48. Brignole M, Alboni P, Benditt D, et al. Guidelines on management (diagnosis and treatment) of syncope. Eur Heart J 22:1256-1306, 2001.

49. Perez-Lugones A, Schweikert R, Pavia S, et al. Usefulness of midodrine in patients with severely symptomatic neurocardiogenic syncope: A randomized control study. J Cardiovasc Electrophysiol 12:935-938, 2001.

50. Raviele A, Brignole M, Sutton R, et al. Effect of etilefrine in preventing syncopal recurrence in patients with vasovagal syncope: A double-blind, randomized, placebo-controlled trial. The Vasovagal Syncope International Study. Circulation 99:1452-1457, 1999.

51. Di Girolamo E, Di Iorio C, Sabatini P, et al. Effects of paroxetine hydrochloride, a selective serotonin reuptake inhibitor, on refractory vasovagal syncope: A randomized, double-blind, placebo-controlled study. J Am Coll Cardiol 33:1227-1230, 1999.

52. Ector H, Reybrouck T, Heidbuchel H, et al. Tilt training: A new treatment for recurrent neurocardiogenic syncope and severe orthostatic intolerance. Pacing Clin Electrophysiol 21:193-196, 1998.

53. Raj SR, Sheldon RS. Role of pacemakers in treating neurocardiogenic syncope. Curr Opin Cardiol 18:47-52, 2003.

54. Connolly SJ, Sheldon R, Thorpe KE, et al. Pacemaker therapy for prevention of syncope in patients with recurrent severe

vasovagal syncope: Second Vasovagal Pacemaker Study (VPS II): A randomized trial. JAMA 289:2224-2229, 2003.

55. Ketch T, Biaggioni I, Robertson R, et al. Four faces of baroreflex failure: Hypertensive crisis, volatile hypertension, orthostatic tachycardia, and malignant vagotonia. Circulation 105: 2518-2523, 2002.

56. Cowley AW Jr, Liard JF, Guyton AC. Role of baroreceptor reflex in daily control of arterial blood pressure and other variables in dogs. Circ Res 32:564-576, 1973.

57. Manger WM, Gifford RW Jr. Pheochromocytoma. New York, Springer Verlag, 1977.

58. Robertson D, Hollister AS, Biaggioni I, et al. The diagnosis and treatment of baroreflex failure. N Engl J Med 329:1449-1455, 1993.

59. Shannon JR, Robertson D. The clinical utility of plasma catecholamines. J Lab Clin Med 128:450-451, 1996.

60. Jordan J, Shannon JR, Black BK, et al. Malignant vagotonia due to selective baroreflex failure. Hypertension 30:1072-1077, 1997.

# SECTION 9

# Individual Drug Classes

## Chapter 61

# How Hypertensive Drugs Get Approved in the United States

## Robert R. Fenichel

This chapter describes the means by which manufacturers gain permission to bring antihypertensive drugs to the U.S. market. Some of the chapter is applicable only to oral antihypertensive formulations intended for long-term use, but much of it applies equally well to intravenous antihypertensive formulations and, indeed, to drugs other than antihypertensives.

Before a drug may be promoted as an antihypertensive on the U.S. market, the claim of antihypertensive efficacy must be approved by the U.S. Food and Drug Administration (FDA). An antihypertensive product might theoretically avoid FDA jurisdiction by never appearing in interstate commerce, but the notion of "interstate commerce" has been so broadly construed that this option is more apparent than real.

Federal regulations do not prevent U.S. physicians from prescribing, or U.S. pharmacists from dispensing, medications (or other substances) for nonapproved uses. Medical insurers, however, frequently refuse to reimburse patients for the cost of such prescriptions. After medical misadventures, physicians may find it difficult to defend a therapeutic choice that was not FDA approved. Perhaps for these reasons, and with the notable exception of immediate-release nifedipine preparations (approved in the United States only for the treatment of chronic stable angina, but widely prescribed as antihypertensives), unapproved products are not frequently prescribed as antihypertensives by U.S. physicians.

Would-be manufacturers have adequate incentives, then, to obtain FDA approval for an antihypertensive claim. To obtain that approval, the sponsor must demonstrate the following:

- The product is of known and stable composition, and can be reliably manufactured and distributed.
- There is an identifiable population in whom the product is reproducibly effective and reasonably safe.
- It is possible to lay out evidence-based instructions for use of the product.

## CHEMISTRY AND BIOPHARMACEUTICS

If a product is not of stable composition, then there is little point in discussing its clinical effects. In general, a drug's manufacturer is required to formalize the work of synthesis, compounding, packaging, and labeling, so that little is left to judg-

mental variation. The manufacturer is also required to establish a system of controls, to verify at various stages of manufacture that things are what they should be. The details of these requirements will not be of interest to most clinicians.

The proposed product must also be studied to determine the pharmacokinetics (absorption, distribution, metabolism, and excretion) of its active ingredient(s). Sometimes development of the to-be-marketed formulation proceeds in parallel with clinical trials; in these cases, special bioavailability trials may need to be done to demonstrate that the to-be-marketed formulation is not substantially different from the formulation(s) tested in clinical trials. In addition, samples of the final product in final packaging must be shown to survive storage for the claimed shelf life.

## TOXICOLOGY

FDA consent is required when a novel chemical substance is given experimentally to a human being in the United States. Before that time, the manufacturer of a new antihypertensive will generally have done studies to demonstrate that the new drug is antihypertensive in animals. Such studies are not required,* but in the case of antihypertensives some such studies are almost always performed, to reassure the manufacturer (and the FDA) that antihypertensive efficacy in humans can be plausibly anticipated, justifying the risks and costs of human trials. Once antihypertensive efficacy has been demonstrated in humans, the animal-efficacy data are no longer of great interest.

Toxicologic studies in animals, unlike studies of antihypertensive efficacy, are strictly required. In general, human trials are permitted only after the FDA has reviewed animal studies in which maximal-tolerated doses were administered for as long as, or longer than, the proposed exposure in human trials. Unlike the efficacy studies in animals, some of these toxicology studies retain their importance throughout the

---

*Because many human illnesses have no animal models, the FDA could not reasonably require demonstrations of efficacy in animals for all drug claims. Even in hypertension (where animal models are available), a drug effective in humans might conceivably not be effective in any nonhuman species.

development process and after approval. In particular, some toxicologic studies (reproductive and carcinogenicity studies) are not analogous to any feasible human trials.

## CLINICAL TRIALS

The earliest human trials are those that are traditionally called *phase 1* trials. These studies may be unblinded and nonrandomized; their purpose is not to demonstrate antihypertensive efficacy, but rather to investigate human pharmacokinetics and metabolic pathways, to detect unanticipated adverse effects, and to begin the search for well-tolerated doses with some evidence of antihypertensive activity in humans. The subjects in phase 1 trials are conventionally healthy young adult volunteers; a typical trial might utilize only a dozen or so such volunteers, each exposed once or a few times to one or two doses. If the product is to be taken orally, there will be at least one study to determine the extent to which the rate and extent of absorption are affected by food. More complexly, if metabolism and elimination of the product's ingredients have been found to be dependent on renal function, or on the function of one or another of the cytochrome P450 pathways in the liver or the gut, or if administration of the product results in induction or inhibition of those pathways, then other studies will need to investigate potential interactions between this product and at least a few of the important other products that interact with the same pathways.

Using the results of the phase 1 studies, the *phase 2* studies are generally double-blind, randomized, placebo-controlled trials. In a typical such trial, each of a few dozen patients is randomized to receive a few weeks of treatment with a regimen of placebo or the new drug. In other trials done around this time or a bit later, investigators recruit patients who are diabetic, who have hepatic or renal dysfunction, or who are receiving various unrelated drugs (e.g., antianginal drugs, cholesterol-lowering drugs, oral contraceptives) that are frequently received by reasonably large numbers of hypertensive patients. These various middle-stage trials greatly increase the total accumulated number of patient-days of exposure to the new drug, and sometimes they reveal adverse effects that were not apparent earlier. If all goes well, they suggest which regimens are most worth examining in the definitive trials.

As the phase 2 studies are completed, the trials that are intended to provide definitive proof of efficacy are designed and begun. These *phase 3* trials are typically randomized, double-blind, placebo-controlled, parallel-group trials comparing two or three regimens of the new drug (different doses, different interdosing intervals) with placebo, with each trial following a few hundred hypertensive patients for 2 or 3 months. In the case of a combination product (say, a combination of an angiotensin-converting enzyme [ACE] inhibitor and a thiazide diuretic), the phase 3 trials are typically of parallel-group "factorial" design, in which patients are randomized to each of the possible combinations of (1) one dose from among several possible doses (including placebo) of the first drug and (2) one dose from among several possible doses (again, including placebo) of the second drug. The primary metric of each of these trials is the placebo-corrected change in blood pressure (BP), usually seated diastolic blood pressure (DBP), although systolic blood pressure (SBP) is increasingly of equal importance. One of these trials is said to have succeeded when analysis shows that one or more regimens have effects that are significantly superior to those seen with placebo. Documentation of the phase 3 trials is usually the last-completed component of the package that an applicant submits to the FDA for marketing approval.

The phase 1/phase 2/phase 3 nomenclature is widely used, but the conventional distinctions are increasingly blurry. In recent years, for example, some investigators have done even their earliest trials using patients, healthy except for hypertension, instead of healthy volunteers.

## SUBMISSION OF THE APPLICATION

A typical complete application comprises about 200,000 pages of text and tables, collected into volumes of about 500 pages each. A little more than half of the application is typically devoted to the clinical trials, which usually have involved a total of 1500 to 3000 patients.* Under the Prescription Drug User Fee Act (1997, amended 2002), the application must be accompanied by a filing fee; for 2004, the fee was $573,500.

Although FDA permission is required for human drug experiments within the United States, there is no requirement that a development program include any U.S. trials at all, so a program based entirely on non-U.S. trials might theoretically not come to the FDA's attention until the moment that the application was submitted. This theoretical possibility has never been realized; sponsors and investigators of new antihypertensives have always availed themselves of the opportunity to meet with the FDA on multiple earlier occasions during development. In an early meeting, the topic might be the order in which various potential claims might best be studied, or what studies might be useful to estimate the importance of a worrisome toxicologic finding. In later meetings, the sponsor and FDA might discuss which drug-drug interactions were most reasonable to explore, or the design of the phase 3 trials. Still later, most sponsors visit the FDA to discuss the formatting of the application and the design of any computer-based aids for the FDA reviewers.

## REVIEW OF THE APPLICATION

Some drug products are approved not on the basis of new toxicologic and clinical data, but rather on the basis of chemical identity (and physical near-identity) to previously approved products. Applications describing such products ("generics") are handled by the FDA's Office of Generic Drugs (OGD). The pertinent chemical and biopharmaceutic criteria used by OGD are sufficient to guarantee that new drug/old drug differences are small compared with the expected interpatient and intrapatient variability. The details of those criteria will probably be of little interest to readers of this volume.

---

*No specific requirement for overall patient exposure is present in FDA regulations, but the FDA has accepted as "guidelines" the notions that there should be at least 1500 patients studied, at least 500 followed for at least 6 months, and at least 100 followed for a year or more. These numbers were the consensus recommendations of "harmonization" discussions among the FDA and its counterparts in Europe and Japan. This patient exposure greatly exceeds what is needed for a demonstration of antihypertensive efficacy, and it is determined by the desire to detect adverse effects that might not be apparent in smaller populations.

Applications for new antihypertensive drug products come to the FDA's Division of Cardio-Renal Drug Products (DCRDP). As of late 2003, the staff of DCRDP included 11 physicians (down from 16 in 1999), 13 toxicologists (down from 15), and 12 administrative and technical personnel (up from 11). In addition, there were at that time 8 chemists, 8 biopharmaceutic reviewers, and 5 statisticians who—although not formally members of DCRDP—were assigned full-time to the support of the DCRDP.

## Filing

Within 60 days of the arrival of a new application, the DCRDP must decide whether the application is capable of being reviewed at all. Rarely, the DCRDP decides that an application is incomplete on its face,* so review would be impossible. In such cases, the DCRDP formally "Refuses To File" the application, and further processing is omitted. The "Refusal to File" action (like all others) is subject to appeal and reversal; in addition, a manufacturer may insist that an application be filed (and reviewed) despite the initial refusal by the DCRDP.

## Criteria of Approvability

Before a product is approved for marketing, the sponsor must have demonstrated to the FDA that the product is produced by a securely repeatable process, and that its bioavailability has been described. The specific requirements in these areas are narrowly technical, and they are probably not of interest to most clinicians.

The clinical and toxicologic requirements are of broader interest. The FDA does not look to the clinical trials for a useful estimate of the magnitude of antihypertensive effect. That magnitude varies, of course, from patient to patient. In the clinical treatment of hypertension, drugs are titrated to effect, and any given drug is used only in patients who appear to respond to it. If a treatment is effective in a given patient, then it is immaterial that its antihypertensive effect in other patients is small or even absent. But because natural variations in BP are often similar in amplitude to the effects of therapy, the clinical trials may be the only setting in which active drugs can reliably be distinguished from placebos, and this distinction is at the center of the clinical review.

To demonstrate superiority to placebo, it is theoretically not necessary to do a placebo-controlled trial. If a new antihypertensive regimen were shown to be unequivocally *superior* to an approved regimen of an approved antihypertensive agent, the new drug could be approved. If, on the other hand, trials seemed to show only that the new drug were *similar* to approved therapy, then interpretation would be much more difficult. Such results might reflect genuine shared superiority to placebo, but they might instead reflect only that the trials had been so poorly executed that even a totally ineffective new drug could not have been distinguished from the approved therapy. In any event, the FDA has never seen an application for approval of an antihypertensive drug in which the major phase 3 trials were not placebo-controlled. The primary met-

ric of each trial is usually the baseline-adjusted seated DBP, but other measurements of BP (seated systolic, supine systolic and diastolic, standing systolic and diastolic) are also performed. Responder rates* are usually recorded, but—in part because of their necessarily arbitrary definitions, in part because of their statistical inefficiency—they have not been used as primary measures. Trials are usually powered to show that each of several doses of test drug is significantly superior to placebo, but sometimes the analysis uses a trend test to show only that taking all of the trial results together, the observed BPs cannot reasonably be believed to have been unrelated to the administered doses of test drug. In factorial trials, where individual cells of the randomization may each receive relatively few patients, a two-dimensional analog of the trend test[1] is especially attractive.

From the widespread adoption of $p \leq .05$ as the threshold of meaningful statistical significance, and from the Federal regulations' requirement (21 CFR §314.126) that approvals be supported by "adequate and well-controlled studies" (note the plural), the FDA has come to expect that any approvable antihypertensive claim would be supported by at least two trials, each successful by the criterion of $p \leq .05$. A single trial with $p \leq .05 \times 0.05 \div 2 = 0.00125$[†] could in principle provide equally strong evidence,[‡] but no antihypertensive application to date has ever rested its case on such an argument.[§]

FDA policy with respect to antihypertensives is derived from the landmark historical placebo-controlled trials that demonstrated the benefits of treatment with respect to the irreversible outcomes of stroke and similar hard endpoints. As described in Chapters 1 and 29 to 35, these trials employed antihypertensive medications of many different classes, always in stepped-therapy schemes, and usually starting with a diuretic or β-blocker. In every such trial with adequate statistical power to show a difference, antihypertensive therapy was seen to be superior to placebo. While the fractional reduction in event rate was consistently large, the absolute benefit—at least in patients with mild or moderate disease—was generally small, typically only a few averted events per thousand years of patient treatment.

Because the benefits of antihypertensive treatment have been so consistent across such a wide range of regimens, the FDA believes (with Dr. Jan Staessen and the Clinical Trialists Collaborative Group; see Chapter 29) that reduction of BP—however achieved—can be expected to be associated with a reduction in the incidence of irreversible vascular events. Accordingly, the FDA considers antihypertensive efficacy to have been demonstrated when the regimen in question is shown to reduce BP.

---

*For example, one application revealed that during a few months of storage, the to-be-marketed product came to contain large quantities of a degradation product whose carcinogenicity had not been studied in any species.

*For example, the fractions of patients whose last measured seated diastolic blood pressure (DBP) was below 90 mm Hg *or* at least 10 mm Hg less than it had been at baseline.

†That is, two trials rejecting the null hypothesis with each $p \leq .05$ ($0.05 \times 0.05$), and both results in the *same* tail of the distribution ($\div 2$).

‡ As could, say, four trials, each successful with $p \approx .3$.

§ A treatment that is nontrivially antihypertensive in patients with mild to moderate hypertension can easily be distinguished from placebo in small, short trials (a few hundred patients for a few weeks), so these statistical thresholds (whatever their exact levels) are not much of a hurdle. They are much more of an issue in other clinical areas (e.g., congestive heart failure), and they may become important in hypertension if claims are sought on the basis of the large, hard-endpoint trials.

On the other hand, the small absolute benefit of antihypertensive treatment could easily be outweighed by a small incidence of unrelated toxic effects, possibly an incidence too small to be reasonably estimated from the total experience in a typical package of clinical trials. The clinical and toxicologic reviewers must be satisfied that a new antihypertensive regimen is unlikely to be more toxic than those that, in the hard-endpoint trials, provided a net positive benefit.

Special additional criteria are imposed on fixed-dose combination products. Because any combination therapy exposes the patient to the potential adverse effects of each component, the FDA requires that each component of a combination product contribute to the antihypertensive effect, and that there be well-defined situations in which the combination offers antihypertensive efficacy that is superior to that provided by monotherapy with one or another of the components. Some additional considerations related to fixed-dose combination products were described in a 1994 editorial.[2]

## Why New Hard-Endpoint Trials Are Not Required

To avoid relying on uncertain predictions of long-term toxicity, the FDA could require that before any new antihypertensive regimens could be approved, net benefit would need to have been demonstrated in new hard-endpoint trials. The FDA's adoption of such a requirement has been proposed from time to time, and some of the difficulties of such a policy were discussed at the Cardio-Renal Advisory-Committee meeting of October 20, 1995.

Because most of the reported hard-endpoint trials were performed before the availability of some currently available drugs, and especially because they predated our current knowledge of effective dosing of diuretics, limiting FDA approval to hard-endpoint-trial–based therapy would not result in treatment recommendations that would be acceptable to most modern clinicians. The regimens tested in the hard-endpoint trials were shown to provide net benefit, but our knowledge of these regimens' toxicity* suggests that current recommendations (although not strictly based on hard-endpoint data) are likely to provide greater net benefit.

Also, the very success of the hard-endpoint trials of the 1970s and 1980s makes it ethically impossible to perform similar placebo-controlled trials today. When interventions have been shown to prevent a substantial incidence of irreversible harm, it is no longer permissible to assign patients to inactive

therapy.† Without placebo controls, and probably without control regimens identical to any of the creaky, now disfavored regimens of the reported hard-endpoint trials, net benefit would be difficult to demonstrate.

Finally, many of the possible hazards of antihypertensive therapy can be reliably estimated from hard-endpoint trials in other clinical areas. Of course, it is always possible that an antihypertensive regimen will turn out to induce obscure organ toxicity (e.g., agranulocytosis, pancreatitis) whose net effect, integrated over the years of treatment, will negate the benefit of pressure reduction. To the extent, however, that the toxicity of antihypertensive therapy is likely to be directly related to cardiovascular effects (e.g., from excessive rate or extent of pressure reduction), that toxicity can often be assessed by looking at the results of relatively short hard-endpoint trials in which the same therapy was given to patients (e.g., those with myocardial infarctions or congestive heart failure) who might be expected to be unusually sensitive to such effects.

## Primary Reviews

In the usual case, the application is formally accepted for filing, and the various sections of the application are reviewed more-or-less independently by specialists from the separate disciplines. In particular, separate primary reviews are contributed by a chemist, a toxicologist, and a biopharmaceutist. If the proposed product is to be administered parenterally, an additional review is provided by a microbiologist. In each of these disciplines, the primary reviewer's work is not considered complete until it has been cosigned by a supervisor. In many cases, the initial nonclinical reviews reveal various gaps in the manufacturer's documentation of its data and control procedures. The reviews lead to correspondence between the agency and the manufacturer, and thereafter to a (usually) convergent series of supplemental submissions and reviews.

Review of the clinical trials is handled differently. Sometimes there are separate reviews by a statistician and a physician, but more often the statistician and a physician (or two or three physicians) jointly produce a single review, dividing the work among themselves under the direction of a team leader who is then responsible for integrating the group's work into a coherent document. In addition to writing their review(s), the clinical reviewers will usually identify a few trial sites for routine audit by FDA field personnel. Like the nonclinical reviews, a clinical review often leads to correspondence intended to fill in gaps in documentation. In their conclusions, primary clinical reviews attempt to identify the clinical data whose interpretation should lead to approval or nonapproval, with suggestions for labeling in the event of approval.

## Secondary Reviews

On average, each volume of an application submitted to DCRDP will cause the generation of about one page of primary review, so the several primary reviews add up to a few hundred pages of text. The primary reviews are then brought together by a team leader (always a physician), who prepares a secondary review of (typically) a few dozen pages, including overall recommendations for approval/nonapproval and labeling. The secondary reviewer's recommendations regarding approval and labeling may differ from those of the primary reviewers, but the primary reviews are not revised on

---

*They often used doses of hydrochlorothiazide and triamterene up to 100 and 300 mg/day, respectively, and often used hydralazine (up to 200 mg/day) and α-methyldopa (up to 2 g/day) as the first add-ons.

† Similar considerations are prominent in other clinical areas in which the goal of treatment is to reduce the incidence of irreversible harm. In congestive heart failure, for example, patients in a typical placebo-controlled trial receive either (an ACE inhibitor and placebo) or (an ACE inhibitor and the test drug). Omission of ACE inhibitors would be impermissible, because ACE inhibitors reduce mortality in this condition.

Despite the use of ACE inhibitors, patients with congestive heart failure have high mortality compared with age-matched controls, so the possibility of additional clinical benefit from an additional drug is not far-fetched. In hypertension, on the other hand, it may be unrealistic to expect that a new drug will provide additional hard-endpoint benefit when it is added to a regimen that is already providing blood pressure control that is thought to be adequate.

this account. In this situation, the secondary reviewer will devote some of the review to discussion of the arguments that were raised by the primary reviewers.

## Advisory Committee

At approximately this point in the review process, issues raised by the application may optionally be brought to a public meeting of the FDA's Cardio-Renal Advisory Committee. The Committee comprises 10 to 12 clinicians and statisticians, appointed for 4-year terms. In most years, the Committee will have three or four 2-day meetings, during which a total of 8 to 10 applications will be discussed. Sometimes the DCRDP turns to the Committee for help in reaching a difficult decision about a specific application, but Committee meetings are more often used to bring complex regulatory issues to public awareness, usually (not always) with initial reference to a pending application. At most meetings, the Committee ultimately discusses and votes on a series of formal questions posed to the Committee by the DCRDP. The decisions of the Committee are not binding upon the FDA, but it is unusual for the FDA to contravert strong recommendations from the Committee.

## Tertiary and Quaternary Reviews

After the Committee meeting (if any), a tertiary review (usually just a few pages long) is written by the DCRDP Director. If the DCRDP Director disagrees with the secondary reviewer or the Advisory Committee, then his or her review will generally explain the disagreement.

With two other divisions, DCRDP is a component of the FDA's Office of Drug Evaluation I (ODE I). The FDA's decision authority about applications that come to DCRDP is held by ODE I, but this decision authority is often, on a case-by-case basis, delegated to DCRDP for applications (new formulations, new fixed-dose combinations, and so on) that do not involve new chemical substances. Applications for products containing new chemical substances are passed to ODE I for quaternary review.

## Action Letters

The tertiary (or quaternary) review describes the FDA's decision as to whether or not the application is approvable, and an "Action Letter" is then sent to the sponsor of the application. An Action Letter describes the application as *Nonapprovable,* *Approvable,* or *Approved.*

A Nonapprovable letter must describe the deficiencies in the application that led to the FDA's negative conclusion. At the other extreme, an Approval letter is usually short and simple. Marketing of the product is not permitted until the issuance of an Approval letter.

The third type of Action Letter, the Approvable letter, was originally used for products that appeared to be safe and effective, but with respect to which there remained minor gaps in the chemistry description, unsettled portions of labeling, or other deficiencies that appeared to be straightforwardly reparable. The typical Approvable letter was then followed by no more than a few weeks of faxes and meetings before the predictable appearance of an Approval letter. More recently, apparently as a response to time constraints imposed upon the FDA by the Prescription Drug User Fee Act, Approvable letters have been less closely coupled to ultimate approval.

The total elapsed time from the DCRDP's receipt of the application to its issuance of the Action Letter averaged about 14 months in the late 1990s. The DCRDP declines to release any newer statistics, and such statistics would in any event be difficult to interpret, in view of recent changes in the use of Approvable letters.

## References

1. Hung HMJ, Chi GYH, Lipicky RJ. On some statistical methods for analysis of combination drug studies. Commun Statist Theory Meth 23:361-376, 1994.
2. Fenichel RR, Lipicky RJ. Combination products as first-line pharmacotherapy. Arch Intern Med 154:1429-1430, 1994.

# Diuretics: Mechanisms of Action

## Mark A. Knepper, Thomas Kleyman, Gerardo Gamba

## INTRODUCTION

The regulation of blood pressure is achieved in part through the control of sodium chloride (NaCl) balance, which is largely dependent on regulation of NaCl excretion by the kidney.[1] Accordingly, many forms of blood pressure are associated with abnormalities in $Na^+$ and $Cl^-$ transport along the renal tubule.[2] Furthermore, an important staple in the treatment of hypertension has been diuretic agents, which work by directly inhibiting $Na^+$ transporters and channels that mediate renal tubule $Na^+$ reabsorption. This chapter reviews the mechanism of diuretic action, focusing on the molecular properties of the $Na^+$ transporters and channels that they inhibit. We focus on diuretic agents that work by blocking transport and specifically do not discuss mineralocorticoid receptor antagonists, angiotensin II receptor antagonists, and blockers of adrenergic receptors, which work in part by increasing NaCl excretion but do so indirectly.

Fundamentally, there are three main groups of direct-acting diuretic agents (Figure 62–1): (1) "loop diuretics" such as furosemide or bumetanide, which block the type 2 $Na^+$, $K^+$-$2Cl^-$ cotransporter (NKCC2) of the thick ascending limb of Henle (TAL); (2) thiazides and related diuretics, which block the $Na^+$-$Cl^-$ cotransporter (NCC) of the distal convoluted tubule (DCT); and (3) amiloride and its congeners, which block the epithelial sodium channel (ENaC) expressed in the connecting tubule and collecting duct (CD) portions of the renal tubule. The major portions of this chapter summarize the properties of these transporters and address the mechanisms involved in blockade of these transporters.

Figure 62–1 and Table 62–1 summarize the major renal tubule segments and the major renal tubule transporters expressed in them. A filtrate of blood plasma generated in the renal glomerulus is delivered sequentially to the proximal tubule, the loop of Henle, the distal convoluted tubule, the connecting tubule, and the collecting duct. Each segment reabsorbs a fraction of NaCl delivered to it. The collecting duct carries out the final adjustments in urinary composition and is the site of fine control of $Na^+$ transport by aldosterone, angiotensin II, and vasopressin.

Renal tubules are epithelial structures that transport NaCl from their lumens to the interstitium and thereby back to the blood. As is true of all epithelial cells, renal tubule epithelial cells consist of two membrane domains (apical and basolateral) separated by a tight junction that connects each cell to its immediate neighbors. Transcellular transport of $Na^+$ across an epithelium therefore requires transport across both the apical and basolateral plasma membranes. The basolateral transport pathway is the same for each renal tubule segment, namely the $Na^+$, $K^+$-ATPase, which trans-

ports three $Na^+$ ions out of the cell and two $K^+$ ions into the cell per adenosine triphosphate (ATP) $\gamma$-phosphate bond hydrolyzed.[3] $Na^+$,$K^+$-ATPase consist of two subunits, a nonglycosylated $\alpha$ subunit and a chaperone-like $\beta$ subunit, which is not directly involved in ion transport but is necessary for normal trafficking of the assembled complex to the plasma membrane.[4] The $Na^+$,$K^+$-ATPase in the kidney tubule consists of $\alpha_1\beta_1$ complexes.[5] Hypothetically, drugs that target the $Na^+$, $K^+$-ATPase such as the cardiac glycoside, ouabain, could serve as diuretics. However, the therapeutic ratio for such drugs is too low for them to be effective diuretics, and they exert toxic effects on the $Na^+$, $K^+$-ATPase isoform in the heart prior to any significant diuretic effect in the kidney.

The diuretic agents considered in this review increase $Na^+$ excretion by blocking $Na^+$ transporters in the apical plasma membrane of renal tubule cells. Their efficacy depends on the process of active transepithelial secretion of the drugs from blood to lumen in the late part of the proximal convoluted tubule and early part of the proximal straight tubule.[6] Because this process concentrates the diuretics at their site of action, the renal tubule lumen, the therapeutic ratio for these agents tends to be very high. Although commonly used diuretics such as the loop diuretics, thiazides, and amiloride can inhibit $Na^+$ transport at extrarenal sites, circulating levels necessary for effective inhibition of renal tubule transporters are usually too low to have extrarenal effects, owing to the proximal tubule secretory mechanism. However, acute or chronic renal failure can result in significant impairment of the proximal secretory mechanism, resulting in relative resistance to these diuretics.[7,8] Under these circumstances, the clinician needs to increase diuretic doses to overcome this resistance, resulting in a greater likelihood of toxicity.

It is interesting that there are no effective diuretics that are targeted to transporters in the proximal tubule, the renal tubule segment that is responsible for two thirds of renal tubule $Na^+$ reabsorption. A major reason for the lack of such agents has been revealed in studies of renal tubule function in mice in which the major proximal $Na^+$ transporter NHE3 (sodium-hydrogen exchanger, type 3) has been deleted.[9] These mice do not manifest high rates of salt and water excretion as might be expected. Instead, increased salt and water delivery to the macula densa results in activation of the tubuloglomerular feedback mechanism, which markedly lowers glomerular filtration rate. Therefore NaCl balance is maintained, despite a marked reduction in proximal NaCl absorption in these mice, through a marked decrease in glomerular filtration rate.

In the remainder of this chapter we focus on the properties of the apical $Na^+$ transporters and channels that are targets for loop diuretics, thiazide diuretics, and amiloride.

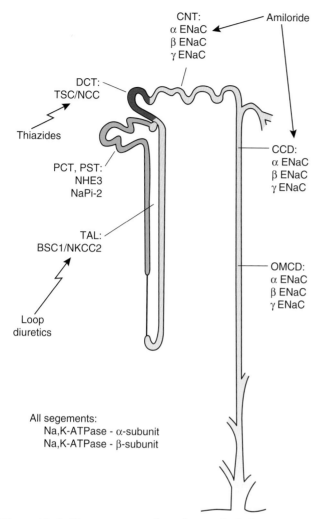

CNT:
α ENaC
β ENaC
γ ENaC

Amiloride

DCT:
TSC/NCC

Thiazides

PCT, PST:
NHE3
NaPi-2

CCD:
α ENaC
β ENaC
γ ENaC

TAL:
BSC1/NKCC2

OMCD:
α ENaC
β ENaC
γ ENaC

Loop
diuretics

All segments:
Na,K-ATPase - α-subunit
Na,K-ATPase - β-subunit

**Figure 62–1** Diuretic targets along the renal tubule. The tubule segments and main transporters are depicted. Tubule segments are: PCT, proximal convoluted tubule; PST, proximal straight tubule; TAL, thick ascending limb of Henle's loop; DCT, distal convoluted tubule; CNT, connecting tubule; CCD, cortical collecting duct; OMCD, outer medullary collecting duct.

## LOOP DIURETICS

### Transport Mechanisms in the Thick Ascending Limb of the Loop of Henle

The TAL is responsible for the reabsorption of about 15% to 20% of the NaCl in the glomerular filtrate. In addition, the TAL also plays important roles in divalent cation ($Ca^{2+}$ and $Mg^{2+}$) and ammonium ion ($NH_4^+$) reabsorption. However, its chief role is regulation of water excretion through the dilution of luminal fluid and the concentration of the surrounding interstitium. Concentration of the interstitium is a result of a process called "countercurrent multiplication"[10] and is critical to the generation of a final urine that is concentrated relative to plasma. This functional capacity is necessary for the survival of land mammals, including humans.

The molecular mechanism of salt reabsorption by TAL is shown in Figure 62–2. As in the rest of the nephron, in TAL the salt is transported from the luminal side to the interstitial space because of the polarized expression of the $Na^+$, $K^+$-ATPase (the "sodium pump") to the basolateral membrane. This pump produces a continuous efflux of sodium ions into the interstitial space, reducing the intracellular sodium concentration, thus generating a gradient for sodium transport in which apical sodium is transported into the TAL cells. As shown in Figure 62–2, the major pathway for sodium reabsorption in the apical membrane of the TAL is the $Na^+$,$K^+$-2$Cl^-$ cotransporter. This is a secondary carrier that takes advantage of the gradient for $Na^+$ transport to translocate $K^+$ and $Cl^-$ from the lumen into the TAL cells against their respective electrochemical gradients. This $Na^+$,$K^+$-2$Cl^-$ cotransporter is the main pharmacologic target of loop diuretics (furosemide, bumetanide, ethacrynic acid, torasemide, and piretanide). Loop diuretics exert their action by direct interaction with the $Na^+$,$K^+$-2$Cl^-$ cotransporter in the TAL.

As shown in Figure 62–2, salt reabsorption in the TAL requires the simultaneous function of at least six proteins produced by different genes. Salt enters the cell across the apical plasma membrane, together with $K^+$, through the $Na^+$,$K^+$-2$Cl^-$ cotransporter. The sodium and chloride ions leave the cell in the basolateral membrane through the $Na^+$,$K^+$-ATPase and the $Cl^-$ channels (CLC-Kb), respectively. The $Na^+$,$K^+$-ATPase is composed of two subunits: the α- and β-subunits that are

**Table 62–1** Major Na Transporter and Na Channel Proteins in the Kidney

| Name | Identification | Location* | No. Amino Acids | Actual MW (kDa)§ |
|------|---------------|-----------|-----------------|------------------|
| NHE3 | Type 3 Na-H exchanger | PT, DL, TAL (apical) | 831 | 84 |
| NKCC2 | Type 2 Na,K-2Cl cotransporter | TAL (apical) | 1095 | 163 |
| NCC | Na-Cl cotransporter | DCT (apical) | 1022 | 165 |
| ENaC-α | α-subunit of epithelial Na channel | CNT, CD (apical) | 699 | 86 |
| ENaC-β | β-subunit of epithelial Na channel | CNT, CD (apical) | 640 | 88 |
| ENaC-γ | γ subunit of epithelial Na channel | CNT, CD (apical) | 649 | 85 |
| NKA-$α_1$ | Na,K-ATPase, $α_1$-subunit | All segments (basolateral) | 1023 | 98 |
| NKA-$β_1$ | Na-,K-ATPase, $β_1$-subunit | All segments (basolateral) | 304 | 50 |

*Tubule segments: Proximal tubule (PT), descending limb of Henle's loop (DL), thick ascending limb of Henle's loop (TAL), distal convoluted tubule (DCT), connecting tubule (CNT), collecting duct (CD).
§Actual molecular weight (MW) determined by immunoblotting.

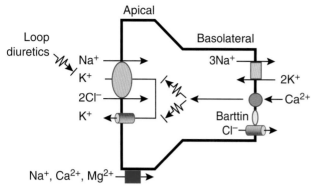

**Figure 62–2** Molecular physiology of ion transport in the thick ascending loop of Henle.

products of two different genes. The α-subunit is not glycosylated and plays a catalytic and transport role. In contrast, the β-subunit is glycosylated and is required for successful targeting of the Na⁺,K⁺-ATPase complex to the plasma membrane. A similar situation occurs with CLC-Kb, since it is also composed of two subunits—CLC-Kb, the pore-forming subunit, and a protein known as *Barttin* that is required to drive CLC-Kb to the basolateral membrane.

Potassium ions entering the cell across the apical plasma membrane are largely returned to the tubular lumen via an inwardly rectifying K⁺ channel known as the renal outer medullary potassium channel (ROMK). Potassium recycling into the lumen is required for NaCl reabsorption by the TAL. Because the potassium concentration in the glomerular ultrafiltrate (4 mEq/L) is much lower than that of sodium (145 mEq/L) or chloride (110 mEq/L), without the recycling pathway for potassium, the concentration of this cation in the lumen of the TAL would be rapidly reduced below the minimum required for transport. As a consequence, the function of the Na⁺,K⁺-2Cl⁻ cotransporter would stop because of depletion of K⁺ from the lumen. The recycling, however, assures that potassium concentration within the TAL lumen will always be enough to allow the proper function of the Na⁺,K⁺-2Cl⁻ cotransporter. The potassium recycling, together with the movement of sodium and chloride to the interstitial space, generates a positive voltage within the TAL lumen that drives the reabsorption of a second cation through the paracellular pathway. Because the tight junctions are permeable to sodium, magnesium, and calcium, all three ions are reabsorbed at rates dependent on their luminal concentrations. Thus the coordinated function of the Na⁺,K⁺-2Cl⁻ cotransporter, the apical K⁺ channels, and the basolateral Cl⁻ channels makes the TAL epithelial cells thermodynamically more efficient, since two cations are reabsorbed at the expense of the ATP needed to pump one.[11]

The functional description of the molecular mechanisms for salt reabsorption in the TAL cells helps us to understand the mechanism by which loop diuretics exert their effects in the kidney. By blocking the function of the Na⁺,K⁺-2Cl⁻ cotransporter, loop diuretics reduce the salt reabsorption rate in the TAL. As a consequence, an increased amount of salt is delivered to the distal nephron, increasing the fractional excretion of salt into urine, thus producing natriuresis and diuresis. Increased delivery of NaCl to the macula densa would normally result in a compensating decrease in

glomerular filtration rate as a result of activation of the tubuloglomerular feedback (TGF) mechanism.[12] Such compensation does not occur when increased NaCl delivery is mediated by loop diuretics because the TGF mechanism is dependent on the function of the bumetanide-sensitive Na⁺,K⁺-2Cl⁻ cotransporter present in the macula densa cells. This cotransporter has been demonstrated to be same one (NKCC2) as that in the TAL cells.[13]

Greater delivery of NaCl to the connecting tubule and collecting duct results in greater Na⁺ reabsorption by the principal cells in these segments, resulting in greater potassium secretion. In addition, the greater rate of sodium transport indirectly cause a greater rate of H⁺ secretion by the intercalated cells of the connecting tubule and outer medullary collecting duct. For these reasons, one potential, undesired consequence of loop diuretic administration can be increased fractional excretion of potassium and hydrogen, resulting in hypokalemia and metabolic alkalosis.

## Molecular Biology of the Apical Na⁺,K⁺-2Cl⁻ Cotransporter

Two genes encoding isoforms of the Na⁺,K⁺-2Cl⁻ cotransporters have been identified. They belong to the family of electroneutral cation-chloride coupled cotransporters, known in the human genome database as SLC12. SLC12A1 gene encodes the renal-specific Na⁺,K⁺-2Cl⁻ (NKCC2) that is exclusively expressed in the TAL of the kidney. This gene is located in human chromosome 15.[14] SLC12A2 gene encodes the ubiquitous Na⁺,K⁺-2Cl⁻ cotransporter (NKCC1), which is expressed in several tissues and cell lines and is located on human chromosome 5.[15,16] NKCC2 shares a basic structural topology with the members of the cation-chloride gene family. As shown in Figure 62–3, *A*, NKCC2 is a glycoprotein of 1095 amino acids with molecular weight of ~165 kDa featuring a central hydrophobic region containing 12 putative transmembrane domains that are flanked by amino and carboxyl-terminal hydrophilic domains, presumably located within the cell. The extracellular hydrophilic loop between putative transmembrane domains S7 and S8 contains two *N*-glycosylation motifs. Several putative protein kinase A (PKA) and protein kinase C (PKC) phosphorylation sites are present within the amino and carboxyl-terminal domains.

At least six isoforms of NKCC2 are expressed in the mouse kidney because of the combination of two alternative splicing mechanisms.[17] As shown in Figure 62–3, on one hand, two isoforms are produced by truncation of the carboxyl-terminal domain. The longer isoform (Figure 62–3, *A*) is the 1095 amino acid residue protein, whereas the shorter isoform (Figure 62–3, *B*) is composed of 770 residues. Interestingly, the longer isoform is the Na⁺,K⁺-2Cl⁻ cotransporter, whereas the truncated isoform encodes a K⁺-independent but nevertheless furosemide-sensitive Na⁺-Cl⁻ cotransporter that is activated by hypotonicity and inhibited by cyclic adenosine monophosphate (cAMP) analogs.[18] This truncated isoform seems to be important in salt reabsorption along TAL during water diuresis states. On the other hand, the SLC12A1 gene contains three 96 bp mutually exclusive cassette exons designated A, B, and F[19,20] that encode for 32 amino acid residues that are part of the transmembrane domain 2 and the connecting segment between transmembrane domains 2 and 3 (see Figure 62–3). Thus this splicing mechanism produces three proteins that are identical,

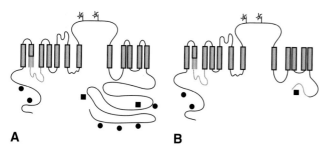

**Figure 62–3** Proposed topology and splice variants of the mouse apical, renal-specific Na+,K+-2Cl− cotransporter. **A,** The long isoform that encodes the Na+,K+-2Cl− cotransporter. **B,** The short isoform that encodes the Na+-Cl− cotransporter contains 55 amino acid residues at the end of the C-terminal domain (highlighted in gray) that are not present in the longer isoform. The region of the transmembrane domain 2 and the interconnecting segment between transmembrane domains 2 and 3 that are highlighted in gray depict the region of the mutually exclusive cassette exons A, B, or F. In this region, both the long and the short isoform can be either A, B, or F. Two glycosylation sites are depicted in the extracellular loop between membrane segments 7 and 8 by two little evergreen bushes. The localization of the putative phosphorylation sites for protein kinase A or C are shown in circles or boxes, respectively.

except in the sequence of these 32 residues that comes from one of the three mutually exclusive exons. Because these two splicing mechanisms can be combined with the carboxyl-terminal domain splicing, six isoforms can be produced: three with long carboxyl-terminal domains (that can be A, B, or F in the second transmembrane domain) and three with short carboxyl-terminal domains (that can be A, B, or F).[17,21]

The splicing event producing three long carboxyl-terminal domain isoforms named A, B, and F has remarkable effects in the TAL physiology. Early studies on isolated cortical or medullary TAL segments by Burg[22] and by Rocha and Kokko[23] clearly showed that medullary TAL transports NaCl more rapidly than the cortical TAL, but the diluting power was greater in the cortical TAL.[24] These observations suggested heterogeneity of the transport properties along the TAL. Supporting this conclusion, a higher apparent affinity for Cl− was observed in cortical than in medullary TALH.[25-29] In this regard, the splicing isoforms A, B, and F exhibit axial distribu-

tion along the TAL (Figure 62–4). The F isoform is absent in the cortical but present in the medullary TAL, with higher expression in the inner stripe of the outer medulla. The A isoform is present in both cortical and medullary TAL, and the B isoform is present only in the cortical TAL.[19,20,30] In agreement with this distribution, the affinity for the cotransported ions varies among the three isoforms. The affinity profile is: B > A > F.[31,32] Thus, at the beginning of the TAL, where salt concentration is high, the main isoform is the F, exhibiting the lower affinity, while at the end of TAL, where further dilution is required, the main isoform is the B that exhibits the highest affinity. The A isoform is expressed along the entire TAL and is also the one with the highest capacity for ion transport.[31] Thus, by producing three isoforms of the Na+,K+-2Cl− cotransporter, alternative splicing of the SLC12A1 gene underlies the heterogeneity of salt transport in the TAL.

## Regulation of the Na+,K+-2Cl− Cotransporter

As discussed previously, the NaCl reabsorption in the TAL plays a central role in the regulation of water balance by driving concentrating and diluting processes. Consistent with this role, NaCl transport in this segment is regulated by the antidiuretic hormone vasopressin. As demonstrated in isolated perfused tubule studies, vasopressin has rapid actions to increase NaCl absorption by the TAL.[33,34] The effect is mediated by cAMP and appears to involve trafficking of the Na+,K+-2Cl− cotransporter, NKCC2, from an intracellular vesicular pool to the apical plasma membrane.[35-37] It may be dependent in part on phosphorylation of the transporter in the amino-terminal tail region.[35] In addition, the stimulatory effect of vasopressin on NKCC2 trafficking appears to be related to inhibition by cAMP of an inhibitory effect of the 770 amino acid short isoform of NKCC2 on trafficking of the full length isoform (vide supra).[36,37] Other hormones, including parathyroid hormone, calcitonin, and glucagon also increase intracellular cAMP in the TAL cell[38] and stimulate concomitant increases in NaCl absorption rate,[39,40] presumably by the same mechanism as demonstrated for vasopressin. Prostaglandin E2 has been demonstrated to have a short-term inhibitory effect on NaCl absorption in the TAL,[41] presumably via its ability to inhibit cAMP production in TAL cells.[42] Another mediator that regulates TAL NaCl transport via effects in NKCC2 is nitric oxide (NO), which directly inhibits NaCl absorption in isolated perfused TALs.[43]

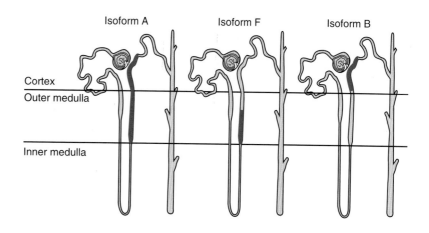

**Figure 62–4** Distribution of the isoforms A, F, and B of the Na+,K+-2Cl− cotransporter along the TALH.

In addition to the short-term effect of vasopressin on NKCC2 trafficking or activity, long-term increases in circulating vasopressin levels have been demonstrated to increase the abundance of the NKCC2 protein in TAL cells.[44] This action results in a long-term potentiation of NaCl transport in the TAL, as demonstrated in isolated perfused tubule studies.[45]

Paralleling the short-term inhibitory effect of prostaglandin E2 on NaCl transport in the TAL, long-term changes in prostaglandin E2 levels appear to modulate NKCC2 expression in the TAL.[46] In these studies, cyclooxygenase inhibitors indomethacin or diclofenac increased NKCC2 abundance, an effect that was reversed by administration of a prostaglandin E2 analog, misoprostol.

In addition to actions of agents that signal predominantly in the TAL via cAMP, regulatory mediators that signal via other mechanisms also regulate NKCC2 expression in the TAL. For example, NO, which increases cyclic guanosine monophosphate in cells, increases NKCC2 expression as evidenced by observed decreases in abundance in response to inhibition of nitric oxide synthases by N-nitro-L-arginine methyl ester (L-NAME).[47] Furthermore, angiotensin II infusion was also found to increase NKCC2 abundance in the TAL,[48] although inhibition of angiotensin II type 1 (AT$_1$) receptors by candesartan[49] or deletion of AT$_{1a}$ receptors in mice[50] did not produce the opposite effects. Quite possibly the effect of angiotensin II infusion on NKCC2 expression is indirect and related to local changes in NO or PGE2 levels.

## Potential Role of the Na$^+$,K$^+$-2Cl$^-$ Cotransporter in Arterial Hypertension

Because of similarities of Bartter's syndrome to Gitelman syndrome, it was speculated that Bartter syndrome, an autosomal-recessive disorder, was due to reduction in the NaCl transport function of the TAL. Bartter's syndrome is characterized by hypokalemic metabolic alkalosis, with hypocalciuria and normomagnesemia,[51] as well as renal salt wasting, polyuria, arterial hypotension, and nephrocalcinosis. Mutations in at least five genes result in Bartter's syndrome.[52] Thus this is a monogenic but heterogeneous disease. In all cases, the function of the TAL is affected. Inactivating mutations in the genes encoding the proteins involved in salt reabsorption in TAL produce Bartter's syndrome types I, II, III, and IV. These are the Na$^+$,K$^+$-2Cl$^-$ cotransporter,[14,53-56] the apical K$^+$ channel ROMK,[57-63] the basolateral Cl$^-$ channel CLC-Kb,[64,65] and the chaperon subunit of the Cl$^-$ channel known as Barttin,[66-68] respectively. In addition, "gain of function" mutations of the calcium-sensing receptor also cause Bartter's syndrome.[69,70] Activation of the calcium-sensing receptor that is expressed in the basolateral membrane of the TAL reduces the activity of the Na$^+$,K$^+$-2Cl$^-$ cotransporter and the ROMK channels. Thus the participation of all these genes, including the Na$^+$,K$^+$-2Cl$^-$ cotransporter, in the genesis of a syndrome that exhibits arterial hypotension shows that they are among the genes involved in defining the blood pressure levels and thus are potentially involved in hypertension.

## Loop Diuretics in the Treatment of Hypertension

Loop diuretics can potentially be used for treatment of hypertension. Because loop diuretics reduce salt reabsorption in the

TAL, their potency as natriuretic agents is superior to thiazides or the K$^+$-retaining diuretics. However, in terms of lowering the blood pressure, loop diuretics are less effective than thiazides. In addition, these diuretics have never been tested in outcome trials, and they must be dosed twice daily or more frequently. For all these reasons, loop diuretics, unlike thiazides, are unsatisfactory for the chronic treatment of hypertension and are not recommended for the treatment of stage 1 or stage 2 uncomplicated hypertension. Instead, loop diuretics are very useful to treat essential hypertension complicated by heart failure, edema and/or renal insufficiency. Thus the more common clinical settings in which loop diuretics are prescribed included edematous states caused by congestive heart failure, chronic renal failure, nephrotic syndrome, or chronic liver disease to induce natriuresis and diuresis.

## THIAZIDE-TYPE DIURETICS

### Transport Mechanisms in the Distal Convoluted Tubule

The distal convoluted tubule (DCT) is a specialized segment of the nephron located between the TALH and the collecting duct in which 5% to 7% of the glomerular filtrate is reabsorbed. As is the TAL, the DCT is also involved in calcium excretion and in concentrating urine, in addition to regulating NaCl balance.[71] The molecular mechanism of salt reabsorption in the DCT is shown in Figure 62–5. Similar to most of the renal epithelium, the sodium gradient from lumen to interstitium is generated and maintained by a very intense activity of the Na$^+$,K$^+$-ATPase that is polarized to the basolateral membrane.[72] The DCT begins a few cells after the macula densa and is divided in two segments known as "early" and "late" segments.[73] Most studies in rat, mouse, rabbit, and human kidney agree that along the whole DCT, the major sodium reabsorption pathway in the apical membrane is the Na$^+$-Cl$^-$ cotransporter NCC. In the early DCT, this is the only Na$^+$ transport pathway identified so far, whereas in late DCT, NCC expression overlaps with that of the ENaC, vide infra.[71,73-77] As shown in Figure 62–5, the apical Na$^+$-Cl$^-$ cotransporter in the DCT is the major target for the thiazide-type diuretics (chlorthalidone, hydrochlorothiazide, bendroflumethiazide, and metolazone).[71,78]

The thiazide-type diuretics were introduced into clinical medicine in 1957[79] and were followed by the more-potent loop diuretics (furosemide, bumetanide, and ethacrynic acid).

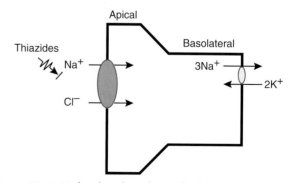

**Figure 62–5** Molecular physiology of salt transport in the early distal convoluted tubule.

Several years later the first clue to the mechanism of action of thiazides was elucidated by Kunau et al.,[80] who demonstrated that thiazides inhibited Cl⁻ reabosrption in the distal nephron and not in the proximal tubule as was originally proposed. Then Stokes et al.[81] showed for the first time that thiazides inhibited a Na⁺-Cl⁻ cotransporter. These authors used a urinary bladder preparation from the winter flounder.[82,83] With this preparation, Stokes et al.[81] unequivocally showed that thiazides competitively inhibited the salt reabsorption by blocking the function of the apical Na⁺-Cl⁻ cotransporter. A few years later, Ellison et al.,[71] using in vivo microperfusion, finally defined the existence of a thiazide-sensitive Na⁺-Cl⁻ cotransporter as the major pathway for salt reabsorption in the DCT. It was later observed that tracer [³H]metolazone was able to bind with high affinity to membrane preparations from rat renal cortex.[84,85] These studies showed that both Na⁺ and Cl⁻ needed to be present for binding of [³H]metolazone to renal cortex. It was observed that cations stimulated the binding of tracer metolazone following a saturation curve compatible with Michaelis-Menten behavior, whereas Cl⁻ produced a biphasic effect: At low Cl⁻ concentration, the binding was stimulated, whereas at higher concentration, it was inhibited. Following these observations, it was proposed that to block the function of the cotransporter, the thiazides probably compete with Cl⁻ for the same binding site on the cotransporters.[85] However, careful analysis of the functional properties of the rat cotransporter has recently revealed that thiazides compete with both Na⁺ and Cl⁻.[86]

In the DCT, salt and Ca²⁺ reabsorption rates are reciprocally related. Blocking or reducing the activity of the Na⁺-Cl⁻ cotransporter increases Ca²⁺ reabsorption, while increased expression or activity of the Na⁺-Cl⁻ cotransporter reduces Ca²⁺ reabsorption.[87] The mechanism by which thiazide diuretics affects calcium reabsorption is still unclear, but most evidence suggests that thiazide action and calcium reabsorption may be functionally linked through an indirect mechanism. Thiazides reduce NaCl entry at the apical membrane, but intracellular Na⁺ is continuously pumped out of the cell by the Na⁺,K⁺-ATPase at the basolateral membrane. Thus intracellular Na⁺ concentration is reduced, and as a consequence, DCT cells become hyperpolarized, increasing the electrochemical driving force for Ca²⁺ entry at the apical membrane through Ca²⁺ channels.[88] This secondary effect of thiazides on Ca²⁺ reabsorption constitutes the basis for their use in the treatment of calcium stone disease and may also explain the protective effect of thiazides in osteoporosis.[89,90]

## Molecular Biology of the Apical Na⁺-Cl⁻ Cotransporter

With a functional expression strategy in *Xenopus laevis* oocytes, the first electroneutral Na⁺-coupled Cl⁻ cotransporter to be identified at the molecular level was the thiazide-sensitive Na⁺-Cl⁻ cotransporter (NCC) from the winter flounder urinary bladder.[91] Then, with a cRNA probe constructed from the fish cDNA, the mammalian cDNA encoding the NCC was isolated by homology.[78] The functional expression of fish and mammalian NCC in *Xenopus* oocytes gives rise to a ²²Na⁺ transport uptake mechanism that is Cl⁻ dependent and inhibitable by thiazide-type diuretics, with an inhibition profile (polythiazide > metolazone > hydrochlorothiazide > chlorothiazide) similar to the clinical potency of thiazides and to that previously shown

for inhibition of Cl⁻–dependent Na⁺ absorption,[92] as well as the thiazide competition for the high-affinity [³H]metolazone binding sites on kidney cortical membranes.[84]

NCCs share a similar secondary topology with the other members of the Na⁺-coupled Cl⁻ cotransporter family, as deduced from the hydrophobicity analysis following the Kyte-Doolittle algorithm.[93] The human NCC is a glycoprotein of 1022 amino acid residues, with core molecular weight of ~120 kDa, that shows the basic structure of 12 putative transmembrane domains flanked by two hydrophilic amino- and carboxyl-terminal domains containing several putative PKC and PKA phosphorylation sites (Figure 62–6). Mutation analysis of rat NCC has shown that there are two N-linked glycosylation sites in the loop between S7 and S8 that are absolutely required for the protein to be functional.[94] The protein is extensively glycosylated, increasing its molecular weight to 163 kDa as measured by immunoblotting studies.[95]

Eight members of the cation-coupled Cl⁻ cotransporter gene family have been identified from vertebrate sources. A phylogenetic tree depicting the relationship between members in this family is shown in Figure 62–7. Two genes encode the NKCC1 and NKCC2 Na⁺,K⁺-2Cl⁻ cotransporters,[78,96] one gene encodes NCC[91] (see later), and there are four genes encoding isoforms of the K⁺-Cl⁻ cotransporters: Three are ubiquitously expressed (KCC1, KCC3, and KCC4),[97] and another gene exhibits brain-specific expression (KCC2).[98] In addition, one gene encodes a member of the family known as CIP (cotransporter interacting protein) for which the function is still unknown.[99,100] As Figure 62–7 shows, two branches are clearly separated. One includes the Na⁺-coupled Cl⁻ cotransporters NKCC1, NKCC2, and NCC, whereas the other includes the Na⁺-independent, K⁺-coupled Cl⁻ cotransporters KCC1 to KCC4. Homology between the Na⁺-coupled Cl⁻ cotransporters and the K⁺-coupled Cl⁻ cotransporters is ~20 %. The degree of identity between NKCC1, NKCC2, and NCC is more than 50%. The strongest homology is observed in the transmembrane domains but is also evident in the interconnecting loops as well as in the C-terminal domain.

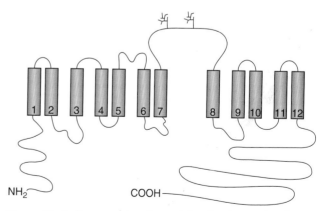

**Figure 62–6** Proposed topology of the distal convoluted tubule thiazide-sensitive Na⁺-Cl⁻ cotransporter. The central hydrophobic domain features 12 membrane spanning domains shown by numbers. Two glycosylation sites are shown in the putative extracellular loop between membrane domains 7 and 8 as two little evergreen bushes.

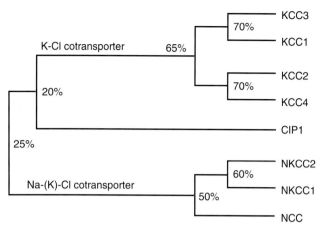

**Figure 62–7** Phylogenetic tree of the electroneutral Na-coupled chloride cotransporter family SLC12.

## Regulation of the Na⁺-Cl⁻ Cotransporter

With the advent of high-quality polyclonal antibodies to all the major Na⁺ transporters expressed along the renal tubule, profiling techniques have been used to investigate the pattern of Na⁺ transporter abundance changes under different physiologic and pathophysiologic circumstances (for review see references 101-103). These studies have been coupled with other approaches to show that NCC expression is highly regulated by multiple factors that are known to modulate the renal excretion of sodium and hence the arterial blood pressure. Such studies have revealed that an important regulator of NCC is the mineralocorticoid aldosterone.

Early micropuncture studies in adrenalectomized rats showed an increase in sodium tubule fluid:plasma concentration ratio in the DCT[104] that was decreased to control levels by aldosterone. In addition, in vivo microperfusion investigations have shown that aldosterone increases thiazide-sensitive salt transport in the DCT.[105] Aldosterone has been shown to increase [³H]metolazone binding in membrane fractions from renal cortex, a measure of NCC abundance,[106] and by immunoblotting with specific anti-NCC antibodies, it has been demonstrated that elevated plasma aldosterone concentration is associated with increase in the NCC abundance in renal cortex, regardless of whether plasma aldosterone is increased by aldosterone infusion[95] or dietary-sodium restriction.[107] The increment in NCC abundance in response to dietary-salt restriction is significantly higher than the increase observed in the subunits of the amiloride-sensitive Na⁺ channel.[107,108] It has been shown that infusions of aldosterone in dexamethasone-replaced adrenalectomized rats clearly increase NCC abundance in renal cortex and that this increment is prevented by spironolactone.[109] Additionally, it has been demonstrated that the furosemide-induced increase in NCC expression can be abrogated with spironolactone.[110] These findings suggest that aldosterone regulation of NCC protein is mediated through the classical mineralocorticoid receptor. Interestingly, however, existing evidence indicates that NCC regulation by mineralocorticoids must be indirect (i.e., unrelated to NCC gene transcription), because there has been a consistent failure to detect changes in NCC mRNA levels in response to dietary-salt restriction[111,112] or furosemide administration.[110,111] Indeed, a study in which NCC mRNA

and protein levels were assessed simultaneously showed that the increase in NCC protein induced by dietary NaCl restriction was not associated with detectable changes in NCC mRNA levels.[108]

In addition to regulation by aldosterone, the abundance of NCC protein in kidney is regulated in several conditions in which aldosterone levels are not affected, indicating that NCC is a target for other hormones and regulators. NCC abundance is moderately increased by vasopressin administration (DDAVP).[113] Furthermore, when the kidney undergoes escape from vasopressin-induced water retention after the development of hyponatremia, NCC abundance is more markedly increased.[114] The authors proposed that this increase in NCC abundance in response to water retention may be associated with inappropriate secretion of antidiuretic hormone.

Despite the positive regulation by aldosterone, NCC is the only transport protein that is decreased during the aldosterone escape phenomenon,[115] suggesting that NCC is one of the principal targets of pressure natriuresis. A similar conclusion has been drawn by Majid and Navar based on measurements of pressure natriuresis in intact dogs.[116] NCC abundance is also increased in hyperinsulinemic conditions such as obesity,[117] streptozotocin administration,[118] or insulin infusions,[119] suggesting that increased sodium reabsorption by NCC could be implicated in the development of hypertension in these conditions (see following).

NCC is positively regulated by estradiol[120] and by the acid-base status[121]: Metabolic acidosis induces a decrease in NCC abundance, whereas metabolic alkalosis increases it. Potassium depletion reduces expression of NCCs by a mechanism not related to aldosterone because a decrease in NCC mRNA levels is involved.[122] Finally, NCC protein expression is up-regulated in an animal model of prenatally programmed hypertension[123] and down-regulated in animal models of chronic liver disease[124] and chronic renal failure,[125] suggesting that NCC is implicated in the development of hypertension and the urinary abnormalities observed in these syndromes. Therefore, regulation of NCC expression appears to be an important cog in the overall mechanism by which the kidney regulates sodium excretion.

## Potential Role of NCC in Arterial Hypertension

Given the important physiologic role for the Na⁺-Cl⁻ cotransporters in the kidney, it was expected that mutations in these genes would play a role in human pathophysiology. Because of the resemblance between the inherited hypokalemic metabolic alkalosis syndromes and the clinical and metabolic picture of chronic diuretic intoxication, the NCC (gene SLC12A3) was a strong candidate gene for such a disease. More than 80 different mutations along the human SLC12A3 gene have been found to be present in patients with Gitelman's syndrome,[126-128] and all Gitelman's patients that have been genotyped have mutations in the SLC12A3 gene, suggesting that no other genes are involved in Gitelman's syndrome. The complete linkage that was observed between Gitelman's syndrome and the locus for NCC, located in human chromosome 16, strongly suggested that inactivating mutations of this gene were associated with Gitelman's disease.[126,127,129] Subsequently, a phenotype resembling Gitelman's syndrome was obtained in mice by targeted disruption of the NCC gene,[130] and heterologous expression in *Xenopus laevis* oocytes of mouse NCC cRNA containing some of the point mutations reported in Gitelman's kindreds revealed that the resulting NCC proteins are nonfunctional.[131,132] Thus, inactivating mutations of NCC are the cause of Gitelman's syndrome. One of the major features of this disease is the reduction in the arterial blood pressure. The study of 199 members of a single large family with Gitelman's syndrome, containing 60 subjects with both alleles normal, 113 with mutation in one allele, and 26 with mutations in both alleles, revealed that Gitelman's patients (those having both alleles mutated) develop arterial hypotension, while heterozygous subjects, those with one normal and one mutated allele, do not exhibit a significant decrease in arterial blood pressure. However, urinary Na+:Cr ratio was significantly higher in homozygous and eterozygous persons, as compared with normal subjects, indicating that a compensatory increase in dietary sodium uptake corrected arterial hypotension in heterozygous subjects.[133]

NCC is implicated in the pathophysiology of a salt-dependent hypertension syndrome known as *pseudohypoaldosteronism type II* (PHAII) or *Gordon's syndrome*. PHAII is an autosomal-dominant disease caused by mutations in the gene encoding a particular serine/threonine kinase named WNK4.[134] PHAII is a mirror image of Gitelman's syndrome because PHAII patients develop arterial hypertension accompanied by hyperkalemic metabolic acidosis. Mayan et al.[135] have shown that the PHA syndrome is particularly sensitive to treatment with thiazide diuretics, because the reduction of mean arterial pressure in response to only 20 mg of hydrochlorothiazide in patients with PHAII is 6 to 7 times greater than in patients with essential hypertension. Thus NCC was proposed as a candidate gene for PHAII, but no linkage was observed between the presence of the disease and the NCC locus in PHAII kindreds.[136] However, it has been shown by two independent groups that one function of wild-type WNK4 is to inhibit activity of the Na-Cl cotransporter NCC via reduced cell surface expression of the cotransporter[137,138] and that WNK4-bearing PHAII-type mutations lose the ability to inhibit NCC expression. These observations suggest that loss of WNK4 negative regulation of NCC activity is at least one of the mechanisms for increasing arterial blood pressure in PHAII patients because of an increased reabsorption of salt in the distal nephron.[139] Thus, by regulating the extracellular fluid volume, NCC is important for the regulation of arterial blood pressure and therefore is a candidate gene in the genesis of essential arterial hypertension.

### Thiazide-Type Diuretics in the Treatment of Hypertension

In 1957, Frederick C. Novello and James M. Sprague synthesized chlorothiazide, the first benzothiadiazine that exhibited a strong diuretic effect and was clinically useful,[79] a major breakthrough in the treatment of hypertension. Almost 50 years after the discovery of thiazide diuretics, these compounds are still considered by many clinicians as the first-line drug in the treatment of hypertension. According to the recommendation of the Seventh Report of the Joint National Committee on Prevention, Detection, Evaluation, and Treatment of High Blood Pressure (JNC 7),[140] thiazide diuretics should be used as the initial drug therapy for most hypertensive patients, either alone or in combination with other antihypertensive agents. Thiazide-type diuretics have been investigated in controlled clinical trials of antihypertensive therapy. In most of these trials, including the Antihypertensive and Lipid-Lowering Treatment to Prevent Heart Attack Trial (ALLHAT), thiazides have been superior to other antihypertensive drugs in preventing at least some of the cardiovascular complications of hypertension.[141] Thus, according to JNC 7, thiazides are the recommended drug for initial therapy in most patients with stage 1 hypertension (systolic blood pressure between class 140 and 159 mm Hg and/or diastolic blood pressure between 90 an 99 mm Hg),[140] although the report makes clear that angiotensin-converting enzyme (ACE) inhibitors, angiotensin receptor blockers, β-blockers, or calcium channel blockers can be considered as acceptable alternatives. In addition, JNC 7 recommendations are that thiazide diuretics should also be included when combination therapy is in order. In patients with stage 2 hypertension (systolic blood pressure >160 mm Hg and/or diastolic blood pressure >100 mm Hg) a two-drug combination is recommended, usually a thiazide-type diuretic plus an ACE inhibitor, an angiotensin receptor blocker, a β-blocker, or a calcium channel blocker. Interestingly, despite the fact that JNC VI and 7 recommend thiazide-type diuretics as first-line therapy for hypertension, they appear to be underutilized.[142]

## AMILORIDE CONGENERS

### Transport Mechanisms in the Collecting Duct

ENaCs are expressed in apical plasma membranes of principal cells in the distal nephron (Figure 62–8), extending from the late distal convoluted tubule through the inner medullary collecting duct. These channels are the major pathway that mediates reabsorptive Na+ transport across epithelial cell layers in conjunction with a basolateral Na+,K+-ATPase and are selectively inhibited by submicromolar concentrations of the diuretic amiloride. Epithelial Na+ channels have a key role in the regulation of urinary Na+ reabsorption, extracellular fluid volume homeostasis, and control of blood pressure and are a major site of action of key volume regulatory hormones such as aldosterone.[143]

### Cloning and Characteristics of ENaC

The epithelial Na+ channel is composed of three structurally related subunits—termed α-, β-, and γ-ENaC—that share limited sequence identity.[144] These channels have a tetrameric

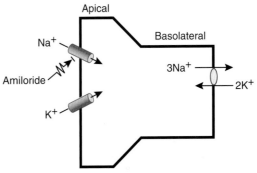

**Figure 62–8** Molecular physiology of sodium reabsorption the principal cells of the collecting duct.

structure consisting of two α-, two β-, and one γ-subunit that surround a central pore.[145] The α-subunits are on opposite sides of the pore, separated by β- and γ-subunits.[146] Figure 62–9 depicts a linear representation of the three subunits. They are polypeptides of 641 to 670 amino acid residues with molecular weight between 72 and 76 kDa. Each subunit has two membrane-spanning domains separated by a large extra-cellular domain and intracellular amino- and carboxyl-termini.[147,148] The extracellular loops are highly glycosylated, increasing the molecular weight of each subunit, and possess several cysteine-rich regions that are conserved in all members of the ENaC family, suggesting that disulfide bridges among isoforms could play an important role in the tertiary structure of the protein. The channel pore is formed by the regions immediately preceding and extending through the second membrane-spanning domain. Sites that restrict K+ perme-ation through the channel and sites where amiloride interacts with the channel are found within the area just preceding the second membrane-spanning domain.[149,150]

ENaCs are members of a growing gene superfamily.[151] Members include genes identified in *Caenorhabditis elegans* based on mutations that result in mechanosensation defects (*mecs*) or neuronal degeneration (*degs*), H+-gated channels (referred to as ASIC) that have a role in nociception, a peptide-gated channel cloned from the marine snail *Helix aspers*, and a family of ion channels found in the fruit fly *Drosophila melanogaster*.

## Regulation of Na+ Channels

ENaC activity is regulated by several hormones that modulate extracellular volume and blood pressure, including aldos-terone, arginine vasopressin, insulin, angiotensin II (via AT₁ receptors in the collecting duct), and endothelin. ENaC activ-ity is also regulated by a variety of factors within the urinary space. For example, serine proteases, such as prostasin, are secreted into the tubular lumen and activate Na+ channels, presumably by cleaving Na+ channel subunits.[152-154] Urinary acidification and mechanical forces, such as shear stress asso-ciated with increases in rates of tubular flow, activate EnaC.[155]

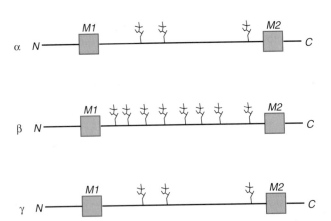

**Figure 62–9** Linear representation of the proposed topology of the epithelial sodium channel α-, β-, and γ-subunits. The boxes in black marked as M1 or M2 are the transmembrane helices. The extracellular loop located between M1 and M2 contains several glycosylation sites (depicted as little evergreen bushes).

Figure 62–10 illustrates the regulation of ENaC surface expression in the apical membrane of collecting duct cells. The C-termini of ENaC subunits have a proline-rich protein interaction module, referred to as a "PY" domain. Nedd4 (neural precursor cells expressed developmentally down-regulated) is a ubiquitin ligase that contains multiple "WW" domains[156] that are protein interaction modules that recog-nize and bind PY domains. WW domains are made up of 35 to 40 amino acid residues containing two conserved trypto-phan (W) residues that are spaced 20 to 22 amino acid residues apart. Nedd4 binds to ENaC β- and γ-subunits through WW-PY interactions and facilitates the transfer of ubiquitin to the ENaC subunits. Channel ubiquitination serves as a signal for internalization of channels from the plas-ma membrane and degradation.[157,158] Mutations described in patients with Liddle's syndrome result in deletions of or muta-tions within the PY domain that disrupt the binding of Nedd4 to ENaC and subsequent channel ubiquitination. Na+ channels with Liddle's syndrome mutations reside at the plasma mem-brane for a significantly longer time than wild-type channels, leading to enhanced Na+ reabsorption by the collecting duct. A number of Nedd4 isoforms have been described, and the role of specific Nedd4 isoforms in the regulation of ENaC is presently being explored.

A number of studies have provided new insights regarding mechanisms by which aldosterone regulates epithelial Na+ channels. Aldosterone increases the expression of the α-subunit of ENaC in specific renal tubular segments, as well as expression of channels at the luminal membrane.[107,159] A grow-ing number of aldosterone-regulated genes have been identi-fied. The serum- and glucocorticoid-regulated kinase (sgk) is an aldosterone-induced protein that, when co-expressed with ENaC, results in an increase in surface expression of Na+ chan-nels.[160] Sgk has a PY motif and binds the protein Nedd4. Subsequent sgk-mediated phosphorylation of Nedd4 prevents the interaction of Nedd4 with ENaC and reduces Nedd4-medi-ated ubiquitination and internalization of ENaC.[161,162]

## Liddle's Syndrome and Pseudohypoaldosteronism Type I

Na+ channel gain-of-function mutations have been identified in patients with Liddle's syndrome, a rare disorder character-ized by volume expansion, hypokalemia, and hypertension. Patients with this disorder have mutations in genes encoding ENaC β- or γ-subunits that result in either truncations of the intracellular carboxyl-termini or amino acid substitutions within the PY motifs of the β- or γ-subunits.[143,163,165] As dis-cussed previously, these mutations are thought to disrupt the binding of Nedd4 to ENaC and prevent Nedd4-dependent inhibition of channel expression. Furthermore, certain com-mon human epithelial Na+ channel polymorphisms segregate with blood pressure (i.e., βT594M), suggesting that these poly-morphisms are associated with altered activity of the chan-nel.[166] Rare mutations of the mineralocortoid receptor that result in receptor activation by progesterone have been associ-ated with early-onset hypertension that is exacerbated by preg-nancy.[167] Specific disorders of mineralocorticoid and glucocor-ticoid metabolism are also associated with hypertension and are reviewed in Chapter 75.

Na+ channel loss-of-function mutations have been identi-fied in patients with an autosomal-recessive variant of type 1

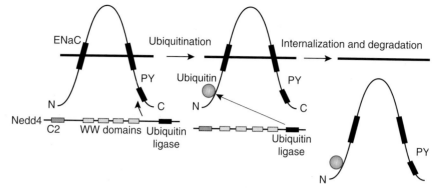

**Figure 62–10** Regulation of ENaC surface expression by Nedd4. (Adapted from Snyder PM.[188])

pseudohypoaldosteronism, a disorder characterized by volume depletion, hypotension, and hyperkalemia.[168] Mutations in the mineralocorticoid receptor have been reported in patients with an autosomal-dominant variant of type 1 pseudohypoaldosteronism, a relatively mild form of pseudohypoaldosteronism that tends to remit with age.[169]

## Amiloride Congeners

Amiloride was discovered during a search for diuretics that could prevent the kaliuresis that was observed with thiazide and loop diuretics.[170] Amiloride induces a mild natriuresis following oral administration while exerting an antikaliuretic effect. Both the natriuresis and antikaliuretic effects are due to inhibition of the epithelial $Na^+$ channel.[171] In the late distal convoluted tubule through the cortical collecting duct, $Na^+$ reabsorption via epithelial $Na^+$ channels is tightly coupled to $K^+$ secretion that is mediated by apical membrane $K^+$ channels. Activation of $Na^+$ channels enhances $K^+$ secretion, whereas inhibition of $Na^+$ channels is associated with an inhibition of $K^+$ secretion. The major apical membrane $K^+$ channel in the distal nephron is a member of the family of inwardly rectifying $K^+$ channels referred to as *Kir1.1* or *ROMK*.[172] Other $K^+$ channels, including a large conductance $Ca^{2+}$-activated $K^+$ channel, commonly referred to as *maxi $K^+$*, also participate in renal $K^+$ secretion in the collecting duct.[173,174]

Increased tubular flow rates in the collecting duct occur with administration of thiazide or loop diuretics. As mentioned previously, increased tubular flow rates in collecting ducts activate epithelial $Na^+$ channels and enhance rates of $Na^+$ reabsorption. Furthermore, an increase in tubular flow rates in collecting ducts activates maxi $K^+$ channels. Thus the kaliuresis observed with thiazide and loop diuretics reflects both flow-dependent activation of epithelial $Na^+$ channels and maxi $K^+$ channels in cortical collecting ducts.

Amiloride is a substituted pyrazinolyguanidine, and it is the charged, or protonated, form of amiloride that blocks the $Na^+$ channel. The pKa of amiloride is 8.8 in water, and amiloride is largely protonated in the distal nephron where urinary acidification occurs.[175] Other organic cations, including triamterene and trimethoprim, inhibit $Na^+$ channels and function as $K^+$-sparing diuretics.[176,177] These organic cations apparently block the channel's pore, and residues that likely participate in amiloride binding have been localized to a region immediately preceding the channel's selectivity filter.[178] Mineralocorticoid antagonists, such as spironolactone and eplerenone, are also $K^+$-sparing diuretics. Spironolactone is often used in the clinical setting of cirrhosis and extracellular fluid volume expansion. Administration of spironolactone in the setting of severe congestive heart failure has been associated with a reduction in mortality.[179] However, side effects associated with administration of spironolactone, including gynecomastia, limit its clinical use. Eplerenone represents a member of a new class of selective mineralocorticoid receptor antagonists that may provide physicians with an alternative to spironolactone that is better tolerated.[180] A recent publication from the Eplerenone Post-Acute Myocardial Infarction Heart Failure Efficacy and Survival Study (EPHESUS) indicated that administration of eplerenone to patients following myocardial infarction complicated by heart failure was associated with a reduction in mortality and morbidity.[181] Eplerenone was extremely well tolerated in the EPHESUS trial.

## Amiloride in the Treatment of Hypertension

Diuretics are used in the treatment of hypertension and edematous states, including congestive heart failure and cirrhosis. Amiloride has been used alone as a diuretic in the treatment of these disorders, although more-potent diuretics that affect different sites in the nephron, including thiazides and loop diuretics, are more frequently used in this setting. Both thiazide and loop diuretics induce kaliuresis, and amiloride is most often administered to prevent kaliuresis, because hypokalemia may lead to further elevations in blood pressure in patients with hypertension.[182,183] In addition, hypokalemia is also associated with insulin resistance, diabetes, arrhythmias, and sudden death.[184-186] Amiloride may be used to prevent hypokalemia and hypertension associated with elevated circulating levels of glucocorticoids or mineralocorticoids and in patients with inherited disorders associated with $Na^+$ channel activation such as Liddle's syndrome. Amiloride also exerts $Mg^{2+}$-sparing effects and the combined use of amiloride and loop diuretics, such as furosemide, may prevent diuretic-induced $Mg^{2+}$ wasting.[187] The major side effect associated with administration of amiloride and other $K^+$-sparing diuretics is hyperkalemia. Although approximately 10% of patients receiving amiloride in the absence of a kaliuretic diuretic may develop hyperkalemia, defined as a serum $K^+$ concentration of greater than 5.5 mEq/L, the incidence of hyperkalemia decreases to a few percent when amiloride is administered with a thiazide diuretic. The incidence of hyperkalemia in patients receiving $K^+$-sparing diuretics increases in patients receiving β-adrenergic blockers or ACE inhibitors. In addition, the incidence of hyperkalemia is increased in patients with renal insufficiency, diabetes mellitus, metabolic or respiratory acidosis, and in the elderly. The use of $K^+$-sparing diuretics is also associated with an increase in urinary pH and decrease in serum bicarbonate concentration, which reflects a decrease in proton secretion in the distal nephron.

# References

1. Guyton AC. Blood pressure control: Special role of the kidneys and body fluids. Science 252(5014):1813-1816, 1991.
2. Lifton RP, Gharavi AG, Geller DS. Molecular mechanisms of human hypertension. Cell 104(4):545-556, 2001.
3. Skou JC. Further investigations on a $Mg^{++}$-$Na^+$-activated adenosintriphosphatase, possibly related to the active, linked transport of $Na^+$ and $K^+$ across the nerve membrane. Biochimica et Biiophysica Acta 42:6-23, 1960.
4. McDonough AA, Farley RA. Regulation of Na,K-ATPase activity. Curr Opin Nephrol Hypertens 2(5):725-734, 1993.
5. Tumlin JA, Hoban CA, Medford RM, et al. Expression of Na-K-ATPase alfa and beta subunit mRNA and protein isoforms in the rat nephron. Am J Physiol (Renal Fluid Electrolyte Physiol) 266:F240-F245, 1994.
6. Berkhin EB, Humphreys MH. Regulation of renal tubular secretion of organic compounds. Kidney Int 59(1):17-30, 2001.
7. Wilcox CS. New insights into diuretic use in patients with chronic renal disease. J Am Soc Nephrol 13(3):798-805, 2002.
8. Brater CD. Diuretic therapy. N Engl J Med 339:387-395, 1998.
9. Lorenz JN, Schultheis PJ, Traynor T, et al. Micropuncture analysis of single-nephron function in NHE3-deficient mice. Am J Physiol 277(3 Pt 2):F447-F453, 1999.
10. Masilamani S, Knepper MA, Burg MB. Urine concentration and dilution. *In* Brenner BM (ed). The Kidney. Philadelphia, Saunders, 2000; pp 595-636.
11. Sun A, Grossman EB, Lombardi M, Hebert SC. Vasopressin alters the mechanism of apical $Cl^-$ entry from $Na^+$:$Cl^-$ to $Na^+$:$K^+$:$2Cl^-$ cotransport in mouse medullary thick ascending limb. J Membrane Biol 120:83-94, 1991.
12. Schnermann J. Juxtaglomerular cell complex in the regulation of renal salt excretion. Am J Physiol (Regulatory Integrative Comp Physiol) 274:R263–R279, 1998.
13. Nielsen S, Maunsbach AB, Ecelbarger CA, et al. Ultrastructural localization of Na-K-2Cl cotransporter in thick ascending limb and macula densa of rat kidney. Am J Physiol 275(6 Pt 2):F885-F893, 1998.
14. Simon DB, Karet FE, Hamdan JM, et al. Bartter's syndrome, hypokalaemic alkalosis with hypercalciuria, is caused by mutations in the Na-K-2Cl cotransporter NKCC2. Nat Genet 13:183-188, 1996.
15. Payne JA, Xu J-C, Haas M, et al. Primary structure, functional expression, and chromosomal localization of the bumetanide-sensitive Na-K-Cl cotransporter in human colon. J Biol Chem 270:17977-17985, 1995.
16. Delpire E, Rauchman MI, Beier DR, et al. Molecular cloning and chromosome localization of a putative basolateral $Na^+$-$K^+$-$2Cl^-$ cotransporter from mouse inner medullary collecting duct (mIMCD-3) cells. J Biol Chem 269:25677-25683, 1994.
17. Mount DB, Baekgard A, Hall AE, et al. Isoforms of the Na-K-2Cl transporter in murine TAL I. Molecular characterization and intrarenal localization. Am J Physiol (Renal Physiol) 276:F347-F358, 1999.
18. Plata C, Meade P, Hall AE, et al. Alternatively spliced isoform of the apical Na-K-Cl cotransporter gene encodes a furosemide sensitive Na-Cl cotransporter. Am J Physiol Renal Physiol 280:F574-F582, 2001.
19. Payne JA, Forbush III B. Alternatively spliced isoforms of the putative renal Na-K-Cl cotransporter are differentially distrib-uted within the rabbit kidney. Proc Natl Acad Sci USA 91:4544-4548, 1994.
20. Igarashi P, Vanden Heuver GB, Payne JA, et al. Cloning, embryonic expression, and alternative splicing of a murine kidney-specific Na-K-Cl cotransporter. Am J Physiol (Renal Fluid Electrolyte Physiol) 269:F406-F418, 1995.
21. Gamba G. Molecular biology of distal nephron sodium transport mechanisms. Kidney Int 56(4):1606-1622, 1999.
22. Burg MB. Thick ascending limb of Henle's loop. Kidney Int 22:454-464, 1982.
23. Rocha AS, Kokko JP. Sodium chloride and water transport in the medullary thick ascending limb of Henle. Evidence for active chloride transport. J Clin Invest 52(3):612-623, 1973.
24. Reeves WB, Molony DA, Andreoli TE. Diluting power of thick limbs of Henle. III. Modulation of in vitro diluting power. Am J Physiol 255(6 Pt 2):F1145-F1154, 1988.
25. Counillon L, Pouyssegur J. The expanding family of eucaryotic $Na(+)/H(+)$ exchangers. J Biol Chem 275(1):1-4, 2000.
26. Hus-Citharel A, Morel F. Coupling of metabolic $CO_2$ production to ion transport in isolated rat thick ascending limbs and collecting tubules. Pflugers Arch 407(4):421-427, 1986.
27. Eveloff J, Bayerdorffer E, Silva P, et al. Sodium-chloride transport in the thick ascending limb of Henle's loop. Oxygen consumption studies in isolated cells. Pflugers Arch 389(3):263-270, 1981.
28. Koenig B, Ricapito S, Kinne R. Chloride transport in the thick ascending limb of Henle's loop: Potassium dependence and stoichiometry of the NaCl cotransport system in plasma membrane vesicles. Pflugers Arch 399(3):173-179, 1983.
29. Burnham C, Karlish SJ, Jorgensen PL. Identification and reconstitution of a $Na^+/K^+/Cl^-$ cotransporter and $K^+$ channel from luminal membranes of renal red outer medulla. Biochim Biophys Acta 821(3):461-469, 1985.
30. Yang T, Huang YG, Singh I, et al. Localization of bumetanide- and thiazide-sensitive Na-K-Cl cotransporters along the rat nephron. Am J Physiol (Renal Fluid Electrolyte Physiol) 271:F931-F939, 1996.
31. Plata C, Meade P, Vazquez N, et al. Functional properties of the apical $Na^+$-$K^+$-$2Cl^-$ cotransporter isoforms. J Biol Chem 277(13):11004-11012, 2002.
32. Gimenez I, Isenring P, Forbush B III. Spatially distributed alternative splice variants of the renal Na-K-Cl cotransporter exhibit dramatically different affinities for the transported ions. J Biol Chem 277(11):8767-8770, 2002.
33. Sasaki S, Imai M. Effects of vasopressin on water and NaCl transport across the in vitro perfused medullary thick ascending limb of Henle's loop of mouse, rat, and rabbit kidneys. Pflugers Arch 383(3):215-221, 1980.
34. Hall DA, Varney DM. Effect of vasopressin on electrical potential difference and chloride transport in mouse medullary thick ascending limb of Henle's loop. J Clin Invest 66(4):792-802, 1980.
35. Gimenez I, Forbush B. Short-term stimulation of the renal Na-K-Cl cotransporter (NKCC2) by vasopressin involves phosphorylation and membrane translocation of the protein. J Biol Chem 278(29):26946-26951, 2003.
36. Plata C, Mount DB, Rubio V, et al. Isoforms of the Na-K-2Cl cotransporter in murine TAL. II. Functional characterization and activation by cAMP. Am J Physiol (Renal Physiol) 276:F359-F366, 1999.
37. Meade P, Hoover RS, Plata C, et al. cAMP-dependent activation of the renal-specific $Na^+$-$K^+$-$2Cl^-$ cotransporter is mediated by regulation of cotransporter trafficking. Am J Physiol Renal Physiol 284(6):F1145-F1154, 2003.
38. Morel F, Chabardes D, Imbert-Teboul M, et al. Multiple hormonal control of adenylate cyclase in distal segments of the rat kidney. Kidney Int 11(Suppl):S55-S62, 1982.

39. Di Stefano A, Wittner M, Nitschke R, et al. Effects of parathyroid hormone and calcitonin on Na⁺, Cl⁻, K⁺, Mg²⁺ and Ca²⁺ transport in cortrical and medullary thick ascending limbs of mouse kidney. Pflugers Arch 417:161-167, 1990.

40. Elalouf JM, Roinel N, de Rouffignac C. Effects of glucagon and PTH on the loop of Henle of rat juxtamedullary nephrons. Kidney Int 29(4):807-813, 1986.

41. Stokes JB. Effect of prostaglandin E2 on chloride transport across the rabbit thick ascending limb of Henle. Selective inhibitions of the medullary portion. J Clin Invest 64(2):495-502, 1979.

42. Torikai S, Kurokawa K. Effect of PGE2 on vasopressin-dependent cell cAMP in isolated single nephron segments. Am J Physiol (Renal Fluid Electrolyte Physiol) 245:F58-F66, 1983.

43. Ortiz PA, Hong NJ, Garvin JL. NO decreases thick ascending limb chloride absorption by reducing Na(+)-K(+)-2Cl(−) cotransporter activity. Am J Physiol Renal Physiol 281(5):F819-F825, 2001.

44. Kim G-H, Ecelbarger CA, Mitchell C, et al. Vasopressin increases Na-K-2Cl cotransporter expression in thick ascending limb of Henle's loop. Am J Physiol (Renal Physiol) 276:F96-F103, 1999.

45. Besseghir K, Trimble ME, Stoner L. Action of ADH on isolated medullary thick ascending limb of the Brattleboro rat. Am J Physiol 251(2 Pt 2):F271-F277, 1986.

46. Fernandez-Llama P, Ecelbarger CA, Ware JA, et al. Cyclooxygenase inhibitors increase Na-K-2Cl cotransporter abundance in thick ascending limb of Henle's loop. Am J Physiol 277(2 Pt 2):F219-F226, 1999.

47. Turban S, Wang XY, Knepper MA. Regulation of NHE3, NKCC2 and NCC abundance in kidney during aldosterone-escape phenomenon: Role of NO. Am J Physiol Renal Physiol 10:1152, 2003.

48. Kwon TH, Nielsen J, Kim YH, et al. Regulation of sodium transporters in the thick ascending limb of rat kidney: Response to angiotensin II. Am J Physiol Renal Physiol 285(1):F152-F165, 2003.

49. Beutler KT, Masilamani S, Turban S, et al. Long-term regulation of ENaC expression in kidney by angiotensin II. Hypertension 41(5):1143-1150, 2003.

50. Brooks HL, Allred AJ, Beutler KT, et al. Targeted proteomic profiling of renal Na(+) transporter and channel abundances in angiotensin II type 1a receptor knockout mice. Hypertension 39(2 Pt 2):470-473, 2002.

51. Bartter FC, Pronove P, Gill JR Jr., et al. Hyperplasia of the juxtaglomerular complex with hyperaldosteronism and hypokalemic alkalosis. A new syndrome. J Am Soc Nephrol 9(3):516-528, 1998.

52. Hebert SC. Bartter syndrome. Curr Opin Nephrol Hypertens 12(5):527-532, 2003.

53. Kurtz CL, Karolyi L, Seyberth HW, et al. A common NKCC2 mutation in Costa Rican Bartter's syndrome patients: Evidence for a founder effect. J Am Soc Nephrol 8(11):1706-1711, 1997.

54. Vargas-Poussou R, Feldman D, Vollmer M, et al. Novel molecular variants of the Na-K-2Cl cotransporter gene are responsible for atenatal Bartter syndrome. Am J Hum Genet 62:1332-1340, 1998.

55. Abdel A, Badawi MH, Yaeesh SA, et al. Bartter's syndrome in Arabic children: Review of 13 cases. Pediatr Int 41(3):299-303, 1999.

56. Bettinelli A, Ciarmatori S, Cesareo L, et al. Phenotypic variability in Bartter syndrome type I. Pediatr Nephrol 14(10-11):940-945, 2000.

57. Simon DB, Karet FE, Rodriguez-Soriano J, et al. Genetic heterogeneity of Bartter's syndrome revealed by mutations in the K⁺ channel, ROMK. Nat Genet 14:152-156, 1996.

58. Karolyi L, Conrad M, Köckerling A, et al. Mutations in the gene encoding the inwardly-rectifying renal potassium channel, ROMK, cause the antenatal variant of Bartter syndrome: Evidence for genetic heterogeneity. International Collaborative Study Group for Bartter-like Syndromes. Hum Mol Genet 6(1):17-26, 1997.

59. Vollmer M, Koehrer M, Topaloglu R, et al. Two novel mutations of the gene for Kir 1.1 (ROMK) in neonatal Bartter syndrome. Pediatr Nephrol 12(1):69-71, 1998.

60. Feldmann D, Alessandri JL, Deschenes G. Large deletion of the 5′ end of the ROMK1 gene causes antenatal Bartter syndrome. J Am Soc Nephrol 9(12):2357-2359, 1998.

61. Derst C, Wischmeyer E, Preisig-Muller R, et al. A hyper-prostaglandin E syndrome mutation in Kir1.1 (renal outer medullary potassium) channels reveals a crucial residue for channel function in Kir1.3 channels. J Biol Chem 273(37):23884-23891, 1998.

62. Schulte U, Hahn H, Konrad M, et al. pH gating of ROMK (K(ir)1.1) channels: Control by an Arg-Lys-Arg triad disrupted in antenatal Bartter syndrome. Proc Natl Acad Sci USA 96(26):15298-15303, 1999.

63. Starremans PF, Der Kemp AM, Knoers NM, et al. Functional implications of mutations in the human renal outer medullary potassium channel (ROMK2) identified in Bartter syndrome. Pflugers Arch 443(3):466-472, 2002.

64. Simon DB, Bindra RS, Mansfield TA, et al. Mutations in the chloride channel gene, CLCNKB, cause Bartter's syndrome type III. Nat Genet 17:171-178, 1997.

65. Konrad M, Vollmer M, Lemmink HH, et al. Mutations in the chloride channel gene CLCNKB as a cause of classic Bartter syndrome. J Am Soc Nephrol 11(8):1449-1459, 2000.

66. Brennan TM, Landau D, Shalev H, et al. Linkage of infantile Bartter syndrome with sensorineural deafness to chromosome 1p. Am J Hum Genet 62(2):355-361, 1998.

67. Vollmer M, Jeck N, Lemmink HH, et al. Antenatal Bartter syndrome with sensorineural deafness: Refinement of the locus on chromosome 1p31. Nephrol Dial Transplant 15(7):970-974, 2000.

68. Birkenhager R, Otto E, Schurmann MJ, et al. Mutation of BSND causes Bartter syndrome with sensorineural deafness and kidney failure. Nat Genet 29(3):310-314, 2001.

69. Vargas-Poussou R, Huang C, Hulin P, et al. Functional characterization of a calcium-sensing receptor mutation in severe autosomal dominant hypocalcemia with a bartter-like syndrome. J Am Soc Nephrol 13(9):2259-2266, 2002.

70. Watanabe S, Fukumoto S, Chang H, et al. Association between activating mutations of calcium-sensing receptor and Bartter's syndrome. Lancet 360(9334):692-694, 2002.

71. Ellison DH, Velazquez H, Wright FS. Thiazide-sensitive sodium chloride cotransport in early distal tubule. Am J Physiol (Renal Fluid Electrolyte Physiol) 253:F546-F554, 1987.

72. Doucet A. Function and control of Na-K-ATPase in single nephron segments of the mammalian kidney. Kidney Int 34:749-760, 1988.

73. Reilly RF, Ellison DH. Mammalian distal tubule: Physiology, pathophysiology, and molecular anatomy. Physiol Rev 80(1):277-313, 2000.

74. Loffing J, Kaissling B. Sodium and calcium transport pathways along the mammalian distal nephron: from rabbit to human. Am J Physiol Renal Physiol 284(4):F628-F643, 2003.

75. Loffing J, Loffing-Cueni D, Valderrabano V, et al. Distribution of transcellular calcium and sodium transport pathways along mouse distal nephron. Am J Physiol Renal Physiol 281(6):F1021-F1027, 2001.

76. Obermuller N, Bernstein P, Velázquez H, et al. Expression of the thiazide-sensitive Na-Cl cotransporter in rat and human kidney. Am J Physiol (Renal Fluid Electrolyte Physiol) 269:F900-F910, 1995.

77. Campean V, Kricke J, Ellison D, et al. Localization of thiazide-sensitive Na(+)-Cl(−) cotransport and associated gene products in mouse DCT. Am J Physiol Renal Physiol 281(6):F1028-F1035, 2001.

78. Gamba G, Miyanoshita A, Lombardi M, et al. Molecular cloning, primary structure and characterization of two members of the mammalian electroneutral sodium-(potassium)-chloride cotransporter family expressed in kidney. J Biol Chem 269:17713-17722, 1994.

79. Novello FC, Sprague JM. Benzothiadiazine dioxides as novel diuretics. J Am Chem Soc 79:2028-2029, 1957.

80. Kunau RT, Weller DR, Webb HL. Clarification of the site of action of chlorothiazide in the rat nephron. J Clin Invest 56:410-407, 1975.

81. Stokes JB, Lee I, D'Amico M. Sodium chloride absorption by the urinary bladder of the winter flounder: A thiazide-sensitive, electrically neutral transport system. J Clin Invest 74:7-16, 1984.

82. Renfro JL. Interdependence of active Na$^+$ and Cl$^-$ transport by the isolated urinary bladder of the teleost, pseudopleuronectes americanus. J Exp Zool 199:383-390, 1977.

83. Renfro JL. Water and ion transport by the urinary bladder of the teleost Pseudopleuronectus americanus. Am J Physiol 228:52-61, 1975.

84. Beaumont K, Vaughn DA, Fanestil DD. Thiazide diuretic receptors in rat kidney: Identification with [$^3$H]metolazone. Proc Natl Acad Sci USA 85:2311-2314, 1988.

85. Tran JM, Farrell MA, Fanestil DD. Effect of ions on binding of the thiazide-type diuretic metolazone to kidney membrane. Am J Physiol (Renal Fluid Electrolyte Physiol) 258:F908-F915, 1990.

86. Monroy A, Plata C, Hebert SC, Gamba G. Characterization of the thiazide-sensitive Na(+)-Cl(−) cotransporter: A new model for ions and diuretics interaction. Am J Physiol Renal Physiol 279(1):F161-F169, 2000.

87. Costanzo LS. Localization of diuretic action in microperfused rat distal tubules: Ca and Na transport. Am J Physiol (Renal Fluid Electrolyte Physiol) 248:F527-F535, 1985.

88. Gesek FA, Friedman PA. Mechanism of calcium transport stimulated by chlorothiazide in mouse distal convoluted tubule cells. J Clin Invest 90:429-438, 1992.

89. Ray WA, Griffin MR, Downey W, Melton III LJ. Long-term use of thiazide diuretics and risk of hip fracture. Lancet I:687-690, 1989.

90. Wasnich R, Davis J, Ross P, Vogel J. Effect of thiazide on rates of bone mineral loss: A longitudinal study. Br Med J 301:1303-1305, 1990.

91. Gamba G, Saltzberg SN, Lombardi M, et al. Primary structure and functional expression of a cDNA encoding the thiazide-sensitive, electroneutral sodium-chloride cotransporter. Proc Natl Acad Sci USA 90:2749-2753, 1993.

92. Li JH, Zuzack JS, Kau ST. Winter flounder urinary bladder as a model tissue for assessing the potency of thiazide diuretics. *In* Puschett JB, Greenberg A (eds). Diuretics III: Chemistry, Pharmacology and Clinical Applications. New York, Elsevier Science Publishing, 1990; pp 107-10.

93. Kyte J, Doolittle RF. A simple method for displaying the hydropathic character of a protein. J Mol Biol 157:105-132, 1982.

94. Hoover RS, Poch E, Monroy A, et al. N-glycosylation at two sites critically alters thiazide binding and activity of the rat thiazide-sensitive Na(+):Cl(−) cotransporter. J Am Soc Nephrol 14(2):271-282, 2003.

95. Kim G-H, Masilamani S, Turner R, et al. The thiazide-sensitive Na-Cl cotransporter is an aldosterone-induced protein. Proc Natl Acad Sci USA 95:14552-14557, 1998.

96. Xu J-C, Lytle C, Zhu TT, et al. Molecular cloning and functional expression of the bumetanide-sensitive Na-K-Cl cotransporter. Proc Natl Acad Sci USA 91:2201-2205, 1994.

97. Gillen CM, Brill S, Payne JA, Forbush III B. Molecular cloning and functional expression of the K-Cl cotransporter from rabbit, rat and human. A new member of the cation-chloride cotransporter family. J Biol Chem 271:16237-16244, 1996.

98. Payne JA, Stevenson TJ, Donaldson LF. Molecular characterization of a putative K-Cl cotransporter in rat brain. A neuronal-specific isoform. J Biol Chem 271:16245-16252, 1996.

99. Caron L, Rousseau F, Gagnon E, Isenring P. Cloning and functional characterization of a cation Cl-cotransporter interacting protein. J Biol Chem 275:32027-32036, 2000.

100. Mount DB, Arias I, Xie Q, et al. Cloning and characterization of SLC12A9, a new member of the cation-chloride cotransporter gene family. FASEB J 16:A807, 2002.

101. Knepper MA, Brooks HL. Regulation of the sodium transporters NHE3, NKCC2 and NCC in the kidney. Curr Opin Nephrol Hypertens 10(5):655-659, 2001.

102. Knepper MA. Proteomics and the kidney. J Am Soc Nephrol 13(5):1398-1408, 2002.

103. Knepper MA, Masilamani S. Targeted proteomics in the kidney using ensembles of antibodies. Acta Physiol Scand 173(1):11-21, 2001.

104. Hierholzer K, Wiederholt M, Stolte H. [The impairment of sodium resorption in the proximal and distal convolution of adrenalectomized rats]. Pflugers Arch Gesamte Physiol Menschen Tiere 291(1):43-62, 1966.

105. Velazquez H, Bartiss A, Bernstein P, et al. Adrenal steroids stimulate thiazide-sensitive NaCl transport by rat renal distal tubules. Am J Physiol (Renal Fluid Electrolyte Physiol) 270:F211-F219, 1996.

106. Fanestil DD. Steroid regulation of thiazide-sensitive transport. Semin Nephrol 12:18-23, 1992.

107. Masilamani S, Kim GH, Mitchell C, et al. Aldosterone-mediated regulation of ENaC alpha, beta, and gamma subunit proteins in rat kidney. J Clin Invest 104(7):R19-R23, 1999.

108. Masilamani S, Wang X, Kim GH, et al. Time course of renal Na-K-ATPase, NHE3, NKCC2, NCC, and ENaC abundance changes with dietary NaCl restriction. Am J Physiol Renal Physiol 283(4):F648-F657, 2002.

109. Nielsen J, Kwon TH, Masilamani S, et al. Sodium transporter abundance profiling in the kidney: Effect of spironolactone. Am J Physiol Renal Physiol 283:F923-F933, 2002.

110. Abdallah JG, Schrier RW, Edelstein C, et al. Loop diuretic infusion increases thiazide-sensitive Na$^+$/Cl$^-$ cotransporter abundance: Role of aldosterone. J Am Soc Nephrol 12(7):1335-1341, 2001.

111. Moreno G, Merino A, Mercado A, et al. Electronuetral Na-coupled cotransporter expression in the kidney during variations of NaCl and water metabolism. Hypertension 31:1002-1006, 1998.

112. Wolf K, Castrop H, Riegger GA, et al. Differential gene regulation of renal salt entry pathways by salt load in the distal nephron of the rat. Pflugers Arch 442(4):498-504, 2001.

113. Ecelbarger CA, Kim GH, Wade JB, Knepper MA. Regulation of the abundance of renal sodium transporters and channels by vasopressin. Exp Neurol 171(2):227-234, 2001.

114. Ecelbarger CA, Knepper MA, Verbalis JG. Increased abundance of distal sodium transporters in rat kidney during vasopressin escape. J Am Soc Nephrol 12(2):207-217, 2001.

115. Wang XY, Masilamani S, Nielsen J, et al. The renal thiazide-sensitive Na-Cl cotransporter as mediator of the aldosterone-escape phenomenon. J Clin Invest 108(2):215-222, 2001.

116. Majid DSA, Navar GL. Blockade of distal nephron sodium transport attenuates pressure natriuresis in dogs. Hypertension 23:1040-1045, 1994.

117. Bickel CA, Verbalis JG, Knepper MA, et al. Increased renal Na-K-ATPase, NCC, and beta-ENaC abundance in obese Zucker rats. Am J Physiol Renal Physiol 281(4):F639-F648, 2001.

118. Ward DT, Yau SK, Mee AP, et al. Functional, molecular, and biochemical characterization of streptozotocin-induced diabetes. J Am Soc Nephrol 12(4):779-790, 2001.

119. Ecelbarger CA, Bickel CA, Verbalis JG, et al. Regulation of Na-dependent cotransporter and Na channel abundance by insulin. J Am Soc Nephrol 11:27A, 2002.

120. Verlander JM, Tran TM, Zhang L, et al. Estradiol enhances thiazide-sensitive NaCl cotransporter density in the apical plasma membrane of the distal convoluted tubule in ovariectomized rats. J Clin Invest 101:1661-1669, 1998.

121. Kim GH, Martin SW, Fernandez-Llama P, et al. Long-term regulation of renal Na-dependent cotransporters and ENaC: Response to altered acid-base intake. Am J Physiol Renal Physiol 279(3):F459-F467, 2000.

122. Amlal H, Wang Z, Soleimani M. Potassium depletion down-regulates chloride-absorbing transporters in rat kidney. J Clin Invest 101:1045-1054, 1998.

123. Manning J, Beutler K, Knepper MA, et al. Upregulation of renal BSC1 and TSC in prenatally programmed hypertension. Am J Physiol Renal Physiol 283(1):F202-F206, 2002.

124. Fernandez-Llama P, Jimenez W, Bosch-Marce M, et al. Dysregulation of renal aquaporins and Na-Cl cotransporter in CCl4-induced cirrhosis. Kidney Int 58(1):216-228, 2000.

125. Kwon TH, Kiaer J, Ndez-Llama P, et al. Altered expression of Na transporters NHE-3, NaPi-II, Na-K-ATPase, BSC-1, and TSC in CRF rat kidneys. Am J Physiol 277(2 Pt 2):F257-F270, 1999.

126. Simon DB, Nelson-Williams C, Johnson-Bia M, et al. Gitelman's variant of Bartter's syndrome, inherited hypokalaemic alkalosis, is caused by mutations in the thiazide-sensitive Na-Cl cotransporter. Nat Genet 12:24-30, 1996.

127. Mastroianni N, Bettinelli A, Bianchetti M, et al. Novel molecular variants of the Na-Cl cotransporter gene are responsible for Gitelman syndrome. Am J Hum Genet 59:1019-1026, 1996.

128. Monnens L, Bindels R, Grünfeld P. Gitelman syndrome comes of age. Nephrol Dial Transplant 13:1617-1619, 1998.

129. Mastroianni N, DeFusco M, Zollo M, et al. Molecular cloning, expression pattern, and chromosomal localization of the human Na-Cl thiazide-sensitive cotransporter (SLC12A3). Genomics 35:486-493, 1996.

130. Schultheis PJ, Lorenz JN, Meneton P, et al. Phenotype resembling Gitelman's syndrome in mice lacking the apical Na$^+$-Cl$^-$ cotransporter of the distal convoluted tubule. J Biol Chem 273:29450-29155, 1998.

131. Kunchaparty S, Palcso M, Berkman J, et al. Defective processing and expression of thiazide-sensitive Na-Cl cotransporter as a cause of Gitelman's syndrome. Am J Physiol 277(4 Pt 2): F643-F649, 1999.

132. De Jong JC, Van Der Vliet WA, van den Heuvel LP, et al. Functional expression of mutations in the human NaCl cotransporter: Evidence for impaired routing mechanisms in Gitelman's syndrome. J Am Soc Nephrol 13(6):1442-1448, 2002.

133. Cruz DN, Simon DB, Nelson-Williams C, et al. Mutations in the Na-Cl cotransporter reduce blood pressure in humans. Hypertension 37(6):1458-1464, 2001.

134. Wilson FH, Disse-Nicodeme S, Choate KA, et al. Human hypertension caused by mutations in WNK kinases. Science 293(5532):1107-1112, 2001.

135. Mayan H, Vered I, Mouallem M, et al. Pseudohypoaldosteronism type II: Marked sensitivity to thiazides, hypercalciuria, normomagnesemia, and low bone mineral density. J Clin Endocrinol Metab 87(7):3248-3254, 2002.

136. Simon DB, Farfel Z, Ellison D, et al. Examination of the thiazide-sensitive Na-Cl cotransporter as a candidate gene in Gordon's syndrome. J Am Soc Nephrol 6:632, 1995.

137. Vazquez N, Monroy A, Dorantes E, et al. Functional differences between flounder and rat thiazide-sensitive Na-Cl cotransporter. Am J Physiol Renal Physiol 282(4):F599-F607, 2002.

138. Yang CL, Angell J, Mitchell R, et al. WNK kinases regulate thiazide-sensitive Na-Cl cotransport. J Clin Invest 111(7): 1039-1045, 2003.

139. Rossier BC. Negative regulators of sodium transport in the kidney: Key factors in understanding salt-sensitive hypertension? J Clin Invest 111(7):947-950, 2003.

140. Chobanian AV, Bakris GL, Black HR, et al. The Seventh Report of the Joint National Committee on Prevention, Detection, Evaluation, and Treatment of High Blood Pressure: The JNC 7 Report. JAMA 289(19):2560-2571, 2003.

141. Major outcomes in high-risk hypertensive patients randomized to angiotensin-converting enzyme inhibitor or calcium channel blocker vs diuretic: The Antihypertensive and Lipid-Lowering Treatment to Prevent Heart Attack Trial (ALLHAT). JAMA 288(23):2981-2997, 2002.

142. Psaty BM, Manolio TA, Smith NL, et al. Time trends in high blood pressure control and the use of antihypertensive medications in older adults: the Cardiovascular Health Study. Arch Intern Med 162(20):2325-2332, 2002.

143. Rossier BC, Pradervand S, Schild L, et al. Epithelial sodium channel and the control of sodium balance: Interaction between genetic and environmental factors. Annu Rev Physiol 64:877-897, 2002.

144. Canessa CM, Schild L, Buell G, et al. Amiloride-sensitive epithelial Na$^+$ channel is made of three homologous subunits. Nature 367:463–467, 1994.

145. Kosari F, Sheng S, Li J, et al. Subunit stoichiometry of the epithelial sodium channel. J Biol Chem 273(22):13469-13474, 1998.

146. Firsov D, Gautschi I, Merillat A-M, et al. The heterotetrameric architecture of the epithelial sodium channel (ENaC). EMBO J 7:344-352, 1998.

147. Snyder PM, McDonald FJ, Stokes JB, et al. Membrane topology of the amiloride-sensitive epithelial sodium channel. J Biol Chem 269(39):24379-24383, 1994.

148. Canessa CM, Merillat A-M, Rossier BC. Membrane topology of the epithelial sodium channel in intact cells. Am J Physiol (Cell Physiol) 267:C1682-C1690, 1994.

149. Sheng S, Li J, McNulty KA, et al. Characterization of the selectivity filter of the epithelial sodium channel. J Biol Chem 275(12):8572-8581, 2000.

150. Snyder PM, Olson DR, Bucher DB. A pore segment in DEG/ENaC Na(+) channels. J Biol Chem 274(40):28484-28490, 1999.

151. Kellenberger S, Schild L. Epithelial sodium channel/degenerin family of ion channels: A variety of functions for a shared structure. Physiol Rev 82(3):735-767, 2002.

152. Vallet V, Chraibi A, Gaeggeler H-P, et al. An epithelial serine protease activates the amiloride-sensitive sodium channel. Nature 389:607-610, 1997.

153. Vuagniaux G, Vallet V, Jaeger NF, et al. Synergistic activation of ENaC by three membrane-bound channel-activating serine proteases (mCAP1, mCAP2, and mCAP3) and serum- and glucocorticoid-regulated kinase (Sgk1) in Xenopus Oocytes. J Gen Physiol 120(2):191-201, 2002.

154. Hughey RP, Mueller GM, Bruns JB, et al. Maturation of the epithelial Na+ channel involves proteolytic processing of the α- and γ-subunits. J Biol Chem 278(39):37073-37082, 2003.

155. Satlin LM, Sheng S, Woda CB, et al. Epithelial Na(+) channels are regulated by flow. Am J Physiol Renal Physiol 280(6): F1010-F1018, 2001.

156. Staub O, Dho S, Henry PC, et al. WW domains of Nedd4 binds to the proline-rich PY motifs in the epithelial Na$^+$ channel deleted in Liddle's syndrome. EMBO J 15:2371-2380, 1996.

157. Staub O, Gautschi I, Ishikawa T, et al. Regulation of stability and function of the epithelial Na$^+$ channel (ENaC) by ubiquitination. EMBO J 16:6325-6336, 1997.

158. Staub O, Abriel H, Plant P, et al. Regulation of the epithelial Na+ channel by Nedd4 and ubiquitination. Kidney Int 57(3):809-815, 2000.

159. Loffing J, Zecevic M, Feraille E, et al. Aldosterone induces rapid apical translocation of ENaC in early portion of renal collecting system: Possible role of SGK. Am J Physiol Renal Physiol 280(4):F675-F682, 2001.

160. Chen S-Y, Bhargava A, Mastroberardino L, et al. Epithelial sodium channel regulated by aldosterone-induced protein sgk. Proc Natl Acad Sci USA 96:2514-2519, 1999.

161. Debonneville C, Flores SY, Kamynina E, et al. Phosphorylation of Nedd4-2 by Sgk1 regulates epithelial Na(+) channel cell surface expression. EMBO J 20(24):7052-7059, 2001.

162. Snyder PM, Olson DR, Thomas BC. Serum and glucocorticoid-regulated kinase modulates Nedd4-2-mediated inhibition of the epithelial Na+ channel. J Biol Chem 277(1):5-8, 2002.

163. Shimkets RA, Warnock DG, Bositis CM, et al. Liddle's syndrome: Heritable human hypertension caused by mutations in the beta subunit of the epithelial sodium channel. Cell 79: 407-414, 1994.

164. Hansson JH, Nelson-Williams C, Suzuki H, et al. Hypertension caused by a truncated epithelial sodium channel gamma subunit: Genetic heterogeneity of Liddle syndrome. Nat Genet 11(1):76-82, 1995.

165. Tamura H, Schild L, Enomoto N, et al. Liddle disease caused by a missense mutation of b subunit of the epithelila sodium channel gene. J Clin Invest 97:1780-1784, 1996.

166. Su YR, Rutkowski MP, Klanke CA, et al. A novel variant of the beta-subunit of the amiloride-sensitive sodium channel in African Americans. J Am Soc Nephrol 7(12):2543-2549, 1996.

167. Geller DS, Farhi A, Pinkerton N, et al. Activating mineralocorticoid receptor mutation in hypertension exacerbated by pregnancy. Science 289(5476):119-123, 2000.

168. Chang SS, Grunder S, Hanukoglu A, et al. Mutations in subunit of the epithelial sodium channel cause salt wasting with hyperkalaemic acidosis, pseudohypoaldosteronism type 1. Nat Genet 12:248-253, 1996.

169. Geller DS, Rodriguez-Soriano J, Vallo BA, et al. Mutations in the mineralocorticoid receptor gene cause autosomal dominant pseudohypoaldosteronism type I. Nat Genet 19(3):279-281, 1998.

170. Bull MB, Laragh JH. Amiloride. A potassium-sparing natriuretic agent. Circulation 37(1):45-53, 1968.

171. Kleyman TR, Cragoe EJ, Jr. The mechanism of action of amiloride. Semin Nephrol 8(3):242-248, 1988.

172. Ho K, Nichols CG, Lederer J, et al. Cloning and expression of an inwardly rectifying ATP-regulated potassium channel. Nature 362:31-38, 1993.

173. Woda CB, Bragin A, Kleyman TR, et al. Flow-dependent K+ secretion in the cortical collecting duct is mediated by a maxi-K channel. Am J Physiol Renal Physiol 280(5):F786-F793, 2001.

174. Woda CB, Miyawaki N, Ramalakshmi S, et al. Ontogeny of flow-stimulated potassium secretion in rabbit cortical collecting duct: Functional and molecular aspects. Am J Physiol Renal Physiol 285(4):F629-F639, 2003.

175. Kleyman TR, Cragoe EJ. Amiloride and its analogs as tools in the study of ion transport. J Membrane Biol 105:1-21, 1988.

176. Li JH, Lindemann B. Competitive blocking of epithelial sodium channels by organic cations: The relationship between macroscopic and microscopic inhibition constants. J Membr Biol 76(3):235-251, 1983.

177. Choi MJ, Fernandez PC, Patnaik A, et al. Brief report: Trimethoprim-induced hyperkalemia in a patient with AIDS. N Engl J Med 328(10):703-706, 1993.

178. Schild L, Schneeberger E, Gautschi I, et al. Identification of amino acid residues in the a, b and g subunits of the epithelial sodium channel (ENaC) involved in amiloride block and ion permeation. J Gen Physiol 109:15-26, 1997.

179. Pitt B, Zannad F, Remme WJ, et al. The effect of spironolactone on morbidity and mortality in patients with severe heart failure. Randomized Aldactone Evaluation Study Investigators. N Engl J Med 341(10):709-717, 1999.

180. Brown NJ. Eplerenone: Cardiovascular protection. Circulation 107(19):2512-2518, 2003.

181. Pitt B, Remme W, Zannad F, et al. Eplerenone, a selective aldosterone blocker, in patients with left ventricular dysfunction after myocardial infarction. N Engl J Med 348(14):1309-1321, 2003.

182. Krishna GG, Shulman MD, Narins RG. Clinical use of the potassium-sparing diuretics. Semin Nephrol 8(4):354-364, 1988.

183. Krishna GG, Kapoor SC. Potassium depletion exacerbates essential hypertension. Ann Intern Med 115(2):77-83, 1991.

184. Freis ED. The efficacy and safety of diuretics in treating hypertension. Ann Intern Med 122:223-226, 1995.

185. Prichard BN, Owens CW, Woolf AS. Adverse reactions to diuretics. Eur Heart J 13(Suppl G):96-103, 1992.

186. Helderman JH, Elahi D, Andersen DK, et al. Prevention of the glucose intolerance of thiazide diuretics by maintenance of body potassium. Diabetes 32(2):106-111, 1983.

187. Ryan MP. Magnesium and potassium-sparing diuretics. Magnesium 5(5-6):282-292, 1986.

188. Snyder PM. The epithelial Na+ channel: Cell surface insertion and retrieval in Na+ homeostasis and hypertension. Endocr Rev 23(2):258-275, 2002.

# β-Adrenergic Blockers
## William H. Frishman

The seventh report of the Joint National Committee on Prevention, Detection, Evaluation, and Treatment of High Blood Pressure (JNC 7) from the National High Blood Pressure Education Program of the National Heart Lung and Blood Institute has reiterated the recommendation of JNC III thru VI that β-adrenergic blockers are appropriate alternatives as first-line treatment for hypertension.[1] These recommendations are based on the reduction of patient morbidity and mortality when these drugs are used in large clinical trials. Although there is no consensus as to the mechanisms by which β-blocking drugs lower blood pressure (BP), it is probable that some or all of the modes of action referred to in Box 63–1 are involved.[2]

Thirteen orally active β-adrenergic blockers are approved in the United States for the treatment of hypertension (Table 63–1). In addition, intravenous labetalol is approved for the management of hypertensive emergencies. Oral bisoprolol in combination with a very-low-dose diuretic is available as a first-line antihypertensive treatment, the first such β-blocker combination so approved for the treatment of hypertension.[3] The various β-blocking agents differ in terms of the presence or absence of intrinsic sympathomimetic activity (ISA), membrane-stabilizing activity (MSA), $\beta_1$-selectivity, α-adrenergic blocking activity, and relative potencies and durations of action. Nevertheless, all β-blockers studied to date appear to have favorable BP-lowering effects when used in appropriate dosages.[4,5]

## PHARMACODYNAMIC PROPERTIES

### Membrane-Stabilizing Activity

At concentrations well above therapeutic levels, certain β-blockers have a quinidine-like or local anesthetic membrane-stabilizing effect on the cardiac action potential. There is no evidence that MSA is responsible for any direct negative inotropic effect of the β-blockers, because drugs with and without this property can depress left ventricular function. However, MSA can manifest itself clinically with massive β-blocker intoxications.[2,4]

### $\beta_1$-Selectivity

When used in low doses, $\beta_1$-selective blocking agents such as acebutolol, betaxolol, bisoprolol, esmolol, atenolol, and metoprolol inhibit cardiac $\beta_2$-receptors but have less influence on bronchial and vascular β-adrenergic receptors ($\beta_2$). In higher doses, however, $\beta_1$-selective blocking agents also block $\beta_2$ receptors. Accordingly, $\beta_1$-selective agents may be safer than nonselective ones in patients with obstructive pulmonary disease, because $\beta_2$ receptors remain available to mediate adrenergic bronchodilation. However, even selective β-blockers may aggravate bronchospasm in certain patients, and so these drugs should generally not be used in patients with bronchospastic disease.[2,4]

A second theoretical advantage is that unlike nonselective β-blockers, $\beta_1$-selective blockers in low doses may not block the $\beta_2$ receptors that mediate dilation of arterioles. It is possible that leaving the $\beta_2$ receptors unblocked and responsive to epinephrine may be functionally important in some patients with asthma, hypoglycemia, hypertension, or peripheral vascular disease treated with β-adrenergic blocking drugs.[2,4]

### Intrinsic Sympathomimetic Activity or Partial Agonist Activity

Certain β-adrenergic receptor blockers possess partial agonist activity at $\beta_1$-adrenergic receptor sites, $\beta_2$-adrenergic receptor sites, or both. In a β-blocker, this property is identified as a slight cardiac stimulation, which can be blocked by propranolol. The β-blockers with this property slightly activate the β receptor in addition to preventing the access of natural or synthetic catecholamines to the receptor. In the treatment of patients with arrhythmias, angina pectoris of effort, or hypertension, drugs with mild-to-moderate partial agonist activity appear to be as efficacious as β-blockers lacking this property. It is still debated whether the presence of partial agonist activity in a β-blocker constitutes an overall advantage or disadvantage in cardiac therapy. Drugs with partial agonist activity cause less slowing of the heart rate at rest than do propranolol and metoprolol, although the increments in heart rate with exercise are similarly blunted. β-Blocking agents with nonselective partial agonist activity reduce peripheral vascular resistance and may also cause less depression or atrioventricular conduction delay compared with drugs lacking this property.[2-6]

### α-Adrenergic Activity

Carvedilol and labetalol are β-blockers with antagonistic properties at both α- and β-adrenergic receptors and direct vasodilator activity. Like other β-blockers, they are useful in the treatment of hypertension and angina pectoris. However, unlike most β-blocking drugs, the additional α-adrenergic blocking actions of carvedilol and labetalol lead to a reduction in peripheral vascular resistance that may maintain cardiac output. Whether concomitant α-adrenergic blocking activity is actually advantageous in a β-blocker remains to be determined.[2,4]

## PHARMACOKINETIC PROPERTIES

Although the β-adrenergic blocking drugs as a group have similar therapeutic effects, their pharmacokinetics are markedly different (Tables 63–2 and 63–3). Their varied aromatic ring structures lead to differences in completeness of

**Box 63-1** Proposed Mechanisms to Explain the Antihypertensive Actions of β-Blockers

1. Reduction in cardiac output
2. Central nervous system effect
3. Inhibition of renin-angiotensin-aldosterone system
4. Reduction in plasma volume
5. Reduction in vasomotor tone
6. Reduction in peripheral vascular resistance
7. Improvement in vascular compliance
8. Resetting of baroreceptor levels
9. Effects on prejunctional β receptors: reduction in norepinephrine release
10. Attenuation of pressor response to catecholamines with exercise and stress

(From Frishman WH. Clinical Pharmacology of the β Adrenoceptor Blocking Drugs, 2nd ed. Norwalk, Appleton-Century-Crofts, 1984. With permission.)

gastrointestinal absorption, amount of first-pass hepatic metabolism, lipid solubility, protein binding, extent of distribution in the body, penetration into the brain, concentration in the heart, rate of hepatic biotransformation, pharmacologic activity of metabolites, and renal clearance of the drugs and their metabolites, which may influence their clinical usefulness in some patients.[2,4,7]

The β-blockers can be divided by their pharmacokinetic properties into two broad categories: those eliminated by hepatic metabolism, which tend to have relatively short plasma half-lives, and those eliminated unchanged by the kidney, which tend to have longer half-lives. Propranolol and metoprolol are both lipid soluble, are almost completely absorbed by the small intestine, and are largely metabolized by the liver. They tend to have highly variable bioavailability and relatively short plasma half-lives. A lack of correlation between the duration of clinical pharmacologic effect and plasma half-life may allow these drugs to be administered once or twice daily.[2,4]

In contrast, agents such as atenolol and nadolol are more water soluble, are incompletely absorbed through the gut, and are eliminated unchanged by the kidney. They tend to have less variable bioavailability in patients with normal renal function, in addition to longer half-lives, allowing one dose a day. The longer half-lives may be useful in patients who find compliance with frequent β-blocker dosing a problem.[2,4]

Extended-release formulations of metoprolol and propranolol are available that allow once-daily dosing of these drugs. Studies have shown that both long-acting propranolol and metoprolol provide much smoother curves of daily plasma levels than do comparable divided doses of conventional propranolol and metoprolol. In addition, a delayed-release/extended-release chronotherapeutic formulation of propranolol has become available, which is dosed at night to address circadian variations in BP in an attempt to blunt early morning elevations while providing 24-hour BP control.[8] Early morning BP peaks have been associated with increased cardiovascular and cerebrovascular events, but the clinical significance of early morning BP blunting with delayed-release drugs has not yet been shown.[9] Sublingual and nasal spray formulations that can provide immediate β-blockade have been tested in clinical trials.[2,4]

Ultra-short-acting β-blockers are now available and may be useful where a short duration of action is desired (e.g., in patients with questionable congestive heart failure [CHF]). One of these compounds, esmolol, a $\beta_1$-selective drug has been shown to be useful in the treatment of perioperative hypertension and supraventricular tachycardias. The short half-life (approximately 15 minutes) relates to the rapid metabolism of the drug by circulating and hepatic esterases. Metabolism does not seem to be altered by disease states.[10]

**Table 63-1** Pharmacodynamic Properties of β-Adrenergic Blocking Drugs Used for Hypertension in the United States

| Drug | $\beta_1$-Blockade Potency Ratio (Propranolol = 1.0) | Relative $\beta_1$-Selectivity | Intrinsic Sympathomimetic Activity | Membrane-Stabilizing Activity |
|---|---|---|---|---|
| Acebutolol | 0.3 | + | + | + |
| Atenolol | 1.0 | ++ | 0 | 0 |
| Betaxolol | 1.0 | ++ | 0 | + |
| Bisoprolol* | 10.0 | ++ | 0 | 0 |
| Carteolol | 10.0 | 0 | + | 0 |
| Carvedilol† | 10.0 | 0 | 0 | ++ |
| Labetalol‡ | 0.3 | 0 | +? | 0 |
| Metoprolol | 1.0 | ++ | 0 | 0 |
| Nadolol | 1.0 | 0 | 0 | 0 |
| Penbutolol | 1.0 | 0 | + | 0 |
| Pindolol | 6.0 | 0 | ++ | + |
| Propranolol | 1.0 | 0 | 0 | ++ |
| Timolol | 6.0 | 0 | 0 | 0 |

(Adapted from Frishman WH. Alpha and beta-adrenergic blocking drugs. In Frishman WH, Sonnenblick EH, Sica DA (eds). Cardiovascular Pharmacotherapeutics, 2nd ed. New York, McGraw Hill, 2003; pp 67-97.)
*Bisoprolol is also approved as a first-line antihypertensive therapy in combination with a very-low-dose diuretic.
†Carvedilol has additional $\alpha_1$-adrenergic blocking activity without peripheral $\beta_2$-agonism.
‡Labetalol has additional $\alpha_1$-adrenergic blocking activity and direct vasodilatory activity ($\beta_2$-agonism); it is available for use in intravenous form for hypertensive emergencies.

**Table 63-2** Pharmacokinetic Properties of β-Adrenoceptor Blocking Drugs Used in Hypertension

| Drug | Extent of Absorption (% of Dose) | Extent of Bioavailability (% of Dose) | Dose-Dependent Bioavailability (Major First-Pass Hepatic Metabolism) | Interpatient Variations in Plasma Levels | β-Blocking Plasma Concentrations | Protein Binding (%) | Lipid Solubility* |
|---|---|---|---|---|---|---|---|
| Acebutolol | ≈90 | ≈40 | Yes | 7-fold | 0.2-2.0 µg/ml | 25 | Low |
| Atenolol | ≈50 | ≈40 | No | 4-fold | 0.2-5.0 µg/ml | <5 | Low |
| Betaxolol | >90 | ≈80 | No | 2-fold | 0.005-0.05 µg/ml | 50 | Low |
| Bisoprolol | >90 | ≈88 | No | | 0.005-0.02 µg/ml | ≈30 | Low |
| Carteolol | ≈90 | ≈90 | No | 2-fold | 40-160 ng/ml | 20-30 | Low |
| Carvedilol | >90 | ≈30 | Yes | 5-10–fold | 10-100 ng/ml | 98 | Moderate |
| Celiprolol | ≈30 | ≈30 | No | 3-fold | | 22-24 | Low |
| Esmolol† | NA | NA | NA | 5-fold | 015-1.0 µg/ml | 55 | Low |
| Labetalol | >90 | ≈33 | Yes | 10-fold | 0.7-3.0 µg/ml | ≈50 | Moderate |
| Metoprolol | >90 | ≈50 | Yes | 10-fold | 50-100 ng/ml | 12 | Moderate |
| Metoprolol LA | >90 | 65-70 | Yes | 10-fold | 35-323 ng/ml | 12 | Moderate |
| Nadolol | ≈30 | ≈30 | No | 7-fold | 50-100 ng/ml | ≈30 | Low |
| Nebivolol | >90 | 12-96 | Yes | 7-fold | 1.5 ng/ml | 98 | High |
| Oxprenolol | ≈90 | 19-74 | Yes | 5-fold | 80-100 ng/ml | 80 | Moderate |
| Penbutolol | >90 | ≈100 | No | 4-fold | 5-15 ng/ml | 80-98 | High |
| Pindolol | >90 | ≈90 | No | 4-fold | 50-100 ng/ml | 57 | Moderate |
| Propranolol | >90 | 30-70 | Yes | 20-fold | 50-100 ng/ml | 93 | High |
| Propranolol LA‡ | >90 | 30-40 | Yes | 20-30–fold | 20-100 ng/ml | 93 | High |
| Sotalol | ≈70 | ≈90 | No | 4-fold | 1-32 µg/ml | 0 | Low |
| Timolol | >90 | ≈75 | Yes | 7-fold | 5-10 ng/ml | ≈10 | Low-Moderate |

(Adapted From Frishman WH. Alpha- and beta-adrenergic blocking drugs. *In* Frishman WH, Sonnenblick EH, Sica DA (eds). Cardiovascular Pharmacotherapeutics, 2nd ed. New York, McGraw Hill, 2003; pp 67-97.)

*Determined by the distribution ratio between octanol and water.

†Ultra-short-acting β-blocker available only in intravenous form.

‡Propranolol is available in both extended-release and delayed-release/extended-release formulations.

**Table 63-3** Elimination Characteristics of β-Adrenoceptor Blocking Drugs Used in Hypertension

| Drug | Elimination Half-Life (hours) | Total Body Clearance (ml/min) | Urinary Recovery of Unchanged Drug (% of Dose) | Total Urinary Recovery (% of Dose) | Predominant Route of Elimination | Active Metabolites | Drug Accumulation in Renal Disease |
|---|---|---|---|---|---|---|---|
| Acebutolol | 3-4* | 480 | ≈40 | >90 | RE (≈40% unchanged and HM) | Yes | Yes |
| Atenolol | 6-9 | 130 | ≈40 | >95 | RE | No | Yes |
| Betaxolol | 15 | 350 | 15 | >90 | HM | No | Yes |
| Bisoprolol | 9-12 | 260 | 50 | >98 | RE + HM | Yes | Yes |
| Carteolol | 5-6 | 497 | 40-68 | 90 | RE | Yes | Yes |
| Carvedilol | 7-10 | 600† | <2 | 16 | HM | Yes | No |
| Celiprolol | 5 | 500 | ≈90 | ≈30 | RE (≈50% unchanged and HM) | Yes | No |
| Esmolol | 9 min | 285 ml/min/kg or 19,950 ml/min | 1-2 | 71-88 | Red blood cells | No | No |
| Labetalol | 3-4 | 2700 | <1 | >90 | HM | No | No |
| Metoprolol | 3-4 | 1100 | ≈3 | >95 | HM | No | No |
| Metoprolol LA | 3-4 | 1100 | ≈3 | >95 | HM | No | Yes |
| Nebiuolol | 8-27 | — | <1 | — | HM | No | No |
| Oxprenolol | 2 | — | ≤3 | — | HM | — | No |
| Penbutolol | 27 | 350 | 50-70 | >90 | RE | No | No |
| Pindolol | 3-4 | 400 | ≈40 | >90 | RE (≈40% unchanged and HM) | No | No |
| Propranolol | 3-4 | 1000 | <1 | >90 | HM | Yes | No |
| Propranolol LA‡ | 10 | 1000 | <1 | >90 | HM | Yes | No |
| Timolol | 4-5 | 660 | ≈20 | 65 | RE (≈20% unchanged and HM) | No | No |

(Adapted from Frishman WH. Clinical Pharmacology of the β-Adrenoceptor Blocking Drugs, 2nd ed. Norwalk, Appleton-Century-Crofts, 1984.)

RE, renal excretion; HM, hepatic metabolism.

*Acebutolol has an active metabolite with elimination half-life of 8 to 13 hours.

†Plasma clearance.

‡Includes the extended-release and delayed-release/extended-release formulations.

## EFFECTS ON BLOOD PRESSURE

β-Adrenergic blockers, alone and in combination with other antihypertensives, reduce BP in patients with combined systolic and diastolic hypertension and with isolated systolic hypertension.[11-14] Uncommonly, there is a paradoxical elevation of systolic blood pressure during β-blockade in persons with severe aortic arteriosclerosis, presumably due to the increased stroke volume caused by rate slowing in the setting of increased impedance. Escalating doses of β-blockers and combined α-β–blockers can induce salt and water retention, making diuretics a common adjunctive therapy.[15] The β-blocking drugs are considered to be an alternative first-line treatment for hypertension and are also indicated for patients having concomitant angina pectoris, arrhythmias, hypertrophic cardiomyopathy, congestive cardiomyopathy, hyperdynamic circulations, essential tremor, and migraine headaches.[2,6,15-21] Some β-adrenergic blockers are also found to reduce the risk of mortality in survivors of acute myocardial infarction (MI), with and without heart failure.[22,23] The drugs can be used with caution in pregnancy, and appear to be especially useful in treating and preventing perioperative hypertension.[24,25]

Most antihypertensive drugs, including β-blockers, may reduce left ventricular mass and wall thickness.[26,27] However, in an outcome study of patients with stage 2 hypertension and ECG evidence of left ventricular hypertrophy (LVH), it was shown that losartan had a greater effect on LVH regression compared with atenolol, despite similar BP control.[28] Using a primary composite endpoint of death, stroke, and cardiovascular morbidity, there was a significant benefit in favor of losartan.[29]

There is evidence that some β-adrenergic blockers (those not having partial agonist activity) may not be as effective as other antihypertensive treatments in Black patients. Similar observations have been made in older patients.[30] However, when combined with a diuretic, β-blockers appear to be as effective as other combination treatment regimens in both Black and elderly patients.[2,4]

The α-β–blocker, labetalol, is the only β-blocker indicated for parenteral management of hypertensive emergencies and for treatment of intraoperative and postoperative hypertension. It can also be used in oral form to treat patients with hypertensive urgencies.[2,4]

## ADVERSE EFFECTS AND CONTRAINDICATIONS

β-Adrenergic blockers should not be used in patients with asthma, chronic obstructive pulmonary disease, unstable CHF with systolic dysfunction, heart block (greater than first degree), or sick sinus syndrome.[2-6] The α-β–blocker carvedilol can be used to reduce morbidity and mortality in those patients having hypertension and stable New York Heart Association (NYHA) class II-IV heart failure who are receiving diuretics, angiotensin-converting enzyme (ACE) inhibitors, and digoxin.[16,31,32] The $\beta_1$-selective agents bisoprolol and long-acting metoprolol used in an extended-release formulation have also been shown to reduce morbidity and mortality in patients with stable NYHA class II-III heart failure.[33,34]

β-Blockers should be used with caution in insulin-dependent diabetes because they may worsen glucose intolerance and mask the symptoms of and prolong recovery from hypoglycemia. There is probably a shorter recovery period from hypoglycemia with $\beta_1$-selective adrenergic blockers.[2,4] β-Blockers should not be discontinued abruptly in patients with known ischemic heart disease.[2-6] In a prospective cohort study, it was found that antihypertensive therapy with β-blockers was associated with a greater incidence of type 2 diabetes than was the use of ACE inhibitors, diuretics, and calcium channel blockers.[35] However, this increased risk of diabetes must be weighed against the proven benefit of β-blockers in reducing the risk of cardiovascular events.[36] Perhaps for this reason, JNC 7 recommended β-blockers as having "compelling indications" for use in patients with diabetes in whom the leading cause of death is cardiovascular disease.

β-Blockers may increase levels of plasma triglycerides and reduce those of high-density lipoprotein cholesterol.[37] Despite this effect, β-blockers without ISA are the only agents conclusively shown to decrease the rate of sudden death, overall mortality, and recurrent MI in survivors of acute MI.[22] β-Blockers with ISA or α-blocking activity have little or no adverse effect on plasma lipids.[37]

Dreams, hallucinations, insomnia, and depression can occur during therapy with β-blockers.[5,38] These symptoms provide evidence of drug entry into the central nervous system (CNS) and may be more common with the highly lipid-soluble β-blockers (propranolol, metoprolol), which presumably penetrate the CNS better. It has been claimed that β-blockers with less lipid-solubility (atenolol, nadolol) cause fewer CNS side effects.[39,40] This claim is intriguing but its validity has not been corroborated by other extensive clinical experiences.[41,42]

There are special considerations when β-blockers are combined with other drugs.[43-45] Combinations of diltiazem or verapamil with β-blockers may have additional sinoatrial and atrioventricular node depressant effects, and may also promote negative inotropy.[43] Combinations of β-blockers and reserpine may cause marked bradycardia and syncope. Combination with phenylpropanolamine, pseudoephedrine, ephedrine, and epinephrine can cause elevations in BP due to unopposed α-receptor–induced vasoconstriction.

## References

1. Chobanian AV, Bakris GL, Black HR, et al. The seventh report of the Joint National Committee on Prevention, Detection, Evaluation and Treatment of High Blood Pressure ( JNC 7). Express version: JAMA 289:2560-2572, 2003; Complete version: Hypertension 42:1206-1252, 2003.
2. Frishman WH, Sonnenblick EH. β-adrenergic blocking drugs and calcium channel blockers. *In* Alexander RW, Schlant RC, Fuster V. Hurst's The Heart, 9th ed. New York, McGraw Hill, 1998; pp 1583-1618.
3. Frishman WH, Bryzinski BS, Coulson LR, et al. A multifactorial trial design to assess combination therapy in hypertension: Treatment with bisoprolol and hydrochlorothiazide. Arch Intern Med 154:1461-1468, 1994.
4. Frishman WH. Alpha and beta-adrenergic blocking drugs. *In* Frishman WH, Sonnenblick EH, Sica DA (eds). Cardiovascular Pharmacotherapeutics, 2nd ed. New York, McGraw Hill, 2003; pp 67-97.

5. Frishman WH. Alpha and beta-adrenergic blocking drugs. *In* Frishman WH, Sonnenblick EH, Sica DA (eds). Cardiovascular Pharmacotherapeutics Manual, 2nd ed. New York, McGraw Hill, 2004; pp 19-57.

6. Frishman WH. Clinical Pharmacology of the β-Adrenoceptor Blocking Drugs, 2nd ed. Norwalk, Appleton-Century-Crofts, 1984.

7. Frishman WH, Alwarshetty M. Beta-adrenergic blockers in systemic hypertension: Pharmacokinetic considerations related to the JNC-VI and WHO-ISH guidelines. Clin Pharmacokinet 41:505-516, 2002.

8. Sica D, Frishman WH, Manowitz N. Pharmacokinetics of propranolol after single and multiple dosing with sustained release propranolol or propranolol CR (Innopran XL™), a new chronotherapeutic formulation. Heart Dis 5:176-181, 2003.

9. Black HR, Elliott WJ, Grandits G, et al. Principal results of the Controlled Onset Verapamil Investigation of Cardiovascular Endpoints (CONVINCE) Trial. JAMA 289:2073-2082, 2003.

10. Frishman WH, Murthy VS, Strom JA, et al. Ultra short-acting β-adrenoreceptor blocking drug: Esmolol. *In* Messerli FH (ed). Cardiovascular Drug Therapy, 2nd ed. Philadelphia, WB Saunders, 1996; pp 507-516.

11. Systolic Hypertension in the Elderly Program Cooperative Research Group. Implications of the Systolic Hypertension in the Elderly Program. Hypertension 21:335-343, 1993.

12. Materson BJ, Reda DJ, Cushman WC, et al. Single-drug therapy for hypertension in men: A comparison of six antihypertensive agents with placebo. The Department of Veterans Affairs Cooperative Study Group on Antihypertensive Agents. N Engl J Med 328:914-921, 1993.

13. Psaty BM, Smith NL, Siscovick DS, et al. Health outcomes associated with antihypertensive therapies used as first-line agents: A systematic review and meta-analysis. JAMA 277:739-745, 1997.

14. ALLHAT Officers and Coordinators. Major outcomes in high risk hypertensive patients randomized to angiotensin converting enzyme inhibitor therapy or calcium channel blocker vs diuretic: The Antihypertensive and Lipid-Lowering Treatment to Prevent Heart Attack Trial (ALLHAT). JAMA 288: 2981-2997, 2002.

15. Frishman WH, Sica DA. β-Adrenergic blockers. *In* Izzo JL Jr., Black HR (eds). Hypertension Primer, 3rd ed. Dallas, American Heart Association, 2003; pp 417-421.

16. Frishman WH. Carvedilol. N Engl J Med 339:1759-1765, 1998.

17. Abrams J, Frishman WH, Bates SM, et al. Pharmacologic options for treatment of ischemic disease. *In* Antman ED (ed). Cardiovascular Therapeutics: A Companion to Braunwald's Heart Disease, 2nd ed. Philadelphia, WB Saunders, 2002; pp 97-153.

18. Fihn SD, Williams SV, Daley J, et al. Guidelines for the management of patients with chronic stable angina: Treatment. Ann Intern Med 135:616-632, 2001.

19. Heidenreich PA, McDonald KM, Hastie T, et al. Meta-analysis of trials comparing β blockers, calcium antagonists and nitrates for stable angina. JAMA 281:1927-1936, 1999.

20. LeJemtel TH, Sonnenblick EH, Frishman WH. Diagnosis and management of heart failure. *In* Fuster V, Alexander RW, O'Rourke RA, et al (eds). Hurst's The Heart, 11th ed. New York, McGraw Hill, 2004; pp 723-762.

21. Frishman WH, Cavusoglu E. β-adrenergic blockers and their role in the therapy of arrhythmias. *In* Podrid PJ, Kowey PR (eds). Cardiac Arrhythmias: Mechanisms, Diagnosis and Management. Baltimore, Williams & Wilkins, 1995; pp 421-433.

22. Frishman WH. Postinfarction survival: Role of β-adrenergic blockade. *In* Fuster V, Ross R, Topol EJ (eds). Atherosclerosis and Coronary Artery Disease. Philadelphia, Lippincott Raven, 1996; pp 1205-1214.

23. CAPRICORN Investigators. Effect of carvedilol on outcome after myocardial infarction in patients with left ventricular dys-function: The CAPRICORN randomized trial. Lancet 357: 1385-1390, 2001.

24. Qasqas SA, McPherson C, Frishman WH, Elkayam U. Cardiovascular pharmacotherapeutic considerations during pregnancy and lactation. Parts 1 and 2. Cardiol Rev 12: 201-221, 240-261, 2004.

25. Auerbach AD, Goldman L. β blockers and reduction of cardiac events in noncardiac surgery. Clinical applications. JAMA 287:1445-1447, 2002.

26. Devereux RB. Do antihypertensive drugs differ in their ability to regress left ventricular hypertrophy? Circulation 95: 1983-1985, 1997.

27. Dahlof B. Left ventricular hypertrophy and angiotensin II antagonists. Am J Hypertens 14:174-182, 2001.

28. Okin PM, Devereux RB, Jern S, et al. Regression of electrocardiographic left ventricular hypertrophy by losartan versus atenolol: The Losartan Intervention for Endpoint reduction in Hypertension (LIFE) Study. Circulation 108:684-690, 2003.

29. Dahlof B, Devereux RB, Kjeldsen SE, et al. Cardiovascular morbidity and mortality in the Losartan Intervention for Endpoint reduction in hypertension study (LIFE): A randomized trial against atenolol. Lancet 359:995-1003, 2002.

30. Messerli FH, Frossman E, Goldbourt U. Are β blockers efficacious as first-line therapy for hypertension in the elderly? JAMA 279:1903-1907, 1998.

31. Packer M, Fowler MB, Roecker EB, et al. Carvedilol Prospective Randomized Cumulative Survival (COPERNICUS) Study Group. Effect of carvedilol on morbidity of patients with severe chronic heart failure: Results of the Carvedilol Prospective Randomized Cumulative Survival (COPERNICUS) Study. Circulation 106:2194-2199, 2002.

32. Poole-Wilson PA, Swedberg K, Cleland JGF, et al. Carvedilol or Metoprolol European Trial Investigators. Comparison of carvedilol and metoprolol on clinical outcomes in patients with chronic heart failure in the Carvedilol or Metoprolol European Trial (COMET): Randomized controlled trial. Lancet 362(9377):7-13, 2003.

33. CIBIS II. The Cardiac Insufficiency Bisoprolol Study II. A randomized trial. Lancet 353:9-13, 1999.

34. Hjalmarson A, Goldstein S, Fagerberg B, et al. Effect of controlled-release metoprolol on total mortality, hospitalizations and well-being in patients with heart failure. The Metoprolol CR/XL Randomized Intervention Trial in Congestive Heart Failure (MERIT-HF). MERIT-HF Study Group. JAMA 283:1295-1302, 2000.

35. Gress TW, Nieto J, Shahar E, et al. Hypertension and antihypertensive therapy as risk factors for type 2 diabetes mellitus. Atherosclerosis Risk in Communities Study. N Engl J Med 342:905-912, 2000.

36. Sowers JR, Bakris GL. Antihypertensive therapy and the risk of type 2 diabetes mellitus (editorial). N Engl J Med 342:969-970, 2000.

37. Schacter NS, Zimetbaum P, Frishman WH. Lipid-lowering drugs. *In* Frishman WH, Sonnenblick EH, Sica DA (eds). Cardiovascular Pharmacotherapeutics, 2nd ed. New York, McGraw Hill, 2003; pp 317-353.

38. Frishman WH, Razin A, Swencionis C, et al. Beta-adrenoceptor blockade in anxiety states: A new approach to therapy. Update. Cardiovasc Rev (Classics of the Decade Series). 13:8-13, 1992.

39. Frishman WH. Atenolol and timolol: Two new systemic adrenoceptor antagonists. N Engl J Med 306:1456-1462, 1982.

40. Frishman WH: Nadolol. A new β adrenoceptor antagonist. N Engl J Med 305:678-684, 1981.

41. Wurzelman J, Frishman MW, Aronson M, et al. Neuropsychiatric effects of antihypertensive drugs in the old old. Cardiol Clin 5:689-699, 1987.

42. Perez-Stable EJ, Halliday R, Gardiner PS, et al. The effects of propranolol on cognitive function and quality of life: A randomized trial among patients with diastolic hypertension. Am J Med 108:359-365, 2000.

43. Frishman WH, Sica DA: Calcium channel blockers. *In* Frishman WH, Sonnenblick EH, Sica DA (eds). Cardiovascular Pharmacotherapeutics, 2nd ed. New York, McGraw Hill, 2003; pp 105-130.

44. Opie LH. Cardiovascular drug interactions. *In* Frishman WH, Sonnenblick EH, Sica DA (eds). Cardiovascular Pharmacotherapeutics, 2nd ed. New York, McGraw Hill, 2003; pp 875-891.

45. Frishman WH, Opie LH, Sica DA. Adverse cardiovascular drug interactions and complications. *In* Fuster V, Alexander RW, O'Rourke RA, et al (eds). Hurst's The Heart, 11th ed. New York, McGraw Hill, 2004; pp 2169-2188.

# Chapter 64

# α-Adrenoceptor Blockers

## James L. Pool

## THE SYMPATHETIC NERVOUS SYSTEM IN BLOOD PRESSURE REGULATION

In the human vasculature, there are two types of adrenoceptors, alpha (α) and beta (β), which are transmembrane receptors initiating biologic signals. Since the discovery of the α- and β-adrenergic receptors (adrenoceptors) more than 50 years ago,[1] α-adrenoceptors (αAR) have been shown to participate in the physiologic regulation of vascular resistance and also play a role in hypertension[2] and other cardiovascular disorders such as myocardial hypertrophy.[3] To understand the role of αAR and the modulation of receptor function in hypertension by pharmacologic antagonists of αAR, it is necessary to be familiar with the contributions of the sympathetic nervous system (SNS) to the development of hypertension (see Chapter 6).[2,4-6]

Effective organ perfusion requires appropriate resistance to blood flow to maintain arterial pressure. The arterial pressure is regulated by changes in cardiac output and/or systemic vascular resistance. The dominant regulator of vascular resistance is smooth muscle tone, which helps regulate the most important determinant of resistance to flow, the cross-sectional area of a vessel. Two major neurohormonal systems—the autonomic nervous system (ANS) and the renin-angiotensin-aldosterone system (RAAS)—regulate smooth muscle tone. The peripheral ANS has three main components: (1) the SNS, which comprises the autonomic outflow from the thoracic and high lumbar segments of the spinal cord; (2) the parasympathetic nervous system (PNS), which includes the outflow from the cranial nerves and the low lumbar and sacral spinal cord; and (3) the enteric nervous system, the intrinsic neurons in the wall of the gut. In addition to the blood vessels, the urinary bladder, penis, and prostate also have smooth muscle cells that are innervated by SNS and PNS neurons to help regulate micturition, erection, and ejaculation.[7,8] As noted later, the SNS influences on lower urinary tract function play an important role in benign prostatic hyperplasia (BPH)[9] and lower urinary tract symptoms (LUTS),[10] both common conditions among older males with hypertension.

## ABNORMALITIES OF THE SYMPATHETIC NERVOUS SYSTEM IN HYPERTENSION

A number of abnormalities have been identified in high blood pressure, most notably increased SNS activity, which contributes to an increase in vasoconstriction and total peripheral vascular resistance. Studies have demonstrated in both borderline and mild hypertension an increased cardiac β-adrenergic drive with increased cardiac output and faster heart rate and an increased vascular α-adrenergic drive. A longitudinal study over 20 years showed the gradual transformation of such patients to established hypertension with normal cardiac output and increased vascular resistance.[11] Mechanisms that underlie this transition from high cardiac output to high vascular resistance involve modifications of SNS receptors and a dominant role for αAR. There is functional down-regulation of β-adrenergic responsiveness in the heart[12] plus alteration of vascular anatomy and function[4] followed by a steady increase in vascular resistance. An exaggerated response of blood vessels to adrenergic and nonadrenergic vasoconstrictors[13] likely contributes to the steady increase in vascular resistance during this evolution of hypertension.

## THE SUBTYPES OF α-ADRENOCEPTORS

Almost all vasomotor neurons are adrenergic, with the neurotransmitter norepinephrine producing vasoconstriction by acting on a specific type of transmembrane receptor on the vascular smooth muscle, the αAR. Within αAR there now identified six subtypes—which are designated $\alpha_{1A}$, $\alpha_{1B}$, $\alpha_{1D}$, $\alpha_{2A}$, $\alpha_{2B}$, and $\alpha_{2C}$—and one other candidate ($\alpha_{1L}$), which may be a conformational state of the $\alpha_{1A}$ adrenoceptor.[14-16] Table 64-1 lists further details about these six subtypes.[17] Furthermore, the vascular endothelium is now known to be more than a passive anatomic barrier that contacts the blood. Instead, the endothelium is an important organ possessing at least two different αAR subtypes ($\alpha_{2A}$, $\alpha_{2C}$) and three β-adrenoceptor subtypes ($\beta_1$, $\beta_2$, and $\beta_3$), which either directly or through the release of nitric oxide actively participate in the regulation of the vascular tone. The precise roles for each of these multiple subtypes of adrenoceptors in the regulation of blood pressure are not completely defined.

## MOLECULAR MECHANISM OF $\alpha_1$-ADRENOCEPTOR ACTIVATION

Stimulation of the αAR complex begins when circulating norepinephrine binds to the postsynaptic $\alpha_1$-adrenoceptor ($\alpha_1$AR), thus activating the receptor.[18] As shown in detail in Figure 64-1, innervation of smooth muscle by sympathetic nerve terminals involves a tight junction (or "synapse"), so there is close proximity of neural membranes to smooth muscle cells. The synaptic gap (or "cleft") between the neural endings and the smooth muscle cells is visible only with an electron microscope. The neural components of these synapses are described as "presynaptic"; the smooth muscle components, including the $\alpha_1$AR, are "postsynaptic." Sympathetic nerve impulses travel down the nerve, depolarize the nerve terminal, and stimulate the release of norepinephrine into the synaptic cleft by exocytosis. Exocytosis occurs when norepinephrine-containing vesicles in the nerve terminals bind to presynaptic neural membranes; the fused vesicles then

**Table 64-1** $\alpha_1$-Adrenoceptor Subtypes (1995 Classification)

| Native Receptors | Cloned Receptors | Cloned Receptors (Historical) | Human Chromosome Location |
|---|---|---|---|
| $\alpha_{1A}$ | $\alpha_{1a}$ | $\alpha_{1a}$ | C8 |
| $\alpha_{1B}$ | $\alpha_{1b}$ | $\alpha_{1b}$ | C5 |
| $\alpha_{1D}$ | $\alpha_{1d}$ | $\alpha_{1a/d'}$ $\alpha_{1a}$ | C20 |

open and empty their neurotransmitter (norepinephrine) into the synaptic cleft, where it is available to bind to postsynaptic adrenoceptors.

The postsynaptic $\alpha_1$AR is a complex structure that spans the width of the smooth muscle cell membrane, with specific topographic features on its outer surface that "recognize" and bind the newly released norepinephrine. This $\alpha_1$AR complex includes (1) the $\alpha_1$AR, (2) a "transducer subunit"—the guanine nucleotide releasing protein (GNRP), (3) a "catalytic subunit"—phospholipase C (PLC), and (4) the dual "second messengers"—inositol 1,4,5-trisphosphate ($IP_3$) and diacylglycerol (DAG). When circulating norepinephrine binds to the transmembrane $\alpha_1$AR, this "activates" the receptor and initi-

ates a cascade of events. The activated $\alpha_1$AR couples with a GNRP to activate PLC, which hydrolyzes phosphatidylinositol 4,5-bisphosphate ($PIP_2$) to generate $IP_3$ and DAG. Release of the newly synthesized $IP_3$ initiates a sharp rise in the cytoplasmic, ionized calcium ($Ca^{2+}$) by releasing intracellular stored $Ca^{2+}$. The large and transient increase in $Ca^{2+}$ activates chloride channels, leading to a membrane depolarization, which opens voltage-gated $Ca^{2+}$ channels, releasing $Ca^{2+}$ into the cytoplasm, resulting in contraction of the smooth muscle cell. In addition, the other "second messenger," DAG, transiently activates protein kinase C (PKC), which increases the opening probability of $Ca^{2+}$ channels through a phosphorylation-dependent process, thus increasing cytoplasmic $Ca^{2+}$.

## α-ADRENOCEPTORS IN THE URINARY BLADDER AND LUMBOSACRAL SPINAL CORD

During the development of BPH and LUTS in males, obstruction to urine flow is attributed to two components: (1) a "static" or anatomic component (enlarged prostate gland) and (2) a "dynamic" or functional component (increased smooth muscle tone in the bladder neck, the prostate capsule, and the fibromuscular stroma of the prostate gland). Up to 40% of

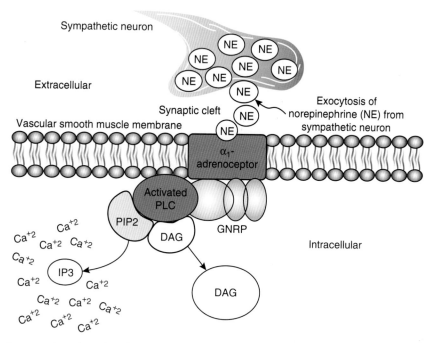

**Figure 64-1** Sympathetic nerve impulses depolarize nerve terminals and stimulate the release of norepinephrine (NE) into the synaptic cleft by the process of exocytosis. NE-containing vesicles in nerve terminals bind to presynaptic neural membranes; then the fused vesicles open, emptying NE into the synaptic cleft, where it is available to bind to adrenoceptors (AR). The active $\alpha_1$AR couples with a guanine nucleotide releasing protein (GNRP) (Gq/G11) to activate phospholipase C (PLC), which hydrolyzes phosphatidylinositol 4,5-bisphosphate (PIP2) to generate inositol 1,4,5-trisphosphate (IP3) and diacylglycerol (DAG). IP3 releases intracellular stored $Ca^{2+}$. Not shown in this figure are two additional intracellular events. The large and transient increase in $Ca^{2+}$ activates chloride channels, leading to a membrane depolarization that opens voltage-gated $Ca^{2+}$ channels. Also, DAG transiently activates protein kinase C (PKC), which increases the opening probability of $Ca^{2+}$ channels through a phosphorylation-dependent process. This complex $\alpha_1$AR pathway causes the physiologic action (contraction) of NE in vascular smooth muscle.

total urethral pressure is due to $\alpha$-adrenergic tone, and the rest is due to static pressure from the enlarged prostate.[19] Relaxation of this smooth muscle tone by $\alpha_1$AR blockers increases urinary flow and improves LUTS in patients with BPH.[20]

Although a simplified explanation of this therapeutic effect was provided initially, the exact role of the SNS in the regulation of micturition in normal and BPH persons remains uncertain. Early findings suggest that two types of spinal $\alpha_1$AR mechanisms are involved in reflex bladder activity.[7] Facilitatory $\alpha_1$AR in bulbospinal pathways from the brainstem to the lumbosacral spinal cord contribute to neural control of the lower urinary tract. In the urinary outflow tract, $\alpha_1$AR are located in smooth muscle cells of the neck of the urinary bladder, capsule of the prostate, and fibromuscular stroma of the prostate. Stimulation of $\alpha_1$AR in the bladder outflow tract increases resistance to urine flow. The frequency of the reflex to urinate is inhibited by afferent $\alpha_1$AR in the spinal cord. The descending limb of the micturition reflex pathway may be facilitated by $\alpha_1$AR. For control of the micturition reflex, selective $\alpha_1$ adrenoceptor antagonists ($\alpha_1$ARA) are used, and it is thought that these drugs have dual sites of action, including both the central nervous system and the smooth muscle of the lower urinary tract.

## SELECTIVE POSTSYNAPTIC $\alpha_1$-ADRENOCEPTOR BLOCKADE

When stimulated, $\alpha_1$AR, located postsynaptically in smooth muscle, produce vasoconstriction of the blood vessels. Sympathetic overactivity in hypertension results in an excess stimulation of postsynaptic $\alpha_1$AR. Consequently, there emerged a sound therapeutic rationale for the use of selective $\alpha_1$ARA in the treatment of hypertension. By selectively inhibiting the vascular $\alpha_1$AR and thereby inhibiting the receptor-mediated response to norepinephrine, these agents reduce blood pressure via a decrease in peripheral vascular resistance (Figure 64-2).[21] The reduction in blood pressure is achieved with little or no change in central hemodynamic parameters such as heart rate, stroke index, or cardiac index. As shown in Figure 64-2, these favorable hemodynamic effects of selective $\alpha_1$ inhibitors are evident during exercise, when cardiac performance is better preserved with $\alpha_1$-blockers than with $\beta$-blockers.

## AN OVERVIEW OF $\alpha$-ADRENOCEPTOR ANTAGONISTS

Nonselective $\alpha$-adrenoceptor antagonists, phentolamine and phenoxybenzamine, which bind to both $\alpha_1$ and $\alpha_2$ receptors, were discovered first. However, three categories of $\alpha$-adrenoceptor blockers have been introduced over the past four decades, including nonselective ($\alpha_1 + \alpha_2$), presynaptic $\alpha_2$, and postsynaptic $\alpha_1$ARA. Table 64-2 lists clinically available and major research drugs available in this class. Selective, postsynaptic $\alpha_1$ARA, often referred to as "$\alpha_1$-blockers" or simply "$\alpha$-blockers," lower blood pressure primarily by post-synaptic $\alpha_1$AR blockade. In this respect, selective $\alpha_1$ARAs differ from nonselective $\alpha$-blockers including the competitive inhibitor phentolamine and the noncompetitive inhibitor phenoxyben-

zamine.[22] Importantly, stimulation of presynaptic $\alpha_2$-adrenoceptors inhibits norepinephrine release. Nonselective $\alpha$-blockade prevents this inhibition and causes $\alpha_2$ receptors to increase norepinephrine release, with resultant $\beta$-adrenoceptor-mediated tachycardia, enhanced renin secretion, and attenuation of postsynaptic $\alpha_1$ inhibition. In fact, selective blockade of these presynaptic $\alpha_2$-adrenoceptors with a drug such as yohimbine can lead to a rise in blood pressure. As a result of these pharmacodynamic consequences of nonselective $\alpha$-adrenoceptor blockade, these agents were unsuccessful in treatment of essential hypertension and symptomatic BPH.

Phentolamine, a parenteral drug, is used almost exclusively for emergent and urgent severe hypertension with excess catecholamine release (see Chapter 78). The oral, nonselective and noncompetitive $\alpha$ inhibitor phenoxybenzamine remains an important agent in the preoperative management of pheochromocytoma and cases of inoperable metastatic pheochromocytoma (see Chapter 76). In contrast to the nonselective drugs, the selective $\alpha_1$ARAs, which include the three major marketed antihypertensive agents doxazosin, prazosin, and terazosin (Figure 64-3), reduce vascular tone in capacitance vessels and resistance vessels to provide a balance of preload and afterload reduction, thus avoiding vasodilation (afterload reduction) without venodilation (preload reduction), which would promote an increase in cardiac output and heart rate.

A unique feature of two of the selective $\alpha_1$ARAs—labetalol and carvedilol—is blockade of $\beta_1$- and $\beta_2$-adrenoceptors. Labetalol is an equal molar mixture of four stereoisomers. One stereoisomer is an $\alpha_1$ARA, which is equivalent to ~10% of $\alpha$-blockade with phentolamine. Another isomer is a nonselective $\beta$-adrenoceptor antagonist with partial agonist activity, and the other two isomers are inactive. The isomer that is a $\beta$-adrenoceptor antagonist was developed separately as a drug (dilevalol) but was removed from world markets because of serious hepatotoxicity. Labetalol lowers arterial pressure by reducing vascular resistance as a consequence of blockade of $\alpha_1$AR and stimulation of peripheral $\beta_2$-adrenoceptors. In contrast, carvedilol is predominately a nonselective $\beta$-blocker and selective $\alpha_1$ARA, which is indicated for the treatment of heart failure and/or hypertension. The ratio of $\alpha_1$- to $\beta$-adrenoceptor antagonist potency for carvedilol is 1:10.

## TREATMENT OF HYPERTENSION WITH $\alpha_1$-ADRENOCEPTOR ANTAGONISTS

Clinical studies have shown $\alpha_1$ARA to lower blood pressure through reduction of vascular resistance without significant effects on heart rate, cardiac output, or central hemodynamic parameters in hypertensive patients.[23] In normotensive persons who have normal sympathetic tone and peripheral vascular resistance, blood pressure effects are not clinically significant, which has contributed to their utility in the treatment of conditions other than hypertension, such as BPH and Raynaud's disease. Prazosin, terazosin, and doxazosin are effective antihypertensive agents, whether used as monotherapy or as part of a regimen of multiple antihypertensive drugs. Because of their longer duration of action, doxazosin and terazosin have generally replaced prazosin in treatment of blood pressure. Their effects are additive to those of angiotensin converting enzyme (ACE) inhibitors, angiotensin receptor

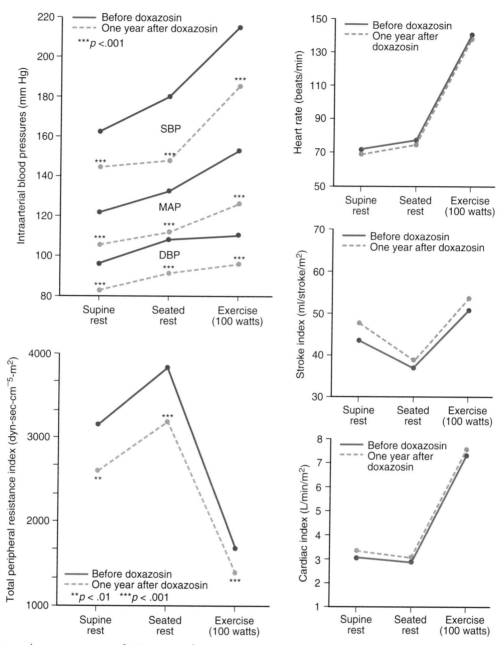

**Figure 64–2** During chronic treatment of 12 patients for 1 year with doxazosin, there is a marked decrease in the total peripheral resistance index at rest and exercise, but maintenance of normal central hemodynamic parameters, including stroke index and cardiac index. (From Lund-Johansen P, Omvik P. Acute and chronic hemodynamic effects of drugs with different actions on adrenergic receptors: A comparison between alpha blockers and different types of beta blockers with and without vasodilating effect [Review]. Cardiovasc Drug Ther 5(3):605-615, 1991. Reprinted with permission of Kluwer Academic Publishers, Boston, MA.)

antagonists, β-blockers, calcium channel blockers, diuretics, and direct-acting vasodilators. About 50% of mild to moderate essential hypertensives treated with monotherapy in placebo-controlled trials achieved diastolic blood pressures <90 mm Hg but lesser systolic blood pressure control <140 mm Hg.[24] In large placebo-controlled hypertension studies, doxazosin or terazosin once daily lowered blood pressure at 24 hours by ~10/8 mm Hg as compared with placebo in the standing position and ~9/5 mm Hg in the supine position.

Age, race, and gender do not influence blood pressure response to selective $α_1$-blockers. In clinical practice for more than a decade, $α_1$-blockers have had their widest application as one component of multiple drug regimens for the treatment of moderate to severe hypertension. Although less pronounced than with potent vasodilators, monotherapy with $α_1$-blockers promotes sodium and water retention. Use of a diuretic prevents fluid retention and can markedly enhance the antihypertensive effect of the drugs.

**Table 64–2** $\alpha_1$-Adrenoceptor Antagonists

| Antagonist Compound | $\alpha_1$ Selective | | | $\alpha_1$ Nonselective + $\alpha_2$ Nonselective | $\alpha_1$ Selective + $\beta_1 + \beta_2$ Nonselective |
|---|---|---|---|---|---|
| | $\alpha_{1A}$ | $\alpha_{1B}$ | $\alpha_{1D}$ | | |
| Alfuzosin | x | x | x | | |
| BMY 7378 | | | x | | |
| Bunazosin | x | x | x | | |
| Carvedilol* | x | x | x | | x |
| Chloroethylclonidine | | x | | | |
| Cyclazosin | | x | | | |
| Doxazosin* | x | x | x | | |
| Indoramin | x | x | x | | |
| Labetalol* | x | x | x | | x |
| MDL 72832 | x | | | | |
| MDL 73005EF | | | x | | |
| Moxisylyte§ | x | x | x | | |
| Naftopidil | x | | | | |
| Phenoxybenzamine* | x | x | x | x | |
| Phentolamine* | x | x | x | x | |
| Prazosin* | x | x | x | | |
| RS 17053 | x | | | | |
| RS 100329 | x | | | | |
| SK&F 105854 | | | x | | |
| SNAP 5150 | x | | | | |
| (+)Niguldipine | x | | | | |
| Tamsulosin* | x | | x | | |
| Terazosin* | x | x | x | | |
| Tolazoline* | x | x | x | | |
| Trimazosin | x | x | x | | |
| 5-methylurapidil | x | | | | |
| WB 4101 | x | | x | | |

*Approved by US Food and Drug Administration.
§Moxisylyte has a second generic name, thymoxamine.
Abbreviations and chemical names: BMY 7378 = 8-[2-[4-(2methoxyphenyl)-1-piperazinyl]ethyl]-8-azaspiro[4,5]decane-7,9 dione dihydrochloride; MDL 72832 = {8-[4-(1,4-benzodioxan-2-ylmethylamino)butyl]-8-azaspirol[4,5]decane-7,9-dione HCl;
MDL 73005EF = {8-[2-(1,4-benzodioxan-2-ylmethylamino)ethyl]-8-azaspirol[4,5]decane-7,9-dione HCl;
RS 17053 = N-[2-(-cyclopropyl methoxy phenoxy)ethyl]-5-chloro-$\alpha$, $\alpha$-dimethyl-1H-indole-3-ethanamine HCl;
RS100329 = 5-methyl-3-[3-[4-[2-(2,2,2,-trifluoroethoxy)phenyl]-1-piperazinyl]propyl]-2,4-(1H)-pyrimidinedione;
SNAP 5150 = 5-(aminocarbonyl)-1,4-dihydro-2,6-dimethyl-4-(4-nitrophenyl)-3-((3-(4,4-diphenylpiperidin-1-yl)propyl)aminocarbonyl)pyridine; WB 4101 = 2-(2-6dimethoxyphenoxyethyl)aminomethyl-1,4-benzodioxane HCl.

## INEFFECTIVE FOR TREATMENT OF HEART FAILURE

$\alpha$-Blockers have not shown sustained benefits in chronic congestive heart failure (CHF). Mortality from left ventricular dysfunction is not improved by selective $\alpha_1$ARA. In the 1986 Veterans Administration Cooperative Study[25] on the effect of vasodilator therapy in chronic CHF, mortality in the prazosin treatment group was similar to that in the placebo group. Furthermore, chronic therapy in heart failure with $\alpha_1$-blocker (doxazosin) plus $\beta$-blocker (metoprolol) produces effects identical to those seen in patients receiving $\beta$-blocker alone.

## METABOLIC EFFECTS

Selective $\alpha_1$ARA have proven beneficial effects on the lipid profiles of hypertensive patients. Several controlled studies have demonstrated reductions in total cholesterol, low-density lipoprotein (LDL) cholesterol and triglycerides and increased levels of high-density lipoprotein (HDL) cholesterol and the ratio of HDL cholesterol:total cholesterol.[26] In hypertensive patients with baseline values similar to the general population, doxazosin produced small reductions in total serum cholesterol (2%-3%), LDL cholesterol (4%), and a similarly small increase in the HDL:total cholesterol ratio (4%). These modifications of the serum lipid profile are the result of several different mechanisms.[27] These include an increase in LDL cholesterol receptor number, a decrease in LDL cholesterol synthesis, stimulation of lipoprotein lipase activity, reduction of very-low-density lipoprotein (VLDL) cholesterol synthesis and secretion, and a reduction in the absorption of dietary cholesterol. In addition, a unique feature of the 6-hydroxy and 7-hydroxy metabolites of doxazosin is the ability to inhibit the oxidation of LDL cholesterol,[28] which has an important role in the initiation and progression of atherosclerosis. In hypertensives with diabetes mellitus that are treated

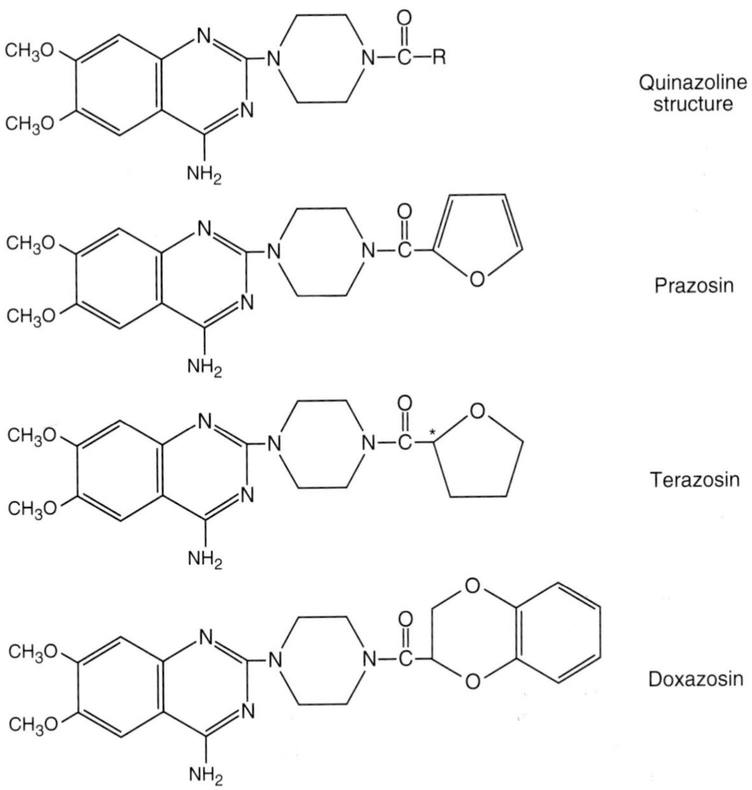

**Figure 64-3** The chemical structure of quinazoline compounds is shown at the top with the three derivatives (prazosin, terazosin, and doxazosin) that are approved by the U.S. Food and Drug Administration for the treatment of hypertension and benign prostatic hyperplasia. The saturated furan configuration of terazosin provides the molecule with one optically active chemical center (*), so terazosin has two enantiomeric forms. The 6'- and 7'-hydroxy metabolites of doxazosin (not shown here) have demonstrated in vitro antioxidant properties.

with $\alpha_1$-blockers, improvements in insulin sensitivity and reductions in elevated serum insulin levels and fasting glucose have been demonstrated.[29]

## ADVERSE DRUG EFFECTS

Selective $\alpha_1$-antagonists are generally well-tolerated, with a few common adverse effects. In placebo-controlled trials, the symptoms that most commonly caused discontinuation of $\alpha_1$-antagonist therapy were asthenia (2%), nasal congestion (2%), and dizziness (1%).[24,30] Generally, there is no drug dose relationship for clinical adverse effects. Dizziness secondary to $\alpha_1$-blockers is not entirely understood, because patients can experience this sensation without documented postural hypotension. However, a major precaution is the so-called "first-dose phenomenon," which is severe, symptomatic orthostatic hypotension that usually occurs within 90 minutes after the first dose or when the dose is increased rapidly. If the patient has concomitant treatment with one or more agents (especially diuretic, β-blocker, or verapamil), additional caution with the first dose is advisable. However, syncope is uncommon, occurring in <1% of patients when an initial, small dose (1 mg or less) was taken at bedtime as monotherapy. Men should be cautioned that the combine of $\alpha_1$-blocker and sildenafil (Viagra), tadalafil (Cialis), or vardenafil (Levitra) could produce marked hypotension. Postmenopausal women with pelvic relaxation syndrome and individuals with certain types of urinary bladder dysfunction can develop urinary incontinence with $\alpha_1$-blocker–mediated relaxation of the bladder outlet.

There are no clinically important adverse effects on laboratory tests. Serum electrolytes, BUN, creatinine, glucose, and uric acid are not altered. There are no significant effects on renal function in hypertensive patients with normal, moderate, or severe renal impairment. In placebo-controlled trials, a greater percentage of $\alpha_1$-blocker patients had small decreases in hematocrit, hemoglobin, white blood cell count, total serum protein, and albumin levels from baseline values. Except for the white blood cell count, these changes have been attributed to hemodilution secondary to mild fluid retention. The reduction of white blood cell counts remains unexplained, but individual reductions have been small, and prolonged drug treatment has not been associated with progressive white blood cell count reductions.

## ALLHAT TRIAL CHANGED $\alpha_1$-BLOCKER USE

The Antihypertensive and Lipid-Lowering Treatment to Prevent Heart Attack Trial (ALLHAT) was a large, randomized, double-blind superiority trial comparing four antihypertensive drugs—chlorthalidone, doxazosin, amlodipine, and lisinopril—with a total of 42,448 recruited patients.[31,32] The participants were men and women aged ≥55 years with hypertension plus an additional risk factor for coronary heart disease. At a median follow-up of 3.3 years in 9067 patients, the doxazosin and chlorthalidone treatment groups had no difference in the primary endpoint of fatal and nonfatal myocardial infarction.[33] However, the doxazosin limb of the study was discontinued because, compared with the chlorthalidone group, there was a 25% higher incidence of significant cardiovascular disease (Figure 64-4),[34] which was predominately the result of twice the incidence of CHF. There was an early divergence of the Kaplan-Meier curves for CHF for doxazosin and chlorthalidone after randomization, which has raised questions about withdrawal of previous drug therapy

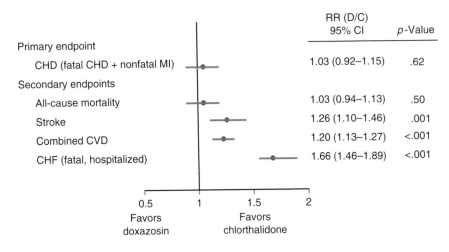

| | RR (D/C) 95% CI | p-Value |
|---|---|---|
| **Primary endpoint** | | |
| CHD (fatal CHD + nonfatal MI) | 1.03 (0.92–1.15) | .62 |
| **Secondary endpoints** | | |
| All-cause mortality | 1.03 (0.94–1.13) | .50 |
| Stroke | 1.26 (1.10–1.46) | .001 |
| Combined CVD | 1.20 (1.13–1.27) | <.001 |
| CHF (fatal, hospitalized) | 1.66 (1.46–1.89) | <.001 |

0.5　1　1.5　2
Favors doxazosin　　Favors chlorthalidone

**Figure 64–4** The principal outcomes of the ALLHAT Trial for the α-blocker (doxazosin) treatment arm versus diuretic (chlorthalidone) treatment arm are shown for the primary CHD endpoint and the four major secondary endpoints.[34] Abbreviations: RR, risk ratio; D/C, doxazosin compared with chlorthalidone; CI, confidence interval.

(i.e., diuretics, ACE inhibitors, or β-blockers) among patients at risk for CHF. ALLHAT has raised a number of questions that cannot be answered because there was no placebo control and systolic blood pressure control was not equal in the doxazosin and chlorthalidone groups. As shown in Figure 64–5, systolic blood pressure throughout the ALLHAT Trial was 2 to 3 mm Hg higher in the doxazosin treatment arm. Nevertheless, this information on the outcomes of long-term antihypertensive treatment with $\alpha_1$ARA has led to $\alpha_1$ARA not being recommended as a first-line treatment for hypertension in several countries. However, ALLHAT was not designed to investigate the use of $\alpha_1$ARA for (1) younger hypertensive subjects or hypertensives with a lesser CHD risk factor profile, (2) diuretic-based combination therapy for the treatment of hypertension, (3) combined treatment of hypertension and BPH, or (4) treatment of normotensive patients with BPH, where $\alpha_1$ARAs remain the best monotherapy for the control of symptoms.

In spring 2000, as a result of early, unfavorable results from ALLHAT, α-blockers were no longer recommended as first-line treatment for hypertension in high-risk patients. Stafford et al.[35] tracked trends in α-blocker prescriptions filled by community pharmacies and reports of α-blocker use in patient encounters with office-based physicians from 1996 to 2002. The authors used U.S. data from two sources: (1) α-blocker prescription orders reported in the National Prescription Audit—a random, computerized sample of about 20,000 of 29,000 pharmacies—and (2) office-based physician α-blocker prescribing patterns reported in the National Disease and Therapeutic Index, a random sample of about 3500 physician offices. The researchers found that there had been steady increases in new α-blocker prescriptions, dispensed prescriptions, and physician prescribing from 1996 through 1999. There was a moderate reversal in these trends following the early termination and subsequent publications of ALLHAT in early 2000. Between 1999 and 2002, new annual α-blocker prescription orders declined by 26%, from 5.15 million to 3.79 million, dispensed prescriptions by 22%, from 17.2 million to 13.4 million, and physician-reported drug use by 54%, from 2.26 million to 1.03 million.

## α-BLOCKERS EXPAND MANAGEMENT OF BENIGN PROSTATIC HYPERPLASIA

For men older than the age of 60 years, LUTS associated with BPH and obstruction occur in up to 70%.[36] Before effective medical management, men with bothersome LUTS were observed for variable lengths of time until they were considered suitable candidates for transurethral prostatectomy (TURP). In the early 1970s, α-blockers emerged as an effective treatment option for LUTS secondary to BPH to relieve bothersome symptoms.[20] Medical therapy evolved into the major clinical option in the management of BPH, including men with mild to severe LUTS. Before α-blockers, there was no suitable treatment option for mild LUTS. There was a dramatic increase in prescriptions for medical therapies and a decline in the use of TURP. Today, medical therapy is the dominant form of treatment for BPH.

The lack of specificity and side effects of nonselective α-blockers limited their use in LUTS patients. Although developed for the treatment of essential hypertension, selective $\alpha_1$-blockers contributed largely to the growth of medical therapy for BPH. In 1987, terazosin was approved in the United States for treatment of hypertension; in 1994, it was

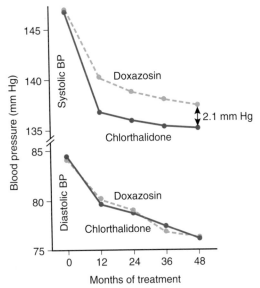

**Figure 64–5** Mean systolic and diastolic blood pressures (BPs) in the ALLHAT Trial are shown at baseline and four annual visits. Diastolic BPs are controlled equally, but there are consistently 2 to 3 mm Hg higher systolic BPs in the doxazosin group at all treatment visits.[34]

approved for treatment of LUTS, followed by approval of doxazosin for both indications. Finasteride, the 5-α-reductase inhibitor that blocks the conversion of testosterone to dihydrotestosterone, was the first drug approved by the FDA in 1992 to treat BPH. However, α-blockers became the predominant medical therapy because of excellent efficacy in relieving LUTS. Generally, 59% to 86% of men using α-blockers will see a decrease in symptoms.[36] Symptoms generally improve in 2 to 3 weeks. Terazosin and doxazosin typically improve urinary flow rate by 2 to 2.5 ml/sec. Tamsulosin introduced the concept of uroselectivity. Targeting the $\alpha_{1a}$- and $\alpha_{1b}$-adrenoceptors in the bladder neck and prostate, tamsulosin achieves a greater effect on the prostate and a similar degree of improvement in both urine flow rates and symptoms with fewer cardiovascular side effects as compared with nonselective agents. Tamsulosin has become the most widely used $\alpha_1$-blocker for BPH in the United States; it eliminates the need for titration and has fewer side effects. However, the incidence of retrograde ejaculation with higher doses of tamsulosin approaches 20%.

The Veterans Affairs (VA) Cooperative BPH Study[37] in 1996 was the first large-scale study (n =1229) to compare an α-blocker (terazosin), a 5-α-reductase inhibitor (finasteride), and the combination of these two agents for the improvement of LUTS and urine flow rate in BPH. This 1-year VA trial showed that terazosin achieved greater improvement in symptoms and flow rate as compared with finasteride, which was similar to placebo. The combination of terazosin and finasteride was not better than α-blocker alone. The 4-year Proscar (finasteride) Long-Term Efficacy and Safety Study (PLESS)[38] with 3040 men reported the impact of finasteride alone as compared with placebo on disease progression defined as acute urinary retention (AUR) and BPH surgery. Finasteride reduced the incidence of AUR by 57% and surgery for BPH by 55% as compared with placebo, which established a role for finasteride in long-term management of BPH. Men with moderate to severe symptoms and an enlarged prostate respond best to finasteride therapy. Men with little or no enlargement of the prostate are less likely to experience improvement in symptoms or reduction in events with finasteride. The size of the prostate does not predict improvements in LUTS symptoms during α-blocker therapy.

In 2003, the Medical Therapy of Prostatic Symptoms (MTOPS) Trial[39] with 3047 men, which lasted 4.5 years, established a role for combination drug therapy with α-blocker and finasteride. The "overall risk of clinical progression"—defined as an increase from baseline of ≥4 points in the American Urological Association (AUA) symptom score, acute urinary retention, urinary incontinence, renal insufficiency, or recurrent urinary tract infections—was significantly reduced by doxazosin by 39%, by finasteride by 34%, and by a combination of doxazosin and finasteride by 66% as compared with placebo. Long-term combination therapy with doxazosin and finasteride was safe and reduced the risk of overall clinical progression of BPH more than did treatment with either drug alone. Combination therapy and finasteride alone reduced the long-term risk of AUR and the need for invasive BPH therapy. The principal effect of doxazosin on progression was prevention of a 4-point rise in AUA symptom score.

These long-term, large clinical trials of medical therapy for BPH have clarified treatment options. α-Blockers offer the best monotherapy for symptom relief of LUTS. The available selective α-blockers have similar effects on symptoms and flow rate. Finasteride prevents disease progression, whether defined by symptoms, AUR, or surgery. Finally, combination therapy with an α-blocker plus finasteride is the most-effective treatment for BPH symptoms and disease progression, and the ideal candidates for combination therapy have moderate or severe symptoms and prostate enlargement.

# References

1. Ahlquist RP. A study of the adrenotropic responses. Am J Physiol 153:586-600, 1948.
2. Somers VK, Anderson EA, Mark AL. Sympathetic neural mechanisms in human hypertension. Curr Opin Nephrol Hypertens 2:96-105, 1993.
3. Yamazaki T, Komuro I, Yazaki Y. Signalling pathways for cardiac hypertrophy. Cell Signal 10:693-698, 1998.
4. Sivertsson R. Structural adaptation in borderline hypertension. Hypertension 6(6 Pt 2):III103-III107, 1984.
5. Anderson EA, Sinkey CA, Lawton WJ, et al. Elevated sympathetic nerve activity in borderline hypertensive humans. Evidence from direct intraneural recordings. Hypertension 14:177-183, 1989.
6. Julius S. Autonomic nervous system dysregulation in human hypertension. Am J Cardiol 67:3B-7B, 1991.
7. Andersson KE. Bladder activation: Afferent mechanisms. Urology 59(5 Suppl 1):43-50, 2002.
8. Andersson KE. Treatment of the overactive bladder: Possible central nervous system drug targets. Urology 59(5 Suppl 1):18-24, 2002.
9. Berry SJ, Coffey DS, Walsh PC, et al. The development of human benign prostatic hyperplasia with age. J Urol 132:474-479, 1984.
10. Chute CG, Panser LA, Girman CJ, et al. The prevalence of prostatism: A population-based survey of urinary symptoms. J Urol 150:85-89, 1993.
11. Lund-Johansen P. Central haemodynamics in essential hypertension at rest and during exercise: A 20-year follow-up study. J Hypertens Suppl 7:S52-S55, 1989.
12. Trimarco B, Volpe M, Ricciardelli B, et al. Studies of the mechanisms underlying impairment of beta-adrenoceptor-mediated effects in human hypertension. Hypertension 5:584-590, 1983.
13. Sivertsson R, Sannerstedt R, Lundgren Y. Evidence for peripheral vascular involvement in mild elevation of blood pressure in man. Clin Sci Mol Med Suppl 3:65s-68s, 1976.
14. Bylund DB, Eikenberg DC, Hieble JP, et al. International Union of Pharmacology nomenclature of adrenoceptors (Review). Pharmacol Rev 46:121-136, 1994.
15. Hieble JP, Ruffolo RR, Jr. Subclassification and nomenclature of alpha 1- and alpha 2-adrenoceptors (Review). Prog Drug Res 47:81-130, 1996.
16. Hieble JP. Adrenoceptor subclassification: An approach to improved cardiovascular therapeutics. Pharm Acta Helv 74:163-171, 2000.
17. Piascik MT, Soltis EE, Piascik MM, et al. Alpha-adrenoceptors and vascular regulation: Molecular, pharmacologic and clinical correlates. Pharmacol Ther 72:215-241, 1996.
18. Piascik MT, Perez DM. Alpha1-adrenergic receptors: New insights and directions. J Pharmacol Exp Ther 298:403-410, 2001.
19. Furuya S, Kumamoto Y, Yokoyama E, et al. Alpha-adrenergic activity and urethral pressure in prostatic zone in benign prostatic hypertrophy. J Urol 128:836-839, 1982.
20. Kirby RS, Pool JL. Alpha adrenoceptor blockade in the treatment of benign prostatic hyperplasia: Past, present and future (Review). Br J Urol 80:521-532, 1997.

21. Lund-Johansen P, Omvik P. Acute and chronic hemodynamic effects of drugs with different actions on adrenergic receptors: A comparison between alpha blockers and different types of beta blockers with and without vasodilating effect (Review). Cardiovasc Drug Ther 5:605-615, 1991.

22. Davey M. Mechanism of alpha blockade for blood pressure control. Am J Cardiol 59:18G-28G, 1987.

23. Lund-Johansen P, Hjermann I, Iversen BM, et al. Selective alpha-1 inhibitors: First- or second-line antihypertensive agents (Review). Cardiology 83:150-159, 1993.

24. Pool JL, Nunez E, Messerli FH, et al. *In:* Messerli FH (ed). Cardiovascular Drug Therapy. Philadelphia, Saunders, 1996; pp 665-673.

25. Cohn JN, Archibald DG, Ziesche S, et al. Effect of vasodilator therapy on mortality in chronic congestive heart failure. Results of a Veterans Administration Cooperative Study. N Engl J Med 314:1547-1552, 1986.

26. Cubeddu LX, Pool JL, Bloomfield R, et al. Effect of doxazosin monotherapy on blood pressure and plasma lipids in patients with essential hypertension. Am J Hypertens 1:158-167, 1988.

27. Pool JL. Effects of doxazosin on serum lipids: A review of the clinical data and molecular basis for altered lipid metabolism. Am Heart J 121(1 Pt 2):251-259, 1991.

28. Chait A, Gilmore M, Kawamura M. Inhibition of low density lipoprotein oxidation in vitro by the 6- and 7-hydroxy-metabolites of doxazosin, an alpha 1-adrenergic antihypertensive agent. Am J Hypertens 7:159-167, 1994.

29. Lithell HO. Insulin resistance and diabetes in the context of treatment of hypertension. Blood Press 3(Suppl):28-31, 1998.

30. Neutel JM, Taylor SH, Smith DGH, et al. Doxazosin. *In* Messerli FH (ed). Cardiovascular Drug Therapy. Philadelphia, Saunders, 1996; pp 681-689.

31. Davis BR, Cutler JA, Gordon DJ, et al. Rationale and design for the Antihypertensive and Lipid Lowering Treatment to Prevent Heart Attack Trial (ALLHAT). ALLHAT Research Group. Am J Hypertens 9(4 Pt 1):342-360, 1996.

32. Major outcomes in high-risk hypertensive patients randomized to angiotensin-converting enzyme inhibitor or calcium channel blocker vs diuretic: The Antihypertensive and Lipid-Lowering Treatment to Prevent Heart Attack Trial (ALLHAT). JAMA 288:2981-2997, 2002.

33. Major cardiovascular events in hypertensive patients randomized to doxazosin vs chlorthalidone: The antihypertensive and lipid-lowering treatment to prevent heart attack trial (ALLHAT). ALLHAT Collaborative Research Group. JAMA 283:1967-1975, 2000.

34. Diuretic versus alpha-blocker as first-step antihypertensive therapy: Final results from the Antihypertensive and Lipid-Lowering Treatment to Prevent Heart Attack Trial (ALLHAT). Hypertension 42:239-246, 2003.

35. Stafford RS, Furberg CD, Finkelstein SN, et al. Impact of clinical trial results on national trends in alpha-blocker prescribing, 1996-2002. JAMA 291:54-62, 2004.

36. Benign Prostatic Hyperplasia: Diagnosis and Treatment. Rockville, MD, AHCPR Publication No. 94-0582, 1994.

37. Lepor H, Williford WO, Barry MJ, et al. The efficacy of terazosin, finasteride, or both in benign prostatic hyperplasia. Veterans Affairs Cooperative Studies Benign Prostatic Hyperplasia Study Group. N Engl J Med 335:533-539, 1996.

38. McConnell JD, Bruskewitz R, Walsh P, et al. The effect of finasteride on the risk of acute urinary retention and the need for surgical treatment among men with benign prostatic hyperplasia. Finasteride Long-Term Efficacy and Safety Study Group. N Engl J Med 338:557-563, 1998.

39. McConnell JD, Roehrborn CG, Bautista OM, et al. The long-term effect of doxazosin, finasteride, and combination therapy on the clinical progression of benign prostatic hyperplasia. N Engl J Med 349:2387-2398, 2003.

# Chapter 65

# Angiotensin-Converting Enzyme Inhibitors

## Domenic A. Sica, Todd W. B. Gehr

## INTRODUCTION

In the management of hypertension and cardiovascular disease, multiple treatment strategies have come and gone over the last four decades. The *stepped care* approach was popular for some time. The diuretic-based stepped care approach to hypertension therapy is supported by sound outcomes data from numerous randomized, controlled trials.[1] However, adopting a *stepped care* approach to the treatment of hypertension neglects the diverse *individualized* pathophysiology of this condition. Its advocates value the clarity of standardization of hypertension treatment, while others are displeased with its inflexible nature.

The concept of individualized *therapy* has gradually evolved, particularly in the context of the recent treatment experience with angiotensin-converting enzyme (ACE) inhibitors. Over the past two decades, the renin-angiotensin-aldosterone (RAA) axis has been increasingly viewed as wielding an important influence on hypertension and target organ disease and thus has emerged as an attractive target for pharmacologic intervention. Of drugs known to interrupt the RAA axis, the treatment experience is greatest for ACE inhibitors.[2]

The ACE inhibitor class has expanded to include 10 ACE agents available in the United States and many more worldwide. In addition to their vasodepressor properties, ACE inhibitors effectively slow the progression of renal, cardiac, and/or vascular disease.[2,3] Thus it was a logical step in their development to seek additional indications for treatment of congestive heart failure (CHF), postmyocardial infarction (post-MI), and diabetic nephropathy (Tables 65-1 and 65-2).[2,3] A therapeutic indication has also been granted for the ACE inhibitor ramipril for the treatment of the high-risk cardiac patient without discernable left ventricular dysfunction.[4]

This chapter broadly discusses the pharmacokinetics, pharmacodynamics, response, and outcomes data for ACE inhibitors. The reader is directed to sources that provide more-comprehensive discussion of particular themes that cannot be discussed because of space constraints, such as the properties and function of ACE (Chapter 9) and outcome trials of ACE inhibitors (Chapter 35).

## PHARMACOLOGY

The first orally active ACE inhibitor was the sulfhydryl-containing compound captopril, which was introduced in 1981. Subsequently, the more long-acting compound enalapril maleate, a prodrug requiring in vivo hepatic and intestinal wall esterolysis to yield the active diacid inhibitor enalaprilat, and lisinopril became available. All orally administered ACE inhibitors are prodrugs with the exception of lisinopril and captopril.[5] It was originally thought that formation of the active diacid metabolites of ACE inhibitors, such as enalapril, would be inhibited in the presence of hepatic impairment, as in advanced CHF. This slowdown in metabolism proved to be inconsequential, however.[6]

ACE inhibitors are structurally heterogeneous. The binding ligand for ACE separates these drugs into three groups: sulfhydryl-, phosphinyl-, and carboxyl-containing moieties. The purported pharmacologic advantages of sulfhydryl-containing ACE inhibitors, such as captopril, are to date clinically unproved, but the sulfhydryl group found on captopril is widely viewed as the source of the more-frequent skin rashes—usually maculopapular in type—and the dysgeusia seen with this compound.[7] The suggestion that the phosphinyl group, found on fosinopril, might favorably alter its penetration into the myocardium and thereby improve myocardial inotropic and lusitropic responses is likewise unproved.[8]

ACE inhibitors can be further distinguished by differences in rate and extent of absorption, plasma protein binding, systemic half-life, and mode of systemic disposition, but they behave quite similarly in how they lower blood pressure (BP) (Table 65-3).[3,5,9,10] Beyond the issue of dosing frequency, these pharmacologic differences are seldom of sufficient consequence to govern selection of an agent.[3,10] Two pharmacologic considerations for the ACE inhibitors, route of systemic elimination and tissue-binding, have recently generated considerable discussion and merit additional comment.[11,12]

## Route of Elimination

In the presence of chronic kidney disease (CKD), the ACE inhibitors ramipril, enalapril, fosinopril, trandolapril, and benazepril do not accumulate with repetitive dosing, suggesting that these prodrugs either undergo biliary clearance directly or that their conversion to an active diacid form is independent of renal function.[13-15] Each of these prodrug ACE inhibitors is marginally active, so the absence of accumulation in CKD should not be viewed as evidence of a clinically relevant dual route of elimination for these drugs. ACE inhibitor accumulation in CKD is most germane for the diacid metabolites (typically the active form) of these compounds. The diacid metabolites of fosinopril and trandolapril, fosinoprilat and trandolaprilat, are the only ones that undergo dual renal and hepatic elimination.[14,15] The systemic clearance of all other ACE inhibitors is largely renal, declining early in the course of CKD and occurring as a function of varying degrees of filtration and tubular secretion.[11] ACE inhibitor accumulation has yet to be associated with known side effects, such as cough or angioneurotic edema. However, elevations in ACE inhibitor concentrations can be accompanied by significantly reduced BP and its organ-directed sequelae.[16]

**Table 65-1** FDA-Approved Indications for ACE Inhibitors

| Drug | HTN | CHF | Diabetic Nephropathy | High-Risk Patients Without Left Ventricular Dysfunction |
|---|---|---|---|---|
| Captopril | ● | ● (post-MI)* | ● | |
| Benazepril | ● | | | |
| Enalapril | ● | ●† | | |
| Fosinopril | ● | ● | | |
| Lisinopril | ● | ● (post-MI)* | | |
| Moexipril | ● | | | |
| Perindopril | ● | | | |
| Quinapril | ● | ● | | |
| Ramipril | ● | ● (post-MI) | | ● |
| Trandolapril | ● | ● (post-MI) | | |

*Captopril and lisinopril are indicated for CHF treatment both postmyocardial infarction and as adjunctive therapy in general heart failure therapy.
†Enalapril is indicated for asymptomatic, left ventricular dysfunction.
ACE, angiotensin-converting enzyme; HTN, hypertension; CHF, congestive heart failure; MI, myocardial infarction.

**Table 65-2** ACE Inhibitors: Dosage Strengths and Treatment Guidelines

| Drug | Trade Name | Usual Total Dose and/ or Range—*Hypertension* (Frequency day) | Usual Total Dose and/ or Range—*Heart Failure* (Frequency day) | Comment | Fixed-Dose Combination* |
|---|---|---|---|---|---|
| Benazepril | Lotensin | 20-40 (1) | Not FDA approved for heart failure | | Lotensin HCT |
| Captopril | Capoten | 12.5-100 (2-3) | 18.75-150 (3) | Generically available | Capozide† |
| Enalapril | Vasotec | 5-40 (1-2) | 5-40 (2) | Available generically and intravenously | Vaseretic |
| Fosinopril | Monopril | 10-40 (1) | 10-40 (1) | Renal and hepatic elimination | Monopril-HCT |
| Lisinopril | Prinivil, Zestril | 2.5-40 (1) | 5-20 (1) | Generically available | Prinizide, Zestoretic |
| Moexipril | Univasc | 7.5-30 (1) | Not FDA approved for heart failure | | Uniretic |
| Perindopril | Aceon | 2-16 (1) | Not FDA approved for heart failure | | |
| Quinapril | Accupril | 5-80 (1) | 10-40 (1-2) | | Accuretic |
| Ramipril | Altace | 2.5-20 (1) | 10 (2) | Indicated in high-risk vascular patients | |
| Trandolapril | Mavik | 1-8 (1) | 1-4 (1) | Renal and hepatic elimination | Tarka |

*Fixed-dose combinations in this class typically contain a thiazide-like diuretic.
†Capozide is indicated for first-step treatment of hypertension.

**Table 65-3** Predominant Hemodynamic Effects of ACE Inhibitors

| Hemodynamic Parameter | Effect | Clinical Significance |
|---|---|---|
| **CARDIOVASCULAR** | | |
| Total peripheral resistance | Decreased | |
| Mean arterial pressure | Decreased | |
| Cardiac output | Increased or no change | These parameters contribute to a |
| Stroke volume | Increased | general decrease in systemic blood |
| Preload and afterload | Decreased | pressure |
| Pulmonary artery pressure | Decreased | |
| Right atrial pressure | Decreased | |
| Diastolic dysfunction | Improved | |
| **RENAL** | | |
| Renal blood flow | Usually increased | Contributes to the renoprotective |
| Glomerular filtration rate | Variable, usually unchanged but may ↓ in renal failure | effect of these agents |
| Efferent arteriolar resistance | Decreased | |
| Filtration fraction | Decreased | |
| **PERIPHERAL NERVOUS SYSTEM** | | |
| Biosynthesis of noradrenaline | Decreased | Enhances blood pressure lowering |
| Reuptake of adrenaline | Inhibited | effect and resets baroreceptor |
| Circulating catecholamines | Decreased | function |

## Tissue Binding

The physicochemical differences among ACE inhibitors, including binding affinity, potency, lipophilicity, and depot effect, allow for the arbitrary classification of ACE inhibitors according to affinity for tissue-ACE.[12,17,18] The extent to which tissue ACE is blocked by an ACE inhibitor is a function of both the inhibitor's intrinsic binding affinity and the free inhibitor concentration found within that tissue. The tissue-based free inhibitor concentration is in a continuous state of flux and at any one time is determined by the sum of ACE inhibitor delivered to tissues and residual ACE inhibitor released from tissues for reentry into the bloodstream. The quantity of ACE inhibitor conveyed to tissues is determined by several pharmacologic variables including dose frequency/amount, absolute bioavailability, plasma half-life, and tissue penetration. When blood levels of an ACE inhibitor are high—typically in the first third to half of the dosing interval—tissue retention per se of an ACE inhibitor is not needed for an enduring level of ACE inhibition. However, as ACE inhibitor blood levels fall during the second half of the dosing interval, two factors—inhibitor binding affinity and tissue retention—take on added importance if functional ACE inhibition is to be maintained.

The question arises as to whether the degree of tissue ACE inhibition may extend to efficacy differences between the various ACE inhibitors. In this regard, there appears to be little difference among the various ACE inhibitors in their capacity to reduce BP. When relative drug-to-drug BP responses differ among ACE inhibitors, it is generally the result of dissimilar half-lives of the compounds under study.

An additional consideration is whether ACE inhibitors with high tissue affinity differ in their ability to provide BP-independent target organ protection, as has been theorized for ramipril in the Heart Outcomes Prevention Evaluation (HOPE).[19] In this regard, endothelial function has been observed to improve more regularly with the higher tissue-ACE affinity compounds, such as quinapril and ramipril. If improvement in endothelial function is accepted as a surrogate for protection from target organ events, then relevant differences may exist among ACE inhibitors.

However, there have been no direct head-to-head outcomes trials comparing ACE inhibitors with different tissue affinity. Results of the limited head-to-head comparisons available do not convincingly support the claim of overall superiority for lipophilic ACE inhibitors.[20,21]

## APPLICATION OF PHARMACOLOGIC DIFFERENCES

Because there is little that truly separates one long-acting ACE inhibitor from another in the treatment of hypertension, cost has assumed increased importance.[22] For pricing to be key in the selection of an ACE inhibitor is not unreasonable if the drug were being used only for the control of BP. ACE inhibitors, however, are also extensively used for their cardiorenal outcomes benefits, and only a limited number of ACE inhibitors have been studied in this context. The term *class effect* has entered into the discussion of both of these aspects of ACE inhibitor use but is relevant to one and not the other.

*Class effect* is a phrase often invoked to legitimatize substitution of one ACE inhibitor for another that has been specifically studied in a disease state, such as CHF or diabetic nephropathy.[19,23-25] The concept of *class effect* is well suited for application to the BP effects of ACE inhibitors, where scant difference exists among the numerous agents in the class. The concept of *class effect*, already vague in its definition, becomes even more ambiguous when "true" dose equivalence for a non-BP endpoint, such as rate of progression to end-stage renal disease (ESRD) or survival in the setting of CHF, is being determined for the various ACE inhibitors. Determining ACE inhibitor dose equivalence from outcomes trials is confounded by differing dose frequency, titration requirements, and level of renal function in individual studies.[26-31] The latter is particular relevant to the elderly, because senescence-related changes in renal function extend the functional half-life of ACE inhibitors (renally cleared) and make it nearly impossible to determine "true" dose equivalence between various drugs in the class. In interpreting the results of outcome studies with ACE inhibitors, it is prudent to assume that the benefits derive from the compound being tested, for the outcome being studied, at the per protocol dose and frequency of dosing. However, despite these caveats about the difficulty in establishing dose equivalence, the clinician can estimate equivalent doses among the various ACE inhibitors *if* ACE inhibitor substitution is planned.

## MECHANISM OF ACTION AND HEMODYNAMIC EFFECTS

The site of ACE inhibitor activity (within the RAA axis) can be pinpointed at the pluripotent ACE, an enzyme known to catalyze the conversion of angiotensin I to angiotensin II, as well as to facilitate the degradation of bradykinin to assorted peptides.[17,32] However, ACE inhibition, as a means to reduce angiotensin II levels has inherent limitations.[17] ACE inhibition fails to suppress production of angiotensin II by alternative enzymatic pathways—such as chymase and other tissue-based proteases.[17,33] These alternative pathways represent the principal mode of angiotensin II generation in several tissues, including the myocardium and the vasculature of humans.[34,35] With long-term administration of an ACE inhibitor, these alternative pathways become involved in a sequence of events culminating in a return of angiotensin-II concentrations to pretherapy levels ("angiotensin II escape").

Substrate for these alternative pathways is obtained from the increase in angiotensin I levels arising from a disinhibition of renin secretion by ACE inhibition–induced reductions in circulating angiotensin II.[35,36] Because ACE inhibitors reduce angiotensin II levels for only a limited period of time (weeks) during chronic administratin, other mechanisms must account for their persistent BP-lowering effect.[36,37] One possibility is that increased concentrations of the vasodilator bradykinin enhance the release of nitric oxide (NO), stimulate the production of endothelium-derived hyperpolarizing factor, and accentuate the release of prostacyclin ($PGI_2$).[38,39] Moreover, ACE is also responsible for the degradation of angiotensin-(1-7), an angiotensin peptide with the capacity to counterbalance a number of the pleitrophic (renal and vascular) effects of angiotensin II (see Chapter 10).[39] The contribution of angiotensin "fragments" (many of which are physiologically active) and prostaglandins/NO to the antihypertensive effect of ACE inhibitors is still debated.[39,40]

Conversely, nonsteroidal antiinflammatory drugs (NSAIDs) and selective cyclooxygenase inhibitors (COXIBs), such as celecoxib and rofecoxib, attenuate the BP-lowering effect of a number of antihypertensive drugs including ACE inhibitors.[41,42] This occurs more commonly in salt-sensitive hypertensives, as in many elderly patients.[42] A question that remains unresolved is the degree to which aspirin (acetylsalicyclic acid [ASA]) administration interferes with the anti-hypertensive and/or cardioprotective effects of an ACE inhibitor.[43-45] Low-dose ASA (100 mg/day or less) appears to minimally affect the BP reduction seen with ACE inhibition.[43,44] For example, in the Hypertension Optimal Treatment (HOT) study, long-term, low-dose ASA did not interfere with the BP-lowering effect of antihypertensive combinations, which in many cases included ACE inhibitors.[44] However, higher doses, generally above 236 mg/day, can blunt the antihypertensive response to an ACE inhibitor and possibly neutralize the clinical benefits of ACE inhibitors in patients with heart failure.[45]

A reduction in both central and peripheral sympathetic nervous system (SNS) activity accounts for a portion of the antihypertensive effect of an ACE inhibitor (Table 65–3).[46,47] ACE inhibitors preserve circulatory reflexes and baroreceptor function; thus they do not reflexly increase heart rate when BP is reduced.[48] The latter property accounts for the low incidence of postural hypotension with ACE inhibitors and provides an important safety benefit in elderly persons, who as a group are typically predisposed to orthostatic hypotension.[49] ACE inhibitors also improve endothelial function, facilitate vascular remodeling, and favorably modify the viscoelastic properties of structurally abnormal blood vessels (see Chapters 14 and 15).[50,51] These vascular effects are the likely explanation for the incremental reduction in BP with the long-term use of ACE inhibitors.

## BLOOD PRESSURE–LOWERING EFFECT

All ACE inhibitors available in the United States are FDA-approved for the treatment of hypertension (see Table 65–2). Based on outcome data, the Seventh Report of the Joint National Committee on the Prevention, Detection, Evaluation, and Treatment of High Blood Pressure (JNC 7); the World Health Organization/International Society of Hypertension; and European Society of Hypertension/European Society of Cardiology now recognize ACE inhibitors as an option for first-line therapy in patients with essential hypertension, especially in those with a high coronary disease risk profile, diabetes with renal disease/proteinuria, CHF, and/or post MI.[1,52-55]

The enthusiasm for the use of ACE inhibitors extends beyond the issue of effectiveness, because they are comparably efficacious as (and no better than) most other drug classes, including diuretics, β-blockers, and calcium channel blockers. Response rates with ACE inhibitors range from 40% to 70% in stage 1 or 2 hypertension, with salt intake and race serving as important variables in determining the response.[56] In interpreting clinical trial results with ACE inhibitors, a distinction should be made between the mean reduction in BP (which is typically highly significant) and the percentage of individuals who are poor, average, and excellent responders (which may vary considerably among studies).

There are few predictors of the vasodepressor response to ACE inhibitors. Although ACE gene polymorphism (and specific genotypes), among other genetic determinants, have been suggested to predict the antihypertensive response to an ACE inhibitor, findings have been sufficiently inconsistent to warrant a wait-and-see attitude for genotyping.[57] There has also been a limited predictive relationship between the pretreatment and/or posttreatment PRA value (used as a marker of RAA axis activity) and the fall in BP with an ACE inhibitor. However, when hypertension is marked by significant elevation of PRA (activation of the RAA axis), as in renal artery stenosis, the response to an ACE inhibitor can be profound.[58]

Certain patient groups, including low-renin, salt-sensitive, volume-expanded individuals such as the diabetic and African American hypertensives, are generally less responsive to ACE inhibitor monotherapy. However, the BP response to an ACE inhibitor can be highly variable in African American and diabetic patients, with some individuals in these groups experiencing significant falls in BP. The low-renin state characteristic of the elderly hypertensive differs from other low-renin forms of hypertension in that it reflects the consequences of senescence-related changes in the RAA axis and not volume expansion.[59] The elderly generally respond well to ACE inhibitors in conventional doses,[60] although senescence-related renal failure, which slows the elimination of most ACE inhibitors, complicates interpretation of dose-specific treatment successes.

Results from a number of head-to-head trials support the comparable antihypertensive efficacy and tolerability of the various ACE inhibitors *if* comparable doses of the individual ACE inhibitors are given (see Table 65–2). However, there are differences among the ACE inhibitors, as to the time to onset and/or duration of effect, which may relate to the absorption and tissue distribution characteristics of a compound.

Enalaprilat is the lone ACE inhibitor available in an intravenous form; however, multiple choices exist for the orally available ACE inhibitors.[3] ACE inhibitors labeled as "once-daily" vary in their ability to reduce BP for a full 24 hours, as defined by a trough:peak ratio >50%.[61] Consequently, in deciding on the dosing frequency for ACE inhibitors, one should bear in mind that response patterns to these drugs are highly individualized, with many patients requiring a second daily dose to maintain effect. However, in the elderly, senescence-related changes in renal function (and reduced renal clearance of the compound) and/or giving a high dose may obviate a second ACE inhibitor dose during the 24-hour treatment period.[62]

A frequent question asked is what steps to take when an ACE inhibitor fails to normalize BP. This question is best answered in the context of the magnitude of the response. If there is a minimal BP-reducing effect, then a switch to an alternative drug class is justified unless continuation of an ACE inhibitor is indicated on the basis of a high cardiac and/or renal risk profile. However, ACE inhibitor nonresponders fairly regularly "respond" on addition of a diuretic or a calcium channel blocker, so very few patients should have an ACE inhibitor discontinued simply based on a failure to "respond" to monotherapy.

If the BP response to an ACE inhibitor is modest, one can increase the daily dose (possibly by reverting to twice-daily administration), understanding that the dose-response curve for ACE inhibitors, like many antihypertensive agents, is fairly steep at the beginning doses and flattens thereafter.[63-64] Increasing the dose of an ACE inhibitor does not generally change the peak effect; rather, it extends the duration of response. In fact, several of the shorter-acting ACE inhibitors, such as enalapril, can behave as once-a-day medications if high-enough daily doses are given to prolong the duration of effect. A final consideration with ACE inhibitor therapy is that of an incremental benefit (over several weeks) on BP relating

to factors such as vascular remodeling and/or improvement in endothelial function.[51]

## ACE INHIBITORS IN COMBINATION WITH OTHER AGENTS

The BP-lowering effect of an ACE inhibitor is improved with the simultaneous administration of a diuretic, particularly in salt-sensitive forms of hypertension.[65] This pattern of response has encouraged the development of fixed-dose combination products, composed of an ACE inhibitor and varying doses (as low as 12.5 mg) of a thiazide-type diuretic.[65,66] The rationale for combining these two drug classes arises from the observation that diuretic-related sodium depletion activates the RAA axis, causing BP to shift to an angiotensin II–dependent mode, a circumstance most responsive to the BP-reducing effect of an ACE inhibitor.

β-Blockers have also been administered in conjunction with ACE inhibitors, an approach that was possible per protocol in the Antihypertensive and Lipid-Lowering Treatment to Prevent Heart Attack Trial (ALLHAT).[53] The β-blocker atenolol was the most commonly added second medication in ALLHAT. A potential physiologic basis for this combination is that β-blockade blunts the reactive rise in PRA that goes along with ACE inhibitor therapy; alternatively, this combination can be considered for use in the setting of coronary artery disease, with any BP gain being a secondary consideration.[67] When a meaningful reduction in BP follows from the addition of a β-blocker to an ACE inhibitor, it is often accompanied by a reduction in pulse rate. Alternatively, adding a peripheral α-antagonist, such as doxazosin, to an ACE inhibitor can further reduce BP, albeit without a clear mechanistic basis.[68]

The BP-lowering effect of an ACE inhibitor is enhanced with the addition of a CCB, either dihydropyridine or non-dihydropyridine, and this has been the basis for several fixed-dose combination products.[69-71] Adding an ACE inhibitor to a CCB is also helpful in attenuating the peripheral edema commonly seen with CCB therapy.[72] In addition, preliminary evidence supports use of CCB-therapy in attenuating the reduction in glomerular filtration rate (GFR) that can accompany ACE inhibitor treatment.[73] This is of particular relevance to the elderly, since one reason for underuse of ACE inhibitors in older persons is fear of inducing a decline in renal function superimposed on preexisting renal dysfunction. This CCB-ACE inhibitor hemodynamic interaction at a renal level may occasionally result in false-positive captopril renography studies.

The efficacy of both ACE inhibitors and angiotensin-receptor blockers (ARBs) as antihypertensive agents is well established. This has fueled the belief that in combination, these two drug classes may provide an incremental benefit in both BP reduction and target organ protection. However, there is insufficient evidence to support a general recommendation for the combination of these two drug classes in BP management.[74,75]

Studies have established the utility of ACE inhibitors in the management of hypertensive patients otherwise unresponsive to multiple drug combinations, such as a diuretic together with minoxidil, a CCB and/or a peripheral α-blocker.[76] If an acute reduction in BP is needed, oral or sublingual captopril—with an onset of action as soon as 15 minutes after administration—can be administered. An additional option for the management of hypertensive emergencies is intravenous enalaprilat, with a dose of 0.625 mg representing a maximal effective dose (higher doses may only extend the duration of action).[77] ACE inhibitors should be administered cautiously in patients suspected of marked activation of the RAA axis (e.g., prior treatment with diuretics and/or immediately post-MI). In such persons, sudden and extreme falls in BP—so-called first dose hypotension—have been observed.[78]

## ACE INHIBITORS IN HYPERTENSION ASSOCIATED WITH OTHER DISORDERS

ACE inhibitors effectively regress left ventricular hypertrophy (LVH).[79] This is an important property of ACE inhibitors, given that LVH portends a significant future risk of sudden death or MI.[80] ACE inhibitors can be safely utilized in patients with coronary artery disease (CAD) and are indicated for secondary prevention after acute MI.[2,3] The ACE inhibitor perindopril has been shown to reduce cardiovascular risk in a low-risk population with stable CAD and no apparent heart failure.[81] Although they are not proven coronary vasodilators, ACE inhibitors improve hemodynamic factors such that myocardial oxygen consumption is reduced with no worsening of angina and possibly some attendant reductions in ischemia (Table 65–3). For example, ACE inhibitors do not reflexively increase myocardial sympathetic tone in hypertensive patients with angina, as can take place with other antihypertensives.[82,83]

ACE inhibitors are useful in the treatment of both isolated systolic hypertension and systolic-predominant forms of hypertension, in part because of their capacity to improve artery compliance.[51,84] They are also of value in the treatment of patients with cerebrovascular disease, because they preserve cerebral autoregulation in the face of reduced BP, a property of particular relevance to the elderly hypertensive.[85] ACE inhibitors dilate both small and large arteries and can be used safely in patients with peripheral arterial disease (PAD). They may favorably modify the pattern and/or the course of intermittent claudication.[86] Of the 9297 patients in the HOPE study, 4051 had PAD—defined by a history of PAD, claudication, or an ankle-brachial index <0.90. These patients had a reduction in the primary endpoint similar to those without PAD, indicating that ACE inhibition lowers the risk of fatal and nonfatal ischemic events in PAD patients.[87]

ACE inhibitors are preferred agents in the hypertensive diabetic patient for both BP reduction and organ protection, a use presumably independent of BP lowering.[88] It is often necessary to coadminister a diuretic, because the BP-lowering effect of ACE inhibitor monotherapy is modest in the low-renin, volume-expanded form of hypertension characteristic of the diabetic. A final consideration in the hypertensive diabetic relates to the effect of ACE inhibitors on lipid parameters and/or insulin resistance. Although an unambiguous effect on serum lipids and/or insulin resistance has yet to be demonstrated for ACE inhibitors,[89] both the CAPtopril Prevention Project (CAPPP) and HOPE studies showed that the ACE inhibitors captopril and ramipril, respectively, decreased the incidence of new-onset type 2 diabetes mellitus.[90,91]

## TARGET ORGAN EFFECTS AND RECENT CLINICAL TRIALS

### Renal

JNC 7 recommends the use of ACE inhibitors in patients with hypertension and CKD to both control hypertension and slow the rate of progression of renal failure.[1,54] However, the renoprotective features of ACE inhibitors should never substitute for tight BP control, which is of paramount importance in the management of the hypertensive CKD patient. In this regard, JNC 7 suggests a goal BP of <130/80 mm Hg in albuminuric patients (>300 mg/day) with or without CKD.[54] In hypertensive CKD patients, ACE inhibitor monotherapy (without related diuretic administration) rarely yields a brisk BP-lowering response—because of the volume dependency of this form of hypertension. For example, in the African American Study of Kidney Disease (AASK), hypertensive African American CKD patients treated with ramipril and randomized to a mean arterial BP of 102 to 107 mm Hg required three additional medications on average to achieve this goal BP range.[92]

Both macroproteinuria and microalbuminuria have emerged as strong markers for the rate of CKD progression.[93] In particular, microalbuminuria foreshadows the progression of diabetic nephropathy and should be routinely measured in all diabetics.[93] The choice of risk terms (macroproteinuria or microalbuminuria) is by no means absolute in that the partition values for urine albumin:creatinine ratio, used to identify microalbuminuria, are without a specific threshold value.[94] Proteinuria also serves as an independent risk factor for fatal and nonfatal cardiovascular events.[94,95] Screening for microalbuminuria is recommended in all diabetics and increasingly in others perceived to be at high risk for renal or cardiovascular disease.[96,97] It is now recommended that proteinuria be therapeutically targeted when present in either diabetic or non diabetic renal disease.[98,99] ACE inhibitors and ARBs effectively reduce protein excretion and thereby are important tools in the treatment of microalbuminuria or macroalbuminuria with or without concomitant hypertension.[99,100]

ACE inhibitors have renoprotective effects in various settings, including established type 1 insulin-dependent diabetic nephropathy,[24] type 2 non–insulin-dependent diabetic nephropathy,[101,102] normotensive type 1 diabetic patients with microalbuminuria,[103] and an assortment of nondiabetic renal diseases.[98,104-106] In some diabetic patients, ACE inhibitor therapy has resulted in the remission of nephrotic range proteinuria and long-term stabilization of renal function.[107,108]

However, aggressive BP control (<130/80 mm Hg) in elderly patients with type 2 diabetes and preserved renal function has been shown to stabilize renal function regardless of whether the initial therapy was with an ACE inhibitor or a calcium channel blocker.[109,110] ACE inhibitor therapy is also beneficial in nondiabetic renal diseases. In AASK, ramipril was more effective than amlopidine in limiting the decline in GFR in patients with hypertensive nephrosclerosis and a urinary protein:creatinine ratio >0.22.[106] Moreover, a meta-analysis of ACE inhibitor use in nondiabetic renal disease concluded that ACE inhibitors conferred renal benefit in nondiabetic patients with >0.5 g/day of proteinuria.[111] In many of the studies making up this meta-analysis, the target BP was <140/90 mm Hg, which is important in that the renoprotective effects of ACE inhibitors (compared with other antihypertensive agents) may not be as conspicuous at lower BP values.

However, positive renal outcomes with ACE inhibitors in nephropathic states are not guaranteed. In the Ramipril Efficacy in Nephropathy (REIN) study, patients with proteinuric chronic nephropathies were assigned randomly to treatment with the ACE inhibitor ramipril or placebo plus conventional antihypertensive therapy. ACE inhibitors significantly reduced the rate of proteinuria, the decline in GFR, and the risk of ESRD in patients with >3 g/day of proteinuria; however, during the study period, those with proteinuria less than 2 g/24 hours, type 2 diabetes, or polycystic kidney disease did not benefit to an appreciable extent from ACE inhibitor therapy.[112]

ACE inhibitor regimens shown to slow the rate of CKD progression include captopril 25 mg three times per day, enalapril 5 to 10 mg/day, benazepril 10 mg/day, and ramipril 2.5 to 5 mg/day.[3] Each of these compounds is renally cleared; thus it can be presumed that reduced renal clearance under the circumstances of CKD extended their pharmacologic effect.[113] Whereas it is accepted that the beneficial effects of ACE inhibition are greatest when urinary protein excretion is excessive (> 3 g/24 hours),[114] the ACE inhibitor dose providing optimal renoprotection is still debated. For example, low-dose ramipril (1.25 mg/day) had no effect on cardiovascular and renal outcomes of patients with type 2 diabetes and albuminuria, despite a slight decrease in BP and urinary albumin,[116] whereas in the HOPE trial, ramipril given at a high-end dose (titrated to 10 mg/day) prevented or delayed the progression of microalbuminuria.[115] Dose titration of an ACE inhibitor should be viewed in the context of the therapeutic endpoint, because reduction in protein excretion, lipid parameters, and BP exhibit differing dose responses to up-titration of an ACE inhibitor.[117,118] For example, in chronic proteinuric nondiabetic nephropathies, up-titration of the ACE inhibitor lisinopril to maximum tolerated doses improves hypertriglyceridemia and hypercholesterolemia (through increases in serum albumin/total protein concentration and thereby oncotic pressure by a direct, dose-dependent effect). These lipid benefits occur with upward dose titration even though the majority of the BP-lowering effect is realized with low-end doses of lisinopril (Figure 65–1).[118]

ACE inhibitor treatment offers a variety of potentially beneficial renal effects involving hemodynamic, cellular, and lipid-related pathways. However, the positive hemodynamic effects of ACE inhibition can sometimes be misconstrued to represent a "nephrotoxic" process. ACE inhibitors transiently reduce GFR in tandem with reductions in glomerular capillary pressures.[119,120] Such falls in GFR are typically inconsequential, generally of the order of 10% to 15% and usually reversible, and in point of fact, predictive of renal protection in the long term.[120] The elderly are more prone to frequent reductions in GFR with ACE inhibitors, at least in part because of their more-extensive microvascular and macrovascular renal disease (see *Side Effects of ACE Inhibitors*).[121] A question commonly put forward, particularly in the elderly, is whether a specific level of renal function exists at which an ACE inhibitor should not be started. There is not a specific level of renal function that prohibits the start of an ACE inhibitor unless clinically important hyperkalemia is anticipated.

Four factors can be viewed as possible modifiers of the renal effects of ACE inhibition. First, a low-sodium intake enhances both the antiproteinuric and antihypertensive response to ACE

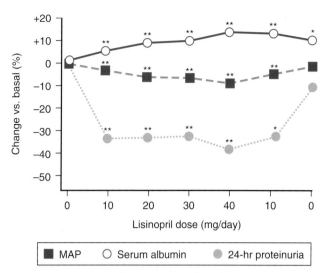

**Figure 65–1** Percent changes versus baseline in mean arterial pressure (MAP), 24-hour urinary protein excretion rate, and serum albumin at different lisinopril treatment periods in 22 patients with nondiabetic proteinuric nephropathies. (*p <.05, **p <.01 vs. baseline). With permission from Ruggenenti P, Mise N, Pisoni R, et al. Diverse effects of increasing lisinopril doses on lipid abnormalities in chronic nephropathies. Circulation 107:586-592, 2003.[118]

inhibition.[122,123] Second, short-term studies indicate that dietary protein restriction adds to the ACE inhibitor effect on protein excretion in nephrotic patients, implying that the combination of ACE inhibition and dietary-protein restriction could prove more effective than ACE inhibition alone in slowing the progression of CKD.[124] A third factor is nocturnal resistance to the antiproteinuric effect of ACE inhibition despite 24-hour persistence of the BP effect.[125] Finally, inherited variations in the activity of ACE exist because of two common polymorphisms of the ACE gene (I [insertion] and D [deletion]), giving rise to three potential genotypes II, ID, and DD. The DD genotype is associated with higher circulating ACE levels and an increased pressor response to infused angiotensin I as compared with the II genotype, with the ID genotype displaying intermediate characteristics.[126]

The observation that DD patients were at increased risk for MI and ischemic cardiomyopathy was the first indication that the inherited variation in ACE activity might be of clinical significance.[127] One observational study has shown that renal function declines more precipitously in diabetic CKD patients with the DD genotype, and when such patients are given ACE inhibitors, they do not show significant reductions in either protein excretion or the rate of CKD progression.[128] Although a promising concept, pharmacogenetic studies to date do not provide a definitive answer as to whether the antiproteinuric effect of ACE inhibition (or renal failure progression rate) is adversely affected (or bettered) by a specific ACE genotype.[129]

## Cardiac

ACE inhibitor therapy provides positive outcome benefits in a number of cardiac scenarios, including CHF,[23,28,130] post-MI,[131-134] and the hypertensive patient with a high definable cardiac risk.[19,52,53,81] This benefit exists both in normotensive[19] and hypertensive[19,52,53] individuals and in those with varying risk profiles.[19,52,53,81] This beneficial effect has been observed with several ACE inhibitors, suggesting that a class effect may be present for the positive cardiac outcome benefits of these compounds.[19,52,53,81] Placebo-controlled and open-label trials suggest that ACE inhibitors improve CHF symptomatology and more importantly, reduce the risk of death and hospitalization from CHF.[23,28,130] These positive outcome results have established ACE inhibitors as first-line therapy in the treatment of CHF.[135,136] ACE inhibitors decrease angiotensin II production (at least in the short term)[34,35] and thereby readjust the neurohumoral imbalance of CHF.[137,138] Low doses of ACE inhibitors are sufficient to improve exercise tolerance and CHF symptoms[27,30] and arrest the weight loss otherwise seen with progressive CHF.[139] However, improvement in CHF mortality requires high-dose ACE inhibitor therapy.[28,31]

The treatment of CHF should include sequential titration of ACE inhibitors to doses proven to favorably affect mortality in randomized clinical trials. The ability to reach these doses in the CHF patient oftentimes proves challenging, because systemic hypotension and/or a decline in GFR often arise with high-dose ACE inhibitor therapy.[140,142] Thus, reaching full ACE inhibitor doses calls for a well-developed understanding of the relationship between volume status, BP, and the sought-after ACE inhibitor dose.[140,141]

Several ACE inhibitors—including captopril, fosinopril, lisinopril, quinapril, ramipril, and trandolapril—now can claim positive outcomes data in various types of CHF.[130,131] Despite these compelling outcomes data, physician prescribing practice has lagged behind. Only a modest fraction (50%-75%) of CHF patients eligible for ACE inhibitor therapy actually receive the therapy.[143,144] Moreover, the ACE inhibitor doses commonly used in real-world practice on average are less than one half the targeted dose proven effective in randomized, controlled trials.[143,144] Factors predicting the use and optimal dosing of ACE inhibitors include the treatment setting (prior hospitalization and/or specialty clinic follow-up), the prescribing physician (cardiology specialty vs. family practitioner/general internist), the patient status (increased severity of symptoms, male, younger), and the drug (lower frequency of administration).[143] Underdosing of ACE inhibitors has a negative economic impact in CHF because it is associated with more frequent CHF hospitalizations.[145]

Enalapril, captopril, lisinopril, and trandolapril have been shown to significantly reduce morbidity and mortality over a wide range of ventricular dysfunction in the post-MI patient.[131,133,134] In a hemodynamically stable patient (systolic BP >100 mm Hg) following an MI, an oral ACE inhibitor should be initiated (generally within the first 24 hours of the event), particularly if the MI is accompanied by depressed left ventricular function.[146] The hemodynamic effects and overall benefit of ACE inhibition are gained early after an MI, with the 30-day survival increasing by 40% in the first day, 45% in days 2 to 7, and approximately 15% thereafter.[147] Recent trends show a promising increase in ACE inhibitor prescriptions for patients discharged following an acute MI.[132]

Captopril, lisinopril, ramipril, and trandolapril are approved for specific post-MI left ventricular dysfunction, and enalapril is indicated for use in asymptomatic left ventricular dysfunction (see Table 65–1).[3] The consistency of these findings suggests a class effect for this facet of ACE

inhibitor use.[134] There are too few data to conclude that there are clinically significant differences among the ACE inhibitors in the post-MI setting, given both the lack of head-to-head trials and the variability of study circumstances for particular ACE inhibitors.[133,134]

Several trials have assessed the utility of ACE inhibitors in modifying cardiac endpoints.[19,52,53,81] These trials have compared ACE inhibitor therapy to either placebo[19,81] or an active comparator such as a thiazide diuretic.[52,53] A number of these trials have been interpreted as showing that ACE inhibitors have particular advantages in reducing cardiovascular disease outcomes. However, available data demonstrate insignificant differences in total major cardiovascular events between regimens based on ACE inhibitors, calcium antagonists, and diuretics or β-blockers, taken in the context of ACE inhibitor–based regimens reducing BP less.[148] Ethnic background of the study participants may also be an important determinant of the efficiency of ACE inhibitors in outcome trials. For example, the ALLHAT trial[53] showed a smaller reduction of total major cardiovascular events with the ACE inhibitor lisinopril than with the diuretic chlorthalidone, in large part because of the large proportion of African American patients in the study and the much smaller reduction in BP achieved with lisinopril in that subgroup.

## Stroke

Given the significant public health impact of stroke and the identification of both nonmodifiable (age, gender, race/-ethnicity) and modifiable (BP, diabetes, lipid profile, and lifestyle) risk factors, early prevention strategies are increasingly being put into practice. When a patient suffers a stroke, the focus of care becomes the prevention of secondary events. This can be accomplished with antiplatelet and lipid-lowering, as well as BP-reduction, strategies. Despite the clear risk reduction with effective realization of these preventative strategies, new approaches are needed. One such "new" approach is to determine whether the stroke benefit gained from BP reduction is unique to the agent employed—such as an ACE inhibitor or an ARB—or a simple consequence of upgrading the hemodynamic profile.[149-151] The data supporting ACE inhibitors in reducing stroke rate have been mixed.[150,152] In the ALLHAT study, stroke incidence was 15% greater with the ACE inhibitor lisinopril (primarily in African Americans) than with the thiazide-type diuretic chlorthalidone.[53] In part, this was related to the less-effective BP reduction in the lisinopril group than in the chlorthalidone group. Similar negative data for ACE inhibitors and stroke arose from the Perindopril Protection Against Recurrent Stroke Study (PROGRESS) of the ACE inhibitor perindopril in the context of secondary stroke prevention.[149] In this study, 6105 hypertensive and non-hypertensive patients who had sustained a stroke without a major disability within the past 5 years were randomized to a 4-mg dose of perindopril with or without a 2.5-mg dose of indapamide (diuretic therapy was at the discretion of the treating physician). BP was reduced by an average of 9/4 mm Hg in the active treatment group, resulting in a 28% reduction in risk of major stroke in all participants. This reduction of risk extended to all forms of stroke (major disabling, hemorrhagic, ischemic, or unknown) to patients with and without hypertension and with and without diabetes. The most beneficial effect was seen in the group receiving perindopril and indapamide, in which BP decreased by 12/5 mm Hg. Surprisingly, patients who received perindopril monotherapy had no reduction in cerebrovascular morbidity and mortality despite a significant 5/3–mm Hg fall in BP.[149] The PROGRESS data are important becasuse it has been debated whether the long-term lowering of BP in patients who have sustained a prior cerebrovascular event reduces recurrent stroke rate comparably with the benefit observed for primary stroke prevention with BP reduction.

The HOPE trial results with the ACE inhibitor ramipril showed that the benefits of lowering BP on the risk of stroke are not confined to patients with hypertension. Compared with placebo, ramipril reduced the risk of any stroke by 32% and that of fatal stroke by 61%. Benefits were consistent across baseline BPs, concomitant drug use, and subgroups defined by the presence or absence of previous stroke, peripheral arterial disease, diabetes, or hypertension.[153] Based on the HOPE study, the American Heart Association guidelines for the primary prevention of stroke recommend ramipril to prevent stroke in high-risk patients and in patients with diabetes and hypertension.[154]

## SIDE EFFECTS OF ACE INHIBITORS

A syndrome of "functional renal insufficiency" has been observed as a class effect with ACE inhibitors.[155] This phenomenon was initially reported in patients with renal artery stenosis and a solitary kidney or bilateral renal artery stenosis. Predisposing conditions include dehydration, CHF, NSAID use, and/or either microvascular or macrovascular renal disease.[142,156] The mechanism common to these conditions is a fall in afferent arteriolar flow. When this occurs, glomerular filtration temporarily declines. In response to this reduction in glomerular filtration, local production of angiotensin II increases. In concert with this increase in angiotensin II, the efferent or postglomerular arteriole constricts, reestablishing hydrostatic pressures in the more proximal glomerular capillary bed.

The abrupt removal of angiotensin II, as occurs with an ACE inhibitor (or an ARB), will acutely dilate the efferent arteriole in tandem with a reduction in systemic BP. In combination, these hemodynamic changes drop glomerular hydrostatic pressure such that glomerular filtration plummets. This type of "functional renal insufficiency" is best treated by discontinuation of the responsible agent, careful volume expansion (if intravascular volume contraction is a contributing factor), and, if warranted on clinical grounds, evelution for the presence of renal artery stenosis (Figure 65–2).[140]

Hyperkalemia is an additional ACE inhibitor–associated side effect.[157] ACE inhibitor–related hyperkalemia occurs infrequently unless a specific predisposition to hyperkalemia exists, such as diabetes or CHF with renal failure (receiving potassium-sparing diuretics or potassium supplements).[158,159] Conversely, ACE inhibitors reduce the potassium loss that ordinarily accompanies diuretic therapy.

A dry, irritating, nonproductive cough is a common complication of ACE inhibitor treatment, with an incidence of up to 44%.[160] Cough is a class effect of ACE inhibitors and has been attributed to an increase in bradykinin and/or other vasoactive peptides such as substance P, which may play a second messenger role in setting off the cough reflex. Although numerous therapies have been tried, few have had any lasting success in eliminating ACE inhibitor–induced cough. The sensible clinical approach for suspected ACE inhibitor–related cough is to reassess the patient several weeks after drug discontinuation. Disappearance of the cough can then be taken as proof of an ACE inhibitor cause.

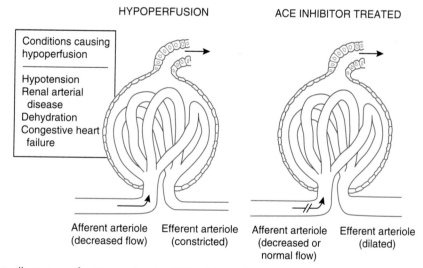

HYPOPERFUSION      ACE INHIBITOR TREATED

Conditions causing hypoperfusion

Hypotension
Renal arterial disease
Dehydration
Congestive heart failure

Afferent arteriole (decreased flow)    Efferent arteriole (constricted)    Afferent arteriole (decreased or normal flow)    Efferent arteriole (dilated)

**Figure 65–2** Schematic illustration of settings wherein ACE inhibitor therapy may worsen renal function. Conditions causing renal hypoperfusion include systemic hypotension, high-grade renal artery stenosis, extracellular fluid volume contraction (simplified as "dehydration" in the figure), administration of vasoconstrictor agents (NSAIDs or cyclosporine, not shown), and CHF. These conditions typically increase renin secretion and angiotensin II production. Angiotensin II constricts the efferent arteriole to a greater extent than the afferent arteriole, such that glomerular hydrostatic pressure and GFR can be maintained despite hypoperfusion. When these conditions occur in ACE inhibitor–treated patients, angiotensin II formation and effect are diminished, and GFR may decrease. (Adapted with permission from Circulation 104:1985-1991, 2001.[140])

Nonspecific side effects of ACE inhibitors are generally uncommon with the exception of taste disturbances, leukopenia, skin rash, and dysgeusia, which are largely seen in captopril-treated patients.[161] ACE inhibitor use has not been associated with headache. In fact, ACE inhibitors have been used for migraine prophylaxis, and they have been proven effective in reducing the risk of nitrate-induced headache.[162] Angioneurotic edema is a potentially life-threatening complication of ACE inhibitors that is more common in Blacks.[163] Angioedema of the intestine (more common in women) can also occur with ACE inhibitor therapy, with a typical presentation of abdominal pain/diarrhea with or without facial and/or oropharyngeal swelling (Figure 65–3).[164] However, the use of ACE inhibitors is not associated with a significantly increased risk of acute pancreatitis.[165] A final side effect of ACE inhibitors is anemia. ACE inhibitors suppress the production of erythropoietin in a dose-dependent manner, which presents a particular problem when they are administered in the presence of renal failure.[166] Alternatively, this aspect of ACE inhibitor effect can be used therapeutically in posttransplant erythrocytosis and high-altitude polycythemia.[167,168]

## SUMMARY

ACE inhibitors are used commonly to reduce BP or to provide cardioprotection and/or renoprotection. They provide the greatest target organ protection in patients with CHF, proteinuric renal disease, or post-MI. Dosing guidelines exist for each of these scenarios, although such guidelines may not be followed as closely in clinical practice as is advised. ACE

inhibitor–related side effects are generally easily recognized and, other than functional renal insufficiency, do not occur more commonly other than in the elderly.

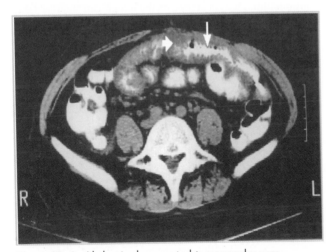

**Figure 65–3** Abdominal computed tomography was performed in a 58-year-old woman with acute abdominal pain, nausea, vomiting, and abdominal distention. The patient had had recurrent swelling of the tongue and pharynx during therapy with lisinopril, but the medication had been continued. On the scan, the mucosa of a loop of small intestine is markedly thickened, and the irregularities within the wall are most consistent with the presence of edema (thick arrow). The valvulae conniventes are prominent and widened (thin arrow), resulting in a severely narrowed lumen. All of the patient's symptoms resolved within 24 hours after the discontinuation of lisinopril. Adapted with permission from N Engl J Med 334:1641, 1996.[164]

## References

1. Chobanian AV, Bakris GL, Black HR, et al. The Seventh Report of the Joint National Committee on Prevention, Detection, Evaluation, and Treatment of High Blood Pressure: The JNC 7 report. JAMA 289:2560-2572, 2003.
2. Sica DA, Gehr TWB. Angiotensin converting enzyme inhibitors. In Oparil S, Weber M (eds). Hypertension: A Companion to the Kidney, 1st edition. Philadelphia, WB Saunders, 2000; pp 599-608.
3. Sica DA, Gehr TWB, Frishman WH. The renin-angiotensin axis: Angiotensin converting enzyme inhibitors and angiotensin-receptor blockers. In Frishman W, Sonnenblick S, Sica DA (eds). Cardiovascular Pharmacotherapeutics, 2nd ed. New York, McGraw-Hill, 2003; pp 131-156.
4. Warner GT, Perry CM. Ramipril: A review of its use in the prevention of cardiovascular outcomes. Drugs 62:1381-405, 2002.
5. White CM. Pharmacologic, pharmacokinetic, and therapeutic differences among ACE inhibitors. Pharmacotherapy 18:588-599, 1998.
6. Cody R. Optimizing ACE inhibitor therapy of congestive heart failure: Insights from pharmacodynamic studies. Clin Pharmacokinet 24:59-70, 1993.
7. Chalmers D, Whitehead A, Lawson DH. Postmarketing surveillance of captopril for hypertension. Br J Clin Pharmacol 34:215-223, 1992.
8. Sica DA. Angiotensin converting enzyme inhibitors: Fosinopril. In Messerli F (ed). Cardiovascular Drug Therapy, 2nd ed. Philadelphia, WB Saunders, 1996; pp 801-809.
9. Brockmeier D. Tight binding influencing the future of pharmacokinetics. Meth Find Exp Clin Pharmacol 20:505-516, 1998.
10. Reid JL. From kinetics to dynamics: Are there differences between ACE inhibitors? Eur Heart J 18(Suppl E):E14-18, 1997.
11. Hoyer J, Schulte K-L, Lenz T. Clinical pharmacokinetics of angiotensin converting enzyme inhibitors in renal failure. Clin Pharmacokinet 24:230-254, 1993.
12. Dzau VJ, Bernstein K, Celermajer D, et al. The relevance of tissue angiotensin-converting enzyme: Manifestations in mechanistic and endpoint data. Am J Cardiol 88(Suppl 9):1L-20L, 2001.
13. Ebihara A, Fujimura A. Metabolites of antihypertensive drugs: An updated review of their clinical pharmacokinetic and therapeutic implications. Clin Pharmacokinet 21:331-343, 1991.
14. Hui KK, Duchin KL, Kripalani KJ, et al. Pharmacokinetics of fosinopril in patients with various degrees of renal function. Clin Pharmacol Ther 49:457-467, 1991.
15. Danielson B, Querin S, LaRochelle P, et al. Pharmacokinetics and pharmacodynamics of trandolapril after repeated administration of 2 mg to patients with chronic renal failure and healthy control subjects. J Cardiovasc Pharmacol 23(Suppl 4):S50-59, 1994.
16. Brunner-La Rocca HP, Weilenmann D, Kiowski W, et al. Plasma levels of enalaprilat in chronic therapy of heart failure: Relationship to adverse events. J Pharmacol Exp Ther 289:565-571, 1999.
17. Brown NJ, Vaughn DE. Angiotensin-converting enzyme inhibitors. Circulation 97:1411-1420, 1998.
18. Johnston CI, Fabris B, Yamada H, et al. Comparative studies of tissue inhibition by angiotensin converting enzyme inhibitors. J Hypertens 7(Suppl):S11-S16, 1989.
19. Yusuf S, Sleight P, Pogue J, et al. Effects of an angiotensin-converting enzyme inhibitor, ramipril, on cardiovascular events in high-risk patients: The Heart Outcomes Prevention Evaluation Study Investigators. N Engl J Med 342:145-153, 2000.

20. Leonetti G, Cuspidi C. Choosing the right ACE inhibitor. A guide to selection. Drugs 49:516-535, 1995.

21. Zeitz CJ, Campbell DJ, Horowitz JD. Myocardial uptake and biochemical and hemodynamic effects of ACE inhibitors in humans. Hypertension 41:482-487, 2003.

22. Huskamp HA, Deverka PA, Epstein AM, et al. The effect of incentive-based formularies on prescription-drug utilization and spending. N Engl J Med 349:2224-2232, 2003.

23. The SOLVD investigators. Effect of enalapril on survival in patients with reduced left ventricular ejection fractions and congestive heart failure. N Engl J Med 325:293-302, 1991.

24. Lewis EJ, Hunsicker LG, Bain RP, et al. The effect of angiotensin converting enzyme inhibition on diabetic nephropathy: The Collaborative Study Group. N Engl J Med 329:1456-1462, 1993.

25. Sica DA. The HOPE Study: ACE inhibitors: Are their benefits a class effect or do individual agents differ? Curr Opin Nephrol Hypertens 10:597-601, 2001.

26. Segura J, Christiansen H, Campo C, et al. How to titrate ACE inhibitors and angiotensin receptor blockers in renal patients: According to blood pressure or proteinuria? Curr Hypertens Rep 5:426-429, 2003.

27. Wilson Tang WH, Vagelos RH, et al. Neurohormonal and clinical responses to high- versus low-dose enalapril therapy in chronic heart failure. J Am Coll Cardiol 39:70-78, 2002.

28. Packer M, Poole-Wilson PA, Armstrong PW, et al. Comparative effects of low and high doses of the angiotensin-converting enzyme inhibitor, lisinopril, on morbidity and mortality in chronic heart failure: ATLAS Study Group. Circulation 100:2312-2318, 1999.

29. Massie B. Neurohormonal blockade in chronic heart failure: How much is enough? Can there be too much? J Am Coll Cardiol 39:79-82, 2002.

30. Tang WH, Vagelos RH, Yee YG, et al. Neurohormonal and clinical responses to high- versus low-dose enalapril therapy in chronic heart failure. J Am Coll Cardiol 39:70-78, 2002.

31. Van Veldhuisen DJ, Genth-Zotz S, Brouwer J, et al. High versus low-dose ACE inhibition in chronic heart failure. A double-blind, placebo-controlled study of imidapril. J Am Coll Cardiol 32:1811-1818, 1998.

32. Carretero OA, Scicli AG. The kallikrein-kinin system as a regulator of cardiovascular and renal function. In Brenner BM, Laragh JH (eds). Hypertension: Pathophysiology, Diagnosis, and Management, 2nd ed. New York, Raven Press, Ltd, 1995; pp 983-999.

33. Urata H, Nishimura H, Ganten D. Chymase-dependent angiotensin II forming system in humans. Am J Hypertens 9:277-284, 1996.

34. Petrie MC, Padmanabhan N, McDonald JE, et al. Angiotensin converting enzyme and non-ACE dependent angiotensin II generation in resistance arteries from patients with heart failure and coronary heart disease. J Am Coll Cardiol 37:1056-1061, 2001.

35. Ennezat PV, Berlowitz M, Sonnenblick EH, et al. Therapeutic implications of escape from angiotensin-converting enzyme inhibition in patients with chronic heart failure. Curr Cardiol Rep 2:258-262, 2000.

36. Mooser V, Nussberger J, Juillerat L, et al. Reactive hyperreninemia is a major determinant of plasma angiotensin II during ACE inhibition. J Cardiovasc Pharmacol 15:276-282, 1990.

37. Swedberg K, Eneroth P, Kjekshus J, et al. Hormones regulating cardiovascular function in patients with severe congestive heart failure and their relation to mortality. CONSENSUS Trial Study Group. Circulation 82:1730-1736, 1990.

38. Gainer JV, Morrow JD, Loveland A, et al. Effect of bradykinin-receptor blockade on the response to angiotensin-converting enzyme inhibitor in normotensive and hypertensive subjects. N Engl J Med 339:1285-1292, 1998.

39. Tom B, Dendorfer A, Danser AH. Bradykinin, angiotensin (1-7), and ACE inhibitors: How do they interact? Int J Biochem Cell Biol 35:792-801, 2003.

40. Rodriguez-Garcia JL, Villa E, Serrano M, et al. Prostacyclin: Its pathogenic role in essential hypertension and the class effect of ACE inhibitors on prostaglandin metabolism. Blood Press 8:279-284, 1999.

41. Johnson AG. NSAIDs and increased blood pressure: What is the clinical significance? Drug Saf 17:277-289, 1997.

42. Morgan T, Anderson A. The effect of nonsteroidal anti-inflammatory drugs on blood pressure in patients treated with different antihypertensive drugs. J Clin Hypertens 5:53-57, 2003.

43. Nawarskas JJ, Townsend RR, Cirigliano MD, et al. Effect of aspirin on blood pressure in hypertensive patients taking enalapril or losartan. Am J Hypertens 12:784-789, 1999.

44. Zanchetti A, Hansson L, Leonetti G, et al. Low-dose aspirin does not interfere with the blood pressure-lowering effects of antihypertensive therapy. J Hypertens 20:1015-1022, 2002.

45. Cleland JG, John J, Houghton T. Does aspirin attenuate the effect of angiotensin-converting enzyme inhibitors in hypertension or heart failure? Curr Opin Nephrol Hypertens 10:625-631, 2001.

46. Lang CC, Stein M, He HB, et al. Angiotensin converting enzyme inhibition and sympathetic activity in healthy subjects. Clin Pharmacol Ther 59:668-674, 1996.

47. Ranadive SA, Chen AX, Serajuddin AT. Relative lipophilicities and structural-pharmacological considerations of various angiotensin-converting enzyme (ACE) inhibitors. Pharm Res 9:1480-1486, 1992.

48. Fagard R, Amery A, Reybrouck T, et al. Acute and chronic systemic and hemodynamic effects of angiotensin converting enzyme inhibition with captopril in hypertensive patients. Am J Cardiol 46:295-300, 1980.

49. Slavachevsky I, Rachmani R, Levi Z, et al. Effect of enalapril and nifedipine on orthostatic hypotension in older hypertensive patients. J Am Geriatr Soc 48:807-810, 2000.

50. Vanhoutte PM. Endothelial dysfunction and inhibition of converting enzyme. Eur Heart J 19(Suppl):J7-J15, 1998.

51. Schiffrin EL. Effects of antihypertensive drugs on vascular remodeling: Do they predict outcome in response to antihypertensive therapy? Curr Opin Nephrol Hypertens 10:617-624, 2001.

52. Wing LM, Reid CM, Ryan P, et al. A comparison of outcomes with angiotensin-converting enzyme inhibitors and diuretics for hypertension in the elderly. N Engl J Med 348:583-592, 2002.

53. The ALLHAT Officers and Co-ordinators for the ALLHAT Collaborative Group. Major outcomes in high-risk hypertensive patients randomized to angiotensin converting enzyme inhibitor or calcium channel blocker vs diuretic: The Antihypertensive and Lipid-Lowering Treatment to Prevent Heart Attack Trial (ALLHAT). JAMA 288:1981-1997, 2002.

54. Chobanian AV, Bakris GL, Black HR, et al. Joint National Committee on Prevention, Detection, Evaluation, and Treatment of High Blood Pressure: Seventh report of the Joint National Committee on Prevention, Detection, Evaluation, and Treatment of High Blood Pressure. Hypertension 42:1206-1252, 2003.

55. Guidelines Committee. 2003 European Society of Hypertension-European Society of Cardiology guidelines for the management of arterial hypertension. J Hypertens 21:1011-1053, 2003.

56. Materson BJ, Reda DJ, Cushman WC, et al. Single-drug therapy for hypertension in men. A comparison of six antihypertensive agents with placebo. N Engl J Med 328:914-921, 1993.

57. Li X, Du Y, Du Y, et al. Correlation of angiotensin-converting enzyme gene polymorphism with effect of antihypertensive therapy by angiotensin-converting enzyme inhibitor. J Cardiovasc Pharmacol Ther 8:25-30, 2003.

58. Smith RD, Franklin SS. Comparison of effects of enalapril plus hydrochlorothiazide versus standard triple therapy on renal function in renovascular hypertension. Am J Med 79(Suppl 3C):14-23, 1985.

59. Weidmann P, De Myttenaere-Bursztein S, Maxwell MH. Effect of aging on plasma renin and aldosterone in normal man. Kidney Int 8:325-333, 1975.

60. Israili ZH, Hall WD. ACE Inhibitors: Differential use in elderly patients with hypertension. Drugs Aging 7:355-371, 1995.

61. Omboni S, Fogari R, Palatini P, et al. Reproducibility and clinical value of the trough-to-peak ratio of the antihypertensive effect. Evidence from the Sample Study. Hypertension 32:424-429, 1998.

62. Morgan TO, Morgan O, Anderson A. Effect of dose on trough peak ratio of antihypertensive drugs in elderly hypertensive males. Clin Exp Pharmacol Physiol 22:778-780, 1995.

63. Sica DA, Gehr TWB. Dose-response relationship and dose adjustments. Hypertension Primer, 2nd ed. Lippincott Williams & Wilkins, Baltimore, 1999; pp 342-344.

64. Elung-Jensen T, Heisterberg J, Kamper AL, et al. Blood pressure response to conventional and low-dose enalapril in chronic renal failure. Br J Clin Pharmacol 55:139-146, 2003.

65. Sica DA. Rationale for fixed-dose combinations in the treatment of hypertension: The cycle repeats. Drugs 62:443-462, 2002.

66. Law MR, Wald NJ, Morris JK, et al. Value of low dose combination treatment with blood pressure lowering drugs: Analysis of 354 randomised trials. BMJ 326:427-434, 2003.

67. Docherty A, Dunn FG. Treatment of hypertensive patients with coexisting coronary arterial disease. Curr Opin Cardiol 18:268-271, 2003.

68. Black HR, Sollins JS, Garofalo JL. The addition of doxazosin to the therapeutic regimen of hypertensive patients inadequately controlled with other antihypertensive medications: A randomized, placebo-controlled study. Am J Hypertens 13:468-474, 2000.

69. Gradman AH, Cutler NR, Davis PJ, et al. Combined enalapril and felodipine extended release for systemic hypertension: Enalapril-Felodipine ER Factorial Study Group. Am J Cardiol 79:431-435, 1997.

70. DeQuattro V, Lee D. Fixed-dose combination therapy with trandolapril and verapamil SR is effective in primary hypertension. Am J Hypertens 10(Suppl 2):138S-145S, 1997.

71. Pool J, Kaihlanen P, Lewis G, et al. Once-daily treatment of patients with hypertension: A placebo-controlled study of amlodipine and benazepril vs amlodipine or benazepril alone. J Hum Hypertens 15:495-498, 2001.

72. Sica DA. Calcium-channel blocker edema: Can it be resolved? J Clin Hypertens 5:291-294, 2003.

73. Zuccala G, Onder G, Pedone C, et al. Use of calcium antagonists and worsening renal function in patients receiving angiotensin-converting-enzyme inhibitors. Eur J Clin Pharmacol 58:695-699, 2003.

74. Sica DA. Combination angiotensin-converting enzyme inhibitor and angiotensin receptor blocker therapy: Its role in clinical practice: Practical aspects of combination therapy with angiotensin-receptor blockers and angiotensin-converting enzyme inhibitors. J Clin Hypertens 5:414-420, 2003.

75. Taylor AA. Is there a place for combining angiotensin-converting enzyme inhibitors and angiotensin-receptor antagonists in the treatment of hypertension, renal disease or congestive heart failure? Curr Opin Nephrol Hypertens 10:643-648, 2001.

76. Pogatsa-Murray G, Varga L, Varga A, et al. Changes in left ventricular mass during treatment with minoxidil and cilazapril in hypertensive patients with left ventricular hypertrophy. J Hum Hypertens 11:149-156, 1997.

77. Hirschl MM, Binder M, Bur A, et al. Clinical evaluation of different doses of intravenous enalaprilat in patients with hypertensive crises. Arch Intern Med 155:2217-2223, 1995.

78. Sica DA. Dosage considerations with perindopril for hypertension. Am J Cardiol 88(Suppl 1):13-18, 2001.

79. Gottdiener JS, Reda DJ, Massie BM, et al. Effect of single-drug therapy on reduction of left ventricular mass in mild to moderate hypertension: Comparison of six antihypertensive agents. Circulation 95:2007-2014, 1997.

80. Koren MJ, Devereux RB, Casale PN, et al. Relation of left ventricular mass and geometry to morbidity and mortality in uncomplicated essential hypertension. Ann Intern Med 114:345-352, 1991.

81. Fox KM. European Trial on Reduction of Cardiac Events with Perindopril in Stable Coronary Artery Disease Investigators. Efficacy of perindopril in reduction of cardiovascular events among patients with stable coronary artery disease: Randomised, double-blind, placebo-controlled, multicentre trial (the EUROPA study). Lancet 362:782-788, 2003.

82. Daly P, Mettauer B, Rouleau JL, et al. Lack of reflex increase in myocardial sympathetic tone after captopril: Potential antianginal mechanism. Circulation 71:317-325, 1985.

83. Pepine CJ, Rouleau JL, Annis K, et al. Effects of angiotensin-converting enzyme inhibition on transient ischemia: The Quinapril Anti-Ischemia and Symptoms of Angina Reduction (QUASAR) trial. J Am Coll Cardiol 42:2049-2059, 2003.

84. Schiffrin EL. Effect of antihypertensive treatment on small artery remodeling in hypertension. Can J Physiol Pharmacol 81:168-76, 2003.

85. Walters MR, Bolster A, Dyker AG, et al. Effect of perindopril on cerebral and renal perfusion in stroke patients with carotid disease. Stroke 32:473-478, 2001.

86. Regensteiner JG, Hiatt WR. Current medical therapies for patients with peripheral arterial disease: A critical review. Am J Med 112:49-57, 2002.

87. Ostergren J, Sleight P, Dagenais G, et al. Impact of ramipril in patients with evidence of clinical or subclinical peripheral arterial disease. Eur Heart J 25:17-24, 2004.

88. Position statement: Hypertension management in adults with diabetes. Diabetes Care 27:S65-S67, 2004.

89. Lithell HO, Pollare T, Berne C. Insulin sensitivity in newly detected hypertensive patients: Influence of captopril and other antihypertensive agents on insulin sensitivity and related biological parameters. J Cardiovasc Pharmacol 15(Suppl 5):S46-S52, 1990.

90. Yusuf S, Gerstein H, Hoogwerf B, et al. Ramipril and the development of diabetes. J Am Med Assoc 286:1882-1885, 2001.

91. Hansson L, Lindholm L, Niskanen L, et al. Effect of angiotensin-converting-enzyme inhibition compared with conventional therapy on cardiovascular morbidity and mortality in hypertension: The Captopril Prevention Project (CAPPP) randomised trial. Lancet 353:611-616, 1999.

92. Wright JT Jr, Agodoa L, Contreras G, et al. Successful blood pressure control in the African American Study of Kidney Disease and Hypertension. Arch Intern Med 162:1636-1643, 2002.

93. Yu HT. Progression of chronic renal failure. Arch Intern Med 163:1417-1429, 2003.

94. Wachtell K, Ibsen H, Olsen MH, et al. Albuminuria and cardiovascular risk in hypertensive patients with left ventricular hypertrophy: The LIFE study. Ann Intern Med 139:901-906, 2003.

95. Donnelly R, Yeung JM, Manning G. Microalbuminuria: A common, independent cardiovascular risk factor, especially but not exclusively in type 2 diabetes. J Hypertens 21(Suppl 1):S7-S12, 2003.

96. Brown WW, Peters RM, Ohmit SE, et al. Early detection of kidney disease in community settings: The kidney early evaluation program (KEEP). Am J Kidney Dis 42:22-35, 2003.

97. Boulware LE, Jaar BG, Tarver-Carr ME, et al. Screening for proteinuria in US adults: A cost-effectiveness analysis. JAMA 290:3101-3014, 2003.

98. Jafar TH, Stark PC, Schmid CH, et al. Progression of chronic kidney disease: The role of blood pressure control, proteinuria, and angiotensin-converting enzyme inhibition: a patient-level meta-analysis. Ann Intern Med 139:244-252, 2003.

99. Laverman GD, Remuzzi G, Ruggenenti P. ACE inhibition versus angiotensin receptor blockade: Which is better for renal and cardiovascular protection? J Am Soc Nephrol 15(Suppl 1):S64-70, 2004.

100. Laverman GD, de Zeeuw D, Navis G. Between-patient differences in the renal response to renin-angiotensin system intervention: Clue to optimising renoprotective therapy? J Renin Angiotensin Aldosterone Syst 3:205-213, 2002.

101. Ravid M, Lang R, Rachmani R, et al. Long-term renoprotective effect of angiotensin converting enzyme inhibition in non-insulin dependent diabetes mellitus. A 7-year follow-up study. Arch Intern Med 156:286-289, 1996.

102. Lebovitz HE, Wiegmann TB, Cnaan A, et al. Renal protective effects of enalapril in hypertensive NIDDM: Role of baseline albuminuria. Kidney Int Suppl 45:S150-S155, 1994.

103. Viberti G, Mogensen CE, Groop LC, et al. Effect of captopril on progression to clinical proteinuria in patients with insulin-dependent diabetes mellitus and microalbuminuria: European Microalbuminuria Captopril Study Group. J Am Med Assoc 271:275-279, 1994.

104. Uhle BU, Whitworth JA, Shahinfar S, et al. Angiotensin-converting enzyme inhibition in nondiabetic progressive renal insufficiency: A controlled double-blind trial. Am J Kidney Dis 27:489-495, 1996.

105. Giatras I, Lau J, Levey As, et al. Effect of angiotensin-converting enzyme inhibitors on the progression of nondiabetic renal disease: A meta-analysis of randomized trials. Ann Intern Med 127:337-347, 1997.

106. Agodoa LY, Appel L, Bakris GL, et al. Effect of ramipril vs amlodipine on renal outcomes in hypertensive nephrosclerosis: A randomized controlled trial. JAMA 285:2719-2728, 2001.

107. Wilmer WA, Hebert LA, Lewis EJ, et al. Remission of nephrotic syndrome in type 1 diabetes: Long-term follow-up of patients in the captopril study. Am J Kidney Dis 34:308-314, 1999.

108. Lewis JB, Berl T, Bain RP, et al. Effect of intensive blood pressure control on the course of type 1 diabetic nephropathy. Am J Kidney Dis 34:809-817, 1999.

109. Estacio RO, Esler A, Mehler P. Effects of aggressive blood pressure control in normotensive type 2 diabetic patients on albuminuria, retinopathy and strokes. Kidney Int 61:1086-1097, 2002.

110. Estacio R, Jeffers R, Gifford N, et al. Effect of blood pressure control on diabetic microvascular complications in patients with hypertension and type 2 diabetes. Diabetes Care 23:B54-B64, 2000.

111. Jafar T, Schmid C, Landa M, et al. The effect of angiotensin-converting-enzyme inhibitors on the progression of non-diabetic renal disease: A pooled analysis of individual patient data from 11 randomized controlled trials. Ann Intern Med 135:73-87, 2001.

112. Ruggenenti P, Perna A, Gherardi G, et al. Chronic proteinuric nephropathies: Outcomes and response to treatment in a prospective cohort of 352 patients with different patterns of renal injury. Am J Kidney Dis 35:1155-1165, 2000.

113. Sica DA. Kinetics of angiotensin converting enzyme inhibitors in renal failure. J Cardiovasc Pharmacol 20(Suppl 10):S13-S20, 1992.

114. Jafar TH, Stark PC, Schmid CH, et al. Angiotensin-converting enzyme inhibition and progression of renal disease: Proteinuria as a modifiable risk factor for the progression of non-diabetic renal disease. Kidney Int 60:1131-1140, 2001.

115. Mann JF, Gerstein HC, Yi QL, et al. Development of renal disease in people at high cardiovascular risk: Results of the HOPE randomized study. J Am Soc Nephrol 14:641-647, 2003.

116. Marre M, Lievre M, Chatellier G, et al. Effects of low dose ramipril on cardiovascular and renal outcomes in patients with type 2 diabetes and raised excretion of urinary albumin: Randomised, double blind, placebo controlled trial (the DIAB-HYCAR study). Br Med J 328:495, 2004.

117. Laverman G, Ruggenenti P, Remuzzi G. Angiotensin-converting enzyme inhibition or angiotensin receptor blockade in hypertensive diabetics? Curr Hypertens Rep 5:364-367, 2003.

118. Ruggenenti P, Mise N, Pisoni R, et al. Diverse effects of increasing lisinopril doses on lipid abnormalities in chronic nephropathies. Circulation 107:586-592, 2003.

119. Bakris GL, Weir MR. Angiotensin-converting enzyme inhibitor-associated elevations in serum creatinine: Is this a cause for concern? Arch Intern Med 160:685-693, 2000.

120. Apperloo AJ, de Zeeuw D, de Jong PE. A short-term antihypertensive-treatment induced drop in glomerular filtration rate predicts long-term stability of renal function. Kidney Int 51:793-797, 1997.

121. Sica DA. Assessment of the role of ACE inhibitors in the elderly. In Prisant M (ed). Hypertension in the Elderly. Totowa, NJ, Humana Press, Inc., 2005.

122. Heeg JE, de Jong PE, van der Hem GK, et al. Efficacy and variability of the antiproteinuric effect of ACE inhibition by lisinopril. Kidney Int 36:272-279, 1989.

123. Buter H, Hemmelder MH, Navis G, et al. The blunting of the antiproteinuric efficacy of ACE inhibition by high sodium intake can be restored by hydrochlorothiazide. Nephrol Dial Transplant 13:1682-1685, 1998.

124. Gansevoort RT, de Zeeuw D, de Jong PE. Additive antiproteinuric effect of ACE inhibition and a low protein diet in human renal disease. Nephrol Dial Transplant 10:497-504, 1995.

125. Buter H, Hemmelder MH, van Paassen P, et al. Is the antiproteinuric response to inhibition of the renin-angiotensin system less effective during the night? Nephrol Dial Transplant 12(Suppl 2):53-56, 1997.

126. Ueda S, Elliott, Morton JJ, et al. Enhanced pressor response to angiotensin I in normotensive men with the deletion genotype (DD) for angiotensin-converting enzyme. Hypertension 25:1266-1269, 1995.

127. Cambien F, Poirier O, Lecerf L, et al. Deletion polymorphism in the gene for angiotensin-converting enzyme is a potent risk factor for myocardial infarction. Nature 359:641-644, 1992.

128. Parving HH, Jacobsen P, Tarnow L, et al. Effect of deletion polymorphism of angiotensin converting enzyme gene on progression of diabetic nephropathy during inhibition of angiotensin converting enzyme. Observational follow-up study. Br Med J 313:591-594, 1996.

129. Rudnicki M, Mayer G. Pharmacogenomics of angiotensin converting enzyme inhibitors in renal disease: Pathophysiological considerations. Pharmacogenomics 4:153-162, 2003.

130. Garg R, Yusuf S, for the Collaborative Group on ACE Inhibitor Trials. Overview of randomized trials of angiotensin-converting enzyme inhibitors on mortality and morbidity in patients with heart failure. J Am Med Assoc 273:1450-1456, 1995.

131. Flather MD, Yusuf S, Kober L, et al. Long-term ACE-inhibitor therapy in patients with heart failure or left-ventricular dysfunction: A systematic overview of data from individual patients: ACE-Inhibitor Myocardial Infarction Collaborative Group. Lancet 355:1575-1581, 2000.

132. Burwen DR, Galusha DH, Lewis JM, et al. National and state trends in quality of care for acute myocardial infarction between 1994-1995 and 1998-1999: The medicare health care quality improvement program. Arch Intern Med 163:1430-1439, 2003.

133. Megarry M, Sapsford R, Hall AS, et al. Do ACE inhibitors provide protection for the heart in the clinical setting of acute myocardial infarction? Drugs 54 (Supplement 5):48-58, 1997.

134. Indications for ACE inhibitors in the early treatment of acute myocardial infarction: Systematic review of individual data from 100,000 patients in randomised trials. Circulation 97:2202-2212, 1998.

135. Liu P, Arnold JM, Belenkie I, et al. The 2002/3 Canadian Cardiovascular Society consensus guideline update for the diagnosis and management of heart failure. Can J Cardiol 19:347-56, 2003.

136. ACC/AHA Guidelines for the Evaluation and Management of Chronic Heart Failure in the Adult: Executive Summary: A Report of the American College of Cardiology/American Heart Association Task Force on Practice Guidelines. Circulation 104:2996-3007, 2001.

137. Massie B. Neurohormonal blockade in chronic heart failure: How much is enough? Can there be too much? J Am Coll Cardiol 39:79-82, 2002.

138. Remme WJ. Effect of ACE inhibition on neurohormones. Eur Heart J 19(Supplement J):J16-J23, 1998.

139. Anker SD, Negassa A, Coats AJ, et al. Prognostic importance of weight loss in chronic heart failure and the effect of treatment with angiotensin-converting-enzyme inhibitors: An observational study. Lancet 361:1077-1083, 2003.

140. Schoolwerth AC, Sica DA, Ballermann BJ, Wilcox CS. Renal considerations in angiotensin converting enzyme inhibitor therapy: A statement for healthcare professionals from the Council on the Kidney in Cardiovascular Disease and the Council for High Blood Pressure Research of the American Heart Association. Circulation 104:1985-1991, 2001.

141. Kittleson M, Hurwitz S, Shah MR, et al. Development of circulatory-renal limitations to angiotensin-converting enzyme inhibitors identifies patients with severe heart failure and early mortality. J Am Coll Cardiol 41:2029-2035, 2003.

142. Agusti A, Bonet S, Arnau JM, et al. Adverse effects of ACE inhibitors in patients with chronic heart failure and/or ventricular dysfunction: Meta-analysis of randomised clinical trials. Drug Saf 26:895-908, 2003.

143. Bungard TJ, McAlister FA, Johnson JA, et al. Underutilization of ACE inhibitors in patients with congestive heart failure. Drugs 61:2021-2033, 2001.

144. Chen YT, Wang Y, Radford MJ, et al. Angiotensin-converting enzyme inhibitor dosages in elderly patients with heart failure. Am Heart J 141:410-417, 2001.

145. Schwartz JS, Wang YR, Cleland JG, et al. High- versus low-dose angiotensin converting enzyme inhibitor therapy in the treatment of heart failure: An economic analysis of the Assessment of Treatment with Lisinopril and Survival (ATLAS) trial. Am J Manag Care 9:417-24, 2003.

146. Ryan TJ, Antman EM, Brooks NH, et al. 1999 Update: ACC/AHA Guidelines for the Management of Patients With Acute Myocardial Infarction: Executive Summary and Recommendations: A report of the American College of Cardiology/American Heart Association Task Force on Practice Guidelines (Committee on Management of Acute Myocardial Infarction). Circulation 100:1016-30, 1999.

147. Naccarella F, Naccarelli GV, Maranga SS, et al. Do ACE inhibitors or angiotensin II antagonists reduce total mortality and arrhythmic mortality? A critical review of controlled clinical trials. Curr Opin Cardiol 17:6-18, 2002.

148. Turnbull F, Blood Pressure Lowering Treatment Trialists' Collaboration. Effects of different blood-pressure-lowering regimens on major cardiovascular events: Results of prospectively-designed overviews of randomised trials. Lancet 362:1527-1535, 2003.

149. Randomised trial of a perindopril-based blood-pressure-lowering regimen among 6,105 individuals with previous stroke or transient ischaemic attack. Lancet 358:1033-1041, 2001.

150. Anderson C. Blood pressure-lowering for secondary prevention of stroke: ACE inhibition is the key. Stroke 34:1333-1334, 2003.

151. Bath P. Blood pressure-lowering for secondary prevention of stroke: ACE inhibition is not the key. Stroke 34:1334-1335, 2003.

152. Davis SM, Donnan GA. Blood pressure reduction and ACE inhibition in secondary stroke prevention: Mechanism uncertain. Stroke 34:1335-1336, 2003.

153. Bosch J, Yusuf S, Pogue J, et al. Use of ramipril in preventing stroke: Double blind randomised trial. BMJ 324:1-5, 2002.

154. Goldstein LB, Adams R, Becker K, et al. Primary prevention of ischemic stroke: A statement for healthcare professionals from the Stroke Council of the American Heart Association. Stroke 32:280-299, 2001.

155. Textor SC. Renal failure related to angiotensin-converting enzyme inhibitors. Semin Nephrol 17:67-76, 1997.

156. Bouvy ML, Heerdink ER, Hoes AW, et al. Effects of NSAIDs on the incidence of hospitalisations for renal dysfunction in users of ACE inhibitors. Drug Saf 26:983-989, 2003.

157. Textor SC, Bravo EL, Fouad FM, et al. Hyperkalemia in azotemic patients during angiotensin-converting enzyme inhibition and aldosterone reduction with captopril. Am J Med 73:719-725, 1982.

158. Juurlink DN, Mamdani M, Kopp A, et al. Drug-drug interactions among elderly patients hospitalized for drug toxicity. J Am Med Assoc 289:1652-1658, 2003.

159. Cruz CS, Cruz AA, Marcilio de Souza CA. Hyperkalaemia in congestive heart failure patients using ACE inhibitors and spironolactone. Nephrol Dial Transplant 18:1814-1819, 2003.

160. Israili ZH, Hall WD. Cough and angioneurotic associated with angiotensin-converting enzyme inhibitor therapy: A review of the literature and pathophysiology. Ann Intern Med 117:234-242, 1992.

161. Chalmers D, Dombey SL, Lawson DH. Post-marketing surveillance of captopril (for hypertension): A preliminary report. Br J Clin Pharmacol 24:343-349, 1987.

162. Onder G, Pahor M, Gambassi G, et al. Association between ACE inhibitors use and headache caused by nitrates among hypertensive patients: Results from the Italian group of pharmacoepidemiology in the elderly. Cephalalgia 23:901-906, 2003.

163. Gibbs CR, Lip GYH, Beevers DG. Angioedema due to ACE inhibitors: Increased risk in patients of African origin. Br J Clin Pharmacol 48:861-865, 1999.

164. Gregory KW, Davis RC. Images in clinical medicine: Angioedema of the intestine. N Engl J Med 334:1641, 1996.

165. Cheng RM, Mamdani M, Jackevicius CA, et al. Association between ACE inhibitors and acute pancreatitis in the elderly. Ann Pharmacother 37:994-998, 2003.

166. Sica DA, Gehr TWB. The pharmacokinetics and pharmacodynamics of angiotensin receptor blockers in end-stage renal disease. J Renin-Angio Aldo Sys 3:247-254, 2002.

167. Trivedi H, Lal SM. A prospective, randomized, open labeled crossover trial of fosinopril and theophylline in post renal transplant erythrocytosis. Ren Fail 25:77-86, 2003.

168. Plata R, Cornejo A, Arratia C, et al. Angiotensin-converting-enzyme inhibition therapy in altitude polycythaemia: A prospective randomised trial. Lancet 359:663-666, 2002.

# Calcium Antagonists

## L. Michael Prisant

Calcium antagonists are commonly used antihypertensive drugs among prescribing physicians.[1-4] In the Cardiovascular Health Study, there was an increase in the use of calcium antagonists from 14% in 1990 to 36% in 1999 among 5775 participants aged 65 years or older (Figure 66–1).[4] The growth of calcium antagonist use has been attributed to increased drug advertising.[5] Their use has not been influenced by the academic controversy involving alleged excess cardiovascular events, gastrointestinal bleeding, and cancer.[6-12] There has been a decline in their use among patients with coronary disease, decreasing from a peak of 57% in 1994 to 43% in 1999 ($p < 0.001$).[4] It remains to be seen whether the report of the Antihypertensive and Lipid-Lowering Treatment to Prevent Heart Attack Trial (ALLHAT) will influence treatment decisions regarding calcium antagonist use.[13]

## PHARMACOLOGY OF CALCIUM ANTAGONISTS

Calcium antagonists are more heterogenous than other classes of antihypertensive drugs (e.g., angiotensin receptor blockers). They are divided into the phenylalkylamine (verapamil); benzothiazepine (diltiazem); and 1,4-dihydropyridine (nifedipine-like) classes.[14] Others prefer simply to divide the calcium antagonists into dihydropyridines (vasodilating) and non-dihydropyridines (myocardial active) to emphasize their relative vascular to cardiac selectivity. The dihydropyridines may be further subdivided based on their tissue selectivity (Figure 66–2). Tissue selectivity refers to the ratio calculated as a 50% inhibition of vascular constriction versus inhibition of the contractility of isolated myocardium.[15] The higher the ratio, the more selective the calcium antagonist is for vascular tissue and the lower the potential for producing a negative inotropic effect. All dihydropyridines other than nifedipine, lacidipine, and lercanidipine have been referred to as second-generation dihydropyridines.[14,16] The third-generation dihydropyridines lercanidipine and lacidipine are hydrophobic, membrane soluble, and have a long duration of action.[17]

All calcium antagonists bind to the $\alpha_{1c}$-subunit of the voltage-dependent L-type calcium channel, although the actual binding sites differ among the three groups.[18] By inhibiting the influx of calcium from outside the cell to inside the cell through the voltage-dependent L-type channel, actin and myosin do not interact and vasodilation occurs. Mibefradil (Posicor), which was withdrawn from the market because of drug-drug interactions, blocked both the low-voltage T and the high-voltage L channels.[14,19] L-type channels are located on cardiac muscle, arteries, and veins, as well as leukocytes, platelets, brain, retina, salivary glands, gastric mucosa, pancreas, adrenal glands, pituitary gland, and other smooth muscle (bronchial, gastrointestinal, genitourinary, and uterine).[18] This explains some side effects and the diverse application of calcium antagonists to systemic hypertension, angina pectoris, supraventricular arrhythmias, subarachnoid hemorrhage, myocardial infarction, Raynaud's disease, esophageal spasm, primary pulmonary hypertension, and migraine headaches.[20] In addition to the smooth muscle relaxation, there are other effects of calcium antagonists that potentially lower blood pressure, including acute and repetitive natriuresis,[21,22] inhibition of aldosterone release,[23] inhibition of growth and proliferation of vascular smooth muscle cells and fibroblasts,[24] and interference with $\alpha_2$-adrenoreceptor- and angiotensin-mediated vasoconstriction.[25,26] Antiatherogenic properties have been documented in animal models (Figure 66–3),[27,28] but results of studies of the vascular effects of calcium antagonists in humans have been mixed.[29-33]

Division of calcium antagonists into dihydropyridines and nondihydropyridines differentiates their effects on myocardial contractility, cardiac conduction, and glomerular hemodynamics. Verapamil and diltiazem depress the sinoatrial (SA) node slightly, decrease conduction through the atrioventricular (AV) node, and reduce myocardial contractility. Unlike the dihydropyridines, there is less vasodilation and related vascular side effects.[34] The dihydropyridines increase or fail to reduce intraglomerular pressure, completely abolish renal autoregulation, and increase proteinuria and glomerulosclerosis.

There are differences in time to peak concentration and elimination half-life among calcium antagonists (Table 66–1. All except amlodipine, lacidipine, and lercanidipine are short-acting in their native form and require novel drug delivery systems to prolong their duration of action.[35-37] The short plasma half-life of lercanidipine is misleading given its long duration of action.[17] The explanation for the discrepancy is that the molecule is attached to the arterial wall and not circulating in plasma. Several calcium antagonists (Covera-HS, Verelan-PM, Cardizem LA) have been designed as chronotherapeutic formulations.[38-41] Because cardiovascular events are more likely to occur in the early morning hours, the delivery system was created to deliver peak plasma levels in the early morning hours when taken at bedtime. Intravenous diltiazem, nicardipine, and verapamil are available.

## PHARMACOKINETICS

After oral dosing, all three classes of calcium antagonist undergo first-pass metabolism by intestinal enterocytes and the liver.[42] Bioavailability is 20% for verapamil, 45% for diltiazem, and 45% to 75% for nifedipine. Amlodipine has a relatively high bioavailability as compared with all other calcium antagonists.[43] All calcium antagonists are highly bound to plasma proteins.

More than 90% of verapamil is absorbed; bioavailability is reduced because of extensive first-pass metabolism[44] but increases with repetitive dosing. Verapamil is a substrate for

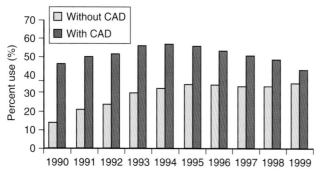

**Figure 66–1** Percent use of calcium antagonist use from 1990-1999. The Cardiovascular Health Study (*n* = 5775). (Data from Psaty BM, Manolio TA, Smith NL, et al. Time trends in high blood pressure control and the use of antihypertensive medications in older adults: The Cardiovascular Health Study. Arch Intern Med 162:2325-2332, 2002.)

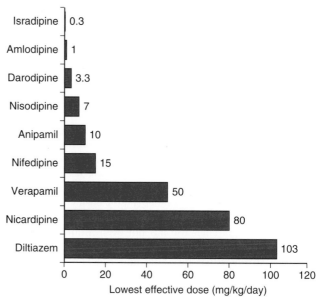

**Figure 66–3** Lowest effective dose of oral administration of a calcium antagonist to reduce aortic cholesterol accumulation in lipid-fed rabbits. (Derived from Weinstein DB, Heider JG. Antiatherogenic properties of calcium antagonists. State of the art. Am J Med 86:27-32, 1989; and Nayler WG. Vascular injury: Mechanisms and manifestations. Am J Med 90:8S-13S, 1991.)

cytochrome P450 CYP3A and P-glycoprotein. *N*-dealkylation and *O*-demethylation are the primary metabolic pathways for verapamil. There are 12 metabolites, but norverapamil has 20% of the pharmacologic activity of verapamil. Urinary excretion accounts for 70% of the drug elimination. Clearance is decreased in cirrhosis, in the elderly, and in women.[45,46] Caution has been sounded for the use of sustained-release verapamil in patients with chronic kidney disease.[47]

More than 90% of diltiazem is absorbed after oral administration. Bioavailability is reduced because of extensive first-pass metabolism.[48] Diltiazem is a substrate for cytochrome P450 CYP3A and P-glycoprotein. O-deacetylation and N-demethylation followed by O-demethylation are the primary metabolic pathways for diltiazem. Deacetyldiltiazem accounts for 15% to 35% of diltiazem levels and has at most 50% of the pharmaco-

logic effect of the parent compound. Clearance is decreased in elderly patients.[48]

Almost 95% of nifedipine is absorbed after oral administration.[49] About 30% to 40% of the drug is eliminated with first-pass metabolism. Oxidation results in three inactive metabolites that are predominately excreted in the urine. Unlike other calcium antagonists, amlodipine does not undergo extensive first-pass metabolism.

## DRUG DELIVERY SYSTEMS

Drug delivery systems for calcium antagonists are intended to prolong the intrinsic duration of action of the drug, to decrease dosing frequency and reduce side effects (Table 66–2). Disadvantages for these drug delivery systems include postponed achievement of pharmacodynamic effect on initiation of therapy, the potential for sustained toxicity, decreased absorption with rapid gastrointestinal tract motility, and adverse reactions caused by the delivery system. Care must be taken when switching from a drug of one delivery system to another by titrating the drug dose.

Plendil, Adalat CC, and Sular use the coat core system, which is a hydrophilic gel surrounding active drug (Figure 66–4). The drug diffuses across the hydrophilic gel matrix coat as it travels throughout the gastrointestinal tract, and the matrix eventually erodes. Crushing or dividing the tablet exposes the patient to the active drug acutely, resulting in flushing, hypotension, and tachycardia.

The osmotic pump or Gastrointestinal Therapeutic System (GITS) provides zero-order drug delivery and is used with Procardia XL, Dynacirc CR, and Covera HS (Figure 66–5).[50,51]

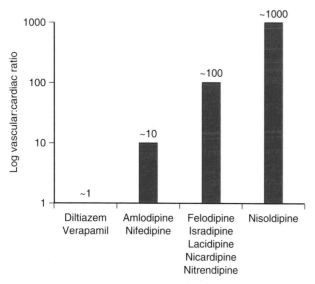

**Figure 66–2** Relative vascular-cardiac selectivity of calcium antagonists. (Derived from Godfraind T, Salomone S, Dessy C, et al. Selectivity scale of calcium antagonists in the human cardiovascular system based on in vitro studies. J Cardiovasc Pharmacol 20(Suppl 5):S34-S41, 1992.)

**Table 66-1** Comparative Pharmacokinetics of Calcium Antagonists

| Drug | Absorption | Bioavailability | Protein Binding | Time to Peak (hours) | Elimination Half-life (hours) |
|------|-----------|-----------------|-----------------|---------------------|------------------------------|
| Diltiazem CD | 95% | 40% | 70-80% | 10-14 | 5-8 |
| Amlodipine | >90% | 60-65% | 95% | 6-12 | 35-45 |
| Felodipine ER | >99% | 20% | 99% | 2.5-5 | 10-17 |
| Isradipine CR | 90-95% | 15-24% | 95% | 7-18 | 8 |
| Lercanidipine | 44% | 10-12% | 98% | 2-3 | 8-10 |
| Nicardipine SR | >90% | 35% | >90% | 1-4 | 8.6 |
| Nifedipine CC | >90% | 84-89% | 92-98% | 2.5-12 | 7 |
| Nisoldipine CC | >80% | 5% | >99% | 6-12 | 7-12 |
| Verapamil SR | >90% | 20-35% | >90% | 5.2-7.7 | 4.5-12 |

CC, coat core; CD, controlled delivery; CR, controlled release; ER, extended release; SR, sustained release.

The osmotic pump contains two compartments, a polymeric push compartment and an osmotic drug core; the entire tablet is surrounded by a cellulosic membrane, which is permeable to water but not to the drug or the osmotic excipients.[52] There is a laser-drilled opening on the drug side of the tablet to allow dispensing of the drug as the polymeric push compartment swells. Covera HS has two laser drill holes for drug release and a special delay coat to time the release of verapamil in the hours prior to awakening. The osmotic pump is very hard, which increases the possibility for chipping teeth, obstructing the gastrointestinal tract where there is a stricture, and the theoretical possibility of eroding through diverticula.[53]

Cardizem SR, Cardizem CD, Cardizem LA, Tiazac, Verelan, Verelan PM, and Cardene SR use encapsulated beads.[37] Cardene SR is a mixture of 25% immediate-release powder and 75% slow-release beads.[54] Cardizem CD consists of two populations of beads: (1) 40% with a thin copolymer coat for the initial 12 hours and (2) 60% with a thicker copolymer coat for the next 12 hours.[55] Tiazac consists of coated beads with a monolayer microporous semipermeable polymer, which controls the rate of drug diffusion in the gastrointestinal tract. Cardizem LA differs from Tiazac in the amount of coating applied to the beads. It is dosed at bedtime and formulated to reach peak plasma levels between 6 A.M. and 12 noon. Verelan is a multiparticulate bead system (Spheroidal Oral Drug Absorption System, SODAS) that consists of 1-mm inert beads surrounded by rate-controlling polymers that allow release of verapamil without regard to pH (Figure 66-6). Similar to Verelan, Verelan PM uses water-soluble and water-insoluble polymers to delay release of verapamil for 4 to 5 hours.[56]

Isoptin SR and Calan SR consist of a mixture of verapamil combined with polysaccharide sodium alginate, which absorbs water and becomes gelatinous in the gastrointestinal tract. Verapamil is released via diffusion through the matrix, and surface erosion of the tablet. Unlike Verelan, this formulation must be taken with food to avoid doubling the peak plasma levels.

Dilacor XR uses the completely biodegradable Geomatrix tablets, which consist of two slow hydrating barriers sandwiching a hydrophilic matrix core (Figure 66-7).[57] Diltiazem diffuses at a constant rate across the unprotected sides of the active layer as the volume of the dry tablet increases from 0.19 to 2.21 ml with complete hydration. Each tablet contains 60 mg of diltiazem; thus three tablets are encapsulated for the 180-mg dose.

**Table 66-2** Novel Drug Delivery Systems for Calcium Antagonists

| Generic Name | Brand Name | Dosing Interval | Delivery System |
|--------------|-----------|-----------------|-----------------|
| Diltiazem | Cardizem SR | 2X/day | Coated beads (Multiple) |
| | Cardizem CD | 1X/day | Coated beads (2 Populations) |
| | Cardizem LA | 1X/day HS | Coated beads (Multiple) |
| | Tiazac | 1X/day | Coated beads (Multiple) |
| | Dilacor | 1X/day | Geomatrix |
| Felodipine | Plendil | 1X/day | Coat core |
| Isradipine | DynaCirc CR | 1X/day | Osmotic pump |
| Nicardipine | Cardene SR | 2X/day | Coated beads and powder |
| Nifedipine | Procardia XL | 1X/day | Osmotic pump |
| | Adalat CC | 1X/day | Coat core |
| Nisoldipine | Sular | 1X/day | Coat core |
| Verapamil | Calan SR | 1-2X/day | Sodium alginate matrix |
| | Isoptin SR | 1-2X/day | Sodium alginate matrix |
| | Verelan | 1X/day | Coated beads (multiple) |
| | Covera HS | 1X/day HS | Osmotic pump with delay coat |
| | Verelan PM | 1X/day HS | Multiple beads with delay coat |

Gel-forming matrix with active drug

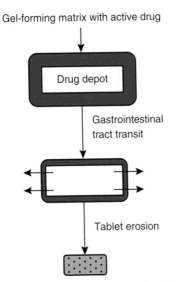

Drug depot

Gastrointestinal
tract transit

Tablet erosion

**Figure 66–4** Coat Core Delivery System. This delivery system is used with nifedipine, nisoldipine, and felodipine.

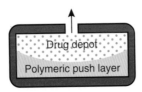

Drug depot
Polymeric push layer

**Figure 66–5** Osmotic Pump Delivery System. This delivery system is used with nifedipine, isradipine, and verapamil.

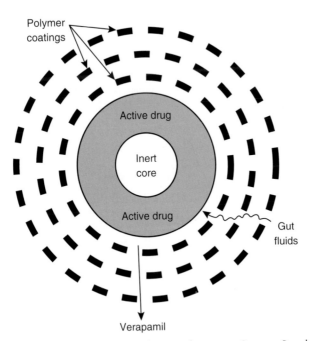

Polymer coatings

Active drug

Inert core

Active drug

Gut fluids

Verapamil

**Figure 66–6** Spheroidal Oral Drug Absorption System. Bead delivery systems are used with verapamil, diltiazem, and nicardipine.

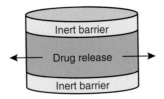

Inert barrier
Drug release
Inert barrier

**Figure 66–7** Geomatrix Delivery System. This delivery system is used with diltiazem.

## DRUG INTERACTIONS

Table 66–3 lists common pharmacokinetic drug-drug interactions. Grapefruit juice inhibits cytochrome P450 CYP3A on enterocytes[58] and increases the bioavailability of felodipine by 200%, of nisoldipine by 150%, and of amlodipine or nifedipine by 20% to 30%. Increases in verapamil levels following grapefruit juice have been reported.[59] Lithium neurotoxicity occurs with verapamil use.[60]

There are several important pharmacodynamic interactions between calcium antagonists and other drug classes. Drugs that slow the heart rate or conduction or reduce contractility can magnify those effects in combination with verapamil or diltiazem. These includes β-blockers, $\alpha_2$-stimulants, digitalis, amiodarone, flecainide, and disopyramide.

## SIDE EFFECTS

Short-acting dihydropyridines are associated with flushing, tachycardia, angina, dizziness, and headache caused by vasodilation. Long-acting dihydropyridines avoid these side effects but are associated with dose-dependent peripheral edema (Figure 66–8).[51] The peripheral edema is caused by a mismatch between arteriolar and venular dilation favoring fluid extravasation.[61,62] This side effect occurs less commonly with the nondihydropyridine calcium antagonists. The peripheral edema is not associated with weight gain and therefore is not responsive to diuretics. There appears to be a lower rate of peripheral edema among the third-generation dihydropyridines. In a multicenter double-blind, parallel trial of 828 elderly hypertensives treated with lacidipine 2 to 4 mg/day, lercanidipine 10 to 20 mg/day, or amlodipine 5 to 10 mg/day, the rate of edema was 4.3%, 9.3%, or 19% ($p$ <.0001), respectively.[63] The prevalence of peripheral edema is reduced when a converting enzyme inhibitor is combined with a dihydropyridine. In an 8-week, double-blind, parallel group trial of 563 hypertensives, the rate of peripheral edema was 4.9% for amlodipine 5 mg, 23.6% for amlodipine 10 mg, 2.2% for amlodipine 5 mg/benazepril 10 mg, and 1.5% for amlodipine 5 mg/benazepril 20 mg ($p$ <.001).[64]

Gingival overgrowth (Figure 66–9) occurs with calcium antagonists, cyclosporin, and phenytoin.[65] The prevalence is higher with nifedipine (38%) than with diltiazem (21%) or verapamil (19%) or in control patients (4%).[66] Attention to plaque control is important. Rarely, gingivectomy is needed.

Figure 66–10 shows common side effects seen with diltiazem in a randomized controlled trial.[55] Sinus bradycardia and peripheral edema were seen with the higher doses of diltiazem. Occasionally headache, dizziness, asthenia, fatigue, rash, and

**Table 66–3** Drug Interactions with Calcium Antagonists

| Verapamil | | | |
| --- | --- | --- | --- |
| **Drug Levels ↑** | **Drug Levels ↓** | **Verapamil Levels ↑** | **Verapamil Levels ↓** |
| Buspirone | Lithium | Ceftriaxone | Diclofenac |
| Carbamazepine | Oxcarbazepine | Cimetidine | Phenobarbital |
| Cyclosporine | | Clindamycin | Phenytoin |
| Digitoxin | | Fluoxetine | Rifampin |
| Digoxin | | Ketoconazole | Sulfinpyrazone |
| Dofetilide | | Terfenadine | |
| Imipramine | | | |
| Metoprolol | | | |
| Midazolam | | | |
| Prazosin | | | |
| Propranolol | | | |
| Quinidine | | | |
| Simvastatin | | | |
| Theophylline | | | |

| Diltiazem | | | |
| --- | --- | --- | --- |
| **Drug Levels ↑** | **Drug Levels ↓** | **Diltiazem Levels ↑** | **Diltiazem Levels ↓** |
| Alfentanil | | Cimetidine | Moricizine |
| Amlodipine | | | Rifampin |
| Buspirone | | | |
| Carbamazepine | | | |
| Cilostazol | | | |
| Cyclosporine | | | |
| Digitoxin | | | |
| Digoxin | | | |
| Imipramine | | | |
| Lovastatin | | | |
| Methylprednisolone | | | |
| Moricizine | | | |
| Nifedipine | | | |
| Propranolol | | | |
| Quinidine | | | |
| Simvastatin | | | |
| Sirolimus | | | |
| Tacrolimus | | | |
| Theophylline | | | |

| Nifedipine | | | |
| --- | --- | --- | --- |
| **Drug Levels ↑** | **Drug Levels ↓** | **Nifedipine Levels ↑** | **Nifedipine Levels ↓** |
| Digoxin | Quinidine | Cimetidine | Rifampin |
| Diltiazem | | Cyclosporine | St. John's Wort |
| Ginseng | | Dalfopristin | |
| Ginkgo biloba | | Fluoxetine | |
| Phenytoin | | Fluconazole | |
| Propranolol | | Quinidine | |
| Tacrolimus | | Quinupristin | |
| Theophyllines | | Ranitidine | |
| Vincristine | | Terfenadine | |

first-degree AV block were also reported. Figure 66–11 emphasizes that constipation occurs as a dose-dependent side effect of verapamil.[67] Dizziness, headache, and nausea also occur. Rarely, hepatotoxicity, complete heart block, or skin eruptions can occur. Calcium antagonists, including diltiazem and verapamil, should be avoided in patients with heart failure (systolic dysfunction), because they are associated with heart failure exacerbations.[68,69]

## CALCIUM ANTAGONISTS AS ANTIHYPERTENSIVES

Table 66–4 lists the calcium antagonists marketed in the United States and their indications according to the Food and Drug Administration. Not listed are nimodipine, which is used for subarachnoid hemorrhage, and bepridil, an antianginal drug that is rarely used.

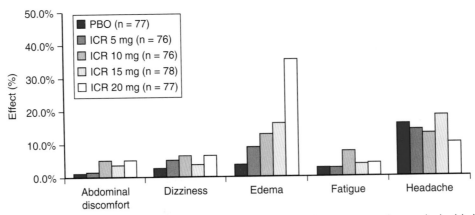

**Figure 67–8** Side effects of the dihydropyridine isradipine controlled-release. This was a randomized, double-blind, placebo-controlled, multicenter 9-week study. The only side effect that was dose-related was edema. PBO, placebo; ICR, isradipine controlled-release. (Derived from data of Chrysant SG, Cohen M. Sustained blood pressure control with controlled-release isradipine (isradipine-CR). J Clin Pharmacol 35:239-243, 1995.)

## EFFICACY

Calcium antagonists are as effective as other antihypertensive agents in lowering blood pressure. Two studies directly compared multiple classes of antihypertensive medications in terms of efficacy and side effects. The Treatment of Mild Hypertension Study was a randomized, double-blind, placebo-controlled trial of 902 men and women 45 to 69 years of age with a diastolic blood pressure less than 100 mm Hg.[70] All participants were advised to reduce sodium and alcohol intake, lose weight, and increase physical exercise. They were randomized to placebo, chlorthalidone 15 mg/day, acebutolol 400 mg/day, doxazosin 2 mg/day, amlodipine 5 mg/day, or enalapril 5 mg/day. If the blood pressure exceeded a prespecified threshold, then enalapril 2.5 to 5 mg/day could be added to the diuretic group or chlorthalidone 15 to 30 mg/day could be added to all other groups. As shown in Figure 66–12, amlodipine was as effective as the representative of any other antihypertensive drug class at the dose of drug used and tended to be more effective than the angiotensin-converting enzyme inhibitor. The greatest decline in left ventricular mass was seen in the

chlorthalidone group, as determined by serial echocardiograms (Figure 66–13).[71] The mean reduction in left ventricular mass of 25 g was nearly identical in all groups (including acebutolol, doxazosin, and enalapril, not shown), except chlorthalidone (34 g, $p = .03$ vs. placebo). Erectile dysfunction was significantly more common with chlorthalidone (Figure 66–14).[72] At 24 months, the incidence of erectile dysunction was greatest with chlorthalidone as compared with placebo ($p = .025$). At 48 months there was no difference among the groups. The average decrease in low-density lipoprotein cholesterol was greater with doxazosin than amlodipine ($-11.3$ mg/dl vs. $-5.1$ mg/dl, $p < .01$), and the decline in triglycerides was greater with amlodipine than acebutolol ($-18.4$ mg/dl vs. $-6.4$ mg/dl, $p < .01$). Amlodipine did not change glucose, potassium, uric acid, or creatinine. The starting dose of amlodipine (81.6%) and acebutolol (77.0%) was more likely to be maintained than placebo (54.6%, $p < .01$).[70]

The only other trial that compared six classes of antihypertensive drugs against placebo is a Veterans Affairs Cooperative Study, a randomized, double-blind study that involved 1292 men with untreated diastolic blood pressure between 95 to 109 mm Hg.[73-75] The following drugs were titrated over a period of 4 to 8 weeks: hydrochlorothiazide 12.5 to 50 mg/day, atenolol 25 to 100 mg/day, clonidine 0.1 to 0.3 mg twice daily, captopril 12.5 to 50 mg twice daily, prazosin 2 to 10 mg twice daily, diltiazem sustained-release 60 to 180 mg twice daily, or placebo. Treatment was deemed successful if the diastolic blood pressure was less than 90 mm Hg after the titration period and at 1 year of treatment (Figure 66–15). Diltiazem was significantly better than captopril, prazosin or placebo ($p < .05$).[75] Diltiazem (21.6%) was less likely to fail to achieve the titration goal of a diastolic blood pressure less than 90 mm Hg as compared with atenolol (29.4%), clonidine (30.7%), prazosin (34.2%), hydrochlorothiazide (38.1%), or placebo (61%).[73] Among younger and older African Americans, diltiazem achieved the highest treatment success rate after 1 year. Figure 66–16 shows the change in left ventricular mass from baseline in subjects whose pretreatment mass was greater than 350 g.[76] At 8 weeks, diltiazem and prazosin significantly reduced left ventricular mass ($p < .01$) to the greatest extent. However, after 1 year, hydrochlorothiazide ($p < .001$), captopril ($p < .01$), and atenolol ($p < .05$) were most effective.

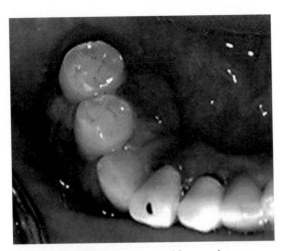

**Figure 66–9** Gingival growth caused by a calcium antagonist.

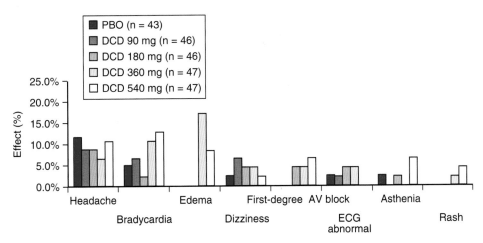

Figure 66–10 Side effects of diltiazem-controlled delivery. This was a multicenter, randomized, double-blind, placebo-controlled parallel design trial with a 4- to 6-week placebo baseline and 4-week treatment period. Sinus bradycardia and edema were treatment-related adverse events. (Derived from data of Felicetta JV, Serfer HM, Cutler NR, et al. A dose-response trial of once-daily diltiazem. Am Heart J 123:1022-1026, 1992.)

## DEMOGRAPHICS

Calcium antagonists are believed to be more effective in elderly and Black patients. Pharmacokinetic studies using verapamil, diltiazem, and amlodipine document a lower clearance and prolonged elimination half-life, as well as greater declines in blood pressure in elderly patients than in younger patients.[45,48,77]

In a double-blind, positively controlled, forced-dose titration study comparing atenolol, captopril, and verapamil sustained release as single agents in the treatment of 394 Black patients with a diastolic blood pressure 95 to 114 mm Hg, verapamil was most effective in controlling blood pressure.[78] Another study showed a slower clearance of nifedipine in Black subjects ($8.9 \pm 0.7$ ml/min/kg) as compared with white subjects ($11.6 \pm 0.8$ ml/min/kg; $p = .00004$).[79] Figure 66–17 shows that in the Veterans Affairs Cooperative Study, diltiazem achieved the highest treatment success rate after 1 year among younger and older African Americans.

Although gender has not generally been viewed as an important factor in the response of antihypertensive agents, data suggest that oral verapamil is not cleared as well and plasma concentrations are higher among women.[46,80] These pharmacokinetic data translate well into differences in blood pressure response, as documented by a metanalysis of three randomized, double-blind, placebo-controlled trials of controlled-onset, extended-release verapamil.[81] When using ambulatory blood pressure, the change in blood pressure was $-15.1/-10.4$ mm Hg for women as compared with $-10.0/-8.2$ mm Hg for men ($p < .001$ for systolic and $p = .003$ for diastolic pressure).

## SODIUM INTAKE AND NONSTEROIDAL ANTIINFLAMMATORY DRUGS

The calcium antagonists differ from the angiotension-converting enzyme inhibitors in that their blood pressure–lowering effect is not augmented by sodium restriction. In one small study, the change in blood pressure in response to verapamil 120 mg dosed three times daily on a low-sodium (9 mEq) diet was $-18/11$ mm Hg and on a high sodium (212 mEq) diet $-19/-14$ mm Hg.[82] Another double-blind study randomized 397 salt-sensitive hypertensive

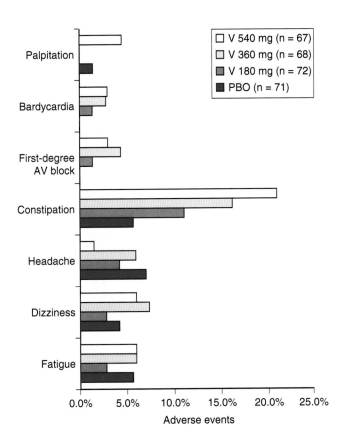

Figure 66–11 Side effects of verapamil chronotherapeutic extended-release. This was a double-blind placebo-controlled parallel-group trial with fixed-dose treatment for 4 weeks. Constipation is a dose-related adverse event. PBO, placebo; V, Verapamil. (Derived from data of Cutler NR, Anders RJ, Jhee SS, et al. Placebo-controlled evaluation of three doses of a controlled-onset extended-release formulation of verapamil in the treatment of stable angina pectoris. Am J Cardiol 75:1102-1106, 1995.)

**Table 66–4** Indications for Calcium Antagonists

| Generic | Brand Name | Stable Angina | Vasospastic Angina | Hypertension | Supraventricular |
|---------|-----------|:---:|:---:|:---:|:---:|
| **Benzothiazepine** | | | | | |
| Diltiazem | Cardizem | X | X | | X |
| Diltiazem | Cardizem-SR | | | X | |
| Diltiazem | Cardizem-CD | X | X | X | |
| Diltiazem | Cardizem LA† | | | X | |
| Diltiazem | Dilacor-XR | X | | X | |
| Diltiazem | Tiazac | | | X | |
| **Dihydropyridine** | | | | | |
| Amlodipine | Norvasc | X | X | X | |
| Felodipine | Plendil | | | X | |
| Isradipine | DynaCirc | X | | X | |
| Isradipine | DynaCirc-CR | | | X | |
| Nicardipine | Cardene | X | | X | |
| Nicardipine | Cardene-SR | | | X | |
| Nifedipine | Adalat/Procardia | X | X | | |
| Nifedipine | Adalat CC | | | X | |
| Nifedipine | Procardia XL | X | X | X | |
| Nisoldipine | Sular | | | X | |
| **Phenylalkylamine** | | | | | |
| Verapamil | Calan/Isoptin | X | X | X | X |
| Verapamil | Calan-SR | | | X | |
| Verapamil | Covera-HS† | X | | X | |
| Verapamil | Isoptin-SR | | | X | |
| Verapamil | Verelan | | | X | |
| Verapamil | Verelan-PM† | | | X | |

†Chronotherapeutic delivery system.

patients to isradipine 2.5 to 20 mg twice daily, enalapril 2.5 to 20 mg twice daily, or placebo to evaluate modulation of blood responses.[83] This study observed that the decline in blood pressure was greater for isradipine on a high- versus low-sodium (−14.9/−10.1 mm Hg vs. −7.6/−4.8 mm Hg) diet, whereas enalapril had a similar effect on both diets.

Nonsteroidal antiinflammatory agents attenuate the antihypertensive effects most classes of blood pressure–lowering drugs, probably because of inhibition of renal prostaglandin production.[84-87] However, calcium antagonists appear to be resistant to this effect. In a randomized, double-blind, study of 162 hypertensive patients treated with sustained-release verapamil hydrochloride 240 to 480 mg/day, participants were randomized to ibuprofen, naproxen, or placebo for 3 weeks.[88] There were no significant differences in sitting, standing, or supine blood pressure with ibuprofen 400 mg dosed three times daily or naproxen 500 mg dosed twice daily as compared with placebo despite increased weight with both nonsteroidal antinflammatory drugs (Figure 66–18). In another study, 100 patients were treated with nicardipine 30 mg three times daily and then randomized to 375 mg of naproxen twice daily or placebo for 4 weeks. Although weight increased by about

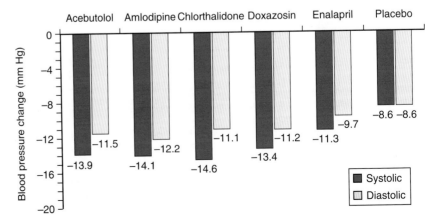

**Figure 66–12** Average Blood Pressure Change from Baseline at 48 Months: The Treatment of Mild Hypertension Study. For systolic or diastolic blood pressure, acebutolol, amlodipine, chlorthalidone, and doxazosin lowered blood pressure more than placebo ($p < .01$). (Data derived from Neaton JD, Grimm RH Jr., Prineas RJ, et al. Treatment of Mild Hypertension Study. Final results. Treatment of Mild Hypertension Study Research Group. JAMA 270:713-724, 1993.)

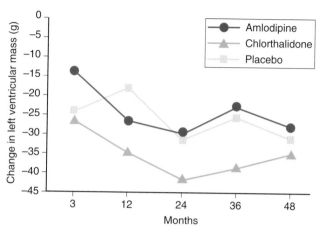

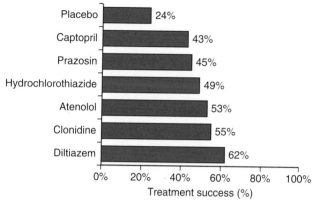

**Figure 66-13** Change in Echocardiographic Left Ventricular Mass: Treatment of Mild Hypertension Study. The mean change in left ventricular mass of 25 g was nearly identical in all groups (including acebutolol, doxazosin, and enalapril not shown), except chlorthalidone (34 g, $p = .03$ versus placebo). (Derived from data of Liebson PR, Grandits GA, Dianzumba S, et al. Comparison of five antihypertensive monotherapies and placebo for change in left ventricular mass in patients receiving nutritional-hygienic therapy in the Treatment of Mild Hypertension Study (TOMHS). Circulation 91:698-706, 1995.)

**Figure 66-15** Comparison of Six Antihypertensive Drugs—Treatment Success: Veterans Administration Cooperative Study. Treatment success is determined by a diastolic blood pressure less than 90 mm Hg after 1 year of treatment. Diltiazem was significantly better than captopril, prazosin, or placebo ($p < .05$). (Derived from data of Materson BJ, Reda DJ, Cushman WC. Department of Veterans Affairs Single-Drug Therapy of Hypertension Study. Revised figures and new data. Department of Veterans Affairs Cooperative Study Group on Antihypertensive Agents. Am J Hypertens 8:189-192, 1995.)

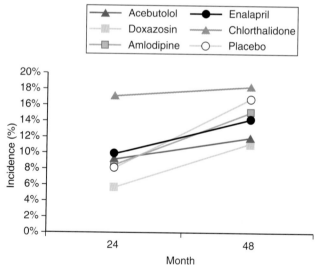

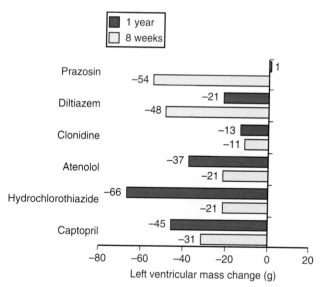

**Figure 66-14** Incidence of Erectile Dysfunction: The Treatment of Mild Hypertension Study. At 24 months, the incidence of erectile dysunction was greatest with chlorthalidone as compared with placebo ($p = .025$). At 48 months, there was no difference among the groups. (Derived from data of Grimm RH Jr., Grandits GA, Prineas RJ, et al. Long-term effects on sexual function of five antihypertensive drugs and nutritional hygienic treatment in hypertensive men and women. Treatment of Mild Hypertension Study (TOMHS). Hypertension 29:8-14, 1997.)

**Figure 66-16** Regression of Left Ventricular Mass with Monotherapy: Veterans Affairs Cooperative Study. The change in left ventricular mass from baseline is shown in subjects whose pretreatment mass was greater than 350 g. At 8 weeks diltiazem and prazosin significantly reduced left ventricular mass ($p < .01$). However, after 1 year hydrochlorothiazide ($p < .001$), captopril ($p < .01$), and atenolol ($p < .05$) were most effective. (Derived from data of Gottdiener JS, Reda DJ, Massie BM, et al. Effect of single-drug therapy on reduction of left ventricular mass in mild to moderate hypertension: Comparison of six antihypertensive agents. The Department of Veterans Affairs Cooperative Study Group on Antihypertensive Agents. Circulation 95:2007-2014, 1997.)

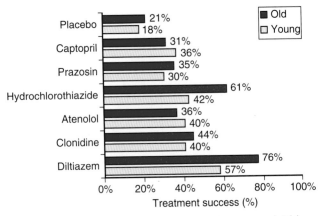

**Figure 66–17** Treatment Success Among Younger and Older African-Americans: Veterans Affairs Cooperative Study. Treatment success is determined by a diastolic blood pressure less than 90 mm Hg after 1 year of treatment. (Derived from data of Materson BJ, Reda DJ, Cushman WC. Department of Veterans Affairs Single-drug Therapy of Hypertension Study. Revised figures and new data. Department of Veterans Affairs Cooperative Study Group on Antihypertensive Agents. Am J Hypertens 8:189-192, 1995.)

0.7 kg in the naproxen-treated subjects, there was no increase in blood pressure.[89] In a double-blind crossover study, indomethacin 50 mg twice daily increased blood pressure in patients treated with enalapril but not in patients treated with amlodipine.[90] The cyclooxygenase-2 (COX-2) inhibitors celecoxib and rofecoxib did not increase systolic blood pressure over 6 weeks in a randomized, double-blind, controlled trial of elderly hypertensive patients receiving a calcium antagonist.[91] Future studies should examine the impact of nons-

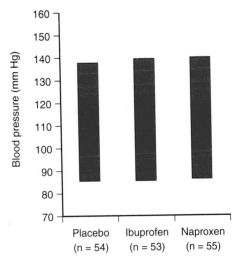

**Figure 66–18** Effect of nonsteroidal drug treatment on sitting antihypertensive response of verapamil. These two nonsteroidal antiinflammatory drugs did not attenuate the antihypertensive effect of verapamil after 3 weeks of treatment. (Derived from data of Houston MC, Weir M, Gray J, et al. The effects of nonsteroidal anti-inflammatory drugs on blood pressures of patients with hypertension controlled by verapamil. Arch Intern Med 155:1049-1054, 1995.)

teroidal treatment in the setting of calcium antagonists in combination with other antihypertensive drugs.

## COMBINATIONS WITH ANTIHYPERTENSIVE DRUGS

Effective blood pressure control usually requires two or more drugs. Figure 66–19 shows that the antihypertensive effects of most drug classes are additive to calcium antagonists.[92] The combination of sustained-release verapamil and trandolapril is additive for lowering blood pressure and reducing proteinuria.[93] The change in 24-hour ambulatory blood pressure in 31 elderly persons treated with felodipine 5 mg/day, candesartan 16 mg/day, and their combination was −11.9/5.7 mm Hg, −12.2/7.5 mm Hg, and −21.0/11.2 mm Hg ($p$ <.005 as compared with either monotherapy).[94] In a double-blind, placebo-controlled, 3 × 4 factorial design trial (n = 707) of placebo; enalapril 5 mg/day or 20 mg/day; felodipine 2.5 mg/day, 5 mg/day, or 10 mg/day; and the various combinations, the antihypertensive effects of the combinations were additive. Also, the combinations had a lower rate of peripheral edema (4.1%) compared with felodipine monotherapy (10.8%) but did not reduce the rate of cough, headache, or dizziness. Diltiazem-extended and enalapril appear to be additive, as are amlodipine and benazepril.[95-98]

Combining a dihydropyridine calcium antagonist with a β-adrenergic antagonist has the benefit of blocking the sympathetic nervous system activation that occurs with short-acting dihydropyridines. In a randomized, double-blind trial, 234 hypertensive patients were randomized to nicardipine 30 mg, propranolol 40 mg, or the combination of each dosed three times daily.[99] The change in average supine blood pressure after 6 weeks was −15.9/−13.8 mm Hg, −15.6/−12.6 mm Hg, and −19.8/−15.7 mm Hg for nicardipine, propranolol, and the combination. Although the combination was less than additive with respect to blood pressure, there were fewer vasodilator side effects with the combination (5%) or propanolol monotherapy (3%) as compared with nicardipine monotherapy (14%, $p$ ≤.05). Adding isradipine 2.5 to 5 mg dosed twice

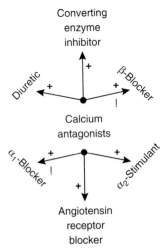

**Figure 66–19** Possible drug combinations with calcium antagonists. + indicates an additive combination; ! indicates that caution is required with the combination.

daily to pindolol, a β-blocker with intrinsic sympathomimetic activity, reduced supine blood pressure by −18/−15 mm Hg ($p$ <.001) after 4 weeks.[100] In a randomized, double-blind, crossover study with 4-week treatment phases, 15 patients received diltiazem 120 mg twice daily, atenolol once daily, both drugs, or placebo.[101] Compared with placebo, either monotherapy reduced blood pressure by −8/−9 mm Hg; the combination reduced blood pressure by −16/−13 mm Hg and was superior to monotherapy ($p$ <.05). The average PR interval 2 hours after drug dosing was 0.164 second for placebo, 0.175 second for diltiazem, 0.174 second for atenolol, and 0.184 second for the combination. Other studies have combined verapamil and propranolol.[102] Combining verapamil or diltiazem with a β-blocker increases the risk of sinus bradycardia or arrest, junctional escape rhythm, AV conduction block, and heart failure.

Combining an $\alpha_1$-blocker with a calcium antagonist may be synergistic.[103] In a randomized, double-blind, crossover study, each of 75 patients received amlodipine 10 mg, doxazosin 4 mg, and the combination of amlodipine 5 mg and doxazosin 2 mg daily for 6 weeks after a 2-week washout period.[104] The change from baseline was −29/−10 mm Hg for amlodipine monotherapy, −28/−8 mm Hg for doxazosin monotherapy, and −41/−15 mm Hg for the half-strength combination. The mechanism for the hypotensive response is unclear. One study observed an increase in bioavailability of terazosin when added to verapamil.[105] The use of this combination requires great care in slowly titrating the dose of the $\alpha_1$-blocker. The patient should be told that his or her prescription must be refilled promptly without any lapse to avoid severe orthostatic hypotension and syncope.

Whether combining calcium antagonists and diuretics has an advantageous effect on blood pressure control is controversial.[106-108] It has been suggested that the sequence of drug administration may be important. Addition of isradipine to hydrochlorothiazide-treated patients has been shown to be as efficacious as adding propranolol,[109] and factorial design trials with verapamil and diltiazem have shown an additive antihypertensive effect.[110,111]

The combination of a dihydropyridine to a nondihydropyridine produces additive antihypertensive effects.[112-114] One study reported a decrease in blood pressure when either diltiazem sustained-release or verapamil sustained-relase was added to nifedipine sustained-release.[115] However, diltiazem more effectively lowered blood pressure than did verapamil. This is because nifedipine levels were higher when the drug was combined with diltiazem (1430 ng•h/ml) than when it was combined with verapamil (1134 ng•h/ml, $p$ = .026) as compared with baseline nifedipine levels (957 ng•h/ml). The combination of verapamil and nifedipine was associated with more side effects than the combination of diltiazem and nifedipine.[115]

## MAJOR CLINICAL TRIALS

Calcium antagonists are effective antihypertensive and antianginal agents. Major prospective clinical trials support their role for treating hypertension without worsening overall mortality. ALLHAT documents that the long-acting calcium antagonist amlodipine does not increase cardiovascular or all-cause mortality as compared with chlorthalidone.[13] This review will consider only hypertension trials (Table 66–5).

## TRIALS OF CAROTID INTIMA-MEDIA PROGRESSION

The Multicenter Isradipine Diuretic Atherosclerosis Study (MIDAS) randomized 883 hypertensive patients to short-acting isradipine or hydrochlorothiazide to assess the rate of progression of carotid thickening over 3 years.[31] Enalapril 2.5 to 10 mg twice daily could be added to attain a diastolic blood pressure goal below 90 mm Hg. Systolic blood pressure was reduced more with the diuretic. There was no difference in the rate of progression of carotid thickening. Although there were more hospitalizations for unstable angina with isradipine treatment, there was no difference in all-cause mortality ($p$ = .81) or any major vascular event ($p$ = .07).

The Verapamil in Hypertension and Atherosclerosis Study (VHAS) randomized 498 patients to either sustained-release verapamil or chlorthalidone over 4 years to assess the impact on carotid intimal-medial thickness at six sites.[32] Captopril 25 to 50 mg could be added if blood pressure remained uncontrolled. For the first 6 months, the study was double-blind and afterward was open-label. Blood pressure control was similar with both drugs. The number of fatal and nonfatal cardiovascular events was similar in the two groups. There was significantly greater plaque regression in the group treated with verapamil as compared with chlorthalidone ($p$ <.02). Furthermore, fatal and nonfatal cardiovascular events occurred in 19 of 224 verapamil-treated and 35 of 232 chlorthalidone-treated patients.

A substudy of the International Nifedipine GITS Study: Intervention as a Goal in Hypertension Treatment (INSIGHT) examined progression of intima-media carotid thickening in 439 patients treated with nifedipine GITS or amiloride with hydrochlorothiazide over 48 months.[116] Atenolol 25 to 50 mg or enalapril 5 to 10 mg could be added if blood pressure was not controlled. There was no difference in blood pressure control, but more progression in carotid thickening was observed with the diuretic than with the calcium antagonist.

The European Lacidipine Study on Atherosclerosis (ELSA) studied 2334 patients randomized to either lacidipine or atenolol to assess the effect on carotid intima-media thickness at four sites over 4 years.[117] A diuretic could be added if blood pressure was not controlled. Clinic blood pressure measurements were similar between the two groups; however, 24-hour blood pressure was lower with atenolol than lacidipine. Despite this difference, there was less progression of intima-media thickness with lacidipine than with atenolol. However, there was no difference in the number cardiovascular events between treatments.

## TRIALS OF RENAL PROTECTION

Small short-term studies show proteinuria reduction with diltiazem and verapamil in hypertensive diabetic patients.[93,118] Many trials with dihydropyridine calcium antagonists do not show similar protection. The Microalbuminuria Reduction with Valsartan Study (MARVAL) reported a greater reduction in urinary albumin excretion rate among diabetics with microalbuminuria treated with valsartan versus amlodipine.[119] The African American Study of Kidney Disease and Hypertension (AASK) randomized 1094 nondiabetic Black

**Table 66–5** Clinical Trials of Hypertension with Calcium Antagonists

| Trial | n | Design | Intervention | Duration | Primary Outcome | Results |
|---|---|---|---|---|---|---|
| AASK | 1094 | R, DB | Amlodipine 5-10 mg vs. ramipril 2.5-10 mg vs. metoprolol 50-200 mg | 3 yr | Rate of change of glomerular filtration rate (amlodipine arm terminated by data safety and monitoring committee) | Ramipril was superior to amlodipine for proteinuria more than 300 mg/day; no difference in deaths |
| ABCD | 470 | R, DB | Nisoldipine 20-60 mg vs. enalapril 10-40 mg ± metoprolol ± HCTZ* | 5 yr | Relative effects of moderate and intensive blood pressure control on the change in creatinine clearance; one secondary outcome included cardiac morbidity and mortality | No difference in primary endpoint, but more fatal and nonfatal myocardial infarctions with nisoldipine, but no difference in cardiovascular death or total mortality |
| ALLHAT | 33,357 | R, DB | Chlorthalidone 12.5-50 mg, amlodipine 2.5-10 mg, lisinopril 10-40 mg, doxazosin 2-8 mg ± reserpine 0.5-0.2 mg, clonidine 0.2-0.6 mg, hydralazine 50-200 mg | 4.9 yr | Fatal coronary heart disease or nonfatal myocardial infarction | No difference in primary endpoint or total mortality, but more heart failure with amlodipine compared to diuretic ± atenolol 25-100 mg |
| CONVINCE | 16,476 | R, DB | Verapamil-COER 180-360 mg vs. HCTZ 12.5-25 mg or atenolol 50-100 mg ± ACE inhibitor or HCTZ | 3 yr | Nonfatal myocardial infarction or stroke or death from cardiovascular disease (terminated prematurely by sponsor) | No difference in the combined endpoint, but fewer myocardial infarctions and more strokes with calcium antagonist; no difference in all-cause mortality |
| ELSA | 2334 | R, DB | Lacidipine 4-6 mg vs. atenolol 50-100 mg | 4 yr | Rate of progression of mean maximum intima media thickness in 6 carotid focal points over 3 years | Less progression with lacidipine than atenolol; no difference in cardiovascular events |
| FACET | 380 | R, SB | Fosinopril 20 mg vs amlodipine 10 mg (or both if blood pressure not controlled) | 2.8 yr | Treatment-related difference in serum lipids and diabetes control Cardiovascular events were a secondary outcome | No difference in the primary endpoint, but there were fewer major vascular events in the fosinopril and combination group than the amlodipine group |
| HOT | 18,790 | PROBE | Felodipine 5-10 mg ± β-blocker or ACE* inhibitor or diuretic | 3.8 yr | Major cardiovascular events and target diastolic blood pressure ≤80, ≤85, and ≤90 mm Hg | Fewer cardiovascular events in patients with diabetes mellitus (n =1501), but not in the overall cohort |
| IDNT | 1715 | R, DB | Irbesartan 300 mg vs. amlodipine 10 mg vs. placebo | 2.6 yr | Doubling of serum creatinine, onset of end-stage renal disease, or all-cause mortality | Irbesartan superior to placebo and amlodipine for composite endpoint; no difference in cardiovascular events |
| INSIGHT | 6321 | R, DB | Nifedipine GITS* 30-60 mg vs. amiloride 2.5-5 mg with HCTZ 25-50 mg ± atenolol 50-100 mg or enalapril 5-10 mg | 4 yr | Cardiovascular death, heart failure, myocardial infarction, and stroke | No difference in primary endpoint, but more fatal myocardial infarctions and nonfatal heart failure in nifedipine GITS group; no difference in overall mortality |

| Trial | N | Design | Treatment | Duration | Endpoint | Results |
|---|---|---|---|---|---|---|
| | 439 | R, DB | As above | 4 yr | Rate of progression of mean maximum intima-media thickness of the carotid | Less progression with nifedipine than the diuretic |
| INVEST | 22,576 | PROBE | Verapamil SR 240-360 mg ± trandolapril 2-4 mg ± HCTZ 25 mg vs. atenolol 50-100 mg ± HCTZ 25-50 mg ± trandolapril 2-4 mg | 2.7 yr | All-cause mortality, nonfatal myocardial infarction, and nonfatal strokes | No difference in primary outcome; lower rate of diabetes in calcium channel blocker arm |
| MARVAL | 332 | R, DB | Valsartan 80-160 mg vs. amlodipine 5-10 mg ± bendrofluazide ± doxazosin | 24 wk | Urinary albumin excretion rate from baseline | Valsartan was more effective than amlodipine |
| MIDAS | 883 | R, DB | Isradipine 2.5-5 mg vs. hydrochlorothiazide 12.5-25 mg ± enalapril | 3 yr | Rate of progression of mean maximum intima-media thickness in 12 carotid focal points over 3 years | No difference in the rate of progression between the isradipine and the diuretic; no difference in mortality, but more admissions for angina |
| NICS-EH | 414 | R, DB | Nicardipine 40 mg vs. trichlormethiazide 2 mg | 5 yr | Cardiovascular complications | No difference in rate of complications |
| NORDIL | 10,881 | PROBE | Diltiazem 180-360 mg vs. diuretic and/or β-blocker ± ACE inhibitor ± $\alpha_1$-blocker | 5 yr | Cardiovascular death or nonfatal stroke or myocardial infarction | No difference in primary endpoint, but fewer strokes in diltiazem group |
| SHELL | 1882 | PROBE | Lacidipine 4-6 mg vs. chlorthalidone 12.5-25 mg ± fosinopril 10 mg | 32 mo | Composite endpoint of sudden death, fatal or nonfatal myocardial infarction, stroke, heart failure, myocardial revascularization, carotid endarterectomy | No difference in the composite or individual cardiovascular or cerebrovascular end points; no difference in total mortality |
| STONE | 1632 | A, DB | Nifedipine 10-60 mg vs. placebo ± captopril 25-50 mg ± HCTZ 25 mg | 30 mo | Stroke, heart failure, myocardial infarction, severe arrhythmia, sudden death | Fewer strokes and severe arrhythmias, but no difference total mortality, cardiovascular deaths, or sudden deaths |
| STOP-2 | 6614 | PROBE | Diuretics ± β-blockers vs. ACE inhibitors ± HCTZ vs calcium antagonists ± β-blocker | | Cardiovascular mortality | ACE inhibitors or calcium antagonists were were not better than diuretics and β-blockers; there were fewer myocardial infarctions and heart failure with ACE inhibitors compared with calcium antagonists; no difference in total mortality among three groups |
| SYST-CHINA | 2394 | A, DB | Nitrendipine 10-40 mg vs. placebo ± captopril 12.5-50 mg ± HCTZ 12.5-50 mg | 2 yr | Fatal and nonfatal stroke | Active treatment reduced strokes and total mortality |

(Continued)

**Table 66-5** Clinical Trials of Hypertension with Calcium Antagonists—cont'd

| Trial | n | Design | Intervention | Duration | Primary Outcome | Results |
|---|---|---|---|---|---|---|
| SYST-EUR | 4695 | R, DB | Nitrendipine 10-40 mg vs. placebo ± enalapril 5-20 mg ± HCTZ 12.5-25 mg | 2 yr | Stroke | Active treatment reduced nonfatal strokes, nonfatal cardiac endpoints, but not total mortality, myocardial infarction or heart failure |
| VALUE | 15,245 | R, DB | Valsartan 80-160 mg vs. amlodipine 5-10 mg ± HCTZ 12.5-25 mg | 4.2 yr | Time to first cardiac event (sudden death and fatal or nonfatal myocardial, infarction, heart failure, revascularization) | No difference in primary endpoint or total mortality; few myocardial infarctions with amlodipine; less new-onset diabetes with valsartan |
| VHAS | 498 | R, SB† | Verapamil SR 240 mg vs. chlorthalidone 25 mg | 4 yr | Slope of change of mean maximal thickness from 6 carotid sites over 4 years | Rate of progression greater with diuretic More cardiovascular events with diuretic |

See text for the abbreviations of trials.
*R, Randomized; A, Alternate allocation; DB, double blind; SB, single blind; PROBE, prospective, randomized, open-label, blinded endpoint; HCTZ, hydrochlorothiazide; ACE, angiotensin-converting enzyme; GITS, gastrointestinal therapeutic system; COER, controlled-onset extended-release.
†For first 3 months, trial was double-blind, then open-labeled.

patients with hypertensive renal insufficiency (20-65 ml/min/1.73 m²) to amlodipine, ramipril, or metoprolol extended-release.[120] This randomized, double-blind trial also included two levels of blood pressure control. The average number of additional drugs needed to control blood pressure was 2.75. The amlodipine arm was terminated early because of greater (50%) worsening of glomerular filtration rate ($p = .03$) and more end-stage renal disease ($p = .01$) as compared with the ramipril arm. Proteinuria also increased with amlodipine. There was no difference in overall mortality.

The Irbesartan Diabetic Nephropathy Trial studied 1715 hypertensive diabetic patients with protein excretion ≥900 mg/24 hour and serum creatinine 1 to 3 mg/dl.[121] Treatment was randomized to irbesartan, amlodipine, or placebo, but 3.0 to 3.3 drugs were needed to achieve the target blood pressure of 135/85 mm Hg or less. The rate of doubling of serum creatinine was 39% lower with irbesartan as compared with amlodipine ($p < .001$), and the rate of end-stage renal disease was 24% lower with irbesartan ($p = .06$). There was no difference in total mortality. The number of cardiovascular events was similar among all three groups (irbesartan, 29.7%; amlodipine, 28.3%; and placebo, 32.5%).[122] However, there were fewer myocardial infarctions with amlodipine as compared with placebo (4.7% vs. 8.1%, $p = .021$) and more cases of heart failure with amlodipine as compared with irbesartan (16.7% vs. 10.4%, $p = .007$). There were no differences among the three groups with respect to cerebrovascular events, although a protective trend was seen in amlodipine-treated patients.

These trials suggest that amlodipine is not protective against hypertensive or diabetic end-stage renal stage disease as compared with ramipril or irbesartan. However, in ALLHAT (see later), the decline in glomerular filtration rate (Figure 66–20) over 4 years was −2.9 ml/min/1.73 m² for amlodipine ($p < .001$ vs. diuretic), −7.6 ml/min/1.73 m² for chlorthalidone, and −7.0 ml/min/1.73 m² for lisinopril ($p = .03$ vs. diuretic).[13] Also, INSIGHT reported less impaired renal function with nifedipine GITS versus hydrochlorothiazide combined with amiloride.[123] These observations merit prospective studies in hypertensive patients that have no evidence of renal insufficiency at baseline. Also, studies that combine a converting enzyme inhibitor with a dihydropyridine have shown reductions in urinary albumin excretion comparable with those seen with a converting enzyme inhibitor alone.[124] Thus, studies are needed that look at the impact of various combinations on diuretic outcomes.

## TRIALS IN ISOLATED SYSTOLIC HYPERTENSION

The Systolic Hypertension in Europe (Syst-Eur) trial was a randomized, double-blind, placebo-controlled study in patients 60 years and older.[125] Participants received placebo or nitrendipine with enalapril and hydrochlorothiazide if needed to achieve blood pressure control. Combination drug therapy was frequently needed to lower the systolic blood pressure to less than 150 mm Hg. The study was stopped prematurely after 2 to 2.5 years because of a 42% reduction in fatal and nonfatal stroke for active as compared with placebo treatment. For fatal and nonfatal myocardial infarctions, however, there was only a nonsignificant 30% reduction in events ($p = .12$). Although not significant individually, when myocardial infarction and heart failure events were combined, there was a reduction in nonfatal cardiac endpoints ($p = .03$).

The role of a calcium antagonist in preventing vascular dementia in older patients was evaluated in Syst-Eur.[126,127] When the Mini-Mental Status Examination and computed tomography of the brain were used as diagnostic criteria, active treatment reduced the rate of dementia from 7.4 to 3.3 cases per 1000 patient years ($p < .001$).[127] Because no other class of antihypertensive drug has documented this finding, the results should be replicated prospectively.

The Systolic Hypertension in China (Syst-China) trial treated 2394 elderly hypertensive patients with placebo or nitrendipine alone or in combination with captopril, hydrochlorothiazide, or both.[128] Treatment assignment was by alternate allocation rather than randomization. The average entry blood pressure was 171/86 mm Hg. With treatment, the blood pressure declined by 11/2 mm Hg in the placebo group and 20/5 mm Hg in the nitrendipine group. Total mortality and stroke were significantly lower with active treatment, but there was no difference between groups. There was no decline in myocardial infarction, heart failure, or sudden death.

## ASSESSMENT OF CHRONOTHERAPEUTICS

The Controlled Onset Verapamil Investigation of Cardiovascular Endpoints (CONVINCE) trial tested whether a chronotherapeutic medication timed to deliver verapamil from 6 A.M. to noon is equivalent to traditional antihypertensive therapy in preventing cardiovascular events.[129-131] A group of 16,602 high-risk subjects 55 years or older with stages 1 to 3 hypertension were randomized to a chronotherapeutic preparation of verapamil or traditional antihypertensive drugs (diuretic or β-blocker). Additional drugs, including diuretics and converting enzyme inhibitors, could be added to achieve blood pressure control. The sponsor terminated the trial prematurely. There was no difference in the combined endpoint of fatal and nonfatal myocardial infarction and stroke at that point, but because of the limited statistical power of the prematurely terminated

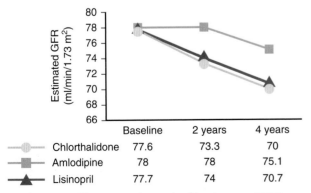

| | Baseline | 2 years | 4 years |
|---|---|---|---|
| Chlorthalidone | 77.6 | 73.3 | 70 |
| Amlodipine | 78 | 78 | 75.1 |
| Lisinopril | 77.7 | 74 | 70.7 |

**Figure 66–20** Change in glomerular filtration rate (GFR) over 4 years. (Graph derived from Major outcomes in high-risk hypertensive patients randomized to angiotensin-converting enzyme inhibitor or calcium channel blocker vs diuretic: The Antihypertensive and Lipid-Lowering Treatment to Prevent Heart Attack Trial (ALLHAT). JAMA 288:2981-2997, 2002.)

trial, it was not possible to demonstrate equivalence of the treatments. The authors concluded that, considered in the context of other trials of calcium antagonists, their data indicate that the effectiveness of calcium antagonist therapy in reducing cardiovascular outcomes is similar to but not better than traditional diuretic or β-blocker treatment.[131]

## TRIALS OF DIABETIC PATIENTS

The Appropriate Blood Pressure Control in Diabetes (ABCD) trial was a prospective, double-blind, randomized study that examined blood pressure control in 950 patients with type 2 diabetes mellitus with a diastolic blood pressure 80 mm Hg or higher.[132] The cohort in this single-center study was stratified into a normotensive (n = 480) and a hypertensive group (n = 470). The hypertensive group was further stratified into treatment goals of 80 to 89 mm Hg and 75 mm Hg.[133] Patients could receive nisoldipine 10 to 60 mg/day or enalapril 5 to 40 mg/day. If titration failed to achieve the target blood pressure, then open-labeled hydrochlorothiazide and metoprolol could be added, as well as other nonstudy medications. The primary endpoint was the effect of blood pressure control on 24-hour creatinine clearance. The secondary endpoints included the incidence of cardiovascular events. There was no difference in blood pressure control between the enalapril and nisoldipine groups, but fewer patients in the calcium antagonist group received a β-blocker (p = .035) or a diuretic (p = .02). There were more fatal and nonfatal myocardial infarctions in the nisoldipine group as compared with the enalapril group (22 vs. 5, p = .001). This was subsequently revised in a follow-up publication to 27 versus 9 (p = .029), reducing the adjusted risk ratio from 7 to 4.2.[134] This article supported the posthoc analysis of the MIDAS trial, suggesting that isradipine was associated with more cardiovascular events in the presence of elevated glycosylated hemoglobin.[9]

The Fosinopril versus Amlodipine Cardiovascular Events Randomized Trial (FACET) compared the effectiveness of amlodipine 10 mg daily with fosinopril 20 mg daily on lipid and diabetes control in a population of 380 hypertensive diabetics.[135] If blood pressure was not controlled in this open-label study, then the opposite drug was added. Although there was no difference in the endpoint of glucose or lipid control, there were more cardiovascular events in the amlodipine monotherapy group (n = 141) than in the fosinopril monotherapy group (n = 131; 27 vs. 10 events (p = .008). However, there were even fewer events in the combination group (n = 108; 4 events, p = .001).

## MISCELLANEOUS TRIALS OF BLOOD PRESSURE CONTROL

The Shanghai Trial of Nifedipine in the Elderly (STONE) was a single-blind trial that used alternate treatment allocation.[136] After a 4-week placebo period, 1632 patients received nifedipine 10 to 30 mg twice daily or placebo. Captopril, dihydrochlorothiazide, or both could be added to either treatment arm to attain blood pressure treatment goals. The average decline in blood pressure was −22/−12 mm Hg for nifedipine and −12/−8 mm Hg for placebo (p ≤ .0001 for both systolic and diastolic blood pressure). There were more strokes and

arrhythmias in the placebo group, but there was no difference in cardiovascular or total mortality.

The Hypertension Optimal Treatment (HOT) Study examined the effects of three levels of diastolic blood pressure control on cardiovascular events among 18,790 study participants with a PROBE design.[137] This international trial enrolled hypertensive patients 50 to 80 years of age with a diastolic blood pressure between 100 and 115 mm Hg. The targets for blood pressure control were ≤90, ≤85, or ≤80 mm Hg. Treatment to achieve each level of blood pressure control included stepwise increments of felodipine; a converting enzyme inhibitor, β-blocker, or both; and hydrochlorothiazide. The primary aim was to assess the relationship between major cardiovascular events (cardiovascular death nonfatal myocardial infarction, and nonfatal stroke) and the target blood pressures. The achieved blood pressures were 144/85, 141/83, and 140/81 mm Hg. There was no significant reduction in major cardiovascular events with the lower blood pressures; however, the trend for all myocardial infarction was significant (p = .05). Among the 1501 diabetic subjects in HOT, there was a significant reduction in cardiovascular events (p = .005) and cardiovascular mortality (p = .045) but no reduction in stroke, myocardial infarction, and total mortality.

## TRIALS OF DRUG COMPARISONS

INSIGHT was a prospective, randomized, double-blind trial of 6321 patients with a blood pressure 150/95 mm Hg or higher or systolic blood pressure 160 mm Hg or higher.[123] Participants were randomized to nifedipine GITS 30 to 60 mg or hydrochlorothiazide 25 to 50 mg with amiloride 2.5 to 5 mg daily. If blood pressure was not lowered by 20/10 mm Hg or was greater than 140/90 mm Hg, then atenolol 25 to 50 mg or enalapril 5 to 10 mg daily could be added. The primary composite endpoint was cardiovascular death, myocardial infarction, stroke, and heart failure. There was no difference in the primary endpoint but there were more cases of fatal myocardial infarction (.05% vs. 02%, p = .017) and nonfatal heart failure (.08% vs. .03%, p = .028) among patients assigned to the calcium antagonist as compared with conventional therapy. There was no difference in all-cause mortality. New-onset diabetes occurred more commonly in the diuretic group (5.6% vs. 4.3%, p = .02). In the diabetic cohort (n = 1302), there was a 24% reduction in the composite of all-cause mortality death from vascular cause and death from nonvascular cause in the nifedipine group (p = .03).[138]

The Swedish Trial in Old Patients with Hypertension-2 (STOP-2) study used the prospective, randomized, open-labeled, blinded endpoint (PROBE) design to compare the effects of calcium antagonists to conventional drugs or converting enzyme inhibition in 6614 elderly hypertensive subjects aged 70 to 84 years. If either component of the blood pressure was 180/105 mm Hg or greater, patients were randomly assigned to one of three arms: conventional drugs (atenolol 50 mg, metoprolol 100 mg, pindolol 5 mg, or hydrochlorothiazide 25 mg plus amiloride 2.5 mg daily), calcium antagonists felodipine 2.5 mg or isradipine 2.5 mg daily, or converting enzyme inhibitors (enalapril 10 mg or lisinopril 10 mg daily).[139] The actual drug choice within the assigned group was not randomized. If blood pressure was not controlled to less than 160/95 mm Hg on hydrochlorothiazide or a β-blocker, the alternative drug was added; for the converting enzyme inhibitor, a diuretic was added, and for the calcium antagonists, a β-blocker was added. There was no difference in the primary endpoint, cardiovascular mortality, according to treatment. However, the converting enzyme inhibitors were associated with a 23% lower rate of myocardial infarction (12.8% vs. 16.7%, $p = .018$) and 22% lower rate of heart failure (13.9% vs. 17.5%, $p = .025$) as compared with the calcium antagonists.

The National Intervention Cooperative Study in Elderly Hypertensives Study Group (NICS-EH) compared the outcomes of a diuretic versus calcium antagonist treatment in preventing cardiovascular events in elderly hypertensive patients in Japan.[140] After a 4-week placebo period, either sustained-release nicardipine 20 to 40 mg or trichlormethiazide 2 to 4 mg daily was given to 414 participants 60 years or older with a systolic blood pressure 160 to 220 mm Hg and a diastolic blood pressure less than 115 mm Hg. Medication was administered by using the double-dummy technique. After 5 years, blood pressure control was similar. There was no difference in the rate of cardiovascular endpoints in the two groups.

The Nordic Diltiazem (NORDIL) study studied 10,881 patients between 50 to 74 years with a diastolic blood pressure 100 mm Hg or higher by using a PROBE design.[141] Patients were titrated with diltiazem or conventional antihypertensive drugs (diuretics, β-blockers, or both) to achieve a diastolic blood pressure less than 90 mm Hg. A converting enzyme inhibitor or $\alpha_1$-blocker could be added to either therapy. The combined primary endpoint was any cardiovascular death and nonfatal myocardial infarction or stroke. There was no difference in the primary endpoint, but there were 20% fewer strokes with diltiazem (6.4% vs. 7.9%, $p = .04$) than with conventional therapy.

ALLHAT was a randomized, double-blind trial of 42,466 high-risk hypertensive patients 55 years or older comparing the effects of treatment with chlorthalidone 12.5 to 25 mg (n = 15,255) to amlodipine 2.5 to 10 mg (n = 9048), lisinopril 10 to 40 mg (n = 9054), and doxazosin 1 to 8 mg daily (n = 9061) on the primary combined endpoint of fatal coronary heart disease and nonfatal myocardial infarction.[13] The primary hypothesis of ALLHAT was that representatives of the newer classes of antihypertensive drugs would be superior to the diuretic in endpoint reduction. If blood pressure was not controlled, atenolol 25 to 100 mg daily, clonidine 0.1 to 0.3 mg twice daily, or reserpine 0.05 to 0.2 mg daily could be titrated. Hydralazine 25 to 100 mg twice daily could be added for additional blood pressure control. The doxazosin arm was stopped early because of higher rates of stroke and heart failure and futility of finding significant advantage over the diuretic with respect to the primary endpoint.[142] However, blood pressure was not as well controlled with doxazosin as with the diuretic. Comparing chlorthalidone and amlodipine, there was no difference for the primary combined outcome, combined coronary heart disease events, or end-stage renal disease. Participants randomized to amlodipine had the lowest all-cause mortality and stroke rates. Rates of cancer and gastrointestinal bleeding were not increased with the calcium antagonist, nor were there increases in hospitalized or treated angina. Only heart failure occurred with a 38% higher incidence ($p < .001$). The rate of heart failure increased very early in the trial. Critics of ALLHAT have suggested that much of the investigator diag-

nosed heart failure in the trial was due to misdiagnosis or secondary to withdrawal of prior diuretics and to unmasking of heart failure.[143] Subsequent publications have validated the diagnosis, at least for hospitalized and fatal cases.[144,145] As previously stated, ALLHAT has disproved many of the criticisms previously directed against calcium channel blockers.

The Systolic Hypertension in the Elderly: Lacidipine Long-term (SHELL) study was designed to compare a diuretic with lacidipine on cardiovascular outcome in elderly patients with isolated systolic hypertension, defined as a systolic blood pressure 160 mm Hg or higher and a diastolic blood pressure 95 mm Hg or less.[146] A composite of cardiovascular and cerebrovascular events was the primary outcome. The study used a PROBE design; however, 12 sites followed a double-blind design for the first year. Patients (n = 1882) were randomly assigned to chlorthalidone 12.5 mg or lacidipine 4 mg dosed once daily after a 2-week washout period. If there was not a reduction in systolic blood pressure 20 mm Hg or greater and systolic blood pressure exceeded 160 mm Hg after 4 weeks, chlorthalidone was titrated to 25 mg or lacidipine to 6 mg daily. If blood pressure control was still not achieved after 1 month, then the dose of the assigned drug was reduced to the starting dose and fosinopril 10 mg once daily was added. The planned sample size of 4800 patients was not achieved. Baseline blood pressure was 178/87 mm Hg. After 32 months, blood pressure was reduced by 36/8 mm Hg in chlorthalidone-treated patients and 35/8 mm Hg in the lacidipine-treated patients. Low-dose monotherapy was taken by 72% of lacidipine-treated and 47% of diuretic-treated patients. The overall incidence of the primary endpoints was 9.3% with no difference according to treatment. There was no significant difference for individual cardiovascular events. Total mortality, a secondary endpoint, was comparable.

The International Verapamil SR/Trandolapril Study (INVEST) enrolled 22,576 hypertensive patients with known coronary artery disease and used a PROBE design.[147] Patients were randomized to sustained-release verapamil 240 mg once daily or atenolol 50 mg once daily.[147] Drugs were titrated to a blood pressure goal of 140/90 mm Hg or 130/85 mm Hg for patients with diabetes mellitus or chronic renal insufficiency. Verapamil was titrated from 240 to 360 mg and trandolapril from 2 to 4 mg with hydrochlorothiazide 25 mg added, if necessary. Atenolol was titrated from 50 to 100 mg and hydrochlorothiazide 25 to 50 mg with trandolapril 2 to 4 mg added if needed. Diastolic and systolic blood pressure was controlled in 91% and 64% of study participants, respectively. The average decline in blood pressure at 24 months was $-18.7/-10$ mm Hg and $-19.0/-10.2$ mm Hg in the calcium antagonist and β-blocker arms, respectively. Greater than 48% of subjects required three or more drugs. The composite primary endpoint was nonfatal myocardial infarction, nonfatal stroke, and total mortality. Blood pressure control was similar over the 4 years of the study. There was no difference between groups for the composite primary endpoint or the individual components, but new-onset diabetes was more common in the β-blocker arm than the calcium antagonist arm (8.2% vs. 7.0%).

The Valsartan Antihypertensive Long-term Use Evaluation (VALUE) trial compared the efficacy of valsartan and amlodipine for reducing first cardiac events.[148] The double-blind trial enrolled 15,245 hypertensive patients. Valsartan 80 to 160 mg or amlodipine 5 to 10 mg was titrated with hydrochlorothiazide 12.5 to 25 mg and other nonstudy medications to achieve a blood pressure less than 140/90 mm Hg. The mean follow-up was 4.2 years. The average reduction in blood pressure was 15.2/8.2 mm Hg and 17.3/9.9 mm Hg for valsartan- and amlodipine-assigned patients, respectively ($p < .0001$). The greatest decline in blood pressure was observed during the first 3 months with amlodipine. There was no difference in overall cardiac morbidity, cardiac mortality, or total mortality. There were fewer myocardial infarctions recorded with amlodipine (4.1%) compared with valsartan (4.8%, $p = .02$). New onset diabetes was reduced by 23% ($p < .0001$) with valsartan. Although there was no overall difference in the primary composite endpoint, there was a benefit favoring amlodipine during the first 3 months, which paralleled the greatest difference between treatment regimens. An exploratory analysis was undertaken using serial median matching to compare similar patients based on demographics and level of systolic blood pressure.[149] Using this technique, there was no difference in the composite endpoint, stroke, death, or myocardial infarction; however, heart failure was 19% less among valsartan-treated patients.

## TRIAL IN PROGRESS

### Anglo-Scandinavian Cardiac Outcomes Trial (ASCOT)

ASCOT is a 2×2-factorial designed trial of 19,342 hypertensive patients with three additional cardiovascular risk factors randomized to receive the calcium antagonist amlodipine 5 to 10 mg with the converting enzyme inhibitor perindopril 4 to 8 mg, if needed or the β-blocker atenolol 50 to 100 mg with bendroflumethiazide 1.25 to 2.5 mg and potassium supplements, if necessary.[150] Doxazosin GITS 4 to 8 mg can be added to either arm if blood pressure is not controlled. The 10,305 participants with nonfasting total cholesterol concentrations ≤6.5 mmol/L (≤207 mg/dl) were randomly assigned to atorvastatin 10 mg or placebo. The primary endpoint of ASCOT is combined fatal coronary heart disease and nonfatal myocardial infarction. The lipid arm (ASCOT-LLA) has been terminated for benefit.[151]

## SUMMARY

Calcium channel blockers will continue to be used by physicians because they are effective in lowering blood pressure. The ALLHAT study has proven their safety in hypertensive patients. There was no increased risk of myocardial infarction, cancer, or overall mortality as compared with chlorthalidone. Care must be taken in using these medications in patients with systolic heart failure or advanced renal insufficiency and patients receiving multiple medications.

## References

1. Nelson CR, Knapp DA. Trends in antihypertensive drug therapy of ambulatory patients by US office-based physicians. Hypertension 36:600-6033, 2000.
2. Siegel D, Lopez J. Trends in antihypertensive drug use in the United States: Do the JNC V recommendations affect prescribing? Fifth Joint National Commission on the Detection, Evaluation, and Treatment of High Blood Pressure. JAMA 278:1745-178, 1997.
3. Manolio TA, Cutler JA, Furberg CD, et al. Trends in pharmacologic management of hypertension in the United States. Arch Intern Med 155:829-837, 1995.
4. Psaty BM, Manolio TA, Smith NL, et al. Time trends in high blood pressure control and the use of antihypertensive medications in older adults: The Cardiovascular Health Study. Arch Intern Med 162:2325-2332, 2002.
5. Wang TJ, Ausiello JC, Stafford RS. Trends in antihypertensive drug advertising, 1985-1996. Circulation 99:2055-7, 1999.
6. Held PH, Yusuf S, Furberg CD. Calcium channel blockers in acute myocardial infarction and unstable angina: An overview. BMJ 299:1187-1192, 1989.
7. Yusuf S, Held P, Furberg C. Update of effects of calcium antagonists in myocardial infarction or angina in light of the second Danish Verapamil Infarction Trial (DAVIT-II) and other recent studies. Am J Cardiol 67:1295-1297, 1991.
8. Furberg CD, Psaty BM, Meyer JV. Nifedipine. Dose-related increase in mortality in patients with coronary heart disease. Circulation 92:1326-1331, 1995.
9. Byington RP, Craven TE, Furberg CD, et al. Isradipine, raised glycosylated haemoglobin, and risk of cardiovascular events. Lancet 350:1075-1076, 1997.
10. Wagenknecht LE, Furberg CD, Hammon JW, et al. Surgical bleeding: Unexpected effect of a calcium antagonist. BMJ 310:776-777, 1995.
11. Pahor M, Guralnik JM, Furberg CD, et al. Risk of gastrointestinal haemorrhage with calcium antagonists in hypertensive persons over 67 years old. Lancet 347:1061-1065, 1996.
12. Pahor M, Guralnik JM, Ferrucci L, et al. Calcium-channel blockade and incidence of cancer in aged populations. Lancet 348:493-497, 1996.
13. Major outcomes in high-risk hypertensive patients randomized to angiotensin-converting enzyme inhibitor or calcium channel blocker vs diuretic: The Antihypertensive and Lipid-Lowering Treatment to Prevent Heart Attack Trial (ALLHAT). JAMA 288:2981-2997, 2002.
14. Triggle DJ. Mechanisms of action of calcium antagonists. In Epstein M (ed). Calcium Antagonists in Clinical Medicine. Philadelphia, Hanley & Belfus, 2002; pp 1-32.
15. Godfraind T, Salomone S, Dessy C, et al. Selectivity scale of calcium antagonists in the human cardiovascular system based on in vitro studies. J Cardiovasc Pharmacol 20(Suppl 5):S34-41, 1992.
16. Herbette LG, Mason PE, Gaviraghi G, et al. The molecular basis for lacidipine's unique pharmacokinetics: Optimal hydrophobicity results in membrane interactions that may facilitate the treatment of atherosclerosis. J Cardiovasc Pharmacol 23(Suppl 5):S16-S25, 1994.
17. Herbette LG, Vecchiarelli M, Sartani A, et al. Lercanidipine: Short plasma half-life, long duration of action and high cholesterol tolerance. Updated molecular model to rationalize its pharmacokinetic properties. Blood Press Suppl 2:10-17, 1998.
18. Abernethy DR, Schwartz JB. Calcium-antagonist drugs. N Engl J Med 341:1447-1457, 1999.
19. Oparil S, Kobrin I, Abernethy DR, et al. Dose-response characteristics of mibefradil, a novel calcium antagonist, in the treatment of essential hypertension. Am J Hypertens 10:735-742, 1997.
20. Schwartz ML, Rotmensch HH, Vlasses PH, et al. Calcium blockers in smooth-muscle disorders. Current status. Arch Intern Med 144:1425-1429, 1984.
21. Krusell LR, Christensen CK, Lederballe Pedersen O. Acute natriuretic effect of nifedipine in hypertensive patients and normotensive controls: A proximal tubular effect? Eur J Clin Pharmacol 32:121-126, 1987.
22. Krusell LR, Jespersen LT, Schmitz A, et al. Repetitive natriuresis and blood pressure. Long-term calcium entry blockade with isradipine. Hypertension 10:577-581, 1987.

23. Terzoli L, Leonetti G, Pedretti R, et al. Nifedipine does not blunt the aldosterone and cardiovascular response to angiotensin II and potassium infusion in hypertensive patients. J Cardiovasc Pharmacol 11:317-320, 1988.

24. Yang Z, Noll G, Luscher TF. Calcium antagonists differently inhibit proliferation of human coronary smooth muscle cells in response to pulsatile stretch and platelet-derived growth factor. Circulation 88:832-836, 1993.

25. van Zwieten PA, van Meel JC, Timmermans PB. Pharmacology of calcium entry blockers: Interaction with vascular alpha-adrenoceptors. Hypertension 5:II8-17, 1983.

26. van Zwieten PA, Timmermans PB, van Heiningen PN. Receptor subtypes involved in the action of calcium antagonists. J Hypertens Suppl 5:S21-8, 1987.

27. Weinstein DB, Heider JG. Antiatherogenic properties of calcium antagonists: State of the art. Am J Med 86:27-32, 1989.

28. Nayler WG. Vascular injury: Mechanisms and manifestations. Am J Med 90:8S-13S, 1991.

29. Lichtlen PR, Hugenholtz PG, Rafflenbeul W, et al. Retardation of angiographic progression of coronary artery disease by nifedipine. Results of the International Nifedipine Trial on Antiatherosclerotic Therapy (INTACT). INTACT Group Investigators. Lancet 335:1109-1113, 1990.

30. Waters D, Lesperance J, Francetich M, et al. A controlled clinical trial to assess the effect of a calcium channel blocker on the progression of coronary atherosclerosis. Circulation 82:1940-1953, 1990.

31. Borhani NO, Mercuri M, Borhani PA, et al. Final outcome results of the Multicenter Isradipine Diuretic Atherosclerosis Study (MIDAS). A randomized controlled trial. JAMA 276: 785-791, 1996.

32. Zanchetti A, Rosei EA, Dal Palu C, et al. The Verapamil in Hypertension and Atherosclerosis Study (VHAS): Results of long-term randomized treatment with either verapamil or chlorthalidone on carotid intima-media thickness. J Hypertens 16:1667-1676, 1998.

33. Pitt B, Byington RP, Furberg CD, et al. Effect of amlodipine on the progression of atherosclerosis and the occurrence of clinical events. PREVENT Investigators. Circulation 102:1503-1510, 2000.

34. Prisant LM. Calcium antagonists: Pharmacologic considerations. Ethn Dis 8:98-102, 1998.

35. Prisant LM, Bottini B, DiPiro JT, et al. Novel drug-delivery systems for hypertension. Am J Med 93:45S-55S, 1992.

36. Elliott WJ, Prisant LM. Drug delivery systems for antihypertensive agents. Blood Press Monit 2:53-60, 1997.

37. Elliott WJ, Prisant LM. Controlled-release formulations of calcium antagonist. In Epstein M (ed). Calcium Antagonists in Clinical Medicine. Philadephia, Hanley & Belfus, 2002; pp 139-150.

38. Neutel JM, Alderman M, Anders RJ, et al. Novel delivery system for verapamil designed to achieve maximal blood pressure control during the early morning. Am Heart J 132:1202-1206, 1996.

39. White WB, Anders RJ, MacIntyre JM, et al. Nocturnal dosing of a novel delivery system of verapamil for systemic hypertension. Verapamil Study Group. Am J Cardiol 76:375-380, 1995.

40. Prisant LM, Devane JG, Butler J. A steady-state evaluation of the bioavailability of chronotherapeutic oral drug absorption system verapamil PM after nighttime dosing versus immediate-acting verapamil dosed every eight hours. Am J Ther 7:345-351, 2000.

41. Glasser SP, Neutel JM, Albert KS, et al. Efficacy and safety of diltiazem HCl extended release (G99) dose at nighttime (10PM) compared to placebo and to morning dosing (8AM) in moderate to severe essential hypertension. Am J Hypertens 15:52A, 2002.

42. McAllister RG Jr., Schloemer GL, Hamann SR. Kinetics and dynamics of calcium entry antagonists in systemic hypertension. Am J Cardiol 57:16D-21D, 1986.

43. Murdoch D, Heel RC. Amlodipine. A review of its pharmacodynamic and pharmacokinetic properties, and therapeutic use in cardiovascular disease. Drugs 41:478-505, 1991.

44. McTavish D, Sorkin EM. Verapamil. An updated review of its pharmacodynamic and pharmacokinetic properties, and therapeutic use in hypertension. Drugs 38:19-76, 1989.

45. Abernethy DR, Schwartz JB, Todd EL, et al. Verapamil pharmacodynamics and disposition in young and elderly hypertensive patients. Altered electrocardiographic and hypotensive responses. Ann Intern Med 105:329-36, 1986.

46. Krecic-Shepard ME, Barnas CR, Slimko J, et al. Gender-specific effects on verapamil pharmacokinetics and pharmacodynamics in humans. J Clin Pharmacol 40:219-230, 2000.

47. Pritza DR, Bierman MH, Hammeke MD. Acute toxic effects of sustained-release verapamil in chronic renal failure. Arch Intern Med 151:2081-2084, 1991.

48. Schwartz JB, Abernethy DR. Responses to intravenous and oral diltiazem in elderly and younger patients with systemic hypertension. Am J Cardiol 59:1111-1117, 1987.

49. Murdoch D, Brogden RN. Sustained release nifedipine formulations. An appraisal of their current uses and prospective roles in the treatment of hypertension, ischaemic heart disease and peripheral vascular disorders. Drugs 41:737-779, 1991.

50. Swanson DR, Barclay BL, Wong PS, et al. Nifedipine gastrointestinal therapeutic system. Am J Med 83:3-9, 1987.

51. Chrysant SG, Cohen M. Sustained blood pressure control with controlled-release isradipine (isradipine-CR). J Clin Pharmacol 35:239-243, 1995.

52. Chung M, Reitberg DP, Gaffney M, et al. Clinical pharmacokinetics of nifedipine gastrointestinal therapeutic system. A controlled-release formulation of nifedipine. Am J Med 83:10-14, 1987.

53. Prisant LM, Carr AA, Bottini PB, et al. Nifedipine GITS (gastrointestinal therapeutic system) bezoar. Arch Intern Med 151:1868-1869, 1991.

54. Webster J, Petrie JC, Jeffers TA, et al. Nicardipine sustained release in hypertension. Br J Clin Pharmacol 32:433-439, 1991.

55. Felicetta JV, Serfer HM, Cutler NR, et al. A dose-response trial of once-daily diltiazem. Am Heart J 123:1022-1026, 1992.

56. Smith DH, Neutel JM, Weber MA. A new chronotherapeutic oral drug absorption system for verapamil optimizes blood pressure control in the morning. Am J Hypertens 14:14-19, 2001.

57. Prisant LM, Bottini B, DiPiro JT, et al. Novel drug-delivery systems for hypertension. Am J Med 93:45S-55S, 1992.

58. Kane GC, Lipsky JJ. Drug-grapefruit juice interactions. Mayo Clin Proc 75:933-42, 2000.

59. Ho PC, Ghose K, Saville D, et al. Effect of grapefruit juice on pharmacokinetics and pharmacodynamics of verapamil enantiomers in healthy volunteers. Eur J Clin Pharmacol 56:693-698, 2000.

60. Price WA, Giannini AJ. Neurotoxicity caused by lithium-verapamil synergism. J Clin Pharmacol 26:717-719, 1986.

61. Messerli FH, Grossman E. Pedal edema: Not all dihydropyridine calcium antagonists are created equal. Am J Hypertens 15:1019-1020, 2002.

62. Pedrinelli R, Dell'Omo G, Melillo E, et al. Amlodipine, enalapril, and dependent leg edema in essential hypertension. Hypertension 35:621-625, 2000.

63. Leonetti G, Magnani B, Pessina AC, et al. Tolerability of long-term treatment with lercanidipine versus amlodipine and lacidipine in elderly hypertensives. Am J Hypertens 15: 932-940, 2002.

64. Messerli FH, Oparil S, Feng Z. Comparison of efficacy and side effects of combination therapy of angiotensin-converting enzyme inhibitor (benazepril) with calcium antagonist (either nifedipine or amlodipine) versus high-dose calcium antagonist monotherapy for systemic hypertension. Am J Cardiol 86:1182-1187, 2000.

65. Prisant LM, Herman W. Calcium channel blocker induced gingival overgrowth. J Clin Hypertens 4:310-311, 2002.

66. Steele RM, Schuna AA, Schreiber RT. Calcium antagonist-induced gingival hyperplasia. Ann Intern Med 120:663-4, 1994.

67. Cutler NR, Anders RJ, Jhee SS, et al. Placebo-controlled evaluation of three doses of a controlled-onset, extended-release formulation of verapamil in the treatment of stable angina pectoris. Am J Cardiol 75:1102-1106, 1995.

68. Tsuyuki RT, McKelvie RS, Arnold JM, et al. Acute precipitants of congestive heart failure exacerbations. Arch Intern Med 161:2337-2342, 2001.

69. Elkayam U, Amin J, Mehra A, et al. A prospective, randomized, double-blind, crossover study to compare the efficacy and safety of chronic nifedipine therapy with that of isosorbide dinitrate and their combination in the treatment of chronic congestive heart failure. Circulation 82:1954-1961, 1990.

70. Neaton JD, Grimm RH Jr., Prineas RJ, et al. Treatment of Mild Hypertension Study. Final results. Treatment of Mild Hypertension Study Research Group. JAMA 270:713-724, 1993.

71. Liebson PR, Grandits GA, Dianzumba S, et al. Comparison of five antihypertensive monotherapies and placebo for change in left ventricular mass in patients receiving nutritional-hygienic therapy in the Treatment of Mild Hypertension Study (TOMHS). Circulation 91:698-706, 1995.

72. Grimm RH Jr., Grandits GA, Prineas RJ, et al. Long-term effects on sexual function of five antihypertensive drugs and nutritional hygienic treatment in hypertensive men and women. Treatment of Mild Hypertension Study (TOMHS). Hypertension 29:8-14, 1997.

73. Materson BJ, Reda DJ, Cushman WC, et al. Single-drug therapy for hypertension in men. A comparison of six antihypertensive agents with placebo. The Department of Veterans Affairs Cooperative Study Group on Antihypertensive Agents. N Engl J Med 328:914-921, 1993.

74. Materson BJ, Reda DJ. Correction: Single-drug therapy for hypertension in men. N Engl J Med 330:1689, 1994.

75. Materson BJ, Reda DJ, Cushman WC. Department of Veterans Affairs Single-drug Therapy of Hypertension Study. Revised figures and new data. Department of Veterans Affairs Cooperative Study Group on Antihypertensive Agents. Am J Hypertens 8:189-192, 1995.

76. Gottdiener JS, Reda DJ, Massie BM, et al. Effect of single-drug therapy on reduction of left ventricular mass in mild to moderate hypertension: Comparison of six antihypertensive agents. The Department of Veterans Affairs Cooperative Study Group on Antihypertensive Agents. Circulation 95:2007-2014, 1997.

77. Abernethy DR, Gutkowska J, Lambert MD. Amlodipine in elderly hypertensive patients: pharmacokinetics and pharmacodynamics. J Cardiovasc Pharmacol 12(Suppl 7):S67-S71, 1988.

78. Saunders E, Weir MR, Kong BW, et al. A comparison of the efficacy and safety of a beta-blocker, a calcium channel blocker, and a converting enzyme inhibitor in hypertensive blacks. Arch Intern Med 150:1707-1713, 1990.

79. Krecic-Shepard ME, Park K, Barnas C, et al. Race and sex influence clearance of nifedipine: Results of a population study. Clin Pharmacol Ther 68:130-142, 2000.

80. Gupta SK, Atkinson L, Tu T, et al. Age and gender related changes in stereoselective pharmacokinetics and pharmacodynamics of verapamil and norverapamil. Br J Clin Pharmacol 40:325-331, 1995.

81. White WB, Johnson MF, Black HR, et al. Gender and age effects on the ambulatory blood pressure and heart rate responses to antihypertensive therapy. Am J Hypertens 14:1239-1247, 2001.

82. Nicholson JP, Resnick LM, Laragh JH. The antihypertensive effect of verapamil at extremes of dietary sodium intake. Ann Intern Med 107:329-334, 1987.

83. Chrysant SG, Weder AB, McCarron DA, et al. Effects of isradipine or enalapril on blood pressure in salt-sensitive hypertensives during low and high dietary salt intake. MIST II Trial Investigators. Am J Hypertens 13:1180-1188, 2000.

84. Webster J. Interactions of NSAIDs with diuretics and beta-blockers mechanisms and clinical implications. Drugs 30:32-41, 1985.

85. Houston MC. Nonsteroidal anti-inflammatory drugs and antihypertensives. Am J Med 90:42S-47S, 1991.

86. Radack KL, Deck CC, Bloomfield SS. Ibuprofen interferes with the efficacy of antihypertensive drugs. A randomized, double-blind, placebo-controlled trial of ibuprofen compared with acetaminophen. Ann Intern Med 107:628-635, 1987.

87. Gurwitz JH, Avorn J, Bohn RL, et al. Initiation of antihypertensive treatment during nonsteroidal anti-inflammatory drug therapy. JAMA 272:781-786, 1994.

88. Houston MC, Weir M, Gray J, et al. The effects of nonsteroidal anti-inflammatory drugs on blood pressures of patients with hypertension controlled by verapamil. Arch Intern Med 155:1049-1054, 1995.

89. Klassen DK, Jane LH, Young DY, et al. Assessment of blood pressure during naproxen therapy in hypertensive patients treated with nicardipine. Am J Hypertens 8:146-153, 1995.

90. Morgan TO, Anderson A, Bertram D. Effect of indomethacin on blood pressure in elderly people with essential hypertension well controlled on amlodipine or enalapril. Am J Hypertens 13:1161-1167, 2000.

91. Whelton A, White WB, Bello AE, et al. Effects of celecoxib and rofecoxib on blood pressure and edema in patients > or =65 years of age with systemic hypertension and osteoarthritis. Am J Cardiol 90:959-963, 2002.

92. Moser M, Prisant LM. Low-dose combination therapy in hypertension. Am Fam Physician 56:1275-6, 1279, 1282, 1997.

93. Bakris GL, Weir MR, DeQuattro V, et al. Effects of an ACE inhibitor/calcium antagonist combination on proteinuria in diabetic nephropathy. Kidney Int 54:1283-1289, 1998.

94. Morgan T, Anderson A. A comparison of candesartan, felodipine, and their combination in the treatment of elderly patients with systolic hypertension. Am J Hypertens 15:544-549, 2002.

95. Applegate WB, Cohen JD, Wolfson P, et al. Evaluation of blood pressure response to the combination of enalapril (single dose) and diltiazem ER (four different doses) in systemic hypertension. Am J Cardiol 78:51-55, 1996.

96. Chrysant SG, Gavras H, Niederman AL, et al. Clinical utility of long-term enalapril/diltiazem ER in stage 3-4 essential hypertension. Long-term Use of Enalapril/Diltiazem ER in Stage 3-4 Hypertension Group. J Clin Pharmacol 37:810-815, 1997.

97. Cushman WC, Cohen JD, Jones RP, et al. Comparison of the fixed combination of enalapril/diltiazem ER and their monotherapies in stage 1 to 3 essential hypertension. Am J Hypertens 11:23-30, 1998.

98. Frishman WH, Ram CV, McMahon FG, et al. Comparison of amlodipine and benazepril monotherapy to amlodipine plus benazepril in patients with systemic hypertension: A randomized, double-blind, placebo-controlled, parallel-group study. The Benazepril/Amlodipine Study Group. J Clin Pharmacol 35:1060-6, 1995.

99. Lessem JN, Barone EJ, Berl T, et al. Nicardipine and propranolol in the treatment of essential hypertension. Am J Hypertens 2:146-153, 1989.

100. Hansson L, Dahlof B. Antihypertensive effect of a new dihydropyridine calcium antagonist, PN 200-110 (isradipine), combined with pindolol. Am J Cardiol 59:137B-140B, 1987.

101. Tonkin AL, Wing LM, Russell AE, et al. Diltiazem and atenolol in essential hypertension: Additivity of effects on blood pressure and cardiac conduction with combination therapy. J Hypertens 8:1015-1019, 1990.

102. McInnes GT, Findlay IN, Murray G, et al. Cardiovascular responses to verapamil and propranolol in hypertensive patients. J Hypertens 3(Suppl 3):S219-S221, 1985.

103. Elliott HL, Meredith PA, Reid JL. Verapamil and prazosin in essential hypertension: Evidence of a synergistic combination? J Cardiovasc Pharmacol 10(Suppl 10):S108-S110, 1987.

104. Nalbantgil S, Nalbantgil I, Onder R. Clinically additive effect between doxazosin and amlodipine in the treatment of essential hypertension. Am J Hypertens 13:921-926, 2000.

105. Lenz ML, Pool JL, Laddu AR, et al. Combined terazosin and verapamil therapy in essential hypertension: Hemodynamic and pharmacokinetic interactions. Am J Hypertens 8: 133-145, 1995.

106. Sever PS, Poulter NR. Calcium antagonists and diuretics as combined therapy. J Hypertens 5:S123-S126, 1987.

107. Frishman WH, Landau A, Cretkovic A. Combination drug therapy with calcium-channel blockers in the treatment of systemic hypertension. J Clin Pharmacol 33:752-755, 1993.

108. Nicholson JP, Resnick LM, Laragh JH. Hydrochlorothiazide is not additive to verapamil in treating essential hypertension. Arch Intern Med 149:125-128, 1989.

109. Prisant LM, Carr AA, Nelson EB, et al. Isradipine vs propranolol in hydrochlorothiazide-treated hypertensives: A multicenter evaluation. Arch Intern Med 149:2453-2457, 1989.

110. Letzel H, Bluemner E. Dose-response curves in antihypertensive combination therapy: Results of a controlled clinical trial. J Hypertens 8:S83-S86, 1990.

111. Burris JF, Weir MR, Oparil S, et al. An assessment of diltiazem and hydrochlorothiazide in hypertension. Application of factorial trial design to a multicenter clinical trial of combination therapy. JAMA 263:1507-1512, 1990.

112. Kaesemeyer WH, Prisant LM, Carr AA. Verapamil and nifedipine in combination for the treatment of hypertrophy heart disease. Am J Hypertens 4:866-867, 1991.

113. Kaesemeyer WH, Carr AA, Bottini PB, et al. Verapamil and nifedipine in combination for the treatment of hypertension. J Clin Pharmacol 34:48-51, 1994.

114. Sica DA. Current concepts of pharmacotherapy in hypertension: Combination calcium channel blocker therapy in the treatment of hypertension. J Clin Hypertens 3:322-327, 2001.

115. Saseen JJ, Carter BL, Brown TE, et al. Comparison of nifedipine alone and with diltiazem or verapamil in hypertension. Hypertension 28:109-114, 1996.

116. Simon A, Gariepy J, Moyse D, et al. Differential effects of nifedipine and co-amilozide on the progression of early carotid wall changes. Circulation 103:2949-2954, 2001.

117. Zanchetti A, Bond MG, Hennig M, et al. Calcium antagonist lacidipine slows down progression of asymptomatic carotid atherosclerosis: Principal results of the European Lacidipine Study on Atherosclerosis (ELSA), a randomized, double-blind, long-term trial. Circulation 106:2422-2427, 2002.

118. Demarie BK, Bakris GL. Effects of different calcium antagonists on proteinuria associated with diabetes mellitus. Ann Intern Med 113:987-988, 1990.

119. Viberti G, Wheeldon NM. Microalbuminuria reduction with valsartan in patients with type 2 diabetes mellitus: A blood pressure-independent effect. Circulation 106:672-678, 2002.

120. Agodoa LY, Appel L, Bakris GL, et al. Effect of ramipril vs amlodipine on renal outcomes in hypertensive nephrosclerosis: A randomized controlled trial. JAMA 285:2719-2728, 2001.

121. Lewis EJ, Hunsicker LG, Clarke WR, et al. Renoprotective effect of the angiotensin-receptor antagonist irbesartan in patients with nephropathy due to type 2 diabetes. N Engl J Med 345:851-860, 2001.

122. Berl T, Hunsicker LG, Lewis JB, et al. Cardiovascular outcomes in the Irbesartan Diabetic Nephropathy Trial of Patients with Type 2 Diabetes and Overt Nephropathy. Ann Intern Med 138:542-549, 2003.

123. Brown MJ, Palmer CR, Castaigne A, et al. Morbidity and mortality in patients randomised to double-blind treatment with a long-acting calcium-channel blocker or diuretic in the International Nifedipine GITS study: Intervention as a Goal in Hypertension Treatment (INSIGHT). Lancet 356:366-372, 2000.

124. Fogari R, Zoppi A, Mugellini A, et al. Effect of benazepril plus amlodipine vs benazepril alone on urinary albumin excretion in hypertensive patients with type II diabetes and microalbuminuria. Clin Drug Invest 13(Suppl 1):50-55, 1997.

125. Staessen JA, Fagard R, Thijs L, et al. Randomised double-blind comparison of placebo and active treatment for older patients with isolated systolic hypertension. The Systolic Hypertension in Europe (Syst-Eur) Trial Investigators. Lancet 350:757-764, 1997.

126. Forette F, Seux ML, Staessen JA, et al. Prevention of dementia in randomised double-blind placebo-controlled Systolic Hypertension in Europe (Syst-Eur) trial. Lancet 352:1347-1351, 1998.

127. Forette F, Seux ML, Staessen JA, et al. The prevention of dementia with antihypertensive treatment: New evidence from the Systolic Hypertension in Europe (Syst-Eur) study. Arch Intern Med 162:2046-2052, 2002.

128. Liu L, Wang JG, Gong L, et al. Comparison of active treatment and placebo in older Chinese patients with isolated systolic hypertension. Systolic Hypertension in China (Syst-China) Collaborative Group. J Hypertens 16:1823-1829, 1998.

129. Black HR, Elliott WJ, Neaton JD, et al. Rationale and design for the Controlled ONset Verapamil Investigation of Cardiovascular Endpoints (CONVINCE) Trial. Control Clin Trials 19:370-390, 1998.

130. Black HR, Elliott WJ, Neaton JD, et al. Baseline characteristics and early blood pressure control in the CONVINCE Trial. Hypertension 37:12-18, 2001.

131. Block HR, Elliot WJ, Grandits G, et al. Principal results of the Controlled Onset Verapamil Investigation of Cardiovascular Endpoints (CONVINCE) trial. JAMA 289:2073-2082, 2003.

132. Schrier RW, Estacio RO, Jeffers B. Appropriate Blood Pressure Control in NIDDM (ABCD) Trial. Diabetologia 39:1646-1654, 1996.

133. Estacio RO, Jeffers BW, Hiatt WR, et al. The effect of nisoldipine as compared with enalapril on cardiovascular outcomes in patients with non-insulin-dependent diabetes and hypertension. N Engl J Med 338:645-652, 1998.

135. Schrier RW, Estacio RO. Additional follow-up from the ABCD trial in patients with type 2 diabetes and hypertension. N Engl J Med 343:1969, 2000.

134. Tatti P, Pahor M, Byington RP, et al. Outcome results of the Fosinopril Versus Amlodipine Cardiovascular Events Randomized Trial (FACET) in patients with hypertension and NIDDM. Diabetes Care 21:597-603, 1998.

136. Gong L, Zhang W, Zhu Y, et al. Shanghai trial of nifedipine in the elderly (STONE). J Hypertens 14:1237-1245, 1996.

137. Hansson L, Zanchetti A, Carruthers SG, et al. Effects of intensive blood-pressure lowering and low-dose aspirin in patients with hypertension: Principal results of the Hypertension Optimal Treatment (HOT) randomised trial. HOT Study Group. Lancet 351:1755-1762, 1998.

138. Mancia G, Brown M, Castaigne A, et al. Outcomes with nifedipine GITS or co-amilozide in hypertensive diabetics and nondiabetics in Intervention as a Goal in Hypertension (INSIGHT). Hypertension 41:431-436, 2003.

139. Hansson L, Lindholm LH, Ekbom T, et al. Randomised trial of old and new antihypertensive drugs in elderly patients: Cardiovascular mortality and morbidity the Swedish Trial in Old Patients with Hypertension-2 study. Lancet 354:1751-1756, 1999.

140. Randomized double-blind comparison of a calcium antagonist and a diuretic in elderly hypertensives. National Intervention Cooperative Study in Elderly Hypertensives Study Group. Hypertension 34:1129-1133, 1999.

141. Hansson L, Hedner T, Lund-Johansen P, et al. Randomised trial of effects of calcium antagonists compared with diuretics and beta-blockers on cardiovascular morbidity and mortality in hypertension: The Nordic Diltiazem (NORDIL) study. Lancet 356:359-365, 2000.

142. Major cardiovascular events in hypertensive patients randomized to doxazosin vs chlorthalidone: The Antihypertensive and Lipid-Lowering treatment to prevent Heart Attack Trial (ALLHAT). ALLHAT Collaborative Research Group. JAMA 283:1967-1975, 2000.

143. Weber MA. Commentary: The ALLHAT report: A case of information and misinformation. J Clin Hypertens 5:9-13, 2003.

144. David BR, Cutler JA, Furberg CD, et al. Relationship of antihypertensive treatment regimens and change in blood pressure to risk for heart failure in hypertensive patients randomly assigned to doxazosin or chlorthalidone: Further analyses from the Antihypertensive and Lipid Lowering Treatment to Prevent Heart Attack Trial. Ann Intern Med 137:313-320, 2002.

145. Piller LB, Davis BR, Cutler JA, et al. Validation of heart failure events in the Antihypertensive and Lipid Lowering Treatment to Prevent Heart Attack Trial (ALLHAT) participants assigned to doxazosin and chlorthalidone. Current Controlled Trials in Cardiovascular Medicine 3:10-18, 2002.

146. Malacco E, Mancia G, Rappelli A, et al. Treatment of isolated systolic hypertension: The SHELL study results. Blood Press 12:160-167, 2003.

147. Pepine CJ, Handberg EM, Cooper-DeHoff RM, et al. A calcium antagonist vs a non-calcium antagonist hypertension treatment strategy for patients with coronary artery disease. The International Verapamil-Trandolapril Study (INVEST): A randomized controlled trial. JAMA 290:2805-2816, 2003.

148. Julius S, Kjeldsen SE, Weber M, et al. Outcomes in hypertensive patients at high cardiovascular risk treated with regimens based on valsartan or amlodipine: The VALUE randomised trial. Lancet 363:2022-2031, 2004.

149. Weber MA, Julius S, Kjeldsen SE, et al. Blood pressure dependent and independent effects of antihypertensive treatment on clinical events in the VALUE Trial. Lancet 363:2049-2051, 2004.

150. Sever PS, Dahlof B, Poulter NR, et al. Rationale, design, methods and baseline demography of participants of the Anglo-Scandinavian Cardiac Outcomes Trial. ASCOT investigators. J Hypertens 19:1139-47, 2001.

151. Sever P, Dohlof B, Poulter NR, et al. Prevention of coronary and stroke events with atorvastatin in hypertensive patients who have average or lower-than-average cholesterol concentrations, in the Anglo-Scandinavian Cardiac Outcomes Trial - Lipid Lowering Arm (ASCOT-LLA): A multicenter randomised controlled trial. Lancet 361:1149-1158, 2003.

# Chapter 67

# Angiotensin II Receptor Antagonists

## Michael C. Ruddy, John B. Kostis

## INTRODUCTION

The main components of the renin-angiotensin system were characterized by the mid-1950s. Leonard Skeggs and his group in Cleveland had used hog renal renin and equine plasma renin substrate to show that there are two forms of the peptide product.[1] The biologically inactive decapeptide angiotensin I was found to be quickly transformed in plasma by a chloride-dependent "converting enzyme" to the vasopressor octapeptide angiotensin II.[2] The same laboratory also determined the nature of the renin substrate molecule from which angiotensin is generated, as well as the function of converting enzyme. They found three important biochemical properties of the converting enzyme: its anion dependence, its metalloprotein nature, and its ability to catalyze the hydrolytic cleavage of a dipeptide from the carboxyl terminus of its decapeptide substrate. By 1956, these investigators had documented the precise amino acid sequence of angiotensin I and II.[3]

Skeggs suggested three possible avenues of therapeutic effect on the renin-angiotensin system. The first possibility, that of direct inhibition of the action of renin on its substrate, remains to this day under study with several renin inhibitors currently undergoing investigation (see Chapter 72). A second proposal was to prevent the formation of the octapeptide hypertenin II (angiotensin II) from its decapeptide precursor by inhibition of the converting enzyme. This strategy has since been extraordinarily successful through the development of orally active angiotensin-converting enzyme (ACE) inhibitors (see Chapters 9 and 65).

A third suggestion was to prevent the vasoconstrictive action of angiotensin II on smooth muscle with inhibitory compounds based on the structure of angiotensin II.[4] Since the mid-1990s, this latter approach has developed into a mainstay of therapy for an increasing number of patients with hypertensive circulatory and renal disorders. This chapter outlines the increasingly important products of Skeggs's amazingly prescient hypotheses.

## ANGIOTENSIN SYSTEM

### Pathways for Angiotensin Generation

All of the known biologic actions of the renin-angiotensin system are mediated by the angiotensin series of peptides. Of these, the octapeptide angiotensin II has the broadest range of activity and the greatest potency in circulatory regulation. Most angiotensin II is formed in two steps through the sequential catalytic action of renin and ACE on the substrate angiotensinogen. In addition, some angiotensin II is formed in cardiac and renal tissue through the action of other proteolytic enzymes, such as chymase and cathepsin on the decapeptide angiotensin I.[5]

## Actions of Angiotensin II

A primary function of the renin-angiotensin system is to maintain perfusion when the circulation is threatened by volume depletion or hypotensive stress.[6] In this respect, acute effects of angiotensin II production include vasoconstriction, increased aldosterone secretion with retention of salt, increased thirst and release of antidiuretic hormone, and amplification of sympathetic nervous system activity.[7,8]

### Blood Vessels

Angiotensin II acts as a potent constrictor of precapillary arterioles and, to a lesser extent, postcapillary venules.[9] The direct action at the vascular smooth muscle site appears to account for most of the increase in peripheral resistance. The vasoconstrictor effect of angiotensin II is mediated primarily through direct binding to angiotensin II type 1 ($AT_1$) receptors on vascular smooth muscle.[10] However, in certain vascular beds, such as those perfusing skeletal muscle of the extremities of humans, it has been demonstrated that α-adrenergic antagonists can appreciably attenuate the vasoconstrictor effect of infused angiotensin II.[11] This finding is consistent with an important role for sympathetic augmentation of the vascular action of angiotensin II. The vasoconstrictor effect of angiotensin II is greatest in the splanchnic, renal, and cutaneous vascular beds and is less in vessels of the brain, lung, heart (coronary), and skeletal muscle. In the latter regions, blood flow may actually increase during low-dose infusions of angiotensin II due to the stronger effect of elevated systemic blood pressure opposing the relatively weak vasoconstrictor response in these areas.[12]

### Adrenal Cortex

The angiotensin system has an important role in the regulation of plasma volume through the actions of angiotensin II on the adrenal gland and the kidney. Angiotensin II is the primary secretagogue for the synthesis and release of aldosterone by cells of the adrenal cortical zona glomerulosa. The cells of the zona glomerulosa have a high density of $AT_1$ receptors.[13] Adrenal secretion of aldosterone can be elicited by concentrations of angiotensin II that are well below the threshold of a systemic pressor response.[13] Aldosterone acts on the distal tubule and collecting duct of the kidney to promote reabsorption of sodium in exchange for secretion of potassium and hydrogen ions. The effect of increasing aldosterone levels is preservation of or expansion of total body sodium and plasma volume.

Aldosterone has important profibrotic and hypertrophic effects in the cardiovascular system (see Chapters 12 and 70).[14] These include direct prosynthetic effects on collagen 1A1, 1A2, and 3A1, and indirect effects via transforming growth factor-$\beta_1$ (TGF-$\beta_1$).[15] Aldosterone has also been shown

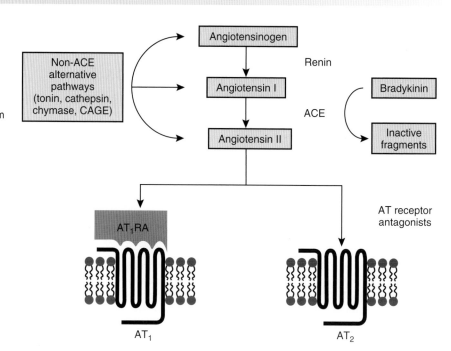

**Figure 67–1** The renin-angiotensin system cascade. ACE, angiotensin-converting enzyme; CAGE, chymostatin-sensitive angiotensin II–generating enzyme; AT, angiotensin II. (From Johnston CI, Risvanis J. Preclinical pharmacology of angiotensin II receptor antagonists: Update and outstanding issues. Am J Hypertens 10:306S-310S, 1997.)

to up-regulate the expression of $AT_1$ receptors, suggesting positive feedback between the actions of angiotensin II and aldosterone.[16]

## Kidney

The rate-limiting step for the production of intrarenal angiotensin II appears to be mostly dependent on renin secreted by the cells of the juxtaglomerular apparatus.[17] The final catalytic step in the formation of renal interstitial angiotensin II from its precursor molecule, angiotensin I, appears to be predominantly via non-ACE pathways.[18] The kidney appears to be especially sensitive to the actions of angiotensin II. Most of the intrarenal effects of angiotensin II can be observed experimentally at circulating levels 10 to 100 times lower than required for its extrarenal actions.[19]

Angiotensin II receptors are found in the efferent and afferent glomerular arterioles, the juxtaglomerular cells, glomerular mesangial cells and podocytes, the basolateral and apical surfaces of proximal and distal tubular cells, the macula densa, the collecting duct, and medullary interstitium.[20] Effects of angiotensin II have been observed in each of the major cellular elements of the kidney, including cells of the microvasculature, the mesangium, the tubular epithelium, and the interstitium.

Autoregulation of glomerular filtration rate in response to variations in renal perfusion pressure is mediated predominantly, although not exclusively, through angiotensin II.[21] At the level of the preglomerular and postglomerular arterioles, angiotensin II acts as a vasoconstrictor. The glomerular efferent arterioles are highly sensitive to even low concentrations of this peptide.[22] The glomerular afferent arterioles are less sensitive to the constrictor effects of angiotensin II, perhaps due to differential production of vasodilator prostaglandins and nitric oxide by these vessels.[23] Also, angiotensin II produces a direct contractile response of the glomerular mesangial cells, which tends to decrease the effective surface area available for glomerular filtration.[24] Modest increases in tissue or circulating angiotensin II levels act to increase glomerular

hydrostatic pressure and filtration rate by the dual additive effects of raised systemic perfusion pressure together with heightened resistance of the postglomerular outflow. At higher levels of angiotensin II, the less sensitive preglomerular afferent arterioles constrict, impeding glomerular perfusion. Thus, reduced glomerular perfusion combined with the direct contractile action of angiotensin II on the glomerular mesangium may result in significant impairment of renal blood flow and glomerular filtration rate. $AT_1$ receptors on the cell surface of the juxtaglomerular apparatus mediate an inhibitory signal for renin release by these cells, thereby providing a key element in the rapid servocontrol of local and systemic production of angiotensin II.

Angiotensin II, through activation of cytokines, such as TGF-β, promotes mesangial cell proliferation and extracellular matrix deposition.[25] Glomerular hypertension and angiotensin II have also been shown to increase the rate of glomerular podocyte loss.[26] In aging and in several disease states, these local actions of angiotensin II are likely to contribute importantly to glomerulosclerosis and progressive decline of filtration rate.

The proximal tubular epithelial cells express a high density of $AT_1$ receptors on both the basolateral and luminal membranes.[27] The density of receptors decreases from the most proximal to distal portions of this segment.[28] Low to moderate concentrations of angiotensin II promote tubular reabsorption of filtered sodium and water.[29] This is mediated primarily through stimulation of the epithelial apical sodium-proton pump.[30] Also, glomerular autoregulation leads to increased filtration fraction and concomitant elevation of peritubular capillary and interstitial oncotic pressure. The latter serves to amplify the more direct, receptor-mediated actions of angiotensin II on tubular sodium and fluid reabsorption. Thus, angiotensin II within the usual physiologic range serves to preserve or enhance net renal sodium retention by at least three mechanisms: (1) direct receptor-mediated actions along the proximal tubule, (2) indirect alterations of peritubular Starling forces, and (3) indirectly through stimulation of adrenal aldosterone release and augmentation of basolateral Na,K-ATPase along the distal tubular epithelium and collecting duct.

## Nervous System

The effects of angiotensin II on the nervous system are complex (see Chapter 6). The earliest described action was the central pressor effect. It has been demonstrated that infusion of angiotensin II into the isolated cerebral circulation of dogs was associated with a rise in systemic blood pressure even though the angiotensin has no access to the systemic blood vessels.[31] Blockade of peripheral α-adrenergic receptors inhibited this central action of angiotensin II, indicating that sympathetic tone plays an important role.[32] Ablation of the area postrema inhibits the effects of centrally administered angiotensin II, indicating that this area mediates angiotensin II induced stimulation of sympathetic outflow.[33]

It has also been demonstrated that angiotensin II enhances the activity of peripheral noradrenergic nerve terminals. Angiotensin II stimulates the release of and inhibits the reuptake of norepinephrine at peripheral sympathetic nerve endings.[7]

Both intravenous and centrally administered angiotensin II has been shown to provoke water intake and salt appetite and also stimulate secretion of vasopressin and adrenocorticotropic hormone.[34] These central actions of angiotensin II are thought to provide short and intermediate-term defense for extracellular fluid volume in the hypovolemic or hypotensive state. Although angiotensin II does not cross the blood-brain barrier, there is evidence that its central actions may be mediated through the subfornical organ.[35] Finally, it has been found that neurons at various locations in the central nervous system are capable of synthesizing angiotensin II, presumably for local release as a neuromodulator.

## Structural Effects of Angiotensin II

Subpressor amounts of angiotensin II, when administered over days to weeks, can produce hypertrophy of the myocardium and vascular smooth muscle.[36] These actions can be attenuated or prevented altogether with ACE inhibitors and angiotensin receptor antagonists. In vascular smooth muscle cell cultures, angiotensin II has been shown to enhance production of extracellular matrix proteins, such as type V collagen and fibronectin.[37] Angiotensin II can also act as a mitogen by promoting a proliferative response in fibroblasts, adrenal cortical cells, and vascular smooth muscle cells.[38] The growth promoting effects of low levels of angiotensin II occur despite down-regulation of the $AT_1$ receptors.

## Distribution of Angiotensin Receptors

Angiotensin II, like other peptidic hormones, elicits its cellular actions by first binding to highly specific receptors located on the cell membrane. In humans, two angiotensin II receptor subtypes have been identified. The $AT_1$ and $AT_2$ receptor subtypes have been cloned and characterized as members of the superfamily of seven-transmembrane-spanning G-protein–coupled receptors (see Chapter 11).[39] The $AT_1$ receptor appears to mediate most of the known actions of the angiotensins.

**Table 67-1** Actions of Angiotensin II

| Tissue | Action |
|---|---|
| Vasculature | Vasoconstriction |
| | Promotes smooth muscle hypertrophy |
| Adrenal cortex | Stimulates synthesis and secretion of aldosterone |
| Adrenal medulla | Increases release of epinephrine |
| Kidney | Vasoconstriction of the efferent and afferent arterioles |
| | Inhibition of renin release by the juxtaglomerular apparatus |
| | Stimulation of sodium reabsorption in the proximal tubule |
| | Promotion of mesangial growth and matrix deposition |
| Heart | Stimulation of myocardial hypertrophy and collagen synthesis |
| Brain | Stimulation of thirst and release of vasopressin |
| | Increase in central sympathetic outflow |
| Peripheral sympathetic nerve terminals | Presynaptic augmentation of norepinephrine release |

$AT_1$ receptors have been demonstrated in a large number of tissues, including vascular smooth muscle, adrenal zona glomerulosa, mesangial and tubular epithelial cells of the kidney, myocardium, neuronal tissue, and choroid plexus.[40] The $AT_2$ receptor subtype has been found in abundance in fetal mesenchymal cells, brain tissue, adrenal medulla, and uterus.[40] The physiologic functions and intracellular signaling mechanisms of the $AT_2$ receptor protein remain incompletely understood. There is evidence that the $AT_2$ receptor subtype can mediate antiproliferative and apoptotic effects of angiotensin II.[41]

With the exception of the adrenal glomerulosa, prolonged exposure of target organs to angiotensin II reduces responsiveness, an effect that has been shown to be associated with internalization and phosphorylation of the $AT_1$ receptor.[42] Comparisons among different cell types reveal that receptor density and magnitude of response to angiotensin II are not always related. For example, vascular smooth muscle cells have a much lower density of $AT_1$ receptors than cells of the adrenal glomerulosa yet have a more rapid and dramatic response to angiotensin II.[43]

## DEVELOPMENT OF ANGIOTENSIN II ANTAGONISTS

### Peptide Analogs of Angiotensin II

Detailed analyses of the structural requirements of angiotensin for binding to its receptors and studies of many analogs of angiotensin II eventually led to the development of saralasin, a potent angiotensin II receptor blocker (ARB).[44] Saralasin is an octapeptide, which differs in structure from angiotensin II at the first (sarcosine) and eighth (alanine) amino acid positions. Sarcosine is a nonmammalian amino acid, which, when located at the N-terminal of angiotensin II, was found to slow the degradation of the molecule. Saralasin was shown to lower blood pressure and aldosterone levels in humans in proportion to the circulating levels of angiotensin II.[45] Due to its peptide nature, saralasin required intravenous administration, was expensive to manufacture, and had a short half-life. Initially, saralasin was approved only as a diagnostic probe for renin-dependent forms of hypertension.[46] Because this agent also possessed weak agonist action, it occasionally produced a significant pressor effect in patients with low renin forms of hypertension.[47] The inconvenience and expense of administration, coupled with the unpredictability of response, markedly limited the application of saralasin in the clinical mainstream. Following the development and approval of the orally active converting enzyme inhibitors in the early 1980s, saralasin was withdrawn from the market.

## Medicinal Chemistry of Nonpeptide Angiotensin II Receptor Antagonists

For several decades investigators struggled to identify potent orally active ARBs. An important breakthrough occurred in 1982, when Furakawa et al. of the laboratories of Takeda Ltd. in Japan identified and patented several 1-benzylimidazole 5 acetic acid derivatives that had specific angiotensin II receptor binding activity.[48] However, these initial compounds possessed only weak antihypertensive effects.[49] Investigators at the Dupont Merck Pharmaceutical Company postulated that the imidazole compounds and angiotensin II bound to the same receptor site, but the test molecules needed enlargement to better mimic angiotensin II at its points of attachment to the receptor. The molecular model employed by these investigators suggested that there was overlap between the imidazole groups with histidine at the 6-position of angiotensin II.[50] The lipophilic N-butyl group at the 2-position was pointed at the leucine at the 5-position of the octapeptide. It was posited that the benzyl group of the Takeda compound extended in the direction of the N-terminal of angiotensin II. Elongation of the compound by building the molecule toward the tyrosine site at the 4-position of angiotensin II might increase potency.[50]

Addition of a carboxylic moiety at the para position of the benzene ring improved receptor binding 10-fold and lowered blood pressure when administered intravenously to renal hypertensive rats. By enlarging the molecule with placement of a second acidic phenyl group linked by a single carbon atom to the first aromatic ring, binding affinity increased another 10-fold, and oral bioavailability was markedly enhanced.[51] A significant and final improvement in bioavailability and receptor binding was obtained when the carboxylic moiety located on the second phenyl group was replaced by a tetrazole at the ortho position.

## BIPHENYL TETRAZOLE DERIVATIVES

Losartan is chemically described as 2-butyl-4-chloro-1-[p-(o-1H-tetrazole-5-ylphenyl)-benzyl] imidazole-5-methanol monopotassium salt and was the first approved nonpeptide orally active antihypertensive agent with specific binding to the AT$_1$ receptor subtype.[52] Maximum pharmacologic action requires the oxidation of the 5-hydroxymethyl group on the imidazole ring to form EXP3174, the carboxylic acid metabolite of losartan.[53]

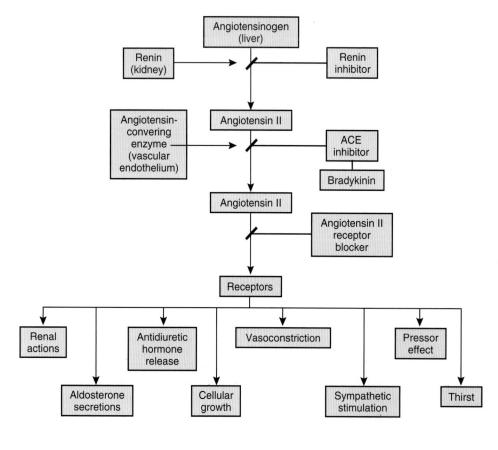

**Figure 67–2** Approaches to regulating the renin-angiotensin system. (From Gibbons G. The pathophysiology of hypertension: The importance of angiotensin II in cardiovascular remodeling. Am J Hypertens 11:177S-181S, 1998.)

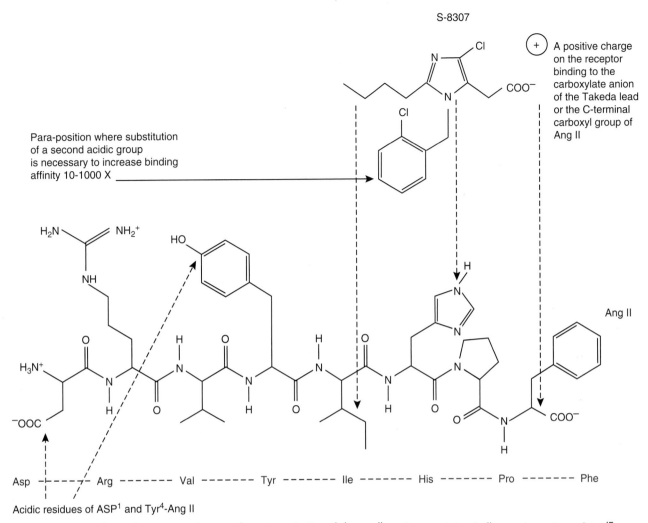

**Figure 67–3** Hypothetical structure relations of angiotensin II and the orally active angiotensin II receptor antagonists. (From Timmerman PB, Duncia JV, Carini D, et al. Discovery of losartan, the first angiotensin II receptor antagonist. J Hum Hypertens 9:S3-S18, 1995.)

The second $AT_1$ subtype ARB to gain approval for clinical use is valsartan. Investigators at Ciba (Novartis) in Switzerland employed a strategy to open up the imidazole ring and replace it with the acylated amino acid valine.[54] The acidic biphenyl tetrazole substituent is preserved. The carboxyl moiety of the valine serves to preserve oral bioavailability with high affinity receptor binding. Thus, valsartan is, like EXP3174 (the active metabolite of losartan), a diacid. Unlike losartan, valsartan does not require metabolic oxidation to achieve maximum pharmacologic effect.[55]

Irbesartan is chemically described as 2-butyl-(1*H*-tetrazol-5-yl) [1,1'-biphenyl]-4-yl [methyl]-1,3-diazespiro [4,4] non-1-en. This compound was discovered by Sanofi Recherche of France and has been jointly developed with Bristol-Myers Squibb in the United States. The French investigators incorporated an imidazolinone moiety in place of the imidazole heterocyclic ring. A carbonyl group functions as the hydrogen bond acceptor in place of the 5-hydroxymethyl group of losartan and the valine carboxylic acid group of valsartan.[56] This agent possesses a high affinity and specificity for $AT_1$ receptors. Irbesartan does not require biotransformation to achieve its effects.[57]

Another successful approach has been to develop fused-ring imidazoles. Candesartan cilexetil is an ester carbonate benzimidazole prodrug that has been designed by Takeda Ltd. and jointly developed with Astra-Zeneca.[58] This agent is rapidly metabolized to CV-11974, a highly potent $AT_1$ receptor antagonist. The latter compound bears a C7 carboxyl group that is positioned in a fashion similar to the imidazole carboxyl moiety of EXP3174, the active metabolite of losartan.[59]

## NONBIPHENYL TETRAZOLE DERIVATIVES

The Boehringer Ingelheim/Thomae research team has followed a similar fused-ring approach but substituted a second phenylimidazole moiety at the 6-position of the primary heterocycle.[60] This compound, telmisartan, incorporates a carboxylic acid as the biphenyl acidic group that achieves greater receptor antagonism than does the tetrazole analog.[61]

Investigators at SmithKline Beecham devised an alternative model for the superimposition of the Takeda benzylimidazole antagonists with angiotensin II. As with the Dupont model, the 2-chlorobenzyl substituent of the Takeda lead was proposed to be spacially equivalent to the Tyr-4 position of angiotensin II, and the aliphatic butyl group pointed toward the Ile-5. However, the equivalence between the imidazole of the Takeda lead and the His-6 of angiotensin II was not assumed. Instead, the imidazole was thought to function as a scaffold for positioning of substituent groups toward the receptor.[62] This led to a different but also successful approach through refining the presentation of the carboxylic acid and greater filling of the binding pocket for the Phe-8 side chain of angiotensin II. Chain extension at the imidazole-5-position via a *trans*-5-acrylic acid group yielded the final product, eprosartan, which is 40,000-fold more potent than the original Takeda lead.[63]

## EFFECTS OF ANGIOTENSIN ANTAGONISTS

### Hemodynamic Effects

Angiotensin II antagonists reduce peripheral resistance and systemic arterial pressure in hypertensive animals.[64] The depressor effect is more potent and more consistent in renin-angiotensin dependent models, such as the 2-kidney 1-clip or angiotensin-infusion forms of hypertension.[65,66] Volume expansion or bilateral nephrectomy appears to attenuate or abolish the antihypertensive effect of the ARBs.[67] In euvolemic normotensive animals and humans, angiotensin II antagonists have little effect. In the majority of hypertensive humans these agents produce a significant reductions in peripheral resistance and blood pressure.[68,69]

Lowering of peripheral resistance is most likely due to several factors, especially direct binding to and antagonism of vascular angiotensin II receptor sites and reversal of the vasoconstrictive action normally mediated by angiotensin II.[67] Augmentation of this effect may occur through binding and blockade of angiotensin II receptors on sympathetic nerve terminals with consequent attenuation of sympathetically mediated vasoconstriction.[70] ARBs have also been demonstrated to enhance nitric oxide–mediated vascular endothelial function.[71] In normotensives ARB-induced declines in arterial compliance and blood pressure have been found to correlate with pretreatment plasma renin activity.[72]

### Cardiac Effects

Despite the angiotensin antagonist–induced decline in peripheral resistance, heart rate is little affected in euvolemic hypertensive animals and humans during ARB treatment. This neutral effect on heart rate in the setting of lowered peripheral resistance may be due to antagonism of angiotensin II receptors at peripheral sympathetic sites, as well as through centrally mediated actions of these agents.[73]

Based on several converging lines of evidence, it has been predicted that $AT_1$ antagonists would have an especially beneficial effect on cardiac and vascular hypertrophy. Plasma angiotensin II levels tend to increase during therapy with these agents, most likely as a result of $AT_1$ receptor–mediated disinhibition of renin release by cells of the renal juxtaglomerular apparatus.[74] Also, it has been found that the cardiac chymase-angiotensin system provides an alternate path

for angiotensin II formation that is independent of converting enzyme.[75] Moreover, there is evidence that the $AT_2$ receptor subtype can mediate an antiproliferative effect on vascular cells.[76] Thus, administration of a selective $AT_1$ antagonist would not only attenuate growth promoting effects mediated by the $AT_1$ receptor but also, as angiotensin II levels rise, may enhance the antiproliferative effect mediated by the unblocked $AT_2$ receptor subtype.[76]

There is evidence that ARBs prevent angiotensin II mediated cardiac growth and remodeling.[78,79] These effects may prove to be of importance in the prevention or treatment of ischemic or hypertensive cardiomyopathies. In experimental models of coronary ischemia, losartan appears to have beneficial effects on survival and on myocardial growth and remodeling.[79,80]

ARBs may also benefit the heart by decreasing collagen deposition and cardiac fibrosis, by blocking angiotensin II effects directly or aldosterone effects indirectly.[81] ARBs may prevent the development of atrial fibrillation by attenuation of structural remodeling of the atrial myocardium.[82]

There is experimental evidence that ARBs may improve coronary reserve in hypertensive animals concomitant with a reduction in cardiac mass.[83,84] Alterations in coronary blood flow are a function of coronary vasomotor tone, diastolic perfusion pressure, and left ventricular end-diastolic pressure, all of which may be affected by ARBs.[85,86] Thus, in the clinical setting, the effects of ARBs on coronary flow are expected to vary.

### Renal Effects

Through binding to $AT_1$ receptor sites, the ARBs inhibit the intrarenal actions of angiotensin II. In healthy persons on a low-salt diet, an orally administered ARB was found to produce a prompt dose-related increase in renal plasma flow and a slightly delayed, but more prolonged, increase in plasma renin activity.[87] In patients with essential hypertension, ARBs generally have no discernible effect on glomerular filtration rate as assessed by creatinine clearance.[88] Renal blood flow is usually unaffected by ARBs in the euvolemic animal or human.[89]

The overall effect of angiotensin II blockade on renal hemodynamics depends on the nature and degree of local and systemic counteracting responses. For example, in healthy men on a very-low-salt diet, it has been found that renal blood flow increases with an ARB administration to an extent that equals or exceeds that following ACE inhibitor infusion.[90] On the other hand, compensatory activation of the sympathetic nervous system may occur in response to a pronounced fall in systemic blood pressure and, in turn, result in net renal vasoconstriction and a decline in renal function.[91] In the clinical setting of salt or volume depletion ARBs may also produce a decline in glomerular filtration rate, perhaps by interference with glomerular blood flow autoregulation.[92]

In experimental models of unilateral renal artery stenosis, ARBs consistently produce a decline in glomerular filtration rate in the affected kidney.[93] Reported effects on glomerular filtration and renal blood flow in the contralateral kidney have been variable.[94] In patients with renal impairment and renovascular occlusive disease, reversible increases in serum creatinine have been reported with ARB treatment.[92,95]

ARBs produce a modest natriuretic action through blockade of proximal tubular $AT_1$ receptor sites that mediate sodium reabsorption.[92] This effect is most evident in the volume depleted state, in which the renin activation and the influence

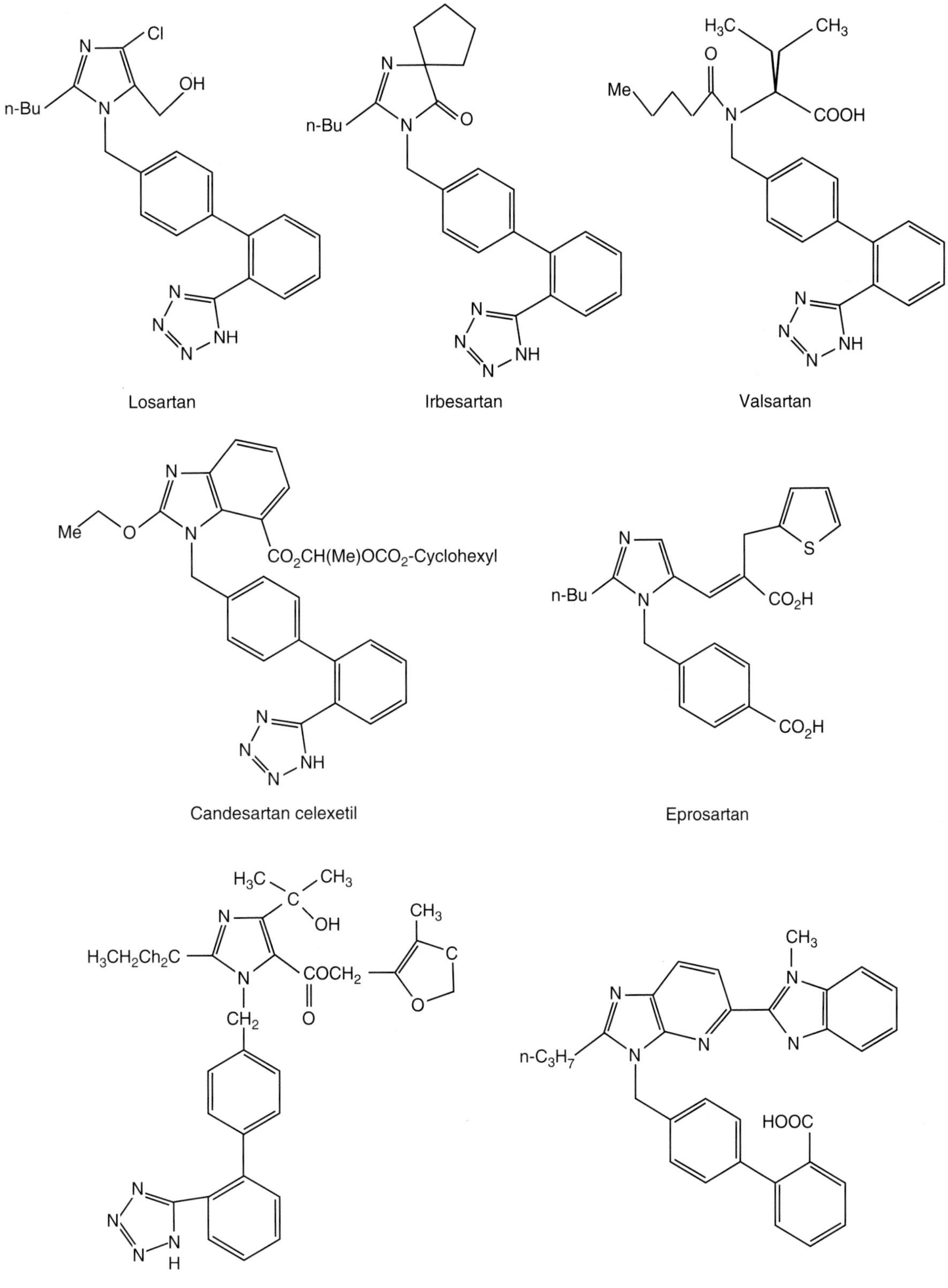

**Figure 67-4** Chemical structures of the angiotensin II receptor antagonists.

of the renin-angiotensin system are greatest.[92,96] An additional natriuretic action occurs through inhibition of aldosterone synthesis and release by the adrenal zona glomerulosa cells.[97,98] Reduced aldosterone-mediated distal tubular sodium reabsorption may contribute to the diuretic effect of the ARBs.

Administration of ARBs to animals with several forms of experimental renal impairment produced a decline of proteinuria in association with attenuated glomerular hydrostatic pressure. Moreover, because angiotensin II has the potential for growth promoting effects at the mesangial tissue level, it has been speculated that angiotensin II receptor blockade may exert additional effects on glomerular filtration at the basement membrane filtration barrier site.[99] In hypertensive patients with proteinuric renal disorders, administration of losartan was associated with a decrease in urinary protein, an increase in effective renal blood flow and stable glomerular filtration rate.[100] A number of clinical studies have found that the administration of ARBs to patients with diabetic and nondiabetic renal disorders is associated with a reduction in proteinuria. The degree and time course of the antiproteinuric response to these agents vary considerably and appear to differ from that of the antihypertensive effect. The peak of the ARB-antiproteinuric dose-response curve has yet to be reported.

Among the ARBs, losartan appears to have the unique property of exerting a modest uricosuric effect.[101] The effect is dose dependent and has been documented in normotensive and hypertensive individuals with and without renal impairment. It does not appear to be dependent on the activity of the renin-angiotensin system and is not affected by changes in salt intake. Infusion of the active metabolite of losartan, EXP3174 has no effect on uric acid excretion, indicating that the effect is specific to the parent drug losartan.[101] The mechanism is not known but may be related to renal tubular anion load competing with urate at the tubular transport sites.

## Nervous System

Angiotensin II antagonism appears to inhibit peripheral sympathetic activity via blockade of presynaptic $AT_1$ receptors that normally amplify release of neurotransmitters.[102] There is also evidence that these agents, when administered intracerebrally to experimental animals, inhibit centrally mediated sympathetic nervous outflow at the level of the paraventricular nucleus.[103] Drinking behavior and release of vasopressin are also suppressed following central administration of these agents.[104]

## Behavior, Affect, and Cognition

In experimental animals ARBs have been shown to improve cognitive function and anxiety-associated deficits.[105] In humans, a randomized trial comparing amlodipine with losartan showed that the ARB treated group had higher mean scores on the Psychological Well-Being Index after 12 weeks of double-blind therapy, despite equivalent blood pressure lowering.[106]

Blockade of the brain $AT_1$ receptors has been shown in animals to reduce the sympathoadrenal and hormonal responses to stress and prevent stress-induced gastric injury.[107] It has been suggested but not yet proven that there may be a role for ARBs in the treatment of stress-related disorders and in the preservation of cognition.[107,108]

The Study on Cognition and Prognosis in the Elderly (SCOPE) was designed to assess the relative effects of candesartan versus placebo on cardiovascular outcomes and cognition scores in 4500 elderly hypertensive patients. The primary endpoint of combined cardiovascular mortality, nonfatal stroke and myocardial infarction was slightly, but not significantly, reduced in the ARB group. Cognitive function was equally well preserved in both treatment groups.[109]

---

**Box 67–1** Hemodynamic and Neurohumoral Effects of $AT_1$ Receptor Antagonists

Arterial vasodilation
Decrease in peripheral resistance
Reduction of serum aldosterone levels
Increase in plasma renin activity
Increase in plasma angiotensin II
Inhibition of peripheral sympathetic activity
Decreased glomerular filtration rate in volume depletion states
Increased glomerular filtration fraction in volume depletion states

---

## CLINICAL PHARMACOLOGY

The angiotensin $AT_1$ receptor antagonists appear to occupy space among the seven transmembrane helices of the receptor protein. Interaction with amino acid residues in these regions of the receptor molecule prevents the binding of angiotensin II to the receptor.[110] All currently available ARBs have been shown to attenuate the circulatory, renal, endocrine, and neurohumoral actions normally mediated by angiotensin II. Unlike the earlier nonselective peptide antagonist, saralasin, these agents are devoid of partial agonist effect. The ARBs have been shown to cause a twofold to threefold rise in plasma renin activity and a consequent rise in angiotensin II concentration.[111]

At this time seven ARBs have U.S. Food and Drug Administration (FDA) approval for the treatment of hypertension. Losartan and irbesartan have also gained approval for use in diabetic nephropathy. Ongoing and completed clinical trials are evaluating various ARBs for treatment of additional hypertension-related circulatory disorders.

It is important to note that ARBs and ACE inhibitors are contraindicated during pregnancy. Several dozen cases of fetal and neonatal morbidity and death have been reported in conjunction with ACE inhibitor administration in the second or third trimester of pregnancy.[112] Fetal abnormalities have included renal failure, oligohydramnios, limb and craniofacial deformities, and hypoplastic lung development.

The ARBs differ from each other in their oral bioavailability, rate of absorption, tissue distribution, metabolism, and rate of elimination. Several of these agents act as prodrugs with conversion to more biologically active metabolites.

## Losartan Potassium

Losartan potassium is the first orally active ARB approved for clinical use.[113] It is chemically described as 2-butyl-4-chloro-1[p-(o-1H-tetrazol-5-ylphenyl)-benzyl]imidazol-5-methanol monopotassium salt. The potassium salt of losartan is well absorbed orally with a systemic bioavailability of approximately 33%.[114-116] It is rapidly absorbed with peak plasma levels achieved in about 1 hour. Losartan has a relatively short terminal half-life of 1.5 to 2.5 hours.[117] Losartan undergoes substantial first pass metabolism by the cytochrome P450 enzymes 2C9 and 3A4.[118,119] The methyl hydroxyl group of losartan located on the imidazole ring undergoes biooxidation to the carboxylated form of the compound, EXP3174.[118] Approximately 50% of orally administered losartan is converted to the active metabolite. EXP3174, with potency 15 to 30 times greater than that of losartan, is responsible for most of the angiotensin receptor antagonism.[117]

The more active metabolite reaches peak concentration in 3 to 4 hours and has a longer terminal half-life of 6 to 9 hours.[117] Food intake slows absorption of losartan and delays the time to peak concentration ($C_{max}$) but has little effect on the total area under the curve (AUC) of either losartan or its principal metabolite.[120]

Losartan is a competitive antagonist of angiotensin II in that it causes a rightward shift of the concentration-contractile curve without depression of the maximum pressor response to the octapeptide. In contrast, EXP3174 is a noncompetitive, so-called insurmountable antagonist in that it produces a nonparallel right shift in the concentration-contractile curve and reduces the maximum response to angiotensin II. The mechanism for the noncompetitive nature of drug-receptor interaction is not yet known. However, it seems likely that tight receptor binding by the active metabolite contributes to the prolonged biologic activity of orally administrated losartan.

In the plasma, losartan and its metabolites are highly protein bound (98.7%-99.8%) in a nonsaturable mode. These compounds have been shown to penetrate the blood-brain barrier poorly, if at all. Biliary excretion plays a major role in the elimination of losartan and its metabolites.[120] A lower starting dose is recommended for patients with hepatic dysfunction. Somewhat less than one third of the absorbed drug and its metabolites are cleared by renal filtration.[120] Dose adjustment is not necessary in patients with renal impairment, including dialysis patients, unless they are volume depleted or have occlusive renovascular disease.[121] Neither losartan nor EXP3174 can be removed by hemodialysis.[119]

Losartan administration does not affect the pharmacokinetics of warfarin or digoxin.[122,123] Coadministration of losartan with cimetidine led to about a 20% increase in the AUC of losartan but not its more potent metabolite.[119] Phenobarbital administration led to a reduction of about 20% in the AUC of both losartan and its carboxylated metabolite.[119] These interactions are not considered to be clinically significant.

In healthy volunteers, administration of fluconazole, an inhibitor of the cytochrome P450 isoenzyme CYP2C9 but not itraconazole, an inhibitor of CYP3A4, was found to inhibit the formation of the active metabolite EXP-3174.[124] This implies that CYP2C9 is a major enzyme for the conversion of losartan to its more active metabolite. It is possible that concomitant use of other agents known to inhibit one of these oxidative enzymes may significantly attenuate the therapeutic effect of losartan.

Losartan is approved by the U.S. FDA for the treatment of hypertension and diabetic nephropathy. It is available in 25- and 50-mg tablets. The usual starting dose is 50 mg once daily and the highest recommended dose is 100 mg/day. For patients with intravascular depletion or on diuretic therapy, the 25-mg dose may be safer.

## Valsartan

Valsartan acts as a competitive antagonist for the AT$_1$ receptor of angiotensin II and is chemically described as $N$-(1-oxopentyl)-$N$[[2′-(1$H$-tetrozol-5-yl)[1,1′-biphenyl]-4-yl]methyl]-L-valine.[55] Unlike losartan, valsartan is not a prodrug, and its activity is independent of hepatic metabolism.[125] Oral bioavailability for the capsule formulation of valsartan is approximately 25% (range 10%-35%).[126] The time to peak concentration in the plasma is 2 to 4 hours. Food intake decreases AUC by approximately 40% and peak plasma concentrations by about 50%.[127] Like losartan, valsartan is highly bound to serum proteins (95%), primarily albumin.[128] The volume of distribution of this compound is only 17 L, indicating that tissue distribution is not very extensive. For most patients the onset of the antihypertensive effect is about 2 hours, with the maximum reduction of blood pressure achieved in about 6 hours.[125,127]

Elimination of valsartan is mainly (80%) in the unchanged form through the gastrointestinal tract.[126] Approximately 9% of the dose is metabolized to valeryl 4-hydroxy valsartan. This process does not appear to be cytochrome P450 dependent. Orally administered valsartan shows a biexponential decay curve with an elimination half-life of about 6 hours. The antihypertensive action of valsartan persists for 24 hours following oral administration. Valsartan does not appear to accumulate in plasma following repeated administration. However, patients with hepatic or biliary tract impairment have an increase in the AUC, indicating a slower plasma clearance rate.[129]

The pharmacokinetics of valsartan do not appear to be appreciably affected by renal impairment. However, as with all agents that affect the renin-angiotensin system, the presence of renal insufficiency warrants careful monitoring of the patients' hemodynamic, renal, and electrolyte status.

Coadministration of valsartan with amlodipine, atenolol, cimetidine, digoxin, furosemide, glibenclamide, hydrochlorothiazide, indomethacin, or warfarin has failed to show any clinically significant pharmacokinetic interactions.[127] Valsartan, like other ARBs and ACE inhibitors, is contraindicated in pregnancy. The extent to which it is excreted in human milk is not yet known. Dose adjustment does not appear to be necessary for the elderly, although careful clinical monitoring is prudent in this group.[130]

Valsartan is approved for the treatment of hypertension in the United States and other countries. It is available in capsule form as the 80- and 160-mg dose formulations. It is recommended to initiate valsartan therapy with 80 mg once daily. The dosage of valsartan may be increased as needed up to a total daily dose of 320 mg. It is prudent to reevaluate patients within 1 month following such a dose adjustment.

## Irbesartan

Irbesartan is chemically described as 2-butyl-3-[[2(1$H$-tetrazo 5yl) [1,1′ biphenyl 4yl] methyl]-1,3 diazaspiro [4,4] non-1 en-4-olone. This compound has an imidazolinone ring in which a carbonyl group functions as the hydrogen bond acceptor in place of the C-5 hydroxymethyl group of losartan.[56] Irbesartan has been shown to be an insurmountable noncompetitive antagonist of the AT$_1$ receptor (Figure 67–5).[57,131] Irbesartan does not require biotransformation for its pharmacologic action.[132]

Oral bioavailability of Irbesartan is relatively high at 60% to 80% and is not affected by food intake.[133] Peak plasma concentrations occur 1.5 to 2 hours following oral administration. Irbesartan is less protein bound than other ARBs and has a plasma half-life of approximately 11 to 15 hours.[133]

Irbesartan is metabolized by oxidation and glucuronide conjugation. Oxidation is mediated primarily through the 2C9 isoenzyme. Metabolism by 3A4 was found to be negligible.[132] Irbesartan had no effect on the function of other cytochrome P450 oxidative isoenzymes, such as 1A1, 1A2, 2A6, 2B6, and 2E1.[112] Irbesartan has no demonstrated effects on the pharmacokinetics or pharmacodynamics of nifedipine, hydrochlorothiazide, warfarin, and digoxin.[132]

Irbesartan is eliminated from the body primarily through biliary excretion (75%) and to a lesser extent through the kidneys.[134] Drug accumulation does not appear to occur in the setting of hepatic or renal insufficiency, and dose adjustment is not required for these conditions.[132] Irbesartan is not dialyzable. In the elderly, $C_{max}$ and AUC are increased by 20% to 50% and elimination half-life unchanged. Dose adjustment of irbesartan has not been found to be necessary in the elderly or for gender or race.[112,132,134]

Irbesartan is approved for use in the treatment of high blood pressure and diabetic nephropathy. It is available in tablets containing 75, 150, and 300 mg. The usual starting dose is 150 mg once daily.[112] However, for patients receiving a diuretic or otherwise volume depleted it may be prudent to begin with a lower initial dose, such as 75 mg/day.

## Candesartan Cilexetil

Candesartan, 2-ethoxy-1-[[2'-(1H-tetrazol-5-yl)biphenyl-4-yl]methyl]-1H-benzimidazole-7-carboxylic acid, is a potent ARB.[135] This structure is a biphenyl imidazole derivative that, like losartan, has a tetrazolyl moiety, a lipophilic side chain, and a carboxyl group. To overcome poor oral absorption, the cilexetil ester prodrug form was synthesized. Candesartan cilexetil has been found to be rapidly and completely converted by hydrolytic cleavage to the active compound, candesartan, during gastrointestinal absorption.

Candesartan has been shown to have a high degree of $AT_1$ receptor affinity and to dissociate slowly from its binding sites.[135] In the presence of angiotensin II, candesartan acts as an insurmountable antagonist for the $AT_1$ receptor. The effects of candesartan at the receptor level have been observed at low doses and found to be of long duration.[136]

The maximal serum concentration of candesartan is reached at approximately 4 hours after oral dosing with a terminal half-life of about 9 hours.[137]

The AUC of candesartan has been found to be linear throughout the dose range of 2 to 16 mg. In elderly healthy volunteers, steady-state concentrations of candesartan are approximately 30% to 50% higher than in younger subjects.[137] Oral bioavailability does not appear to be affected by food intake.[138] Most of the drug is excreted in the urine as candesartan with a smaller fraction as an inactive metabolite.[139] Excretion through the biliary tract accounts for less than 40% of total drug elimination.

The pharmacokinetic profile of candesartan has been shown to not be altered in patients with mild to moderate hepatic dysfunction.[140] In patients with renal impairment, the AUC, $C_{max}$, and terminal half-life were significantly greater than in healthy subjects. It may be prudent to employ lower starting doses in patients with severe renal dysfunction. The drug is not dialyzable.[140]

Coadministration of candesartan cilexetil with hydrochlorothiazide has caused a small but significant decrease in the AUC of the latter agent and a slightly higher bioavailability and $C_{max}$ for candesartan itself.[141] Candesartan produces a small decrease in warfarin trough concentration but does not affect prothrombin time. No significant interactions have been found when candesartan cilexetil was coadministered with nifedipine, glibenclamide, digoxin, or estrogen-containing oral contraceptives.[141]

Candesartan cilexetil is approved in the United States and in other countries for the treatment of hypertension. It is available as 4-, 8-, 16-, and 32-mg tablets.

## Eprosartan

Eprosartan is a nonphenyl, nontetrazole ARB with a high degree of affinity for $AT_1$ receptor sites.[142] This compound is chemically described as (E)-α-[[2-butyl-1-[(4-carboxyphenyl)-methyl]-1H-imidazol-5-yl]methylene]-2-thiophenepropanoic acid. Eprosartan has incomplete oral absorption, with an oral bioavailability of 13% to 15%.[143] Maximum plasma concentrations of the drug are reached in 1 to 3 hours. Food intake appears to have unpredictable effects on $C_{max}$ and time to $C_{max}$.[144] The bioavailability of eprosartan has been shown to increase with age.[144]

Approximately 90% of orally administered eprosartan is found in the feces and the remainder found in the urine.[145] Of the excreted drug only 20% undergoes metabolism to its glucuronide form.[145] Both renal insufficiency and hepatic impairment have been found to delay the elimination of eprosartan. Eprosartan is not metabolized by the cytochrome P450 system and has not been shown to have significant drug interactions with glyburide and digoxin.[146] Eprosartan, like most of the current ARBs, is highly protein bound in plasma (98%) but does not appear to affect the anticoagulant activity of warfarin.[146]

Eprosartan has been approved for use in the United States and in other countries in the treatment of high blood pressure. It is available in 200-, 300-, and 400-mg tablets for once-daily administration.

## Telmisartan

Telmisartan, 4'-[(1,4'-dimethyl-2'-propyl[2,6'-bi-1H-benzimidazol]-1'-yl)methyl]-[1,1'-biphenyl]-2-carboxylic acid, is an orally active ARB with competitive affinity for the $AT_1$ receptor subtype.[147] Approximately one half of an orally administered dose is absorbed.[148] Oral bioavailability is somewhat dose-dependent. Peak plasma concentrations of telmisartan are reached relatively rapidly, within 0.5 to 1.0 hours following oral ingestion. Food intake reduces the AUC by 6% to 20%. Unlike losartan and candesartan, telmisartan is not a prodrug. Approximately 87% of an orally administered dose is eventually excreted unchanged through the biliary tract. A very small proportion of telmisartan undergoes metabolism to the glucuronide form. The cytochrome P450 isoenzymes are not involved in the metabolism of telmisartan.

Telmisartan is highly protein bound in plasma (>99.5%) and has a very large volume of distribution of approximately 500 L, indicating additional tissue binding. The terminal elimination half-life is approximately 24 hours.[147] Due to its biliary route of elimination, telmisartan should be used with caution in patients with hepatic insufficiency. Telmisartan and digoxin coadministration has been shown to be associated with significant increases in levels of the later agent. It is recommended that digoxin levels be monitored when initiating, adjusting and discontinuing telmisartan to avoid possible over-digitalization. Telmisartan does not appear to affect the anticoagulant effect of warfarin.

The antihypertensive effect of telmisartan has been found to be greater in hypertensive patients with higher plasma renin activity.[149] In the United States and in other countries telmisartan is approved for the treatment of hypertension. It is available in the United States as 40- and 80-mg tablets for once-daily administration. The recommended starting-dose for telmisartan is 40 mg once daily.

## Olmesartan Medoxomil

Olmesartan medoxomil is chemically described as 2,3-dihydroxy-2-butenyl 4-(1-hydroxy-1-methylethyl)-2-propyl-1-[*p*-(*o*-1 *H*-tetrazol-5-ylphenyl)benzyl]imidazole-5-carboxylate, cyclic 2,3-carbonate. It is an orally active $AT_1$ receptor antagonist that is rapidly and completely deesterified in vivo in the intestinal wall to the active diacid metabolite, olmesartan.[150] It is selective for the $AT_1$ receptor without partial agonist activity and, as expected, suppresses the pressor response to angiotensin II in rats. Olmesartan has higher affinity for the $AT_1$ receptor than losartan in that 50% inhibition of angiotensin II binding to the $AT_1$ receptor of bovine adrenocortical cells was 7.7 nanomolar, approximately 8% of the concentration of losartan needed to achieve the same degree of binding inhibition. It lowers SBP and DBP and increases renin and angiotensin II concentrations in humans.

After oral administration, olmesartan medoxomil is rapidly absorbed and deesterified during absorption to the pharmacologically active compound olmesartan with peak plasma concentrations between 1 and 3 hours and an elimination half-life of 12 to 18 hours.[151] The absolute bioavailability of olmesartan medoxomil after oral administration is 26% to 28.6%. Steady-state plasma concentrations are reached within the first few daily doses, and accumulation is not noted on long-term dosing. The volume distribution after intravenous administration is 15 to 25 L. Olmesartan is not metabolized, and 35% to 50% of the systemically available active compound is excreted unchanged in the urine and the remainder in the bile. Olmesartan medoxomil has minimal or no inhibitory activity on human cytochrome P450. Coadministration of olmesartan medoxomil with digoxin or warfarin did not result in clinically significant steady-state pharmacokinetic interaction.[151]

Data from seven randomized, multicenter, double-blind, placebo-controlled Phase II and III trials with similar designs, eligibility criteria, and efficacy endpoints were pooled in a single integrated analysis of efficacy for olmesartan medoxomil (2.5-80 mg/day) (n = 2693).[152] Reductions in cuff seated systolic blood pressure (SeSBP) and seated diastolic blood pressure (SeDBP) (SeSBP by 15.1 and 17.6 mm Hg and SeDBP by 12.2 and 13.1 mm Hg for the 20- to 40-mg dose), as well as in 24-hour ambulatory blood pressure were observed. Placebo-corrected trough/peak ratios were 64% to 79% for DBP and 52% to 72% for SBP, indicating a more than appropriate diurnal profile for once-daily dosing.[152] Minor changes in heart rate were observed (−0.5 to −1.1 beats/min compared with −0.3 beats/min with placebo). In both older and younger individuals, the only adverse experience reported more frequently in the olmesartan medoxomil treated subjects compared with placebo-treated subjects was dizziness, usually mild.

The ARBs olmesartan medoxomil, losartan potassium, valsartan, and irbesartan were compared in a 588 patient multicenter randomized double-blind trial with once-a-day therapy with the recommended starting doses.[153] Sitting DBP reduction at 24 hours postdosing, the primary efficacy variable, was 11.5 mm Hg with olmesartan medoxomil 20 mg, 8.2 mm Hg with losartan potassium 50 mg, 7.9 mm Hg with valsartan 80 mg, and 9.9 mm Hg with irbesartan 150 mg. The more pronounced reduction with olmesartan medoxomil with respect to the other three agents was statistically significant. In addition, the reduction in mean 24-hour DBP on ambulatory blood pressure monitoring was significantly larger with olmesartan medoxomil (8.5 mm Hg) than with losartan potassium (6.2 mm Hg) and valsartan ( 5.6 mm Hg) but not significantly different from irbesartan (7.4 mm Hg). Systolic blood pressure trough/peak ratio was highest for olmesartan medoxomil (0.69), lowest for valsartan (0.55), and intermediate for losartan potassium and irbesartan (0.64 and 0.62, respectively). Adverse event rates were comparable among the four treatment groups.

As with other ARBs, the antihypertensive effect of olmesartan medoxomil is enhanced with the addition of low-dose hydrochlorothiazide.[154]

## Safety and Adverse Effects of the Angiotensin II Receptor Antagonists

ARBs are generally very well tolerated. With two important exceptions, these agents have a side effect profile that is similar to that of the ACE inhibitors. Like the ACE inhibitors, ARBs may produce excessive and too rapid fall of blood pressure in the volume depleted or otherwise highly renin-dependent forms of hypertension. In patients with renal impairment there is an increased risk of hyperkalemia due to inhibition of aldosterone release. As with ACE inhibitors, patients with bilateral renovascular and renal parenchymal disease who are treated with ARBs are at increased risk of deterioration of renal function, which is usually but not always reversible.

ARBs do not appear to have adverse effects on glucose or lipid metabolism. Losartan is unique among this class in its uricosuric effect.

Of special note is that the incidence of cough with ARBs is similar to that of placebo.[155-157] The incidence of angioedema appears to be very low, although cases have been reported.[158,159] Indeed, among the currently available antihypertensive drug classes, ARBs appear to have the lowest incidence of adverse effects.[160,161]

## CLINICAL USES OF THE ANGIOTENSIN II RECEPTOR ANTAGONISTS

### Hypertension

All of the currently approved ARBs have been demonstrated in randomized, placebo-controlled clinical trials to lower blood pressure in hypertensive individuals. Approximately 50% to 60% of hypertensive patients have a clinically significant response to these agents.[69,162] This is comparable to monotherapy with diuretics, β-blockers, ACE inhibitors, and calcium antagonists.[163,164]

**Table 67–2** Pharmacologic Characteristics of Angiotensin Receptor Antagonists

| | Candesartan Cilexetil | Eprosartan | Irbesartan | Losartan Potassium | Olmesartan Medoxomil | Telmisartan | Valsartan |
|---|---|---|---|---|---|---|---|
| U.S. proprietary name | Atacand | Teveten | Avapro | Cozaar | Benicar | Micardis | Diovan |
| Prodrug | Yes | No | No | Yes | Yes | No | No |
| Bioavailability (%) | 15 | 13 | 60-80 | 33 | 26 | 42-58 | 25 |
| Peak effect (hour) | 3-4 | 3 | 1.5-2 | 3-4 | 1-2 | 0.5-1 | 2-4 |
| Food effect | None | Yes | None | Minimal | None | Minimal | Yes |
| Half-life (hour) | 9 | 5-9 | 11-15 | 2 | 12-18 | 24 | 6 |
| Trough/peak ratio (%) | 80 | 67 | >60 | 58-78 | 52-79 | >97 | 69-76 |
| $AT_1/AT_2$ affinity | >10,000 | 1000 | 8500 | 1000 | 12,500 | >3000 | 20,000 |
| Protein binding (%) | >99 | 98 | 90 | 99 | 99 | >99.5 | >95 |
| Urinary elimination (%) | 33 | 7 | 20 | 35 | 35-50 | <1 | 13 |
| CYP450 metabolism | No | No | 2C9 | 2C9, 3A4 | No | No | No |
| Drug interactions | No | No | No | Rifampin, fluconazole | No | Digoxin | No |
| Dosages available (mg) | 4, 8, 16, 32 | 400, 600 | 75, 150, 300 | 25, 50, 100 | 5, 20, 40 | 20, 40, 80 | 80, 160 |

The antihypertensive efficacy of the ARBs seems to depend at least partially on the activity of the renin-angiotensin system.[72] Approximately 80% of patients demonstrate a significant blood pressure lowering response when losartan is combined with a thiazide diuretic.[154] The antihypertensive response can be abolished in experimental animals following nephrectomy and is attenuated in humans following volume expansion.[165] The full therapeutic profile of the ARBs has yet to be completely elucidated. The effects of age, race, and concomitant medical conditions on the antihypertensive efficacy of these agents await further clarification.

Several studies have compared the relative efficacy among the currently available ARBs. In general, the observed differences have been modest. In one double-blind, parallel group study of 8 weeks' duration, candesartan cilexetil 8 mg/day was found to produce an antihypertensive effect equal to

**Box 67–2** Antihypertensive Mechanisms of the Angiotensin II Receptor Antagonists

Vascular actions
    Direct blockade of angiotensin II–mediated vasoconstriction
    Reversal of vascular hypertrophy
    Augmentation of nitric oxide–mediated endothelial function
Renal actions
    Augmentation of renal blood flow
    Direct and indirect enhancement of proximal tubular natriuresis
    Inhibition of aldosterone release and distal tubular sodium
Reabsorption
Central and sympathetic nervous system actions
    Attenuation of presynaptic norepinephrine release
    Inhibition of central all-mediated sympathetic outflow
    Inhibition of all-mediated thirst and vasopressin release

that of losartan 50 mg/day.[166] The 16-mg dose of candesartan cilexetil was found to be more effective than losartan 50 mg administered once daily. However, the use of microcrystalline cellulose back-filled gelatin capsules in the losartan group has been debated.[167,168] In a double-masked, elective dose titration study of 8 weeks' duration, irbesartan 150 to 300 mg once daily was found to produce a greater decline in trough seated diastolic BP than did losartan 50 to 100 mg/day.[169] Also, a smaller proportion of patients taking the starting dose of irbesartan (53%) as compared with the losartan group (61%) required up-titration at 4 weeks to reach the goal DBP of 90 mm Hg. Adding hydrochlorothiazide to both study drugs produced further reductions in blood pressure, with the greater effect seen in the irbesartan group compared with the losartan group.[169] The incidence of adverse effects in patients receiving either candesartan cilexetil or irbesartan was similar to that experienced by the patients receiving losartan.[166,169]

It has been suggested that the highly insurmountable receptor antagonists may have a greater amplitude and duration of action.[170] As outlined earlier, the recommended daily starting dose of olmesartan 20 mg has been observed to have a somewhat greater effect on DBP than losartan 50 mg, valsartan 80 mg, or irbesartan 150 mg.[153] A meta-analysis of 43 controlled trials involving the use of losartan, valsartan, irbesartan, and candesartan concluded that within the ARB class of antihypertensive drugs, there is comparable antihypertensive efficacy and a flat-dose response.[171] All of the agents studied showed substantial augmentation of the antihypertensive effect with the addition of thiazide diuretics.

## ARBs in Cardiac Disease

Angiotensin II exerts many actions on the heart and the coronary circulation. In the vasculature, angiotensin II causes vasoconstriction, as well as smooth muscle cell hypertrophy, and enhances norepinephrine release further potentiating vasoconstriction. Angiotensin II also causes increased contractility and facilitates the development of left ventricular hypertrophy. Angiotensin II effects on plasminogen activator inhibitor I, smooth muscle proliferation, and extracellular matrix formation may enhance the development of atherosclerosis.

The rationale for the use of ARBs in heart failure is based on several factors.[172] Because these agents reduce peripheral resistance, it has been posited that concomitant reduction in cardiac impedance would promote cardiac emptying with less left ventricular wall stress. Also, blockade of the direct hypertrophic action of angiotensin II on the myocardium by the ARBs might augment the benefit. Furthermore, there is evidence that some intracardiac angiotensin II is formed via a non–ACE-dependent mechanism. The latter effect might be expected to provide an advantage over ACE inhibitor therapy for treatment of heart failure.

In young healthy adults, plasma angiotensin II, lean body mass, and systemic blood pressure are related to left ventricular mass.[173] Moreover, in patients with heart failure, those who are on ACE inhibitor therapy have been shown to have higher plasma angiotensin II levels than controls, a finding consistent with non–ACE-mediated angiotensin II production in patients with failing hearts.[174]

In a study of the acute effects of ARBs in patients with heart failure, ARB treatment has been found to improve hemodynamic indices, such as blood pressure, pulmonary wedge pressure, systemic vascular resistance, and cardiac output.[175] In patients with ischemic or idiopathic dilated cardiomyopathy, exercise $VO_2$ and exercise tolerance were found to increase during treatment with both the ACE inhibitor enalapril and the ARB losartan.[176] In contrast to enalapril, the effect of losartan was not antagonized by aspirin.[176] In an earlier study, oral administration of losartan to patients with symptomatic heart failure resulted in beneficial hemodynamic effects with short-term administration and more enhanced benefits after 12 weeks of therapy.[177]

The ELITE (Evaluation of Losartan in the Elderly) study was designed to determine whether the ARB, losartan, offered advantages over the ACE inhibitor captopril in older patients with heart failure.[178] The primary endpoint of the study was persistent increase in serum creatinine equal to or greater than 0.3 mg/dl on therapy. The secondary endpoint was death or hospital admission for heart failure. In this randomized, double-blind study of 722 patients with heart failure and ejection fraction equal to or lower than 40%, losartan was titrated to 50 mg once a day and captopril was titrated to 50 mg three times a day for 48 weeks. The occurrence of the primary endpoint (persistent increase in serum creatinine) was the same in the two groups. For the secondary endpoints, the losartan treatment group had a 46% lower risk of death, 64% reduction in sudden death, and a 26% reduction in total hospitalization rate compared with the captopril treated group. Improvement in symptoms was similar for the two groups, as was the rate of hospitalization for progressive heart failure. Fewer losartan patients than captopril patients discontinued therapy because of adverse experiences (12.2% vs. 20.8%). It remains unclear why the relative beneficial effect of losartan was so dramatic for sudden death and less so for symptoms of and hospitalization rates for heart failure. This unexpected lowering in mortality with losartan compared to captopril may have been due to better suppression of the effects of angiotensin II, the absence of bradykinin effects during losartan therapy, or to the better compliance of patients on losartan.

To confirm this, ELITE II was carried out in a larger number of patients (3152) with similar characteristics and with a protocol similar to ELITE. All cause mortality was slightly but not significantly higher for losartan (11.7%) compared with 10.4% for captopril.[179] Losartan was again somewhat better tolerated than captopril. In another study, where the effects of losartan and enalapril were compared in patients with moderate or severe chronic heart failure, no significant differences between the groups in terms of exercise capacity or neurohormonal activation (plasma levels of N-terminal atrial natriuretic factor and norepinephrine) were observed.[180]

In patients with symptomatic heart failure receiving maximally prescribed or tolerated ACE inhibitors, the effects of add-on therapy with ARBs have been studied.[181] The combination was found to be safe and to lead to a further decrease in cardiac afterload. It has been hypothesized that the combination will produce a greater suppression of angiotensin II effects by blocking both ACE and non–ACE-dependent pathways. At the same time the potentially beneficial effects of ACE inhibition in preventing bradykinin degradation should be maintained.

In the Val-Heft (Valsartan Heart Failure Trial), valsartan 160 mg twice daily was compared with placebo in patients with heart failure treated with digitalis, diuretics, and ACE inhibitors in the majority and β-blockers in some.[182,183] The combined endpoint of worsening heart failure, resuscitated cardiac arrest, or mortality occurred 13% less frequently in the valsartan group, primarily because of a decrease in heart failure hospitalizations. Significant improvements in heart failure symptoms, ejection fraction, and quality-of-life indices were observed. The beneficial effect of valsartan on patients who were not on background ACE inhibitor therapy was marked.

The effects of ARBs in patients with left ventricular hypertrophy have also been studied. Findings from experimental and clinical studies suggest that the pharmacodynamic profile of the antihypertensive agent plays a role in addition to that of blood pressure lowering in decreasing left ventricular mass. Losartan has been found to decrease cardiac mass and improve coronary flow reserve in spontaneously hypertensive rats and to decrease left ventricular hypertrophy due to volume overload induced by aortic insufficiency in Wistar rats.[184,185]

In a 10-month study of 89 hypertensive patients, losartan given as monotherapy or in association with hydrochlorothiazide produced not only a significant reduction in blood pressure but also a decrease in left ventricular mass studied by echocardiography.[186] The Losartan Intervention for Endpoint Reduction in Hypertension study (LIFE) was designed to compare the effects of losartan with the β-blocker atenolol in a double-blind, parallel design on more than 9000 patients with electrocardiographic evidence of left ventricular hypertrophy.[187] The primary endpoint of cardiovascular morbidity and mortality (i.e., stroke, myocardial, infarction, and cardiovascular death) occurred significantly less frequently in the losartan group. Also, new-onset diabetes was less common with losartan than with the β-blocker.[188]

The CHARM clinical trial (Candesartan in Heart failure Assessment of Reduction in Mortality and Morbidity) compared candesartan titrated to 32 mg once daily to placebo in three distinct populations: (1) patients with left ventricular ejection fraction less than or equal to 40% who were not receiving ACE inhibitors (CHARM-Alternative Trial, 2028 patients), (2) patients with left ventricular ejection fraction less than or equal to 40% who were receiving ACE inhibitors (CHARM-Added Trial, 2548 patients), and (3) patients with left ventricular ejection fraction higher than 40% (CHARM-Preserved Trial, 3023 patients). Overall, when all three studies were analyzed together, candesartan was generally well tolerated and significantly reduced cardiovascular deaths and hospital admissions for heart failure.[189-192]

The OPTIMAAL (Optimal Trial in Myocardial Infarction with the Angiotensin II Antagonist Losartan) compared losartan, target dose 50 mg daily, to captopril 50 mg three times daily in 4577 patients with acute myocardial infarction.[193] At an average follow-up 2.7 years, mortality was 17% in the losartan group and 16% in the captopril group ($p = .07$). In the VALIANT study of 14,703 patients, with myocardial infarction complicated by left ventricular systolic dysfunction, heart failure, or both, valsartan treatment was equivalent to captopril for the composite endpoint of fatal and nonfatal cardiovascular events.[194] Of note is that the combination of valsartan and captopril increased the rate of adverse events without improving survival.

Taken together, these trials indicate that ARBs confer benefits similar to ACE inhibitors in patients with coronary heart disease, left ventricular hypertrophy, and heart failure. The combination of ARBs with ACE inhibitors may convey additional benefits, especially in preventing hospitalization for heart failure.

## Renal Disease

ARBs, like the ACE inhibitors, have multiple hemodynamic and nonhemodynamic actions that contribute to renoprotection. The ELITE trial was among the first clinical trials to assess the relative effects of ARB therapy on renal function. The study found that in humans with heart failure, long-term therapy with losartan has a comparable effect with that of captopril on renal function, as assessed by serum creatinine levels.[178]

In nonhemodynamically mediated experimental renal disease, the evidence is less consistent. For example, experimental puromycin nephrosis does not appear to be affected by the administration of ARBs.[195] In passive Heymann nephritis, a rat model of membranous nephropathy with proteinuria, angiotensin blockade had virtually no effect on urinary albumin excretion, as opposed to a markedly beneficially effect observed with enalapril.[196] However, in a model of antithymocyte serum-induced mesangioproliferative glomerulonephritis, angiotensin II blockade was found to be attenuate histopathologic changes and reduce renal TGF-$\beta$ mRNA.[197]

Several randomized clinical trials have recently demonstrated the renal protective effect of angiotensin II receptor blockade in proteinuric diabetics. The Reduction of Endpoints in NIDDM with the Angiotensin II Antagonist Losartan (RENAAL) study and the Irbesartan Diabetic Nephropathy Trial (IDNT) were similarly designed comparisons of the long-term effects of ARB therapy with conventional antihypertensive therapy on the composite primary endpoint of doubling of serum creatinine, occurrence of end-stage renal failure, or death.[198,199] Both of the ARB-treated groups showed a significant reduction in composite risk of 16% to 20%. The relative risk reductions experienced by the ARB groups in both studies were also significant for the renal-specific outcomes of doubling of serum creatinine (33% for IDNT and 25% for RENAAL) and end-stage renal disease (28% for IDNT and 25% for RENAAL). Losartan and irbesartan have been approved for use in diabetic nephropathy.

In most cases diabetic proteinuria (urinary albumin excretion >300 mg/24 hour) is preceded by microalbuminuria (urinary albumin excretion 30-300 mg/24 hour). Furthermore, microalbuminuria is a strong predictor of all-cause mortality and cardiovascular mortality in type 2 diabetes. Although the mechanism underlying the association between microalbuminuria and mortality is not well understood, the presence of microalbuminuria may reflect a generalized defect in vascular permeability leading to atherogenesis. Therapy with ARBs is associated with a reduction of microalbuminuria and a slowing of progression to macroalbuminuria.[200-202] In humans with nondiabetic renal disease and proteinuria, therapy with ARBs has been found to significantly reduce protein excretion in a dose-dependent manner comparable with that of ACE inhibitors.[203-206]

## Rationale for the Use of ARBs in Combination with ACE Inhibitors

ACE inhibitors and ARBs have been found to slow the progression of renal impairment in experimental animals and in humans with diabetic and nondiabetic chronic kidney disease.[207] Both classes of antihypertensive agent inhibit the vasoconstrictive effects of angiotensin II at the efferent arteriole, by either reducing the concentration of angiotensin II (ACE inhibitors) or by blocking its receptor site (ARBs). ARBs and ACE inhibitors have both been observed to exert nonhemodynamic actions as well. Treatment with ACE inhibitors also increases the level of bradykinin and other small peptides that are normally degraded by ACE. There is evidence that this action may contribute to the renoprotective effect of the ACE inhibitors, a property not shared with the ARBs. On the other hand, renal production of angiotensin II is not completely

---

**Box 67–3** Clinical Effects of Angiotensin II Receptor Antagonists Results from Randomized Clinical Trials

Uncomplicated hypertension
  Decreased blood pressure
Hypertension with left ventricular hypertrophy
  Decreased mortality
  Decreased incidence of new-onset diabetes
Chronic heart failure
  Improved hemodynamic profile
  Improved exercise tolerance
  Decreased hospitalization rate
  Decreased cardiovascular mortality rate
Acute myocardial infarction with and without left ventricular dysfunction
  Beneficial effect on cardiovascular mortality similar to that of the ACE inhibitors
Proteinuric chronic kidney disease
  Decreased proteinuria
Hypertension with type 2 diabetes and proteinuria
  Preservation of renal function

blocked by ACE inhibition due to the presence of chymase and other non-ACE peptidases. Furthermore, the currently available ARBs are selective for the $AT_1$ receptor subtype, leaving the $AT_2$ receptors available to the effects of higher levels of angiotensin II. The $AT_2$ receptors have been shown to mediate production of nitric oxide and attenuate cell proliferation in a number of organs, including the kidney.[208,209] Thus, it seems apparent that ACE inhibitors and ARBs have both overlapping and complementary mechanisms of action.

Several reports have shown that the combination of ACE inhibitor with ARB therapy is associated with a greater antiproteinuric effect than with either agent alone.[210,211] In the recent COOPERATE trial carried out in Japan, 263 patients with nondiabetic proteinuric renal disease were randomized to receive either losartan 100 mg/dl, the ACE inhibitor trandolapril 3 mg/day, or combination therapy at the same doses.[212] During a 3-year follow-up, the ACE inhibitor-ARB combination group achieved a highly significant 49% to 50% relative risk reduction for reaching the combined renal endpoint of doubling of serum creatinine or end-stage renal failure. Many of the patients in the COOPERATE trial had IgA nephropathy, a less common cause of renal failure in North America. Whether the findings of COOPERATE hold promise for the treatment of other forms of glomerular and nonglomerular renal disease remains to be determined.

## SUMMARY

The ARBs are effective antihypertensive agents in a broad range of patients and appear to have a lower incidence of adverse effects than other currently available drugs. As a class, these ARBs have a high degree of specificity for the $AT_1$ receptor subtype and also have become valuable pharmacologic probes for studying the role of the renin-angiotensin system in a number of circulatory and renal disorders.

Seven ARBs have gained U.S. FDA approval for the treatment of hypertension and several for the treatment of diabetic renal disease.[213] The Seventh Report of the Joint National Committee on Prevention, Detection, Evaluation, and Treatment of High Blood Pressure (JNC 7) has recognized that hypertension often exists with other serious conditions for which, based on clinical trials data, there are "compelling" indications for use of a particular drug or class of drugs, including the ARBs.[214] Such high-risk conditions for which ARBs are indicated include congestive heart failure, chronic kidney disease, and diabetes mellitus. Absence of a positive "compelling" indication for any disorder does not exclude the potential efficacy of ARBs or any other drug class for that disorder, if clinical trials data are lacking or are inconclusive.

Studies are underway to assess whether ARB therapy is equally or more effective than other agents in decreasing cardiovascular morbidity and mortality in hypertensives with comorbidities, such as diabetes, smoking, hyperlipidemia obesity, left ventricular hypertrophy, renal disease, and proteinuria.[215,216] Promising results from a number of clinical trials suggest that ARBs may confer important benefit for patients with other serious conditions, such as chronic coronary artery disease, acute coronary syndromes, and nondiabetic chronic kidney disease, as well as for primary and secondary prevention of cerebrovascular events.[165]

## References

1. Skeggs LT, Marsh WH, Kahn JR, Shumway NP. The existence of two forms of hypertensin. J Exp Med 99:275-282, 1954.
2. Skeggs LT, Kahn JR, Shumway NP: The preparation and function of hypertensin converting enzyme. J Exp Med 103: 295-299, 1956.
3. Skeggs LT, Lentz KE, Kahn JR, et al. The amino acid sequence of hypertensin II. J Exp Med 104:193-197, 1956.
4. Gibbons G. The pathophysiology of hypertension: The importance of angiotensin II in cardiovascular remodeling. Am J Hypertension 11:177S-181S, 1998.
5. Urata H, Kinoshita A, Misono K, et al. Identification of a highly specific chymase as the major angiotensin II-forming enzyme in the human heart. J Biol Chem 265:22348-22357, 1990.
6. Sancho J, Re R, Burton J. The role of the renin-angiotensin-aldosterone system in cardiovascular homeostasis in normal human subjects. Circulation 53:400-412, 1976.
7. Ganong W. Neuropeptides in cardiovascular control. J Hypertens 2(suppl 3):15-22, 1984.
8. Zimmerman B, Sybertz E, Wong P. Interaction between sympathetic and renin-angiotensin system. J Hypertens 2: 581-588, 1984.
9. Wood J. Peripheral venous and arteriolar responses to infusions of angiotensin in normal and hypertensive subjects. Circ Res 9: 768-774, 1961.
10. Catt K. Angiotensin II receptors. In Robertson J, Nichols M (eds). The Renin-Angiotensin System. London, Gower Medical, 1993; pp 12.1-12.14.
11. Forsyth R, Hoffbrand B, Melmon K. Hemodynamic effects of angiotensin in normal and environmentally stressed monkeys. Circulation 44:119-125, 1971.
12. Fleming J, Joshua I. Mechanisms of the biphasic effect of angiotensin II on arteriolar response. Am J Physiol 247: H88-H98, 1984.
13. Quinn S, Williams G. Regulation of aldosterone secretion. In James VT (ed). The Adrenal Gland. New York, Raven Press, 1992; pp 159-189.
14. Brewster U, Setaro J, Perazella M. The renin-angiotensin-aldosterone system: Cardiorenal effects and implications for renal and cardiovascular disease states. Am J Med Sci 326:15-24, 2003.
15. Tsybouleva N, Zhang L, Chen S, et al. Aldosterone, through novel signaling proteins, is a fundamental molecular bridge between the genetic defect and the cardiac phenotype of hypertrophic cardiomyopathy. Circulation 109:1284-1291, 2004.
16. Lijnen P, Petrov V. Role of intracardiac renin-angiotensin-aldosterone system in extracellular matrix modeling. Methods Exp Clin Pharmacol 25:541-564, 2003.
17. Hollenberg N, Fisher N, Price D. Pathways for angiotensin generation in intact human tissue: Evidence from comparative pharmacologic interruption of the renin system. Hypertension 32:387-392, 1998.
18. Nishiyama A, Seth DB, Navar LG. Renal interstitial fluid angiotensin I and angiotensin II concentration during local angiotensin converting enzyme inhibition. J Am Soc Nephrol 13:2207-2212, 2002.
19. Hall JE. Control of sodium excretion by angiotensin II: Intrarenal mechanisms and blood pressure regulation. Am J Physiol 250:R960-R972, 1986.
20. Harrison-Bernard LM, Navar LG, Ho M, et al. Immunohistochemical localization of ANG II $AT_1$ receptor in adult rat kidney using a monoclonal antibody. Am J Physiol 273:F170-F177, 1997.
21. Dworkin L, Ichikawa I, Brenner B. Hormonal modulation of glomerular filtration function. Am J Physiol 244:F95-F106, 1983.

22. Edwards R. Segmental effects of norepinephrine and angiotensin II on isolated renal microvessels. Am J Physiol 244: F526-F535, 1983.

23. Hura C, Kunau R. Angiotensin II-stimulated prostaglandin production by canine renal afferent arterioles. Am J Physiol 254: F734-F745, 1983.

24. Andrews P. Investigations of cytoplasmic contractile and cytoskeletal elements in the kidney glomerulus. Kidney Int 20: 549-559, 1981.

25. Wolf G, Ziyadeh FN. The role of angiotensin II in diabetic nephropathy: Emphasis on non-hemodynamic mechanisms. Am J Kidney Dis 29:153-163, 1997.

26. Durvasula R, Peterman A, Hiromura K, et al. Activation of a local tissue angiotensin system in podocytes by mechanical strain. Kidney Int 65:30-39, 2004.

27. Mujais S, Kauffman S, Katz A. Angiotensin II binding sites in individual segments of the rat nephron. J Clin Invest 77:315-327, 1986.

28. Cogan MG. Angiotensin II: Powerful controller of sodium transport in the early proximal tubule. Hypertension 15: 451-458, 1990.

29. Schuster V, Kokko J, Jacobson H. Angiotensin II directly stimulates sodium transport in rabbit proximal convoluted tubules. J Clin Invest 73:507-516, 1984.

30. Liu F, Cogan M. Angiotensin II stimulation of hydrogen ion secretion in rat early proximal tubule. J Clin Invest 82: 601-610, 1988.

31. Sweet C, Kadowitz P, Brody M. Arterial hypertension elicited by prolonged intervertebral infusion of angiotensin II in conscious dog. Am J Physiol 221:1640-1651, 1971.

32. Reid J, Rubin P. Peptides and central neural regulation of the circulation. Physiol Rev 67:725-749, 1987.

33. Joy M, Lowe R. Evidence that the area postrema mediates the central cardiovascular response to angiotensin II. Nature 228: 1303, 1970.

34. Simpson JB. The circumventricular organs and the central actions of angiotensin II. Neuroendocrinol 32:248-256, 1981.

35. Pardridge MW. Neuropeptides and the blood-brain barrier. Ann Rev Phyiol 45:73-82, 1983.

36. Schelling P, Fischer H, Ganten D. Angiotensin and cell growth: a link to cardiovascular hypertrophy. J Hypertens 9:3-15, 1991.

37. Kjato H, Suzuki H, Tajima S, et al. Angiotensin II stimulates collagen synthesis in cultured vascular smooth muscle cells. J Hypertens 9:17-22, 1991.

38. Zachary I, Woll P, Rozengurt E. A role for neuropeptides in the control of cell proliferation. Dev Biol 124:295-311, 1987.

39. Sandberg K. Structural analysis and regulation of angiotensin receptors. Trends Endocrinol Metab 5:28-35, 1994.

40. Griedling K, Lasegue B, Alexander R. Angiotensin receptors and their therapeutic implications. Annu Rev Pharmacol Toxicol 36:281-306, 1996.

41. Dzau V, Horiuchi M. Differential expression of angiotensin receptor subtypes in the myocardium: A hypothesis. Eur Heart J 17:978-980, 1996.

42. Schieffer B, Paxton W, Marrero M, Bernstein K. Importance of tyrosine phosphorylation in angiotensin II type I receptor signaling. Hypertension 27:476-480, 1996.

43. Goodfriend TL. Angiotensin receptors: History and mysteries. Am J Hypertens 13:442-449, 2000.

44. Pals D, Masucci F, Sipos F, Denning G. A specific competitive antagonist of the vascular action of angiotensin II. Circ Res 29: 664-672, 1971.

45. Rosei E, Trust P. The effects of the angiotensin II antagonist on blood pressure and plasma aldosterone in man in relation to the prevailing plasma angiotensin II concentration. Prog Biochem Pharmacol 12:230-241, 1976.

46. Streeten D, Anderson G, Freiberg J, Dalakos T. Use of an angiotensin II antagonist (saralasin) in the recognition of angiotensinogenic hypertension. N Engl J Med 292:657-662, 1975.

47. Keeton TK, Campbell WB. The pharmacologic alteration of renin release. Pharmacol Rev 32:81-227, 1980.

48. Furakawa Y, Kishimoto S and Nishikawa K. Hypotensive imidazole derivatives and hypotensive imidazole 5-acetic acid derivatives. Patents issued to Takeda Chemical Industries Ltd. On July 20, 1982 and October 19, 1982, respectively, US Patents 4,340,598 and 4,355,040, Osaka, Japan, 1982.

49. Wong PC, Chiu AT, Price WA, et al. Nonpeptide ARBs. I. Pharmacological characterization of 2-n-butyl-4-chloro-1 (2-chlorobenzyl)imidazole-5-acetic acid, sodium salt (S-8307). J Pharmacol Exp Ther 247:1-7, 1988.

50. Chiu AT, Duncia JV, McCall DE, et al. Nonpeptide ARBs. III. Structure-function studies. J Pharmacol. Exp Ther 250:867-874, 1989.

51. Carini DJ, Duncia JV, Aldrich PE, et al. Nonpeptide ARBs: The discovery of a series of N-biphenylmethylimidazoles as potent orally active antihypertensives. J Med Chem 34:2525-2547, 1991.

52. Wexler RR, Greenlee WJ, Irvin JD, et al. Nonpeptide ARBs: The next generation in antihypertensive therapy. J Med Chem 39: 626-656, 1996.

53. Wong PC, Price WA, Chiu AT, et al. Nonpeptide angiotensin antagonists. IX. Pharmacology of EXP3174: An active metabolite of DuP 753, an orally active antihypertensive agent. J Pharmacol Exp Ther 255(1):211-217, 1990.

54. Buhlmeyer P, Furet P, Criscione L, et al. Valsartan, a potent, orally active angiotensin II antagonist developed from the structurally new amino acid series. Bioorg Med Chem Lett 4:29-34, 1994.

55. Criscione L, de Gasparo M, Buhlmeyer P, et al. Pharmacologic profile of CGP-48933, a novel, nonpeptide antagonist of AT1 angiotensin II receptor subtype. Br J Pharmacol 110:761-771, 1993.

56. Bernhart CA, Perreaut PM, Ferrari BP, et al. A new series of imidazolones: Highly specific and potent nonpeptide AT1 ARB. J Med Chem 36:3371-3380, 1993.

57. Cazaubon C, Gougat J, Bouscet F, et al. Pharmacologic characterization of SR 47436: A new nonpeptide AT1 subtype ARB. J Pharmacol Exp Ther 265:826-834, 1993.

58. Kobo K, Kohara Y, Imamya E, et al. Nonpeptide ARBs. Synthesis and biologic activity of benzimidazolecarboxylic acids. J Med Chem 36:2182-2195, 1993.

59. Kubo K, Kohara Y, Yoshimura Y, et al. Nonpeptide ARBs. Synthesis and biologic activity of potential prodrugs of benzimidazole-7-carboxylic acids. J Med Chem 36:2343-2349, 1993.

60. Ries UJ, Mihm G, Narr B, et al. 6-Substituted benzimidazoles as new nonpeptide ARBs: synthesis, biological activity, and structure activity relationships. J Med Chem 36:4040-4051, 1993.

61. Wienen W, Hauel N, Van Meel JC, et al. Pharmacologic characterization of the novel nonpeptide ARB, BIBR 277. Br J Pharmacol 110:245-252, 1993.

62. Samamen JM, Peishoff CE, Keenan RM, Weinstck J. Refinement of a molecular model of angiotensin II employed in the discovery of potent nonpeptide antagonists. Bioorg Med Chem Lett 3:909-914, 1993.

63. Keenan RM, Weinstock J, Finkelstein JA, et al. Potent nonpeptide ARBs. 1-(carboxybenzyl)imidazole-5-acrylic acids. J Med Chem 36:1880-1892, 1993.

64. Cody RJ, Haas GJ, Binkley PF, Brown DM. Hemodynamic and vascular characteristics of Dup 753: A specific angiotensin II antagonist in the spontaneously hypertensive rat (SHR). J Am Coll Cardiol 17(Suppl A):202A, 1991.

65. Timmermans PB, Duncia JV, Carini DJ, et al. Discovery of losartan, the first ARB. J Human Hypertension 9(Suppl 5):S3-S18, 1995.

66. Lacour C, Canals F, Galindo G, et al. Efficacy of SR 47436 (BMS-186295), a nonpeptide angiotensin AT1 receptor antagonist in hypertensive rat models. Eur J Pharmacol 264:307-316, 1994.

67. Messerli FH, Weber MA, Brunner HR. Angiotensin II receptor inhibition: A new therapeutic principle. Arch Intern Med 156:1957-1965, 1996.

68. Brunner HR, Delacretaz E, Nussberger J, et al. Angiotensin II antagonists DuP 753 and TCV 116. J Hypertension Suppl 12:S29-S34, 1994.

69. Gradman AH, Arcuri KE, Goldberg AI, et al. A randomized, placebo controlled, double-blind, parallel study of various doses of losartan potassium compared with enalapril maleate in patients with essential hypertension. Hypertension 25:1345-1350, 1995.

70. Wong PC, Hart SD, Timmermans PB. Effect of angiotensin II antagonism on canine renal sympathetic nerve function. Hypertension 17(Part 2):1127-1134, 1991.

71. Schiffrin E. Vascular changes in hypertension in response to drug treatment: Effects of angiotensin receptor blockers. Can J Cardiol 18(suppl A):15A-18A, 2002.

72. Resnick L, Catanzaro D, Sealey J, Laragh J. Acute vascular effects of the angiotensin II receptor antagonist olmesartan in normal subjects: Relation to the renin aldosterone system. Am J Hypertension 17:203-208, 2004.

73. Reid IA. Interactions between ANG II, sympathetic nervous system, and baroreceptor reflexes in regulation of blood pressure. Am J Physiol 262:E763-E778, 1992.

74. Goldberg M, Tanaka W, Burchowsky A, et al. Effects of losartan on blood pressure, plasma renin activity and angiotensin II in volunteers. Hypertension 21:704-713, 1993.

75. Husain A. The chymase-angiotensin system in humans. J Hypertension 11:1155-1159, 1993.

76. Dzau VJ, Sasamura H, Hein L. Heterogeneity of angiotensin synthetic pathways and receptor subtypes: Physiological and pharmacological implications. Curr Opin Hypertens 1:3-9, 1993.

77. Bunkenburg B, van Amelsvoort T, Roog H, Wood JM. Receptor-mediated effects of angiotensin II on growth of vascular smooth muscle cells from spontaneously hypertensive rats. Hypertension 20:746-754, 1992.

78. Raya TE, Morkin E, Goldman S. Angiotensin antagonists in models of heart failure. In Saavedra JM, Timmermans PB (eds). Angiotensin Receptors. Plenum Press, New York, London, 1994; pp 309-318.

79. Schieffer B, et al. Comparative effect of chronic angiotensin inhibition and angiotensin II type I receptor blockade on cardiac remodeling after myocardial infarction in the rat. Circulation 89:2273-2282, 1994.

80. Smits JF, van Krimpen C, Schoemaker RG, et al. Angiotensin II receptor blockade after myocardial infarction in rats: Effects on hemodynamics, myocardial DNA synthesis, and interstitial collagen content. J Cardiovasc Pharmacol 20:772-778, 1992.

81. Hayashi M, Tsutamoto T, Wada A, et al. Immediate administration of mineralocorticoid receptor antagonist spironolactone prevents post-infarct left ventricular remodeling associated with suppression of a marker of myocardial collagen synthesis in patients with first anterior acute myocardial infarction. Circulation 107:2559-2565, 2003.

82. Kumagai K, Nakashima H, Urata H, et al. Effects of angiotensin II type 1 receptor antagonist on electrical and structural remodeling in atrial fibrillation. J Am Coll Card 41:2197-2204, 2003.

83. Dahlof B. Effect of angiotensin II blockade on cardiac hypertrophy and remodeling: A review. J Human Hypertens 9(Suppl 5): S37-S44, 1995.

84. Kaneko K, Susic D, Nunez E, Frolich E. Losartan reduces cardiac mass and improves coronary flow reserve in the spontaneously hypertensive rat. J Hypertension 14:645-654, 1996.

85. Braunwald E, Sarnoff SJ, Case RB. Hemodynamic determinants of coronary flow: Effect of changes in aortic pressure and cardiac output on the relationship between myocardial oxygen consumption and coronary flow. Am J Physiol 192:157-163, 1958.

86. Diets R, et al. Modulation of coronary circulation and the cardiac matrix by the renin-angiotensin system. Eur Heart J 12(Suppl F):107-111, 1991.

87. Lansang M, Osei S, Price D, et al. Renal hemodynamic and hormonal responses to the angiotensin II antagonist candesartan. Hypertension 36:834-838, 2000.

88. Burnier MJ, Brunner HR. Angiotensin receptor antagonists and the kidney. Opin Nephrol Hypertens 3:537-545, 1994.

89. Bauer JH, Reams GP. The angiotensin II type I receptor antagonists: A new class of antihypertensive drugs. Arch Intern Med 155:1361-1368, 1995.

90. Price DA, De'Oliveira JM, Fisher ND, Hollenberg NK. Renal hemodynamic response to an angiotensin antagonist, eprosartan, in healthy men. Hypertension 30:240-246, 1997.

91. Takishita S, Muratani H, Sesoko S. Short-term effects of angiotensin II blockade on renal blood flow and sympathetic activity in awake rats. Hypertension 24:445-450, 1994.

92. Burnier M, Roch-Ramel F, Brunner HR. Renal effects of angiotensin II receptor blockade in normotensive subjects. Kidney Int 49:1787-1790, 1996.

93. El Amrani AI, Philippe M, Michel JB. Bilateral renal responses to the ARB losartan, in 2K-1C Goldblatt hypertensive rats. J Hypertens 10(Suppl 4):206, 1992.

94. Lee JY, Blaufox MD. Renal effect of DuP 753 in renovascular hypertension. Am J Hypertens 4(Part 2):84A, 1991.

95. Saine DR, Ahrens ER. Renal impairment associated with losartan. Ann Intern Med 124:775, 1996.

96. Fenoy FJ, Milicic I, Smith RD, et al. Effects of DuP 753 on renal function of normotensive and spontaneously hypertensive rats. Am J Hypertens 4(Part 2):321S-326S, 1991.

97. Balla T, Bankal AJ, Eng S, Catt KJ. Angiotensin II receptor subtypes and biological responses in the adrenal cortex and medulla. Mol Pharmacol 40:401-406, 1991.

98. Goldberg MR, Bradstreet TE, McWilliams EJ, et al. Biochemical effects of losartan, a nonpeptide ARB, on the renin-angiotensin-aldosterone system in hypertensive patients. Hypertension 25:37-46, 1995.

99. Burnier M, Brunner H. ARBs and the kidney. Curr Opin Hypertens 1:92-100, 1995.

100. Gansevoort RT, de Zeeuw D, Shahinfar S, et al. Effects of the angiotensin II antagonist losartan in hypertensive patients with renal disease. J Hypertens Suppl 12:S37-S42, 1994.

101. Nakashima M, Uematsu T, Kosuge K, Kanamaru M. Pilot study of the uricosuric effect of DuP-753, a new ARB in healthy subjects. Eur J Clin Pharmacol 42:333-335, 1992.

102. Moan A, Hoieggen A, Nordby G, et al. Effects of losartan on insulin sensitivity in severe hypertension: Connections through sympathetic nervous activity? J Human Hypertens 9(Suppl 5):S45-S50, 1995.

103. Stadler T, Veltmar A, Qadri F, Unger T. Angiotensin II evokes noradrenaline release from the paraventricular nucleus in conscious rats. Brain Res 569:117-122, 1992.

104. Blair-West JR, Carey K, Denton DA, et al. Evidence that brain angiotensin II is involved in both thirst and sodium appetite in baboons. Am J Physiol 275:R1639-1646, 1998.

105. Braszko J. The contribution of $AT_1$ and $AT_2$ angiotensin receptors to its cognitive effects. Acta Neurobiol Exp 56:49-54, 1996.

106. Dahlof B, Lindholm L, Carney S, et al. Main results of the losartan versus amlodipine (LOA) study on drug tolerability and psychological well-being. J Hypertens 15:1327-1335, 1997.

107. Armando I, Seltzer A, Bregonzio C, Saavedra J. Stress and angiotensin II: Novel therapeutic opportunities. Curr Drug Target Neurol Disord 2:413-419, 2003.

108. Ferder L, Inserra F, Basso N. Advances in our understanding of aging: Role of the renin-angiotensin system. Curr Opin Pharmacol 2:189-194, 2002.

109. Lithell H, Hansson L, Skoog I, et al., for SCOPE Study Group. The Study on Cognition and Prognosis in the Elderly (SCOPE): Principal results of a randomized double-blind intervention trial. J Hypertens 21:875-886, 2003.

110. Ji H, Leung M, Zhang Y, Catt K, Sandberg K. Differential structural requirements for specific binding of nonpeptide and peptide antagonists to the AT1 angiotensin receptor: Identification of amino acid residues that determine binding of the antihypertensive drug losartan. J Biol Chem 269:16533-16536, 1994.

111. Azizi M, Chatellier G, Guyene T, et al. Additive effects of combined angiotensin converting enzyme inhibition and angiotensin II antagonism on blood pressure and renin release in sodium depleted normotensives. Circulation 92:825-834, 1995.

112. Medical Economics: Avapro (irbesartan), US product information. In Physicians Desk Reference, 52nd ed. Montvale, New Jersey, 1998.

113. Beevers D. Losartan: The first angiotensin receptor antagonist in clinical use. J Human Hypertension 9(Suppl 5): S1-S3, 1995.

114. Munafo A, Christen Y, Nussberger J, et al. Drug concentration response relationships in normal volunteers after oral administration of losartan, an angiotensin antagonist. Clin Pharmacol Ther 51:513-521, 1992.

115. Weber MA. Clinical experience with the angiotensin receptor antagonist losartan: A preliminary report. Am J Hypertens 5:247S-251S, 1992.

116. Ohtawa M, Takayama F, Saitoh K, Yoshinaga T, Nakashima M. Pharmacokinetics and biochemical efficacy after single and multiple oral administration of losartan, an orally active nonpeptide angiotensin receptor antagonist, in humans. Br J Pharmacol 35:290-297, 1993.

117. Burnier M, Waeber B, Brunner H. Clinical pharmacology of the ARB losartan in healthy subjects. J Hypertension 13(Suppl 1):S23-S28, 1995.

118. Stearns R, Chakravarty P, Chen R, Chiu S. Biotransformation of losartan to its active carboxylic acid metabolite in human liver microsomes. Role of cytochrome P450C and 3A subfamily members. Drug Metab Dispos 23:207-215, 1995.

119. Medical Economics: Cozaar (losartan potassium), US product information. In Physicians Desk Reference, 52nd ed. Montvale, New Jersey, 1998.

120. Lo M, Goldberg M, McCrea J, et al. Pharmacokinetics of losartan, an ARB, and its active metabolite EXP3174 in humans. Clin Pharmacol Ther 58:641-649,1995.

121. Sica D, Lo M, Shaw W, et al. The pharmacokinetics of losartan in renal insufficiency. J Hypertension 13(suppl 1):S49-S52, 1995.

122. Kong A, Tomasko L, Waldman S, et al. Losartan does not affect the pharmacokinetics and pharmacodynamics of warfarin. J Clin Pharmacol 35:1008-1015, 1995.

123. De Smet M, Schoors D, De Meyer G, et al. Effect of multiple doses of losartan on the pharmacokinetics of single doses of digoxin in healthy volunteers. Br J Clin Pharmacol 40:571-575, 1995.

124. Kaukonen K, Olkkola K, Neuvonen P. Fluconazole but not itraconazole decreases the metabolism of losartan to E-3174. Eur J Clin Pharmacol 53:445-449, 1998.

125. Muller P, Flesch G, de Gasparo M, et al. Pharmacokinetics and pharmacodynamic effects of the angiotensin I antagonist valsartan at steady state in healthy, normotensive subjects. Eur J Clin Pharmacol 52(6):441-449, 1997.

126. Flesch G, Muller P, Lloyd P. Absolute bioavailability and pharmacokinetics of valsartan, an angiotensin II antagonist, in man. Eur J Clin Pharmacol 52(2):115-120, 1997.

127. Markham A, Goa K. Valsartan. A review of its pharmacology and therapeutic use in essential hypertension. Drugs 54:299-311, 1997.

128. Colussi D, Parisot C, Rossolino M, et al. Protein binding in plasma of valsartan, a new ARB. J Clin Pharmacol 37:214-221, 1997.

129. Brookman L, Rolan P, Benjamin I, et al. Pharmacokinetics of valsartan in patients with liver disease. Clin Pharmacol Ther 62:272-278,1997.

130. Sioufi A, Marfil F, Jaouen A, et al. The effect of age on the pharmacokinetics of valsartan. Biopharm Drug Dispos 19:237-244, 1998.

131. Johnston CL, Risvanis J. Preclinical pharmacology of ARBs. Am J Hypertens 10(part 2):306S-310S, 1997.

132. Ruilope L. Human pharmacokinetic/pharmacodynamic profile of irbesartan: A new potent ARB. J Hypertens 15(suppl 7):S15-S20, 1997.

133. Marino M, Langenbacher K, Ford N, Uderman H. Pharmacokinetics and pharmacodynamics of irbesartan in healthy subjects. J Clin Pharmacol 38:246-255, 1998.

134. Brunner H. The new ARB, irbesartan pharmacokinetic and pharmacodynamic considerations. Am J Hypertens 10(part 2): 311S-317S, 1997.

135. Nishikawa K, Naka T, Chatani F, Yoshimura Y. Candesartan cilexetil: A review of its preclinical pharmacology. J Human Hypertension 11(Suppl 2):S9-S17, 1997.

136. Sever P. Candesartan cilexetil: A new, long-acting, effective angiotensin II type 1 receptor blocker. J Human Hypertens 11(Suppl 2):S91-S95, 1997.

137. Hubner R, Hogemann A, Sunzel M, Riddel J. Pharmacokinetics of candesartan after single and repeated doses of candesartan cilexetil in young and elderly healthy volunteers. J Human Hypertens 11(Suppl 2):S19-S25, 1997.

138. Riddell JG. Bioavailability of candesartan is unaffected by food in healthy volunteers administered candesartan cilexetil. J Human Hypertens 11(Suppl 2):S29-30, 1997.

139. van Lier JJ, van Heiningen PNM, Sunzel M. Absorption, metabolism and excretion of 14C-candesartan and 14C-candesartan cilexetil in healthy volunteers. J Human Hypertens 11(Suppl 2):S27-S28, 1997.

140. de Zeeuw D, Remuzzi G, Kirch W. Pharmacokinetics of candesartan cilexetil in patients with renal or hepatic impairment. J Human Hypertens 11(Suppl 2):S37-42, 1997.

141. Jonkman JHG, van Lier JJ, van Heiningen PNM, et al. Pharmacokinetic drug interaction studies with candesartan cilexetil. J Human Hypertens 11(Suppl 2):S31-S35, 1997.

142. Edwards RM, Aiyar N, Ohlstein EH, et al. Pharmacological characterization of the nonpeptide ARB, SK&F 108566. J Pharmacol Exp Ther 260:175-181, 1992.

143. Cox PJ, Bush BD, Gorycki PD, et al. The metabolic fate of eprosartan in healthy subjects. Exp Toxicol Pathol 48(Suppl II):75-82, 1996.

144. Martin D, Chapelsky MC, Ilson B, et al. Pharmacokinetics and protein binding of eprosartan in healthy volunteers and in patients with varying degrees of renal impairment. J Clin Pharmacol 38:129-137, 1998.

145. Tenero D, Martin D, Miller A, et al. Effect of age and gender on the pharmacokinetics and plasma protein binding of eprosartan (Abstract). Pharmacotherapy 17:114, 1997.

146. McClellan KJ, Balfour JA. Eprosartan. Drugs 55:713-718, 1998.

147. Wienen W, Hauel N, vanMeel JC, et al. Pharmacologic characterization of the novel nonpeptide ARB BIBR 277. Br J Pharmacol 110:245-252, 1993.

148. Micardis prescribing information. Boehringer Ingelheim Pharmaceuticals, Inc., 1999.

149. Neutel JM, Smith DHG. Dose-response and pharmacokinetics of telmisartan, a new angiotensin II receptor blocker. J Hypertension 16(Suppl 2):S210-S214, 1998.

150. Schwocho L, Masonson H. Pharmacokinetics of CS-866, a new angiotensin II receptor blocker, in healthy subjects. J Clin Pharmacol 41:515-527, 2001.

151. Laeis P, Puchler K, Kirch W. The pharmacokinetic and metabolic profile of olmesartan medoxomil limits the risk of clinically relevant drug interaction. J Hypertens 19:S21-S32, 2001.

152. Neutel J. Clinical studies of CS-866, the newest angiotensin II receptor antagonist. Am J Coll Cardiol 87:37C-43C, 2001.

153. Oparil S, Williams D, Chrysant S, Marbury T, Neutel J. Comparative efficacy of olmesartan, losartan, valsartan and Irbesartan in the control of essential hypertension. J Clin Hypertens 3:283-291, 2001.

154. Chrysant S, Weber M, Wang A, Hinman D. Evaluation of antihypertensive therapy with the combination of olmesartan medoxomil and hydrochlorothiazide. Am J Hypertension 17:252-259, 2004.

155. Benz J, Oshrain C, Henry D, et al. Valsartan, a new ARB: A double-blind study comparing the incidence of cough with lisinopril and hydrochlorothiazide. J Clin Pharmacol 37:101-107, 1997.

156. Ramsay L, Yeo W. ACE inhibitors, angiotensin II antagonists and cough. The losartan cough study group. J Hum Hypertens 9(Suppl 5):S51-S54, 1995.

157. Pouleur HG. Clinical overview of irbesartan. Am J Hypertens 10:318S-324S, 1997.

158. Acker CG, Greenberg A. Angioedema induced by the angiotensin II blocker losartan. N Engl J Med 333:1572, 1995.

159. Frye C, Pettigrew T. Angioedema and photosensitive rash induced by valsartan. Pharmacotherapy 18:866-868, 1998.

160. Smith R, Aurup P, Goldberg A, Snavely D. Long term safety of losartan in open label trials with mild to moderate essential hypertension. Am J Hypertens 11(part 2):43A, 1998.

161. Moore M: Efficacy of AT1 receptor blockade in hypertension. Am J Hypertens 11(part 2):251A, 1998.

162. Oparil S, Dyke S, Harris F, et al. The efficacy and safety of valsartan compared with placebo in the treatment of patients with essential hypertension. Clin Ther 18:797-810, 1996.

163. Oparil S, Barr E, Telkins M, et al. Efficacy, tolerability, and effects on quality of life of losartan, alone or with hydrochlorothiazide, versus amlodipine, alone or with hydrochlorothiazide, in patients with essential hypertension. Clin Ther 18:608-625, 1996.

164. Holwerda N, Fofari R, Angeli P, et al. Valsartan, a new angiotensin II antagonist for the treatment of essential hypertension: Efficacy and safety compared with placebo and enalapril. J Hypertension 14:1147-1151,1996.

165. Corvol P, Plouin P. Angiotensin II receptor blockers: current status and future prospects. Drugs 62:53-64, 2002.

166. Andersson OK, Neldam S. The antihypertensive effect and tolerability of candesartan cilexetil, a new generation angiotensin II antagonist, in comparison with losartan. Blood Pressure 7:53-59, 1998.

167. Bunt T, Dumswala A. Candesartan vs. losartan. J Human Hypertens 12:419, 1998.

168. Nyman L, Quintiles A, Cullberg K, et al. Encapsulation of commercially available losartan does not influence its bioavailability. Am J Hypertens 11(part 2):77A, 1998.

169. Oparil S, Guthrie R, Lewin A, et al. An elective-titration study of the comparative effectiveness of two angiotensin II-receptor blockers, irbesartan and losartan. Clin Ther 20:398-409, 1998.

170. Gradman AH. AT1-receptor blockers: Differences that matter. J Human Hypertens 16:S9-S16, 2002.

171. Conlin P, Spence D, Williams B, et al. Angiotensin II antagonists for hypertension: Are there differences in efficacy? Am J Hypertens 13:418-426, 2000.

172. Cody R. The clinical potential of renin inhibitors and angiotensin antagonists. Drugs 47:586-598, 1994.

173. Harrap SB, Dominiczak AF, Fraser R, et al. Plasma angiotensin II, predisposition to hypertension, and left ventricular size in healthy young adults. Circulation 93:1148-1154, 1994.

174. Pitt B. ACE inhibitors in heart failure: prospects and limitations. Cardiovasc Drugs Ther 11(Suppl 1):285-290, 1997.

175. Regitz-Zagrosek V, Neuss M, Fleck E. Effects of angiotensin receptor antagonists in heart failure: Clinical and experimental aspects. Eur Heart J 16(Suppl N):86-91, 1995.

176. Guazzi M, Melzi G, Agostoni P. Comparison of changes in respiratory function and exercise oxygen uptake with losartan versus enalapril in congestive heart failure secondary to ischemic or idiopathic dilated cardiomyopathy. Am J Cardiol 80:1572-1576, 1997.

177. Crosier I, Ikram H, Awan N, et al. Losartan in heart failure. Hemodynamic effects and tolerability. Losartan Hemodynamic Study Group. Circulation 91:691-697, 1995.

178. Pitt B, Segal R, Martinez FA, et al. Randomized trial of losartan versus captopril in patients over 65 with heart failure (Evaluation of Losartan in the Elderly Study, ELITE). Lancet 349(9054):747-752, 1997.

179. Pitt B, Poole-Wilson P, Segal R, et al., on behalf of the ELITE II Investigators. Effect of losartan compared with captopril on mortality in patients with symptomatic heart failure: Randomized trial—the Losartan Heart Failure Survival Study ELITE II. Lancet 355:1582-1587, 2000.

180. Dickstein K, Chang P, Willenheimer R, et al. Comparison of the effects of losartan and enalapril on clinical status and exercise performance in patients with moderate or severe chronic heart failure. J Am Coll Cardiol 26:438-445, 1995.

181. Hamroff G, Blaufarb I, Mancini D, et al. Angiotensin II-receptor blockade further reduces afterload safely in patients maximally treated with angiotensin-converting enzyme inhibitors for heart failure. J Cardiovasc Pharmacol 30:533-611, 1997.

182. Cohn J, Tognoni G., for the Valsartan Heart Failure Trial Investigators. A randomized trial of the angiotensin-receptor blocker valsartan in chronic heart failure. N Engl J Med 345:1667-1675, 2001.

183. Carson P, Tognoni G, Cohn J. Effect of valsartan on hospitalization: Results of the Val-HeFt. J Cardiac Fail 3:164-171, 2003.

184. Kaneko K, Susic D, Nunez E, Frohlich ED. Losartan reduces cardiac mass and improves coronary flow reserve in the spontaneously hypertensive rat. J Hypertens 14:645-653, 1996.

185. Ishiye M, Umemura K, Uematsu T, Nakashima M. Effects of losartan, an angiotensin II antagonist, on the development of cardiac hypertrophy due to volume overload. Biol Pharm Bull 18:700-704, 1995.

186. Tedesco MA, Ratti G, Aquino D, et al. The effectiveness and tolerability of losartan and effect on left ventricular mass in patients with essential hypertension. Cardiologia 43:53-59, 1998.

187. Dahlof B, Devereux R, de Faire U, et al. The Losartan Intervention For Endpoint Reduction (LIFE) in Hypertension study: Rationale, design, and methods. The LIFE Study Group. Am J Hypertens 10(7 Pt1):705-713, 1997.

188. Dahlof B, Devereux R, Kjeldsen S, et al., for the LIFE study group. Cardiovascular morbidity and mortality in the Losartan Intervention for Endpoint reduction in hypertension study (LIFE): A randomized trial against atenolol. Lancet 359: 995-1003, 2002.

189. Pfeffer M, Swedberg K, Granger C, et al., for CHARM investigators. Effects of candesartan on mortality and morbidity in patients with chronic heart failure. Lancet 362:759-766, 2003.

190. McMurray J, Ostergren J, Swedberg K, et al., for the CHARM investigators. Effects of candesartan in patients with chronic heart failure and reduced left ventricular systolic function intolerant to angiotensin-converting enzyme inhibitors: The CHARM-alternative trial. Lancet 362:772-776, 2003.

191. Granger C, McMurray J, Yusuf S, et al., for CHARM Investigators and Committees. Effects of Candesartan in patients with chronic heart failure and reduced left ventricular systolic function intolerant to angiotensin converting enzyme inhibitors: The CHARM-Alternative trial. Lancet 362: 772-776, 2003.

192. Yusuf S, Pfeffer M, Swedberg K, et al., Charm Investigators and Committees. Effects of candesartan in patients with chronic heart failure and preserved left ventricular ejection fraction: The CHARM-Preserved trial. Lancet 362:777-781, 2003.

193. Dickstein K, Kjekshus J. OPTIMAAL steering committee of the OPTIMAAL study group. Effects of losartan and captopril on mortality and morbidity in high-risk patients after acute myocardial infarction: The OPTIMAAL randomized trial. Optimal Trial in Myocardial Infarction with Angiotensin II Antagonist Losartan. Lancet 360:752-760, 2002.

194. Pfeffer M, McMurray J, Velazquez E, et al., for the VALIANT trial investigators. Valsartan, captopril, or both in myocardial infarction complicated by heart failure, left ventricular dysfunction or both. N Engl J Med 249:1893-1906, 2003.

195. Tarif N, Bakris GL. Angiotensin II receptor blockade and progression of nondiabetic-mediated renal disease. Kidney Int Suppl 63:S67-S70, 1997.

196. Hutchison FN, Webster SK. Effect of AII receptor antagonist on albuminuria and renal function in passive Heymann nephritis. Am J Physiol 263:F311-F318, 1992.

197. Zoja C, Abbate M, Corna D, et al. Pharmacologic control of angiotensin II ameliorates renal disease while reducing renal TGF-beta in experimental mesangioproliferative glomerulonephritis. Am J Kidney Dis 31:453-463, 1998.

198. Brenner B, Cooper M, de Zeeuw D, et al., for the RENAAL Study Investigators. Effects of losartan on renal and cardiovascular outcomes in patients with type II diabetes and nephropathy. N Engl J Med 345:861-869, 2001.

199. Lewis E, Hunsicker L, Clarke W, et al., for the Collaborative Study Group. Renoprotective effect of the angiotensin receptor antagonist Irbesartan in patients with nephropathy due to type 2 diabetes. N Engl J Med 345:851-860, 2001.

200. Parving H, Lehnert H, Brochner-Mortensen J, et al., for the Irbesartan in patients with Type II Diabetes and Microalbuminuria Study group. N Engl J Med 345:870-878, 2001.

201. Morgensen C, Neldam S, Tikkanen I, et al., for the CALM study group. Br Med J 321:1440-1444, 2000.

202. Viberti G, Wheeldon NM. Microalbuminuria Reduction With VALsartan (MARVAL) Study Investigators. Microalbuminuria reduction in patients with type 2 diabetes mellitus: A blood pressure independent effect. Circulation 106:672-678, 2002.

203. Gansevoort R, de Zeeuw D, de Jong P. Is the antiproteinuric effect of ACE inhibition mediated by interference in the renin-angiotensin system? Kidney Int 45:861-886, 1994

204. Kurokawa K. Effects of candesartan on the proteinuria of chronic glomerulonephritis. J Hum Hypertens 13:S57-60, 1999.

205. Plum J, Bunten B, Grabenese B. Effects of the angiotensin II antagonist valsartan on blood pressure, proteinuria, and renal hemodynamics in patients with chronic renal failure and hypertension. J Am Soc Nephrol 9:2223-2234, 1998.

206. Franscini LM, Von Vigier R, Pfister R, et al. Effectiveness and safety of the angiotensin II antagonist irbesartan in children with chronic kidney diseases. Am J Hypertens 15:1057-1063, 2002.

207. Taal MW, Brenner BM. Renoprotective benefits of RAS inhibition: From ACEI to angiotensin II antagonists. Kidney Int 57:1803-1817, 2000.

208. Delles C, Jacobi J, John S, Effects of enalapril and eprosartan on the renal vascular nitric oxide system in human essential hypertension. Kidney Int. 61:1462-1468, 2002.

209. Noris M, Remuzzi G. ACE inhibitors and $AT_1$ receptor antagonists: Is two better than one? Kidney Int 61:1545-1547, 2002.

210. Segura J, Praga M, Campo C, et al. Combination is better than monotherapy with ACE inhibitor or angiotensin receptor antagonist at recommended doses. J Renin Angiotensin Aldosterone Syst 4:43-47, 2003.

211. Campbell R, Sangalli F, Perticucci E, et al. Effects of combined ACE inhibitor and angiotensin II antagonist treatment in human chronic nephropathies. Kidney Int 63:1094-1103, 2003.

212. Nakao N, Yoshimura A, Morita H, et al. Combination treatment of angiotensin-II receptor blocker and angiotensin converting enzyme inhibitor in non-diabetic renal disease (COOPERATE): A randomized controlled trial. Lancet 361:117-124, 2003.

213. Ruddy M. Angiotensin II receptor blockade in diabetic nephropathy. Am J Hypertens 15:468-471, 2002.

214. Seventh Report of the Joint National Committee on Prevention, Detection, Evaluation, and Treatment of High Blood Pressure. Hypertension 42:1206-1252, 2003.

215. Mann J, Julius S, for the VALUE Trial group. The Valsartan Antihypertensive Long-term Use Evaluation (VALUE) Trial of Cardiovascular Events in Hypertension. Rationale and Design. Blood Pressure 7:176-183, 1998.

# Direct-Acting Smooth Muscle Vasodilators and Adrenergic Inhibitors

## Edward D. Frohlich

Since the early 1970s, antihypertensive drug therapy has made a tremendous impact on morbidity and mortality from cardiovascular diseases. Nevertheless, despite the introduction of newer modalities of treatment and the claims of adverse effects related to the adrenergic inhibitors and the direct-acting smooth muscle vasodilators, improvement in cardiovascular outcomes seems to have stalled. End-stage renal disease (ESRD) and congestive heart failure, both related to hypertension, continue to increase unabated.

Whereas use of many of the agents discussed in this chapter has drastically decreased in the United States in favor of newer agents with different mechanisms of action, the older agents continue to be used broadly elsewhere around the world. No doubt this is related to availability of generic formulations of these agents and their lower cost. Moreover, one subclass of the adrenergic inhibitors, the α-adrenergic receptor blockers, continue to be employed widely for the treatment of benign prostatic hyperplasia (BPH).

Among the more-potent antihypertensive drugs are those that inhibit sympathetic activity. This inhibition may be achieved at practically any anatomic level of adrenergic function. However, for these compounds to maintain their effectiveness over time, for the most part, they must be used in conjunction with diuretics. The following discussion reviews these adrenolytic agents, describing their mechanisms of action, hemodynamic effects, clinical uses, and adverse effects.

Every direct-acting smooth muscle vasodilator and adrenergic inhibitor except the β-adrenergic receptor blockers and, perhaps, the α-adrenergic blockers, will induce compensatory sodium and water retention and extracellular fluid volume expansion following reduction of arterial pressure.[1-3] The clinician must therefore recognize the need for concomitant diuretic therapy. The type of diuretic is relatively unimportant: Drastic dietary-sodium restriction, a thiazide diuretic, or a loop diuretic can be employed. However, because it is most important to minimize potassium wastage and maintain persistent and steady contraction of the intravascular volume, a thiazide is generally the best choice for patients with relatively normal renal function because it has a longer duration of action than the loop diuretic. The diuretic enhances the antihypertensive action of the adrenergic inhibitor by maintaining the contraction of the extracellular and intravascular compartments characteristic of most hypertensive diseases.

## ADRENERGIC INHIBITORS

Stress and anxiety can alter cardiovascular function, producing transient increases in heart rate and arterial blood pressure. However, these stimuli are generally not sufficient to cause hypertension, which requires persistent increased tension or tone of the arteriolar vascular smooth muscle for its

maintenance. Confusion in terminology can confound any discussion of agents that inhibit neural function. The present discussion does not concern itself with agents that sedate, tranquilize, or minimize psychic stress through higher centers.

Central adrenergic efferent impulses pass through major cardiovascular centers in the hypothalamic, medullary, and other subcortical areas to the spinal cord to synapse with second neurons located in sympathetic ganglia at the thoracolumbar level of the spinal column. These more distal neurons are stimulated at the ganglion level by the release of acetylcholine from the terminals of the central neurons, thereby propagating the peripheral outflow of adrenergic impulses. Neural impulses, passing distally via the adrenergic neurons, reach the heart or blood vessels, where they release norepinephrine from nerve terminals. Norepinephrine stimulates the effector organ—heart, venule, or arteriole—by attachment to specific binding sites identified as either α- or β-adrenergic receptors.

Norepinephrine and other neurohumoral mediators, including epinephrine and dopamine, are synthesized in the adrenal gland and adrenergic neurons, but norepinephrine is the major neurotransmitter that is released from postganglionic nerve terminals. Norepinephrine synthesis begins with the essential amino acid L-tyrosine by hydroxylation with tyrosine hydroxylase to form L-hydroxyphenylalanine and then L-hydroxyphenylethylamine (dopamine). Dopamine β-hydroxylase and phenylethanolamine-N-methyl-transferase continue the biosynthesis of the catecholamines to form L-norepinephrine and L-epinephrine, respectively. Norepinephrine is the major neurotransmitter and is most responsible for adrenergic receptor stimulation. Norepinephrine is found in the axon sheath and stored in the nerve terminals in vesicles that release it on nerve stimulation.

Norepinephrine is metabolized within the nerve terminal, by monoamine oxidase (MAO) in the mitochondria via a deamination process to form, initially, dihydroxymandelic acid and later, vanillylmandelic acid. In contrast, the norepinephrine that finds its way extraneuronally is metabolized by the enzyme catechol O-methyltransferase to form 3-methoxy,4-hydroxymandelic acid or vanillylmandelic acid. These metabolic products can be measured in the laboratory as metanephrines and normetanephrines or vanillylmandelic acid, respectively. Consideration of these metabolic processes is important in the interpretation of laboratory tests utilized in the diagnosis of pheochromocytoma, particularly in the identification of therapeutic agents that may be responsible for false-positive or false-negative test results.

With the arrival of the adrenergic impulse at the postganglionic nerve terminal, there is release of free norepinephrine. The neurotransmitter may bind to myocardial and/or vascular smooth muscle receptor sites, producing the adrenergic cardiovascular response. It may also be taken up by the nerve terminal (so-called reuptake) for conservation and release at a later time or may be acted on by the extraneuronal enzymatic system to form the metabolites or to circulate freely within the vascular system. The normal circulating levels of epinephrine and norepinephrine are less than 100 pg/ml and less than 500 pg/ml, respectively; the daily urinary excretion rates of catecholamines and metabolites are shown in Table 68–1.

With the binding of norepinephrine at the effector receptor site, several possible processes may occur. Stimulation of the β-adrenergic receptor will produce vasoconstriction of the arteriole and venule. Stimulation of the α-adrenergic receptor will promote peripheral vasodilation and increased heart rate, myocardial contractility, and myocardial metabolism.

There are many loci at which antihypertensive agents may inhibit the adrenergic nerve stimulus, including afferent sensory pathways from the heart, vessels, and mechanoreceptors; centrally at the ganglion level; or at the nerve terminal. Certain antihypertensive agents may also inhibit norepinephrine biosynthesis or block its action at the adrenergic receptor. The following discussion concerns the specifics of each class of adrenergic inhibitors.

## Ganglion Blocking Drugs

### Mechanism of Action

When the adrenergic preganglionic impulse arrives at the ganglion, acetylcholine is released from the nerve terminals, crosses the synaptic gap, and stimulates the postganglionic axons. The physiochemical action on the axon membrane is complex, but in simplest terms, involves the alteration of axon permeability. Thus, when acetylcholine attaches to receptor sites on the axon membrane, transmembrane ion flux is permitted, by which potassium ions move extracellularly and sodium ions intracellularly. When this depolarization process reaches an optimal rate, transmission of the neural impulse down the postganglionic neuron continues.[4]

One of the first major classes of antihypertensive drugs was the ganglion blockers.[5] These agents act by occupying receptor sites on the postganglionic axon to stabilize the membrane against acetylcholine stimulation; they have no effect on preganglionic neuronal acetylcholine release, cholinesterase activity, postganglionic neuronal catecholamine release, or

**Table 68–1** 24-Hour Urinary Excretion Rate of Catecholamines and Metabolites

| CATECHOLAMINES | |
| --- | --- |
| 50–650 µg | |
| CATECHOLAMINES | |
| Norepinephrine | 0.100 µg |
| Epinephrine | 0–25 µg |
| Dopamine | 60–440 µg |
| METABOLITES | |
| HVA | 0–15.0 mg |
| VMA | 0–7.0 mg |
| Metanephrine | 30–350 µg |
| Normetanephrine | 50–650 µg |

HVA, homovanillic acid; VMA, vanillylmandelic acid.

vascular smooth muscle contractility.[4-6] Tetraethylammonium chloride was the first agent used; later, other compounds were synthesized, including hexamethonium chloride, pentolinium tartrate, mecamylamine hydrochloride, pempidine hydrochloride, and chlorisondamine chloride. In a controlled, prospective, double-blind study involving three of the more commonly used ganglion-blocking drugs (at the time of their popular use), when equivalent doses of these agents were employed, all three agents were equally efficacious in reducing arterial pressure.[7]

Because interference with transmission of the autonomic impulse at the ganglion level impairs adrenergic and parasympathetic impulse transmission, clinical use of ganglion blockers was associated with severe side effects of unwanted parasympathetic inhibition. With the advent of more-specific adrenergic-blocking drugs, such as guanethidine sulfate and methyldopa, the ganglion-blocking drugs were less frequently used, until at present they are mostly of academic interest.

The exception is trimethaphan camsylate, which is still useful as an antihypertensive agent because of its intravenous formulation and mode of action. Trimethaphan is infused by slow intravenous drip (1 mg in a 1-L solution with the addition of one or two additional 1000-mg ampules, if necessary).[8] Reduction of arterial pressure is immediate, and careful monitoring of pressure is essential. When the infusion is discontinued, return of arterial pressure to preinfusion levels is prompt. Therefore, when administering this agent to the severely hypertensive patient, the physician must initiate long-acting antihypertensive therapy before discontinuing the infusion. Furthermore, as with any adrenergic inhibitor, volume contraction is associated with augmented hypotensive responses, and norepinephrine administration is associated with an enhanced pressor response. This phenomenon of denervation supersensitivity is extremely important in patients treated with sympatholytic agents.[9]

### Hemodynamic Effects

Adrenergic transmission to the heart and vessels is impaired by ganglion-blocking drugs, and reduced heart rate, myocardial contractility, and total peripheral resistance result. The fall in arterial pressure and vascular resistance is not as great in the supine as in the upright position because the adrenergic venomotor effect is enhanced by the gravitational effect of pooling of blood when the patient is upright. As a result of a reduction in venomotor tone, the patient treated with ganglion-blocking drugs or any other sympatholytic therapy will pool blood in the capacitance vessels of the dependent areas of the body. As a result, venous return to the heart is reduced in proportion to the degree of adrenergic inhibition and the degree of upright posture. This effect explains the phenomenon of orthostatic hypotension that, if carried to the extreme, can be associated with syncope.[10] Thus the orthostatic fall in cardiac output is not primarily the result of direct adrenergic inhibition of myocardial function but of reduced venous return. Because the orthostatic effect on arterial pressure is so important with sympatholytic therapy, the knowledgeable physician should measure blood pressure in the supine or sitting, as well as in the standing, position. The orthostatic hypotension should be considered an effect of treatment rather than a side effect. To enhance the antihypertensive effect of sympatholytic agents in the supine position, it is necessary to reduce intravascular (and extracellular fluid) volume and prevent reexpansion of blood volume.[2,3,11] Furthermore, to artificially produce this orthostatic response, elevation of the head of the bed is a worthwhile maneuver. Because cardiac output is reduced with ganglion-blocking therapy, there is at least a proportionate reduction of renal blood flow, which may be associated with a reduced creatinine clearance.[12,13] Cerebral[14] and splanchnic[15] blood flows are also reduced.

### Side Effects

It is often stated that with prolonged hypotensive therapy with trimethaphan (48 to 72 hours), the patient often becomes refractory (or tachyphylactic) to the treatment.[14] Although this may occur, expansion of intravascular volume is a more likely explanation, and better control of pressure may be achieved with introduction of a diuretic or more vigorous use of diuretics already prescribed.[1,2] Moreover, contraction of intravascular volume produces exaggerated hypotension and adrenergic stimulation (e.g., with norepinephrine). Because parasympathetic inhibition also results from ganglion blockade, tonic activity to the gastrointestinal tract will occur, and the physician is cautioned to consider development of a paralytic ileus or acute urinary retention as possible side effects. Thus, abdominal pain with reduced bowel sounds, constipation, or reduced urinary output during ganglion-blocking therapy in a patient with aortic dissection may not reflect extension of the dissecting aneurysm into the mesenteric or renal arteries but instead may be a side effect of the medication.

### Clinical Uses

Although several other potent and rapidly acting parenteral antihypertensive agents are available, there is still a role for trimethaphan in the treatment of hypertensive emergencies. Thus, in producing controlled hypotension during surgery, in arteriography, or in acute aortic dissection, trimethaphan-induced hypotension may be more manageable than hypotension induced by an agent with a more-prolonged action. Under these circumstances, ganglion blockade will not be associated with the secondary reflective stimulation of the heart that is found with other vasodilator therapy.

## Postganglionic Adrenergic Inhibitors

When acetylcholine stimulates the postganglionic axon at the ganglion level, the impulse is propagated distally and culminates in the release of norepinephrine at the nerve terminal with stimulation of adrenergic receptors on the vascular smooth muscle membrane. This impulse can be interfered with pharmacologically by a variety of mechanisms, including depletion of neurohumoral stores at the nerve terminal, prevention of norepinephrine reuptake by the nerve terminal, inhibition of catecholamine biosynthesis, therapeutic introduction of false neurohumoral transmitters that bind to the adrenergic receptors on vascular smooth muscle, or blockade of the latter receptors. The following discussion concerns sympathetic blocking drugs that act through one or a combination of these mechanisms.

### Rauwolfia Alkaloids

These agents, including reserpine and more than 20 related compounds, were initially introduced for the treatment of hypertension in the early 1950s. They deplete the myocardium, blood vessels, adrenergic nerve terminals, adrenal medulla, and brain of catecholamines and serotonin.[16,17] By depleting the nerve terminal of norepinephrine stores and inhibiting norepinephrine reuptake, adrenergic transmission is altered so that vascular resistance falls. With prolonged treatment, the persistent arterial hypotension is associated with slight decreases in renal blood flow and glomerular filtration rate. This may be related to the reduction in cardiac output or a venodilator effect similar to that of ganglion-blocking drugs.[17,18] Although arterial dilation with increased blood flow has been considered greatest in the skin, other vascular beds are also involved (e.g., nasal stuffiness, a frequent complaint, is ameliorated by nasally administered vasoconstrictors).[19,20]

### Side Effects

Because the inhibitory effect of the rauwolfia alkaloids is selective for adrenergic function, parasympathetic activity remains unopposed. Thus, bradycardia, prolonged atrioventricular conduction, nasal dilation and stuffiness, increased gastric acid secretion with possible secondary peptic ulceration, and frequency of bowel movements are adverse effects of these drugs.[20] These effects may be counteracted by parasympathetic inhibitors or by intranasally administered vasoconstrictors. However, prolonged use of those latter agents may produce a chemical rhinitis. As a result of depletion of brain catecholamines and serotonin, there may be behavioral alterations and subtle or overt depression, sometimes leading to suicide.[21]

### Clinical Uses

Reserpine and similar alkaloids are efficacious in reducing arterial pressure to normal levels when used with diuretics and/or hydralazine.[22,23] When reserpine is used in doses of 0.10 to 0.50 mg/day (or with whole-root preparations, 50-100 mg), it synergizes the antihypertensive action of these two agents. Reserpine and other sympatholytic agents have been useful in treating hypertensive emergencies and the cardiovascular manifestations of thyrotoxicosis without altering thyroid function.[24,25]

### Guanethidine and Bretylium

These agents interfere with adrenergic neurotransmission at the postganglionic nerve terminals. Like reserpine, these compounds deplete nerve terminals, blood vessels, and myocardium of catecholamine stores. However, unlike reserpine, they have little effect on catecholamine stores in the adrenal gland and brain. Furthermore, even though they fail to deplete normal adrenal medullary catecholamines, they can release these substances from a pheochromocytoma, producing an alarming and dramatic hypertensive crisis. With catecholamine depletion and impairment of chemical neurotransmission, denervation supersensitivity of effector cells is achieved.[26,27]

### Hemodynamic Effects

After injection of guanethidine or bretylium, there is a transitory pressor phase associated with an increased heart rate and cardiac output related to catecholamine release.

A prolonged period of cardiac, vascular, and nerve terminal catecholamine depletion follows, associated with progressive reductions in systemic and pulmonary arterial pressure. The arterial pressure reduction, brought about through an interference in chemical neurotransmission, can be explained by a reduction in vascular resistance. This hypotension is not as great in the supine position as in the upright posture or with agents that simultaneously contract or prevent reexpansion of plasma volume.[1-3] Because of the coincidental inhibition of venous tone,[19] venous return to the heart is reduced by peripheral pooling of blood in dependent areas of the body with upright posture. As a result, cardiac output falls and enhances the hypotensive action of guanethidine by this effect (not a side effect) of orthostatic hypotension.[28,29] Associated with the resulting fall in cardiac output, there is a proportionate reduction in organ blood flows.[29-32] The renal and splanchnic areas may receive a smaller proportion of the total cardiac output, but glomerular filtration rate and renal function appear to return toward normal with time.[30-33] With reduced skeletal muscle blood flow and adrenergic innervation to skeletal muscle, resting muscle weakness may result that can be exacerbated by diuretic treatment.[34,35] This muscle weakness may be aggravated still further during or immediately after exercise when, because of arteriolar dilation, increased muscle flow, and passively increased peripheral pooling of blood, cardiac output becomes so reduced that the patient becomes symptomatic.[36]

### Side Effects

Many of the side effects of guanethidine (orthostatic hypotension, exercise hypotension, bradycardia, increased gastric secretion) result from unopposed parasympathetic activity and impaired adrenergic function. Similarly, diarrhea, retrograde ejaculation, and fluid retention may also be explained by reduced adrenergic transmission. Many of these side effects may be counteracted by reduced guanethidine dosage, addition of parasympatholytic agents, or addition of a diuretic.[37] Because guanethidine acts by entering the nerve terminal and interfering with neurohumoral transmission, any agent that prevents this will block the action of guanethidine. This is the means by which the tricyclic antidepressants—imipramine, desipramine, and protriptyline compounds—act.[38,39] Therefore guanethidine, guanadrel, and bretylium should not be prescribed for any patient receiving these psychoactive agents (and the converse also obtains).

### Clinical Uses

Because of the prolonged action of guanethidine, it need be prescribed only once daily (25-150 mg). Moreover, because sympathetic inhibition is usually maximal with bedrest, there is little to be gained by prescribing it in divided doses. Furthermore, because fluid retention and expanded intravascular and extracellular fluid volumes are most pronounced with potent adrenolytic agents, a diuretic is indicated for use with guanethidine with the caveat that patients should be observed carefully for hypokalemia and impaired renal excretory function. This phenomenon of fluid reexpansion explains most of the refractoriness to guanethidine and other sympatholytic therapy, since impairment in drug absorption over time seems unlikely.[37] Moreover, when a diuretic is added to guanethidine, care should be exercised to determine development of symptomatic orthostatic hypotension.

## Methyldopa, Clonidine, Guanabenz, and Guanfacine

The mechanisms of the antihypertensive effects of these adrenergic inhibitors are different from those of the foregoing agents. Originally, the antihypertensive action of methyldopa was believed to be exerted through tissue depletion of biogenic amines via inhibition of dopa decarboxylase.[40] However, although methyldopa does inhibit dopa decarboxylase, that mechanism contributes minimally to its blood pressure–lowering effect. Instead, methyldopa lowers blood pressure by being converted to $\alpha$-methyl-norepinephrine, a metabolite that displaces norepinephrine from the $\alpha$-adrenergic receptor site, thereby preventing the neurotransmitter from producing vascular smooth muscle stimulation (e.g., the concept of false neurotransmission). Even more importantly, this metabolite of methyldopa, as well as clonidine and the other agents in this group stimulates adrenergic receptors in central vasomotor centers (e.g., nucleus tractus solitarii), thereby inhibiting sympathetic outflow from the brain.[41-47]

### Hemodynamic Effects

Shortly after their administration (by mouth or by injection), these agents cause a progressive decrease in arterial pressure and heart rate that is associated with a reduction in cardiac output or total peripheral resistance, or both.[37,48] With time, the reduction in cardiac output becomes less apparent, and the renal blood flow is maintained.[49]

### Clinical Uses

Methyldopa has been useful in all types and degrees of severity of hypertension. It is effective in reducing supine pressure without associated orthostatic hypotension in doses from 250 mg to 2.0 g daily. This antihypertensive effect may diminish if methyldopa is used as monotherapy; its effectiveness can be restored and enhanced with a diuretic. Similar indications apply to clonidine and the other centrally active $\alpha$-adrenergic receptor blockers. Another use for clonidine is in the diagnosis of pheochromocytoma. When 0.1 mg of clonidine is administered hourly for three doses, the plasma norepinephrine levels fall in patients with essential hypertension but remain elevated in those with pheochromocytoma.[50] Furthermore, clonidine can be administered via transdermal patches.

### Side Effects

As with any antihypertensive agent that inhibits sympathetic nervous system activity, most anticipated side effects (postural hypotension, weakness, fluid expansion, gastrointestinal symptoms) may be related to its adrenolytic action or the resultant overriding of parasympathetic function, or both. Additional side effects characteristic of methyldopa, including somnolence and depressive reactions, may be related to its action on biogenic amine stores in the brain.[37] Methyldopa also may produce a flulike syndrome characterized primarily by a fever as high as 41°C (105°F)[51]; when therapy is discontinued, the fever disappears. This problem may be related to hepatocellular damage without jaundice or development of a positive direct Coombs' test that, rarely, may be associated with hemolytic anemia.[37,52] In general, therapy may be maintained with methyldopa in the presence of a positive direct Coombs' test; however, if anemia occurs, the therapy should be discontinued.[53] Other side effects attributable to agents of this class include dry mouth, somnolence, and depression.[54]

Sudden withdrawal of clonidine therapy has been associated with severe rebound hypertension. This can be treated with intravenous α-adrenergic blockers.[55]

## Monoamine Oxidase Inhibitors

Although still prescribed by some physicians as antihypertensive agents, their inclusion in this discussion is merited only because of their potentially dangerous side effects. The first therapeutic use of MAOs was administration of iproniazid for tuberculosis. It was soon learned that these compounds had mood-elevating effects[56] and ameliorated chest pain of coronary arterial insufficiency.[54] At present, their major role is in the treatment of mental depression,[54] but one compound, pargyline hydrochloride, was introduced primarily as an antihypertensive agent.[37] MAOs may actually aggravate hypertension by inhibiting norepinephrine metabolism.[54] Because MAO is inhibited in the postganglionic nerve terminal, several weakly pressor amines (e.g., dopamine, octopamine) accumulate at this site. These substances are believed to act as false neurohumoral transmitters, tending to elevate blood pressure.[57]

### Hemodynamic Effects

Only a relatively few hypertensive patients have been studied, and the results have not been striking. One report claimed marked reduction in arterial pressure and vascular resistance and a moderate impairment in glomerular filtration.[58]

### Side Effects

The major side effects are centrally medicated mental/emotional reactions including euphoria, insomnia, and acute psychoses. In addition, hepatocellular necrosis, blood dyscrasias, and symptoms of adrenergic inhibition occur.[37] Most important is the severe acute hypertensive crisis that has been observed repeatedly following the ingestion of certain foods containing tyramine (e.g., aged cheeses, beer, sherry, Chianti wine, and herring) while the patient is receiving MAOs (e.g., pargyline hydrochloride, tranylcypromine sulfate, phenelzine sulfate, nialamide, iproniazid).[59-61]

### Clinical Uses

Because of the potentially severe hypertensive crises that may be associated with these antihypertensive drugs, they should be considered primarily of academic interest in the treatment of hypertension.[37]

## Veratrum Alkaloids

These compounds are of importance because of their availability, potent antihypertensive efficacy, and unusual mode of action. They alter the responsiveness of the vagal afferent nerve fibers in the coronary sinus, left ventricle, and carotid sinus so that any pressure stimulus will result in increased nerve traffic. This stimulus is interpreted in the medullary vasomotor centers as reflecting a higher pressure than actually exists as a result of an induced delay in the vagal repolarization process.[62,63]

### Hemodynamic Effects

As a result of this altered afferent input to the central vasomotor centers, there is a reflexive fall in systolic and diastolic pressure and heart rate; the latter response may be abolished by atropine sulfate. Because adrenergic function is not blocked, only reset at a different pressure level, the usual postural and adrenergic reflective responses are not altered. The result is a significant fall in total peripheral resistance with little change in cardiac output despite the rather marked bradycardia. Cerebral and renal blood flow and glomerular filtration rate remain normal unless the hypotensive response is excessive.[63]

### Side Effects

Because of the narrow therapeutic index, the effective control of arterial pressure by the veratrum alkaloids is not infrequently associated with side effects, including nausea, vomiting, excessive salivation and diaphoresis, blurred vision, and mental confusion. These effects have been reduced slightly by combined use with other antihypertensives.

### Clinical Uses

Clinical use of the veratrum alkaloids has been restricted severely by their side effects. A parenteral agent (cryptenamine tannate [Unitensin], 1.0 mg) has been useful in the treatment of certain hypertensive emergencies, including eclampsia.

## α-Adrenergic Receptor Blocking Agents

Members of the class of α-adrenergic blocking agents including doxazosin, prazosin, and terazosine block adrenergic type 1 receptors localized on the vascular smooth muscle cell membrane so that the release of norepinephrine from the postganglionic nerve ending is inhibited in its action at the end-organ receptor. Consequently, peripheral adrenergic activity is diminished.

### Hemodynamic Effects

As a result of the foregoing action, vascular smooth muscle tone in the arteriolar wall and total peripheral resistance is decreased. Initially, there may be a reflex increase in cardiac stimulation; but within a short period of time, the increase in heart rate is less. For this reason, the postural hypotension observed after the initial dosing of these compounds becomes less obvious with continuous drug use. As with all other agents described previously that inhibit adrenergic activity or reduce vascular smooth muscle tone by direct relaxation of the arteriolar myocyte, intravascular (plasma) volume expands. The net effect may be a lesser control of arterial pressure associated with some intravascular volume expansion with peripheral edema. The drug-induced hypotension can be restored with the addition of a diuretic.

### Clinical Uses

Of the adrenergic inhibitors discussed in this chapter, the α-adrenergic blocking agents are the most commonly prescribed and yet are among the most controversial. Many of the early national consensus reports and guidelines did not recommend these agents for the initial treatment of patients with hypertension. In more recent reports they were included, but in the Joint National Committee's most recent report (JNC 7), α-adrenergic blocking drugs were excluded from initial therapeutic recommendations based on results of the large Antihypertensive and Lipid-Lowering Treatment to Prevent Heart Attack Trial (ALLHAT).[64] In ALLHAT, one of the agents in this class was found to be associated with a higher prevalence of cardiac failure (CHF) as compared with the diuretic chlorthalidone. While these agents may not be among the more important for therapy of most patients with hypertension, there still is a very definite place for them.

The α receptor inhibitors have been of greatest value in elderly men with hypertension who also have benign prostatic hyperplasia (BPH) or in normotensive elderly men with BPH. These agents are also useful for patients who have had adverse effects (bronchospasm, negative chronotropic and inotropic cardiac effects, greater than second-degree heart block, bronchoconstriction, depression, cold-induced peripheral vasoconstriction) from a β-adrenergic blocker or other adrenergic inhibitors. The α receptor inhibitors are also of value in patients with metabolic abnormalities associated with other antihypertensive agents, because they produce no metabolic alterations.

### Side Effects

As a result of the hemodynamic actions of the α-blockers, postural hypotension is not infrequent, and as a result, measurement of blood pressures should be obtained in the erect posture as well as the sitting or standing positions. When postural hypotension is documented (or even suspected by clinical symptoms), it is wise to advise these patients to assume the upright position cautiously—particularly when awakening during the night because of nocturia. The second most important side effect, as suggested previously, is apparent fluid retention. In reality, this is not true fluid retention but (as stated previously) edema associated with restoration of intravascular (plasma) volume as a result of reexpanded volume in consequence to reduced capillary hydrostatic pressure.

CHF has been identified as a major consequence of α receptor inhibition, particularly in elderly patients. This concept has been advocated in reports of increased CHF from the ALLHAT study.[64] The criteria for CHF in patients receiving doxazosin were not detailed in that report, but it was explicitly stated that the patients receiving this agent had greater risk of CHF and stroke than in those patients receiving chlorthalidone.[64] In subsequent reports, "symptomatic heart failure" was defined "as clear-cut signs or symptoms of left or right ventricular dysfunction that cannot be attributed to other causes. A patient had to have at least one symptom (paroxysmal nocturnal dyspnea, dyspnea at rest, New York Heart Association class II dyspnea, other symptoms [on less-than-ordinary exertion], or orthoponea) and one sign (rales, ankle edema, tachycardia, cardiomegaly or characteristic pulmonary pattern on chest radiography, S3 gallop, or jugular venous distension)."[65,66] Thus, because of the apparent fluid retention that results from the intrinsic hemodynamic effects of doxazosin and other α-adrenergic blockers, the elderly hypertensive patients randomized to doxazosin in ALLHAT very well may have demonstrated some degree of dyspnea, weight gain, peripheral edema, some evidence of cardiac enlargement, and expanded intravascular volume—even if true CHF did not supervene. These patients (by study design) could not receive a diuretic to reverse the edema. Nevertheless, when prescribing an α-adrenergic inhibitor to an elderly high-risk patient, care must be exercised to follow-up not only for signs of postural hypotension but also for potential intravascular volume expansion manifested by edema and dyspnea to prevent the development of CHF.

## DIRECT-ACTING VASCULAR SMOOTH MUSCLE RELAXANTS

With the introduction of β-adrenergic blocking therapy, a resurgence in interest in direct-acting smooth muscle vasodilating drugs for hypertension occurred. These agents have also been used with varying success in patients with cardiac failure. Hydralazine and minoxidil act by decreasing arteriolar resistance. With the fall in total peripheral resistance and arterial pressure, a reflex stimulation of the heart occurs so that tachycardia and palpitations frequently result unless these cardiac reflexive responses are offset by an adrenergic inhibitor (e.g., a β-adrenergic receptor blocking drug). These agents should not be administered to patients with hypertension who have myocardial infarction, angina pectoris, or aortic dissection because the reflexive cardiac effects will aggravate these underlying cardiac conditions. Other side effects include headaches and nasal stuffiness—attributable to the local vasodilation—and fluid retention and edema (i.e., pseudotolerance), which occurs more frequently with minoxidil.

A unique side effect of hydralazine is precipitation of a lupus erythematosus–like syndrome, which occurs more frequently in patients who are receiving more than 400 mg/day of hydralazine. A common side effect from minoxidil is hirsutism, which is particularly bothersome to women. When hydralazine is administered by injection (10-15 mg intravenously), a prompt reduction in pressure occurs.

Another parenteral vasodilator, diazoxide, is a nonnatriuretic thiazide congener that must be injected rapidly (in single-bolus doses of 300 mg or in successive pulsed-bolus divided doses) to prevent binding to circulating albumin. Diazoxide should not be administered to the patient with hypertension who has cardiac failure, angina pectoris, myocardial infarction, or an active aortic dissection. However, it has been useful for the patient with hypertensive encephalopathy, intracranial hemorrhage, and severe malignant or accelerated hypertension (without cardiac failure) in whom rapid and immediate reduction in arterial pressure is mandatory.

## References

1. Weil JV, Chidsey CA. Plasma volume expansion resulting from interference with adrenergic function in normal man. Circulation 37:54-61, 1968.
2. Dustan HP, Tarazi RC, Bravo EL. Dependence of arterial pressure on intravascular volume in treated hypertensive patients. N Engl J Med 286:861-866, 1972.
3. Dustan HP, Cumming GR, Corcoran AC, et al. A mechanism of chlorothiazide-enhanced effectiveness of antihypertensive ganglioplegic drugs. Circulation 19:360-365, 1959.
4. Patton WDM. Transmission and block in autonomic ganglia. Pharmacol Rev 6:59-67, 1954.
5. Smirk FH. Methonium compounds in hypertension. Lancet 2:477, 1950.
6. Patton WDM, Zaimis EJ. The methonium compounds. Pharmacol Rev 4:219–253, 1952.
7. Veterans Administration Cooperative Study on Antihypertensive Agents. Double-blind control study of antihypertensive agents. II: Further report on the comparative effectiveness of reserpine, reserpine and hydralazine, and three ganglion blocking agents, chlorisondamine, mecamylamine, and pentolinium tartrate. Arch Intern Med 110:222-229, 1962.

8. Bhatia S, Frohlich ED. A hemodynamic comparison of agents useful in hypertensive emergencies. Am Heart J 85:367-373, 1973.

9. Cannon WB, Rosenbleuth A. The Supersensitivity of Denervation Structures: A Law of Denervation. New York, Macmillan, 1949.

10. Freis ED, Rose JC, Partenope EA, et al. The hemodynamic effects of hypotensive drugs in man. II: Hexamethonium. J Clin Invest 32:1285-1298, 1953.

11. Takagi H, Dustan HP, Page IH. Relationship among intravascular volume, total body sodium, arterial pressure, and vasomotor tone. Circ Res 9:1233-1239, 1961.

12. Ford RV, Moyer JH, Spurr CL. Hexamethonium in the chronic treatment of hypertension: Its effects on renal hemodynamics and on the excretion of water and electrolytes. J Clin Invest 32:1133-1139, 1953.

13. Ullmann TD, Menczel J. The effect of a ganglion blocking agent (hexamethonium) on renal function and on excretion of water and electrolytes in hypertension and in congestive heart failure. Am Heart J 52:106-120, 1956.

14. Finnerty FA, Witkin L, Fazekas JF. Cerebral hemodynamics in acute hypotension. J Clin Invest 33:933, 1954.

15. Reynolds TB, Paton A, Freeman M, et al. The effect of hexamethonium bromide in splanchnic blood flow, oxygen consumption and glucose output in man. J Clin Invest 32:793-800, 1953.

16. Pletschet A, Shore PA, Brodie BB. Serotonin release as a possible mechanism of reserpine action. Science 122:374-375, 1955.

17. Brest AN, Onesti G, Swartz C, et al. Mechanisms of antihypertensive drug therapy. JAMA 211:480-484, 1970.

18. Moyer JH. Cardiovascular and renal hemodynamic response to reserpine (Serpasil) and clinical results of using this agent for treatment of hypertension. Ann N Y Acad Sci 59:82-94, 1954.

19. Gaffney TE, Bryant WM, Braunwald E. Effects of reserpine and guanethidine on venous reflexes. Circ Res 11:889-894, 1962.

20. Frohlich ED. Inhibition of adrenergic function in the treatment of hypertension. Arch Intern Med 133:1033-1048, 1974.

21. Freis ED. Mental depression in hypertensive patients treated for long periods with large doses of reserpine. N Engl J Med 251:1006-1008, 1954.

22. Veterans Administration Cooperative Study Group on Antihypertensive Agents. Effects of treatment in morbidity in hypertension: Results in patients with diastolic blood pressures averaging 115 through 129 mm Hg. JAMA 202:116-122, 1967.

23. Veterans Administration Cooperative Study Group on Antihypertensive Agents. Effects of treatment in morbidity in hypertension. II: Results in patients with diastolic blood pressure averaging 90 through 114 mm Hg. JAMA 213:1143-1152, 1970.

24. Canary JJ, Schaaf M, Duffy BJ Jr, et al. Effects of oral and intramuscular administration of reserpine in thyrotoxicosis. N Engl J Med 257:435-442, 1957.

25. Waldstein SS, West GH Jr, Lee WLY, et al. Guanethidine in hyperthyroidism. JAMA 189:609-612, 1964.

26. McCubbin JW, Kaneko Y, Page IH. The peripheral cardiovascular actions of guanethidine in dogs. J Pharmacol Exp Ther 181:346-354, 1961.

27. Emmelin N, Engstrom J. Supersensitivity of salivary glands following treatment with bretylium or guanethidine. Br J Pharmacol Chemother 16:315-319, 1961.

28. Frohlich ED, Freis ED. Clinical trial of guanethidine: A new type of antihypertensive agent. Med Ann D C 28:419-423, 1959.

29. Cohn JN, Liptak TE, Freis ED. Hemodynamic effect of guanethidine in man. Circ Res 12:298-307, 1963.

30. Villarreal H, Exaire JB, Rubio V, et al. Effects of guanethidine and bretylium tosylate on systemic and renal hemodynamics in essential hypertension. Am J Cardiol 14:633-640, 1964.

31. Gaffney TE, Braunwold E, Cooper T. Analysis of the acute circulatory effects of guanethidine and bretylium. Circ Res 10:83-88, 1962.

32. Novack P. The effect of guanethidine on renal, cerebral, and cardiac hemodynamics. In Brest AN, Moyer JH (eds). Hypertension, Recent Advances. Philadelphia, Lea & Febiger, 1961; pp 444-448.

33. Williams RL, Mains JE III, Pearson JE. Direct and systemic effects of guanethidine on renal function. J Pharmacol Exp Ther 177:69-77, 1971.

34. Bowman WC, Notts MW. Actions of sympathomimetic amines and their antagonists on skeletal muscle. Pharmacol Rev 21:27-72, 1969.

35. Chrysant S, Frohlich ED. Antihypertensive drugs: The pathophysiology of their side effects. Am Fam Physician 9:94-101, 1974.

36. Khatri IM, Cohn HN. Mechanism of exercise hypotension after sympathetic blockade. Am J Cardiol 25:329-338, 1970.

37. Page LB, Sidd JJ. Medical management of primary hypertension. N Engl J Med 287:967-967, 1018-1023, 1074-1081, 1972.

38. Mitchell JR, Arias L, Oates JA. Antagonism of the antihypertensive action of guanethidine sulfate by desipramine hydrochloride. JAMA 202:149-152, 1967.

39. Mitchell JR, Cavanaugh JH, Arias L, et al. Guanethidine and related agents. III: Antagonism by drugs which inhibit the norepinephrine pump in man. J Clin Invest 49:1596-1604, 1970.

40. Oates JA, Gillespie L, Undenfriend S, et al. Decarboxylase, inhibition and blood pressure reduction by α-methyl-3,4-dihydroxy-DL-phenylalanine. Science 131:1890-1891, 1960.

41. Kopin IJ. False adrenergic transmitters. Ann Rev Pharmacol 8:377-394, 1968.

42. Henning M, van Zwieten PA. Central hypotensive effect of α-methyldopa. J Pharm Pharmacol 20:409-417, 1968.

43. Ingenito AJ, Barrett JP, Procita L. A centrally mediated peripheral hypotensive effect of α-methyldopa. J Pharmacol Exp Ther 175:593-599, 1970.

44. Sattler RW, van Zwieten PA. Acute hypotensive action of 2-(2,6-dichlorophenylamino)-2-imidazoline hydrochloride (ST 155) after infusion into the cat's vertebral artery. Eur J Pharmacol 2:9-13, 1967.

45. Schmitt H, Boissier JR, Giudicelli JF. Centrally mediated decrease in sympathetic tone induced by 2-(2,6-dichlorophenylamine)-2-imidazoline (ST 155, Catapressan). Eur J Pharmacol 2:147-148, 1967.

46. Katie F, Lavery H, Lowe RD. The central action of clonidine and its antagonism. Br J Pharmacol 44:779-787, 1972.

47. Kobinger W, Walland A. Investigations into the mechanism of the hypotensive effect of 2-(2,6-dichlorophenylamine)-2-imidazoline HCl. Eur J Pharmacol 2:155-161, 1967.

48. Dollery CT, Harington M, Hodge JV. Haemodynamic studies with methyldopa: Effect on cardiac output and response to pressor amines. Br Heart J 25:670-676, 1963.

49. Mohammed S, Hanenson IB, Magenheim HG, et al. The effects of α-methyldopa on renal function in hypertensive patients. Am Heart J 76:21-27, 1968.

50. Bravo EL, Tarazi RC, Fouad FM, et al. Clonidine suppression test: A useful aid in the diagnosis of pheodermocytoma. N Engl J Med 305:623-626, 1981.

51. Glontz GE, Saslaw S. Methyldopa fever. Arch Intern Med 122:445-447, 1968.

52. Norlledge SM, Carstairs KC, Dacie JV. Autoimmune haemolytic anemia associated with α-methyldopa therapy. Lancet 2:135-139, 1966.

53. Finnerty FA Jr. Drugs in the treatment of hypertension. Mod Concepts Cardiovasc Dis 42:33-36, 1973.

54. Jarvik MD. Drugs used in the treatment of psychiatric disorders. In Goodman LS, Gilman A (eds). The Pharmacological Basis of Therapeutics. New York, Macmillan, 1968; pp 159-214.

55. Hansson L, Hunyor SN, Julius S, et al. Blood pressure crisis following withdrawal of clonidine (Catapres, Catapresan) with special reference to arterial and urinary catecholamine levels,

and suggestions for acute management. Am Heart J 85:605-610, 1973.

56. Cohen RA, Kopin IJ, Creveling CR, et al. False neurochemical transmitters: Combined clinical staff conference at the National Institutes of Health. Ann Intern Med 65:347-362, 1966.

57. Onesti G, Novack P, Ramirez O, et al. Hemodynamic effects of pargyline in hypertensive patients. Circulation 30:830-835, 1964.

58. Richards DW. Paradoxical hypertension from tranylcypromine sulfate. Report of the Council on Drugs. JAMA 186:854, 1963.

59. Blackwell B. Hypertensive crisis due to monoamine oxidase inhibitors. Lancet 2:849-851, 1963.

60. Goldberg LI. Monoamine oxidase inhibitors: Adverse reactions and possible mechanisms. JAMA 190:456-462, 1964.

61. Dawes GS, Comroe JH Jr. Chemoreflexes from the heart and lungs. Physiol Rev 34:167-201, 1954.

62. Wang SC, Ngai SH, Grossman RG. Mechanism of vasomotor action of veratrum alkaloids: Extravagal sites of action of veriloid, protoveratrine, germitrine, neogermitrine, germerine, veratridine and veratramine. J Pharmacol Exp Ther 113:100-114, 1955.

63. Freis ED, Stanton JR, Partenope EA, et al. The hemodynamic effects of hypotensive drugs in man. I: Veratrum viride. J Clin Invest 28:353-368, 1949.

64. Major Cardiovascular Events in Hypertensive Patients Randomized to Doxazosin vs Chlorthalidone: The Antihypertensive and Lipid-Lowering Treatment to Prevent Heart Attack Trial (ALLHAT). JAMA 283:1967-1975, 2000.

65. Davis BA, Cutler JA, Furberg CD, et al. Relationship of antihypertensive treatment regimens and change in blood pressure to risk for heart failure in hypertensive patients randomly assigned to doxazosin or chlorthalidone: Further analyses from the Antihypertensive and Lipid-Lowering Treatment to prevent Heart Attack Trial. Ann Intern Med 137:313-320, 2002.

66. ALLHAT Officers and Coordinators for the ALLHAT Collaborative Research Group. Diuretic versus $\alpha$ blocker as first-step antihypertensive therapy. Final results from the Antihypertensive and Lipid-Lowering Treatment to Prevent Heart Attack Trial (ALLHAT). Hypertension 42:239-246, 2003.

# Chapter 69

# Endothelin Antagonists

## Ernesto L. Schiffrin

## ROLE OF ENDOTHELINS IN EXPERIMENTAL HYPERTENSION

The endothelins (ET), potent 21-amino acid vasoconstrictor peptides produced in many different tissues, particularly in the endothelium of blood vessels, have already been described in Chapter 17. ET-1 is the main endothelin secreted by the endothelium, and acts in a paracrine or autocrine fashion on adjacent cells (endothelial or smooth muscle). ET-1 may act on $ET_A$ and $ET_B$ smooth muscle receptors to induce contraction, proliferation, and cell hypertrophy and on endothelial $ET_B$ receptors to induce release of nitric oxide (NO) and prostacyclin to elicit vasorelaxation. It is not known whether the vasoconstrictor or the vasorelaxant action of endothelins is their most important physiologic function, and this probably varies from one vascular bed to another. In the coronary circulation, the virtual absence of endothelial $ET_B$ receptors[1] results in endothelins behaving as coronary vasoconstrictors. In other vascular beds it is possible that ET-1 acts on smooth muscle cells as a paracrine constrictor and growth promoter only when it is overexpressed in endothelial cells under pathologic conditions.

In the heart, ET-1 is produced by various cell types, including endothelial cells, smooth muscle cells, fibroblasts, and cardiomyocytes. Up-regulation of the ET-1 gene may occur in these cells in response to angiotensin II, wall stretch, and ischemia. The $ET_A$ subtype is the predominant receptor present in cardiomyocytes, whereas a mixed population of $ET_A$ and $ET_B$ receptors is found in cardiac fibroblasts.[2] Endothelins stimulate expression of fetal genes, protein synthesis, and growth in cardiomyocytes.

In relation to the kidney, the expression of endothelins, the presence of $ET_A$ and $ET_B$ receptors and the vasoconstrictor and salt-retaining effects of these peptides have already been described in detail in Chapter 17.

Antagonists that are highly selective for the $ET_A$ or for the $ET_B$ receptor have been developed, have agents that have high affinity for both $ET_A$ and $ET_B$ receptors, the so-called balanced or nonselective $ET_A/ET_B$ receptor antagonists (Table 69–1). It is unclear as yet whether the balanced or nonselective antagonists act through blockade of both receptor subtypes, or by predominantly blocking endothelin actions mediated via the $ET_A$ receptor. Although some of these agents can be administered only intravenously (e.g., TAK-044, BQ-123, BQ-610, FR139317, IPI-725, BQ-788, RES-701-1), others are orally active and have at some point undergone clinical development for primary pulmonary hypertension, heart failure, subarachnoid hemorrhage, and have been considered potentially for systemic hypertension. The availability of subtype-selective and nonselective antagonists of endothelin receptors has allowed the dissection of the physiologic and pathophysiologic roles of endothelins mediated through these receptor subtypes in both experimental animals and humans.

Activation of the endothelin system has been demonstrated in salt-dependent models of hypertension, such as the deoxycorticosterone (DOCA)-salt hypertensive rat and the DOCA-salt–treated spontaneously hypertensive rat (SHR). These models overexpress ET-1 in the vascular endothelium,[3,4] and respond with blood pressure (BP) lowering to endothelin antagonism with bosentan, an $ET_A/ET_B$ endothelin antagonist.[5] In contrast, the endothelin system appears not to be activated in SHR.[3] When the activity of the vascular endothelin system is enhanced, growth is accentuated in resistance arteries, and administration of endothelin antagonists lowers BP and induces regression of hypertrophic arterial remodeling.[5,6] Endothelin effects in the kidney of some of these hypertensive models may contribute to water and sodium retention, renal vasoconstriction and hypertension, and eventually, renal failure.[7] In rats infused with angiotensin II (Ang II), a known stimulant of ET-1 expression, endothelin antagonists lowered BP and reduced cardiac and small artery hypertrophic remodeling.[8] Thus the endothelin system seems to be activated more often in low-renin, salt-sensitive, and severe forms of hypertension, but may be also stimulated by exogenous Ang II, and therefore presumably under certain conditions by endogenous Ang II. Cyclosporine-induced hypertension may also exhibit an endothelin-dependent component, and bosentan lowers BP in this model in rats and primates.[9] Endothelin may also play a role in hypertensive models with hyperinsulinemia and insulin resistance, in which chronic administration of bosentan reduces BP.[10]

In all these salt-sensitive, severe, or exogenous Ang II-infused models of hypertension in which ET-1 expression has been shown to be enhanced, severe hypertrophy of small arteries is often a characteristic feature.[11] In those models in which overexpression of ET-1 occurs, bosentan or other endothelin antagonists reduced BP and hypertrophic remodeling of small arteries and protected the kidney.[12] In some experimental models of hypertension enhanced expression of ET-1 may be local rather than generalized, and the endothelium of coronary arteries appears to be particularly vulnerable in this regard.[13] Enhanced production of ET-1, without compensatory vasodilation because of absence of endothelial $ET_B$ receptors,[1] could result in vasoconstriction of the coronary circulation and a significant role of endothelin in myocardial ischemia in hypertension. In the absence of endothelin tissue overexpression, the endothelin system may still play a role, if not in BP elevation, in perivascular fibrosis of the heart and in deterioration of renal function, as shown by the response to chronic bosentan treatment in SHR.[14] Cardiac endothelin expression increases in animal models of cardiac hypertrophy, and chronic administration of either selective $ET_A$ or mixed antagonists may reduce the development of left ventricular hypertrophy (LVH). Norepinephrine administered for 7 days increased expression of ET-1 in the heart in rats, mainly in cardiomyocytes and endothelial cells, and bosentan administration has blunted

**Table 69-1** Endothelin Antagonists

| ET$_A$/ET$_B$ | ET$_A$ | ET$_B$ |
|---|---|---|
| TAK-044 | BQ-123 | BQ-788 |
| Bosentan* | BQ-610 | RES-701-1 |
| PD145065 | FR139317 | RO-468443 |
| L-744,453 | IPI-725 | |
| L-751281 | A-127722.5 | |
| L-754,142 | LU135252 | |
| SB209670 | (darusentan) | |
| SB217242 | PD155080 | |
| (enrasentan) | PD156707 | |
| | BMS-182874 | |
| | TBC11251 | |
| | (sitaxsentan) | |

*Approved for use in primary pulmonary hypertension.

manifestations of cardiac hypertrophy.[15] The endothelin system is activated in heart failure in rats, and infusion of the ET$_A$ antagonist BQ-123 for a short period of time decreased the rate and force of contraction of the heart, indicating an inotropic action of the activated endothelin system in this model.[16] Prolonged infusion of BQ-123 significantly reduced mortality in the same rat model of heart failure.[17] Deterioration of cardiac function mediated by pathophysiologic activation of the cardiac endothelin system, as well as endothelin-dependent vasoconstriction and increased afterload in advanced heart failure, may therefore respond favorably to ET receptor antagonism, as has been demonstrated in humans.[18]

## PATHOPHYSIOLOGY OF THE CARDIOVASCULAR ENDOTHELIN SYSTEM IN HUMANS AND INVESTIGATIONAL USE OF ENDOTHELIN

Plasma endothelin levels are usually normal in human hypertension, although in some severely hypertensive patients, elevated endothelin immunoreactivity may be found in plasma.[11] The acute intravenous administration of the mixed ET$_A$/ET$_B$ endothelin receptor antagonist TAK-044 induced an increase in forearm blood flow and lowered BP slightly in healthy subjects.[19] This suggests that endothelin-dependent vascular tone may be present in normotensive humans. Enhanced plasma endothelin responses to mental stress have been reported in normotensive offspring of hypertensive parents,[20] which could indicate a genetically determined endothelial dysfunction preceding the development of hypertension. In patients with moderate to severe hypertension, the expression of preproET-1 mRNA in the endothelium of small arteries obtained from gluteal subcutaneous biopsies was significantly greater than in normotensive subjects or patients with mild hypertension.[21] This is in agreement with the report of increased ET-1 production by the endothelium of small arteries in experimental models with severe hypertension.

Enhanced production of ET-1 could play a role in small artery hypertrophic remodeling in patients with moderate to severe hypertension in addition to contributing to elevation of BP. In African Americans, in whom hypertension is often severe and salt-sensitive, activation of the endothelin system has been

described.[22] Other studies suggest that in Blacks, activation of the endothelin system is mainly associated with the more severe forms of hypertension.[23] It has also been shown that endothelin levels in plasma are associated with salt sensitivity in human subjects. In these subjects, abnormalities in the relation of endothelin, renin, and the sympathetic nervous system as measured by plasma catecholamines have been documented, which could contribute to activation of the endothelin system in response to a salt load. Other forms of hypertension in which endothelins may play a role are those associated with chronic renal failure, erythropoietin, and cyclosporine administration, pheochromocytoma, and pregnancy.[11]

The definitive place of endothelins in the pathophysiology of hypertension is still unclear, and its place in the therapeutic armamentarium awaits clinical trials with the different endothelin antagonists currently developed or in development. Bosentan given to patients with mild hypertension over a period of 4 weeks at a dose of 0.5 g once or twice daily was equally effective as 20 mg of enalapril daily, and well tolerated.[24] In the same study, a blunting of reflex neurohormonal vasoconstrictor activation was reported following administration of bosentan.[25] However, elevation of liver enzymes reported with the use of large doses of bosentan has stopped the development of this agent for a chronic condition such as systemic hypertension, which is associated with long life and for which many effective treatments are available. Bosentan has been approved for use in pulmonary hypertension, a rapidly fatal condition for which few other therapeutic alternatives exist.[26,27] The ET$_A$-selective endothelin antagonist LU135252 (darusentan) has been shown to lower BP in hypertensive subjects with few if any adverse effects.[28] Interestingly, headache was present more often in normal controls than in hypertensive persons with darusentan. This may depend on activation of NO synthase and production of NO in response to stimulation of unblocked ET$_B$ receptors. Because there is impairment of endothelial function in hypertensive subjects, fewer nitroglycerin-like effects are expected in hypertensive (for the reasons mentioned just previously) than in normotensive subjects. However, it does not seem that endothelin antagonists will be developed in the near future for the treatment of systemic hypertension.

## SUMMARY

We believe based on the data summarized in this chapter that it is likely that ET-1 is mainly involved in BP elevation and vascular hypertrophy in moderate to severe hypertension, and particularly in salt-sensitive forms and perhaps in special populations.[23] Worsening endothelial damage in hypertension may activate expression of endothelin in vessels and in the heart. Endothelin activation may be initially beneficial because (1) the vessel wall is thickened and wall stress is reduced, and (2) there are positive inotropic effects on the heart. However, progression of these changes may eventually result in pathophysiologically significant deleterious effects on the cardiovascular system. Endothelin antagonists may prove useful at this point, particularly in moderate to severe hypertension and in certain subsets of patients such as salt-sensitive hypertensives or African Americans. Endothelin antagonists may also prove to be useful in prevention of progression of nephroangiosclerosis and renal failure in hypertension, protection from ischemic heart disease and stroke,[29] as well as treatment of heart failure.[18] Endothelin antagonists may function in these conditions as disease-modifying agents, perhaps more than as BP-lowering agents.

Bosentan has been approved for the treatment of primary pulmonary hypertension,[26,27] a rapidly fatal disease for which few therapeutic alternatives are available and in which activation of the endothelin system has been well documented. In acute and chronic heart failure, in which there was great hope for successful utilization of endothelin antagonists based on studies in experimental animals, results of clinical trials have been disappointing.[30] However, new studies with different agents are currently being performed that may offer greater hope for the use of these agents in heart failure.

Whether balanced $ET_A/ET_B$ antagonists, selective $ET_A$ antagonists or endothelin converting enzyme inhibitors[31] will prove to be the preferred agents is as yet unclear. Further clinical evaluation of these drugs will allow us to learn more about their therapeutic utility and about the pathophysiologic implication of the endothelin system in human disease, as well as its role in the short- and long-term regulation of cardiovascular function.

# References

1. Russell FD, Skepper JN, Davenport AP. Detection of endothelin receptors in human coronary artery vascular smooth muscle cells but not endothelial cells by using electron microscope autoradiography. J Cardiovasc Pharmacol 29:820-826, 1997.
2. Fareh J, Touyz RM, Schiffrin EL, et al. Endothelin-1 and angiotensin II receptors in cells from rat hypertrophied heart. Receptor regulation and intracellular $Ca^{2+}$ modulation. Circ Res 78:302-311, 1996.
3. Larivière R, Thibault G, Schiffrin EL. Increased endothelin-1 content in blood vessels of deoxycorticosterone acetate-salt hypertensive but not in spontaneously hypertensive rats. Hypertension 21:294-300, 1993.
4. Day R, Larivière R, Schiffrin EL. In situ hybridization shows increased endothelin-1 mRNA levels in endothelial cells of blood vessels of deoxycorticosterone acetate-salt hypertensive rats. Am J Hypertens 8:294-300, 1995.
5. Li J-S, Larivière R, Schiffrin EL. Effect of a nonselective endothelin antagonist on vascular remodeling in DOCA-salt hypertensive rats. Evidence for a role of endothelin in vascular hypertrophy. Hypertension 24:183-188, 1994.
6. Schiffrin EL, Larivière R, Li J-S, et al. Enhanced expression of endothelin-1 gene in blood vessels of DOCA-salt hypertensive rats: Correlation with vascular structure. J Vasc Res 33:235-248, 1996.
7. Benigni A, Zoja C, Corna D, et al. Specific endothelin subtype A receptor antagonist protects against injury in renal disease progression. Kidney Int 44:440-444, 1993.
8. D'Uscio LV, Moreau P, Shaw S, et al. Effects of chronic $ET_A$-receptor blockade in angiotensin II-induced hypertension. Hypertension 29:435-441, 1997.
9. Bartholomeusz B, Hardy KJ, Nelson AS, et al. Bosentan ameliorates cyclosporin A-induced hypertension in rats and primates. Hypertension 27:1341-1345, 1996.
10. Verma S, Bhanot S, McNeill JH. Effect of chronic endothelin blockade in hyperinsulinemic hypertensive rats. Am J Physiol 269(6-pt 2):H207-H2021, 1995.
11. Schiffrin EL. Endothelin: Potential role in hypertension and vascular hypertrophy. Brief invited review Hypertension 25:1135-1143, 1995.
12. Li J-S, Schürch W, Schiffrin EL. Renal and vascular effects of chronic endothelin receptor antagonism in malignant hypertensive rats. Am J Hypertens 9:803-811, 1996.
13. Deng LY, Schiffrin EL. Endothelin-1 gene expression in blood vessels and kidney of spontaneously hypertensive rats (SHR), L-NAME-treated SHR, and renovascular hypertensive rats. J Cardiovasc Pharmacol 31(Suppl 1):S380-S383, 1998.
14. Karam H, Heudes D, Bruneval P, et al. Endothelin antagonism in end-organ damage of spontaneously hypertensive rats - Comparison with angiotensin-converting enzyme inhibition and calcium antagonism. Hypertension 28:379-385, 1996.
15. Kaddoura S, Firth JD, Boheler KR, et al. Endothelin-1 is involved in norepinephrine-induced ventricular hypertrophy in vivo. Acute effects of bosentan, an orally active, mixed endothelin $ET_A$ and $ET_B$ receptor antagonist. Circulation 93:2068-2079, 1996.
16. Sakai S, Miyauchi T, Sakurai T, et al. Endogenous endothelin-1 participates in the maintenance of cardiac function in rats with congestive heart failure. Circulation 93:1214-1222, 1996.
17. Sakai S, Miyauchi T, Kobayashi M, et al. Inhibition of myocardial endothelin pathway improves long-term survival in heart failure. Nature 384:353-355, 1996.
18. Kiowski W, Sütsch G, Hunziker P, et al. Evidence for endothelin-1-mediated vasoconstriction in severe chronic heart failure. Lancet 346:732-736, 1995.
19. Haynes WG, Ferro CJ, O'Kane KPJ, et al. Systemic endothelin receptor blockade decreases peripheral vascular resistance and blood pressure in humans. Circulation 93:1860-1870, 1996.
20. Noll G, Wenzel RR, Schneider M, et al. Increased activation of sympathetic nervous system and endothelin by mental stress in normotensive offspring of hypertensive parents. Circulation 93:866-869, 1996.
21. Schiffrin EL, Deng LY, Sventek P, et al. Enhanced expression of endothelin-1 gene in endothelium of resistance arteries in severe human essential hypertension. J Hypertens 15:57-63, 1997.
22. Ergul S, Parish DC, Puett D, et al. Racial differences in plasma endothelin-1 concentrations in individuals with essential hypertension. Hypertension 1996; 28:652-655.
23. Elijovich F, Laffer CL, Amador E, et al. Regulation of plasma endothelin by salt in salt-sensitive hypertension. Circulation 103, 263-268, 2001.
24. Krum H, Viskoper RJ, Lacourière Y, et al. The effect of endothelin-receptor antagonist, bosentan, on blood pressure in patients with hypertension. N Engl J Med 338:784-790, 1998.
25. Krum H, Budde M, Charlon V. Effect of endothelin receptor antagonism on reflex neurohormonal vasoconstrictor activation in patients with essential hypertension. Circulation Suppl I:I-406, 1997 (Abstract).
26. Williamson DJ, Wallman LL, Jones R, et al. Hemodynamic effects of bosentan, an endothelin receptor antagonist, in patients with pulmonary hypertension. Circulation 102:411-418, 2000.
27. Channick RN, Simonneau G, Sitbon O, et al. Effects of the dual endothelin-receptor antagonist bosentan in patients with pulmonary hypertension: A randomised placebo-controlled study. Lancet 358:1119-1123, 2001.
28. Nakov R, Pfarr E, Eberle S, et al. An effective endothelin A receptor antagonist for treatment of hypertension Am J Hypertens 15:583-589, 2002.
29. Schiffrin EL, Intengan HD, Thibault G, et al. Clinical significance of endothelin in cardiovascular disease. Curr Opin Cardiol 12:354-367, 1997.
30. Lüscher TF, Enseleit F, Pacher R, et al. Hemodynamic and neurohumoral effects of selective endothelin A ($ET_A$) receptor blockade in chronic heart failure: The Heart Failure ETA Receptor Blockade Trial (HEAT). Circulation 106:2666-2672, 2002.
31. Jeng AY, Mulder P, Kwan AL, Battistini B. Nonpeptidic endothelin-converting enzyme inhibitors and their potential therapeutic applications. Can J Physiol Pharmacol 80(5):440-449, 2002.

# Mineralocorticoid Receptor Antagonists

## Ellen G. McMahon

Over the last several decades, the widespread use of new therapeutic agents to treat hypertension, dyslipidemia, and heart disease has reduced the morbidity and mortality associated with cardiovascular diseases. However, the incidence of end-stage renal disease and congestive heart failure continues to rise despite improvements in control of blood pressure and lipids.[1,2] This is most likely due to the fact that, despite the availability of a vast array of agents to lower blood pressure, only 31% of treated patients reach target blood pressures.[3] Typically, patients with uncontrolled hypertension have markedly elevated systolic blood pressure, diabetes, or evidence of target organ damage (left ventricular hypertrophy [LVH] or microalbuminuria). The annual risk of life-threatening cardiovascular events is estimated to be 2% to 3% per annum in these difficult to control patients.[4] Thus the number of cardiovascular events that might be prevented with improved blood pressure control in these patients is correspondingly large.

For many years, activation of the renin-angiotensin-aldosterone system (RAAS) has been associated with unsatisfactory outcomes in patients with heart failure and hypertension. In severe heart failure patients, plasma aldosterone levels are positively correlated with mortality and, in hypertensive patients, there is a positive correlation between LVH and plasma aldosterone.[5,6] An inverse correlation that was independent of blood pressure or age has been reported between plasma aldosterone levels and arterial compliance in a population of essential hypertensives.[7] Patients with primary aldosteronism have increased incidence and severity of cardiovascular complications compared to essential hypertensives with similar blood pressure elevation.[8,9] Thus, several studies have demonstrated that aldosterone correlates with the severity of target organ damage and is likely an independent risk factor for cardiovascular events.

Upstream blockers of the RAAS (angiotensin-converting enzyme [ACE] inhibitors and the angiotensin receptor blockers [ARBs]) have been available for many years. Why, then, is aldosterone blockade needed, since upstream blockers of this pathway should negate all of the negative effects of aldosterone by inhibiting aldosterone production? The answer lies in a phenomenon known as "aldosterone rebound," which occurs during chronic treatment with ACE is such that aldosterone levels rise over time despite maximal blockade at proximal sites in the pathway. Aldosterone rebound has been reported in patients treated with ACE inhibitors and ARBs for hypertension, heart failure, and diabetic nephropathy.[10-12] In the Randomized Evaluation of Strategies for Left Ventricular Dysfunction (RESOLVD) Pilot Study, in which heart failure patients were administered enalapril and the ARB candesartan, either alone or in combination for a period of 43 weeks, aldosterone levels return to pretreatment values with prolonged therapy even in patients treated with both enalapril and candesartan.[13]

Aldosterone rebound is expected because we know that there are multiple modulators of aldosterone secretion, in addition to angiotensin II (Ang II). Potassium, adrenocorticotropic hormone, the neurotransmitters norepinephrine and serotonin, endothelin and nitric oxide are all known modulators of aldosterone secretion, independent of Ang II.[14] Thus, it is not surprising that aldosterone rebound occurs with blockade of the Ang II pathway. Patients treated with upstream RAAS blockers remain unprotected from the deleterious effects of aldosterone.

## ALDOSTERONE AND CARDIOVASCULAR INJURY

The classical mineralocorticoid effect of aldosterone on transporting epithelium in the kidney has long been thought to be the predominant cardiovascular effect of the hormone. However, there is now compelling evidence that aldosterone mediates significant cardiovascular effects via the actions on mineralocorticoid receptors outside the kidney, namely in the brain, heart, and blood vessels.[15] Moreover, the enzymes responsible for aldosterone biosynthesis are present outside of the adrenal gland in the same tissues.[16-20] It is now postulated that many of the effects of aldosterone on the cardiovascular system are mediated through activation of nonepithelial mineralocorticoid receptors in these tissues (Figure 70–1).

Brilla and Weber were the first to suggest that aldosterone may play a deleterious role via its action on mineralocorticoid receptors in nonepithelial tissues. These investigators identified a link between activation of the RAAS and the development of myocardial fibrosis in both left and right ventricles, using experimental models of hypertension.[21] Subsequent studies have confirmed and extended these original observations using the Nω-nitro-L-arginine methyl ester (L-NAME/Ang II/salt, Ang II/salt, deoxycorticosterone (DOCA)/salt, and aldosterone/salt models of hypertension.[22-25] It is clear from these studies that elevated levels of aldosterone correlate strongly with the development of ventricular fibrosis. However, work from Rocha et al.[25] suggests that the primary damaging effect of aldosterone may be the induction of vascular inflammation and injury of the small arteries and arterioles in target organ tissues, preceding a reactive and reparative fibrotic process.

Aldosterone has also been implicated as a mediator of the aortic collagen accumulation that often occurs during the development of hypertension in animal models. Lacolley et al.[26] have demonstrated that mineralocorticoid receptor blockade in aldosterone/salt hypertensive rats prevents increased arterial stiffness and pulse pressure increases, even at doses that do not significantly reduce blood pressure. Similar reductions in aortic collagen accumulation with mineralocorticoid receptor antagonism were reported in the spontaneously hypertensive rat (SHR).[27] These animal studies are supported by clinical evidence

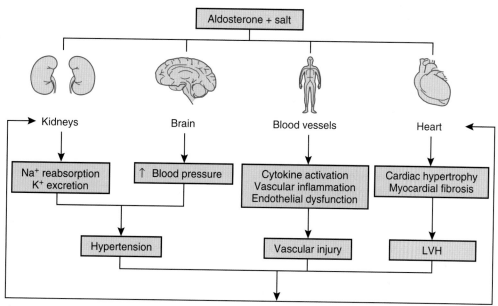

**Figure 70-1** Deleterious effects of aldosterone in the presence of high salt intake leading to cardiovascular disease. (With permission from McMahon EG. Eplerenone, a new selective aldosterone blocker. Curr Pharm Des 9(13):1065-1075, 2003.)

of an inverse relationship between plasma levels of aldosterone and large artery compliance in hypertensive patients.[28]

Aldosterone also appears to disrupt fibrinolytic balance. Brown et al. have demonstrated that aldosterone up-regulates plasminogen activator inhibitor type-1 (PAI-1), the major physiologic inhibitor of plasminogen activation.[29] Up-regulation of PAI-1 may shift thrombotic/thrombolytic balance to favor clot formation. Aldosterone may also be a mediator of endothelial dysfunction because blockade of aldosterone in patients with congestive heart failure improves endothelial function and increases nitric oxide bioactivity.[30] Aldosterone blockade improves endothelial dysfunction in animal models of heart failure and hypertension.[31,32]

Aldosterone produces proarrhythmogenic effects in cardiomyocytes in that exposure of adult rabbit cardiomyocytes to aldosterone produced inhibitory effects on $Na^+$-$K^+$ pump activity.[33] In rabbits, elevated aldosterone levels induce a decrease in cardiac sarcolemmal $Na^+$,$K^+$-ATPase, which is blocked by mineralocorticoid receptor antagonism and thought to be due to direct activation of cardiomyocyte mineralocorticoid receptors (MR) by aldosterone.[34] Inhibition of $Na^+$,$K^+$-ATPase is also associated with the activation of key growth-related genes in cardiomyocytes and thus, this direct effect of aldosterone on cardiomyocytes may contribute to LVH in hypertension and heart failure.[35]

Nonepithelial effects of aldosterone have also been demonstrated in the brain. Gomez-Sanchez et al. have shown that intracerebroventricular administration of aldosterone in rats, at doses too low to have effects when administered systemically, slowly induces hypertension over a period of several weeks.[36] In Dahl inbred salt-sensitive rats on a high-salt diet, blood pressure rises slowly over time, despite suppression of the RAAS with high salt intake. When these animals are administered either a mineralocorticoid receptor antagonist (RU28318) or high levels of corticosterone (the physiologic glucocorticoid in the rat into the brain), the rise in blood pressure is attenuated.[37] Mineralocorticoid receptors have been identified in human

brain, but it is not known whether activation of these receptors by aldosterone contributes to hypertension in humans.

## Nongenomic Effects of Aldosterone

On binding MR, aldosterone initiates a transcriptional response that culminates in cellular and physiologic events. Nongenomic effects of aldosterone in vascular tissues that do not require gene transcription have also been described.[38] These effects occur within minutes of aldosterone exposure and are typically unresponsive to the nonselective aldosterone receptor antagonist, spironolactone.[39] The vascular effect of eplerenone, a selective mineralocorticoid receptor antagonist,[40] on aldosterone-stimulated nongenomic activation of the $Na^+$,$K^+$-ATPase, was evaluated using rat aorta and rat mesenteric arteries. Aldosterone inhibited $Na^+$,$K^+$-ATPase (as measured by ouabain-sensitive $^{86}Rb$ uptake) in rat aortic rings 20 to 25 minutes after exposure to aldosterone and eplerenone prevented this rapid effect of aldosterone on $Na^+$,$K^+$-ATPase activity.[41] Inhibition of gene transcription with actinomycin D and of protein synthesis with cycloheximide had no effect on the short-term aldosterone inhibition of the $Na^+$-$K^+$ pump, indicating that the rapid effects are mediated via MR but involve nongenomic mechanisms. These observations suggest that aldosterone is directly involved in cellular ionic homeostasis in rat arteries and provide evidence that eplerenone is able to antagonize nongenomic aldosterone effects in vascular tissues. However, the contribution of nongenomic effects to the detrimental action of aldosterone on the cardiovascular system remains controversial.[42-44]

## Spironolactone and Eplerenone

Simpson and Tait initially isolated aldosterone in 1953. It was some years before an aldosterone antagonist was developed and made available for the treatment of hypertension. Scientists at Searle Laboratories in Skokie, IL, synthesized spironolactone in 1958 and reported on the aldosterone-blocking and oral activity of this agent in 1959.[45] Spironolactone was approved in 1962 as a potassium-sparing diuretic for the management of primary aldosteronism, edematous conditions, essential hypertension, and hypokalemia. When used for prolonged periods of time at high doses, spironolactone use is associated with endocrine side effects, such as loss of libido, menstrual irregularities, gynecomastia, and impotence.[46] These side effects are due to the affinity of spironolactone for androgen and progesterone receptors.

Eplerenone (Inspra) was synthesized by J. Grob of Ciba-Geigy back in the mid-1980s as a more selective mineralocorticoid receptor antagonist.[47] Eplerenone was approved in the United States for use in hypertension in 2002. In 2003, eplerenone was approved to improve survival in postmyocardial infarction patients with left ventricular (LV) systolic dysfunction and clinical evidence of congestive heart failure. As shown in Figure 70–1, the critical feature of the eplerenone molecule conferring enhanced selectivity is the presence of the 9,11-epoxide group in the lactone ring. Eplerenone is the first mineralocorticoid antagonist that acts at the MR to prevent its activation by aldosterone in a highly selective manner. Unlike previous aldosterone blockers (spironolactone), eplerenone possesses very low activity at the human androgen, progesterone, and glucocorticoid receptors (hAR, hPR and hGR, respectively).[48]

The activity of eplerenone at human steroid receptors was measured in vitro using recombinant human steroid receptors. These assays measure the ability of a compound to stimulate receptor transcriptional transactivation function and/or to antagonize a full agonist transcriptional response at steroid receptors. Eplerenone antagonized hMR transcriptional activation by aldosterone in a concentration-dependent manner with a calculated $IC_{50}$ of 0.081 μM (Table 70–1). The potency of eplerenone at other steroid receptors was significantly reduced, with no activity measured at progesterone and glucocorticoid receptors, even when eplerenone was tested at concentrations up to 100 uM. At human androgen receptors, eplerenone blocking activity was measurable but was only one-sixtieth of the blocking activity measured at the MR. In contrast, the earlier MR antagonist spironolactone demonstrated significant activity at all human steroid receptors tested. In particular, spironolactone possesses significant blocking

activity at the androgen receptor; the $IC_{50}$ for androgen blockade with spironolactone is one-sixth the activity at the mineralocorticoid receptor. In addition, the spironolactone molecule is a reasonably potent agonist at progesterone receptors. These new data using human steroid receptor preparations confirm earlier studies using steroid receptor preparations from animal tissues[47] and demonstrate that eplerenone is a significantly more selective aldosterone receptor antagonist compared with spironolactone.[48]

The improved selectivity of eplerenone was confirmed in clinical studies, which demonstrated that eplerenone provides continuous blockade of aldosterone for at least 1 year without tolerability issues.[49]

In addition to improved steroid receptor selectivity, the pharmacokinetic properties of eplerenone in humans are different from those of spironolactone. Although both spironolactone and eplerenone are rapidly cleared from plasma, several long-lived active metabolites are produced from spironolactone that contribute to its pharmacologic activity in humans.[50] Canrenone and 6-β-OH-7-α-thiomethylspirolactone (TMS) are the major circulating metabolites in human plasma, and both demonstrate binding to MRs and antimineralocorticoid activity in animals. Both of these active metabolites have long half-lives—16.5 and 13.8 hours mean post–steady-state half-lives, respectively, for canrenone and TMS in normal, healthy volunteers dosed with spironolactone at 100 mg/day each day for 15 days.[50] In contrast, the two major metabolites of eplerenone in humans, 6-β-OH eplerenone and the open lactone ring form of eplerenone are both inactive when tested using human mineralocorticoid receptors.[51]

Spironolactone has a very high degree of first-pass metabolism in humans, with metabolites that undergo a high degree of enterohepatic cycling.[52] Spironolactone is also an inducer of hepatic microsomal drug metabolizing enzymes in humans.[50] In patients with congestive heart failure, the log-linear phase half-life of canrenone was substantially prolonged compared with the half-life in healthy subjects.[53] In contrast, eplerenone does not undergo extensive first-pass metabolism and is not an inducer of cytochrome P450 isoforms in humans.[51]

It is well documented that upstream blockers of the RAAS stimulate renin release and elevate angiotensin II levels due to disruption of the short feedback loop, whereby angiotensin II

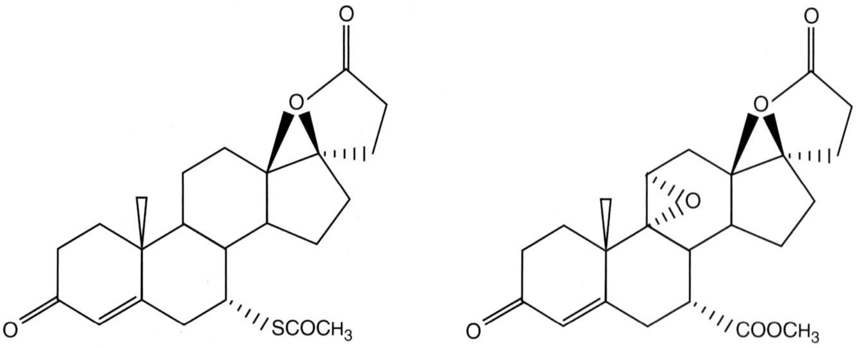

Spironolactone
SC-09420
$C_{24}H_{32}O_4S$
(416.58)

Eplerenone
SC-66110
$C_{24}H_{30}O_6$
(414.50)

**Figure 70–2** Chemical structures of spironolactone and eplerenone, the two mineralocorticoid receptor antagonists currently available in the United States. (With permission from Garthwaite SM, McMahon EG. The evolution of aldosterone antagonists. Mol Cell Endocrinol 217:27-31, 2004.)

**Table 70–1** Comparison of Spironolactone and Eplerenone Selectivity at Human Steroid Receptors

| | Eplerenone (uM) | Spironolactone (uM) |
|---|---|---|
| MR (IC$_{50}$) | 0.081 | 0.002 |
| AR (IC$_{50}$) | 4.827 | 0.013 |
| GR (IC$_{50}$) | >100 | 2.899 |
| PR (EC$_{50}$) (agonist) | >100 | 2.619 |

IC$_{50}$, the concentration of antagonist required to inhibit by 50% activation by 0.5 nM aldosterone for MR, mineralocorticoid receptor, 10 nM dihydrotestosterone for AR, androgen receptor and 5 nM dexamethasone for GR, glucocorticoid receptor. EC$_{50}$, the concentration of ligand to achieve 50% activation of the PR, progesterone receptor compared with the full agonist progesterone (50 nM). (With permission from Garthwaite SM, McMahon EG. The evolution of aldosterone antagonists. Mol Cell Endocrinol 217:27-31, 2004.).

inhibits renin release.[54] In a similar manner, blockade of aldosterone action at MR in the distal nephron by eplerenone or spironolactone stimulates renin release and increases aldosterone levels via disruption of the long feedback loop. Thus a predicted pharmacodynamic response to mineralocorticoid blockade with spironolactone or eplerenone is a rise in plasma renin and aldosterone levels.[55] The rise in aldosterone levels in response to chronic MR blockade does not produce detrimental effects because the MR is not available for activation by aldosterone. Rather, the elevation in serum aldosterone in response to MR blockade with spironolactone or eplerenone is a useful biomarker of efficacious MR blockade in vivo. It is important to note that neither spironolactone or eplerenone, at clinically relevant concentrations, inhibits the key enzymes in the biosynthetic pathway for aldosterone production.[47]

## Blood Pressure–Lowering Activity of Eplerenone in Humans

The blood pressure–lowering activity of eplerenone was assessed in mild-to-moderate hypertensives in a double-blind, randomized, placebo-controlled trial of 8 weeks' duration.[55]

Blood pressure lowering with eplerenone (50, 100, and 400 mg once daily or 25, 50, or 200 mg twice daily) was compared with the response achieved with spironolactone administered at 50 mg twice daily or placebo. Seated and standing systolic and diastolic blood pressure reductions were significantly greater at all eplerenone doses compared with placebo ($p < .05$). The blood pressure lowering with eplerenone was dose dependent, and no consistent, clinically significant differences in lowering of blood pressure were observed when comparing once-daily with twice-daily dosing. Blood pressure lowering with eplerenone at 100 mg (50 mg twice daily or 100 mg once daily) was approximately 50% to 75% of that achieved with spironolactone, consistent with the greater potency of spironolactone for binding to the MR.

A more thorough dose-response study was conducted with once-daily dosing of eplerenone in a double-blind, placebo-controlled, parallel-arm, fixed-dose study in essential hypertensive patients studied for 12 weeks.[56] After single-blind placebo treatment for 3 to 4 weeks to obtain baseline measurements, patients were randomized to receive placebo or eplerenone at 25, 50, 100, or 200 mg once daily. As shown in Figure 70–3, after 12 weeks of treatment, reductions in clinic blood pressures showed a significant dose response in which 25 mg of eplerenone achieved statistical significance compared with placebo for systolic blood pressure. Maximum reductions in blood pressure were achieved with the 100-mg dose, and eplerenone was well tolerated in this 400+ patient study, with no difference in adverse event profiles in the eplerenone-treated groups compared with placebo.[56]

As expected, eplerenone treatment produced dose-dependent elevations in both active renin and aldosterone levels in plasma, consistent with disruption of the normal feedback loop by downstream effectors of the pathway (Figure 70–4). It is important to note that these measurements of renin and aldosterone were obtained 24 hours after the last dose of eplerenone. Therefore, the pharmacodynamic effect of eplerenone persists for 24 hours, even though the terminal plasma half-life of the molecule is only 4 to 6 hours. This dissociation between plasma half-life and the pharmacodynamic effect of eplerenone is expected based on the mechanism of action of the compound. The MR is a cytosolic protein, which binds aldosterone and translocates into the nucleus. In the nucleus, the

**Figure 70–3** Mean changes from baseline in seated blood pressure after 12 weeks of therapy with eplerenone (25-200 mg once daily) and placebo in essential hypertensive patients. Baseline seated systolic blood pressure (SBP) averaged 151-155 mm Hg, and seated diastolic blood pressure (DBP) averaged 100-101 mm Hg. (Redrawn from White WB, Carr AA, Krause S, et al. Assessment of the novel selective aldosterone blocker eplerenone using ambulatory and clinical blood pressure in patients with systemic hypertension. Am J Cardiol 92:38-42, 2003.)

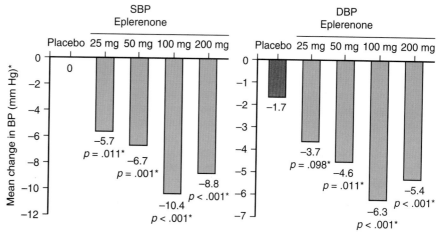

*p-Value vs. placebo based on ANCOVA using baseline as covariate and treatment and center as factors.

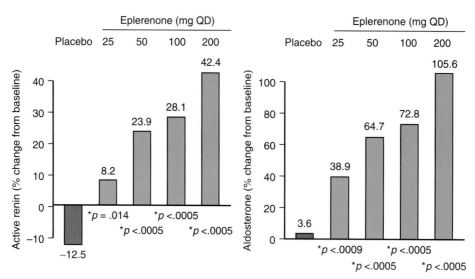

*p-Value vs. placebo based on ANCOVA using baseline as covariate and treatment and center as factors.

**Figure 70–4** Changes from baseline in active plasma renin and serum aldosterone in essential hypertensive patients after 12 weeks of eplerenone treatment (25-200 mg once daily) and placebo. (Redrawn with permission from White WB, Carr AA, Krause S, et al. Assessment of the novel selective aldosterone blocker eplerenone using ambulatory and clinical blood pressure in patients with systemic hypertension. Am J Cardiol 92:38-42, 2003.)

hormone-receptor complex functions as a transcription factor, whereby it binds to DNA, activating gene transcription and new protein synthesis. Therefore, the physiologic effects of aldosterone, like all steroid hormones, take hours to develop, and the response persists long after aldosterone has been cleared from plasma.[57] Likewise, blockade of this response by eplerenone can persist long after eplerenone has disappeared from the plasma. Thus, the prolonged biologic effect of eplerenone is due to this molecular mechanism of action.

The majority of patients with hypertension require two or more antihypertensive medications to achieve blood pressure treatment goals.[58] Because ACE inhibitors and ARBs often do not adequately suppress aldosterone, it was of interest to determine the efficacy and tolerability of eplerenone in patients not adequately controlled on these agents.[59] Hypertensive patients whose blood pressure was not controlled despite ACE inhibitor and ARB use, were randomized in a double-blinded fashion to receive either placebo once daily or eplerenone (50 mg once daily, increasing to 100 mg, if needed) for a period of 8 weeks. Mean seated diastolic blood pressure was significantly reduced ($-12.7 \pm 0.81$ mm Hg) at 8 weeks in patients receiving ARB/eplerenone compared with those on ARB/placebo ($-9.3 \pm 0.83$ mm Hg), as was systolic blood pressure ($-16.0 \pm 1.37$ vs. $-9.2 \pm 1.41$ mm Hg). For the ACE inhibitor–treated patients, systolic blood pressure was reduced significantly by the addition of eplerenone ($-13.4 \pm 1.35$ vs. $-7.5 \pm 1.31$ mm Hg), although diastolic blood pressure was not ($-9.9 \pm 0.88$ vs. $-8.0 \pm 0.86$ mm Hg). Thus selective aldosterone blockade with eplerenone may be useful as add-on therapy in hypetensive patients who are not adequately controlled on an ACE inhibitor or an ARB alone.

It is well known that hypertension and its complications disproportionately affect African Americans compared with whites.[60] Mortality risk from hypertensive heart disease and renal disease is twofold higher in African Americans compared with whites.[61] In addition, African-American hypertensives are more likely to have low renin levels and therefore are less responsive to monotherapy with blockers of the renin-angiotensin system.[62] A recent study compared the efficacy of eplerenone treatment versus losartan in hypertensive Black patients (study population included Blacks living in South Africa as well as Black African Americans). The effects of these two agents were also compared in white patients.[63] In a randomized, double-blind, placebo- and active-controlled, placebo run-in, parallel-group design, patients with mild-to-moderate hypertension were randomized to placebo, eplerenone (starting at 50 mg once daily up to 200 mg once daily), or losartan (starting at 50 mg once daily up to 100 mg once a day, the maximal recommended dose) to achieve a blood pressure of less than 140/90 mm Hg. Duration of treatment was 16 weeks. Eplerenone was more efficacious at lowering both diastolic (Figure 70–5) and systolic blood pressure (Figure 70–6) in Black hypertensives compared with losartan and placebo. In white patients, losartan and eplerenone were equally efficacious at lowering both systolic and diastolic blood pressure. The incidence of adverse events was similar in the three treatment groups (placebo, losartan, and eplerenone), and no clinically relevant differences in laboratory values were observed, with small increases in serum potassium concentrations within the normal range noted with eplerenone treatment.

Isolated systolic hypertension, primarily in the elderly, is another difficult-to-treat form of hypertension that is increasing in prevalence because the elderly (>60 years of age) are the most rapidly growing segment of our population. Improved treatment of systolic hypertension is an important goal because systolic blood pressure is a stronger predictor of cardiovascular risk that elevated diastolic blood pressure.[64] The effects of eplerenone and amlodipine on isolated systolic hypertension in the elderly have been compared to assess the usefulness of aldosterone blockade with eplerenone in older patients.[65] Eplerenone was highly effective at lowering systolic

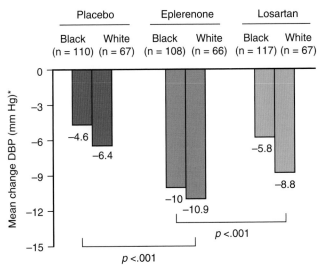

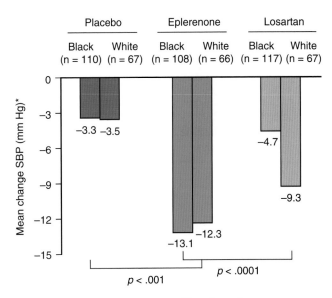

**Figure 70-5** Mean changes in diastolic blood pressure (DBP) for placebo-, eplerenone-, and losartan-treated patients with essential hypertension after 16 weeks of therapy. Treatment was initiated with daily doses of eplerenone 50 mg, losartan 50 mg, or matching placebo. If DBP was ≥90 mm Hg or if systolic blood pressure was ≥140 mm Hg at weeks 4, 8, or 12, the dose was increased to 100 mg/day of losartan and eplerenone. If blood pressure remained above 140/90 mm Hg, the dose was increased to eplerenone 200 mg/day or continued at losartan 100 mg/day, the maximal recommended dose. (Redrawn with permission from Flack JM, Oparil S, Pratt JH, et al. Efficacy and tolerability of eplerenone and losartan in hypertensive black and white patients. J Am Coll Cardiol 41:1148-1155, 2003.)

**Figure 70-6** Mean changes in systolic blood pressure (SBP) for placebo-, eplerenone-, and losartan-treated patients with essential hypertension after 16 weeks of therapy. Treatment was initiated with daily doses of eplerenone 50 mg, losartan 50 mg, or matching placebo. If diastolic blood pressure was ≥90 mm Hg or if SBP was ≥140 mm Hg at weeks 4, 8, or 12, the dose was increased to 100 mg/day of losartan and eplerenone. If blood pressure remained above 140/90 mm Hg, the dose was increased to eplerenone 200 mg/day or continued at losartan 100 mg/day, the maximal recommended dose. (Redrawn with permission from Flack JM, Oparil S, Pratt JH, et al. Efficacy and tolerability of eplerenone and losartan in hypertensive black and white patients. J Am Coll Cardiol 41:1148-1155, 2003.)

blood pressure in this group of patients. After 24 weeks of treatment in patients with a baseline blood pressure of 168/86 mm Hg, eplerenone lowered systolic blood pressure by $20.5 \pm 1.1$ mm Hg compared with $20.1 \pm 1.1$ mm Hg with amlodipine. Diastolic blood pressure was slightly lower with amlodipine ($-6.9 \pm 0.7$ mm Hg) compared with eplerenone ($-4.5 \pm 0.7$ mm Hg [$p = .014$]). The effects of eplerenone and amlodipine treatment on arterial pulse wave velocity were assessed in a subset of patients in the study. Interestingly, reductions in baseline carotid-femoral and carotid-radial pulse wave velocity were significant in the eplerenone and amlodipine groups, and both compounds lowered pulse wave velocity similarly. This suggests that both compounds are effective in improving vascular compliance or reducing vessel wall stiffness. Both amlodipine and eplerenone had good tolerability and safety profiles in this older-patient population.

LVH is associated with a markedly increased risk of cardiovascular events in essential hypertensive patients, independent of blood pressure.[66] In essential hypertensive patients, LV mass index correlated strongly with serum aldosterone levels even after adjustments for blood pressure.[6] These data suggest that aldosterone blockade in hypertension may lead to regression of LVH. A 9-month double-blind, randomized study was performed to determine whether aldosterone blockade with

eplerenone, alone or in combination with an ACE inhibitor, could lead to regression of LVH in essential hypertensive patients.[67] Patients with LVH were randomly assigned to receive eplerenone (200 mg once daily), enalapril (40 mg once daily), or eplerenone (200 mg once daily) with enalapril (10 mg once daily). Changes in LV mass were measured using magnetic resonance imaging (MRI). Eight weeks into the study, hydrochlorothiazide or amlodipine could be added, if diastolic blood pressure remained above 90 mm Hg. As shown in Figure 70-7, eplerenone and enalapril monotherapies significantly reduced LV mass, and the combination resulted in a reduction in LV mass that was greater than the effect of eplerenone-alone and numerically not statistically greater than the enalapril alone response. LVH regression achieved with aldosterone blockade was additive to that seen with ACE inhibition alone. Reductions in diastolic blood pressure were similar in the three treatment groups, as were reductions in systolic blood pressure, although the fall in systolic pressure was somewhat greater in the enalapril/eplerenone group compared to the eplerenone-alone group (Figure 70–8). When the relationship between changes in LV mass and changes in blood pressure was examined, blood pressure reduction alone did not account for the LVH regression. This conclusion is similar to those reached by investigatiors in the LIFE study

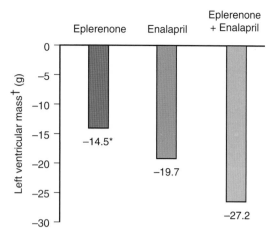

†Adjusted to treatment, center, and baseline value.
*p-Value eplerenone vs. eplerenone + enalapril: p = .007

**Figure 70–7** Adjusted mean change in LV mass from baseline as measured by cardiac MRI after 9 months of treatment in hypertensive patients with LVH treated with eplerenone, enalapril, or the combination of enalapril and eplerenone. LVH was diagnosed by either ECG or echocardiogram. After withdrawal of antihypertensive medications, patients took placebo for a 14-day, single-blind, run-in period. Patients were then randomly assigned to receive once-daily eplerenone (200 mg), enalapril (40 mg), or eplerenone (200 mg) with enalapril (10 mg). These doses were reached after a 4-week forced titration schedule. If blood pressure was not controlled (diastolic blood pressure ≥90 mm Hg or systolic blood pressure >180 mm Hg at week 8), patients received open-label hydrochlorothiazide 12.5-25 mg and/or amlodipine 10 mg. (Redrawn with permission from Pitt B, Reichek N, Willenbrock R, et al. Effects of eplerenone, enalapril, and eplerenone/enalapril in patients with essential hypertension and left ventricular hypertrophy. The 4E-left ventricular hypertrophy study. Circulation 108: 1831-1838, 2003.)

(Losartan Intervention For Endpoint Reduction), in which LV mass reduction was independent of blood pressure reduction.[68] Additional studies are required to understand the optimal dose-response relationship of eplerenone with an ACE inhibitor in this patient population and to establish that the combination of ACE inhibitor and eplerenone reduces morbidity and mortality in patients with essential hypertension and LVH.

Numerous preclinical studies support the notion that aldosterone blockade is renal protective in hypertensive animal models, independent of blood pressure lowering.[69] Rocha et al. demonstrated that removal of aldosterone, either by adrenalectomy or through administration of the selective aldosterone receptor antagonist eplerenone, markedly reduced renal damage, independent of blood pressure reduction, in the L-NAME/Ang II/salt-hypertensive rat model.[22] In this study, adrenalectomy or eplerenone treatment prevented the development of proteinuria in L-NAME/Ang II/salt-treated rats, and the add back of aldosterone to the adrenalectomized rats restored the proteinuria associated with L-NAME/Ang II/salt treatment. These studies suggest that aldosterone, rather than

Ang II, may be the important mediator of renal damage in hypertensive models produced via activation of the RAAS.

A clinical study has been conducted to determine whether aldosterone blockade with eplerenone is as effective as enalapril in reducing microalbuminuria in type 2 diabetic hypertensive patients and whether the combination may be more effective than either monotherapy.[70] Type 2 diabetic patients with mild-to-moderate hypertension and microalbuminuria (urinary albumin/creatinine ratio [UACR] ≥100 mg/g) were randomly assigned to receive initially once-daily treatment with eplerenone 50 mg, enalapril 10 mg, or the combination of both. Study medications were force-titrated up at week 2 and week 4, regardless of blood pressure level, to the maximum doses (200 mg of eplerenone, 40 mg of enalapril, or eplerenone 200 mg/enalapril 10 mg). At week 8 or later, if blood pressure remained uncontrolled (≥90 mm Hg), hydrochlorothiazide (12.5-25 mg) could be added, if needed. Treatment effects on UACR and blood pressure are shown in Table 70–2. Eplerenone reduced proteinuria significantly (by 62%) after 6 months of treatment, compared with 45% in the enalapril group and 74% in the eplerenone/enalapril group (p<.001 vs. baseline for all treatments). Interestingly, the combination of eplerenone/enalapril reduced proteinuria to a greater extent than either monotherapy, suggesting that the renoprotective effects of aldosterone blockade are additive to the ACE inhibitor effects. Blood pressure reductions were similar in all treatment groups except that diastolic blood pressure was reduced more in the eplerenone/enalapril combination group compared with the eplerenone monotherapy group (−16.2 ± 0.86 vs. −13.2 ± 0.84 mm Hg; p=.015). Systolic blood pressure was reduced similarly in all three groups, suggesting that the antiproteinuric effects of these treatments are somewhat independent of blood pressure lowering. Elevated serum potassium was noted because maximal doses of eplerenone and enalapril were used, but potassium elevations were comparable with what has been reported with ACE inhibitors in similar patient populations.[71,72] However, additional studies are required to explore the dose range of eplerenone and enalapril that would mitigate the risk of elevated potassium but still preserve the renoprotective effects of these two therapeutic interventions.

Analysis of the relationship between blood pressure lowering and serum potassium concentration with eplerenone in essential hypertensives has produced some surprising results.[73] Two titration-to-effect clinical trials with similar study designs were used to determine whether the blood pressure–lowering response to eplerenone was related to changes in serum potassium. One would presume that serum potassium changes are a marker of eplerenone inhibition of aldosterone effects on sodium and potassium excretion in the distal tubule, a classic epithelial target tissue of aldosterone. A total of 397 patients from two double-blind, randomized, multicenter, placebo-controlled, lead-in, parallel-group, titration-to-effect studies were included in the analysis. After a 4-week placebo run-in, patients were given 50 mg of eplerenone once daily. If after 4 weeks any participant did not meet blood pressure goals, he or she was up-titrated to 100 mg. After 8 weeks, patients not achieving goals were further up-titrated to 200 mg once daily. Antihypertensive response status was defined by diastolic blood pressure (<90 mm Hg were responders; ≥90 mm Hg were nonresponders). Figure 70–9 shows the reduction in systolic blood pressure in "responders"

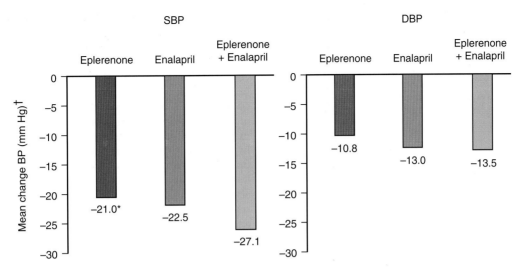

†Adjusted to treatment, center, and baseline value.
*p-Value eplerenone vs. eplerenone + enalapril: p = .017

**Figure 70-8** Systolic and diastolic blood pressure after 9 months of treatment in hypertensive patients with LVH treated with eplerenone, enalapril, or the combination of enalapril plus eplerenone. LVH was diagnosed by either ECG or echocardiogram. After withdrawal of antihypertensive medications, patients took placebo for a 14-day, single-blind, run-in period. Patients were then randomly assigned to receive once-daily eplerenone (200 mg), enalapril (40 mg), or eplerenone (200 mg) with enalapril (10 mg). These doses were reached after a 4-week forced titration schedule. If blood pressure was not controlled (diastolic blood pressure ≥90 mm Hg or systolic blood pressure >180 mm Hg at week 8), patients received open-label hydrochlorothiazide 12.5-25 mg and/or amlodipine 10 mg. (Redrawn with permission from Pitt B, Reichek N, Willenbrock R, et al. Effects of eplerenone, enalapril, and eplerenone/enalapril in patients with essential hypertension and left ventricular hypertrophy. The 4E-left ventricular hypertrophy study. Circulation 108:1831-1838, 2003.)

**Table 70-2** Antiproteinuric and Blood Pressure–Lowering Effect of Eplerenone Monotherapy, Enalapril Monotherapy, and Enalapril with Enalapril in Hypertensive Patients with Type II Diabetes

| | EPL | ENAL | EPL + ENAL |
|---|---|---|---|
| **UACR** | | | |
| N | 74 | 74 | 67 |
| Baseline UACR (mg/g) | 611 | 483 | 471 |
| Δ UACR (week 24 vs. baseline) | -62% | -45% | -74% |
| p-Values vs. ENAL | .015 | | |
| p-Values vs. EPL + ENAL | .018 | <.001 | |
| **BP** | | | |
| N | 89 | 83 | 85 |
| Δ SBP/DBP (week 8 vs. baseline) | -13.5/10.2 | -15.4/11.6 | -16.5/12.8 |
| Δ SBP/DBP (week 24 vs. baseline) | -19.5/-13.2* | -20.4/-15.0 | -21.8/-16.2 |

For UACR (urinary albumin:creatinine ratio), results are expressed as mean percent change from baseline at the week-24 endpoint. For blood pressure (BP), results are expressed as mean decreases at week 24 from baseline systolic (SBP) or diastolic blood pressure (DBP). (With permission from Epstein M, Buckalew V, Martinez F, et al. Antiproteinuric efficacy of eplerenone, enalapril, and eplerenone/enalapril combination therapy in diabetic hypertensives with microalbuminuria (Abstract). Am J Hypertens 15:24A, 2002.)
*p = .015 vs. EPL + ENAL.
EPL, eplereone; ENAL, enalapril; UACR, urinary albumin:creatinine ratio; SBP, systolic blood pressure; DBP, diastolic blood pressure.

and "nonresponders" and changes in serum potassium over time. Interestingly, the change in serum potassium did not predict the antihypertensive response to eplerenone at any dose. Such findings suggest that the antihypertensive action of eplerenone is linked to blockade of aldosterone effects on nonclassic, nonepithelial target tissues (brain, heart, vascular smooth muscle) rather than classic, epithelial, electrolyte transporting target tissues, such as the kidney.

## SUMMARY

There is now compelling evidence that aldosterone mediates significant deleterious effects on the cardiovascular system by binding and activating MR in the heart, brain, and blood vessels. These effects include vascular inflammation and injury, endothelial dysfunction, myocardial and vascular fibrosis, proarrhythmogenic, and hypertrophic effects on cardiomy-

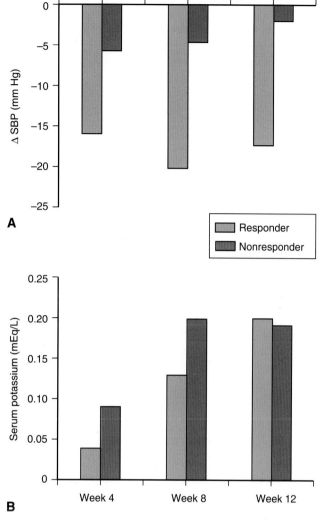

**A**

**B**

**Figure 70–9** Changes in systolic blood pressure **(A)** as a function of changes in serum potassium concentration **(B)** for responders and nonresponders at each week/dose interval in patients from two clinical studies conducted as part of the eplerenone Phase III hypertension development program. Data from essential hypertensive patients in the two double-blind, randomized, multicenter, placebo-controlled, titration-to-effect studies were pooled for analysis. Patients were given 50 mg of eplerenone once daily, and if after 4 weeks, blood pressure goals were not met, these patients were up-titrated to 100 mg of eplerenone once daily. An additional up-titration to 200 mg once dialy occurred, if necessary. (With permission from Levy DG, Rocha R, Funder JW. Distinguishing the antihypertensive and electrolyte effects of eplerenone. J Clin Endocrinol Metab 89:2736-2749, 2004.)

ocytes and centrally mediated hypertensive effects. In addition to the classic genomic effects of aldosterone, nongenomic actions have been identified in vascular tissue. Blockade of aldosterone at MR produces target organ protective effects in hypertensive patients by reducing LVH and microalbuminuria. Eplerenone is significantly more selective for MR than spironolactone, and this improved selectivity measured in vitro has translated into improved tolerability compared

with spironolactone. Interestingly, preliminary studies suggest that eplerenone blocks nongenomic effects of aldosterone in vascular tissues, whereas spironolactone does not. However, it is not clear whether nongenomic effects of aldosterone contribute to the detrimental action of aldosterone on the cardiovascular system. Eplerenone lowers blood pressure quite effectively in essential hypertensive patients, irrespective of race, age, or gender. This could be due to the fact that primary aldosteronism is a substantially more common cause of hypertension than was previously appreciated.[74-76] although this hypothesis remains somewhat controversial.[77] Nonetheless, with only a minority of treated hypertensive patients actually reaching target blood pressures, eplerenone (Inspra) represents an important addition to the armamentarium of agents to treat this disorder.

## References

1. United States Renal Data System. 2003 Annual Data Report.
2. American Heart Association. 2003 Heart and Stroke Statistical update. Dallas, American Heart Association, 2004.
3. Hajjar I, Kotchen T. Trends in prevalence, awareness, treatment and control of hypertension in the United States, 1988-2000. JAMA 290:199-206, 2003.
4. 1999 World Health Organization-International Society of Hypertension-Guidelines for the Management of Hypertension. J Hypertens 17:151-183, 1999.
5. Swedberg K, Eneroth P, Kjekshus J, et al. Hormones regulating cardiovascular function in patients with severe congestive heart failure and their relation to mortality. CONSENSUS Trial Study Group. Circulation 82:1730-1736, 1990.
6. Duprez DA, Bauwens FR, De Buyzere ML, et al. Influence of arterial blood pressure and aldosterone on left ventricular hypertrophy in moderate essential hypertension. Am J Cardiol 71:17A-20A, 1993.
7. Duprez DA, De Buyzere ML, De Backer T, et al. Influence of systemic arterial blood pressure and nonhemodynamic factors on the brachial artery pulsatility index in mild to moderate essential hypertension. Am J Cardiol 71:350-353, 1993.
8. Rossi GP, Sacchetto A, Visentin P, et al. Changes in left ventricular anatomy and function in hypertension and primary aldosteronism. Hypertension 27:1039-1045, 1996.
9. Halimi J-M, Mimram A. Albuminuria in untreated patients with primary aldosteronism or essential hypertension. J Hypertens 13:1801-1802, 1995.
10. Staessen J, Lijnen P, Fagard R, et al. Rise in plasma aldosterone concentration during long-term angiotensin II suppression. J Endocrinol 91:457-465, 1981.
11. Jorde UP, Ennezat PV, Lisker J, et al. Maximally recommended doses of angiotensin-converting enzyme (ACE) inhibitors do not completely prevent ACE-mediated formation of angiotensin II in chronic heart failure. Circulation 101:844-846, 2000.
12. Sato A, Hayashi K, Naruse M, et al. Effectiveness of aldosterone blockade in patients with diabetic nephropathy. Hypertension 41:64-68, 2003.
13. McKelvie RS, Yusuf S, Pericak D, et al. Comparison of candesartan, enalapril, and their combination in congestive heart failure: Randomized Evaluation of Strategies for Left Ventricular Dysfunction (RESOLVD) pilot study. The RESOLVD Pilot Study Investigators. Circulation 100:1056-1064, 1999.
14. Quinn SJ, Williams GH. Regulation of aldosterone secretion. Annu Rev Physiol 50:409-426, 1988.
15. Lombes M, Farman N, Bonvalet JP, et al. Identification and role of aldosterone receptors in the cardiovascular system. Ann Endocrinol (Paris) 61:41-46, 2000.

16. Silvestre J-S, Heymes C, Oubénaïssa A, et al. Activation of cardiac aldosterone production in rat myocardial infarction: effect of angiotensin II receptor blockade and role in cardiac fibrosis. Circulation 99:2694-2701, 1999.

17. Mizuno Y, Yoshimura M, Yasue H, et al. Aldosterone production is activated in failing ventricle in humans. Circulation 103:72-77, 2001.

18. Yamamoto N, Yasue H, Mizuno Y, et al. Aldosterone is produced from ventricles in patients with essential hypertension. Hypertension 39:958-962, 2002.

19. Roland BL, Krozowski ZS, Funder JW. Glucocorticoid receptor, mineralocorticoid receptors, 11 beta-hydroxysteroid dehydrogenase-1 and -2 in rat brain and kidney: In situ studies. Mol Cell Endocrinol 111:R1-R7, 1995.

20. Kornel L, Smoszna-Fonaszewska B. Aldosterone (ALDO) increases transmembrane influx of $Na^+$ in vascular smooth muscle (VSM) cells through increased synthesis of $Na^+$ channels. Steroids 60:114-119, 1995.

21. Brilla CG, Weber KT. Mineralocorticoid excess, dietary sodium and myocardial fibrosis. J Lab Clin Med 120:893-901, 1992.

22. Rocha R, Stier CT Jr, Kifor I, et al. Aldosterone: A mediator of myocardial necrosis and renal arteriopathy. Endocrinology 141:3871-3878, 2000.

23. Rocha R, Martin-Berger CL, Yang P, et al. Selective aldosterone blockade prevents angiotensin II/salt-induced vascular inflammation in the rat heart. Endocrinology 143:4828-4836, 2002.

24. Young MJ, Funder JW. The renin-angiotensin-aldosterone system in experimental mineralocorticoid-salt induced cardiac fibrosis. Am J Physiol 271:E883-E888, 1996.

25. Rocha R, Rudolph AE, Frierdich GE, et al. Aldosterone induces a vascular phenotype in the rat heart. Am J Physiol 283:H1802-H1810, 2002.

26. Lacolley P, Labat C, Pujol A, et al. Increased carotid wall elastic modulus and fibronectin in aldosterone-salt-treated hypertensive rats. Effects of eplerenone. Circulation 106:2848-2853, 2002.

27. Benetos A, Lacolley P, and Safar ME. Prevention of aortic fibrosis by spironolactone in spontaneously hypertensive rats. Arterioscler Thromb Vasc Biol 17:1152-1156, 1997.

28. Blacher J, Amah G, Girerd X, et al. Association between increased plasma levels of aldosterone and decreased systemic arterial compliance in subjects with essential hypertension. Am J Hypertens 10:1326-1334, 1997.

29. Brown NJ, Nakamura S, Ma L, et al. Aldosterone modulates plasminogen activator inhibitor-1 and glomerulosclerosis in vivo. Kidney Int 58:1219-1227, 2000.

30. Farquharson CAJ, Struthers AD. Spironolactone increases nitric oxide bioactivity, improves endothelial vasodilator dysfunction, and suppresses vascular angiotensin I/angiotensin II conversion in patients with chronic heart failure. Circulation 101:594-597, 2000.

31. Schafer A, Fraccarollo D, Hildeman SK, et al. Addition of the selective aldosterone receptor antagonist eplerenone to ACE inhibition in heart failure: effect on endothelial dysfunction. Cardiovasc Res 58:655-662, 2003.

32. Quaschning T, Ruschitzka F, Shaw S, et al. Aldosterone receptor antagonism normalizes vascular function in liquorice-induced hypertension. Hypertension 37:801-805, 2001.

33. Mihailidou AS, Bundgaard J, Mardini M, et al. Hyperaldosteronemia in rabbits inhibits the cardiac sarcolemmal $Na^+$-$K^+$ pump. Circ Res 86:37-42, 2000.

34. Mihailidou AS, Mardini M, Funder JW, et al. Mineralocorticoid and angiotensin receptor antagonism during hyperaldosteronemia. Hypertension 40:124-129, 2002.

35. Komentiani P, Li J, Gnudi L, et al. Multiple signal transduction pathways link $Na^+/K^+$-ATPase to growth-related genes in cardiac myocytes. J Biol Chem 24:15249-15256, 1998.

36. Gomez-Sanchez EP. Intracerebroventricular infusion of aldosterone induces hypertension in rats. Endocrinology 118:819-823, 1986.

37. Gomez-Sanchez EP, Fort C, Thwaites D. Central mineralocorticoid receptor antagonism blocks hypertension in Dahl J/JR rats. Am J Physiol 262:E96-E99, 1992.

38. Funder JW. Non-genomic actions of aldosterone: Role in hypertension. Curr Opin Nephrol Hypertens 10:227-230, 2001.

39. Alzamora R, Michea L, Marusic ET. Role of 11beta-hydroxysteroid dehydrogenase in nongenomic aldosterone effects in human arteries. Hypertension 35:1099-1104, 2000.

40. McMahon EG. Eplerenone, a new selective aldosterone blocker. Curr Pharm Des 1065-1075, 2003.

41. Alzamora R, Marusic ET, Gonzalez M, et al. Nongenomic effect of aldosterone on $Na^+$-$K^+$-adenosine triphosphatase in arterial vessels. Endocrinology 144:1266-1272, 2003.

42. Gunaruwan P, Schmitt M, Taylor J, et al. Lack of rapid aldosterone effects on forearm resistance vasculature in health. J Renin Angiotensin Aldosterone Syst 3:123-125, 2002.

43. Romagni P, Rossi F, Guerrini L, et al. Aldosterone induces contraction of the resistance arteries in man. Atherosclerosis 166:345-349, 2003.

44. Schmidt BMW, Oehmer S, Delles C, et al. Rapid nongenomic effects of aldosterone on human forearm vasculature. Hypertension 42:156-160, 2003.

45. Cella J, Brown EA, Burtner RR. Steroidal aldosterone blockers. Int J Org Chem 24:743-748, 1959.

46. Greenblatt DJ, Koch-Weser J. Adverse reactions to spironolactone: a report from the Boston Collaborative Drug Surveillance Program. JAMA 225:40-43, 1973.

47. deGasparo M, Joss U, Ramjoue HP, et al. Three new epoxyspironolactone derivatives: characterization in vivo and in vitro. J Pharm Exp Ther 240:650-656, 1987.

48. Garthwaite SM, McMahon EG. The evolution of aldosterone antagonists. Mol Cell Endocrinol 217:27-31, 2004.

49. Burgess ED, Lacourciere Y, Ruilope LM, et al. Long-term safety and efficacy of the selective aldosterone blocker eplerenone in patients with essential hypertension. Clin Ther 25(9):2388-2404, 2003.

50. Karim A. Spironolactone: disposition, metabolism, pharmacodynamics and bioavailability. Drug Metab Rev 8:151-188, 1978.

51. U.S. Package Insert for Inspra.

52. Abshagen U, von Grodzicki U, Hirschberger U, et al. Effect of enterohepatic circulation on the pharmacokinetics of spironolactone in man. Naunyn Schmiedebergs Arch Pharmacol 300:281-287, 1977.

53. Sadee W, Schroder R, vonLeitner E, et al. Multiple dose kinetics of spironolactone and canrenoate-potassium in cardiac and hepatic failure. Eur J Clin Pharmacol 7(3):195-200, 1974.

54. Davis JO, Freeman RH. Mechanisms regulating renin release. Physiol Rev 56:1-56, 1976.

55. Weinberger MH, Roniker B, Krause SL, et al. Eplerenone, a selective aldosterone blocker, in mild-to-moderate hypertension. Am J Hypertens 15:709-716, 2002.

56. White WB, Carr AA, Krause S, et al. Assessment of the novel selective aldosterone blocker eplerenone using ambulatory and clinical blood pressure in patients with systemic hypertension. Am J Cardiol 92:38-42, 2003.

57. Stockand JD. New ideas about aldosterone signaling in epithelia. Am J Physiol Renal Physiol 282:F559-F576, 2002.

58. Chobanian AV, Bakris GL, Black HR, et al. National high blood pressure education program coordinating committee. The seventh report of the Joint National Committee on Prevention, Detection, Evaluation and Treatment of High Blood Pressure: The JNC 7 report. Hypertension 42:1206-1252, 2003.

59. Krum H, Nolly H, Workman D, et al. Efficacy of eplerenone added to renin-angiotensin blockade in hypertensive patients. Hypertension 40:117-123, 2002.

60. Coresh J, Jaar B. Further trends in the etiology of end-stage renal disease in African-Americans. Curr Opin Nephrol Hypertens 6:243-249, 1997.

61. Hoyert DL, Kochanek KD, Murphy SL. Deaths: Final data for 1997. Natl Vital Stat Rep 47:1-104, 1999.

62. Flack JM, Saunders E, Gradman M, et al. Antihypertensive efficacy and safety of losartan alone and in combination with hydrochlorothiazide in adult African Americans with mild to moderate hypertension. Clin Ther 23:1193-1208, 2001.

63. Flack JM, Oparil S, Pratt JH, et al. Efficacy and tolerability of eplerenone and losartan in hypertensive black and white patients. J Am Coll Cardiol 41:1148-1155, 2003.

64. Stamler J, Stamler R, Neaton J. Blood pressure, systolic and diastolic, and cardiovascular risks: U.S. population data. Arch Intern Med 153:598-615, 1993.

65. White WB, Duprez D, St. Hillaire R, et al. Effects of the selective aldosterone blocker eplerenone versus the calcium antagonist amlodipine in systolic hypertension. Hypertension 41:1021-1026, 2003.

66. Benjamin EJ, Levy D. Why is left ventricular hypertrophy so predictive of morbidity and mortality? Am J Med Sci 317:168-175, 1999.

67. Pitt B, Reichek N, Willenbrock R, et al. Effects of eplerenone, enalapril, and eplerenone/enalapril in patients with essential hypertension and left ventricular hypertrophy. The 4E-left ventricular hypertrophy study. Circulation 108:1831-1838, 2003.

68. Dahlof B, Devereux RB, Kjeldsen SE, et al. LIFE study group. Cardiovascular morbidity and mortality in the Losartan Intervention For Endpoint reduction in hypertension study (LIFE): A randomized trial against atenolol. Lancet 359:995-1003, 2002.

69. Stier CT, Chander PN, Rocha R. Aldosterone as a mediator in cardiovascular injury. Cardiol Rev 10:97-107, 2002.

70. Epstein M, Buckalew V, Martinez F, et al. Antiproteinuric efficacy of eplerenone, enalapril, and eplerenone/enalapril combination therapy in diabetic hypertensives with microalbuminuria (Abstract). Am J Hypertens 15:24A, 2002.

71. Lewis EJ, Hunsicker LG, Bain RP, et al. The effect of angiotensin-converting enzyme on diabetic nephropathy. The Collaborative Study Group. N Engl J Med 329:1456-1462, 1993.

72. Maschio G, Alberti D, Janin G, et al. The angiotensin-converting-enzyme inhibition in progressive renal insufficiency study group. N Engl J Med 334:939-945, 1996.

73. Levy DG, Rocha R, Funder JW. Distinguishing the antihypertensive and electrolyte effects of eplerenone. J Clin Endocrinol Metab 89:2736-2740, 2004.

74. Calhoun DA, Nishizaka MK, Zaman MA, et al. Hyperaldosteronism among black and white subjects with resistant hypertension. Hypertension 40:892-896, 2002.

75. Lim PO, MacDonald TM. Primary aldosteronism, diagnosed by the aldosterone to renin ratio, is a common cause of hypertension. Clin Endocrinol 59:427-530, 2003.

76. Mosso L, Carvajal C, Gonzalez A, et al. Primary aldosteronism and hypertensive disease. Hypertension 42:161-165, 2003.

77. Kaplan NM. Cautions over the current epidemic of primary aldosteronism. Lancet 357:953-954, 2001.

# Chapter 71

# Vasopeptidase Inhibitors

## Luis Miguel Ruilope

## INTRODUCTION

Studies performed in the past 50 years have clearly documented that hypertension is a major risk factor for cardiovascular morbidity and mortality.[1] Furthermore, the reduction of diastolic and systolic blood pressure with drugs is associated with a reduction of almost all hypertension-related diseases, such as stroke, myocardial infarction (MI), heart failure, and vascular mortality.[2-6] Treatment with any commonly used regimen reduces the risk of total major cardiovascular events, and larger reductions in blood pressure produce larger reductions in risk.[6] These findings have made research on antihypertensive drugs extremely active, with the development of a wide range of agents that act through different mechanisms and thus attack high blood pressure from different angles.

Vasopeptidase inhibitors are a class of drugs that simultaneously inhibit both angiotensin-converting enzyme (ACE) and neutral endopeptidase (NEP). ACE inhibitors have a well-established clinical role in hypertension and heart failure[7] (see Chapter 35).

NEP is a membrane-bound metalloprotease found principally in the brush-border membrane of renal tubules, in the lungs, intestine, adrenal, brain, heart, and peripheral blood vessels.[8,9] NEP plays a role in the initial enzymatic degradation of the bioactive carboxyterminal portions of the natriuretic peptides and has many other substrates, for example, adrenomedullin, angiotensins I and II, endothelin, bradykinin, substance P, chemotactic peptide, enkephalins, and the amyloid ($\beta$) peptide.[10,11]

The natriuretic peptides constitute a family of peptides involved in the regulation of blood pressure and plasma volume.[12] The atrial and brain-derived natriuretic peptides are produced principally in the myocardium in response to atrial distention. C-type natriuretic peptide, found in the kidney, heart, lung, and vascular endothelium, is released in response to shear stress.[9] These peptides bind to specific, high-affinity cell-surface receptors. Natriuretic peptides exert physiologic effects at several sites, resulting in vasodilation, natriuresis, diuresis, decreased aldosterone release, decreased cell growth, and inhibition of the sympathetic nervous system and the renin-angiotensin-aldosterone system.[12] Atrial natriuretic peptide also inhibits production of endothelin.[13]

## NEUTRAL ENDOPEPTIDASE INHIBITION

Because inhibition of NEP protects the natriuretic peptides and bradykinin from catabolism, it should be beneficial in hypertension and congestive heart failure treatments. However, discordant findings have been reported in hypertensive patients.[14-17] The variable effect of NEP inhibition on blood pressure and systemic vascular resistance is likely to be due to increased levels of some vasoconstrictors such as Ang II and endothelin and to reduced levels of the vasodilator Ang-(1-7). Increased blood pressure during NEP inhibition in healthy volunteers was associated with an increase in plasma endothelin levels.[17] Both animal and clinical studies show that NEP inhibition increases the plasma levels of angiotensins I and II, aldosterone, and catecholamines.[14,15,18,19]

In patients with congestive heart failure, NEP inhibitors have beneficial hemodynamic effects. NEP inhibition is associated with reduced cardiac filling pressures and decreased indices of the renin axis.[20] NEP inhibition may also directly protect endothelial function and reduce atheromatous changes in the vascular wall.[21]

## Vasopeptidase Inhibitors: Rationale for Combining ACE and NEP Inhibitors

Like ACE, NEP is a peptidase found in both endothelial and epithelial cells, mainly in the lungs, kidneys, and blood vessels,[8,9] that blocks the renin system at different levels (see Chapter 9). Therefore, NEP inhibition protects natriuretic peptides from inactivation, whereas ACE inhibition attenuates the formation of angiotensin II, which acts as a physiologic antagonist of the atrial natriuretic peptide. ACE inhibition[22,23] not only interrupts the renin-angiotensin system, but also increases bradykinin, nitric oxide, and prostacyclin. Potential benefits of bradykinin include natriuretic, vasodilator, and cardioprotective effects; antihypertrophic and antiarrhythmogenic effects; and improved glucose uptake by myocytes.[24]

Simultaneous inhibition of both ACE and NEP lowers blood pressure more than inhibition of either enzyme alone in both animals and humans. For example, in patients given candoxatril (a NEP inhibitor) for a month, the blood pressure was unchanged,[25] and in healthy volunteers, candoxatril administration was followed by a rise in systolic pressure in association with an increase in the plasma concentration of endothelin.[17] However, in spontaneously hypertensive rats the combination of a NEP inhibitor (SCH 42495) and the ACE inhibitor captopril, as well as the dual NEP/ACE inhibitor S21402, reduced systolic blood pressure more effectively than the ACE inhibitor or the NEP inhibitor alone.[26] Favrat et al.[16] compared a NEP inhibitor (sinorphan) with captopril and with the two drugs in combination in patients with essential hypertension. Neither agent alone produced significant day-long blood pressure changes, but there were substantial decreases with the combination treatment.

Inhibition of NEP and ACE results in vasodilator effects and, possibly, tissue protective effects, at least in part to reduced formation of angiotensin II and reduced degradation of natriuretic peptides (Figure 71–1). Because NEP and ACE inhibitors are intimately concerned with regulating structural and functional properties of the heart and blood vessels, the term *vasopeptidase inhibitor* has been coined for this new drug class.

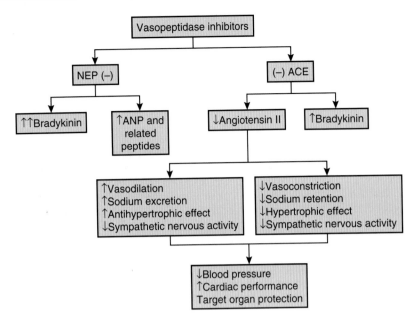

**Figure 71–1** Functional effects of vasopeptidase inhibition. NEP, neutral endopeptidase; ACE, angiotensin-converting enzyme; ANP, atrial natriuretic peptide.

## VASOPEPTIDASE INHIBITORS: AVAILABLE COMPOUNDS

Several dual ACE/NEP inhibitors have been developed; some have been assessed clinically, and others have not. The most studied vasopeptidase inhibitor is omapatrilat. After preclinical and preliminary clinical studies, omapatrilat was considered a very promising agent for treating patients with hypertension and congestive heart failure, the two main indications for which vasopeptidase inhibitors were targeted. However, an unacceptable high incidence of angioedema,[27] threefold higher than that of ACE inhibitors, has likely stopped the development of this new class of agents.

A description of some vasopeptidase inhibitors follows.

### Sampatrilat

Sampatrilat is a dual inhibitor of NEP and ACE, developed by Pfizer and Shire for the potential treatment of hypertension.[28] Sampatrilat reduced mean arterial pressure, improved daily sodium excretion, increased renal blood flow, and decreased left ventricular mass in a dog model of heart failure. In hypercholesterolemic rabbits, sampatrilat suppressed atherogenesis and improved endothelial function.[29] In rats with congestive heart failure following left coronary artery ligation (CAL), sampatrilat improved hemodynamic function and cardiac remodeling through a direct action on the failing heart.[30] Sampatrilat (30 mg/kg/day) was administered orally from the first to sixth week after the operation. Sampatrilat reduced the mortality of the rats with CAL (20% vs. 57% for untreated rats). Treatment with sampatrilat for 5 weeks suppressed tissue ACE and NEP activities. Sampatrilat did not affect arterial blood pressure but attenuated CAL-induced increases in the left ventricular end-diastolic pressure, heart weight, and collagen content of the viable left ventricle. The mechanism by which sampatrilat improved cardiac remodeling may be attributable to direct inhibition of cardiac fibrosis, possibly through the cardiac natriuretic peptide system. In humans, sampatrilat was tested clinically in a comparison with lisinopril in 120 patients with mild-to-moderate essential hypertension.[31] By day 10, 200 mg sampatrilat was nearly as effective as lisinopril 20 mg in lowering systolic pressure but was less effective in lowering diastolic pressure. ACE activity decreased by only 40% to 50%, and plasma renin activity during sampatrilat treatment was unchanged. In a study of African American patients with hypertension,[32] sampatrilat produced a sustained decrease in mean ambulatory blood pressure over the 56-day treatment period, with a greater treatment effect on diastolic blood pressure than lisinopril at day 56. Treatment-emergent adverse events were similar in both treatment groups.

### MDL 100,240

MDL 100,240 is a prodrug that, on conversion to MDL 100,173, acts as a potent dual inhibitor of ACE and NEP with a balanced effect on both enzymes. Studies in experimental models of hypertension and congestive heart failure confirmed the vasodilator and natriuretic effects of MDL, which appear to be independent of the degree of activation of the renin-angiotensin-aldosterone system. In addition, MDL 100,240 was effective both in preventing and regressing hypertension-induced vascular remodeling and cardiac hypertrophy.[33] In a transgenic rat model of hypertension[34] with severe cardiovascular damage due to enhanced tissue synthesis of angiotensin II both MDL 100,240 and ramipril significantly lowered blood pressure compared with placebo. Both drugs regressed left ventricular hypertrophy. MDL 100,240 also prevented aortic dilation and hypertrophy of the mesenteric arterioles and reduced constrictor responses to phenylephrine and endothelin-1, as well as plasma aldosterone and creatinine levels. Thus, severe hypertension and related cardiovascular disease were regressed by MDL 100,240. In 12 healthy volunteers, single 25-mg (intravenous) doses of the drug reduced systolic blood pressure, provided the diet contained no more than 80 mg sodium per day. Urinary flow rate increased significantly during the first 2 hours after dosing, together with an increase in sodium excretion. MDL 100,240 also increased excretion of uric acid.[35] In normal volunteers, MDL 100,240 had a half-life of about 7.5 hours during once daily administration.[36] There was no evidence of accumulation when it was administered over an 8-day period.

## Gemopatrilat

This azepinone derivative BMS-189921 showed blood pressure–lowering properties similar to omapatrilat in animal models of hypertension.[37] In normotensive Wistar nephrotic rats, the renoprotective actions of gemopatrilat were dependent on dietary-sodium intake: During a low-sodium diet, gemopatrilat was renoprotective but less effective than lisinopril. However, its therapeutic efficacy was completely abolished by a high-sodium diet.[38]

## Fasidotril

This compound also proved to be effective in animal models of hypertension.[39] Fasidotril treatment (100 mg/kg twice daily for 3 weeks) resulted in a progressive and sustained decrease in systolic blood pressure (−20 to −30 mm Hg) in spontaneously hypertensive and Goldblatt (renovascular) rats compared with vehicle-treated rats and prevented the progressive rise in blood pressure in DOCA-salt hypertensive rats.[39] At a dose of 100 mg twice daily, it was studied in a placebo-controlled trial in 57 patients with essential hypertension. After 42 days, supine and standing systolic and diastolic blood pressures were 7.4/5.4 mm Hg and 7.6/6.8 mm Hg lower, respectively, in the drug-treated than in the placebo group.[39]

## Mixanpril

Mixanpril is a benzotylthioacetate prodrug of S21402, which has been studied extensively in various rat rodent models.[40] S21402 decreased blood pressure similarly in DOCA-salt and renovascular hypertensive rats, indicating that the antihypertensive effect is independent of the renin-angiotensin system. In diabetic spontaneously hypertensive rats, mean systolic blood pressure (200 ± 5 mm Hg) was reduced by mixanpril (176 ± 2 mm Hg) as it was by captopril (162 ± 5 mm Hg), valsartan (173 ± 5 mm Hg), and amlodipine (159 ± 4 mm Hg), and was further reduced by the combination of captopril with valsartan (131 ± 5 mm Hg). Only mixanpril and the combination of captopril and valsartan significantly reduced mesenteric weight. The mesenteric wall:lumen ratio was reduced by all drugs but to a greater extent by the combination of captopril and valsartan.[41]

## Z-13752A

This drug has been studied in a canine model of coronary-artery occlusion, where it proved to be protective against the adverse consequences of intervention.[42] This protection was largely due to potentiation of released bradykinin.[43] Pharmacokinetic studies in healthy volunteers suggested that a once-daily dosing could be appropriate.[43]

## Omapatrilat

The most extensively investigated ACE/NEP inhibitor is omapatrilat (Bristol Myers Squibb). This compound has similar inhibitory activity against both ACE and NEP.[44]

## ANIMAL STUDIES

As reviewed by Weber[44] and more recently by Campbell,[45] multiple experimental studies have demonstrated that omapatrilat lowers blood pressure in animals. The major characteristic of omapatrilat is that it lowers blood pressure in all models of hypertension whatever the degree of activity of the renin-angiotensin system.[46] In Dahl salt-sensitive rats, a high-sodium diet significantly impaired endothelium-dependent relaxation. When these animals were treated with omapatrilat, there was a far greater return toward normal responsiveness than there was with captopril.[47] Relaxation was reduced to 31% of baseline by the high-salt diet, and was then increased to 86% by omapatrilat, and to only 56% by captopril. In spontaneously hypertensive rats, omapatrilat induced a sustained lowering of systolic blood pressure (−68 mm Hg) without change in cardiac rate. Blood pressure normalization was accompanied by increases in plasma angiotensins I, II, and (1-7) levels, with important increases in urinary excretion rates of angiotensin I and (1-7) but not angiotensin II.[48] On the other hand, in conscious dogs made hypertensive by bilateral renal wrapping, intravenous administration of omapatrilat reduced peak left ventricular pressure through arterial vasodilation and preload reduction. Omapatrilat increased plasma levels of adrenomedullin, whereas levels of the natriuretic peptides and cyclic guanosine monophosphate were unchanged.[49]

Experimental studies have also reported that omapatrilat has beneficial cardiorenal and humoral actions in different models of congestive heart failure.[45,46] In a cardiomyopathic hamster model, treatment with omapatrilat decreased left-ventricular end-diastolic pressure and left-ventricular systolic pressure. The changes were associated with a 40% increase in cardiac output, a 47% decrease in peripheral vascular resistance, and a decrease in mean arterial pressure. In rats, survival 24 hours after MI improved with omapatrilat.[50] Omapatrilat reduced infarct size 24 hours after MI and reduced ventricular arrhythmia score 1 to 12 hours after. Rats treated with omapatrilat had reduced left ventricular diastolic and systolic dimensions and left and right ventricular weights compared with controls, indicating a decrease in reactive hypertrophy. Improvement in cardiac remodeling was accompanied by improved ventricular function.[50] Cardiomyocyte apoptosis occurs at a high level late after MI and contributes to adverse cardiac remodeling.[51] Myocardial apoptosis was reduced by ACE inhibition, but vasopeptidase inhibition was even more effective in preventing adverse cardiac remodeling after myocardial infarction.[51]

In insulin-resistant Zucker fatty rats, omapatrilat resulted in a lower rate of endogenous glucose production than placebo both at baseline and after insulin administration at low and high doses. The insulin-sensitizing effects of omapatrilat were blocked by HOE-140 (a bradykinin, B$_2$ receptor antagonist) and NG-nitro L-arginine methyl ester (a nitric oxide synthase inhibitor) in all tissues except myocardium. This insulin-sensitizing effect was greater than that of ramipril.[52] Furthermore, a greater attenuation of albuminuria was afforded by omapatrilat than perindopril in diabetic spontaneously hypertensive rats. Omapatrilat reduced renal NEP binding by 33%, associated with a reduction in albuminuria and prevention of renal structural injury (assessed by glomerulosclerotic index and tubulointerstitial area).[53]

# PHARMACOLOGY

Omapatrilat has a plasma half-life of 14 to 19 hours at the 10- to 80-mg/day dose.[54] It is absorbed rapidly, and peak concentrations are reached in only 0.5 to 2.0 hours. The ratio of the area under the curve on day 10 to that of day 1 when this drug was given constantly during a 10-day period was 1.65. The drug has a prolonged elimination profile. There is only a small tendency to accumulation, and accumulation seems to not be increased in the presence of reduced renal function.[55] Omapatrilat reduces serum ACE activity by more than 80% during the full 24-hour dosing interval at all doses. NEP is also inhibited.[54] Changes in urinary atrial natriuretic peptide excretion during chronic (7 weeks) treatment with omapatrilat were dose-dependent,[54] and were sustained for more than 24 hours postdose.

## Preliminary Human Studies

Omapatrilat lowers blood pressure dose dependently[56,57] at doses ranging between 1 and 80 mg/dl in normotensive persons and in patients with mild to moderate hypertension, regardless of age, race, or gender.

In patients with hypertension, omapatrilat produces greater decreases in systolic, diastolic, and pulse pressure than ACE inhibition alone.[44,45,58] Omapatrilat (80 mg/dl) was a more effective hypotensive agent than was enalapril (40 mg/dl) over 12 weeks of therapy in hypertensive persons studied 24 hours after the last administration. Comparison with the calcium channel blocker amlodipine also revealed more pronounced antihypertensive effects of omapatrilat.[59]

## Clinical Trials in Hypertension

The Omapatrilat Cardiovascular Treatment Assessment Versus Enalapril (OCTAVE)[27] study randomized 25,302 hypertensive patients to either omapatrilat titrated up to 80 mg daily or enalapril titrated up to 40 mg/day for a period of 24 weeks. Compared with enalapril, omapatrilat reduced blood pressure further (3 mm Hg, systolic and 2 mm Hg, diastolic). Although antihypertensive efficacy was an important outcome, the chief interest in this study was to assess the relative incidence of angioedema in the two treatment groups. Angioedema was reported in 2.17% of the patients who received omapatrilat and in 0.68% of those receiving enalapril. Individual episodes of angioedema with omapatrilat were more severe and occurred earlier, the majority within the first few hours after the initial dose. The overall relative risk for angioedema was 3.1 times higher in the omapatrilat group, and the risk for angioedema requiring hospitalization was 9.5 times higher. However, most patients did not require aggressive treatment: 59% and 76% of persons experiencing angioedema with omapatrilat and enalapril, respectively, received either no treatment or were treated with antihistamines only. Risk factors predisposing to angioedema included Black race and smoking. In Black patients, the rate of angioedema was increased approximately threefold with both omapatrilat and enalapril (5.54% and 1.62%, respectively) compared with other racial/ethnic groups. The rate of angioedema was also increased in current smokers receiving omapatrilat (3.93%) but not enalapril (0.81%). The cause of angioedema in patients taking omapatrilat is not known, although mediation by bradykinin has been suggested, because inhibition of ACE and of NEP can each produce increases in bradykinin.

A large international placebo-controlled trial was proposed to study the effects of omapatrilat in elderly patients with isolated stage 1 systolic hypertension.[60] OPERA (Omapatrilat in Persons with Enhanced Risk of Atherosclerotic Events) was designed to study 12,600 participants in a 5-year multinational, randomized, double-blind, placebo-controlled trial. The primary objective of OPERA was to test the hypothesis that omapatrilat significantly enhances survival and reduces cardiovascular outcomes in older (>65 years) men and women with enhanced risk of atherosclerotic events due to stage 1 isolated systolic hypertension. OPERA would also determine whether treatment was justified in older patients with mild systolic hypertension because there is no clear evidence that any therapeutic intervention is of clinical value in this patient group. The OPERA study, which was planned before OCTAVE, was dropped when the results of OCTAVE became available.

## Clinical Trials in Congestive Heart Failure

Omapatrilat produces an acute dose-related hemodynamic improvement in heart failure patients that is maintained for at least 12 weeks.[61,62] Omapatrilat not only reduced blood pressure in patients with heart failure but also reduced the augmentation index and increased postobstructive brachial artery reactive hyperemia.[63] In 48 patients in New York Heart Association (NYHA) functional class II or III, with left ventricular ejection fraction less than or equal to 40% and in sinus rhythm, omapatrilat improved functional status at 12 weeks. Dose-dependent improvements in left ventricular ejection fraction and left ventricular end-systolic wall stress (sigma) were seen, together with a reduction in systolic blood pressure. There was evidence of a natriuretic effect, and total blood volume decreased. Omapatrilat induced an increase in postdose plasma atrial natriuretic peptide levels in the high-dose groups, with a reduction in predose plasma brain natriuretic peptide and epinephrine levels after 12 weeks of therapy.[64]

The IMPRESS (Inhibition of Metallo Protease by BMS-186716 in a Randomized Exercise and Symptoms Study in Subjects with Heart Failure) trial[65] compared 289 patients treated with omapatrilat (target dose 40 mg daily) and 284 patients given lisinopril (target dose 20 mg daily). All patients had previously been on an ACE inhibitor. Omapatrilat was more effective in producing improvements in class III/IV patients. By the end of the 7-month observation period, omapatrilat had a significant advantage in the combined endpoint of mortality, admission for worsening heart failure, and discontinuation of study medication because of worsening heart failure.

These promising findings led to a large clinical trial: Omapatrilat Versus Enalapril Randomized Trial of Utility in Reducing Events (OVERTURE). The OVERTURE study[66] assigned 5770 patients with NYHA classes II to IV heart failure to treatment with either enalapril (10 mg twice daily) or omapatrilat (40 mg once daily) for a mean of 14.5 months. Enalapril or omapatrilat was added to conventional therapy that included β-blockers in 50% patients. The primary endpoint of combined risk of death or hospitalization for heart failure was not different for the two treatment groups, fulfilling prespecified criteria for noninferiority but not for superiority.[66]

Analysis of secondary outcomes showed that the omapatrilat group had a 9% lower risk of cardiovascular death or hospitalization and a 6% lower risk of death. Posthoc analysis showed an 11% lower risk for hospitalization for heart failure in patients treated with omapatrilat.

Although angioedema was reported more commonly with omapatrilat than enalapril, the absolute frequency, incremental risk, and severity in the OVERTURE study was lower than that reported in hypertensive patients. This was attributed to the possibility that patients with heart failure may be resistant to the ability of bradykinin to produce cutaneous exudation, as it was reported in dogs with experimental heart failure.[67] Hypotension and dizziness were more frequent with omapatrilat (19.5% and 19.4%, respectively) than with enalapril (11.5% and 13.9%), but heart failure and renal impairment were less frequent with omapatrilat (22.6% and 6.8%) than with enalapril (25.6% and 10.1%). The incidence of cough was similar for omapatrilat and enalapril therapy (9.7% and 9.0%, respectively). In conclusion, the OVERTURE trial demonstrated that omapatrilat reduced morbidity and mortality in patients with moderate-to-severe heart failure but was not more effective than ACE inhibition alone in reducing the risk of a primary clinical event. Secondary and posthoc analyses focused on all cardiovascular events suggested the possibility of between-group differences in favor of omapatrilat. Furthermore, omapatrilat treatment has been shown to increase endothelin-1 and antiinflammatory cytokine levels in patients with chronic heart failure.[68] Sheth et al.[68] randomized 107 patients with ischemic or dilated cardiomyopathy, NYHA functional classes II to III, with left ventricular ejection less than 40%, and on ACE inhibitor therapy either to omapatrilat 40 mg daily or lisinopril 20 mg/day. C-terminal atrial natriuretic peptide levels decreased with lisinopril but not with omapatrilat. Endothelin-1 levels increased in both groups, but the increase reached statistical significance only with omapatrilat. Levels of the proinflammatory cytokine interleukin-6 tended to decrease, and the anti-inflammatory cytokine interleukin-10 increased in both groups but with statistical significance only for omapatrilat therapy. These effects of omapatrilat on endothelin-1 and antiinflammatory cytokines may provide potential explanations for differences in clinical outcomes in heart failure patients.

## PERSPECTIVES

The natriuretic peptides have actions that might be considered beneficial for hypertensive patients—vasodilation, natriuresis, and inhibition of the sympathetic nervous system and the renin-angiotensin-aldosterone system.[45,69] Several studies with omapatrilat have shown that it is a highly potent antihypertensive agent, more potent than some of the leading antihypertensives, such as losartan, amlodipine, and lisinopril.[44] One factor that may give vasopeptidases the edge over ACE inhibitors because antihypertensives may be their greater potentiation of bradykinin is perhaps their Achilles' heel, as well. The angioedema risk with omapatrilat has cast a shadow over the entire ACE/NEP inhibitor class.

The future of the vasopeptidase inhibitors will depend on the ability to improve the risk:benefit ratio either by developing agents that produce less angioedema, or by defining more precisely a high-risk population that could benefit from dual ACE/NEP inhibition. The NEP drug class probably does have a role in hypertension, although probably only in otherwise difficult-to-manage patients, where the risk of angioedema is counterbalanced by having effected blood pressure control. Furthermore, omapatrilat reduced albuminuria, prevented renal structural injury, and increased insulin sensitivity in diabetic spontaneously hypertensive rats.[53] Patients with diabetic renal failure represent a rapidly growing population with high cardiovascular and renal risk. Whether vasopeptidase inhibitors would help in retarding the progression of renal failure in these patients is not known. Additional studies are warranted in this high-risk population.

## References

1. Kannel WB, Gordon T, Schwartz MJ. Systolic versus diastolic blood pressure and risk of coronary heart disease: the Framingham Study. Am J Cardiol 27:335-346, 1971.
2. Neal B, MacMahon S, Chapman N. Effects of ACE inhibitors, calcium antagonists, and other blood pressure-lowering drugs. Lancet 356:1955-1964, 2000.
3. Suarez C, Cucala M, Coca A, et al. Spanish contribution to the HOT (Hypertension Optimal Treatment) study. Final results. Spanish investigators in the HOT study. Med Clin (Barc) 113:361-365, 1999.
4. Coca A, Ruilope LM, Calvo C, et al. Effect of anti-hypertensive therapy with irbesartan on the absolute cardiovascular risk. Rev Clin Esp 203:183-188, 2003.
5. Brown MJ, Palmer CR, Castaigne A, et al. Morbidity and mortality in patients randomized to double-blind treatment with a long-acting calcium-channel blocker or diuretic in the International Nifedipine GITS study: Intervention as a Goal in Hypertension Treatment (INSIGHT). Lancet 356:366-372, 2000.
6. Blood Pressure Lowering Treatment Trialists' Collaboration. Effects of different blood pressure lowering regimens on major cardiovascular events: Results of prospectively designed overviews of randomised trials. Lancet 362:1527-1535, 2003.
7. Dzau VJ, Bernstein K, Celermajer D, et al. Pathophysiologic and therapeutic importance of tissue ACE: a consensus report. Cardiovasc Drugs Ther 16:149-160, 2002.
8. Wilkins MR, Unwin RJ, Kenny AJ. Endopeptidase-24.11 and its inhibitors: potential therapeutic agents for edematous disorders and hypertension. Kidney Int 43:273-285, 1993.
9. Gonzalez W, Soleilhac JM, Fournie-Zaluski MC, et al. Characterization of neutral endopeptidase in vascular cells, modulation of vasoactive peptide levels. Eur J Pharmacol 345:323-331, 1998.
10. Burnett JC Jr. Vasopeptidase inhibition. A new concept in blood pressure management. J Hypertens 17:S37-S43, 1999.
11. Robl JA, Sun CQ, Stevenson J, et al. Dual metalloprotease inhibitors: mercaptoacetyl-based fused heterocyclic dipeptide mimetics as inhibitors of angiotensin-converting enzyme and neutral endopeptidase. J Med Chem 40:1570-1577, 1997.
12. Levin ER, Gardner DG, Samson WK. Natriuretic peptides. N Engl J Med 339:321-328, 1998.
13. Ruschitzka F, Corti R, Noll G, et al. A rationale for treatment of endothelial dysfunction in hypertension. J Hypertens 17:S25-S35, 1999.
14. Richards AM, Wittert GA, Crozier IG, et al. Chronic inhibition of endopeptidase 24.11 in essential hypertension: evidence for enhanced atrial natriuretic peptide and angiotensin II. J Hypertens 11:407-416, 1993.
15. McDowell G, Coutgie W, Shaw C, et al. The effect of the neutral endopeptidase inhibitor drug, candoxatril, on circulating levels of two of the most potent vasoactive peptides. Br J Clin Pharmacol 43:329-332, 1997.

16. Favrat B, Burnier M, Nussberger J, et al. Neutral endopeptidase versus angiotensin converting enzyme inhibition in essential hypertension. J Hypertens 13:797-804, 1995.

17. Ando S, Rahman MA, Butler GC, et al. Comparison of candoxatril and atrial natriuretic factor in healthy men. Effects on hemodynamics, sympathetic activity, heart rate variability, and endothelin. Hypertension 26:1160-1166, 1995.

18. Richards AM, Wittert GA, Crozier IG, et al. Chronic inhibition of endopeptidase 24.11 in essential hypertension: evidence for enhanced atrial natriuretic peptide and angiotensin II. J Hypertens 11:407-416, 1993.

19. Campbell DJ, Anastasopulos F, Duncan AM, et al. Effects of neutral endopeptidase inhibition and combined angiotensin converting enzyme and neutral endopeptidase inhibition on angiotensin and bradykinin peptides in rats. J Pharmacol Exp Ther 287:567-577, 1998.

20. Munzel T, Kurz S, Holtz J, et al. Neurohormonal inhibition and hemodynamic unloading during prolonged inhibition of ANF degradation in patients with severe chronic heart failure. Circulation 86:1089-1098, 1992.

21. Schirger JA, Grantham JA, Kullo IJ, et al. Vascular actions of brain natriuretic peptide: modulation by atherosclerosis and neutral endopeptidase inhibition. J Am Coll Cardiol 35:796-801, 2000.

22. Blais C, Drapeau G, Raymond P, et al. Contribution of angiotensin converting enzyme to the cardiac metabolism of bradykinin: an interspecies study. Am J Physiol 273:H2263-H2271, 1997.

23. Ishida H, Scicli AG, Carretero OA. Role of angiotensin converting enzyme and other peptidases in in-vivo metabolism of kinins. Hypertension 14:322-327, 1989.

24. Gavras I. Bradykinin mediated effects of ACE inhibition. Kidney Int 42:1020-1029, 1992.

25. Bevan EG, Connell JM, Doyle J, et al. Candoxatril, a neutral endopeptidase inhibitor: efficacy and tolerability in essential hypertension. J Hypertens 10:607-613, 1992.

26. Tikkanen T, Tikkanen I, Rockell MD, et al. Dual inhibition of neutral endopeptidase and angiotensin-converting enzyme in rats with hypertension and diabetes mellitus. Hypertension 32:778-785, 1998.

27. Kostis JB, Packer M, Black HR, et al. Omapatrilat and enalapril in patients with hypertension: The Omapatrilat Cardiovascular Treatment vs. Enalapril (OCTAVE) trial. Am J Hypertens 17:103-111, 2004.

28. Allikmets K. Sampatrilat Shire. Curr Opin Investig Drugs 3:578-581, 2002.

29. Kullo IJ, Miller VM, Lawson GM, et al. Dual inhibition of neutral endopeptidase (NEP) and angiotensin converting enzyme (ACE) suppresses atherogenesis and improved endothelial function in hypercholesterolemic rabbits. J Am Coll Cardiol 272:164A, 1996.

30. Maki T, Nasa Y, Tanonaka K, et al. Beneficial effects of sampatrilat, a novel vasopeptidase inhibitor, on cardiac remodeling and function of rats with chronic heart failure following left coronary artery ligation. J Pharmacol Exp Ther 305:97-105, 2003.

31. Wallis EJ, Ramsay LE, Hettiarachchi J. Combined inhibition of neutral endopeptidase and angiotensin-converting enzyme by sampatrilat in essential hypertension. Clin Pharmacol Ther 64:439-449, 1998.

32. Norton GR, Woodiwiss AJ, Hartford C, et al. Sustained antihypertensive actions of a dual angiotensin-converting enzyme neutral endopeptidase inhibitor, sampatrilat, in black hypertensive subjects. Am J Hypertens 12:563-571, 1999.

33. Rossi GP. Dual ACE and NEP inhibitors: a review of the pharmacological properties of MDL 100240. Cardiovasc Drug Rev 21:51-66, 2003.

34. Rossi GP, Bova S, Sacchetto A, et al. Comparative effects of the dual ACE-NEP inhibitor MDL-100,240 and ramipril on hyper-

tension and cardiovascular disease in endogenous angiotensin II-dependent hypertension. Am J Hypertens 15:181-188, 2002.

35. Rousso P, Buclin T, Nussberger J, et al. Effects of a dual inhibitor of angiotensin converting enzyme and neutral endopeptidase, MDL 100-240, on endocrine and renal functions in healthy volunteers. J Hypertens 17:427-437, 1999.

36. Rousso P, Buclin T, Nussberger J, et al. Bioavailability of repeated oral administration of MDL 100240, a dual inhibitor of angiotensin-converting enzyme and neutral endopeptidase in healthy volunteers. Eur J Clin Pharmacol 55:749-754, 2000.

37. Robl JA, Sulsky R, Sieber-McMaster E, et al. Vasopeptidase inhibitors: incorporation of geminal and spirocyclic substituted azepinones in mercaptoacyl dipeptides. J Med Chem 42:305-311, 1999.

38. Laverman GD, Van Goor H, Henning RH, et al. Renoprotective effects of VPI versus ACEI in normotensive nephrotic rats on different sodium intakes. Kidney Int 63:64-71, 2003.

39. Laurent S, Boutouyrie P, Azizi M, et al. Antihypertensive effects of fasidotril, a dual inhibitor of neprilysin and angiotensin-converting enzyme, in rats and humans. Hypertension 35:1148-1153, 2000.

40. Gonzalez W, Beslot F, Laboulandine I, et al. Inhibition of both angiotensin-converting enzyme and neutral endopeptidase by D21402 (RB105) in rats with experimental myocardial infarction. J Pharmacol Exp Ther 278:573-578, 1996.

41. Lassila M, Davis BJ, Allen TJ, et al. Cardiovascular hypertrophy in diabetic spontaneously hypertensive rats: optimizing blockade of the renin-angiotensin system. Clin Sci (Lond) 104:341-347, 2003.

42. Rastegar MA, Marchini F, Morazzoni G, et al. The effects of Z13752A, a combined ACE/NEP inhibitor, on responses to coronary artery occlusion: a primary protective role for bradykinin. Br J Pharmacol 129:671-680, 2000.

43. Bani M, Colantoni A, Guillaume M, et al. A double-blind, placebo-controlled study to assess tolerability, pharmacokinetics and preliminary pharmacodynamics of single escalating doses of Z13752A, a novel dual inhibitor of metalloproteases ACE and NEP, in healthy volunteers. Br J Clin Pharmacol 50:338-349, 2000.

44. Weber MA. Vasopeptidase inhibitors. Lancet 358:1525-1532, 2001.

45. Campbell DJ. Vasopeptidase inhibition: a double-edged sword? Hypertension 41:383-389, 2003.

46. Trippodo NC, Robl JA, Asaad MM, et al. Effects of omapatrilat in low, normal, and high renin experimental hypertension. Am J Hypertens 11:363-372, 1998.

47. Quaschning T, d'Uscio LV, Lüscher TF. Greater endothelial protection by the vasopeptidase inhibitor omapatrilat compared to the ACE-inhibitor captopril in salt induced hypertension. J Am Coll Cardiol 35:248-249, 2000.

48. Ferrario CM, Averill DB, Brosnihan KB, et al. Vasopeptidase inhibition and Ang-(1-7) in the spontaneously hypertensive rat. Kidney Int 62:1349-1357, 2002.

49. Maniu CV, Meyer DM, Redfield MM. Hemodynamic and humoral effects of vasopeptidase inhibition in canine hypertension. Hypertension 40:528-534, 2002.

50. Lapointe N, Ngguyen QT, Desjardins JF, et al. Effects of pre-, peri-, and postmyocardial infarction treatment with omapatrilat in rats: survival, arrhythmias, ventricular function, and remodeling. Am J Physiol Heart Physiol 285:H398-H405, 2003.

51. Backlund T, Palojoki E, Saraste A, et al. Effect of vasopeptidase inhibitor omapatrilat on cardiomyocyte apoptosis and ventricular remodeling in rat myocardial infarction. Cardiovasc Res 57:727-737, 2003.

52. Wang Ch, Leung N, Lapointe N, et al. Vasopeptidase inhibitor omapatrilat induces profound insulin sensitization and increases myocardial glucose uptake in Zucker fatty rats: studies comparing a vasopeptidase inhibitor, angiotensin-converting

enzyme inhibitor, and angiotensin II type I receptor blocker. Circulation 107:1923-1929, 2003.

53. Davies BJ, Johnston CI, Burrell LM, et al. Renoprotective effects of vasopeptidase inhibition in an experimental model of diabetic nephropathy. Diabetologia 46:961-971, 2003.

54. Liao WC, Vesterqvist O, Delaney C, et al. Pharmacokinetics and pharmacodynamics of the vasopeptidase inhibitor, omapatrilat in healthy subjects. Br J Clin Pharmacol 56:395-406, 2003.

55. Sica DA, Liao W, Gehr TW, et al. Disposition and safety of omapatrilat in subjects with renal impairment. Clin Pharmacol Ther 68:261-269, 2000.

56. Massien C, Azizi M, Guyene TT, et al. Pharmacodynamic effects of dual neutral endopeptidase-angiotensin-converting enzyme inhibition in humans. Clin Pharmacol Ther 65:448-459, 1999.

57. Azizi M, Lamarre-Cliché M, Labatide-Alanore A, et al. Physiologic consequences of vasopeptidase inhibition in humans: effect of sodium intake. J Am Soc Nephrol 13: 2454-2463, 2002.

58. Nathisuwan S, Talbert RL. A review of vasopeptidase inhibitors: a new modality in the treatment of hypertension and chronic heart failure. Pharmacotherapy 22:27-42, 2002.

59. Ruilope LM, Plantini P, Grossman E, et al. Randomized, double-blind comparison of omapatrilat with amlodipine in mild-to-moderate hypertension. Am J Hypertens 13:134A, 2000.

60. Kostis JB, Cobbe S, Johnston C, et al. Design of the Omapatrilat in Persons with Enhanced Risk of Atherosclerotic events (OPERA) trial. Am J Hypertens 15:193-198, 2002.

61. Klapholz M, Thomas I, Eng C, et al. Effects of omapatrilat on hemodynamics and safety in patents with heart failure. Am J Cardiol 88:657-661, 2001.

62. McClean DR, Ikram H, Mehta S, et al. Vasopeptidase inhibition with omapatrilat in chronic heart failure: acute and long-term hemodynamic and neurohumoral effects. J Am Coll Cardiol 39:2034-2041, 2002.

63. McClean DR, Ikram H, Garlick AH, et al. Effects of omapatrilat on systemic arterial function in patients with chronic heart failure. Am J Cardiol 87:565-569, 2001.

64. McClean DR, Ikram H, Garlick AH, et al. The clinical, cardiac, renal, arterial and neurohormonal effects of omapatrilat, a vasopeptidase inhibitor, in patients with chronic heart failure. J Am Coll Cardiol 36:479-486, 2000.

65. Rouleau JL, Pfeffer MA, Stewart DJ, et al. Comparison of vasopeptidase inhibitor, omapatrilat, and lisinopril on exercise tolerance and morbidity in patients with heart failure: IMPRESS randomized trial. Lancet 356:615-620, 2000.

66. Packer M, Califf RM, Konstam MA, et al. Comparison of omapatrilat and enalapril in patients with chronic heart failure: the Omapatrilat Versus Enalapril Randomized Trial of Utility in Reducing Events (OVERTURE). Circulation 106:920-926, 2002.

67. Rubinstein I, Muns G, Zucker IH. Plasma exudation in conscious dogs with experimental heart failure. Basic Res Cardiol 89:487-498, 1994.

68. Sheth T, Parker T, Block A, et al. Comparison of the effects of omapatrilat and lisinopril on circulating neurohormones and cytokines in patients with chronic heart failure. Am J Cardiol 90:496-500, 2002.

69. Zanchi A, Maillad M, Burnier M. Recent clinical trials with omapatrilat: new developments. Curr Hypertens Rep 5:346-352, 2003.

# Chapter 72

# Renin Inhibitors

## Jürg Nussberger

## PRINCIPLES

One century after the discovery of renin by Tigerstedt and Bergman,[1] it is well established that antagonizing the renin-angiotensin-aldosterone system is a successful treatment for cardiovascular and renal disease. This system maintains cardiovascular homeostasis by up- and down-regulating receptor-mediated effects of the key hormone angiotensin II (Ang II). It appears to primarily regulate the renal Ang II concentration.[2] Ang II is an octapeptide with potent vasoconstrictor and sodium-retaining activity. It also stimulates adrenal aldosterone release, pituitary vasopressin release, and endothelial endothelin-1 release; it centrally stimulates sympathetic activity; and it promotes growth and inflammation. Any means to reduce the activity of Ang II would therefore tend to vasodilate, to reduce body sodium and water and hence decrease blood pressure, (BP), to reduce cardiac afterload and cell hypertrophy, and to be antiinflammatory and antifibrotic and favorably influence atherosclerotic and fibrotic disease.

The action of Ang II can be antagonized by blocking Ang II at the receptor site or by reducing the generation of Ang II (Figure 72–1). The receptor blockade was first clinically tested by infusion of peptide analogs of Ang II such as saralasin[3] and then more recently and very successfully by the orally active Ang II receptor blockers such as losartan.[4] Reduced generation of Ang II can also be obtained by β-adrenergic receptor blocking drugs that reduce the β-adrenergic receptor-mediated release of renin from the kidneys.[5,6] The renal enzyme renin catalyzes the rate-limiting step of the renin-angiotensin cascade, and its key product Ang II inhibits renal renin secretion. Human active renin is an aspartyl protease of 340 amino acids and 40,000 Dalton molecular weight with two $N$-glycosylation sites. It is secreted by the renal juxtaglomerular granular epithelioid cells. Human renin cleaves at optimal pH 6.0 from its natural substrate angiotensinogen (Ang-N), a mainly hepatogenic $\alpha_2$-globulin, the physiologically inactive aminoterminal decapeptide angiotensin I (Ang I). Ang I is activated by the dicarboxypeptidase converting enzyme (angiotensin-converting enzyme [ACE], kininase II) into the octapeptide Ang II. Active renin levels are highly correlated with Ang II levels both in circulating plasma and at tissue sites.[7,8]

Renin secretion from the renal juxtaglomerular cells does not exclusively depend on β-adrenergic receptor activity. Chloride transport across the renal macula densa cells, as well as Ang II receptor activity and renal perfusion pressure, also play important roles in renin release. β-Adrenergic blockade alone can therefore only partially decrease the secretion of renin and reduce the generation of Ang II. Specific blockade of secreted renin was therefore attempted early on with analogs of the renin substrate Ang-N.[9-13]

However, the most-successful drugs in reducing the generation of Ang II were the converting enzyme inhibitors.[8,14] The enzyme converting the inactive decapeptide Ang I into the active octapeptide Ang II is identical with the kininase II that inactivates bradykinin. The discovery in the venom of the snake *Bothrops jararaca* of a peptide that blocked kininase II[15,16] led to the synthesis of potent orally active inhibitors of the enzyme that were soon better known under the name ACE.[17] ACE inhibitors are well documented to decrease Ang II generation, and large clinical trials have established their clinical benefit in hypertension, heart failure, and protection of renal function (see Chapters 9 and 65). ACE inhibitors also cause cough in 10% of patients and angioedema in 1% of patients, side effects that are attributed to accumulation of substance P and bradykinin rather than to the decrease in Ang II levels.

Taken together, there is good clinical evidence that antagonizing Ang II favorably influences cardiovascular and renal disease. Both reduced generation of Ang II and blockade of the Ang II effects at the receptor site appear successful. However, β-adrenergic receptor blocking agents provide incomplete suppression of renal renin secretion and generation of Ang II; ACE inhibitors cause side effects and Ang II receptor antagonists block only a single subtype of Ang receptors, exposing other unprotected Ang receptors to feedback-enhanced circulating Ang levels. Extreme experimental and clinical conditions indicate that renal renin secretion and peripheral renin activation are never fully turned off by feedback mechanisms[18] and that very small amounts of circulating renin still participate in BP regulation.[19] Therefore specific inhibitors of active renin remained a goal of pharmaceutical research over the last three decades.

## WHY RENIN INHIBITION?

In the 1970s, the regulatory role of the renin-angiotensin-aldosterone system in cardiovascular homeostasis was well known.[20] However, the debate continued on whether this system is more a marginal phylogenetic leftover from several hundred million years ago when vertebrates evolved out of the sea into fresh water and later on land and then needed to defend their salt and water balance or whether renin in modern humans is of key importance in normal physiology as well as in many disease states. Renin acts on a unique and species-specific substrate (Ang-N) and is the rate-limiting enzyme for the generation of Ang II, an octapeptide with both potent vasoconstrictor and sodium- and water-retaining capacities. It was therefore tempting to test the blockade of this hormonal system that controlled both vasoconstrictor and volume components of the blood pressure equation. In early clinical tests, Ang II analog peptides with receptor-blocking properties did indeed decrease elevated blood pressure and thus proved the concept that antagonizing the renin-angiotensin system was of pharmacologic interest.[3] However, partial agonistic properties of the Ang II analog peptides and lack of biooral avail-

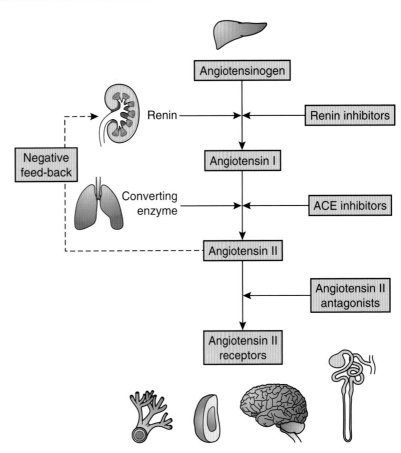

**Figure 72–1** The renin-angiotensin system and the levels of its pharmacologic inhibition. Activation of the Ang II receptor of the subtype 1 inhibits secretion of active renin from renal juxtaglomerular cells (feedback regulation of renal Ang II concentration). Specific renin inhibitors, ACE inhibitors, or Ang II receptor antagonists increase renin secretion by reducing feedback suppression of renin secretion. Renin inhibitors and ACE inhibitors decrease, whereas Ang II antagonists increase circulating levels of Ang II.

ability placed the Ang II receptor blockers on ice for another decade.

Even more extended—over almost three decades—was the development of specific renin inhibitors. It made sense to block renin and stem the tide of the renin-angiotensin cascade at the source, since renin is rate limiting for the generation of all angiotensins. Blockade of renin activity would not enhance the activation of unprotected angiotensin receptor subtypes as seen with selective Ang II receptor antagonists. The exclusive specificity of renin for its substrate Ang-N made it unlikely that the blockade of this enzyme's activity would produce unwanted effects by cumulating other peptides as with ACE inhibitors. Finally, in contrast to β-adrenergic receptor blockers, specific renin inhibitors should antagonize all active renin independent of the mechanism of its generation or release. Thus, even constitutive (unregulated) renal secretion of renin could be blocked.[18]

## RENIN-SPECIFIC ANTIBODIES

Renin-specific purified antibodies, or their Fab fragments, have been demonstrated in sodium-depleted dogs to decrease circulating Ang II levels and BP.[21] However, parenteral administration of these short-lived proteins was necessary, and immunologic complications (antigenic properties, cross-reactions of antibodies, inflammation) were to be expected, as with active immunization against the renin-angiotensin system.[22] The hypotensive effect of a crude renin antiserum that had been tested in animals half a century earlier was never fully accepted as a proof of concept.[23]

## PEPSTATIN AND STATIN DERIVATIVES

Pepstatin is a strong inhibitor of aspartyl proteases such as pepsin, cathepsin D, and renin. This natural pentapeptide isolated from actinomycetes was for many years the classic renin inhibitor in vitro.[24] Pepstatin is not specific for renin and is poorly soluble in water. Structural derivatives of pepstatin increased its solubility and specificity for renin by several orders of magnitude.[25-27] Pepstatin contains the unusual γ amino acid statin that may substitute for the two amino acids at the scissile bond of the protein substrate and block substrate cleavage because of the structural analogy to a transition state of the peptide bond hydrolysis by aspartyl proteases[27] (see later). However, none of these compounds was used clinically. Structural formulas and published potencies of these and subsequent early renin inhibitors were summarized by Hui and Haber.[28]

## ANGIOTENSINOGEN ANALOGS

Several specific renin inhibitors were synthesized as of the 1970s, but low efficacy, lack of oral availability, or high costs of synthesis prevented them from becoming successful drugs. Early renin inhibitors were modified analogs of the octapeptide from Ang-N that had previously been shown to be the minimal substrate for renin.[29] The cleavage site in human renin substrate Ang-N is between residues Leu-10 and Val-11, which differs from the Leu-10–Leu-11 scissile bond sequence in nonprimate species.[30] The replacement or addition of single amino acids around the scissile P1-P1' bond of the substrate led to oligopeptides that were weak renin inhibitors.[9,29,31-33] Nevertheless it could be demonstrated that such a renin-inhibiting decapeptide (RIP) administered intravenously decreased BP in monkeys[34] and humans.[12]

## PRORENIN FRAGMENTS

Prosegment peptidic fragments of pepsinogen are known to inhibit pepsin. By analogy, several attempts were made to inhibit renin with peptidic analogs of prorenin fragments.[35,36] Such renin inhibitors were found to reach low micromolar affinities, but this was not sufficient for compounds administered parenterally. Although innovative, the prorennin fragments approach to renin inhibition was abandoned.

## TRANSITION-STATE ANALOGS

The hypothesis that peptide bond hydrolysis by aspartyl proteinases such as renin proceeds through a tetrahedral transition state is supported by conformational studies of the pepstatin-enzyme complex.[37] A substrate analog that would bind tightly to the active site of renin but could not be cleaved was expected to be a good renin inhibitor. Accordingly, Szelke and colleagues replaced in a minimal renin substrate decapeptide the scissile peptide bond (-CO-NH-) between the Leu-10 and Val-11 positions with a reduced and nonscissile bond (-CH$_2$-NH-) mimicking the hypothetical transition state conformation; they thus founded a new family of renin inhibitors.[38] The reduced bond peptide renin inhibitor H142 was clinically tested: In normal volunteers on a low-salt diet, 30-minute infusions of H142 (1 mg/kg/hr and 2.5 mg/kg/hr) decreased diastolic BP by 19% and 23%, respectively, and plasma renin activity as well as levels of Ang I and II were decreased, while a reactive rise in circulating active renin was documented.[39]

Following the same hypothesis about nonscissile transition state analogs of renin substrate, the pepstatin derivatives and the statin-containing renin inhibitory peptides (SCRIP) were tested, since statin mimicked the transition state of the scissile bond of the renin substrate but did also not contain a dihydroxyl species required for the amide bond hydrolysis (see above). Numerous other substitutions at the scissile bond have subsequently been tested, including dihydroxyethylene[40] and stabilized peptides such as CGP 29287[41] or shorter dipeptides or peptide-like compounds.[28,40,42,43]

## EVALUATION OF RENIN INHIBITORS

Renin inhibitors are designed to decrease the generation of Ang II. In contrast to ACE inhibitors, generation of the inactive decapeptide Ang I rather than its conversion into the active octapeptide Ang II is inhibited. Both renin inhibitors and ACE inhibitors reduce concentrations of Ang II in body fluids and at tissue sites close to the specific Ang II receptors, and both drug classes stimulate renin secretion by the same mechanism as the Ang II receptor blockers: They interrupt the negative feedback of Ang II at the juxtaglomerular cells of the kidneys. Circulating levels of active renin are therefore expected to be increased by any of the currently used specific inhibitors of the renin-angiotensin system. The beneficial cardiovascular effects of these specific inhibitors are primarily due to reduced activation of the Ang II type 1 receptor AT$_1$. Any additional vasodilator, natriuretic, diuretic, or growth-inhibiting effects of ACE inhibitors or Ang II antagonists mediated by other Ang peptides or receptors would necessarily be enhanced by increased Ang I generation as a consequence of the increased active renin levels. ACE inhibitors (kininase II inhibitors) may have additional effects related to the accumulation of kinins.

Effective renin inhibitors must decrease Ang II levels. A reliable measurement of plasma and tissue concentrations of Ang-(1-8)octapeptide is therefore required for evaluation of renin inhibitors.[7,44,45] Changes in plasma Ang II levels during renin inhibition with different renin inhibitors are well correlated with BP changes in hypertensive patients,[46] monkeys,[47] and sheep.[48] Misleading conclusions have often been drawn about decreasing Ang II levels and hypotensive effects of renin inhibitors versus ACE inhibitors because of blood-sampling artifacts[49]: ACE inhibitors cause high Ang I levels and therefore tend to generate Ang II in vitro after blood sampling. Renin inhibitors cause low Ang I levels, and Ang II generation in vitro is prevented.[50] Unless Ang II generation in vitro is prevented by adding sufficient renin inhibitor to the blood-sampling cocktail, Ang II levels during ACE inhibition may be falsely elevated. This contrasts with ACE inhibitor-induced hypotensive effects, which may be greater than those found during a weak renin inhibition, where no Ang II is generated in vitro and plasma levels are found to be accurately decreased. Interestingly, Ang II levels, if accurately measured, are decreased to a greater extent during potent ACE inhibition than during weak renin inhibition. Blood pressure effects of both drug classes are well predictable from accurately measured Ang II levels.

Another flaw in the screening of renin inhibitors was the surprising unreliability of conventional and well-established assays for measurement of plasma renin activity.[51,52] Renin assays that have been in use for decades are not reliable for testing renin inhibitors. They may overestimate the potency of renin inhibitors by several orders of magnitude because of chemicals added to the assays to protect generated Ang I from degradation during plasma incubation or because of pH changes. More renin-inhibiting activity is found in the assay than in vivo, and renin may appear fully inhibited for several hours after administration of a renin inhibitor, while plasma angiotensin levels and BP increase immediately after discontinuation of the drug[46] (Figure 72–2). Methods that protect Ang I generated during plasma incubation by trapping antibodies provide accurate estimations of the IC$_{50}$s of renin inhibitors.[53] Few publications describing renin inhibitors took account of this observation, and promising IC$_{50}$s and overestimated potencies of certain renin inhibitors after oral administration brought inappropriate molecules into clinical testing and led to disappointing results, particularly when these renin inhibitors were compared with potent ACE inhibitors, which did effectively decrease Ang II levels. Adding to the confusion was the fact that artifactually measured plasma Ang II levels were minimally decreased during ACE inhibition, while marginal decreases in Ang II levels during renin inhibition were less prone to artifacts and therefore appeared greater than those obtained with the ACE inhibitors (see earlier). Since the artifact of the renin activity measurement falsely labeled the renin inhibitors as potent and underestimated the potency of the ACE inhibitors, it was not surprising that investi-

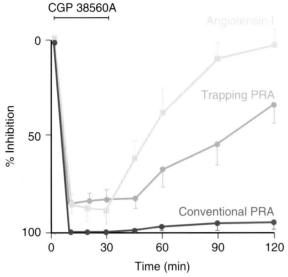

**TRAPPING VERSUS CONVENTIONAL PRA DURING RENIN INHIBITION**

**Figure 72–2** Artifactual overestimation of renin inhibition by conventional measurement of plasma renin activity (PRA) after a 30-minute infusion of the renin inhibitor CGP 38560A in hypertensive patients. PRA appears completely suppressed for hours when measured by the conventional PRA assay. The more-physiologic PRA assay using Ang I trapping antibodies and the circulating immunoreactive Ang I levels indicate shorter effects of the renin inhibitor. (From Jeunemaître X, Ménard J, Nussberger J, et al. Plasma angiotensins, renin and blood pressure during acute renin inhibition by CGP 38560A in hypertensive patients. Am J Hypertens 2:819-827, 1989.)

gators hypothesized additional, non–Ang II–mediated hypotensive effects of ACE inhibitors. The supposedly strong renin inhibitors that supposedly decreased Ang II levels more than ACE inhibitors had less BP effect than ACE inhibitors. Actually, weak renin inhibitors were compared with strong ACE inhibitors. The confusion based on biased biochemical evaluation discredited renin inhibition as a therapeutic principle. More than a dozen pharmaceutical companies abandoned their research on renin inhibitors over the last two decades.

The classic hormonal profiles during renin inhibition show parallel dose-related decreases in plasma renin activity and Ang I and Ang II levels and a slightly delayed increase in plasma active renin concentration (Figures 72–3 and 72–4). Based on accurately measured hormone profiles and knowledge of the inhibition constant Ki of a renin inhibitor, enzyme kinetic considerations allow calculation of the necessary (minimal) plasma inhibitor concentration to be reached for any hypothetical plasma active renin concentration to achieve a desired plasma Ang II level[54] (Box 72–1, Figure 72–5). Assuming Michaelis-Menten kinetics for competitive inhibition and steady state conditions, the formula of Box 72–1 calculates the Ang I generation rate (V) in plasma from the measured plasma drug (I) and renin levels (E). The measured plasma Ang I concentrations are in excellent correlation with the theoretical angiotensin I generation rate (Figure 72–5).[54] The decrease in plasma renin activity induced by renin inhibitor therapy is also correlated with the decreases in blood pressure,[55] since plasma renin activity and angiotensin concentrations are related. Since the renin-angiotensinogen reaction is exquisitely specific to species, animal models for evaluation of renin inhibitors are of limited value. Tests in primates such as the marmoset monkeys are preferred. Ultimately, clinical testing with accurate methodology is mandatory.

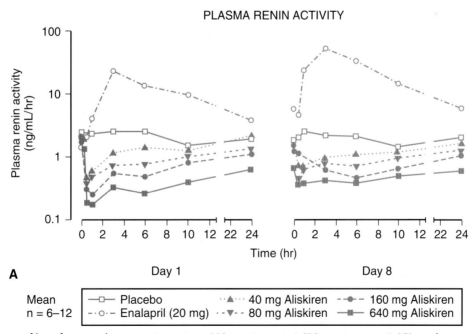

**Figure 72–3** Time profiles of mean plasma renin activity **(A)**, angiotensin I **(B)**, angiotensin II **(C)**, and active renin **(D)** in 9 healthy men after acute (Day 1) and sustained (Day 8) inhibition of the renin-angiotensin system by the orally active renin inhibitor aliskiren and by the ACE inhibitor enalapril. Aliskiren dose-dependently decreases plasma renin activity, Ang I, and Ang II and increases active renin. Enalapril decreases plasma Ang II but increases renin and Ang I. (From Nussberger J, Wuerzner G, Jensen C, et al. Angiotensin II suppression in humans by the orally active renin inhibitor aliskiren [SPP100]. Hypertension 39:e1-e8, 2002.)

*Continued*

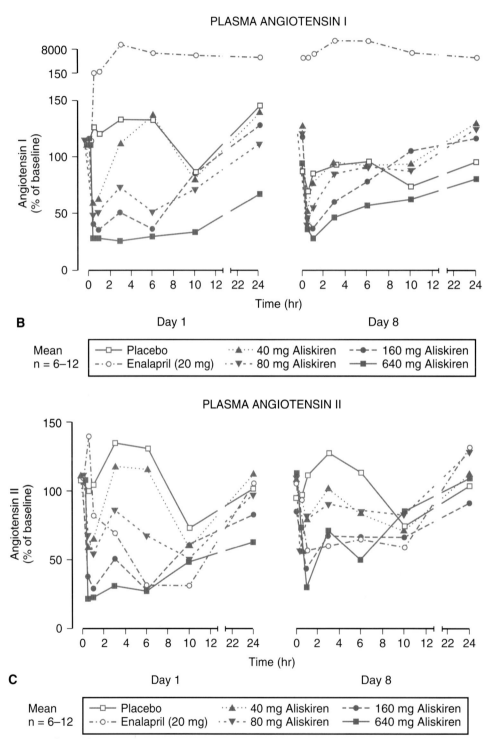

PLASMA ANGIOTENSIN I

**B** Day 1    Day 8

Mean
n = 6–12

| □ Placebo | ▲ 40 mg Aliskiren | ● 160 mg Aliskiren |
| ○ Enalapril (20 mg) | ▼ 80 mg Aliskiren | ■ 640 mg Aliskiren |

PLASMA ANGIOTENSIN II

**C** Day 1    Day 8

Mean
n = 6–12

| □ Placebo | ▲ 40 mg Aliskiren | ● 160 mg Aliskiren |
| ○ Enalapril (20 mg) | ▼ 80 mg Aliskiren | ■ 640 mg Aliskiren |

**Figure 72–3, cont'd** For legend see previous page.

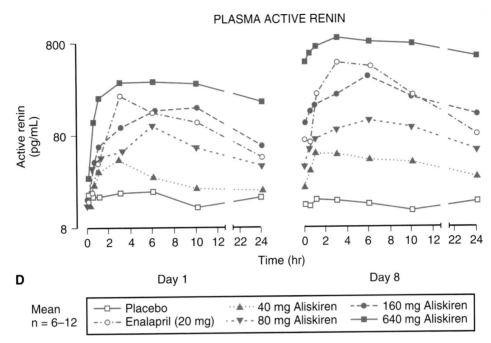

**PLASMA ACTIVE RENIN**

**Figure 72–3, cont'd**

## CLINICAL EXPERIENCE

Over the last two decades, several renin inhibitors have been tested in human subjects. The first clinical experience with a specific renin inhibitor was obtained with the angiotensinogen analog decapeptide RIP.[12] This renin-inhibiting peptide did indeed decrease BP during intravenous administration in humans, but there was evidence for a direct cardiodepressing effect unrelated to the renin inhibition, and the compound was abandoned. The first successful clinical testing of a renin inhibitor was obtained with H142, a reduced peptide bond transition state analog.[39] This peptide was infused into slightly salt-depleted healthy male volunteers. The H142 decreased BP in parallel with decreases in plasma renin activity and Ang I and II levels, and plasma active renin concentrations were increased. Heart rate effects were inconsistent, but heart rate increased when BP fell with the higher doses of H142. Generally, renin inhibitors do not change heart rate in salt-replete individuals. This is in agreement with observations for Ang II antagonists or ACE inhibitors, since Ang II mediates reflex tachycardia during hypotension by increasing central sympathetic outflow and by resetting of the baroreflex.

Subsequent clinical testing of other inhibitors of renin (suffix -kiren) in healthy volunteers even on mild salt restriction did not show BP or heart rate changes but did evoke dose-dependent decreases in plasma renin activity, Ang I, and Ang II that were rapidly reversed after termination of infusion of enalkiren[56] or CGP 38560A[57] or oral dosing of remikiren.[54] A massive and long-lasting rise in plasma active renin concentrations was consistently observed. In renin-dependent hypertension, the transition state analog renin inhibitor CGP 38560A was infused for 30 minutes[46] (Figures 72–1, 72–6, and 72–7): BP fell dose-dependently in parallel with the decreases in plasma renin activity and Ang I and II levels while active renin increased. Antihypertensive action in essential hypertensives was demonstrated for high intravenous bolus doses of enalkiren, particularly in salt-depleted patients, while heart rate remained unchanged[55] (Figure 72–8). Similarly, a weak antihypertensive effect of orally administered remikiren was reported, but these results were never confirmed.[58] Promising early clinical testing has also been reported for the strong peptidic renin inhibitor R-PEP-27[59] and for the orally active renin inhibitors zankiren[60] and FK 906,[61] but no follow-up has been published, and the compounds appear to have been abandoned.

All of these renin inhibitors provided the classic hormonal profile when tested with valid methods. However, the peptides or peptide-like renin inhibitors generally required parenteral administration and were therefore without great clinical potential. Few renin inhibitors have been tested with oral administration, and so far only one, aliskiren[62] (Figure 72–9), appears to become a commercially viable therapeutic agent.

## ORALLY ACTIVE RENIN INHIBITORS

Several renin inhibitors have been tested after oral administration,[54,58,60-63] In humans, no renin inhibitor has been more than 3% absorbed. Nevertheless, even with low bioavailability, significant and long-lasting decreases in BP can be obtained in hypertensive patients[63] (Figure 72–10).

## ALISKIREN

Clinical testing of the orally active renin inhibitor aliskiren indicates that renin inhibitors have therapeutic potential similar to that of other antagonists of the renin-angiotensin system. Early observations indicate that tolerability should be comparable to or better than that of established drugs. Aliskiren is a low-molecular-weight (MW 552, free base) non-peptidic renin

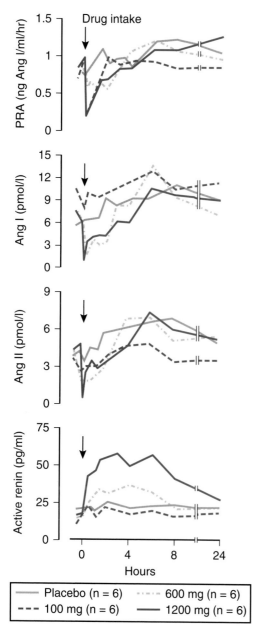

### EFFECTS OF THE RENIN INHIBITOR (RO 42-5892) ON THE RENIN-ANGIOTENSIN SYSTEM AFTER ORAL ADMINISTRATION

Placebo (n = 6) ······ 600 mg (n = 6)
--- 100 mg (n = 6) ——— 1200 mg (n = 6)

**Figure 72–4** Time profiles of mean plasma renin activity (PRA), Ang I, Ang II, and active renin in 6 healthy men after oral single administration of the renin inhibitor remikiren at three doses or placebo. Remikiren decreases in a dose-related manner PRA, Ang I, and Ang II, and it increases active renin. The decreases in plasma levels of Ang I and Ang II remain significant for maximally 2 hours, and the increase in active renin lasts for 8 hours. (From Camenzind E, Nussberger J, Juillerat L, et al. Effect of the renin response during renin inhibition: Oral Ro 42-5892 in normal humans. J Cardiovasc Pharmacol 18:299-307, 1991.)

**Box 72–1** Calculation of Angiotensin I Generation Rate

$$V = \frac{kp \times [E] \times [S]}{K_M \, (1+[I]/K_i) + [S]}$$

V = angiotensin I generation rate
$kp \approx k_{cat}$ = rate constant = 0.6/s
[E] = active renin concentration
[S] = angiotensinogen = 1.35 μM
$K_M$ = Michaelis-Menten constant = 0.4 μM
[I] = drug concentration
$K_i$ = inhibitor constant = 0.4 nM

Formula for the calculation of the generation rate of angiotensin I (and Ang II) during renin inhibition assuming Michaelis-Menten kinetics for competitive inhibition and assuming steady state conditions. $K_M$ and $k_{cat}$ for renin and $K_i$ of any renin inhibitor of interest are known constants. Concentrations of the inhibitor (I), the enzyme active renin (E), and the substrate angiotensinogen (S) can be measured. (From Camenzind E, Nussberger J, Juillerat L, et al. Effect of the renin response during renin inhibition: Oral Ro 42-5892 in normal humans. J Cardiovasc Pharmacol 18:299-307, 1991.)

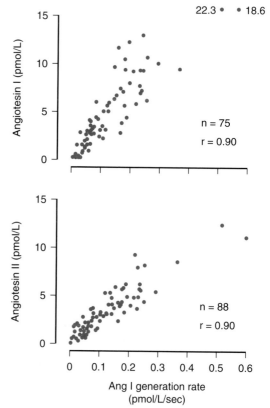

**Figure 72–5** Correlation between the actually measured plasma Ang I (upper panel) and Ang II (lower panel) levels and the calculated Ang I generation rates according to the formula of Box 72–1 applied to the renin inhibitor study of Figure 72–4. $K_M$ = 0.4 μM, $k_{cat}$ = 0.6/s, $K_i$ = 0.4 nM, angiotensinogen (S) = 1.35 μM. The good correlation allows the prediction of levels of renin inhibitor to be achieved at a given renin concentration to obtain a required reduction in angiotensin concentrations. (From Camenzind E, Nussberger J, Juillerat L, et al. Effect of the renin response during renin inhibition: Oral Ro 42-5892 in normal humans. J Cardiovasc Pharmacol 18:299-307, 1991.)

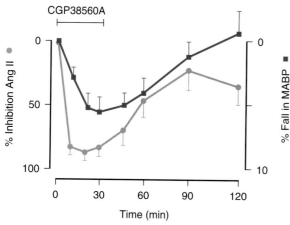

**Figure 72–6** Parallel changes in plasma angiotensin II concentrations and mean arterial BP (MABP) in hypertensive patients during and following a 30-minute infusion of the renin inhibitor CGP 38560A. Maximal effects are reached by the end of the infusion, and a return toward baseline conditions occurs within the following hour (see also Figure 72–2). (From Jeunemaître X, Ménard J, Nussberger J, et al. Plasma angiotensins, renin and blood pressure during acute renin inhibition by CGP 38560A in hypertensive patients. Am J Hypertens 2:819-827, 1989.)

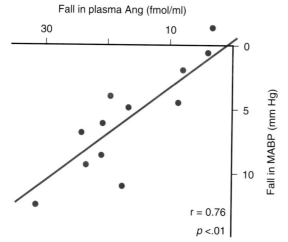

**Figure 72–7** Correlation between the maximal fall in plasma angiotensin concentrations and the maximal fall in mean arterial BP (MABP) in 12 hypertensive patients during infusion of the renin inhibitor CGP 38560A (see also Figure 72–6). Angiotensin II concentrations may control the BP of these patients.[46]

inhibitor that consists of a substituted octanamid (see Figure 72–9). It is a competitive transition state analog and specific inhibitor of human renin. After acute and repeated ingestion by healthy volunteers, aliskiren causes the classical decreases in plasma renin activity and Ang I and Ang II levels and an increase in plasma active renin[62] (see Figure 72–3). It decreases urinary aldosterone excretion as much as enalapril (see Figure 72–11) and has a natriuretic effect.[62] In hypertensive patients, aliskiren at a daily oral dose of 300 mg was at least as effective as 150 mg irbesartan or 100 mg losartan in reducing BP[63] (Figure 72–10).

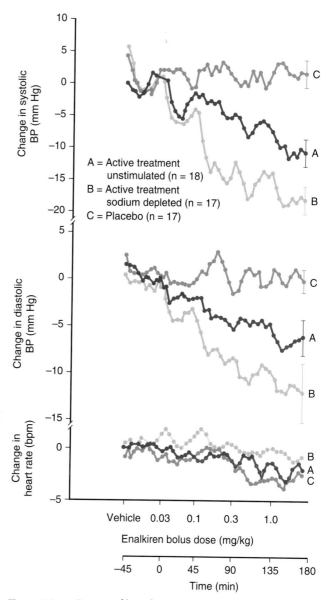

**Figure 72–8** Time profiles of systolic (upper panel) and diastolic BP (middle panel) and heart rate (lower panel) in patients with essential hypertension receiving increasing bolus doses of the renin inhibitor enalkiren at 45-min intervals. Dose-related antihypertensive effects of the renin inhibitor are enhanced after diuretic pretreatment with hydrochlorothiazide (**B vs. A**). Heart rate remains unchanged and placebo has no effect (**C**). (From Weber MA, Neutel JM, Essinger I, et al. Assessment of renin dependency of hypertension with a dipeptide renin inhibitor. Circulation 61:1768-1774, 1990.)

## OUTLOOK

Although it took three decades to reach today's insight into the utility of renin inhibition, it now appears that renin inhibitors could become, after ACE inhibitors and AT$_1$-receptor blockers, yet another class of useful drugs antagonizing the renin-angiotensin system. Renin inhibition does exactly what investigators anticipated some 30 years ago: It decreases Ang II

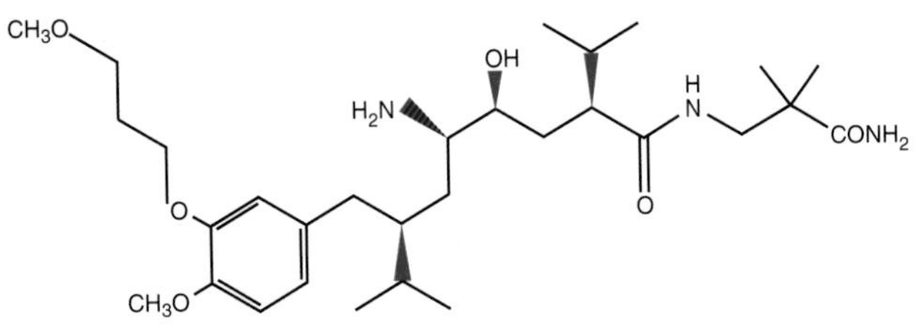

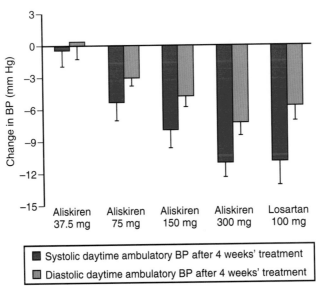

SPP 100 (Aliskiren)

**Figure 72-9** Structural formula of aliskiren, the first clinically successful orally active renin inhibitor. This substituted octanamid is a competitive transition state analog and specific inhibitor of human renin.[62]

generation with all the physiologic consequences, including decreasing BP and cardiac afterload. Improved bioavailability should reduce the cost of renin inhibitors. Early results with combination therapy including both a renin inhibitor and an ACE inhibitor, $AT_1$ receptor blocker or mineralocorticoid receptor antagonist, suggest synergistic rather than additive effects, and more-complete blockade of the renin-angiotensin system appears advantageous in most forms of hypertension. With favorable low incidences of side effects, renin inhibitors combined with $AT_1$ receptor blockers or mineralocorticoid receptor antagonists may become widely used cardiovascular drugs.

HYPOTENSIVE EFFECT OF ALISKIREN AND LOSARTAN

**Figure 72-10** Antihypertensive effect of aliskiren and losartan in patients with essential hypertension. Mean (SEM) change in daytime ambulatory systolic and diastolic BPs after 4 weeks of treatment with losartan and different doses of the orally active renin inhibitor aliskiren. The higher doses of the renin inhibitor are similarly hypotensive as the angiotensin receptor antagonist. (From Stanton A, Jensen C, Nussberger J, et al. Blood pressure lowering in essential hypertension with an oral renin inhibitor, aliskiren. Hypertension 42:1137-1143, 2003.)

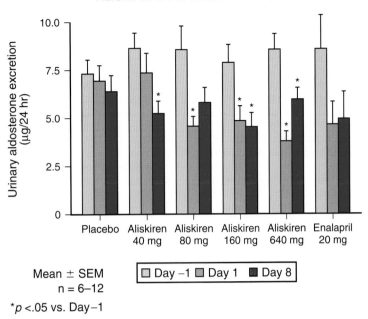

ALISKIREN AND URINARY ALDOSTERONE

Mean ± SEM
n = 6–12

*p <.05 vs. Day−1

□ Day −1  ▨ Day 1  ■ Day 8

**Figure 72–11** Urinary aldosterone excretion in healthy men after acute (Day 1) and sustained (Day 8) inhibition of the renin-angiotensin system by the renin inhibitor aliskiren and by the ACE inhibitor enalapril. All treatments reduce aldosterone excretion as compared with pretreatment (Day −1), but enalapril with only n = 6 does not reach significance. (From Nussberger J, Wuerzner G, Jensen C, et al. Angiotensin II suppression in humans by the orally active renin inhibitor aliskiren (SPP100). Hypertension 39:e1-e8, 2002.)

# References

1. Tigerstedt R, Bergman PG. Niere und Kreislauf. Skand Arch Physiol 8:223-271, 1898.
2. Mazzolai L, Pedrazzini T, Nicoud F, et al. Increased cardiac angiotensin II levels induce right and left ventricular hypertrophy in normotensive mice. Hypertension 35:985-991, 2000.
3. Brunner HR, Gavras H, Laragh JH, et al. Angiotensin II blockade in man by sar1-ala8-angiotensin II for understanding and treatment of high blood pressure. Lancet II:1045-1048, 1973.
4. Christen Y, Waeber B, Nussberger J, et al. Oral administration of DuP753, a specific angiotensin II receptor antagonist, to normal male volunteers. Inhibition of pressure response to exogenous angiotensin I and II. Circulation 83:1333-1342, 1991.
5. Bühler FR, Laragh JH, Vaughan ED, et al. Antihypertensive action of propranolol: Specific anti-renin responses in high and normal renin forms of essential, renal, renovascular and malignant hypertension. Am J Cardiol 32:511-522, 1973.
6. Michelakis AM, McAllister RG. The effect of chronic adrenergic receptor blockade on plasma renin activity in man. J Clin Endocrinol Metab 34:386-394, 1972.
7. Nussberger J. Circulating versus tissue angiotensin II. In Epstein M, Brunner HR (eds). Angiotensin II Receptor Antagonists. Philadelphia, Hanley and Belfus, 2000; pp 69-78.
8. Juillerat L, Nussberger J, Ménard J, et al. Determinants of angiotensin II generation during converting enzyme inhibition. Hypertension 16:564-572, 1990.
9. Kokubu T, Ueda E, Fujimoto S, et al. Peptide inhibitors of the renin-angiotensin system. Nature 217:456-457, 1968.
10. Poulsen K, Burton J, Haber E. Competitive inhibitors of renin: A review. Prog Biochem Pharmacol 12:135-141, 1976.
11. Haber E. Specific inhibitors of renin. Clin Sci 59(Suppl 6):7-19, 1980.
12. Zusman RM, Burton J, Christensen D, et al. Hemodynamic effects of a competitive renin in inhibitory peptide in humans. Evidence for multiple mechanisms of action. Trans Assoc Am Physicians 96:365-374, 1983.
13. Pals DT, DeGraaf DL, Kari WM, et al. Cardiovascular effects of a renin inhibitor in relation to posture in nonhuman primates. Clin Exp Hypertens A7:105-121, 1985.
14. Waeber B, Nussberger J, Brunner HR. Angiotensin-converting enzyme inhibitors in hypertension. In Laragh JH, Brenner BM (eds). Hypertension: Pathophysiology, Diagnosis and Management. New York, Raven Press, 1995; pp 2861-2875.
15. Ferreira SH. A bradykinin-potentiating factor present in the venom of Bothrops jararaca. Br J Pharmacol 24:163-169, 1965.
16. Ferreira SH, Greene X. Isolation of bradykinin-potentiating peptides from Bothrops jararaca venom. Biochemistry 9:2583-2593, 1970.
17. Cushman DW, Ondetti MA. Inhibitors of angiotensin converting enzyme. Prog Med Chem 17:41-104, 1980.
18. Bohlender J, Nussberger J, Bader M, et al. Feedback-control of renin and angiotensin levels in rats transgenic for wild-type angiotensinogen. Hypertension, submitted.
19. Azizi M, Bissery A, Bura-Rivière A, et al. Dual renin-angiotensin system blockade restores blood pressure-renin dependency in individuals with low renin concentrations. J Hypertens 21:1887-1895, 2003.
20. Oparil S, Haber E. The renin-angiotensin system. N Engl J Med 291:389-401, 1974.
21. Dzau V, Kopelman RI, Barger AC, et al. Comparison of renin-specific IgG and antibody fragment in studies of blood pressure regulation. Am J Physiol 246:H404-H409 and 247:XXXII, 1984.
22. Michel JB, Galen FX, Guettier C, et al. Immunological approach to blockade of the renin-substrate reaction. J Hypertens 7(Suppl 2):S63-S70, 1989.

23. Johnson CA, Wakerlin GE. Antiserum for renin. Proc Soc Exp Biol Med 44:277-281, 1940.
24. Gross F, Lazar J, Orth H. Inhibition of the renin-angiotensinogen reaction by pepstatin. Science 175:656, 1972.
25. Evin G, Gardes J, Kreft C, et al. Soluble pepstatins: A new approach to blockade in vivo of the renin angiotensin system. Clin Sci 55:167s-171s, 1978.
26. Eid M, Evin G, Castro B, et al. New renin inhibitors homologous with pepstatin. Biochem J 197:465-471, 1981.
27. Boger J, Lohr NS, Ulm EH, et al. Novel renin inhibitors containing the amino acid statine. Nature 303:81-84, 1983.
28. Hui K, Haber E. Renin inhibitors. In Robertson JIS, Nicholls MG (eds). The Renin-Angiotensin System. New York, Raven Press, 1993; pp 85.1-85.14.
29. Skeggs LT, Lentz KE, Kahn JR, et al. Kinetics of the action of renin with nine synthetic peptide substrates. J Exp Med 128:13-34, 1968.
30. Tewksbury DA, Dart RA, Travis J. The amino terminal amino acid sequence of human angiotensinogen. Biochem Biophys Res Commun 99:1311-1315, 1981.
31. Poulsen K, Burton J, Haber E. Competitive inhibitors of renin. Biochemistry 12:3877-3882, 1973.
32. Burton J, Poulsen K, Haber E. Competitive inhibitors of renin. Inhibitors effective at physiological pH. Biochemistry 14:3892-3898, 1975.
33. Haber E. Peptide inhibitors of renin in cardiovascular studies. Fed Proc 42:3155-3161, 1983.
34. Burton J, Cody RJ, Herd JA, et al. Specific inhibition of renin by an angiotensinogen analog: Studies in sodium depletion and renin-dependent hypertension. Proc Natl Acad Sci USA 77:5476-5479, 1980.
35. Evin G, Devin J, Castro B, et al. Synthesis of peptides related to the prosegment of mouse submaxillary gland renin precursor: A new approach to renin inhibitors. Proc Natl Acad Sci USA 81:48-52, 1984.
36. Cumin F, Evin G, Fehrentz JA, et al. Inhibition of human renin by synthetic peptides derived from its prosegment. J Biol Chem 260:9154-9157, 1985.
37. James MNG, Sielecki A, Salituro F, et al. Conformational flexibility in the active site of aspartyl proteinases revealed by a pepstatin fragment binding to penicillopepsin. Proc Natl Acad Sci USA 79:6137-6141, 1982.
38. Szelke M, Leckie B, Hallett A, et al. Potent new inhibitors of human renin. Nature 299:555-557, 1982.
39. Webb DJ, Manhem PJO, Ball SG, et al. A study of the renin inhibitor H142 in man. J Hypertens 3:653-658, 1985.
40. Luly JR, BaMaung N, Soderquist J, et al. Renin inhibitors. Dipeptide analogues of angiotensinogen utilizing a dihydroxyethylene transition-state mimic at the scissile bond to impart greater inhibitory potency. J Med Chem 31:2264-2276, 1988.
41. Wood JM, Gulati N, Forgiarini P, et al. Effects of a specific and long-acting renin inhibitor in the marmoset. Hypertension 7:797-803, 1985.
42. Toda N, Miyazaki M, Etoh Y, et al. Human renin inhibiting dipeptide. Eur J Pharmacol 129:393-396, 1986.
43. Hanson GJ, Baran JS, Lowrie HS, et al. Dipeptide glycols: A new class of renin inhibitors. Biochem Biophys Res Commun 132:155-161, 1985.
44. Nussberger J, Brunner D, Waeber B, et al. True versus immunoreactive angiotensin II in human plasma. Hypertension 7(Suppl I): I1-I7, 1985.
45. Nussberger J, Brunner HR. Measurement of angiotensins in plasma. In Robertson JIS, Nicholls MG (eds). The Renin-Angiotensin System. New York, Raven Press, 1993; pp 15.1-15.13.
46. Jeunemaître X, Ménard J, Nussberger J, et al. Plasma angiotensins, renin and blood pressure during acute renin inhibition by CGP 38560A in hypertensive patients. Am J Hypertens 2:819-827, 1989.
47. Hui KY, Knight DR, Nussberger J, et al. Effects of renin inhibition in the conscious primate Macaca fascicularis. Hypertension 14:480-487, 1989.
48. Fitzpatrick MA, Rademaker MT, Charles CJ, et al. Comparison of the effect of renin inhibition and angiotensin-converting enzyme inhibition in ovine heart failure. J Cardiovasc Pharmacol 19:169-175, 1992.
49. Blaine E, Schorn T, Boger J. Statine-containing renin inhibitor: Dissociation of blood pressure lowering and renin inhibition in sodium-deficient dogs. Hypertension 6(Suppl I):I111-I118, 1984.
50. Nussberger J, Brunner D, Waeber B, et al. In vitro renin inhibition to prevent generation of angiotensins during determination of plasma angiotensin I and II. Life Sci 42:1683-1688, 1988.
51. Haber E, Koerner T, Page LB, et al. Application of a radioimmunoassay for angiotensin I to the physiologic measurements of plasma renin activity in normal human subjects. J Clin Endocrinol Metab 29:1349-1355, 1969.
52. Sealey JE, Gerten-Banes J, Laragh JH. The renin system. Variations in man measured by radioimmunoassay or bioassay. Kidney Int 1:240-253, 1972.
53. Poulsen K, Joergensen J. An easy radioimmunological microassay of renin activity, concentration and substrate in human and animal plasma and tissues based on angiotensin I trapping by antibody. J Clin Endocrinol Metab 39:816-825, 1974.
54. Camenzind E, Nussberger J, Juillerat L, et al. Effect of the renin response during renin inhibition: Oral Ro 42-5892 in normal humans. J Cardiovasc Pharmacol 18:299-307, 1991.
55. Weber MA, Neutel JM, Essinger I, et al. Assessment of renin dependency of hypertension with a dipeptide renin inhibitor. Circulation 61:1768-1774, 1990.
56. Delabays A, Nussberger J, Porchet M, et al. Hemodynamic and humoral effects of the new renin inhibitor enalkiren in normal humans. Hypertension 13:941-947, 1989.
57. Nussberger J, Delabays A, de Gasparo M, et al. Hemodynamic and biochemical consequences of renin inhibition by infusion of CGP 38560A in normal volunteers. Hypertension 13:948-953, 1989.
58. Van den Meiracker AH, Admiraal PJJ, Man in't Veld AJ, et al. Prolonged blood pressure reduction by orally active renin inhibitor RO-42-5892 in essential hypertension. Br Med J 301:205-210, 1990.
59. Zusman RM, Hui KY, Nussberger J, et al. R-PEP-27, a potent renin inhibitor, decreases plasma angiotensin II and blood pressure in normal volunteers. Am J Hypertens 7:295-301, 1994.
60. Boger RS, Glassman HN, Thys R, et al. Absorption and blood pressure response to the new orally active renin inhibitor, A-72517, in hypertensive patients. Am J Hypertens 6:103A, 1993.
61. Ogihara T, Nagano M, Higaki J, et al. Antihypertensive efficacy of FK 906, a novel human renin inhibitor. Clin Ther 15:539-548, 1993.
62. Nussberger J, Wuerzner G, Jensen C, et al. Angiotensin II suppression in humans by the orally active renin inhibitor aliskiren (SPP100). Hypertension 39:e1-e8, 2002.
63. Stanton A, Jensen C, Nussberger J, et al. Blood pressure lowering in essential hypertension with an oral renin inhibitor, aliskiren. Hypertension 42:1137-1143, 2003.

# Secondary Hypertension

## Chapter 73

# Obstructive Sleep Apnea and Hypertension
## Apoor S. Gami, Virend K. Somers

## INTRODUCTION AND EPIDEMIOLOGY

Obstructive sleep apnea (OSA) is common in men and women of varied ethnic and geographic origins.[1-4] In general, about 25% of men and 10% of women have pathologic OSA, whereas 4% of men and 2% of women actually experience symptoms consistent with the OSA syndrome.[3,4] A prospective, population-based, cohort study has estimated that the 5-year cumulative incidence of OSA in American adults is about 16%.[5]

In 2003, the Joint National Committee on Prevention, Detection, Evaluation, and Treatment of High Blood Pressure acknowledged that OSA is an important secondary cause of systemic hypertension.[6] This causal link is substantiated by studies of integrated physiology and a preponderance of epidemiologic data[2,7-10] that have been substantiated by a large prospective population-based study.[10] Cross-sectional studies show that about half of patients with OSA have hypertension,[8,9] and the strong association exists regardless of gender, age, race, and body mass index.[8] The most compelling evidence comes from a study of more than 700 patients followed over 4 years after OSA diagnosis, in whom there was a direct linear relationship between the severity of OSA and the *incidence* (i.e., new cases) of hypertension (Figure 73-1).[10] Patients with mild OSA had twice the risk, and patients with moderate-severe OSA had almost three times the risk of developing hypertension as persons without OSA. This relationship was independent of obesity, smoking, alcohol, age, gender, and baseline blood pressure.[10]

## OBSTRUCTIVE SLEEP APNEA

Patients with OSA experience recurrent occlusions of the pharyngeal airway during sleep, resulting in partial or total cessation of airflow and hypoxemia.[11] This is followed by arousal to a lighter stage of sleep (usually without overt awakening) and restoration of airflow. This sequence of apneas and arousals can occur hundreds of times during the night.[12] Risk factors for OSA include male gender; middle age; retroposition of the mandible; decreased palatal height; and increased body mass index, waist circumference, and neck circumference.[4,13-15] Polysomnography is the gold standard to diagnose and assess the severity of OSA. Full polysomnography includes the simultaneous measurement during sleep of the electrocardiogram, electrooculogram, electroencephalogram, electromyogram, thoracoabdominal movements by strain belts, and nasooral airflow (Figure 73-2). An obstructive apnea is defined as the absence of airflow for at least 10 seconds in the presence of thoracoabdominal movements. An obstructive hypopnea is defined as at least a 50% decrease in airflow associated with either a decrease in oxygen saturation greater than 4% or evidence of arousal on the electroencephalogram. The apnea-hypopnea index (AHI), the number of apneic and hypopneic events per hour of sleep, is used to quantify the severity of OSA. An AHI less than 5 is normal; 5 to 15 is classified mild OSA; 15 to 30, moderate OSA; and greater than 30, severe OSA.[16]

## BLOOD PRESSURE IN NORMAL SLEEP

Normally, in patients without OSA, rapid eye movement (REM) sleep is characterized by marked fluctuations in blood pressure and heart rate, as well as increased sympathetic activity to muscle blood vessels. In general, however, heart rate and blood pressure are lower during sleep than during waking hours.[17-21] Decreases in blood pressure are mild and due to reductions in both cardiac output and systemic vascular resistance.[22,23] These normal changes are most apparent during deep non-REM sleep, and they appear to be related to cardiovascular autonomic function during sleep,[19] characterized by increased vagal activation and decreased sympathetic drive.[17,19,24]

## BLOOD PRESSURE IN OBSTRUCTIVE SLEEP APNEA

### Acute Nocturnal Changes in Blood Pressure

The sleep stage–dependent changes of normal sleep are disrupted in patients with OSA, in whom blood pressure markedly increases during sleep.[25-27] The mechanisms responsible for this increase include sympathetic activation due to chemoreflex excitation and the effects of circulating vasoconstrictors. Sympathetic activity and blood pressure

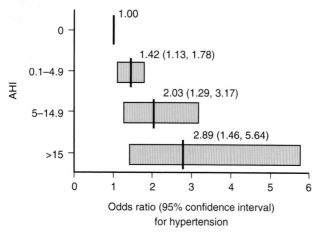

**Figure 73–1** Odds ratio for presence of hypertension at 4 years, based on baseline apnea-hypopnea index (AHI), after adjustment for baseline hypertension status, body mass index, neck and waist circumference, age, sex, and weekly use of alcohol and cigarettes. An AHI of 0 is used as the reference category. The odds ratios for the presence of hypertension at follow-up were 1.42 with an AHI 0.1 to 4.9, 2.03 with an AHI 5.0 to 14.9, and 2.89 with an AHI 15.0 or greater. (Data from Peppard PE, Young T, Palta M, et al. Prospective study of the association between sleep-disordered breathing and hypertension. N Engl J Med 342:1378–1384, 2000.)

progressively increase during an apnea.[25] At termination of apnea, blood pressure surges, sometimes to levels as high as 240/130 mm Hg, and sympathetic activity is abruptly inhibited.[25] The numerous repetitive apneic episodes result in large fluctuations in sympathetic activity and blood pressure throughout the night (Figure 73–3). These changes occur more often during stage II and REM sleep, when apnea severity is greatest. In addition, the normal nocturnal decrease in blood pressure may not occur or is blunted in patients with OSA (i.e., they are often "nondippers").[25,28] The increases in sympathetic activity during apneic episodes are due to the synergistic effects of hypoxemia and hypercapnia on peripheral and central chemoreceptors,[29-32] the effects of which are further augmented by the apnea-related absence of sympathetic inhibitory signals from the thoracic afferents.[33,34]

## Chronic Daytime Changes in Blood Pressure

The development of hypertension may be due to the daytime carryover of various nocturnal mechanisms of increased blood pressure in patients with OSA, in addition to other factors that are not directly related to the sleep-wake cycle.

### Sympathetic Activity

Increases in sympathetic activity, evident during sleep, persist during daytime normoxic wakefulness in patients with OSA.[25,31,35-37] Abnormalities in both baroreflex function[32,38,39] and chemoreceptor activation[31,32] may contribute to this sustained daytime sympathetic excitation.

### Cardiovascular Variability

In otherwise healthy patients with OSA, heart rate variability is decreased and blood pressure variability is increased in parallel with the severity of the sleep disorder.[40] In individuals without high blood pressure, decreased heart rate variability confers an increased risk of developing hypertension.[41] Increased blood pressure variability in patients with hypertension and decreased heart rate variability in patients with cardiovascular disease are both associated with adverse outcomes.[42-46] Thus, abnormalities in cardiovascular variability may be related to the development of hypertension and other cardiovascular diseases in patients with OSA.

### Endothelial Dysfunction

Patients with hypertension have impaired endothelium-dependent vascular relaxation,[47] and this may be partly explained by associations with OSA. Endothelium-dependent vasodilation of conductance and resistance vessels is abnormal in otherwise healthy patients with OSA.[48-50] Increased sympathetic drive, decreased nitric oxide production, inflammation, and humoral factors may mediate or contribute to endothelial dysfunction and hypertension in patients with OSA. Patients with OSA have lower endothelial nitric oxide synthase activity, and OSA may also be accompanied by lower circulating levels of nitric oxide.[51,52]

### Humoral Factors

Endothelin-1 is a potent vasoconstrictor with sustained activity and may be partly responsible for daytime hypertension associated with OSA. Endothelin-1 is elevated in patients with untreated OSA but not in patients with normal sleep.[53] Hypoxia is a strong stimulus for endothelin-1 production. In an animal model, intermittent hypoxia (such as in OSA) increases endothelin-1 and blood pressure, whereas treatment with an endothelin-1 blocker lowers blood pressure.[54] Leptin, an adipocyte-derived hormone with effects in various organ systems, may be associated with an increased risk of cardiovascular events.[55] Leptin levels are increased in obese patients and are even higher in patients with OSA.[56] In an animal model, administration of leptin increases blood pressure and renal sympathetic drive.[57,58] As such, in addition to its associations with obesity and cardiovascular disease events, leptin may contribute to sustained daytime hypertension in patients with OSA.

### Inflammation

OSA is characterized by marked local and systemic inflammation, independent of obesity and other comorbidities. Pharyngeal airway tissues of patients with OSA are congested with inflammatory cells, which may result in anatomic narrowing and functional impairments of the airway that predispose to apneas.[59] Systemic inflammation is evidenced by elevated circulating levels or activity of C-reactive protein,[60,61] cytokines such as interleukin-6 and tumor necrosis factor-α,[61,62] adhesion molecules,[63-66] and reactive oxygen species.[67-69] Hypertension, is also independently associated with elevated plasma concentrations of C-reactive protein.[70] Middle-aged individuals with higher C-reactive protein levels, even those with low blood

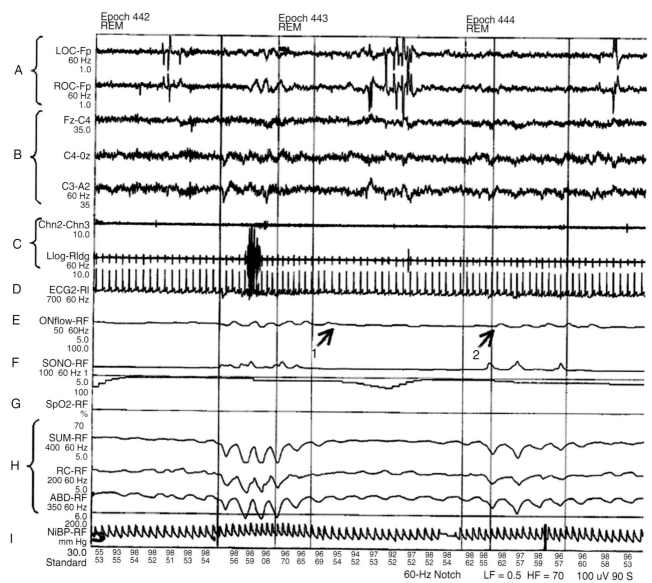

**Figure 73-2** Polysomnographic tracing with obstructive apneas. Shown are **(A)** electrooculography, **(B)** electroencephalography, **(C)** electromyography, **(D)** electrocardiography, **(E)** thermistor measures of airflow, **(F)** sonography, **(G)** pulse oximetry, **(H)** measures of thoracoabdominal movements via excursion belts, and **(I)** blood pressure *measurements* during 90 seconds of REM sleep. *Arrow 1* marks the initiation of an obstructive apnea, and *arrow 2* marks its termination. (From Gami AS, Caples SM, Somers VK. Obesity and obstructive sleep apnea. Endocrinol Metab Clin N Am 32(4):869-894, 2003; with permission.)

pressure and no comorbidities, have a significantly increased risk of developing incident hypertension in less than a decade.[71] The inflammatory milieu in these conditions is likely related to endothelial dysfunction and may have potential implications for related cardiovascular complications.

### Predisposition to Obesity

The relationship between obesity and hypertension is likely mediated by multiple interacting factors, including genetics, neural and metabolic abnormalities, fat distribution, and OSA.[72] Obesity is thought to be the most powerful risk factor for OSA. About 70% of patients with OSA are obese, and a 10% weight gain is associated with a sixfold increase in the risk of OSA.[10] Although numerous mechanisms are implicated in the causal pathway from obesity to OSA, it is possible, conversely, that OSA itself is a risk factor for obesity. Patients with newly diagnosed OSA have reported weight gain in the time before the diagnosis.[53,56] As discussed later, treatment of OSA results in weight loss and redistribution of fat.[73,74] Multiple mechanisms may explain this relationship (such as decreased activity due to daytime somnolence, resistance to the satiety signal of the leptin hormone,[56] and effects of leptin on respiratory control during sleep).[75] Thus, although obesity may cause OSA in some patients, in others OSA may lead to weight gain. This is important because the combination of OSA and obesity synergistically increase the risk of hypertension.[8,76,77]

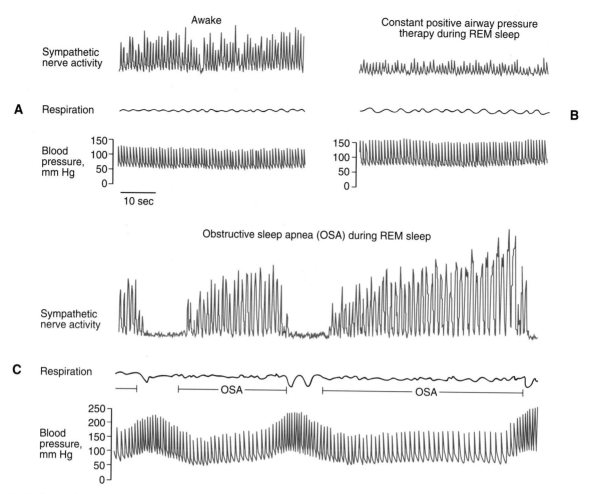

**Figure 73–3** Sympathetic nerve activity (SNA), respirations, and intraarterial blood pressure (BP) in an individual with obstructive sleep apnea **(A)** when awake, **(B)** during rapid eye movement (REM) sleep with obstructive apneas, and **(C)** during REM sleep with continuous positive airway pressure (CPAP) therapy. SNA is increased when awake, and it is higher during REM sleep. BP is normal when awake and exceeds 250/110 mm Hg at termination of the apneas during REM sleep. CPAP therapy during REM sleep abolishes apneas, resulting in decreased SNA and elimination of BP fluctuations. (Republished with permission of Journal of Clinical Investigations, from Somers VK, Dyken ME, Clary MP, et al. Sympathetic neural mechanisms in obstructive sleep apnea. J Clin Invest 96:1897–1904, 1995; permission conveyed through Copyright Clearance Center, Inc.)

## OBSTRUCTIVE SLEEP APNEA THERAPY

### Weight Loss

Weight loss can potentially cure OSA and may also attenuate associated comorbidities, especially hypertension.[78-82] Even a small weight reduction can elicit significant improvements in symptoms and severity of OSA.[83,84] Due to generally poor success in obesity treatment, other therapies for OSA are often necessary.

### Positive Airway Pressure

Continuous positive airway pressure (CPAP) is most commonly administered via a nasal mask. Applied during sleep, the pressurized air exerts an outward force and essentially splints the airway open, preventing obstruction during ventilation.[85] In most patients without specific indications for surgical treatments (i.e., craniofacial abnormalities), CPAP is the most effective therapy for OSA and improves daytime symptoms and function in patients with moderate or severe OSA.[86-88] The main obstacle to treating patients with CPAP is poor compliance, due to discomfort or inconvenience of the apparatus. Only half of patients accept the recommendation for its use, and a small fraction are compliant.[89-92] Strategies to increase its use include more comfortable masks,[93] humidified air,[94] different inspiratory and expiratory pressures (bilevel positive airway pressure, or BiPAP),[95,96] and team-based approaches to managing patients.[89] Treatment with CPAP has been shown to significantly lower nocturnal and daytime blood pressure levels (discussed later).

### Oral Appliances

Oral appliances are intended to alleviate OSA by repositioning the tongue and/or mandible to prevent airway occlusion during sleep. Results are fair (up to 60% efficacious) with various designs,[97-100] and they may be more useful for patients with supine OSA.[101] Patients prefer oral appliances to other modes of treatment,[97] and they should be offered to patients who do not tolerate or are not candidates for other therapies. It is unknown whether use of oral appliances results in decreased daytime blood pressure.

## Surgery

Surgery can cure OSA when specific craniofacial abnormalities, such as severe retrognathia, tonsillar hypertrophy, or deviated nasal septum, cause airway obstruction.[102,103] Despite its popularity, uvulopalatoplasty (UPP) is often ineffective, and more than half of patients will still have severe OSA (AHI >20) 2 years after surgery.[104] Patients who may benefit more from UPP are those with milder OSA and those who weigh less.[104] Bariatric surgery, including the Roux-en-Y gastric bypass, gastroplasty, and gastric banding, results in substantial weight loss in patients who are severely obese. This usually results in improvement or cure of OSA and many associated comorbidities.[82,105-110] However, as in nonsurgical weight loss, OSA returns when weight is regained.[109] The definitive and immediate treatment of OSA, reserved for debilitating cases that are unresponsive to other therapies or during medical illnesses that preclude their use, is tracheostomy, which allows ventilation to completely bypass the collapsible airway.[111]

## BLOOD PRESSURE EFFECTS OF OBSTRUCTIVE SLEEP APNEA THERAPY

### Positive Airway Pressure

The widely used, titratable, and effective therapy for OSA, nasal CPAP, has beneficial effects on numerous mechanisms of hypertension, acute nocturnal blood pressure surges, daytime hypertension, and the complications of hypertension.

Both short- and long-term use of CPAP attenuate many of the mechanisms related to hypertension in patients with OSA. It has been shown to markedly decrease sympathetic activity acutely during the night[25] and during daytime wakefulness.[112] Its use is also associated with decreased production of superoxide by polymorphonuclear neutrophils,[51] increased nitric oxide,[67] and attenuated white cell adhesion to cultured endothelial cells,[65] which may improve endothelial function. Sustained CPAP therapy reduces circulating levels of angiotensin II[113] and leptin.[52,74,114,115] There is even evidence that long-term use of CPAP aids weight loss[73,116] and changes the distribution of fat (decreasing visceral adiposity),[74] both of which have important effects on hypertension.[117,118]

There are unequivocal beneficial effects of CPAP on blood pressure and hypertension. During sleep, CPAP decreases acute nocturnal blood pressure surges[25,119,120] and helps reestablish the normal dip in nocturnal blood pressure.[25] The carryover of these effects into the daytime has been shown by numerous observational studies[120-125] and now more randomized controlled trials.[92,125] Becker et al. randomized 60 patients with moderate or severe OSA to either effective CPAP or subtherapeutic CPAP for 9 weeks. Although only 32 patients completed the study (again highlighting technical and compliance issues related to CPAP), the results showed a significant decrease of about 10 mm Hg in mean, systolic, and diastolic blood pressures during the night and daytime in patients using effective CPAP (Figure 73–4).[92]

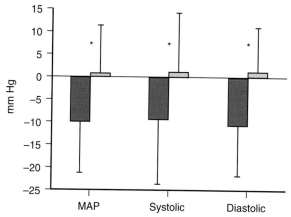

**Figure 73–4** Changes in mean arterial pressure (MAP), systolic pressure, and diastolic pressure with use of effective continuous positive airway pressure (CPAP) therapy *(closed bars)* and subtherapeutic CPAP therapy *(open bars)*. Blood pressures were measured continuously and noninvasively in an ambulatory setting before and after an average of 2 months of effective or subtherapeutic CPAP therapy in a predominantly hypertensive group of patients with moderate to severe obstructive sleep apnea syndrome. Asterisks indicate p <.05. (From Becker HF, Jerrenstrup A, Ploch T, et al. Effect of nasal continuous positive airway pressure treatment on blood pressure in patients with obstructive sleep apnea. Circulation 107:68–73, 2003; with permission.)

The magnitude of blood pressure reduction with CPAP therapy appears to be greatest in patients using antihypertensive medications.[125] It also appears that the magnitude of blood pressure reduction correlates with the severity of OSA.[125] These data add to the evidence that OSA may be a cause of resistant hypertension,[126-130] which may be more responsive to pharmacologic therapy after initiation of CPAP (see Chapter 59 for a discussion of resistant hypertension).

In addition to direct effects on hypertension, OSA therapy may conceivably decrease the incidence and the severity of complications of hypertension, such as left ventricular hypertrophy,[131] congestive heart failure,[132-135] atrial fibrillation,[136] and ischemic heart disease.[137] Of special note are the beneficial effects of CPAP therapy on several components (in addition to hypertension) of the metabolic syndrome, including visceral adiposity,[74] insulin resistance,[138-141] and dyslipidemia.[142,143]

## SUMMARY

1. OSA is a secondary cause of systemic hypertension.
2. OSA is prevalent in patients with hypertension.
3. Risk factors for OSA include male gender, age, body mass index, waist circumference, neck circumference, and oral cavity dimensions.
4. Patients with resistant hypertension (patients whose blood pressure is not at goal while taking adequate doses of two or more appropriately chosen medications) should be considered for polysomnography to rule out OSA.

5. Polysomnography is the gold standard for diagnosing and assessing the response to therapy for OSA.

6. Effective therapies for most patients with OSA include sustained weight loss (ideal) and CPAP (most widely used).

7. Treatment of OSA with CPAP may have important beneficial effects for treatment of hypertension and mitigating its serious complications, including arrhythmias, congestive heart failure, and ischemic heart disease.

# References

1. Ohayon MM, Guilleminault C, Priest RG, et al. Is sleep-disordered breathing an independent risk factor for hypertension in the general population (13,057 subjects)? J Psychosom Res 48:593-601, 2000.

2. Bixler EO, Vgontzas AN, Lin HM, et al. Association of hypertension and sleep-disordered breathing. Arch Intern Med 160:2289-2295, 2000.

3. Young T, Palta M, Dempsey J, et al. The occurrence of sleep-disordered breathing among middle-aged adults. N Engl J Med 328:1230-1235, 1993.

4. Young T, Shahar E, Nieto FJ, et al. Predictors of sleep-disordered breathing in community-dwelling adults: The Sleep Heart Health Study. Arch Intern Med 162:893-900, 2002.

5. Tishler PV, Larkin EK, Schluchter MD, et al. Incidence of sleep-disordered breathing in an urban adult population: The relative importance of risk factors in the development of sleep-disordered breathing. JAMA 289:2230-2237, 2003.

6. Chobanian AV, Bakris GL, Black HR, et al. The Seventh Report of the Joint National Committee on Prevention, Detection, Evaluation, and Treatment of High Blood Pressure: The JNC 7 report. JAMA 289:2560-2572, 2003.

7. Dart RA, Gregoire JR, Gutterman DD, et al. The association of hypertension and secondary cardiovascular disease with sleep-disordered breathing. Chest 123:244-260, 2003.

8. Nieto FJ, Young TB, Lind BK, et al. Association of sleep-disordered breathing, sleep apnea, and hypertension in a large community-based study. Sleep Heart Health Study. JAMA 283:1829-1836, 2000.

9. Millman RP, Redline S, Carlisle CC, et al. Daytime hypertension in obstructive sleep apnea. Prevalence and contributing risk factors. Chest 99:861-866, 1991.

10. Peppard PE, Young T, Palta M, et al. Prospective study of the association between sleep-disordered breathing and hypertension. N Engl J Med 342:1378-1384, 2000.

11. Guilleminault C, Tilkian A, Dement WC. The sleep apnea syndromes. Annu Rev Med 27:465-484, 1976.

12. Guilleminault C, Kim YD, Horita M, et al. Power spectral sleep EEG findings in patients with obstructive sleep apnea and upper airway resistance syndromes. Electroencephalogr Clin Neurophysiol Suppl 50:113-120, 1999.

13. Davies RJ, Stradling JR. The relationship between neck circumference, radiographic pharyngeal anatomy, and the obstructive sleep apnoea syndrome. Eur Respir J 3:509-514, 1990.

14. Katz I, Stradling J, Slutsky AS, et al. Do patients with obstructive sleep apnea have thick necks? Am Rev Respir Dis 141:1228-1231, 1990.

15. Kushida CA, Efron B, Guilleminault C. A predictive morphometric model for the obstructive sleep apnea syndrome. Ann Intern Med 127:581-587, 1997.

16. Sleep-related breathing disorders in adults: Recommendations for syndrome definition and measurement techniques in clinical research. The Report of the American Academy of Sleep Medicine Task Force. Sleep 22:667-689, 1999.

17. Hornyak M, Cejnar M, Elam M, et al. Sympathetic muscle nerve activity during sleep in man. Brain 114(Pt 3):1281-1295, 1991.

18. Okada H, Iwase S, Mano T, et al. Changes in muscle sympathetic nerve activity during sleep in humans. Neurology 41:1961-1966, 1991.

19. Somers V, Dyken M, Mark A, et al. Sympathetic-nerve activity during sleep in normal subjects. N Engl J Med 328:303-307, 1993.

20. Khatri IM, Freis ED. Hemodynamic changes during sleep. J Appl Physiol 22:867-873, 1967.

21. Coccagna G, Mantovani M, Brignani F, et al. Laboratory note. Arterial pressure changes during spontaneous sleep in man. Electroencephalogr Clin Neurophysiol 31:277-281, 1971.

22. Miller JC, Helander M. The 24 hour cycle and nocturnal depression of human cardiac output. Aviat Space Environ Med 50:1139-1144, 1979.

23. Coote JH. Respiratory and circulatory control during sleep. J Exp Biol 100:223-244, 1982.

24. Furlan R, Guzzetti S, Crivellaro W, et al. Continuous 24-hour assessment of the neural regulation of systemic arterial pressure and RR variabilities in ambulant subjects. Circulation 81:537-547, 1990.

25. Somers VK, Dyken ME, Clary MP, et al. Sympathetic neural mechanisms in obstructive sleep apnea. J Clin Invest 96:1897-1904, 1995.

26. Tilkian AG, Guilleminault C, Schroeder JS, et al. Hemodynamics in sleep-induced apnea. Studies during wakefulness and sleep. Ann Intern Med 85:714-719, 1976.

27. Motta J, Guilleminault C, Schroeder JS, et al. Tracheostomy and hemodynamic changes in sleep-inducing apnea. Ann Intern Med 89:454-458, 1978.

28. Portaluppi F, Provini F, Cortelli P, et al. Undiagnosed sleep-disordered breathing among male nondippers with essential hypertension. J Hypertens 15:1227-1233, 1997.

29. Somers VK, Mark AL, Zavala DC, et al. Contrasting effects of hypoxia and hypercapnia on ventilation and sympathetic activity in humans. J Appl Physiol 67:2101-2106, 1989.

30. Somers VK, Mark AL, Zavala DC, et al. Influence of ventilation and hypocapnia on sympathetic nerve responses to hypoxia in normal humans. J Appl Physiol 67:2095-2100, 1989.

31. Hedner J, Wilcox I, Laks L, et al. A specific and potent pressor effect of hypoxia in patients with sleep apnea. Am Rev Respir Dis 146:1240-1245, 1992.

32. Narkiewicz K, van de Borne PJ, Pesek CA, et al. Selective potentiation of peripheral chemoreflex sensitivity in obstructive sleep apnea. Circulation 99:1183-1189, 1999.

33. Somers V, Mark A, Abboud F. Potentiation of sympathetic nerve responses to hypoxia in borderline hypertensive subjects. Hypertension 11:608-612, 1988.

34. Somers V, Mark A, Abboud F. Interaction of baroreceptor and chemoreceptor control of sympathetic nerve activity in normal humans. J Clin Invest 87:1953-1957, 1991.

35. Carlson JT, Hedner J, Elam M, et al. Augmented resting sympathetic activity in awake patients with obstructive sleep apnea. Chest 103:1763-1768, 1993.

36. Narkiewicz K, van de Borne PJ, Cooley RL, et al. Sympathetic activity in obese subjects with and without obstructive sleep apnea. Circulation 98:772-776, 1998.

37. Hedner J, Ejnell H, Sellgren J, et al. Is high and fluctuating muscle nerve sympathetic activity in the sleep apnea syndrome of pathogenetic importance for the development of hypertension? J Hypertens 6:S529-S531, 1988.

38. Carlson J, Rangemark C, Hedner J. Attenuated endothelium-dependent vascular relaxation in patients with sleep apnoea. J Hypertens 14:577-584, 1996.

39. Narkiewicz K, van de Borne P, Montano N, et al. Contribution of tonic chemoreflex activation to sympathetic activity and blood pressure in patients with obstructive sleep apnea. Circulation 97:943-945, 1998.

40. Narkiewicz K, Montano N, Cogliati C, et al. Altered cardiovascular variability in obstructive sleep apnea. Circulation 98, 1998.

41. Singh JP, Larson MG, Tsuji H, et al. Reduced heart rate variability and new-onset hypertension: Insights into pathogenesis of hypertension: the Framingham Heart Study. Hypertension 32:293-297, 1998.

42. Ghuran A, Reid F, La Rovere MT, et al. Heart rate turbulence-based predictors of fatal and nonfatal cardiac arrest (the Autonomic Tone and Reflexes After Myocardial Infarction substudy). Am J Cardiol 89:184-190, 2002.

43. La Rovere MT, Bigger JT Jr, Marcus FI, et al. Baroreflex sensitivity and heart-rate variability in prediction of total cardiac mortality after myocardial infarction. ATRAMI (Autonomic Tone and Reflexes After Myocardial Infarction) Investigators. Lancet 351:478-484, 1998.

44. Saul JP, Arai Y, Berger RD, et al. Assessment of autonomic regulation in chronic congestive heart failure by heart rate spectral analysis. Am J Cardiol 61:1292-1299, 1988.

45. Kleiger RE, Miller JP, Bigger JT Jr, et al. Decreased heart rate variability and its association with increased mortality after acute myocardial infarction. Am J Cardiol 59:256-262, 1987.

46. Frattola A, Parati G, Cuspidi C, et al. Prognostic value of 24-hour blood pressure variability. J Hypertens 11:1133-1137, 1993.

47. Panza JA, Quyyumi AA, Brush JE Jr, et al. Abnormal endothelium-dependent vascular relaxation in patients with essential hypertension. N Engl J Med 323:22-27, 1990.

48. Nieto FJ, Herrington DM, Redline S, et al. Sleep apnea and markers of vascular endothelial function in a large community sample of older adults. Am J Respir Crit Care Med 169:354-360, 2004.

49. Ip MS, Tse HF, Lam B, et al. Endothelial function in obstructive sleep apnea and response to treatment. Am J Respir Crit Care Med 169:348-353, 2004.

50. Kato M, Roberts-Thomson P, Phillips B. Impairment of endothelium-dependent vasodilation of resistance vessels in patients with obstructive sleep apnea. Circulation 102:2607-2610, 2000.

51. Schulz R, Schmidt D, Blum A. Decreased plasma levels of nitric oxide derivatives in obstructive sleep apnoea: Response to CPAP therapy. Thorax 55:1046-1051, 2000.

52. Ip MS, Lam B, Chan LY, et al. Circulating nitric oxide is suppressed in obstructive sleep apnea and is reversed by nasal continuous positive airway pressure. Am J Respir Crit Care Med 164:1997-1998, 2000.

53. Phillips B, Narkiewicz K, Pesek C, et al. Effects of obstructive sleep apnea on endothelin-1 and blood pressure. J Hypertension 17:61-66, 1999.

54. Kanagy NL, Walker BR, Nelin LD. Role of endothelin in intermittent hypoxia-induced hypertension. Hypertension 37:511-515, 2001.

55. Wallace AM, McMahon AD, Packard CJ, et al. Plasma leptin and the risk of cardiovascular disease in the west of Scotland coronary prevention study (WOSCOPS). Circulation 104:3052-3056, 2001.

56. Phillips BG, Kato M, Narkiewicz K, et al. Increases in leptin levels, sympathetic drive, and weight gain in obstructive sleep apnea. Am J Physiol Heart Circ Physiol 279:H234-H237, 2000.

57. Haynes WG, Morgan DA, Walsh SA, et al. Receptor-mediated regional sympathetic nerve activation by leptin. J Clin Invest 100:270-278, 1997.

58. Shek E, Brands M, Hall J. Chronic leptin infusion increases arterial pressure. Hypertension 31:409-414, 1998.

59. Hatipoglu U, Rubinstein I. Inflammation and obstructive sleep apnea syndrome pathogenesis: a working hypothesis. Respiration 70:665-671, 2003.

60. Shamsuzzaman AS, Winnicki M, Lanfranchi P, et al. Elevated C-reactive protein in patients with obstructive sleep apnea. Circulation 105:2462-2464, 2002.

61. Teramoto S, Yamamoto H, Ouchi Y. Increased C-reactive protein and increased plasma interleukin-6 may synergistically affect the progression of coronary atherosclerosis in obstructive sleep apnea syndrome. Circulation 107:E40-0, 2003.

62. Vgontzas AN, Papanicolaou DA, Bixler EO, et al. Sleep apnea and daytime sleepiness and fatigue: relation to visceral obesity, insulin resistance, and hypercytokinemia. J Clin Endocrinol Metab 85:1151-1158, 2000.

63. Ohga E, Nagase T, Tomita T, et al. Increased levels of circulating ICAM-1, VCAM-1, and L-selectin in obstructive sleep apnea syndrome. J Appl Physiol 87:10-14, 1999.

64. El-Solh AA, Mador MJ, Sikka P, et al. Adhesion molecules in patients with coronary artery disease and moderate-to-severe obstructive sleep apnea. Chest 121:1541-1547, 2002.

65. Dyugovskaya L, Lavie P, Lavie L. Increased adhesion molecules expression and production of reactive oxygen species in leukocytes of sleep apnea patients. Am J Respir Crit Care Med 165:934-939, 2002.

66. Dyugovskaya L, Lavie P, Lavie L. Phenotypic and functional characterization of blood gammadelta T cells in sleep apnea. Am J Respir Crit Care Med 168:242-249, 2003.

67. Schulz R, Mahmoudi S, Hattar K, et al. Enhanced release of superoxide from polymorphonuclear neutrophils in obstructive sleep apnea. Impact of continuous positive airway pressure therapy. Am J Respir Crit Care Med 162:566-570, 2000.

68. Lavie L, Lotan R, Hochberg I, et al. Haptoglobin polymorphism is a risk factor for cardiovascular disease in patients with obstructive sleep apnea syndrome. Sleep 26:592-595, 2003.

69. Lavie L. Obstructive sleep apnoea syndrome—an oxidative stress disorder. Sleep Med Rev 7:35-51, 2003.

70. Schillaci G, Pirro M, Gemelli F, et al. Increased C-reactive protein concentrations in never-treated hypertension: The role of systolic and pulse pressures. J Hypertens 21:1841-1846, 2003.

71. Sesso HD, Buring JE, Rifai N, et al. C-reactive protein and the risk of developing hypertension. JAMA 290:2945-2951, 2003.

72. Wolk R, Shamsuzzaman AS, Somers VK. Obesity, sleep apnea, and hypertension. Hypertension 2003.

73. Loube DI, Loube AA, Erman MK. Continuous positive airway pressure treatment results in weight less in obese and overweight patients with obstructive sleep apnea. J Am Diet Assoc 97:896-897, 1997.

74. Chin K, Shimizu K, Nakamura T, et al. Changes in intra-abdominal visceral fat and serum leptin levels in patients with obstructive sleep apnea syndrome following nasal continuous positive airway pressure therapy. Circulation 100:706-712, 1999.

75. O'Donnell CP, Tankersley CG, Polotsky VP, et al. Leptin, obesity, and respiratory function. Respir Physiol 119:163-170, 2000.

76. Kiselak J, Clark M, Pera V, et al. The association between hypertension and sleep apnea in obese patients. Chest 104:775-780, 1993.

77. Garrison RJ, Kannel WB, Stokes J III, et al. Incidence and precursors of hypertension in young adults: The Framingham Offspring Study. Prev Med 16:235-251, 1987.

78. Harman EM, Wynne JW, Block AJ. The effect of weight loss on sleep-disordered breathing and oxygen desaturation in morbidly obese men. Chest 82:291-294, 1982.

79. Suratt PM, McTier RF, Findley LJ, et al. Effect of very-low-calorie diets with weight loss on obstructive sleep apnea. Am J Clin Nutr 56:182S-184S, 1992.

80. Pasquali R, Colella P, Cirignotta F, et al. Treatment of obese patients with obstructive sleep apnea syndrome (OSAS): Effect of weight loss and interference of otorhinolaryngoiatric pathology. Int J Obes 14:207-217, 1990.

81. Kansanen M, Vanninen E, Tuunainen A, et al. The effect of a very low-calorie diet-induced weight loss on the severity of obstructive sleep apnoea and autonomic nervous function in obese patients with obstructive sleep apnoea syndrome. Clin Physiol 18:377-385, 1998.

82. Dixon JB, O'Brien PE. Changes in comorbidities and improvements in quality of life after LAP-BAND placement. Am J Surg 184:51S-54S, 2002.

83. Browman CP, Sampson MG, Yolles SF, et al. Obstructive sleep apnea and body weight. Chest 85:435-438, 1984.

84. Smith PL, Gold AR, Meyers DA, et al. Weight loss in mildly to moderately obese patients with obstructive sleep apnea. Ann Intern Med 103:850-855, 1985.

85. Sullivan CE, Issa FG, Berthon-Jones M, et al. Reversal of obstructive sleep apnoea by continuous positive airway pressure applied through the nares. Lancet 1:862-865, 1981.

86. Davies RJ, Stradling JR. The efficacy of nasal continuous positive airway pressure in the treatment of obstructive sleep apnea syndrome is proven. Am J Respir Crit Care Med 161:1775-1776, 2000.

87. Montserrat JM, Ferrer M, Hernandez L, et al. Effectiveness of CPAP treatment in daytime function in sleep apnea syndrome: A randomized controlled study with an optimized placebo. Am J Respir Crit Care Med 164:608-613, 2001.

88. Jenkinson C, Davies RJ, Mullins R, et al. Comparison of therapeutic and subtherapeutic nasal continuous positive airway pressure for obstructive sleep apnoea: A randomised prospective parallel trial. Lancet 353:2100-2105, 1999.

89. Engleman HM, Wild MR. Improving CPAP use by patients with the sleep apnoea/hypopnoea syndrome (SAHS). Sleep Med Rev 7:81-99, 2003.

90. Meurice JC, Dore P, Paquereau J, et al. Predictive factors of long-term compliance with nasal continuous positive airway pressure treatment in sleep apnea syndrome. Chest 105:429-433, 1994.

91. Grote L, Hedner J, Grunstein R, et al. Therapy with nCPAP: Incomplete elimination of sleep related breathing disorder. Eur Respir J 16:921-927, 2000.

92. Becker HF, Jerrentrup A, Ploch T, et al. Effect of nasal continuous positive airway pressure treatment on blood pressure in patients with obstructive sleep apnea. Circulation 107:68-73, 2003.

93. Malhotra A, Ayas NT, Epstein LJ. The art and science of continuous positive airway pressure therapy in obstructive sleep apnea. Curr Opin Pulm Med 6:490-495, 2000.

94. Massie CA, Hart RW, Peralez K, et al. Effects of humidification on nasal symptoms and compliance in sleep apnea patients using continuous positive airway pressure. Chest 116:403-408, 1999.

95. Littner M, Hirshkowitz M, Davila D, et al. Practice parameters for the use of auto-titrating continuous positive airway pressure devices for titrating pressures and treating adult patients with obstructive sleep apnea syndrome. An American Academy of Sleep Medicine report. Sleep 25:143-147, 2002.

96. Berry RB, Parish JM, Hartse KM. The use of auto-titrating continuous positive airway pressure for treatment of adult obstructive sleep apnea. An American Academy of Sleep Medicine review. Sleep 25:148-173, 2002.

97. Ferguson KA, Ono T, Lowe AA, et al. A randomized crossover study of an oral appliance vs nasal-continuous positive airway pressure in the treatment of mild-moderate obstructive sleep apnea. Chest 109:1269-1275, 1996.

98. O'Sullivan RA, Hillman DR, Mateljan R, et al. Mandibular advancement splint: An appliance to treat snoring and obstructive sleep apnea. Am J Respir Crit Care Med 151:194-198, 1995.

99. Schmidt-Nowara WW, Meade TE, Hays MB. Treatment of snoring and obstructive sleep apnea with a dental orthosis. Chest 99:1378-1385, 1991.

100. Mehta A, Qian J, Petocz P, et al. A randomized, controlled study of a mandibular advancement splint for obstructive sleep apnea. Am J Respir Crit Care Med 163:1457-1461, 2001.

101. Cartwright RD. Predicting response to the tongue retaining device for sleep apnea syndrome. Arch Otolaryngol 111:385-388, 1985.

102. Sher AE, Schechtman KB, Piccirillo JF. The efficacy of surgical modifications of the upper airway in adults with obstructive sleep apnea syndrome. Sleep 19:156-177, 1996.

103. Heimer D, Scharf SM, Lieberman A, et al. Sleep apnea syndrome treated by repair of deviated nasal septum. Chest 84:184-185, 1983.

104. Larsson LH, Carlsson-Nordlander B, Svanborg E. Four-year follow-up after uvulopalatopharyngoplasty in 50 unselected patients with obstructive sleep apnea syndrome. Laryngoscope 104:1362-1368, 1994.

105. Sugerman HJ, Fairman RP, Lindeman AK, et al. Gastroplasty for respiratory insufficiency of obesity. Ann Surg 193:677-685, 1981.

106. Victor DW Jr, Sarmiento CF, Yanta M, et al. Obstructive sleep apnea in the morbidly obese. An indication for gastric bypass. Arch Surg 119:970-972, 1984.

107. Sugerman HJ, Fairman RP, Baron PL, et al. Gastric surgery for respiratory insufficiency of obesity. Chest 90:81-86, 1986.

108. Dixon JB, Schachter LM, O'Brien PE. Sleep disturbance and obesity: Changes following surgically induced weight loss. Arch Intern Med 161:102-106, 2001.

109. Charuzi I, Lavie P, Peiser J, et al. Bariatric surgery in morbidly obese sleep-apnea patients: Short- and long-term follow-up. Am J Clin Nutr 55:594S-596S, 1992.

110. Peiser J, Lavie P, Ovnat A, et al. Sleep apnea syndrome in the morbidly obese as an indication for weight reduction surgery. Ann Surg 199:112-115, 1984.

111. Mickelson SA. Upper airway bypass surgery for obstructive sleep apnea syndrome. Otolaryngol Clin North Am 31:1013-1023, 1998.

112. Hedner J, Darpo B, Ejnell H, et al. Reduction in sympathetic activity after long-term CPAP treatment in sleep apnoea: Cardiovascular implications. Eur Respir J 8:222-229, 1995.

113. Moller DS, Lind P, Strunge B, et al. Abnormal vasoactive hormones and 24-hour blood pressure in obstructive sleep apnea. Am J Hypertens 16:274-280, 2003.

114. Harsch IA, Konturek PC, Koebnick C, et al. Leptin and ghrelin levels in patients with obstructive sleep apnoea: Effect of CPAP treatment. Eur Respir J 22:251-257, 2003.

115. Saarelainen S, Lahtela J, Kallonen E. Effect of nasal CPAP treatment on insulin sensitivity and plasma leptin. J Sleep Res 6:146-147, 1997.

116. Sullivan CE, Issa FG, Berthon-Jones M, et al. Home treatment of obstructive sleep apnoea with continuous positive airway pressure applied through a nose-mask. Bull Eur Physiopathol Respir 20:49-54, 1984.

117. Peiris AN, Sothmann MS, Hoffmann RG, et al. Adiposity, fat distribution, and cardiovascular risk. Ann Intern Med 110:867-872, 1989.

118. Hayashi T, Boyko EJ, Leonetti DL, et al. Visceral adiposity and the prevalence of hypertension in Japanese Americans. Circulation 108:1718-1723, 2003.

119. Mayer J, Becker H, Brandenburg U, et al. Blood pressure and sleep apnea: Results of long-term nasal continuous positive airway pressure therapy. Cardiology 79:84-92, 1991.

120. Jennum P, Wildschiodtz G, Christensen NJ, et al. Blood pressure, catecholamines, and pancreatic polypeptide in obstructive sleep apnea with and without nasal Continuous Positive Airway Pressure (nCPAP) treatment. Am J Hypertens 2:847-52, 1989.

121. Wilcox I, Grunstein RR, Hedner JA, et al. Effect of nasal continuous positive airway pressure during sleep on 24-hour blood pressure in obstructive sleep apnea. Sleep 16:539-544, 1993.

122. Akashiba T, Kurashina K, Minemura H, et al. Daytime hypertension and the effects of short-term nasal continuous positive

airway pressure treatment in obstructive sleep apnea syndrome. Intern Med 34:528-532, 1995.

123. Voogel AJ, van Steenwijk RP, Karemaker JM, et al. Effects of treatment of obstructive sleep apnea on circadian hemodynamics. J Auton Nerv Syst 77:177-183, 1999.

124. Faccenda JF, Mackay TW, Boon NA, et al. Randomized placebo-controlled trial of continuous positive airway pressure on blood pressure in the sleep apnea-hypopnea syndrome. Am J Respir Crit Care Med 163:344-348, 2001.

125. Pepperell JC, Ramdassingh-Dow S, Crosthwaite N, et al. Ambulatory blood pressure after therapeutic and subtherapeutic nasal continuous positive airway pressure for obstructive sleep apnoea: A randomised parallel trial. Lancet 359:204-210, 2002.

126. Lavie P, Hoffstein V. Sleep apnea syndrome: A possible contributing factor to resistant hypertension. Sleep 24:721-725, 2001.

127. Logan AG, Perlikowski SM, Mente A, et al. High prevalence of unrecognized sleep apnoea in drug-resistant hypertension. J Hypertens 19:2271-2277, 2001.

128. Isaksson H, Svanborg E. Obstructive sleep apnea syndrome in male hypertensives, refractory to drug therapy. Nocturnal automatic blood pressure measurements—An aid to diagnosis? Clin Exp Hypertens A 13:1195-1212, 1991.

129. Zelveian PA. Possible contributing factors of sleep apnea syndrome to resistant hypertension. Sleep 26:12; author reply 12, 2003.

130. Logan AG, Tkacova R, Perlikowski SM, et al. Refractory hypertension and sleep apnoea: Effect of CPAP on blood pressure and baroreflex. Eur Respir J 21:241-247, 2003.

131. Cloward TV, Walker JM, Farney RJ, et al. Left ventricular hypertrophy is a common echocardiographic abnormality in severe obstructive sleep apnea and reverses with nasal continuous positive airway pressure. Chest 124:594-601, 2003.

132. Malone S, Liu PP, Holloway R, et al. Obstructive sleep apnoea in patients with dilated cardiomyopathy: Effects of continuous positive airway pressure. Lancet 338:1480-1484, 1991.

133. Laaban JP, Pascal-Sebaoun S, Bloch E, et al. Left ventricular systolic dysfunction in patients with obstructive sleep apnea syndrome. Chest 122:1133-1138, 2002.

134. Kaneko Y, Floras JS, Usui K, et al. Cardiovascular effects of continuous positive airway pressure in patients with heart failure and obstructive sleep apnea. N Engl J Med 348:1233-1241, 2003.

135. Mansfield DR, Gollogly NC, Kaye DM, et al. Controlled Trial of Continuous Positive Airway Pressure in Obstructive Sleep Apnea and Heart Failure. Am J Respir Crit Care Med 2003.

136. Kanagala R, Murali NS, Friedman PA, et al. Obstructive sleep apnea and the recurrence of atrial fibrillation. Circulation 107:2589-2594, 2003.

137. Peled N, Abinader EG, Pillar G, et al. Nocturnal ischemic events in patients with obstructive sleep apnea syndrome and ischemic heart disease: Effects of continuous positive air pressure treatment. J Am Coll Cardiol 34:1744-1749, 1999.

138. Brooks B, Cistulli PA, Borkman M, et al. Obstructive sleep apnea in obese noninsulin-dependent diabetic patients: Effect of continuous positive airway pressure treatment on insulin responsiveness. J Clin Endocrinol Metab 79:1681-1685, 1994.

139. Elmasry A, Lindberg E, Berne C, et al. Sleep-disordered breathing and glucose metabolism in hypertensive men: A population-based study. J Intern Med 249:153-161, 2001.

140. Ip M, Lam B, Ng M, et al. Obstructive sleep apnea is independently associated with insulin resistance. Am J Respir Crit Care Med 165:562-563, 2002.

141. Harsch IA, Pour Schahin S, Radespiel-Troger M, et al. CPAP treatment rapidly improves insulin sensitivity in patients with OSAS. Am J Respir Crit Care Med 2003.

142. Ip MS, Lam KS, Ho C, et al. Serum leptin and vascular risk factors in obstructive sleep apnea. Chest 118:580-586, 2000.

143. Punjabi NM, Sorkin JD, Katzel LI, et al. Sleep-disordered breathing and insulin resistance in middle-aged and overweight men. Am J Respir Crit Care Med 165:677-682, 2002.

# Chapter 74

# Renovascular Hypertension: Diagnosis and Treatment

## Samuel Spitalewitz, Ira W. Reiser

## SIGNIFICANCE

Renovascular hypertension results from renal ischemia and is usually caused by a partially or completely occlusive lesion of one or both renal arteries. It may affect up to 5% of patients with hypertension and is the most common cause of correctable (secondary) hypertension. Renovascular hypertension may lead to ischemic nephropathy and even end-stage renal disease (ESRD) in a significant proportion of affected patients.[1,2] It is a major public health problem.

## INCIDENCE AND CAUSE

Most patients with renovascular disease present with moderate to severe hypertension, although blood pressure may be normal or only mildly elevated. Renovascular disease is less common in African Americans than in Caucasians, in whom it may cause accelerated or malignant hypertension in as many as 10% to 45% of affected patients.[3,4] In African American patients with clinical features, suggestive of renovascular disease, the incidence of accelerated or malignant hypertension may be as high as 20%.[4]

Hypertension may result from any form of ischemic renal disease (e.g., scleroderma, vasculitis of the kidney or renal artery, atheroembolic disease, aneurysms, or other extrinsic compression of the renal arteries). Atherosclerotic renal artery disease accounts for more than two thirds of cases of renovascular hypertension, but most of the remainder are caused by fibromuscular dysplasia.[1] Atherosclerotic renovascular disease typically presents in patients older than 40 years of age, most commonly involves the renal ostium (extending from an aortic atherosclerotic plaque) or the proximal third of the renal artery, and has a male:female ratio of 2:1.[1,5] Fibromuscular dysplasia, of which there are four types (medial fibroplasia, perimedial fibroplasia, medial hyperplasia, and intimal fibroplasia), is more commonly seen in younger patients, usually Caucasian females. Medial fibroplasia is the most common type and accounts for approximately two thirds of cases. The lesions of fibromuscular dysplasia are generally bilateral and, unlike those seen with atherosclerotic renovascular disease, affect the more distal portion of the renal artery.[6]

## CLINICAL SIGNS AND SYMPTOMS

Because of its low incidence in uncomplicated hypertensives, screening all hypertensive patients for renovascular disease is not cost-effective.[7] The clinician should screen those hypertensive patients who present with one or more of the following signs or symptoms[1,8-14]:

1. Severe or refractory hypertension, with evidence of grade 3 or 4 hypertensive retinopathy (particularly in Caucasian patients)
2. Abrupt onset of moderate to severe hypertension, particularly in a previously well-controlled hypertensive or normotensive patient
3. Onset of hypertension before age 20 (early onset) or after age 50 (late onset), particularly in the absence of a family history of hypertension
4. Unexplained significant deterioration in renal function with or without hypertension or proteinuria (which may be in the nephrotic range)
5. A rise in serum creatinine concentration of greater than 20% to 30% in association with the administration of angiotensin-converting enzyme (ACE) inhibitors or angiotensin II receptor blockers (ARBs), or with a reduction of blood pressure to "normal" with other antihypertensive agents
6. Paradoxical worsening of hypertension with diuretic therapy
7. Spontaneous hypokalemia
8. Recurrent "flash" pulmonary edema or otherwise unexplained episodes of congestive heart failure
9. Generalized vascular disease
10. The presence of a systolic-diastolic abdominal bruit that lateralizes to one or both flanks (a systolic bruit alone is more sensitive but less specific)
11. Stigmata of cholesterol emboli

To better predict which patients should be selected for renal angiography, Krijnen et al. have weighted some of the aforementioned and other signs and symptoms to derive a clinical assessment score for patients.[15] At best, each score assigned to a patient had only a 72% sensitivity and 90% specificity in predicting which patients had renovascular disease. In addition, their cohort excluded African Americans and their definition of renal artery disease (greater than a 50% lesion by angiography) was independent of a response to treatment.[16] Similarly, a prospective method utilizing ACE inhibition to predict the presence and severity of renal artery disease and other predictive efforts are too nonspecific to rule out its presence or absence.[9,17-20] Therefore, a suggestive history remains the best and most practical criterion to determine whether to proceed with the screening tests described later.

## SCREENING TESTS

There are several screening tests for renal artery disease, each with its own advantages and disadvantages. The tests we find most useful are radioisotope scanning, magnetic resonance angiography (MRA), and spiral (helical) computed axial tomography (CT).[21] Because a negative screening test does not entirely preclude the presence of a renal artery lesion, if our clinical suspicion is high and a radiologic or a surgical intervention is deemed emergent, we proceed directly to angiography (Figure 74–1).

## Radioisotope Scanning

Renal scintigraphy, with and without ACE inhibition, is our most frequently used initial screening test in patients without renal insufficiency (Figure 74–2).[1,22] A scintigraphic study without ACE inhibition (nonstimulated), using either I[131] orthoiodohippurate (OIH) or [99m]Tc diethylenetriamine pentaacetic acid (DTPA) as the radioisotope, is only as sensitive and specific as an intravenous pyelogram (see later) and is, therefore, of limited value as a screening test.[22-24] However, both the sensitivity and the specificity of the study can be greatly improved (90%-95%) with a stimulated (captopril) scan.[25-28] When the precaptopril and postcaptopril (nonstimulated vs. stimulated) renograms are compared, a decrement in renal function may be seen in the involved kidney. This occurs because ACE inhibition attenuates the angiotensin-mediated vasoconstriction (in the efferent arteriole more so than the afferent arteriole) distal to the renovascular lesion, thereby reducing intraglomerular capillary pressure and, as a consequence, the glomerular filtration rate (GFR). Less often, an improvement in function may be demonstrated on the uninvolved side.[24,29,30] The sensitivity of ACE-enhanced renography appears to be better than that of an ARB enhanced scan. Angiotensin receptor blockade results in efferent arteriole vasodilation through its action on angiotensin II type 1 (AT$_1$) receptors, as well as afferent arteriole vasodilation via angiotensin II–induced stimulation of AT$_2$ receptors. As a result of the physiologic effects of angiotensin II and its receptors, GFR is more likely to be maintained distal to a renal artery lesion with an ARB when compared with an ACE inhibitor, thereby diminishing the scan's sensitivity.[14,31,32] In addition to its high sensitivity and specificity, ACE inhibition renography is easy to perform, does not require discontinuing antihypertensive medications (except ACE inhibitors and ARBs at least 48 hours prior to the study), and may predict the blood pressure response to revascularization.[25,26,28,33-37] The following are consistent with a positive study:

1. Decreased relative uptake by the involved kidney, which in turn contributes less than 40% of the total renal function
2. Almost twice the usual time (5 minutes to peak uptake of the isotope on the affected side
3. Delayed washout of the radioisotope of more than 5 minutes on the involved side compared with the contralateral kidney

The radionuclides of choice are DTPA, a marker of glomerular filtration, and OIH, a marker of renal plasma flow. No statistically significant difference in quantitative or qualitative accuracy has been demonstrated between the two markers in the absence of significant renal insufficiency.[38] However, in the presence of moderate renal insufficiency, OIH is more sensitive.[33] Mercaptoacetyltriglycine (Mag$_3$), a radionuclide with transport properties similar to those of hippuran, has also been utilized and is particularly useful when colabeled with [99]Tc, with which it better delineates renal anatomy and can estimate renal blood flow.[39]

Although uncommon, an occasional patient, when given captopril prior to renal scintigraphy, may experience a hypotensive episode, which is unrelated to the presence of

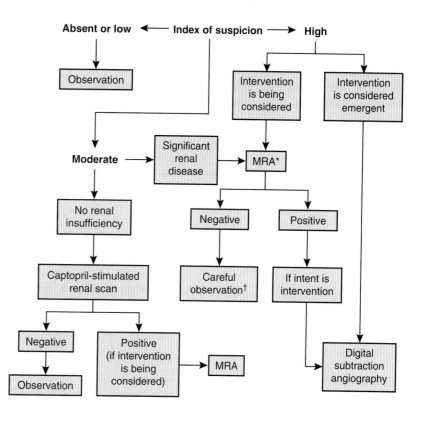

**Figure 74–1** Schematic approach to the diagnostic investigation of renal artery stenosis. *A spiral computed tomography scan may be substituted for an MRA if there is no renal insufficiency or if an MRA is contraindicated or both. †If a patient's renal function significantly deteriorates or blood pressure cannot be controlled medically, proceed to angiography.

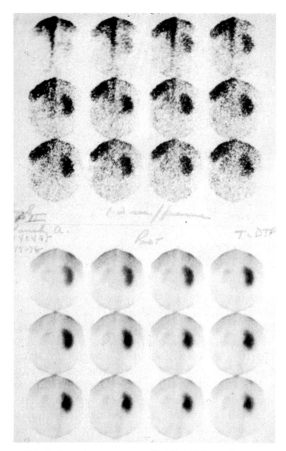

**Figure 74–2** Renal scan, using $^{99m}$TC DPTA as the radionuclide, demonstrates reduced and delayed blood flow to the left kidney due to renovascular disease of the left renal artery.

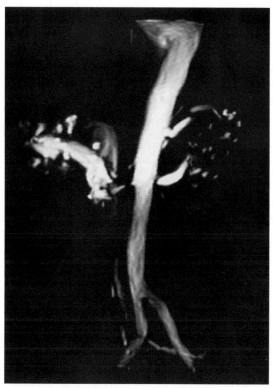

**Figure 74–3** Time-of-flight MRA demonstrates a small area of narrowing 6 mm from the origin of the right renal artery and a severe occlusion of the left renal artery at its origin with poststenotic dilation.

significant renal artery stenosis (RAS).[40] Because prostaglandin metabolism may play a pathophysiologic role in renovascular hypotension, to avoid hypotension, an alternative method to increase the sensitivity of renal scintigraphy may be by inhibiting prostaglandin synthesis.[41] Preliminary experience utilizing acetylsalicylic acid in place of captopril indicates that it may be an acceptable alternative to ACE inhibition.[42,43] Thus far, no patient studied with this procedure has had a clinically significant episode of hypotension.

Stimulated renal scintigraphy is a practical screening test with high sensitivity and specificity, but its use is limited in patients with advanced azotemia or bilateral renovascular disease. It has been suggested that stimulated renal scans not be used in patients with creatinine clearances of less than 20 ml/min because of diminished accuracy at this level of renal dysfunction.[23,24,28,30,44-46] However, furosemide when combined with OIH in stimulated scintigraphy has been found to be both sensitive (96%) and specific (95%) in screening patients with varying degrees of renal insufficiency (serum creatinine concentrations 1.8 to 5.3 mg/dl). This study was done in only a small number of patients and must be confirmed by larger trials.[33]

Radioisotope scanning is most useful in patients with normal renal function and "resistant" or difficult-to-control hypertension. If the scan is negative, and the patient's moderate to severe hypertension is likely to be due to inadequate

therapy or noncompliance, we will not proceed with any further screening tests. If the scan is positive, we usually proceed with MRA.

## Magnetic Resonance Angiography

Prospective studies indicate that three-dimensional phase contrast MRA with the paramagnetic contrast material gadopentetate dimeglumine (gadolinium), which is nonnephrotoxic, may be more sensitive than other screening tests (Figure 74–3).[21,47,48] As an example, 80 patients were studied in trials comparing MRA with digital subtraction angiography (DSA) (see later) or conventional renal angiography.[49,50] A sensitivity approaching 100% and a specificity of 71% to 96% was found with MRA. A meta-analysis of studies comparing MRA with conventional angiography has confirmed these findings and notes the superiority of gadolinium-enhanced studies compared with nonenhanced studies.[51] When combined with cardiac synchronization, three-dimensional MRA can sharply delineate virtually the entire length of the major renal arteries. However, the visualization of distal, intrarenal, and accessory renal arteries that may have hemodynamically significant occlusive lesions remains suboptimal but has improved with the use of breath-hold high-spatial resolution, three-dimensional MRA with gadolinium.[52-62] In a study by Thornton et al. comparing MRA with breath-holding with conventional DSA, 2 of 10 (20%) accessory renal arteries were missed by MRA but detected by conventional DSA.[58] Although the percentage of nondemonstrable accessory renal arteries by MRA in this study appears high, it must be noted that these arteries were less than 2 mm in size and clinically insignificant. The demonstration of stenoses and/or occlusions of arteries *with clinical significance* was therefore 100%, with one false positive. In another study by Shetty et al., all 11 accessory arteries were successfully detected using this MRA technique.[60] Results similar to these have also been obtained in patients with renal occlusive disease resulting in renal insufficiency. False-negative studies are rare, but overestimation of the degree of RAS because of overlying atherosclerotic plaques or tortuous vessels remains problematic and may lead to a false positive diagnosis in a small percentage of patients.

Despite these shortcomings, MRA is the single most reliable noninvasive method of detecting RAS and may soon, if negative, obviate the need for conventional angiography.[51,63-65] MRA can also noninvasively determine both the absolute renal blood flow and the GFR and thus assess the functional significance of renovascular lesions.[54,55] Furthermore, preliminary data suggest that the use of triple dose gadolinium may result in better imaging resolution and a greater confidence in diagnosis when compared with the conventional dose.[66] However, its safety in patients with renal insufficiency is unknown and, therefore, the role of high-dose gadolinium is not yet established.

MRA is extremely valuable in providing a noninvasive method of visualizing the arterial anatomy and is often the decisive factor in determining whether reperfusion is warranted. This excellent screening modality remains limited by its expense, its lack of general availability, and its contraindication in patients with metallic clips and implants, such as pacemakers and defibrillators.

## Computed Axial Tomography

Spiral (helical) CT angiography with intravenous contrast administration has been used as a screening test for detecting renovascular lesions in patients with normal renal function. With this technique, the diagnostic accuracy in detecting renal artery lesions is quite good, with some investigators reporting a 98% sensitivity and a 94% specificity.[67] In a prospective study comparing spiral CT angiography and intraarterial DSA in 50 patients with normal renal function suspected of having RAS and in potential kidney donors, spiral CT angiography demonstrated 27 of 28 accessory renal arteries and 100% of stenoses of 50% or more in the main renal arteries.[68] These results were reconfirmed in a larger study by Wittenberg et al.[69] In this study, 197 arteries were examined in 82 patients and only one significant renal occlusive lesion was missed. In another prospective study comparing it with Doppler ultrasound, spiral CT angiography was the more accurate screening technique.[70] If these initial observations are confirmed by larger studies in patients without renal insufficiency, spiral CT angiography may become the noninvasive screening technique of choice. However, both the sensitivity and the specificity of this test decline (to 93% and 81%, respectively) in the presence of renal insufficiency (serum creatinine concentration >1.7 mg/dl).[67] Furthermore, the risk of radiocontrast-induced nephrotoxicity is significant because the volume of radiocontrast required is large (approximately 100 ml). These shortcomings have been the major limitations to its usefulness in our patient population, many of whom have significant renal insufficiency at presen-

tation. We use spiral CT angiography, if an MRA is contraindicated and there is no renal insufficiency nor an emergent need for nonmedical intervention.

## Angiography

Negative screening tests do not totally exclude the presence of a renal artery lesion, especially in the distal vessels.[21] Therefore, the clinical index of suspicion should determine which screening tests, if any, should be done. The clinician may opt to proceed immediately with conventional renal angiography or an intraarterial DSA, both of which remain the diagnostic gold standards (Figure 74–4).[23,24,29] This is done when emergent percutaneous or surgical intervention is deemed appropriate. Because intraarterial DSA requires the administration of less radiocontrast (25-50 ml) than conventional angiography (100 ml), it is preferred, especially in patients with compromised renal function.

Carbon dioxide ($CO_2$) digital angiography has been used as an effective alternative to iodinated contrast agents in patients with renal insufficiency. When used in combination with digital subtraction, intraarterial $CO_2$ angiography provides diagnostic imaging similar to that achieved using standard contrast studies, while eliminating the potential nephrotoxicity of radiocontrast.[71,72] Despite the absence of renal toxicity with $CO_2$ angiography, it may not provide adequate visualization of the more distal vasculature and requires an experienced technician, as well as sophisticated programming with electronic enhancement. In addition, the procedure may be complicated by air embolization, neurotoxicity, and renal ischemia due to "vapor lock." It still remains an investigational tool. Spinosa et al. have established the usefulness of gadolinium-enhanced $CO_2$ angiography when compared with $CO_2$-enhanced renal angiography.[73,74] Gadolinium appears to be nonnephrotoxic even when given intraarterially and can also be used to

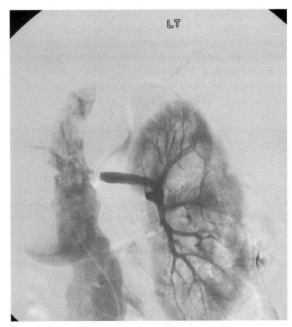

**Figure 74–4** Selective renal angiography of the left renal artery demonstrates a 99% stenosis of the artery at its origin.

supplement $CO_2$ angiograms or, when necessary, confirm $CO_2$-enhanced angiographic findings. Although promising, the results of these studies were not directly compared with conventional angiography in the same patients, making it impossible to determine whether areas of arterial occlusion were missed with this technique.

Compared with intraarterial injection, *intravenous* DSA is less invasive and does not pose a risk of cholesterol embolization. However, the renal vasculature is not as well delineated as with intraarterial injection; the amount of radiocontrast required is greater (150-200 ml); and the sensitivity and specificity are 90% or less, compared with arterial studies.[75,76] In addition, it requires more dye and is less reliable than a spiral CT scan. Therefore, we no longer use this test.

## Duplex Doppler Ultrasonography

Similar to scintigraphy with $Mag_3$ colabeled with $^{99}$Tc, ultrasonic duplex scanning of the renal arteries can provide both anatomic and functional information. This technique combines direct visualization of the main renal arteries via B-mode ultrasound imaging with Doppler measurements of various hemodynamic parameters characteristic of renal artery lesions. Stenotic lesions are detected by comparing the acceleration time, the resistive indexes of each kidney and artery, and the systolic or end-diastolic flow in the involved renal artery to that in the aorta. Early experience with this technique demonstrated a significant false-negative rate of 8% to 20%. However, studies have demonstrated greatly improved sensitivity and specificity when sonography was performed before and then compared with the results of angiography.[77-84] As with radioisotope scanning, captopril (stimulated) Doppler ultrasound studies have further increased the sensitivity of the technique. The specific Doppler wave forms distal to the vascular lesion are enhanced by captopril and the sensitivity of the study may increase significantly and may approach 100% following captopril administration.[85]

Duplex ultrasonography by utilizing intrarenal echo-Doppler velocimetric indexes (particularly the acceleration time and index) have been used to assess the success of dilation procedures, predict re-stenosis, and detect re-stenosis in arteries previously revascularized by angioplasty, stent placement, or surgery.[29,79-81] A prospective study compared duplex Doppler scanning with captopril-stimulated renography in terms of their ability to detect hemodynamically significant renovascular lesions and to predict the fall in blood pressure following percutaneous transluminal angioplasty. No significant difference between the two tests was found, and the positive predictive value of both for blood pressure cure or improvement approached 90%.[86] Radermacher et al.[87] utilized the Doppler determined renal resistive index, a measure of structural alterations in distal smaller renal arteries and arterioles, to predict which of 138 patients with 50% or greater stenosis of unilateral or bilateral renal arteries would have an improvement in blood pressure and/or renal function following revascularization. Although specific information about individual patients regarding the degree of stenosis, whether the lesions were unilateral or bilateral and the type of procedure performed was not given, a resistance index (1 minus end-diastolic velocity divided by maximal systolic velocity × 100) of greater than 80 identified with reasonable accuracy (80%-97%) those patients in whom angioplasty and/or sur-

gery did not improve blood pressure, renal function, or kidney survival. Patients with a resistance index less than 80 were likely to have a successful intervention. The resistance index is potentially a useful guideline but should not be the sole factor in determining which patients should undergo interventional procedures.[88]

Duplex Doppler scanning is noninvasive, does not require discontinuing any antihypertensive medications, and does not involve exposure to radiation or radiocontrast. Unlike the other screening tests described, it may be used with accuracy in patients with renal failure, and it provides information regarding the presence of bilateral disease.

Despite these advantages, the usefulness of duplex Doppler ultrasonography as a screening tool is limited because it is very time-consuming, operator-dependent, and technically difficult to perform, and extensive training in the procedure is necessary for an accurate study to be performed. In addition, intrarenal vascular lesions and multiple (and even main) renal arteries may be missed, particularly in obese patients or in those with overlying intestinal gas.[29,77,84,86] MRA is also considerably more sensitive and specific than duplex sonography, particularly in detecting accessory renal arteries (96% vs. 5%).[89] Therefore, sonography's major use at present is to follow lesions in patients in whom an MRA is contraindicated and who have significant renal insufficiency, precluding a spiral CT scan.

## SCREENING TESTS OF LITTLE CLINICAL USEFULNESS

### Intravascular Ultrasonography

This invasive sonographic procedure provides structural detail of the renal vascular lesion and, therefore, can distinguish between fibromuscular dysplasia and atherosclerotic renal artery lesions.[90] Compared with noninvasive sonography, it can more accurately assess the severity of occlusion and closely correlates with angiographic findings.[90,91] Because it estimates volumetric flow, it has also been used to assess the patency of renal arteries before and after angioplasty and stent placement.[92,93] Intravascular ultrasonography is invasive and requires radiocontrast to guide the placement of the intraarterial ultrasound probe. Therefore, its usefulness as a screening test is limited, especially in patients with impaired renal function.

### Intravenous Pyelography

Decreased function of the kidney with renovascular disease may be detected by conventional intravenous pyelography (IVP), but greater sensitivity is achieved with a "hypertensive" IVP. With the latter technique, additional radiographs are taken at 1, 2, 3, 4, and 5 minutes. Thus, the hypertensive IVP is more likely to demonstrate a delay in the calyceal appearance or nephrogram of the affected kidney, which may be missed if only later films are viewed, as in a conventional IVP. Other IVP findings suggestive of renal artery disease include discrepancy in renal size or cortical thickness, hyperconcentration of the radiocontrast in the involved kidney, ureteral notching due to collateral circulation, and a prolonged nephrogram effect in the later films.[1] An IVP is now seldom used as a screening test for renovascular hypertension because of its low sensitivity and specificity (both approximately 75%), the risk of radiocontrast-induced nephrotoxicity, and its relatively high radiation dose.[29,94] Furthermore, in the presence of bilateral renal artery disease, many of the previously mentioned findings may be absent, especially if there is little difference in function between the two kidneys.[23]

## Plasma Renin Activity

Elevated baseline plasma renin activity (PRA) is found in only 50% to 80% of patients with renovascular hypertension and may be observed in 16% of patients with essential hypertension. Thus, an elevated baseline PRA is of limited diagnostic significance, and its absence in no way excludes renovascular hypertension. The predictive value of PRA may be enhanced by measuring its increase 1 hour after the ingestion of 25 to 50 mg of captopril.[23,29,30] This "captopril test" improves the diagnostic accuracy of PRA, but the reported sensitivity and specificity of the procedure vary widely (63%-100% and 72%-100%, respectively), even when strict criteria for a positive result are met.[23,30,95,96] In addition, to perform this test accurately, antihypertensive agents affecting PRA must be discontinued, which may be dangerous in these patients, most of whom have moderate to severe hypertension. The usefulness of the captopril test is further limited because it is impractical and requires strict standardization; its accuracy is reduced in the presence of mild renal insufficiency (serum creatinine concentration >1.5-2.0 mg/dl), and its predictive value is less than that of a renogram obtained following ACE inhibition (see later).[22,25-27,97]

Because ACE inhibition may impair renal function in patients with bilateral renal artery disease, van de Van et al.[9] utilized the effects of ACE inhibition on the plasma creatinine concentration in 108 patients at high risk for bilateral atherosclerotic renal artery disease to predict its presence prior to undergoing angiography. An increase in the plasma creatinine concentration of 20% or greater identified all patients who on angiography had severe bilateral disease (defined as 50% or more bilateral stenosis). As could be anticipated, many patients with unilateral and/or less severe disease also had an increase in serum creatinine concentration. Thus, although highly sensitive, this test yielded a specificity of only 70%, giving it little clinical usefulness.

## DOES A RENAL ARTERY LESION CAUSE HYPERTENSION?

The mere presence of a renal artery lesion does not mean that it is the cause of hypertension. Therefore, prior to any intervention aimed at eliminating or controlling hypertension, the physiologic significance of a lesion should be proven.[1] ACE inhibitor scans, renal vein renin (RVR) measurements, and the pressure gradient across the renal artery lesion have been used to determine whether a stenosis is cause for hypertension.[98] If a lesion is the cause of "renin-dependent" hypertension, renin secretion by the kidney distal to the renal vascular lesion should be increased, and secretion by the contralateral kidney should be suppressed, resulting in an RVR ratio of 1.5 or more (affected:nonaffected side). When the RVR ratio is used to predict reduction in blood pressure following inter-

vention, a sensitivity of only 80% and a specificity of 62% have been reported.[75] However, the predictive accuracy of the RVR can be improved with the administration of ACE inhibitors prior to testing.[23] With unilateral renal artery disease and a captopril-stimulated lateralizing RVR, an improvement in blood pressure after revascularization is seen in up to 90% of patients.[24] However, the absence of lateralization does not necessarily mean that there will be no fall in blood pressure after intervention, for as many as 60% of these patients may still have an improvement in their blood pressures following revascularization.[24] Because of its low predictive value, the need for renal vein catheterization with radiocontrast injection, and the need to discontinue medications that may affect renin secretion, RVR measurements are no longer commonly used. More predictive than RVR measurements is the pressure gradient across the renal artery lesion as determined by intraarterial renal angiography. The absence of a significant pressure gradient (10-15 mm Hg) suggests that the lesion is of little physiologic significance and that revascularization in this setting will be of little benefit.

Because no single test is reliable enough to determine a causal relationship between a renal artery lesion and hypertension, the signs and symptoms previously described (items 1 through 8 under the Clinical Signs and Symptoms section), if present, should alert the clinician that it is highly likely that the lesion is causing hypertension. Once the diagnosis of renovascular hypertension is made, the clinician may attempt to control the patient's blood pressure with medical therapy alone and/or with percutaneous transluminal renal angioplasty (PTRA), placement of a vascular endoprosthesis (a stent), or surgery. The therapeutic approach is determined by the type of lesion causing the hypertension, the site and extent of renal artery involvement, the overall medical status of the patient, and the perceived risks which are, in part, based on the interventionist's skills in performing the procedures. The effectiveness of each approach in controlling hypertension as well as the role of revascularization in preserving renal function (many of these patients have associated ischemic nephropathy and renal insufficiency) are reviewed later.

## MEDICAL THERAPY FOR HYPERTENSION

Medical therapy for renovascular hypertension is similar to that for essential hypertension, but because severe hypertension is more common in patients with renovascular disease, combination drug therapy is frequently necessary in that group. Nevertheless, blood pressure control is usually achieved in more than 90% of cases. Because the hypertension may be dependent on angiotensin II, antihypertensives that inhibit renin or angiotensin II production or block their actions are especially useful in renovascular hypertension. Therefore, β-blockers, ACE inhibitors, and ARBs have been extensively utilized, with ACE inhibitors being especially efficacious.[99-102] Studies have demonstrated control of blood pressure in 80% of patients when ACE inhibitors are used alone and in up to 90% when they are combined with diuretic therapy.[100,101] However, ACE inhibitors should be used with caution, particularly in patients with bilateral RAS (see later). Although there is less clinical experience with the newer ARBs, in experimental models of renovascular hypertension, they are as potent as ACE inhibitors.[103]

Despite control of blood pressure with medical therapy, several studies have demonstrated that atherosclerotic renal artery lesions progress in 40% to 60% of patients within 7 years (with half of these lesions progressing within 2 years).[104-106] Patients with an initial stenosis of more than 75% have the fastest rate of progression, with total occlusion occurring in 40% of these lesions.[104] Renal function, however, may not necessarily decline concomitantly. In addition to the "natural" progression of the atherosclerotic vascular lesion, medical therapy, by reducing blood pressure, may result in chronic hypoperfusion distal to the lesion and may hasten tubular atrophy, interstitial fibrosis, and glomerulosclerosis in the affected kidney or kidneys.[107-109] Some investigators have demonstrated in animal models that at a given level of blood pressure, ACE inhibitors are more likely than other antihypertensive agents to induce these structural changes.[107,108] However, to date, there are no clinical studies suggesting that ACE inhibitors or ARBs irreversibly hasten the loss of renal function when given on a long-term basis to patients with unilateral or bilateral atherosclerotic renovascular disease.[110] Nevertheless, when these drugs are used, especially when they are combined with diuretic therapy, patients' renal function should be monitored frequently. In addition to monitoring renal function with serum creatinine concentrations and 24-hour creatinine clearances, it has also been suggested that renal size and renal cortical blood flow velocity also be monitored using duplex scanning, because these parameters may provide earlier signs of irreversible renal function loss.[111] In a study of 122 patients, persistent stenosis increased the risk of long-term loss of renal mass, but this loss was more closely associated with the degree of RAS and the level of systolic blood pressure than with the use of ACE inhibitors. In addition to a possible association with *chronic* hypoperfusion and nephron loss, ACE inhibitors, as well as the ARBs, may result in *acute* (usually reversible) renal failure in 10% to 20% of patients with bilateral RAS or with RAS affecting a solitary kidney. This is most likely to occur when patients are volume-contracted.

Compared with atherosclerotic RAS, the risk of progressive occlusion and renal ischemia with medial fibroplasia, the predominant form of fibrous renal artery disease, is low.[103,104] In contrast, the lesions of perimedial fibroplasia, medial hyperplasia, and intimal fibroplasia frequently progress and may result in a deterioration of renal function similar to that seen with atherosclerotic RAS.[112,113] Therefore, renal function must be carefully monitored in these patients.[104]

## ANGIOPLASTY AND STENTING FOR HYPERTENSION

PTRA is an angiographic technique by which stenotic renal arteries are dilated with a catheter containing a cylindric inflatable balloon at its tip (Figure 74–5). The success rate of PTRA is dependent on the site and type of the vascular lesion; it is most likely to be successful in lesions in which there is incomplete arterial occlusion, the length of the stenosis is less than 10 mm, and in lesions which do not involve the renal os.[114,115]

Most studies of PTRA in patients with fibromuscular dysplasia report a high technical success rate (87%-100%), an improvement in or cure of the hypertension in as many as 90% of patients, and a low incidence (10%) of re-stenosis.[113,115-119] In contrast to fibromuscular dysplasia, the technical success rate of PTRA when performed for unilateral atherosclerotic renovascular lesions may be as low as 70%, and long-term improvement in or cure rates of the hypertension vary widely.[113,115-119] The improvement in or cure of hypertension depends in large part on the location of the lesion. In a study of 100 patients, Canzanello et al. demonstrated an improvement in blood pressure of 86% in patients with nonostial unilateral lesions compared with 46% for patients with ostial unilateral lesions.[119] Acute reversible renal insufficiency complicated 21% of the procedures, and mechanical complications, such as thrombosis, perforation, or dissection of renal arteries or diffuse atheroembolism occurred in 14% of the patients.

The preceding data were generated in uncontrolled trials. A randomized prospective trial comparing medical therapy (in 26 patients) with PTRA (in 23 patients) for unilateral RAS demonstrated that PTRA reduced the number of drugs necessary for blood pressure control at 6 months.[120] At baseline, 54% of the medically treated patients needed more than two antihypertensive medications, compared with 34% in the angioplasty group. With time, 88% of the medically treated group required two or more medications, compared with 35% of those who were postangioplasty. PTRA was complicated by one case of dissection with segmental renal infarction, and by re-stenosis in 18%. It should be noted, however, that more patients with ostial lesions at baseline (46% vs. 30%) were treated medically. Thus, the more favorable outcome observed with PTRA may reflect this selection bias. Of the medically managed patients, 27% were terminated from the study and subsequently underwent angioplasty because of refractory hypertension. It was not specified whether these "refractory" patients had ostial lesions and whether PTRA was successful. The results of this study are therefore difficult to interpret, and others are needed for a better comparison of these two approaches.

In contrast, no improvement in blood pressure was observed in a group of 13 patients with unilateral RAS randomized to PTRA as compared with 14 treated with medical therapy and followed for up to 54 months (range, 3-54 months).[121] Major outcome events, such as death, myocardial infarction, heart failure, stroke, and dialysis, did not differ between the two groups. In addition, 28% of the patients who underwent angioplasty experienced complications attributable to the procedure, the most common of which was bleeding at the arterial puncture site (8 patients). Thus, it appears that when PTRA is used to control hypertension due to unilateral RAS, the potential gain, if any, is often outweighed by the risk and the discomfort of the procedure. Similarly, in the largest prospective blood pressure control study thus far, unimpressive results were obtained by van Jaarsveld et al.[122] As defined by the presence of RAS 50% or greater, 75% of the patients had unilateral disease and 25% had bilateral disease. One hundred seven patients with similar clinical characteristics and a serum creatinine concentration 2.3 mg/dl or less at baseline were randomly assigned to medical therapy or PTRA (all but two without stenting). Based on an intent-to-treat analysis, the angioplasty group demonstrated only minimal improvement in blood pressure control at 3 months, but none at 12 months' follow-up. Although 50% of the PTRA group reoccluded at 12 months, the lack of response in blood

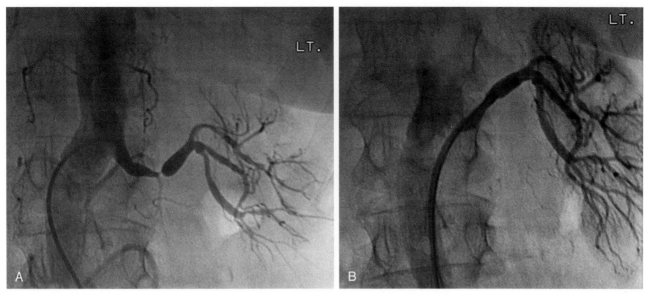

**Figure 74-5** Nonostial renal artery lesion before **(A)** and after **(B)** percutaneous transluminal angioplasty.

pressure control was unrelated to either re-stenosis (proven by repeat angiography) at 12-month follow-up or to worsening of renal function. Blood pressure in the reoccluded group was similar to the group that did not reocclude and to the medically treated group. Although renal function appeared to be better in the angioplasty group than in the medical therapy group at 3 months, it was similar in both groups at 1-year follow-up. These apparent "negative" results with PTRA, however, must be taken in context. It is important to note that approximately 50% of the patients who were assigned to receive antihypertensive drug therapy alone subsequently underwent "rescue" angioplasty because of inadequate blood pressure control. These patients, however, were analyzed as "medical therapy" patients. The success or at least the need of angioplasty may, therefore, have been significantly greater than reported. In addition, 25% of the patients had bilateral renal artery disease, which is considered to be less easily treated (by either method) than unilateral, but the results of their treatment is not separately reported. Successful treatment of unilateral disease both with regard to blood pressure control and/or preservation of renal function may have been better than bilateral disease. These data, however, cannot be gleaned from this study. The authors' conclusion that it is still prudent to "restrict" PTRA seems justified, although their study is inconclusive and does little to clarify the issues it was designed to study.[123]

The results of PTRA in patients with bilateral RAS are equally unimpressive, due, at least in part, to the high incidence of ostial or completely occluding lesions, both of which are more difficult to dilate and are associated with a high complication rate.[114,116,119] Ramsay and Waller have reviewed 10 series of patients who underwent PTRA for treatment of atherosclerotic RAS.[116] In general, the selection criteria were ill-defined, and the patients chosen for the PTRA were carefully selected, which probably biased the findings in favor of angioplasty. The studies cited had significant variations in the technical failure rates and the estimates of cure or improvement in blood pressure. Furthermore, the types of lesions treated were often not characterized. Despite the limitations of these stud-

ies, it appears that in bilateral atherosclerotic lesions, the technical failure rate may be as high as 60% and the cure rate for hypertension as low as 8%, with improvement in blood pressure in only 43%.[116] The results are especially disappointing when the bilateral disease is associated with an atrophic kidney, because total renal artery occlusion of the atrophic kidney is observed in half of the cases.[115] As demonstrated by Geyskes, PTRA in a patient with an atrophic kidney resulted in an improvement in blood pressure in only 8 of 57 (14%) and in a cure of the hypertension in only 5 patients (9%).[115]

In view of these data, it is reasonable to attempt PTRA only in the patients in whom medical therapy has failed and in whom an incomplete but high-grade (75%-90%) unilateral RAS distal to the os is present. Even with an initial successful therapeutic outcome, the incidence of re-stenosis following PTRA for RAS is significant (30% for nonostial lesions and 50% for ostial lesions) and may occur soon after the procedure (15%-30% by 2 years). Reocclusion, however, does not preclude a repeat PTRA.[99]

To prevent or treat re-stenosis and improve blood pressure control with PTRA for atheromatous ostial lesions, intravascular stents have been placed during angioplasty (Figure 74-6).[124-126] One group of investigators has now performed this procedure without nephrotoxic radiocontrast by using a combination of intraarterial carbon dioxide and gadopentetate dimeglumine, avoiding the risk of contrast-induced acute renal failure.[127] Initial studies of intravascular stenting reported a success rate of 65% to 70% and a risk of re-stenosis ranging from 13% to 39%.[124,125] More encouraging results were demonstrated in 68 patients with ostial lesions after stent placement for unsuccessful PTRA.[126] The technical success rate was 100%; re-stenosis (defined as reocclusion of more than 50% of the vessel diameter) occurred in only 11% during a mean follow-up time of 27 months, and either cure or improvement of the hypertension was noted in 78%. No major complications were reported in this study. It is important to note that the majority of the patients (64%) were followed for only 12 months, with only 9% followed long-term (60 months). Furthermore, patients with a residual stenosis of

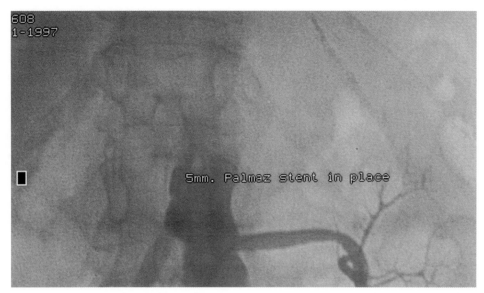

**Figure 74–6** The renal ostial lesion depicted in Figure 74–5 is shown after placement of an intravascular stent.

up to 50% of the arterial lumen were classified as complete technical successes, even though they remain at a substantial risk for reocclusion. The study demonstrates the safety and short-term efficacy of the procedure but does not provide sufficient evidence to support long-term efficacy of endovascular stenting.[128] Nevertheless, it appears that renal arterial stenting may prove to be most useful in patients with ostial disease, restenosis after PTRA, or complications due to PTRA, such as dissection.[113]

Primary renal artery stenting (i.e., without antecedent PTRA) has also been performed in atherosclerotic RAS.[129] Most radiologists propose primary stent placement for those lesions within the aortic wall or within 10 mm of the aortic lumen, or if there is elastic recoil with PTRA with a residual stenosis of 30% or greater. The technical success rate is high and the rate of serious complications is low. Although the investigators do not specify what percentage of the patients had nonstial lesions, approximately 60% demonstrated cure or improvement of their blood pressure (regardless of whether there was unilateral or bilateral disease) at 6 months. At 1 and 4 years' follow-up, the improvement rate fell to 42%, and only 1% remained cured of their hypertension.[130,131] At 6 months, 25% of the lesions were re-stenosed (proven angiographically), but longer-term patency rates of the stents are unknown because of lack of angiographic follow-up.[129-131]

Two other studies have been done in patients who have undergone primary and/or secondary stenting.[132,133] In both studies, no clinically significant improvement in blood pressure was observed. In the study with the longest follow-up (5 years), despite an initial diminution in the number of antihypertensive medications required at 3 to 6 months, the number increased subsequently and was no different from before stent placement. Patency was angiographically determined at a mean of 8 months ± 5 months (range 2-24 months). A restenosis rate of 50% or more occurred in 14%.[133]

A prospective study directly compared the outcomes of angioplasty alone versus primary angioplasty plus stent placement for ostial atherosclerotic RAS.[134] In this trial, 85 patients were randomized to one or the other intervention, with stent placement if angioplasty alone failed within 6 months. Angioplasty plus stent was associated with a significantly higher initial success rate (88% vs. 57%), a much higher patency rate at 6 months (75% vs. 29%), and a lower restenosis rate (14% vs. 48%). Twelve patients underwent secondary stenting for primary or late failure within the 6 months' follow-up period with a similar success rate to primary stenting. Regarding control of hypertension, the combined procedure and angioplasty alone lowered blood pressure to the same extent, but was not compared with medical therapy. These results, at least for the short-term follow-up at 6 months, suggest that primary stenting for atherosclerotic lesions is superior to angioplasty alone because it eliminates the need for reintervention. No conclusions, however, can be drawn regarding blood pressure control (by either intervention) versus medical therapy.

Based on these data, stenting for control of blood pressure alone is not generally recommended. To date, no investigators have cited criteria that clearly define which patients with nonstial lesions should undergo primary renal artery stenting. We perform primary renal artery stenting in nonstial lesions in the patients in whom angiography demonstrates a very high-grade stenosis (90%) and/or a stenosis of 7 to 10 mm or longer, because the probability of success with PTRA alone is low.

Following successful PTRA, a reduction in blood pressure may be seen as early as 4 to 6 hours after the procedure, but the maximal antihypertensive effect is commonly achieved well after 48 hours.[99,118] In some cases, the full antihypertensive benefit may not be observed until after several weeks. The absence of an early decline in blood pressure suggests that significant long-term improvement of the hypertension is unlikely.[118]

Although PTRA and stenting are generally safe procedures, complication rates of approximately 5% to 15% have been reported. Most of these complications, such as hematoma formation at the puncture site and renal artery spasm, are of minor clinical significance. However, if it is severe, renal artery spasm can lead to local thrombosis and renal infarction. This can be prevented or reversed by the administration of intraarterial nitroglycerin. Major complications frequently include reversible, contrast-induced acute tubular necrosis (approximately 20%) and, infrequently (<5%), renal artery perforation, dissection, or irreversible acute renal failure due to atheroembolization.

## SURGERY FOR HYPERTENSION

Surgical revascularization for renovascular hypertension involves bypassing the site of the arterial lesion by grafting or anastomosing another vessel distal to the lesion and/or removing an atrophic kidney. Because PTRA is highly successful in patients with fibromuscular dysplasia, is less invasive, and is associated with lower morbidity and mortality rates than is surgical revascularization, surgery is not recommended as primary therapy for these patients. It is done, however, when PTRA is unsuccessful or is technically not feasible, as is the case when branch renal artery disease is present (30% of patients with fibrous renal artery disease).[135,136] When surgery is performed, 90% to 95% of patients with fibromuscular dysplasia are cured or see substantial improvement of their hypertension.[75,113,136-138]

Although surgical revascularization in patients with atherosclerotic RAS may result in cure or improvement of the hypertension in as many as 80% to 90% of patients, surgery other than a simple nephrectomy of an atrophic kidney is not recommended for blood pressure control alone in patients with unilateral or with bilateral atherosclerotic renal artery disease. These patients are generally older and commonly have extensive extrarenal vascular disease. Their long-term survival rate following surgery, particularly if they have bilateral RAS and diffuse atherosclerosis, is poor. Furthermore, their hypertension can usually be controlled with medical therapy. If surgery becomes the only option, the probability of successful control of blood pressure in unilateral RAS is inversely related to the duration of and vascular damage caused by preexisting essential hypertension, as well as to the degree that the renin angiotensin system is activated in the contralateral kidney (see later). In the presence of underlying contralateral RAS with renal ischemia, parenchymal small-vessel disease, or both, the antihypertensive response to surgery is significantly diminished.[113,136-140]

The morbidity and mortality with surgical revascularization is significant. As with any major intraabdominal vascular surgery, complications include those due to manipulation of the aorta (thrombosis, dissection, and atheroembolization), acute renal failure due to renal ischemia, pancreatitis, hemorrhage, splenic infarction, renal graft aneurysm formation, and postoperative RAS or renal artery thrombosis. Because of their younger age and absence of extrarenal vascular disease, mortality rates are very low in patients with fibromuscular disease. In contrast, mortality rates are significantly higher in patients with atherosclerotic disease unless they are carefully selected, in which case mortality rates may be as low as 3% to 5%. Mortality rates increase in patients older than 65 years of age, particularly if generalized atherosclerosis (coronary or cerebral vascular disease), congestive heart failure or significant renal disease is present. To decrease mortality, screening for and surgical correction of significant carotid or coronary artery disease should be accomplished before revascularization.[135]

Hypertension may recur after surgery and is most often due to either recurrent atherosclerotic disease or anastomotic neointimal hyperplasia. Although recurrent lesions are generally clinically silent, in as many as 15%, either PTRA or another surgical procedure may be required. In approximately 10% of patients, bypass graft re-stenosis will occur and may be seen as late as 10 years after surgical revascularization.[99]

To date, no prospective randomized trials have been done comparing medical therapy, PTRA, and surgery in controlling atherosclerotic renovascular hypertension. However, the results of several nonrandomized studies have suggested that surgery is the most successful, whereas other studies have demonstrated no difference in control of blood pressure among the three approaches.[99,141-143] Many of these studies were done prior to the widespread use of ACE inhibitors, and recent advances in surgical techniques make these earlier comparisons irrelevant to current management strategies.

In a more recent prospective randomized trial comparing PTRA and surgical revascularization in a group of patients with unilateral RAS, a higher success rate and a lower incidence of re-stenosis were found in the surgical group after 2 years. However, the effect on blood pressure was not different when both interventions were successful.[144]

### Recommendations for the Management of Hypertension in Patients with Renal Artery Stenosis

Consistent with current data, we manage hypertension in patients with RAS as follows:

1. Because of its low risk:benefit ratio, high success rate, and low rate of re-stenosis, PTRA is the treatment of choice for fibromuscular dysplasia uncomplicated by branch renal artery disease. If PTRA is unsuccessful, or if branch renal artery disease is present, surgical revascularization should be undertaken, because these patients are generally young and have excellent responses to surgery, obviating the need for long-term medical therapy.

2. Medical therapy should be the primary management in patients with atherosclerotic RAS with mild, controllable hypertension or with comorbid conditions such as diffuse atherosclerosis that place them at high operative risk. Because renal function may decline with progression of the underlying atherosclerotic lesions or with the medical therapy itself, we monitor renal function closely in these patients. In addition, a renal scan can be performed soon after goal blood pressure is attained to assess the degree to which treatment has lowered the filtration rate in the stenotic kidney. If therapy includes ACE inhibitors or ARBs, and if there is a significant decrement in renal function, treatment may be switched to a calcium channel blocker and/or other agents less likely to impair autoregulation. If after alteration in the medical regimen renal functional deterioration persists, or if renal size(s) over time begin(s) to diminish significantly, PTRA or surgery should be performed in an attempt to preserve or improve renal function. As discussed later, the modality chosen is highly individualized.

3. In the absence of diffuse vascular disease or other comorbid conditions that may increase operative risk, revascularization should be undertaken in those generally younger

(age 50-60) patients with atherosclerotic RAS and moderate to severe hypertension (particularly if associated with episodes of flash pulmonary edema) only if blood pressure is not well controlled by medical therapy or if deterioration of renal function occurs with blood pressure control. PTRA, with or without intravascular stenting, should then be done in the presence of a nonostial, partially occluding vascular lesion. In view of more technically successful results with intravascular stenting, we attempt this procedure in patients with ostial lesions, with nonostial lesions that have re-stenosed after PTRA, and with lesions that have more than 90% stenosis or are 7 to 10 mm in length or longer, particularly in patients in whom the surgical risk is considerable. If the above approach is unsuccessful, surgical revascularization is performed, particularly in patients with unilateral RAS or when concomitant aortic surgery is required, as for an abdominal aortic aneurysm.

## PRESERVATION OF RENAL FUNCTION

As previously discussed, atherosclerotic renal artery lesions may progress. However, it is not known how many patients with bilateral renovascular disease develop ischemic nephropathy or ESRD, and it is not known over what time period this occurs and which, if any, factors exist which may help reliably predict its incidence.[145,146] Two retrospective studies examined these issues.[147,148] In the first study, the investigators reviewed the medical records of 51 patients with particularly severe bilateral RAS (total occlusion or stenosis of 90% or more in one renal artery, with at least 50% stenosis on the opposite side).[147] Only medical therapy had been offered to these patients because of physician or patient preference, because the lesions were not amenable to angioplasty, because the kidneys were too small to salvage, or because the patient was not clinically suitable for surgical intervention. The overall mortality rate was high—38% within 2 years of renal angiography and 45% at 5 years. The incidence of ESRD was 12% at 5 years. The rate of decline of the GFR for all patients was 4 ml/min/year (range 1-16 ml/min/year). Those most likely to reach ESRD were those with more advanced renal failure (GFR <25 ml/min) at the time of angiography and those whose renal function showed a decline in GFR of greater than 8 ml/min/year. It is impressive that in a large percentage of patients, little or no serial change in renal function was observed despite the presence of severe bilateral disease. Progressive renal dysfunction and narrowing of the arterial lumen does not inevitably occur, and the development of collateral circulation to the kidneys may offset the reduction in flow in the major renal arteries. Hence, even in the presence of severe RAS, collateral circulation may maintain renal viability and function.[149,150]

In the second study, a cohort of 593 consecutive patients underwent DSA because of peripheral vascular disease.[148] Of this group, the presence of RAS (defined as an occlusion ≥50%) could be assessed in 397 patients and was found coincidentally in 126. These "incidentally found" lesions were unilateral in 70% and bilateral in the remainder. Although renal function varied widely within this group (the creatinine clearance as estimated by the Cockroft Gault formula was 58.2 ± 22.3 ml/min), none of these patients required renal replacement therapy during a 10-year follow-up. Remarkably, no dif-

ferences in renal function were found between patients with unilateral and bilateral RAS. Nevertheless, the group with bilateral disease, although at higher risk of ESRD, did not progress. It is important to note, however, that many renal arteries were not visualized and a significant number of "incidental" renal artery lesions may have been excluded from follow-up. These favorable results are not always the case, however, and it is clear that with medical therapy alone, progressive and/or rapid decline in renal function can result from renal artery disease. Renal failure is potentially reversible, perhaps more so in those with a more rapid decline in renal function.[151]

It has been estimated that ischemic nephropathy is the cause of renal failure in 5% to 15% of patients older than the age of 50 years, and it may account for 10% to 20% of all patients with ESRD. Despite dialytic therapy, mortality rates are high (>50% over 3 years), and 5- and 10-year survival rates are only 18% and 5%, respectively. In view of these grim statistics, restoration of renal function (either by surgery or by PTRA with or without stenting) is critically important and should be attempted whenever indicated.[106,112,152-154]

PTRA in patients with renal dysfunction due to ischemic nephropathy improves renal function in 40% of patients and stabilizes function in an additional 30% to 40%.[106,119,152,155,156] The majority of patients included in these studies had nonostial lesions. Because the success rate is reasonable and is comparable to that of surgical revascularization, which has a higher morbidity and mortality rate, PTRA should be the initial intervention in patients with nonostial atherosclerotic lesions who have deteriorating renal function.[157] Re-stenosis occurs in 10% to 30% of these patients, and many of them are amenable to repeat PTRA.[152]

Only 15% to 20% of atherosclerotic lesions are nonostial.[157] With ostial atherosclerotic lesions, PTRA without stenting has been largely ineffective because of the high technical failure rate due to elastic recoil of the artery and because of neointimal hyperplasia or recurrent atherosclerosis, both of which commonly result in eventual failure.[157] As previously discussed, the placement of intravascular stents for ostial atherosclerotic lesions is a promising new technique to improve the safety and possibly the long-term patency rate and efficacy of PTRA.

Studies have examined the role of intravascular stenting in the preservation of renal function.[126,130,132,158-160] Following unsuccessful angioplasty, 68 patients with ostial lesions underwent stenting. None of the 48 patients with normal renal function at baseline (serum creatinine concentration <1.4 mg/dl) had worsening of renal function at a mean follow-up of 27 months. Similarly, no deterioration of renal function was observed in the 30% of patients who had significant renal insufficiency at baseline.[126] In another study, 32 patients with a median serum creatinine concentration of 2.9 mg/dl underwent renal artery stenting and were followed for a mean of 8 months (range 0-29 months). Of the 32 patients, 11 (34%) showed significant improvement in renal function, 11 (34%) stabilized, and 9 (28%) worsened. In a subset of 23 patients, in whom the level of renal function prior to stenting was known for a sufficient time period that the reciprocal of the serum creatinine versus time could be plotted, the rate of progression of renal failure was slowed in 18 (78%) following the procedure. Patients with baseline serum creatinine levels of less than 4.5 mg/dl were most likely to benefit from stenting.[132] Similar data were reported by Beutler et al. who followed 63 patients (46% of whom "failed" PTRA) who were stented and followed for a mean of 23 months.[158] Data for at least 1 year prior to study were available regarding renal function. Twenty-eight patients had stable renal function (<20% change in serum creatinine) prior to stenting. One patient died at 6 months with ESRD and 1 became dialysis-dependent at 5 months. Of the remaining 26 patients within this group, renal function was unchanged in 18 (69%) and improved in only 2 (8%) after the procedure. However, 6 patients (23%) showed worsening of their previously stable renal (dys)function. Of those 35 patients who had declining renal function prior to study (>20% rise in serum creatinine), after stenting 13% continued to deteriorate, but 66% stabilized with 20% more improved. Further analysis of the data revealed that of all patients who exhibited deterioration of renal function after stenting, those with baseline serum creatinine concentration of greater than 3.4 mg/dl were far more likely to do so (5 of 10 patients). However, only 10 of 53 patients (19%) whose serum creatinine concentrations at baseline were less than 3.4 mg/dl had deterioration of renal function during follow-up. Based on the aforementioned data, it can be concluded that renal artery stenting for bilateral disease is likely to at least stabilize or improve renal function in those patients with initial mild renal failure who manifested significant worsening of their renal function prior to the procedure. It is unlikely to reverse advanced renal failure, particularly if renal sizes are less than 8.0 cm.[140]

Although their study was not designed to specifically examine preservation of renal function, Burket et al. demonstrated an improvement in renal function in 43%, no change in 24%, and worsening in 32% of the 37 patients with baseline renal insufficiency (serum creatinine concentration >1.6 mg/dl) stented for primarily ostial lesions.[160] The follow-up ranged from 1 to 52 months (mean 15 ± 14 months).

A meta-analysis of 10 studies done by Isles et al. demonstrated results consistent with those previously cited.[161] The average follow-up for these patients, however, was less than 1 year. Results of stenting for ischemic nephropathy in patients followed for longer periods have been reported.[131,133,159,162] Of 163 patients who underwent primary stenting, Dorros et al. followed 145 for approximately 4 years.[131] The outcome of renal function was stratified according to whether the lesion was initially bilateral or unilateral. The baseline serum creatinine concentration in both groups was approximately 2.0 mg/dl. Of those with unilateral disease, 67% experienced improved or stable renal function, and the remainder progressed as reflected by an increase in the serum creatinine concentration of more than 0.2 mg/dl above baseline. Of those with bilateral disease, 75% had stable or improved renal function, and 25% deteriorated. Overall survival, however, was worse for those with poorer renal function at baseline, regardless of whether stenting was successful. Survival at 4 years was good in patients with normal baseline renal function (92% ± 4%), fair (74% ± 7%) in those with mildly impaired renal function (serum creatinine concentration 1.5-1.9 mg/dl), and poor (52% ± 7%) in patients with serum creatinine levels of 2.0 mg/dl or more. The rate of restenosis is not reported in this study. These authors have also published the results of a larger series of patients (1058) followed for up to 4 years.[162] Their results were more promising and demonstrated that stabilization or improved renal function could be achieved in 70% of those with unilateral lesions and 92% of those with bilateral lesions. It is important to note, how-

ever, that there was no comparison with medical therapy alone and no prior knowledge of stability of renal function and that the mean baseline serum creatinine concentration was less than 2.0 mg/dl (1.7 ± 1.1 mg/dl).

Tuttle et al. followed 129 patients after primary or secondary stenting for a mean of 24 months.[133] During this follow-up time, renal function, as assessed by creatinine clearances, remained stable, but no improvement in renal function was demonstrated regardless of baseline creatinine clearance (range 23 ± 3-53 ± 3 ml/min). However, of the 129 patients studied, 4 of the 8 who were initially dialysis-dependent recovered renal function after stenting. Their mean serum creatinine concentration was 2.3 ± 0.5 mg/dl at 15 ± 6 months (range 9-24 months). As demonstrated by angiography in 46 patients with a total of 49 stents, the re-stenosis rate was 14% at 8 ± 5 months.[133] Rundback et al. followed 45 patients with azotemia (serum creatinine concentration >1.5 mg/dl) and atheromatous RAS untreatable by, or recurrent after, PTRA for a mean of 54 months. Similar to the findings of Tuttle et al., renal function remained stable (serum creatinine concentration approximately 2.1 mg/dl).[159]

These reports are limited by the absence of a control group treated with medical therapy alone and by the fact that (except in two studies cited above 132,158) no data are provided about whether intervention was performed because of ongoing deterioration of renal function prior to stenting.[126] Nevertheless, PTRA with intravascular stenting may prove to be the best therapeutic option for patients with ostial atherosclerotic RAS who are deemed poor surgical risks or have refused surgery and are demonstrating worsening renal function or are on dialysis. In the presence of renal insufficiency, when possible, stent placement should be performed with $CO_2$ and/or gadolinium guidance.[117]

The results of *surgical* revascularization for the preservation of renal function in patients with atherosclerotic RAS have been similar to or slightly better than results with PTRA and, on occasion, have even reversed ESRD.* Improvement in renal function has been observed in approximately 50%, and stabilization of renal function has occurred in approximately 35%.†

Prospective randomized studies comparing medical therapy with surgical treatment of RAS are rare. Uzzo et al. prospectively randomized 52 patients with atherosclerotic RAS affecting their entire nephron mass to medical versus surgical management.[166] All patients had angiographic confirmation of bilateral RAS involving greater than 75% of the luminal diameter, high-grade (>75%) disease involving a solitary kidney, or unilateral high-grade (>75%) stenosis with azotemia (serum creatinine concentration >1.5 mg/dl and a GFR of <70 ml/min). Patients were excluded if the serum creatinine concentration was greater than 4.0 mg/dl, if their blood pressure was poorly controlled despite attempts at adequate medical management, or if there were comorbid conditions precluding surgery. The primary aim was a comparison of stop-point events between the medical and surgical groups. Four stop-points were defined: (1) development of poorly controlled hypertension (diastolic blood pressure >100 mm Hg); (2) reduction of GFR 50% or greater from baseline, an increase in serum creatinine concentration to greater than 4 mg/dl

---

*References 106, 112, 137, 152, 157, 163, 164.
†References 106, 112, 137, 152, 157, 159, 163, 165.

(5 mg/dl if baseline serum creatinine concentration was between 2 and 4 mg/dl), doubling of the serum creatinine from baseline or the development of ESRD; (3) intercurrent myocardial infarction or cerebrovascular accident; and (4) death. There was no statistically significant difference in the endpoints reached between the groups, and the time to reach an endpoint was not dissimilar. Overall survival, dialysis free survival and/or blood pressure control were not significantly different between the two groups. Patients with baseline azotemia (serum creatinine concentration 2-4 mg/dl), however, when surgically revascularized were less likely to die or to develop uncontrollable hypertension. Due to its small sample size, firm conclusions cannot be drawn from this study, but it underscores the need for further large-scale prospective studies.[166]

Because the operative morbidity and mortality rates (11% and 3%-6%, respectively) are significant, careful patient selection is imperative.[106,138,140,163] If the disease is progressing, if PTRA with or without stenting has failed, and if other patient-specific risk factors favor long-term survival, and the patient fulfills the strict criteria outlined subsequently, surgical revascularization should be undertaken before advanced renal failure is evident. The best window of opportunity for renal survival achieved by surgical revascularization is when the serum creatinine concentration is between 1.5 and 3.0 mg/dl.[140] Patients with diffuse atherosclerotic disease and congestive heart failure, or those undergoing simultaneous bilateral renal artery repair or revascularization in combination with another major vascular procedure, pose the greatest surgical risk.[157] As with surgical correction for renovascular hypertension, underlying coronary or cerebrovascular disease needs to be corrected prior to surgery in order to reduce operative risk. Although balloon angioplasty can be performed for in-stent re-stenosis, stenting does not preclude future surgical revascularization but does make it more difficult because the stent becomes endothelialized and difficult to remove.

Successful surgical revascularization depends on the degree of renal insufficiency present, the rate at which renal function has deteriorated preoperatively, and the anatomy of the renal vasculature distal to the renoocclusive lesion or lesions. In the presence of advanced renal failure (serum creatinine concentration above 4.0 mg/dl), revascularization offers little benefit because significant irreversible renal parenchymal disease is invariably present.[135,140] In addition to the absolute level of renal function, it appears that patients with the most rapid decline in renal function in the 6 months prior to surgery have the greatest recovery of renal function following revascularization.[167] Adequate collateral renal circulation is critical for surgical revascularization because it is necessary for maintaining viable glomeruli. Therefore, recovery or stabilization of renal function is more likely postoperatively when one or more of the following is present preoperatively[135,168-170]:

1. Visualization of the collecting system on an IVP or during the pyelogram phase of the arteriogram
2. Renal length greater than 9.0 cm
3. Demonstration of retrograde filling of the distal renal vasculature from collateral circulation on the side of total renal artery occlusion during angiography
4. The presence of viable glomeruli on renal biopsy (performed before or at the time of revascularization)

Because of the higher attendant risk of surgery, and comparable results with PTRA and stenting, and perhaps with

medical therapy, we adhere very strictly to these guidelines and patient selection before recommending surgery and have become more inclined to attempt percutaneous intervention.

## Recommendations for the Management of Chronic Renal Failure Due to Ischemic Renal Disease (RAS)

1. Medical therapy should be the primary management, particularly in older patients who are poor operative risks and especially if renal dysfunction is stable. Careful follow-up is indicated because progressive atherosclerosis can lead to worsening hypertension and renal insufficiency.
2. PTRA with intravascular stenting is the best therapeutic option for older patients who have demonstrated deterioration of their mild to moderate renal insufficiency (serum creatinine concentration 1.5 to ≤3.5 mg/dl), who are generally considered to be poor operative risks. Whenever possible, PTRA with stenting should be attempted with $CO_2$ and/or gadolinium guidance to avoid nephrotoxicity.[127]
3. As success with PTRA with stenting is improving, the role of surgical intervention is declining. We and others reserve it for the occasional "younger" patient with an overall more favorable prognosis with high-grade ostial lesions in whom PTRA and stenting have failed.[171] These patients should have minimal or insignificant untreated extrarenal vascular disease and exhibit declining mild to moderate renal dysfunction (serum creatinine concentration 1.5 to ≤3.5 mg/dl). In addition, they should fulfill the strict criteria previously outlined. Surgical revascularization is suggested, if concomitant aortic surgery is required, such as an abdominal aortic aneurysm repair.
4. If there is far advanced renal failure (serum creatinine concentration >4.0 mg/dl) both PTRA with or without stenting and surgical revascularization are unlikely to significantly reverse renal failure. However, because of the occasional patient who may respond, we may offer PTRA with stenting, particularly if the procedure can be done with $CO_2$ and/or gadolinium guidance, in a final effort to avoid dialysis.[127,159]

It is important to note that although the methods for diagnosis and treatment of RAS have improved, the use of invasive diagnostic techniques and treatment early in the course of the disease still have no proven benefit.[172] The effects of revascularization (surgical and percutaneous) on long-term renal and cardiovascular outcomes should be compared with those of comprehensive pharmacologic treatment. Until such a comparison is made, the immediate risks versus the potential, unproven long-term benefits must be carefully considered and individualized to each patient.[171] Until then, the emphasis should be on identifying those patients at risk for renal failure and treating and preventing those factors which accelerate their atherosclerosis and progression to more advanced stages of renal failure. Particular attention should be directed toward lowering lipid levels, which may restore vessel patency in atherosclerotic RAS through regression of the stenotic plaque, similar to the regression demonstrated in coronary, carotid, and peripheral arteries.[173]

Renal artery disease is a major health problem and is the cause of high rates of morbidity and mortality. Appropriate management requires the combined expertise of nephrologists, interventional angiographers, and vascular surgeons. The correct therapeutic approach, which is highly individualized, may lead to better management of blood pressure, stabilization, or restoration of renal function and, perhaps, improved patient survival; it represents a continuing challenge to those caring for these patients. Large-scale trials that will determine the best therapeutic modality for patients with the clinical consequences of RAS are long overdue.[146,174]

# References

1. Ploth DW. Renovascular hypertension. *In* Jacobson HR, Striker GE, Klahr S (eds). The Principles and Practice of Nephrology, 2nd ed. St Louis, Mosby, 1995; pp 379-386.
2. Kaplan NM, Rose BD. Who should be screened for renovascular or secondary hypertension? Uptodate Nephrol Hypertens 10: 1-3, 2002.
3. Davis BA, Crook JE, Vestal RE, et al. Prevalence of renovascular hypertension in patients with grade III or IV retinopathy. N Engl J Med 301:1273-1276, 1979.
4. Svetkey LP, Kadir S, Dunnick NR, et al. Similar prevalence of renovascular hypertension in selected blacks and whites. Hypertension 17:678-683, 1991.
5. Wollenweber J, Sheps SG, Davis GD. Clinical course of atherosclerotic renovascular disease. Am J Cardiol 21:60-71, 1968.
6. Pohl MA, Novick AC. Natural history of atherosclerotic and fibrous renal artery disease: Clinical implications. Am J Kidney Dis 5:120-130, 1985.
7. Zierler RE. Screening for renal artery stenosis: Is it justified? Mayo Clin Proc 77:307-308, 2002.
8. Rose BD. Pathophysiology of Renal Disease, 2nd ed. New York, McGraw-Hill, 1987; pp 512-515.
9. van de Ven PJG, Beutler JJ, Kaatee R, et al. Angiotensin converting enzyme inhibitor-induced renal dysfunction in atherosclerotic renovascular disease. Kidney Int 53:986-993, 1998.
10. Missouris CG, Belli A-M, MacGregor GA. "Apparent" heart failure: A syndrome caused by renal artery stenoses. Heart 83:152-155, 2000.
11. Mansoor S, Shah A, Scoble JE. "Flash pulmonary oedema"—A diagnosis for both the cardiologist and the nephrologist? Nephrol Dial Transplant 16:1311-1313, 2001.
12. Bhandari S, Kalowski S. Surgical correction of nephrotic syndrome. Nephron 87:291-292, 2001.
13. Rossignol P, Chatellier G, Azizi M, et al. Proteinuria in renal artery occlusion is related to active renin concentration and contralateral kidney size. J Hypertens 20:139-144, 2002.
14. Palmer BF. Renal dysfunction complicating the treatment of hypertension. N Engl J Med 347: 1256-1261, 2002.
15. Krijnen P, van Jaarsveld BC, Steyerberg EW, et al. A clinical prediction rule for renal artery stenosis. Ann Intern Med 129: 705-711, 1998.
16. Wilcox CS. Screening for renal artery stenosis: are scans more accurate than clinical criteria (Editorial)? Ann Intern Med 129:738-740, 1998.
17. Hollenberg NK. Medical therapy of renovascular hypertension: efficacy and safety of captopril in 269 patients. Cardiovasc Rev Rep 4:852-876, 1983.
18. Shurrab AE, Mamtora H, O'Donoghue D, et al. Increasing the diagnostic yield of renal angiography for the diagnosis of atheromatous renovascular disease. Br J Radiol 74:213-218, 1983.
19. Jackson B, Matthews PG, McGrath BP, et al. Angiotensin converting enzyme inhibition in renovascular hypertension: Frequency of reversible renal failure. Lancet 323:225-226, 1984.
20. van Jaarsveld BC, Krijnen P, Derkx FHM, et al. Resistance to antihypertensive medication as predictor of renal artery stenosis: Comparison of two drug regimens. J Hum Hypertens 15:669-676, 2001.
21. Vasbinder GBC, Nelemans PJ, Kessels AGH, et al. Diagnostic tests for renal artery stenosis in patients suspected of having renovascular hypertension: A meta-analysis. Ann Intern Med 135:401-411, 2001.
22. Nally JV. Provocative captopril testing in the diagnosis of renovascular hypertension. Urol Clin North Am 21:227-234, 1994.
23. Mann SJ, Pickering TG. Detection of renovascular hypertension. State of the art. Ann Intern Med 117:845-853, 1992.
24. Canzanello VJ, Textor SC. Noninvasive diagnosis of renovascular disease. Mayo Clin Proc 69:1172-1181, 1994.
25. Pederson EB. Angiotensin-converting enzyme inhibitor renography. Pathophysiological, diagnostic and therapeutic aspects in renal artery stenosis. Nephrol Dial Transplant 9:482-492, 1994.
26. Elliot WJ, Martin WB, Murphy MB. Comparison of two noninvasive screening tests for renovascular hypertension. Arch Int Med 153:755-764, 1993.
27. Wilcox CS. Ischemic nephropathy: Noninvasive testing. Semin Nephrol 16:43-52, 1996.
28. Setaro JF, Saddler MC, Chen CC, et al. Simplified captopril renography in diagnosis and treatment of renal artery stenosis. Hypertension 18:289-298, 1991.
29. Kaplan NM, Rose BD. Screening for renovascular hypertension. Uptodate Nephrol Hypertens 10:1-6, 2002.
30. Wilcox CS. Use of angiotensin-converting enzyme inhibitors for diagnosing renovascular hypertension. Kidney Int 44:1379-1390, 1993.
31. Karanikas G, Becherer A, Weisner K, et al. ACE inhibition is superior to angiotensin receptor blockade for renography in renal artery stenosis. Eur J Nucl Med 29:312-318, 2002.
32. Demeilliers B, Jover B, Mimran A. Contrasting renal effects of chronic administration of enalapril and losartan on one-kidney, one clip hypertensive rats. J Hypertens 16:1023-1029, 1998.
33. Erbsloh-Moller B, Dumas A, Roth D, et al. Furosemide-I$^{131}$ hippuran renography after angiotensin-converting enzyme inhibition for the diagnosis of renovascular hypertension. Am J Med 90:23-29, 1991.
34. Mann SJ, Pickering TG, Sos TA, et al. Captopril renography in the diagnosis of renal artery stenosis: Accuracy and limitations. Am J Med 90:30-40, 1991.
35. Dondi M, Fanti S, De Fabritiis A, et al. Prognostic value of captopril renal scintigraphy in renovascular hypertension. J Nucl Med 33:2040-2044, 1992.
36. Chen CC, Hoffer PB, Vahjen G, et al. Patients at high risk for renal artery stenosis: A simple method of renal scintigraphic analysis with Tc-99m DTPA and captopril. Radiology 176:365-370, 1990.
37. Ugur O, Serdengecti M, Karacalioglu D, et al. Prediction of response to revascularization in patients with renal artery stenosis by Tc-99m-ethylenedicysteine captopril scintigraphy. Ann Nucl Med 13:77-81, 1999.
38. Blaufox MD, Fine EJ, Heller S, et al. Prospective study of simultaneous orthoiodohippurate and diethylenetriaminepentaacetic acid and captopril renography. The Einstein/Cornell Collaborative Hypertension Group. J Nucl Med 39:522-528, 1998.
39. Dondi M, Monetti N, Fanti S, et al. Use of technetium-99m-MAG$_3$ for renal scintigraphy after angiotensin-converting enzyme inhibition. J Nucl Med 32:424-428, 1991.
40. Stavropoulos SW, Sevigny SA, Ende JF, et al. Hypotensive response to captopril: a potential pitfall of scintigraphic assessment for renal artery stenosis. J Nucl Med 40:406-411, 1999.
41. Imanishi M, Tsuji T, Nakamura S, et al. Prostaglandin I (2)/E(2) ratios in unilateral renovascular hypertension of different severities. Hypertension 38:23-29, 2001.

42. Ergun EL, Caglar M, Erdem Y, et al. Tc-99m DTPA acetylsalicylic acid (aspirin) renography in the detection of renovascular hypertension. Clin Nucl Med 25:682-690, 2000.

43. Maini A, Gambhir S, Singhal M, et al. Aspirin renography in the diagnosis of renovascular hypertension: A comparative study with captopril renography. Nucl Med Commun 4:325-331, 2000.

44. Scoble JE, McClean A, Stansby G, et al. The use of captopril-DTPA scanning in the diagnosis of atherosclerotic renal artery stenosis in patients with impaired renal function. Am J Hypertens 4(Suppl):721S-723S, 1991.

45. Fernandez P, Morel D, Jeandot R, et al. Value of captopril renal scintigraphy in hypertensive patients with renal failure. J Nucl Med 40:412-417, 1999.

46. Svetkey LP, Wilkinson R Jr, Dunnick NR, et al. Captopril renography in the diagnosis of renovascular disease. Am J Hypertens 4(Suppl):711S-715S, 1991.

47. Townsend RR, Cohen DL, Katholi R, et al. Safety of intravenous gadolinium (Gd-BOPTA) infusion in patients with renal insufficiency. Am J Kidney Dis 36:1207-1212, 2000.

48. Tombach B, Bremer C, Reimer P, et al. Renal tolerance of a neutral gadolinium chelate (gadobutrol) in patients with chronic renal failure: Results of a randomized study. Radiology 218:651-657, 2001.

49. Postma CT, Joosten FB, Rosenbusch G, et al. Magnetic resonance angiography has a high reliability in the detection of renal artery stenosis. Am J Hypertens 10:957-963, 1997.

50. Rieumont MJ, Kaufman JA, Geller SC, et al. Evaluation of renal artery stenosis with dynamic gadolinium-enhanced MR angiography. Am J Roentgenol 169:39-44, 1997.

51. Tan KT, van Beek EJR, Brown PWG, et al. Magnetic resonance angiography for the diagnosis of renal artery stenosis: A meta-analysis. Clin Radiol 57:617-624, 2002.

52. Schoenberg SO, Knopp MV, Londy F, et al. Morphologic and functional magnetic resonance imaging of renal artery stenosis: A multireader tricenter study. J Am Soc Nephrol 13:158-169, 2002.

53. Schoenberg SO, Prince MR, Knopp MV, et al. Renal MR angiography. MRI Clin North Am 6:351-370, 1998.

54. Sommer G, Noorbehesht B, Pelc N, et al. Normal renal blood flow measurement using phase-contrast cine magnetic resonance imaging. Invest Radiol 27:465-470, 1992.

55. Vallee JP, Lazeyras F, Khan HG, et al. Absolute renal blood flow quantification by dynamic MRI and Gd-DTPA. Eur Radiol 10:1245-1252, 2000.

56. Klatzburg RW, Dumoulin CL, Buonocore MA, et al. Noninvasive measurement of renal hemodynamic functions using gadolinium-enhanced magnetic resonance imaging. Invest Radiol 29:5123-5126, 1994.

57. de Haan MW, Kouwenhoven M, Thelissen GRP, et al. Renovascular disease in patients with hypertension: Detection with systolic and diastolic gating in three-dimensional phase contrast MR angiography. Radiology 198:449-456, 1996.

58. Thornton MJ, Thornton F, O'Callaghan J, et al. Evaluation of dynamic gadolinium-enhanced breath-hold MR angiography in the diagnosis of renal artery stenosis. Am J Roentgenol 173:1279-1283, 1999.

59. De Cobelli F, Vanzulli A, Sironi S, et al. Renal artery stenosis: Evaluation with breath-hold, three-dimensional, dynamic, gadolinium-enhanced versus three-dimensional, phase-contrast MR angiography. Radiology 205:689-695, 1997.

60. Shetty AN, Bis KG, Kirsch M, et al. Contrast-enhanced breath-hold three-dimensional magnetic resonance angiography in the evaluation of renal arteries: Optimization of technique and pitfalls. J Magn Reson Imaging 12:912-923, 2000.

61. Fain SB, King BF, Breen JF, et al. High-spatial-resolution contrast-enhanced MR angiography of the renal arteries: A prospective comparison with digital subtraction angiography. Radiology 218:481-490, 2001.

62. Urban BA, Ratner LE, Fishman EK. Three-dimensional volume-rendered CT angiography of the renal arteries and veins: Normal anatomy, variants and clinical applications. Radiographics 21:373-386, 2001.

63. Ghantous VE, Eisen TD, Sherman AH, et al. Evaluating patients with renal failure for renal artery stenosis with gadolinium-enhanced magnetic resonance angiography. Am J Kidney Dis 33:36-42, 1999.

64. Olbricht CJ, Arlart IP. Magnetic resonance angiography—The procedure of choice to diagnose renal artery stenosis? Nephrol Dial Transplant 13:1620-1622, 1998.

65. Qanadli SD, Soulez G, Therasse E, et al. Detection of renal artery stenosis: Prospective comparison of captopril-enhanced Doppler sonography, captopril-enhanced scintigraphy, and MR angiography. AJR AM J Roentgenol 177:1123-1129, 2001.

66. Thurner SA, Capelastegui A, Del Olmo FH, et al. Safety and effectiveness of single-versus triple-dose gadodiamide injection-enhanced MR angiography of the abdomen: A phase III double-blind multicenter study. Radiology 219:137-146, 2001.

67. Olbricht CJ, Paul K, Prokop M, et al. Minimally invasive diagnosis of renal artery stenosis by spiral computed tomography angiography. Kidney Int 48:1332-1337, 1995.

68. Kim TS, Chung JW, Park JH, et al. Renal artery evaluation: Comparison of spiral CT angiography to intra-arterial DSA. J Vasc Interv Radiol 9:553-559, 1998.

69. Wittenberg G, Kenn W, Tschammler A, et al. Spiral CT angiography of renal arteries: comparison with angiography. Eur Radiol 9:546-551, 1999.

70. Halpern EJ, Rutter CM, Gardiner GA Jr, et al. Comparison of Doppler US and CT angiography for evaluation of renal artery stenosis. Acad Radiol 5:524-532, 1998.

71. Hawkins IF, Wilcox CS, Kerns SR, et al. $CO_2$ digital angiography: A safer contrast agent for renal vascular imaging. Am J Kidney Dis 24:685-694, 1994.

72. Caridi JG, Stavropoulos SW, Hawkins IF Jr. $CO_2$ digital subtraction angiography for renal artery angioplasty in high-risk patients. Am J Roentgenol 173:1551-1556, 1999.

73. Spinosa DJ, Matsumoto AH, Angle JF, et al. Renal insufficiency: usefulness of gadodiamide-enhanced renal angiography to supplement $CO_2$-enhanced renal angiography for diagnosis and percutaneous treatment. Radiology 210:663-672, 1999.

74. Spinosa DJ, Matsumoto AH, Angle JF, et al. Safety of $CO_2$- and gadodiamide-enhanced angiography for the evaluation and percutaneous treatment of renal artery stenosis in patients with chronic renal insufficiency. Am J Roentgenol 176:1305-1311, 2001.

75. Working Group on Renovascular Hypertension. Detection, evaluation and treatment of renovascular hypertension. Final Report. Arch Int Med 147:820-829, 1987.

76. Dunnick NR, Svetkey LP, Cohan RH, et al. Intravenous digital subtraction renal angiography: Use in screening for renovascular hypertension. Radiology 171:219-222, 1989.

77. Olin JW, Piedmonte MR, Young JR, et al. The utility of duplex ultrasound scanning of the renal arteries for diagnosing renal artery stenosis. Ann Intern Med 122:833-838, 1995.

78. Kliewer MA, Tupler RH, Hertzberg BS, et al. Doppler evaluation of renal artery stenosis: Interobserver agreement in the interpretation of wave form morphology. AJR 162:1371-1376, 1994.

79. Starvos T, Harshfield D. Renal Doppler, renal artery stenosis, and renovascular hypertension: Direct and indirect duplex sonographic abnormalities in patients with renal artery stenosis. Ultrasound Q 12:217-263, 1994.

80. Marana I, Airoldi F, Burdick L, et al. Effects of balloon angioplasty and stent implantation on intrarenal echo-Doppler velocimetric indices. Kidney Int 53:1795-1800, 1998.

81. Sharafuddin MJ, Raboi CA, Abu-Yousef M, et al. Renal artery stenosis: Duplex US after angioplasty and stent placement. Radiology 220:168-173, 2001.

82. Hua HT, Hood DB, Jensen CC, et al. The use of colorflow duplex scanning to detect significant renal artery stenosis. Ann Vasc Surg 14:118-124, 2000.

83. Johansson M, Jensen G, Aurell M, et al. Evaluation of duplex ultrasound and captopril renography for detection of renovascular hypertension. Kidney Int 58:774-782, 2000.

84. Hoffman U, Edwards JM, Carter S, et al. Role of duplex scanning for the detection of atherosclerotic renal artery disease. Kidney Int 39:1232-1239, 1991.

85. Reneá PC, Oliva VL, Bui BT, et al. Renal artery stenosis: Evaluation of Doppler US after inhibition of angiotensin-converting enzyme with captopril. Radiology 196:675-679, 1995.

86. Kaplan-Pavlovcic S, Nadja C. Captopril renography and duplex Doppler sonography in the diagnosis of renovascular hypertension. Nephrol Dial Transplant 13:313-317, 1998.

87. Radermacher J, Chavan A, Bleck J, et al. Use of doppler ultrasonography to predict the outcome of therapy of renal artery stenosis. N Engl J Med 344:410-417, 2001.

88. Mukherjee D, Bhatt DL, Robbins M, et al. Renal artery end-diastolic velocity and renal artery resistance index as predictors of outcome after renal stenting. Am J Cardiol 88:1064-1066, 2001.

89. Leung DA, Hoffmann U, Pfammatter T, et al. Magnetic resonance angiography versus duplex sonography for diagnosing renovascular disease. Hypertension 33:726-731, 1999.

90. Sheikh KH, Davidson CJ, Newman GE, et al. Intravascular ultrasound assessment of the renal artery. Ann Int Med 115:22-25, 1991.

91. Chavan A, Hausmann D, Brunkhorst R. Intravascular ultrasound to establish the indication for renal angioplasty. Nephrol Dial Transplant 13:1583-1584, 1998.

92. Savader SJ, Lund GB, Venbrux AC. Doppler flow wire evaluation of renal artery blood flow before and after PTA: Initial results. J Vasc Interv Radiol 9:451-460, 1998.

93. Carlier SG, Li W, Cespedes I, et al. Images in cardiovascular medicine. Simultaneous morphologic and functional assessment of a renal artery stent intervention with intravascular ultrasound. Circulation 97:2575-2576, 1998.

94. Nally JV, Olin JW, Lammert GK. Advances in non-invasive screening for renovascular disease. Cleve Clin J Med 61:328-336, 1994.

95. Frederickson ED, Wilcox CS, Bucci CM, et al. A prospective evaluation of a simplified captopril test for the detection of renovascular hypertension. Arch Intern Med 150:569-572, 1990.

96. Lenz T, Kia T, Rupprecht G, et al. Captopril test: Time over? J Hum Hypertens 13:431-435, 1999.

97. Muller FB, Sealey JE, Case DB. The captopril test for identifying renovascular disease in hypertensive patients. Am J Med 80:633-644, 1986.

98. Derkx FH, Schalekamp MA. Renal artery stenosis and hypertension. Lancet 344:237-239, 1994.

99. Ram CVS, Clagett GP, Radford LR. Renovascular hypertension. Semin Nephrol 15:152-174, 1995.

100. Hollenberg NK. The treatment of renovascular hypertension: Surgery, angioplasty and medical therapy with converting enzyme inhibitors. Am J Kidney Dis 10(suppl 1):52-60, 1987.

101. Franklin SS, Smith RD. Comparison of the effects of enalapril plus hydrochlorothiazide versus standard triple therapy on renal function in renovascular hypertension. Am J Med 79:14-23, 1985.

102. Tullis MJ, Caps MT, Zierler RE, et al. Blood pressure, antihypertensive medication and atherosclerotic renal artery stenosis. Am J Kidney Dis 33:675-681, 1999.

103. Imamura A, Mackenzie HS, Lacy ER. Effects of chronic treatment with an angiotensin converting enzyme inhibitor or an angiotensin receptor antagonist in two-kidney, one-clip hypertensive rats. Kidney Int 47:1394-1402, 1995.

104. Pohl MA, Novick AC. Natural history of atherosclerotic and fibrous renal artery disease: clinical implications. Am J Kidney Dis 5:120-130, 1985.

105. Schreiber MJ, Pohl MA, Novick AC. The natural history of atherosclerotic and fibrous renal artery disease. Urol Clin North Am 11:383-392, 1984.

106. Rimmer JM, Gennari FJ. Atherosclerotic renovascular disease and progressive renal failure. Ann Int Med 118:712-719, 1993.

107. Hricik DE, Dunn MJ. Angiotensin-converting-enzyme inhibitor-induced renal failure: Causes, consequences and diagnostic uses. J Am Soc Nephrol 1:845-858, 1990.

108. Michel JB, Dussaule JC, Choudat L. Effects of antihypertensive treatment in one-clip, two-kidney hypertension in rats. Kidney Int 29:1011-1020, 1986.

109. Veniant M, Heudes D, Clozel JP. Calcium blockade versus ACE inhibition in clipped and unclipped kidneys of 2K-1C rats. Kidney Int 46:421-429, 1994.

110. van de Ven P, Beutler JJ, Kaatee R, et al. Angiotensin converting enzyme inhibitor-induced renal dysfunction in atherosclerotic renovascular disease. Kidney Int 53:986-993, 1998.

111. Caps MT, Zierler ER, Polissar NL, et al. Risk of atrophy in kidneys with atherosclerotic renal artery stenosis. Kidney Int 53:735-742, 1998.

112. Jacobson HR. Ischemic renal disease: An overlooked clinical entity? Kidney Int 134:729-743, 1988.

113. Aurell M, Jensen G. Treatment of renovascular hypertension. Nephron 75:373-383, 1997.

114. Marshall FI, Hagen S, Mahaffy RG, et al. Percutaneous transluminal angioplasty for atheromatous renal artery stenosis: Blood pressure response and discriminant analysis of outcome predictors. Q J Med 75:483-489, 1990.

115. Geyskes GG. Treatment of renovascular hypertension with percutaneous transluminal renal angioplasty. Am J Kidney Dis 12:253-265, 1988.

116. Ramsay LE, Waller PC. Blood pressure response to percutaneous angioplasty: An overview of published series. BMJ 300:569-572, 1990.

117. Libertino JA, Beckmann CF. Surgery and percutaneous angioplasty in the management of renovascular hypertension. Urol Clin North Am 21:235-243, 1994.

118. Bonelli FS, McKusick MA, Textor SC. Renal artery angioplasty: Technical results and clinical outcome in 320 patients. Mayo Clin Proc 70:1041-1052, 1995.

119. Canzanello VJ, Millan VG, Spiegel JE. Percutaneous transluminal angioplasty in management of atherosclerotic renovascular hypertension: Results in 100 patients. Hypertension 13:163-172, 1989.

120. Plouin PF, Chatellier BD, Raynaud A, for the ESSAI Multicentrique Medicaments vs. Angioplastie (EMMA) Study Group. Blood pressure outcome of angioplasty in atherosclerotic renal artery stenosis. A randomized trial. Hypertension 31:823-829, 1998.

121. Webster J, Marshall F, Abalalla M, et al. Randomized comparison of percutaneous angioplasty vs. continued medical therapy for hypertensive patients with atheromatous renal artery stenosis: Scottish and Newcastle Renal Artery Stenosis Collaborative Group. J Hum Hypertens 12:329-335, 1998.

122. van Jaarsveld BC, Krijnen P, Pieterman H, et al. The effect of balloon angioplasty on hypertension in atherosclerotic renal artery stenosis. N Engl J Med 342:1007-1014, 2000.

123. Ritz E, Mann JFE. Renal angioplasty for lowering blood pressure (Editorial). N Engl J Med 342:1042-1043, 2000.

124. Rees CR, Palmaz JC, Becker GJ. Palmaz stent in atherosclerotic renal arteries involving the ostia of the renal arteries: Preliminary report of a multicenter study. Radiology 181:507-514, 1991.

125. van de Ven PJ, Beutler JJ, Kaatee R. Transluminal vascular stent for ostial atherosclerotic renal artery stenosis. Lancet 346:672-674, 1995.

126. Blum U, Krumme B, Flugel P. Treatment of ostial renal-artery stenoses with vascular endoprostheses after unsuccessful balloon angioplasty. N Engl J Med 336:459-465, 1997.

127. Spinosa DJ, Matsumoto AH, Angle JH, et al. Use of gadopentetate dimeglumine as a contrast agent for percutaneous transluminal renal angioplasty and stent placement. Kidney Int 53:503-507, 1998.

128. Novick AC. Treatment of ostial renal-artery stenoses with vascular endoprosthesis after unsuccessful balloon angioplasty (Editorial comment). J Urol 158:983, 1997.

129. Dorros G, Jaff M, Jain A. Follow-up of primary Palmaz-Schatz stent placement for atherosclerotic renal artery stenosis. Am J Cardiol 75:1051-1055, 1995.

130. Dorros G, Jaff MR, Mathiak L, et al. Stent revascularization for atherosclerotic renal artery stenosis. One-year clinical follow-up. Tex Heart Inst J 25:40-43, 1998.

131. Dorros G, Jaff M, Mathiak L, et al. Four-year follow-up of Palmaz-Schatz stent revascularization as treatment for atherosclerotic renal artery stenosis. Circulation 98:642-647, 1998.

132. Harden PN, MacLeod MJ, Rodger RS, et al. Effect of renal-artery stenting on progression of renovascular renal failure. Lancet 349:1133-1136, 1997.

133. Tuttle KR, Chouinard RF, Webber JT, et al. Treatment of atherosclerotic ostial renal artery stenosis with the intravascular stent. Am J Kidney Dis 32:611-622, 1998.

134. van de Ven PJ, Kaatee R, Beutler JJ, et al. Arterial stenting and balloon angioplasty in ostial atherosclerotic renovascular disease: A randomised trial. Lancet 353:282-286, 1999.

135. Novick AC. Surgical correction of renovascular hypertension. Surg Clin North Am 68:1007-1025, 1988.

136. Novick AC. Current concepts in the management of renovascular hypertension and ischemic renal failure. Am J Kidney Dis 13(suppl 1):33-37, 1989.

137. Hansen KJ, Starr SM, Sands RE. Contemporary surgical management of renovascular disease. J Vasc Surg 16:319-331, 1992.

138. Stanley JC. The evolution of surgery for renovascular occlusive disease. Cardiovasc Surg 2:195-202, 1994.

139. Lawrie GM, Morris GC, Glaeser DH. Renovascular reconstruction: factors affecting long-term prognosis in 919 patients followed up to 31 years. Am J Cardiol 63:1085-1092, 1989.

140. Textor SC. Revascularization in atherosclerotic renal artery disease. Kidney Int 53:799-811, 1998.

141. Olin JW, Vidt DG, Gifford RW Jr. Renovascular disease in the elderly: An analysis of 50 patients. J Am Coll Cardiol 5:1232-1238, 1985.

142. Greminger P, Luscher TF, Zuber J. Surgery, transluminal dilatation and medical therapy in the management of renovascular hypertension. Nephron 44(suppl 1):36-39, 1986.

143. Zech P, Finaz de Villaine J, Pozet N. Surgical versus medical treatment in renovascular hypertension. Restrospective study of 166 cases. Nephron 44(suppl 1):105-108, 1986.

144. Weibull H, Bergqvist D, Bergentz SE. Percutaneous transluminal angioplasty versus reconstruction of atherosclerotic renal artery stenosis. Prospective randomized study. J Vasc Surg 18:841-852, 1993.

145. Wright JR, Shurrab AE, Cheung C, et al. A prospective study of the determinants of renal functional outcome and mortality in atherosclerotic renovascular disease. Am J Kidney Dis 39:1153-1161, 2002.

146. Tuttle KR. Renal parenchymal injury as a determinant of clinical consequences in atherosclerotic renal artery stenosis. Am J Kidney Dis 39:1321-1322, 2002.

147. Baboolal K, Evans C, Moore RH. Incidence of end-stage renal disease in medically treated patients with severe bilateral atherosclerotic renovascular disease. Am J Kidney Dis 31:971-977, 1998.

148. Leertouwer TC, Pattynama PMT, van den Berg-Huysmans A. Incidental renal artery stenosis in peripheral vascular disease: A case for treatment? Kidney Int 59:1480-1483, 2001.

149. Caps MT, Perissinotto C, Zierler RE, et al. Prospective study of atherosclerotic disease progression in the renal artery. Circulation 98:2866-2872, 1998.

150. Meyrier A, Hill GS, Simon P. Ischemic renal diseases: New insights into old entities. Kidney Int 54:2-13, 1998.

151. Muray S, Martin M, Amoedo ML, et al. Rapid decline in renal function reflects reversibility and predicts the outcome after angioplasty in renal artery stenosis. Am J Kidney Dis 39:60-66, 2002.

152. Greco BA, Breyer JA. Atherosclerotic ischemic renal disease. Am J Kidney Dis 29:167-187, 1997.

153. Middleton JP. Ischemic disease of the kidney: How and why to consider revascularization. J Nephrol 3:123-136, 1998.

154. Mailloux LU, Napolitano B, Bellucci AG. Renal vascular disease causing end-stage renal disease, incidence, clinical correlates, and outcomes: A 20-year clinical experience. Am J Kidney Dis 24:622-629, 1994.

155. O'Donovan RM, Gutierrez OH, Izzo JL Jr. Preservation of renal function by percutaneous renal angioplasty in high-risk elderly patients: Short-term outcome. Nephron 60:187-192, 1992.

156. Sos TA. Angioplasty for the treatment of azotemia and renovascular hypertension in atherosclerotic renal artery disease. Circulation 83(Suppl I):162-166, 1991.

157. Novick AC. Options for therapy of ischemic nephropathy: Role of angioplasty and surgery. Semin Nephrol 16:53-60, 1996.

158. Beutler JJ, van Ampting JMA, van de Ven PJG, et al. Long-term effects of arterial stenting on kidney function for patients with ostial atherosclerotic renal artery stenosis and renal insufficiency. J Am Soc Nephrol 12:1475-1481, 2001.

159. Rundback JH, Gray RJ, Rozenblit G, et al. Renal artery stent placement for the management of ischemic nephropathy. J Vasc Interv Radiol 9:413-420, 1998.

160. Burket MW, Cooper CJ, Kennedy DG, et al. Renal artery angioplasty and stent placement: Predictors of a favorable outcome. Am Heart J 139:64-71, 2000.

161. Isles CG, Robertson S, Hill D. Management of renovascular disease: A review of renal artery stenting in ten studies. Q J Med 92:159-167, 1999.

162. Dorros G, Jaff M, Mathiak L, et al. Multicenter Palmaz stent renal artery stenosis revascularization registry report: Four year follow-up of 1,058 successful patients. Cathet Cardiovasc Intervent 55:182-188, 2002.

163. Libertino JA, Bosco PJ, Ying CY. Renal vascularization to preserve and restore renal function. J Urol 147:1485-1487, 1992.

164. Kaylor WM, Novick AC, Ziegelbaum M. Reversal of end-stage renal failure in patients with atherosclerotic renal occlusion. J Urol 141:486-488, 1989.

165. van Rooden CJ, van Bockel JH, De Backer GG, et al. Long-term outcome of surgical revascularization in ischemic nephropathy: Normalization of average decline in renal function. J Vasc Surg 29:1037-1049, 1999.

166. Uzzo RG, Novick AC, Goormastic M, et al. Medical versus surgical management of atherosclerotic renal artery stenosis. Transplant Proc 34:723-725, 2002.

167. Dean RH, Tribble RW, Hansen KJ. Evolution of renal insufficiency in ischemic nephropathy. Ann Surg 213:446-456, 1991.

168. Novick AC, Ziegelbaum M, Vidt DG. Trends in surgical revascularization for renal artery disease: ten years experience. JAMA 257:498-501, 1987.

169. Schefft P, Novick AC, Stewart BH. Renal revascularization in patients with total occlusion of the renal artery. J Urol 124:184-186, 1980.

170. Rose BD, Mailloux LU, Kaplan NM. Chronic renal failure due to ischemic renal disease. Uptodate Nephrol Hypertens 10:1-6, 2002.

171. Plouin PF, Rossignol P, Bobrie G. Atherosclerotic renal artery stenosis: To treat conservatively, to dilate, to stent or to operate? J Am Soc Nephrol 12:2190-2196, 2001.

172. Safian RD, Textor SC. Renal artery stenosis. N Engl J Med 344:431-442, 2001.

173. Khong TK, Missouris CG, Belli AM, et al. Regression of atherosclerotic renal artery stenosis with aggressive lipid lowering therapy. J Hum Hypertens 15:431-433, 2001.

174. Conlon PJ, O'Riordan E, Kalra PA. New insights into the epidemiologic and clinical manifestations of atherosclerotic renovascular disease. Am J Kidney Dis 35:573-587, 2000.

# Adrenal Cortex Hypertension

## William F. Young, Jr.

Adrenal cortex–dependent hypertension is not common in the general population of hypertensives, but an accurate diagnosis provides clinicians with a unique treatment opportunity, that is, to render a surgical cure or to achieve a dramatic response with pharmacologic therapy. Forms of adrenal cortical hypertension that may be amenable to surgery include overproduction of aldosterone, deoxycorticosterone, and cortisol, resulting in the syndromes of primary aldosteronism, hyperdeoxycorticosteronism, and Cushing's syndrome, respectively. In this chapter the key features of the clinical presentation, diagnosis, and treatment of each of these disorders are reviewed.

## PRIMARY ALDOSTERONISM

Hypertension, hypokalemia, suppressed plasma renin activity (PRA), and increased aldosterone excretion characterize the syndrome of primary aldosteronism, first described in 1955.[1] Aldosterone-producing adenoma (APA) and bilateral idiopathic hyperaldosteronism (IHA) and are the most common subtypes of primary aldosteronism (Box 75–1). A much less common form, unilateral hyperplasia or primary adrenal hyperplasia (PAH), is caused by hyperplasia of the zona glomerulosa of predominantly one adrenal gland. Familial hyperaldosteronism (FH) is also rare, and two types have been described: FH type I and FH type II. FH type I, or glucocorticoid-remediable aldosteronism (GRA), is autosomal dominant in inheritance and associated with variable degrees of hyperaldosteronism, high levels of hybrid steroids (e.g., 18-hydroxycortisol and 18-oxocortisol), and suppression with exogenous glucocorticoids.[2] FH type II was reported initially in five families (13 patients) and refers to the familial occurrence of APA or IHA or both.[3]

### Prevalence

In the past, clinicians would not consider the diagnosis of primary aldosteronism unless the patient presented with spontaneous hypokalemia, and then the diagnostic evaluation would require discontinuing antihypertensive medications for 2 weeks. The "spontaneous hypokalemia/no antihypertensive drug" diagnostic approach resulted in predicted prevalence rates of less than 0.5% of hypertensive patients.[4-9] However, it is now recognized that most patients with primary aldosteronism are not hypokalemic[10-13] and that screening can be completed with a simple blood test (plasma aldosterone concentration [PAC]:plasma renin activity [PRA] ratio) while the patient is taking antihypertensive drugs.[14-20] Using the PAC:PRA ratio as a screening test followed by aldosterone suppression confirmatory testing has resulted in much higher prevalence estimates (5%-13% of all patients with hypertension) for primary aldosteronism.[10,21-27]

## Clinical Presentation

The diagnosis of primary aldosteronism is usually made in patients who are in the third to sixth decade of life. Few symptoms are specific to the syndrome. Patients with marked hypokalemia may have muscle weakness, cramping, headaches, palpitations, polydipsia, polyuria, or nocturia, or a combination of these. There are no specific physical findings. The degree of hypertension is usually moderate to severe and may be resistant to usual pharmacologic treatments.[28-29] (See Chapter 59 for a discussion of primary aldosteronism in the setting of resistant hypertension.) Hypokalemia is frequently absent; thus, all patients with hypertension are candidates for this disorder. Several studies have shown that patients with primary aldosteronism may be at higher risk than other patients with hypertension for target organ damage of the heart and kidney.[30-41]

## Diagnosis

The diagnostic approach to primary aldosteronism can be considered in three phases: screening tests, confirmatory tests, and subtype evaluation tests.

### Screening Tests

Spontaneous hypokalemia is uncommon in patients with uncomplicated hypertension and, when present, strongly suggests associated mineralocorticoid excess. However, normokalemia does not exclude primary aldosteronism. Several studies have shown that most patients with primary aldosteronism have baseline serum levels of potassium in the normal range.[21,42,43] Therefore, hypokalemia is not required to make the diagnosis of primary aldosteronism. Patients with hypertension and hypokalemia, regardless of presumed cause (e.g., diuretic treatment), and most patients with treatment-resistant hypertension should undergo screening for primary aldosteronism (Figure 75–1).

In patients with suspected primary aldosteronism, screening can be accomplished by measuring a morning, nonfasting (preferably 8 A.M.) ambulatory paired random PAC and PRA (see Figure 75–1). This test may be performed while the patient is taking antihypertensive medications and without postural stimulation.[19,44] Hypokalemia reduces the secretion of aldosterone, and it is optimal to restore the serum level of potassium to normal before performing diagnostic studies. Aldosterone receptor antagonists (e.g., spironolactone and eplerenone) are the only medications that will absolutely interfere with interpretation of the ratio. Angiotensin-converting enzyme (ACE) inhibitors and antiotension receptor blockers (ARBs) have the potential to "falsely elevate" PRA. Therefore, in a patient treated with an ACE inhibitor or an ARB, the findings of a detectable PRA level or a low PAC:PRA ratio do not exclude the diagnosis

**Box 75-1** Adrenocortical Causes of Hypertension

**Primary Aldosteronism**
Aldosterone-producing adenoma (APA)
Bilateral idiopathic hyperplasia (IHA)
Primary (unilateral) adrenal hyperplasia (PAH)
Aldosterone-producing adrenocortical carcinoma
Familial hyperaldosteronism (FH)
Glucocorticoid-remediable aldosteronism (FH type I)
FH type II (APA or IHA)

**Hyperdeoxycorticosteronism**
Congenital adrenal hyperplasia
11β-Hydroxylase deficiency
17α-Hydroxylase deficiency
Deoxycorticosterone-producing tumor
Primary cortisol resistance

**Apparent Mineralocorticoid Excess (AME)/11β-Hydroxysteroid Dehydrogenase Deficiency**
Genetic
Type I AME
Type II AME
Acquired
Licorice or carbenoxolone ingestion (type I AME)
Cushing's syndrome (type II AME)

**Cushing's Syndrome**
Exogenous glucocorticoid administration—most
common cause
Endogenous
ACTH-dependent (85%)
Pituitary
Ectopic
ACTH-independent (15%)
Unilateral adrenal disease
Bilateral adrenal disease
Massive macronodular hyperplasia (rare)
Primary pigmented nodular adrenal disease
(rare)

ACTH, adrenocorticotropic hormone.

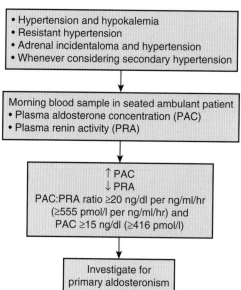

WHEN TO CONSIDER SCREENING
FOR PRIMARY ALDOSTERONISM

- Hypertension and hypokalemia
- Resistant hypertension
- Adrenal incidentaloma and hypertension
- Whenever considering secondary hypertension

Morning blood sample in seated ambulant patient
• Plasma aldosterone concentration (PAC)
• Plasma renin activity (PRA)

↑ PAC
↓ PRA
PAC:PRA ratio ≥20 ng/dl per ng/ml/hr
(≥555 pmol/l per ng/ml/hr) and
PAC ≥15 ng/dl (≥416 pmol/l)

Investigate for
primary aldosteronism

**Figure 75-1** Use of the plasma aldosterone concentration: plasma renin activity ratio to screen for primary aldosteronism.

the PAC:PRA ratio is widely accepted as the screening test of choice for primary aldosteronism.[53,54]

It is important to understand that the lower limit of detection varies among different PRA assays and can have a dramatic effect on the PAC:PRA ratio.[55-57] As an example, a very different ratio is obtained if the lower limit of detection for PRA is 0.6 ng/ml/hour rather than 0.1 ng/ml/hour; for a PAC of 16 ng/dl, the PAC:PRA ratio would be 27 and 160, respectively. Thus, the cutoff for a "high" PAC:PRA ratio is laboratory dependent and, more specifically, PRA assay-dependent. Weinberger et al.[18] found that the combination of a PAC:PRA ratio greater than 30 and PAC greater than 20 ng/dl had a sensitivity of 90% and a specificity of 91% for APA. Hirohira et al.[57] found that a PAC:PRA ratio greater than 32 had a sensitivity of 100% and a specificity of 61% for APA. At the Mayo Clinic, a PAC (in ng/dl):PRA (in ng/ml/hour) ratio 20 or greater *and* PAC 15 or greater are found in more than 90% of patients with surgically confirmed APA. In patients without primary aldosteronism, most of the variation occurs within the normal range. A high PAC:PRA ratio is a positive screening test result, a finding that warrants further testing.

### Confirmatory Testing

An increased PAC:PRA ratio is not diagnostic by itself, and primary aldosteronism must be confirmed by demonstrating inappropriate aldosterone secretion. The list of drugs and hormones capable of affecting the renin-angiotensin-aldosterone axis is extensive, and frequently in patients with severe hypertension, a "medication-contaminated" evaluation is unavoidable. Calcium channel blockers, $\alpha_1$-adrenergic receptor blockers, and β-adrenergic receptor blockers do not affect the diagnostic accuracy in most cases.[58] It is impossible to interpret data obtained from patients receiving treatment with aldosterone receptor antagonists (e.g., spironolactone, eplerenone) when PRA is not suppressed. Therefore, treatment with an

of primary aldosteronism. In addition, a strong predictor for primary aldosteronism is a PRA level undetectably low in a patient taking an ACE inhibitor or an ARB.

The PAC:PRA ratio, first proposed as a screening test for primary aldosteronism in 1981,[14] is based on the concept of paired hormone measurements.[16] For example, in a hypertensive hypokalemic patient (1) secondary hyperaldosteronism should be considered when both PRA and PAC are increased and the PAC:PRA ratio is less than 10 (e.g., renovascular disease), (2) an alternate source of mineralocorticoid receptor agonism should be considered when both PRA and PAC are suppressed (e.g., hypercortisolism), and (3) primary aldosteronism should be suspected when PRA is suppressed and PAC is increased (Figure 75-2). Fourteen prospective studies have been published on the use of the PAC:PRA ratio in screening for primary aldosteronism.* Although there is some uncertainty about test characteristics and lack of standardization,[20]

*References 14, 19, 21, 23-26, 42-52.

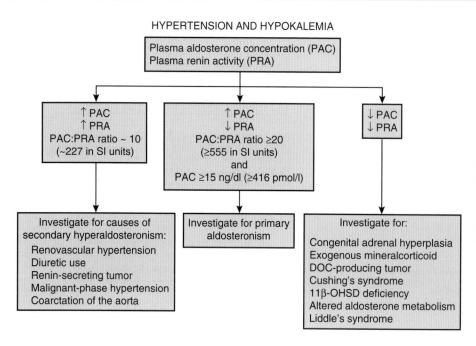

HYPERTENSION AND HYPOKALEMIA

**Figure 75–2** Use of the plasma aldosterone concentration:plasma renin activity ratio to differentiate among different causes of hypertension and hypokalemia. SI units, international system of units. (Modified from Young WF Jr, Hogan MJ. Renin-independent hypermineralocorticoidism. Trends Endocrinol Metab 5:97-106, 1994.)

aldosterone receptor antagonist should not be initiated until the evaluation has been completed and the final decisions about treatment have been made. If primary aldosteronism is suspected in a patient receiving treatment with spironolactone or eplerenone, the treatment should be discontinued for at least 6 weeks before further diagnostic testing.

Aldosterone suppression testing can be performed with orally administered sodium chloride and measurement of urinary aldosterone or with intravenous sodium chloride loading and measurement of PAC.[42,58,59] After hypertension and hypokalemia are controlled, patients should receive a high-sodium diet (supplemented with sodium chloride tablets if needed) for 3 days. The risk of increasing dietary sodium in patients with severe hypertension must be assessed in each case. Because the high-salt diet can increase kaliuresis and hypokalemia, vigorous replacement of potassium chloride may be needed, and the serum level of potassium should be monitored daily. On the third day of the high-sodium diet, a 24-hour urine specimen is collected for measurement of aldosterone, sodium, and potassium. To document adequate sodium repletion, the 24-hour urinary sodium excretion should exceed 200 mEq. Urinary aldosterone excretion greater than 12 μg/24 hours in this setting is consistent with autonomous aldosterone secretion.[60]

### Subtype Studies

Following screening and confirmatory testing, the third management issue guides the therapeutic approach by distinguishing APA and PAH from IHA and GRA. Unilateral adrenalectomy in patients with APA or PAH results in normalization of hypokalemia in all; hypertension is improved in all and is cured in approximately 30% to 60% of these patients.[61] In IHA and GRA, unilateral or bilateral adrenalectomy seldom corrects the hypertension.[58] IHA and GRA should be treated medically.

Primary aldosteronism subtype evaluation may require one or more tests, the first of which is imaging the adrenal glands with computed tomography (CT) (Figure 75–3). When a solitary unilateral macroadenoma (>1 cm) and normal contralat-

eral adrenal morphology are found on CT in a young patient (<40 years) with primary aldosteronism, unilateral adrenalectomy is a reasonable therapeutic option (Figure 75–3). However, in many cases, CT may show normal-appearing adrenals, minimal unilateral adrenal limb thickening, unilateral microadenomas (≤1 cm), or bilateral macroadenomas (Figure 75–4). In these cases, additional testing is required to determine the source of excess aldosterone secretion. Small APAs may be labeled incorrectly as "IHA" on the basis of CT findings of bilateral nodularity or normal-appearing adrenals. Also, apparent adrenal microadenomas may represent areas of hyperplasia, and unilateral adrenalectomy would be inappropriate. In addition, nonfunctioning unilateral adrenal macroadenomas are not uncommon, especially in older patients (>40 years) (Figure 75–4).[62]

In general, patients with APAs have more severe hypertension, more frequent hypokalemia, and higher plasma (>25 ng/dl) and urinary (>30 μg/24 hour) levels of aldosterone and are younger (<50 years) than those with IHA.[58,63] Patients fitting these descriptors are considered to have a "high probability of APA" (Figure 75–3). However, these factors are not absolute predictors of unilateral versus bilateral adrenal disease. With the addition of adrenal venous sampling, we have found unilateral APAs in 36% of those with clinically "high-probability" APA who had normal findings or unilateral adrenal limb thickening on CT.[64] Gordon et al.[65] reported that CT contributed to lateralization in only 59 of 111 patients with surgically proven APA; CT detected fewer than 25% of the APAs that were less than 1 cm in diameter. Magill et al.[66] reported that in 38 patients who had both CT and adrenal venous sampling, CT findings were either inaccurate or provided no additional information for 68% of patients with primary aldosteronism. Therefore, adrenal venous sampling is essential to direct appropriate therapy in patients with primary aldosteronism who have a high probability of APA and seek a potential surgical cure.

Adrenal venous sampling is the reference standard test to differentiate unilateral from bilateral disease in patients with primary aldosteronism.[67] Adrenal venous sampling is a difficult

CONFIRMED PRIMARY ALDOSTERONISM

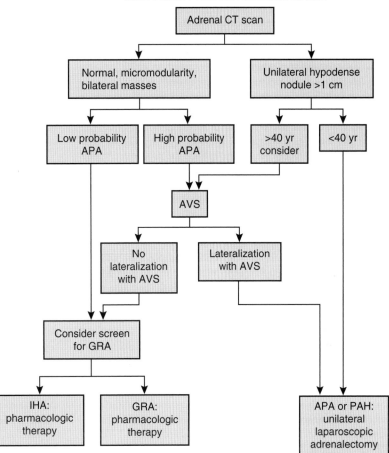

**Figure 75–3** Subtype evaluation of primary aldosteronism. See text for details. APA, aldosterone-producing adenoma; AVS, adrenal venous sampling; CT, computed tomography; GRA, glucocorticoid-remediable aldosteronism; IHA, idiopathic hyperaldosteronism; PAH, primary adrenal hyperplasia. (Modified from Young WF Jr, Hogan MJ. Renin-independent hypermineralocorticoidism. Trends Endocrinol Metab 5:97-106, 1994.)

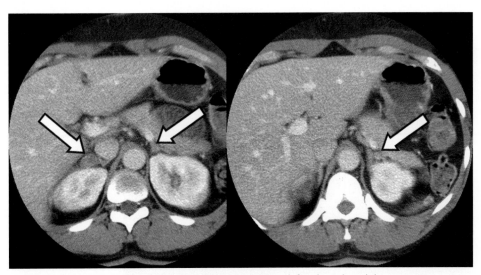

**Figure 75–4** Appearance of a 1.8-cm right adrenal nodule and 0.7-cm left adrenal nodule *(arrows)* on contrast-enhanced CT in a 49-year-old man. The patient had been hypertensive for 20 years, with poor control for the last 4 years; his antihypertensive medication program included an ACE inhibitor, a calcium channel blocker, thiazide diuretic, and a β-adrenergic blocker. The screening test for primary aldosteronism was positive, with a plasma aldosterone concentration (PAC) of 53 ng/dl and low plasma renin activity (PRA) at <0.6 ng/ml/hr (PAC:PRA ratio >88). The 24-hour urinary excretion of aldosterone was increased at 40 μg (urinary sodium = 236 mEq/24 hr).

procedure because the right adrenal vein is small; the success rate depends on the proficiency of the angiographer (Figure 75–5).[65] According to a review of 47 reports, the success rate for cannulating the right adrenal vein in 384 patients was 74%.[58] With experience, the success rate increased to 90% to 93%.[64,65] Some centers perform adrenal venous sampling in all patients with the diagnosis of primary aldosteronism.[65] A more practical approach is the selective use of adrenal venous sampling outlined in Figure 75–3. To minimize stress-induced fluctuations in aldosterone secretion, an infusion of 50 μg of cosyntropin per hour is initiated 30 minutes before adrenal vein catheterization and continued throughout the procedure.[64] The adrenal veins are catheterized through the percutaneous femoral vein approach, and the position of the catheter tip is verified by gentle injection of a small amount of nonionic contrast medium and radiographic documentation (Figure 75–5). Blood is obtained from both adrenal veins and the inferior vena cava (IVC) below the renal veins and assayed for aldosterone and cortisol concentrations. The venous sample from the left side typically is obtained from the inferior phrenic vein immediately adjacent to the entrance of the adrenal vein. The right adrenal vein may be especially difficult to catheterize because it is short and enters the IVC at an acute angle.[67] The cortisol concentrations from the adrenal veins and IVC are used to confirm successful catheterization. The adrenal vein:IVC cortisol ratio is typically greater than 10:1 (mean values at Mayo Clinic are 32:1 on the right and 22:1 on the left).

Dividing the right and left adrenal vein PACs by their respective cortisol concentrations corrects for the dilutional effect of the inferior phenic vein flow into the left adrenal vein; these are termed "cortisol-corrected ratios" (Table 75–1). In patients with APA, the mean cortisol-corrected aldosterone ratio (APA-side PAC/cortisol:normal adrenal PAC/cortisol) is 18:1 (range, 3.7:1-79:1).[64] A cutoff of the cortisol-corrected aldosterone ratio from high side to low side greater than 4:1 is used to indicate unilateral aldosterone excess.[64] Usually in patients with unilateral aldosterone excess, the contralateral aldosterone:cortisol ratio is less than the IVC aldosterone:cortisol ratio, reflecting a lower proportional contribution of aldosterone from the contralateral adrenal gland (Table 75–1).[64,67] In patients with IHA, the mean cortisol-corrected aldosterone ratio is 2:1 (high side:low side; range, 1:0-3:5); a ratio less than 3:1 is suggestive of bilateral aldosterone hypersecretion.[64] In patients with IHA, the "low-side" aldosterone:cortisol ratio is usually greater than in the IVC. Adrenal venous sampling is essential to direct appropriate therapy for patients with primary aldosteronism who have a high probability of APA and CT findings of unilateral adrenal limb thickening.

## Principles of Treatment

Normalization of blood pressure should not be the only goal in managing the patient with primary aldosteronism. In addition to the kidney and colon, mineralocorticoid receptors are present in the heart, brain, and blood vessels. A number of animal studies indicate that aldosterone exerts deleterious effects when plasma concentrations are inappropriate for salt status.[68-70] In experimental models of hypertension and heart failure, the nonepithelial effects of aldosterone are mediated via classical mineralocorticoid receptors, and are largely or completely abolished by administration of an aldosterone receptor blocker or by reduction of circulating aldosterone by adrenalectomy.[68,71] It has been demonstrated that selective aldosterone blockade (at doses that do not alter blood pressure) markedly reduces tissue (brain, heart, kidney) damage in saline-drinking spontaneously hypertensive rats.[68] Aldosterone induces myocardial fibrosis by either stimulation of cardiac fibroblasts and/or vascular fibrinoid necrosis.[72] A clinical correlate of these laboratory studies was the Randomized Aldactone Evaluation Study (RALES) where spironolactone produced a 30% reduction in mortality in patients with stage IV congestive heart failure.[73,74] Increased risk of ischemic cardiac events is associated with activation of the renin-angiotensin-aldosterone system.[75] Plasminogen activator inhibitor-1 (PAI-1) is a major physiologic inhibitor

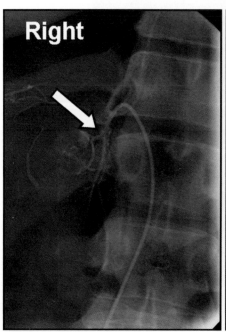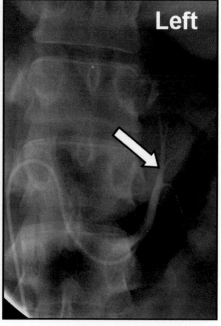

**Figure 75–5** Adrenal venous sampling radiographs from the patient described in Figure 75–4. Adrenal veins are noted by arrows.

**Table 75-1** Adrenal Vein Sampling

| Vein | Aldosterone (A) ng/dl | Cortisol (C) μg/dl | A:C Ratio | Aldosterone Ratio |
|------|------|------|------|------|
| RT Adrenal Vein | 782 | 1105 | 0.7 | |
| LT Adrenal Vein | 8504 | 700 | 12.1 | 17.3:1* |
| IVC | 87 | 31 | 2.8 | |

*Left adrenal vein A:C ratio divided by right adrenal vein A:C ratio; IVC, inferior vena cava.

Adrenal venous sampling (AVS) data from the 49-year-old man with primary aldosteronism described in Figure 75–4. Because of bilateral adrenal abnormalities on CT and the patient's desire for surgically induced improved blood pressure control, AVS was completed. AVS localized the tumor to the left adrenal gland. He had laparoscopic left adrenalectomy, and an 0.8-cm cortical adenoma was found. The postoperative PAC was <1.0 ng/dl. Hypertension was subsequently controlled with one antihypertensive agent.

of fibrinolysis.[76,77] Aldosterone increases PAI-1 expression in vascular smooth muscle and endothelial cells[78] and levels correlate with plasma concentrations of aldosterone[79]—a correlation inhibited by spironolactone.[80]

It has been reported that patients with primary aldosteronism, when matched for age, blood pressure, and duration of hypertension, have greater left ventricular (LV) mass measurements when compared with patients with other types of hypertension (e.g., pheochromocytoma, Cushing's syndrome, and essential hypertension).[81] In addition, when 26 APA patients were matched (age, sex, race, body mass index, blood pressure, duration of hypertension) with 26 essential hypertension patients, it was found that aldosterone excess was associated with both increased LV wall thickness and mass, as well as decreased early diastolic LV filling indexes.[82] The LV hypertrophy in primary aldosteronism appears to be asynchronous with other sites of target organ damage. In essential hypertensive patients, it has been shown that there is a strong correlation between LV mass and the severity of hypertensive retinopathy and renal involvement.[83] However, in patients with primary aldosteronism, the LV hypertrophy was found to be markedly advanced despite mild extracardiac target organ damage.[83] The LV wall thickness and mass decreased markedly by 1 year following adrenalectomy for APA, but not in those on medical therapy.[84] It should be noted that other studies have been unable to find differences in the degree of LV hypertrophy in patients with primary aldosteronism when compared with patients with renovascular and essential hypertension.[85]

The results of studies on small resistance arteries in fat biopsies from patients with primary aldosteronism suggest that there may be some unique vascular remodeling. For example, in patients with primary aldosteronism and renovascular hypertension, a marked increase in the media-lumen ratio has been found when compared with patients with essential hypertension or pheochromocytoma.[86,87] Therefore, normalization of circulating aldosterone or aldosterone recep-

tor blockade should be part of the management plan for all patients with primary aldosteronism.

The cause of the primary aldosteronism determines the appropriate treatment. Although the hypertension in patients with APA and unilateral hyperplasia is frequently cured with unilateral adrenalectomy, the average cure rate for IHA is only 19% after unilateral or bilateral adrenalectomy.[58] IHA and GRA should be treated medically.[55]

### Surgical Treatment of Aldosterone-Producing Adenoma and Unilateral Hyperplasia

The treatment of choice for APA and unilateral hyperplasia is unilateral total adrenalectomy. Laparoscopic adrenalectomy is the preferred surgical approach and is associated with shorter hospital stays and less long-term morbidity.[88] The blood pressure response to aldosterone receptor blockade preoperatively often predicts the blood pressure response to unilateral adrenalectomy in patients with APA. To decrease the surgical risk, hypokalemia should be corrected with spironolactone or eplerenone preoperatively; treatment with this drug should be discontinued postoperatively.

Aldosterone concentrations in blood or urine should be measured shortly after the operation. For the first few weeks postoperatively, a generous sodium diet should be followed to avoid the hyperkalemia of hypoaldosteronism that may occur because of the chronic suppression of the renin-angiotensin-aldosterone axis. Typically, the hypertension resolves in 1 to 3 months postoperatively. Although blood pressure control improves in nearly 100% of patients postoperatively, average long-term cure rates after unilateral adrenalectomy for APA are 30% to 60%.[61] Persistent hypertension following adrenalectomy for APA is correlated directly with having more than one first-degree relative with hypertension, use of more than two antihypertensive agents preoperatively, older age, and duration of hypertension, and is most likely due to coexistent primary hypertension.[61,89]

### Pharmacologic Treatment of Idiopathic Hyperaldosteronism

Dietary sodium restriction (<100 mEq sodium/day), maintenance of ideal body weight, avoidance of alcohol, and regular aerobic exercise contribute significantly to the success of pharmacologic treatment. Potassium supplementation either as a medication or a diet rich in potassium (in the absence of severe sodium restriction) is ineffective for correcting the hypokalemia of primary aldosteronism. No placebo-controlled randomized trials have evaluated the relative efficacy of drugs in the treatment of primary aldosteronism.[90] For more than three decades, spironolactone has been the drug of choice to treat primary aldosteronism. However, it is not selective for the aldosterone receptor. For example, antagonism at the testosterone receptor may result in painful gynecomastia, impotence, and menstrual irregularity. The incidence of gynecomastia in 699 patients treated with spironolactone was dose-dependent (6.9% at doses <50 mg/day and 52% at doses >150 mg/day).[91] The starting dose of spironolactone is 25 to 50 mg once daily with food; the dose may be increased weekly to a maximum of 200 mg twice daily. Blood pressure and the serum levels of potassium and creatinine should be monitored frequently. Treatment goals are normotension without the aid of other antihypertensive drugs and normokalemia without potassium supplementation.

Eplerenone is a new steroid-based antimineralocorticoid that acts as a competitive and selective aldosterone receptor antagonist that has been approved by the U.S. Food and Drug Administration for the treatment of uncomplicated essential hypertension and post myocardial infarction congestive heart failure. The 9,11-epoxide group in eplerenone results in a significant reduction of the progestational and antiandrogenic actions of the molecule compared with spironolactone.[92] Compared with spironolactone, eplerenone has 0.1% of the binding affinity to androgen receptors and less than 1% of the binding affinity to progesterone receptors.[93] Eplerenone has been effective in the treatment of mild to moderate essential hypertension and was well tolerated with the incidence of adverse events similar to placebo.[94,95] The doses used ranged from 50 to 400 mg once daily. In a separate study, the addition of eplerenone to an ACE inhibitor or an ARB resulted in significant lowering of blood pressure in patients with suboptimally controlled essential hypertension.[96]

For primary aldosteronism it is anticipated that the starting dose of eplerenone will be 25 to 50 mg twice daily. Potency studies with eplerenone show 25% to 50% less milligram-per-milligram potency compared with spironolactone. Treatment trials comparing the efficacy of eplerenone versus spironolactone for the treatment of primary aldosteronism have not been published. Presumably eplerenone will be the superior drug if it is shown to be as effective as spironolactone for the treatment of mineralocorticoid-dependent hypertension and if it lacks the limiting antiandrogen side effects of spironolactone. Because of the higher cost of eplerenone and lack of data in patients with primary aldosteronism, spironolactone should remain the aldosterone receptor antagonist of choice. Eplerenone should be considered in the spironolactone intolerant patient. As with spironolactone, blood pressure and the serum levels of potassium and creatinine need to be monitored closely.

For patients who are intolerant of eplerenone or spironolactone, amiloride may be prescribed for its potassium-sparing properties. The starting dose of amiloride is usually 5 mg once or twice daily and increased up to 15 mg twice daily if needed to correct the hypokalemia. Amiloride is not an effective antihypertensive agent for patients with primary aldosteronism, and if hypertension persists, a second-step agent (e.g., a thiazide diuretic) should be added.

Hypervolemia is a major reason for drug resistance in patients with primary aldosteronism. Low doses (e.g., 12.5-25 mg of hydrochlorothiazide daily) of a thiazide or a related sulfonamide diuretic potentiate the control of blood pressure when given in combination with a potassium-sparing diuretic.[97] ACE inhibitors, by inhibiting the generation of angiotensin II, may preferentially decrease blood pressure in patients with IHA because of their enhanced adrenal sensitivity to angiotensin II in secreting aldosterone.[98] However, the blood pressure–lowering effect of ACE inhibitors in patients with primary aldosteronism is not marked.[99,100] Angiotensin receptor antagonists should be similar to ACE inhibitors in decreasing blood pressure in patients with primary aldosteronism caused by IHA.

### Pharmacologic Treatment of GRA

Typically, GRA is diagnosed in the first to third decades of life. Of interest is that most of these patients are normokalemic, a finding likely explained by the diurnal character of the disorder.[43] Also, the patients usually have a family history of onset of hypertension at a young age. Although GRA is an unusual cause of primary aldosteronism, it is important that it be diagnosed because of the risk of hemorrhagic stroke. Of 167 patients with proven GRA, 18% had cerebrovascular complications at an average age of 32 years.[43] The cerebrovascular event was hemorrhagic stroke in 70% of the patients and was fatal in 61% of them. It appears that patients with GRA, like those with polycystic kidney disease, are at risk for cerebrovascular aneurysms. Glucocorticoids administered in physiologic to suppressive doses to patients with GRA correct the hypertension and hypokalemia. For example, dexamethasone at doses of 0.125 to 0.5 mg daily suppresses pituitary corticotropin secretion. However, because of the risk of subclinical iatrogenic Cushing's syndrome, aldosterone receptor antagonists may be preferred.

### Surgical and Pharmacologic Therapy for Patients with Aldosterone-Producing Adrenal Malignancy

Adrenal carcinoma should be suspected if a patient has an aldosterone-producing tumor larger than 3 cm in diameter. Malignancy is difficult to diagnose histologically. The only absolute criterion is the presence of local invasion or metastatic lesions. The treatment of choice for adrenocortical carcinoma is complete surgical resection with the anterior abdominal approach.[101] Even if the resection is apparently complete, the recurrence rate is high, and the 5-year survival rate for all patients with adrenocortical carcinoma is approximately 16% to 30%.[102,103] Mitotane should be given to patients with incompletely resected tumors. This drug is an adrenal cytolytic agent that inhibits adrenal steroid synthesis and destroys normal and neoplastic adrenocortical cells. The initial dosage is one 500-mg tablet with food twice daily. The total dosage is increased by 500 mg every 3 days until the maximal tolerated dosage or a maximal dose of 10 g daily is attained. In most patients, the dosage is limited by nausea, anorexia, diarrhea, somnolence, skin rash, and pruritus. Mitotane is lipophilic and has a long half-life (0.5 to 6 months). Therefore, it is contraindicated for women desiring fertility within 2 to 5 years after treatment. This drug also destroys the normal contralateral adrenal gland, and concomitant therapy with dexamethasone 0.5 mg daily should be administered.

Because of the high recurrence rate of adrenocortical carcinoma, adjuvant treatment with mitotane should be considered even for patients who appear to have had a surgical cure. The patient's condition is reevaluated with CT or magnetic resonance imaging (MRI) at 3, 6, and 12 months postoperatively. If recurrent disease is not evident at 12 months postoperatively, adjuvant mitotane therapy may be discontinued. Aldosterone receptor antagonists are effective in blocking the effects of excessive aldosterone secretion.

## HYPERDEOXYCORTICOSTERONISM

Deoxycorticosterone (DOC) is a mineralocorticoid receptor agonist. Hypersecretion of DOC is found in two forms of congenital adrenal hyperplasia (CAH), DOC-secreting tumors, and primary cortisol resistance (see Box 75–1).

## Congenital Adrenal Hyperplasia

CAH is caused by enzymatic defects in adrenal steroidogenesis that result in deficient secretion of cortisol. The lack of inhibitory feedback by cortisol on the hypothalamus and pituitary produces an adrenocorticotropic hormone (ACTH)-driven buildup of cortisol precursors proximal to the enzymatic deficiency. A deficiency of both 11β-hydroxylase and 17α-hydroxylase causes hypertension and hypokalemia because of hypersecretion of the mineralocorticoid 11-DOC. The mineralocorticoid effect of increased circulating levels of DOC also decreases PRA and aldosterone excretion. These defects are autosomal recessive in inheritance and are typically diagnosed in childhood. However, partial enzymatic defects have been shown to cause hypertension in adults.[104]

### 11β-Hydroxylase Deficiency

Approximately 5% of all cases of CAH are due to 11β-hydroxylase deficiency; the prevalence in whites is 1 in 100,000.[105] In addition to high levels of DOC and 11-deoxycortisol, the substrate mass effect results in increased levels of adrenal androgens. Females present in childhood with hypertension, hypokalemia, and virilization, and pseudoprecocious puberty appears in males. Approximately two thirds of patients have mild to moderate hypertension.[106] The clinical scenario in combination with markedly increased levels of DOC, 11-deoxycortisol, and adrenal androgens (dehydroepiandrosterone and androstenedione) confirm the diagnosis. Glucocorticoid replacement normalizes the steroid abnormalities and hypertension. Glucocorticoid replacement options in adults include dexamethasone (0.5-0.75 mg daily), prednisone (5 mg in the A.M. and 2.5 mg in the P.M.), or hydrocortisone (20 mg in the A.M. and 10 mg in the P.M.). For screening, family members should have the cosyntropin stimulation test for cortisol and 11-deoxycortisol.[105]

### 17α-Hydroxylase Deficiency

The 17α-hydroxylase deficiency form of CAH is rare.[107] The deficiency results in decreased production of cortisol and sex hormones. Genetic 46,XY males present with either pseudohermaphroditism or as phenotypic females, and 46,XX females present with primary amenorrhea. Therefore, a person with this form of CAH may not come to medical attention until puberty. The biochemical findings include low concentrations of plasma adrenal androgens, plasma 17α-hydroxyprogesterone, aldosterone, and cortisol and increased plasma concentrations of DOC, corticosterone, and 18-hydroxycorticosterone, which suppress PRA. As with 11β-hydroxylase deficiency, glucocorticoid replacement normalizes the steroid abnormalities and hypertension. Sex steroids also need to be replaced. For screening, family members should have the cosyntropin stimulation test for cortisol and 17-hydroxypregnenolone.[107]

## Deoxycorticosterone-Producing Tumor

DOC-producing adrenal tumors are usually large and malignant.[108,109] Some of them secrete androgens and estrogens in addition to DOC, which may cause virilization in women and feminization in men. A high level of plasma DOC or urinary tetrahydrodeoxycorticosterone and a large adrenal tumor seen on CT confirm the diagnosis. Optimal treatment is complete surgical resection.

## Primary Cortisol Resistance

Increased cortisol secretion and plasma cortisol concentrations without evidence of Cushing's syndrome are found in patients with primary cortisol resistance, a rare familial syndrome.[110] The syndrome is characterized by hypokalemic alkalosis, hypertension, increased plasma concentrations of DOC, and increased adrenal androgen secretion, which are probably caused by several defects in glucocorticoid receptors and the steroid-receptor complex. The treatment for mineralocorticoid-dependent hypertension is blockade of the mineralocorticoid receptor with an aldosterone receptor antagonist or suppression of ACTH secretion with dexamethasone at the same dosages as mentioned previously for primary aldosteronism and CAH, respectively.[111]

## APPARENT MINERALOCORTICOID EXCESS SYNDROMES

Cortisol can be a potent mineralocorticoid. The microsomal enzyme 11β-hydroxysteroid dehydrogenase (11β-OHSD; EC 1.1.1.146) is responsible for the renal metabolism of cortisol to the metabolically inactive cortisone. Deficiency of this enzyme results in a high intrarenal concentration of cortisol as well as hypertension, hypokalemia, suppressed PRA, and low aldosterone levels.[112,113] An increased ratio of urinary metabolites of cortisol (tetrahydrocortisol [THF] + 5α-tetrahydrocortisol [allo-THF]) to those of cortisone (tetrahydrocortisone [THE]) confirms the diagnosis. The ratio of (THF + alloTHF) to THE is approximately 1:1 in normal subjects but is greater than 7:1 in patients with 11β-OHSD deficiency. Two types of defects have been described in the renal metabolism of cortisol (see Box 75–1). Type I apparent mineralocorticoid excess (AME) syndrome refers to deficiency in the 11β-OHSD enzyme. Type II AME is due to a deficiency in the A-ring reduction metabolic pathway.[113] Treatment includes blockade of the mineralocorticoid receptor with an aldosterone receptor antagonist or suppression of endogenous cortisol secretion with dexamethasone. The congenital forms are rare autosomal-recessive disorders.[113]

The acquired forms are more common and include licorice-induced hypertension and Cushing's syndrome. Glycyrrhetinic acid in licorice is a potent inhibitor of the 11β-HSD enzyme.[114] Analyses of urinary F to E ratios in patients with licorice-induced hypertension have documented a reversible acquired 11β-HSD deficiency (type I AME).[114,115]

## CUSHING'S SYNDROME

Hypertension occurs in 75% to 80% of patients with Cushing's syndrome.[116] The mechanisms of hypertension include increased production of DOC, increased vascular reactivity to catecholamines, and cortisol inactivation overload with stimulation of the mineralocorticoid receptor. Deficient cortisol ring-A reduction caused by overload of metabolizing enzymes results in a functional type II AME in patients with severe hypercortisolism.[117] Cushing's syndrome is a symptom complex that results from prolonged exposure to supraphysiologic concentrations of glucocorticoids.[118] The source of excess glucocorticoids may be exogenous (iatrogenic) or endogenous. Endogenous Cushing's syndrome is caused by (1) hypersecretion of corticotropin (ACTH), referred to as *ACTH-dependent Cushing's syndrome,* or (2) primary adrenal hypersecretion of glucocorticoids, referred to as *ACTH-independent Cushing's syndrome.* The overall treatment program for patients with Cushing's syndrome includes the resolution of hypercortisolism, the concomitant treatment of the complications of the syndrome (e.g., hypertension, osteoporosis, and diabetes mellitus), and after definitive treatment, the management of glucocorticoid withdrawal and hypothalamic-pituitary-adrenal (HPA) axis recovery.

## Presentation

Typical signs and symptoms of Cushing's syndrome include weight gain with central obesity, facial rounding and plethora, dorsocervical fat pad, easy bruising, fine "cigarette paper skin," poor wound healing, purple striae, proximal muscle weakness, emotional and cognitive changes (e.g., irritability, crying, depression, restlessness), hypertension, osteoporosis, opportunistic and fungal infections (e.g., mucocutaneous candidiasis, tinea versicolor, pityriasis), altered reproductive function, and hirsutism.

Iatrogenic Cushing's syndrome, more common than the endogenous forms, is usually due to the known administration of glucocorticoids orally, intraarticularly, epidurally, or topically (inhaled, nasal, dermal).[119,120] Excess ACTH secretion by a pituitary tumor or a neoplastic source elsewhere is the cause of endogenous Cushing's syndrome in 85% of patients. ACTH-independent forms of Cushing's syndrome (adrenal adenoma, adrenal carcinomas, and adrenal nodular hyperplasias) are responsible for the other 15% of the endogenous cases.

## Diagnosis

Accurate diagnosis of Cushing's syndrome and subtype is essential to direct the appropriate treatment program. Because of the known manifestations of the disorder, hypercortisolism must be suspected and then confirmed with measurement of the serum and 24-hour urine concentrations of cortisol. Autonomous hypercortisolism is confirmed with the low-dose dexamethasone suppression test (dexamethasone 0.5 mg orally every 6 hours for 48 hours); a 24-hour urinary cortisol excretion of 20 µg or greater confirms the diagnosis. The plasma ACTH concentration classifies the subtype of hypercortisolism as either ACTH-dependent ("normal" to high levels of ACTH) or ACTH-independent (undetectable ACTH) (Figure 75–6).

The pituitary of patients with ACTH-dependent Cushing's syndrome should be examined with MRI. If a pituitary tumor is not found on computed imaging, further evaluation is indicated, with imaging of the lung and sampling of the inferior petrosal sinuses for ACTH with ovine corticotropin-releasing hormone stimulation.

In patients with ACTH-independent hypercortisolism, the high-dose dexamethasone suppression test shows no suppression in urinary cortisol excretion. In these patients, computed imaging of the adrenal glands usually indicates the type of adrenal disease (Figure 75–6).

## Principles of Treatment

Selective pituitary adenectomy by transsphenoidal surgery (TSS) is the treatment of choice for pituitary-dependent disease. The long-term surgical cure rate for ACTH-secreting microadenomas is approximately 90%.[121,122] If pituitary surgery is not curative, bilateral laparoscopic adrenalectomy, pituitary irradiation, or both are adjunctive treatment options.[123,124] Surgical extirpation of an adrenal adenoma or carcinoma or the source of ectopic ACTH production is the treatment of choice for primary adrenocortical disease or ectopic ACTH production. Bilateral laparoscopic adrenalectomy is the preferred treatment for ACTH-independent bilateral macronodular or micronodular hyperplasia.[125] Pharmacologic therapy is reserved for patients with disease not cured by these surgical approaches.

## Iatrogenic Cushing's Syndrome

Iatrogenic Cushing's syndrome is usually the result of the appropriate treatment of a life-threatening or debilitating inflammatory disorder (e.g., vasculitis or severe asthma) with supraphysiologic doses of glucocorticoids. The most frequently used preparation is prednisone. It has been suggested, but not proven, that alternate-day steroid therapy results in fewer side effects and less suppression of the HPA axis. HPA axis suppression can occur with high-dose (>25 mg prednisone or equivalent per day) glucocorticoid therapy for more than 1 week or lower doses (>12.5 mg prednisone or equivalent per day) for more than 4 weeks. If glucocorticoid therapy must be continued, the lowest possible dose that effectively treats the underlying disorder should be sought.

## Pituitary-Dependent Cushing's Syndrome

The treatment of choice for pituitary-dependent Cushing's syndrome is transsphenoidal selective adenectomy by an experienced neurosurgeon. Inferior petrosal sinus sampling for ACTH should be considered in patients without an obvious pituitary tumor found on MRI examination of the sella. If no tumor is obvious intraoperatively, lateralization of ACTH secretion from the preoperative inferior petrosal sinus sampling study guides the surgeon in performing a hemihypophysectomy. The goal is to remove the adenoma selectively and preserve normal pituitary tissue. At pituitary surgery centers, the mortality of TSS is 1% or less.[122,126] The incidence of perioperative morbidity is approximately 10% and includes transient diabetes insipidus, hyponatremia (due to inappropriate secretion of antidiuretic hormone), cerebrospinal fluid leak, and meningitis.[126] Potential permanent complications are infrequent (<5%) and include diabetes insipidus, partial or complete anterior pituitary failure, and injury to the carotid arteries, optic nerve, or cranial nerves in the cavernous sinus.[126]

### Postoperative Management

Patients whose disease is cured by TSS develop sudden secondary adrenal insufficiency. For this reason, all our patients receive a glucocorticoid preparation preoperatively on the morning of

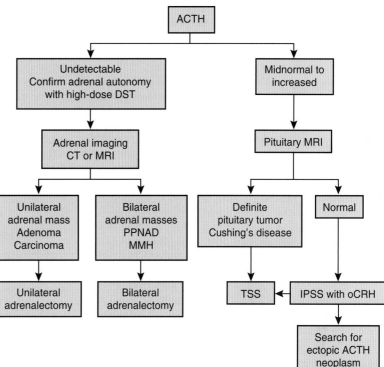

CONFIRMED CUSHING'S SYNDROME

**Figure 75-6** Subtype evaluation of Cushing's syndrome. See text for details. ACTH, adrenocorticotropic hormone; CT, computed tomography; DST, dexamethasone suppression test; IPSS, inferior petrosal sinus sampling; MMH, massive macronodular hyperplasia; MRI, magnetic resonance imaging; oCRH, ovine corticotropin-releasing hormone; PPNAD, primary pigmented nodular adrenal disease; TSS, transsphenoidal surgery.

the operation and again on the evening of the operation. Plasma cortisol concentrations are measured at 8 A.M. and 4 P.M. on the day after the operation. Most patients whose disease is cured develop symptoms of adrenal insufficiency 24 to 36 hours after the last dose of glucocorticoid. Patients are warned about these symptoms and advised to report them promptly; a blood sample is then obtained for cortisol measurement, and glucocorticoid is promptly administered intramuscularly. If the plasma cortisol concentrations are less than 3 µg/dl, a short-term cure is ensured.[127] Some patients with long-term cures have had postoperative plasma cortisol concentrations between 3 and 20 µg/dl.[127] Observation and reevaluation several weeks later with baseline 24-hour urinary cortisol excretion is indicated for these patients.

Most patients have been exposed to endogenous hypercortisolism for many years, and abrupt postoperative institution of replacement doses of glucocorticoid results in prominent withdrawal symptoms. Typically, patients are dismissed from the hospital on a regimen of prednisone 5 mg orally in the morning and 5 mg orally before the evening meal; 1 to 2 weeks later, the dosage is decreased to 5 mg in the morning and 2.5 mg in the afternoon. Even with this cautious tapering program, all patients have withdrawal (recovery) symptoms of myalgias, depression, and fatigue. Perioperative counseling about the anticipated recovery phase is necessary.

Full recovery of the HPA axis may require 6 to 24 months. The recovery of hypothalamic corticotrophin-releasing hormone secretion is the primary and limiting determinant for recovery. Some degree of adrenal insufficiency must occur during recovery from suppression of the HPA axis. By 2 to 3 months postoperatively, it is important to change the dosing to a single morning dose of a short-acting glucocorticoid (e.g., 20 mg hydrocortisone). This lower dosage facilitates HPA recov-

ery by causing relative cortisol deficiency in the afternoon and evening. If the symptoms of adrenal insufficiency cannot be tolerated, 5 to 10 mg of hydrocortisone may be added at 4 P.M. daily for 2 to 3 weeks. Morning plasma cortisol concentrations are measured every 1 to 2 months to assess recovery of the HPA axis. When the daily dosage of hydrocortisone is 20 mg, it is rarely necessary to taper the dose further. When the basal level of plasma cortisol is 10 µg/dl or greater, therapy may be discontinued. Depending on the degree of HPA suppression, it may take up to 2 years before the plasma cortisol concentration normalizes. Cosyntropin stimulation testing is superfluous in this setting. Also, alternate-day glucocorticoid administration is not usually necessary or helpful in the withdrawal process. Patients should receive stress glucocorticoid coverage and wear medical alert identification for 1 year after they have stopped taking exogenous glucocorticoids. Also, it is important to assess the status of the pituitary-thyroid and pituitary-gonadal axes 6 to 12 weeks postoperatively.

### Failed Transsphenoidal Surgery

If TSS fails to cure Cushing's syndrome, a second operation should be considered. The role of total hypophysectomy in this situation is controversial, and many factors, such as hypopituitarism and the desire for future reproductive function, should be considered. In patients with severe Cushing's syndrome that TSS has failed to cure (and in certain patients with mild-to-moderate persistent disease), a quick and definitive cure of hypercortisolism with bilateral laparoscopic adrenalectomy can be lifesaving.[123] Nelson's syndrome (an aggressive ACTH-secreting tumor) correlates with preoperative invasive features of the pituitary tumor and is not caused by adrenalectomy.

In patients with mild Cushing's syndrome who have persistent disease after TSS, combined sellar radiation and pharmacotherapy may be considered. If the residual adenoma can be identified on MRI, gamma-knife radiosurgery is preferred because it is more rapidly effective and associated with less hypopituitarism than conventional radiotherapy.[128,129]

Until radiotherapy is effective, some form of pharmacotherapy must be continued. Drugs directed at decreasing pituitary tumor ACTH secretion (e.g., cyproheptadine, bromocriptine, valproic acid, and octreotide) are rarely effective. The two agents most commonly used to inhibit steroidogenesis are ketoconazole and mitotane (1,1-dichloro-2[o-chlorophenyl]-2-[P-chlorophenyl]-ethane, o,p′ DDD [Lysodren]). Ketoconazole is an imidazole-derivative antimycotic agent that inhibits 17,20-desmolase, 11β-hydroxylase, and other enzymes in the adrenal cortex. Dosages range from 200 to 600 mg administered twice daily on an empty stomach. Because drug absorption requires an acidic environment, antacids and agents that decrease stomach acidity should be avoided. Side effects include liver dysfunction, renal dysfunction, gynecomastia, and gastrointestinal upset. Liver function tests, serum creatinine, and urinary cortisol excretion should be followed every 6 to 8 weeks. The use of mitotane is discussed subsequently (see Adrenocortical Carcinoma).

## Ectopic ACTH Syndrome

The optimal treatment for ectopic ACTH production ("ectopic ACTH syndrome") is resection of the ACTH- or corticotrophin-releasing hormone-secreting tumor. However, this may not be possible for two reasons: (1) inability to localize the source of ectopic ACTH production (in 20% of cases at time of presentation) and (2) inability to completely resect the ectopic ACTH-secreting tumor (unresectable or metastatic disease). Ectopic ACTH syndrome was diagnosed in 106 patients at the Mayo Clinic between 1956 and 1998.[130] Bronchial carcinoid was the most frequent cause (25%), followed by islet cell cancer (16%), small cell lung carcinoma (11%), medullary thyroid cancer (8%), disseminated neuroendocrine tumor of unknown primary source (7%), thymic carcinoid (5%), pheochromocytoma (3%), disseminated gastrointestinal carcinoid (1%), and other tumors (8%). No tumor was found in 16% of patients. Twenty-eight patients were managed medically, and the others had either curative tumor resection (13 patients) or bilateral adrenalectomy (65 patients). The diagnoses of Cushing's syndrome and ACTH-secreting neoplasm were usually made concurrently; however, there were remarkable cases in which the two conditions were diagnosed several years apart.

In patients with an occult ectopic source of ACTH, a quick definitive cure with bilateral adrenalectomy can be lifesaving. Pharmacotherapy in these patients rarely completely controls the hypercortisolism, and the associated morbidity and risk of mortality persist.

### Metastatic or Unresectable ACTH-Secreting Tumor

For an unresectable or metastatic ACTH-secreting tumor, bilateral laparoscopic adrenalectomy offers a quick definitive cure and is the treatment of choice.[123] Pharmacotherapy is rarely effective in controlling hypercortisolism because of the markedly elevated levels of plasma ACTH. In some cases, such as small cell lung carcinoma, tumor-specific chemotherapy may produce a hormonal cure.

The perioperative glucocorticoid therapy for bilateral adrenalectomy is the same as discussed above for patients having TSS. However, prednisone at a dosage of 5 to 7.5 mg daily (or an equivalent of hydrocortisone) is required lifelong. In many cases, the full replacement dosage is not needed because of a small amount of residual functioning adrenocortical tissue. Patients are instructed about stress steroid coverage and the need to wear medical identification. In addition, orally administered mineralocorticoid replacement in the form of fludrocortisone at a dosage of 0.05 to 0.1 mg/day is started before dismissal from the hospital. The proper dosage is determined by serum electrolytes and supine and standing blood pressures.

## Adrenocortical Carcinoma

The treatment of choice for adrenocortical carcinoma is complete surgical resection by the anterior abdominal approach.[103] This malignant tumor should be suspected in patients with marked hypercortisolism (24-hour urinary cortisol >1000 μg) and adrenal tumors greater than 6 cm in the largest lesional diameter on computed imaging. Even if resection is apparently complete, the recurrence rate is high and the 5-year survival rate is 20% to 30%.[103] Treatment with mitotane should be administered, if tumor resection is incomplete. This drug is an adrenal cytolytic agent that inhibits adrenal steroid synthesis and destroys normal and neoplastic adrenocortical cells. Treatment is started 3 to 6 weeks after adrenalectomy. The initial dosage is one 500-mg tablet with food twice daily. The total dosage is increased by 500 mg weekly until the maximal tolerated dosage or a maximal dose of 10 g daily is attained. In most patients, the dosage is limited by nausea, anorexia, diarrhea, somnolence, skin rash, and pruritus. Mitotane is lipophilic and has a long half-life (0.5 to 6 months). Therefore, mitotane is contraindicated for women desiring fertility within 2 to 5 years after treatment. This drug may also destroy the normal contralateral adrenal gland, and concomitant therapy with dexamethasone (0.5 mg daily) or prednisone (5 mg daily) should be administered. In addition, low-dose mineralocorticoid replacement may be needed, and this is determined by periodic measurement of the serum concentration of potassium. If hyperkalemia develops, treatment is started with fludrocortisone 0.05 mg daily and adjusted to maintain the serum level of potassium in the normal range.

Because of the high recurrence rate of adrenocortical carcinoma, adjuvant treatment with mitotane should be considered for patients with apparent surgical cure.

## Adrenal Adenoma

Cushing's syndrome caused by an adrenal adenoma is cured by unilateral adrenalectomy. This operation is usually performed laparoscopically. The patient should be told that it may take 4 to 18 months before the HPA axis recovers. The rate-limiting step in axis recovery is the hypothalamic corticotropin-releasing hormone neuron or higher regulatory inputs or both. At approximately 6 weeks after the operation, treatment is switched to a shorter-acting glucocorticoid (e.g., hydrocortisone 20 mg in the A.M. and 10 mg in the P.M.). The afternoon dose is tapered and discontinued over 2 to 8 weeks.

The single morning dosage allows for relative nocturnal glucocorticoid insufficiency and stimulation of the hypothalamic neurons. The concentration of plasma cortisol at 8 A.M. (before hydrocortisone administration) is measured every 6 to 8 weeks. Hydrocortisone treatment may be discontinued when the plasma cortisol concentration is 10 µg/dl or greater. Patients are instructed about the need for stress steroid coverage for approximately 1 year after exogenous treatment is discontinued. Mineralocorticoid replacement is usually not required for patients after unilateral adrenalectomy.

## Hypertension and Cushing's Syndrome

The hypertension associated with Cushing's syndrome should be treated until a surgical cure is achieved.[131] Spironolactone, at dosages used to treat primary aldosteronism, is effective in reversing the hypokalemia. Second-step agents include thiazide diuretics, β-adrenergic receptor blockers, ACE inhibitors, and calcium antagonists. The hypertension associated with the hypercortisolism usually resolves over several weeks after the surgical cure, and treatment with antihypertensive agents can be tapered and withdrawn.

## References

1. Conn JW. Presidential address: Part I. Painting background, Part II. Primary aldosteronism, a new clinical syndrome. J Lab Clin Med 45:3-15, 1955.
2. Lifton RP, Dluhy RG, Powers M, et al. A chimeric 11β-hydroxylase/aldosterone synthase gene causes glucocorticoid-remediable aldosteronism and human hypertension. Nature 355:262-265, 1992.
3. Stowasser M, Gordon RD, Tunny TJ, et al. Familial hyperaldosteronism type II: five families with a new variety of primary aldosteronism. Clin Exp Pharmacol Physiol 19:319-322, 1992.
4. Andersen GS, Toftdahl DB, Lund JO, et al. The incidence rate of phaeochromocytoma and Conn's syndrome in Denmark, 1977-1981. J Hum Hypertens 2:187-189, 1988.
5. Gifford RW Jr. Evaluation of the hypertensive patient with emphasis on detecting curable causes. Milbank Mem Fund Q 47:170-186, 1969.
6. Kaplan NM. Hypokalemia in the hypertensive patient, with observations on the incidence of primary aldosteronism. Ann Intern Med 66:1079-1090, 1967.
7. Sinclair AM, Isles CG, Brown I, et al. Secondary hypertension in a blood pressure clinic. Arch Intern Med 147:1289-1293, 1987.
8. Abdelhamid S, Muller-Lobeck H, Pahl S, et al. Prevalence of adrenal and extra-adrenal Conn syndrome in hypertensive patients. Arch Intern Med 156:1190-1195, 1996.
9. Anderson G, Blakeman N, Streeten D. The effect of age on prevalence of secondary forms of hypertension in 4429 consecutively referred patients. J Hypertens 12:609-615, 1994.
10. Rossi E, Regolisti G, Negro A, et al. High prevalence of primary aldosteronism using postcaptopril plasma aldosterone to renin ratio as a screening test among Italian hypertensives. Am J Hypertens 15:896-902, 2002.
11. Young WF Jr. Primary aldosteronism: management issues. Ann N Y Acad Sci 970:61-76, 2002.
12. Stowasser M, Gordon RD, Gunasekera TG, et al. High rate of detection of primary aldosteronism, including surgically treatable forms, after "non-selective" screening of hypertensive patients. J Hypertens 21:2149-2157, 2003.
13. Lim PO, MacDonald TM. Primary aldosteronism, diagnosed by the aldosterone to renin ratio, is a common cause of hypertension. Clin Endocrinol 59:427-430, 2003.
14. Hiramatsu K, Yamada T, Yukimura Y, et al. A screening test to identify aldosterone-producing adenoma by measuring plasma renin activity. Results in hypertensive patients. Arch Intern Med 141:1589-1593, 1981.
15. Vallotton MB. Screening and diagnosis of hypertension forms secondary to excess of mineralocorticoid. Rev Fr Endocrinol Clin 39:109-118, 1998.
16. McKenna TJ, Sequeira SJ, Hefferanan A, et al. Diagnosis under random conditions of all disorders of the renin-angiotensin-aldosterone axis, including primary hyperaldosteronism. J Clin Endocrinol Metab 73:952-957, 1991.
17. Ignatowska-Switalska H, Chodakowska J, Januszewicz W, et al. Evaluation of plasma aldosterone to plasma renin activity ratio in patients with primary aldosteronism. J Hum Hypertens 11:373-378, 1997.
18. Weinberger MH, Fineberg NS. The diagnosis of primary aldosteronism and separation of two major subtypes. Arch Int Med 153:2125-2129, 1993.
19. Gallay BJ, Ahmad S, Xu L, et al. Screening for primary aldosteronism without discontinuing hypertensive medications: Plasma aldosterone-renin ratio. Am J Kidney Dis 37:699-705, 2001.
20. Montori VM, Young WF Jr. Use of plasma aldosterone concentration-to-plasma renin activity ratio as a screening test for primary aldosteronism: A systematic review of the literature. Endocrinol Metab Clin North Am 31:619-632, 2002.
21. Gordon RD, Stowasser M, Tunny TJ, et al. High incidence of primary aldosteronism in 199 patients referred with hypertension. Clin Exp Pharmacol Physiol 21:315-318, 1994.
22. Kumar A, Lall SB, Ammini A, et al. Screening of a population of young hypertensives for primary hyperaldosteronism. J Hum Hypertens 8:731-732, 1994.
23. Kreze A, Okalova D, Vanuga P, et al. Occurrence of primary aldosteronism in a group of ambulatory hypertensive patients. Vnitr Lek 45:17-21, 1999.
24. Lim P, Dow E, Brennan G, et al. High prevalence of primary aldosteronism in the Tayside hypertension clinic population. J Hum Hypertens 14:311-315, 2000.
25. Loh KC, Koay ES, Khaw MC, et al. Prevalence of primary aldosteronism among Asian hypertensive patients in Singapore. J Clin Endocrinol Metab 85:2854-2859, 2000.
26. Fardella C, Mosso L, Gomez-Sanchez C, et al. Primary hyperaldosteronism in essential hypertensives: prevalence, biochemical profile, and molecular biology. J Clin Endocrinol Metab 85:1863-1867, 2000.
27. Schwartz GL, Turner ST. Prevalence of unrecognized primary aldosteronism in essential hypertension. Am J Hypertens 15:18A, 2002.
28. Young WF Jr, Hogan MJ. Renin-independent hypermineralocorticoidism. Trends Endocrinol Metab 5:97-106, 1994.
29. Ganguly A. Primary aldosteronism. N Engl J Med 339:1828-1834, 1998.
30. Tanabe A, Naruse M, Naruse K, et al. Left ventricular hypertrophy is more prominent in patients with primary aldosteronism than in patients with other types of secondary hypertension. Hypertens Res 20:85-90, 199.
31. Rossi GP, Sacchetto A, Pava E, et al. Remodeling of the left ventricle in primary aldosteronism due to Conn's adenoma. Circulation 95:1471-1478, 1997.
32. Shigematsu Y, Hamada M, Okayama H, et al. Left ventricular hypertrophy precedes other target-organ damage in primary aldosteronism. Hypertension 29:723-727, 1997.
33. Yoshihara F, Nishikimi T, Yoshitomi Y, et al. Left ventricular structural and functional characteristics in patients with renovascular hypertension, primary aldosteronism and essential hypertension. Am J Hypertens 9:523-528, 1996.
34. Rizzoni D, Porteri E, Castellano M, et al. Vascular hypertrophy and remodeling in secondary hypertension. Hypertension 28:785-790, 1996.

35. Rizzoni D, Muiesan ML, Porteri E, et al. Relations between cardiac and vascular structure in patients with primary and secondary hypertension. J Am Coll Cardiol 32:985-992, 1998.

36. Abe M, Hamada M, Matsuoka H, et al. Myocardial scintigraphic characteristics in patients with primary aldosteronism. Hypertension 23:164-167, 1994.

37. Halimi JM, Mimran A. Albuminuria in untreated patients with primary aldosteronism or essential hypertension. J Hypertens 13:1801-1802, 1995.

38. Torres VE, Young WF Jr, Offord KP, et al. Association of hypokalemia, aldosteronism, and renal cysts. N Engl J Med 322:345-351, 1990.

39. Ogasawara M, Nomura K, Toraya S, et al. Clinical implications of renal cyst in primary aldosteronism. Endocr J 43:261-268, 1996.

40. Duprez D, De Buyzere M, Reitzchel ER, et al. Aldosterone and vascular damage. Curr Hypertens Rep 2:327-334, 2000.

41. Nishimura M, Uzu T, Fujii T, et al. Cardiovascular complications in patients with primary aldosteronism. Am J Kidney Dis 33:261-266, 1999.

42. Streeten DHP, Tomycz N, Anderson GH Jr. Reliability of screening methods for the diagnosis of primary aldosteronism. Am J Med 67:403-413, 1979.

43. Rich GM, Ulick S, Cook S, et al. Glucocorticoid-remediable aldosteronism in a large kindred: Clinical spectrum and diagnosis using a characteristic biochemical phenotype. Ann Intern Med 116:813-820, 1992.

44. Calhoun DA, Nishizaka MK, Zaman MA, et al. Hyperaldosteronism among black and white subjects with resistant hypertension. Hypertension 40:892-896, 2002.

45. Brown MA, Cramp HA, Zammit VC, et al. Primary hyperaldosteronism: a missed diagnosis in "essential hypertensives"? Aust NZ J Med 26:533-538, 1996.

46. Gordon RD, Ziesak MD, Tunny TJ, et al. Evidence that primary aldosteronism may not be uncommon: 12% incidence among antihypertensive drug trial volunteers. Clin Exp Pharmacol Physiol 20:296-298, 1993.

47. Hamlet SM, Tunny TJ, Woodland E, et al. Is aldosterone/renin ratio useful to screen a hypertensive population for primary aldosteronism? Clin Exp Pharmacol Physiol 12:249-252, 1985.

48. Kumar A, Lall SB, Ammini A, et al. Screening of a population of young hypertensives for primary hyperaldosteronism. J Hum Hypertens 8:731-732, 1994.

49. Lazurova I, Schwartz P, Trejbal D, et al. Incidence of primary hyperaldosteronism in hospitalized hypertensive patients. Bratisl Lek Listy 100:200-203, 1999.

50. Lim PO, Rodgers P, Cardale K, et al. Potentially high prevalence of primary aldosteronism in a primary-care population. Lancet 353:40, 1999.

51. Mosso L, Fardella C, Montero J, et al. High prevalence of undiagnosed primary hyperaldosteronism among patients with essential hypertension [Alta prevalencia de hiperaldosteronismo primario no diagnosticado en hipertension catalogados como esenciales]. Rev Med Chile 127:800-806, 1999.

52. Rossi GP, Rossi E, Pavan E, et al. Screening for primary aldosteronism with a logistic multivariate discriminant analysis. Clin Endocrinol 49:713-723, 1998.

53. Moneva MH, Gomez-Sanchez CE. Establishing a diagnosis of primary aldosteronism. Curr Opin Endocrinol Diabetes 8:124-129, 2001.

54. Gordon RD, Stowasser M, Rutherford JC. Primary aldosteronism: are we diagnosing and operating too few patients? World J Surg 25:941-947, 2001.

55. Young WF Jr. Primary aldosteronism: A common and curable form of hypertension. Cardiol Rev 7:207-214, 1999.

56. Stowasser M. Primary aldosteronism: Rare bird or common cause of secondary hypertension? Curr Hypertens Rep 3:230-239, 2001.

57. Hirohara D, Nomura K, Okamoto T, et al. Performance of the basal aldosterone to renin ratio and of the renin stimulation test by furosemide and upright posture in screening for aldosterone-producing adenoma in low renin hypertensives. J Clin Endocrinol Metab 86:4292-4298, 2001.

58. Young WF Jr, Klee GG. Primary aldosteronism: Diagnostic evaluation. Endocrinol Metab Clin North Am 17:367-395, 1988.

59. Holland O, Brown H, Kuhnert L, et al. Further evaluation of saline infusion for the diagnosis of primary aldosteronism. Hypertension 6:717-723, 1984.

60. Bravo EL, Tarazi RC, Dustan HP, et al. The changing clinical spectrum of primary aldosteronism. Am J Med 74:641-651, 1983.

61. Sawka AM, Young WF Jr, Thompson GB, et al. Primary aldosteronism: Factors associated with normalization of blood pressure after surgery. Ann Intern Med 135:258-261, 2001.

62. Kloos RT, Gross MD, Francis IR, et al. Incidentally discovered adrenal masses. Endocr Rev 16:460-484, 1995.

63. Blumenfeld JD, Sealey JE, Schlussel Y, et al. Diagnosis and treatment of primary aldosteronism. Ann Intern Med 121:877-885, 1994.

64. Young WF Jr, Stanson AW, Grant CS, et al. Primary aldosteronism: Adrenal venous sampling. Surgery 120:913-920, 1996.

65. Gordon RD, Stowasser M, Rutherford JC. Primary aldosteronism: Are we diagnosing and operating too few patients? World J Surg 25:941-947, 2001.

66. Magill SB, Raff H, Shaker JL, et al. Comparison of adrenal vein sampling and computed tomography in the differentiation of primary aldosteronism. J Clin Endocrinol Metab 86:1066-1071, 2001.

67. Doppman JL, Gill JR Jr. Hyperaldosteronism: Sampling the adrenal veins. Radiology 198:309-312, 1996.

68. Rocha R, Rudolph AE, Frierdich GE, et al. Aldosterone induces a vascular inflammatory phenotype in the rat heart. Am J Physiol Heart Circ Physiol 283:H1802-H1810, 2002.

69. Rocha R, Funder JW. The pathophysiology of aldosterone in the cardiovascular system. Ann N Y Acad Sci 970:89-100, 2002.

70. Stier CT Jr, Chander PN, Rocha R. Aldosterone as a mediator in cardiovascular injury. Cardiol Rev 10:97-107, 2002.

71. Martinez DV, Rocha R, Matsumura M, et al. Cardiac damage prevention by eplerenone: comparison with low sodium diet or potassium loading. Hypertension 39:614-618, 2002.

72. Brilla CG, Pick R, Tan LB, et al. Remodeling of the rat right and left ventricles in experimental hypertension. Circ Res 67:1355-1364, 1990.

73. Pitt B, Zannad F, Remme WJ, et al. The effect of spironolactone on morbidity and mortality in patients with severe heart failure. N Engl J Med 341:709-717, 1999.

74. Rocha R, Williams GH. Rationale for the use of aldosterone antagonists in congestive heart failure. Drugs 62:723-731, 2002.

75. Alderman MH, Madhavan S, Ooi WL, et al. Association of the renin-sodium profile with the risk of myocardial infarction in patients with hypertension. N Engl J Med 324:1098-1104, 1991.

76. Vaughan DE, Lazos SA, Tong K. Angiotensin II regulates the expression of plasminogen activator inhibitor-1 in cultured endothelial cells. A potential link between the renin-angiotensin system and thrombosis. J Clin Invest 95:995-1001, 1995.

77. Kerins DM, Hao Q, Vaughan DE. Angiotensin induction of PAI-1 expression in endothelial cells is mediated by the hexapeptide angiotensin IV. J Clin Invest 96:2515-2520, 1995.

78. Brown NJ, Kim KS, Chen YQ, et al. Synergistic effect of adrenal steroids and angiotensin II on plasminogen activator inhibitor-1 production. J Clin Endocrinol Metab 85:336-344, 2000.

79. Brown NJ, Agirbasli MA, Williams GH, et al. Effect of activation and inhibition of the renin angiotensin system on plasma PAI-1. Hypertension 32:965-971, 1998.

80. Sawathiparnich P, Kumar S, Vaughan DE, et al. Spironolactone abolishes the relationship between aldosterone and plasminogen activator inhibitor-1 in humans. J Clin Endocrinol Metab 87:448-452, 2002.

81. Tanabe A, Naruse M, Naruse K, et al. Left ventricular hypertrophy is more prominent in patients with primary aldosteronism than in patients with other types of secondary hypertension. Hypertens Res 20:85-90, 1997.

82. Rossi GP, Sacchetto A, Pava E, et al. Remodeling of the left ventricle in primary aldosteronism due to Conn's adenoma. Circulation 95:1471-1478, 1997.

83. Shigematsu Y, Hamada M, Okayama H, et al. Left ventricular hypertrophy precedes other target-organ damage in primary aldosteronism. Hypertension 29:723-727, 1997.

84. Rossi GP, Sacchetto A, Visentin P, et al. Changes in left ventricular anatomy and function in hypertension and primary aldosteronism. Hypertension 27:1039-1045, 1996.

85. Yoshihara F, Nishikimi T, Yoshitomi Y, et al. Left ventricular structural and functional characteristics in patients with renovascular hypertension, primary aldosteronism and essential hypertension. Am J Hypertens 9:523-528, 1996.

86. Rizzoni D, Porteri E, Castellano M, et al. Vascular hypertrophy and remodeling in secondary hypertension. Hypertension 28:785-790, 1996.

87. Rizzoni D, Muiesan ML, Porteri E, et al. Relations between cardiac and vascular structure in patients with primary and secondary hypertension. J Am Coll Cardiol 32:985-992, 1998.

88. Young WF Jr. Laparoscopic adrenalectomy. Curr Opin Endocrinol Diabetes 6:199-203, 1999.

89. Celen O, O'Brien MJ, Melby JC, et al. Factors influencing outcome of surgery for primary aldosteronism. Arch Surg 131:646-650, 1996.

90. Lim PO, Young WF, MacDonald TM. A review of the medical treatment of primary aldosteronism. J Hypertens 19:353-361, 2001.

91. Jeunemaitre X, Chatellier G, Kreft-Jais C, et al. Efficacy and tolerance of spironolactone in essential hypertension. Am J Cardiol 60:820-825, 1987.

92. Zillich AJ, Carter BL. Eplerenone—A novel selective aldosterone blocker. Ann Pharmacother 36:1567-1576, 2002.

93. De Gasparo M, Joss U, Ramjoue HP, et al. Three new epoxy-spironolactone derivatives: Characterization in vivo and in vitro. J Pharmacol Exp Ther 240:650-656, 1987.

94. Weinberger MH, Roniker B, Krause SL, et al. Eplerenone, a selective aldosterone blocker, in mild-to-moderate hypertension. Am J Hypertens 15:709-716, 2002.

95. Burgess ED, Lacourciere Y, Ruilope-Urioste LM, et al. Long-term safety and efficacy of the selective aldosterone blocker eplerenone in patients with essential hypertension. Clin Ther 25:2388-2404, 2003.

96. Krum H, Nolly H, Workman D, et al. Efficacy of eplerenone added to renin-angiotensin blockade in hypertensive patients. Hypertension 40:117-123, 2002.

97. Bravo EL, Fouad-Tarazi FM, Tarazi RC, et al. Clinical implications of primary aldosteronism with resistant hypertension. Hypertension 11:I207-I211, 1988.

98. Wisgerhof M, Carpenter PC, Brown RD. Increased adrenal sensitivity to angiotensin II in idiopathic hyperaldosteronism. J Clin Endocrinol Metab 47:938-943, 1978.

99. Mantero F, Fallo F, Opocher G, et al. Effect of angiotensin II and converting enzyme inhibitor (captopril) on blood pressure, plasma renin activity and aldosterone in primary aldosteronism. Clin Sci 61:289s-293s, 1981.

100. Griffing GT, Melby JC. The therapeutic effect of a new angiotensin-converting enzyme inhibitor, enalapril maleate, in idiopathic hyperaldosteronism. J Clin Hypertens 1:265-276, 1985.

101. Stratakis CA, Chrousos GP. Adrenal cancer. Endocrinol Metab Clin North Am 29:15-25, 2000.

102. Henley DJ, van Heerden JA, Grant CS, et al. Adrenal cortical carcinoma: a continuing challenge. Surgery 94:926-931, 1983.

103. Kendrick ML, Curlee K, Lloyd R, et al. Aldosterone-secreting adrenocortical carcinomas are associated with unique operative risks and outcomes. Surgery 132:1008-1012, 2002.

104. Guthrie GP, Wilson EA, Quillen DL, et al. Adrenal androgen excess and defective 11β-hydroxylation in women with idiopathic hirsutism. Arch Intern Med 142:729-735, 1982.

105. Pang S. Congenital adrenal hyperplasia. Endocrinol Metab Clin North Am 26:853-891, 1997.

106. White PC, Speiser PW. Steroid 11β-hydroxylase deficiency and related disorders. Endocrinol Metab Clin North Am 23:325-339, 1994.

107. Biglieri EG, Kater CE. 17α-hydroxylation deficiency. Endocrinol Metab Clin North Am 20:257-268, 1991.

108. Kelly WF, O'Hare MJ, Loizou S. Hypermineralocorticism without excessive aldosterone secretion: An adrenal carcinoma producing deoxycorticosterone. Clin Endocrinol (Oxf) 17:353-361, 1982.

109. Powell-Jackson JD, Calin A, Fraser R, et al. Excess deoxycorticosterone secretion from adrenocortical carcinoma. Br Med J 2:32-33, 1974.

110. Brandon DD, Markwick AJ, Chrousos GP, et al. Glucocorticoid resistance in humans and non-human primates. Cancer Res 49(suppl):2203s-2213s, 1989.

111. Javier EC, Reardon GE, Malchoff CD. Glucocorticoid resistance and its clinical presentations. Endocrinologist 1:141-148, 1991.

112. Walker BR, Edwards CRW. Dexamethasone-suppressible hypertension. Endocrinologist 3:87-97, 1993.

113. Ulick S, Tedde R, Mantero F. Pathogenesis of the type 2 variant of the syndrome of apparent mineralocorticoid excess. J Clin Endocrinol Metab 70:200-206, 1990.

114. Walker BR, Edwards CRW. Licorice-induced hypertension and syndromes of apparent mineralocorticoid excess. Endocrinol Metab Clin North Am 23:359-377, 1994.

115. Farese RV Jr, Biglieri EG, Shackleton CHL, et al. Licorice-induced hypermineralocorticoidism. N Engl J Med 325:1223-1227, 1991.

116. Walker BR, Edwards CRW. Cushing's syndrome. In James VHT (ed). The Adrenal Gland, 2nd ed. New York, Raven Press, 1992; pp 289-318.

117. Ulick S, Wang JZ, Blumenfeld JD, et al. Cortisol inactivation overload: a mechanism of mineralocorticoid hypertension in the ectopic adrenocorticotropin syndrome. J Clin Endocrinol Metab 74:963-967, 1992.

118. Raff H, Findling JW. A physiologic approach to diagnosis of the Cushing syndrome. Ann Intern Med 138:980-991, 2003.

119. Cizza G, Nieman LK, Doppman JL, et al. Factitious Cushing syndrome. J Clin Endocrinol Metab 81:3573-3577, 1996.

120. Raff H. Suppression of the hypothalamic-pituitary-adrenal axis and other systemic effects of inhaled corticosteroids in asthma. Endocrinologist 8:9-14, 1998.

121. Yap LB, Turner HE, Adams CB, et al. Undetectable postoperative cortisol does not always predict long-term remission in Cushing's disease: A single centre audit. Clin Endocrinol (Oxf) 56:25-31, 2002.

122. Reitmeyer M, Vance ML, Laws ER Jr. The neurosurgical management of Cushing's disease. Mol Cell Endocrinol 197:73-79, 2002.

123. Vella A, Thompson GB, Grant CS, et al. Laparoscopic adrenalectomy for adrenocorticotropin-dependent Cushing's syndrome. J Clin Endocrinol Metab 86:1596-1599, 2001.

124. Mahmoud-Ahmed AS, Suh JH. Radiation therapy for Cushing's disease: A review. Pituitary 5:175-180, 2002.

125. Swain JM, Grant CS, Schlinkert RT, et al. Corticotropin-independent macronodular adrenal hyperplasia: A clinico-pathologic correlation. Arch Surg 133:541-546, 1998.

126. Barker FG II, Klibanski A, Swearingen B. Transsphenoidal surgery for pituitary tumors in the United States, 1996-2000:

Mortality, morbidity, and the effects of hospital and surgeon volume. J Clin Endocrinol Metab 88:4709-4719, 2003.

127. Laws ER, Reitmeyer M, Thapar K, et al. Cushing's disease resulting from pituitary corticotrophic microadenoma. Treatment results from transsphenoidal microsurgery and gamma knife radiosurgery. Neurochirurgie 48:294-299, 2002.

128. Kobayashi T, Kida Y, Mori Y. Gamma knife radiosurgery in the treatment of Cushing disease: Long-term results. J Neurosurg 97(5 suppl):422-428, 2002.

129. Pollock BE, Young WF Jr. Stereotactic radiosurgery for patients with ACTH-producing pituitary adenomas after prior adrenalectomy. Int J Radiat Oncol Biol Phys 54:839-841, 2002.

130. Aniszewski JP, Young WF Jr, Thompson GB, et al. Cushing syndrome due to ectopic adrenocorticotropic hormone secretion. World J Surg 25:934-940, 2001.

131. Torpy DJ, Mullen N, Ilias I, et al. Association of hypertension and hypokalemia with Cushing's syndrome caused by ectopic ACTH secretion: A series of 58 cases. Ann N Y Acad Sci 970:134-144, 2002.

# Pheochromocytoma: Detection and Management

## Marion R. Wofford, Daniel W. Jones

## INTRODUCTION

Pheochromocytomas are catecholamine-secreting tumors that arise from chromaffin cells. Although extremely rare, the recognition and localization of these tumors are critical to the cure of hypertension, which may be paroxysmal and lethal to the patients that harbor them. The incidence of pheochromocytoma is estimated to be 2 to 8 in 100,000 per year among hypertensive patients.[1,2] The Mayo Clinic reported that only 13 of 54 autopsy-proven pheochromocytomas had been diagnosed prior to death.[3] Pheochromocytomas are classically associated with paroxysmal hypertension. Patients present with a wide variety of signs, symptoms, and potentially life-threatening consequences of catecholamine excess. Clinicians must maintain a high index of suspicion and perform an evaluation when pheochromocytoma is suspected. Most pheochromocytomas are sporadic, but familial forms should be considered a possibility in all patients. The evaluation for pheochromocytoma includes establishment of catecholamine excess, genetic analysis in many patients, and localization of the tumor. Treatment is usually surgical resection.

## PATHOPHYSIOLOGY

In embryonic development, primitive stem cells migrate from the neural crest giving rise to chromaffin cells. Chromaffin bodies regress in the prenatal period, but remnants may remain. In adults most chromaffin cells are found in the adrenal medulla, the predominant site of pheochromocytomas, but may occur along the sympathetic ganglia or in chromaffin body remnants in other locations.[4] The term *pheochromocytoma* refers to adrenal chromaffin tissues, whereas *paraganglioma* refers to extraadrenal chromaffin bodies.[5,6] Pheochromocytoma generally refers to tumors in both locations.

Chromaffin cells of pheochromocytomas produce catecholamines from tyrosine. The intermediate metabolites dopa and dopamine are converted to norepinephrine, the end-product of extraadrenal pheochromocytomas. In the adrenal medulla norepinephrine is metabolized to epinephrine; however, epinephrine is rarely the sole catecholamine secreted by pheochromocytomas. Norepinephrine and epinephrine are subsequently converted to the *O*-methylated metabolites, normetanephrine and metanephrine.[7] Dopamine and the urinary metabolite, homovanillic acid, are uncommonly secreted by pheochromocytomas and occur most often in malignant forms.[8]

The clinical manifestations of pheochromocytoma are variable and related to the heterogeneous secretion of catecholamines and their metabolites. In addition to catecholamines, pheochromocytomas may secrete a variety of peptides including opioids, endothelin, erythropoietin, parathyroid hormone–related protein, neuropeptide Y, and chomogranin A.[9] It is not known why some pheochromocytomas secrete catecholamines intermittently, causing paroxysmal signs and symptoms, while others release neurohormones continuously, causing refractory hypertension without paroxysms.[4]

In general, patients with tumors that secrete predominantly epinephrine have more β receptor–mediated tachycardia, systolic hypertension, hyperhydrosis, flushing, and anxiety.[10] Tumors producing epinephrine alone may present with hypotensive symptoms.[11] Patients with norepinephrine-secreting tumors have α-adrenergic receptor–mediated vasoconstriction with related diastolic hypertension and generally have fewer symptoms classically associated with pheochromocytomas.[3,10]

## Clinical Features

A high index of suspicion for pheochromocytoma is critical in making the diagnosis as the presentation is variable (Box 76-1). The classic triad of global headache, tachycardia, and diaphoresis usually associated with hypertension should prompt a consideration of pheochromocytoma. Two of the three symptoms are usually present. The Mayo Clinic reported results of 54 autopsy-proven pheochromocytoma cases. Hypertension had been diagnosed in 54% of the cases: 27% had headaches, and 17% had diaphoresis and palpitations.[12]

Paroxysmal hypertension should generate a suspicion for pheochromocytoma, although most patients with this history do not have this tumor. Patients with signs and symptoms of pheochromocytoma may have essential hypertension or other forms of secondary hypertension, such as renovascular hypertension; hypertension of pregnancy; hypertensive crises associated with withdrawal of β-blockers, clonidine, or drugs of abuse; anxiety and panic attacks; intracranial tumors; or self-administration of sympathomimetic amines.

There is no correlation between levels of circulating catecholamines and blood pressure in patients with pheochromocytoma.[12] Some pheochromocytoma patients may have episodic hypertension with normal levels of catecholamines, whereas others have high circulating catecholamines but are without symptoms. Ninety percent of patients with pheochromocytoma have hypertension. Paroxysmal hypertension often prompts the search for a catecholamine-secreting tumor, but the hypertension is more often sustained, leading to the misdiagnosis of primary hypertension.[4] Patients with sporadic pheochromocytomas may present in hypertensive crisis that is often severe and resistant to standard antihypertensive medications. Hypertension related to pheochromocytoma in children is more likely to be sustained.[13] Patients who should be considered for evaluation of pheochromocytoma have

**Box 76–1** Clinical Features Associated with Pheochromocytoma

**Signs and Symptoms**
Hypertension:* Paroxysmal or sustained, refractory
Headaches
Tachycardia
Diaphoresis
Pallor or flushing
Tremors
Anxiety
Chest or abdominal pain
Hemodynamic changes during surgery, pregnancy,
    coitus, micturition

**Endocrine**
Hypercalcemia
Diabetes mellitus
Cushing's syndrome
Thyroid carcinoma

**Cardiovascular**
Myocardial infarction
Arrhythmia
Cardiomyopathy
Congestive heart failure
Orthostatic hypotension

**Neurologic**
Seizure
Stroke
Encephalopathy

*A small percentage (10%) of patients with pheochromocytoma are normotensive.

hypertension resistant to conventional therapy, hypertension of new onset, paroxysmal hypertension, or a familial syndrome associated with pheochromocytoma.

Orthostatic hypotension is common among patients with pheochromocytoma and is often related to a reduced plasma volume.[14] It has been postulated that prolonged catecholamine exposure alters normal sympathetic nervous system (SNS) reflex responses to upright blood pressure, contributing to the postural hypotension. Animal models of pheochromocytoma,[15] as well as clinical studies,[16] suggest that the SNS is intact and may play a role in increasing the blood pressure in pheochromocytoma patients but is not related to orthostasis. Levenson reported that orthostasis in patients with pheochromocytoma was related to decreased stroke volume and impaired adaptation of total peripheral resistance during tilt maneuvers.[17]

The cardiac manifestations of pheochromocytomas include tachycardia, cardiac arrhythmias, angina, and myocardial infarction in the absence of coronary disease.[18] Hypertrophic or congestive cardiomyopathy and noncardiogenic pulmonary edema have been reported.[19]

Crises due to catecholamine secretion may cause hypertensive retinopathy, stroke, dissecting aortic aneurysm, renal failure, disseminated intravascular coagulation, rhabdomyolysis, or tumor hemorrhage. Other presentations include pallor or flushing, sweating, paroxysmal symptoms suggesting seizure disorder, anxiety attacks, tremulousness, weakness, fatigue, weight loss, and paresthesias.[12]

Although lower levels of plasma catecholamines may be present between crises, there may be an increase in metabolic rate and weight loss. Hyperglycemia may occur due to elevated catecholamines that suppress insulin production and increase hepatic gluconeogenesis. Vascular constriction with diminished plasma volume or the formation of erythropoietin by the tumor may cause an elevated hematocrit.

Catecholamine release from a pheochromocytoma is not mediated by neuronal activity but can occur with physical stimuli, tumor necrosis, or changes in blood flow. Classic presentations are an acute hypertensive crisis during surgery, physical activity, abdominal trauma, or in patients with bladder pheochromocytoma, voiding. A number of drugs have provocative effects on pheochromocytomas, including imaging agents, glucagon, histamine, guanethidine, metoclopramide, and phenothiazines.[12]

Pseudopheochromocytoma refers to a condition that causes paraoxysmal hypertension in the absence of biochemical evidence of excess catecholamines consistent with pheochromocytoma. Patients with pseudopheochromocytoma are characterized by abrupt elevation of blood pressure; abrupt symptoms of nausea, palpitations, chest pain, and dizziness; and absence of triggers related to fear or panic. The denial of emotional stress is misleading, so the consideration of a psychosocial relationship is often delayed. In one series, 21 patients referred for evaluation of extreme fluctuations in blood pressure were found to have labile blood pressure related to unrecognized emotional stress. These patients were treated effectively with antihypertensive drugs, psychopharmacotherapeutic agents, and counseling, either alone or in combination.[20]

## Tumor Location

About 85% of pheochromocytomas are found in the adrenal medulla. In adults, up to 18% of pheochromocytomas are extraadrenal locations such as the organ of Zuckerkandl at the aortic bifurcation, carotid body, glomus jugulare of cranial nerves IX and X, aortic chemoreceptors, the urinary bladder, or other sites along the sympathetic chain of the abdomen or pelvis.[6] Approximately 10% of the extraadrenal tumors are intrathoracic, usually in the posterior mediastinum. There are reported cases in the heart,[21] neck, base of the skull, or exotic sites such as the middle ear.[6] Thirty percent of pheochromocytomas in children are extraadrenal.[22]

After the age of 60 years, the most common location for pheochromocytomas is the adrenal gland. When associated with familial syndromes, adrenal tumors are often bilateral. Extraadrenal pheochromocytomas are rarely associated with familial syndromes and are more likely to be found in persons younger than 20 years of age.[23]

Malignant pheochromocytomas, accounting for 19% of tumors, are more likely to be >5.0 cm in size. These tumors cannot be distinguished from benign pheochromocytomas by histology. Malignancy is defined as local extension or the presence of metastasis.[24] The most common sites for metastasis include liver, lung, bone, and lymph nodes.[25]

## Familial Syndromes

Most pheochromocytomas are sporadic and noninherited (Box 76–2).[4] Sporadic pheochromocytomas are usually diagnosed in the fourth through sixth decades, whereas familial

**Box 76–2** Molecular Genetics Associated with Familial Pheochromocytoma

| Genetic Disorder | Associated Syndrome |
|---|---|
| VHL gene on chromosome 3p | VHL syndrome |
| *RET* protooncogene on chromosome 1 | MEN types 2A and 2B |
| NF1 gene on chromosome 17q | Neurofibromatosis |
| SDHD and SDHB on mitochondrial DNA | Paraganglioma of head and neck |

VHL, von Hippel-Lindau; MEN, multiple endocrine neoplasm; NF1, neurofibromatosis 1; SDHD, succinate dehydrogenase subunit D; SDHB, succinate dehydrogenase subunit B.

tumors are often detected early in life by surveillance in high-risk patients. Patients with sporadic tumors characteristically have a negative family history, a unilateral extraadrenal tumor, and lack the characteristics of neuroendocrine syndromes. In some series of patients with pheochromocytoma, only 10% had a familial disorder, including the multiple endocrine neoplasm (MEN) syndromes, von Hippel-Lindau (VHL) syndrome, or neurofibromatosis.[26,27]

With advances in molecular genetics, patients with apparent sporadic tumors have been found to have mutations.[28] In a cohort of 277 patients with sporadic pheochomocytoma, Neumann et al.[28] found that 66 patients (25%) had a mutation of one of four autosomal-dominant genes associated with pheochromocytoma. Thirty percent had the VHL gene and 12% had protooncogene *RET* associated with MEN syndromes. Two susceptibility genes associated with pheochromocytomas and glomus tumors, known as SDHD and SDHB (succinate dehydrogenase subunit D and subunit B), were found in 17% and 18%, respectively.[28]

A careful family history, higher index of suspicion for familial syndrome, and careful physical examination in patients with "presumed" sporadic tumors might lead to detection of genetic disorders. Molecular testing for the *RET* mutation is available and recommended in patients with sporadic pheochromocytoma. Tests for other mutations related to pheochromocytoma are not commercially available.[29]

Familial pheochromocytoma is inherited in an autosomal-dominant pattern with variable penetrance.[27,28] The components of MEN type 2A (Sipple's syndrome) include pheochromocytoma, medullary thyroid carcinoma (MTC), and parathyroid hyperplasia or neoplasia. The MEN type 2B syndrome may present with pheochromocytoma, MTC, and mucosal neuromas. The syndromes are the result of a "gain-of-function" mutation of the *RET* protooncogene on chromosome 10, which activates the tyrosine kinase receptor causing hyperplasia and possibly neoplastic change.[30] Pheochromocytoma occurs in 40% to 50% of affected individuals in MEN 2A families. The tumors are usually due to adrenomedullary hyperplasia causing multicentric and bilateral epinephrine-secreting tumors. Extraadrenal pheochromocytomas are rare in the MEN syndromes.[28] Although rarely associated with familial syndromes, 4.4 % of MEN 2A patients in one series had a malignant form of pheochromocytoma.[31]

Thyroid carcinoma associated with MEN is a high-grade malignancy and may present in the first years of life.

Associated pheochromocytomas present later in life and rarely metastasize. Fifty percent of patients with MEN2 syndromes are asymptomatic, so early detection and surveillance for MTC and pheochromocytoma is important.[27]

In the VHL syndrome, a "loss-of-function" mutation of the VHL suppressor gene on chromosome 3p causes alterations in the normal degradation of proteins, including hypoxia-inducible factor.[32] This mutation results in tumor formation with variable penetrance and expression.[33] The syndrome consists of a variety of neoplasms and masses, including cerebellar and retinal hemangioblastomas, renal cell carcinoma, pancreatic and renal cysts, and pheochromocytoma.[34] The pheochromocytomas of VHL secrete norepinephrine, but the levels may not be high enough to cause hypertension or other symptoms.[35]

The SDHD and SDHB genes, as with the VHL mutation, cause a defect in the oxygen-sensing pathways. These susceptibility genes are part of the mitochondrial complex II.[36] Alterations in the respiratory chain may result in malignant hyperplasia.[32] The SDHD and SDHB are associated with hereditary paragangliomas of the head and neck.[29]

Neurofibromatosis type 1 (NF1) is rarely associated with pheochromocytoma. Although pheochromocytomas are extremely rare in neurofibromatosis, among hypertensive patients with this syndrome the prevalence may be higher than 50%.[37] The effect of these tumors becomes apparent at a later age than pheochromocytomas in MEN and VHL. Although patients may not have symptoms of catecholamine excess, the presence of neurofibromas, café-au-lait spots, and hypertension should prompt a search of pheochromocytoma. The NF1 tumor suppressor gene has been isolated to chromosome 17q and encodes for the protein neurofibromin.[38] Type 2 neurofibromatosis is not associated with pheochromocytoma.

## Diagnosis

Screening for pheochromocytoma should be conducted in any patient with signs, symptoms, or family history that suggests the disorder. Failure to make a diagnosis may result in catastrophic outcomes.

Consideration should be given in patients with the classic triad of tachycardia, diaphoresis, and headaches, and also in those with paroxysmal symptoms; unexplained hemodynamic changes during surgery, pregnancy, coitus, or micturition; or after use of certain drugs.

The choice of diagnostic tests may be limited by the availability of certain assays (Box 76–3). Although a number of tests are available, there is no single test with absolute accuracy.[39,40] Further complicating the diagnostic approach are the variability of catecholamines and metabolites produced by pheochromocytomas and the intermittent secretion and possibly low levels of catecholamines associated with symptoms. The measurement of urine or plasma catecholamines is diagnostic in 95 % of patients. Most patients can be identified with a single test when abnormal values are several-fold higher than the normal range. However, in a few patients values are only slightly elevated, yet clinical suspicion may be high.[24] In these cases the diagnosis is most challenging.

Biochemical tests used to measure catecholamines and metabolites include plasma catecholamines and metanephrines, urinary catecholamines and metanephrines, and urinary vanillylmandelic acid.[23,24] Urinary "fractionated" metanephrines provide more information than "total' metanephrines. The

**Box 76–3** Recommended Tests for Diagnosis of Pheochromocytoma

Plasma-free metanephrines*
24-hour urine fractionated metanephrines*
Clonidine suppression test†
Glucagon provocation test†

---

*Liquid chromatographic measurement.
†Tests to be performed by experienced clinician.

development of liquid chromotographic measurement of plasma metanephrines provides a more convenient assessment of catecholamine production.[41] False-negative tests may result with any of these methods leading to missed diagnosis. Because pheochromocytoma is so rare and all of these tests lack 100% specificity, false-positive tests are also possible.

Plasma-free metanephrines measured by liquid chromatography has been recommended as the best initial test.[39] In a multicenter cohort of patients tested for pheochromocytoma, 214 patients of 644 tested had confirmation of the diagnosis. The sensitivity of plasma-free metanephrines was 99%. In those patients with pheochromocytoma, the concentration of plasma-free metanephrines was 21-fold higher in sporadic and 7-fold higher in familial pheochromocytomas compared with those without a pheochromocytoma. In hereditary syndromes and sporadic forms, plasma-free metanephrines had a specificity of 96% and 82%, respectively.[39]

A retrospective chart review of patients seen at the Mayo Clinic for evaluation of pheochromocytoma was recently conducted to determine the diagnostic efficacy of plasma-free metanephrines and 24-hour urine total metanephrines and catecholamines taken from patients with confirmed pheochromocytoma.[40] The investigators found that plasma metanephrines had a high sensitivity but lacked specificity compared with 24-hour urine collections for metanephrines and catecholamines. False-negative 24-hour urine results were found in asymptomatic patients or in patients at high risk for familial syndromes. These investigators suggest that in patients with familial syndromes, a measure of fractionated plasma metanephrines is the best approach. For patients tested for sporadic tumors, measures of 24-hour urinary catecholamines and metanephrines provide 98% specificity with a low false-positive rate.

The clonidine-suppression test is rarely needed to diagnose pheochromocytoma but helps distinguish patients with pheochromocytoma from those with false-positive biochemical tests.[42] Clonidine decreases the release of norepinephrine from the brain and terminal sympathetic axons. Failure to suppress norepinephrine levels is consistent with pheochromocytoma, whereas a fall of >50% supports sympathetic activation. This test is helpful when the biochemical measures of plasma catecholamines or metabolites are not diagnostic.[43,44] Provocation of catecholamine release with glucagon may be used with caution when patients have symptoms of pheochromocytoma but blood pressure is near normal and the plasma catecholamine level is not very high (500-1000 pg/ml).[26]

Consideration should be given to the possibility of false positives if the results of biochemical tests are equivocal. Acetaminophen has been shown to interfere with catecholamine assays, so patients should avoid this agent for 5 days prior to testing.[23] Tricyclic antidepressants, labetolol,

and phenoxybenzamine have been shown to cause false-positive plasma metanephrines.[44] Collection of plasma for testing is optimized if patients have been fasting overnight and avoided caffeinated beverages, are supine for 20 minutes prior to collection, and are taking no interfering medications.

A combination of tests may be required in centers where plasma-free metanephrines are not available. Sensitivity and specificity increase when multiple tests are carried out. Plasma catecholamines (norepinephrine and epinephrine) greater than 2000 pg/ml and urinary metanephrines (metanephrine and normetanephrine) of at least 1.8 mg/24 hours are diagnostic in sporadic and familial pheochromocytomas 98% of the time.[23] Additional studies are needed to determine the best biochemical test for different risk groups.

## Imaging

Computed tomography (CT) (Figure 76–1) or magnetic resonance imaging (MRI) should be obtained to determine the location of a pheochromocytoma only after biochemical confirmatory tests have been performed. Special attention should be given to the adrenal glands and the sympathetic chain. About 95% of the tumors are located in the abdomen and 90% are adrenal.[45] The most common extraadrenal sites are paraaortic (75%), bladder (10%), thoracic (10%), and pelvic (5%).[6] Sporadic tumors are located with either CT or MRI, because they tend to be >3 cm in size. CT may miss small tumors of familial syndromes.[45]

If further imaging is thought necessary, an MIBG (131-I-metaiodobenzylguanidine) scan may detect tumors missed by CT or MRI. The National Institutes of Health consensus report recommends that even if CT or MRI is positive, an MIBG scan should be obtained to detect multiple lesions. This test has a specificity of 100% but a sensitivity of 78%.[24]

## Medical Management

Medical management of pheochromocytoma must always precede surgical resection, and surgery is needed to remove the potentially lethal tumor. The goal of antihypertensive therapy is to control blood pressure, treat symptomatic tachycardia, and avoid hypertensive emergency. The α-adrenergic blocker phenoxybenzamine has been recommended as the treatment of choice during the preoperative period.[46] However, intraoperative reports do not confirm a benefit of this adrenergic blocker in patients undergoing surgical removal of pheochromocytoma and, in fact, suggest more complications with phenoxybenzamine.[47,48] With the development of improved surgical and anesthetic techniques, it may not be necessary to treat a patient with phenoxybenzamine in the absence of hemodynamic instability.

Selective α-adrenergic blockers may be used to control blood pressure. Doxazosin, prazosin, and terazosin do not cause the reflex tachycardia that may result from nonselective α-adrenergic blockade. Calcium channel blockers have also been used safely in patients with pheochromocytoma alone or combined with α-adrenergic blockers. Nifedipine GITS has been used to control blood pressure even during glucagon provocative testing.[49]

β-Blockers should be used only after α-blockade. A hypertensive crisis may occur due to unopposed α-mediated vasoconstriction if β-blockers are used alone. β-Blockade may be

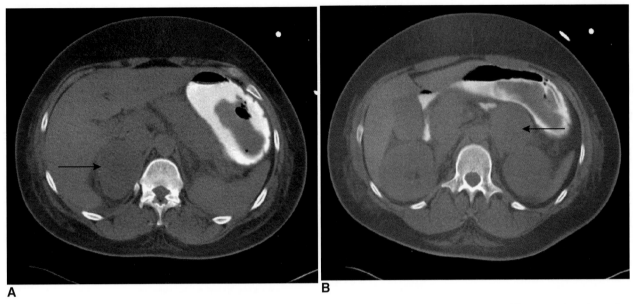

**Figure 76-1** CT scan without contrast showing bilateral adrenal pheochomocytomas in a 27-year-old man with a thyroid mass who presented with cardiomyopathy and hypoxic respiratory failure. He was found to have meduallary thyroid carcinoma consistent with MEN2. *Arrows* represent pheochromocytoma of adrenal glands.

added to control tachycardia related to catecholamine secretion, but when used alone may result in pulmonary edema caused by decreased cardiac output.[50]

## Surgery

Surgical excision of pheochromocytoma can be performed with low mortality and morbidity and may result in a high cure rate for hypertension. Although the surgical approach and outcome have changed dramatically with the development of laproscopic techniques for removal of pheochromocytoma,[51] perioperative complications may be severe.[52]

The management of hypovolemia prior to and during surgery is critical to a successful outcome. Surges in the blood pressure may occur with tumor manipulation, requiring the use of intraoperative phentolamine, labetolol, or nicardipine.[50]

The postoperative complications include orthostatic hypotension due to decreased intravascular volume. Postoperative hypertension may occur with vigorous volume repletion, underlying primary hypertension, or the presence of residual tumor.[51]

## References

1. Beard CM, Sheps SG, Kurland LT, et al. Occurrence of pheochromocytoma in Rochester, Minnesota, 1950 through 1979. Mayo Clin Proc 58:802-804, 1983
2. Stenstorm G, Svardsudd K: Phaeochromocytoma in Sweden, 1958-81: An analysis of the National Cancer Registry Data. Acta Med Scand 220(suppl):225, 1986.
3. Sutton MG, Sheps SG, Lie JT. Prevalence of clinically unsuspected pheochromocytoma. Review of a 50-year autopsy series. Mayo Clin Proc 56:354-360, 1981.
4. Manger WM, Gifford RW Jr. Clinical and Experimental Pheochromocytoma. Cambridge, MA, Blackwell Science, 1996.
5. Erickson D, Kudva YC, Ebersold MJ, et al. Benign paragangliomas: Clinical presentation and treatment outcomes in 236 patients. J Clin Endocrinol Metab 86:5210-5216, 2001.
6. Whalen RK, Althausen AF, Daniels GH. Extra-adrenal pheochromocytoma. J Urol 147:1-10, 1992.
7. Eisenhofer D, Huynh T-T, Hiroi M, et al. Understanding catecholamine metabolism as a guide to the biochemical diagnosis of pheochromocytoma. Rev Endocrinol Metab Dis 2:297-311, 2001.
8. Goldstein RE, O'Neill JA Jr, Holcomb GW III, et al. Clinical experience over 48 years with pheochromocytoma. Ann Surg 229:755-764, 1999.
9. Bravo EL. Evolving concepts in the pathophysiology, diagnosis, and treatment of pheochromocytoma. Endocr Rev 15:356-368, 1994.
10. Ito Y, Fujimoto Y, Obara T. The role of epinephrine, norepinephrine, and dopamine in blood pressure disturbances in patients with pheochromocytoma. World J Surg 16:759-764, 1992.
11. Page LB, Raker JW, Berberich FR. Pheochromocytoma with predominant epinephrine secretion. Am J Med 47:648-652, 1969.
12. Bravo EL, Tarazi RC, Gifford RW, et al. Circulatory and urinary catecholamines in pheochromcytoma: Diagnostic and pathophysiologic implications. N Engl J Med 301:682-686, 1994.
13. Stackpole RH, Melicow MM, Uson AC. Pheochromocytoma in children. Report of 9 cases and review of the first 100 published cases with follow-up studies. J Pediatr 63:315-330, 1963.
14. Bravo E, Fouad-Tarazi F, Rossi G, et al. A reevaluation of the hemodynamics of pheochromocytoma. Hypertension 15(2 Suppl):I128-131, 1990.
15. Johnson MD, Smith PG, Mills E, et al. Paradoxical elevation of sympathetic activity during catecholamine infusion in rats. J Pharmacol Exp Ther 227:254-259, 1983.
16. Prokocimer PG, Maze M, Hoffman BB. The role of the sympathetic nervous system in the maintenance of hypertension in rats harboring pheochromocytoma. J Pharmacol Exp Ther 241(3):870-874, 1987.
17. Levenson JA, Safar ME, London BM, et al. Hemodynamics in patients with pheochromocytoma. Clin Sci 58:349-356, 1980.

18. Cohen CD, Dent DM. Pheochromocytoma and acute cardiovascular death (with special reference to myocardial infarction). Postgrad Med J 60:111-115, 1984.

19. de Leeuw PW, Waltman FL, Birkenhager WH. Noncardiogenic pulmonary edema as sole manifestation of pheochromocytoma. Hypertension 8:810-812, 1986.

20. Mann SJ. Severe paroxysmal hypertension (Pseudopheochromocytoma). Arch Intern Med 159:670-674, 1999.

21. Lin JC, Palafox BA, Jackson HA, et al. Cardiac pheochromocytoma: Resection after diagnosis by 111-indium octreotide scan. Ann Thorac Surg 67:555-558, 1997.

22. Januszewicz P, Wieteska-Klimczak A, Wyszynska T. Pheochromocytoma in children: Difficulties in diagnosis and localization. Clin Exp Hypertens [A] 12:571-579, 1990.

23. Bravo EL, Tagle R. Pheochromocytoma: State-of-the-art and future prospects. Endocr Rev 24:539-553, 2003.

24. Pacak K, Linehan WM, Eisenhofer G, et al. Recent advances in genetics, diagnosis, localization, and treatment of pheochromocytoma. Ann Intern Med 134:315-329, 2001.

25. Pattarino F, Bouloux PM. The diagnosis of malignancy in phaeochromocytoma. Clin Endocrinol (Oxf) 44:239-241, 1996.

26. Bravo EL, Gifford RW Jr. Current concepts. Pheochromocytoma: Diagnosis, localization and management. N Engl J Med 311(20):1298-1303, 1984.

27. Koch CA, Vortmeyer AO, Zhuang Z, et al. New insights into the genetics of familial chromaffin cell tumors. Ann N Y Acad Sci 970:11-28, 2002.

28. Neumann, HP, Bausch, B, McWhinney, SR, et al. Germ-line mutations in nonsyndromic pheochromocytoma. N Engl J Med 346:1459-1466, 2002.

29. Dluhy, RG. Pheochromocytoma death of an axiom. N Engl J Med 346:1486-1488, 2002.

30. Santoro M, Carlomagno F, Romano, et al. Activation of RET as a dominant transforming gene by germline mutations of MEN2A and MEN2B. Science 267:381-383, 1995.

31. Gagel RF, Tashjian AH Jr, Cummings T, et al. The clinical outcome of prospective screening for multiple endocrine neoplasia type 2a. An18-year experience. N Engl J Med 318:478-484, 1988.

32. Maxwell PH, Wiesener MS, Chang GW, et al. The tumour suppressor protein VHL targets hypoxia-inducible factors for oxygen-dependent proteolysis. Nature 399:271-275, 1999.

33. Eng C, Clayton D, Schuffenecker I, et al. The relationship between specific RET proto-oncogene mutations and disease phenotype in multiple endocrine neoplasia type 2. International RET mutation consortium analysis. JAMA 276:1575-1579, 1996.

34. Neumann HP, Berger DP, Sigmund G. Pheochromocytomas, multiple endocrine neoplasia type 2 and von Hippel-Lindau disease. N Engl J Med 329:1531-1538, 1993.

35. Eisenhofer G, Walther MM, Huynh TT, et al. Pheochromocytomas in von Hippel-Lindau syndrome and multiple endocrine neoplasia type 2 display distinct biochemical and clinical phenotypes. J Clin Endocrinol Metab 86:1999-2008, 2001.

36. Baysal BE, Ferrell RE, Willett-Brozick JE, et al. Mutations in SDHD, a mitochondrial complex II gene, in hereditary paraganglioma. Science 287:848-851, 2000.

37. Kalff V, Shapiro B, Lloyd R, et al. The spectrum of pheochromocytoma in hypertensive patients with neurofibromatosis. Arch Intern Med 142:2092-2098, 1982.

38. Walther MM, Herring J, Enquist E, et al. von Recklinghausen's disease and pheochromocytomas. J Urol 162:1582-1586, 1999.

39. Lenders JW, Pacak K, Walther MM, et al. Biochemical diagnosis of pheochromocytoma: which test is best? JAMA 287:1427-1434, 2002.

40. Sawka AM, Jaeschke R, Singh RJ, et al. A comparison of biochemical tests for pheochromocytoma: Measurement of fractionated plasma metanephrines compared with the combination of 24-hour urinary metanephrines and catecholamines. J Clin Endocrinol Metab 88:553-558, 2003.

41. Lenders JW, Eisenhofer G, Armando I, et al. Determination of metanephrines in plasma by liquid chromatography with electrochemical detection. Clin Chem 39:97-103, 1993.

42. Bravo EL, Tarazi RC, Fouad FM, et al. Clonidine-suppression test: A useful aid in the diagnosis of pheochromocytoma. N Engl J Med 305:623-626, 1983.

43. Grossman E, Goldstein DS, Hoffman A, Keiser HR. Glucagon and clonidine testing in the diagnosis of pheochromocytoma. Hypertension 17:733-741, 1991.

44. Eisenhofer G, Goldstein DS, Walther MM, et al. Biochemical diagnosis of pheochromocytoma: How to distinguish true-from false-positive test results. J Clin Endocrinol Metab 88:2656-2666, 2003.

45. Bravo EL. Pheochromocytoma: New concepts and future trends. Kidney Int 40:544-556, 1991.

46. Ross EJ, Prichard BN, Kaufman L, et al. Preoperative and operative management of patients with phaeochromocytoma. Br Med J 1:191-198, 1967.

47. Boutros AR, Bravo EL, Zanettin G, et al. Perioperative management of 63 patients with pheochromocytoma. Cleve Clin J Med 57:613-617, 1990.

48. Ulchaker JC, Goldfarb DA, Bravo EL, et al. Successful outcomes in pheochromocytoma surgery in the modern era. J Urol 161:764-767, 1999.

49. Proye C, Thevenin D, Cecat P, et al. Exclusive use of calcium channel blockers in preoperative and intraoperative control of pheochromocytomas: Hemodynamics and free catecholamine assays in ten consecutive patients. Surgery 106:1149-1154, 1989.

50. Prys-Roberts C. Phaeochromocytoma—Recent progress in its management. Br J Anaesth 85:44-57, 2000.

51. Walther MM. New therapeutic and surgical approaches for sporadic and hereditary pheochromocytoma. Ann N Y Acad Sci 970:41-53, 2002.

52. Plouin PF, Duclos JM, Soppelsa F, et al. Factors associated with perioperative morbidity and mortality in patients with pheochromocytoma: Analysis of 165 operations at a single center. J Clin Endocrinol Metab 86:1480-1486, 2001.

# Chapter 77

# Anesthesia and Hypertension

## Scott T. Reeves, J. G. Reves

## INTRODUCTION

This chapter reviews the current knowledge of anesthesia and surgery in the hypertensive patient. It is hoped that internists, surgeons, and anesthesiologists will be able to use this information to better prepare patients for surgery by understanding how hypertension, its treatment, and anesthesia interact. Emphasis is placed on the cardiovascular pharmacology of anesthetic drugs, anesthetic techniques, the preoperative evaluation of the patient, and the implications of the operative procedure for management strategies. The risks of perioperative hypertension and the best way to minimize those risks are also discussed.

Elsewhere in this book the pathophysiology and treatment of hypertension are discussed in detail. This chapter reviews the effects of anesthesia and surgery on the hypertensive patient from a physiologic, pharmacologic, and clinical outcome perspective. Hypertension (blood pressure [BP] >140/90 mm Hg) and surgery are both prevalent, particularly in the elderly.[1]

It is important to have an understanding of the effect that hypertension has on anesthesia and surgery, as well as the effect that surgery and anesthesia have on hypertensive patients. It has been estimated that severe hypertension (BP ≥180/110 mm Hg) is found in 11% of surgical patients.[2] The prevalence of hypertension depends on the surgical population; it is increased in older patients and in those undergoing vascular and cardiac surgery.[3] Hypertension is common during surgery, occurring in 57% of patients undergoing abdominal aortic surgery, in 29% of those undergoing peripheral vascular surgery, and in 8% of those undergoing intraperitoneal procedures.[4] In patients having carotid artery or open heart surgery, the incidence of hypertension varies between 40% and 80%.[5,6]

Patients who develop hypertension in the perioperative period can be divided into four classes of hypertensive patients (Table 77–1). The first includes normotensive patients who respond to the many stresses of the perioperative period, such as anxiety, pain, or a distended bladder, that evoke catecholamine release and the subsequent development of hypertension.[7] This form of hypertension is usually transient (self-limited) and can be successfully treated by removing the precipitating stimulus. The second class includes those with a history of hypertension controlled (BP ≤140/90 mm Hg) by pharmacologic therapy. These patients are likely to respond to the multiple perioperative stressors of surgery with hypertension, but to a lesser degree than the third and fourth classes of patients. The third class includes those with undiagnosed or uncontrolled hypertension (BP 160/90 to 180/110 mm Hg). These patients are likely to have recurrent hypertension in the perioperative period. The fourth class includes hypertensive patients who may or may not be treated, but who present for anesthesia with uncontrolled hypertension (BP ≥180/110 mm Hg). This class is at highest risk for perioperative hypertension, hypotension, and a labile hemodynamic course, as well as morbid events. They should generally have surgery delayed until the hypertension can be better controlled.[4,8]

It is important to recognize that hypertensive patients often have comorbid diseases, such as diabetes, renal disease, cerebrovascular disease, peripheral vascular disease, and cardiac disease, including coronary artery disease, left ventricular hypertrophy, and congestive heart failure (CHF). Hypertensive patients are at increased risk of hemodynamic fluctuations during the perioperative course,[9-12] which may result in myocardial ischemia,[9-11,13] myocardial infarction,[4,14] postoperative renal dysfunction,[15,16] and an increased incidence of postoperative neurologic deficits.[16-18] Hypertension generally confers added risk to anesthesia and surgery, as discussed later in the chapter.

Figure 77–1 illustrates the effects of hypertension on the heart and identifies the important determinants of BP that are affected by anesthetic and antihypertensive drugs. The hypertensive patient is likely to have elevated systemic vascular resistance (SVR), reduced total blood volume, impaired cardiac contractility, and a hypertrophied myocardium. The hypertrophied left ventricle (which by its very pathology has higher oxygen requirements and potentially less oxygen supply) is vulnerable to subendocardial ischemia,[9,19] particularly if there is tachycardia and/or if the coronary perfusion pressure decreases during anesthesia. Almost all anesthetic drugs and most anesthetic techniques will produce vasodilation (see the next section), and most inhalation anesthetics are direct negative inotropic drugs. Thus, hypertensive patients who may be volume depleted,[20] who have high SVR, and who may have depressed ventricular function commonly experience hypotension with the induction of anesthesia. This hypotension can compromise myocardial oxygen delivery, which may lead to ischemic ventricular dysfunction.

The treatment of hypertension is particularly important for patients undergoing anesthesia and surgery for two reasons. It is well documented that hypertensive patients whose BP is controlled have fewer hemodynamic fluctuations in the perioperative period.[16,19-21] The fewer the hemodynamic fluctuations (particularly tachycardia), the less likely patients are to have myocardial ischemia.[9,22] Also, many of the drugs commonly used in the treatment of hypertension have pharmacologic interactions with anesthetics. Anesthetic drugs and techniques (general, spinal, epidural) require a complex set of homeostatic reflexes to maintain cardiac output and BP, as illustrated in Figure 77–2.[23] Antihypertensive drugs that lower plasma volume (e.g., diuretics),[24] vasodilators, and β-adrenergic antagonists accentuate the hypotensive effects of anesthesia and impair the autoregulatory responses of increased heart rate (HR), contractility, and vasoconstriction that are triggered by anesthesia.

**Table 77–1** Perioperative Hypertensive Patients

| Classification* | BP† (mm Hg) | Commentary‡ | Disposition |
|---|---|---|---|
| 1. Normotensive | <140/90 | Controlled, resolves with removal of stressor | Treat q.s. |
| 2. Controlled hypertensives | <140/90 | Adequately controlled | Treat q.s. |
| 3. Poorly controlled or undiagnosed hypertensives | 140/90 ≤180/110 | Poorly controlled | Dx and Rx; better Rx; arrange appropriate medical follow-up |
| 4. Uncontrolled or undiagnosed hypertensives | ≥110 diastolic | Uncontrolled | Dx and Rx; better Rx; arrange appropriate medical management; *delay elective surgery* |

BP, blood pressure; q.s., as needed during the perioperative period; Dx, diagnose; Rx, treat.
*Classification adapted from literature review and definitions of the Joint National Committee on Prevention, Detection, Evaluation, and Treatment of High Blood Pressure. The sixth report. Arch Intern Med 157:2413-2446, 1997.
†BP at preoperative evaluation or before anesthesia induction.
‡Hypertensive response (≥140/90 mm Hg) during the preoperative or perioperative period in patients who are diagnosed as hypertensive or not diagnosed as hypertensive but who develop hypertension during the perioperative period.

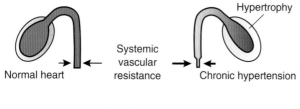

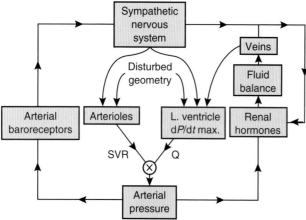

**Figure 77–1** Schema of the hemodynamic perturbations induced in the hypertensive patient demonstrates the interactions of adaptive hypertrophy of the arteriolar media and of the left ventricle, with sympathetic nervous activity. SVR, systemic vascular resistance. (From Prys-Roberts C. Anaesthesia and hypertension. Br J Anaesth 56:711-724, 1984.)

Two classes of antihypertensive drugs that are especially helpful in the perioperative management of hypertensive patients are the β-adrenergic antagonists and the $\alpha_2$-agonists. β-Blockers attenuate the hypertensive and tachycardiac responses to perioperative stress and reduce myocardial ischemia.[9,25,26] $\alpha_2$-Agonists, such as clonidine, reduce the incidence of hypertension and tachycardia, as well as the need for additional anesthesia.[27] Patients whose hypertension is treated with these classes of drugs will likely have smoother perioper-

ative courses. The failure of diuretics to provide smooth hemodynamics during anesthesia is attributed to the lower total blood volume, increased circulating vasoactive substances, and potassium depletion.[9] There is insufficient information on the many new antihypertensive drug classes, such as angiotensin II receptor, II-imidazoline receptor, and selective aldosterone receptor antagonists, to know how these agents affect the perioperative course.

## CARDIOVASCULAR PHARMACOLOGY OF SEDATIVE AND ANESTHETIC DRUGS

To better understand the hemodynamic effects of sedative, inhalation, and intravenous anesthetics, we review the major cardiovascular effects of drugs used in anesthesia, as well as the cardiovascular effects of common anesthetic techniques. This section is a synopsis of material presented in earlier reviews of the pharmacology of anesthetic drugs.[23,28-31] The cardiovascular effects of the various drugs and anesthetic techniques are summarized in Table 77–2.

### Anesthetic Techniques

Anesthetic techniques can be divided into four categories. The first is general anesthesia, which is accomplished with a wide variety of intravenous and inhalation anesthetic drugs. The majority of general anesthetics are given with a hypnotic (usually a barbiturate or a benzodiazepine), an analgesic (an opioid and/or an inhalation drug), and a muscle relaxant (neuromuscular blocking drugs). A second form of anesthesia is neuraxial block, which is accomplished by placing a local anesthetic in the spinal or epidural space. A third technique is regional nerve block with a local anesthetic. The final anesthetic technique involves sedation of the patient and local anesthetic infiltration at the site of the surgery. This is called *monitored anesthesia care* (MAC).

We have examined the effect of anesthetic technique on hypertensive patients.[32] General and neuraxial techniques result in the greatest hypotension because both result in vasodilation (Figure 77–3). Loss of consciousness, as seen in

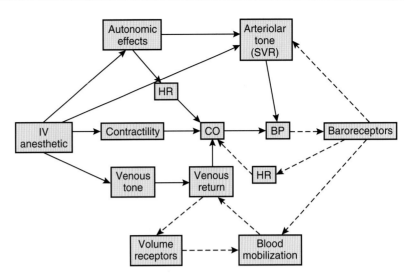

**Figure 77-2** The multiple effects of anesthetic drugs on the cardiovascular system are shown. Direct *(solid arrows)* and indirect *(broken arrows)* effects of intravenous (IV) anesthetics on cardiovascular function. SVR, systemic vascular resistance; HR, heart rate; CO, cardiac output; BP, blood pressure. (From Reves JG, Gelman S. Cardiovascular effects of intravenous anesthetic drugs. *In* Covino F, Rehdel K, Strichartz GR [eds]. Effects of Anesthesia. Bethesda, MD, American Physiological Society, 1985; pp 179-193.)

**Table 77-2** Anesthesia Drugs/Techniques/Effects on Hemodynamic Variables

| Variable | Intravenous | Inhalation | Neuraxial | Regional Nerve Block |
|---|---|---|---|---|
| Cardiac output | 0 to ↓ | ↓ | ↓ to 0 | 0 |
| SVR | ↓ to 0 | ↓ | ↓ | 0 |
| Contractility | 0 | ↓ | 0 | 0 |
| Heart rate | 0 | ↓ | 0 | 0 |
| Stroke volume | 0 | ↓ | 0 | 0 |

SVR, systemic vascular resistance.
Neuraxial, spinal or epidural anesthesia.
Key: 0 = no change, ↓ = decrease.

normal sleep,[33] reduces HR, cardiac output, and BP. Most drugs used for general anesthesia have hemodynamic effects that, together with loss of consciousness, cause hypotension. Neuraxial block produces hypotension by creating a complete sympathectomy to (or slightly above) the dermatome level of the anesthesia. This causes profound vasodilation, reduced preload, lower cardiac output, and hypotension. The use of epidural anesthesia with general anesthesia significantly lowers the incidence of operative hypertension, but is associated with greater hypotension and can evoke hypertension when it is withdrawn postoperatively.[34] Regional block and MAC have minimal hemodynamic effects and are less likely to cause hypotension in hypertensive patients. Hypertensive patients often have hypertensive responses during anesthesia, and all anesthetic techniques are associated with similar peak incidences of hypertension (Figure 77-4; see also Figure 77-3).

## CARDIOVASCULAR PHARMACOLOGY OF GENERAL ANESTHETICS

### General Anesthetic Induction Drugs

#### Thiopental

Thiopental (Pentothal) has survived the test of time as an intravenous anesthetic drug. Since Lundy introduced it in 1934, thiopental has become the most widely used induction agent because of the rapid hypnotic effect (one arm-brain circulation time), highly predictable effect, lack of vascular irri-

tation, and general overall safety.[35] The principal hemodynamic change produced by thiopental is a decrease in myocardial contractility[36-38] due to reduced availability of calcium to myofibrils.[39] There is also an increase in HR.[37-41] The cardiac index (CI) is unchanged[41,42] or reduced,[37] whereas the mean arterial pressure (MAP) is maintained[41,43] or slightly reduced.[44] When thiopental is given to hypovolemic patients, which could include poorly controlled hypertensive patients, there is a significant reduction in cardiac output and an important decrease in BP. Thus, patients without adequate compensatory mechanisms may have serious hemodynamic depression with a thiopental induction.[45] This probably explains the disastrous results of thiopental administration at Pearl Harbor,[46] where many wounded men who were hypovolemic experienced shock with the rapid administration of the newly released anesthetic thiopental.

#### Diazepam

Diazepam (Valium) is probably the most widely used benzodiazepine in the world. It was introduced in the United States in 1963 and is used for sedation and anesthesia induction. The presumed mechanism of action of diazepam and other benzodiazepines in the central nervous system is by potentiation of the inhibitory effect of γ-aminobutyric acid on neuronal transmission.[47] All benzodiazepines have hypnotic, anticonvulsant, muscle relaxant, amnesic, and anxiolytic properties. Induction with diazepam is characterized by hemodynamic stability. Filling pressures and CI remain unchanged,[48-53] with

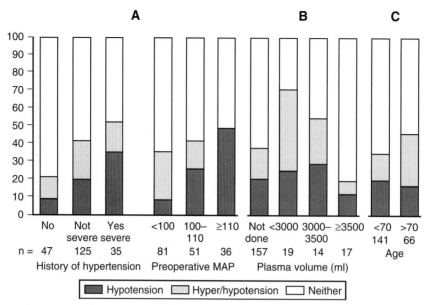

**Figure 77–3** Percentage of patients with intraoperative hypotension (black), hypertension/hypotension (cross-hatched), or neither high-risk pattern (white), according to preoperative characteristics. **(A)** Patients are compared based on their history of hypertension and preoperative mean arterial pressure (MAP). A preoperative MAP >110 mm Hg was a significant ($p$ <.001) predictor of intraoperative hypotension. **(B)** Patients are compared based on their initial plasma volume as determined using Evans blue. Decreased plasma volume was a significant ($p$ = .03) predictor of intraoperative hypotension and was associated with a higher incidence of intraoperative hypertension/hypotension. **(C)** Patients are compared based on age. Age >70 years was a significant ($p$ <.006) predictor of intraoperative hypertension/hypotension. Age alone did not significantly increase the incidence of intraoperative hypotension. *Preoperative hypertension* was defined as a systolic BP >160 mm Hg or a diastolic BP >95 mm Hg. Severe preoperative hypertension was defined as diastolic BP ≥120 mm Hg. *Intraoperative hypotension* was defined as a decrease of >20 mm Hg from preoperative MAP lasting 1 hour or longer. *Intraoperative hypertension/hypotension* was defined as an increase of ≥20 mm Hg above the usual MAP lasting >15 minutes combined with a decrease of >20 mm Hg in MAP lasting <1 hour. (*A-C* From Charlson MD, MacKenzie CR, Gold JP, et al. Preoperative characteristics predicting intraoperative hypotension and hypertension among hypertensives and diabetics undergoing noncardiac surgery. Ann Surg 212[1]:66-81, 1990.)

variable but modest changes in HR.[48-54] Although diazepam may be safely combined with other anesthetic drugs, there is some potential for hemodynamic depression.[55] The effect of the combination of diazepam and morphine (indeed of any benzodiazepine and opioid) in patients who have ischemic heart disease[56,57] and valvular heart disease[58] has been reported. The combination of diazepam (0.125-0.5 mg/kg) and fentanyl (50 μg/kg) used to induce anesthesia in patients for coronary artery bypass graft surgery[59] led to a supra-additive fall in BP was more pronounced in hypovolemic hypertensive patients. The authors concluded from this that diazepam ablates normal sympathetic tone.[59]

### Midazolam

Midazolam (Versed) is a water-soluble benzodiazepine synthesized in the United States in 1975. It is unique among benzodiazepines with its rapid onset and short duration of action and relatively rapid plasma clearance.[60] It is the most commonly used benzodiazepine in anesthetic practice. The hemodynamic changes that result from the intravenous administration of midazolam (0.2 mg/kg) in premedicated patients who have coronary artery disease are usually minor.[53,61] Changes of potential importance include a decrease in MAP of 20% and

an increase in HR of 15%.[61] The CI is maintained.[53,61] Filling pressures are either unchanged or decreased in patients who have normal ventricular function[53,61] but are significantly decreased in patients who have an elevated pulmonary capillary wedge pressure (≥18 mm Hg).[62] Interactions between midazolam and other drugs are relatively mild and predictable. The combination of nitrous oxide ($N_2O$) (50%) with midazolam (0.2 mg/kg) does not cause increased cardiovascular depression.[53] The safe combination of $N_2O$ and midazolam contrasts with the well-known additive depression of $N_2O$ and narcotic agents.[63] Midazolam is routinely combined with fentanyl for induction and maintenance of general anesthesia during cardiac surgery without adverse hemodynamic sequelae.[64-66] However, if midazolam is given to patients who have received fentanyl, significant hypotension may occur, as seen with diazepam and fentanyl.[59]

### Ketamine

Although ketamine (Ketalar) produces rapid hypnosis and profound analgesia, respiratory and cardiovascular functions are not depressed as much as with most other induction agents. Disturbing psychotomimetic activity (described as vivid dreams, hallucinations, or other mental disturbances on

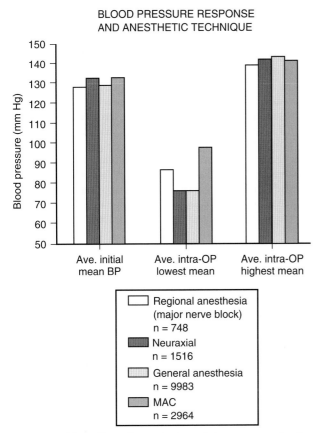

BLOOD PRESSURE RESPONSE
AND ANESTHETIC TECHNIQUE

**Figure 77–4** The effect of anesthetic technique on maximal changes in BP is shown. BP drops (average intraoperative [Intra-OP] lowest mean vs. average preoperative mean) are significantly (*p* <.001) greater with general and neuraxial anesthetic techniques compared with regional (major nerve block) and monitored anesthetic care (MAC) techniques. The average intra-OP highest mean BP was similar among anesthetic techniques. *Regional anesthesia* refers to major peripheral nerve blocks, such as brachial plexus blocks, lumbar plexus blocks, sciatic nerve blocks, and paravertebral blocks; *general anesthesia* refers to general anesthesia; *neuraxial anesthesia* refers to spinal, epidural, or combined spinal/epidural anesthesia. See text for more details on anesthetic technique. (From Gould JD, Reves JG, D'Ercole FJ, et al. Effect of anesthetic technique on blood pressure response in hypertensive patients. Anesth Analg 88:SCA62, 1999.)

emergence from ketamine anesthesia) as well as undesirable increases in myocardial oxygen consumption have limited the use of ketamine. One unique feature of ketamine is stimulation of the cardiovascular system. The most prominent hemodynamic changes are significant increases in HR, CI, SVR, and systemic and pulmonary artery pressures. Because of the hypertension after ketamine, this drug is seldom used in hypertensive patients.

## Propofol

Propofol (Diprivan) was introduced into clinical practice in 1977.[67] It is an alkylphenol (substituted derivative of phenol) with hypnotic properties. The hemodynamic effects of propo-

fol have been compared with the most commonly used induction drugs, including the thiobarbiturates and etomidate.[68-72] Systolic pressure falls 15% to 40% after intravenous induction with ±2 mg/kg and maintenance infusion of ±100 µg/kg/min propofol. Similar changes are seen in both diastolic pressure and MAP. The effect of propofol on HR is variable. Despite a significant decrease in MAP, some studies have shown no change in HR,[73] a decrease in HR,[72] or an increase in HR.[74] The majority of studies have demonstrated significant reductions in SVR (9%-30%), CI, stroke volume, and left ventricular stroke work index after propofol. In summary, propofol alone or in combination causes significant decreases in arterial pressure and CI secondary to increased venodilation with decreased myocardial contractility. Its use in uncontrolled hypertensives could be problematic.

## Drugs for Maintenance of Anesthesia

### Inhalation Anesthesia

Contemporary inhalation anesthesia includes the use of six drugs—the volatile liquids halothane, enflurane, sevoflurane, desflurane, and isoflurane, and the inert gas $N_2O$. Each inhalation anesthetic has a specific cardiovascular profile, but all except $N_2O$ are vasodilators and negative inotropes. As with the intravenous agents, their hemodynamic effects depend on several factors that include the drug per se, the cardiovascular status of the patient, and concurrent pharmacologic therapy. Unlike the intravenous drugs, the cardiovascular effects of the inhalation agents are more similar to one another than they are different. The inhalation anesthetics often reduce cardiac output. All of the inhalation agents exert a direct, dose-dependent negative inotropic effect on the myocardium in humans.[75-77] There are small differences among agents in the degree of myocardial depression and in the mechanism of myocardial suppression. In general, halothane and enflurane reduce cardiac output to a greater degree than isoflurane in healthy patients. Volatile anesthetics further depress myocardial contractility in disease states, such as ischemic heart disease.[78] The influences of age, myocardial disease, premedication, and adjuvant drugs are important additive depressant factors. Inhalation anesthetics must be used judiciously in hypertensive patients because of their propensity to cause hypotension.

### Narcotics

Opioids are also used to provide analgesia during general anesthesia and postoperatively. The drugs commonly used are morphine, fentanyl, sufentanil, alfentanil, and remifentanil. Morphine causes more hemodynamic perturbations than the others. Morphine, because of release of histamine, causes vasodilation that may produce hypotension. The other synthetic opioids are devoid of this action, and their administration is marked by maintenance of SVR. All opioids tend to be vagomimetic, causing a decrease in HR. Opioids have little effect on cardiac output, stroke volume, cardiac filling, or baroreflex function. They are used in hypertensive patients to blunt sympathetic responses to painful stimuli. They are useful in this setting because they tend to minimize hemodynamic fluctuation, but they must be combined with other anesthetic drugs to accomplish total anesthesia. The hemodynamic interactions with these drugs can cause vasodilation and hypotension.

## EVALUATION AND PREPARATION OF THE HYPERTENSIVE SURGICAL PATIENT

There is no area in medicine where the collaborative team approach to patient care can be better employed than in evaluating and preparing the hypertensive patient for surgery. The internist (cardiologist, generalist), the surgeon, and the anesthesiologist all have important roles in the optimal care of these high-risk patients.[79] The objectives of the evaluation are listed in Box 77–1. Each specialist has a specific role: The surgeon must determine the appropriate operation; the internist must optimize the medical therapy; and the anesthesiologist must choose the appropriate monitoring, anesthetic technique, and postoperative pain strategy.

Table 77–1 lists the categories into which hypertensive patients fall when presenting for surgery. Patients who are optimally medically managed before, during, and after surgery have a smoother hemodynamic course. Patients in groups 3 and 4 of Table 77–1 have more labile courses than patients in groups 1 and 2.[2-4,16,20,80] It is important when evaluating the hypertensive patient that comorbid conditions be detected (Table 77–3) and that antihypertensive therapy be optimized (BP ≤140/90 mm Hg).

The preoperative evaluation listed in Box 77–1, including relevant history and physical examination (see Table 77–3), can be made by the internist, the surgeon, or the anesthesiologist. It does not matter who has the initial responsibility. What is vital is that all of the objectives in Box 77–1 are successfully attained before surgery. The cause of hypertension should be determined, remembering that essential hypertension is most common. Knowing, wherever possible, the causes and pathophysiology of the hypertension (see Figure 77–1) is critical to proper perioperative management. It is important to determine what antihypertensive medications the patient is taking, what the dosing regimen is, and whether this regimen should be continued or changed during the perioperative period. If the regimen cannot be continued, an alternative strategy must be developed. Studies support the continuation of the patient's antihypertensive medicines until the morning of surgery.[2-4,9,16,19,79-81] The discontinuation of antihypertensive medication, especially β-blockers and/or clonidine, may precipitate rebound hypertension, tachycardia, or myocardial ischemia,[19,81] which will be problematic in the perioperative management of the patient. In patients unable to take oral medications, intravenous β-blockade or transdermal clonidine can be utilized.[81] Antihypertensive therapy should be

continued after surgery and throughout the perioperative period as the patient's course dictates. Occasionally, patients with newly diagnosed mild hypertension (type I or II) may have the institution of therapy delayed until after surgery to avoid the creation of instability in HR or BP.[81]

The single most important and most obvious preoperative assessment (see Table 77–3) is the adequacy of BP control. If BP is greater than 110 mm Hg diastolic at the preoperative evaluation, it is generally recommended to delay elective surgery until BP can be better controlled.* The introduction of a β-blocker preoperatively minimizes BP fluctuations and decreases the number and duration of perioperative coronary ischemic events.[81] Unless the surgery is emergent or urgent, it is best to get the resting BP as close to the normal range as possible, or at least to less than 110 mm Hg diastolic. It should be remembered that many patients who are faced with the prospect of surgery have conditions that may artifactually raise their BP, for example, anxiety or pain. Therefore, a preoperative BP that is above the "normal" range, as defined by office readings in relaxed patients, is acceptable for the preoperative patient. It is also useful to obtain a supine and a standing BP as an assessment of the orthostatic component of BP control. This measurement can also indirectly gauge the blood volume.

Routine perioperative evaluation of the newly diagnosed hypertensive patient includes a comprehensive physical examination searching for target organ damage and evidence of associated cardiovascular pathology. A few simple tests, including an electrocardiogram and chest radiograph (looking for evidence of left ventricular hypertrophy), serum electrolytes (especially in patients treated with diuretics), blood urea nitrogen/creatinine to evaluate renal status, and a baseline hematocrit should be performed.[81] Additional tests may be indicated based on the results of the patient's history and physical examination and initial studies. According to American College of Cardiology/American Heart Association guidelines, if the initial evaluation of the patient undergoing noncardiac surgery establishes hypertension as mild or moderate and there are no associated metabolic or cardiovascular abnormalities, there is no reason to delay surgery.[81]

Preoperative evaluation of the surgical patient may reveal not only hypertension but also other important coexisting diseases (cardiac, renal, cerebrovascular). Each of these requires lifelong management, and one benefit of routine preoperative evaluation may be the discovery of these potentially life-threatening diseases.[79] Medical consultation should be obtained to be certain that the extent of the comorbid disease is fully understood and that a long-term plan for management after surgery is put into place.

Consultations have an important role in the preoperative evaluation of the hypertensive patient. To be most informative to the professionals involved, as well as to provide optimal patient care, consultations should include a number of important elements.[79-84] Box 77–2 lists suggestions to make the consultative process most effective.[79] It is generally unproductive for professionals to stray from their own realm of expertise, no matter how great the temptation. Thus, medical consultants who "clear patients for surgery" encroach on the surgeon's ultimate decision. Likewise, internists' advice to anesthesiologists regarding monitoring or anesthetic techniques is noncontributory. The four key questions that

**Box 77–1** Objectives of the Preoperative Evaluation of Hypertensive Patients

Diagnosis of hypertension (cause)
Ascertain antihypertensive medical therapy
Determine adequacy (optimization) of therapy
Identify comorbid diseases (see Table 77–4)
Obtain appropriate consultative services
Devise appropriate postoperative antihypertensive plan

---

*References 2, 3, 8, 16, 20, 81.

**Table 77–3** Identifying Comorbidity in the Hypertensive Patient

| System | Effect of Hypertension | History | Physical | Tests |
|---|---|---|---|---|
| Cardiovascular | CAD | Angina, MI | | ECG, ETT (other functional study), coronary angiography |
| | LVH (diastolic/systolic dysfunction), pulmonary edema, ischemia | Dyspnea, orthopnea, PND, exercise tolerance, edema | $S_3$, $S_4$, rales, JVD, HJR, peripheral edema | ECG, CXR, Echo |
| | Hypovolemia | Syncope, near-syncope | Orthostatic BP | Orthostatic BP |
| | PVD | Claudication | Peripheral pulses, ABI | Angiography |
| Renal | Renal impairment | Symptoms occur late in process | | HCT, BUN, Cr, electrolytes, UA |
| Central nervous | Cerebrovascular disease | TIA, CVA, syncope | Carotid bruits, neurologic deficits | Carotid Doppler, angiography, CT scan, MRI |

CAD, coronary artery disease; MI, myocardial infarction; ECG, electrocardiogram; ETT, exercise tolerance test; LVH, left ventricular hypertrophy; PND, paroxysmal nocturnal dyspnea; $S_3$, $S_4$, third and fourth heart sounds; JVD, jugular venous distention; HJR, hepato-jugular reflux; CXR, chest radiography; Echo, two-dimensional echocardiography; BP, blood pressure; PVD, peripheral vascular disease; ABI, ankle/brachial index; HCT, hematocrit; BUN, blood urea nitrogen; Cr, creatinine; UA, urinalysis; TIA, transient ischemic attack; CVA, cerebrovascular accident; CT, computed tomography; MRI, magnetic resonance imaging.

surgeons and anesthesiologists have for their medical consultants follow:

1. What diseases does the patient have?
2. Are the diseases being appropriately treated?
3. Is there any further medical therapy that should be instituted?
4. Who will be responsible for the postoperative treatment of the medical conditions that are identified?

## HYPERTENSION, ANESTHESIA, AND SURGERY

After the preoperative evaluation, the anesthetic plan is made. It must include choice of anesthetic technique; monitoring strategy; method of anesthesia induction, maintenance, and emergence; and postoperative disposition. The patient's coexisting diseases, the planned operative procedure, and the duration of the procedure all influence the anesthetic plan.

In general, anesthetic technique falls into one of four categories: centroneuraxial anesthesia, regional (major nerve block) anesthesia, MAC, and general anesthesia. *Centroneuraxial* anesthesia includes spinal and epidural anesthesia. *Major nerve block* anesthesia includes, but is not limited to, brachial plexus blocks

**Box 77–2** Essentials of Effective Perioperative Consultation

Establish clear communication.
Ask specific questions in the realm of consultant's expertise.
Avoid general statements on "clearance for surgery."
Avoid specific advice on matters for which another professional has ultimate decision.
Specify whether anything can be done to improve patient status.

A condensation of the authors' thoughts and those of Kleinman et al.[79] and Lee et al.[83]

(interscalene, supraclavicular, and axillary) for upper extremity surgery, lumbar plexus blocks and femoral-sciatic nerve blocks for lower extremity surgery, and paravertebral blocks for trunk surgery. In simplest terms, *MAC* involves intravenous sedation, patient monitoring, and local anesthetic infiltration at the operative site. *Regional* anesthesia provides profound analgesia and muscle relaxation to a limited portion of the body, allowing the patient to maintain normal respiratory control, easy assessment of neurologic status, and minimal physiologic disturbance. *General* anesthesia involves inducing a state of unconsciousness with analgesia, amnesia, and immobility. Frequently, endotracheal intubation, mechanical ventilation, complete paralysis, and hemodynamic support are part of a general anesthetic.

### Choice of Technique in Hypertensive Patients

With regard to anesthetic technique, two main questions need to be addressed:

1. How does the choice of anesthetic technique affect perioperative cardiovascular, neurologic, and renal morbidity and mortality in the hypertensive patient?
2. What effect (consequence) does the chosen anesthetic technique have on the incidence of perioperative hypertension, hypotension, hemodynamic lability, and myocardial ischemia?

### General Anesthesia

Most of the literature evaluating the cardiovascular responses of hypertensive patients to anesthetic techniques relates to use of general anesthesia. The cardiovascular responses of hypertensive patients undergoing general anesthesia tend to be labile.[2,9,10,13] Hypertensive patients become hypotensive with induction and have hypertensive responses to laryngoscopy, intubation, noxious stimuli, and emergence. Their response to rapid changes in anesthetic depth is also exaggerated.

Intraoperative BP lability, hypertension, and hypotension place hypertensive patients at increased risk of myocardial ischemia,[9] myocardial reinfarction,[14] and perioperative renal dysfunction.[16,20] Charlson et al.[20] have looked at the association between preoperative patient characteristics and intraoperative hemodynamics. Figure 77–3 shows these results. Patients older than 70 years (see Figure 77–3,C) with a preoperative MAP 110 or greater (see Figure 77–3,A) are at greatest risk for intraoperative hemodynamic lability (hypertensive/hypotensive episodes). Charlson et al.'s data[20] also support a role for appropriate fluid management in decreasing hemodynamic lability; patients with a plasma volume greater than 3500 ml had a decreased incidence of intraoperative hypotension and hypertension episodes (see Figure 77–3,B).

Other than a few studies of spinal anesthesia,[16,21] there have been no studies comparing anesthetic effects (MAC, regional, centroneuraxial, and general) on BP response in hypertensive patients. To this end, we analyzed more than 120,000 anesthetic records stored in the Duke Anesthesia Database compiled by an automated anesthesia information system used at Duke University.[32] From the database 15,211 hypertensive patients where identified; their mean BP was recorded before initiating an anesthetic technique (MAC, centroneuraxial, major nerve block, or general) and then compared with their intraoperative highest and lowest mean BPs. Figure 77–4 shows the differences in change in MAP after induction of anesthesia among the anesthetic techniques. Reductions in BP are significantly ($p < .001$) greater with general and centroneuraxial anesthetics compared with MAC and major nerve block. The maximal mean BP intraoperatively was similar with all techniques. Patients with higher initial MAP had larger intraoperative reductions in BP after initiating anesthesia, regardless of the choice of techniques, confirming previous studies (see Figure 77–3,A).[20] These data support the notion that better BP control intraoperatively may be achieved with major nerve block anesthesia compared with general or centroneuraxial techniques. Many operations cannot be performed with nerve block anesthesia, however.

## Regional Anesthesia (Neuraxial and Major Nerve Blocks)

Regional anesthesia has theoretic advantages in the high-risk patient.[85] Because regional techniques do not involve intubation, paralysis, or mechanical ventilation with positive pressure, they are less physiologically intrusive and therefore may be better tolerated in patients predisposed to hemodynamic lability. Furthermore, the dense block provided by regional techniques almost eliminates the hypertensive response to surgical stimuli, and excellent postoperative analgesia (with major nerve block or epidural) may prevent hypertensive or ischemic responses to postoperative pain.[34]

Epidural and spinal anesthesia involve the injection of local anesthetic in or around the spinal cord to interrupt afferent impulses. The result is usually a dense sensory and motor block to the lower half of the body (T4-T10 dermatomal level and below depending on dose and technique). This block also produces a profound sympathectomy to the lower extremities and part of the splanchnic circulation, with resultant vasodilation and venodilation of these vascular beds. This reduction in preload, particularly in a hypertensive patient with mild

hypovolemia, left ventricular hypertrophy, and diastolic dysfunction, can cause a marked drop in cardiac output and BP. Racle et al.[21] compared the cardiovascular responses of normotensive and hypertensive patients after spinal anesthesia and found that hypertensive patients, on average, had a significantly larger drop in systolic, diastolic, and mean BPs compared with normotensive patients.

In general, patients with well-controlled hypertension tolerate lumbar and thoracic epidural block without unpredictable or profound decreases in arterial pressure. In contrast, a small group (n = 5) of patients with untreated hypertension showed an average decrease of 44% in systolic BP. Three of these patients required active intervention to correct the problem.[86] Finally, in a study by Garnett et al.[34] of patients (42% hypertensive) undergoing elective aortic surgery, epidural anesthesia in combination with general anesthesia reduced the risk of intraoperative hypertension compared with general anesthesia alone. Epidural anesthesia did not prevent, and possibly intensified, hypotension during the procedure. The hypotension was associated with a higher incidence of electrocardiographic evidence of myocardial ischemia.

Hypertensive patients have perioperative hemodynamic characteristics that are associated with increased perioperative complications. Untreated patients and those with severe hypertension are at particularly high risk. The hemodynamic patterns of the various anesthetic techniques in hypertensive patients are different, and improved perioperative outcome has not been demonstrated unequivocally for any of them. Each anesthetic technique has certain benefits and risks, as well as certain desirable and undesirable characteristics. For example, a technique that prevents hypertensive responses may make the patient prone to hypotension and ischemia. Rather than anesthetic technique, it is more likely that acute, aggressive treatment of perioperative hypotension, hypertension, tachycardia and ischemia is the key to improving perioperative outcomes. Brief periods of hypertension, hypotension, tachycardia or ischemia, if treated appropriately and promptly, are unlikely to have negative sequelae, whereas prolonged periods place the patient at increased risk.[20] Thus, an anesthesiologist familiar with the consequences of the anesthetic technique, appropriate intraoperative monitoring to detect rapid hemodynamic changes and ischemia, and aggressive correction of the hemodynamic disturbances, are more important than the choice of anesthetic technique alone.

## Outcome Studies

The majority of studies evaluating the effects of anesthetic technique (centroneuraxial, regional, or general) on cardiac morbidity and mortality were carried out in patients undergoing peripheral vascular surgery[87-90] or carotid endarterectomy.[91-94] The studies in patients undergoing peripheral vascular surgery all compare a centroneuraxial technique with general anesthesia. The largest study by Bode[87] randomly assigned 423 patients scheduled for elective femoral-distal vessel bypass surgery to one of three anesthetic techniques (spinal, epidural, or general). Using an intent-to-treat analysis, they reported no statistically significant differences between groups with regard to in hospital mortality, nonfatal myocardial infarction, angina, or CHF. Other studies comparing general anesthesia with combined epidural-general anesthesia for abdominal aortic surgery found no differences in perioperative cardiovascular outcome.[95,96] The carotid endarterectomy literature comparing regional anesthesia with general anesthesia has also failed to demonstrate a significant difference in cardiac outcome between techniques. Charlson,[20] looking at patients at risk for postoperative renal dysfunction (hypertensives and diabetics), concluded that patients whose MAP fell below the preoperative baseline (<20 mm Hg) for 60 minutes or greater or rose above baseline (>20 mm Hg) for greater than 30 minutes and received less than 3000 ml/hour of fluids had significantly increased postoperative renal dysfunction. Postoperative renal dysfunction varied with the anesthetic technique. The incidence of renal dysfunction was higher in patients receiving regional or centroneuraxial anesthesia than in those receiving general anesthesia. However, after further analysis, taking into account the occurrence of the three significant predictors of renal dysfunction listed previously, the type of anesthesia was not an independent predictor of postoperative renal dysfunction in these patients.

The incidence of perioperative stroke in the general surgery population is low, and it is unlikely that a study comparing the effects of different anesthetic techniques on stroke rate in hypertensive patients would show significant differences among techniques. A prospective study of this issue by Larsen[18] found that anesthetic technique was not a significant predictor of postoperative cerebrovascular accidents. Furthermore, the carotid endarterectomy literature has failed to demonstrate a difference in neurologic outcome between regional and general anesthetic techniques. There are no particular anesthetic techniques or specific drug combinations that have been shown to be better than others for the hypertensive patient. *The choice of general or regional anesthesia, or a combination of both, depends primarily on the skill and experience of the anesthesiologist rather than on the apparent suitability of any technique in the hands of others.*[16]

## Choice of Monitoring in Hypertensive Patients

Monitoring is a decision the anesthesiologist must make. A history of hypertension, by itself, is not a indication for additional hemodynamic monitoring. Rather, the patient's coexisting diseases (coronary artery disease, CHF, renal insufficiency, cerebrovascular disease), the planned operative procedure, and the duration of the procedure weigh more heavily into monitoring decisions. Routine monitoring for anesthesia includes noninvasive BP cuff, pulse oximetry, capnography, continuous electrocardiographic monitoring, and temperature monitoring. Invasive hemodynamic monitors (arterial line, central venous pressure, or pulmonary artery catheter) should not be used without considering the risks. Five-lead electrocardiographic monitoring should be used in hypertensive patients, because it enhances ischemia detection with no additional patient risk. Bladder catheterization should be considered for longer procedures to monitor urine output.

Intracranial, intrathoracic, major vascular, and cardiac surgery require invasive monitoring based on the hemodynamic insults and hemodynamic requirements of the procedure alone. Whereas a patient with severe renal disease, hypertension, angina, and a history of CHF could undergo the creation of a primary arteriovenous fistula under MAC with routine monitors, the same patient would require invasive arterial and central venous monitoring for a total hip replacement. For major or prolonged operations, it is preferable to monitor BP through an arterial line. When an arterial line is planned, it should be inserted before induction, because induction is one of the phases when cardiovascular lability is greatest.[2] In extensive surgeries, procedures with large intravascular volume shifts, hypertensive emergencies, and in the presence of severe myocardial dysfunction, central monitoring with a central venous or pulmonary artery catheter should be undertaken.[2,16,19] When uncertainty exists regarding monitoring, it is probably safer to err in favor of the monitoring device. Increased monitoring of high-risk cardiac patients during the perioperative period has been shown to decrease postoperative morbidity.[97]

In summary, although various monitoring approaches can be recommended, we believe that there is no preponderant evidence to support any particular anesthetic approach over another in the hypertensive patient.

## OPERATIVE COURSE

Before inducing anesthesia, the anesthesiologist must have a plan for managing intraoperative hemodynamics. This plan includes setting certain hemodynamic limits that will be tolerated intraoperatively. What are the safe levels for hypertension and hypotension? Some anesthesiologists attempt to maintain a patient's BP within 20% of the "preoperative baseline." Others review the medical record and pick a range of pressures at which the patient "normally lives" symptom free. For example, if a patient has a BP of 180/100 mm Hg during the daytime and 100/60 mm Hg at night, with neither causing physiologic insult, the patient should be able to tolerate these extremes under anesthesia. A patient's coexisting disease(s), the effect of hypertension on cerebral autoregulation, and the operative procedure are all considered. Thresholds may be lowered to prevent rupture of vascular anastomoses and may be raised to prevent cerebral ischemia during carotid endarterectomy.

The goal of this section is to not define acceptable limits or give management strategies based on certain procedures, but rather to illustrate some of the issues involved in the decision-making process. After setting the physiologic parameters, the pharmacologic means to achieve these goals must be considered. Again, the operative procedure is a major factor. For example, aortic and cardiac surgery demand precise hemodynamic control, and the use of a sodium nitroprusside infusion is routine. The management of cerebrovascular surgery also demands strict hemodynamic control. In this instance, the choice of pharmacologic intervention must take into account effects on cerebroautoregulation and intracranial pressure. Other procedures, such as resection of a carcinoid tumor or pheochromocytoma, have unique perioperative management strategies based on the pathophysiology of the hemodynamic derangement. For the majority of patients undergoing general surgical or orthopedic procedures, intermittent intravenous boluses of appropriate vasoactive drugs are used to control hemodynamics, whereas continuous infusion is used if the causes of hemodynamic perturbation are judged to be persistent.

## Induction and Intubation

Induction of anesthesia with rapidly acting intravenous drugs is acceptable, recognizing that an exaggerated decrease in BP may occur. The choice of induction agent is not as critical as the method of administration. A large initial bolus is more likely to cause hypotension than a slower, titrated induction. Use of pharmacologic agents that cause peripheral vasodilation in a population with elevated SVR and mild hypovolemia explains the common occurrence of hypotension. Giving a small volume load before induction may help attenuate this hypotensive response.

Laryngoscopy and intubation of the trachea can result in a hypertensive and tachycardic response in normotensive patients. The response in hypertensive patients, even those considered to be well treated, can be exaggerated. There are many ways of controlling the hemodynamic response to laryngoscopy and intubation.[98] Preoperative clonidine, topical treatment of the airway with lidocaine, intravenous lidocaine, intravenous nitroprusside, and intravenous esmolol before intubation are some of the reported methods.[25,99-101] Using a modest dose of narcotic (fentanyl 5-8 $\mu$g/kg) before intubation and limiting laryngoscopy to 15 seconds or less are also very effective in reducing the hemodynamic response. After intubation, the patient is often placed on mechanical, positive-pressure ventilation. This can cause a reduction in preload with a resultant drop in cardiac output and BP. Usually, gentle volume expansion resolves this problem.

## Maintenance and Emergence

The goal during maintenance of anesthesia is to anticipate surgical stimuli and adjust the anesthetic depth to minimize hemodynamic responses. This can be accomplished with any of a number of techniques. Often, a "balanced" technique is used. The combination of $N_2O$, a narcotic, and a low-dose inhalation agent provides a technique that is rapidly titratable to operative stimuli and hemodynamic responses. Both inhalation and intravenous drugs should be given to maintain therapeutic levels; thus, continuous administration is the most rational method.[102] Appropriate fluid management to minimize direct and indirect intravascular volume change also limits hemodynamic lability during maintenance. Preoperative treatment with clonidine improves intraoperative hemodynamics in hypertensive patients,[103,104] and perioperative β-blocker administration can blunt the hypertensive and tachycardic response to noxious stimuli.[12,105] The benefits of perioperative β-blocker treatment in reducing perioperative ischemia[9] and decreasing cardiovascular morbidity and mortality in high-risk patients[26] cannot be overemphasized.

Hypertension that occurs during maintenance of anesthesia can be treated by increasing anesthetic depth or by administering an intravenous antihypertensive agent. Drugs commonly used intraoperatively include labetalol, esmolol, metoprolol, and hydralazine. Intravenous calcium channel blockers and angiotensin-converting enzyme inhibitors are also available. Severe, resistant hypertension is usually managed with intravenous infusions of sodium nitroprusside or nitroglycerin, or a combination of both. Fenoldopam, a selective dopamine $D_1$-agonist, is useful in the management of resistant/emergent hypertensive episodes. Administered by a continuous infusion, fenoldopam has efficacy and titratability similar to those of nitroprusside. In addition to lowering BP, fenoldopam significantly increases urine flow, sodium excretion, and creatinine clearance.[105-108] Fenoldopam may be the antihypertensive drug of choice in certain patient populations (i.e., those with renal insufficiency).

Intraoperative hypotension can be treated by decreasing anesthetic depth, increasing intravenous fluids, or giving a sympathomimetic drug, such as phenylephrine or ephedrine. Although phenylephrine and ephedrine usually resolve hypotension and help preserve vital organ perfusion, this treatment should be considered a temporizing measure until the underlying problem is identified and corrected.

Emergence from anesthesia involves turning off the anesthetic agent and allowing the patient to awaken. Tracheal stimulation from the endotracheal tube and operative pain can cause severe hypertension at this point secondary to catecholamine responses.[7] Pharmacologic means of blunting the pressor responses are options for managing emergence.

## POSTOPERATIVE MANAGEMENT

Perioperative hypertension is associated with many adverse outcomes (Box 77–3) and should be prevented. Aggressive treatment to prevent myocardial ischemia, CHF, stroke, bleeding, and rupture of vascular suture lines is necessary. One of the most significant predictors of postoperative hypertension is a history of preoperative hypertension.[109] Although the hypertension may not have an identifiable cause, secondary etiologies should be considered. Excluding postoperative pain, hypoxia, and hypercarbia should be routine. Iatrogenic hypervolemia can cause hypertension, as can a distended bladder. Aggressive postoperative pain management may decrease the incidence of postoperative hypertension and cardiac morbidity.[110] Management of hypertension in the immediate postoperative period should be an extension of the intraoperative plan. Invasive monitoring should be continued until the patient becomes hemodynamically stable. The same intravenous agents used intraoperatively can be used postoperatively until the patient can return to his or her oral regimen, which should be restarted as soon as possible.[111] In some settings, it is appropriate to have an internist and/or cardiologist consultant assist in the postoperative control of BP.

---

**Box 77–3** Consequences of Perioperative Hypertension

Mortality
Myocardial ischemia
Myocardial infarction
Increased hemorrhage (surgical bleeding)
Intracranial hemorrhage
Disruption of vascular surgical incision sites
Congestive heart failure
Increased intracranial pressure
Hypertensive encephalopathy
Prolonged hospital stay
Added hospital costs

From Skarvan K. Perioperative hypertension: New strategies for management. Curr Opin Anaesthesiol 11:29-35, 1998.

## SUMMARY

Hypertension is the most prevalent circulatory disorder in the United States, affecting approximately 60 million people. Surgical patients with hypertension are at increased risk for perioperative hemodynamic lability, myocardial ischemia, myocardial infarction, CHF, renal failure, and stroke (see Box 77–3). Hypertensive patients often have significant coexisting disease, and appropriate preoperative evaluation and use of consultants are necessary to optimize these patients' medical management and minimize their perioperative risk. Patients with well-controlled hypertension have a lower risk for perioperative complications than patients with uncontrolled hypertension. Elective procedures should be postponed and appropriate medical management initiated when uncontrolled hypertension is evident (BP ≥110 mm Hg diastolic). No particular anesthetic technique (general, centroneuraxial, major nerve block, MAC) has been shown to improve morbidity and mortality in the hypertensive patient. However, familiarity with the hemodynamic consequences of the various anesthetic techniques; knowledge of the interactions between antihypertensive medications and anesthetic agents; appropriate hemodynamic monitoring; and early recognition and treatment of intraoperative hypertension, hypotension, tachycardia, and ischemia are necessary. The development of postoperative hypertension also requires swift detection and treatment to prevent perioperative complications. In short, the hypertensive surgical patient is at increased risk for perioperative morbidity and mortality. These risks can be minimized with optimal preoperative preparation and prompt assessment and treatment of adverse hemodynamic changes in the intraoperative and postoperative period.

## References

1. Barker WH, Mullcoly JP, Linton KLP. Trends in hypertension prevalence, treatment, and control in a well-defined older population. Hypertension 31:552-559, 1998.
2. Foex P. Anesthesia for the hypertensive patients. Cleve Clin Q 48:63-67, 1981.
3. Skarvan K. Perioperative hypertension: New strategies for management. Curr Opin Anaesthesiol 11:29-35, 1998.
4. Goldman L, Caldera DL. Risks of general anesthesia and elective operation in the hypertensive patient. Anesthesiology 50:285-292, 1979.
5. Estafanous FG, Tarazi RC, Viljonan JR, et al. Systemic hypertension following myocardial revascularization. Am Heart J 85:732-738, 1973.
6. Hans SS, Glover JL. The relationship of cardiac and neurological complications to blood pressure changes following carotid endarterectomy. Am Surg 61:356-359, 1995.
7. Wallach R, Karp RB, Reves JG, et al. Pathogenesis of paroxysmal hypertension developing during and after coronary artery bypass surgery: A study of hemodynamic and humoral factors. Am J Cardiol 46:559-565, 1980.
8. Joint National Committee on Detection, Evaluation, and Treatment of High Blood Pressure. The fifth report. Arch Intern Med 153:154-183, 1993.
9. Stone JG, Foex P, Sear JW, et al. Risk of myocardial ischaemia during anaesthesia in treated and untreated hypertensive patients. Br J Anaesth 61:675-679, 1988.
10. Prys-Roberts CV, Meloche R, Foex P, et al. Studies of anaesthesia in relation to hypertension. I: Cardiovascular responses of treated and untreated patients. Br J Anaesth 43:122-137, 1971.
11. Bedford RF, Feinstein B. Hospital admission blood pressure: A predictor of hypertension following endotracheal intubation. Anesth Analg 59:367-370, 1980.
12. Prys-Roberts C, Foex P, Biro GP, et al. Studies of anaesthesia in relation to hypertension. Adrenergic beta-receptor blockade. Br J Anaesth 45:671-680, 1973.
13. Prys-Roberts C, Greene LT, Meloche R, et al. Studies of anaesthesia in relation to hypertension. Haemodynamic consequences of induction and endotracheal intubation. Br J Anaesth 43:531-546, 1971.
14. Steen PA, Tinker, JH, Tarhan S. Myocardial reinfarction after anesthesia and surgery. JAMA 239:2566-2570, 1978.
15. Charlson ME, MacKenzie CR, Gold JP, et al. Postoperative renal dysfunction can be predicted. Surg Gynecol Obstet 169:303-309, 1989.
16. Prys-Roberts C. Anaesthesia and hypertension. Br J Anaesth 56:711-724, 1984.
17. Asiddao CB, Donegan JH, Whitsell RC, et al. Factors associated with perioperative complications during carotid endarterectomy. Anesth Analg 61:631-637, 1982.
18. Larsen SF, Zaric D, Boysen G. Postoperative cerebrovascular accidents in general surgery. Acta Anaesthesiol Scand 32:698-701, 1988.
19. Estafanous F. Hypertension in the surgical patient: Management of blood pressure and anesthesia. Cleve Clin J Med 56:385-393, 1989.
20. Charlson ME, MacKenzie CR, Gold JP, et al. Preoperative characteristics predicting intraoperative hypotension and hypertension among hypertensives and diabetics undergoing noncardiac surgery. Ann Surg 212:66-81, 1990.
21. Racle JP, Poy JY, Haberer JP, et al. A comparison of cardiovascular responses of normotensive and hypertensive elderly patients following bupivacaine spinal anesthesia. Reg Anesth 14:66-71, 1989.
22. Slogoff S, Keats AS. Does perioperative myocardial ischemia lead to postoperative myocardial infarction? Anesthesia 62:107-114, 1985.
23. Reves JG, Gelman S. Cardiovascular effects of intravenous anesthetic drugs. In Covino F, Rehder K, Strichartz GR (eds). Effects of Anesthesia. Bethesda, MD, American Physiological Society, 1985; pp 179-193.
24. Freis ED. Salt in hypertension and the effects of diuretics. Annu Rev Pharmacol Toxicol 19:13-23, 1979.
25. Sharma S, Mitra S, Grover VK, et al. Esmolol blunts the haemodynamic responses to tracheal intubation in treated hypertensive patients. Can J Anaesth 43:778-782, 1996.
26. Mangano DT, Layug EL, Wallace A, et al. Effect of atenolol on mortality and cardiovascular morbidity after noncardiac surgery. N Engl J Med 335:1713-1720, 1996.
27. Quintin L, Bouilloc X, Butin E, et al. Clonidine for major vascular surgery in hypertensive patients: a double-blind, controlled randomized study. Anesth Analg 83:687-695, 1996.
28. Reves J, Sladen R, Newman F. Multicenter study of target-controlled infusion of propofol-sufentanil or sufentanil-midazolm for coronary artery bypass graft surgery. Anesthesiology 85:522-535, 1996.
29. Reves JG, Hill S, Berkowitz D. Pharmacology of intravenous anesthetic induction drugs. In Kaplan J, Reich DL, Konstadt SN (eds). Cardiac Anesthesia, 4th ed. Philadelphia, WB Saunders, 1999; pp 611-634.
30. Reves JG, Greeley WJ, Grichnik K, et al. Anesthesia and supportive care for cardiothoracic surgery. In Sabiston DC Jr, Spencer FC (eds). Surgery of the Chest, 6th ed. Philadelphia, WB Saunders, 1995; pp 117-152.
31. Dentz ME, Grichnik KP, Sibert KS, et al. Anesthesia and postoperative analgesia. In Sabiston DC Jr (ed). Textbook of Surgery. Philadelphia, WB Saunders, 1996; pp 186-206.

32. Gould JD, Reves JG, D'Ercole FJ, et al. Effect of anesthetic technique on blood pressure response in hypertensive patients. Anesth Analg 88:SCA62, 1999.

33. Khatri I, Freis E. Hemodynamic changes during sleep. J Appl Physiol 22:867, 1967.

34. Garnett RL, MacIntyre A, Lindsay P, et al. Perioperative ischaemia in aortic surgery: combined epidural/general anesthesia and epidural analgesia vs. general anaesthesia and IV analgesia. Can J Anaesth 43:769-777, 1996.

35. Olesen A, Huttel M, Hole P. Venous sequelae following the injection of etomidate or thiopentone IV. Br J Anaesth 56:171-173, 1984.

36. Seltzer J, Gerson J, Allen F. Comparison of the cardiovascular effects of bolus v. incremental administration of thiopentone. Br J Anaesth 52:527-530, 1980.

37. Sonntag H, Hellberg K, Schenk H, et al. Effects of thiopental (trapanal) on coronary blood flow and myocardial metabolism in man. Acta Anaesthesiol Scand 19:69-78, 1975.

38. Toner W, Howard P, McGowan W, et al. Another look at acute tolerance to thiopentone. Br J Anesth 52:1005-1008, 1980.

39. Frankl W, Poole-Wilson P. Effects of thiopental on tension development, action potential, and exchange of calcium and potassium in rabbit ventricular myocardium. J Cardiovasc Pharmacol 3:554-565, 1981.

40. Christensen J, Andreasen F, Jansen J. Pharmacokinetics and pharmacodynamics of thiopentone. A comparison between young and elderly patients. Anaesthesia 37:398, 1982.

41. Filner B, Karliner J. Alterations of normal left ventricular performance by general anesthesia. Anesthesiology 45:610-621, 1976.

42. Reiz S, Balfors E, Friedman A, et al. Effects of thiopentone on cardiac performance, coronary hemodynamics and myocardial oxygen consumption in chronic ischemic heart disease. Acta Anaesthesiol Scand 25:103-110, 1981.

43. White P. Comparative evaluation of intravenous agents for rapid sequence induction—Thiopental, ketamine and midazolam. Anesthesiology 57:279-284, 1982.

44. Flickinger H, Fraimow W, Cathcart R, et al. Effect of thiopental induction on cardiac output in man. Anesth Analg 40:693-700, 1961.

45. Pedersen T, Engback J, Klausen N, et al. Effects of low-dose ketamine and thiopentone on cardiac performance and myocardial oxygen balance in high-risk patients. Acta Anaesthesiol Scand 26:235-239, 1982.

46. King E. The treatment of army casualties in Hawaii. Army Med Bull 61:18, 1942.

47. Richter J. Current theories about the mechanisms of benzodiazepines and neuroleptic drugs. Anesthesiology 54:66-72, 1981.

48. Rao S, Sherbanuik R, Prasad K, et al. Cardiopulmonary effects of diazepam. Clin Pharmacol Ther 14:182-189, 1973.

49. Prakash R, Thurer R, Vargas A, et al. Cardiovascular effects of diazepam induction in patients for aortocoronary saphenous vein bypass grafts. Abstracts of Scientific Papers. ASA Annual Meeting. San Francisco, October 1976.

50. Jackson A, Dhadphale P, Callaghan M, et al. Haemodynamic studies during induction of anaesthesia for open-heart surgery using diazepam and ketamine. Br J Anaesth 50:375-377, 1978.

51. McCammon R, Hilgenberg J, Stoelting R. Hemodynamic effects of diazepam and diazepam-nitrous oxide in patients with coronary artery disease. Anesth Analg 59:438-441, 1980.

52. Samuelson P, Leil W, Kouchoukos N, et al. Hemodynamics during diazepam induction of anesthesia for coronary artery bypass grafting. South Med J 73:332-334, 1980.

53. Samuelson P, Reves J, Kouchoukos N, et al. Hemodynamic responses to anesthetic induction with midazolam or diazepam in patients with ischemic heart disease. Anesth Analg 60:802-809, 1981.

54. D'Amelio G, Volta S, Stritoni P, et al. Acute cardiovascular effects of diazepam in patients with mitral valve disease. Eur J Clin Pharmacol 6:61-65, 1973.

55. Bailey P, Stanley T. Pharmacology of intravenous narcotic anesthetics. In Miller R (ed). Anesthesia. London, Churchill Livingstone, 1986; pp 745-798.

56. Hoar P, Nelson N, Mangano D, et al. Adrenergic response to morphine-diazepam anesthesia for myocardial revascularization. Anesth Analg 60:406-411, 1981.

57. Melsom M, Andreassen P, Melsom H, et al. Diazepam in acute myocardial infarction. Clinical effects and effects on catecholamines, free fatty acids and cortisol. Br Heart J 38:804-808, 1976.

58. Stanley T, Bennett G, Loeser E, et al. Cardiovascular effects of diazepam and droperidol during morphine anesthesia. Anesthesiology 44:255-258, 1976.

59. Tomichek R, Rosow C, Schneider R, et al. Cardiovascular effects of diazepam-fentanyl anesthesia in patients with coronary artery disease. Anesth Analg 61:217-218, 1982.

60. Reves J, Fragen R, Vinik H, et al. Midazolam: Pharmacology and uses. Anesthesiology 62:310-321, 1985.

61. Reves J, Samuelson P, Lewis S. Midazolam maleate induction in patients with ischemic heart disease. Haemodynamic observations. Can Anaesth Soc J 26:402-409, 1979.

62. Reves J, Samuelson P, Linnan M. Effects of midazolam maleate in patients with elevated pulmonary artery occluded pressure. In Aldrete J, Stanley T (eds). Trends in Intravenous Anesthesia. Chicago, Year Book Medical, 1980; pp 253-257.

63. Lunn J, Stanley T, Eisele J, et al. High-dose fentanyl anesthesia for coronary artery surgery. Plasma fentanyl concentrations and influence of nitrous oxide on cardiovascular responses. Anesth Analg 58:390-395, 1979.

64. Melvin M, Johnson B, Quasha A, et al. Induction of anesthesia with midazolam decreases halothane MAC in humans. Anesthesiology 57:238-241, 1982.

65. Newman M, Reves J. Pro: midazolam is the sedative of choice to supplement narcotic anesthesia (Review). J Cardiothorac Vasc Anesth 7:615-619, 1993.

66. Theil D, Stanley T, White W, et al. Midazolam and fentanyl continuous infusion anesthesia for cardiac surgery: A comparison of computer-assisted versus manual infusion systems. J Cardiothorac Vasc Anesth 7:300-306, 1993.

67. Kay B, Rolly G. ICI 35 868, a new intravenous induction agent. Acta Anaesth Belg 28:303-307, 1977.

68. Profeta J, Guffin A, Mikula S, et al. The hemodynamic effects of propofol and thiamylal sodium for induction in coronary artery surgery. Anesth Analg 66:S142, 1987.

69. De Hert S, Vermeyen K, Adrensen H. Influence of thiopental, etomidate and propofol on regional myocardial function in the normal and acute ischemic heart segment in dogs. Anesth Analg 70:600-607, 1990.

70. Mulier J, Wouters P, Van Aken H, et al. Cardiodynamic effects of propofol in comparison with thiopental: Assessment with a transesophageal echocardiographic approach. Anesth Analg 72:28-35, 1991.

71. Brussel T, Theissen J, Vigfusson G, et al. Hemodynamic and cardiodynamic effects of propofol and etomidate: Negative inotropic properties of propofol. Anesth Analg 69:35-40, 1989.

72. Patrick M, Blair I, Feneck R, et al. Comparison of the hemodynamic effects of propofol (diprivan) on thiopentone in patients with coronary artery disease. Postgrad Med J 61:23-27, 1985.

73. Vermeyen K, Erpels F, Janssen L, et al. Propofol-fentanyl anaesthesia for coronary bypass surgery in patients with good left ventricular function. Br J Anaesth 59:1115-1120, 1987.

74. Stephan H, Sonntag H, Schenk H, et al. Effects of propofol on cardiovascular dynamics, myocardial blood flow and myocardial metabolism in patients with coronary artery disease. Br J Anaesth 58:969-975, 1986.

75. Brown B, Crout R. A comparative study of the effects of five general anesthetics on myocardial contractility. Anesthesiology 34:236-245, 1971.

76. Merin RG, Basch S. Are the myocardial functional and metabolic effects of isoflurane really different from those of halothane and enflurane? Anesthesiology 55:398-408, 1981.

77. Price ML, Price HL. Effect of general anesthetics on contractile response of rabbit aorta strips. Anesthesiology 23:16-20, 1962.

78. Mallow JE, White RD, Cucchiara RF. Hemodynamic effects of isoflurane and halothane in patients with coronary artery disease. Anesth Analg 55:135-138, 1976.

79. Kleinman B, Szinn E, Shah K, et al. The value to the anesthesia-surgical care team of the preoperative cardiac consultation. J Cardiothorac Anesth 3:682-687, 1989.

80. Wells PH, Kaplan JA. Optimal management of patients with ischemic heart disease for noncardiac surgery by complementary anesthesiologist and cardiologist interaction. Am Heart J 102:1029-1037, 1981.

81. Eagle KA, Berger PB, Calkins H, et al. ACC/AHA guideline update for perioperative cardiovascular evaluation for noncardiac surgery—Executive summary. J Am Coll Cardiol 39:542-553, 2002.

82. Goldman L, Lee T, Rudd P. Ten commandments for effective consultations. Arch Intern Med 143:1753-1755, 1983.

83. Lee T, Pappius EM, Goldman L. Impact of inter-physician communication on the effectiveness of medical consultations. Am J Med 74:106-112, 1983.

84. Rudd P. Contrasts in academic consultation. Ann Intern Med 94:537-538, 1981.

85. Yaeger MP, Glass DD, Neff RK, et al. Epidural anesthesia and analgesia in high-risk surgical patients. Anesthesiology 66:729-736, 1987.

86. Dagnino J, Prys-Roberts C. Evaluation of beta-adrenoceptor responsiveness during anesthesia in humans. Anesth Analg 62:255, 1983.

87. Bode RH, Lewis KP, Zarich SW, et al. Cardiac outcome after peripheral vascular surgery. Anesthesiology 84:3-13, 1996.

88. Cook PT, Davies MJ, Cronin KD, et al. A prospective randomized trial comparing spinal anaesthesia using hyperbaric cinocaine with general anaesthesia for lower limb vascular surgery. Anaesth Intensive Care 14:373-380, 1986.

89. Rivers SP, Scher LA, Sheehan E, et al. Epidural versus general anesthesia for intrainguinal arterial reconstruction. J Vasc Surg 14:764-770, 1991.

90. Christopherson R, Beattie C, Frank SM, et al. Perioperative morbidity in patients randomized to epidural or general anesthesia for lower extremity vascular surgery. Anesthesiology 79:422-434, 1993.

91. CASANOVA Study Group. Carotid surgery versus medical therapy in asymptomatic carotid stenosis. Stroke 22:1229-1235, 1991.

92. Executive Committee for the Asymptomatic Carotid Atherosclerosis Study. Endarterectomy for asymptomatic carotid artery stenosis. JAMA 273:1421-1428, 1995.

93. Godin MS, Bell WH, Schwedler M, et al. Cost effectiveness of regional anesthesia in carotid endarterectomy. Am Surg 55:656-659, 1989.

94. Shah DM, Darling RC, Chang BB, et al. Carotid endarterectomy in awake patients: Its safety, acceptability, and outcome. J Vasc Surg 19:1015-1020, 1994.

95. Haku E, Hayashi M, Kato H. Anesthetic management of abdominal aortic surgery: A retrospective review of perioperative complications. J Cardiothorac Anesth 3:587-591, 1989.

96. Baron JF, Bertrand M, Barre E, et al. Combined epidural and general anesthesia versus general anesthesia for abdominal aortic surgery. Anesthesiology 75:611-618, 1991.

97. Rao TLK, Jacobs KH, El-Etr AA. Reinfarction following anesthesia in patients with myocardial infarction. Anesthesiology 59:499-505, 1983.

98. Kovac AL. Controlling the hemodynamic response to laryngoscopy and endotracheal intubation. J Clin Anesth 8:63-79, 1996.

99. Stoelting RK. Circulatory response to laryngoscopy and tracheal intubation with or without prior oropharyngeal viscous lidocaine. Anesth Analg 56:618-621, 1977.

100. Stoelting RK. Circulatory changes during direct laryngoscopy and tracheal intubation: Influence of duration of laryngoscopy with or without prior lidocaine. Anesthesiology 47:381-384, 1977.

101. Stoelting RK. Attenuation of blood pressure response to laryngoscopy and tracheal intubation with sodium nitroprusside. Anesth Analg 58:116-119, 1979.

102. Smith BE, Reves JG. Computer-assisted continuous infusion of intravenous anesthesia drugs. Int Anesthesiol Clin 33:3, 1995.

103. Ghignone M, Calvillo O, Quintin L. Anesthesia and hypertension: The effect of clonidine on perioperative hemodynamics and isoflurane requirements. Anesthesiology 67:3-10, 1987.

104. Flacke JW, Bloor BC, Flacke WE, et al. Reduced narcotic requirement by clonidine with improved hemodynamic and adrenergic stability in patients undergoing coronary bypass surgery. Anesthesiology 67:11-19, 1987.

105. Prys-Roberts C. Interactions of anesthesia and high preoperative doses of beta-receptor antagonists. Acta Anaesthesiol Scand 74:447-453, 1982.

106. Elliott WJ, Weber RR, Nelson KS, et al. Renal and hemodynamic effects of intravenous fenoldopam versus nitroprusside in severe hypertension. Circulation 81:970-977, 1990.

107. Murphy MB, McCoy CE, Weber RR, et al. Augmentation of renal blood flow and sodium excretion in hypertensive patients during blood pressure reduction by intravenous administration of the dopamine-1 agonist fenoldopam. Circulation 76:1312-1318, 1987.

108. Panacek EA, Bednarczyk EM, Dunbar LM, et al. Randomized prospective trial of fenoldopam vs sodium nitroprusside in the treatment of acute severe hypertension. Acad Emerg Med 2:959-965, 1995.

109. Gal TJ, Cooperman LH. Hypertension in the immediate postoperative period. Br J Anaesth 47:70-74, 1975.

110. Weiss SJ, Longnecker DE. Perioperative hypertension: An overview. Coron Artery Dis 4:401-406, 1993.

111. Joint National Committee on Prevention, Detection, Evaluation, and Treatment of High Blood Pressure. The sixth report. Arch Intern Med 157:2413-2446, 1997.

# Chapter 78

# Management of Hypertensive Emergencies and Urgencies

## Donald G. Vidt

The term *hypertensive crisis* includes a spectrum of clinical situations with different severities of blood pressure (BP) elevation and variable degrees of urgency of initial treatment. Hypertensive crisis affects upward of 500,000 Americans each year. Although the incidence of hypertensive crisis is low, affecting fewer than 1% of hypertensive adults, more than 50 million American adults suffer from hypertension. Hypertensive crises are classified as hypertensive emergencies or hypertensive urgencies, based on the presence or absence of progressive target organ dysfunction.[1]

Hypertensive emergencies are severe elevations in BP that are complicated by evidence of progressive target organ dysfunction such as coronary ischemia, disordered cerebral function, a cerebrovascular event, pulmonary edema, or renal failure.[2,3] These patients warrant immediate admission to an intensive care unit (ICU) for parenteral administration of antihypertensive agents. Hypertensive urgencies are severe elevations in BP, without evidence of progressive target organ dysfunction and can usually be managed by orally administered medications initiated in the emergency department (ED) with appropriate follow-up within 24 hours to several days, depending on individual characteristics of the patient.

Most hypertensive urgencies or emergencies are preventable and are the result of inadequate treatment of mild-to-moderate hypertension or nonadherence to antihypertensive therapy. Improved treatment of hypertension in the United States, despite suboptimal control rates, has resulted in progressive decline in patients presenting with crisis levels of BP. Hypertensive crises continue to be a major problem in many other parts of the world and, in the United States, may still represent approximately 5% of patients seen in the EDs of large urban hospitals.[4] Previously unrecognized forms of secondary hypertension, such as renovascular hypertension, renal parenchymal disease, or pheochromocytoma, and rarely, primary hyperaldosteronism, may be responsible and will require early recognition if a specific therapy is to be initiated. Prompt, thorough assessment by ED staff will identify the clinical status of the patient, provide clues to an underlying etiology for the hypertension, assess the degree of target organ involvement, and assist in selecting the most appropriate pharmacologic agent and method of administration.

## Etiology

The manifestations seen in patients presenting with hypertensive crises are due to an extreme, or sometimes rapid elevation in BP. Such emergencies may present as progressive worsening of long-standing chronic hypertension as represented by the syndrome of accelerated or malignant hypertension, or as a rapid or sudden rise in BP in a previously normotensive patient.[5,6] Examples of this latter presentation may be associated with conditions, such as acute glomerulonephritis, preeclampsia, or scleroderma renal disease, in which the rapid progress of the disease is associated with sudden onset and rapid acceleration of hypertension. Further risk to target organ function results from vascular damage or circulatory disturbances caused by the extreme elevation of BP.

Hypertensive emergencies occur in association with underlying target organ complications, such as acute myocardial infarction or acute aortic dissection, or in association with progressive deterioration in target organ function, such as hypertensive encephalopathy, acute congestive heart failure, or rapidly deteriorating renal function. Although these conditions require immediate antihypertensive therapy, keep in mind that the presenting level of BP alone does not determine the presence or absence of a hypertensive emergency. Rather, BP must be viewed together with other comorbidities and the degree of target organ dysfunction. The patient with a long history of hypertension who presents with malignant hypertension and hypertensive encephalopathy is likely to have a markedly elevated BP in the range of 220 to 240 over 140 mm Hg. In contrast, a patient presenting with an aortic dissection or acute pulmonary edema may have only modest elevations of BP in the range of 150 to 160 over 100 mm Hg. Yet, both represent hypertensive emergencies and require immediate therapy.

## Accelerated or Malignant Hypertension

Malignant hypertension constitutes a syndrome of severe elevations of mean arterial pressure (MAP) often to or exceeding 140 mm Hg, manifested clinically by retinal hemorrhages, exudates, and papilledema. The term *malignant* hypertension was formerly reserved for those patients who exhibited advanced funduscopic changes, including papilledema, whereas the term *accelerated* hypertension was used when the syndrome was observed without papilledema.

The distinction between accelerated and malignant hypertension has been deemphasized because the short- and long-term prognoses are independent of the presence or absence of papilledema, and both the pathogenesis and clinical management of accelerated and malignant hypertension are the same.[7,8] In addition, the presence of papilledema may be difficult to detect on funduscopic examination and is subject to observer interpretation.[9]

Vascular damage is believed to relate both to the duration and severity of the elevated MAP. Untreated or inadequately treated essential hypertension represents the most common antecedent of malignant hypertension and has been observed to be more common among smokers.[10] With improved hypertension control efforts, progression to the malignant phase of hypertension is seen less commonly. Secondary etiologies of hypertension are more prevalent among patients who do progress to accelerated or malignant hypertension.

## Pathophysiology

The vascular lesions of accelerated-malignant hypertension consist predominately of myointimal proliferation and fibrinoid necrosis.[11] The myointimal proliferation is a common feature of sustained hypertension, and its severity will vary with the severity and duration of the hypertension. The combination of medial thickening and cellular intimal proliferation contribute to the "onion skin" appearance of small arteries. These changes reduce lumen diameter over time.[5,11]

The accelerated phase of hypertension is characterized by fibrinoid necrosis, which can further compromise the lumen and small vessels. Fibrinoid necrosis within the kidney contributes to rapid progression of renal insufficiency, but these changes may be reversible with aggressive lowering of BP.

In Caucasians, essential hypertension accounts for only 20% to 30% of malignant hypertension, whereas among African Americans, essential hypertension is the predominant cause of malignant hypertension, accounting for upward of 80% of all cases. Hypertension-related morbidity and mortality from causes such as stroke, end-stage renal disease (ESRD), and heart failure are three to five times higher among African Americans. Interaction of genetic and environmental factors appears to play a role, as does low socioeconomic status.

Renal parenchymal disease and renovascular hypertension account for the majority of secondary causes of accelerated-malignant hypertension in all populations. Vascular changes within the kidney correlate well with the development of renal failure, and impaired perfusion caused by occlusion of renal vessels leads to ischemic damage, renal scarring, and glomerulosclerosis.

Endocrine and paracrine mediators and the renin-angiotensin system are activated in accelerated-malignant hypertension, and increased angiotensin II can lead to further renal vasoconstriction and ischemia.[12-14] Volume depletion due to pressure natriuresis stimulates further renin release and worsens the hypertension. Stimulation of other humoral factors, such as catecholamines and vasopressin, contributes to the pathophysiologic process of accelerated-malignant hypertension, although much of the documentation relating levels of BP elevation to vascular changes is drawn from animal models. Whether these animal models are applicable to all human accelerated-malignant hypertension remains uncertain. Experimental models of renal artery stenosis share some pathophysiologic features with renovascular hypertension in humans, a well-documented cause of accelerated-malignant hypertension.

## Initial Assessment

Early triage is critical in an effort to assure the most timely and appropriate therapy for each patient. Prompt evaluation by the ED is designed to establish the clinical status of the patient, provide clues to a possible underlying etiology of the hypertension, assess the degree of target organ involvement, and facilitate selection of the most suitable pharmacologic agent and method of administration.[15]

## Initial History

A brief but thorough history should address the duration and the severity of hypertension, all current medications, including prescription and nonprescription drugs, and the use of recreational drugs. A history of other comorbid conditions and prior cardiovascular or renal disease is critical to the initial evaluation.

Patients should be questioned directly regarding the level of compliance with current antihypertensive medications in an effort to establish current adequacy of therapy. Frequent or continuous monitoring of BP should be established during this evaluation. Historical information about neurologic, cardiovascular, and/or renal symptoms and specific manifestations, such as headache, seizures, chest pain, dyspnea, and edema, should be sought. In patients with encephalopathic symptoms and impaired cognitive function, the availability of a close family member may be critical to obtaining part or all of the history.

## Physical Examination

Begin with an assessment of BP, using an appropriate sized cuff, in both upper extremities. Careful funduscopic examination should detect any hemorrhages, exudates, and/or papilledema. Verify brachial, femoral, and carotid pulses. A careful cardiovascular examination and a thorough neurologic examination, including mental status assessment, should be conducted. Your physical assessment should help determine the degree of involvement of affected target organs and will often provide clues to the possible existence of a secondary form of hypertension, such as renovascular hypertension. If a secondary cause of hypertension is suspected, appropriate blood and urine samples should be obtained before aggressive therapy is initiated.

## Initial Laboratory Studies

A urinalysis with sediment examination, a stat chemistry profile, and an electrocardiogram should be obtained immediately. The urinalysis may show significant proteinuria, red blood cells, and/or cellular casts. Cellular casts are suggestive of renal parenchymal disease. Electrolyte abnormalities, particularly hypokalemia or hypomagnesemia, increase the risk of cardiac arrhythmias, and the chemistry profile may also provide evidence of renal dysfunction. The electrocardiogram can provide evidence of coronary ischemia or left ventricular hypertrophy. A computed tomography (CT) scan of the head should be obtained when the physical examination suggests stroke, or in the comatose patient.

This initial evaluation should identify the patient with a hypertensive emergency as opposed to a hypertensive urgency or severe elevated BP.[15] The algorithm outlined in Table 78–1 will assist the clinician in distinguishing the characteristics of the hypertensive emergency from those of a hypertensive urgency or elevated BP. In the case of a hypertensive emergency, BP reduction should not be delayed until the results of all diagnostic tests are available, but should be initiated as soon as the patient's clinical status is established. Initial therapy will often be based on a presumptive diagnosis made during the initial triage evaluation.

**Table 78-1** Algorithm: Triage Evaluation

| BP (mm Hg) | Group I—High BP >180/100 | Group II—Urgency ≥180/110 | Group III—Emergency Usually >220/140 |
|---|---|---|---|
| Symptoms | • Headache <br> • Anxiety <br> • Often asymptomatic | • Severe headache <br> • Shortness of breath <br> • Edema | • Shortness of breath <br> • Chest pain <br> • Nocturia <br> • Dysarthria <br> • Weakness <br> • Altered consciousness |
| Examination | • No target organ damage (TOD) <br><br> • No clinical cardiovascular (CV) disease | • TOD <br><br> • Clinical CV disease present or stable | • Encephalopathy <br> • Pulmonary edema <br> • Renal insufficiency <br> • Cerebrovascular accident <br> • Cardiac ischemia |
| Therapy | • Observe 1-3 hours <br> • Initiate/resume medication(s) <br><br> • Increase dosage of inadequate agent | • Observe 3-6 hours <br> • Lower BP with short-acting oral agents <br> • Adjust current therapy | • Baseline laboratory tests <br> • Intravenous line <br> • Monitor BP <br> • May initiate parenteral therapy in the emergency department |
| Plan | • Arrange follow-up >72 hours <br><br> • If no prior evaluation, schedule appointment | • Arrange follow-up evaluation <24 hours | • Immediate admission to ICU <br> • Treat to initial goal BP <br> • Additional diagnostic studies |

BP, blood pressure; ICU, intensive care unit. (From Vidt DG. Emergency room management of hypertensive urgencies and emergencies. J Clin Hypertens [Greenwich] 3:158-164, 2001.)

## Hypertensive Emergencies

The clinical characteristics of a hypertensive emergency are listed in Box 78–1. Keep in mind the important caveat that the level of BP alone does not determine a hypertensive emergency; rather, it is the degree of target organ involvement that determines the rapidity with which BP should be treated and reduced to a safer level to prevent or limit further target organ damage.

In both hypertensive and normotensive individuals, cerebral blood flow is effectively autoregulated, enabling the brain to maintain a constant blood flow, despite changes in perfusion pressure. A rightward shift in autoregulation is seen in patients with chronic hypertension.[16,17] As a result, the lowest tolerated BP at which symptoms of hypoperfusion develop is higher in hypertensive than in normotensive individuals (Figure 78–1).[17] Thus, caution must be used in both the rate of reduction of BP and in setting the initial BP goal to protect against the risk of cerebral hypoperfusion. It is recommended that the initial reduction in MAP not exceed 20% to 25% of the pretreatment BP, or to an initial diastolic BP goal of 100 to 110 mm Hg.

## Ruling Out Secondary Causes of Hypertension

Renal parenchymal disease; renovascular hypertension; or one of the endocrine forms of hypertension, particularly pheochromocytoma, Cushing's syndrome, or rarely, primary aldosteronism, may be associated with progressive hypertension.[18] Renal parenchymal disease may, of course, be primary and be associated with hypertension as the disease progresses

**Box 78–1** Clinical Characteristics of the Hypertensive Emergency

> Blood pressure
>   Usually >220/140 mm Hg
> Funduscopic findings
>   Hemorrhages, exudates, papilledema
> Neurologic status
>   Headache, confusion, somnolence, stupor, visual loss, seizures, focal neurologic deficits, coma
> Cardiac findings
>   Prominent apical pulsation, cardiac enlargement, congestive heart failure, S₃ gallop, arrhythmia
> Renal symptoms
>   Azotemia, proteinuria, oliguria, hematuria
> Gastrointestinal symptoms
>   Nausea, vomiting

$S_3$, third heart sound. (Adapted from Vidt DG. Emergency room management of hypertensive urgencies and emergencies. J Clin Hypertens [Greenwich] 3:158-164, 2001.)

or may be secondary to long-standing, poorly controlled arterial hypertension. In either case, a vicious cycle of worsening hypertension may accompany progressive renal insufficiency.

Renovascular hypertension, often of sudden onset, may be observed with renal artery stenosis due to fibromuscular disease among younger patients, particularly women. The most common subgroup of fibromuscular disease, medial fibroplasia

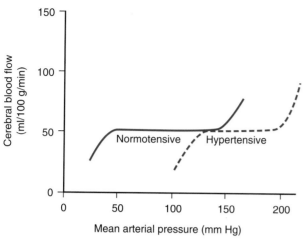

**Figure 78-1** Idealized curves of cerebral blood flow at varying levels of systemic blood pressure in normotensive and hypertensive subjects. (Appeared in Kaplan NM. Lancet 344:1335, 1994, but originally from Strandgaard et al. BMJ 1:507-510, 1973.)

with aneurysm formation, rarely progresses to loss of a kidney.[19] In contrast, medial hyperplasia and perimedial fibroplasia are both progressive lesions, frequently associated with severe hypertension, and may lead to sudden renal artery obstruction and kidney loss.

Atherosclerotic renal vascular disease is much more common than fibromuscular disease, usually involves the ostium of one or both renal arteries, and is often associated with progressive renal insufficiency and severe or refractory hypertension because it is frequently a manifestation of generalized vascular disease.[20] It often presents with refractory hypertension, complicated by renal insufficiency or acute congestive heart failure.[20]

Characteristic symptoms or "spells" usually suggest the diagnosis of pheochromocytoma, whereas body habitus changes offer valuable clues to Cushing's syndrome. Few clinical clues other than hypokalemia suggest the diagnosis of primary aldosteronism, but this diagnosis is likely in the patient who presents with accelerated-malignant hypertension with low plasma renin activity. Box 78–2 outlines the clinical clues that may suggest one of the previously mentioned secondary causes of hypertension during initial evaluation.

## Oral Agents for Hypertensive Urgencies

Several antihypertensive agents provide a rapid onset of action following oral administration and can be used in the ED when it is deemed that a patient requires therapy and reduction of BP before being discharged (Table 78–2).[15] Caution should be exerted to avoid overly aggressive initial reductions in BP. A goal BP in the range of 160/100 to 110 mm Hg would be appropriate. The patient can then be discharged on a long-acting agent, and medication can be titrated at subsequent scheduled outpatient visits.

Most readers remember the problems experienced with short-acting oral nifedipine, which was formerly a widely used initial therapy for hypertensive emergencies and urgencies.[21] Even modest doses of 10 to 20 mg of nifedipine, given orally or sublingually, were often accompanied by precipitous reduc-

**Box 78-2** Clinical Clues to Selected Secondary Causes of Hypertension

**Cushing's syndrome**
- Recent change in appearance and weight gain
- Extreme weakness, muscle wasting
- Typical body habitus with moon facies and hirsutism
- Skin changes: bruising, plethora, purplish skin strias
- Glucose intolerance, diabetes
- Neutrophilia with relative lymphocytopenia

**Pheochromocytoma**
- Symptomatic spells, including headaches, tachycardia, palpitations, pallor, tremor, perspiration
- Unusual lability of BP or orthostatic hypotension
- Substandard weight or recent weight loss
- Pressor response to antihypertensive drugs or during reduction of anesthesia
- History of neurocutaneous syndromes or multiple endocrine neoplasia
- Abnormal glucose tolerance

**Primary aldosteronism**
- Hypokalemia, spontaneous or diuretic-induced
- History of inordinate weakness of proximal muscle groups
- History of paresthesias, periodic paralysis (rare)
- Polyuria, nocturia

**Renovascular disease**
- Systolic-diastolic epigastric bruit
- Onset of hypertension age <30 or >50
- Unilateral small kidney discovered by any investigative study
- Azotemia, cigarette smoking, extensive vascular disease
- Renal insufficiency in response to ACE inhibitors
- Any unexplained impairment in renal function
- Any history of arterial thrombus or emboli, trauma, retroperitoneal fibrous or neurofibromatosis

**Renal parenchymal disease**
- Renal insufficiency, proteinuria, hematuria
- Prior renal ultrasound, KUB showing a small kidney
- Urine light chains (by sulfosalicylic acid)
- Family history of renal disease
- Long history of untreated or uncontrolled hypertension

ACE, angiotensin-converting enzyme; KUB, kidney, ureter, bladder.

tions in BP within 15 to 30 minutes after administration. As reports accumulated regarding ischemic cardiac and cerebral events following short-acting nifedipine administration, a moratorium was placed on use of this agent for the treatment of hypertensive urgencies or emergencies. Unfortunately, a few centers still use this agent in their EDs and do so at their own risk because short-acting nifedipine is not approved by the U.S. Food and Drug Administration for the treatment of hypertension.

*Captopril*, an angiotensin-converting enzyme (ACE) inhibitor, is well tolerated and has effectively reduced BP in hypertensive urgencies. Given by mouth, captopril is usually

**Table 78-2** Oral Agents for Hypertensive Emergencies

| Agent | Dose | Onset/Duration of Action (after discontinuation) | Precautions |
|---|---|---|---|
| Captopril | 25 mg PO, repeat as needed SL, 25 mg | 15-30 min/6-8 hr SL<br>15-30 min/2-6 hr | Hypotension, renal failure in bilateral renal artery stenosis |
| Clonidine | 0.1-0.2 mg PO, repeat hourly as required to total dose of 0.6 mg | 30-60 min/8-16 hr | Hypotension, drowsiness, dry mouth |
| Labetalol | 200-400 mg PO, repeat every 2-3 hr | 30 min-2 hr/2-12 hr | Bronchoconstriction, heart block, orthostatic hypotension |

effective within 15 to 30 minutes and may be repeated in 1 to 2 hours, depending on the response.[22] The drug has been administered sublingually with an observed onset of action within 10 to 20 minutes and a maximum effect within 1 hour.[23] Captopril has been very effective in the initial therapy of patients with malignant hypertension, particularly when responsiveness is enhanced by the administration of a loop diuretic, such as furosemide.[24] For patients who respond to captopril, you may wish to change to a long-acting ACE inhibitor at the time of release from the ED. Medication can be added or up-titrated at scheduled outpatient visits.

*Clonidine* is a centrally-acting, α-adrenergic agonist with onset of action within 30 to 60 minutes following oral administration. Maximal effects are seen within 2 to 4 hours. Although most commonly administered in a loading regimen of 0.1 to 0.2 mg followed by 0.1 mg/hour for several hour,[25,26] evidence suggests that a comparable response may be seen with a single 0.2-mg dose. The most common adverse effects of clonidine are drowsiness and dryness of the mouth, affecting upward of 50% of patients. If clonidine is to be continued, efforts should be made to limit the average daily dosage to 0.2 mg twice daily, in view of adverse effects that are clearly dose related. Diuretics and/or other agents can be used in combination to minimize the daily dosage of clonidine and provide optimal BP control.

*Labetalol* is a combined α- and β-adrenergic blocking agent, which is effective orally in a dose of 200 to 400 mg, which may be repeated after several hours. The onset of effect is usually observed within 1 to 2 hours.[27,28] Like other β-blocking agents, labetalol carries a potential to induce heart block and worsen symptoms of bronchospasm in the patient with established asthma. It is best avoided in patients with more than first-degree heart block, symptomatic bradycardia, or congestive heart failure. Antihypertensive effects of labetalol can be potentiated by the use of an oral diuretic or other add-on agents.

*Urapidil* is available for the treatment of hypertensive emergencies in Europe but is not yet approved for the treatment of hypertension in the United States. Urapidil is a peripheral $\alpha_1$ receptor blocker and a central 5-hydroxytriptamene$_{1a}$ receptor antagonist.[29] Intravenous urapidil has been proven useful in the management of hypertensive crises and hypertension during and after surgery.[30, 31] Oral administration of urapidil following intravenous administration can maintain lower BPs for periods of 12 hours or longer in patients with severe hypertension. This approach has been shown both to facilitate early discharge and reduce the risk of further hypertensive episodes within 12 hours.[32] Extensive clinical experience with urapidil has been reported from other parts of the world over the past decade.

For the majority of patients with elevated BP, most of whom are noncompliant with medications or inadequately treated, the addition or initiation of a long-acting antihypertensive agent in the ED is appropriate. You may wish to consider utilizing a long-acting, fixed-combination product, the dosage of which can then be modified or up-titrated at subsequent outpatient visits.

## Parenteral Agents for Hypertensive Emergencies

The following parenteral agents are effective in treating hypertensive emergencies (see Table 78–3). They act primarily as peripheral vasodilators or adrenergic inhibitors.

## Peripheral Vasodilation

*Sodium nitroprusside* is a potent vasodilator that is exceptionally predictable when administered in a hypertensive crisis of any etiology. It has an extremely rapid onset of action, within seconds of initiating an infusion, and a very rapid offset of effect within 1 to 2 minutes, which necessitates constant supervision of BP.[33] Its popularity relates in part to its effectiveness in reducing both preload and afterload, as well as decreasing myocardial oxygen demand, and the ability to achieve a controlled titration of BP. Nitroprusside does not cause sedation or somnolence but is rapidly degraded by light, requiring periodic exchange of solutions. One of the major concerns in using sodium nitroprusside is its metabolism to cyanagen and to thiocyanate.[34] In patients with significant impairment in renal function, accumulation of thiocyanate may occur over several days, with toxic effects, including encephalopathic symptoms. In patients with impaired hepatic function and poor renal perfusion, cyanide poisoning has been reported. Nitroprusside may also increase intracranial pressure, which can be a concern in patients with cerebrovascular emergencies.

*Nitroglycerin* may be of particular efficacy in hypertensive emergencies with coexistent coronary ischemia.[35] Nitroglycerin dilates collateral coronary vessels and, like nitroprusside, has a rapid onset and offset of effect, requiring close monitoring. Nitroglycerin dilates capacitance vessels primarily when infused at low doses of 5 to 10 µg/min, whereas much higher infusion rates effect arteriolar vasodilation. The infusion rate of nitroglycerin may be increased at 3- to 5-minute intervals until the desired effect is achieved. BP effects of nitroglycerin are neither as predictable nor as large as those seen with nitroprusside. Nitroglycerin may be particularly useful

**Table 78–3** Parenteral Agents for Hypertensive Emergencies

| Agent | Dose | Onset/Duration of Action (after discontinuation) | Precautions |
|---|---|---|---|
| **Parenteral Vasodilators** | | | |
| Sodium nitroprusside | 0.25-10 $\mu g \cdot kg^{-1} \cdot min^{-1}$ as IV infusion | Immediate/2-3 min after infusion | Nausea, vomiting, muscle twitching; with prolonged use cause thiocyanate intoxication, methemoglobinemia acidosis, cyanide poisoning; bags, bottles, and delivery sets must be light resistant |
| Nitroglycerine | 5-100 $\mu g$ as IV infusion* | 2-5 min/5-10 min | Headache, tachycardia, vomiting, flushing, methemoglobinemia; requires special delivery systems due to the drug's binding to PVC tubing |
| Nicardipine | 5-15 mg/hr IV infusion | 1-5 min/15-30 min, but may exceed 12 hr after prolonged infusion | Tachycardia, nausea, vomiting, headache, increased intracranial pressure; hypotension may be protracted after prolonged infusions |
| Verapamil | 5-10 mg IV; can follow with infusion of 3-25 mg/hr | 1-5 min/30-60 min | Heart block (1, 2, and 3 degrees), especially with concomitant digitalis or β-blockers, bradycardia |
| Diazoxide | 50-150 mg as IV bolus, repeated or 15-30 mg/min | 2-5 min/3-12 hr | Hypotension, tachycardia, aggravation of angina pectoris, nausea and vomiting, hyperglycemia with repeated injections |
| Fenoldopam mesylate | 0.1-0.3 $mg \cdot kg^{-1} \cdot min^{-1}$ IV infusion | <5 min/30 min | Headache, tachycardia, flushing, local phlebitis |
| Hydralazine | 10-20 mg as IV bolus or 10-40 mg IM, repeat every 4-6 hr | 10 min IV/>1-4 hr (IV), 20-30 min IM/4-6 hr (IM) | Tachycardia, headache, vomiting, aggravation of angina pectoris |
| Enalaprilat | 0.625-1.25 mg every 6 hr IV | 15-60 min/12-24 hr | Renal failure in patients with bilateral artery stenosis, hypotension |
| **Parenteral Adrenergic Inhibitors** | | | |
| Labetalol | 20-80 mg as IV bolus every 10 min; up to 2 mg/min as IV infusion | 5-10 min/2-6 hr | Bronchoconstriction, heart block, orthostatic hypotension |
| Esmolol | 500 $\mu g$/kg IV bolus injection or 25-100 $\mu g \cdot kg^{-1} \cdot min^{-1}$ by infusion; may repeat bolus after 5 min or increase infusion rate to 300 $\mu g \cdot kg^{-1} \cdot min^{-1}$ | 1-5 min/15-30 min | First-degree heart block, congestive heart failure, asthma |
| Phentolamine | 5-15 mg as IV bolus | 1-2 min/10-30 min | Tachycardia, orthostatic hypotension |

*Requires special delivery system.
IV, intravenous; PVC, polyvinyl chloride; IM, intramuscularly.

in patients with severe coronary ischemia in whom BPs are only modestly elevated or in patients with post–coronary artery bypass hypertension. Tolerance to intravenous nitroglycerin may occur within 24 to 48 hours of initiating an infusion, and unpredictable absorption in polyvinyl chloride containers and tubing necessitates the use of glass containers.

Both nitroprusside and nitroglycerin release nitric oxide and are considered nitric oxide donors, an important mechanism for the vasodilation induced by these agents. Isosorbide dinitrate is also a nitric oxide donor, and when administered in aerosol form to the oral mucosa, has a rapid onset of action. It has proved effective in the treatment of myocardial ischemia and hypertensive emergencies. In one study, the efficacy of isosorbide dinitrate was compared to sublingual nifedipine in patients with severe hypertension. While nifedipine produced a precipitous fall in BP, the isosorbide dinitrate aerosol produced a more gradual and predictable decline in BP over a period of 60 to 90 minutes.[36]

*Nicardipine* is an intravenous dihydropyridine calcium antagonist that has proved effective in a high percentage of hypertensive emergencies, particularly at higher infusion rates. The growing popularity of this agent can be attributed to its ease of administration as a continuous infusion, starting at 5 mg/hour. The infusion rate is increased by 2.5 mg/hour at intervals of 15 to 20 minutes until a maximum recommended infusion rate of 15 mg/hour is obtained, or until the desired reduction in BP is achieved. An excellent correlation has been demonstrated between plasma concentration and dose response of BP, and the dosing of nicardipine does not appear dependent on the patient's body weight.[37] Although nicardipine has been shown to reduce both cerebral and coronary ischemia, headache, nausea and vomiting may accompany its use, and modest tachycardia and increased myocardial oxygen demand limit its use in patients with severe coronary ischemia.

*Diazoxide* is rarely used today in the treatment of hypertensive emergencies. Although a potent vasodilator, large doses of 300 mg were associated with severe hypotension. Smaller mini-boluses of 50 mg administered every 10 to 15 minutes can provide a controlled reduction in BP but lead to reflex tachycardia, hyperglycemia, hyperuricemia, and sodium and water retention.[38] Diazoxide is contraindicated in patients with coronary ischemia or suspected aortic dissection and offers no advantage over several other agents that have more acceptable adverse effect profiles.

*Fenoldopam mesylate* is a selective, peripherally acting dopamine-1 receptor agonist that provides systemic vasodilation, particularly in the renal circulation, and it also has effects on renal proximal and distal tubules.[39,40] It does not bind to dopamine-2 receptors or β-adrenergic receptors and has no α-adrenergic agonist effects, but is an $\alpha_1$-antagonist and does not cross the blood-brain barrier. Fenoldopam lowers BP by causing peripheral arterial vasodilation with little to no effect on preload.

The onset of clinical effect is usually seen within 5 minutes and effects dissipate within 30 minutes following discontinuation of the infusion. Side effects include headache, flushing, tachycardia, and dizziness. Bradycardia has occasionally been noted, and a dose-related increase in intraocular pressure has been observed in normotensive and hypertensive patients. Inactive metabolites are eliminated primarily in the urine, and

no dosage adjustments are required for patients with renal or hepatic impairment.

In contrast to other parenteral antihypertensive agents, fenoldopam's unique effects on the kidney provide increased urine flow rate, sodium and potassium excretion, and creatinine clearance, making this agent especially attractive in hypertensive emergencies with renal impairment.[41] Nitroprusside has opposite effects on renal urodynamics. In congestive heart failure, incremental doses of fenoldopam have been shown to increase cardiac index in association with decreased BP, variable effects on pulmonary capillary or wedge pressure, and no change in right atrial pressure.

*Hydralazine*, a direct arterial vasodilator, has no significant effects on venous tone. Reductions in arterial BP are accompanied by reflex increases in heart rate, increased myocardial oxygen demand, sodium, and water retention. Hydralazine use has also been associated with increases in intracranial pressure. The use of hydralazine today is restricted to pregnant women with preeclampsia, because hydralazine can improve uterine blood flow.[42] Five to ten mg may be effective intravenously as a bolus injection and may be repeated. Flushing and headache may be observed.

*Enalaprilat*, the active metabolite of enalapril, can be administered intravenously in a dose of 1.25 mg at 6-hour intervals. The onset of action is usually seen within 30 minutes, but the response to enalaprilat in hypertensive emergencies can be unpredictable, partially due to variations in volume status and in plasma renin concentration.[43] Enalaprilat may be particularly useful in hypertensive emergencies associated with congestive heart failure or high plasma angiotensin II concentrations.

## Parenteral Adrenergic Inhibitors

*Labetalol* is an α-blocker and noncardioselective β-blocker, which has proved especially effective when used in bolus intravenous injections in the initial treatment of hypertensive emergencies. It can provide controlled reduction in BP to a predetermined goal.[44] Once a goal pressure is achieved, injections are stopped and the long duration of action facilitates conversion to effective oral therapy. Infusion of labetalol at a rate of 2 mg/minute offers an alternative method of administration and is associated with a gradual yet controlled reduction in BP.[45] Because β-blocking effects predominate, bradycardia or heart block may occur in patients with intrinsic heart disease, and bronchospasm can limit its usefulness in patients with asthma.

*Esmolol* is an intravenous, ultra-short-acting β-adrenergic blocker. Onset of effect is seen between 1 and 5 minutes, with a rapid offset of effect within 15 to 30 minutes following discontinuation.[46,47] Esmolol is administered as a 500-µg/kg/min bolus injection, which may be repeated after 5 minutes. Alternatively, an infusion of 50 to 100 µg/kg/min may be initiated and increased to 300 µg/kg/min as needed. It is most often used in surgical units for the intraoperative or postoperative short-term control of BP and can also be useful in the setting of myocardial ischemia or infarction. Adverse effects include heart block, congestive heart failure, and bronchoconstriction.

*Phentolamine*, a nonselective α-adrenergic blocking agent, is reserved for use in suspected excess catecholamine states, such as pheochromocytoma or cocaine withdrawal. It may be useful as a diagnostic agent administered as a bolus injection of 5 to 10 mg in patients with suspected high circulating levels of catecholamines.[3,48] Acute BP lowering will be seen within several minutes and may last 10 to 30 minutes in the setting of catecholamine excess. Tachycardia is common and may precipitate myocardial ischemia in high-risk patients. Nitroprusside and labetalol are more easily titrated in the management of hypertensive emergencies associated with high circulating levels of catecholamines; therefore, phentolamine is rarely used therapeutically today.

## Management of Specific Hypertensive Emergencies (see Table 78–4)

*Hypertensive encephalopathy* is a lethal complication of severe hypertension and occurs when an increase in BP exceeds the brain's autoregulatory ability to maintain constant cerebral perfusion, resulting in disruption of the blood-brain barrier and diffuse cerebral edema.[49] This diagnosis should be suspected when a severe elevation in BP is accompanied by neurologic signs and symptoms characteristic of encephalopathy. Clinical signs include obtundation or confusion, focal neurologic deficits, retinopathy with papilledema, and occasional focal seizures. This is a diagnosis of exclusion and requires that stroke, intracranial hemorrhage, seizure disorder, other mental disorders, mass lesions, vasculitis, and encephalitis be considered. When suspected, BP should be promptly lowered as recommended in the management of a hypertensive emergency. A CT scan or magnetic resonance imaging (MRI) of the head should be obtained as soon as it is feasible.

Agents with a rapid onset of effect that can be titrated to a desirable initial BP goal are preferred.[50] Sodium nitroprusside is an agent of choice because its rapid onset of action and short half-life allow for minute-to-minute control of BP and because it has minimal effects on cerebral blood flow.

**Table 78–4** A Quick Reference for Preferred Parenteral Drugs for Selected Hypertensive Emergencies

| Emergency | *Preferred Drugs | Drugs to Avoid |
|---|---|---|
| Hypertensive encephalopathy | Nitroprusside Nicardipine Labetalol Fenoldopam | Diazoxide (rapid decrease in cerebral blood flow) |
| Malignant hypertension (when IV therapy is indicated) | Labetalol Nicardipine Nitroprusside Fenoldopam Enalaprilat | |
| Cerebrovascular accidents | Nicardipine Labetalol Nimodipine (in SAH) Nitroprusside | Diazoxide, hydralazine (may increase intracerebral pressure) |
| Myocardial infarction, unstable angina | Nitroglycerin Nitroprusside Nicardipine Nitroprusside | Diazoxide, hydralazine (increase heart rate, myocardial oxygen demand) Labetalol and esmolol (decrease cardiac output) |
| Congestive heart failure | Nitroglycerin Enalaprilat Loop diuretics | |
| Aortic dissection | Nitroprusside Esmolol Labetalol | Diazoxide Hydralazine Nicardipine |
| Adrenergic crisis | Phentolamine Nitroprusside Labetalol | Labetalol (in cocaine crisis) |
| Postoperative hypertension | Nitroglycerin Nitroprusside Labetalol Nicardipine Fenoldopam | |
| Preeclampsia, eclampsia of pregnancy | Hydralazine Labetalol Nicardipine | Nitroprusside Enalaprilat |

*The "Preferred Drugs" are listed in the order of preference for use.
IV, intravenous; SAH, subarachnoid hemorrhage.

Nicardipine and labetalol have also proved to be particularly effective in the management of hypertensive encephalopathy. Fenoldopam proves an appropriate alternative in view of its rapid onset of action and lack of adverse cerebral effects. Frequent neurologic assessments during the period of titration are imperative. BP reduction is often associated with dramatic improvement in sensorial function in the patient with hypertensive encephalopathy. Further deterioration in neurologic function in the face of effective BP reduction requires consideration of other possible diagnoses.

*Cerebrovascular Accidents*—Optimal treatment of severe hypertension in the presence of cerebrovascular accidents, such as intracerebral and subarachnoid hemorrhage or cerebral infarction, remains debatable.[51] Keep in mind that high BP may be a contributor to or the result of the acute neurologic event. The risks of elevated BP causing cerebral edema or possible rebleeding must be weighed against the risks of worsening cerebral ischemia with too rapid or excessive BP reduction.

The protective rise in BP immediately following a stroke is an attempt to maintain adequate perfusion to ischemic cerebral tissue. The benefits to be derived from acute reductions in BP are not well founded in controlled clinical studies. One recent study has shown no significant relationship between admission systolic and diastolic BP and the outcome at 3 months. They also observed that high nighttime systolic and low nighttime diastolic values were identified as independent predictors of stroke outcome. Their data suggested that a spontaneous BP decrease in the first 5 days poststroke may be independently related to poor outcome. These findings warn against a too rigorous lowering of early poststroke BP.[52]

Following a thrombotic stroke, BP rises acutely but tends to decline without any specific therapy over the next 24 to 48 hours. An acute rise in BP may not occur following an intracerebral hemorrhage. Our recommendation is that acute therapy be considered only for severely elevated BP (diastolic BP >130 mm Hg). Even then, BP should be very cautiously reduced with a rapid-acting agent to an initial goal of no more than 20% to 25% below the pretreatment BP, or to a diastolic pressure level of 100 to 110 mm Hg during the initial 24 hours. Nicardipine by continuous infusion or labetalol given by repeated small boluses or by continuous infusion are both appropriate agents and have been used effectively in this setting. Nitroprusside is attractive because of its rapid onset and offset of effect, but it could further increase intracranial pressure. A cerebroselective dihydropyridine calcium antagonist, nimodipine, has proven beneficial following subarachnoid hemorrhage to reduce cerebral vasospasm.[53] The effects of nimodipine on BP in this setting are negligible. Agents such as diazoxide or hydralazine should be avoided because they raise intracranial pressure.

*Myocardial Infarction and Unstable Angina*—In the patient with severe ischemic coronary disease, nitroglycerin is the agent of choice if BPs are only modestly elevated.[54] Nitroglycerin has the advantages of improving collateral coronary blood flow and myocardial oxygen utilization. The major effect of nitroglycerin at lower infusion rates is on preload, whereas much higher infusion rates are required to induce arteriolar vasodilation and reduce afterload. Intravenous labetalol can also be effective and when hypertension is severe, use of nitroprusside should be considered.[55] β-Blockers have little acute antihypertensive effect, but their early use may reduce infarct size and provide significant secondary cardioprotection, including reduced in-hospital mortality. Vasodilator drugs, such as diazoxide and hydralazine, can induce reflex increases in heart rate and increase myocardial oxygen demand. To assist in the management of acute pain and anxiety, narcotic analgesics and/or modest sedation should be considered. When BP has been lowered, thrombolytic therapy can be considered.

*Congestive Heart Failure*—Acute left ventricular failure is often precipitated by an acute rise in systemic vascular resistance and further compromise in left ventricular compliance. In patients with typical systolic heart failure, intravenous nitroprusside or nitroglycerin is appropriate therapy. Intravenous enalaprilat can be used, but responses are not as predictable as those observed with nitroprusside. The importance of concomitant use of oxygen, intravenous loop diuretics, and morphine should not be underestimated. β-Blockers, including labetalol, should be avoided because they may worsen cardiac function. Once the patient has been stabilized and is ready for discharge, the addition of a β-blocker may be considered, as recommended for chronic congestive heart failure.

A bedside echocardiogram may be useful to evaluate global left ventricular function, because diastolic dysfunction may contribute to congestive heart failure in the setting of severe hypertension. Although patients with diastolic dysfunction benefit from reductions in systolic and diastolic BP, diastolic dysfunction provides an indication for considering a β-blocker or a nondihydropyridine calcium antagonist, such as verapamil.[56]

*Acute aortic dissection* is the most lethal of the diseases involving the aorta. Hypertension is found in more than 90% of patients with acute aortic dissection. Typically, a patient with acute aortic dissection is an elderly male with a long history of hypertension who presents with severe acute chest pain. Chest pain is present in 94% of patients, is severe, excruciating, and abrupt at onset.[57] Often described as a "ripping or tearing" pain in the anterior chest, it occasionally extends to the back and radiates down toward the abdomen or flank areas. BP is elevated in most cases, particularly those with distal dissection. Hypotension may be a prominent feature in patients with proximal aortic dissection. Absent or unequal pulses in the extremities are seen in 35% to 50%, and new aortic insufficiency can be an important clinical sign. Neurologic manifestations may include ischemic neuropathy, stroke, paraplegia, and paresis. Involvement of the mesenteric artery can cause nausea, vomiting, abdominal pain, or hematemesis.

Medical treatment aims at decreasing the velocity and the slope of the pulse wave (dP/dt max) and lowering BP, using intensive drug therapy in an effort to prevent progression of the dissection.[58] Emergency reduction of BP to the lowest tolerated level (systolic, 100-110 mm Hg), with drugs that do not increase heart rate and contractility, is required. The treatment of choice for acute aortic dissection is nitroprusside, in combination with a β-blocker, such as esmolol or propranolol. β-Blockade must be established early to avoid reflex cardiac stimulation following acute reduction in BP. Labetalol is a useful alternative, particularly in patients with coronary artery disease because it also reduces myocardial oxygen consumption and enhances coronary artery perfusion. It may be administered as repeated miniboluses or as a continuous intravenous infusion. Agents, such as hydralazine, diazoxide, and nicardipine are best avoided because they may lead to reflexive cardiac stimulation. If an aortic dissection is suspected, definitive diagnostic studies must be accomplished as soon as BP is controlled. The aortogram is the most definitive method to confirm a dissection because it shows the intimal tear and reveals false channels. CT scanning with contrast enhancement, transesophageal echocardiography, and MRI are also useful in establishing the diagnosis. Dissections of the ascending aorta and aortic arch require immediate surgical repair, whereas dissections distal to the left subclavian artery can usually be managed medically, unless complicated by leaking or vascular compromise of an organ or limb, continued or recurrent pain, or extension of dissection, despite optimal BP control.

*Adrenergic Crisis*—Although pheochromocytoma is the classic example of a catecholamine excess–induced hypertensive emergency, markedly elevated catecholamines are more frequently seen with cocaine or amphetamine overdose, withdrawal from agents such as clonidine or β-blockers, or an interaction with tyramine-containing compounds and monamine oxidase inhibitors. Excessive circulating catecholamines and severe hypertension are also associated with acute spinal cord injuries.

*Phentolamine*, with and without a β-blocker, can be used in initial management. In view of the hypertensive risk of unopposed α-adrenergic receptor stimulation in the setting of catecholamine excess, β-blockers should not be initiated until adequate α-blockade has been established. Sodium nitroprusside or labetalol are more easily titrated in the management of hypertensive emergencies caused by high circulating levels of catecholamines. Although increased experience with labetalol suggests that early reports of paradoxical hypertension may have been exaggerated, this risk must be considered.[59,60] This response presumably relates to the fact that the β-blocking effects of labetalol tend to predominate in clinical usage. In cocaine-induced hypertensive crisis, the use of β-blockers may enhance cocaine-induced coronary vasoconstriction, further increase BP, and enhance the risk of both seizures and reduced survival. Furthermore, labetalol does not reverse cocaine-induced coronary vasoconstriction.[61] In this condition, nicardipine, verapamil, or fenoldopam can be used.[62,63]

*Postoperative Hypertension*—Early postoperative hypertension due to increased sympathetic tone and vascular resistance is common, particularly following vascular surgical procedures. Hypertension has been reported in upward of 30% to 50% of patients following coronary artery bypass graft surgery. The treatments of choice are nitroglycerin and sodium nitroprusside. Significant vascular bleeding postoperatively in a patient with uncontrolled hypertension may necessitate immediate lowering of BP. A number of easily titratable agents, including nitroprusside, labetalol, nicardipine, and possibly, fenoldopam, can be useful in this situation. Nicardipine, in particular, has shown efficacy in controlling postoperative hypertension in both cardiac and noncardiac surgical patients.[64] In one study, intravenous nicardipine was as effective as sodium nitroprusside and achieved BP control more rapidly and with fewer dose adjustments than sodium nitroprusside.[37]

*Preeclampsia and Eclampsia in Pregnancy*—The syndrome of preeclampsia features the onset of hypertension after the twentieth week of pregnancy, edema, and proteinuria, and occurs almost exclusively during a first pregnancy. Preeclampsia must be differentiated from chronic hypertension that preceded the onset of pregnancy. An abrupt increase in BP at the onset of labor or during delivery may herald the onset of eclampsia, defined by the occurrence of seizures due to hypertensive encephalopathy.[65]

Parenteral magnesium sulfate is the drug of choice for preventing eclamptic convulsions. Treatment should be continued for 12 to 24 hours postpartum because of the significant risk of seizures in the early postpartum period. For acutely lowering BP, hydralazine is the drug of choice. An initial dose of 5 mg intravenously can be followed by subsequent boluses of 5 to 10 mg at 20- to 30-minute intervals. Side effects include tachycardia and headache. For patients already in a hospital ICU, intravenous labetalol or nicardipine have also become preferred agents because of their effectiveness and ease of administration.[66,67] Diazoxide, a potent vasodilator, previously recommended for women with hypertension refractory to hydralazine, is rarely used today. If using calcium channel blockers, keep in mind that magnesium sulfate may potentiate the effects of calcium channel blockers, resulting in precipitous and profound hypotension.[68] Oral or sublingual nifedipine is no longer recommended for the treatment of severe hypertension in pregnancy because of the risks of precipitous hypotension. Sodium nitroprusside is not recommended because of the potential risk of fatal cyanide poisoning, demonstrated primarily in animal models. Limited experience with intravenous prostacyclin has shown it to be as effective as hydralazine with less risk of tachycardia.[69]

Careful attention must be paid to salt and water metabolism to minimize the risk of fluid overload or severe hyponatremia, which can precipitate cerebral edema. The clinical findings of severe preeclampsia or eclampsia can be expected to clear rapidly following delivery.

## SUMMARY

Hypertensive emergencies and urgencies demand prompt recognition and management because they may represent a threat to organ function and life. Early triage in ED is necessary to identify the true hypertensive emergency for immediate admission and in-hospital management, whereas most hypertensive urgencies can be managed in ED followed by appropriate follow-up in the outpatient department. Initial evaluation of the hypertensive emergency should establish the degree of target organ damage, possibly identify any readily recognized secondary causes of hypertension, should facilitate selection of initial therapy, and determine the goal BP for treatment. Initial treatment should achieve a partial reduction in BP to a safer, noncritical level, although not necessarily to achieve normotension. Most hypertensive urgencies can be managed in the outpatient setting, if appropriate follow-up can be provided.

## References

1. Joint National Committee. The Sixth Report of the Committee on the Prevention, Detection, Evaluation, and Treatment of High Blood Pressure (JNC VI). Arch Intern Med 157:2413-2446, 1997.
2. Garcia JY Jr, Vidt DG. Current management of hypertensive emergencies. Drugs 34:263-278, 1987.
3. Calhoun DA. Hypertensive crisis. *In* Oparil S, Weber MA (eds). Hypertension: A Companion to Brenner and Rector's The Kidney. Philadelphia, WB Saunders, 2000; pp 715-718.

4. Preston RA, Baltodano NM, Cienki J, et al. Clinical presentation and management of patients with uncontrolled, severe hypertension: Results from a public teaching hospital. J Hum Hypertens 13:249-255, 1999.

5. Kincaid-Smith P. Complications and survival of 315 patients with malignant hypertension. J Hypertens 9:245-269, 1980.

6. Lip GY, Beevers M, Beevers DG. Complications and survival of 315 patients with malignant-phase hypertension. J Hypertens 13:915-924, 1995.

7. Ahmed ME, Walker JM, Beevers DG, et al. Lack of difference between malignant and accelerated hypertension. Br Med J (Clin Res Ed) 292:235-237, 1986.

8. Yu SH, Whitworth JA, Kincaid-Smith PS. Malignant hypertension: aetiology and outcome in 83 patients. Clin Exp Hypertens A8:1211-2330, 1986.

9. McGregor E, Isles CG, Jay JL, et al. Retinal changes in malignant hypertension. Br Med J (Clin Res Ed) 292:233-234, 1986.

10. Bloxham CA, Beevers DG, Walker JM. Malignant hypertension and cigarette smoking. Br Med J 1:581-583, 1979.

11. Kincaid-Smith P, McMichael J, Murphy EA. Clinical course and pathology of hypertension with papilledema (malignant hypertension). Q J Med 27:117-154, 1958.

12. Beilin LJ, Goldby FS, Mohring J. High arterial pressure versus humoral factors in the pathogenesis of the vascular lesions of malignant hypertension. Clin Sci Mol Med 52:111-117, 1977.

13. Koch-Weser J. Hypertensive emergencies. N Engl J Med 290:211-214, 1974.

14. Yoshida M, Nonoguchi H, Owada A, et al. Three cases of malignant hypertension: the roles of endothelin-1 and the renin-angiotensin-aldosterone system. Clin Nephrol 42:295-299, 1994.

15. Vidt DG. Emergency room management of hypertensive urgencies and emergencies. J Clin Hypertens (Greenwich) 3:158-164, 2001.

16. Strandgaard S. Autoregulation of cerebral blood flow in hypertensive patients. The modifying influence of prolonged antihypertensive treatment on the tolerance to acute, drug-induced hypotension. Circulation 53:720-727, 1976.

17. Strandgaard S, Olesen J, Skinhoj E, et al. Autoregulation of brain circulation in severe arterial hypertension. Br Med J 3:507-510, 1973.

18. Vidt DG. Resistant hypertension. *In* Oparil S, Weber MA (eds). Hypertension: A Companion to Brenner and Rector's The Kidney. Philadelphia, WB Saunders, 2000; pp 564-572.

19. Working Group on Renovascular Hypertension. Detection, evaluation, and treatment of renovascular hypertension. Final report. Arch Intern Med 147:820-829, 1987.

20. Conlon PJ, O'Riordan E, Kalra PA. New insights into the epidemiologic and clinical manifestations of atherosclerotic renovascular disease. Am J Kidney Dis 35:573-587, 2000.

21. Grossman E, Messerli FH, Grodzicki T, et al. Should a moratorium be placed on sublingual nifedipine capsules given for hypertensive emergencies and pseudoemergencies? JAMA 276: 1328-1331, 1996.

22. Biollaz J, Waeber B, Brunner HR. Hypertensive crisis treated with orally administered captopril. Eur J Clin Pharmacol 25:145-149, 1983.

23. Castro del Castillo A, Rodriguez M, Gonzalez E, et al. Dose-response effect of sublingual captopril in hypertensive crises. J Clin Pharmacol 28:667-670, 1988.

24. Ramos O. Malignant hypertension: The Brazilian experience (clinical conference). Kidney Int 26:209-217, 1984.

25. Houston MC. Treatment of hypertensive emergencies and urgencies with oral clonidine loading and titration. A review. Arch Intern Med 146:586-589, 1986.

26. Zeller KR, Von Kuhnert L, Matthews C. Rapid reduction of severe asymptomatic hypertension. A prospective, controlled trial. Arch Intern Med 149:2186-2189, 1989.

27. Ghose RR. Acute management of severe hypertension with oral labetalol. Br J Clin Pharmacol 8:189S-193S, 1979.

28. Catapano MS, Marx JA. Management of urgent hypertension: A comparison of oral treatment regimens in the emergency department. J Emerg Med 4:361-368, 1986.

29. Van Zwieten PA, Mathy MJ, Thoolen MJ. Deviating central hypotensive activity of urapidil in the cat. J Pharm Pharmacol 37:810-811, 1985.

30. van der Stroom JG, van Wezel HB, Vergroesen I, et al. Comparison of the effects of urapidil and sodium nitroprusside on haemodynamic state, myocardial metabolism and function in patients during coronary artery surgery. Br J Anaesth 76: 645-651, 1996.

31. Hirschl MM, Binder M, Bur A, et al. Safety and efficacy of urapidil and sodium nitroprusside in the treatment of hypertensive emergencies. Intensive Care Med 23:885-888, 1997.

32. Hirschl MM, Herkner H, Bur A, et al. Course of blood pressure within the first 12 h of hypertensive urgencies. J Hypertens 16:251-255, 1998.

33. Page IH, Corcoran AL, Dustan HP, et al. Cardiovascular actions of sodium nitroprusside in animals and hypertensive patients. Circulation 11:188-198, 1995.

34. Bedoya LA, Vidt DG. Treatment of the hypertensive emergency. *In* Jacobson HR, Striker GE, Klahr S (eds). The Principles and Practice of Nephrology. Philadelphia, BC Decker, 1991; pp 547-557.

35. Flaherty JT, Magee PA, Gardner TL, et al. Comparison of intravenous nitroglycerin and sodium nitroprusside for treatment of acute hypertension developing after coronary artery bypass surgery. Circulation 65:1072-1077, 1982.

36. Rubio-Guerra AF, Vargas-Ayala G, Lozano-Nuevo JJ, et al. Comparison between isosorbide dinitrate aerosol and nifedipine in the treatment of hypertensive emergencies. J Hum Hypertens 13:473-476, 1999.

37. IV Nicardipine Study Group. Efficacy and safety of intravenous nicardipine in the control of postoperative hypertension. Chest 99:393-398, 1991.

38. Miller WE, Gifford RW Jr, Humphrey DC, et al. Management of severe hypertension with intravenous injections of diazoxide. Am J Cardiol 24:870-875, 1969.

39. Post JB IV, Frishman WH. Fenoldopam: A new dopamine agonist for the treatment of hypertensive urgencies and emergencies. J Clin Pharmacol 38:2-13, 1998.

40. Murphy MB, Murray C, Shorten GD. Fenoldopam: A selective peripheral dopamine-receptor agonist for the treatment of severe hypertension. N Engl J Med 345:1548-1557, 2001.

41. Murphy MB, Murray C, Shorten GD. Fenoldopam: A selective peripheral dopamine-receptor agonist for the treatment of severe hypertension. N Engl J Med 345:1548-1557, 2001.

42. Paterson-Brown S, Robson SC, Redfern N, et al. Hydralazine boluses for the treatment of severe hypertension in preeclampsia. Br J Obstet Gynaecol 101:409-413, 1994.

43. DiPette DJ, Ferraro JC, Evans RR, et al. Enalaprilat, an intravenous angiotensin-converting enzyme inhibitor, in hypertensive crises. Clin Pharmacol Ther 38:199-204, 1985.

44. Cressman MD, Vidt DG, Gifford RW Jr, et al. Intravenous labetalol in the management of severe hypertension and hypertensive emergencies. Am Heart J 107:980-985, 1984.

45. Lebel M, Langlois S, Belleau LJ, et al. Labetalol infusion in hypertensive emergencies. Clin Pharmacol Ther 37:615-618, 1985.

46. Oxorn D, Knox JW, Hill J. Bolus doses of esmolol for the prevention of perioperative hypertension and tachycardia. Can J Anaesth 37:206-209, 1990.

47. Lowenthal DT, Porter RS, Saris SD, et al. Clinical pharmacology, pharmacodynamics and interactions with esmolol. Am J Cardiol 56:14F-18F, 1985.

48. Gifford RW Jr. Management of hypertensive crises. JAMA 266:829-835, 1991.

49. Strandgaard S, Paulson OB. Cerebral blood flow and its pathophysiology in hypertension. Am J Hypertens 2:486-492, 1989.

50. Vaughan CJ, Delanty N. Hypertensive emergencies. Lancet 356:411-417, 2000.

51. Brown RD Jr. Management of hypertensive patients with cerebrovascular disease. *In* Izzo JL, Black HR (eds). Hypertension Primer, 2nd ed. Baltimore, Lippincott Williams & Wilkins, 1999; pp 6-397.

52. Boreas AM, Lodder J, Kessels F, et al. Prognostic value of blood pressure in acute stroke. J Hum Hypertens 16:111-116, 2002.

53. Wong MC, Haley EC Jr. Calcium antagonists: Stroke therapy coming of age. Stroke 21:494-501, 1990.

54. Flaherty JT, Reid PR, Kelly DT, et al. Intravenous nitroglycerin in acute myocardial infarction. Circulation 51:132-139, 1975.

55. Lau J, Antman EM, Jimenez-Silva J, et al. Cumulative meta-analysis of therapeutic trials for myocardial infarction. N Engl J Med 327:248-254, 1992.

56. Frohlich ED. Management of hypertensive patients with left ventricular hypertrophy and diastolic dysfunction. *In* Izzo JL, Black HR (eds). Hypertension Primer, 2nd ed. Baltimore, Lippincott Williams & Wilkins, 1999; pp 402-404.

57. Asfoura JY, Vidt DG. Acute aortic dissection [published erratum appears in Chest 1991 Nov;100(5):1480]. Chest 99:724-729, 1991.

58. Wheat MW Jr. Acute dissection of the aorta. Cardiovasc Clin 17:241-262, 1987.

59. Reach G, Thibonnier M, Chevillard C, et al. Effect of labetalol on blood pressure and plasma catecholamine concentrations in patients with phaeochromocytoma. Br Med J 280:1300-1301, 1980.

60. Feek CM, Earnshaw PM. Hypertensive response to labetalol in phaeochromocytoma. Br Med J 281:387, 1980.

61. Lange RA, Cigarroa RG, Flores ED, et al. Potentiation of cocaine-induced coronary vasoconstriction by beta-adrenergic blockade. Ann Intern Med 112:897-903, 1990.

62. Pitts WR, Lange RA, Cigarroa JE, et al. Cocaine-induced myocardial ischemia and infarction: pathophysiology, recognition, and management. Prog Cardiovasc Dis 40:65-76, 1997.

63. Boehrer JD, Moliterno DJ, Willard JE, et al. Influence of labetalol on cocaine-induced coronary vasoconstriction in humans. Am J Med 94:608-610, 1993.

64. Halpern NA, Goldberg M, Neely C, et al. Postoperative hypertension: A multicenter, prospective, randomized comparison between intravenous nicardipine and sodium nitroprusside. Crit Care Med 20:1637-1643, 1992.

65. Cunningham FG, Lindheimer MD. Hypertension in pregnancy. N Engl J Med 326:927-932, 1992.

66. August P. Management of pregnant hypertensive patients. *In* Izzo JL, Black HR (eds). Hypertension Primer, 2nd ed. Baltimore, Lippincott Williams & Wilkins, 1999; pp 427-429.

67. Mabie WL, Gonzalez AR, Sibai BM, et al. A comparative trial of labetalol and hydralazine in the acute management of severe hypertension complicating pregnancy. Obstet Gynecol 70:328-333, 1987.

68. Corbonne B, Jannet D, Touboul C, et al. Nicardipine treatment of hypertension during pregnancy. Obstet Gynecol 81:908-914, 1993.

69. Moodley J, Gousus E. A comparative study of the use of epoprostenol and dihydralazine in pregnancy. Br J Obstet Gynaecol 99:727-730, 1992.

# Aggressive Blood Pressure Targets: Developing Effective Algorithms

## Myron H. Weinberger

## INTRODUCTION

The decision of when and how to begin antihypertensive therapy is a complex one. Some of the factors influencing the "when" are discussed in Chapter 48 of this book. The reader is referred to that chapter and to the specific chapters dealing in detail with each of the lifestyle interventions for information concerning nonpharmacologic therapy when that is deemed the initial choice for a specific patient. After deciding that drug therapy is required because the blood pressure is above the "prehypertension" range or because of failure of nonpharmacologic approaches to reduce blood pressure adequately, the selection of the most appropriate agent(s) is a challenging one in view of the large number of drugs currently available and the massive amount of information available attesting to the efficacy of all of these agents. The results of numerous recent studies have led experts to recommend a variety of different drugs and different therapeutic approaches, all with scientific support. This has created a great deal of confusion and in many cases misinterpretation of study results and consternation in the minds of physicians regarding the optimal treatment approach for a given patient.

This chapter addresses the rationale for making this selection, alternative approaches, adverse effects associated with specific classes of drugs, and most importantly, the enhancement of efficacy obtained by combining different classes of agents. One of the fundamental precepts, bolstered by the results of virtually all of the outcome studies, is that hypertensive patients are not all the same. The mechanisms responsible for their blood pressure elevations, as well as their responses to specific classes of antihypertensive drugs are diverse. Hypertensive persons may have different comorbidities that influence the selection of antihypertensive therapy, and the effects of the drugs used to treat these concomitant conditions on blood pressure must be considered. Finally, the selection of antihypertensive drug regimens may have an impact on other cardiovascular risk factors that are often found in hypertensive patients. An extensive discussion of therapeutic approaches for those with secondary forms of hypertension is beyond the scope of this chapter and can be found in Chapters 73 through 76.

The choice of initial drug therapy is influenced by the level of blood pressure; comorbid risk factors; and diseases and issues related to feasibility of patient adherence to medication, such as insurance and related financial status, lifestyle effects, psychological factors, and the potential impact of minor or serious side effects of drugs. In addition, information is available that may provide a clue regarding the therapeutic approach most likely to be beneficial in a given patient. As mentioned in Chapter 48, the decision to begin drug therapy is usually made when the office blood pressure is above 140 mm Hg systolic and/or 90 mm Hg diastolic on several measurements or when the average daytime ambulatory blood pressure exceeds 135 mm Hg systolic and/or 85 mm Hg diastolic and the nighttime average is greater than 120 mm Hg systolic and/or 75 mm Hg diastolic. The reason for dependence of these threshold values on time of day is related to the normal nocturnal decline in blood pressure that is often absent in those with hypertension. When the nocturnal decline is less than normal, this presents a greater pressure load on the cardiovascular system and has recently been shown to be related to an increased risk of cardiovascular events. In persons with diabetes mellitus, in whom the blood pressure goal recommended by the American Diabetes Association is below 130/80 mm Hg; in patients with renal disease, in whom the American Society of Nephrology recommends blood pressure levels of 125/75 mm Hg or lower to preserve renal function; or in those with congestive heart failure, in whom values lower than the traditional 140/90 mm Hg are usually preferred to reduce the workload of the heart, antihypertensive drug therapy is often begun at levels less than 140/90 mm Hg. Detailed information regarding preferred agents and approaches for each of these comorbidities is addressed in Chapters 24, 25, 52, 53, and 54. It is important to recognize that in virtually every study involving patients with these disorders, multiple drug therapy has been required to achieve the lower blood pressure goals. Indeed, even in uncomplicated hypertensive patients, multiple therapy is usually required to reach goals of less than 140/90 mm Hg.

The identification of an increased risk for cardiovascular disease in persons designated as "prehypertensive" (i.e., those having systolic pressures between 120 and 139 mm Hg and/or diastolic pressures between 80-89 mm Hg)[1] has raised an intriguing question regarding the potential benefit of drug therapy for this group. This issue remains to be addressed in the future. The recommendations in the Seventh Report of the Joint National Committee on Prevention, Detection, Evaluation, and Treatment of High Blood Pressure (JNC 7)[2,3] have indicated that in individuals with blood pressure above 160/100 mm Hg, monotherapy does usually not suffice to achieve the blood pressure goals. Thus JNC 7 recommends beginning treatment with two drugs having differing mechanisms of action when the pressure is this high. This chapter does not deal with the severe, accelerated, or resistant forms of hypertension, because they are the topics of Chapters 59 and 78.

Patients may not always be as willing to wait for blood pressure reduction as their healthcare providers. It is important for the patient to realize that the decrease in blood pressure may be gradual and that it may be necessary to try several agents, alone or in combination, to achieve the target blood pressure with a minimum of side effects. The patient should be encouraged to report side effects when they occur and to understand the blood pressure goals and the time frame for achieving them.

## THE USE OF PLASMA RENIN ACTIVITY TO GUIDE THERAPEUTIC CHOICES: THE "LARAGH" METHOD

Dr. John Laragh and his group working at the Cornell University Medical Center have been pioneers in elucidating the role of the renin-angiotensin-aldosterone system in human hypertension and its associated disorders. The results of their voluminous body of work have led to an approach to selecting antihypertensive therapy based on measurement of plasma renin activity (Figure 79–1).[4] This group demonstrated more than 30 years ago the inverse relationship between plasma renin activity, measured by the production of angiotensin from endogenous renin substrate, and urinary sodium excretion, a

surrogate for dietary-sodium intake. They found that plasma renin activity was markedly reduced when dietary-sodium intake exceeded 150 to 200 mmol/day, the typical range for most free-living individuals. Plasma renin activity begins to rise at levels of dietary-sodium intake below 50 to 100 mmol/day.

The "Laragh" concept is based on measuring plasma renin activity to determine whether an individual has a blood pressure elevation that is primarily due to increased vasoconstriction from endogenous pressor agents (renin-dependent, "R," i.e. plasma renin activity >0.65 ng/ml/hr) or due to increased extracellular fluid volume ("V," sodium or salt dependent; plasma renin activity <0.65 ng/ml/hr).[4] However, the accuracy of this measurement requires reduction of salt intake to levels below the threshold for the stimulation of renin (i.e., <50-100

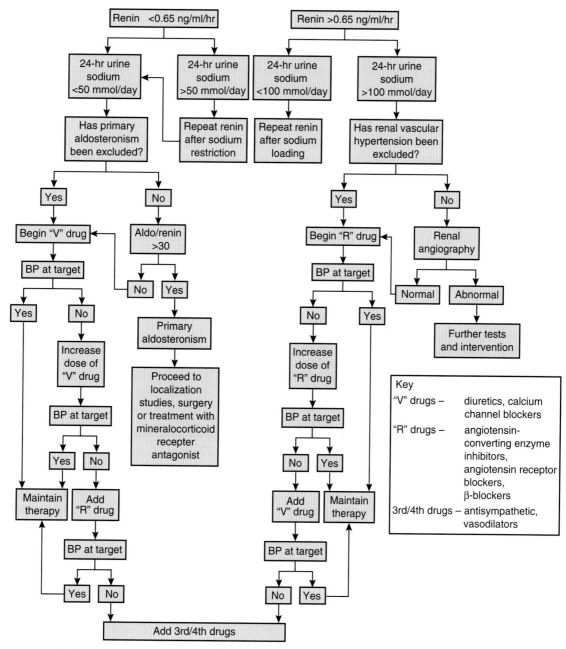

**Figure 79–1** Treatment algorithm based on plasma renin activity.

mmol/day to identify the "low-renin" or "V" individual). This requires collection of a 24-hour urine sample for measurement of sodium and creatinine to verify the completeness of the collection. Additional studies are required to rule out renin suppression as the result of primary aldosteronism or other mineralocorticoid excess syndromes. Similarly, when renin levels are >0.65 ng/ml/hr, the presence of renal vascular hypertension and other disorders of the kidney manifest by excessive renin release must be excluded by having the individual consume a high-sodium intake, verified by 24-hour urine measurement of sodium and creatinine. Even when these precautions are taken, about 20% of the patients will fail to reproduce their initial renin status on repeat examination. The logistics and expense involved in extra appointments for the measurements of renin and urinary sodium excretion and the cost for these laboratory tests must also be taken into consideration.

Initial antihypertensive therapy is selected on the basis of the apparent physiologic abnormality revealed by the renin measurements. Patients are then separated into "V" (volume and salt-dependent) or "R" (renin or vasoconstrictor-dependent) forms of hypertension, and drugs are selected on that basis. The "V" subjects, who comprise 30% to 60% of most hypertensive populations, have been shown to have the greatest initial blood pressure response to agents that reduce extracellular fluid volume, such as diuretics, aldosterone antagonists (spironolactone [Aldactone], eplerenone [Inspra]), and calcium channel entry blockers. For the "R" subgroup, typically comprising 10% to 30% of the essential hypertensive population, drugs that block the effects of vasoconstrictors such as β-adrenergic blocking agents, angiotensin-converting enzyme inhibitors, angiotensin receptor blockers, the experimental renin inhibitors, and sympatholytic agents are initially prescribed. A large segment, likely the majority, of the hypertensive population, based on the results of clinical trials, will not be controlled with a single agent,[2,3] presumably because their blood pressure elevation is influenced by more than a single physiologic mechanism. These patients will require the addition of an agent from the "class" opposite that initially prescribed. When no response is noted to the initial drug and patient adherence to the prescribed medication is presumed to be likely, three options should be considered: (1) determining whether there is some interfering or confounding element, (2) deciding whether the renin measurement should be repeated, and (3) discontinuing the initial agent and substituting a drug from the opposite class. The "Laragh" method, despite its simplicity and sophisticated physiologic rationale, requires confirmation by other studies employing a larger number of subjects under conditions of ordinary office practice before widespread adoption is reasonable.

## CHOOSING ANTIHYPERTENSIVE DRUG THERAPY BASED ON DEMOGRAPHIC FACTORS

A large number of studies have examined the blood pressure response to monotherapy as well as to multiple-drug approaches in many different hypertensive subpopulations. These studies have provided valuable information regarding blood pressure responses based on demographic characteristics as well as differences in the impact of specific therapeutic agents on cardiovascular events and the adverse effects of specific drugs. This information has proven to be useful in the selection of initial and additive drugs (Figure 79–2).

## AGE

Age is related to the prevalence of hypertension, mechanisms for blood pressure elevation, risk factors for cardiovascular disease, cardiovascular events, response to specific antihypertensive drug therapy, and side effects of these drugs. The prevalence of hypertension increases with age such that the majority of individuals over the age of 60 have an elevation of blood pressure. In the older population the systolic pressure is more likely to be elevated than the diastolic pressure. In younger persons both systolic and diastolic or occasionally, only diastolic pressure is elevated. The rise in systolic blood pressure with aging may be related to reduced arterial compliance and increased pulse wave velocity (see Chapters 15 and 22). In older individuals there are physiologic changes that also influence the response to blood pressure medication. Cardiac output decreases and β-adrenergic receptor and baroreceptor sensitivity are diminished. Thus β-adrenergic blocking drugs, which lower blood pressure primarily by reducing cardiac output, are less effective in older than in younger individuals, in whom there is often an enhancement of adrenergic responsiveness and a resting tachycardia, clues to the likelihood of response to β-adrenergic blocking drugs. The renin-angiotensin system appears to be more sluggish in responding to changes in sodium and volume in older compared with younger persons, and thus the blood pressure response to angiotensin-converting enzyme inhibitors and angiotensin receptor blockers is less in older compared with younger individuals when these agents are given alone. In older persons there is often a decrease in glomerular filtration rate and renal function, contributing to an expanded extracellular fluid volume. This is often manifest by relative suppression of renin and an increased blood pressure response to diuretic therapy. Because of the reduced sympathetic responsiveness in the elderly, protection against volume depletion is less vigorous than in younger individuals and thus orthostatic hypotension, falls, and even syncope are more likely, particularly when diuretics are given.

For this reason I favor using low doses of diuretics (6.25-12.5 mg/day of hydrochlorothiazide or its equivalent in other intermediate- to long-acting agents) in the older population if diuretics are chosen as initial therapy. The Systolic Hypertension in the Elderly Program (SHEP) trial demonstrated no reduction of cardiovascular events despite blood pressure reduction in older subjects receiving chlorthalidone in whom hypokalemia occurred.[5] The popularity of furosemide as a diuretic agent because of its potency and its preferential selection in acute pulmonary edema and renal failure has led to its widespread and inappropriate use in uncomplicated hypertensives. Because of its short duration of action (4-5 hours) and potency, administration of furosemide causes a prompt and often precipitous diuresis and natriuresis, followed by marked stimulation of the renin-angiotensin-aldosterone system and resultant salt and water retention equal to that recently excreted until the next dose is given. Thus furosemide must be given three to four times daily if effective blood pressure control is desired. This requirement for frequent dosing is associated with markedly reduced

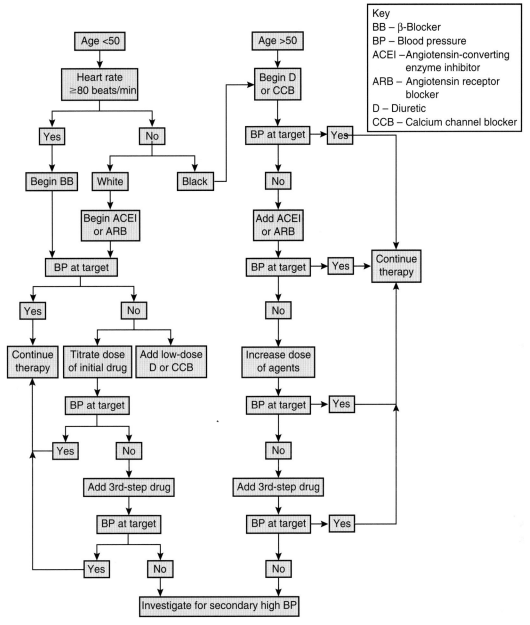

**Figure 79-2** Treatment algorithm based on age and ethnicity.

patient adherence and a variety of metabolic complications for those able to maintain the schedule. For this reason, furosemide should be reserved for use in the complicated hypertensive patient (i.e., the patient with chronic kidney disease or heart failure).

In older persons, particularly women, diuretics may occasionally cause profound and life-threatening hyponatremia. The risk of this idiosyncratic reaction may be reduced by avoiding administration of diuretics to patients in whom serum sodium is low-normal at baseline and by monitoring the serum sodium levels soon after beginning diuretic therapy in these patients. Hyponatremia is not a dose-dependent adverse effect and may even occur with the first dose of the drug. Hypokalemia is a much more frequent concomitant of diuretic therapy and usually requires weeks or months of administration to become apparent. Diuretic-associated

potassium loss is dependent on sodium intake, because it is mediated by the aldosterone response to sodium and volume depletion and the resultant potassium-for-sodium exchange in the distal segment of the kidney. Therefore, it can be reduced or prevented by reducing sodium intake, which will also enhance the efficacy of diuretic therapy in lowering the blood pressure.

Alternatively, potassium-sparing agents can be combined with the diuretic. Several are currently available, most in combination form with hydrochlorothiazide. Triamterene is frequently prescribed in combination with hydrochlorothiazide (Dyazide, Maxzide), but this combination is less effective in preventing potassium loss than others because the potassium-conserving duration of action of the triamterene component is shorter than the potassium-losing duration of hydrochlorothiazide. Amiloride (Midamor) is a longer-acting potassium-sparing agent that is usually combined with hydrochlorothiazide (Moduretic). It is available in the United States only in doses of 5 mg amiloride and 50 mg hydrochlorothiazide, which is a much higher diuretic dose than is preferable for most patients. Triamterene and amiloride are available as single agents but are relatively ineffective as diuretics when used without a thiazide or other more-effective diuretic. The oldest potassium-sparing agent, spironolactone (Aldactone), is the most-potent agent of this group in terms of both blood pressure reduction and potassium conservation. Its mechanism of action is different from those of the other potassium-sparing agents because spironolactone specifically antagonizes the effect of aldosterone at the level of the renal mineralocorticoid receptor. The appeal of spironolactone waned because of the frequent occurrence of sex-hormone–related side effects caused by its interaction with the estrogen receptor. This was manifest by impotence, gynecomastia, and breast tenderness in males and menstrual irregularities in females. Spironolactone is also available combined with hydrochlorothiazide (Aldactazide). A new and more selective mineralocorticoid receptor blocker, eplerenone[6] (Inspra) has become available (see Chapters 12 and 70). This agent has virtually no sex-hormone–related side effects and appears to be better tolerated than spironolactone. It also will be available in combination form with hydrochlorothiazide.

A word of caution should be voiced regarding the use of potassium-sparing agents. In patients with renal impairment, in some elderly diabetics with hyporeninemic hypoaldosteronism, in some patients receiving nonsteroidal antiinflammatory drugs (NSAIDs), and occasionally, in patients when combined with angiotensin-converting enzyme inhibitors or angiotensin receptor blockers, these agents can cause problematic hyperkalemia. If a diuretic is selected as the initial choice for an older hypertensive, lower doses are prudent. In addition, monitoring for and correction of the commonly encountered metabolic side effects of diuretic therapy other than hypokalemia and hyponatremia—such as hyperuricemia and gout, hyperglycemia, and hyperlipidemia—is appropriate. While some have contended that these metabolic effects of diuretic therapy are trivial and transient, the results of the recent Antihypertensive and Lipid-Lowering Treatment to Prevent Heart Attack Trial (ALLHAT)[7] suggest otherwise, because the group assigned to initial therapy with chlorthalidone, a thiazide-type diuretic, had a significantly greater incidence of new-onset diabetes mellitus at the end of the study as compared with the groups assigned to amlodipine or lisinopril. Furthermore, the changes in potassium, glucose, and lipids were found to persist at the end of 5 years of study, and thus are hardly transient.

Calcium channel entry blockers provide an alternative to diuretics for the older hypertensive, because these agents lower blood pressure by inducing a diuresis and natriuresis in addition to their vasodilator effect.[8] This rarely recognized action of calcium channel blockers provides a dual mechanism of action for reducing blood pressure and probably accounts for the very broad spectrum of antihypertensive efficacy demonstrated by this class of drugs. The calcium channel blocker class can be separated on the basis of chemical structure and actions into three distinct groups: the benzothiazepines (diltiazem), phenylalkylamines (verapamil), and the dihydropyridines (amlodipine, felodipine, isradipine, nicardipine, nifedipine, and nisoldipine are currently available in the United States). For blood pressure reduction the dihydropyridines appear to be the most potent.

The antihypertensive dose of diltiazem is typically much higher than the antianginal dose. Early studies indicated that the average effective antihypertensive dose of diltiazem was more than 300 mg/day. Verapamil also requires an average dose of 240 to 480 mg/day for antihypertensive efficacy. The greatest use of the nordihydropyridine calcium channel blockers is in individuals in whom slowing of heart rate is desired, because they reduce heart rate by their effect on cardiac conduction. In addition, they are useful in the treatment of patients with atrial fibrillation, a not uncommon finding in older hypertensives. However, because of this negative chronotropic effect, they should be used cautiously in patients receiving β-adrenergic blocking drugs because of risk of profound, symptomatic bradycardia and heart block. Other side effects include edema (about which more will be said later), constipation, and skin rash.

The dihydropyridines are devoid of heart-rate slowing effects. In fact, the initial short-acting forms of these drugs, which are no longer widely used, caused reflex activation of the sympathetic nervous system as a result of their precipitous and rapid blood pressure–lowering effect. However, the current generations of these agents, generally sufficiently long-acting for once-daily administration, do not have any demonstrable effect on heart rate. The most commonly prescribed agent of the group, amlodipine (Norvasc), is frequently given for the treatment of angina as well as hypertension. The dihydropyridines are generally the most potent in reducing blood pressure but also may cause edema. The edema seen with calcium channel entry blockers appears to be somewhat paradoxical in view of the extensive documentation of their diuretic and natriuretic actions. The edema seems to be due to the potent vasodilation of the capillary bed, increasing the capillary pressure with leakage of fluid into the interstitial tissues and, by the effect of gravity, to pooling in the legs. This can typically be remedied by antigravitational maneuvers such as elevating the legs periodically, wearing support stockings, or if those techniques are not adequate, by the addition of small doses of an angiotensin-converting enzyme inhibitor or an angiotensin receptor antagonist, which appears to correct the increased capillary pressure responsible for the edema.

Cognitive decline and dementia of all forms are more frequent among older persons than younger and in hypertensives as compared with normotensives. In fact, elevated blood pressure has emerged as a major risk factor for the development of dementia. Importantly, trials in elderly hypertensives have demonstrated, prospectively, a reduction in the development of dementia in this susceptible group when systolic blood pressure is lowered with a dihydropyridine calcium channel entry blocker.[9] It is likely that other agents will show a similar benefit, but no data on this issue are presently available.

When the initial agent chosen for the older hypertensive, typically a low-dose diuretic or a calcium channel entry blocker, does not reduce blood pressure to goal (systolic pressure below 140 mm Hg), the addition of an angiotensin-converting enzyme inhibitor or angiotensin receptor blocker will usually produce a further decrease in pressure because of the additive effects of such agents to diuretics and calcium channel blockers. I prefer not to use β-blocking drugs in this population unless there is another compelling indication for their use (such as atrial fibrillation, angina, congestive heart failure, benign tremor, or migraine headaches) because of their low antihypertensive efficacy and their adverse effects on cardiac output and lipids.[10]

When essential hypertension is diagnosed at a younger age, typically less than 40 years, the etiology is more typically the result of an increase in vasoconstriction induced by catecholamines or angiotensin II via the renin system. In addition to the increase in blood pressure, a resting tachycardia or hyperdynamic chest wall may be observed. Such individuals are typically more responsive to β-adrenergic blocking agents, to which they may exhibit a reduction of blood pressure at relatively low doses, thus making dose-related side effects less likely, or to agents interfering with the renin-angiotensin system, such as angiotensin-converting enzyme inhibitors or angiotensin II receptor blockers. When β-adrenergic blocking agents are prescribed, there is often concern regarding the occurrence of bradycardia. Because the main mechanism by which β-blockers reduce blood pressure is by reducing heart rate and thereby decreasing cardiac output, a reduction in heart rate is a good way to evaluate the efficacy of the agent. For this reason, asymptomatic bradycardia, even with pulse rates as low as 40 beats/min, should not necessarily be a reason for discontinuation of a β-blocker if the blood pressure is responsive and the patient does not exhibit other side effects. β-Adrenergic blocking agents are less effective in cigarette smokers, presumably because of the increase in catecholamine release in such individuals.

With angiotensin-converting enzyme inhibitor treatment, the major life-threatening side effect is angioedema. This is a relatively rare event but does appear to be more prevalent in Blacks, who generally are less responsive than Caucasians to monotherapy with angiotensin-converting enzyme inhibitors in terms of blood pressure reduction. This side effect does not seem to be dose-dependent and may occur at any time during treatment, not necessarily with the initial dose. Cough is another much more frequently encountered side effect of this drug class that, although not dose-dependent, appears to be duration-dependent, more likely to occur the longer the patient takes the drug. Cough also seems to be more prevalent among African American and Asian American hypertensives, as well as women and smokers. The incidence of both angioedema and cough with angiotensin II receptor blockers is much lower than that with angiotensin-converting enzyme inhibitors, providing a rationale for preferring the former in many patients.

## ETHNIC BACKGROUND

A variety of studies have reported on differential responsiveness to antihypertensive agents among patients separated on the basis of ethnic background or race (see Chapter 56).[7,11-13] One of the earliest such reports concerned the decreased responsiveness of Black hypertensives to treatment with β-adrenergic blocking drugs.[12] These studies failed to demonstrate a blood pressure response to 160 mg/day of propranolol but demonstrated that 640 mg/day did lower pressure in a small group of Black hypertensives. Similar observations have been made with angiotensin-converting enzyme inhibitors and angiotensin receptor blockers when used alone in this subgroup. On the other hand, diuretics and calcium channel entry blockers generally are effective in reducing pressure in Black hypertensives.[11,12] Because the elevation of pressure in this population is often greater than in other subgroups, multiple medications are more frequently required. The addition

of angiotensin-converting enzyme inhibitors and angiotensin II receptor blockers to initial therapy with diuretics[13] or calcium channel entry blockers usually provides additional blood pressure reduction.

There have been a paucity of studies in the United States to provide information regarding the blood pressure responses of Hispanic Americans, Native Americans, or Asian Americans to different antihypertensive agents given as monotherapy. Some of the large "outcome" trials such as ALLHAT[7] and the International Verapamil-Trandolapril Study (INVEST)[14] can provide that information, because they had a very substantial representation of minority hypertensives.

## GENDER

Despite a large number of studies that have included women as well as men as participants, there is no consistent evidence of gender differences in the response to antihypertensive drugs when other factors such as age and ethnicity are considered.[2,3] Having said that, several gender-specific concerns may influence the choice of antihypertensive drug therapy in women. Because angiotensin-converting enzyme inhibitors and angiotensin II receptor antagonists are contraindicated in pregnancy, they should probably be avoided in women with childbearing potential unless a very effective form of contraception is utilized. When hypertensive women are found to be taking oral contraceptives or hormone replacement therapy, a trial of several months of withdrawal of such agents may be rewarded by a reduction in blood pressure. Women appear to experience a cough with angiotensin-converting enzyme inhibitors, hypokalemia with diuretics, and edema with calcium channel entry blockers more frequently than do men.

## WHAT TO DO WHEN INITIAL THERAPY IS NOT ENOUGH

Several large trials have provided evidence that the majority of uncomplicated hypertensives require more than two drugs to achieve the current blood pressure goal recommendations.[2,3,7,14] As previously mentioned, the JNC 7 report advocates beginning with two agents when the blood pressure is above 160/100 mm Hg, because a single drug is not likely to achieve the targeted blood pressure reduction. In the "Laragh" method, when the initial "V" or "R" drug, chosen on the basis of the renin measurement, in full doses does not lower blood pressure sufficiently, a drug from the opposite class is recommended. When demographic characteristics are used as a clue to initial therapy, a similar approach of adding drugs with a differing mechanism of action from that initially prescribed is usually effective. It should be emphasized that when calcium channel blocking drugs are given initially, the addition of a diuretic is unlikely to produce a significant further blood pressure reduction, although the opposite sequence may demonstrate a further drop in pressure, presumably owing to the dual antihypertensive mechanisms of calcium channel entry blockers.[15] Similarly, combining a β-blocker with an angiotensin-converting enzyme inhibitor or angiotensin receptor blocker, or combining the latter two agents, in the absence of a diuretic or calcium channel blocker, is not likely to produce an additive antihypertensive effect.

The very limited studies demonstrating the benefit of combining angiotensin-converting enzyme inhibitors with angiotensin receptor blockers, to date, have not compared the response to full or increased doses of either agent alone to satisfy the concern that the response to the combination simply reflects greater inhibition of the renin-angiotensin system. Such studies should be available in the future. When two agents, working by different mechanisms, fail to reduce blood pressure adequately, third-step agents—for example, sympatholytic drugs such as clonidine (Catapres), guanfacine (Tenex), guanabenz (Wytensin), methyl-dopa (Aldomet), doxazosin (Cardura), terazosin (Hytrin), prazosin (Minipress) or reserpine—may be appropriate. Alternatively, direct-acting vasodilators such as hydralazine (Apresoline), or rarely, minoxidil (Loniten), may be added.

## SUMMARY

Given the large number of antihypertensive drugs available, it is often bewildering to decide how to begin treatment in a given individual. Essentially there are two rational approaches, one based on a cumbersome and sometimes inconsistent method of measuring plasma renin activity in relationship to 24-hour urinary sodium excretion, which often requires a manipulation of dietary-sodium intake to ensure accuracy, and another based on demographic characteristics. Neither of these approaches is fool-proof, nor have they been consistently and reproducibly subjected to rigorous randomized clinical trial examination to compare their relative costs, efficacies, advantages, and disadvantages. Nonetheless, both offer a way to begin drug treatment in specific patients, recognizing that the overwhelming majority of hypertensives will require more than a single drug to achieve adequate blood pressure control. The use of these algorithms should make the tough choices a little easier.

## References

1. Vasan RS, Larson MG, Leip EP, et al. Impact of high-normal blood pressure on the risk for cardiovascular disease. N Engl J Med 345:1291-1297, 2001.
2. Chobanian AV, Bakris GL, Black HR, et al. The Seventh Report of the Joint National Committee on Prevention, Detection, Evaluation, and Treatment of High Blood Pressure: The JNC 7 (Express) Report. JAMA 289:2560-2572, 2003.
3. Chobanian AV, Bakris GL, Black HR, et al. The Seventh Report of the Joint National Committee on Prevention, Detection, Evaluation, and Treatment of high blood pressure: JNC 7 Complete Report. Hypertension 42:1206-1252, 2003.
4. Laragh JH. Laragh's Lessons in Renin System Pathophysiology for Treating Hypertension and Its Fatal Consequences. Elsevier Science, New York, 2002; pp 1-174.
5. Franse LV, Pahor M, Di Bari M, et al. Hypokalemia associated with diuretic use and cardiovascular events in the Systolic Hypertension in the Elderly Program. Hypertension 35: 1025-1030, 2000.
6. Weinberger MH, Roniker B, Krause SL, et al. Eplerenone, a selective aldosterone blocker (SAB) in mild to moderate hypertension. Am J Hypertens 15:358-363, 2002.
7. The ALLHAT Officers and Coordinators for the ALLHAT Collaborative Research Group. Major outcomes in high-risk hypertensive patients randomized to angiotensin-converting enzyme inhibitor or calcium channel blocker vs diuretic: The Antihypertensive and Lipid-Lowering Treatment to Prevent Heart Attack Trial (ALLHAT). JAMA 288:2981-2997, 2002.
8. Luft FC, Aronoff GR, Slaon RS, et al. Calcium channel blockade with nitrendipine. Hypertension 7:438-442, 1985.
9. Forette F, Seux ML, Staessen JA, et al. The prevention of dementia with antihypertensive treatment: New evidence from the Systolic Hypertension in Europe (Syst-Eur) study. Arch Intern Med 162:2046-2052, 2002.
10. Weinberger MH. Antihypertensive therapy and lipids: Evidence, mechanisms and implications. Arch Intern Med 145:1102-1105, 1985.
11. Cushman WC, Reda DJ, Perry HM, et al. Regional and racial differences in response to antihypertensive medication use in a randomized controlled trial of men with hypertension in the United States. Department of Veterans Affairs Cooperative Study Group on Antihypertensive agents. Arch Intern Med 160:825-831, 2000.
12. Saunders E, Weir MR, Kong BW, et al. A comparison of the efficacy and safety of a beta-blocker, a calcium channel blocker, and a converting enzyme inhibitor in hypertensive blacks. Arch Intern Med 150:1707-1713, 1990.
13. Weinberger MH. Blood pressure and metabolic responses to hydrochlorothiazide, captopril and the combination in black and white mild-to-moderate hypertensive patients. J Cardiovasc Pharm 7:S52-S55, 1985.
14. Pepine CJ, Handberg EM, Cooper-Dehoff RM, et al. A calcium antagonist vs a non-calcium antagonist hypertension treatment strategy for patients with coronary artery disease: The International Verapamil-Trandolapril Study (INVEST): A randomized controlled trial. JAMA 290:2805-2816, 2003.
15. Weinberger MH. Additive effects of diuretics or sodium restriction with calcium channel blockers in the treatment of hypertension. J Cardiovasc Pharm 12:S72-S75, 1988.

# Appendix

Oral Antihypertensive Drugs

| Class | Drug (trade name) | Usual Dose Range, mg/day | Usual Daily Frequency* |
|---|---|---|---|
| Thiazide diuretics | Chlorthalidone | 12.5-25 | 1 |
| | Hydrochlorothiazide | 12.5-50 | 1 |
| | Indapamide (Lozol†) | 1.25-2.5 | 1 |
| | Metolazone (Mykrox) | 0.5-1.0 | 1 |
| | Metolazone (Zaroxolyn) | 2.5-5 | 1 |
| Other diuretics | Bumetanide (Bumex†) | 0.5-2 | 2 |
| | Furosemide (Lasix†) | 20-80 | 2 |
| | Torsemide (Demadex†) | 2.5-10 | 1 |
| Aldosterone receptor blockers | Eplerenone (Inspra) | 50-100 | 1 |
| | Spironolactone (Aldactone†) | 25-50 | 1 |
| β-Blockers | Atenolol (Tenormin†) | 25-100 | 1 |
| | Betaxolol (Kerlone†) | 5-20 | 1 |
| | Bisoprolol (Zebeta†) | 2.5-10 | 1 |
| | Metoprolol | 50-100 | 1-2 |
| | Metoprolol extended release | 50-100 | 1 |
| | Nadolol (Corgard†) | 40-120 | 1 |
| | Propranolol | 40-160 | 2 |
| | Propranolol long-acting (Inderal LA†) | 60-180 | 1 |
| | Timolol (Blocadren†) | 20-40 | 2 |
| β-Blockers with intrinsic sympathomimetic activity | Acebutolol (Sectral†) | 200-800 | 2 |
| Combined α- and β-blockers | Carvedilol (Coreg) | 12.5-50 | 2 |
| | Labetalol (Normodyne, Trandate†) | 200-800 | 2 |
| ACEIs | Benazepril (Lotensin†) | 10-40 | 1 |
| | Captopril (Capoten†) | 25-100 | 2 |
| | Enalapril (Vasotec†) | 5-40 | 1-2 |
| | Fosinopril (Monopril) | 10-40 | 1 |
| | Lisinopril (Prinivil, Zestril†) | 10-40 | 1 |
| | Moexipril (Univasc) | 7.5-30 | 1 |
| | Perindopril (Aceon) | 4-8 | 1 |
| | Quinapril (Accupril) | 10-80 | 1 |
| | Ramipril (Altace) | 2.5-20 | 1 |
| | Trandolapril (Mavik) | 1-4 | 1 |
| Angiotensin II antagonists | Candesartan (Atacand) | 8-32 | 1 |
| | Eprosartan (Teveten) | 400-800 | 1-2 |
| | Irbesartan (Avapro) | 150-300 | 1 |
| | Losartan (Cozaar) | 25-100 | 1-2 |
| | Olmesartan (Benicar) | 20-40 | 1 |
| | Telmisartan (Micardis) | 20-80 | 1 |
| | Valsartan (Diovan) | 80-320 | 1-2 |
| CCBs—Nondihydropyridines | Diltiazem extended release (Cardizem CD, Dilacor XR, Tiazac†) | 180-420 | 1 |
| | Diltiazem extended release (Cardizem LA) | 120-540 | 1 |
| | Verapamil immediate release (Calan, Isoptin†) | 80-320 | 2 |
| | Verapamil long acting (Calan SR, Isoptin SR†) | 120-480 | 1-2 |
| | Verapamil (Coer, Covera HS, Verelan PM) | 120-360 | 1 |

*Continued*

Oral Antihypertensive Drugs—cont'd

| Class | Drug (trade name) | Usual Dose Range, mg/day | Usual Daily Frequency* |
|---|---|---|---|
| CCBs—Dihydropyridines | Amlodipine (Norvasc) | 2.5-10 | 1 |
| | Felodipine (Plendil) | 2.5-20 | 1 |
| | Isradipine (Dynacirc CR) | 2.5-10 | 2 |
| | Nicardipine sustained release (Cardene SR) | 60-120 | 2 |
| | Nifedipine long-acting (Adalat CC, Procardia XL) | 30-60 | 1 |
| | Nisoldipine (Sular) | 10-40 | 1 |
| $\alpha_1$-Blockers | Doxazosin (Cardura) | 1-16 | 1 |
| | Prazosin (Minipress[†]) | 2-20 | 2-3 |
| | Terazosin (Hytrin) | 1-20 | 1-2 |
| Central $\alpha_2$ agonists and other centrally acting drugs | Clonidine (Catapres[†]) | 0.1-0.8 | 2 |
| | Clonidine patch (Catapres-TTS) | 0.1-0.3 | 1 weekly |
| | Reserpine (generic) | 0.1-0.25 | 1 |
| Direct vasodilators | Hydralazine (Apresoline[†]) | 25-100 | 2 |
| | Minoxidil (Loniten[†]) | 2.5-80 | 1-2 |

From the National Heart, Lung, and Blood Institute (NHLBI). From Physicians' Desk Reference. 57th ed. Montvale, NJ: Thomson PDR; 2003.

ACEI, Angiotensin-converting enzyme inhibitors; CCBs, calcium channel blockers.

*In some patients treated once daily, the antihypertensive effect may diminish toward the end of the dosing interval (trough effect). BP should be measured just prior to dosing to determine if satisfactory BP control is obtained. Accordingly, an increase in dosage or frequency may need to be considered. These dosages may vary from those listed in the Physician's Desk Reference, 57th ed.

[†]Available now or soon to become available in generic preparations.

Combination Drugs for Hypertension

| Combination Type | Fixed-Dose Combination, mg | Trade Name |
|---|---|---|
| ACEIs and CCBs | Amlodipine-benazepril hydrochloride (2.5/10, 5/10, 5/20, 10/20) | Lotrel |
| | Enalapril-felodipine (5/5) | Lexxel |
| | Trandolapril-verapamil (2/180, 1/240, 2/240, 4/240) | Tarka |
| ACEIs and diuretics | Benazepril-hydrochlorothiazide (5/6.25, 10/12.5, 20/12.5, 20/25) | Lotensin HCT |
| | Captopril-hydrochlorothiazide (25/15, 25/25, 50/15, 50/25) | Capozide |
| | Enalapril-hydrochlorothiazide (5/12.5, 10/25) | Vaseretic |
| | Fosinopril-hydrochlorothiazide (10/12.5, 20/12.5) | Monopril/HCT |
| | Lisinopril-hydrochlorothiazide (10/12.5, 20/12.5, 20/25) | Prinzide, Zestoretic |
| | Moexipril-hydrochlorothiazide (7.5/12.5, 15/25) | Uniretic |
| | Quinapril-hydrochlorothiazide (10/12.5, 20/12.5, 20/25) | Accuretic |
| ARBs and diuretics | Candesartan-hydrochlorothiazide (16/12.5, 32/12.5) | Atacand HCT |
| | Eprosartan-hydrochlorothiazide (600/12.5, 600/25) | Teveten-HCT |
| | Irbesartan-hydrochlorothiazide (150/12.5, 300/12.5) | Avalide |
| | Losartan-hydrochlorothiazide (50/12.5, 100/25) | Hyzaar |
| | Olmesartan medoxomil-hydrochlorothiazide (20/12.5, 40/12.5, 40/25) | Benicar HCT |
| | Telmisartan-hydrochlorothiazide (40/12.5, 80/12.5) | Micardis-HCT |
| | Valsartan-hydrochlorothiazide (80/12.5, 160/12.5, 160/25) | Diovan-HCT |
| β-Blockers and diuretics | Atenolol-chlorthalidone (50/25, 100/25) | Tenoretic |
| | Bisoprolol-hydrochlorothiazide (2.5/6.25, 5/6.25, 10/6.25) | Ziac |
| | Metoprolol-hydrochlorothiazide (50/25, 100/25) | Lopressor HCT |
| | Nadolol-bendroflumethiazide (40/5, 80/5) | Corzide |
| | Propranolol LA-hydrochlorothiazide (40/25, 80/25) | Inderide LA |
| | Timolol-hydrochlorothiazide (10/25) | Timolide |
| Other combinations | Amiloride-hydrochlorothiazide (5/50) | Moduretic |
| | Spironolactone-hydrochlorothiazide (25/25, 50/50) | Aldactazide |
| | Triamterene-hydrochlorothiazide (37.5/25, 75/50) | Dyazide, Maxzide |

From the National Heart, Lung, and Blood Institute (NHLBI). From Physicians' Desk Reference. 57th ed. Montvale, NJ, Thomson PDR; 2003.
ACEI, Angiotensin-converting enzyme inhibitors; CCBs, calcium channel blockers; ARBs, angiotensin receptor blockers.

# Index

Note: Page numbers followed by f refer to figures, t refer to tables, and b refer to boxes.